COMPREHENSIVE TEXTBOOK OF GENITOURINARY ONCOLOGY

THIRD EDITION

COMPREHENSIVE TEXTBOOK OF GENITOURINARY ONCOLOGY

THIRD EDITION

Editors

Nicholas J. Vogelzang, MD
Director, Nevada Cancer Institute
Las Vegas, Nevada

Peter T. Scardino, MD
Florence and Theodore Baumritter/Enid Ancell Chair
Chairman, Department of Urology
Memorial Sloan-Kettering Cancer Center
New York, New York

William U. Shipley, MD
Andres Soriano Professor of Radiation Oncology
Harvard Medical School
The Claire and John Bertucci Center for Genitourinary Cancers
Head, Genitourinary Oncology Unit
Department of Radiation Oncology
Massachusetts General Hospital
Boston, Massachusetts

Frans M.J. Debruyne, MD, PhD
Professor and Chairman, Department of Urology
Radboud University Nijmegen Medical Centre
Nijmegen, The Netherlands

W. Marston Linehan, MD
Chief, Urologic Oncology Branch
Center for Cancer Research
National Cancer Institute
National Institutes of Health
Bethesda, Maryland

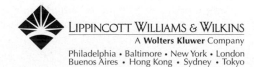
LIPPINCOTT WILLIAMS & WILKINS
A **Wolters Kluwer** Company
Philadelphia • Baltimore • New York • London
Buenos Aires • Hong Kong • Sydney • Tokyo

Acquisitions Editor: Jonathan W. Pine, Jr.
Managing Editor: Anne E. Jacobs
Project Manager: Alicia Jackson
Senior Manufacturing Manager: Benjamin Rivera
Associate Director of Marketing: Adam Glazer
Cover Designer: Andrew Gatto
Production Service: Laserwords Private Limited
Printer: Edwards Brothers

© 2006 by LIPPINCOTT WILLIAMS & WILKINS
530 Walnut Street
Philadelphia, PA 19106
LWW.com

1st Edition, © 1996 Williams & Wilkins
2nd Edition, © 2000 Lippincott Williams & Wilkins

Printed in the United States

Library of Congress Cataloging-in-Publication Data

Comprehensive textbook of genitourinary oncology / editors,
  Nicholas J. Vogelzang ... [et al.].-- 3rd ed.
    p. ; cm.
  Includes bibliographical references and index.
  ISBN 0-7817-4984-0
  1. Genitourinary organs--Cancer. I. Vogelzang, Nicholas J.
  [DNLM: 1. Urogenital Neoplasms. WJ 160 C738 2005]
  RC280.U74C665 2005
  616.99'46--dc22

                    2005015077

Care has been taken to confirm the accuracy of the information presented and to describe generally accepted practices. However, the authors, editors, and publisher are not responsible for errors or omissions or for any consequences from application of the information in this book and make no warranty, expressed or implied, with respect to the currency, completeness, or accuracy of the contents of the publication. Application of this information in a particular situation remains the professional responsibility of the practitioner.

The authors, editors, and publisher have exerted every effort to ensure that drug selection and dosage set forth in this text are in accordance with current recommendations and practice at the time of publication. However, in view of ongoing research, changes in government regulations, and the constant flow of information relating to drug therapy and drug reactions, the reader is urged to check the package insert for each drug for any change in indications and dosage and for added warnings and precautions. This is particularly important when the recommended agent is a new or infrequently employed drug.

Some drugs and medical devices presented in this publication have Food and Drug Administration (FDA) clearance for limited use in restricted research settings. It is the responsibility of health care providers to ascertain the FDA status of each drug or device planned for use in their clinical practice.

To purchase additional copies of this book, call our customer service department at (800) 638-3030 or fax orders to (301) 824-7390. International customers should call (301) 714-2324. Lippincott Williams & Wilkins customer service representatives are available from 8:30 AM to 6:30 PM, EST, Monday through Friday, for telephone access.

Visit Lippincott Williams & Wilkins on the Internet: http://www.lww.com.

10 9 8 7 6 5 4 3 2 1

WE DEDICATE THIS BOOK TO THE BRAVE MEN AND WOMEN
AFFECTED WITH THE MANY AND DIVERSE FORMS OF GENITOURINARY CANCERS.

THEY WERE—AND ARE—OUR INVALUABLE PARTNERS IN THE RESEARCH EFFORTS
TO DEVELOP MORE EFFECTIVE FORMS OF THERAPY FOR THESE DISEASES.

CONTENTS

PART I ■ PROSTATE CANCER

PART III ■ TESTIS CANCER

PART IV ■ KIDNEY CANCER

PART V ■ PENILE CANCER

PART VI ■ OTHER UROLOGIC MALIGNANCIES

Sidney C. Abreu, MD
Chief
Section of Laparoscopy and Endourology
Hospital Urologico de Brasilia
Brasilia, Brazil

Nasser M. Albqami, MD
Fellow of Laparoscopy and Endourology
Urologist, Department of Urology
Elisabethinen Hospital
Linz, Austria

Christopher L. Amling, MD, FACS
Assistant Professor
Chairman and Program Director
Department of Urology
Naval Medical Center San Diego
San Diego, California

Andrew Artz, MD, MS
Instructor
Department of Medicine, Section of Hematology/Oncology
University of Chicago Pritzker School of Medicine
Chicago, Illinois

Micheal B. Atkins, MD
Professor
Department of Medicine
Harvard Medical School

Deputy Chief
Division of Hematology/Oncology
Beth Israel Deaconess Medical Center
Boston, Massachusetts

Gustavo Ayala, MD
Associate Professor
Department of Pathology and Scott Department of Urology
Baylor College of Medicine
Houston, Texas

Dean F. Bajorin, MD, FACP
Professor
Department of Medicine
Weill Medical College of Cornell University

Attending Physician
Department of Medicine
Memorial Sloan-Kettering Cancer Center
New York, New York

Georg Bartsch, MD
Chief, Chairman and Professor
Department of Urology
Innsbruck Medical University
Innsbruck, Austria

Stephen D. W. Beck, MD
Assistant Professor
Department of Urology
Indiana University
Indianapolis, Indiana

Kathleen Beekman, MD
Fellow
Genitourinary Oncology
Memorial Sloan-Kettering Cancer Center
New York, New York

Arie S. Belldegrun, MD
Professor of Urology
Roy and Carol Doumani Chair in Urologic Oncology
Chief of Urologic Oncology
Department of Urology
David Geffen School of Medicine at University
    of California—Los Angeles
Los Angeles, California

Richard Bihrle, MD
Professor of Urology
Department of Urology
Indiana University School of Medicine
Indianapolis, Indiana

Michael L. Blute, MD
Anson L. Clark Professor of Urology
Department of Urology
Mayo Medical School

Chairman
Department of Urology
Mayo Clinic
Rochester, Minnesota

Bernard H. Bochner, MD
Department of Urology
Memorial Sloan-Kettering Cancer Center
New York, New York

Michel Bolla, MD
Professor, Radiation Oncology
Center Hospitalier Regional Universitaire de Grenoble
Grenoble, France

George J. Bosl, MD
Professor of Medicine
Department of Medicine
Weill Medical College of Cornell University

Chairman
Department of Medicine
Memorial Sloan-Kettering Cancer Center
New York, New York

Peter Boyle, MD
Director
International Agency for Research on Cancer
Lyon, France

Grant Buchanan, PhD
Research Fellow
Department of Medicine
University of Adelaide

Research Fellow
Hanson Institute
Royal Adelaide Hospital
Adelaide, Australia

Ronald M. Bukowski, MD
Professor
Department of Medicine
Cleveland Clinic of Medicine of CWRU

Director, Experimental Therapeutics
Cleveland Clinic Taussig Cancer Center
Cleveland Clinic Foundation
Cleveland, Ohio

George P. Canellos, MD
William Rosenberg Professor of Medicine
Department of Medicine
Harvard Medical School

Senior Physician
Department of Medical Oncology
Dana Farber Cancer Institute
Boston, Massachusetts

Stefan Carllson, MD
Professor
Section of Urology
Department of Surgical Science
Karolinska Institutet
Stockholm, Sweden

Peter R. Carroll, MD
Professor and Chair
Department of Urology
University of California

Surgeon-in-Chief
UCSF Comprehensive Cancer Center
San Francisco, California

R. S. K. Chaganti, PhD
Member & Professor, William E. Snee Chair
Medicine and Cell Biology Program
Memorial Sloan-Kettering Cancer Center

Attending Geneticist and Chief, Cytogenetics Service
Department of Medicine
Memorial Hospital for Cancer & Allied Diseases
New York, New York

Thomas Chi, MD
Resident
Department of Urology
University of California

Resident
Department of Urology
San Francisco Hospitals
San Francisco, California

Richard W. Childs, MD
Senior Investigator, Stem Cell Transplantation
Hematology Branch, NHLBI
National Institutes of Health
Bethesda, Maryland

Wong-Ho Chow, PhD
Senior Epidemiologist
Division of Cancer Epidemiology and Genetics
National Cancer Institute, National Institute of Health,
    Department of Health and Human Services
Bethesda, Maryland

Peter L. Choyke, MD
Chief, Molecular Imaging Program
Center for Cancer Research
National Cancer Institute
Bethesda, Maryland

Ralph V. Clayman, MD
Chairman and Professor
Department of Urology
University of California, Irvine
Orange, California

Jonathan A. Coleman, MD
Staff Clinician
Urologic Oncology Branch, National Cancer Institute
Clinical Research Center
Bethesda, Maryland

Richard J. Cote, MD, FRCPath
Professor of Pathology and Urology
Director, Genitourinary Cancer Program
Director, Laboratory of Immuno and Molecular Pathology
University of Southern California, Keck School of Medicine
USC/Norris Comprehensive Cancer Center
Los Angeles, California

E. David Crawford, MD
Professor of Surgery and Radiation Oncology
Department of Radiation Oncology
University of Colorado
Denver Health Sciences Center
Aurora, Colorado

Juanita M. Crook, MD, FRCP(C)
Professor
Department of Radiation Oncology
University of Toronto

Staff Radiation Oncologist
Department of Radiation Oncology
Princess Margaret Hospital/ University Health Network
Ontario, Canada

Zoran Culig, MD
Associate Professor
Department of Urology
Innsbruck Medical University
Innsbruck, Austria

Stéphane Culine, MD, PhD
Professor
Department of Medical Oncology
Montpellier University

Department of Medical Oncology
CRLC Val d'Aurelle
Montpellier, France

Guido Dalbagni, MD, FACS
Associate Professor
Department of Urology
Weill Medical College of Cornell University

Associate Attending
Department of Urology
Memorial Sloan-Kettering Cancer Center
New York, New York

Anthony V. D'Amico, MD, PhD
Professor and Chair of Genitourinary
    Radiation
Department of Oncology
Harvard Medical School

Professor and Chair of Genitourinary
    Radiation
Department of Oncology
Brigham and Women's Hospital
Dana Farber Cancer Institute
Boston, Massachusetts

Ram H. Datar, PhD
Assistant Professor of Clinical Pathology
Department of Pathology
University of Southern California
Los Angeles, California

John W. Davis, MD
Assistant Professor
Department of Urology
Eastern Virginia Medical School

Active Staff
Department of Urology
Sentara Norfolk General Hospital
Norfolk, Virginia

Jose D. Debes, MD
Instructor
Department of Biochemistry and
    Molecular Biology
Mayo Clinic College of Medicine

Senior Research Fellow
Department of Urology
Mayo Clinic College of Medicine
Rochester, Minnesota

Frans M.J. Debruyne, MD, PhD
Professor and Chairman, Department of Urology
Radboud University Nijmegen Medical Centre
Nijmegen, The Netherlands

Susan S. Devesa, PhD
Chief, Descriptive Studies
Division of Cancer Epidemiology and Genetics
National Cancer Institute
National Institute of Health
Bethesda, Maryland

Colin P. N. Dinney, MD
Professor and Chairman
Department of Urology
The University of Texas M.D. Anderson
    Cancer Center
Houston, Texas

S. Machele Donat, MD, FACS
Associate Professor
Department of Urology
Weill Medical College of Cornell University

Associate Attending Surgeon
Department of Urology
Memorial Sloan-Kettering Cancer Center
New York, New York

John P. Donohue, MD
Distinguished Professor Emeritus
Department of Urology
Indiana University Medical Center
Indianapolis, Indiana

Jenny L. Donovan, PhD
Professor of Social Medicine
Department of Social Medicine
University of Bristol
Bristol, United Kingdom

Robert Dreicer, MD, MS, FACP
Professor
Department of Internal Medicine
Cleveland Clinic Lerner College of Medicine

Director, Genitourinary Medical Oncology
Department of Hematology/Oncology
Cleveland Clinic Taussig Cancer Center
Cleveland Clinic Foundation
Cleveland, Ohio

James A. Eastham, MD
Associate Member
Department of Urology
Memorial Sloan-Kettering Cancer Center
New York, New York

Antonio Finelli, MD, MSC, FRCSC
Assistant Professor of Surgery
Department of Surgical Oncology
University of Toronto

Department of Urology/Minimally Invasive Surgery
Princess Margaret Hospital
Ontario, Canada

Robert C. Flanigan, MD
Professor and Albert J. Speh, Jr. and Claire R. Speh
    Chair in Urology
Loyola University Medical Center
Maywood, Illinois

Richard Foster, MD
Professor
Department of Urology
Indiana University
Indianapolis, Indiana

Igor Frank, MD
Department of Urology
Mayo Clinic College of Medicine
Rochester, Minnesota

Zvi Fuks, MD
Alfred P. Sloan Chair
Head, Metastatic Cell Biology Laboratory
Memorial Sloan-Kettering Cancer Center
New York, New York

Matthew D. Galsky, MD
Assistant Member
Genitourinary Oncology Service
Department of Medicine
Memorial Sloan-Kettering Cancer Center
New York, New York

Inderbir S. Gill, MD
Professor of Surgery
Head, Section of Robotic and
    Laparoscopic and Robotic Surgery
Department of Urology
Cleveland Clinic Foundation
Cleveland, Ohio

Timothy David Gilligan, MD, MS
Assistant Professor
Department of Medicine
Case Western Reserve University

Genitourinary Oncologist
Department of Hematology and
    Medical Oncology
Cleveland Clinic
Cleveland, Ohio

Edward Giovannucci, MD, ScD
Professor
Department of Nutrition and Epidemiology
Harvard School of Public Health

Associate Professor
Department of Medicine
Channing Laboratory
Brigham and Women's Hospital
Boston, Massachusetts

S. Larry Goldenberg, MD, FRCS(C), FACS
Professor and Head
Department of Surgery (Urology)
University of British Columbia

Director
Prostate Research Center Vancouver
    General Hospital
British Columbia, Canada

Edward M. Gong, MD
Fellow
Department of Urology
The Pritzker School of Medicine
University of Chicago
Chicago, Illinois

Arthur C. Grabowski, MD
Clinical Fellow
Department of Surgery
University of Toronto

Staff Urologist
Department of Surgery
Rouge Valley Health System – Ajax Site
Ontario, Canada

Mark H. Greene, MD
Chief
Clinical Genetics Branch
National Cancer Institute
Rockville, Maryland

H. Barton Grossman, MD
W.A. "Tex" and Deborah Moncrief, Jr. Distinguished
    Chair in Urology
Professor and Deputy Chairman
Department of Urology
The University of Texas M.D. Anderson
    Cancer Center
Houston, Texas

Robert L. Grubb III
Urologic Oncology Fellow
Urologic Oncology Branch
National Cancer Institute
Bethesda, Maryland

Bertrand D. Guillonneau, MD
Head
Department of Urology
Section of Minimally Invasive Surgery
Memorial Sloan-Kettering Cancer Center
New York, New York

Alexander R. Guimaraes, MD, PhD
Instructor
Department of Radiology
Center for Molecular Imaging Research
Clinical Discovery Program
Harvard Medical School

Instructor
Division of Abdominal Imaging
Department of Radiology
Massachusetts General Hospital
Boston, Massachusetts

Freddie C. Hamdy, MD, FRCSEd Urol
Professor of Urology
Academic Urology Unit
University of Sheffield
Royal Hallamshire Hospital

Honorary Consultant Urologist
Academic Urology Unit
Sheffield Teaching Hospitals NHS Foundation Trust
Sheffield, United Kingdom

Mukesh G. Harisinghani, MD
Assistant Professor
Department of Radiology
Harvard Medical School

Assistant Radiologist
Department of Abdominal Imaging
    and Intervention
Massachusetts General Hospital
Boston, Massachusetts

Jillian A. Harrison, PhD
Post Doctoral Scientist
Department of Morphology
University of Geneva Medical Center
University of Geneva
Geneva, Switzerland

Richard E. Hautmann, MD
Professor and Chief
Department of Urology
University of Ulm
Ulm, Germany

Niall M. Heney, MD, FRCS
Clinical Assistant Professor
Department of Surgery
Harvard University

Urologist
Department of Urology
Massachusetts General Hospital
Boston, Massachusetts

Javier Hernandez, MD
Urology Oncology Fellow/Instructor
Department of Urology
University of Texas Health Science Center
San Antonio, Texas

Harry W. Herr, MD, FRCS
Professor
Department of Urology
Weill Medical College of Cornell University

Attending Surgeon
Department of Urology
Memorial Sloan-Kettering Cancer Center
New York, New York

Simon Horenblas, MD, PhD, FEBU
Professor
Department of Urologic Oncology
Free University Medical Center

Chief
Department of Urology
Netherlands Cancer Institute-Antoni
    van Leeuwenhoek Hospital
Amsterdam, The Netherlands

Wolfgang Horninger, MD
Associate Professor
Department of Urology
Medical University Innsbruck
Innsbruck, Austria

Chief
Prostate Cancer Center
Medical University Innsbruck

Alan Horwich, MBBS, FRCP, FRCR, PhD
Professor
Department of Radiotherapy
The Institute of Cancer Research
University of London
London, United Kingdom

Consultant
Department of Clinical Oncology
The Royal Marsden Hospital, Sutton
Surrey, United Kingdom

Jane Houldsworth, PhD
Associate Laboratory Member
Cell Biology Program
Sloan-Kettering Institute

Associate Attending Geneticist
Department of Medicine
Memorial Sloan-Kettering Cancer Center
New York, New York

Hedvig Hricak, MD, PhD
Carroll and Milton Petrie Chair
Professor of Radiology
Department of Radiology
Weill Medical College of Cornell University

Chairman
Department of Radiology
Memorial Sloan-Kettering Cancer Center
New York, New York

Thomas E. Hutson, DO, PharmD
Director
Oncology Program
Texas Oncology, PA Baylor Sammons
    Cancer Center

Associate Staff
Department of Oncology
Baylor Sammons Medical Center
Dallas, Texas

William B. Isaacs, PhD
Professor
Department of Urology and Oncology
The Johns Hopkins University School of Medicine
Baltimore, Maryland

Günter Janetschek, MD
Professor
Department of Urology
Teaching Hospital University of Innsbruck
    and Vienna
Vienna, Austria

Head
Department of Urology
Elisabethinen Hospital
Linz, Austria

Philip Kantoff, MD
Professor
Department of Medicine
Harvard Medical School

Director of the Lank Center for
    Genitourinary Oncology
Chief, Division of Solid Tumor Oncology
Dana Farber Cancer Institute
Boston, Massachusetts

Michael W. Kattan, PhD
Chairman, Quantitative Health Sciences
The Cleveland Clinic Foundation
Cleveland, Ohio

Donald S. Kaufman, MD
Clinical Professor of Medicine,
Harvard Medical School

Director
The Claire and John Bertucci Center for
    Genitourinary Cancers
Hematology/Oncology Unit
Department of Medicine
Massachusetts General Hospital
Yawkey Center for Outpatient Care
Boston, Massachusetts

Hyung L. Kim, MD
Assistant Professor
Department of Urology
State University of New York
University of Buffalo School of Medicine
  and Biomedical Sciences

Attending Surgeon
Department of Urologic Oncology
Roswell Park Cancer Institute
Buffalo, New York

Isaac Yi Kim, MD, PhD
Department of Urology
UCI Medical Center
Orange, California

Laurence Klotz, MD
Professor, Department of Surgery
University of Toronto

Chief, Division of Urology
Sunnybrook and Women's Health Sciences Centre
Toronto, Ontario, Canada

Gnanamba Varuni Kondagunta, MD
Clinical Assistant Attending
Department of Genitourinary Oncology
Solid Tumor Division
Memorial Sloan-Kettering Cancer Center

Clinical Assistant Attending Physician
Department of Medicine, Genitourinary Oncology
Memorial Hospital for Cancer and Allied Diseases

Instructor in Medicine
Department of Medicine
Weill Medical College of Cornell University
New York Presbyterian Hospital
New York, New York

Theresa M. Koppie, MD
Oncology Fellow
Memorial Sloan-Kettering Cancer Center
New York, New York

Joan L. Kramer, MD
Staff Clinician
Clinical Genetics Branch
Division of Cancer Epidemiology and Genetics
National Cancer Institute
Rockville, Maryland

Ann S. LaCasce, MD
Instructor in Medicine
Department of Medical Oncology
Harvard Medical School

Attending Physician
Department of Medical Oncology
Dana Farber Cancer Institute
Boston, Massachusetts

John S. Lam, MD
Clinical Instructor
Department of Urology
David Geffen School of Medicine at University
  of California—Los Angeles
Los Angeles, California

W. Robert Lee, MD, MS
Vice Chairman, Professor
Department of Radiation Oncology
Wake Forest University
Winston-Salem, North Carolina

Steven A. Leibel, MD
Professor, Medical Director
Department of Radiation Oncology
Stanford University
Stanford, California

Bradley C. Leibovich, MD
Associate Professor
Department of Urology
Mayo Clinic
Rochester, Minnesota

Seth P. Lerner, MD, FACS
Associate Professor
Department of Urology
Baylor College of Medicine
Houston, Texas

Michael M. Lieber, MD
Professor
Department of Urology
Mayo Clinic College of Medicine
Rochester, Minnesota

Hans Lilja, MD, PhD
Attending Research Clinical Chemist
Departments of Clinical Labs, Urology, & Medicine
Memorial Sloan-Kettering Cancer Center
New York, New York

Visiting Professor,
Department of Laboratory Medicine
Division of Clinical Chemistry
Lund University,
Malmö, Sweden

W. Marston Linehan, MD
Chief, Urologic Oncology Branch
Center for Cancer Research
National Cancer Institute
National Institutes of Health
Bethesda, Maryland

Mark S. Litwin, MD, MPH
Professor
Department of Urology and Health Services
University of California
Los Angeles, California

Massimo Loda, MD
Associate Professor of Pathology
Department of Pathology
Dana Farber Cancer Institute/Harvard Medical School

Senior Pathologist
Department of Pathology
Dana Farber Cancer Institute/Brigham & Women's Hospital
Boston, Massachusetts

Sereena Malhi, MD
Staff Physician
Hematology and Medical Oncology
Vanatchee Valley Medical Center
Vanatchee, Washington

Paul D. Maroni, MD
Resident in Urology
Department of Surgery, Division of Urology
University of Colorado at Denver Health Sciences Center
Denver, Colorado

Viraj A. Master, MD, PhD
Clinical Instructor
Urology and UCSF Comprehensive Cancer Center
University of California

Attending Surgeon
Department of Urology
University of California, San Francisco Hospital
San Francisco, California

David F. McDermott, MD
Instructor in Medicine
Department of Medicine
Harvard Medical School

Clinical Director, Bridge Therapy Program
Department of Hematology/Oncology
Beth Israel Deaconess Medical Center
Boston, Massachusetts

W. Scott McDougal, MD
Professor of Urology
Department of Urology
Harvard Medical School

Chief of Urology
Department of Urology
Massachusetts General Hospital
Boston, Massachusetts

Grace T. McKee, MD
Staff Cytopathologist
Associate Professor
Department of Cytopathology
Massachusetts General Hospital
Boston, Massachusetts

Maria J. Merino, MD
Laboratory of Pathology
National Cancer Institute
Bethesda, Maryland

M. Dror Michaelson, MD, PhD
Instructor in Medicine
Department of Medicine
Harvard Medical School

Clinical Associate in Medicine
Department of Hematology/Oncology
Massachusetts General Hospital
Boston, Massachusetts

Jeff Michalski, MD
Radiation Oncologist
Mallinckrodt Institute of Radiology
Washington University
St. Louis, Missouri

David C. Miller, MD
Professor
Department of Urology
University of Michigan
Ann Arbor, Michigan

Alireza Moinzadeh, MD
Fellow
Laparoscopic and Minimally
  Invasive Surgery
Glickman Urological Institute
Cleveland Clinic Foundation
Cleveland, Ohio

James E. Montie, MD
Chairman and Professor
Department of Urology
University of Michigan
Ann Arbor, Michigan

Lee E. Moore, PhD, MPH
Investigator
Occupational and Environmental
  Epidemiology Branch
Division of Cancer Epidemiology
  and Genetics
Bethesda, Maryland

Robert J. Motzer, MD
Attending Physician
Department of Medicine
Memorial Sloan-Kettering Cancer Center
New York, New York

Michael Mullerad, MD
Department of Urology
Bnai-Zion Medical Center
Haifa, Israel

Mari Nakabayashi, MD, PhD
Research Fellow in Medicine
Department of Medicine
Harvard Medical School

Research Associate
Lank Center for Genitourinary Oncology
Dana Farber Cancer Institute
Boston, Massachusetts

Tohru Nakagawa, MD
Researcher
National Cancer Center Research
  Institute
Tokyo, Japan

David E. Neal, FmedSci. FRCS, MS, BSc
Professor of Surgical Oncology
Department of Oncology and Surgery
University of Cambridge

Honorary Consultant Urological Surgeon
Department of Urology
Addenbrooke's Hospital
Cambridge, United Kingdom

Andrew C. Novick, MD
Professor
Department of Surgery
Cleveland Clinic Lerner College of Medicine

Chairman
Glickman Urological Institute
Cleveland Clinic Foundation
Cleveland, Ohio

Michael O'Donnell, MD
Professor
Department of Urology
The University of Iowa

Professor
Department of Urology
The University of Iowa Hospitals and Clinics
Iowa City, Iowa

William K. Oh, MD
Assistant Professor of Medicine
Department of Medicine
Harvard Medical School

Clinical Director
Lank Center for Genitourinary Oncology
Dana Farber Cancer Institute
Boston, Massachusetts

R. T. D. Oliver, MD, FRCP
Professor
Institute of Cancer
Queen Mary University of London

Professor
Department of Medical Oncology
Cancer Services
Barts and the London NHS Trust
London, United Kingdom

Bradley G. Orris, MD
Chief Resident
Department of Urology
Loyola University Medical Center
Maywood, Illinois

J. Kellogg Parsons, MD, MHS
Assistant Professor of Surgery/Urology
Department of Surgery
University of California
San Diego, California

Alan W. Partin, MD, PhD
Professor, Chairman and Urologist-in-Chief
Department of Urology
Johns Hopkins University School of Medicine
James Buchanan Brady Urological Institute
Baltimore, Maryland

Kenneth J. Pienta, MD
Professor
Department of Internal Medicine and Urology
University of Michigan
Ann Arbor, Michigan

Giorgio Pizzocaro, MD
Director,
Division of Urology
Istituto Nazionale Tumori
Milan, Italy

Elizabeth A. Platz, ScD, MPH
Associate Professor
Department of Epidemiology
Johns Hopkins Bloomberg School of Public Health
Baltimore, Maryland

Alan Pollack, MD, PhD
Senior Member and Chairman
Department of Radiation Oncology
Fox Chase Cancer Center
Philadelphia, Pennsylvania

Arnold L. Potosky, MHS, PhD
Health Services Researcher
Applied Research Program
Division of Cancer Control and Population Sciences
National Cancer Institute
Bethesda, Maryland

Victor E. Reuter, MD
Professor of Pathology
Department of Pathology
Weill Medial College of Cornell University

Attending Pathologist and Vice Chair
Department of Pathology
Memorial Sloan-Kettering Cancer Center
New York, New York

Jerome P. Richie, MD
Elliott C. Cutler Professor of Urological Surgery
Department of Urology
Harvard Medical School

Chairman
Harvard Program in Urology
Department of Urology
Brigham & Women's Hospital
Boston, Massachusetts

Mack Roach III, MD, FACR
Professor, Vice Chair, Director of Clinical Research
Department of Radiation Oncology and Urology
UCSF Comprehensive Cancer Center
San Francisco, California

Ronald K. Ross, MD
Professor and Chair
Department of Preventive Medicine
University of Southern California
Los Angeles, California

Mark A. Rubin, MD
Associate Professor
Department of Pathology
Harvard Medical School

Chief, Urologic Pathology
Department of Pathology
Brigham & Women's Hospital
Boston, Massachusetts

Anthony H. Russell, MD, FACR
Associate Professor
Department of Radiation Oncology
Harvard Medical School

Chief, Gynecologic Radiation Oncology
Department of Radiation Oncology
Massachusetts General Hospital
Boston, Massachusetts

Paul Russo, MD, FACS
Associate Attending Surgeon
Department of Urology
Memorial Sloan-Kettering Cancer Center
New York

Howard M. Sandler, MD
Professor and Senior Associate
Chair, Department of Radiation Oncology
University of Michigan
Ann Arbor, Michigan

Peter T. Scardino, MD
Florence and Theodore Baumritter/Enid Ancell Chair
Chairman, Department of Urology
Memorial Sloan-Kettering Cancer Center
New York, New York

Paul F. Schellhammer, MD
Professor
Department of Urology
Eastern Virginia Medical School

Surgeon
Department of Urology
Sentara Norfolk General Hospital
Norfolk, Virginia

Gregory S. Schenk, MD
Department of Urology
Mayo Clinic
Rochester, Minnesota

Howard I. Scher, MD
Professor
Department of Medicine
Joan and Sanford Weill College of Medicine of
    Cornell University

Chief, Genitourinary Oncology Service
Department of Medicine
Memorial Sloan-Kettering Cancer Center
New York, New York

Joel Sheinfeld, MD
Professor
Department of Urology
Weill Medical College of Cornell University

Vice-chairman
Department of Urology
Memorial Sloan-Kettering Cancer Center
New York, New York

Katsuto Shinohara, MD
Professor
Department of Urology
University of California

Attending Surgeon
Department of Urology
University of California, San Francisco
Mt. Zion Comprehensive Cancer Center
San Francisco, California

William U. Shipley, MD
Andres Soriano Professor of Radiation Oncology
Harvard Medical School

The Claire and John Bertucci Center for Genitourinary
    Cancers
Head, Genitourinary Oncology Unit
Department of Radiation Oncology
Massachusetts General Hospital
Boston, Massachusetts

Amita Shukla-Dave, PhD
Instructor
Department of Medical Physics and Radiology
Memorial Sloan-Kettering Cancer Center
New York, New York

Donald G. Skinner, MD
Professor, Chair
Department of Urology
University of Southern California Keck School of Medicine

Chief of Surgery
Norris Comprehensive Cancer Center
Los Angeles, California

Kevin M. Slawin, MD
Professor and Dan L. Duncan Family Chair in Prostate
    Disease
Director, The Baylor Prostate Center
Scott Department of Urology
Baylor College of Medicine

Attending Urologist
Department of Urology
The Methodist Hospital
Houston, Texas

Stefan Sleijfer, MD, PhD
Staff Member
Department of Medical Oncology
Erasmus University Medical Center
Rotterdam, The Netherlands

Stephen R. Smalley, MD
Clinical Professor
Department of Radiation Oncology
University of Kansas
Kansas City, Kansas

Matthew R. Smith, MD, PhD
Assistant Professor
Harvard Medical School

Assistant Physician
Medicine/Hemotology and Oncology Division
Massachusetts General Hospital
Boston, Massachusetts

Alan So, MD, FRCSC
The Prostate Centre
Vancouver General Hospital
Vancouver, British Columbia, Canada

Walter M. Stadler, MD, FACP
Associate Professor
Department of Medicine
Section of Hematology/Oncology
University of Chicago
Chicago, Illinois

Graeme S. Steele, MD, FCS, FACS
Assistant Professor Surgery
Department of Surgery, Division of Urology
Harvard Medical School

Associate Surgeon
Surgery, Division of Urology
Brigham and Women's Hospital
Boston, Massachusetts

John Peter Stein, MD, FACS
Associate Professor
Department of Urology
University of Southern California

Associate Professor
Department of Urology
Norris Comprehensive Cancer Center
Los Angles, California

Gary D. Steinberg, MD
Associate Professor
Department of Urology
University of Chicago
Chicago, Illinois

Jordan R. Steinberg, MD, CM
Assistant Professor
Department of Urology
McGill University

Attending Urologist
Department of Urology
McGill University Health Center
Montreal, Quebec, Canada

Andrew J. Stephenson, MD
Fellow
Department of Urology
Sidney Kimmel Center for Prostate
  and Urologic Cancers
Memorial Sloan-Kettering Cancer Center
New York, New York

Thomas Steuber, MD
Department of Urology
University of Hamburg

Assistant Attending Urologist
Department of Urology
University-Hospital, Hamburg Eppendorf
Hamburg, Germany

Cora N. Sternberg, MD, FACP
Adjunct Professor
Department of Medicine
Tufts University School of Medicine
Boston, Massachusetts

Chief,
Department of Medical Oncology
San Camillo-Forlanini Hospital
Rome, Italy

Shahin Tabatabaei, MD
Instructor in Surgery
Department of Surgery
Harvard University

Urology Surgeon
Department of Urology
Massachusetts General Hospital
Boston, Massachusetts

Satoru Takahashi, MD
Associate Professor
Department of Urology
University of Tokyo
Tokyo, Japan

Winston W. Tan, MD
Assistant Professor
Department of Medicine
Mayo Medical School

Senior Consultant
Department of Hematology and Oncology
St. Luke's Hospital
Jacksonville, Florida

Miah-Hiang Tay, MRCP
Clinical Tutor
Medical Faculty
National University of Singapore
Department of Medical Oncology
National Cancer Center Singapore
Singapore

R. Houston Thompson, MD
Instructor
Department of Urology
Mayo Clinic
Rochester, Minnesota

Ian M. Thompson Jr., MD
Chairman
Department of Urology
The University of Texas Health Science Center at
  San Antonio
San Antonio, Texas

J. Brantley Thrasher, MD, FACS
Professor and William L. Valk Chair
Department of Urology
University of Kansas Medical Center
Kansas City, Kansas

Wayne D. Tilley, PhD
Chair,
Department of Medicine
Dame Roma Mitchell Cancer Research
  Laboratories
University of Adelaide

Director, Hanson Center for Cancer Research
Hanson Institute
Royal Adelaide Hospital
Adelaide, Australia

Donald J. Tindall, PhD
Professor, Director, Vice-Chair
Department of Urology Research
Mayo Clinic
Rochester, Minnesota

Carlos A. Torres-Cabala, MD
Clinical Fellow
Laboratory of Pathology
National Cancer Institute
Bethesda, Maryland

Karim A. Touijer
Department of Urology
Memorial Sloan-Kettering Cancer Center
New York, New York

Taiji Tsukamoto, MD
Department of Urology
Sapporo Medical University School of Medicine
Sapporo, Japan

Nicholas J. Vogelzang, MD
Director, Nevada Cancer Institute
Las Vegas, Nevada

McClellan M. Walther, MD
Attending Urologic Surgeon
Urologic Oncology Branch
National Cancer Institute
Bethesda, Maryland

Padraig R. Warde, MD
Professor
Department of Radiation Oncology
University of Toronto

Associate Director
Radiation Medicine Program
Princess Margaret Hospital
University Health Network
Toronto, Ontario, Canada

Erik S. Weise, MD
Endourology Fellow
Department of Urology
The University of Iowa and
The University of Iowa Hospitals and Clinics
Iowa City, Iowa

Thomas M. Wheeler, MD
Professor and Interim chairman
Department of Pathology
Baylor College of Medicine
Houston, Texas

Peter N. Wiklund, MD, PhD
Professor
Department of Surgical Sciences, Section of Urology
Karolinska Institute

Chief
Department of Urology
Karolinska University Hospital
Stockholm, Sweden

Howard N. Winfield, MD
Professor of Urology
Department of Urology
The University of Iowa

Director of Endourology and Laproscopic Surgery
Department of Urology
The University of Iowa Hospitals and Clinics
Iowa City, Iowa

Ronald de Wit, MD, PhD
Department of Medical Oncology
Erasmus University Medical Center
Daniel den Hoed Cancer Center
Rotterdam, The Netherlands

J.A. Witjes, MD
Department of Urology
University Medical Center Nijmegen
Nijmegen, The Netherlands

Jianfeng Xu, MD, PhD
Professor of Public Health and Cancer Biology
Associate Director
Center for Human Genomics
Wake Forest University School of Medicine
Winston-Salem, North Carolina

Robert H. Young, MD
Director of Surgical Pathology
Massachusetts General Hospital

Professor of Pathology
Harvard Medical School
Boston, Massachusetts

Mimi C. Yu, PhD
Professor
Cancer Center
University of Minnesota
Minneapolis, Minnesota

Jian-Min Yuan, MD, PhD
Associate Professor
Cancer Center
University of Minnesota
Minneapolis, Minnesota

Berton Zbar, MD
Chief
Laboratory of Immunobiology
National Cancer Institute
Frederick, Maryland

Michael J. Zelefsky, MD
Chief, Brachytherapy Service
Professor of Radiation Oncology
Department of Radiation Oncology
Memorial Sloan-Kettering Cancer Center
New York, New York

Anthony Zietman, MD
Professor of Radiation Oncology
Department of Radiation Oncology
Harvard Medical School

Attending Radiation Oncologist
Department of Radiation Oncology
Massachusetts General Hospital
Boston, Massachusetts

Horst Zincke, MD, PhD
Department of Urology
Mayo College of Medicine

Director of Uro-Oncologic Surgery Program
   and Consultant of Urologic Surgery
Department of Urology
Mayo Clinic
Rochester, Minnesota

This third edition of the *Comprehensive Textbook of Genitourinary Oncology* is arriving almost 10 years after its first edition published in 1996, thus testifying to the continued need for a "comprehensive" text in this particular area of oncology. The first edition was managed by the person who is also the current edition's Senior Executive Editor, Jonathan W. Pine, Jr., who has shared our vision for the book and who has patiently guided us to address the ongoing need for it over the past 10 years. Thank you, Jonathan!

The 2005 edition of the *Comprehensive Textbook of Genitourinary Oncology* retains three of its four original editors, Drs. Vogelzang, Scardino, and Shipley, and introduces two new editors, W. Marston Linehan, MD, of the National Cancer Institute, who brings expertise in both renal cancer and molecular biology, and Frans M.J. Debruyne, MD, PhD, who brings added expertise in genitourinary surgery. With this new team of editors, we have stayed true to the intent of the book's first edition—namely, to apply different areas of scientific knowledge to the goal of eradicating genitourinary cancers—and we continue to believe that the goal of disease eradication and life prolongation can be achieved only through intense multidisciplinary care and cooperation between all clinical fields.

As each clinical field in oncology grows and new knowledge is created, it necessitates a regular updating of the literature in that field. A look back at the 1996 edition of this book reveals that significant changes have occurred in each of the three clinical areas, but that surgery has continued to be the strongest component of the text. Significant advances in surgery since the first edition's publication include robotic-assisted laparoscopic surgery, cryoablation, and radio frequency ablation techniques. Intensity-modulated radiation therapy, particle beam radiation therapy, and computer-based planning have allowed the field of radiation oncology to evolve to high levels of precision with ever-lower rates of toxicity. The youngest clinical field, medical oncology, has shown surprising and continued growth in the area of genitourinary cancers and has seen the introduction of anti-angiogenic agents for metastatic renal cell carcinoma—proof that docetaxel-based chemotherapy extends the quantity and quality of life of patients with hormone refractory prostate cancer and that the regimen of MVAC (methotrexate, vinblastine, Adriamycin, and cisplatin) given neoadjuvantly for muscle invasive bladder cancer adds a survival advantage to patients with this disease. Clearly, in the past 10 years, each field in oncology has grown individually and contributed to furthering the goal of eliminating the scourge of genitourinary cancer.

The first edition of this book was also intended to serve as a multidisciplinary focal point for case management and genitourinary case conferences. It (and the second edition) served that purpose over the past 10 years, and we hope that this current edition will continue to serve the purposes of surgeons, radiation oncologists, pathologists, and medical oncologists involved in the care of patients and their many different and challenging neoplasms. Ray Abbratt, one of our colleagues in Cape Town, South Africa, who is both a medical and a radiation oncologist, sent us a picture of the *Comprehensive Textbook of Genitourinary Oncology* placed on a table surrounded by a multidisciplinary genitourinary cancer care team. It is just that sort of multidisciplinary interaction that this book aims to stimulate.

The mutual goal of the National Cancer Institute and the American Cancer Society—as articulated by a noted genitourinary oncologist, Andrew von Eschenbach, MD, Director of the National Cancer Institute of the United States—is to eliminate suffering and death from cancer by 2015. This noble goal may seem distant (and, some would say, unachievable), but nevertheless we hope that the *Comprehensive Textbook of Genitourinary Oncology* will contribute to its eventual achievement by assisting physicians around the world in their work.

Nicholas J. Vogelzang, MD
Peter T. Scardino, MD
William U. Shipley, MD
Frans M.J. Debruyne, MD, PhD
W. Marston Linehan, MD

We represent the evolution of four different areas of scientific knowledge, each born (in part) of the human desire to rid itself of the scourge of cancer. Surgical treatment is the oldest child of the four areas tracing its roots to ancient civilizations. Radiation oncology, the competitive second child, began 100 years ago with the discovery of x-rays by Conrad Roentgen in 1985. Medical oncology, the adolescent in the group, can trace its origins to the use of hormonal therapy and chemotherapy (with the invention of nitrogen mustard) in the 1940s. The youngest child, the field of molecular and cell biology, has taken its early steps toward cancer treatment with gene therapy and growth factor inhibition. At times, these fields have been antagonistic and hostile to one another, as siblings will often be. Yet they have also been firmly supportive of each other. Each of the older siblings has helped to raise the baby of the family, which someday may be the biggest and strongest of all four. Our germ line, however, remains the same: namely, a desire to find better ways to alleviate and, if possible, cure the patient with cancer.

Genitourinary cancers are a wonderfully diverse and challenging set of neoplasms for physicians and scientists to diagnose and manage. The field of genitourinary oncology has been the subject of numerous textbooks over the past 15 years (1–11). These books and many other texts have shaped, refined, and molded the field of genitourinary cancer. Using this broad base of knowledge, we began the task of editing *Comprehensive Textbook of Genitourinary Oncology*.

This book is an attempt to summarize, collate, and display this rapidly changing field, which encompasses medicine, surgery, radiation oncology, basic science, pathology, and supportive care. After a gestation period of several years, the editors came together as a unit in October 1993, and the organization and planning of the book was achieved with remarkable harmony from our personal opinions and philosophies regarding management and evaluation of patients with these diseases. Any omissions or excesses are our responsibility alone.

Comprehensive Textbook of Genitourinary Oncology is intended for physicians and scientists with a clinical or basic science interest in cancers of the genitourinary tract. Recognizing that such cancers occur in close to 300,000 patients within the United States each year and in another 600,000 to 700,000 patients in other countries, we have tried to be international in our selection of contributors. We have also tried to produce a textbook that can be read and used by practicing physicians, be they academic or nonacademic. Our second goal was to produce a textbook that basic scientists working in this diverse and divergent field would be able to reference and read as an authoritative source. Our third goal was to interpret the field for trainees in surgery, medicine, radiation oncology, and pathology. In the past, these trainees have not necessarily had broad cross-specialty exposure, but increasingly trainees spend elective time in the various complementary fields. We hope that this book will reflect the cross-fertilization that increasingly pervades the field of genitourinary oncology.

Nicholas J. Vogelzang, MD
Peter T. Scardino, MD
William U. Shipley, MD
Donald S. Coffey, PhD

References

1. Culp DA, Loening SA, eds. Genitourinary oncology. Philadelphia: Lea & Febiger, 1985.
2. Skinner DG, Lieskovsky G, eds. Genitourinary cancer: the diagnosis and management of genitourinary cancer. Philadelphia: WB Saunders, 1988.
3. Catalona WJ, Ratliff TTL, eds. Urologic oncology. In: McGuire WL, ed. *Cancer treatment and research*. The Hague, Netherlands: Martinus Nijhoff, Cower Academic Publishing Group, 1984.
4. Raghavan D, ed. *The management of bladder cancer*. Baltimore: Edward Arnold Publishers, 1988.
5. Splinter TAW, Scher HI, eds. *Neoadjuvant chemotherapy of invasive bladder cancer. Progress in clinical and biological research*, vol 535. New York: Wiley-Liss, 1990.
6. Horwich A, ed. *Testicular cancer: investigation and management*. London: Chapman and Hall, 1991.
7. Johnson DE, Logothetis CJ, Von Eschenbach AC, eds. *Systemic therapy for genitourinary cancers*. Chicago: Year Book, 1989.
8. Dawson NA, Vogelzang NJ, eds. *Prostate cancer*. New York: Wiley-Liss, 1994.
9. Walsh PC, Retik AB, Stamey TA, Vaughn ED Jr, eds. *Campbell's urology*. Philadelphia: WB Saunders, 1992.
10. Denis L, Niijima T, Prout G Jr, Schroder F, eds. *Developments in bladder cancer*. New York: AR Liss, 1986.
11. Smith PH, ed. *Combination therapy in urologic malignancy*. London: Springer-Verlag, 1989.

We thank all of the authors for their contributions and hard work that have resulted in this third edition. We also appreciate the commitment continuously offered by the outstanding staff at Lippincott Williams & Wilkins. In particular, we thank Senior Executive Editor Jonathan W. Pine, Jr., for his encouragement and thoughtful direction in guiding us through this third edition, and Managing Editors Raymond E. Reter, for the initial stages of the project, Stacey L. Sebring, for the middle stages, and especially Anne E. Jacobs, for managing the project's final stages of editing and production. For their outstanding and tireless efforts in coordinating our individual editorial responsibilities, we thank our assistants and support staff. We are also grateful for the insight and tireless effort of Lisa Errington, Editorial Assistant at the National Cancer Institute. Finally, the editors acknowledge Hope J. Lafferty, Medical Editor at Memorial Sloan-Kettering Cancer Center, whose outstanding organizational and interpersonal skills were integral to this effort throughout the entire process.

Nicholas J. Vogelzang, MD
Peter T. Scardino, MD
William U. Shipley, MD
Frans M.J. Debruyne, MD, PhD
W. Marston Linehan, MD

COMPREHENSIVE TEXTBOOK OF GENITOURINARY ONCOLOGY

THIRD EDITION

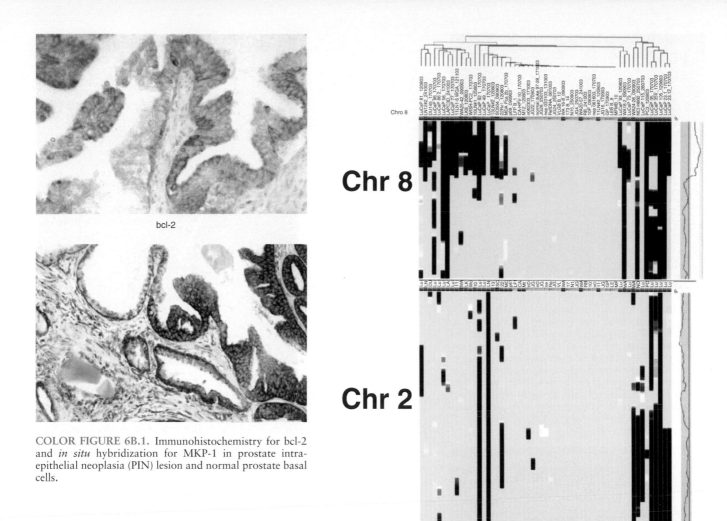

COLOR FIGURE 6B.1. Immunohistochemistry for bcl-2 and *in situ* hybridization for MKP-1 in prostate intraepithelial neoplasia (PIN) lesion and normal prostate basal cells.

COLOR FIGURE 6B.3. Regions of loss of heterozygosity (LOH) in tumors and xenografts compared to normal samples. dChipSNP was used to generate inferred LOH maps, which were then used in hierarchical clustering. The group of samples in the center without LOH are normal germ-line samples. Two distinct tumor clusters can be seen that differ with respect to LOH patterns on chromosomes 2 and 8.

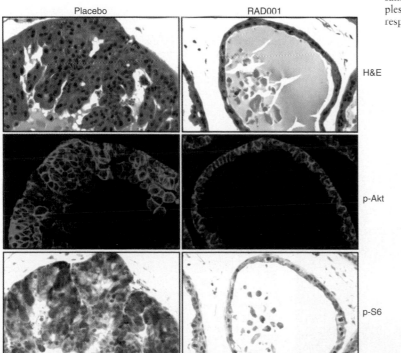

COLOR FIGURE 6B.4. Reversal of the prostate intraepithelial neoplasia (PIN) phenotype with mammalian target of rapamycin (mTOR) inhibition. Phospho-Akt is unaffected while phospho-S6 kinase staining is abolished.

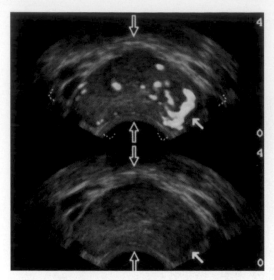

COLOR FIGURE 9.3. Comparison of traditional TRUS versus power Doppler ultrasonography of the prostate. The patient is a 63-year-old man with an elevated PSA and abnormal left-side prostate exam. The bottom panel shows traditional gray-scale ultrasonographic image of the prostate and the top panel shows the power Doppler image of the same area. The hypervascular areas corresponded well to geographically directed biopsies, which showed the extent of prostate cancer to be greater than that detected by conventional gray-scale ultrasound.

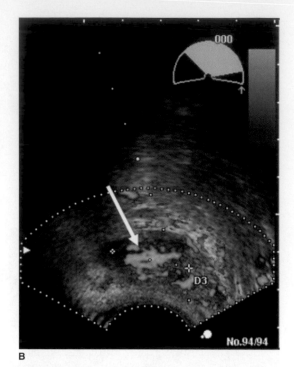

B

COLOR FIGURE 12.1B. The use of Doppler ultrasound in the detection of prostate cancer: Doppler transverse transrectal ultrasound image demonstrates a hyperechoic region (*arrow*) in the right side of the peripheral zone (PZ) suspicious for cancer. Doppler ultrasonography identifies hypervascular areas in the lesion, indicating cancer. (Courtesy of Dr. Fred Lee, University of Wisconsin.)

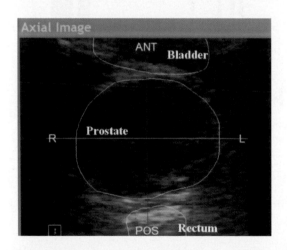

COLOR FIGURE 13F.1. Transabdominal ultrasound taken at the linear accelerator just prior to treatment. Contours from the planning CT scan of the prostate, bladder, and rectum are superimposed on the ultrasound images (*white lines*) to allow alignment of the isocenter (*green and red line intersection*) to the treatment plan.

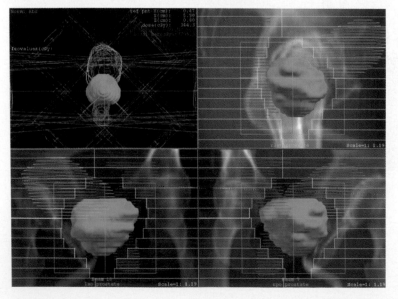

COLOR FIGURE 13F.2. Beam's eye view displays on lateral (*upper right panel*) and two obliquely oriented (*lower panels*) digital reconstructed radiographs. Graphic representations of multileaf collimator leaves demonstrate beam shaping relative to the contour of the PTV (*solid light blue*) and shielding of the rectum (*brown wire cage*) and bladder (*yellow wire cage*). The left upper panel displays a six-field 3D conformal beam arrangement viewed along the superior-inferior axis.

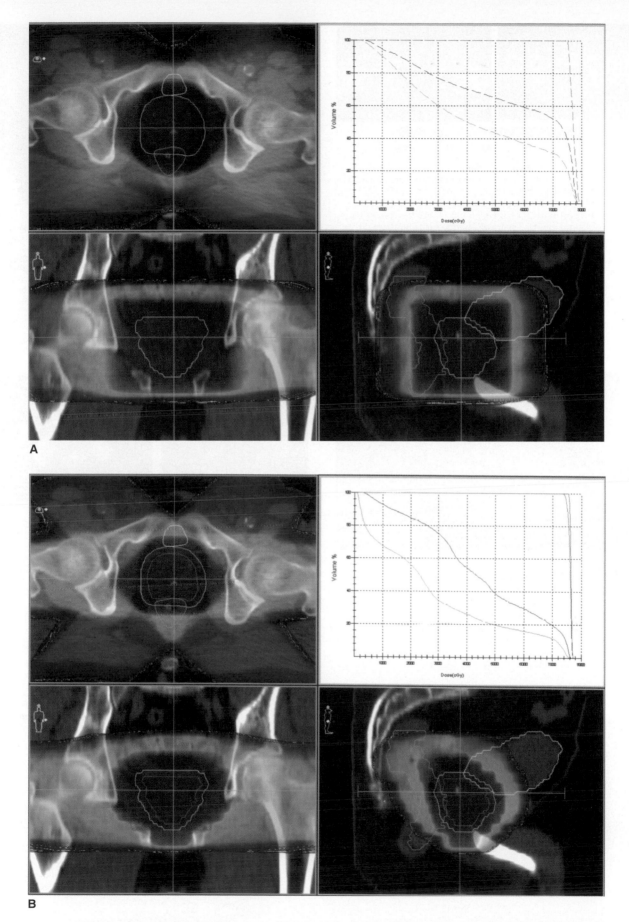

COLOR FIGURE 13F.3. Radiation dose distribution is represented by a color-wash display on axial, sagittal, and coronal CT reconstructions for (**A**) 2-D "arc" plan and (**B**) 3-D six field conformal plan. The upper-right panel in each group is a DVH of the bladder, rectum, and PTV.

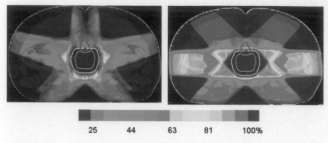

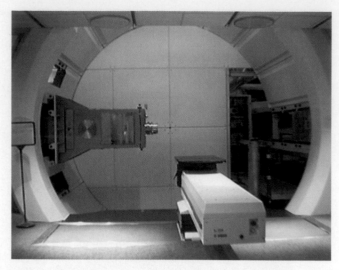

COLOR FIGURE 13G.1. **Left:** Midplane axial color wash dose distribution display of a five-field coplanar prostate IMRT plan for 15 MV x-rays, consisting of fields placed at angles of 0°, 75°, 135°, 225°, and 285°. **Right:** Midplane axial color wash dose distribution display of a six-field coplanar prostate 3D-CRT plan for 15 MV x-rays, consisting of one pair of lateral and two pairs of oblique fields. In these displays a band of the color spectrum corresponds to a range of doses. The prescription dose is normalized to 100%. The red region corresponds to the prescription isodose distribution (100% to 105%). The PTV contour is yellow, the clinical target volume is green, and the rectum is magenta. (From Leibel SA, Fuks Z, Zelefsky MJ, et al. Technological advances in external beam radiation therapy for the treatment of localized prostate cancer. *Semin Oncol* 2003;30: 596–615, with permission.)

COLOR FIGURE 13G.5. Gantry and treatment couch for the delivery of proton beam therapy at the Massachusetts General Hospital.

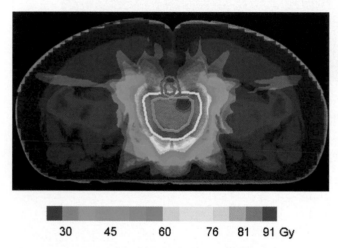

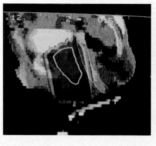

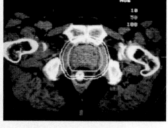

COLOR FIGURE 13G.6. **Left:** Sagittal CT reconstruction showing a perineal proton boost. The patient is in the lithotomy position. Note the rectal probe displacing the posterior rectal wall from the path of the proton beam. **Right:** Transverse CT slice showing the tightly conformal proton radiation isodose distribution encircling the prostate gland.

COLOR FIGURE 13G.3. Midplane axial color wash dose distribution display of a 9-field coplanar prostate IMRT plan for 15 MV x-rays with dose painting. In this plan the planning target volume (*contour in yellow*) is treated to a dose of 81 Gy and the image-detected target volume (*contour in blue*) simultaneously receives 91 Gy.

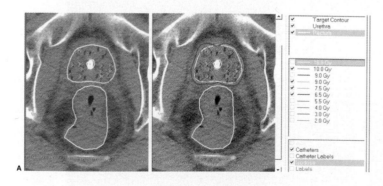

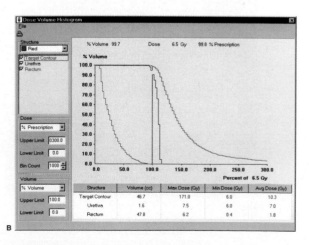

COLOR FIGURE 13H.7. **A:** HDR dose distribution. **B:** Dose volume histogram illustrating dose to target urethra and rectum.

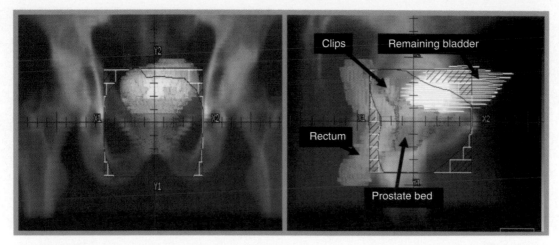

COLOR FIGURE 15D.3. The fields used at M.D. Anderson Cancer Center (MDACC) (82) were typically 10 × 10 cm anterior-posterior fields with the inferior border at the ischial tuberosities. This would place the inferior extent usually below the bulb of the penis. The rectum was split posteriorly, and some of the bladder above the prostatic bed was blocked anteriorly. The prostate bed is shown in tomato, the rest of the bladder in yellow, surgical clips in blue (*green when overlaying yellow*), and the rectum in green. Left, anterior-posterior; right, right lateral.

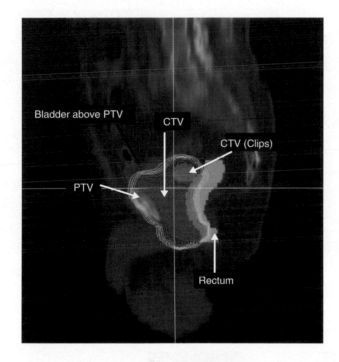

COLOR FIGURE 15D.4. An example of a patient planned using intensity-modulated radiotherapy (IMRT). A sagittal image is shown. An 8 mm planning target volume (PTV) was placed around the clinical target volumes (CTVs).

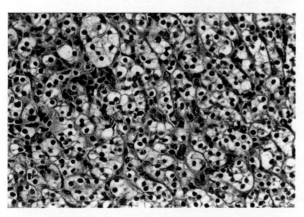

COLOR FIGURE 44B.1. Clear cell renal cell carcinoma (hematoxylin and eosin, original magnification ×100).

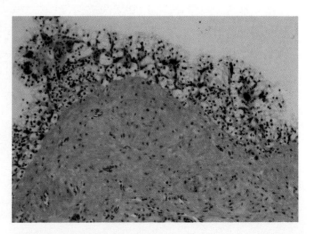

COLOR FIGURE 44B.2. Simple renal cyst (hematoxylin and eosin, original magnification ×100).

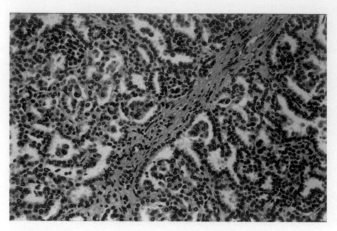

COLOR FIGURE 44B.3. Papillary renal cell carcinoma type I (hematoxylin and eosin, original magnification ×100).

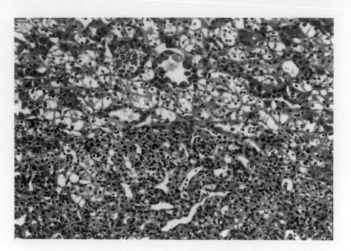

COLOR FIGURE 44B.4. Hybrid tumor composed of oncocytic and chromophobe cells (hematoxylin and eosin, original magnification ×100).

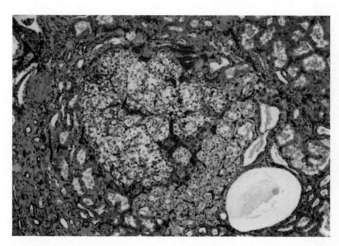

COLOR FIGURE 44B.5. Oncocytosis (hematoxylin and eosin, original magnification ×100).

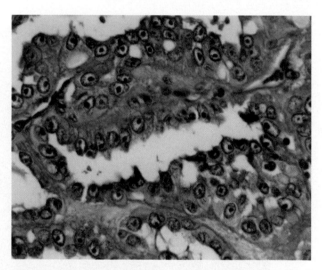

COLOR FIGURE 44B.6. Hereditary leiomyomatosis and renal cell carcinoma with papillary configuration (hematoxylin and eosin, original magnification ×100).

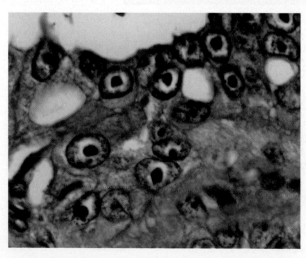

COLOR FIGURE 44B.7. Characteristic prominent nucleoli (hematoxylin and eosin, original magnification ×100).

Human renal epithelial neoplasms

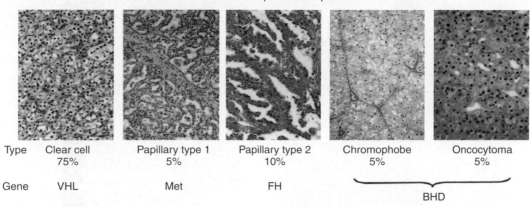

Type	Clear cell 75%	Papillary type 1 5%	Papillary type 2 10%	Chromophobe 5%	Oncocytoma 5%
Gene	VHL	Met	FH	BHD	

COLOR FIGURE 45.1. Kidney cancer is made up of a number of different types of cancer, each with a different histology, a different course, responding differently to therapy, and caused by alteration of a different gene. (From Linehan WM, Walther MM, Zbar B. The genetic basis of cancer of the kidney. *J Urol* 2003;170:2163, with permission.)

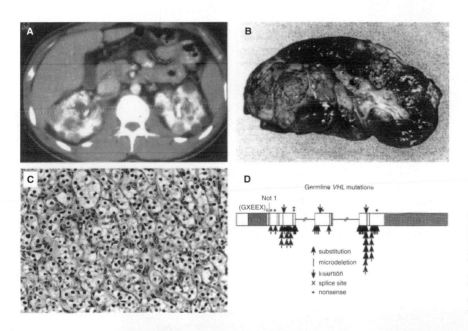

COLOR FIGURE 45.3. Von Hippel-Lindau (VHL)–associated renal carcinoma may be bilateral and multifocal and may appear as early as the second decade. Affected individuals in VHL kindreds are characterized by germline mutation of the *VHL* gene (3). (From Linehan WM, Walther MM, Zbar B. The genetic basis of cancer of the kidney. *J Urol* 2003;170: 2163, with permission.)

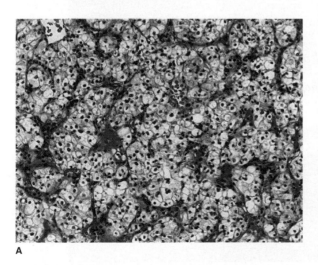

COLOR FIGURE 45.5A. *Von Hippel-Lindau (VHL)* gene: clear cell renal carcinoma. (From Gnarra JR, Tory K, Weng YW, et al. Mutation of the VHL tumour suppressor gene in renal carcinoma. *Nat Genet* 1994;7: 85, with permission.)

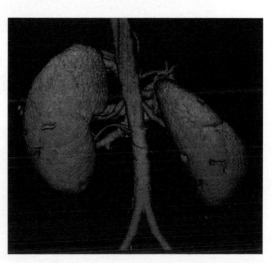

COLOR FIGURE 46.1. Three-dimensional volume rendering of the kidneys from a high-resolution computed tomography (CT) scan of the kidneys made possible by helical acquisition of the data. Note that an accessory right renal artery is seen.

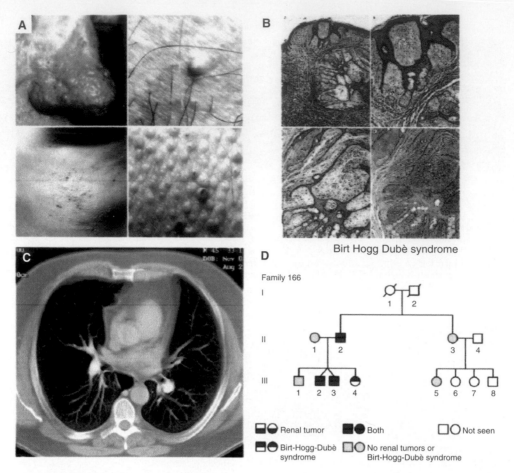

COLOR FIGURE 45.9. Birt-Hogg-Dubé (BHD) is a hereditary cancer syndrome in which affected individuals are at risk for the development of cutaneous fibrofolliculomas (**A, B**), pulmonary cysts (**C**), and renal tumors. BHD is inherited in an autosomal dominant fashion (**D**); that is, offspring have a 50/50 chance of carrying the gene. (From Linehan WM, Walther MM, Zbar B. The genetic basis of cancer of the kidney. *J Urol* 2003; 170:2163, and Toro J, Duray PH, Glenn GM, et al. Birt-Hogg-Dubé syndrome: a novel marker of kidney neoplasia. *Arch Dermatol* 1999;135: 1195, with permission.)

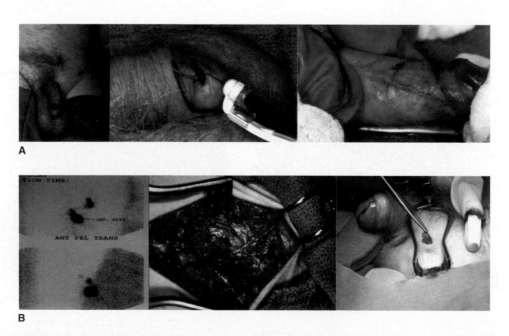

COLOR FIGURE 50.4. **A:** Technique of lymphoscintigraphy: injection of primary tumor site and absorption by local lymphatics. **B:** Lymphoscintigram, blue dye in lymphatics, and identification of sentinel lymph.

CHAPTER 1 ■ CLINICAL PRESENTATION OF PROSTATE CANCER IN THE 21ST CENTURY: WHERE HAVE ALL THE SIGNS AND SYMPTOMS GONE?

JOHN W. DAVIS AND PAUL F. SCHELLHAMMER

INTRODUCTION

As any physician with even a peripheral interest in prostate cancer recognizes, the local manifestations and the far-ranging systemic manifestations associated with this disease that were common two decades ago are now relegated to old texts and history. The tumor marker prostate-specific antigen (PSA) came on the scene in 1986 (1). When it was approved by the FDA for posttreatment monitoring, it also became routinely used as a strategy for earlier disease detection. As a result, prostate cancer has gradually become a disease for which the diagnosis and post-therapy follow-up is almost exclusively determined by a laboratory test. Therefore, the patient who has presented with prostate cancer during the past decade has been essentially free of signs and symptoms. In fact, a frequent statement by the patient when he is informed of the diagnosis of prostate cancer can be paraphrased as follows: "How could anything be wrong when I feel so well and have not experienced any discomfort or problems?" This picture is in marked contrast to the pre-PSA era, where the cardinal sign of prostate cancer was a distinctly palpable abnormality within the prostate, and the cardinal symptoms included a constellation of voiding difficulties, localized or diffuse back or bone pain, and systemic symptoms of weight loss, anorexia, fatigue, weakness, and a host of other disease-related illnesses (Figs. 1.1–1.9). As a result of serum PSA determinations and the radiologic tests they prompt, there is now less experience with clinical signs and symptoms and less emphasis placed on their recognition because, indeed, they are often not operational in providing meaningful diagnostic information. Furthermore, because treatment is so often directed by an abnormal laboratory or radiologic evaluation in an asymptomatic patient, the time frame for manifestation of disease symptomatology, even in the most advanced stages of disease, has been compressed. The result has been the truncation of a prolonged and morbid disease process, and this has been a blessing indeed for the patient.

The future predicts that diagnosis, prognostic assessment, and assignment of one of a number of treatments will be based on further laboratory advances in molecular genomics, proteomic profiling, or both (2,3). Nevertheless, attention to a patient's complaints and physical diagnosis is still relevant. On occasion, one or both will aid in establishing a diagnosis and clarifying the disease process, and even as progress makes some of the information less immediately important, an appreciation of signs and symptoms provides a historical perspective.

DIGITAL RECTAL EXAMINATION

Prior to the PSA era, the digital rectal examination (DRE) provided critical information, not only to raise suspicion of the presence of prostate cancer but also to determine operability for cure. The following description of the DRE is taken from Hugh Hampton Young's monograph (4).

"The rectal examination, which is usually made on the first visit of the patient, is of the greatest importance. After noting the condition of the anal sphincter (for fissures, hemorrhoids, etc.) and the rectal wall, adhesions, thickening, ulceration, compression of lumen, stricture, etc., the prostate is itself examined with the gloved finger. In all cases, it is well to make a drawing with the right hand upon a diagrammatic chart of the conditions found with the gloved left finger in the rectum. The exact size and shape of the prostatic contour should be noted and careful estimations at cardinal points made so as to get the prostatic area accurately depicted. The cross sections through the profile are made at various points, in order to show the changes from normal. The surface conditions of the prostate, smoothness, roughness, lobulation adhesions, etc. are appropriately indicated and the consistence of various portions of the prostate should be accurately shown. First-degree induration is shown by parallel lines in one direction; firmer induration known as second degree is shown by parallel lines at right angles to the first; third-degree induration is indicated by parallel lines running obliquely across the lines of second-degree induration. Areas of very extreme induration, stony in character, may be indicated by solid black areas. The presence of nodules is indicated by circles and the cross section shows their elevation and location above the normal surface of the prostate (Fig. 1.10). Adhesions are shown by parallel lines running off into the periprostatic tissues adjacent to the sides of the prostate or seminal vesicles. Invasion of the space above the prostate, in and about the ampulla and vesicles, is indicated in extent and degree just as it is done in the prostate. Lines of lymphatics and lymph glands are noted (Fig. 1.11). The condition of the rectal wall as to compression or stricture may also be indicated, and the involvement of the membranous urethra, the region of the triangular ligament, bulb, and corpora may also be drawn." A urologist in training today will rarely encounter these abnormalities as an individual finding and rarely, if ever, will they be found as a constellation.

Clearly, a great deal of emphasis was placed on accurately establishing the presence of and extent of the area of induration, and understandably so, as all treatment decisions were

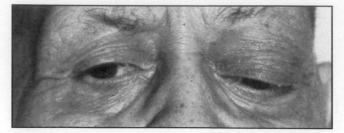

FIGURE 1.1. The patient presented with bone pain and weight loss together with visual impairment and exophthalmus. Osseous metastatic disease was found. A retroorbital mass lesion consistent with metastatic prostate cancer explained the ocular findings.

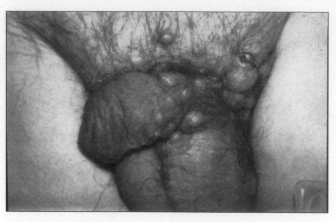

FIGURE 1.2. Numerous subcutaneous inguinal and scrotal nodules that were biopsy-proved as adenocarcinoma of the prostate.

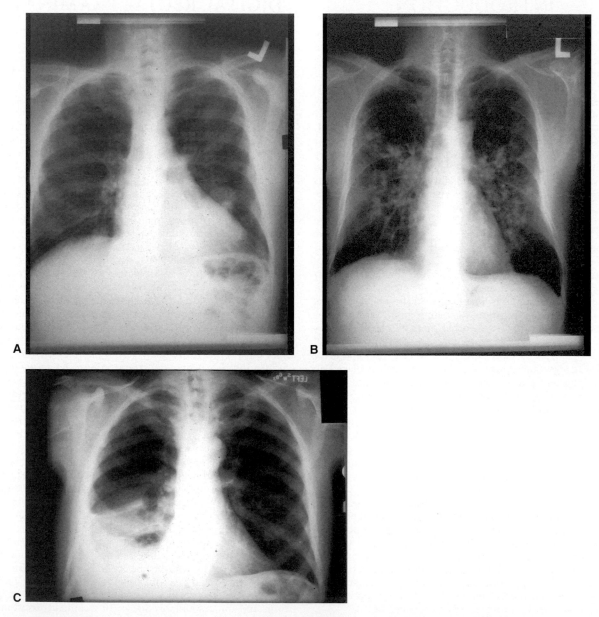

FIGURE 1.3. Various pulmonary lesions that are associated widely with metastatic prostate cancer including (**A**) nodular densities, (**B**) interstitial infiltrate or lymphangetic metastases, and (**C**) pleural effusion.

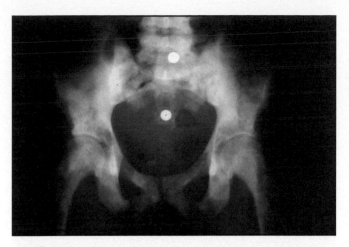

FIGURE 1.4. Plain film of pelvis demonstrating blastic lesions.

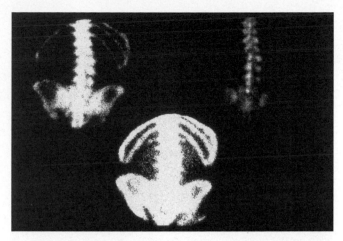

FIGURE 1.6. "Super scan" showing diffuse white-out and no renal excretion.

based on these findings. As experience with clinical-pathologic correlations was obtained, the so-called favorable lesion described and pictured by Young, which included rather extensive prostatic induration occupying the entire prostate (Fig. 1.12), gave way to a much more limited area of induration, the 1-cm nodule, that would allow successful extirpation. Jewett defined the B1 nodule in 1968 as "a palpably discrete nodule

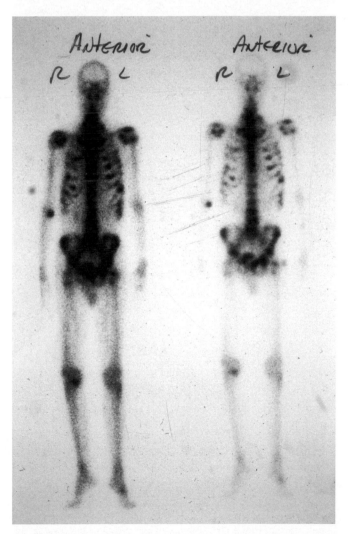

FIGURE 1.5. Bone scan with multiple areas of axial and appendicular metastases.

of firm or stony consistency limited to a part of one lateral lobe, averaging 1 cm or a little more in diameter, with compressible tissue always on two and sometimes on three sides (5) (Fig. 1.13)." That same year, Culp reported data that concurred that the 1-cm nodule was ideally amenable to cure by surgical excision (6). These landmark studies from Johns Hopkins and the Mayo Clinic confirmed that patients with a B1 nodule could expect a reasonable chance of cure by radical prostatectomy. The definitions of induration greater than the 1-cm nodule, though still confined to the prostate (i.e., B1, B2, B3, or T2a, T2b, T2c), have not been consistent, and depending on what definition is assumed, substage-specific outcomes will vary (7). Currently, the majority of prostate cancer is diagnosed as a result of PSA-prompted biopsy of prostate glands that are palpably normal and designated stage T1c. As an example, 67% of the 621 new prostate cancers diagnosed at Eastern Virginia Medical School in 2000 and 2001 were staged T1c. This figure is in agreement with the experience of the CaPSURE database (8). To illustrate further how PSA has

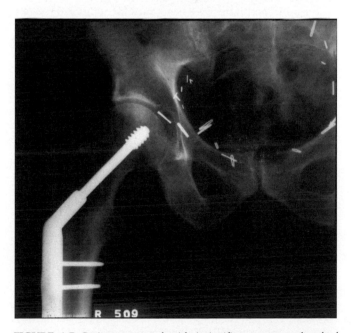

FIGURE 1.7. Patient presented with insignificant trauma that had caused an intratrochanteric fracture in an area of known metastatic involvement. Immediate internal fixation to provide ambulation was accomplished. Bone curettings demonstrated prostate cancer.

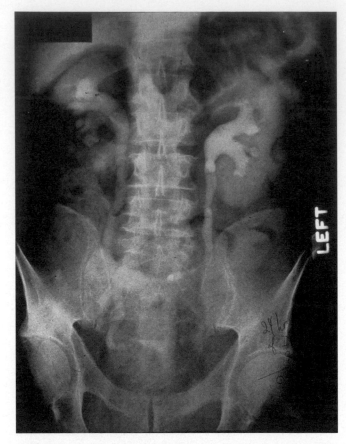

FIGURE 1.8. Bilateral ureteral obstruction secondary to advanced local prostate cancer invading trigone.

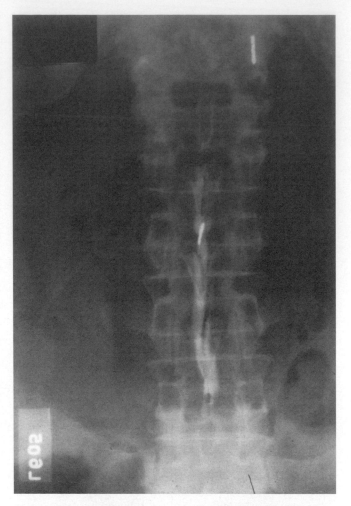

FIGURE 1.9. Myelogram demonstrating cord compression.

supplanted the DRE in prostate cancer diagnosis, a large study of 6,630 men compared their utility (9). PSA detected significantly more cancers than did DRE. Forty five percent of cancers were missed by DRE and detected by PSA, whereas only 18% were missed by PSA and detected solely by DRE (10). The significance of the DRE has waned for additional reasons. The examination, though presumably internally consistent within a physician's practice and experience, is fraught with inter observer variability. In addition, with the exception of the 1-cm B1 nodule, other clinical B or T2 staging relates induration to the prostate rather than to a specifically measured reference point. Obviously, a T2a lesion in a very large prostate volumetrically will surely be larger than a T2a lesion residing in a small prostate. Although the clinical staging of prostate cancer is important and a factor in many of the treatment algorithms and treatment nomograms, there are objective parameters available that are readily measured and are more pertinent to tumor biology. Thus, the number and/or percentage of cores that are positive, the Gleason grade, and the serum PSA level are included as important prognostic features to determine risk (11–13). They are not currently included in the TNM staging system for primary prostate cancer. The inclusion of these parameters has been the subject of ongoing discussion and, in the future, clearly will need to be recognized to construct a staging system that provides optimal risk stratification. It is understandable then that attention previously paid to the DRE has become less critical. However, it can never be disregarded for the information it can sometimes provide. Ten percent to 20% of prostate cancer diagnosis is based on abnormal DRE findings in the presence of PSA levels at or below the "universal" cut point of 4.0 (8,12).

In the past, prostate biopsy was always integrally linked with the DRE. A gloved finger in the rectum guided placement of a hand-operated needle apparatus, often a 14- to 18-gauge Vim Silverman needle, to the area of suspicion. The needle was directed either transperineally [after lidocaine (Xylocaine) analgesia of the perineal skin and subcutaneous tissue] or transrectally. Using the contralateral hand to operate the obturator

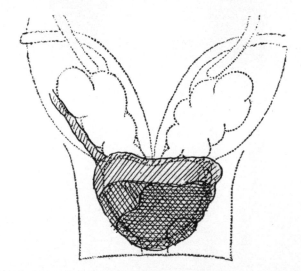

FIGURE 1.10. Rectal chart in Case 15. Membranous urethra involved. Prognosis not good. Single, double, triple X hatching with nodule. (From Young HH. Tumors of the prostate. In Lewis D, ed. *Practice of surgery*, Vol. IX, Chapter XXI. Hagerstown, MD: W.F. Prior Company, Inc., 1928, with permission.)

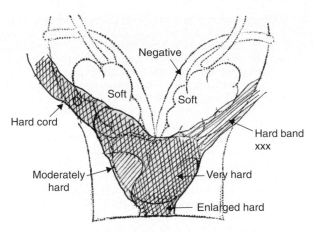

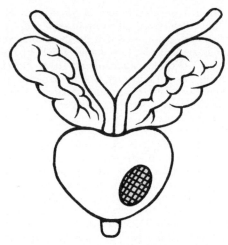

Stage B(1): Localized Nodule

FIGURE 1.11. Rectal chart in Case 12. Membranous urethra is markedly indurated. Lymphatics extend upward on the right side and are more indurated on the left. This would indicate unfavorable prognosis. (From Young HH. Tumors of the prostate. In Lewis D, ed. *Practice of surgery*, Vol. IX, Chapter XXI. Hagerstown, MD: W.F. Prior Company, Inc., 1928, with permission.)

FIGURE 1.13. The B1 nodule, defined by Jewett in 1968 as "a palpably discrete nodule of firm or stony consistency limited to a part of one lateral lobe, averaging 1 cm or a little more in diameter, with compressible tissue always on two and sometimes on three sides."

over grasper, biopsy cores were obtained by tissue shear. The number of cores with such maneuvers rarely exceeded three or four and were often fragmented and associated with crush artifact. Procurement was a relatively "slow" operation that produced patient discomfort. Counseling a patient for a repeat biopsy session was difficult, and the concept of serial outpatient biopsies taken at a 3- or 6-month interval was resisted. Therefore, the strategy to substantiate a diagnosis in a suspicious prostate with prior negative biopsy might include an anesthetic in the operating room, which permitted multiple biopsies continuously submitted for frozen section until the presence of cancer was confirmed.

Currently, prostate biopsy is linked to prostatic ultrasound. In 1990, Dr. William Conner introduced the novel concept of cancer diagnosis based on a three-legged stool of evidence: DRE, PSA, and prostate ultrasound (14). He perhaps might have extended the imagery to include a fourth leg: the automated biopsy gun. It has already been noted that PSA revolutionized the early detection of prostate cancer. Two advances in technology that also contributed to this revolution,

the prostatic ultrasound and the automated biopsy gun, were introduced into practice almost simultaneously with PSA (15, 16). When a PSA elevation raised the suspicion of cancer in a palpably normal prostate gland, ultrasound imaging could visualize changes in echo patterns, often hypoechoic, within the gland (Fig. 1.14). It was toward these cancer-suspect targets that the biopsy needle could be visually directed. The automated gun apparatus permitted procurement of numerous cores of tissue with less discomfort and more precision than had previously been possible. Of interest is the fact that local anesthesia was temporarily "forgotten" in view of the more tolerable automated biopsy procedure. Alavi et al. (17) reintroduced the use of ultrasound-directed local anesthesia to block the neural bundle bilaterally, thereby permitting multiple core and biopsy sessions in the office.

Prior to the introduction of the automated gun, the target for biopsy was the area of prostatic induration detected by DRE. Normal areas of the prostate were infrequently biopsied. Sample error was, thereby, magnified in view of our current

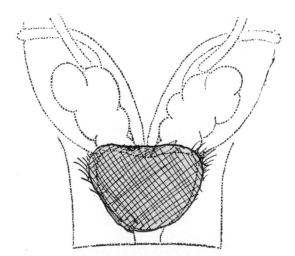

FIGURE 1.12. Rectal chart in Case 17. Prostate only slightly enlarged and induration only moderate. Membraneous urethra and vesicles not involved. No glands. Prognosis good. (From Young HH. Tumors of the prostate. In Lewis D, ed. *Practice of surgery*, Vol. IX, Chapter XXI. Hagerstown, MD: W.F. Prior Company, Inc., 1928, with permission.)

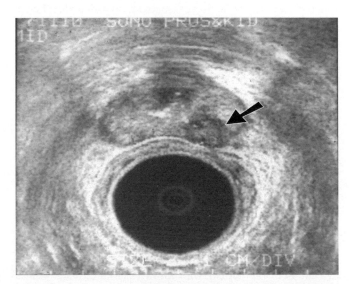

FIGURE 1.14. When a PSA elevation raises the suspicion of cancer in a palpably normal prostate gland, ultrasound imaging can visualize changes in echo patterns, often hypoechoic, within the gland.

knowledge that a positive biopsy is often recovered from a prostate that is considered palpably normal (i.e., stage T1c). Further, it has been recognized that prostatic induration is not specific for cancer. In 1956, Jewett analyzed 211 palpable nodules and found 103 to be malignant and 108 to be benign (18). Included in the benign category was hyperplasia, prostatitis, calculi, tuberculosis, infarction, nonspecific granuloma, and squamous metaplasia. A study in 1988 reexamined the specificity of DRE for cancer in 193 detected nodules (19). Consistent with the earlier study, it was 53%. A provocative analysis by McNaughton Collins et al. entitled "Serendipity strikes again" illustrates that this specificity is further reduced when the geographic location of a positive biopsy is correlated with the geographic location of induration (20). In a review of two series where this distinction was possible, 28% of DRE-detected cancers were found by serendipity; that is, in geographic areas other than where DRE detected induration. Keech, reporting on the Washington University screening experience, confirmed that the site-specific positive predicted value for DRE was lower than the overall positive predicted value (21).

SYMPTOMS

In the pre-PSA era, systemic symptoms were frequently the initial manifestation of prostate cancer. Back pain might be associated with ureteral obstruction and uremia or bone metastasis. Involvement of the vertebrae might also lead to cord compression with the consequences of lower extremity weakness and the sudden onset of hemiplegia or paraplegia. Weakness and lassitude might be caused by myeloplastic anemia. As already mentioned, the dramatic advances in the early detection and diagnosis of prostate cancer is clearly evident by the vanishing picture of an emaciated patient with incapacitating bone pain. With PSA detection of advancing disease and the judicious early application of hormone therapy, radiation, and chemotherapy and other supportive measures (i.e., bisphosphates, erythropoietic stimulating factor, radiopharmaceuticals), the pattern of advanced prostate cancer has remarkably changed from morbid disease progression to effective palliative control. Nevertheless, the words of a prominent prostate cancer surgeon, Dr. Hugh Jewett, touch on the morbidity that can be experienced. He stated, "I never understood the disease I've studied, and am dying of now. My CT scan is fine. My bone scan is littered. My organs all work, but I am being poisoned to death by something along with my rising PSA. I have pain with no fractures, and no energy. Study this painful, sapping poisoning by this strange cancer, and do some patients some good" (22).

It is revealing and sobering to read the earliest descriptions of the prostate cancer population, again as presented in the monograph authored by Hugh Hampton Young: "The initial symptoms are usually frequency of urination, associated often and with slight difficulty, and sometimes with irritation and urgency. With the progression of the disease, the lumen of the urethra was more encroached upon [there was] difficulty, smallness of stream, increasing frequency of urination and irritation and the gradual onset of pain. In some cases complete retention of urine occurred requiring catheterization. In some of these cases, in attempting to pass the instrument, the prostatic urethra was found so greatly contracted that the usual instruments would not pass, dilatation with filiforms and followers being necessary (4)."

Locally advanced prostate cancer with the above-mentioned symptoms will be encountered in the nonscreened population, as well as in the patient with known prostate cancer whose local disease cannot be controlled. However, they are rarely encountered in the screened population in the United States, where voiding symptoms are now detected through quality-of-

life (QOL) questionnaires to identify often minor alterations in voiding symptoms. Lehrer et al. (23) studied the relationship between American Urologic Association (AUA) urinary scores in 265 men with newly diagnosed localized prostate cancer. According to the AUA classification, 55.6% of prostate cancer patients had mild symptoms, 37% had intermittent symptoms, and 7% had severe symptoms. There was a significant difference in AUA symptom score between clinical stages T1/T2 and T3 cancers but no difference between T1 and T2 cancers. Interestingly, with better public education, men have become concerned that urinary symptoms are associated with prostate cancer, and this concern has prompted self-referral to early detection clinics. Brown et al. (24) studied a group of men who presented with lower urinary tract symptoms and found high anxiety about their chances of prostate cancer despite no evidence of the relationship. Weinrich et al. (25) found a high rate of urinary symptoms among African-American men responding to free prostate cancer screenings. In Australia, where the Australian Cancer Society recommends against screening, men requesting a PSA test were more likely to have urologic symptoms and to express more worry about prostate cancer (25). Nijs et al. performed a study in the Netherlands exploring the reasons why men attend or refuse to attend population-based screening for prostate cancer (26). Refusers listed absence of urologic symptoms (57%) and anticipated discomfort (18%). They had worse general health but fewer urologic complaints. Attendees of screening cited personal benefit (82%), contribution to science (49%), and presence of urologic complaints (25%). These studies in multiple settings provide evidence that lower urinary tract symptoms, although not specific for prostate cancer, raise concern and often lead to screening and, therefore, early diagnosis. The AUA has recently published guidelines on the evaluation of men with benign prostatic hyperplasia (BPH) and now states that PSA screening is no longer required in the initial evaluation. PSA screening is still reasonable in a man with a life expectancy greater than 10 years, but a DRE alone is sufficient to evaluate for the presence of locally advanced prostate cancer causing urinary obstructive symptoms (27).

In addition to the local and systemic symptoms already described, cancer may be associated with a varied spectrum of unique signs, symptoms, and syndromes. These have been very completely categorized in the prior edition of this text (28). Table 1.1 is reproduced for reference.

SURVEILLANCE OF PROSTATE CANCER NATURAL HISTORY, OR WATCHFUL WAITING FOR THE APPEARANCE OF SIGNS AND SYMPTOMS

Observation, surveillance, and expectant management, or watchful waiting, has always been an option after prostate cancer diagnosis. The intent is to monitor any changes in status by DRE, appearance of disease-related symptoms, and PSA level.

In a European study by Jonler et al. (29), men who chose watchful waiting were surveyed: 31% had subsequent transurethral resection for obstructive symptoms, 8% had radiation therapy for suspected or proven metastatic disease (i.e., none for curative intent), and 44% began androgen deprivation. In the study of immediate versus deferred treatment for advanced prostate cancer conducted by Medical Research Council (MRC), 465 patients with M0 (locally advanced) or M1 were randomized to deferred treatment (30). In the deferred treatment arm, indications and incidence for subsequent

TABLE 1.1

CLINICAL SYMPTOMS AND SIGNS OF PROSTATE CANCER

Disease type	Description	
	Common	Uncommon
Local disease	Abnormal digital rectal examination Lower urinary tract obstruction Hematuria Ureteral obstruction	Rectal obstruction Priapism (corporal body invasion)
Distant disease	Bone pain Neurologic: cord compression	Neurologic: metastases to brain, cranial nerve, temporal bone, skull base, pituitary Visceral: lung, liver, stomach, adrenal, GI bleeding, testes Cutaneous Paraneoplastic: Cushing, SIADH, hyper- or hypocalcemia Hematologic: disseminated intravascular coagulopathy

SIADH, syndrome of inappropriate antidiuretic hormone.
From Kim ED, Grayhack JT. Clinical symptoms and signs of prostate cancer. In Vogelzang NJ, et al., eds. *Comprehensive textbook of genitourinary oncology*, 2nd ed. Philadelphia: Lippincott Williams and Wilkins, 2000.

treatment included (more than one indication in some patients) pain from bony metastases (39%), local progression (34%), rising PSA (5%), general systemic effects (5%), patient preference (1%), and unknown (1%). A US pre-PSA era study of 75 men with stage T2 tumors who chose surveillance or expectant therapy showed a median time to clinical progression of 6.5 years and a median time to therapy of 9 years (31,32).

Currently the intent, more often than not, is to monitor for the appearance of any sign or symptom of cancer when the diagnosis is made in the absence of both as a result of PSA screening. Zietman et al. studied the records of 199 men with stages T1-2 prostate cancer and a PSA < 20 ng/mL who elected watchful waiting between 1990 and 1999 at two US institutions (33). Sixty-three men decided to initiate therapy. The therapy trigger was a PSA increase in 71%, nodule progression in 6%, PSA and nodule progression in 6%, positive bone scan in 4%, symptoms in 2%, and change of philosophy in 11%. The vast majority of men were treated in delayed fashion for an asymptomatic rise in PSA rather than appearance of signs and symptoms. Thus, comparing the MRC study to Zietman's exclusively PSA-era study, men on a watchful waiting protocol are unlikely to await clinical progression when PSA monitoring reveals a rising profile. This was confirmed in a study by Carter et al. (34) who suggested that watchful waiting may be better termed "temporarily delayed active therapy."

SUMMARY

PSA testing has dramatically changed the face of prostate cancer. What was once a disease that severely impaired urinary function by local invasion and imparted crippling disability secondary to skeletal system metastases and multiorgan failure has been replaced by a laboratory vigil with treatment applied based on PSA level prior to signs and symptoms. As a result, when they do appear, progression events are compressed into a shorter time frame and are better controlled. These factors, together with stage migration and therapeutic advances, have reduced prostate cancer mortality and morbidity.

References

1. Vessella RL, Lange PH. Issues in the assessment of prostate specific antigen immunoassays. An update. *Urol Clin North Am* 1997;24:261–268.
2. Wright GL Jr, Cazares LH, Leung S-M, et al. A protein chip surface enhanced laser desorption/ionization (SELDI) mass spectrometry: A novel proteomic technology for detection of prostate cancer biomarkers in complex protein mixture. *Prostate Cancer Prostatic Dis* 1999;2:264–267.
3. Adam B-L, Qu Y, Davis JW, et al. Serum protein fingerprinting coupled with a pattern-matching algorithm distinguishes prostate cancer from benign prostate hyperplasia and healthy men. *Cancer Res* 2002;62:3609–3614.
4. Young HH. Tumors of the prostate. In Lewis D, ed. *Practice of surgery*, Vol. IX, Chapter XXI. Hagerstown, MD: W.F. Prior Company, Inc., 1928.
5. Jewett HJ, Bridge RW, Gray GF Jr, et al. The palpable nodule of prostatic cancer: Results 15 years after radical excision. *JAMA* 1968;203:403.
6. Culp OS. Radical perineal prostatectomy: its past and possible future. *J Urol* 1968;98:618.
7. Glick AJ, Philput CB, El Mahdi A, et al. Are three substages of clinical B prostate carcinoma useful in predicting disease free survival? *Urology* 1990;36:483–487.
8. Cooperberg MR, Lubeck DP, Mehta SS, et al. Time trends in clinical risk stratification for prostate cancer: implications for outcomes (data from CaPSURE). *J Urol* 2003;17:S21–S27.
9. Catalona WJ, Richie JP, Ahmann FR, et al. Comparison of digital rectal examination and serum prostate specific antigen in the early detection of prostate cancer: results of a multimember clinical trial of 6,630 men. *J Urol* 1995;151:1283–1290.
10. Basle JW, Thompson IM. Lest we abandon digital rectal examination as a screening test for prostate cancer. *J Natl Cancer Inst* 1998;90:1761–1763.
11. Parting AW, Kitten MW, Subbing EN, et al. Combination of prostate-specific antigen, clinical stage, and Gleason score to predict pathological stage of localized prostate cancer: a multi-institutional update. *JAMA* 1997;277:1445–1451.
12. Nelson CP, Dunn RL, Wei JT, et al. Contemporary preoperative parameters predict cancer-free survival after radical prostatectomy: a tool to facilitate treatment decisions. *Urol Oncol* 2003;21:213–218.
13. D'Amico AV, Whittingon R, Malkowicz SB, et al. Clinical utility of the percentage of positive prostate biopsies in defining biochemical outcome after radical prostatectomy for patients with clinically localized prostate cancer. *J Clin Oncol* 2000;18:1164.
14. Cooner WH, Mosley BR, Rutherford CL, et al. Prostate cancer detection in a clinical urological practice by ultrasonography, digital rectal examination and prostate specific antigen. *J Urol* 1990;143:1146–1154.
15. Torp-Pedersen S, Juul N, Jakobsen H. Transrectal prostatic ultrasonography. Equipment, normal findings, benign hyperplasia and cancer. *Scan J Urol Nephrol Suppl* 1988;107:19–25.

16. Ragde H, Aldape HC, Bagley CM. Ultrasound-guided prostate biopsy. Biopsy gun superior to aspiration. *Urol* 1988;32:503–508.

17. Alavi AS, Soloway MS, Vaidya A, et al. Local anesthesia for ultrasound-guided prostate biopsy: A prospective randomized trial comparing 2 methods. *J Urol* 2001;166:1343–1345.

18. Jewett HJ. Significance of the palpable prostatic nodule. *JAMA* 1956;160: 838–839.

19. Clements R, Griffiths GJ, Peeling WB, et al. How accurate is the index finger? A comparison of digital and ultrasound examination of the prostatic nodule. *Clin Radiol* 1988;39:87–89.

20. McNaughton Collins M, Ransohoff DR, Barry MJ. Early detection of prostate cancer. Serendipity strikes again. *JAMA* 1997;278:1516–1519.

21. Keech DW, Androile GL. Prostate cancer screening: what are physicians to do? What have we learned? *Monogr Urol* 1996;17:31–48.

22. Chou E, Simons JW. The molecular biology of prostate cancer morbidity and mortality: accelerated death from ejaculate poisoning? *Urol Oncol* 1997;3:79–84.

23. Lehrer S, Stone NN, Droller MJ, et al. Association between American Urologic Association (AUA) urinary symptom score and disease stage in men with localized prostate cancer. *Urol Oncol* 2002;7:73–76.

24. Brown CT, O'Flynn E, Van Der Meulen J, et al. The fear of prostate cancer in men with lower urinary tract symptoms: should symptomatic men be screened? *BJU Int* 2003;91:30–32.

25. Weinrich SP, Weinrich M, Mettlin C, et al. Urinary symptoms as a predictor for participation in prostate cancer screening among African-American men. *Prostate* 1998;37:215–222.

26. Nijs HG, Essink-Bot ML, DeKoning HJ, et al. Why do men refuse or attend population-based screening for prostate cancer? *J Public Health Med* 2000;22:312–316.

27. AUA Practice guidelines Committee. AUA guidelines on management of benign prostatic hyperplasia (2003). Chapter 1: diagnosis and treatment recommendations. *J Urol* 2003;170:530–547.

28. Kim ED, Grayhack JT. Clinical symptoms and signs of prostate cancer. In Vogelzang NJ, Scardino PT, Shipley WU, Coffey DS, eds. *Comprehensive textbook of genitourinary oncology*, 2nd ed. Philadelphia: Lippincott Williams and Wilkins, 2000.

29. Jonler M, Lund L, Danielsen HB. Urinary symptoms, potency, and quality of life in patients with localized prostate cancer followed up with deferred treatment. *Urology* 1998;52:1055–1062.

30. The Medical Research Council Prostate Cancer Working Party Investigators Group. Immediate versus deferred treatment for advanced prostatic cancer: initial results of the medical research council trial. *Br J Urol* 1997; 79:235–246.

31. Whitmore WF Jr, Warner JA, Thompson IM Jr. Expectant management of localized prostate cancer. *Cancer* 1991;67:1091.

32. Warner J, Whitmore WF Jr. Expectant management of clinically localized prostate cancer. *J Urol* 1994;152:1761.

33. Zietman AL, Thermal H, Wilson L, et al. Conservative management of prostate cancer in the prostate specific antigen era: the incidence and time course of subsequent therapy. *J Urol* 2001;166:1702–1706.

34. Carter CA, Donahue T, Sun L, et al. Temporarily deferred therapy (watchful waiting) for men younger than 70 years and with low-risk localized prostate cancer in the prostate-specific antigen era. *J Clin Oncol* 2003; 21:4001–4008.

CHAPTER 2 ■ EPIDEMIOLOGY OF PROSTATE CANCER

EDWARD GIOVANNUCCI AND ELIZABETH A. PLATZ

INTRODUCTION

Prostate cancer is the most commonly diagnosed cancer in American men and is among the most common cancers diagnosed in many developed countries. The classic risk factors for this cancer are older age, African-American racial group, and family history of prostate cancer. Otherwise, few established risk factors have emerged, despite recent interest and intensive study of this cancer. Nonetheless, the wide variation in incident rates among countries and the increases in prostate cancer rates in groups that have migrated from countries that have low rates to those countries with high rates strongly suggest the importance of environmental factors in its etiology. A number of leads have emerged, though the evidence for each has generally not been consistent or conclusive enough to allow for definitive conclusions at this time. A strong research focus has been on nutritional and hormonal factors, and recently, an interest in inflammatory or infectious etiologies has reemerged. This chapter will outline demographic patterns of prostate cancer, major environmental and host risk factors, and the primary prevention strategies for prostate cancer.

DEMOGRAPHIC PATTERNS

Mortality and Incidence in the United States

Prostate cancer is the second most common cause of cancer death in men in the United States, accounting for about 29,000 deaths annually. The introduction of widespread screening for prostate-specific antigen (PSA) in the early to mid-1990s has caused the prostate cancer detection rate to soar in the Unites States (1). Excluding skin cancer, prostate cancer is now the most commonly diagnosed cancer in American men by far and accounts for an estimated 220,900 new cases annually or about one-third of all new cancer diagnoses in men (2). The lifetime risk of a male in the United States being diagnosed with prostate cancer is 1 in 6 (2). After decades of a slightly increasing mortality rate, beginning around 1992 the prostate cancer mortality rate has declined. The reasons for this decline remain controversial but may be attributable, at least in part, to earlier detection through PSA screening and subsequent treatment and to better treatment for advanced-stage prostate cancer (3). Not surprisingly, given the dramatically increasing incidence and the stable or reducing mortality, the 5-year survival rates increased markedly during 1974–1976, 1983–1985, and 1992–1998, from 68% to 76% to 98%, respectively, among whites in the United States (2). Increases in survival have also been observed in other racial groups. This increased survival is likely mostly due to detection at an earlier stage of the disease and to an overdiagnosis by PSA of prostate cancers with little biological potential

to progress, although an actual improvement due to early detection and treatment may have contributed to this improvement. Overall, 5-year disease-specific survival rates are close to 100% for men diagnosed with localized prostate cancer but only 34% for men diagnosed with distant metastases (2).

Age

The strongest risk factor for prostate cancer is age. The characteristic logarithmic rise in the incidence rate with log age that is observed for many cancers is steepest for prostate cancer. The majority of men are diagnosed with prostate cancer at an age older than 65 years, and the vast majority of prostate cancer deaths occur in this older age group. The median age at prostate cancer diagnosis in the United States is 71 years in whites and 69 years in blacks (4). In recent years, the average age at diagnosis has dropped after the earlier detection of cancers due to the widespread use of PSA screening. However, the average age of death from prostate cancer, the late 70s, has remained relatively stable. The relatively old age at diagnosis coupled with the variable rates of progression for prostate cancer results in a number of dilemmas regarding what efforts should be put into diagnosis and treatment.

Race and Ethnicity

One of the well-recognized risk factors for prostate cancer is race. In the United States, African-Americans have the highest prostate incidence rate (standardized to the 2000 United States population age standard, 1992–1999: 275.3 per 100,000 men annually) and mortality rate (75.1 per 100,000 men annually) among any racial or ethnic group. The incidence rate is 1.6-fold higher than in whites (172.9 per 100,000 men), and the disparity in mortality is even greater at 2.3 times that for whites (32.9 per 100,000 men). Both incidence and mortality rates of prostate cancer for Asian/Pacific Islanders, American Indian/Alaskan Natives, or Hispanics are substantially lower than those for white Americans (2).

The underlying cause(s) for this disparity in rates among races remains of great interest for both societal reasons and for the potential to provide insights into the etiology of prostate cancer. Not only do African-American men experience a higher incidence of this cancer, they appear to experience a more aggressive form of the disease. For example, among whites in the United States, 10% of prostate cancers are diagnosed with distant metastases, compared with 18% for African-American men. Reduced access to health care may contribute to the more advanced stage distribution at diagnosis among African-Americans, but this factor may not account entirely for the difference. In a study conducted among men in the US military medical system, a population

9

without economic barriers to screening, diagnosis, and treatment, the risk of being diagnosed with advanced stage prostate cancer remained higher in African-American men compared with non-Hispanic white men after adjusting for socioeconomic factors (5). Moreover, in a study of male health professionals, risk of total and advanced prostate cancer remained elevated even after adjusting for known and suspected dietary and lifestyle risk factors and screening behaviors (6). Further, because these men were all highly educated health professionals, differences due to socioeconomic status were minimized.

International Patterns of Mortality and Incidence

Prostate cancer incidence rates vary dramatically among countries. However, some of the disparity in prostate cancer incidence rates between countries is likely due to differences in medical practice leading to differential rates of detection of subclinical tumors. For example, PSA screening has caused a great increase in the incidence of prostate cancer diagnosed in the United States, as well as in some other countries to a lesser degree. Prostate cancer mortality rates around the world also vary dramatically, more than 30-fold between the highest and lowest rate countries (2). Developed or "Westernized" countries have substantially higher prostate cancer rates than do developing countries (7). The lowest prostate cancer incidence and mortality rates are observed in the Far East and on the Indian subcontinent, and the highest rates occur in Western Europe, Australia, and North America. Even adjusting for age, the mortality rate in the United States for prostate cancer is 18-fold that of China (8). Although issues such as variable attribution of cause of death and treatment may contribute to the differences in mortality rates, these factors alone are unlikely to account for such a dramatic difference in mortality rates among these countries.

Given the high rates of prostate cancer in African-Americans, it is of interest to examine rates among men of African descent elsewhere in the world. Among the highest prostate cancer rates are those on Caribbean islands, including Trinidad and Tobago, which has the highest mortality rate among 45 countries evaluated (2), and Jamaica (9). In comparison, prostate cancer incidence and mortality rates in African countries such as Nigeria appear to be substantially lower than these (10). However, it remains questionable whether cancer incidence and mortality information is sufficiently comprehensive in African countries to make valid comparisons. In addition, there could be genetic differences in men from these different areas. Nonetheless, the overall evidence indicates that factors related to industrialization contribute to higher incidence and mortality rates of prostate cancer. Identifying these factors could lead to prevention strategies.

Migration Studies

Men of Asian heritage living in the United States are at lower risk for prostate cancer than white Americans but are at greater risk than men of similar ancestries living in Asia (11,12). Japanese immigrants living in Los Angeles County, California have prostate cancer rates that are more comparable to individuals with similar ancestry but who were born in the United States than to Japanese men living in Japan (13). Moreover, these rate differences do not appear to be entirely due to differences in detection of early stage tumors between the United States and Japan (14). The changing rates of clinical prostate cancer among migrants suggest that factors affecting tumor growth or progression may vary between countries. A number of hypotheses attempting to address these rate differences have been generated.

Family History of Prostate Cancer

Another of the few clearly established risk factors for prostate cancer is a family history of prostate cancer. The relationship between family history and prostate cancer has been confirmed in population-based case-control (15–20), record linkage (21–23), and prospective cohort (24–26) studies. In general, men with either a father or a brother with the diagnosis of prostate cancer are at approximately two to three times greater risk of developing prostate cancer than are men without a family history of the disease (15,16). The magnitude of this association is modified by at least three factors. First, a man's risk of prostate cancer is higher if a brother rather than father is affected, compared to neither first-degree relative being affected (15,17,18,27). Second, risk is higher with increasing number of first-degree relatives with prostate cancer [for two or more affected relatives, the relative risk (RR) = 3 to 5] (16,18,24). Third, risk is higher if the first-degree relative was younger at diagnosis (under about 65 years, RR = 1.5 to 6.0) (18,21,22,24). Not surprisingly, the proportion of prostate cancer attributable to family history is greater for younger ages at diagnosis (18,22,28). With advancing years, more and more prostate cancers are considered sporadic, and fewer are due to a strong genetic component.

Family history may be a surrogate of hereditary factors, although to some extent it may reflect common environmental factors (including the *in utero* environment). Further support for an inherited component to prostate cancer risk is that twin studies show higher concordance for prostate cancer diagnosis between monozygotic than dizygotic twins of 18% and 3%, respectively, in a combined analysis of Swedish, Danish, and Finnish twins (29). In a similar comparison of US veteran twins, the respective concordances were 27.1% and 7.1% (30). The observation of a higher risk if a man's brother compared to his father is affected has been postulated to indicate that the underlying genetic inheritance of susceptibility is either X-linked or recessive (27). However, a nongenetic explanation for the higher risk if a brother is affected may result from brothers sharing a more similar environment *in utero* and in childhood than fathers and sons. Segregation analyses in prostate cancer kindreds support an autosomal dominant mode of inheritance (28,31,32), with the attributable risk for the yet unidentified gene(s) ranging from 43% in men diagnosed under age 55 years, to 34% under age 70, to 9% under age 85 years (28).

DIET AND NUTRITION

Some dietary factors have been suggested to increase risk of prostate cancer, whereas others are believed to be potentially protective against this disease. The potential role of energy balance, composition of macronutrients, micronutrients, and phytochemicals are discussed in this section.

Energy Intake and Obesity

Energy balance remains an obvious candidate to influence prostate carcinogenesis because animal studies consistently show that diets with restricted total energy reduce tumor burden relative to *ad libitum* feeding, including for prostate cancer (33–35). In addition, obesity has been shown to be related to a number of cancers in humans (36). Energy intake has been evaluated in relation to prostate cancer risk in more than

20 studies, but findings have not been consistent across these studies (37). However, energy intake is not a straightforward variable to consider in epidemiologic studies; for example, men with higher physical activity levels or inactive men who overeat will tend to have high energy intakes, but one would imagine the influence of energy intake could be quite different in these two groups. A large prospective study showed a positive association between energy intake and advanced prostate cancer primarily in leaner men but not in obese men (38). This finding suggests that men who remain lean despite having a relatively high energy intake may have a metabolic or hormonal profile that is related to a higher risk of prostate cancer progression. The specific factors or profiles underlying this association remain to be identified.

If excessive energy intake alone increased the risk of prostate cancer, then it would be predicted that obesity would be associated with prostate cancer risk. However, no consistent association of high body mass index (BMI) with prostate cancer risk is apparent in epidemiologic studies (39). Prospective studies have reported conflicting results, with some showing a positive relation for BMI or body weight (36,40–46), whereas others are not supportive (47–56). A 34% higher risk of prostate cancer death for a very high BMI of >35 kg/m^2 (>30 kg/m^2 is considered obese) compared to normal BMI (<25 kg/m^2) was reported in a large prospective study in the United States (36). Case-only studies suggest that risk of more aggressive prostate cancer in men who had clinically organ-confined disease is greater with higher BMI (57,58). Thus, obesity could be related to the progression rate, and possibly to mortality from prostate cancer, but does not appear to have a simple relationship with incidence.

Attained height reflects factors that characterize the growth phase of adolescence, including energy balance and related changes in circulating concentrations of steroid hormones, growth hormone, and insulin-like growth factors (these are discussed below). On an individual basis, height is positively associated with prostate cancer risk in some studies (17,49,51,52,54,59–62), particularly with advanced disease (51), although several do not support such an association (44–46,48,53,63). In a case-control study, childhood height was positively associated with prostate cancer risk in American whites but not in African-Americans (62). Tallness may not be a consistent risk factor in all populations because the relative importance of nutritional and genetic factors of height may vary across populations, depending on underlying nutritional status during the growth period. Thus, some heterogeneity in results is not unexpected. Interestingly, when comparing populations, those with taller average heights have higher rates of prostate cancer. Nonetheless, given that most studies do suggest a positive association and none have found an inverse association, it is unlikely that chance alone is the underlying factor. These data suggest that factors related to nutritional status, hormonal status, or both during the growth period influence prostate cancer risk.

Macronutrients and Related Factors

Fat and Fatty Acid Consumption

Fat intake, in particular from animal sources, has been considered to be a modifiable risk factor for prostate cancer. Support for this hypothesis was initiated by the observation that per-capita fat consumption is strongly correlated with prostate cancer incidence and mortality rates internationally (64,65). An association between dietary fat or higher fat foods, especially animal foods such as red meat and dairy products, and prostate cancer has been further supported in several case-control studies conducted in several different populations (66).

Associations with fat persisted, even after adjusting for potentially confounding factors in many of these studies (66). For example, a multiethnic case-control study found an association between higher saturated fat intake and prostate cancer risk, particularly for advanced cancers, separately among African-Americans, whites, Chinese Americans, and Japanese Americans (67). In addition, a case-control study reported positive associations for foods high in animal fat and total and advanced prostate cancer in blacks and in whites (62). Other case-control studies, in contrast, have shown no association for total fat or saturated fat (68,69).

Findings for dietary fat and prostate cancer from prospective cohort studies, which are less prone to bias, are not as consistent. Many have not supported an association (70–72), whereas other studies have supported an association for total fat or fat from animal products (49) or only for advanced prostate cancer (73). Some studies noted stronger relations for fat intake and advanced disease than for total prostate cancer, with relative risks of the order 1.6 to 2.9 between high- and low-intake categories (62,67,73,74). The stronger findings for advanced disease suggest that diet influences late stages of carcinogenesis. Some evidence, though not consistent, has suggested that α-linolenic acid, an omega-3 polyunsaturated fatty acid, increases risk of prostate cancer. This fatty acid is found in vegetable oils such as soy and canola and less so in leafy green vegetables (75), as well as in red meat and dairy fat (76–80). Fatty fish such as salmon and tuna contain long-chain omega-3 polyunsaturated fatty acids such as eicosapentaenoic acid (EPA) and docosahexaenoic acid (DHA). Curiously, EPA and DHA have been either unrelated or inversely associated with risk of prostate cancer in contrast to α-linolenic acid (77–83). Because α-linolenic acid is a precursor to the longer chain omega-3 fatty acids, the positive association between α-linolenic acid and prostate cancer risk remains an enigma. Because only a small proportion of α-linolenic acid is converted to long-chain omega-3 fatty acids, perhaps other breakdown products of this fatty acid are deleterious. Alternatively, this fatty acid may be acting as a surrogate of another factor.

The essential fatty acid linoleic acid, an omega-6 fatty acid found in vegetable and soy oils, is a precursor to arachidonic acid and ultimately to the proinflammatory prostaglandins of the 2 series. No consistent associations between intake of (73,77) or circulating concentration of (78,79) linoleic acid and prostate cancer risk have been observed. Higher concentration of erythrocyte and adipose linoleic acid, a marker of intake, was associated with a nonstatistically significant higher risk of prostate cancer in a small case-control study (81). Dietary intake (77) and circulating concentration (78,79) of arachidonic acid, the immediate precursor to prostaglandins, were not associated with prostate cancer in prospective studies.

Meat Consumption

It is possible that the frequent associations with prostate cancer observed with animal fat in many (though not all) studies is not related directly to fat but to other components in animal foods. Besides being sources of fat, red meat and processed meat are sources of iron and protein, as well as added nitrites and by-products of cooking, such as heterocyclic amines. Across countries, total meat intake is positively correlated with prostate cancer mortality rates (64,65). In some cohort studies, consumption of red meat is associated with a higher risk of prostate cancer (46,49,73,78,84); this association was stronger for processed or cured meats in a few studies (84,85). A large case-control study also supported an association of red meat with advanced prostate cancer in both blacks and whites (62), but other studies are not supportive (50,70,72). In general, intake of poultry has not been a risk factor for prostate cancer in most studies (49,62,70,72,84,85), suggesting that some factor specific to red meat or processed meat is most relevant for prostate carcinogenesis. Recently, interest has arisen in heterocyclic amines—mutagenic compounds formed during high-temperature cooking of meat and fish through the condensation of amino acids with creatinine (86). A case-control study reported no consistent associations for estimated intake of total or specific heterocyclic amines, although a 1.7-times higher risk of prostate cancer was noted for those who consume well-done beefsteak that was fried/grilled or barbequed compared to noneaters/other cooking methods (87). However, a case-control study did not show an association for roasted or grilled meat (68).

Dairy Products and Calcium

Higher consumption of dairy products has been associated with a higher risk of prostate cancer in various types of epidemiologic studies. Countries with greater per-capita consumption of milk tend to have higher prostate cancer mortality rates (64,65,88). In many case-control studies, men consuming high levels of milk and other dairy products are at an either statistically significant increased risk (89–95) or borderline significant ($P \leq .1$) increased risk of prostate cancer (62,96–98). In contrast, several case-control studies have not supported this association (99,100). In addition, most prospective studies (41,49,84,85,101,102) but not all (50,72,103,104) have found an association between higher intake of milk or dairy products and greater risk of total prostate or advanced cancer. The magnitude of the relative risks comparing the high and low categories of milk intakes has varied across studies. The relative risk comparing the high- to low-intake categories has been 2-fold or higher in some studies (89,91,92,95,102,105,106), from about 1.5-fold to less than 2-fold in others (90,93,94,98,107), and about 1.3- to 1.4-fold in still others (41,49,62,101). Thus, overall the evidence supports a positive association between dairy product intake and prostate cancer risk. This conclusion is supported by a recent meta-analysis of case-control studies (108), as well as a subsequent case-control study in Italy (109).

The mechanism underlying the association between milk and prostate cancer risk has been unclear. A recent hypothesis is that high intakes of calcium, for which milk is the main source, may increase risk. In fact, some case-control (95,106) and prospective cohort (101,102,105,107) studies have shown positive associations between calcium intake and prostate cancer risk, especially for advanced disease (95, 105–107). The risk may be even stronger at higher doses of calcium when calcium supplements are taken into account (for example, >1500 or >2000 mg/day) (105,107). However, other studies are nonsupportive (72,85,110,111) or only suggestive of an association between calcium and prostate cancer risk (62,98). Although the association with calcium remains controversial, this hypothesis needs to be resolved because many men in the United States take calcium supplements with expectations of health benefits. Whether higher calcium intake has deleterious effects on prostate cancer risk needs to be determined.

Fruits, Vegetables, Legumes, and Micronutrients

Fruits, Vegetables, and Legumes Including Soy Products

Fruits and vegetables are known to possess a wide spectrum of phytochemicals; some of these compounds may protect against cancer, in general, or prostate cancer, specifically. The relevant compounds include antioxidants, which have received most interest, other vitamins and essential minerals, and nonessential but bioactive compounds. Total fruit and vegetable intakes, which have been related to lower risk of some cancers, have generally not been associated with lower prostate cancer risk in most studies (20,49,50,62,70–72,112,113), but there have been some exceptions that have suggested some benefits (114,115). Overall, the evidence to date does not suggest that total fruits and vegetables will be strongly associated with a reduced risk of prostate cancer.

Although total fruit and vegetable consumption may incorporate a wide spectrum of potentially beneficial compounds, examining total fruits and vegetables may be too simplistic an approach if there is some benefit from a specific subgroup of these items. Four botanical families or groups of vegetables are of special interest. Inverse associations are supported by some studies for tomato-based foods (50,116), brassica vegetables, soy and other legumes, and allium vegetables such as garlic and onions (68,113,117). Each of these groups has major characterizing nutrients. Tomatoes are a particularly good source of lycopene, an efficient antioxidant (118) that is the most abundant carotenoid in the plasma (119,120) and in the prostate (mean of 30% of total carotenoids in a US population) (121). The bioavailability of lycopene is greatly enhanced by heating with oil (122), which is of interest given that cooked tomatoes (especially tomato sauce) rather than raw tomatoes have been most consistently associated with reduced risk of prostate cancer (116). An inverse association with lycopene has also been supported by studies of circulating concentrations of lycopene in relation to prostate cancer risk (123–127), though the association was weak in one study (128) and nonexistent in another study (129). In the latter study (129), the overall levels were much lower than in the supporting studies, suggesting that relatively high concentrations of lycopene need to be achieved to show a benefit.

Brassica, or cruciferous vegetables, which include broccoli, brussels sprouts, and cabbage, are of interest because they contain glucosinolates, which induce phase I and II detoxification enzymes. Higher activity of these enzymes may protect against DNA damage from carcinogens. Whether this mechanism is relevant for prostate cancer is unknown, but several studies have found an inverse association between brassica vegetables and prostate cancer risk (113–115, 130,131). Not all studies are supportive, though. Variability in findings may be due to differences in the amount and the specific type of brassica vegetables consumed in a given population and to the nature and extent of exposure to the putatively carcinogenic agents metabolized by biotransformation enzymes induced by brassica vegetables in various populations.

Consumption of soy products is high in Asian countries, which tend to have low rates of prostate cancer, leading to the hypothesis that soy lowers risk of prostate cancer. Common soy phytoestrogens, including genistein and daidzein, induce growth arrest and apoptosis, inhibit hormone metabolizing enzymes such as 5 α-reductase and 17 β-hydroxysteroid dehydrogenase, and have antioxidant properties (132). Relatively few studies have examined the relation of phytoestrogens and soy products with prostate cancer risk. A large multiethnic case-control study found an inverse association between soy food intake and risk of prostate cancer (115), but other studies have not supported this hypothesis (20,71). Although most interest has focused on soybeans, some studies have suggested inverse associations between intake of legumes in general and prostate cancer risk; these include ecologic (for prostate cancer mortality $r = -0.59$) (65), cohort (50,113), and large case-control (68,114,115) studies. However, one large case-control study was not confirmatory of this association (20). Soybeans, and legumes in general, deserve further study in relation to prostate cancer risk.

Vitamin E

Recent interest in the prevention of prostate cancer by vitamin E arose from the publication of the results from the Alpha-Tocopherol, Beta-Carotene (ATBC) Trial in Finnish smokers. This randomized study did not support a benefit of a 50-mg vitamin E supplement (α-tocopherol) on the main study outcome: lung cancer (133). However, in a secondary analysis, a statistically significant 32% reduction in prostate cancer incidence and a 41% reduction in prostate cancer mortality was observed among men receiving α-tocopherol supplementation relative to those who received a placebo (134). Risk of prostate cancer decreased early in the trial, within several years, suggesting that vitamin E influences the promotional or progression phases of this cancer (134). However, after an additional 6 years of follow-up, the overall reduction in prostate cancer incidence was reduced to a nonsignificant 12% (135).

Epidemiologic studies for vitamin E have not been as promising as the early results from this trial, but evidence of benefit of vitamin E among smokers or for more aggressive disease has been suggested in several studies. In a large cohort study, use of a vitamin E supplement of at least 100 IU/day was associated with a 54% lower risk of metastatic and fatal prostate cancer, but this benefit was apparent only in men who currently smoked or who had recently quit smoking (136). In another study, male smokers with low prediagnostic serum concentrations of vitamin E were at an increased risk for fatal prostate cancer (137). Plasma α-tocopherol was inversely associated with about half the risk of aggressive prostate cancer among current and ex-smokers in another prospective study (124). Another study found an inverse association for γ-tocopherol rather than α-tocopherol (128,138). In part because of the intriguing findings for α-tocopherol in the ATBC trial, α-tocopherol in the prevention of prostate cancer is being tested along with selenium in the SELECT trial. Overall, the data suggest that vitamin E may be more important for smokers than for nonsmokers.

Selenium

Selenium status is important for antioxidant defenses because it is essential for the activity of glutathione peroxidase (139), a critical antioxidant enzyme. As for vitamin E, strong interest in selenium was stimulated from secondary findings from a randomized trial. The Nutritional Prevention of Cancer Study was a randomized trial of selenium supplementation (brewer's yeast that provided 200 μg/day, approximately 3 times the RDA) for 10 years in the prevention of a second skin cancer among skin cancer patients who lived in low soil selenium regions (140). Although the study showed no beneficial effect on skin cancer recurrence, the main end point, a 65% reduction in both local and advanced stage prostate cancer among men randomized to a selenium supplement was found (140). Notably, the effect of selenium on prostate cancer was apparent after only a few years of supplementation (141). Several prospective studies have supported inverse associations between selenium levels in toenails (138,142,143), a marker of selenium intake during the past year, or in the plasma or serum (144–146). A recent study (146) suggested that selenium may be important in inhibiting progression of prostate cancers.

In contrast to these findings, a prospective study in Finland, a country with low selenium intake during the period of follow-up, showed no relation between serum selenium levels and prostate cancer risk (147). In that study, men had circulating selenium levels that were almost 3 times lower (~50 vs. ~150 μg/L) than in the studies conducted in the United States that showed a benefit. Beginning in 1984, fertilizers were fortified with selenium in Finland. Despite marked elevations in blood selenium, during the next decades prostate cancer incidence rates continued to rise in Finland, possibly due to enhanced detection, while prostate cancer mortality rates have been relatively unchanged. It is unclear why studies in the United States indicated a benefit of selenium (138,140,142, 143,145,146), whereas data from Finland based on the prospective study (147) and on the experience with fortification do not support a lowering of prostate cancer risk with higher selenium intake. One could argue that high levels of selenium must be achieved to induce a benefit, but in the Nutritional Prevention of Cancer Trial, the benefit was observed mostly in men with initially lower selenium levels. Resolving the potential role of selenium as a preventive agent against prostate cancer is currently being evaluated in the SELECT chemoprevention trial.

Vitamin A, β-carotene, and Retinol

Vitamin A, found in animal sources primarily as retinol and in vegetable sources as β-carotene and some other carotenoids, is required to maintain normal cellular proliferation and differentiation (148). Retinoids inhibit carcinogenesis in some animal models (148), including prostate cancer (149), but have been shown to have stimulatory effects in other experimental systems (150,151). Prospective dietary (70,112,152) and plasma-based (123,126,128,129) studies and randomized trials with a β-carotene arm (134,153) show no consistent association between β-carotene and prostate cancer risk. Numerous other carotenoids found in the US diet, such as α-carotene in carrots, lutein in dark green vegetables, and β-cryptoxanthin in oranges, have not been consistently related to risk of prostate cancer (112,114,124,126,128,129). For retinol, the literature has been puzzling, with one prospective study showing an inverse association of prostate cancer with intake of vitamin A in older men but a positive association in younger men (70) and other prospective studies (70,112) and large case-control studies (62,68,154) finding no consistent association. Some studies found positive associations for retinol intake and prostate cancer risk (69) particularly among older men (69,74,112,155,156). In addition, prediagnostic serum vitamin A levels were inversely related to prostate cancer risk in two studies (123,157), positively related in a prospective study (both in younger and older men) (124), and not associated in other cohorts (128,129,137). The interpretation of these results is unclear, given that blood retinol levels are tightly regulated (158), and thus not substantially influenced by the normal range of dietary retinol intake observed in epidemiologic studies. Why higher retinol intake could increase risk of prostate cancer is unclear. Of note, high levels of retinol have antagonistic effects on vitamin D (159–162), a putative protective agent (see below).

Zinc

Zinc has received considerable interest in prostate cancer because of its high concentration in the prostate (163,164). Zinc is a necessary component of numerous metalloproteins, including those important for DNA synthesis, immune function, and antioxidant activity (165). *In vitro*, zinc inhibits growth of androgen-sensitive and androgen-independent prostate cancer cell lines via cell cycle arrest, apoptosis, and necrosis (166, 167). Zinc also has antimicrobial activity. However, findings for zinc intake and risk of prostate cancer incidence and mortality have been inconsistent. Studies have suggested moderate inverse associations (68,168,169), no association (69,74,170, 171), or even an increased risk when zinc supplements are taken at high, supraphysiologic doses (172). The increased risk observed with higher supplementary doses observed in a prospective study (172) suggests caution in the level of zinc ingested through supplements.

Vitamin D

Vitamin D has numerous anticancer properties *in vitro* and in animal models (173). However, based on epidemiologic studies on prostate cancer, the results regarding vitamin D are generally nonsupportive of a benefit. In populations in the United States, where severe vitamin D deficiency is uncommon, higher 25(OH) vitamin D, the major circulating form of vitamin D, has not been associated with a reduced risk of prostate cancer (174–178). However, two studies (179,180), which were conducted in Nordic countries, supported an inverse association between 25(OH) vitamin D level and prostate cancer risk. One of these studies also found an increased cancer risk in men with high 25(OH) vitamin D concentrations, suggesting a U-shaped dose-response relationship (180). Not surprisingly, because of reduced sunshine exposure in Nordic countries, 25(OH) vitamin D levels were quite low in these studies. Synthesis of $1,25(OH)_2$ vitamin D, the active component of vitamin D, impaired only when 25(OH) vitamin D is seriously deficient (181,182), perhaps accounts for the inverse association observed only in Nordic countries. For circulating $1,25(OH)_2$ vitamin D, one study (174) is supportive, whereas another is suggestive (176) of an inverse association with aggressive prostate cancer, perhaps only for older-onset prostate cancers. In a case-control study conducted in the United Kingdom, where vitamin D deficiency is relatively common in the elderly (183), regular foreign holidays, higher sunbathing scores, and higher exposure to UV radiation were associated with a reduced risk of prostate cancer (184). None of the four studies that have evaluated whether dietary or supplemental vitamin D is related to risk of prostate cancer found evidence of a protective association (72,95,105,106). Thus, although biological data on vitamin D are intriguing, epidemiologic data thus far have been only weakly supportive of the vitamin D hypothesis.

LIFESTYLE FACTORS

Physical Activity

The role of physical activity on prostate cancer risk remains unestablished. Whereas many studies have noted a modest inverse relation among occupational and/or leisure-time physical activity (44,185–192) or cardiorespiratory fitness (193) with prostate cancer risk, others have found no association (53,67,71,194,195). The study on cardiorespiratory fitness (193) assessed activity in part but also genetic factors related to fitness. Some studies have even suggested positive associations with prostate cancer risk (26,45), particularly with greater physical activity in young adulthood (47,196,197). Another study found more physical activity in young adulthood as potentially beneficial (59). In contrast, high levels of physical activity later in life, particularly in older men, have been found to decrease risk of advanced prostate cancer (198,199). Several reasons may have contributed to these inconsistencies, including the difficulty in accurately assessing physical activity in epidemiologic studies, different roles of moderate- and high-intensity exercise, and a differential effect of exercise depending on time of life. In addition, there may be differences in prostate carcinogenic factors among young men and older men, and activity levels may have varying effects for early and late stages of carcinogenesis. Of note, despite the complexities in measuring physical activity, a strong, unambiguous inverse association for physical activity has been observed for colon cancer (200). This finding for colon cancer suggests that while accurate measurement of activity remains an important issue, poor measurement alone probably is not entirely accounting for the inconsistencies in the prostate cancer literature.

Cigarette Smoking

The majority of cohort studies do not support an association between cigarette smoking and overall prostate cancer incidence (42,44,47,49,50,71,201–206), although there have been a few exceptions that have supported a modest positive association (53,191). In contrast, for metastatic or fatal prostate cancer, a number of cohort studies have reported higher risks in smokers (45,70,202,204,207–210); however, not all studies have found an association (44,49,50,203, 205,206). Some evidence suggests that risk for advanced or fatal prostate cancer may be greater for recent smoking rather than for cumulative exposure (210). In addition, smoking appears to enhance the aggressiveness of prostate cancers, as measured by advanced stage or poorer differentiation at the time of diagnosis (57, 211–214). Tobacco use has also been shown to correlate independently with lower time to development of hormone refractory prostate cancer and with poorer survival in a dose-dependent manner in men with advanced prostate cancer on androgen deprivation therapy (215). It is possible that differences in diagnosis-seeking between smokers and nonsmokers account for the apparently more aggressive behavior of prostate cancer in smokers, but some studies have attempted to control for these factors and still found excessive advanced stage and fatal disease in recent smokers (210). The possibility that carcinogens in cigarette smoke, or other effects of smoking, may promote tumor progression should be considered in future studies. Thus, although tobacco use has been relatively ignored as a relevant factor for prostate carcinogenesis, the worse prognosis in smokers warrants further study.

Alcohol Drinking

Nearly 60 epidemiologic studies have evaluated the association between alcohol consumption and risk of prostate cancer. Most of these studies indicate that alcohol consumption does not appear to be a strong risk factor for prostate cancer incidence or mortality (216). The possibility that a modestly higher risk of prostate cancer may occur in heavier drinkers has been suggested by recent prospective studies (53,217,218). However, given the small magnitude, even if real, public health ramifications are unclear considering the numerous other risks and benefits associated with varying levels and patterns of alcohol drinking. Thus, risk of prostate cancer should probably not be a major factor when considering recommendations related to alcohol drinking.

HORMONAL FACTORS

Sex Steroid Hormones

Given the importance of androgens in the development of the prostate gland and in the progression of prostate cancer at late stages, a long-standing hypothesis has been that normal variation in androgen levels among men may influence risk of prostate cancer. Variation in hormones has been used to account for regional and racial differences in risk and as a mechanism to explain how dietary factors may influence risk. A number of prospective studies have examined the association between circulating sex steroid hormone concentrations and risk of prostate cancer (219–231). Perhaps of some surprise, most studies have not found a significant association. Only one prospective study found that testosterone and androstanediol glucuronide, a metabolite of dihydrotestosterone, were statistically significant positively associated with prostate cancer; this study additionally found that estradiol and sex hormone binding globulin (SHBG) were inversely associated with risk (224). Three prospective studies have suggested a higher risk of prostate cancer associated with a higher ratio of testosterone to either dihydrotestosterone or androstanediol glucuronide (219,221,228). A meta-analysis of the prospective studies conducted up to 1999 did not find case-control differences in androgenic hormones, except possibly for slightly higher concentrations of androstanediol glucuronide in the cases (232). In the meta-analysis, most studies did not adjust for SHBG.

A complementary line of evidence concerns the androgen receptor, which mediates the effect of testosterone and dihydrotestosterone in androgen-responsive tissues (233). The androgen receptor gene, located on the long arm of the X chromosome, contains a variable-length CAG repeat (encodes polyglutamine) in exon 1, which encodes the transcriptional regulatory region of the receptor (234). In experimental constructs, fewer repeats increase the transactivational ability of the receptor (234,235). The normal range of CAG repeats is 11 to 31 (236), and men with longer repeats, even within the normal range, experience reduced androgenicity (237). The mean number of androgen receptor CAG repeats is shorter in African-American men (~20 repeats) than in white men (~22 repeats), suggesting a role for CAG repeats in the higher rates of prostate cancer in African-American men (6,236,238). Some (238–243), but not all (244–251), epidemiologic studies find that shorter androgen receptor gene CAG repeats are associated with a higher risk of prostate cancer. Greater consistency is found when considering only advanced cases, cases diagnosed in the pre-PSA era (which tended to be more advanced than those in the PSA era), and when considering a young age at onset (252).

The role of estrogens in prostate cancer carcinogenesis is controversial, with some groups suggesting the estrogens protect against prostate cancer (224) and others suggesting that estrogens may be positively associated given that levels of estrogen relative to testosterone increase with age as the risk of prostate cancer increases with age. Because age represents cumulative exposure of many factors, the latter argument is not compelling. However, shifting the estrogen-to-testosterone ratio may enhance the immune response and perhaps increase inflammation in the prostate. A case-control study found that higher urinary excretion of 2-hydroxyestrone relative to 16α-hydroxyestrone was associated with a lower risk of prostate cancer (253). 2-hydroxyestrone has no estrogenic activity, whereas α-hydroxyestrone is estrogenic (253), suggesting a deleterious role for estrogen activity. However, one study (254) suggested a protective role of higher circulating levels of estrogen.

The study of the relation of sex steroid hormones to prostate cancer risk has had several limitations that may account for the inconsistent results. Most importantly, studies have tended to evaluate single or only several components of the hormonal pathway, but the hormonal pathway is complex, and many interrelated factors are relevant. Additionally, the study of sex steroid hormones has been limited by measurement issues, such as poor precision in the laboratory assays or reliance on a single measurement in adulthood to characterize long-term exposure. Most of the studies, except those by Gann et al. (224) and Dorgan et al. (228) (which did not observe an association), did not adjust for SHBG levels when examining androgen levels. Adjusting for SHBG levels may provide a better measure of bioavailable testosterone. To what extent a single determination of circulating concentrations of steroid hormones is representative of time-averaged or maximum levels in the blood or of prostatic levels remains unsettled. Also, it is unknown when during the course of a man's life androgens may influence prostate cancer risk; possibly, effects earlier in life, as during the growth period, are crucial. Future studies focused on genetic polymorphisms in hormonal

pathway genes may provide information regarding this important hypothesis. The recent finding that finasteride, a 5-α reductase type 2 inhibitor (blocking the conversion of testosterone to the more active DHT), reduces risk of prostate cancer confirms a role of androgens (255). However, the implications are complicated, because although overall prostate cancer risk was reduced by finasteride, the incidence of high-grade lesions was actually increased by finasteride. Whether this finding was real or represented a histologic artifact remains to be determined.

Insulin-like Growth Factor-1 and Insulin-like Growth Factor Binding Protein-3

Recent studies confirm a role of the insulin-like growth factor (IGF) axis. IGF-1 promotes proliferation and inhibits apoptosis in many cell types, including normal prostate and tumor cells (256,257). Most of the circulating IGF-1 is produced by the liver; IGF-1 secretion is stimulated by growth hormone and requires adequate levels of insulin. IGF-1 is also produced locally in tissues, including the prostate gland, and has paracrine effects. In the circulation, IGF-1 is bound to binding proteins, including insulin-like growth factor binding protein (IGFBP)-3, which has the highest concentration among the binding proteins. High circulating concentrations of IGFBP-3 may reduce bioavailability of IGF-1, and additionally IGFBP-3 appears to promote apoptosis (258,259). Thus, biologically, it can be predicted that high IGF-1 levels would increase cancer risk, whereas high levels of IGF binding proteins would lower risk.

Several studies have found that higher circulating concentrations of IGF-1 and lower circulating concentrations of IGFBP-3 are associated with increased risk of prostate cancer (260–266). The findings among studies for IGFBP-3 are not consistent, although in most of those studies in which IGFBP-3 concentration was statistically adjusted for IGF-1 concentration, an inverse association was found (260,263,264,266–268). In one study, the risk associated with higher IGF-1 level was limited to advanced prostate cancer, suggesting that the IGF-1 axis influences primarily progression rather than initiation of cancer (267). Two meta-analyses confirmed that men with high IGF-1 concentrations had about a 50% higher risk of prostate cancer than men with low IGF-1 concentrations (269,270). However, in these meta-analyses, no clear inverse association was found for IGFBP-3. Some of the discrepancies for IGFBP-3 might relate to differences in assays and whether IGF-1 level was adjusted for in the analysis. Levels of IGF-1 are strongly determined by genetics, but nutritional factors, including energy intake, are also important. Thus, IGF-1 may explain in part the lower risk of prostate cancer in shorter men, as IGF-1 is a determinant of height, and in less developed countries where energy and protein intakes are limited.

INFECTION AND INFLAMMATION

Interest in the role of chronic intraprostatic inflammation in the etiology of prostate cancer has been renewed recently by the awareness of infection and inflammation in the etiology of cancers of the liver, stomach, bladder, and colon (271). Chronic inflammatory infiltrates are common in resected prostate glands. These included regions of focal atrophy, also called proliferative inflammatory atrophy (PIA), a possible cancer precursor (272). The cause(s) of chronic prostatic inflammation is unknown, but this hypothesis opens up avenues for epidemiologic research for factors such as sexually transmitted infections (STIs) and other agents, prostatitis, cytokines and genes encoding cytokines, and factors involved in the response to infection.

The suggestion that STIs may increase the risk of prostate cancer is not new. Three decades ago, Heshmat et al. reported a positive correlation between prostate cancer mortality rates and incidence rates in Denmark for gonorrhea when lagged by 45 years (273). In a meta-analysis of the literature between 1971 and 2000, statistically significant summary estimates (relative risks) from 23 case-control studies of 1.44 for any history of STI, 2.30 for syphilis, and 1.34 for gonorrhea were found (274). However, all of these studies ascertained STI history retrospectively and usually without blinding to case-control status. In addition, possibly history of STIs may not be causally associated with prostate cancer but may be acting as a surrogate for androgenicity-associated libido or lifestyle risk factors for prostate cancer. Interestingly, recent studies (275), including a prospective study (276), found that ejaculation frequency was inversely associated with risk of prostate cancer. These studies suggest that the consequences of reduced or suppressed ejaculation might enhance risk of prostate cancer. Enhanced ejaculation may help clear infectious agents and carcinogens in the seminal fluid or prevent seminal fluid precipitates.

Regarding prostatitis, a meta-analysis of 11 case-control studies reported a statistically significant summary estimate for prostate cancer of 1.57 for men who had ever had a diagnosis of prostatitis (277). These case-control studies potentially suffer from various limitations, including recall bias, variable quality confirmation of prostatitis, and inability to classify type of prostatitis or to detect asymptomatic prostatitis. In addition, detection bias of prostate cancer is a concern, because men who are seeking treatment for prostatitis may have increased opportunity for detection of prostate cancer. Despite these limitations, the positive association in the meta-analysis indicates that this is a promising area for research.

FUTURE RESEARCH INTO PRIMARY PREVENTION

Understanding the epidemiology of prostate cancer remains a major challenge. Study of this malignancy has not produced consistent results to date. A number of factors may have contributed to this mixed literature. First, the natural history of prostate cancer may be unusually long; precursor lesions are common quite early in adulthood, but the clinical manifestations of this disease tend to occur rather late in life. Many factors, including hormones, have been typically examined relatively late in the life course, so the role of early effects have not been well studied. Second, prostate cancer displays an unusually wide range of aggressive biological potential, and risk factors may have diverse influences for different types of prostate cancer. The widespread use of PSA screening in the United States has enriched the pool of diagnosed cases with early lesions that may be less related to factors that influence promotion and progression. Third, some evidence suggests etiologic variability of prostate cancer by age-at-onset; factors related to genetic susceptibility are more important for early onset cancer, and some studies suggest that exogenous factors, such as diet, may be more important for older men.

Despite the complexities, understanding the epidemiology of prostate cancer has promise in providing leads that can be ultimately established as preventive strategies. Four areas hold promise for primary prevention and merit special research attention. These include energy imbalance, inflammation, micronutrients and phytochemicals as protective agents, and dietary and lifestyle factors that may enhance risk. The prevalence of overweight and obesity now exceeds 61% in the United States, and obesity is a major risk factor for many conditions, including heart disease, type 2 diabetes, and several cancers. Research is needed to clarify the relation of adiposity, energy intake, and physical activity and related metabolic and hormonal perturbations through life on risk of prostate cancer incidence and progression. As reviewed earlier, the role of energy intake may be complex and perhaps counterintuitive, with highest risk observed in men who consume high levels of calories but nonetheless remain lean rather than in obese men. Whether this represents a specific metabolic or hormonal profile needs to be evaluated.

In recent years, increasing interest has centered on the role of chronic intraprostatic inflammation in prostate carcinogenesis. Inflammation merits attention because of the recognition of the potential significance of proliferative inflammatory atrophy lesions in the prostate, and because inflammation may be targeted for prevention and intervention. The identification of potential causative infectious agents could lead to treatments that could decrease the risk of prostate cancer. It is possible that the apparent benefit of some antioxidants such as selenium, lycopene, and vitamin E could be related to their utility in a highly oxidative environment associated with inflammation. Some early evidence already suggests a potential benefit of aspirin and NSAIDs use on prostate cancer incidence or progression (278). Many nonspecific and selective COX-2 inhibitors have been in use and could be evaluated in relation to risk of prostate cancer.

A third important area regards the potential use of micronutrients, antioxidants, and phytochemicals as potential nutritional or chemopreventive agents for prostate cancer. A number of candidates exist, though the evidence is not yet compelling for them. The most promising candidates include selenium, alpha and gamma tocopherol, lycopene, marine omega-3 fatty acids, vitamin D, and components in cruciferous vegetables. It is important to note that current epidemiologic evidence for many of these is based primarily on food sources (e.g., tomato products for lycopene, fish for omega-3 fatty acids). For items that have other established health benefits or at least that are unlikely to be harmful, it may be reasonable to make prudent recommendations indicating potential, though not established, benefits on prostate cancer risk based on the best available data. Before recommendations can be made regarding concentrated forms of putative protective agents in pills (e.g., lycopene as the active agent in tomatoes), intervention studies must confirm their benefits. The effects of high doses of concentrated forms of a phytochemical delivered as a pill (e.g., lycopene) may be quite unpredictable.

Finally, the reasons explaining basic epidemiologic patterns in prostate cancer, including the higher risk in African-Americans, lower risk in Asian populations, and higher risk in Western countries (especially those in northern Europe), remain unexplained. It appears that energy imbalance, intake of red meat and dairy products, and low intake of soy products and fish and of important micronutrients could contribute to higher risk in some populations. Hormonal factors may also play a role. It is important to note that hormonal factors are influenced both by genetics and environmental factors, particularly nutritional factors. Already some potential has been established for chemoprevention targeting hormonal factors, such as 5α-reductase type 2 inhibitors (finasteride) (255), though the clinical ramifications remain unestablished. Ideally, hormonal factors could be targeted by nutritional and lifestyle approaches, such as exercise and diet to control insulin resistance and hyperinsulinemia as a strategy to reduce diabetes risk. From the perspective of primary prevention, behaviors that are beneficial against a wide range of common chronic diseases need to be emphasized.

References

1. Potosky AL, Miller BA, Albertsen PC, et al. The role of increasing detection in the rising incidence of prostate cancer. *J Am Med Assoc* 1995;273: 548–552.
2. American Cancer Society. *Cancer facts & figures, 2003.* Atlanta, GA: American Cancer Society, 2003.
3. Chu KC, Tarone RE, Freeman HP. Trends in prostate cancer mortality among black and white men in the United States. *Cancer* 2003;97: 1507–1516.
4. Stanford JL, Stephenson RA, Coyle LM, et al. *Prostate cancer trends 1973–1995.* Bethesda, MD: SEER Program, National Cancer Institute, NIH Pub. No. 99-4543, 1999.
5. Hoffman RM, Gilliland FD, Eley JW, et al. Racial and ethnic differences in advanced-stage prostate cancer: The Prostate Cancer Outcomes Study. *J Natl Cancer Inst* 2001;93:388–395.
6. Platz EA, Rimm EB, Willett WC, et al. Racial variation in prostate cancer incidence and in hormonal system markers among male health professionals. *J Natl Cancer Inst* 2000;92:2009–2017.
7. Parkin DM, Whelan SL, Ferlay J, et al. *Cancer incidence in five continents.* Lyon: International Agency for Research on Cancer, IARC Scientific Publications No. 155, 2003.
8. Parkin DM, Muir CS, Whelan SL, et al. *Cancer incidence in five continents.* Lyon: International Agency for Research on Cancer, 1992.
9. Glover FE Jr, Coffey DS, Douglas LL, et al. The epidemiology of prostate cancer in Jamaica. *J Urol* 1998;159:1984–1986.
10. Ahluwalia B, Jackson MA, Jones GW, et al. Blood hormone profiles in prostate cancer patients in high-risk and low-risk populations. *Cancer* 1981;48:2267–2273.
11. Haenszel W, Kurihara M. Studies of Japanese migrants. I. Mortality from cancer and other diseases among Japanese in the United States. *J Natl Cancer Inst* 1968;40:43–68.
12. Yu H, Harris RE, Gao YT, et al. Comparative epidemiology of cancers of the colon, rectum, prostate and breast in Shanghai, China versus the United States. *Int J Epidemiol* 1991;20:76–81.
13. Shimizu H, Ross RK, Bernstein L, et al. Cancers of the prostate and breast among Japanese and white immigrants in Los Angeles county. *Br J Cancer* 1991;63:963–966.
14. Shimizu H, Ross RK, Bernstein L. Possible underestimation of the incidence rate of prostate cancer in Japan. *Jpn J Cancer Res* 1991;82: 483–485.
15. Hayes RB, Liff JM, Pottern LM, et al. Prostate cancer risk in U.S. blacks and whites with a family history of cancer. *Int J Cancer* 1995;60:361–364.
16. Whittemore AS, Wu AH, Kolonel LN, et al. Family history and prostate cancer risk in black, white, and Asian men in the United States and Canada. *Am J Epidemiol* 1995;141:732–740.
17. Andersson SO, Baron J, Bergström R, et al. Lifestyle factors and prostate cancer risk: A Case-control Study in Sweden. *Cancer Epidemiol Biomarkers Prev* 1996;5:509–513.
18. Lesko SM, Rosenberg L, Shapiro S. Family history and prostate cancer. *Am J Epidemiol* 1996;144:1041–1047.
19. Ghadirian P, Howe GR, Hislop TG, et al. Family history of prostate cancer: A multi-center case-control study in Canada. *Int J Cancer* 1997;70: 679–681.
20. Villeneuve PJ, Johnson KC, Kreiger N, et al. The Canadian Cancer Registries Epidemiology Research Group. Risk factors for prostate cancer: Results from the Canadian National Enhanced Cancer Surveillance System. *Cancer Causes Control* 1999;10:355–367.
21. Cannon L, Bishop DT, Skolnick M, et al. Genetic epidemiology of prostate cancer in Utah Mormon genealogy. *Cancer Surv* 1982;1:47–69.
22. Grönberg H, Damber L, Damber JE. Familial prostate cancer in Sweden. A nationwide register based study. *Cancer* 1996;77:138–143.
23. Goldgar DE, Easton DF, Cannon-Albright LA, et al. Systematic population-based assessment of cancer risk in first-degree relatives of cancer probands. *J Natl Cancer Inst* 1994;86:1600–1608.
24. Rodríguez C, Callee EE, Miracle-McMahill HL, et al. Family history and risk of fatal prostate cancer. *Epidemiology* 1997;8:653–657.
25. Kalish LA, McDougal WS, McKinlay JB. Family history and the risk of prostate cancer. *Urology* 2000;56:803–806.
26. Clarke G, Whittemore AS. Prostate cancer risk in relation to anthropometry and physical activity: The National Health and Nutritional Examination Survey I Epidemiological Follow-Up Study. *Cancer Epidemiol Biomarkers Prev* 2000;9:875–881.
27. Monroe KR, Yu MC, Kolonel LN, et al. Evidence of an X-linked or recessive genetic component to prostate cancer risk. *Nat Med* 1995;1:827–829.
28. Carter BS, Beaty TH, Steinberg GD, et al. Mendelian inheritance of familial prostate cancer. *Proc Natl Acad Sci U S A* 1992;89:3367–3371.
29. Lichtenstein P, Holm NV, Verkasalo PK, et al. Environmental and heritable factors in the causation of cancer: Analyses of cohorts of twins from Sweden, Denmark, and Finland. *N Engl J Med* 2000;343:78–85.
30. Page WF, Braun MM, Partin AW, et al. Heredity and prostate cancer: A study of World War II veteran twins. *Prostate* 1997;33:240–245.
31. Grönberg H, Damber L, Damber JE, et al. Segregation analysis of prostate cancer in Sweden: Support for dominant inheritance. *Am J Epidemiol* 1997;146:552–557.
32. Gong G, Oakley-Girvan I, Wu AH, et al. Segregation analysis of prostate cancer in 1,719 white, African-American and Asian-American families in the United States and Canada. *Cancer Causes Control* 2002;13:471–482.
33. Kritchevsky D. Caloric restriction and experimental carcinogenesis. *Toxicol Sci* 1999;52(Suppl):13–16.
34. Thompson HJ, Jiang W, Zhu Z. Mechanisms by which energy restriction inhibits carcinogenesis. *Adv Exp Med Biol* 1999;470:77–84.
35. Mukherjee P, Sotnikov AV, Mangian HJ, et al. Energy intake and prostate tumor growth, angiogenesis, and vascular endothelial growth factor expression. *J Natl Cancer Inst* 1999;91:512–523.
36. Calle EE, Rodriguez C, Walker-Thurmond K, et al. Overweight, obesity, and mortality from cancer in a prospectively studied cohort of U.S. adults. *N Engl J Med* 2003;348:1625–1638.
37. Platz E. Energy imbalance and prostate cancer. *J Nutr* 2002;132(Suppl): 3471S–3481S.
38. Platz EA, Leitzmann MF, Michaud DS, et al. Interrelation of energy intake, body size, and physical activity with prostate cancer in a large prospective cohort study. *Cancer Res* 2003;63:8542–8548.
39. Nomura AM. Body size and prostate cancer. *Epidemiol Rev* 2001;23: 126–131.
40. Lew EA, Garfinkel L. Variations in mortality by weight among 750,000 men and women. *J Chronic Dis* 1979;32:563–576.
41. Snowdon DA, Phillips RL, Choi W. Diet, obesity, and risk of fatal prostate cancer. *Am J Epidemiol* 1984;120:244–250.
42. Thompson MM, Garland C, Barrett-Connor E, et al. Heart disease risk factors, diabetes, and prostatic cancer in an adult community. *Am J Epidemiol* 1989;129:511–517.
43. Chyou PH, Nomura AM, Stemmermann GN. A prospective study of weight, body mass index and other anthropometric measurements in relation to site-specific cancers. *Int J Cancer* 1994;57:313–317.
44. Thune I, Lund E. Physical activity and the risk of prostate and testicular cancer: A cohort study of 53,000 Norwegian men. *Cancer Causes Control* 1994;5:549–556.
45. Cerhan JR, Torner JC, Lynch CF, et al. Association of smoking, body mass, and physical activity with risk of prostate cancer in the Iowa 65+ Rural Health Study (United States). *Cancer Causes Control* 1997;8: 229–238.
46. Veierod MB, Laake P, Thelle DS. Dietary fat intake and risk of prostate cancer: A prospective study of 25,708 Norwegian men. *Int J Cancer* 1997; 73:634–638.
47. Whittemore AS, Paffenbarger RS, Anderson K Jr, et al. Early precursors of site-specific cancers in college men and women. *J Natl Cancer Inst* 1985;74:43–51.
48. Greenwald P, Damon A, Kirmss V, et al. Physical and demographic features of men before developing cancer of the prostate. *J Natl Cancer Inst* 1974;53:341–346.
49. Le Marchand L, Kolonel LN, Wilkens LR, et al. Animal fat consumption and prostate cancer: A prospective study in Hawaii. *Epidemiology* 1994;5: 276–282.
50. Mills PK, Beeson WL, Phillips RL, et al. Cohort study of diet, lifestyle, and prostate cancer in Adventist men. *Cancer* 1989;64:598–604.
51. Giovannucci E, Rimm EB, Stampfer MJ, et al. Height, body weight, and risk of prostate cancer. *Cancer Epidemiol Biomarkers Prev* 1997;6:557–563.
52. Nilsen TI, Vatten LJ. Anthropometry and prostate cancer risk: A prospective study of 22,248 Norwegian men. *Cancer Causes Control* 1999;10: 269–275.
53. Putnam S, Cerhan J, Parker A, et al. Lifestyle and anthropometric risk factors for prostate cancer in a cohort of Iowa men. *Ann Epidemiol* 2000; 10:361–369.
54. Habel LA, Van Den Eeden SK, Friedman GD. Body size, age at shaving initiation, and prostate cancer in a large, multiracial cohort. *Prostate* 2000; 43:136–143.
55. Schuurman AG, Goldbohm RA, Dorant E, et al. Anthropometry in relation to prostate cancer risk in the Netherlands Cohort Study. *Am J Epidemiol* 2000;151:541–549.
56. Gapstur SM, Gann PH, Colangelo LA, et al. Postload glucose concentration and 27-year prostate cancer mortality (United States). *Cancer Causes Control* 2001;12:763–772.
57. Spitz MR, Strom SS, Yamamura Y, et al. Epidemiologic determinants of clinically relevant prostate cancer. *Int J Cancer* 2000;89:259–264.
58. Rohrmann S, Roberts WW, Walsh PC, et al. Family history of prostate cancer and obesity in relation to high-grade disease and extraprostatic extension in young men with prostate cancer. *Prostate* 2003;55: 140–146.
59. Andersson SO, Baron J, Wolk A, et al. Early life risk factors for prostate cancer: A population-based case-control study in Sweden. *Cancer Epidemiol Biomarkers Prev* 1995;4:187–192.
60. Andersson SO, Wolk A, Bergström R, et al. Body size and prostate cancer: A 20-year follow-up study among 135,006 Swedish construction workers. *J Natl Cancer Inst* 1997;89:385–389.
61. Herbert PR, Ajani U, Cook N, et al. Adult height and incidence of total malignant neoplasms and prostate cancer: The Physicians' Health Study. *Am J Epidemiol* 1996;143S:78, 309.
62. Hayes RB, Ziegler RG, Gridley G, et al. Dietary factors and risks for prostate cancer among blacks and whites in the United States. *Cancer Epidemiol Biomarkers Prev* 1999;8:25–34.

18 Part I: Prostate Cancer

63. Albanes D, Jones DY, Schatzkin A, et al. Adult stature and risk of cancer. *Cancer Res* 1988;48:1658–1662.
64. Armstrong B, Doll R. Environmental factors and cancer incidence and mortality in different countries, with special reference to dietary practices. *Int J Cancer* 1975;15:617–631.
65. Rose DP, Boyar AP, Wynder EL. International comparisons of mortality rates for cancer of the breast, ovary, prostate, and colon, and per capita food consumption. *Cancer* 1986;58:2263–2271.
66. Kushi L, Giovannucci E. Dietary fat and cancer. *Am J Med* 2002;113 (Suppl 9B):63S–70S.
67. Whittemore AS, Kolonel LN, Wu AH, et al. Prostate cancer in relation to diet, physical activity, and body size in blacks, whites, and Asians in the United States and Canada. *J Natl Cancer Inst* 1995;87:652–661.
68. Key TJA, Silcocks PB, Davey GK, et al. A case-control study of diet and prostate cancer. *Br J Cancer* 1997;76:678–687.
69. Andersson SO, Wolk A, Bergstrom R, et al. Energy, nutrient intake and prostate cancer risk: A population-based case-control study in Sweden. *Int J Cancer* 1996;68:716–722.
70. Hsing AW, McLaughlin JK, Schuman LM, et al. Diet, tobacco use, and fatal prostate cancer: Results from the Lutheran Brotherhood Cohort Study. *Cancer Res* 1990;50:6836–6840.
71. Severson RK, Nomura AMY, Grove JS, et al. A prospective study of demographics, diet, and prostate cancer among men of Japanese ancestry in Hawaii. *Cancer Res* 1989;49:1857–1860.
72. Chan JM, Pietinen P, Virtanen M, et al. Diet and prostate cancer risk in a cohort of smokers, with a specific focus on calcium and phosphorus (Finland). *Cancer Causes Control* 2000;11:859–867.
73. Giovannucci E, Rimm EB, Colditz GA, et al. A prospective study of dietary fat and risk of prostate cancer. *J Natl Cancer Inst* 1993;85:1571–1579.
74. West DW, Slattery ML, Robison LM, et al. Adult dietary intake and prostate cancer risk in Utah: A case-control study with special emphasis on aggressive tumors. *Cancer Causes Control* 1991;2:85–94.
75. Groff JL, Gropper SS. *Advanced nutrition and human metabolism*, 3rd ed. Belmont, CA: Wadsworth, 2000.
76. Giovannucci E, Rimm EB, Colditz GA, et al. A prospective study of dietary fat and risk of prostate cancer. *J Natl Cancer Inst* 1993;85:1571–1579.
77. Schuurman AG, van den Brandt PA, Dorant E, et al. Association of energy and fat intake with prostate carcinoma risk: Results from the Netherlands Cohort Study. *Cancer* 1999;86:1019–1027.
78. Gann PH, Hennekens CH, Sacks FM, et al. Prospective study of plasma fatty acids and risk of prostate cancer. *J Natl Cancer Inst* 1994;86:281–286.
79. Harvei S, Bjerve KS, Tretli S, et al. Prediagnostic level of fatty acids in serum phospholipids: Omega-3 and omega-6 fatty acids and the risk of prostate cancer. *Int J Cancer* 1997;71:545–551.
80. Leitzmann MF, Stampfer MJ, Michaud DS, et al. Dietary intake of omega-3 and omega-6 fatty acids and the risk of prostate cancer. *Am J Clin Nutr* 2004;80:204–216.
81. Godley PA, Campbell MK, Gallagher P, et al. Biomarkers of essential fatty acid consumption and risk of prostatic carcinoma. *Cancer Epidemiol Biomarkers Prev* 1996;5:889–895.
82. Norrish AE, Jackson RT, Sharpe SJ, et al. Men who consume vegetable oils rich in monounsaturated fat: Their dietary patterns and risk of prostate cancer (New Zealand). *Cancer Causes Control* 2000;11:609–615.
83. Terry P, Lichtenstein P, Feychting M, et al. Fatty fish consumption and risk of prostate cancer [Letter]. *Lancet* 2001;357:1764–1766.
84. Michaud DS, Augustsson K, Rimm EB, et al. A prospective study on intake of animal products and risk of prostate cancer. *Cancer Causes Control* 2001;12:557–567.
85. Schuurman AG, van den Brandt PA, Dorant E, et al. Animal products, calcium and protein and prostate cancer risk in the Netherlands Cohort Study. *Br J Cancer* 1999;80:1107–1113.
86. Nagao M. A new approach to risk estimation of food-borne carcinogens—heterocyclic amines—based on molecular information. *Mutat Res* 1999;43:3–12.
87. Norrish AE, Ferguson LR, Knize MG, et al. Heterocyclic amine content of cooked meat and risk of prostate cancer. *J Natl Cancer Inst* 1999;91:2038–2044.
88. Grant WB. An ecologic study of dietary links to prostate cancer. *Altern Med Rev* 1999;4:162–169.
89. Talamini R, La Vecchia C, Decarli A, et al. Nutrition, social factors, and prostatic cancer in a Northern Italian population. *Br J Cancer* 1986;53:817–821.
90. Talamini R, Franceschi S, La Vecchia C, et al. Diet and prostatic cancer: A case-control study in Northern Italy. *Nutr Cancer* 1992;18:277–286.
91. Mettlin C, Selenskas S, Natarajan NS, et al. Beta-carotene and animal fats and their relationship to prostate cancer risk: A case-control study. *Cancer* 1989;64:605–612.
92. La Vecchia C, Negri E, D'Avanzo B, et al. Dairy products and the risk of prostatic cancer. *Oncology* 1991;48:406–410.
93. Jain MG, Hislop GT, Howe GR, et al. Plant foods, antioxidants, and prostate cancer risk: Findings from case-control studies in Canada. *Nutr Cancer* 1999;34:173–184.
94. De Stefani E, Fierro L, Barrios E, et al. Tobacco, alcohol, diet and risk of prostate cancer. *Tumori* 1995;81:315–320.
95. Kristal AR, Cohen JH, Qu P, et al. Associations of energy, fat, calcium, and vitamin D with prostate cancer risk. *Cancer Epidemiol Biomarkers Prev* 2002;11:719–725.
96. Rotkin ID. Studies in the epidemiology of prostatic cancer: Expanded sampling. *Cancer Treat Rep* 1977;61:173–180.
97. Schuman LM, Mandel JS, Radke A. Some selected features of the epidemiology of prostatic cancer: Minneapolis-St. Paul, Minnesota Case-Control Study, 1976–1979. In: Magnus K, ed. *Trends in cancer incidence: Causes and practical implications*. Washington, DC: Hemisphere Publishing Corp, 1982:345–354.
98. Tzonou A, Signorello LB, Lagiou P, et al. Diet and cancer of the prostate: A case-control study in Greece. *Int J Cancer* 1999;80:704–708.
99. Ewings P, Bowie C. A case-control study of cancer of the prostate in Somerset and East Devon. *Br J Cancer* 1996;74:661–666.
100. Deneo-Pellegrini H, De Stefani E, Ronco A, et al. Foods, nutrients and prostate cancer: A case-control study in Uruguay. *Br J Cancer* 1999;80:591–597.
101. Chan JM, Stampfer MJ, Ma J, et al. Dairy products, calcium, and prostate cancer risk in the Physicians' Health Study [Comment]. *Am J Clin Nutr* 2001;74:549–554.
102. Tseng M, Breslow R, Babb J, et al. Dairy, calcium, and prostate cancer in the NHANES I Epidemiologic Followup Study cohort. *Am J Epidemiol* 2002;155:S55.
103. Hsing AW, McLaughlin JK, Schuman LM, et al. Diet, tobacco use, and fatal prostate cancer: Results from the Lutheran Brotherhood Cohort Study. *Cancer Res* 1990;50:6836–6840.
104. Veierod MB, Laake P, Thelle DS. Dietary fat intake and risk of prostate cancer: A prospective study of 25,708 Norwegian men. *Int J Cancer* 1997;73:634–638.
105. Giovannucci E, Rimm EB, Wolk A, et al. Calcium and fructose intake in relation to risk of prostate cancer. *Cancer Res* 1998;58:442–447.
106. Chan JM, Giovannucci E, Andersson S-O, et al. Dairy products, calcium, phosphorous, vitamin D, and risk of prostate cancer. *Cancer Causes Control* 1998;9:559–566.
107. Rodriguez C, McCullough ML, Mondul AM, et al. Calcium, dairy products, and risk of prostate cancer in a prospective cohort of United States men. *Cancer Epidemiol Biomarkers Prev* 2003;12:597–603.
108. Qin LQ, Xu JY, Wang PY, et al. Milk consumption is a risk factor for prostate cancer: Meta-analysis of case-control studies. *Nutr Cancer* 2004;48:22–27.
109. Bosetti C, Micelotta S, Dal Maso L, et al. Food groups and risk of prostate cancer in Italy. *Int J Cancer* 2004;110:424–428.
110. Berndt SI, Carter HB, Landis PK, et al. Calcium intake and prostate cancer risk in a long-term aging study: The Baltimore Longitudinal Study of Aging. *Urology* 2002;60:1118–1123.
111. Tavani A, Gallus S, Franceschi S, et al. Calcium, dairy products, and the risk of prostate cancer. *Prostate* 2001;48:118–121.
112. Giovannucci E, Ascherio A, Rimm EB, et al. Intake of carotenoids and retinol in relation to risk of prostate cancer. *J Natl Cancer Inst* 1995;87:1767–1776.
113. Schuurman AG, Goldbohm A, Dorant E, et al. Vegetable and fruit consumption and prostate cancer risk: A cohort study in the Netherlands. *Cancer Epidemiol Biomarkers Prev* 1998;7:673–680.
114. Cohen JH, Kristal AR, Stanford JL. Fruit and vegetable intakes and prostate cancer risk. *J Natl Cancer Inst* 2000;92:61–68.
115. Kolonel LN, Hankin JH, Whittemore AS, et al. Vegetables, fruits, legumes and prostate cancer: A multiethnic case-control study. *Cancer Epidemiol Biomarkers Prev* 2000;9:795–804.
116. Giovannucci E, Rimm EB, Liu Y, et al. A prospective study of tomato products, lycopene, and prostate cancer risk. *J Natl Cancer Inst* 2002;94:391–398.
117. Hsing AW, Chokkalingam AP, Gao YT, et al. Allium vegetables and risk of prostate cancer: A population-based study. *J Natl Cancer Inst* 2002;94:1648–1651.
118. Sies H, Stahl W. Vitamins E and C, ß-carotene, and other carotenoids as antioxidants. *Am J Clin Nutr* 1995;62(Suppl):1315S–1321S.
119. Ascherio A, Stampfer MJ, Colditz GA, et al. Correlations of vitamin A and E intakes with the plasma concentrations of carotenoids and tocopherols among American men and women. *J Nutr* 1992;122:1792–1801.
120. Kaplan LA, Stein EA, Willett WC, et al. Reference ranges of retinol, tocopherols, lycopene and alpha- and beta-carotene in plasma by simultaneous high-performance liquid chromatographic analysis. *Clin Physiol Biochem* 1987;5:297–304.
121. Clinton SK, Emenhiser C, Schwartz SJ, et al. cis-trans lycopene isomers, carotenoids, and retinol in the human prostate. *Cancer Epidemiol Biomarkers Prev* 1996;5:823–833.
122. Stahl W, Sies H. Uptake of lycopene and its geometrical isomers is greater from heat-processed than from unprocessed tomato juice in humans. *J Nutr* 1992;122:2161–2166.
123. Hsing AW, Comstock GW, Abbey H, et al. Serologic precursors of cancer. Retinol, carotenoids, and tocopherol and risk of prostate cancer. *J Natl Cancer Inst* 1990;82:941–946.
124. Gann PH, Ma J, Giovannucci E, et al. Lower prostate cancer risk in men with elevated plasma lycopene levels: Results of a prospective analysis. *Cancer Res* 1999;59:1225–1230.

125. Lu TW, Hung JC, Heber D, et al. Inverse association between plasma lycopene and other carotenoids and prostate cancer. *Cancer Epidemiol Biomarkers Prev* 2001;10:749–756.

126. Vogt TM, Mayne ST, Graubard BI, et al. Serum lycopene, other serum carotenoids, and risk of prostate cancer in US blacks and whites. *Am J Epidemiol* 2002;155:1023–1032.

127. Wu K, Erdman JWJ, Schwartz SJ, et al. Plasma and dietary carotenoids, and the risk of prostate cancer: A nested case-control study. *Cancer Epidemiol Biomarkers Prev* 2004;13:260–269.

128. Huang HY, Alberg AJ, Norkus EP, et al. Prospective study of antioxidant micronutrients in the blood and the risk of developing prostate cancer. *Am J Epidemiol* 2003;157:335–344.

129. Nomura AM, Stemmermann GN, Lee J, et al. Serum micronutrients and prostate cancer in Japanese Americans in Hawaii. *Cancer Epidemiol Biomarkers Prev* 1997;6:487–491.

130. Kristal AR, Lampe JW. Brassica vegetables and prostate cancer risk: A review of the epidemiologic evidence. *Nutr Cancer* 2002;42:1–9.

131. Giovannucci E, Rimm EB, Liu Y, et al. A prospective study of cruciferous vegetables and prostate cancer. *Cancer Epidemiol Biomarkers Prev* 2003;12:1403–1409.

132. Morrissey C, Watson RW. Phytoestrogens and prostate cancer. *Curr Drug Targets* 2003;4:231–241.

133. The Alpha-Tocopherol Beta Carotene Cancer Prevention Study Group. The effect of vitamin E and beta carotene on the incidence of lung cancer and other cancers in male smokers. *N Engl J Med* 1994;330:1029–1035.

134. Heinonen OP, Albanes D, Virtamo J, et al. Prostate cancer and supplementation with α-tocopherol and β-carotene: incidence and mortality in a controlled trial. *J Natl Cancer Inst* 1998;90:440–446.

135. ATBC Study Group. Incidence of cancer and mortality following alpha-tocopherol and beta-carotene supplementation: A postintervention follow-up. *JAMA* 2003;290:476–485.

136. Chan JM, Stampfer MJ, Ma J, et al. Supplemental vitamin E intake and prostate cancer risk in a large cohort of men in the United States. *Cancer Epidemiol Biomarkers Prev* 1999;8:893–899.

137. Eichholzer M, Stahelin HB, Gey KF, et al. Prediction of male cancer mortality by plasma levels of interacting vitamins: 17-year follow up of the prospective Basel study. *Int J Cancer* 1996;66:145–150.

138. Helzlsouer KJ, Huang H-Y, Alberg AJ, et al. Association between a-tocopherol, g-tocopherol, selenium and subsequent prostate cancer. *J Natl Cancer Inst* 2000;92:2018–2023.

139. Combs GF Jr, Combs SB. The nutritional biochemistry of selenium. *Annu Rev Nutr* 1984;4:257–280.

140. Clark LC, Combs GF Jr, Turnbull BW, et al. Nutritional Prevention of Cancer Study Group. Effects of selenium supplementation for cancer prevention in patients with carcinoma of the skin. A randomized controlled trial. *J Am Med Assoc* 1996;276:1957–1963.

141. Clark LC, Dalkin B, Krongrad A, et al. Decreased incidence of prostate cancer with selenium supplementation: Results of a double-blind cancer prevention trial. *Br J Urol* 1998;81:730–734.

142. Yoshizawa K, Willett WC, Morris SJ, et al. A study of prediagnostic selenium level in toenails and the risk of advanced prostate cancer. *J Natl Cancer Inst* 1998;90:1219–1224.

143. Vogt TM, Ziegler RG, Graubard BI, et al. Serum selenium and risk of prostate cancer in U.S. blacks and whites. *Int J Cancer* 2003;103:664–670.

144. Nomura AMY, Lee J, Stemmermann GN, et al. Serum selenium and subsequent risk of prostate cancer. *Cancer Epidemiol Biomarkers Prev* 2000;9:883–887.

145. Brooks JD, Metter EJ, Chan DW, et al. Plasma selenium level before diagnosis and the risk of prostate cancer development. *J Urol* 2001;166:2034–2038.

146. Li H, Stampfer MJ, Giovannucci EL, et al. A prospective study of plasma selenium levels and prostate cancer risk. *J Natl Cancer Inst* 2004;96:696–703.

147. Knekt P, Aromaa A, Maatela J, et al. Serum selenium and subsequent risk of cancer among Finnish men and women. *J Natl Cancer Inst* 1990;82:864–868.

148. Sporn MB, Roberts AB. Role of retinoids in differentiation and carcinogenesis. *J Natl Cancer Inst* 1984;73:1381–1386.

149. Pollard M, Luckert PH. The inhibitory effect of 4-hydroxyphenyl retinamide (4-HPR) on metastasis of prostate adenocarcinoma-III cells in Lobund-Wistar rats. *Cancer Lett* 1991;59:159–163.

150. Schroder EW, Black PH. Retinoids: Tumor preventers or tumor enhancers?. *J Natl Cancer Inst* 1980;65:671–674.

151. Mayne ST, Graham S, Zheng T. Dietary retinol: Prevention or promotion of carcinogenesis in humans?. *Cancer Causes Control* 1991;2:443–450.

152. Daviglus ML, Dyer AR, Persky V, et al. Dietary beta-carotene, vitamin C, and risk of prostate cancer: Results from the Western Electric Study. *Epidemiology* 1996;7:472–477.

153. Cook NR, Lee IM, Manson JE, et al. Effects of beta-carotene supplementation on cancer incidence by baseline characteristics in the Physicians' Health Study (United States). *Cancer Causes Control* 2000;11:617–626.

154. Ross RK, Shimizu H, Paganini-Hill A, et al. Case-control studies of prostate cancer in blacks and whites in Southern California. *J Natl Cancer Inst* 1987;78:869–874.

155. Graham S, Haughey B, Marshall J, et al. Diet in the epidemiology of carcinoma of the prostate gland. *J Natl Cancer Inst* 1983;70:687–692.

156. Kolonel LN, Hankin JH, Yoshizawa CN. Vitamin A and prostate cancer in elderly men: Enhancement of risk. *Cancer Res* 1987;47:2982–2985.

157. Reichman ME, Hayes RB, Ziegler RG, et al. Serum vitamin A and subsequent development of prostate cancer in the first National Health and Nutrition Examination Survey Epidemiologic Follow-up Study. *Cancer Res* 1990;50:2311–2315.

158. Willett WC, Stampfer MJ, Underwood BA, et al. Vitamin A supplementation and plasma retinol levels: A randomized trial among women. *J Natl Cancer Inst* 1984;73:1445–1448.

159. Rohde CM, Manatt M, Clagett-Dame M, et al. Vitamin A antagonizes the action of vitamin D in rats. *J Nutr* 1999;129:2246–2250.

160. Johansson S, Melhus H. Vitamin A antagonizes calcium response to vitamin D in man. *J Bone Miner Res* 2001;16:1899–1905.

161. Melhus H, Michaelsson K, Kindmark A, et al. Excessive dietary intake of vitamin A is associated with reduced bone mineral density and increased risk for hip fracture. *Ann Intern Med* 1998;129:770–778.

162. Feskanich D, Singh V, Willett WC, et al. Vitamin A intake and hip fractures among postmenopausal women. *JAMA* 2002;287:47–54.

163. Bertrand G, Vladesco R. Intervention probable du zinc dans les phenomenes de fecondations chez les animaux vertebres. *C R Seances Soc Biol Fil* 1921;173:176–180.

164. Mawson CA, Fischer MI. The occurrence of zinc in the human prostate gland. *Can J Med Sci* 1952;30:336–339.

165. Prasad AS. Zinc: An overview. *Nutrition* 1995;11(Suppl 2):93–99.

166. Iguchi K, Hamatake M, Ishida R, et al. Induction of necrosis by zinc in prostate carcinoma cells and identification of proteins increased in association with this induction. *Eur J Biochem* 1998;253:766–770.

167. Liang JY, Liu YY, Zou J, et al. Inhibitory effect of zinc on human prostatic carcinoma cell growth. *Prostate* 1999;40:200–207.

168. Kristal AR, Stanford JL, Cohen JH, et al. Vitamin and mineral supplement use is associated with reduced risk of prostate cancer. *Cancer Epidemiol Biomarkers Prev* 1999;8:887–892.

169. Platz EA, Hoffman SC, Morris JS, et al. Prediagnostic toenail cadmium and zinc and subsequent prostate cancer risk. *Proc Am Assoc Cancer Res* 2001;42:151.

170. Kolonel LN, Yoshizawa CN, Hankin JH. Diet and prostatic cancer: A case-control study in Hawaii. *Am J Epidemiol* 1988;127:999–1012.

171. Vlajinac HD, Marinkovic JM, Ilic MD, et al. Diet and prostate cancer: A case-control study. *Eur J Cancer* 1997;33:101–107.

172. Leitzmann MF, Stampfer MJ, Wu K, et al. Zinc supplement use and risk of prostate cancer. *J Natl Cancer Inst* 2003;95:1004–1007.

173. Lokeshwar BL, Schwartz GG, Selzer MG, et al. Inhibition of prostate cancer metastasis in vivo: A comparison of 1,23-dihydroxyvitamin D (calcitriol) and EB1089. *Cancer Epidemiol Biomarkers Prev* 1999;8:241–248.

174. Corder EH, Guess HA, Hulka BS, et al. Vitamin D and prostate cancer: A prediagnostic study with stored sera. *Cancer Epidemiol Biomarkers Prev* 1993;2:467–472.

175. Braun MM, Helzlsouer KJ, Hollis BW, et al. Prostate cancer and prediagnostic levels of serum vitamin D metabolites (Maryland, United States). *Cancer Causes Control* 1995;6:235–239.

176. Gann PH, Ma J, Hennekens CH, et al. Circulating vitamin D metabolites in relation to subsequent development of prostate cancer. *Cancer Epidemiol Biomarkers Prev* 1996;5:121–126.

177. Nomura AM, Stemmermann GN, Lee J, et al. Serum vitamin D metabolite levels and the subsequent development of prostate cancer. *Cancer Causes Control* 1998;9:425–432.

178. Platz EA, Leitzmann MF, Hollis BW, et al. Plasma 1,25-dihydroxy- and 25-hydroxyvitamin D and subsequent risk of prostate cancer. *Cancer Causes Control* 2004;15:255–265.

179. Ahonen MH, Tenkanen LT, Hakama M, et al. Prostate cancer risk and prediagnostic serum 25-hydroxyvitamin D levels (Finland). *Cancer Causes Control* 2000;11:847–852.

180. Tuohimaa P, Tenkanen L, Ahonen M, et al. Both high and low levels of blood vitamin D are associated with a higher prostate cancer risk: A longitudinal, nested case-control study in the Nordic countries. *Int J Cancer* 2004;108:104–108.

181. Dubbelman R, Jonxis JHP, Muskiet FAJ, et al. Age-dependent vitamin D status and vertebral condition of white women living in Curaçao (The Netherlands Antilles) as compared with their counterparts in The Netherlands. *Am J Clin Nut* 1993;58:106–109.

182. Dandona P, Menon RK, Shenoy R, et al. Low 1,25-dihydroxyvitamin D, secondary hyperparathyroidism, and normal osteocalcin in elderly subjects. *J Clin Endocrinol Metab* 1986;63:459–462.

183. Hegarty V, Woodhouse P, Khaw KT. Seasonal variation in 25-hydroxyvitamin D and parathyroid hormone concentrations in healthy elderly people. *Age Ageing* 1994;23:478–482.

184. Luscombe CJ, Fryer AA, French ME, et al. Exposure to ultraviolet radiation: Association with susceptibility and age at presentation with prostate cancer. *Lancet* 2001;358:641–642.

185. Vena JE, Graham S, Zielezny M, et al. Occupational exercise and risk of cancer. *Am J Clin Nutr* 1987;45:318–327.

186. Yu H, Harris RE, Wynder EL. Case-control study of prostate cancer and socioeconomic factors. *Prostate* 1988;13:317–325.

187. Albanes D, Blair A, Taylor PR. Physical activity and risk of cancer in the NHANES I population. *Am J Public Health* 1989;79:744–750.

188. Brownson RC, Chang JC, Davis JR, et al. Physical activity on the job and cancer in Missouri. *Am J Public Health* 1991;81:639–642.

189. Hartman TJ, Albanes D, Rautalahti M, et al. Physical activity and prostate cancer in the Alpha-Tocopherol, Beta-Carotene (ATBC) Cancer Prevention Study (Finland). *Cancer Causes Control* 1998;9:11–18.

190. Hsing AW, McLaughlin JK, Zheng W, et al. Occupation, physical activity, and risk of prostate cancers in Shanghai, People's Republic of China. *Cancer Causes Control* 1994;5:136–140.

191. Lund Nilsen TI, Johnsen R, Vatten LJ. Socio-economic and lifestyle factors associated with the risk of prostate cancer. *Br J Cancer* 2000;82:1358–1363.

192. Norman A, Moradi T, Gridley G, et al. Occupational physical activity and risk for prostate cancer in a nationwide cohort study in Sweden. *Br J Cancer* 2002;86:70–75.

193. Oliveria SA, Kohl III HW, Trichopoulos D, et al. The association between cardiorespiratory fitness and prostate cancer. *Med Sci Sports Exerc* 1996;28:97–104.

194. Liu S, Lee I-M, Linson P, et al. A prospective study of physical activity and risk of prostate cancer in US physicians. *Int J Epidemiol* 2000;29:29–35.

195. Lacey JV, Deng J, Dosemeci M, et al. Prostate cancer, benign prostatic hyperplasia and physical activity in Shanghai, China. *Int J Epidemiol* 2001;30:341–349.

196. Polednak AP. College athletics, body size, and cancer mortality. *Cancer* 1976;38:382–387.

197. Paffenbarger RS Jr, Hyde RT, Wing AL. Physical activity and incidence of cancer in diverse populations: A preliminary report. *Am J Clin Nutr* 1987;45(Suppl):312–317.

198. Lee IM, Paffenbarger RS Jr, Hsieh CC. Physical activity and risk of prostatic cancer among college alumni. *Am J Epidemiol* 1992;135:169–179.

199. Giovannucci E, Leitzmann M, Spiegelman D, et al. A prospective study of physical activity and prostate cancer in male health professionals. *Cancer Res* 1998;58:5117–5122.

200. Giovannucci E. Diet, body weight, and colorectal cancer: A summary of the epidemiological evidence. *J Women's Health* 2003;12:173–182.

201. Ross RK, Bernstein L, Paganini-Hill A, et al. Effects of cigarette smoking on "hormone related" disease in a Southern California retirement community. In: Wald N, Baron J. eds. *Smoking and hormone related disorders*. Oxford: Oxford University Press, 1990:183–196.

202. Hiatt RA, Armstrong MA, Klatsky AL, et al. Alcohol consumption, smoking, and other risk factors and prostate cancer in a large health plan cohort in California (United States). *Cancer Causes Control* 1994;5:66–72.

203. Doll R, Peto R, Wheatley K, et al. Mortality in relation to smoking: 40 years' observations on male British doctors. *Br Med J* 1994;309:901–911.

204. Adami HO, Bergström R, Engholm G, et al. A prospective study of smoking and risk of prostate cancer. *Int J Cancer* 1996;67:764–768.

205. Engeland A, Andersen A, Haldorsen T, et al. Smoking habits and risk of cancers other than lung cancer: 28 years' follow-up of 26,000 Norwegian men and women. *Cancer Causes Control* 1996;7:497–506.

206. Lotufo PA, Lee I-M, Ajani UA, et al. Cigarette smoking and risk of prostate cancer in the Physicians' Health Study (United States). *Int J Cancer* 2000;87:141–144.

207. Hsing AW, McLaughlin JK, Hrubec Z, et al. Tobacco use and prostate cancer: 26-year follow-up of US veterans. *Am J Epidemiol* 1991;133:437–441.

208. Coughlin SS, Neaton JD, Sengupta A. Cigarette smoking as a predictor of death from prostate cancer in 348,874 men screened for the multiple risk factor intervention trial. *Am J Epidemiol* 1996;143:1002–1006.

209. Rodriguez C, Tatham LM, Thun MJ, et al. Smoking and fatal prostate cancer in a large cohort of adult men. *Am J Epidemiol* 1997;145:466–475.

210. Giovannucci E, Rimm EB, Ascherio A, et al. Smoking and risk of total and fatal prostate cancer in United States health professionals. *Cancer Epidemiol Biomarkers Prev* 1999;8:277–282.

211. Daniell HW. A worse prognosis for smokers with prostate cancer. *J Urol* 1995;154:153–157.

212. Roberts WW, Platz EA, Walsh PC. Association of cigarette smoking with extraprostatic prostate cancer in young men. *J Urol* 2003;169:512–516.

213. Kobrinsky NL, Klug MG, Hokanson PJ, et al. Impact of smoking on cancer stage at diagnosis. *J Clin Oncol* 2003;21:907–913.

214. Pickles T, Liu M, Berthelet E, et al. The effect of smoking on outcome following external radiation for localized prostate cancer. Prostate Cohort Outcomes Initiative. *J Urol* 2004;171:1543–1546.

215. Oefelein MG, Resnick MI. Association of tobacco use with hormone refractory disease and survival of patients with prostate cancer. *J Urol* 2004;171:2281–2284.

216. Dennis L. Meta-analysis for combining relative risks of alcohol consumption and prostate cancer. *Prostate* 2000;42:56–66.

217. Sesso H, Paffenbarger R, Lee I. Alcohol consumption and risk of prostate cancer: The Harvard Alumni Health Study. *Int J Epidemiol* 2001;30:749–755.

218. Platz EA, Leitzmann MF, Rimm EB, et al. Alcohol intake, drinking patterns, and risk of prostate cancer in a large prospective cohort study. *Am J Epidemiol* 2004;159:444–453.

219. Nomura A, Heilbrun LK, Stemmermann GN, et al. Prediagnostic serum hormones and the risk of prostate cancer. *Cancer Res* 1988;48:3515–3517.

220. Barrett-Connor E, Garland C, McPhillips JB, et al. A prospective, population-based study of androstenedione, estrogens, and prostatic cancer. *Cancer Res* 1990;50:169–173.

221. Hsing AW, Comstock GW. Serological precursors of cancer: Serum hormones and risk of subsequent prostate cancer. *Cancer Epidemiol Biomarkers Prev* 1993;2:27–32.

222. Comstock GW, Gordon GB, Hsing WW. The relationship of serum dehydroepiandrosterone and its sulfate to subsequent cancer of the prostate. *Cancer Epidemiol Biomarkers Prev* 1993;2:219–221.

223. Carter HB, Pearson JD, Metter EJ, et al. Longitudinal evaluation of serum androgen levels in men with and without prostate cancer. *Prostate* 1995;27:25–31.

224. Gann PH, Hennekens CH, Ma J, et al. Prospective study of sex hormone levels and risk of prostate cancer. *J Natl Cancer Inst* 1996;88:1118–1126.

225. Nomura AMY, Stemmermann GN, Chyou PH, et al. Serum androgens and prostate cancer. *Cancer Epidemiol Biomarkers Prev* 1996;5:621–625.

226. Guess HA, Friedman GD, Sadler MC, et al. 5a-reductase activity and prostate cancer: A case-control study using stored sera. *Cancer Epidemiology Biomarkers Prev* 1997;6:21–24.

227. Vatten LJ, Ursin G, Ross RK, et al. Androgens in serum and the risk of prostate cancer: A nested case-control study from the Janus Serum Bank in Norway. *Cancer Epidemiol Biomarkers Prev* 1997;6:967–969.

228. Dorgan JF, Albanes D, Virtamo J, et al. Relationships of serum androgens and estrogens to prostate cancer risk: Results from a prospective study in Finland. *Cancer Epidemiol Biomarkers Prev* 1998;7:1069–1074.

229. Heikkila R, Aho K, Heliovaara M, et al. Serum testosterone and sex hormone-binding globulin concentrations and the risk of prostate carcinoma: A longitudinal study. *Cancer* 1999;86:312–315.

230. Stattin P, Rinaldi S, Stenman UH, et al. Plasma prolactin and prostate cancer risk: A prospective study. *Int J Cancer* 2001;92:463–465.

231. Mohr BA, Feldman HA, Kalish LA, et al. Are serum hormones associated with risk of prostate cancer? Prospective results from the Massachusetts Male Aging Study. *Urology* 2001;57:930–935.

232. Eaton NE, Reeves GK, Appleby PN, et al. Endogenous sex hormones and prostate cancer: A quantitative review of prospective studies. *Br J Cancer* 1999;80:930–934.

233. Jänne OA, Palvimo JJ, Kallio P, et al. Androgen receptor and mechanisms of androgen action. *Ann Med* 1993;25:83–89.

234. Chamberlain NL, Driver ED, Miesfeld RL. The length and location of CAG trinucleotide repeats in the androgen receptor N-terminal domain affect transactivation function. *Nucleic Acids Res* 1994;22:3181–3186.

235. Kazemi-Esfarjani P, Trifiro MA, Pinsky L. Evidence for a repressive function of the long polyglutamine tract in the human androgen receptor: Possible pathogenic relevance for the (CAG)n-expanded neuropathies. *Hum Mol Genet* 1995;4:523–527.

236. Edwards A, Hammond HA, Jin L, et al. Genetic variation at five trimeric and tetrameric tandem repeat loci in four human population groups. *Genomics* 1992;12:241–253.

237. Tut TG, Ghadessy FJ, Trifiro MA, et al. Long polyglutamine tracts in the androgen receptor are associated with reduced trans-activation, impaired sperm production, and male infertility. *J Clin Endocrinol Metab* 1997;82:3777–3782.

238. Irvine RA, Yu MC, Ross RK, et al. The CAG and GGC microsatellites of the androgen receptor gene are in linkage disequilibrium in men with prostate cancer. *Cancer Res* 1995;55:1937–1940.

239. Ingles SA, Ross RK, Yu MC, et al. Association of prostate cancer risk with genetic polymorphisms in vitamin D receptor and androgen receptor. *J Natl Cancer Inst* 1997;89:166–170.

240. Stanford JL, Just JJ, Gibbs M, et al. Polymorphic repeats in the androgen receptor gene: Molecular markers of prostate cancer risk. *Cancer Res* 1997;57:1194–1198.

241. Giovannucci E, Stampfer MJ, Krithivas K, et al. The CAG repeat within the androgen receptor gene and its relationship to prostate cancer. *Proc Natl Acad Sci U S A* 1997;94:3320–3323.

242. Hsing AW, Gao YT, Wu G, et al. Polymorphic CAG and GGN repeat lengths in the androgen receptor gene and prostate cancer risk: A population-based case-control study in China. *Cancer Res* 2000;60:5111–5116.

243. Xue W, Irvine RA, Yu MC, et al. Susceptibility to prostate cancer: Interaction between genotypes at the androgen receptor and prostate-specific antigen loci. *Cancer Res* 2000;60:839–841.

244. Edwards SM, Badzioch MD, Minter R, et al. Androgen receptor polymorphisms: Association with prostate cancer risk, relapse and overall survival. *Int J Cancer* 1999;84:458–465.

245. Bratt O, Borg A, Kristofferson U, et al. CAG repeat length in the androgen receptor gene is related to age at diagnosis of prostate cancer and response to endocrine therapy, but not to prostate cancer risk. *Br J Cancer* 1999;81:672–676.

246. Correa-Cerro L, Wohr G, Haussler J, et al. (CAG)nCAA and GGN repeats in the human androgen receptor gene are not associated with prostate cancer in a French-German population. *Eur J Hum Genet* 1999;7:357–362.

247. Beilin J, Harewood L, Frydenberg M, et al. A case-control study of the androgen receptor gene CAG repeat polymorphism in Australian prostate carcinoma subjects. *Cancer* 2001;92:941–949.

248. Latil AG, Azzouzi R, Cancel GS, et al. Prostate carcinoma risk and allelic variants of genes involved in androgen biosynthesis and metabolism pathways. *Cancer* 2001;92:1130–1137.

249. Miller EA, Stanford JL, Hsu L, et al. Polymorphic repeats in the androgen receptor in high-risk sibships. *Prostate* 2001;48:200–205.

250. Chen C, Lamharzi N, Weiss NS, et al. Androgen receptor polymorphisms and the incidence of prostate cancer. *Cancer Epidemiol Biomarkers Prev* 2002;11:1033–1040.

251. Li C, Gronberg H, Matsuyama H, et al. Difference between Swedish and Japanese men in the association between AR CAG repeats and prostate cancer suggesting a susceptibility-modifying locus overlapping the androgen receptor gene. *Int J Mol Med* 2003;11:529–533.

252. Giovannucci E. Is the androgen receptor CAG repeat length significant for prostate cancer? *Cancer Epidemiol Biomarkers Prev* 2002;11:985–986.

253. Muti P, Westerlind K, Wu T, et al. Urinary estrogen metabolites and prostate cancer: A case-control study in the United States. *Cancer Causes Control* 2002;13:947–955.

254. Gann PH, Hennekens CH, Ma J, et al. A prospective study of sex hormone levels and risk of prostate cancer. *J Natl Cancer Inst* 1996;88: 1118–1126.

255. Thompson IM, Goodman PJ, Tangen CM, et al. The influence of finasteride on the development of prostate cancer. *N Engl J Med* 2003;349: 215–224.

256. Cohen P, Peehl DM, Rosenfeld RG. The IGF axis in the prostate. *Horm Metab Res* 1994;26:81–84.

257. Cohen P, Peehl DM, Lamson G, et al. Insulin-like growth factors (IGFs), IGF receptors, and IGF-binding proteins in primary cultures of prostate epithelial cells. *J Clin Endocrinol Metab* 1991;73:401–407.

258. Rajah R, Valentinis B, Cohen P. Insulin-like growth factor (IGF)-binding protein-3 induces apoptosis and mediates the effects of transforming growth factor-b1 on programmed cell death through a p53- and IGF-independent mechanism. *J Biol Chem* 1997;272:12181–12188.

259. Liu B, Lee HY, Weinzimer SA, et al. Direct functional interactions between insulin-like growth factor-binding protein-3 and retinoid X receptor-a regulate transcriptional signaling and apoptosis. *J Biol Chem* 2000;275: 33607–33613.

260. Chan JM, Stampfer MJ, Giovannucci E, et al. Plasma insulin-like growth factor-I and prostate cancer risk: A prospective study. *Science* 1998;279: 563–566.

261. Mantzoros CS, Tzonou A, Signorello LB, et al. Insulin-like growth factor 1 in relation to prostate cancer and benign prostatic hyperplasia. *Br J Cancer* 1997;76:1115–1118.

262. Wolk A, Mantzoros CS, Andersson SW, et al. Insulin-like growth factor I and prostate cancer risk: A population-based, case-control study. *J Natl Cancer Inst* 1998;90:911–915.

263. Stattin P, Bylund A, Rinaldi S, et al. Plasma insulin-like growth factor-I, insulin-like growth factor-binding proteins, and prostate cancer risk: A prospective study. *J Natl Cancer Inst* 2000;92:1910–1917.

264. Harman SM, Metter EJ, Blackman MR, et al. Serum levels of insulin-like growth factor I (IGF-I), IGF-II, IGF-binding protein-3, and prostate-specific antigen as predictors of clinical prostate cancer. *J Clin Endocrinol Metab* 2000;85:4258–4265.

265. Khosravi J, Diamandi A, Mistry J, et al. Insulin-like growth factor-I (IGF-I) and IGF-binding protein-3 in benign prostatic hyperplasia and prostate cancer. *J Clin Endocrinol Metab* 2001;86:694–699.

266. Chokkalingam A, Pollak M, Fillmore C, et al. Insulin-like growth factors and prostate cancer: A population-based case-control study in China. *Cancer Epidemiol Biomarkers Prev* 2001;10:421–427.

267. Chan JM, Stampfer MJ, Ma J, et al. Insulin-like growth factor-I (IGF-1) and IGF binding protein-3 as predictors of advanced-stage prostate cancer. *J Natl Cancer Inst* 2002;94:1099–1109.

268. Stattin P, Rinaldi S, Biessey C, et al. High levels of circulating insulin-like growth factor-I increase prostate cancer risk: A prospective study in a population-based non-screened cohort. *J Clin Oncol* 2004;22:3104–3112.

269. Shi R, Berkel HJ, Yu H. Insulin-like growth factor-I and prostate cancer: A meta-analysis. *Br J Cancer* 2001;85:991–996.

270. Renehan AG, Zwahlen M, Minder C, et al. Insulin-like growth factor (IGF)-1, IGF binding protein-3, and cancer risk: Systematic review and meta-regression analysis. *Lancet* 2004;363:1346–1353.

271. Coussens LM, Werb Z. Inflammation and cancer. *Nature* 2002;420: 860–867.

272. De Marzo AM, Marchi VL, Epstein JI, et al. Proliferative inflammatory atrophy of the prostate: Implications for prostatic carcinogenesis. *Am J Pathol* 1999;155:1985–1992.

273. Heshmat MY, Kovi J, Herson J, et al. Epidemiologic association between gonorrhea and prostatic carcinoma. *Urology* 1975;6:457–460.

274. Dennis LK, Dawson DV. Meta-analysis of measures of sexual activity and prostate cancer. *Epidemiology* 2002;13:72–79.

275. Giles GG, Severi G, English DR, et al. Sexual factors and prostate cancer. *BJU Int* 2003;92:211–216.

276. Leitzmann MF, Platz EA, Stampfer MJ, et al. Ejaculation frequency and subsequent risk of prostate cancer. *JAMA* 2004;291:1578–1586.

277. Dennis LK, Lynch CF, Torner JC. Epidemiologic association between prostatitis and prostate cancer. *Urology* 2002;60:78–83.

278. Mahmud S, Franco E, Aprikian A. Prostate cancer and use of nonsteroidal anti-inflammatory drugs: Systematic review and meta-analysis. *Br J Cancer* 2004;90:93–99.

CHAPTER 3 ■ FAMILIAL PROSTATE CANCER

WILLIAM B. ISAACS AND JIANFENG XU

INTRODUCTION

Positive family history of prostate cancer is one of the strongest and most consistently observed risk factors for prostate cancer. Approximately 10% to 15% of men with prostate cancer have at least one relative affected with the disease, and men with a positive family history of prostate cancer have approximately two to three times greater risk of developing the disease. Multiple twin studies have suggested that this familial aggregation of prostate cancer is largely due to shared genetic components. A number of segregation studies further suggest that the genetic component of prostate cancer is consistent with the hypothesis of rare mutations in a limited number of major susceptibility genes and common sequence variants in many prostate cancer risk modifier genes. Significant efforts have been devoted to identifying these major susceptibility genes and modifier genes using family-based linkage and population-based association studies, respectively. Genetic linkage studies in families with multiple prostate cancer patients have identified several chromosomal regions that likely harbor such major susceptibility genes. Mutation analyses of genes in several of these linkage regions among affected individuals have led to the identification of a number of candidate prostate cancer susceptibility genes. Population-based association studies have also identified a number of sequence variants that modify prostate cancer risk in genes that play important roles in diverse cellular pathways including androgen metabolism, growth factor action, DNA repair, and inflammation. However, compared to the reproducible findings of positive family history and overall genetic susceptibility to prostate cancer, there is currently a lack of consistent findings among studies of mutations and sequence variants in these candidate prostate cancer risk genes. The availability of more complete information about the human genome and its variability, combined with technologies enabling high-capacity sequencing and genotyping analyses of large collections of prostate cancer families and case-control study populations, will undoubtedly hasten the identification of genes harboring mutations and sequence variants that are responsible for the well-observed genetic risk for this common disease.

CASE-CONTROL AND COHORT STUDIES OF PROSTATE CANCER: CONSISTENT FINDINGS

The first and critical step to assess whether there is a genetic determinant of a disease is an epidemiologic study using either case-control or cohort design. A case-control is a retrospective and observational study in which the proportion of cases with a potential risk factor (e.g., positive family history) is compared to the proportion of controls (individuals without the disease) with the same risk factor. The common association measure for a case-control study is the odds ratio (OR). This study design is commonly used for initial, economical evaluation of risk factors and is particularly useful for rare conditions or for risk factors with long induction periods. Unfortunately, due to the potential for many forms of bias in this study design, case-control studies provide relatively weak empirical evidence even when properly executed. Sources of bias in the study of prostate cancer family history include differential recall bias and detection bias between cases and controls. Regarding recall bias, prostate cancer patients may be more likely to be aware of the diagnosis of prostate cancer in relatives than healthy controls. For detection bias, prostate cancer in cases may prompt a screening test in their relatives, increasing the likelihood of an additional diagnosis in the family. This bias is extremely important in light of the increased sensitivity of disease detection using prostate-specific antigen (PSA) screening.

A cohort study, also referred to as a longitudinal study, is a prospective and observational study based on data from a follow-up period of a group in which some have had, have, or will have the exposure of interest to determine the association between that exposure and an outcome. Cohort studies are susceptible to bias by differential loss to follow-up. Because of their prospective nature, cohort studies are typically stronger than case-control studies when well executed but they are also more resource intensive. Both genetic and shared environmental risk factors among relatives may lead to familial aggregation of a disease.

A systematic literature review by Johns and Houlston (1) identified at least 22 reported studies on the risk of positive family history to prostate cancer risk from either case-control or cohort study design (2–23). These authors performed a meta-analysis of these published studies to obtain an overall estimate of this risk (1). Four major conclusions can be drawn from these studies (Fig. 3.1).

First, the risk to prostate cancer is significantly higher among men having at least one first-degree relative (father, brother, or son) affected with the disease. Among 13 studies reporting this risk (1,6,8–18), all studies found a significantly positive relationship, with estimates of OR ranging from 2.0 to 3.9. The pooled meta-analysis of these 13 studies gave an estimatated OR of 2.5, with the 95% confidence interval (95% CI) of 2.2 to 2.8. These data argue for a consistent tendency for prostate cancer to cluster in families.

Second, the risk of prostate cancer is even greater among men having more than one affected first-degree relative. Among five studies evaluating this risk (8,10,13,15,18), all but one (15) found an increase, with estimates ranging from 2.8 to 9.4. The pooled meta-analysis of these five studies gave

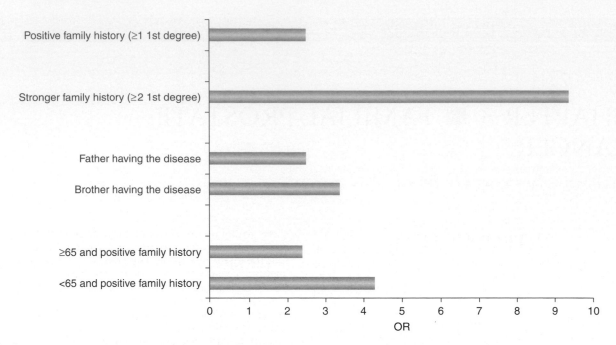

FIGURE 3.1. Estimates of risk for prostate cancer having positive family history meta-analysis. (Adapted from Johns LE, Houlston RS. A systematic review and meta-analysis of familial prostate cancer risk. *BJU Int* 2003;91:789–794, with permission.)

an estimate of OR (95% CI) of 9.4 (5.8 to 14.0). This *dosage effect* of positive family history provides further evidence for a familial aggregation of prostate cancer.

Third, the risk for prostate cancer is greater among men with affected brothers than with affected father or sons. Among eight studies reporting separate risks for these two types of relationships, all but one (15) found higher OR in brothers (range from 2.6 to 5.3) than in fathers and sons (range 1.9 to 3.8). The pooled meta-analysis of these eight studies gave an estimated OR (95% CI) of 3.4 (2.9 to 4.1) in brother-brother relationships and 2.5 (2.1 to 3.1) in father-son relationships. Several factors such as a better detection of prostate cancer in recent years, secular changes in environmental exposures, and recessive or X-linked patterns of inheritance, individually or in any combination, may lead to this observation.

Fourth, the risk for prostate cancer is greater among men with a first-degree relative diagnosed with prostate cancer at an early age. All four studies reporting such risk found this trend (10,12,14,17). The pooled meta-analysis of these four studies gave an estimate of OR (95% CI) of 4.3 (2.9 to 6.3) for men with an affected first-degree relative diagnosed under 65 years of age and an OR (95% CI) of 2.4 (2.0 to 2.9) for men with an affected first-degree relative diagnosed over 65 years of age.

Evidence of positive family history and estimates of the magnitude of this risk factor are important in genetic counseling and provide a basis for further genetic studies. However, it is important to bear in mind that both genetic components and common environmental risk factors shared within a family can lead to familial aggregation. Dissection of genetic and environmental contributions to the familial aggregation can be determined through other approaches including twin studies and segregation analyses.

TWIN STUDIES OF PROSTATE CANCER: CONSISTENT FINDINGS

The goal of twin studies is to dissect the genetic and environmental components of a familial aggregation by comparing

the similarities (concordance rate) of a trait or disease between monozygotic (MZ) and dizygotic (DZ) twins. This ability to dissect genetics from shared environment is based on two assumptions: (a) MZ twins share 100% of genetic factors, whereas DZ twins share, on average, 50%; and (b) MZ and DZ twins share the same or at least similar amounts of environmental factors. A greater concordance rate of a disease among MZ twins compared to DZ twins provides evidence for genetic disease determinants. An estimate of heritability, the proportion that genetics contributes to the cause of a disease, can be obtained using twin studies.

All three large twin studies of prostate cancer published to date reported higher concordance rates of prostate cancer among MZ twins compared to that of DZ twins. Gronberg et al. (24) studied an unselected Swedish twin population. Among 4,840 male twin pairs, 458 prostate cancers were identified; although the rate of concordance was very low in general, MZ twin pairs were concordant for prostate cancer at a higher rate than DZ twin pairs (1.0% vs. 0.2%, respectively). Using a cohort of 31,848 veteran twins born in the period 1917 to 1927, Page et al. (25) identified 1,009 prostate cancer cases. There was a significantly higher concordance rate among monozygotic twin pairs, 27.1%, than among dizygotic twin pairs, 7.1%. Most recently, in an analysis of 44,788 pairs of twins from the Swedish, Danish, and Finnish twin registries, Lichtenstein et al. (26) found concordance rates for prostate cancer of 21% in MZ twin pairs and 6% in DZ twin pairs. Importantly, the authors concluded that 42% (95% CI: 29% to 50%) of prostate cancer risk may be accounted for by heritable factors, an estimate that is highest among all common cancers.

The consistent findings from these twin studies suggest that much of the observed familial aggregation of prostate cancer can be explained by shared genetic components among relatives. Although this is an important finding and provides a basis for further genetic study of prostate cancer, twin studies cannot provide additional information regarding the mechanisms or possible modes of inheritance. Other study designs such as segregation and linkage studies are designed to address these questions.

SEGREGATION ANALYSIS OF PROSTATE CANCER: CONSISTENT FINDINGS

By fitting patterns of familial aggregation of a disease in the general population with several alternative modes of inheritance (e.g., a major gene model, an environmental model, and/or a polygene model), segregation analysis can provide inferences about the specific model that best describes the transmission of the disease in families. The major gene model hypothesizes the existence of a gene with large effects on disease causality, whereas a polygenic model refers to the action of many genes, each having small but additive effects on disease development. Within the major gene model, specific modes of inheritance, such as dominant, recessive, or codominant, can be modeled. In addition, allele frequency and penetrance of disease alleles of a major gene can be estimated as additional unique features of segregation analysis. These analyses begin by identifying probands (index cases) that can be either clinic-based or from a more general population. All relatives of the probands (either nuclear family or extended families) are included in the study regardless of their affected status. Because segregation analysis compares gene models to environmental models, it is another valuable study approach to dissect genetic influences from environment influences. In the case of gene models, the inferred mode and estimates of allele frequency and penetrance are extremely useful for further genetic linkage studies.

The first segregation analysis of prostate cancer was reported by Carter et al. in 1992 (27), and seven additional segregation analyses have been reported to date (28–34). Results from these studies have been reviewed by Schaid (35). Five major findings can be inferred from these studies. First, all these studies found genetic models fit the aggregation of prostate cancer better than environmental models alone, suggesting genetic contribution in familial aggregation of prostate cancer. Second, among several fitted genetic models, all studies found an autosomal dominant model to be the best, although the estimated allele frequencies and penetrance for such a dominant disease allele are different among these studies. Lower allele frequencies are estimated in study populations ascertained from hospital-based radical prostatectomy patients, ranging from 0.006 to 0.0007 (27,29–31), and higher estimates are found in study populations ascertained from population cancer registries, ranging from 0.017 to 0.024 (28,32,33). On the other hand, the estimates of penetrance appear higher in hospital-based studies (88% to 97%), as compared to those in the population-based studies (44% to 75%). Third, other major gene models, such as autosomal recessive model and X-linked models, are also supported in some studies. The study in an Australian population suggests a rare autosomal dominant allele confers large risk at younger ages and a more common allele that is either autosomal recessive or X-linked in effect at older ages (32). One important caveat regarding these studies is that, in general, the structure of prostate cancer families reduces the ability to discriminate between genetic models in segregation analyses—most of these families are small with prostate cancer information primarily coming from fathers and brothers because sons are often too young to be at risk. Fourth, models invoking multiple major genes together may better account for the familial aggregation. This important conclusion is often overlooked because most segregation analyses only tested single major gene models due to computational constraints. However, in a study of highly selected pedigrees that were ascertained for linkage studies, Conlon et al. (34) found the best-fitting model included two or three susceptibility loci, and the two loci with largest effect were autosomal dominant. Fifth, in addition to

major genes, a residual polygenic component may also account for familial aggregation of prostate cancer. In the study by Gong et al., a genetic model allowing for multiple genes, each having low penetrance, fit just as well as an autosomal dominant model (33).

Although the results of these segregation analyses are somewhat varied, it is clear that they implicate both major genes having rare, highly penetrant, disease-causing alleles and multiple modifier genes with more common disease-associated sequence variants as reasonable explanations for familial aggregation of prostate cancer. As such, these studies provide a strong basis for genetic linkage studies to identify the major prostate cancer susceptibility genes in families with multiple affected members and for case-control studies to identify prostate cancer modifier genes in case-control populations.

GENETIC LINKAGE STUDIES OF PROSTATE CANCER: PROMISING BUT INCONSISTENT FINDINGS

When two loci (markers or genes) are located near each other on the same chromosome, they tend to be inherited together and are termed *linked*. The linkage between two nearby loci will break if a recombination occurs during meiosis, the chance of which largely depends on the physical distance between these two loci. Only loci that are very close to each other will remain together after many meioses occurring in a large family. If two loci can be unequivocally tracked (as by the use of polymorphic markers in determining genotype) among parents and offspring in families, linkage studies can test whether two loci are linked and, if linked, measure the extent of linkage. Gene mapping by genetic linkage is based on this property, where the location of a gene can be inferred if it is linked to a marker with known chromosomal position. In the case of searching for a disease gene, which obviously cannot be directly tracked before it is identified, we infer alleles of the disease gene in question from disease phenotype (affected or not) and assume certain modes of inheritance such as dominant or recessive based on segregation analysis as outlined above. The success of gene mapping largely depends on the accuracy of inferring the presence of disease gene alleles from disease phenotype. In Mendelian diseases where the mode of inheritance is certain and alleles of disease genes can be correctly inferred from disease phenotype, linkage studies have been very successful; more than 1,200 disease-causing genes have been identified (36). In complex diseases such as many cancers where mode of inheritance is uncertain or not uniform and alleles of disease genes cannot be unambiguously inferred from disease phenotype, linkage studies are in general less successful. However, if the mode of inheritance is better understood and more well defined for a subset of cancer cases or families, for example, early age of onset of breast cancer, sources of heterogeneity can be reduced, and linkage studies can successfully identify disease-causal genes, as demonstrated for BRCA1 (37,38).

With strong evidence for a genetic component in the etiology of prostate cancer and evidence for a major susceptibility gene, mapping the gene(s) using linkage approaches is a natural next step. In the past decade, numerous prostate cancer family study populations, with various numbers of families ranging from tens to ~400, have been recruited for linkage studies. An exciting moment in the genetic linkage study of prostate cancer was the report of the first genome-wide screen in 66 hereditary prostate cancer (HPC) families ascertained at Johns Hopkins Hospital, each having at least three first-degree relatives affected with prostate cancer (39). A total of 341 microsatellite markers, covering the genome with ~10 cM resolution, were genotyped in these families. Two-point parametric linkage analysis identified seven regions with logarithm of the odds ratio in favor of linkage versus no linkage (LOD) scores >1. The highest LOD score observed was 2.75 at chromosome 1q24-25. Further linkage studies at this region using additional fine mapping markers and in 25 additional HPC families provided stronger support for linkage: This locus was termed HPC1. Initially, there was a high expectation of identifying a prostate cancer gene at HPC1 within a short time period because of the strength of the linkage finding, readily available genomic information at this region, and ability of large-scale sequencing and genotyping. However, the reality was disappointing. In the first several years after the identification of HPC1 linkage, no convincing candidate of prostate cancer gene at this region was identified. In addition, the replication studies from several independent study populations produced conflicting results; more than half of these studies failed to replicate the HPC1 linkage (28,40–48). Facing the difficulty in comprehension of these conflicting results, a combined analysis at the 1q24-25 region was performed in 772 HPC families ascertained by members of the International Consortium for Prostate Cancer Genetics (ICPCG) from several countries (49). Overall, there was some evidence for linkage, with a peak parametric multipoint LOD score assuming heterogeneity (HLOD) of 1.40 ($P = .01$). Although this overall evidence was not particularly convincing, the combined analysis found stronger evidence for linkage at HPC1 in several subsets of HPC families, including families with a male-to-male disease transmission, with mean early age of onset, or families with five and more affected members.

Shortly after the identification of HPC1, other prostate cancer linkages were reported, including loci at 1q42-43 (46), Xq27-28 (HPCX) (50), 1p36 (51), and 20q13 (HPC20) (52). Similar to the status of HPC1, results from multiple replication studies were inconsistent. Combined linkage analysis was recently performed for HPC20 and HPCX, using all the prostate cancer families available in the ICPCG. Among the 1,076 pedigrees not included in the original study reporting HPC20, the maximum HLOD score was 0.06 at the HPC20 region, indicating a failure to replicate linkage (53). In comparison, among the 920 pedigrees not included in the original study reporting HPCX, the maximum HLOD score was 0.83 at HPCX region, providing a weak confirmation of linkage to this region.

These difficulties in identifying and replicating prostate cancer linkages are not unexpected considering the complexity of prostate cancer. Many factors, such as multiple modes of inheritance (autosomal dominant, recessive, and X-linked), potentially multiple genes (i.e., genetic locus heterogeneity), incomplete penetrance, and phenocopies (disease caused by nongenetic risk factors), independently or together may contribute to the inability of inferring disease alleles from disease phenotype. The extremely high prevalence of prostate cancer in the population compounds these issues. Although these factors are the characteristics of prostate cancer and cannot be eliminated, some efforts can be taken to minimize the impact of these factors. One such effort is to increase the sample size (number of families) to achieve a better power. The combined linkage analysis among a large number of families within the ICPCG represents a major step toward such an effort.

Nine groups within the ICPCG have performed genome-wide linkage analysis for prostate cancer susceptibility genes individually in their study populations (54–62). The number of families in each study population range from 13 to 388. Eleven linkage peaks with LOD scores greater than two were identified from these nine genome-wide screens (63). However, no chromosomal region was reported as significant at this level by more than one study, demonstrating a lack of confirmation among studies. The nonreplicable linkage results among these individual genome-wide screens suggest either there is a lack of statistical power to detect linkages of small magnitude or the observed linkage peaks in some study populations are false positives due to the small number of families. To overcome these two potential problems, the ICPCG recently performed a genome-wide screen by combining linkage data from 10 individual study populations (64). The large number of prostate cancer families within the ICPCG study makes it possible to perform a stratified analysis, with reasonably large numbers of families in each substratum, to search for prostate cancer genes in more homogeneous subsets of families. Further efforts within this group are focused at narrowing the phenotype under study on the basis of clinical and pathologic parameters such as tumor stage and grade. By emphasizing cases with some indication of poor prognosis, it may be possible to distinguish more clinically relevant prostate cancers from more indolent and much more common prostate cancers that may be present in the majority of aged men. Whether such a distinction will result in a reduction of heterogeneity sufficient to facilitate gene identification remains an open question.

Results from genetic linkage studies are extremely helpful to identify chromosomal regions that are likely to harbor susceptibility genes. However, even in the case of a reproducible linkage signal, the linked region typically spans 10 to 20 Mb where hundreds of genes reside. Other types of study designs and approaches, such as mutation screening, family-based association studies, and population-based association studies, are needed to ultimately identify disease susceptibility genes that account for linkage signals.

FAMILY-BASED AND POPULATION-BASED ASSOCIATION STUDIES OF PROSTATE CANCER: PROMISING BUT INCONSISTENT FINDINGS

When a mutation or sequence variant confers a strong risk to a disease (i.e., is highly penetrant), it will likely lead to a familial aggregation of the disease, as most individuals who inherit this change will develop the disease; parents who carry the risk allele will have preferentially transmitted this allele to affected offspring. By assessing the overtransmission of the allele to affected offspring (>50%) from parents who are heterozygotes for the allele among different families, family-based association tests can detect such disease-associated alleles. There are several different formats of family-based association tests, including the transmission disequilibrium test (TDT) in trio family structures of two parents and one child and family-based association tests (FBAT) in more general nuclear or extended family structures. On the other hand, when a sequence variant confers a small risk to a disease (low penetrance), it will not necessarily lead to a strong familial aggregation of the disease; however, affected individuals will more likely have the allele than individuals from a general population. By comparing allele or genotype frequencies of the variant between cases and controls, population-based association tests can detect such disease-associated alleles. Furthermore, the magnitude of the risk associated with the allele can be estimated using ORs. It is important to note that population-based association can also detect alleles that confer strong risk. Population-based association tests are susceptible to population stratification when the difference in allele or genotype frequencies between cases and controls is due in part to the different genetic backgrounds of these two groups rather than its true association with disease (65). Family-based association testing is not susceptible to the population stratification.

After the identification of multiple prostate cancer linkages at several chromosomal regions, significant efforts have been devoted to identify genes that account for the linkage using positional cloning approaches. This approach typically begins with a fine mapping linkage analysis using a denser set of markers within the linked region to confirm linkage and to resolve any positional information that may be present from individual recombination events occurring in linked families. This is typically followed by screening probands of linked families for mutations in genes residing in the region of interest refined by fine mapping. When mutation and sequence variants are identified, family-based and population-based association studies are performed to assess their association with prostate cancer. To date, three candidate prostate cancer genes have been reported using this positional cloning approach. The first was a gene with homology to metal-dependent hydrolases, ELAC2/HPC2, at a prostate cancer linkage region of 17p11 (66). Two rare mutations, a frameshift mutation 1641insG and a missense mutation Arg781His, were found to segregate independently in two high-risk pedigrees from Utah. In addition, two common missense variants, Ser271Leu and Ala541Thr, were shown to be associated with prostate cancer risk (66). In a study that was unselected for family history, Rebbeck (67) confirmed the increased risk for men carrying the Leu217/Thr541 allele (OR = 2.37; P = .04). Results from replication studies are inconsistent [reviewed by Schaid (35)].

The second gene identified in this fashion was RNASEL (68). This gene was identified after almost 6 years of intensive positional cloning aimed at the HPC1 gene at 1q24-25. RNASEL regulates cell proliferation and apoptosis through the interferon-regulated 2-5A antiviral pathway and has been suggested to be a candidate tumor suppressor gene. Two inactivating mutations, a rare truncating mutation Glu265X and a rare initiation codon mutation Met1Ile, were found to segregate independently in two HPC1-linked families. In addition, several missense mutations were also identified in HPC probands. Furthermore, loss of wild-type allele was found in the microdissected tumor tissue of a Glu265X mutation carrier, and RNASEL activity was found to be reduced in lymphoblasts from heterozygous Glu265X individuals. Although several independent studies confirmed the findings and identified novel mutations in RNASEL, other studies failed to replicate the findings [reviewed by Schaid (35)].

The third was the macrophage scavenger receptor 1 (MSR1) gene at 8p22-23 linkage region (69,70). Seven rare nonsynonymous mutations, including one nonsense mutation (Arg293X), were identified in 13 of the 190 (6.8%) HPC families studied, including four of the 14 (28.5%) African-American families. A missense change (Asp174Tyr) was exclusively observed in African-American men. These mutations cosegregate with prostate cancer in nuclear families where one parent is an obligate carrier. Furthermore, several of these mutations were also associated with sporadic prostate cancer. Curiously, this gene, like RNASEL, plays an important role in the innate immune response system, possibly implicating genetic variability in pathogen response as a determinant of prostate cancer risk (71). Although several subsequent studies provided additional support for these findings, others failed to replicate these results in their study populations [reviewed by Schaid (35)].

In addition to the identification of genes in prostate cancer linkage regions, several genes that play important roles in other cancers, particularly breast cancer, have also been reported to be associated with prostate cancer risk. Men younger than 65 years who are carriers of BRCA2 mutations have about a sevenfold increased risk for prostate cancer compared with those without mutations (72). Germ-line mutations in BRCA2 account for up to 5% of cases of prostate cancer in familial clusters (73). In another study of 263 men with prostate cancer who were age 55 years or younger, protein truncating mutations in BRCA2 were present in six men (2%), four of whom did not have a family history of breast or ovarian cancer (74). Although the risk of prostate cancer is lower in carriers of BRCA1 mutations than in those with BRCA2 mutations, there is still around a twofold increased relative risk in men younger than 65 years compared with the general population (75). BRCA1 and BRCA2 mutations appear to play an important role in prostate cancer risk among men of Ashkenazi Jewish descent, at least in some studies (76,77).

The CHEK2 gene encodes a G2 checkpoint kinase that plays a critical role in DNA damage repair. A number of mutations in this gene, including two frameshift and three missense mutations, have been identified among sporadic and familial prostate cancer (78). Most of these mutations are only observed in cases or are observed more frequently in cases than in controls. The frequency of the frameshift mutation 1100delC was significantly elevated among 120 patients with HPC from Finland. In addition, another missense mutation Ile157Thr had significantly higher frequency among HPC patients (79). These two mutations were also significantly associated with familial and sporadic prostate cancer in Polish study populations (80). Along with CHEK2, BRCA1, and −2, another gene involved in DNA repair has been implicated as a prostate cancer susceptibility gene in the same Polish study population. An inactivating founder mutation in nibrin, the NBS1 gene product, was observed to segregate with prostate cancer in this collection of familial and sporadic cases (81). Nibrin is a component of the hMRE11/hRAD50/NBS1 nuclease complex that plays a role in BRCA1-associated DNA repair. Taken together, these studies provide a rather strong indication that, as in many other human cancers, inherited defects in genome maintenance are important in conferring risk for at least some fraction of prostate cancers, although the magnitude of this fraction is currently unknown.

WHY ALL THE INCONSISTENT FINDINGS?

As described above, some significant progress has been made in identifying genes that may account for familial prostate cancer. However, there is much left to be learned, and consistent findings in this area are almost the exception rather than the rule. Why is this so? Although no definitive answers exist, there are a number of possibilities to consider. In general, prostate cancer is a very heterogeneous disease, with a complex etiology involving both genetic influences, as discussed above, as well as strong, well-documented environmental influences and, inevitably, interactions between the two. As discussed, the fraction of prostate cancer that may be due to any single factor, such as a single gene, may be quite small and hard to detect, particularly in the midst of many competing etiologies.

Another factor that undoubtedly complicates the analysis and characterization of prostate cancer is its prevalence—it is a very common disease. Autopsy studies indicate that the majority of men over age 60 have prostate cancer. Most of these cancers are small, low-grade lesions that, if left undetected, would have no impact on the life of the host. Although most of these lesions are undetected, more and more of these clinically irrelevant cancers are detected as a result of greater interest in screening for disease and better methods for early diagnosis (e.g., serum PSA testing). Current estimates from the Prostate Cancer Prevention Trial suggest that as many as one in four American men over age 63, if biopsied, would be diagnosed as having prostate cancer (82). At this frequency in the population, many familial clusters of prostate cancer are due simply to chance alone. Thus, in any collection of prostate cancer families, there will be families resulting from shared genetics, shared environmental factors, shared genetics interacting with shared environmental factors, as well as those due to chance and those due to some combination of these factors. Only upon some ability to refine the phenotype under study can we reasonably have hope of simplifying this situation. For example, having large enough study populations so that well-defined subsets of prostate cancer can be emphasized is a possible solution. As opposed to families where two or more relatives have positive biopsies, which is quite a common occurrence, families with multiple first-degree relatives with prostate cancers having poor prognostic features are relatively rare. Will focusing on this type of prostate cancer simplify the picture? Only in a study population that is large enough and well-enough characterized can such a question be addressed. As prostate cancer stands to become an even larger medical burden as the world's populations ages, it is imperative that a better understanding of the molecular genetics of prostate cancer be acquired. Indeed, if the promise of the revolution in molecular medicine is to be realized with respect to prostate cancer, increased efforts using better methodologies, technologies, and larger, well clinically characterized study populations are urgently needed to effectively confront this research problem.

SUMMARY

Although molecular genetics may yet have a major impact on prostate cancer in the clinic, the same cannot be said for the demonstration of family history as a risk factor for prostate cancer. Family history information is now widely used in counseling individuals with respect to prostate cancer screening, and both the American Cancer Society and the American Urological Association recommend beginning disease screening earlier in men with a family history. Much evidence is consistent with an important role for genetic factors in accounting for this familial clustering of prostate cancer. This evidence has provided the basis for large-scale efforts to collect prostate cancer families as the substrate for genome-wide searches for prostate cancer susceptibility alleles. These efforts have led to the identification of multiple loci and candidate genes and, above all, to an increased appreciation of the complex nature of familial prostate cancer. Through the pooling of resources and the international collaborative efforts of multiple groups interested in this question, it is anticipated that the barriers that this complexity presents can be overcome and the genetics of familial prostate cancer clarified.

References

1. Johns LE, Houlston RS. A systematic review and meta-analysis of familial prostate cancer risk. *BJU Int* 2003;91:789–794.
2. Goldgar DE, Easton DF, Cannon-Albright LA, et al. Systematic population-based assessment of cancer risk in first-degree relatives of cancer probands. *J Natl Cancer Inst* 1994;86:1600–1608.
3. Ghadirian P, Cadotte M, Lacroix A, et al. Family aggregation of cancer of the prostate in Quebec: The tip of the iceberg. *Prostate* 1991;19:43–52.
4. Morgani G, Gianferrari L, Cresseri A, et al. Recherches clinco-statistiques et genetiques sur les neoplasmies de la prostate. *Acta Genet* 1956;6: 304–305.
5. Steele R, Lees REM, Kraus AS, et al. Sexual factors in the epidemiology of cancer of the prostate. *J Chron Dis* 1971;24:29–37.
6. Schuman LM, Mandel J, Blackard C, et al. Epidemiologic study of prostatic cancer: preliminary report. *Cancer Treat Rep* 1977;61:181–186.
7. Cannon L, Bishop DT, Skolnick M, et al. Genetic epidemiology of prostate cancer in the Utah Mormon geneology. *Cancer Sur* 1982;1:47–69.
8. Steinberg GD, Carter BS, Beaty TH, et al. Family history and the risk of prostate cancer. *Prostate* 1990;17:337–347.
9. Spitz MR, Currier RD, Fueger JJ, et al. Familial patterns of prostate cancer: a case-control analysis. *J Urol* 1991;146:1305–1307.
10. Whittemore AS, Wu AH, Kolonel LN, et al. Family history and prostate cancer risk in black, white, and Asian men in the United States and Canada. *Am J Epidemiol* 1995;141:732–740.
11. Keetch DW, Rice JP, Suarez BK, et al. Familial aspects of prostate cancer: a case control study. *J Urol* 1995;154:2100–2102.
12. Hayes RB, Liff JM, Pottern LM, et al. Prostate cancer risk in U.S. blacks and whites with a family history of cancer. *Int J Cancer* 1995;60:361–364.
13. Isaacs SD, Kiemeney LA, Baffoe-Bonnie A, et al. Risk of cancer in relatives of prostate cancer probands. *J Natl Cancer Inst* 1995;87:991–996.
14. Lesko SM, Rosenberg L, Shapiro S. Family history and prostate cancer risk. *Am J Epidemiol* 1996;144:1041–1047.
15. Ghadirian P, Howe GR, Hislop TG, et al. Family history of prostate cancer: a multi-center case-control study in Canada. *Int J Cancer* 1997;70: 679–681.
16. Glover FE Jr, Coffey DS, Douglas LL, et al. Familial study of prostate cancer in Jamaica. *Urology* 1998;52:441–443.
17. Bratt O, Kristoffersson U, Lundgren R, et al. Familial and hereditary prostate cancer in southern Sweden. A population-based case-control study. *Eur J Cancer* 1999;35:272–277.
18. Hemminki K, Czene K. Age specific and attributable risks of familial prostate carcinoma from the family-cancer database. *Cancer* 2002;95: 1346–1353.
19. Hemminki K, Dong C. Familial prostate cancer from the family-cancer database. *Eur J Cancer* 2000;36:229–234.
20. Krain LS. Some epidemiologic variables in prostatic carcinoma in California. *Prev Med* 1974;3:154–159.
21. Woolf CM. An investigation of the familial aspects of carcinoma of the prostate. *Cancer* 1960;13:739–744.
22. Meikle AW, Smith JA, West DW. Familial factors affecting prostatic cancer risk and plasma sex-steroid levels. *Prostate* 1985;6:121–128.
23. Gronberg H, Damber L, Damber JE. Familial prostate cancer in Sweden: a nationwide register cohort study. *Cancer* 1996;77:138–143.
24. Gronberg H, Damber L, Damber JE. Studies of genetic factors in prostate cancer in a twin population. *J Urol* 1994;152:1484–1487.
25. Page WF, Braun MM, Partin AW, et al. Heredity and prostate cancer: A study of World War II veteran twins. *Prostate* 1997;33:240–245.
26. Lichtenstein P, Holm NV, Verkasalo PK, et al. Environmental and heritable factors in the causation of cancer: analyses of cohorts of twins from Sweden, Denmark, and Finland. *N Eng J Med* 2000;343:78–85.
27. Carter BS, Beaty TH, Steinberg GD, et al. Mendelian inheritance of familial prostate cancer. *Proc Natl Acad Sci U S A* 1992;89:3367–3371.
28. Gronberg H, Damber L, Damber JE, et al. Segregation analysis of prostate cancer in Sweden: support for dominant inheritance. *Am J Epidemiol* 1997;146:552–557.
29. Schaid DJ, McDonnell SK, Blute ML, et al. Evidence for autosomal dominant inheritance of prostate cancer. *Am J Hum Genet* 1998;62:1425–1438.
30. Verhage BA, Baffoe-Bonnie AB, Baglietto L, et al. Autosomal dominant inheritance of prostate cancer: a confirmatory study. *Urology* 2001;57: 97–101.
31. Valeri A, Briollais L, Azzouzi R, et al. Segregation analysis of prostate cancer in France: Evidence for autosomal dominant inheritance and residual brother-brother dependence. *Ann Hum Genet* 2003;67:125–137.
32. Cui J, Staples MP, Hopper JL, et al. Segregation analyses of 1,476 population-based Australian families affected by prostate cancer. *Am J Hum Genet* 2001; 68:1207–1218.
33. Gong G, Oakley-Girvan I, Wu AH, et al. Segregation analysis of prostate cancer in 1,719 white, African-American and Asian-American families in the United States and Canada. *Cancer Causes Control* 2002;13:471–482.
34. Conlon EM, Goode EL, Gibbs M, et al. Oligogenic segregation analysis of hereditary prostate cancer pedigrees: evidence for multiple loci affecting age at onset. *Int J Cancer* 2003;105:630–635.
35. Schaid DJ. The complex genetic epidemiology of prostate cancer. *Hum Mol Genet* 2004;13(Spec no 1):R103–R121.
36. Botstein D, Risch N. Discovering genotypes underlying human phenotypes: past successes for Mendclian disease, future approaches for complex disease. *Nat Genet* 2003;33:228–237.
37. Hall JM, Lee MK, Newman B, et al. Linkage of early-onset familial breast cancer to chromosome 17q21. *Science* 1990;250(4988):1684–1689.
38. Miki Y, Swensen J, Shattuck-Eidens D, et al. A strong candidate for the breast and ovarian cancer susceptibility gene BRCA1. *Science* 1994; 266(5182): 66–71.
39. Smith JR, Freije D, Carpten JD, et al. Major susceptibility locus for prostate cancer on chromosome 1 suggested by a genome-wide search. *Science* 1996;274:1371–1374.
40. Xu J, Zheng SL, Chang B, et al. Linkage of prostate cancer susceptibility loci to chromosome 1. *Human Genet* 2001;108:335–345.

41. Cooney KA, McCarthy JD, Lange E, et al. Prostate cancer susceptibility locus on chromosome 1q: a confirmatory study. *J Natl Cancer Inst* 1997; 89:955–959.

42. Hsieh CL, Oakley-Girvan I, Gallagher RP, et al. Re: prostate cancer susceptibility locus on chromosome 1q: A confirmatory study. *J Natl Cancer Inst* 1997;89:1893–1894.

43. Neuhausen SL, Farnham JM, Kort E, et al. Prostate cancer susceptibility locus HPC1 in Utah high-risk pedigrees. *Hum Mol Genet* 1999;8: 2437–2442.

44. Goddard KA, Witte JS, Suarez BK, et al. Model-free linkage analysis with covariates confirms linkage of prostate cancer to chromosomes 1 and 4. *Am J Hum Genet* 2001;68:1197–1206.

45. Suarez BK, Lin J, Witte JS, et al. Replication linkage study for prostate cancer susceptibility genes. *Prostate* 2000;45:106–114.

46. Berthon P, Valeri A, Cohen-Akenine A, et al. Predisposing gene for early-onset prostate cancer, localized on chromosome 1q42.2-43. *Am J Hum Genet* 1998;62:1416–1424.

47. Goode EL, Stanford JL, Chakrabarti L, et al. Linkage analysis of 150 high-risk prostate cancer families at 1q24-25. *Genet Epidemiol* 2000;18: 251–275.

48. Eeles RA, Durocher F, Edwards S, et al. Linkage analysis of chromosome 1q markers in 136 prostate cancer families: The Cancer Research Campaign/British Prostate Group U.K. Familial Prostate Cancer Study collaborators. *Am J Hum Genet* 1998;62:653–658.

49. Xu J, International Consortium for Prostate Cancer Genetics (ICPCG). Combined analysis of hereditary prostate cancer linkage to 1q24-25: results from 772 hereditary prostate cancer families from the International Consortium for Prostate Cancer Genetics. *Am J Hum Genet* 2000;66: 945–957.

50. Xu J, Meyers D, Freije D, et al. Evidence for a prostate cancer susceptibility locus on the X chromosome. *Nat Genet* 1998;20:175–179.

51. Gibbs M, Stanford JL, McIndoe RA, et al. Evidence for a rare prostate cancer-susceptibility locus at chromosome 1p36. *Am J Hum Genet* 1999; 64:776–787.

52. Berry R, Schroeder JJ, French AJ, et al. Evidence for a prostate cancer-susceptibility locus on chromosome 20. *Am J Hum Genet* 2000;67:82–91.

53. Schaid DJ, Chang B-L. Description of the International Consortium for Prostate Cancer Genetics, and failure to replicate linkage of hereditary prostate cancer to 20q13. *Prostate* 2005;63:276–290.

54. Hsieh Cl, Oakley-Girvan I, Balise RR, et al. A genome screen of families with multiple cases of prostate cancer: evidence of genetic heterogeneity. *Am J Hum Genet* 2001;69:148–158.

55. Edwards S, Meitz J, Eles R, et al. Results of a genome-wide linkage analysis in prostate cancer families ascertained through the ACTANE consortium. *Prostate* 2003;57:270–279.

56. Cunningham JM, McDonnell SK, Marks A, et al. Genome linkage screen for prostate cancer susceptibility loci: results from the Mayo Clinic Familial Prostate Cancer Study. *Prostate* 2003;57:335–346.

57. Janer M, Friedrichsen DM, Stanford JL, et al. Genomic scan of 254 hereditary prostate cancer families. *Prostate* 2003;57:309–319.

58. Lange EM, Gillanders EM, Davis CC, et al. Genome-wide scan for prostate cancer susceptibility genes using families from the University of Michigan Prostate Cancer Genetics Project finds evidence for linkage on chromosome 17 near BRCA1. *Prostate* 2003;57:326–334.

59. Schleutker J, Baffoe-Bonnie AB, Gillanders E, et al. Genome-wide scan for linkage in Finnish hereditary prostate cancer (HPC) families identifies novel susceptibility loci at 11q14 and 3p25-26. *Prostate* 2003;57:280–289.

60. Wiklund F, Gillanders EM, Albertus JA, et al. Genome-wide scan of Swedish families with hereditary prostate cancer: suggestive evidence of linkage at 5q11.2 and 19p13.3. *Prostate* 2003;57:290–297.

61. Witte JS, Suarez BK, Thiel B, et al. Genome-wide scan of brothers: replication and fine mapping of prostate cancer susceptibility and aggressiveness loci. *Prostate* 2003;57:298–308.

62. Xu J, Gillanders EM, Isaacs SD, et al. Genome-wide scan for prostate cancer susceptibility genes in the Johns Hopkins Hereditary Prostate Cancer Families. *Prostate* 2003;57:320–325.

63. Easton DF, Schaid DJ, Whittemore AS, et al. Where are the prostate cancer genes? A summary of eight genome wide searches. *Prostate* 2003; 57: 261–269.

64. Xu J, Dimitrov L, Chang BL et al. A combined genome-wide linkage scan for prostate cancer susceptibility genes in 1,233 families conducted by the ICPCG. *Am J Hum Genet* 2005 (in press).

65. Freedman ML, Reich D, Penney KL, et al. Assessing the impact of population stratification on genetic association studies. *Nat Genet* 2004;36: 388–393.

66. Tavtigian SV, Simard J, Teng DH, et al. A candidate prostate cancer susceptibility gene at chromosome 17p. *Nat Genet* 2001;27:172–180.

67. Rebbeck TR, Walker AH, Zeigler-Johnson C, et al. Association of HPC2/ELAC2 genotypes and prostate cancer. *Am J Hum Genet* 2000;67: 1014–1019.

68. Carpten J, Nupponen N, Isaacs S, et al. Germline mutations in the ribonuclease L gene in families showing linkage with HPC1. *Nat Genet* 2002;30: 181–184.

69. Xu J, Zheng SL, Komiya A, et al. Germline mutations and sequence variants of the macrophage scavenger receptor 1 gene are associated with prostate cancer risk. *Nat Genet* 2002;32:321–325.

70. Xu J, Zheng SL, Komiya A, et al. Common sequence variants of the macrophage scavenger receptor 1 gene are associated with prostate cancer risk. *Am J Hum Genet* 2003;72:208–212.

71. Nelson WG, De Marzo AM, Isaacs WB. Prostate cancer. *N Engl J Med* 2003;349:366–381.

72. The Breast Cancer Linkage Consortium. Cancer risks in BRCA2 mutation carriers. *J Natl Cancer Inst* 1999;91:1310–1316.

73. Gayther SA, de Foy KA, Harrington P, et al. The frequency of germ-line mutations in the breast cancer predisposition genes BRCA1 and BRCA2 in familial prostate cancer. *Cancer Res* 2000;60:4513–4518.

74. Edwards SM, Kote-Jarai Z, Meitz J, et al. Two percent of men with early-onset prostate cancer harbor germline mutations in the BRCA2 gene. *Am J Hum Genet* 2003;72:1–12.

75. Thompson D, Easton DF. Cancer incidence in BRCA1 mutation carriers. *J Natl Cancer Inst* 2002;94:1358–1365.

76. Giusti RM, Rutter JL, Duray PH, et al. A twofold increase in BRCA mutation related prostate cancer among Ashkenazi Israelis is not associated with distinctive histopathology. *J Med Genet* 2003;40:787–792.

77. Kirchhoff T, Kauff ND, Mitra N, et al. BRCA mutations and risk of prostate cancer in Ashkenazi Jews. *Clin Cancer Res* 2004;10:2918–2921.

78. Dong X, Wang L, Taniguchi K, et al. Mutations in CHEK2 associated with prostate cancer risk. *Am J Hum Genet* 2003;72:270–280.

79. Seppala EH, Ikonen T, Mononen N, et al. CHEK2 variants associate with hereditary prostate cancer. *Br J Cancer* 2003;89:1966–1970.

80. Cybulski C, Huzarski T, Gorski B, et al. A novel founder CHEK2 mutation is associated with increased prostate cancer risk. *Cancer Res* 2004;64: 2677–2679.

81. Cybulski C, Gorski B, Debniak T, et al. NBS1 is a prostate cancer susceptibility gene. *Cancer Res* 2004;64:1215–1219.

82. Thompson IM, Goodman PJ, Tangen CM, et al. The influence of finasteride on the development of prostate cancer. *N Engl J Med* 2003;349: 215–224.

CHAPTER 4 ■ THE ROLE OF THE ANDROGEN RECEPTOR IN THE PATHOPHYSIOLOGY OF PROSTATE CANCER

ZORAN CULIG, JOSE D. DEBES, GEORG BARTSCH, AND DONALD J. TINDALL

INTRODUCTION

Development, growth, and maintenance of the prostate depend on androgens. Androgen production is regulated through the hypothalamic-pituitary-gonadal axis (Fig. 4.1). This regulatory axis involves the secretion of gonadotropin-releasing hormone (GnRH) from the basal region of the hypothalamus into the vascular system in a pulsatile manner every 60 to 90 minutes. GnRH is carried by the hypothalamic-hypophyseal portal system to the anterior lobe of the pituitary gland (adenohypophysis) where it induces the release of luteinizing hormone (LH) and follicle-stimulating hormone (FSH). LH stimulates Leydig cells in the testis to synthesize testosterone, the major circulating androgen in men. FSH acts on Sertoli cells to induce spermatogenesis. Other androgens such as androstanediol, androstenedione, and dehydroepiandrosterone are also produced in the Leydig cells; however, the concentration of these androgens is much lower than that of testosterone (1). LH binds to its receptor on the Leydig cell of the testis and stimulates cyclic adenosine monophosphate (cAMP). This initiates transfer of cholesterol from the outer into the inner mitochondrial membrane where it is converted to pregnenolone. Metabolic conversion of pregnenolone to testosterone occurs in the smooth endoplasmic reticulum (1). Circulating testosterone (611 ng/dL ±186) is bound primarily by sex-hormone binding globulin (57%) and to a lesser extent by albumin (40%) and corticosteroid-binding globulin (<1%). Less than 3% of testosterone is bioavailable in an unbound form (2). Because of its lipophilic properties, unbound testosterone enters the prostate cell by passive diffusion. Once in the prostate cell, 5α-reductase enzymes convert testosterone into the more potent androgen dihydrotestosterone (DHT), which has a 3- to 10-fold higher affinity for its target, the androgen receptor (AR). There are two types of 5α-reductase enzymes: type 1 is present in most tissues, whereas type 2 is more specific for prostate tissue. Inhibitors of these enzymes, like finasteride and dutasteride, are being evaluated for their therapeutic potential in benign prostate hyperplasia (BPH) and prostate cancer (3). In the prostate, DHT is metabolized to 3-α-androstenediol, which can be reconverted to DHT or to 3-β-androstenediol, which is inactive. Testosterone inhibits GnRH secretion from the hypothalamus and LH secretion from the pituitary through a negative feedback loop, thus modulating its own production.

Extraprostatic metabolic pathways for testosterone include hepatic conjugation to nonandrogenic steroids and peripheral aromatization to estrogen (Fig. 4.1). Indeed, most of the estrogen in males is derived from peripheral conversion of androgens in fat tissue. Estrogen also initiates a negative feedback on LH release, reducing further testicular testosterone production.

Thus, estrogens have been used to induce "chemical castration" in men with prostate cancer (4, 5). In contrast, estrogens induce prostate growth and are related to the development of BPH. However, their role in carcinogenesis is still uncertain (6, 7). Prolactin also appears to have a direct effect on prostate growth (8). Prolactin receptors, which are regulated by androgens, have been reported in prostatic tissue, and transgenic mice that overexpress prolactin show increase in the size of the prostates (9). However, there is no clear evidence of prolactin being a cause of prostatic pathology.

More than 95% of androgen is produced by the testes. Additionally, a small fraction (less than 5%) of androgen is produced by the adrenal glands, where synthesis and secretion is regulated by adrenocorticotropin (ACTH), produced in the adenohypophysis (Fig. 4.1). ACTH induces conversion of cholesterol to pregnenolone, which results in synthesis of androstenedione through a pathway similar to that in the testes (10). Even though the androgenic activity of androstenedione is not very high, it can be converted to testosterone and dihydroepiandrosterone (DHEA) in peripheral tissue, including the prostate. The effect of adrenal androgens on the normal prostate does not appear to be significant. However, the presence of this nontesticular source of androgens may be instrumental in promoting prostate cancer growth and has led to the concept and practice of total androgen blockade as a treatment of advanced prostate cancer. In this treatment, GnRH analogs are combined with antiandrogens to block not only testicular androgen but also any action of adrenal-derived androgens (4).

ANDROGEN RECEPTOR BASIC STRUCTURAL AND FUNCTIONAL ASPECTS

The AR is a member of the nuclear receptor superfamily, which includes the progesterone, estrogen, mineralocorticoid, retinoic acid, thyroid, and vitamin D receptors.

The AR is expressed in nearly all prostate cancer cells, even after androgen-ablation therapy (11). The 90 Kb *AR* gene is located on the X chromosome between q11 and q12. It consists of eight exons that encode three domains: the transcriptional activation domain, which contains the activation function 1 (AF-1) region, the DNA-binding domain (DBD), and the ligand-binding domain (LBD) in the C-terminal end, which contains the activation function subdomain (AF-2). In addition, the AR contains a nuclear localization signal in the hinge region, between the DBD and the LBD, which is responsible for nuclear translocation after the receptor binds its ligand (12). The first exon encodes the entire N-terminal domain,

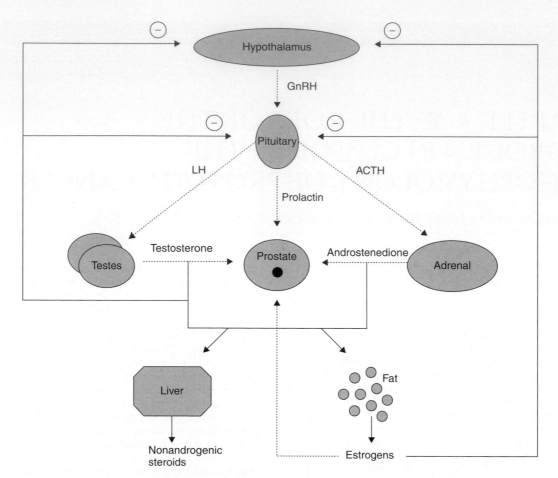

FIGURE 4.1. Hypothalamic-pituitary-gonadal axis. Gonadotropin-releasing hormone (GnRH) induces luteinizing hormone (LH) secretion from the pituitary gland. LH acts on the testes to produce testosterone, which interacts with the androgen receptor in the prostate. The pituitary gland also secretes prolactin, which acts on the prostate, and adrenocorticotropin (ACTH), which stimulates the adrenal glands to secrete androstenedione. Testosterone inhibits its own production by inhibiting GnRH and LH secretion. Androgens are metabolized to nonandrogenic steroids in the liver or to estrogen in fat tissue. Estrogens stimulate prostate growth and induce negative feedback by inhibiting GnRH secretion.

which comprises approximately half of the AR protein (~500 aa) and is the most diverse among the steroid receptor family. The AF-1 transactivation domain is located in this region and is thought to interact with different proteins conferring specificity for the targeted genes. This domain also interacts with the C-terminal region of the AR during homo-dimerization. Two polymorphic regions of trinucleotide repeats (CAG and GGN) in this transactivation domain have been associated with prostate cancer, and one (CAG) has been associated with Kennedy disease (13). The second and third exons encode the DBD (~67 aa), which is composed of two zinc fingers. The first zinc finger is encoded by exon 2 and confers receptor-specificity for androgen-response elements; the second zinc finger is encoded by exon 3 and plays a role in the dimerization of the receptor when binding to DNA. The first zinc finger is conserved among the androgen, glucocorticoid, and progesterone receptors and is thought to be important in recognition of hormone-response elements (14). The fourth exon encodes the hinge region that facilitates nuclear translocation (nuclear targeting sequence 617–633 aa). The remaining four exons encode for the LBD (~250 aa). The LBD forms a stable complex with the ligand, DHT being the most potent, and also interacts with the heat-shock proteins. More than 100 different mutations in the LBD region have been described to date. Many of these mutations, which cause loss-of-function in the AR, are present in patients with androgen insensitivity syndrome. Other mutations that cause

gain-of-function, such as altered steroid specificity, are found in prostate cancers (2).

The AR is a 918 aa protein with a molecular weight of 110 kDa. When it is inactive (not binding its ligand), the AR is bound to heat-shock proteins (hsp90, hsp70, and hsp56) in the cytosol (15). After binding to its ligand, the receptor is phosphorylated and dissociates from the heat-shock proteins. A series of conformational changes take place, and the nuclear localization signal in the hinge region is exposed. The receptor translocates to the nucleus, where dimerization, DNA binding to response elements, and interaction with different transcription factors occur. Six different phosphorylation sites in the N-terminal domain and one in the hinge region appear to facilitate dimerization of the receptor (16).

The AR is important for the growth and differentiation of the male urogenital structures, as well as maintenance of spermatogenesis. However, the AR is also involved in a variety of other biologic processes. The AR is expressed in the skin and is involved in the development of acne and in the suppression of hair growth. Androgens are also involved in modulation of hematopoiesis in the bone marrow. Mutations in the AR are associated with Kennedy disease (spinal and bulbar muscular atrophy), a genetic disorder characterized by muscular weakness, testicular atrophy, reduced fertility, and gynecomastia (17). Importantly, the AR has been linked to the development and progression of prostate cancer. In this regard, several mutations in the receptor have been related to prostate cancer incidence and aggressiveness. The role of these mutations and evidence of their involvement in prostate cancer are discussed later in the chapter.

ANDROGEN RECEPTOR TRANSCRIPTIONAL REGULATION AND COREGULATORY PROTEINS

Regulation of transcription by the AR is a complex process. Chromatin structure, general transcription machinery, coactivators, and corepressors play essential roles. For a clear understanding of transcription, it is important to recognize the difference between general transcription factors and coregulatory proteins (coactivators/corepressors). General transcription factors are required for basal transcription, whereas coregulatory proteins interact with specific DNA elements and induce expression of target genes. In order to initiate transcription after receptor dimerization, RNA polymerase II, as well as general transcription factors (TFIIA, TFIIB, TFIIH, TFIIF, TFIIE), need to be recruited to the promoter region, where transcription is initiated. In brief, TFIID initiates the binding of TATA-binding protein (TBP) to the TATA-box, and TFIIA stabilizes the binding of TBP to DNA. TBP induces DNA bending, which brings the upstream sequences into proximity. Then, TFIIB interacts with TBP and recruits RNA polymerase II and TFIIF to the promoter. RNA polymerase II is the enzyme responsible for synthesizing mRNA, using DNA as a template. TFIIF prevents interaction with nonspecific DNA. TFIIE and TFIIH are then recruited and initiate DNA unwinding around the transcription site (18). Different coactivators form complexes to ultimately regulate specific genes.

This generalized version of the transcription process can be applied to the AR. The AR interacts with TFIIB, TFIIF, TFIIH, and a variety of coactivators that regulate transcription (18). Many of these coactivators are involved in alteration of chromatin structure. Chromatin plays a major role in the transcriptional regulation of receptors. Histones are tightly bound to DNA, forming "compacted" chromatin, also known as heterochromatin, which is inactive. Acetylation of histones is thought to loosen the DNA-histone interaction, forming a less compact DNA fiber known as euchromatin, which is more accessible to DNA-binding proteins. Histones consist of positive amino acids, which bind to negatively charged DNA. Thus, when negatively charged acetyl groups are bound to histones, which is known as acetylation, the loss of the positive charge repels the interaction with DNA (19). After binding its ligand, the AR recruits the coactivator CREB-binding protein (CBP), a histone acetylator, to the promoter to finally induce androgen response elements (AREs) (Fig. 4.2). However, when antiandrogens bind to the AR, histone deacetylators HDAC1 and HDAC2, which have the opposite action of acetylators, are recruited (20). Thus, *acetylation-deacetylation* plays a major role in the regulation of AR transcription.

A number of AR coactivators are thought to play a role in prostate cancer progression. The coactivators belonging to the steroid receptor coactivator family (SRC) are among the most extensively characterized, including SRC-1 (NcoA-1), SRC-2 (GRIP1, TIF2), and SRC-3 (Rac3, ACTR, TRAM1). These coactivators interact with the general transcription factors and are able to recruit additional coregulators like CBP, p300, and p300 and CBP associated factor (PCAF) (21). For example, GRIP1 (glucocorticoid receptor interacting protein 1) is recruited after AR binding to androgens but not to antiandrogens (20). SRC2 and SRC1 can increase AR activation by adrenal androgens and

Activators

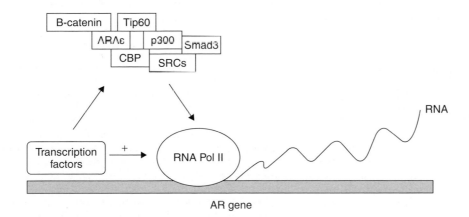

Repressors

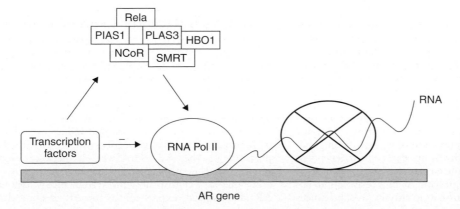

FIGURE 4.2. Androgen receptor transcriptional activity. Activators are recruited to the promoter region to induce RNA synthesis. Repressors are recruited to induce inhibition of RNA synthesis.

are upregulated in advanced prostate cancer (22). Other coactivators like CBP, p300, Rb, Smad3, steroid receptor RNA activator (SRA), Tip60, Cdk activating kinase (CAK), Cyclin E, and B-catenin interact with the AR (Fig. 4.2) (21). CBP and p300, which share more than 80% homology, have been shown to acetylate the AR. Overexpression of CBP induces AR activation by the antiandrogen hydroxyflutamide (23). p300 mediates androgen-independent activation of the AR by IL-6 (24). Moreover, p300 is associated with prostate cancer proliferation and progression after prostatectomy (25). Tip60 can induce androgen-independent activation of the AR and accumulates in the nucleus in androgen-independent prostate cancer, suggesting a role for this coactivator in refractory disease (26). Other coactivators that are specific for the AR include the AR activator proteins (ARAs) ARA24, ARA54, ARA55, ARA160, and ARA267, which enhance AR transcription. ARA24, ARA160, and ARA267 interact with the N-terminal domain of the AR, whereas ARA54, ARA55, and ARA70 interact with the ligand-binding domain. Some of these coactivators (e.g., ARA70 and ARA160) act synergistically to induce transcription. ARA70 induces agonistic effects of nonsteroidal antiandrogens and enhances AR activation by estradiol (21).

Corepressors function as negative regulators and induce silencing of transcriptional activity. Several AR corepressors have been described (Fig. 4.2). Some bind to the same region of the AR as that of coactivators, thus forming nonproductive interactions. Others recruit histone deacetylators to repress the active state of chromatin. Corepressors include histone acetyltransferase binding to ORC (HBO1), ReIa, p53, the protein inhibitor of activated STAT (PIAS) 1 and 3, nuclear corepressor (NCoR), and silencing mediator of retinoic acid and thyroid hormone receptor (SMRT) (17). Most of these corepressors interact with the N-terminal domain of the AR. Moreover, NCoR and SMRT are recruited when the AR binds antiandrogens (20).

The ability of coregulatory proteins to interact with the AR and general transcription factors indicates that they play a major role in the transcriptional regulation of the AR in normal prostate and in prostate cancer.

ANDROGEN RECEPTOR REGULATION OF APOPTOSIS, CELL CYCLE, AND ANGIOGENESIS

Apoptosis

Apoptosis plays a major role in the development of the normal prostate, as well as in cancer. Androgens and the AR are important for inhibiting apoptosis in the prostate. Androgens inhibit caspases through AR-mediated mechanisms, thus blocking apoptosis (27). Also, androgens upregulate the antiapoptotic factor p21 (28). Interestingly, p21 is upregulated in prostate cancers with high Gleason scores (29). The *PTEN* gene is often mutated with subsequent alteration of the PTEN/PI3K/AKT pathway in advanced prostate cancer. PTEN functions as a tumor suppressor due to its ability to reverse PI3K-mediated activation of the survival factor AKT, which suppresses proapoptotic targets such as BAD and caspase 9. Therefore, mutations of PTEN result in an activated form of AKT that constitutively inhibits apoptosis (30,31). The transcription factor FKHR (FOXO1) is another proapoptotic protein that is inhibited by AKT. Activated AR forms a complex with FOXO1, leading to the suppression of its activity and ability to induce apoptosis. This pathway appears to be independent of AKT and indicates that in some environments (e.g., cancer), a more active AR may lead to suppression of apoptosis (32). In addition, AKT induces inhibition of AR activity in prostate cancer

cells. Mitogen-activated pathways are also involved in apoptosis of prostate cells. The protein kinase mitogen endogenous activated kinase kinase1 (MEKK1) regulates apoptosis in prostate cancer. This effect is dependent on the AR, as MEKK1 is able to induce apoptosis in cells that express AR but not in AR-negative cells. Moreover, reconstitution of AR signaling pathways in AR-negative cells restores MEKK1-mediated apoptosis (33,34).

Cell Cycle

Androgen-mediated regulation of the cell cycle is a complex process that involves cell cycle stimulation at low androgen concentrations (<1 nM) and cell cycle inhibition at high androgen concentrations (>10 nM) (11). Transition through the different phases of the cell cycle is dependent on the activity of cyclin-dependent kinases (CDKs), which are the regulatory units that phosphorylate the proteins involved in this process. The activity of CDK2 and CDK4 increases upon androgen stimulation. Also, androgen depletion results in decreased levels of these kinases, suggesting that CDKs are important targets for cell cycle regulation by androgens (28,35). In addition, androgen-stimulated proliferation is associated with an increase of the S-phase kinase associated protein-2 (Skp-2), which is involved in the degradation of E2F1. This factor is a key element in the transition from S to G1 phase. Cell cycle inhibitors are also involved in this process (11). Cells treated with doses of androgens that inhibit proliferation show increased expression of the cell cycle inhibitor p27. Moreover, androgen deprivation results in increased levels of p27 and p16 (36,37). These inhibitors block the action of CDK2 and CDK4/6, respectively. Androgens also regulate the expression of the cell cycle inhibitor p21, which blocks the action of several CDKs. Blocking of the AR with antisense oligonucleotides induces upregulation of p21. Moreover, high androgen concentrations also induce p21 expression, thus inhibiting cell proliferation (38).

Angiogenesis

After castration, apoptosis occurs preferentially in endothelial cells of rat ventral prostate rather than in epithelial cells, suggesting that the AR plays a role in angiogenesis. Two growth factors involved in the regulation of angiogenesis are vascular endothelial growth factor (VEGF) and basic fibroblast growth factor (bFGF). Inhibition of prostate cancer growth after androgen ablation is associated with a marked reduction in levels of VEGF (39). Androgens regulate VEGF mRNA and protein in prostate stromal cells (40). In contrast, androgens do not regulate VEGF receptor. Androgenic regulation of VEGF is a complex process that involves activation of an autocrine loop of tyrosine kinase receptor/AkT pathway leading to induction of hypoxia inhibitory factor-1α and VEGF (41).

Androgen Receptor Expression in Prostate Cancer Models and Clinical Specimens

Many concepts of development and progression of prostate cancer have been based on studies of animal models and human cell lines. In Dunning rat tumors and the two human cell lines PC-3 and DU-145, there is a correlation between an aggressive phenotype and lack of AR expression (42,43). Therefore, it has been assumed that failure of endocrine therapy in prostate cancer is associated with a diminished or lost expression of the AR. However, it became evident from immunohistochemical studies that recurrent prostate cancers and bone and central nervous system metastases express the AR (44). Indeed, expression of the AR in clinical material is

TABLE 4.1

ANDROGEN RECEPTOR EXPRESSION AND FUNCTIONALITY IN FREQUENTLY USED PROSTATE CANCER MODELS

Tumor model	AR expression	AR function
Dunning rat[a]	Decreased in aggressive sublines	Not investigated (42)
LNCaP human[b]	Mutated receptor	Promiscuous activation by steroids and antiandrogens (59,48)
		AR activity increases during long-term androgen ablation
PC-3 human[b]	Very low expression	Transfected receptor cDNA (55)
		Decrease in malignancy
DU-145 human[b]	AR not expressed	Transient transfection assays (69)
MDA PCa2a human[b]	Double AR mutation	Stimulation by glucocorticoids (63)
CWR22 human[a]	Mutated receptor	Promiscuous activation by steroids (68)
		Second mutation appears in relapsed xenograft
LAPC-4 human[a]	Wild-type receptor	Ligand-independent activation by HER-2/neu (71)

AR, androgen receptor.
[a]Xenograft.
[b]Cell line.

heterogeneous. Some tumor cells lose AR expression due to promoter methylation (45). In contrast, AR upregulation, as a result of gene amplification, occurs in a subgroup of patients who fail endocrine therapy (46). The consequence of AR amplification for the clinical course of prostate cancer is not clear, and the mechanism responsible for unfavorable prognosis in patients who lack stromal AR is not known. It is thought that the AR in stromal cells is required for regulation of differentiation of epithelial cells in response to androgenic stimulation.

Both *in vitro* and *in vivo* models have been useful for studying the role of the AR in prostate carcinogenesis (Table 4.1). Valuable information on regulation of AR expression and activity has been obtained from xenografts, such as CWR22. Prostate cancer xenografts that express the AR regress dramatically after castration and regrow after a lag period of time. Expression of the AR decreases after androgen withdrawal but becomes elevated in the relapsed tumors. In the recurrent CWR22 xenograft, increased expression of the AR after castration results from stabilization of the protein (47). The fact that expression of several AR target genes is also elevated indicates that the AR is functional in this tumor model.

In some prostate cancer xenografts, castration and subsequent loss of the AR are observed in parallel with neuroendocrine differentiation, a process characterized morphologically by elongation of cells, and expression of various neuropeptides that influence growth of adjacent cells. Increased expression of neuroendocrine cells in prostate cancer patients is associated with an advanced stage of the disease.

AR-positive cell lines are useful models for studies on AR regulation during long-term androgen withdrawal. Growth of parental LNCaP cells is regulated by androgens in a biphasic manner being stimulated by low concentrations and inhibited by high concentrations of androgens. In contrast, regulation of prostate-specific genes, such as prostate-specific antigen (PSA), is dose-dependent, where maximal induction is observed at higher androgen concentrations.

Prostate cancer cells adapt to endocrine therapy. After continuous androgen ablation, AR expression and activity gradually increase in LNCaP and MDA PCa 2b cells (48,49). However, after prolonged steroid depletion, androgen acts as a negative growth factor by stimulation of the cell cycle

inhibitor p27 (36). Such effects of androgens are observed both *in vitro* and *in vivo* (50). Moreover, finasteride, an inhibitor of the enzyme 5α-reductase, stimulates growth of long-term androgen-ablated cells. Thus, prostate cancer cells appear to adapt to an environment of low androgen supply by increasing expression and activity of the AR. Interestingly, increased AR activity is not associated with elevated expression of the AR-regulated PSA protein because of methylation of the gene promoter (38). Indeed, many high-grade prostate cancers strongly downregulate PSA expression. Long-term androgen-depleted cells are increasingly resistant to induction of apoptosis, as shown after treatment with retinoic acid and taxol (51). Phenotypic changes that occur during long-term androgen ablation are reversed by administration of AR antisense oligonucleotides, which cause an increase in levels of the cell cycle inhibitor p21WAF1 and partial reestablishment of androgen dependence in LNCaP cells (38).

The pivotal role of the AR in prostate cancer suggests that it might be a target for therapy. Several compounds that inhibit AR expression also inhibit cancer cell proliferation. For example, resveratrol (an ingredient of red wine and various foods), nonsteroidal anti-inflammatory drugs, interleukin-1β, conditioned medium from activated T lymphocytes, and vitamin E show an inhibitory effect on the AR (12). Antisense oligonucleotides targeted to destroy polyglutamine repeats in the N-terminal region of the AR also cause a retardation of LNCaP cell growth and diminish PSA expression (52). Microinjection of an anti-AR antibody, but not control antibodies, leads to a significant inhibition of growth of androgen-refractory LNCaP derivatives, suggesting an important role of the AR in regulation of growth of advanced prostate cancer (53). In contrast, vitamin D increases AR levels but inhibits proliferation of LNCaP cells (54).

Moreover, AR reexpression in PC-3 cells is associated with growth arrest and apoptosis (55). Parental PC-3 cells, which are AR-negative, are highly aggressive. However, they acquire a less malignant phenotype after AR transfection, while the integrins α6β4 and α5β1 and mucin 1 are downregulated (56). AR expression in the ARCaP cell line yields reduced growth, migration, and invasion (57). Thus, expression of the AR appears to have a modulating effect on prostate cancer cells.

ANDROGEN RECEPTOR MUTATIONS IN PROSTATE CANCER

The significance of AR mutations in human prostate cancer is controversial, in particular because of differences in reported frequencies of mutated receptors. For example, few if any AR mutations are detected in organ-confined prostate cancer, whereas a number of mutations are found in stage D1 disease (58). The first AR point mutation (T877A) was discovered in the LNCaP cell line (59). In addition to androgens, the mutated AR binds estrogen, progestin, and the antiandrogen hydroxyflutamide. These compounds upregulate activity of the AR to a higher level than that of the wild-type AR and stimulate proliferation in the LNCaP cell line. An interesting question is whether antiandrogens commonly used in prostate cancer therapy may select for cells with mutations. For example, LNCaP cells cultured in androgen-depleted medium with bicalutamide show mutations in the AR ligand-binding domain (60). In this subline, bicalutamide acts as an AR agonist, and hydroxyflutamide acts as an antagonist, in contrast to parental LNCaP cells. Similar mutations have been described in patients undergoing androgen ablation therapy with bicalutamide (61). Also, AR mutations are found in some patients who receive combined treatment with androgen ablation and flutamide (62). Several mutations impart increased AR activity with hydroxyflutamide rather than with bicalutamide. Thus, some AR mutations appear to be induced by antiandrogens. This may explain why some prostate cancer patients respond to second-line androgen ablation therapy. Another potential mechanism relevant to prostate cancer progression is activation of a mutated AR by other steroids. The AR in the MDA PCa 2a cell line has a double mutation; one is the same as that in LNCaP cells (T877A) and the second is a substitution of leucine with histidine at position 701 (63). This double mutation in the cell line leads to an enhanced stimulation by the glucocorticoid hormone dexamethasone but not by the glucocorticoid receptor analog triamcinolone. Activation of the mutated AR in MDA PCa 2a cells is suppressed by bicalutamide. Thus, adrenal androgens and metabolic products of dihydrotestosterone may accelerate natural tumor progression through activation of mutated AR. Other mutations

(e.g., AR 715 val → met, 735 val → met, and 874 hys → tyr) alter the binding specificity to steroids, such that adrenal androgens will activate the AR (64). In the case of mutated AR 715 val → met, enhanced activation by progesterone or metabolites of dihydrotestosterone is not associated with increased binding affinity (65).

Germ-line mutations in the AR are rarely associated with increased risk for prostate cancer. An exception is a mutation in exon E of the AR gene (726 arg → leu) that leads to an enhanced activation of the AR by estradiol. This mutation is associated with an increased risk for prostate cancer in Finnish families (66). Although AR mutations in prostate cancer are, in most cases, associated with gain of function, some mutations induce inactivation of the receptor. For example, the 619 cys → tyr mutation alters the nuclear localization of the AR. A mutation in helix 5 of the AR ligand-binding domain is associated with a weakened interaction with heat-shock proteins and impaired interactions between the N- and carboxy-termini at lower androgen concentrations (67). Another mutation in the AR DNA-binding domain produces a premature stop codon, which results in a truncation of the COOH-terminus (68). This change is associated with constitutive nuclear localization and ligand binding, a fact that might explain lower levels of PSA in a relapsed xenograft. Specific point mutations may be relevant to an inappropriate response to antiandrogens in antiandrogen withdrawal syndrome. However, a direct relationship between antiandrogen withdrawal syndrome and changes in AR has not been proven conclusively.

LIGAND-INDEPENDENT ACTIVATION OF THE ANDROGEN RECEPTOR

During prostate cancer progression, cross-talk between signaling pathways of androgenic and peptide hormones is of particular importance (Fig. 4.3). Although some mechanistic details of interaction between signaling cascades are not well understood, it is clear that AR activity is modulated by a number of nonsteroidal factors. Several studies provide evidence that the AR can be activated in a ligand-independent and

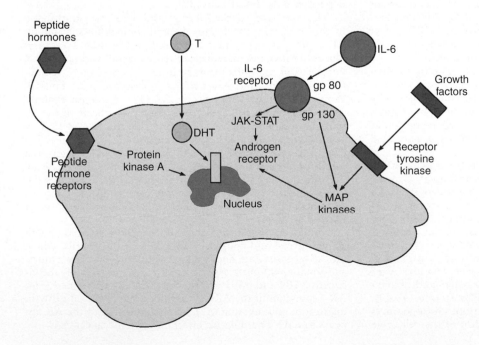

FIGURE 4.3. Activation of the androgen receptor. Dihydrotestosterone (DHT) binds and activates the androgen receptor (AR). Interleukin 6 (IL-6) activates the AR through the JAK-STAT pathway or by phosphorylation of the mitogen-activated protein kinases (MAPKs) ERK-1. This last pathway is involved in the growth factor–dependent activation of the AR.

synergistic manner with low concentrations of androgens (69, 70). The AR can be activated by insulin-like growth factor-I (IGF-I), keratinocyte growth factor, epidermal growth factor (EGF), and the EGF receptor-related molecule Her-2/neu (69, 71). Interestingly, IGF-I expression has been associated with increased risk of prostate cancer, and blockade of its signaling inhibits prostate cancer growth *in vitro* and *in vivo* (72). After binding to membrane receptors, growth factors activate, via phosphorylation, the signaling pathway of mitogen-activated protein kinases (MAPKs) (Fig. 4.3), which are increasingly phosphorylated in patients with high-grade prostate cancer (73). Under conditions in which low androgen levels are present, growth factors can significantly lower the threshold needed for maximal activation of AR by androgens. Constitutive activation of the Ras/MAPK pathway is sufficient to reduce concentration of androgen needed for maximal AR activation (74). In this regard, the HER-2/neu tyrosine kinase receptor not only activates the AR pathway in the absence of androgens but also has a synergistic effect on this pathway with low levels of androgens (71). In addition, some androgen-independent tumors overexpress HER-2/neu, making it an attractive target for therapy. Besides growth factors, agents that increase intracellular cAMP levels also cause a ligand-independent and synergistic activation of the AR. AR activation by cAMP is not necessarily associated with proliferation because of the multifunctional responses induced by this second messenger. Ligand-independent activation of the AR by Her-2/neu appears to be important for *in vivo* progression of prostate cancer, as demonstrated in the LAPC-4 xenograft (71). The neuropeptide bombesin also potentiates AR activity in combination with low doses of androgen (75).

Interaction of interleukin-6 (IL-6) with AR signaling is of special interest (Fig. 4.3). IL-6 levels are elevated in sera of patients with prostate cancer. Expression of IL-6 and its receptor is upregulated in patients with organ-confined prostate disease. IL-6 is also present in PC-3 and DU-145 cells, suggesting that tumor cells are a rich source of the cytokine (76). IL-6 causes multifunctional responses in prostate cancer cells, ranging from growth arrest to protection from apoptosis. The IL-6-related cytokine oncostatin M also activates the AR (77). However, in the case of oncostatin M, hydroxyflutamide acts as an agonist, whereas bicalutamide is not capable of inhibiting AR activation. This is of interest because similar signaling pathways are used by IL-6 and oncostatin M. A suitable model for changes that may occur during prostate cancer progression is represented by the LNCaP–IL-6+ cell line, derived after prolonged exposure to IL-6. These cells exhibit elevated levels of endogenous IL-6, acquire a growth advantage *in vitro* and *in vivo*, and lack expression of tumor suppressors p27 and pRb (78). The AR is expressed and activated in LNCaP–IL-6+ cells. AR activity is also upregulated by IL-4, another cytokine whose levels are elevated in prostate cancer (79). Activation by IL-4 is mediated through the antiapoptotic Akt signaling pathway. AR activity is also modulated by thyroid hormone, caveolin, and cadmium (80–82). Caveolin, a component of caveolae membranes, acts as a scaffold protein in several signaling pathways. Increased expression of caveolin is associated with prostate cancer progression. Cadmium causes increased expression of the AR target genes PSA and the homeobox gene *NKX* 3.1. In addition, prostate weight is higher after cadmium treatment, and this action is blocked by antiandrogens.

The AR plays an important role in prostate cancer. Androgens can act as tumor promoters through AR-mediated mechanisms, leading to cell proliferation and decreased apoptosis. All these processes are influenced by a variety of factors involved in the metabolism and action of steroid hormones. AR function is also affected by mutations, amplification, and polymorphisms in the gene. Some of these events enhance the activation of the AR by growth factors, cytokines, and antiandrogens. Importantly, enhanced AR activation appears to induce proliferation and progression of prostate cancer. Additional work is needed in order to clarify the mechanisms involved in the AR-mediated modulation of prostate cancer.

References

1. Amory JK, Bremner W. Endocrine regulation of testicular function in men: implications for contraceptive development. *Mol Cell Endocrinol* 2001; 182:175–179.
2. Debes JD, Tindall DJ. The role of androgens and the androgen receptor in prostate cancer. *Cancer Lett* 2002;187:1–7.
3. Thompson IM, Goodman PJ, Tangen CM, et al. The influence of finasteride on the development of prostate cancer. *N Engl J Med* 2003;349:215–224.
4. McLeod DG. Hormonal therapy: historical perspective to future directions. *Urology* 2003;61:3–7.
5. Hedlund PO, Ala-Opas M, Brekkan E, et al. Parenteral estrogen versus combined androgen deprivation in the treatment of metastatic prostatic cancer—Scandinavian Prostatic Cancer Group (SPCG) study no. 5. *Scand J Urol Nephrol* 2002;36:405–413.
6. Weihua Z, Warner M, Gustafsson JA. Estrogen receptor beta in the prostate. *Mol Cell Endocrinol* 2002;193:1–5.
7. Taplin ME, Ho SM. Clinical review 134: the endocrinology of prostate cancer. *J Clin Endocrinol Metab* 2001;86:3467–3477.
8. Nevalainen MT, Valve EM, Ingleton PM, et al. Prolactin and prolactin receptors are expressed and functioning in human prostate. *J Clin Invest* 1997;99:618–627.
9. Wennbo H, Kindblom J, Isaksson OG, et al. Transgenic mice overexpressing the prolactin gene develop dramatic enlargement of the prostate gland. *Endocrinology* 1997;138:4410–4415.
10. Partin A, Rodriguez R. The molecular biology, endocrinology, and physiology of the prostate and seminal vesicles. In: Wash PC, ed. *Campbell's urology*, 8th ed. Philadelphia: Saunders, 2002:1237–1296.
11. Huang H, Tindall DJ. The role of the androgen receptor in prostate cancer. *Crit Rev Eukaryot Gene Expr* 2002;12:193–207.
12. Culig Z, Klocker H, Bartsch G, et al. Androgen receptors in prostate cancer. *J Urol* 2003;170:1363–1369.
13. Cude KJ, Dixon SC, Guo Y, et al. The androgen receptor: genetic considerations in the development and treatment of prostate cancer. *J Mol Med* 1999;77:419–426.
14. Schoenmakers E, Alen P, Verrijdt G, et al. Differential DNA binding by the androgen and glucocorticoid receptors involves the second Zn-finger and a C-terminal extension of the DNA-binding domains. *Biochem J* 1999; 341(Pt 3):515–521.
15. Haendler B. Androgen-selective gene regulation in the prostate. *Biomed Pharmacother* 2002;56:78–83.
16. Gioeli D, Ficarro SB, Kwick JJ, et al. Androgen receptor phosphorylation. Regulation and identification of the phosphorylation sites. *J Biol Chem* 2002;277:29304–29314.
17. Lee HJ, Chang C. Recent advances in androgen receptor action. *Cell Mol Life Sci* 2003;60:1613–1622.
18. Lee DK, Chang C. Molecular communication between androgen receptor and general transcription machinery. *J Steroid Biochem Mol Biol* 2003; 84:41–49.
19. Vo N, Goodman RH. CREB-binding protein and p300 in transcriptional regulation. *J Biol Chem* 2001;276:13505–13508.
20. Shang Y, Myers M, Brown M. Formation of the androgen receptor transcription complex. *Mol Cell* 2002;9:601–610.
21. Heinlein CA, Chang C. Androgen receptor (AR) coregulators: an overview. *Endocr Rev* 2002;23:175–200.
22. Gregory CW, He B, Johnson RT, et al. A mechanism for androgen receptor-mediated prostate cancer recurrence after androgen deprivation therapy. *Cancer Res* 2001;61:4315–4319.
23. Comuzzi B, Lambrinidis L, Rogatsch H, et al. The transcriptional co-activator cAMP response element-binding protein-binding protein is expressed in prostate cancer and enhances androgen- and anti-androgen-induced androgen receptor function. *Am J Pathol* 2003;162:233–241.
24. Debes JD, Schmidt LJ, Huang H, et al. p300 mediates androgen-independent transactivation of the androgen receptor by interleukin 6. *Cancer Res* 2002; 62:5632–5636.
25. Debes JD, Sebo TJ, Lohse CM, et al. p300 in prostate cancer proliferation and progression. *Cancer Res* 2003;63:7638–7640.
26. Halkidou K, Gnanapragasam VJ, Mehta PB, et al. Expression of Tip60, an androgen receptor coactivator, and its role in prostate cancer development. *Oncogene* 2003;22:2466–2477.
27. Kimura K, Markowski M, Bowen C, et al. Androgen blocks apoptosis of hormone-dependent prostate cancer cells. *Cancer Res* 2001;61:5611–5618.
28. Lu S, Tsai SY, Tsai MJ. Regulation of androgen-dependent prostatic cancer cell growth: androgen regulation of CDK2, CDK4, and CKI p16 genes. *Cancer Res* 1997;57:4511–4516.

29. Baretton GB, Klenk U, Diebold J, et al. Proliferation- and apoptosis-associated factors in advanced prostatic carcinomas before and after androgen deprivation therapy: prognostic significance of p21/WAF1/CIP1 expression. *Br J Cancer* 1999;80:546–555.

30. Nelson WG, De Marzo AM, Isaacs WB. Prostate cancer. *N Engl J Med* 2003;349:366–381.

31. Wang S, Gao J, Lei Q, et al. Prostate-specific deletion of the murine Pten tumor suppressor gene leads to metastatic prostate cancer. *Cancer Cell* 2003;4:209–221.

32. Li P, Lee H, Guo S, et al. AKT-independent protection of prostate cancer cells from apoptosis mediated through complex formation between the androgen receptor and FKHR. *Mol Cell Biol* 2003;23:104–118.

33. Abreu-Martin MT, Chari A, Palladino AA, et al. Mitogen-activated protein kinase kinase kinase 1 activates androgen receptor-dependent transcription and apoptosis in prostate cancer. *Mol Cell Biol* 1999;19:5143–5154.

34. Fu M, Wang C, Wang J, et al. Androgen receptor acetylation governs trans activation and MEKK1-induced apoptosis without affecting in vitro sumoylation and trans-repression function. *Mol Cell Biol* 2002;22:3373–3388.

35. Gregory CW, Johnson RT Jr, Presnell SC, et al. Androgen receptor regulation of G1 cyclin and cyclin-dependent kinase function in the CWR22 human prostate cancer xenograft. *J Androl* 2001;22:537–548.

36. Kokontis JM, Hay N, Liao S. Progression of LNCaP prostate tumor cells during androgen deprivation: hormone-independent growth, repression of proliferation by androgen, and role for p27Kip1 in androgen-induced cell cycle arrest. *Mol Endocrinol* 1998;12:941–953.

37. Agus DB, Cordon-Cardo C, Fox W, et al. Prostate cancer cell cycle regulators: response to androgen withdrawal and development of androgen independence. *J Natl Cancer Inst* 1999;91:1869–1876.

38. Wang LG, Ossowski L, Ferrari AC. Overexpressed androgen receptor linked to p21WAF1 silencing may be responsible for androgen independence and resistance to apoptosis of a prostate cancer cell line. *Cancer Res* 2001;61:7544–7551.

39. Joseph IB, Nelson JB, Denmeade SR, et al. Androgens regulate vascular endothelial growth factor content in normal and malignant prostatic tissue. *Clin Cancer Res* 1997;3:2507–2511.

40. Levine AC, Liu XH, Greenberg PD, et al. Androgens induce the expression of vascular endothelial growth factor in human fetal prostatic fibroblasts. *Endocrinology* 1998;139:4672–4678.

41. Mabjeesh NJ, Willard MT, Frederickson CE, et al. Androgens stimulate hypoxia-inducible factor activation via autocrine loop of tyrosine kinase receptor/phosphatidylinositol 3'-kinase/protein kinase B in prostate cancer cells. *Clin Cancer Res* 2003;9:2416–2425.

42. Isaacs JT, Isaacs WB, Feitz WFJ, et al. Establishment and localization of seven dunning rat prostatic cell lines and their use in developing methods for predicting metastatic abilities of prostatic cancers. *Prostate* 1986;9:261–281.

43. Quarmby VE, Beckman WCJ, Cooke DB, et al. Expression and localization of androgen receptor in the R-3327 dunning rat prostatic adenocarcinoma. *Cancer Res* 1990;50:735–739.

44. Hobisch A, Culig Z, Radmayr C, et al. Distant metastases from prostatic carcinoma express androgen receptor protein. *Cancer Res* 1995;55:3068–3072.

45. Jarrard DF, Kinoshita H, Shi Y, et al. Methylation of the androgen receptor promoter CpG island is associated with loss of androgen receptor expression in prostate cancer cells. *Cancer Res* 1998;58:5310–5314.

46. Visakorpi T, Hyytinen E, Koivisto P, et al. In vivo amplification of the androgen receptor gene and progression of human prostate cancer. *Nat Genet* 1995;9:401–406.

47. Gregory CW, Johnson RTJ, Mohler JL, et al. Androgen receptor stabilization in recurrent prostate cancer is associated with hypersensitivity to low androgen. *Cancer Res* 2001;61:2892–2898.

48. Kokontis J, Takakura K, Hay N, et al. Increased androgen receptor activity and altered c-myc expression in prostate cancer cells after long-term androgen deprivation. *Cancer Res* 1994;54:1566–1573.

49. Hara T, Nakamura K, Araki H, et al. Enhanced androgen receptor signaling correlates with the androgen-refractory growth in a newly established MDA PCa 2b-hr human prostate cancer cell subline. *Cancer Res* 2003;63:5622–5628.

50. Umekita Y, Hiipakka RA, Kokontis JM, et al. Human prostate tumor growth in athymic mice: inhibition by androgens and stimulation by finasteride. *Proc Natl Acad Sci USA* 1996;93:15152–15157.

51. Gao M, Ossowski L, Ferrari AC. Activation of Rb and decline in androgen receptor protein precede retinoic acid-induced apoptosis in androgen-dependent LNCaP cells and their androgen-independent derivative. *J Cell Physiol* 1999;179:336–346.

52. Eder IE, Culig Z, Ramoner R, et al. Inhibition of LNCaP prostate cancer cells by means of androgen receptor antisense oligonucleotides. *Cancer Gene Therapy* 2000;7:997–1007.

53. Zegarra-Moro OL, Schmidt LJ, Huang H, et al. Disruption of androgen receptor function inhibits proliferation of androgen-refractory prostate cancer cells. *Cancer Res* 2002;62:1008–1013.

54. Zhao XY, Ly LH, Peehl DM, et al. Induction of androgen receptor by 1alpha, 25-dihydroxyvitamin D3 and 9-cis retinoic acid in LNCaP human prostate cancer cells. *Endocrinology* 1999;140:1205–1212.

55. Heisler LE, Evangelou A, Lew AM, et al. Androgen-dependent cell cycle arrest and apoptotic death in PC-3 prostatic cell cultures expressing a full-length human androgen receptor. *Mol Cell Endocrinol* 1997;126:59–73.

56. Bonaccorsi L, Carloni V, Muratori M, et al. Androgen receptor expression in prostate carcinoma cells suppresses alpha6beta4 integrin-mediated invasive phenotype. *Endocrinology* 2000;141:3172–3182.

57. Cinar B, Koeneman KS, Edlund M, et al. Androgen receptor mediates the reduced tumor growth, enhanced androgen responsiveness, and selected target gene transactivation in a human prostate cancer cell line. *Cancer Res* 2001;61:7310–7317.

58. Marcelli M, Ittmann M, Mariani S, et al. Androgen receptor mutations in prostate cancer. *Cancer Res* 2000;60:944–949.

59. Veldscholte J, Ris-Stalpers C, Kuiper GGJM, et al. A mutation in the ligand binding domain of the androgen receptor of human LNCaP cells affects steroid binding characteristics and response to anti-androgens. *Biochem Biophys Res Commun* 1990;17:534–540.

60. Hara T, Miyazaki J, Araki H, et al. Novel mutations of androgen receptor—a possible mechanism of bicalutamide withdrawal syndrome. *Cancer Res* 2003;63:149–153.

61. Haapala K, Hyytinen ER, Roiha M, et al. Androgen receptor alterations in prostate cancer relapsed during a combined androgen blockade by orchiectomy and bicalutamide. *Lab Invest* 2001;81:1647–1651.

62. Taplin ME, Bubley GJ, Ko YJ, et al. Selection for androgen receptor mutations in prostate cancers treated with androgen antagonist. *Cancer Res* 1999;59:2511–2515.

63. Zhao XY, Malloy PJ, Krishman AV, et al. Glucocorticoids can promote androgen-independent growth of prostate cancer cells through a mutated androgen receptor. *Nat Med* 2000;6:703–706.

64. Culig Z, Klocker H, Bartsch G, et al. Mutations of androgen receptor in carcinoma of the prostate—significance for endocrine therapy. *Am J Pharmacogenomics* 2001;1:241–249.

65. Culig Z, Hobisch A, Cronauer MV, et al. Mutant androgen receptor detected in an advanced stage of prostatic carcinoma is activated by adrenal androgens and progesterone. *Mol Endocrinol* 1993;7:1541–1550.

66. Mononen N, Syrjakoski K, Matikainen M, et al. Two percent of Finnish prostate cancer patients have a germ-line mutation in the hormone-binding domain of the androgen receptor gene. *Cancer Res* 2000;60:6479–6481.

67. James AJ, Agoulnik IU, Harris JM, et al. A novel androgen receptor mutant, A748T, exhibits hormone concentration-dependent defects in nuclear accumulation and activity despite normal hormone-binding affinity. *Mol Endocrinol* 2002;16:2692–2705.

68. Tepper CG, Boucher DL, Ryan PE, et al. Characterization of a novel androgen receptor mutation in a relapsed CWR22 prostate cancer xenograft and cell line. *Cancer Res* 2002;62:6606–6614.

69. Culig Z, Hobisch A, Cronauer MV, et al. Androgen receptor activation in prostatic tumor cell lines by insulin-like growth factor-I, keratinocyte growth factor, and epidermal growth factor. *Cancer Res* 1994;54:5474–5478.

70. Hobisch A, Eder IE, Putz T, et al. Interleukin-6 regulates prostate-specific protein expression in prostate carcinoma cells by activation of the androgen receptor. *Cancer Res* 1998;58:4640–4645.

71. Craft N, Shostak Y, Carey M, et al. A mechanism for hormone-independent prostate cancer through modulation of androgen receptor signaling by the HER-2/neu tyrosine kinase. *Nat Med* 1999;5:280–285.

72. Grossmann ME, Huang H, Tindall DJ. Androgen receptor signaling in androgen-refractory prostate cancer. *J Natl Cancer Inst* 2001;93:1687–1697.

73. Gioeli D, Mandell JW, Petroni GR, et al. Activation of mitogen-activated protein kinase associated with prostate cancer progression. *Cancer Res* 1999;59:279–284.

74. Bakin RE, Gioeli D, Sikes RA, et al. Constitutive activation of the ras/mitogen-activated protein kinase signaling pathway promotes androgen hypersensitivity in LNCaP prostate cancer cells. *Cancer Res* 2003;63:1981–1989.

75. Dai J, Shen R, Sumitomo M, et al. Synergistic activation of the androgen receptor by bombesin and low-dose androgen. *Clin Cancer Res* 2002;8:2399–2405.

76. Smith PC, Hobisch A, Lin DL, et al. Interleukin-6 and prostate cancer progression. *Cytokine Growth Factor Rev* 2001;12:33–40.

77. Godoy-Tundidor S, Hobisch A, Pfeil K, et al. Acquisition of agonistic properties of nonsteroidal antiandrogens after treatment with oncostatin M in prostate cancer cells. *Clin Cancer Res* 2002;8:2356–2361.

78. Steiner H, Godoy-Tundidor S, Rogatsch H, et al. Accelerated in vivo growth of prostate tumors that up-regulate interleukin-6 is associated with reduced retinoblastoma protein expression and activation of the mitogen-activated protein kinase pathway. *Am J Pathol* 2003;162:655–663.

79. Lee SO, Lou W, Hou M, et al. Interleukin-4 enhances prostate-specific antigen expression by activation of the androgen receptor and Akt pathway. *Oncogene* 2003;22:6037–6044.

80. Zhang S, Hsieh ML, Zhu W, et al. Interactive effects of triiodothyronine and androgens on prostate cell growth and gene expression. *Endocrinology* 1999;140:1665–1671.

81. Lu ML, Schneider MC, Zheng Y, et al. Caveolin-1 interacts with androgen receptor. A positive modulator of androgen receptor mediated transactivation. *J Biol Chem* 2001;276:13442–13451.

82. Martin MB, Voeller HJ, Gelmann EP, et al. Role of cadmium in the regulation of AR gene expression and activity. *Endocrinology* 2002;143:264–275.

CHAPTER 5 ■ BIOLOGY OF BONE METASTASES IN MEN WITH PROSTATE CANCER

MATTHEW R. SMITH

INTRODUCTION

Bone is a rigid yet dynamic organ that is continuously shaped and repaired by a process termed *remodeling*. Bone remodeling is the predominant metabolic process regulating bone structure and function during adult life. Bone remodeling involves the breakdown and formation of bone by the coordinated action of osteoclasts and osteoblasts (Fig. 5.1). Bone remodeling occurs in discrete microscopic units throughout the skeleton. Remodeling of each unit is geographically and temporally separated from other remodeling units. The process is initiated by migration of osteoclasts to these sites, resorption of bone, apoptosis of osteoclasts, and then new bone formation by osteoblasts.

Osteoclasts are tissue-specific macrophages derived from hematopoietic stem cells from the monocyte/macrophage lineage. Bone resorption is a multistep process initiated by proliferation of immature osteoclast precursors, commitment of these cells to the osteoclast phenotype, and finally degradation of the bone matrix by mature multinucleated osteoclasts. Osteoclasts attach to the bone matrix and develop a specialized cytoskeleton or ruffled border. A process involving proton transport degrades the matrix in the isolated microenvironment at the ruffled border. The bone matrix is a storehouse of growth factors, and normal bone resorption releases a variety of factors that activate osteoblasts including transforming growth factor β (TGF-β), basic fibroblast growth factor (bFGF), Platelet-derived growth factor (PDGF), and insulin-like growth factor (IGF) I and II. Osteoblasts are derived from stromal stem cells. Osteoblasts synthesize and secrete the organic matrix. Mineralization begins soon after the organic matrix is secreted and is completed within several weeks.

The receptor activator of NFκB (RANK) signaling pathway regulates the activation, differentiation, proliferation, and apoptosis of osteoclasts (1). This pathway consists of receptor activator of NFκB ligand (RANKL), its receptor RANK, and its decoy receptor osteoprotegerin (OPG). RANKL binds and activates RANK, a transmembrane receptor expressed on hematopoietic stem cells and osteoclasts. RANK expression on stem cells is required for osteoclast differentiation and activation. Hormones and other factors that stimulate bone resorption induce the expression of RANKL by bone stromal cells. RANKL expression by osteoblasts coordinates bone remodeling by stimulating bone resorption by osteoclasts, which in turn stimulates new bone formation by adjacent osteoblasts in a process termed *coupling*. RANKL signaling pathway is negatively regulated by OPG. OPG is a soluble protein produced by osteoblasts in response to anabolic agents including estrogen and bone morphogenic proteins. OPG acts as a decoy receptor

that blocks RANKL binding to RANK. OPG also acts as a decoy receptor for tumor necrosis factor (TNF)-related apoptosis-inducing ligand (TRAIL).

CLINICAL MANIFESTATIONS OF BONE METASTASES

Prostate cancer preferentially spreads to the skeleton (Fig. 5.2). More than 80% of men who die from prostate cancer have bone metastases at autopsy (2). In contrast to most other cancers, prostate cancer forms predominantly osteoblastic metastases. The vertebral column, pelvis, ribs, and proximal long bones are the most common sites of skeletal metastases. These sites correspond to the most abundant regions of bone marrow in the skeleton.

Pain is the most common symptom of metastatic prostate cancer. Metastases to the vertebrae may cause spinal cord compression, nerve root compression, or cauda equina syndrome. Metastases to the base of the skull can impinge on cranial nerves. Clinical fractures are common with most fractures involving the vertebral bodies. In contrast to osteolytic bone disease, pathologic fractures of long bones are unusual. Hypocalcemia due to excess deposition of calcium in newly formed bone is commonly observed but rarely associated with symptoms. Most men with metastatic prostate cancer have normochromic normocytic anemia.

PATHOPHYSIOLOGY OF OSTEOBLASTIC METASTASES

Most bone metastases in men with prostate cancer appear osteoblastic by radiographic imaging. Osteolytic and osteoblastic lesions represent two extremes of a spectrum, however, and morphologic studies suggest that most bone metastases from prostate cancer are characterized by both excess bone formation and bone resorption. Pathologic acceleration of bone remodeling results in disorganized bone with impaired biomechanical properties.

Osteoblastic metastases from prostate cancer have increased osteoblast number and activity, increased bone volume, and increased bone mineralization rate (3). Osteoclast number and activity are increased in osteoblastic metastases, at bone adjacent to metastases, and at distant uninvolved bone (3,4). Biochemical markers of osteoclast activity are elevated in men with osteoblastic metastases from prostate cancer (5). Although osteoclast activity is increased in men with prostate cancer, it is unclear whether osteoclast activation precedes bone formation as in normal bone remodeling or if

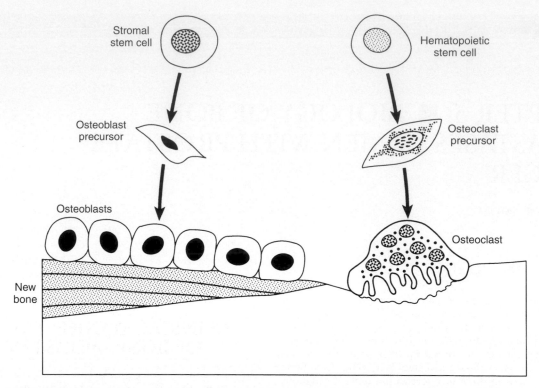

FIGURE 5.1. Normal bone remodeling. Bone remodeling involves the breakdown and formation of bone by the coordinated action of osteoclasts and osteoblasts. Osteoclasts are tissue-specific macrophages derived from hematopoietic stem cells from the monocyte/macrophage lineage. Osteoblasts are derived from stromal stem cells.

osteoclast activation is secondary to excessive osteoblast activity in the metastases. Markers of osteoclast activity predict independently the risk for subsequent skeletal complications (6), suggesting that cancer-mediated osteoclast activation not only accompanies bone metastases but also contributes to the clinical complications of metastatic disease.

Hyperparathyroidism is common in men with metastatic prostate cancer. Serum concentrations of calcium are typically normal or low, suggesting that excessive parathyroid hormone secretion is secondary to increased calcium phosphate deposition in osteoblastic metastases (7). Secondary hyperparathyroidism may propagate a vicious cycle involving parathyroid hormone activation of osteoclasts, release of bone-derived growth factors, tumor cell proliferation, osteoblast activation, and further calcium phosphate deposition.

Hormone therapy also contributes to osteoclast activation in men with prostate cancer. Androgen deprivation therapy, the cornerstone of treatment for advanced prostate cancer, accelerates normal bone turnover and increases biochemical markers of osteoclast activity by approximately twofold in men without bone metastases (8). The unintended skeletal effects of androgen deprivation therapy increase fracture risk in men with prostate cancer (9). In addition, treatment-related increases in osteoclast activity may promote progression of bone metastases by increasing the release of bone-derived growth factors.

Zoledronic acid is a potent bisphosphonate that inhibits osteoclast attachment, differentiation, and survival (10). In a randomized placebo-controlled trial, zoledronic acid decreased the risk of skeletal complications in men with bone metastases and progressive disease after first-line hormonal therapy (11). The efficacy of zoledronic acid supports the concept that excessive osteoclast activity has a causal role in skeletal complications from metastatic prostate cancer.

MECHANISMS OF BONE METASTASES

The concept that interactions between "seed" (circulating tumor cells) and "soil" (metastatic site) determine the metastatic potential of a cancer was first proposed by Stephen Paget more than a century ago (12). Consistent with the *seed and soil* hypothesis, reciprocal interactions between prostate cancer cells and bone stroma appear to account for both the predominant skeletal localization of metastases and the characteristic osteoblastic response (Fig. 5.3).

The bone extracellular matrix supports cellular adhesion and may contribute to the preferential skeletal localization of prostate cancer metastases. Adhesion to the extracellular matrix increases androgen responsiveness and increased expression of androgen-responsive genes (13,14). In addition, adhesion to the extracellular matrix increases androgen-independent expression of some androgen-responsive homeobox genes (15), suggesting that interactions with the extracellular matrix contributes to androgen-independent growth.

Several bone-derived growth factors, including transforming growth factor β, epidermal growth factor, and basic fibroblast growth factor, promote prostate cancer growth and differentiation.

Bone-derived growth factors may also contribute to the preferential skeletal localization of prostate cancer metastases. TGF-β facilitates adhesion to the extracellular matrix (16). Epidermal growth factor (EGF) promotes migration of prostate cancer cells (17).

Many tumor-derived factors have been implicated in the pathogenesis of osteoblastic metastases, including endothelin-1,

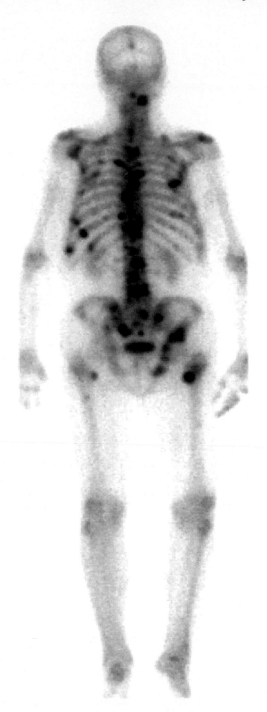

FIGURE 5.2. Bone metastases from prostate cancer. Radionuclide bone scan demonstrates multiple areas of increased tracer uptake at multiple sites in a man with progressive metastatic prostate cancer. Prostate cancer preferentially metastasizes to the vertebrae, pelvis, ribs, and proximal long bones. In contrast to most other malignancies, prostate cancer tends to form osteoblastic metastases.

bone morphogenic proteins, insulin-like growth factors, osteoprotegerin, transforming growth factor β, and serine proteases prostate-specific antigen and urokinase-type plasminogen activator.

Endothelin-1

The endothelin family consists of three paracrine/autocrine peptide factors (ET-1, ET-2, and ET-3) that act as modulators of vasomotor tone, nociception, hormone production, and cell proliferation (18). Endothelins are produced by a variety of normal tissues. ET-1 is the predominant circulating endothelin and is uniformly produced by endothelial cells and normal prostate epithelium. Two endothelin receptors have been identified: the ET_A receptor has a high affinity for ET-1 and ET-2, and the ET_B receptor has equal affinity for all the endothelin-related polypeptides. The growth promoting effects of ET-1 are mediated by the ET_A receptor (19). The ETB receptor attenuates the activity of endothelin-1 by decreasing endothelin-1 secretion, increasing endothelin-1 clearance, and activating inhibitory pathways.

Endothelin-1 has important roles in both the prostate and skeleton. ET-1 is produced by normal and malignant prostate epithelium and has been implicated in prostate cancer progression and bone metastases. ET-1 inhibits osteoclast-mediated bone resorption and promotes the proliferation of osteoblasts (20). Prostate-derived ET-1 promotes new bone formation (21), suggesting that ET-1 contributes to the osteoblastic phenotype of prostate cancer metastases.

Selective ET_A receptor antagonists are in development for the treatment of prostate cancer. Atrasentan is an orally available, highly potent, and selective ET_A receptor antagonist that blocks the effects of ET-1 (22). In a double-blind, placebo-controlled, phase II study of men with hormone refractory prostate cancer, Atrasentan tended to delay time to progression (23).

Bone Morphogenic Proteins

Bone morphogenic proteins (BMPs) constitute a large family of developmentally regulated proteins involved in mesoderm formation and organ patterning. Both normal human prostate and prostate cancer cell lines express a variety of BMPs (24). BMP-6 expression in primary tumors is also associated with radiographic evidence of bone metastases, suggesting a potential role in the pathogenesis of metastases (25).

Insulin-like Growth Factors

Insulin-like growth factors promote the proliferation of both prostate cancer cells and osteoblasts by interactions with specific IGF receptors (26). The biologic activity of IGFs appears to be regulated by the level of IGF-binding proteins (IGFBPs) and IGF receptors of target cells. Men with metastatic prostate cancer have elevated serum levels of IGFs (27). Cleavage of IGF-binding proteins by several IGF-binding protein proteases may contribute to the elevated expression of IGFs in men with prostate cancer. In addition, prostate-specific antigen (PSA) specifically cleaves IGF-binding protein-3 (28).

Osteoprotegerin

The RANK signaling pathway regulates osteoclast activation, differentiation, proliferation, and apoptosis. Bone metastases but not primary prostate tumors consistently express RANKL and its decoy receptor OPG (29). Serum OPG levels are elevated in men with metastatic prostate cancer (30). OPG prevents TRAIL-induced apoptosis of prostate cancer cell lines *in vitro*, suggesting that OPG is a prostate cancer survival factor (31).

Transforming Growth Factor β

Transforming growth factor β is secreted by osteoblasts in a latent, inactive form that is incorporated into the extracellular

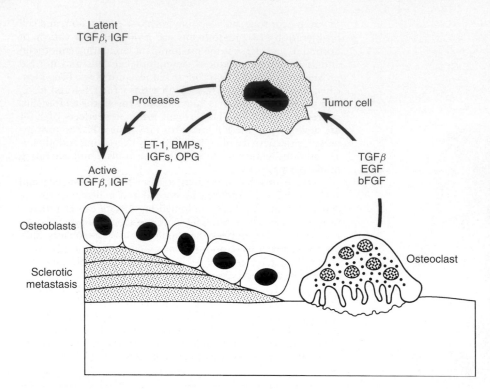

FIGURE 5.3. Model of osteoblastic metastases: Osteoblastic metastases from prostate cancer are characterized by excess activity of both osteoblasts and osteoclasts. Several tumor-derived factors, including endothelin-1 (ET-1), bone morphogenic proteins (BMPs), insulin-like growth factors (IGFs), and transforming growth factor β (TGF-β), directly activate osteoblasts. In addition, tumor-derived proteases stimulate osteoclasts indirectly though activation of latent TGF-β and IGFs by cleaving them from their binding proteins. Osteoclast-mediated bone resorption releases TGF-β, epidermal growth factor (EGF), and basic fibroblast growth factor (bFGF) from the bone extracellular matrix. These bone-derived factors promote prostate cancer growth and propagate a vicious cycle of reciprocal tumor-bone interactions.

matrix. Latent TGF-β is a composed of TGF-β, the amino terminal part of the TGF-β precursor, and latent TGF-β binding protein. Latent TGF-β can be activated by proteolytic cleavage. TGF-β promotes new bone formation by a variety of mechanisms including osteoclast differentiation and maturation. Primary human prostate cancer and prostate cancer cell lines express TGF-β (32,33). The importance of TGF-β in normal bone physiology suggests that tumor-derived TGF-β may have a central role in the development and progression of osteoblastic metastases.

Serine Proteases

Most tumor-derived factors implicated in the pathogenesis of osteoblastic metastases directly stimulate osteoblast activity. In contrast, proteases activate osteoblasts by indirect mechanisms. Prostate-specific antigen and urokinase-type plasminogen activator (uPA) are serine proteases expressed in human prostate cancers. Both PSA and uPA may activate TGF-β and IGF-1 by cleaving them from their binding proteins (34). These proteases may also contribute to the osteoblastic phenotype by cleavage of tumor-derived parathyroid hormone–related protein.

CONCLUSION

Bone metastases are a major cause of morbidity from prostate cancer. Prostate cancer spreads preferentially to the skeleton. Although most bone metastases in men with prostate cancer appear osteoblastic by radiographic imaging, osteoblastic metastases are characterized by abnormal activation of both osteoblasts and osteoclasts. This pathologic acceleration of bone remodeling results in disorganized bone with impaired biomechanical properties. Complex reciprocal interactions between tumor and bone account for both the preferential spread to skeleton and characteristic osteoblastic phenotype. Several tumor-derived factors have been implicated in the pathogenesis

of osteoblastic metastases, including endothelin-1, bone morphogenic proteins, insulin-like growth factors, osteoprotegerin, and transforming growth factor β. Several bone-derived growth factors, including transforming growth factor β, epidermal growth factor, and basic fibroblast growth factor, promote prostate cancer growth and differentiation. Greater understanding of these tumor-host interactions may provide future therapeutic opportunities.

References

1. Boyle WJ, Simonet WS, Lacey DL. Osteoclast differentiation and activation. *Nature* 2003;423:337–342.
2. Harada M, Iida M, Yamaguchi M, et al. Analysis of bone metastasis of prostatic adenocarcinoma in 137 autopsy cases. *Adv Exp Med Biol* 1992; 324:173–182.
3. Clarke NW, McClure J, George NJ. Osteoblast function and osteomalacia in metastatic prostate cancer. *Eur Urol* 1993;24:286–290.
4. Clarke NW, McClure J, George NJ. Morphometric evidence for bone resorption and replacement in prostate cancer. *Br J Urol* 1991;68:74–80.
5. Garnero P, Buchs N, Zekri J, et al. Markers of bone turnover for the management of patients with bone metastases from prostate cancer. *Br J Cancer* 2000;82:858–864.
6. Berruti A, Dogliotti L, Bitossi R, et al. Incidence of skeletal complications in patients with bone metastatic prostate cancer and hormone refractory disease: predictive role of bone resorption and formation markers evaluated at baseline. *J Urol* 2000;164:1248–1253.
7. Murray RM, Grill V, Crinis N, et al. Hypocalcemic and normocalcemic hyperparathyroidism in patients with advanced prostatic cancer. *J Clin Endocrinol Metab* 2001;86:4133–4138.
8. Smith MR, McGovern FJ, Zietman AL, et al. Pamidronate to prevent bone loss in men receiving gonadotropin releasing hormone agonist therapy for prostate cancer. *N Engl J Med* 2001;345:948–955.
9. Higano CS. Management of bone loss in men with prostate cancer. *J Urol* 2003;170:S59–S63; discussion S64.
10. Green JR. Preclinical pharmacology of zoledronic acid. *Semin Oncol* 2002; 29:3–11.
11. Saad F, Gleason DM, Murray R, et al. A randomized, placebo-controlled trial of zoledronic acid in patients with hormone-refractory metastatic prostate carcinoma. *J Natl Cancer Inst* 2002;94:1458–1468.
12. Paget S. The distribution of secondary growths of cancer in cancer of the breast. *Lancet* 1889;1:571–573.

13. Fong CJ, Sherwood ER, Braun EJ, et al. Regulation of prostatic carcinoma cell proliferation and secretory activity by extracellular matrix and stromal secretions. *Prostate* 1992;21:121–131.
14. Murphy BC, Pienta KJ, Coffey DS. Effects of extracellular matrix components and dihydrotestosterone on the structure and function of human prostate cancer cells. *Prostate* 1992;20:29–41.
15. Robbins SE, Shu WP, Kirschenbaum A, et al. Bone extracellular matrix induces homeobox proteins independent of androgens: possible mechanism for androgen-independent growth in human prostate cancer cells. *Prostate* 1996;29:362–370.
16. Kostenuik PJ, Singh G, Orr FW. Transforming growth factor beta upregulates the integrin-mediated adhesion of human prostatic carcinoma cells to type I collagen. *Clin Exp Metastasis* 1997;15:41–52.
17. Rajan R, Vanderslice R, Kapur S, et al. Epidermal growth factor (EGF) promotes chemomigration of a human prostate tumor cell line, and EGF immunoreactive proteins are present at sites of metastasis in the stroma of lymph nodes and medullary bone. *Prostate* 1996;28:1–9.
18. Battistini B, Chailler P, D'Orleans-Juste P, et al. Growth regulatory properties of endothelins. *Peptides* 1993;14:385–399.
19. Nelson JB, Chan-Tack K, Hedican SP, et al. Endothelin-1 production and decreased endothelin B receptor expression in advanced prostate cancer. *Cancer Res* 1996;56:663–668.
20. Nelson JB, Carducci MA. The role of endothelin-1 and endothelin receptor antagonists in prostate cancer. *BJU Int* 2000;85(Suppl 2):45–48.
21. Nelson JB, Nguyen SH, Wu-Wong JR, et al. New bone formation in an osteoblastic tumor model is increased by endothelin-1 overexpression and decreased by endothelin A receptor blockade. *Urology* 1999;53:1063–1069.
22. Carducci MA, Nelson JB, Bowling MK, et al. Atrasentan, an endothelin-receptor antagonist for refractory adenocarcinomas: safety and pharmacokinetics. *J Clin Oncol* 2002;20:2171–2180.
23. Carducci MA, Padley RJ, Breul J, et al. Effect of endothelin-A receptor blockade with atrasentan on tumor progression in men with hormone-refractory prostate cancer: a randomized, phase II, placebo-controlled trial. *J Clin Oncol* 2003;21:679–689.
24. Harris SE, Harris MA, Mahy P, et al. Expression of bone morphogenetic protein messenger RNAs by normal rat and human prostate and prostate cancer cells. *Prostate* 1994;24:204–211.
25. Bentley H, Hamdy FC, Hart KA, et al. Expression of bone morphogenetic proteins in human prostatic adenocarcinoma and benign prostatic hyperplasia. *Br J Cancer* 1992;66:1159–1163.
26. Peehl DM, Cohen P, Rosenfeld RG. The insulin-like growth factor system in the prostate. *World J Urol* 1995;13:306–311.
27. Kanety H, Madjar Y, Dagan Y, et al. Serum insulin-like growth factor-binding protein-2 (IGFBP-2) is increased and IGFBP-3 is decreased in patients with prostate cancer: correlation with serum prostate-specific antigen. *J Clin Endocrinol Metab* 1993;77:229–233.
28. Cohen P, Graves HC, Peehl DM, et al. Prostate-specific antigen (PSA) is an insulin-like growth factor binding protein-3 protease found in seminal plasma. *J Clin Endocrinol Metab* 1992;75:1046–1053.
29. Brown JM, Corey E, Lee ZD, et al. Osteoprotegerin and rank ligand expression in prostate cancer. *Urology* 2001;57:611–616.
30. Brown JM, Vessella RL, Kostenuik PJ, et al. Serum osteoprotegerin levels are increased in patients with advanced prostate cancer. *Clin Cancer Res* 2001;7:2977–2983.
31. Holen I, Croucher PI, Hamdy FC, et al. Osteoprotegerin (OPG) is a survival factor for human prostate cancer cells. *Cancer Res* 2002;62:1619–1623.
32. Marquardt H, Lioubin MN, Ikeda T. Complete amino acid sequence of human transforming growth factor type beta 2. *J Biol Chem* 1987;262:12127–12131.
33. Muir GH, Butta A, Shearer RJ, et al. Induction of transforming growth factor beta in hormonally treated human prostate cancer. *Br J Cancer* 1994;69:130–134.
34. Mundy GR. Metastasis to bone: causes, consequences and therapeutic opportunities. *Nat Rev Cancer* 2002;2:584–593.

CHAPTER 6 ■ ANATOMY AND PATHOLOGY OF PROSTATE CANCER

CHAPTER 6A
Anatomy of the Prostate and the Pathology of Prostate Cancer

Gustavo Ayala and Thomas M. Wheeler

INTRODUCTION

Interest in the anatomy of the prostate and how anatomic considerations relate to the origin, development, and evolution of prostate cancer has enjoyed a renaissance in urology and pathology in the past several decades. This renewed interest was made possible primarily by the availability of whole prostates from radical prostatectomy, a procedure that began to replace irradiation therapy as the treatment of choice for clinically localized prostate cancer in men with a reasonable life expectancy. This chapter focuses on general anatomic considerations as well as the concept of zonal anatomy of the prostate as developed by McNeal. A wide variety of interrelated anatomic features affect not only the overall morphologic assessment by the pathologist but also the natural history of prostate cancer.

EMBRYOLOGY AND DEVELOPMENT OF THE ADULT PROSTATE

The human prostate develops from epithelial invaginations from the prostatic urethra during the third month of gestation under the influence of the underlying mesenchyme (1). Indeed, this specialized mesenchyme may induce prostatic development if transplanted at the proper stage of development underneath the epithelium of another site (2). This inductive effect of the mesenchyme is analogous to that in the development of the human breast. Normal prostatic development requires the presence of 5α-dihydrotestosterone, which is produced from testosterone by the action of the enzyme 5α-reductase. This enzyme is localized in the urogenital sinus and external genitalia of humans (3). Men with an inherited deficiency of 5α-reductase have a rudimentary or undetectable prostate in addition to severe abnormalities of the external genitalia, although the epididymides, vasa deferentia, and seminal vesicles are normal (4).

The structure of the prostate remains relatively unchanged in the prepubertal period but begins to undergo the morphologic changes necessary to transform the organ into the adult phenotype at the time of puberty; from this time, the organ increases steadily in size to reach the adult weight of approximately 20 g by 25 to 30 years of age (1).

NORMAL ANATOMY AND HISTOLOGY OF THE PROSTATE

For the better part of this century, the gross anatomic interrelationships in the prostate have been a matter of controversy. Various investigators, in comparing the human prostate to those of laboratory animals, developed the concept of distinct lobes (1,5). This concept became popular despite the fact that no distinct lobes can be seen in the normal adult prostate. More recently, McNeal has championed the concept of zones rather than lobes (6–8), a theory that is currently the most widely accepted. In this model, the prostate is divided into four distinct zones: the peripheral zone, which comprises the bulk of the normal adult prostate (70% of glandular tissue); the central zone (20% of the glandular tissue); the transition zone (5% of the glandular tissue); and the nonglandular anterior fibromuscular stroma (AFMS) (Figs. 6A.1 and 6A.2).

The peripheral zone comprises all of the prostatic glandular tissue at the apex and essentially all of the prostatic tissue located posteriorly near the capsule. This is the region of the prostate most susceptible to carcinoma, chronic prostatitis, and postinflammatory atrophy. The columnar epithelium lining the glands and ducts in this zone becomes flattened in elderly men, which has been referred to as *age-related atrophy*. The central zone is a cone-shaped zone, with the apex of the cone at the confluence of the ejaculatory ducts and the prostatic urethra at the verumontanum, a ridge of tissue on the posterior aspect of the lower third of the prostatic urethra. The central zone surrounds the ejaculatory duct complex (ejaculatory ducts, specialized loose stroma, and, sometimes, the utricle) all the way from the verumontanum up to the origin of the seminal vesicles and ampulla of the vas, which comprises the base of the cone. Well-defined tissue planes separating the peripheral zone from the central zone are not clearly visible on sections of the prostate taken in a plane perpendicular to the rectal surface by pathologists for diagnostic purposes.

The transition zone consists of two equal portions of glandular tissue lateral to the urethra in the midprostate, just superior to the point at which the urethra angles anteriorly by approximately 35 degrees. This is the portion of the prostate most susceptible to the development of age-related glandular-stromal hyperplasia and the site of a minority of all clinical carcinomas [although the majority of carcinomas are detected as incidental findings on transurethral resection of the prostate (TURP)] (9). The boundary of the transition zone and the peripheral zone is the surgical capsule, a coalition of fibromuscular stroma that becomes more and more apparent as the transition zone is increasingly affected with nodular hyperplasia. The AFMS accounts for the convexity of the anterior external surface. The apical half of the AFMS is rich in striated muscle, which blends into the glandular prostate and the muscle of the pelvic diaphragm. Toward the bladder neck, however, the striated muscle gives way to smooth muscle, which blends

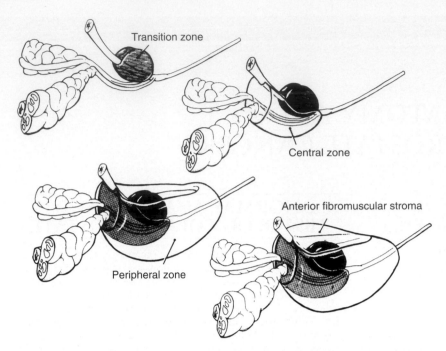

FIGURE 6A.1. Zonal anatomy of the normal prostate as described by McNeal. The transition zone comprises only 5% to 10% of the glandular tissue in the young male. The central zone forms part of the base of the prostate and is traversed by the ejaculatory ducts. The greatest portion of the glandular tissue of the prostate is constituted by the peripheral zone, particularly distal to the verumontanum. (From Greene DR, Shabsigh R, Scardino PT. Urologic ultrasonography. In: Walsh PC, Retik AB, Stamey TA, et al., eds. *Campbell's urology*, 6th ed. Philadelphia: WB Saunders, 1992:342–393, with permission.)

into the fibers of the bladder neck (10). Presumably, the distal portion of the AFMS is important in voluntary sphincter functions, and the proximal portion of the AFMS is important in involuntary sphincter functions.

The histology of the prostate is that of a branched duct gland. Each gland or duct is lined by two cell layers: a luminal secretory columnar cell layer, which is adorned with antibodies to prostate-specific antigen (PSA) and prostate-specific acid phosphatase (PSAP), and an underlying basal cell layer, which probably constitutes a reserve cell function. These cells are decorated specifically by an antibody to high-molecular-weight keratin (clone 34β-E12) (11). The normal prostatic glands and ducts also contain scattered neuroendocrine cells, which are embellished by a variety of antibodies (e.g., serotonin and other neuroendocrine markers)

(12–14). The precise function of these cells is unknown, although they presumably serve a paracrine function. In the adult prostate, the ducts cannot be distinguished from the acini except by location or in the presence of certain disease states (e.g., postinflammatory atrophy) (7). The acini of the transition zone and the peripheral zone are similar to each other morphologically. The acini of the central zone, however, particularly at the base of the prostate, tend to be much larger (up to 0.6 mm) and have delicate papillary infoldings (7). The lining of the prostatic urethra is frequently columnar, similar to that of the ducts and acini. Less commonly, it is transitional in type, similar to that of the urinary bladder. After TURP, the lining of the urethra usually is converted to nonkeratinizing squamous epithelium. Periurethral glands are scattered along the prostatic urethra and the most proximal portions of the large ducts, draining the peripheral zone and the most proximal portions of the ejaculatory duct complex. The periurethral glands consist of tiny ducts and acini that drain directly into the prostatic urethra. These glands may undergo hyperplasia in the region of the verumontanum, a process that has been called *verumontanum mucosal gland hyperplasia* (15). This microacinar proliferation is distinct from nodular hyperplasia but is only a microscopic curiosity—clinical symptoms and signs do not develop because the area of abnormality is so small.

The lumens of otherwise normal prostatic glands and ducts frequently contain multilaminated eosinophilic concretions, termed *corpora amylacea*, that become more common in older men. Calculi are much larger than corpora amylacea and have a predilection for the ducts that traverse the length of the surgical capsule, separating the transition and peripheral zones. Intraluminal crystalloids and acid mucin may be seen in benign glands but are much more common in carcinoma (16). Myoepithelial cells are not present in the normal prostate and functionally should not be required, because the prostatic stroma is in itself contractile fibromuscular tissue.

The prostate is partially invested by a coalition of fibrous tissue, most apparent posteriorly and posterolaterally, that historically has been called the *capsule*. Although the term seems embedded in the literature and common parlance, some investigators doubt the presence of a true capsule (17). The smooth muscle of the prostatic stroma only gradually

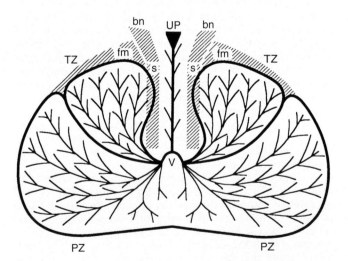

FIGURE 6A.2. Oblique coronal section diagram of prostate, showing location of peripheral zone (PZ) and transition zone (TZ) in relation to proximal urethral segment (UP), verumontanum (V), preprostatic sphincter (s), fibromuscular tissue (fm), bladder neck (bn), and periurethral region with periurethral glands. Branching pattern of prostatic ducts is indicated. The medial transition-zone ducts penetrate into the sphincter. (From McNeal JE. Normal histology of the prostate. *Am J Surg Pathol* 1988;12:621, with permission.)

and not abruptly fades into this fibrous tissue called the capsule. On the other side of this capsule is either a very loose connective tissue or adipose tissue. All investigators agree, however, that no such capsule exists at the apex of the gland or anteriorly. In these locations, the determination of extraprostatic spread of cancer is somewhat arbitrary. McNeal's group devised a classification system to describe the invasiveness of prostate cancer with respect to the capsule (18). Epstein's group added subclassifications for extraprostatic extension (19). The author has modified it somewhat, as shown in (Fig. 6A.3) (20). The levels of prostatic capsular invasion are L0, L1, L2, L3 focal (L3F), and L3 established (L3E) and are defined as follows:

Confined

Level 0 (L0): tumor confined to prostatic stroma within the boundary of normal prostatic acini.

Level 1 (L1): tumor confined to prostatic stroma but outside the boundary of normal prostatic acini.

Level 2 (L2): tumor confined to the prostate but within a layer more fibrous than muscular (capsule).

Not confined

Level 3 (L3): tumor invasive into the periprostatic adipose tissue or smooth muscle of the bladder neck.

Level 3 focal (L3F): tumor outside the prostate to a depth of less than one high-power field on no more than two separate sections.

Level 3 established (L3E): any amount of extraprostatic tumor more than L3F.

According to the staging of the International Union Against Cancer (UICC) and American Joint Commission on Cancer (AJCC), tumors at levels 0 to 2 are considered pathologically *confined* and level 3 is considered pathologically *not confined* to the prostate (21).

The seminal vesicles are located superior to the base of the prostate and undergo confluence with the vas deferens on each side to form the ejaculatory ducts. The seminal vesicles are resistant to most of the disease processes that affect the prostate. Invasion of the seminal vesicles by prostate cancer is one of the most important prognostic indicators in this disease

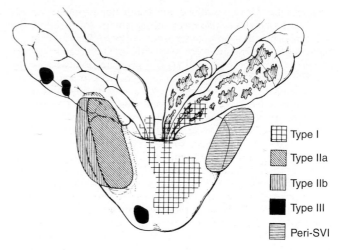

Type I
Type IIa
Type IIb
Type III
Peri-SVI

FIGURE 6A.4. Diagrammatic representation of the three patterns of seminal vesicle involvement (SVI) and peri-SVI. The combination of types I and II is categorized as type I + II. (From Ohori M, Scardino PT, Lapin SL, et al. The mechanisms and prognostic significance of seminal vesicle involvement by prostate cancer. *Am J Surg Pathol* 1993;17:1253, with permission.)

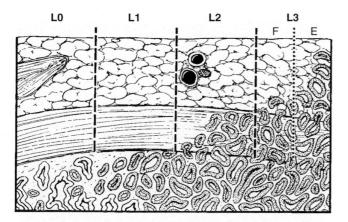

FIGURE 6A.3. Levels of prostatic capsular invasion. (See text for definitions.) Extraprostatic extension designated as L3 signifies extension of tumor into periprostatic soft tissue, which may be subclassified as focal (L3F) or established (L3E). The sharpness of the boundaries between prostatic stroma, capsule, and adipose tissue is exaggerated for clarity. (From Stamey TA, McNeal JE, Freiha FS, et al. Morphometric and clinical studies on 68 consecutive radical prostatectomies. *J Urol* 1988;139:1235–1241; from Wheeler TM. Anatomic considerations in carcinoma of the prostate. *Urol Clin North Am* 1989;16:623–634, with permission.)

and is defined as involvement of the muscularis layer (not simply of the fat adjacent to the seminal vesicles) by tumor (22,23). Most commonly, prostate cancer involves the seminal vesicles by extension up the loose connective tissue of the ejaculatory ducts (type I). The second most common mechanism of involvement is from across the base of the prostate directly into the seminal vesicles (type IIa) or retrograde extension of tumor into the seminal vesicles along nerves in the periprostatic fat (type IIb). Many tumors are large enough to involve the seminal vesicles by more than one mechanism (type I + II). Both type I and type II are the result of spread of tumor in direct contiguity to tumor in the prostate. Rarely, tumor may appear in the seminal vesicles as isolated deposits (type III); in these cases, it is considered to represent metastases or, perhaps, regression of tumor between the prostatic primary site and the focus in the seminal vesicles (Fig. 6A.4). Surprisingly, in one series, seminal vesicle involvement by a type III mechanism had the best prognosis and was associated with tumors of generally smaller volume (23).

NEUROANATOMY OF THE PROSTATE

The prostate is a richly innervated organ, but only the recognition by Walsh and Donker of the importance of these nerves in penile erection and their promotion of operative techniques designed to spare these nerves during radical prostatectomy renewed interest in the surgical treatment of prostate cancer (24). McNeal has described a large superior and smaller inferior pedicle of nerves that supply the nerves entering the prostate at the base and apex of the gland, respectively (8). The superior pedicle also includes many autonomic ganglia. These nerves penetrate the prostate on the posterolateral surface. Within the prostate, the nerves travel along the inner face of the capsule for a small distance and then arborize into the prostatic parenchyma (25).

The prostate receives dual autonomic innervation through the hypogastric and pelvic nerves. The sympathetic innervation derives from short adrenergic neurons from a peripherally located hypogastric ganglion. Ganglia containing acetylcholinesterase (AchE) activity and numerous neuropeptide reactivity have also been observed in and around the prostate. The autonomic innervations of peripheral and central regions of the prostate were very similar. The greatest density of nerves is in the proximal central prostate, followed by the anterior capsule and the least in the peripheral portions of the prostate (26). The nerve fibers associated with smooth muscle were immunoreactive with neuropeptide Y (NPY) and noradrenergic nerves, whereas those found in the subepithelial plexi were AchE (cholinergic) and vasointestinal polypeptide (VIP) positive (26–31). The most common types of fibers were AchE fibers followed by VIP. Jungblut et al. reported that the density of innervation decreases with age (32), and Chapple (27) found a similar phenomenon in benign prostatic hyperplasia (BPH) with decrease in most areas except for the peripheral zone.

Nerves are involved in the development of the organ, its morphology, and its functional maintenance (33–39). The autonomic nervous system plays a role in the growth maturation and secretory functions of the prostate. Several authors have shown that mechanical and/or chemical denervation (35) of the pelvic plexus of Sprague-Dawley and Wistar rats causes morphologic and functional changes of the prostate (40). With light microscopy, histologic features of the denervated prostate showed an overall decrease in cell height and a reduction of secretory changes (41,42). These findings strongly suggest that prostate function is not subject solely to the regulatory influence of the hormonal milieu: "It is also dependent on the anatomical and, quite possibly functional, integrity of the nervous system" (43–45). While unilateral sympathectomy leads to decreases in ventral prostate weight, DNA, and protein content in the lesioned side, unilateral parasympathectomy leads to increases in the intact side (46).

PATHOLOGY OF PROSTATE CARCINOMA

Cancer of the prostate is now the most commonly diagnosed nonskin cancer in men in the United States and is the second leading cause of cancer death. Between 1985 and 1995, the number of cases of prostate cancer identified in the United States increased by a dramatic 50%, due largely to improved detection using screening for serum PSA levels (47). Adenocarcinoma and its variants account for at least 98% of all prostate cancers and therefore command nearly all of the discussion in the rest of this section (48).

Morphologic Diagnosis of Prostate Adenocarcinoma

In the authors' experience, prostate cancers must be at least 5 mm in diameter for reliable gross identification, although much larger tumors may be difficult or impossible to see with the naked eye. Although the color of most cancers is tan-white, the minority of tumors that are yellow are the most distinctive. In the author's experience, such tumors are more common in the transition zone and, as such, may be seen on gross inspection of chips of prostatic tissue removed transurethrally or by open suprapubic prostatectomy. Most grossly recognized tumors are firm to palpation, but a minority are fleshy and soft; these latter tumors are usually very high grade. Most palpable tumors are easy to identify grossly. Nonpalpable tumors diagnosed because of elevated serum PSA levels, however, may not be grossly apparent.

The microscopic diagnosis of adenocarcinoma on histologic sections is based on both architectural criteria (from low magnification) and cytologic criteria (morphology of the individual cell under high magnification) (49). This is an important point because some lesions, such as atypical adenomatous hyperplasia, may fulfill architectural criteria for malignancy as a microacinar proliferation with back-to-back glands and minimally infiltrative borders (50,51) and yet the individual cells may lack the cytologic criteria of malignancy. On the other hand, other lesions, such as prostatic intraepithelial neoplasia (PIN), may fulfill the cytologic criteria of malignancy without satisfying the architectural criteria (52,53). These cytologically dysplastic or even malignant-appearing nuclei are confined by a basement membrane and basal cell layer of a preexisting benign duct or acinus. PIN is discussed in detail in Chapter 6B.

Well-differentiated adenocarcinoma is characterized by a proliferation of microacinar structures lined by prostatic luminal cells without an accompanying basal cell layer. At least some of the neoplastic cells contain prominent nucleoli, defined as at least 1 μm in diameter by Gleason but as larger by other investigators (49,54,55). Epstein, however, believes that, in certain circumstances, the diagnosis of adenocarcinoma in biopsy material may be made without nucleoli if the lesion is otherwise typical of cancer in its infiltrative growth pattern and the nuclei are sufficiently hyperchromatic to obscure underlying nucleoli (56). An infiltrative growth pattern is difficult to define precisely because it may involve only a subtle departure from the normal stromal-glandular relationships. At the apex of the gland, skeletal muscle fibers interweave into a somewhat disorganized prostatic stroma that in normal prostate glands may appear to have an invasive growth pattern. This can make evaluation of the apical surgical margin by frozen section at the time of surgery problematic in cases of well-differentiated adenocarcinoma. In the rest of the gland, however, the normal stromal-glandular relationships usually are reasonably straightforward. Small foci of well-differentiated adenocarcinoma show microacini that appear to split the fibromuscular stromal cells. The leading edge of the tumor may show microacini with a rounded profile on the trailing edge and a pointed profile on the leading edge (Fig. 6A.5).

Another helpful feature in low magnification is a haphazard or random distribution of the individual glands in the microacinar proliferation, as seen in well-differentiated adenocarcinoma. Many benign microacinar proliferations that can be confused with carcinoma have a nonrandom appearance

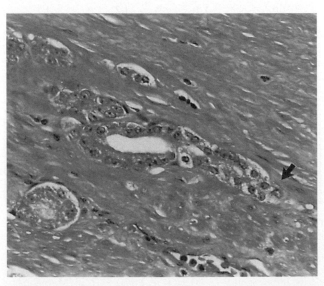

FIGURE 6A.5. Photomicrograph of prostate adenocarcinoma demonstrating an invasive growth pattern with respect to the stroma. Leading edge of infiltration is noted by an arrow. (Hematoxylin and eosin, ×200.)

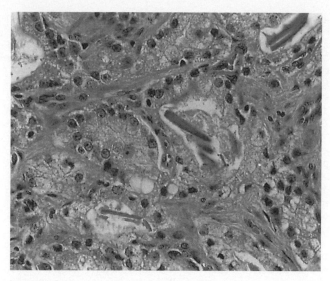

FIGURE 6A.6. Photomicrograph of prostate adenocarcinoma demonstrating intraluminal crystalloids and pale-staining mucin within the lumens of the malignant glands. (Hematoxylin and eosin, ×200.)

under low magnification and normal glandular-stromal relationships under high magnification. Skeletal muscle fibers at the apex or anteriorly in the apical half of the gland frequently are juxtaposed to or surrounded by nonneoplastic glands. Intraluminal acidic mucin or eosinophilic crystalloids or both are supportive but not diagnostic of well-differentiated adenocarcinoma because they may sometimes be encountered in benign glands (56–64) (Fig. 6A.6).

Perineural Invasion

The most common interaction between nerves and prostate epithelium is perineural invasion (PNI). PNI is a very common phenomenon in human prostate cancer, as it is found in more than 85% of cases radical prostatectomy specimens (25). Complete surrounding of a nerve by a glandular structure is diagnostic of adenocarcinoma, although a benign gland occasionally may be located immediately adjacent to a nerve (65). Its biological significance is related to offering a pathway for prostate cancer (PCa) expansion through the thick prostatic capsule. However, the mechanisms involved in PNI are poorly understood. During most of this century, PNI was thought to represent invasion of perineural lymphatics. This concept was later discredited when no lymphatics were found in the perineural space (66). These authors then concluded that the "spread of malignant tumors along nerves in the prostate and elsewhere is not within preformed lymphatics but within tissue planes of least resistance." It is now known that PNI is a symbiotic relationship between the nerves and the cancer cells, which results in growth and survival advantage for both (67). It is likely that a series of biological and molecular events result in interactions between nerves and cancer cells, which end in perineural invasion. The stimulation of growth is further enhanced in the presence of prostatic stroma (68). This survival advantage was based on a decrease in apoptotic rate and increased proliferation in PCa in perineural locations as compared to PCa away from the nerve (69).

The clinical significance of perineural invasion and its prognostic capabilities are questioned in the literature. In 1972, Mostofi found that "perineural invasion had no significant effect on prognosis" (70). Thereafter, numerous other authors have found varying degrees of clinical prognostic significance to perineural invasion. Ravery and van den Ouden reported that perineural invasion in radical prostatectomy

specimens predicts progression as demonstrated by univariate analysis, but not multivariate analysis (71,72). De la Taille found that presence of perineural invasion in biopsies is correlated with PSA progression after radical prostatectomy treatment (73,74), and Anderson found that it is also a predictor of failure in patients treated with conformal external beam radiation therapy (75). Bastacky (76) and Epstein (77) found that the presence of perineural invasion in biopsies is correlated with capsular penetration in clinical stage B adenocarcinoma of the prostate. McNeal found that large volumes of perineural tumor diameters (>0.5 mm) showed an adverse effect on recurrence when the volume of Gleason pattern 4 or 5 elements was <1.8 mL (78,79).

In a retrospective study of clinical and pathologic features in 640 consecutive patients with clinical stage T1a-T3bNXM0 prostate cancer treated with radical prostatectomy, we demonstrated that the volume of tumor around the nerve, labeled as the PNI diameter, was an independent predictor of survival. The perineural invasion diameter was defined as the diameter of perineural cancer cells in the largest focus of perineural invasion and was measured using an ocular micrometer perpendicular to the long axis of the Schwann cell nuclei in the nerve. PNI invasion was observed in 75% of the patients, but the presence of PNI was not an independent predictor of progression. However, PNI diameter was not only associated with other established prognostic parameters but also with recurrence-free survival as an independent predictor with a hazard ratio of 2.4. Patients with PNI <0.25 mm had a good survival, whereas recurrence-free survival diminished progressively with increased PNI diameter (80).

The larger the PNI diameter, the greater the risk of recurrence is, suggesting that not all perineural invasions are equal and that proximity to the nerve might provide advantage for PCa cell growth and survival to different degrees. Those that are most successful show more growth and aggressiveness. Some cancers can make better use of the growth and survival advantage mechanism provided by the perineural microenvironment, the manifestation of which is increased tumor volume around the nerve.

Perineural invasion may be very useful in confirming a diagnosis of adenocarcinoma in small biopsy specimens (56).

Immunohistochemistry

Immunohistochemical analysis may at times be a valuable adjunct in the diagnosis of prostate adenocarcinoma. The two most commonly used primary antibodies are those to PSA and to high-molecular-weight, basal cell–specific keratin (clone 34β-E12). PSA immunohistochemical analysis is most often used to distinguish prostate adenocarcinoma from other types of cancer. The most common scenario in which a pathologist uses PSA staining in the prostate would be to distinguish poorly differentiated adenocarcinoma from transitional cell carcinoma extending down the prostatic ducts. More commonly, however, PSA immunohistochemical analysis is used on deposits of metastatic tumor to confirm the origin of the tumor in the prostate. Fortunately, PSA immunohistochemical analysis is both highly sensitive and highly specific in the applications mentioned (81,82). PSAP also is useful in immunohistochemical analysis, but occasional false-positive results are seen with various neuroendocrine tumors, such as islet cell tumors or rectal carcinoids (83–85). Basal cell–specific keratin immunohistochemical analysis is sometimes used to differentiate various benign small acinar proliferations (e.g., atypical adenomatous hyperplasia) from well-differentiated adenocarcinoma (51).

By definition, adenocarcinoma of the prostate does not show basal cell differentiation, in contrast to most of the microacinar proliferations with which it can be confused. By definition, a focus of PIN shows at least some preservation of the basal cell layer, which may be difficult to appreciate on the hematoxylin and eosin (H&E)-stained section. Basal cell–specific keratin immunohistochemical analysis may be used to distinguish a focus of high-grade PIN from a focus of infiltrating cribriform adenocarcinoma of the prostate (52).

The use of immunohistochemical analysis in diagnosing prostate cancer and determining its prognosis of PCa has grown recently. p63 has been added to the markers of basal cells (86,87). Alpha-methylacyl-CoA racemase (AAMCR) was identified using expression profiling as preferentially expressed in prostate cancer as compared to normal prostate and confirmed using tissue microarrays (88–90). Combinations of high molecular weight cytokeratin (HMWK), p63, and AAMCR have been proposed to distinguish small foci of prostate cancer in prostate biopsies (91).

Grading of Prostate Adenocarcinoma

In the United States, the most widely used and generally accepted grading system is that proposed by Gleason (Fig. 6A.7) (92). This grading system is architectural and is performed under low to medium magnification without specific regard to the high-magnification cytologic features of the individual cancer cells. For the most part, the architectural grade roughly parallels the cytologic grade; however, it is much more rapidly determined, because the different Gleason patterns can be recognized quickly under low magnification. Because prostate cancer is usually heterogeneous, with two or more grades in a given cancer, Gleason chose to incorporate both a primary (most prevalent) and secondary (next most prevalent) grade into his system. The primary grade or pattern is added to the secondary grade or pattern to arrive at a Gleason score. If the tumor is homogeneous with respect to Gleason grade, as may happen not infrequently in needle-biopsy material, the primary and secondary grades are the same, and they would be added together to obtain the Gleason score. Because five distinct grades or patterns are recognized on a scale from 1 to 5 (from well differentiated to poorly differentiated), the total score possibilities range from 2 (1 + 1) to 10 (5 + 5). A problem arises, however, when multiple grades of cancer exist within a single prostate. Byar and Mostofi reported multifocal tumor in 85% of 208 step-sectioned radical prostatectomy specimens, and this has been the authors' experience as well (70). Aihara et al. in a study of 101 completely embedded radical prostatectomy specimens, found that the average number of grades was 2.7 (range, 1 to 5) (93). More than 50% of the prostates contained at least three different grades of cancer. The larger tumors were more likely to contain multiple grades than were the smaller tumors.

This system is the most widely used, but problems have arisen because the majority of patients fall within Gleason 7 category, an intermediate prognostic category. In order to address this, numerous authors have looked at the most prevalent grade within the score, either 3 or 4.

Patients with a Gleason score of 4 + 3 have reduced biochemical free survival as compared to those with Gleason 3 + 4 (94,95). This is probably a manifestation of high-grade tumor burden relative to low-grade tumor burden. However, it seems that even small amounts of high-grade tumor (less than 5% Gleason score 4 or 5) have an impact on prognosis (96). The tertiary Gleason increases risk for progression in PCa.

Another grading system that relies on architecture alone is that proposed in 1982 by Brawn et al. which has become known as the M.D. Anderson grading system, after the institution in which it was first applied (97). This system recognizes four grades based on the percentage of the total tumor that shows glandular differentiation and is only a slight modification of the original Broders grading system (98,99).

In 1975, Mostofi et al. recommended a grading system that takes into account both low-power architectural considerations and high-power assessment of nuclear anaplasia (100). In a subsequent study of nearly 1000 patients, they demonstrated good stratification of death rates from each of the separate components of this grading system (101). This grading system has been adopted by the World Health Organization (WHO), the UICC, and the AJCC. For approved cancer programs in the United States, the grade of the tumor must be reported according to this system. In point of fact, most tumor registrars attempt to translate the Gleason scores into three groups: well, moderately, and poorly differentiated. Unfortunately, the precise cut points in the scale of Gleason scores used to make these three divisions is not uniform from center to center and remains a point of debate.

A new system to grade prostate cancer has recently been introduced. This system is based on the quantification of reactive stroma within the PCa. Although reactive stroma is easy to quantify in other organs, PCa has remained an exception. Reactive stroma is easily detectable in most organs because the transformation from a fibroblast to a myofibroblast has obvious morphologic consequences. The cells become plumper, the cytoplasm denser, and the inorganic fibrillar compartment expands. Because the stroma in the prostate is already muscular, the reverse process occurs: dedifferentiation of smooth muscle cells give rise to myofibroblasts that have the plasticity and production capability to support cancer growth (102,103). These functional changes have little morphologic translation at the H&E level but become obvious on trichrome stains.

The relative volume of intratumoral stroma was graded as 0 if less than 5% of the tumor was stroma, grade 1 if 5% to 15%, grade 2 if 15% to 50%, and grade 3 if more than 50% of the tumor was stroma. Stroma volume grading was an independent predictor in tumors containing stroma, defined as Gleason 7 and lower grades. Of interest, tumors with either little to no stroma (grade 0) or tumors with abundant stroma (grade 3) each showed reduced recurrence-free survival as compared to those with intermediate amounts of stroma (104). Because the stroma has support function for cancer growth (growth factor production through paracrine axis), the more stroma a tumor has, the more aggressive it behaves. Once epithelial mesenchymal-epithelial transformation occurs and the tumor produces the factors that the stroma was previously producing, the cancer also has an aggressive behavior.

Attempts to further refine grading systems have largely given way to exploration of other surrogate markers, such as ploidy and proliferation markers, nuclear morphometry, and various immunohistochemical markers. At this time, however, these markers appear to be only adjuncts to grading and are therefore unlikely to replace histologic grading in the foreseeable future.

Zonal Anatomy and Prostate Adenocarcinoma

Since the late 1980s, attention has been focused on the zonal anatomy and its relationship to prostate adenocarcinoma. Previously, nearly all prostate cancers had been thought to arise posteriorly in close proximity to the prostatic capsule (105, 106). Franks considered that these cancers arose from areas of small-gland atrophy (105). Later, however, McNeal focused attention on high-grade duct-acinar dysplasia (now known as *high-grade PIN*) as the probable precursor lesion for most adenocarcinomas of the prostate (53,107–114). This lesion is

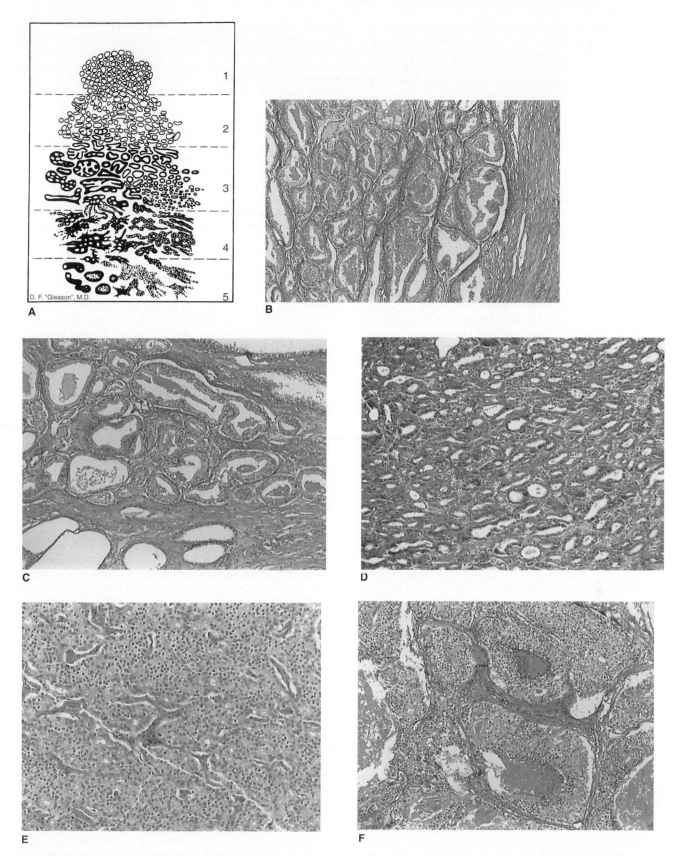

FIGURE 6A.7. A: Simplified drawing of histologic patterns of prostatic adenocarcinoma, emphasizing the degree of glandular differentiation and relation to stroma. All black in the drawing represents tumor tissue, with all cytologic detail obscured except in the right side of pattern 4, where tiny structures are intended to suggest the hypernephroid pattern. **B:** Photomicrograph of representative examples of Gleason grade 1. **C:** Gleason grade 2. **D:** Gleason grade 3. **E:** Gleason grade 4. **F:** Gleason grade 5. (Hematoxylin and eosin, ×100.) (From Gleason DF. Histologic grading of prostatic adenocarcinoma. In: Tannenbaum M, ed. *Urologic pathology: The prostate.* Philadelphia: Lea & Febiger, 1977:181, with permission.)

nearly always present in prostates removed for adenocarcinoma and is frequently located topographically within or adjacent to clinical adenocarcinomas arising in the peripheral zone (20,52,53,114). High-grade PIN is rare in the transition zone, however, and therefore may not be the usual precursor lesion for adenocarcinomas arising in this location (110,114).

Recently, De Marzo has revived the concept of atrophic glands (inflammatory atrophy) as preneoplastic lesions of the prostate (115–118). Although hypermethylation of the human *glutathione-S-transferase-pi* gene (*GSTP1*) CpG island is present in a subset of proliferative inflammatory atrophy lesions, it is absent in normal or hyperplastic epithelium of the prostate (119). However, differences in nomenclature and standardization of diagnostic criteria have made it difficult to confirm the results. In our experience, the frequency of atrophy (postatrophic hyperplasia) in radical prostatectomy specimens is similar in areas of cancer compared to their mirror image in the specimen (120).

When TURP led to the discovery of clinically unsuspected adenocarcinoma of the prostate, many investigators assumed that these cancers had begun near the prostatic capsule and had subsequently invaded the inner aspects of the gland. The inner prostate had been considered to be resistant to the development of cancer, although it was quite susceptible to the development of nodular hyperplasia. Subsequent systematic study of radical prostatectomy specimens, however, revealed that a substantial minority of clinically detected prostate adenocarcinomas actually began in the transition zone, not infrequently within a nodule of nodular hyperplasia. In a series of 108 radical prostatectomy specimens, McNeal et al. were able to assign a zone of origin of the cancer as follows: 68% peripheral zone, 24% transition zone, and 8% central zone (9). It had been noted earlier that most cancers detected by TURP were located anteriorly in the gland, a fact partly responsible for the nonpalpability of these tumors (121). McNeal, however, showed that nearly all of these tumors detected by TURP were, in fact, cancers that had their origin in the transition zone, although very large nonpalpable peripheral-zone cancers may be detected in this way as well. In comparing the histopathology of transition-zone versus nontransition-zone cancers, McNeal et al. noted that transition-zone tumors frequently showed a distinctive morphology composed of individual glands having a single layer of tall columnar cells with pale cytoplasm and basally placed nuclei and would fit into Gleason patterns 1 and 2 (9). Pattern 1 is the result of the growth of these well-differentiated tumors within preexisting nodules of nodular hyperplasia. The condensed fibromuscular stroma separating these nodules confines the tumor somewhat to give it a pushing margin.

Greene et al. confirmed McNeal's findings concerning the distinctive morphology of transition-zone tumors and, in addition, showed that these tumors were significantly better differentiated than tumors in the peripheral zone of the prostate, whether from the same prostate or from a series of prostates removed with clinical stage T2 cancer (the latter nearly always contained peripheral-zone cancer as the index tumor) (114). These transition-zone tumors also were shown to less frequently give rise to lymph node metastases and rarely to be associated with capsular penetration or seminal vesicle involvement. McNeal and his group argued that this was the result of prostate architecture alone because the transition-zone tumors were located anteriorly and the anterior fibromuscular stroma was considerably thicker than the posterior capsule, and the tumors were located away from the ejaculatory duct complex, the most common route by which prostate cancers involve the seminal

vesicles. They concluded that clinical stage T1a, T1b, and T2 cancers were "biologically similar tumors, distinguished only by their site of origin" (9). Greene and Wheeler, however, believed that these tumors were inherently different, because transition-zone tumors tended to be better differentiated, even though these were frequently large tumors and were much more likely to be diploid than peripheral-zone tumors (122). In comparing clinical stage T1a and T1b cancers with T2 cancers, Greene et al. noted that the majority of clinical stage T1a and T1b tumors arose in the transition zone, and nearly all T2 cancers arose in the peripheral zone. However, transition-zone tumors within the T1a and T1b subset nearly always had a clinically silent peripheral-zone cancer (93%), which, although smaller, was of significantly higher grade than the index transition-zone cancer (114). In contrast, peripheral-zone cancers in the T2 subset were associated with transition-zone tumors in only 43% of cases. Greene et al. argued that perhaps the main significance of transition-zone cancers detected by TURP lies in the great likelihood of an associated higher grade peripheral-zone cancer (114). Indeed, the progression of untreated clinical T1a or T1b cancer possibly may be due to growth of the unrecognized peripheral-zone cancer rather than growth of any transition-zone cancer left behind after the TURP. For this reason, a restaging TURP after the discovery of T1a or T1b cancer is considered useless because the residual tumor is located posteriorly or at the apex: sites not removed during the procedure.

Treatment Effects on Primary Prostate Adenocarcinoma

Definitive radiation therapy for prostate cancer may induce changes in the residual nonneoplastic ducts and acini that may be confused with adenocarcinoma histologically by the uninitiated (123). The nonneoplastic ducts and acini have nuclei that may be greatly enlarged and hyperchromatic, with conspicuous nucleoli. The basal cell layer usually becomes very prominent, however, thus precluding a consideration of adenocarcinoma (Fig. 6A.8A). Squamous metaplasia is common. The tumor may show a marked irradiation-induced cytopathic effect, which may make a few widely scattered tumor cells difficult to recognize, particularly when the nuclei have become shrunken and the cytoplasm is feathery and finely vacuolated (Fig. 6A.8B). Also, the irradiation may cause the residual tumor to appear artifactually to be of a higher Gleason score because of loss of architectural features of the gland-forming tumor. Often, the individual tumor cells appear so damaged by the radiation therapy that one could wonder whether such tumor cells are viable or capable of proliferation. In a large series of patients treated with definitive irradiation, Scardino et al. found that the presence of any tumor on biopsy 1 year or more after treatment carried with it a substantially increased likelihood of distant relapse, whether or not the tumor appeared viable (124). One study, however, has demonstrated that the morphologic appearance of the tumor after radiation therapy does correlate with prognosis (125).

Endocrine therapy may take several forms: orchiectomy, estrogen administration, or androgen ablation therapy (126–129). The resulting changes are similar histologically. The nonneoplastic ducts and acini show flattening of the epithelium with shrunken nuclei, giving the cells an atrophic appearance, although the basal cell layer may become more prominent. The residual tumor may show loss of luminal architecture, cytoplasmic vacuolization, nuclear pyknosis, and decreased prominence or absence of nucleoli. This type of treatment may also cause artifactual progression of the Gleason score. Estrogen

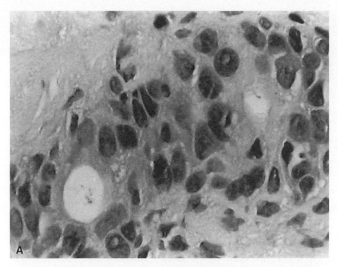

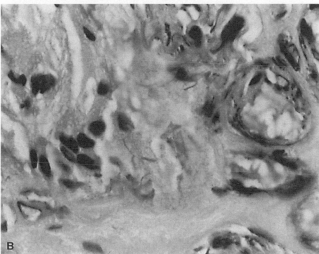

FIGURE 6A.8. **A:** Photomicrograph of postirradiation residual non-neoplastic gland with marked nuclear enlargement and pleomorphism, with focally prominent nucleoli. (Hematoxylin and eosin, ×400.) **B:** Photomicrograph of postirradiation, markedly degenerated residual adenocarcinoma showing nuclear pyknosis, cytoplasmic vacuolization, and loss of glandular architecture. (Hematoxylin and eosin, ×400.)

administration may cause squamous metaplasia in the nonneoplastic glands.

Neoadjuvant total androgen ablation therapy has been used in an attempt to downstage the tumor before radical prostatectomy. In a series from Memorial Hospital in New York, 3 months of neoadjuvant total androgen ablation therapy was followed by radical prostatectomy (130). Residual tumor was identified histologically in all 27 patients in the radical prostatectomy specimen, although it was extremely focal and difficult to recognize in 7 cases (26%). If this becomes an accepted preoperative therapy, pathologists will have to become proficient at recognizing adenocarcinoma that has been altered in this way.

Different types of gene therapy have been used in prostate cancer with varying success. However, morphologic changes associated with therapy have only been described associated to HSV-tk/gancicolvirsuicide gene therapy. Loss of glandular architecture (fusion or dissolution), increased apoptosis/necrosis, as well as groups of degenerating cells in a dense hyalinized stroma were described. Loss of nuclear detail and nucleoli

and nuclear pyknosis were identified at higher magnification. An increased inflammatory response was also identified (131).

Differential Diagnosis of Prostate Adenocarcinoma

Although most investigators consider PIN, and some investigators consider atypical adenomatous hyperplasia, to be a precursor lesion to prostate adenocarcinoma, a number of completely benign lesions may be mistaken for adenocarcinoma under the microscope. Detailed discussion of the recognition and differential diagnosis of PIN is presented in Chapter 6B.

Whatever the mimic, however, the likelihood that the pathologist will overdiagnose malignancy probably decreases as the size of the biopsy material increases; for example, the likelihood is probably lower for a TURP specimen than for a cytologic smear obtained by fine-needle aspiration.

The two most common reasons for confusing benign conditions with carcinoma in biopsy material are the presence of small-gland atrophy (postatrophic hyperplasia) and the presence of seminal vesicle epithelium in the specimen. Small-gland atrophy consists of a wedge-shaped area in the peripheral zone, with the apex of the wedge pointing toward the urethra and the base of the wedge situated along the capsular surface. It appears to be caused by or associated with damage to the draining duct of this area of the peripheral zone due to a pre-existing inflammatory process (8). This duct is surrounded by a variable cuff of small lymphocytes in a densely sclerotic fibrous stroma. The acini distal to the duct show small-gland atrophy in a lobular distribution under low magnification. The nuclei of the latter may show some nuclear enlargement and small nucleoli and thus may manifest PIN-like changes. A basal cell layer is usually apparent, but when it is inconspicuous, this lesion may be difficult to distinguish from adenocarcinoma on a needle biopsy sample (Fig. 6A.9). The small glands always decorate with antibodies to high-molecular-weight cytokeratin (clone 34β E12) (132). Seminal vesicle epithelium normally displays a rather marked degree of nuclear pleomorphism in adult men. Nucleoli may also be conspicuous. The architectural features may be equally troublesome—the arborizing of small glands most distant from the lumen of the seminal vesicle imparts a pseudo-invasive growth pattern (Fig. 6A.10). Most prostate cancers, however, lack the range of nuclear pleomorphism within a single gland-like structure. In addition, the lipofuscin-like pigment in the cytoplasm of seminal vesicle epithelium is a welcome landmark for the pathologist, although occasionally a similar-looking pigment may appear in the cytoplasm of nonneoplastic prostatic epithelium (133).

Less commonly, a number of other microacinar proliferations may mimic well-differentiated adenocarcinoma in biopsy material. Discussion of these is beyond the scope of this chapter but many have been tabulated in one publication (15).

Variants

Mucinous Adenocarcinoma

A small amount of intraluminal mucin is frequently encountered in prostate adenocarcinoma, but tumors showing lakes of extracellular mucin are uncommon (58–60). Diagnosis of this histologic subtype requires that at least 25% of the tumor show this histologic pattern. This entity comprises approximately 0.4% of all prostatic carcinomas (134–136) (Fig. 6A.11). Prostate cancers making any degree of mucin

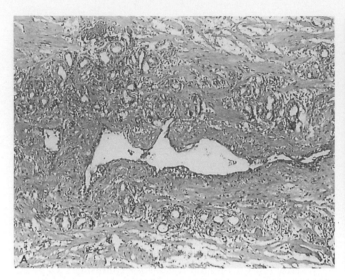
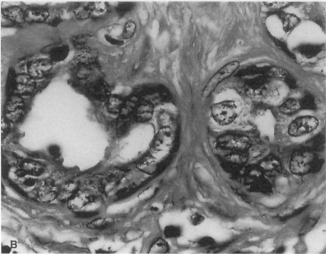

FIGURE 6A.9. Postinflammatory sclerotic atrophy. **A:** Low-power photomicrograph showing fibrosis around the central duct and a lobular distribution of numerous small, crowded glands. (Hematoxylin and eosin, ×100.) **B:** High-power photomicrograph of (**A**), showing two of the small glands of atrophy with enlarged nuclei and a few small nucleoli. Basal cells appear to be present. (Hematoxylin and eosin, ×400.)

may be associated with a peculiar stromal reaction around the malignant glands that has been termed *collagenous micronodules*. These are a specific but infrequent finding in prostate cancer (143). Of course, an extraprostatic primary tumor site should be excluded if warranted. These tumors are almost always associated with the usual acinar adenocarcinoma if the entire tumor is examined. The difficulty arises when only a small portion of tumor is sampled on needle biopsy. Fortunately, these tumors retain cytoplasmic PSA and are negative for carcinoembryonic antigen, a helpful adjunct in difficult cases. Although abundant mucin is produced, intracytoplasmic mucin is not seen, as might be expected, from mucinous tumors arising in other sites. In the author's experience, these tumors arise in the peripheral zone or perhaps the central zone as well. Tumors discovered

on TURP, therefore, probably have their origin outside the transition zone. The prognosis appears to be the same or slightly worse than that associated with the conventional adenocarcinoma of similar grade (137). This entity should not be confused with an extremely rare variant of prostate carcinoma: signet-ring cell type. The tumor cells in this entity are positive for PSA and PSAP and usually are negative for mucin stains (138–142).

Prostatic Duct Adenocarcinoma

Prostatic duct adenocarcinoma was described by Melicow and Pachter in 1967 under the term *endometrial carcinoma of the prostate utricle* (144,145). The pattern of prostatic duct adenocarcinoma is characterized by a papillary or villoglandular

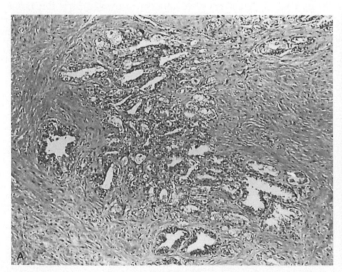
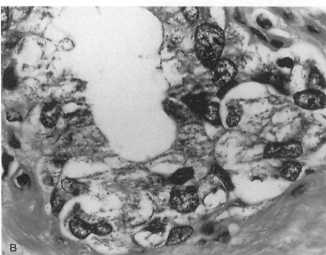

FIGURE 6A.10. Seminal vesicle. **A:** Low-power photomicrograph demonstrating numerous small glandular structures adjacent to the parent duct (not shown) with pseudoinfiltrative appearance. (Hematoxylin and eosin, ×100.) **B:** High-power photomicrograph of (**A**), showing marked nuclear pleomorphism and prominent nucleoli. Golden cytoplasmic pigment is not seen on black and white photomicrograph. (Hematoxylin and eosin, ×400.)

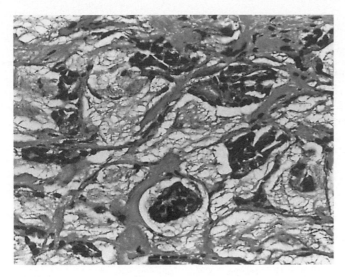

FIGURE 6A.11. Photomicrograph of mucinous adenocarcinoma, demonstrating small morules of tumor cells floating in extracellular pale-staining mucin. (Hematoxylin and eosin, ×200.)

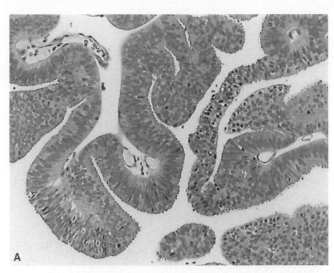

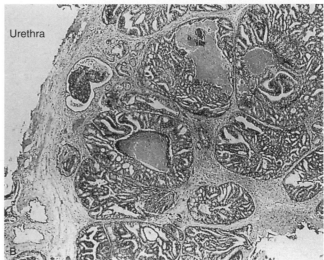

FIGURE 6A.12. Prostatic duct adenocarcinoma. A: Photomicrograph of villoglandular growth pattern of endometrioid subtype that was growing in the lumen of the prostatic urethra and was thought to represent a papillary transitional cell carcinoma by the urologist. (Hematoxylin and eosin, ×200.) B: Photomicrograph of large-duct variant, showing large ducts underlying the prostatic urethra (U) filled with high-grade adenocarcinoma exhibiting comedo-type necrosis. Microacinar invasive adenocarcinoma is also shown adjacent to involved ducts. (Hematoxylin and eosin, ×100.)

growth pattern similar to that of adenocarcinomas of the endometrium and comprises 0.4% to 0.8% of prostate adenocarcinomas (146–150). Because many of these tumors were seen endoscopically to protrude into the prostatic urethra at the level of the verumontanum, the tumors were considered possibly to have arisen from the utricle, which was thought to be an analogue of the uterus in the man. Indeed, the urologist is frequently convinced that these tumors are papillary transitional cell carcinomas of the prostatic urethra because the papillary appearance is easily recognized through the cystoscope. The papillary fronds of the tumor are lined by a single or stratified tall columnar epithelium with basally placed nuclei (Fig. 6A.12A). If the cells have pale-staining cytoplasm, they more closely resemble prostate adenocarcinoma cytologically. Many of these tumors are composed of cells with a more granular eosinophilic cytoplasm and therefore more closely resemble the usual endometrial adenocarcinoma. If the entire prostate is examined, these tumors usually can be seen distending some of the main prostatic ducts posterior and lateral to the urethra. Within the ducts, these tumors may show a cribriform or solid growth pattern, frequently exhibiting comedo-type necrosis (Fig. 6A.12B). The tumor may also show this latter growth pattern as an invasive component in the prostatic stroma or an extraprostatic site. In the authors' experience, this variant is commonly associated with the usual acinar adenocarcinoma if the entire prostate is examined. In the literature, the reported frequency of such an association ranges from 5% to 51%. By definition, however, to be classified as a prostatic duct adenocarcinoma, this component must comprise at least 50% of the volume of the tumor. The prognostic significance of a minor component of prostatic duct carcinoma is unknown (56).

Although prostatic duct adenocarcinomas originally were considered to be low-grade tumors, more recent studies have shown that they are aggressive tumors associated with a 5-year survival rate of 15% to 30%. One series showed that, at radical prostatectomy, nearly all these tumors were associated with capsular penetration, 50% with positive margins, 40% with seminal vesicle invasion, and 27% with positive pelvic lymph nodes (151). Immunohistochemical decoration of the tumor cells is similar to that of other prostate adenocarcinomas: positive for PSA and negative for carcinoembryonic antigen. This is very helpful because the solid variant with

comedo-type necrosis in prostatic ducts must be differentiated from ductal extension of a transitional cell carcinoma.

Small Cell Carcinoma

Small cell carcinoma is a rare variant of prostate carcinoma but is preceded by usual acinar adenocarcinoma in at least one-half of the cases (152,153). Because of this frequent association with acinar adenocarcinoma and the variation in immunohistochemical profile and ultrastructural findings from one tumor to another, this tumor is thought to arise from multipotential prostatic epithelium, not necessarily from neuroendocrine cells of the prostate (137,153–155). Nearly all of the specimens that the authors have observed personally have been from patients who developed recurrence several years after definitive radiation therapy for acinar adenocarcinoma of the

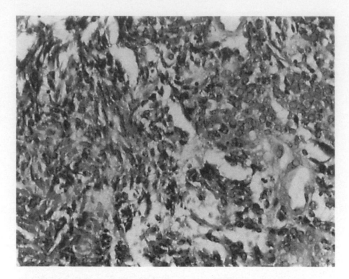

FIGURE 6A.13. Photomicrograph of small cell carcinoma showing absence of glandular growth pattern. Tumor cells have small nuclei and scant cytoplasm. (Hematoxylin and eosin, ×200.)

prostate and, as such, may represent dedifferentiation of the original tumor. The small cell component resembles the more common counterpart within the lung and may have the oat cell–type or intermediate cell–type morphology (Fig. 6A.13). Ultrastructural examination of these tumors may show neurosecretory-type granules, which may explain why many of these tumors decorate with immunohistochemical stains for various neuroendocrine markers. The small cell component is not decorated with immunostains for PSA.

Only rarely do patients exhibit one of the paraneoplastic syndromes more commonly observed with small cell carcinoma of the lung. The prognosis is exceptionally poor, and patients are refractory to androgen ablation or estrogen administration. Cytotoxic chemotherapy, however, may prolong survival time in these patients.

Squamous and Adenosquamous Carcinomas

Squamous and adenosquamous carcinomas are quite rare and comprise approximately 0.2% of malignant tumors of the prostate (156–164). Nearly all of these tumors, in the authors' experience and as described in the literature, are preceded by the usual acinar adenocarcinoma that has been treated with irradiation or hormonal therapy or both (157–159, 164). Florid squamous metaplasia adjacent to an infarct in nodular hyperplasia may occasionally simulate squamous carcinoma, and confusing these two is probably more common than the occurrence of squamous carcinoma itself. The squamous component does not decorate with immunohistochemical stains for PSA. The prognosis is exceptionally poor, with essentially no response to hormonal or other therapies. Bone metastases are usually osteolytic rather than osteoblastic (165,166).

Sarcomatoid Carcinoma (Carcinosarcoma)

Sarcomatoid carcinoma is an extremely uncommon variant of prostate carcinoma that is a high-grade malignant tumor with biphasic epithelioid and sarcomatous areas (167–170). The carcinomatous areas are usually high-grade adenocarcinoma that decorate with immunohistochemical staining for PSA.

The sarcomatous-appearing areas are also high grade and may have the appearance of malignant fibrous histiocytoma, fibrosarcoma, or, less commonly, leiomyosarcoma, chondrosarcoma, osteosarcoma, or rhabdomyosarcoma (167–170). These sarcomatous areas may decorate immunohistochemically like their soft tissue sarcoma counterparts. Therefore, some think of these tumors as carcinosarcomas rather than metaplastic carcinomas. Mostofi et al. believe that the majority of tumors in this category represent spindle cell metaplasia in the carcinoma or a cellular desmoplastic reaction of the stroma. They designate as carcinosarcoma only lesions that contain heterologous components (e.g., neoplastic cartilage, bone) (171). The largest series was reported from the Mayo Clinic (21 cases). The mean age was 68 years. Ten of the patients had a previous diagnosis of prostatic acinar adenocarcinoma, and eight of these had been treated with androgen deprivation or irradiation or both. The 5-year survival rate was 41%; the 7-year survival rate was 14% (170). All patients in the M. D. Anderson Cancer Center series died of their disease at a median time of 12 months (167).

Transitional Cell Carcinoma

Transitional cell carcinoma is the most common of the variants of carcinoma occurring in the prostate and represents 1% to 5% of all such carcinomas (137,172). Many of these tumors are extensions of transitional cell carcinoma into the prostatic ducts from the urinary bladder by way of the prostatic urethra. Cases are reported, however, with no extraprostatic primary site (172–176). Of course, a deeply invasive transitional cell carcinoma in the base of the bladder may directly invade the prostate across tissue planes, but this scenario seldom presents a clinical dilemma. Transitional cell carcinoma that extends far out into the prostatic ducts is invariably high grade. The tumor cells may show pagetoid spread or may represent solid or near-solid filling of the affected ducts and be associated with comedo-type necrosis. In the latter circumstance, this lesion may be difficult to distinguish from prostatic duct adenocarcinoma. In such a situation, immunohistochemical analysis may be very useful. Transitional cell carcinomas are usually high-molecular-weight–keratin positive and PSA negative, in contrast to adenocarcinoma of the prostate. This distinction is critical because the therapy given for metastatic disease differs greatly between these two. If the transitional cell carcinoma is confined to the prostatic ducts, it is essentially an *in situ* carcinoma and is cured with radical surgery, provided no foci of invasion exist elsewhere in the urinary tract. Extensive invasion of the prostatic stroma, however, carries with it an ominous prognosis.

Adenoid Basal Cell Tumor (Basaloid Carcinoma, Adenoid Cystic Carcinoma)

Adenoid basal cell tumor is a very rare tumor with unknown malignant potential because the number of reported cases is so small (177–181). Two histologic patterns are recognized: adenoid cystic and basaloid (177). The two patterns may coexist or each may exist in pure form. Although some of these tumors show considerable resemblance to adenoid cystic carcinoma of other sites, these tumors lack cytoplasmic myofilaments and have an inconsistent basal lamina proliferation around cell nests (177). In that series, the authors reported a case with perineural invasion and extraprostatic spread treated by radical prostatectomy. The lymph nodes were negative, and the patient has remained free of disease with short fol-low-up. Distant metastases from this tumor have not been reported, however. The spectrum of this tumor overlaps somewhat with basal cell hyperplasia and basal cell adenoma. To be accepted as carcinoma, the tumor must also exhibit such features as a desmoplastic stromal response, necrosis, perineural invasion, or infiltration of surrounding tissues. This tumor possesses both basal cells and luminal cells, which can be verified by immunohistochemical analysis (181).

OTHER HISTOLOGIC VARIANTS

Many new histologic variants of prostate cancer have been described in recent years. Most are histologic entities whose significance lies in permitting an accurate diagnosis but generally lack any prognostic significance. In 1996, Nelson and Epstein described a new morphologic variant of PCa which they termed *prostatic carcinoma* with abundant xanthomatous cytoplasm, or foamy gland carcinoma (182). The cancer has abundant foamy cytoplasm, pink secretions, and nuclei with sometimes inconspicuous nucleoli. They stress the low-grade nuclear features and the potential for misdiagnosis when Cowper glands are found in needle biopsies (183). Pseudohyperplastic (184) and atrophic (185) variants have also been described. Adequate knowledge of distinguishing features are important to recognize foci of cancer that carry these characteristics. Fortunately, it is very rare to find these variants alone, as they are frequently associated with the more common acinar form of PCa.

Malignant Mesenchymal Neoplasms

Malignant mesenchymal neoplasms are quite rare compared with tumors with epithelial origin, except in children, in whom they constitute the majority of malignant neoplasms of the prostate (171). Overall, they represent between 0.1% and 0.2% of malignant prostate tumors. The two most commonly encountered sarcomas in pure form are leiomyosarcoma and rhabdomyosarcoma, which respectively are the most commonly occurring sarcomas of the prostate in adults and children (171). These tumors resemble their soft tissue counterparts. They are often quite large at the time of diagnosis, so that their origin, whether in the prostate or in contiguous structures, may be difficult to determine. The prognosis for high-grade sarcomas is not good, with most patients succumbing to widespread hematogenous metastases.

References

1. Lowsley OS. The development of the human prostate gland with reference to the development of other structures at the neck of the urinary bladder. *Am J Anat* 1912;13:299–350.
2. Cunha GR, Chung LWK, Shannon JM, et al. Hormonal induced morphogenesis and growth: role of the mesenchymal-epithelial interactions. *Recent Prog Horm Res* 1983;39:559–598.
3. Wilson JD, Griffin JE, Leskin M, et al. Role of gonadal hormones in development of the sexual phenotypes. *Hum Genet* 1981;58:78–84.
4. Imperato-McGinley J, Guerrero L, Gautier T, et al. Steroid 5-alpha-reductase deficiency in man: an inherited form of male pseudohermaphroditism. *Science* 1974;186:1213–1215.
5. Franks LM. Atrophy and hyperplasia in the prostate proper. *J Pathol Bacteriol* 1954;68:617–622.
6. McNeal JE. Anatomy of the prostate: an historical survey of divergent views. *Prostate* 1980;1:3–13.
7. McNeal JE. Normal and pathologic anatomy of the prostate. *Urology* 1981; 17(Suppl 3):11–16.
8. McNeal JE. Normal histology of the prostate. *Am J Surg Pathol* 1988;12:619–633.
9. McNeal JE, Redwine EA, Freiha FS, et al. Zonal distribution of prostate adenocarcinoma: correlation with histological pattern and direction of spread. *Am J Surg Pathol* 1988;12:897–906.
10. McNeal JE. The prostate and prostatic urethra: a morphologic synthesis. *J Urol* 1972;107:1008–1016.
11. Bostwick DG, Brawer MK. Prostatic intra-epithelial neoplasia and early invasion in prostatic cancer. *Cancer* 1987;59:788–794.
12. di Sant'Agnese PA, de Mesy Jensen KL. Somatostatin and/or somatostatin-like immunoreactive endocrine-paracrine cells in the human prostate gland. *Arch Pathol Lab Med* 1984;108:693–696.
13. di Sant'Agnese PA, de Mesy Jensen KL, Churukian CJ, et al. Human prostatic endocrine-paracrine (APUD) cells: distributional analysis with a comparison of serotonin and neuron-specific enolase immunoreactivity and silver stains. *Arch Pathol Lab Med* 1985;109:607–612.
14. di Sant'Agnese PA. Calcitonin-like immunoreactive and bombesin-like immunoreactive endocrine-paracrine cells of the human prostate. *Arch Pathol Lab Med* 1986;110:412–415.
15. Gagucas RJ, Brown R, Wheeler TM. Verumontanum mucosal gland hyperplasia. *Am J Surg Pathol* 1995;19:30–36.
16. Anton RC, Chakraborty S, Wheeler TM. The significance of intraluminal prostatic crystalloids in benign needle biopsies. *Am J Surg Pathol* 1998;22:446–449.
17. Ayala AG, Ro JY, Babaian R, et al. The prostatic capsule: does it exist? *Am J Surg Pathol* 1989;13:21–27.
18. Stamey TA, McNeal JE, Freiha FS, et al. Morphometric and clinical studies on 68 consecutive radical prostatectomies. *J Urol* 1988;139:1235–1241.
19. Epstein JI, Carmichael MJ, Pizov G, et al. Influence of capsular penetration on progression following radical prostatectomy: a study of 196 cases with long-term follow-up. *J Urol* 1993;150:135–141
20. Wheeler TM, Dilioglugil O, Kattan MW, et al. Clinical and pathologic significance of the level and extent of capsular invasion in clinical stage T1-2 prostate cancer. *Hum Pathol* 1998;29:856–862.
21. American Joint Committee on Cancer. *AJCC Cancer Staging Manual*, 5th ed. Philadelphia: JB Lippincott Co; 1997:219–224.
22. Villers AA, McNeal JE, Redwine EA. Pathogenesis and biological significance of seminal vesicle invasion in prostatic adenocarcinoma. *J Urol* 1990;143:1183–1187.
23. Ohori M, Scardino PT, Lapin SL, et al. The mechanisms and prognostic significance of seminal vesicle involvement by prostate cancer. *Am J Surg Pathol* 1993;17:1252–1261.
24. Walsh PC, Donker PJ. Impotence following radical prostatectomy: insight into etiology and prevention. *J Urol* 1982;128:492–497.
25. Villers A, McNeal JE, Redwine EA, et al. The role of perineural space invasion in the local spread of prostatic adenocarcinoma. *J Urol* 1989;142:763–768.
26. Crowe R, Chapple CR, Burnstock G. The human prostate gland: a histochemical and immunohistochemical study of neuropeptides, serotonin, dopamine beta-hydroxylase and acetylcholinesterase in autonomic nerves and ganglia. *Br J Urol* 1991;68:53–61.
27. Chapple CR, Crowe R, Gilpin SA, et al. The innervation of the human prostate gland—the changes associated with benign enlargement. *J Urol* 1991;146:1637–1644.
28. Higgins JR, Gosling JA. Studies on the structure and intrinsic innervation of the normal human prostate. *Prostate Suppl* 1989;2:5–16.
29. Vaalasti A, Hervonen A. Autonomic innervation of the human prostate. *Invest Urol* 1980;17:293–297.
30. Vaalasti A, Hervonen A. Nerve endings in the human prostate. *Am J Anat* 1980;157:41–47.
31. Vaalasti A, Linnoila I, Hervonen A. Immunohistochemical demonstration of VIP, [Met5]- and [Leu5]-enkephalin immunoreactive nerve fibres in the human prostate and seminal vesicles. *Histochemistry* 1980;66:89–98.
32. Jungblut T, Aumuller G, Malek B, et al. Age-dependency and regional distribution of enkephalinergic nerves in human prostate. *Urol Int* 1989;44:352–356.
33. Kato T, Watanabe H, Shima M, et al. Studies on the innervation of prostate. 2. Histological changes of the dog prostate after transsection of its innervating nerves. *Nippon Hinyokika Gakkai Zasshi* 1971;62:704–707.
34. McVary KT, Razzaq A, Lee C, et al. Growth of the rat prostate gland is facilitated by the autonomic nervous system. *Biol Reprod* 1994;51:99–107.
35. Doggweiler R, Zermann DH, Ishigooka M, et al. Botox-induced prostatic involution. *Prostate* 1998;37:44–50.
36. Watanabe H, Kato H, Kato T, et al. Studies on the innervation of the prostate. I. Tissue respiration of the dog prostate after the cutting off of the various innervating nerves. *Nippon Hinyokika Gakkai Zasshi* 1967;58:381–385.
37. Watanabe H. Tissue respiration of the partially denervated dog prostate. *Tohoku J Exp Med* 1968;95:193–199.
38. Watanabe H, Shima M, Kojima M, et al. Dynamic study of nervous control on prostatic contraction and fluid excretion in the dog. *J Urol* 1988; 140:1567–1570.

39. Lujan M, Paez A, Llanes L, et al. Role of autonomic innervation in rat prostatic structure maintenance: a morphometric analysis. *J Urol* 1998; 160:1919–1923.

40. Wang JM, McKenna KE, McVary KT, et al. Requirement of innervation for maintenance of structural and functional integrity in the rat prostate. *Biol Reprod* 1991;44:1171–1176.

41. Lujan Galan M, Paez Borda A, Fernandez Gonzalez I, et al. Macroscopic and histologic analysis of the rat prostate after denervation. *Arch Esp Urol* 1998;51:219–225.

42. Lujan Galan M, Paez Borda A, Hernandez Lopez C, et al. Ultrastructural morphometric study of the prostate of the rat after microsurgical denervation. *Actas Urol Esp* 1998;22:388–394.

43. Wang JM, McKenna KE, Lee C. Determination of prostatic secretion in rats: effect of neurotransmitters and testosterone. *Prostate* 1991;18:289–301.

44. Lujan Galan M, Paez Borda A, Llanes Gonzalez L, et al. Effect of sacral roots block in the prostatic structure of the rat. *Actas Urol Esp* 2000;24: 516–521.

45. Martinez-Pineiro L, Dahiya R, Nunes LL, et al. Pelvic plexus denervation in rats causes morphologic and functional changes of the prostate. *J Urol* 1993;150:215–218.

46. McVary KT, McKenna KE, Lee C. Prostate innervation. *Prostate Suppl* 1998;8:2–13.

47. Landis SH, Murray T, Bolden S, et al. Cancer statistics. *CA Cancer J Clin* 1999;49:8–31.

48. Peterson RO. *Urologic pathology.* Philadelphia: JB Lippincott Co; 1986: 618.

49. Gleason DF. Atypical hyperplasia, benign hyperplasia, and well-differentiated adenocarcinoma of the prostate. *Am J Surg Pathol* 1985;9(Suppl 5-6): 53–67.

50. Bostwick DG, Srigley J, Grignon D, et al. Atypical adenomatous hyperplasia of the prostate: morphologic criteria for its distinction from well-differentiated carcinoma. *Hum Pathol* 1993;24:819–832.

51. Gaudin PB, Epstein JI. Adenosis of the prostate: histologic features in transurethral resection specimens. *Am J Surg Pathol* 1994;18:863–870.

52. Bostwick DG. Prostatic intraepithelial neoplasia (PIN): current concepts. *J Cell Biochem* 1992;16H:10–19.

53. McNeal JE, Bostwick DG. Intraductal dysplasia: a premalignant lesion of the prostate. *Hum Pathol* 1986;17:64–71.

54. Kelemen PR, Buschmann RJ, Weisz-Carrington P. Nucleolar prominence as a diagnostic variable in prostatic carcinoma. *Cancer* 1990;65:1017–1020.

55. Böcking A, Auffermann W, Schwartz H, et al. Cytology of prostatic carcinoma: quantification and validation of diagnostic criteria. *Anal Quant Cytol Histol* 1984;6:74–88.

56. Epstein JI. The prostate and seminal vesicles. In: Sternberg SS, ed. *Pathology,* 2nd ed. New York: Raven Press; 1994:1807–1853.

57. Humphrey PA, Walther PJ. Adenocarcinoma of the prostate I: tissue sampling considerations. *Am J Clin Pathol* 1993;99:746–759.

58. Hukill PB, Vidone RA. Histochemistry of mucus and other polysaccharides in tumors II: carcinoma of the prostate. *Lab Invest* 1967;16:395–406.

59. Franks LM, O'Shea JP, Thompson AER. Mucin in the prostate: histochemical study in normal glands, latent, clinical and colloid cancers. *Cancer* 1964;17:983–991.

60. Epstein JI, Fynheer J. Acidic mucin in the prostate: can it differentiate adenosis from adenocarcinoma? *Hum Pathol* 1992;23:1321–1325.

61. Grignon DJ, O'Malley FP. Mucinous metaplasia in the prostate gland. *Am J Surg Pathol* 1993;17:287–290.

62. Holmes EJ. Crystalloids of prostatic carcinoma: relationship to Bence-Jones crystals. *Cancer* 1977;39:2073–2080.

63. Ro JY, Ayala AG, Ordóñez NG, et al. Intraluminal crystalloids in prostatic adenocarcinoma: immunohistochemical, electron microscopic, and x-ray microanalytic studies. *Cancer* 1986;57:2397–2407.

64. Bennett B, Gardner WA Jr. Crystalloids in prostatic hyperplasia. *Prostate* 1980;1:31–35.

65. Carstens PHB. Perineural glands in normal and hyperplastic prostates. *J Urol* 1980;123:686–688.

66. Rodin AE, Larson DL, Roberts DK. Nature of the perineural space invaded by prostatic carcinoma. *Cancer* 1967;20:1772–1779.

67. Ayala GE, Wheeler TM, Shine HD, et al. In vitro dorsal root ganglia and human prostate cell line interaction: redefining perineural invasion in prostate cancer. *Prostate* 2001;49:213–223.

68. Cornell RJ, Rowley D, Wheeler T, et al. Neuroepithelial interactions in prostate cancer are enhanced in the presence of prostatic stroma. *Urology* 2003;61:870–875.

69. Yang G, Wheeler TM, Kattan MW, et al. Perineural invasion of prostate carcinoma cells is associated with reduced apoptotic index. *Cancer* 1996; 78:1267–1271.

70. Byar DP, Mostofi FK. Carcinoma of the prostate: prognostic evaluation of certain prognostic features in 208 radical prostatectomies. *Cancer* 1972; 30:5–13.

71. Ravery V, Boccon-Gibod LA, Meulemans A, et al. Predictive value of pathological features for progression after radical prostatectomy. *Eur Urol* 1994;26:197–201.

72. van den Ouden D, Kranse R, Hop WC, et al. Microvascular invasion in prostate cancer: prognostic significance in patients treated by radical prostatectomy for clinically localized carcinoma. *Urol Int* 1998;60: 17–24.

73. de la Taille A, Katz A, Bagiella E, et al. Perineural invasion on prostate needle biopsy: an independent predictor of final pathologic stage. *Urology* 1999;54:1039–1043.

74. de la Taille A, Rubin MA, Bagiella E, et al. Can perineural invasion on prostate needle biopsy predict prostate specific antigen recurrence after radical prostatectomy? *J Urol* 1999;162:103–106.

75. Anderson PR, Hanlon AL, Patchefsky A, et al. Perineural invasion and Gleason 7-10 tumors predict increased failure in prostate cancer patients with pretreatment PSA <10 ng/ml treated with conformal external beam radiation therapy. *Int J Radiat Oncol Biol Phys* 1998;41: 1087–1092.

76. Bastacky SI, Walsh PC, Epstein JI. Relationship between perineural tumor invasion on needle biopsy and radical prostatectomy capsular penetration in clinical stage B adenocarcinoma of the prostate. *Am J Surg Pathol* 1993; 17:336–341.

77. Epstein JI. The role of perineural invasion and other biopsy characteristics as prognostic markers for localized prostate cancer. *Semin Urol Oncol* 1998;16:124–128.

78. McNeal JE, Haillot O. Patterns of spread of adenocarcinoma in the prostate as related to cancer volume. *Prostate* 2001;49:48–57.

79. McNeal JE, Yemoto CE. Spread of adenocarcinoma within prostatic ducts and acini. Morphologic and clinical correlations. *Am J Surg Pathol* 1996; 20:802–814.

80. Maru N, Ohori M, Kattan MW, et al. Prognostic significance of the diameter of perineural invasion in radical prostatectomy specimens. *Hum Pathol* 2001;32:828–833.

81. Nadji M, Tabei SZ, Castro A, et al. Prostate-specific antigen: an immunohistologic marker for prostatic neoplasms. *Cancer* 1981;48:1229–1232.

82. Nadji M, Tabei SZ, Castro A, et al. Prostatic origin of tumors: an immunohistochemical study. *Am J Clin Pathol* 1980;73:735–739.

83. Choe BK, Pontes EJ, Rose NR, et al. Expression of human prostatic acid phosphatase in a pancreatic islet cell carcinoma. *Invest Urol* 1978;15: 312–318.

84. Cohen C, Bentz MS, Budgeon LR, Prostatic acid phosphatase in carcinoid and islet cell tumors [Editorial]. *Arch Pathol Lab Med* 1983;107:277.

85. Sobin LH, Hjermstad BM, Sesterhenn IA, et al. Prostatic acid phosphatase activity in carcinoid tumors. *Cancer* 1986;58:136–138.

86. Signoretti S, Waltregny D, Dilks J, et al. p63 is a prostate basal cell marker and is required for prostate development. *Am J Pathol* 2000;157: 1769–1775.

87. Parsons JK, Gage WR, Nelson WG, et al. p63 protein expression is rare in prostate adenocarcinoma: implications for cancer diagnosis and carcinogenesis. *Urology* 2001;58:619–624.

88. Luo J, Zha S, Gage WR, et al. Alpha-methylacyl-CoA racemase: a new molecular marker for prostate cancer. *Cancer Res* 2002;62:2220–2226.

89. Magi-Galluzzi C, Luo J, Isaacs WB, et al. Alpha-methylacyl-CoA racemase: a variably sensitive immunohistochemical marker for the diagnosis of small prostate cancer foci on needle biopsy. *Am J Surg Pathol* 2003; 27:1128–1133.

90. Ernst T, Hergenhahn M, Kenzelmann M, et al. Gene expression profiling in prostatic cancer. *Verh Dtsch Ges Pathol* 2002;86:165–175.

91. Sanderson SO, Sebo TJ, Murphy LM, et al. An analysis of the p63/alphamethylacyl coenzyme A racemase immunohistochemical cocktail stain in prostate needle biopsy specimens and tissue microarrays. *Am J Clin Pathol* 2004;121:220–225.

92. Gleason DF, The Veterans Administration Cooperative Research Group. Histologic grading and clinical staging of prostatic carcinoma. In: Tannenbaum M, ed. *Urologic pathology: The prostate.* Philadelphia: Lea & Febiger; 1977:171–174.

93. Aihara M, Wheeler TM, Ohori M, et al. Heterogeneity of prostate cancer in radical prostatectomy specimens. *Urology* 1993;43:60–67.

94. Chan TY, Partin AW, Walsh PC, et al. Prognostic significance of Gleason score 3 + 4 versus Gleason score 4 + 3 tumor at radical prostatectomy. *Urology* 2000;56:823–827.

95. Makarov DV, Sanderson H, Partin AW, et al. Gleason score 7 prostate cancer on needle biopsy: is the prognostic difference in Gleason scores 4 + 3 and 3 + 4 independent of the number of involved cores? *J Urol* 2002; 167:2440–2442.

96. Pan CC, Potter SR, Partin AW, et al. The prognostic significance of tertiary Gleason patterns of higher grade in radical prostatectomy specimens: a proposal to modify the Gleason grading system. *Am J Surg Pathol* 2000; 24:563–569.

97. Brawn PN, Ayala AA, Eschenbach AC, et al. Histologic grading study of prostatic adenocarcinoma: development of a new system and comparison with other methods. *Cancer* 1982;49:525–532.

98. Broders AC. Epithelioma of the genitourinary organs. *Ann Surg* 1922;75: 574–604.

99. Broders AC. Carcinoma: grading and practical application. *Arch Pathol* 1926;2:376–381.

100. Mostofi FK, Sesterhenn IA, Sobin LH. Histological typing of prostate tumors, #22. In: *International Histological Classification of Tumors.* Geneva: World Health Organization; 1980:17–21.

101. Harada M, Mostofi FK, Corle DK, et al. Preliminary studies of histological prognosis in cancer of the prostate. *Cancer Treat Rep* 1977;61:223–225.

102. Tuxhorn JA, Ayala GE, Rowley DR. Reactive stroma in prostate cancer progression. *J Urol* 2001;166:2472–2483.

103. Tuxhorn JA, McAlhany SJ, Dang TD, et al. Stromal cells promote angiogenesis and growth of human prostate tumors in a differential reactive stroma (DRS) xenograft model. *Cancer Res* 2002;62:3298–3307.

104. Ayala G, Tuxhorn JA, Wheeler TM, et al. Reactive stroma as a predictor of biochemical-free recurrence in prostate cancer. *Clin Cancer Res* 2003; 9:4792–4801.

105. Moore RA. The morphology of small prostatic carcinoma. *J Urol* 1935; 33:224–234.

106. Kahler JE. Carcinoma of the prostate gland: a pathologic study. *J Urol* 1939;41:557–574.

107. McNeal JE. Morphogenesis of prostatic carcinoma. *Cancer* 1965;18: 1659–1666.

108. McNeal JE. Origin and development of carcinoma in the prostate. *Cancer* 1969;23:24–34.

109. Epstein JI, Cho KR, Quinn BD. Relationship of severe dysplasia to stage A (incidental) adenocarcinoma. *Cancer* 1990;65:2321–2327.

110. Troncoso P, Babaian RJ, Ro JY, et al. Prostatic intraepithelial neoplasia and invasive prostatic adenocarcinoma in cystoprostatectomy specimens. *Urology* 1989;34(suppl 6):52–56.

111. Quinn BD, Cho KR, Epstein JI. Relationship of severe dysplasia to stage B adenocarcinoma of the prostate. *Cancer* 1990;65:2328–2337.

112. Kastendieck H. Correlations between atypical primary hyperplasia and carcinoma of the prostate: a histological study of 180 total prostatectomies. *Pathol Res Pract* 1980;169:366–387.

113. De La Torre M, Häggman M, Bränstedt S, et al. Prostatic intraepithelial neoplasia and invasive carcinoma in total prostatectomy specimens: distribution, volumes, and DNA ploidy. *Br J Urol* 1993;72:207–213.

114. Greene DR, Wheeler TM, Egawa S, et al. A comparison of the morphological features of cancer arising in the transition zone and in the peripheral zone of the prostate. *J Urol* 1991;146:1069–1076.

115. De Marzo AM, Meeker AK, Zha S, et al. Human prostate cancer precursors and pathobiology. *Urology* 2003;62:55–62.

116. Billis A, Magna LA. Inflammatory atrophy of the prostate. Prevalence and significance. *Arch Pathol Lab Med* 2003;127:840–844.

117. Nelson WG, De Marzo AM, Deweese TL, et al. Preneoplastic prostate lesions: an opportunity for prostate cancer prevention. *Ann N Y Acad Sci* 2001;952:135–144.

118. De Marzo AM, Marchi VL, Epstein JI, et al. Proliferative inflammatory atrophy of the prostate: implications for prostatic carcinogenesis. *Am J Pathol* 1999;155:1985–1992.

119. Nakayama M, Bennett CJ, Hicks JL, et al. Hypermethylation of the human glutathione S-transferase-pi gene (GSTP1) CpG island is present in a subset of proliferative inflammatory atrophy lesions but not in normal or hyperplastic epithelium of the prostate: a detailed study using laser-capture microdissection. *Am J Pathol* 2003;163:923–933.

120. Anton RC, Kattan MW, Chakraborty S, et al. Postatrophic hyperplasia of the prostate: lack of association with prostate cancer. *Am J Surg Pathol* 1999;23:932–936.

121. Wheeler TM, Scardino PT, Cantini M. Whole organ mapping of radical prostatectomy specimens. *J Urol* 1987;137(Pt 2):224A (Abstract 483).

122. Greene DR, Wheeler TM. Clinical relevance of the individual prostate cancer focus. *Cancer Invest* 1994;12:425–437.

123. Bostwick DG, Egbert BM, Fajardo LF. Radiation injury of the normal and neoplastic prostate. *Am J Surg Pathol* 1982;6:541–551.

124. Scardino PT, Frankel JM, Wheeler TM, et al. The prognostic significance of postirradiation biopsy results in patients with prostate cancer. *J Urol* 1986;135:510–516.

125. Crook JM, Bahadur YA, Robertson SJ, et al. Evaluation of radiation effect, tumor differentiation, and prostate specific antigen staining in sequential prostate biopsies after external beam radiotherapy for patients with prostate carcinoma. *Cancer* 1997;79:79–81.

126. Franks LM. Estrogen-treated prostatic cancer. *Cancer* 1960;13:490–501.

127. Mostofi FK, Price EB Jr. Tumors of male genital system. In: *Atlas of tumor pathology*, Fascicle 8, 2nd series. Washington, DC: Armed Forces Institute of Pathology; 1973:236–338.

128. Murphy WM, Soloway MS, Barrows GH. Pathologic changes associated with androgen deprivation therapy for prostate cancer. *Cancer* 1991;68: 821–828.

129. Tetu B, Srigley JR, Boivin JC, et al. Effect of combination endocrine therapy (LHRH agonist and flutamide) on normal prostate and prostatic adenocarcinoma: a histopathologic and immunohistochemical study. *Am J Surg Pathol* 1991;15:111–120.

130. Armas OAL, Aprikan AG, Melamed J, et al. Clinical and pathological effects of neoadjuvant total androgen ablation therapy on clinically localized prostatic adenocarcinoma. *Am J Surg Pathol* 1994;18:979–991.

131. Ayala G, Wheeler TM, Shalev M, et al. Cytopathic effect of in situ gene therapy in prostate cancer. *Hum Pathol* 2000;31:866–870.

132. Cheville JC, Bostwick DG. Postatrophic hyperplasia of the prostate: a histologic mimic of prostatic adenocarcinoma. *Am J Surg Pathol* 1995;19: 1068–1076.

133. Brennick JB, O'Connell JX, Dickersin GR, et al. Lipofuscin pigmentation (so-called melanosis) of the prostate. *Am J Surg Pathol* 1994;18: 446–454.

134. Epstein JI, Lieberman PH. Mucinous adenocarcinoma of the prostate gland. *Am J Surg Pathol* 1985;9:299–308.

135. Odom DG, Donatucci CF, Deshon GE. Mucinous adenocarcinoma of the prostate. *Hum Pathol* 1986;17:863–865.

136. Elbadawi A, Craig W, Linke CA, et al. Prostate mucinous carcinoma. *Urology* 1979;13:658–666.

137. Amin MB, Ro JY, Ayala AG. Clinical relevance of histologic variants of prostate cancer. *Cancer Bull* 1993;45:403–410.

138. Ro JY, El-Naggar A, Ayala AG, et al. Signet-ring cell carcinoma of the prostate: electron-microscopic and immunohistochemical studies of eight cases. *Am J Surg Pathol* 1988;12:453–460.

139. Hejka AG, England DM. Signet-ring cell carcinoma of prostate: immunohistochemical and ultrastructural study of a case. *Urology* 1989;34: 155–158.

140. Remmele W, Weber A, Harding P. Primary signet-ring cell carcinoma of the prostate. *Hum Pathol* 1988;19:478–480.

141. Giltman LI. Signet-ring adenocarcinoma of the prostate. *J Urol* 1981;126: 134–135.

142. Uchijima Y, Ito H, Takahashi M, et al. Prostate mucinous adenocarcinoma with signet-ring cell. *Urology* 1990;36:267–268.

143. Bostwick DG, Wollan P, Adlakha K. Collagenous micronodules in prostate cancer: a specific but infrequent diagnostic finding. *Arch Pathol Lab Med* 1995;119:444–447.

144. Melicow MM, Pachter MR. Endometrial carcinoma of prostatic utricle (uterus masculinus). *Cancer* 1967;20:1715–1722.

145. Melicow MM, Tannenbaum M. Endometrial carcinoma of uterus masculinus (prostatic utricle): report of 6 cases. *J Urol* 1971;106:892–902.

146. Bostwick DG, Kindrachuk RW, Rouse RV. Prostatic adenocarcinoma with endometrioid features: clinical, pathologic, and ultrastructural findings. *Am J Surg Pathol* 1985;9:595–609.

147. Epstein JI, Woodruff JM. Adenocarcinoma of the prostate with endometrioid features: a light microscopic and immunohistochemical study of ten cases. *Cancer* 1986;57:111–119.

148. Greene LF, Farrow GM, Ravits JM, et al. Prostatic adenocarcinoma of ductal origin. *J Urol* 1979;121:303–305.

149. Dube VE, Farrow GM, Greene LF. Prostatic adenocarcinoma of ductal origin. *Cancer* 1973;32:402–409.

150. Dube VE, Joyce GT, Kennedy E. Papillary primary duct adenocarcinoma of the prostate. *J Urol* 1972;107:825–826.

151. Christensen WN, Steinberg G, Walsh PC, et al. Prostatic duct adenocarcinoma: findings at radical prostatectomy. *Cancer* 1991;67:2118–2124.

152. Tetu B, Ro JY, Ayala AG, et al. Small-cell carcinoma of the prostate I: a clinicopathologic study of 20 cases. *Cancer* 1987;59:1803–1809.

153. Schron DS, Gipson T, Mendelsohn G. The histogenesis of small-cell carcinoma of the prostate: an immunohistochemical study. *Cancer* 1984;53: 2478–2480.

154. Hagood PG, Johnson FE, Bedrossian CW, et al. Small-cell carcinoma of the prostate. *Cancer* 1991;67:1046–1050.

155. Ro JY, Tetu B, Ayala AG, et al. Small-cell carcinoma of the prostate II: immunohistochemical and electron microscopic study of 18 cases. *Cancer* 1987;59:977–982.

156. Accetta PA, Gardner WA. Squamous metastases from prostatic adenocarcinoma [Abstract]. *Lab Invest* 1982;46:2.

157. Moyana TN. Adenosquamous carcinoma of the prostate. *Am J Surg Pathol* 1987;11:403–407.

158. Saito R, Davis BK, Ollapally EP. Adenosquamous carcinoma of the prostate. *Hum Pathol* 1984;15:87–89.

159. Lager DJ, Goeken JA, Kemp JD, et al. Squamous metaplasia of the prostate: an immunohistochemical study. *Am J Clin Pathol* 1988;90:597–601.

160. Bennett RS, Edgerton EO. Mixed prostatic carcinoma. *J Urol* 1973;110: 561–563.

161. Gray GF, Marshall VF. Squamous carcinoma of the prostate. *J Urol* 1975; 113:736–738.

162. Sieracki JC. Epidermoid carcinoma of the human prostate: report of three cases. *Lab Invest* 1955;4:232–240.

163. Sarma DP, Weilbaecher TG, Moon TD. Squamous cell carcinoma of prostate. *Urology* 1991;37:260–262.

164. Wernert N, Goebbels R, Bonkhoff H, et al. Squamous cell carcinoma of the prostate. *Histopathology* 1990;17:339–344.

165. Mott LJM. Squamous cell carcinoma of the prostate: report of 2 cases and review of the literature. *J Urol* 1979;121:833–835.

166. Thompson GJ, Albers DD, Broders AC. Unusual carcinomas involving the prostate gland. *J Urol* 1953;69:416–425.

167. Shannon RL, Ro JY, Grignon DJ, et al. Sarcomatoid carcinoma of the prostate: a clinicopathologic study of 12 cases. *Cancer* 1992;69:2676–2682.

168. Wick MR, Young RH, Malvesta R, et al. Prostatic carcinosarcomas: clinical, histologic, and immunohistochemical data on two cases, with a review of the literature. *Am J Clin Pathol* 1989;92:131–139.

169. Ogawa K, Kim YC, Nakashima Y, et al. Expression of epithelial markers in sarcomatoid carcinoma: an immunohistochemical study. *Histopathology* 1987;11:511–522.

170. Dundore PA, Cheville JC, Nascimento AG, et al. Carcinosarcoma of the prostate: report of 21 cases. *Cancer* 1995;76:1035–1042.
171. Mostofi FK, Davis CJ Jr, Sesterhenn IA. Histopathology of prostate cancer. In: Lepor H, Lawson RK, eds. *Prostate diseases*. Philadelphia: WB Saunders, 1993:229–256.
172. Goebbels R, Amberger L, Wernert N, et al. Urothelial carcinoma of the prostate. *Appl Pathol* 1985;3:242–254.
173. Greene LF, O'Dea MJ, Dockerty MB. Primary transitional cell carcinoma of the prostate. *J Urol* 1976;116:761–763.
174. Rubinstein AB, Rubnitz ME. Transitional cell carcinoma of the prostate. *Cancer* 1969;24:543–546.
175. Wendelken JR, Schelhammer PF, Ladaga LE, et al. Transitional cell carcinoma: cause of refractory cancer of the prostate. *Urology* 1979;13: 557–560.
176. Mahadevia PS, Koss LG, Tar IJ. Prostatic involvement in bladder cancer: prostate mapping in 20 cystoprostatectomy specimens. *Cancer* 1986;58: 2096–2102.
177. Devaraj LT, Bostwick DG. Atypical basal cell hyperplasia of the prostate: immunophenotypic profile and proposed classification of basal cell proliferations. *Am J Surg Pathol* 1993;17:645–659.
178. Reed RJ. Consultation case. *Am J Surg Pathol* 1984;8:699–704.
179. Young RH, Frierson HF Jr, Mills SE, et al. Adenoid cystic-like tumor of the prostate gland: a report of two cases and review of the literature on "adenoid cystic carcinoma" of the prostate. *Am J Clin Pathol* 1988;89: 49–56.
180. Denholm SW, Webb JN, Howard GCW, et al. Basaloid carcinoma of the prostate gland: histogenesis and review of the literature. *Histopathology* 1992;20:151–155.
181. Grignon DJ, Ro JY, Ordóñez NG, et al. Basal cell hyperplasia, adenoid basal cell tumor, and adenoid cystic carcinoma of the prostate gland: an immunohistochemical study. *Hum Pathol* 1988;19:1425–1433.
182. Nelson RS, Epstein JI. Prostatic carcinoma with abundant xanthomatous cytoplasm. Foamy gland carcinoma. *Am J Surg Pathol* 1996;20: 419–426.
183. Cina SJ, Silberman MA, Kahane H, et al. Diagnosis of Cowper's glands on prostate needle biopsy. *Am J Surg Pathol* 1997;21:550–555.
184. Levi AW, Epstein JI. Pseudohyperplastic prostatic adenocarcinoma on needle biopsy and simple prostatectomy. *Am J Surg Pathol* 2000;24: 1039–1046.
185. Egan AJ, Lopez-Beltran A, Bostwick DG. Prostatic adenocarcinoma with atrophic features: malignancy mimicking a benign process. *Am J Surg Pathol* 1997;21:931–935.

CHAPTER 6B
Prostate Cancer: Molecular Pathology and Biologic Determinants

Mark A. Rubin and Massimo Loda

INTRODUCTION

The prevalence of pathologic prostate cancer is extremely high and increases with age. Pathologic prostate cancer is seen in autopsy series in men in their 20s and 30s and increases to greater than 80% in men over the age of 70 (1). The adoption of screening based on the measurement of the serum prostate-specific antigen (PSA) has led to earlier detection of prostate cancer. As a result, most tumors now appear confined to the prostate at presentation. The clinical and pathologic features used for tumor staging include preoperative PSA level, clinical stage, and the state of tumor differentiation (Gleason score) detected at biopsy. These parameters can stratify patients into subgroups differing with respect to outcome after surgery and are widely used to

guide clinical decision-making. However, precisely because of PSA-based cancer detection, patients are increasingly presenting within a narrow range of these parameters, which, as such, are beginning to lose their discriminatory power. In fact, among all patients undergoing prostatectomy for organ-confined disease, more than one third will relapse, demonstrating that the tumor was not confined to the prostate (2). PSA testing has greatly facilitated the detection of prostate cancer, which may have contributed to the decline in mortality from prostate cancer during the past few years. In turn, however, there has likely been an increase in the probability of detecting clinically insignificant disease. The evidence for this is increasing (3–5). The challenge is to identify those patients at risk for relapse as well as those with indolent tumors not requiring further intervention. Given the prevalence of the disease, the ease of diagnosis, the aging of the population, and the morbidity of treatment, the ability to distinguish aggressive versus indolent forms of cancer is critical.

Further improvements in staging beyond tumor size and state of cellular differentiation requires the identification of new predictors of tumor behavior. The molecular oncology paradigm is based on the belief that the behavior of a tumor is ultimately dependent on certain key molecular characteristics. The goal of molecular staging of prostate cancer is to identify genes involved in pathways relevant to prostate cancer pathogenesis and to use them as prognostic and/or predictive markers in both serum- and tissue-based assays. Molecular approaches to this problem have focused on candidate gene analysis in tissue-based assays (discussed in detail later). The loss of expression of genes with tumor suppressor activities such as *p27*, *PTEN*, and *E-cadherin* has been associated with disease progression or with higher grade tumors, while overexpression or amplification of putative oncogenes including *Her-2/neu*, *Bcl-2*, *myc*, and *cyclin D1* has been noted in aggressive androgen-independent disease. However, none of these has yet gained widespread use in clinical practice as an adjunct to the canonical pathologic parameters.

GENETICS OF HEREDITARY PROSTATE CANCER

Currently, the evidence for a strong genetic component of prostate cancer is compelling. Observations made in the 1950s by Morganti and colleagues suggested a strong familial predisposition for prostate cancer (6). Strengthening the genetic evidence is the high frequency for prostate cancer in monozygotic as compared to dizygotic twins in a study of twins from Sweden, Denmark, and Finland (7). However, unlike the successful mapping and cloning of *BRCA1* and *BRCA2*, which explain a large proportion of hereditary breast cancers, genes conferring susceptibility to prostate cancer have been more elusive. Work during the past decade using genome-wide scans in prostate cancer families has identified high-risk alleles, displaying either an autosomal dominant or X-linked mode of inheritance from at least seven candidate genetic loci (Table 6B.1). From these loci, three candidate genes have emerged, *HPC2/ELAC2* on 17p (8,9), *RNASEL* on 1q25 (10), and *MSR1* on 8p22-23 (11). Although an initial attempt to confirm these findings was promising (12), more recent reports find little evidence that *ELAC2* is linked to hereditary or sporadic prostate cancer (8,13–15). *RNASEL* (encoding ribonuclease L) is a ubiquitously expressed latent endoribonuclease involved in the mediation of the antiviral and proapoptotic activities of the interferon-inducible 2-5A system

TABLE 6B.1

PROSTATE CANCER SUSCEPTIBILITY LOCI IDENTIFIED BY LINKAGE ANALYSIS

Susceptibility locus	Locus	Mode	Putative gene	Reference
HPC1	1q24-25	AD	RNASEL (10)	Smith et al. (24)
PCAP	1q42.2-43	AD	?	Berthon et al. (25)
CAPB	1p36	AD	?	Gibbs et al. (26)
HPCX	Xq27-28	X-linked/AR	?	Xu et al. (27)
HPC20	20q13	AD	?	Berry et al. (28)
HPC2	17p	AD	HPC2/ELAC2 (9)	Tavtigian et al. (9)
	8p22-23	AD	MSR1	Xu et al. (11)

Mode, suggested mode of inheritance; AD, autosomal dominant; AR, autosomal recessive.

(16,17). Work from several groups demonstrates that *RNASEL* mutations lead to decreased enzymatic activity rather than gene inactivation (10,18–20). Although approximately 13% of prostate cancer cases in the population have been reported to carry a mutation in this gene (10), another study only found mutations in hereditary cases of prostate cancer (21). Mutations in *RNASEL* predispose men to an increased incidence of prostate cancer, which in some cases appear to behave more aggressively and/or are diagnosed at an earlier age compared with non-*RNASEL* linked cases (22). However, an *RNASEL* knockout mouse exists, which is devoid of any prostate-related phenotype. Interestingly, this mouse is susceptible to infections, an intriguing observation given the increasing interest in proliferative inflammatory atrophy (PIA) as a putative precursor lesion in the development of prostate cancer (see below). One may speculate that mutations in this gene might reduce the ability to eradicate certain infectious agents within the prostate. The resultant chronic inflammation may play a role in prostate cancer pathogenesis (23).

The other putative hereditary gene, *MSR1*, is a macrophage specific receptor, which can bind polyanionic ligands including gram-negative and gram-positive bacteria. *MSR1* knockout mice also have a reduced capacity to eradicate pathogens but no particular prostatic phenotype (11).

It is clear, however, that these three genes do not account for the majority of hereditary prostate cancer cases. The discovery of highly penetrant prostate cancer genes has been particularly difficult for at least two main reasons. First, due to the advanced age of onset (median 60 years), identification of more than two generations to perform molecular studies on is difficult. Second, given the high frequency of prostate cancer, it is likely that cases considered to be hereditary during segregation studies actually represent phenocopies. Currently, it is not possible to distinguish sporadic (phenocopies) from hereditary cases in families with high rates of prostate cancer. In addition, hereditary prostate cancer does not occur in any of the known cancer syndromes and does not have any clinical (other than a somewhat early age of onset at times) or pathologic characteristics to allow researchers to distinguish it from sporadic cases (29). It is hoped that the formation of large international consortia that are collaborating and pooling families will provide some relief to these problems. Perhaps even more important in terms of inherited susceptibility for prostate cancer are common polymorphisms in a number of low-penetrance alleles of other genes—the so-called genetic modifier alleles. The list of these variants is long, but the major pathways currently under examination include those involved in androgen action, DNA repair, carcinogen metabolism, and inflammation pathways (10,30). It is widely assumed that

the specific combinations of these variants, in the proper environmental setting, can profoundly affect the risk of developing prostate cancer.

MODELS OF ADVANCED PROSTATE CANCER FOR MOLECULAR ANALYSIS

Since the original work by Huggins and Hodges published in the first volume of *Cancer Research* in 1941 [recently reprinted as a classic article (31)], there have been few clinical advances in the treatment of hormone refractory prostate cancer, mostly because the mechanisms by which prostate cancer becomes androgen independent are unknown (32,33). The lack of well-characterized tissue resources from men with metastatic prostate cancer remains one of the major limitations to studying advanced disease. Three groups (i.e., University of Michigan, Ann Arbor, MI; University of Washington, Seattle, WA; and Johns Hopkins University, Baltimore, MD) have developed rapid autopsy programs with the goal of procuring metastatic osseous and nonosseous prostate cancer samples for research purposes (34,35).

One of the most important observations is the morphologic heterogeneity of metastatic prostate cancer. Standard descriptions of prostate cancer pathology rarely make attempts to subclassify metastatic tumors based on their morphology and have discouraged grading of these lesions (36,37). From the clinical perspective, no strong evidence exists supporting that the grading of metastatic prostate cancer has any clinical utility. However, Cheville et al. found that of various pathologic features associated with cancer-specific survival in men with hormone naive metastatic disease, degree of tumor differentiation was strongly associated with cancer-specific survival (38).

One important observation from autopsy series examining hormone refractory metastatic prostate cancer is that unlike many of the animal models, these human tumors are not often characterized by a neuroendocrine phenotype (35,39). It is true, however, that when hormone refractory prostate cancer does express neuroendocrine markers (particularly in association with a small cell phenotype), this is associated with an adverse outcome (35,40–42). However, well-defined quantitative criteria are needed to make this a more useful biomarker. Importantly, novel cell lines and xenograft models are being derived from these primary tumors (43–45). The morphologic observation of the rarity of neuroendocrine differentiation in human hormone refractory, metastatic prostate cancer should be considered when using cell lines such as the neuroendocrine ones derived from transgenic adenocarcinoma mouse prostate (TRAMP) model metastases (46) as being representative of advanced prostate cancer.

EARLY MOLECULAR ALTERATIONS IN PROSTATE CANCER PROGRESSION: PROSTATE INTRAEPITHELIAL NEOPLASIA AND PROLIFERATIVE INFLAMMATORY ATROPHY

Prostate Intraepithelial Neoplasia

Most carcinomas arise from preinvasive intraepithelial precursor lesions (47). These lesions show morphologic features and molecular alterations characteristic of malignancy, including genetic instability (48), but occur within preexisting epithelia and are confined within the basement membrane. The frequency of proliferating cells and of apoptotic bodies increases from normal prostate through prostate intraepithelial neoplasia (PIN) to adenocarcinoma. However, apoptotic cells increase by approximately an eighth to a tenth compared to proliferating ones (49).

Several genes have been implicated in the earliest development of prostate cancer (Table 6B.2).

Mitogen-activated protein (MAP) kinases transduce extracellular signals into cellular responses. Serum and growth factors activate extracellular signal-regulated protein kinases (ERKs) by dual tyrosine and threonine phosphorylation and trigger cell proliferation or differentiation. In contrast, cellular stresses activate c-jun N-terminal kinases (JNKs) and reactivating kinase (p38/RK) and result in growth arrest and induction of apoptosis. Mitogen-activated protein kinase phosphatase-1 (MKP-1)

inactivates preferentially the proapoptotic MAP kinases JNK and p38 and is therefore antiapoptotic (50,51). The percent of apoptosis is significantly higher in PIN lesions that do not express MKP-1 (and/or bcl-2) protein compared to those that do (50). Thus, MKP-1 shifts the balance existing between cell proliferation and death in PIN by inhibiting, when expressed, pathways leading to apoptosis (Fig. 6B.1).

Prostate intraepithelial neoplasias, both in humans and in rats, show low to absent levels of the cell cycle inhibitor p27 (51), suggesting that they may derive from (and persist as) the p27 negative, proliferating compartment of basal cells (52).

p53 mutations have been found in normal prostate tissue of prostate cancer patients and in prostatic intraepithelial neoplasia. Such a finding contrasts with the common belief that p53 mutation or loss is a late event in prostate carcinogenesis and implicates p53 inactivation as an early event in prostate tumorigenesis (53).

Hepsin is a differentially expressed gene when prostate cancer is compared to normal tissue. By immunohistochemistry, hepsin was found to be highly expressed in PIN, suggesting that dysregulation of hepsin is an early event in the development of prostate cancer (54).

If genetic instability helps to drive cancer formation, and telomere shortening is a major mechanism leading to genetic instability, then telomere shortening should occur in the intraepithelial phase of carcinoma. In fact, an in situ telomere fluorescence in situ hybridization (FISH) technique was employed to demonstrate telomere shortening in the majority of high-grade PIN lesions (55).

Estrogen receptor beta (ERβ) is the second major type of estrogen receptor and, contrary to the alpha isoform, is expressed by epithelial cells in the prostate. Although its role as a facilitator or as a suppressor of prostatic tumorigenesis is still debated (56), low-grade but not high-grade PIN expresses ERβ (57), raising the attractive possibility that lack of expression of ERβ may contribute to the initial phases of epithelial tumorigenesis.

TABLE 6B.2

SELECTED GENES ASSOCIATED WITH PROSTATE CANCER PROGRESSION

Abbreviation	Gene name(s)	Locus	Functional role	Molecular alteration
GST-pi	Glutathione-S-transferase pi	11q13	Caretaker gene	Hypermethylation
NKX3.1	NK3 transcription factor homologue A	8p21	Homeobox gene	No mutations
PTEN	Phosphatase and tensin homologue (mutated in multiple advanced cancers)	10q23.3	Tumor suppressor gene	Mutations and haplotype insufficiency
AMACR	Alpha-methylacyl-CoA racemase	5p13.2-q11.1	β-oxidation of branched-chain fatty acids	Overexpressed in PIN/PCa
Hepsin	Hepsin	19q11-q13.2	Transmembrane protease, serine 1	Overexpressed in PIN/PCa
KLF-6	Kruppel-like factor 6/ COPEB	10p15	Zinc finger transcription factor	Mutations and haplotype insufficiency
EZH2	Enhancer of zeste homologue 2	7q35	Transcriptional memory	Overexpressed in aggressive PCa
p27	Cyclin-dependent kinase inhibitor 1B (p27, Kip1)	12p13	Cyclin-dependent kinases 2 and 4 inhibitor	Downregulated with PCa progression
E-cadherin	E-cadherin	16q22.1	Cell adhesion molecule	Downregulated with PCa progression

PCa, prostate cancer; PIN, prostatic intraepithelial neoplasia.

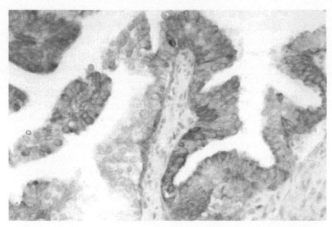

bcl-2

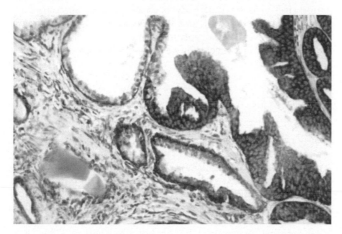

FIGURE 6B.1. Immunohistochemistry for bcl-2 and *in situ* hybridization for MKP-1 in prostate intraepithelial neoplasia (PIN) lesion and normal prostate basal cells. (See color insert.)

Proliferative Inflammatory Atrophy

Pathologists have long recognized focal areas of epithelial atrophy in the prostate (58–60). These, distinct from the diffuse atrophy seen after androgen deprivation, most often appear in the periphery of the prostate, where prostate cancers typically arise (59,61–65). Epithelial atrophy may be associated with acute or chronic inflammation, contain proliferative epithelial cells, and may show morphologic transitions in continuity with high-grade PIN (64,66). A direct transition from these atrophic lesions to carcinoma with little or no recognizable PIN component can also be observed (49,60,67). Focal atrophy of the prostate exists as a spectrum of morphologies and can be quite extensive. Because these lesions have also been shown to have a high proliferation index (61,64,65,68), they have been termed proliferative inflammatory atrophy (PIA) lesions (64). In support of PIA as a prostate cancer precursor, chromosome 8 gain, detected by FISH with a chromosome 8 centromere probe, was found in human PIA, PIN, and prostate cancer (68,69). Others have recently documented rare *p53* mutations in one variant of PIA (70), and recent work from Nakayama et al. shows that approximately 6% of PIA lesions show evidence of somatic methylation of the *GSTP1* gene promoter (71). The pi-class of glutathione-*S*-transferase (*GST*), which plays a caretaker role by normally preventing stress-related damage, demonstrates hypermethlyation in a high percentage of invasive prostate cancers as well (72–74). Thus, expression of this protective gene occurs early and persists throughout prostatic carcinogenesis. Focal atrophy lesions may arise either as a consequence of epithelial damage from infection, ischemia, or toxin exposure or as a direct consequence of inflammatory oxidant damage to the epithelium (64). Regardless of the etiology of PIA, the epithelial cells in these lesions exhibit molecular signs of stress, expressing high levels of GSTP1, GSTA1, and cyclo-oxygenase 2 (COX-2) (64,66,75,76). There is also mounting evidence that the atrophic luminal cells in PIA represent a form of intermediate epithelial cell (77) similar to cells postulated to be the targets of neoplastic transformation in the prostate (52,78–80). Therefore, both PIA and high-grade PIN may represent steps along a pathway in the progression to invasive prostate cancer. However, it is not clear if they represent separate pathways or steps along the same pathway. Ongoing work sponsored by the National Cancer Institute (NCI) is focusing on developing a consensus definition of PIA so that future studies can be optimally compared.

TECHNOLOGIES FOR THE DISCOVERY AND ASSESSMENT OF BIOMARKERS

Tissue Microarray Technology

Analysis of candidate biomarkers of response or prognosis has mostly been done at the tissue level by staining selected slides from individual cases. More recently, the tissue microarray (TMA) technology has allowed for the placement of several hundred tissue samples into a single standard tissue block. The advantage of this technology is that multiple tumors can be evaluated simultaneously by immunohistochemistry or *in situ* hybridization on a single slide. Test conditions are similar for all elements on the slide, providing more uniformity than standard experiments, while conservation of resource is maximized. One limitation of TMA technology is that due to tumor (tissue) heterogeneity, sampling may miss areas of protein expression. By redundant sampling, one can minimize this problem.

There are screening arrays that are used for the evaluation and development of biomarkers. These TMAs tend to be small (100 to 200 samples) and are used to test new antibodies or work out the optimal test conditions. Larger outcome TMAs are used to evaluate putative biomarkers. The use of automated arrayers allows the production of multiple replicate blocks. This is ideal for studying large cohorts among multiple institutions.

Laser Capture Microdissection

Laser capture microdissection (LCM) represents an important improvement on standard microdissection techniques, which are limiting in the study of prostate cancer due to their heterogeneous nature (81). LCM offers laser precision and can achieve transfer and isolation of single cells from which DNA, RNA, and proteins can be extracted. Coupled with immunohistochemistry, it allows the isolation of nucleic acids from subpopulations of cells not identifiable by morphology alone (82). LCM was developed by Emmert-Buck and colleagues at the NCI (83). LCM was born out of a need to isolate pure populations of tumor, normal, and dysplastic tissues as part of the Cancer Genome Anatomy Project (CGAP) project (http://cgap.nci.nih.gov) (84,85). LCM now allows the investigator to ask questions regarding individual cells and the relationship between tumor cells and the surrounding stromal tissues.

Gene Expression Arrays

The lack of progress in defining useful molecular markers and in understanding the deregulated biologic processes driving prostate cancer cell transformation has led to the application of genomic approaches to this problem, such as the cDNA and oligonucleotide microarray technology. cDNA microarrays consist of thousands of different cDNA clones spotted onto known locations on glass microscope slides (86). These are then hybridized with differentially labeled cDNA populations made from the mRNAs of two different samples. The primary data obtained are the ratios of fluorescence intensity (red/green), representing the ratio of concentrations of mRNA molecules that hybridized to each of the cDNAs represented on the array. The oligonucleotide technology involves the hybridization of fluorescently labeled RNAs to oligonucleotides of known sequence that are photolithographically synthesized on a solid surface (87). The relative expression levels of thousands of genes can be determined by these large-scale expression assays. Microarray expression experiments have identified a number of additional molecular markers useful either in diagnosis or prognosis including *hepsin* and *AMACR* (54,88) or expression-based models as potential predictors of disease or disease progression (89) (see below).

Large-scale Genomic Analysis: Single Nucleotide Polymorphism and Array-comparative Genomic Hybridization

One of the most important tools in the molecular analysis of human tumors is the genome-wide assessment of chromosomal and genetic alterations such as regions of amplification or chromosome loss. In order to do this, several techniques have become available in recent years such as comparative genomic hybridization (CGH) and single nucleotide polymorphism (SNP) arrays. One important advantage of these techniques is the fact that they work in formalin-fixed, paraffin-embedded archived material allowing retrospective screening of unlimited numbers of tumors. One of the challenges in exploring the biology of solid tumors is the extent of cellular heterogeneity. Most tumor samples contain a mixture of malignant epithelial cells, normal epithelial cells, and an admixture of stromal cells. DNA for SNP or CGH analysis can be obtained from DNA prepared from prostate tumors after laser capture microdissection (LCM), circumventing the difficult problem of heterogeneity in solid tumors.

The molecular patterns obtained by gene expression profiling can be compared to genetic analysis of the same tumors by chip-based SNPs or array-comparative genomic hybridization (array-CGH). Such comparisons allow expression signatures to be linked with genetic activation or inactivation of pathways known to be important in cancer. The ultimate goal would then be to identify genomic/expression signatures directly in prostate biopsy specimens by means of multiplexed *in situ* hybridization or immunohistochemistry for the relevant genes in the altered pathway.

Bioinformatics

A rapidly emerging field, bioinformatics, is starting to alter the way research is being conducted. Using information from large databases, *in silico* studies can be conducted to discover and validate new candidate genes and pathways significant in areas such as the development of prostate cancer.

Bioinformatics is the mainstay of analysis in experiments of expression profiling or large-scale genomic analysis. Rhodes et al. identified lists of significant prostate cancer–related genes by performing a meta-analysis on publicly available cDNA expression array data sets (90). This study was also able to extrapolate prostate cancer–related pathways by piecing together data from multiple studies. This approach has now become available on an Internet-based Web site called ONCOMINE (www.oncomine.org) that allows the user to perform a meta-analysis on genes of interest and contains links to other Web sites that provide information regarding their genes of interest. Pathologists will play an important role in this field due to the central role they play in the interpretation of tissue specimens, as gatekeepers of pathology databases, and because of the need for appropriate protection of patient-sensitive information available on pathology data systems.

Bioinformatics platforms for use in the Internet-based evaluation of TMAs have already been developed. Such applications need no special client software, as any Java-compliant browser will work. Encryption of the data passing between the client and the server allows for patient confidentiality to be maintained.

Clinical Databases

In order to identify the prognostically meaningful genes that are involved in cancer progression, large databases of tumor samples with clinical follow-up need to be examined. All the technologies outlined above that are being used to interrogate such databases are complementary. Combined, these technology platforms are beginning to identify molecular signatures predictive of tumor behavior and will soon be used routinely as an adjunct to canonical morphologic analysis. The challenge ahead is to conclusively determine the role some of these genes play as prognostic and or/predictive markers using large, retrospective, possibly multi-institutional databases with long-term follow-up. An additional level of complexity to be overcome is the use of such markers as prognosticators in needle biopsies, prior to any therapy. Unfortunately, the extreme heterogeneity of prostate cancer currently precludes their use as predictors in the initial assessment by needle biopsy. However, interesting data are beginning to emerge from gene expression analysis of tumor cells that have been laser-microdissected from biopsy specimens (91). Potential therapeutic targets are also beginning to surface concomitant to novel therapeutic agents designed to interfere with specific molecules in critical pathways. Construction of databases associated with tissue specimens from patients undergoing novel treatment modalities will prove invaluable in the interpretation of drug targeting.

SERUM- AND TISSUE-BASED BIOMARKERS

Prostate-specific Antigen

PSA is a serine protease produced by the epithelial cells lining the acini and ducts of the prostate gland. Under normal conditions, it is secreted into the lumina of prostatic ducts and can be detected in high concentrations in seminal plasma.

PSA expression, while highly restricted and confined mainly to benign and malignant prostatic luminal epithelial cells, can also be elevated in prostatitis, benign prostatic hyperplasia (BPH), and after prostate manipulation, thus making this marker not absolutely cancer specific.

Pretreatment serum PSA is related to clinical stage, Gleason grade, tumor volume, and pathologic stage (92). Serum PSA is currently used as a tumor marker for prostate cancer and also for the early detection, staging, and post-treatment follow-up of patients. Immunohistochemical staining for PSA is useful in the identification as prostate carcinoma of metastatic tumor of unknown origin. Interestingly, prostate cancers with poor differentiation express inferior amounts of immunologically detectable PSA compared to well-differentiated tumors and behave more aggressively (93).

Prostate-specific Membrane Antigen

Prostate-specific membrane antigen (PSMA) is a well-established prostate cancer cell surface antigen and constitutes an antigenic target in prostate cancer. Importantly, PSMA expression appears to be elevated in poorly differentiated, metastatic, and hormone refractory carcinomas, although it has been detected in nonprostatic tissues as well (94). It is expressed at high density on the cell membrane of all prostate cancers, and after antibody binding, the PSMA-antibody complex is rapidly internalized. Anti PSMA monoclonal antibodies can be used to target delivery of highly cytotoxic agents to the cancer cells without affecting normal cells (95,96). PSMA is used as an immunoscintigraphic target using the antibody conjugate CYT-356 (ProstaScint; Cytogen, Princeton, NJ) and has been shown to have clinical value, particularly in detecting occult prostate cancer (94).

p53

The *p53* tumor suppressor gene plays a central role in key regulatory pathways as cell cycle control, DNA repair, and apoptosis. Loss of heterozygosity (LOH) of chromosome 17p, where *p53* is located, occurs in about one-fifth of prostate cancers [(97) and reviewed in (98)]. Most *p53* missense mutations prolong its half-life, facilitating detection by immunohistochemistry so that detection of nuclear p53 almost always signifies a mutant form of this gene (95). p53 protein overexpression is correlated with higher Gleason score, nuclear grade, pathologic stage, and proliferation in localized primary prostate carcinomas. p53 overexpression is an adverse prognostic indicator and an independent prognostic marker for disease-free survival after radical prostatectomy [for review, see (96) and references therein]. More recently, the human tumor suppressor *RTVP-1* gene has been shown to be regulated by *p53* and to induce apoptosis in human prostate cancer cell lines. In addition, *RTVP-1* is downregulated and epigenetically modified in human prostate cancer specimens compared with normal human prostate tissue at the mRNA and protein levels (99). Mutations in the *p53* tumor suppressor gene are generally believed to be a late event in the progression of prostate cancer and are associated with androgen-independence, increased angiogenesis, metastasis, recurrence, and a worse prognosis. However, *p53* mutations have been demonstrated in approximately one third of early-stage prostate cancers, and expression of human papilloma virus (HPV) E6 or overexpression of mdm2 contributes to loss of p53 function in an additional 25% of organ-confined disease (53). The existence of *p53* mutations seems to predict resistance to radiation therapy or systemic treatment (100). Interestingly, targeting of MDM2, the ubiquitin ligase responsible for p53 degradation, has

yielded some interesting results, at least *in vitro*. MDM2 inhibitors may thus provide novel approaches to therapy of prostate cancer (101).

bcl-2

The *bcl-2* gene is the prototype of a class of oncogenes that modulate apoptosis. The regulation of cell death by members of this gene family may be achieved through competing dimerization of different family members.

Although initially discovered via the translocation in follicular lymphomas (t14; 18), *bcl-2* has subsequently been found to be involved in the carcinogenesis of various epithelial tumors including prostate carcinoma [see (102,103) and references therein].

Normally *bcl-2* is expressed in the basal cells of the prostate glandular epithelium, which are resistant to the effects of androgen withdrawal. In contrast, the bcl-2 negative secretory glandular epithelial cells undergo apoptotic cell death in response to androgen deprivation. High levels of *bcl-2* expression are seen with greater frequency as prostate cancers progress to androgen-independent tumor (104–106). *bcl-2* may confer survival advantage to prostate cancer cells in an androgen-depleted environment. Thus, hormonal ablation may select *bcl-2* positive cells, which fail to undergo apoptosis after androgen withdrawal. Expression of *bcl-2* correlates inversely with clinical outcome in patients with both clinically localized tumors and locally advanced or metastatic prostate cancer receiving hormonal therapy (107,108). Interestingly, expression of *bcl-2* within prostate carcinoma cells is associated with resistance to cell death induction by various chemotherapeutic agents. A mechanism whereby *bcl-2* induces its antiapoptotic effect may be via regulation of microtubule integrity (109). Anticancer drugs that inhibit microtubule function (e.g. paclitaxel and vinblastine) also induce *bcl-2* phosphorylation, which leads to its inactivation and then apoptotic cell death. Inactivation of *p53* and expression of *bcl-2* each confers a growth advantage to prostate cancer cells predicting an aggressive clinical course and resistance to therapeutic cell death induction. The observations of an inverse correlation between *p53* and *bcl-2* expression in advanced, androgen-independent tumors and the lack of genetic complementation between these two genes in animal models of multistep carcinogenesis suggests an effector and repressor role, respectively, in a common cell death pathway (110). It is no surprise that targeting the *bcl-2* family has become an important new tool in prostate cancer therapeutics with additive effects after irradiation (111,112).

The Cyclin-dependent Kinase Inhibitor *p27* and Its Executioner, skp2

p27 is a cyclin-dependent kinase inhibitor (CKI) and a tumor suppressor gene. The *p27* gene regulates progression of the cell cycle from G1 to S phase by predominantly binding to and inhibiting the cyclinE/cdk2 complex (113). In the normal adult prostate, *p27* protein is expressed primarily by secretory cells. Cells lacking *p27* and expressing basal cell–specific cytokeratin are present between the basal and luminal cells and appear to be increased in prostate tissue previously subjected to androgen blockade and in benign prostatic hyperplasia. The lack of nuclear *p27* expression in the suprabasal epithelial cells may therefore delineate a subcompartment of cells that proliferate in the absence of androgens (52). As mentioned previously (see "Prostate Intraepithelial Neoplasia"), dysregulation of *p27* expression may be a critical early event in the development of prostatic neoplasia. In addition, loss of expression of *p27* by immunohistochemistry in invasive prostatic adenocarcinoma has been shown to be a powerful indicator of poor prognosis independent of the traditional predictive parameters such as preoperative PSA levels and Gleason score, particularly in organ-confined disease (114,115). p27 protein expression in the preoperative prostate needle biopsy has also been shown to correlate with subsequent radical prostatectomy *p27*, Gleason grade, and pathologic stage (116).

p27 expression in the prostate is regulated, at least in part, by androgens. In the rat prostate, androgens regulate *p27* levels by inducing its proteosome-mediated degradation during proliferation as well as its stabilization during terminal differentiation (104). Thus, *p27*, when expressed, probably shifts androgen action from a proliferative to a differentiating one.

skp2 (S-phase kinase-associated protein 2) is a member of the F-box protein family and specifically recognizes phosphorylated *p27* and targets it for degradation (105). The oncogenic potential of skp2 has been demonstrated by co-transfecting skp2 and H-ras^{G12V} into primary rat embryo fibroblasts. Transfected fibroblasts showed increase in colony formation in soft agar and tumor formation in nude mice (106). In addition, transgenic mice expressing both skp2 and N-ras induce T-cell lymphomas with shorter latency and decreased survival when compared with N-ras transgenic animals (107).

Recently, increased skp2 expression has been observed in several human cancers (106–108) and generally inversely correlates with decreased *p27* levels. In addition, skp2 expression inversely correlates with *p27* expression in prostatic adenocarcinoma (117,118). In addition, it is overexpressed in a subset of androgen-independent prostate carcinomas metastatic to bone that display high proliferative growth rates, and its expression is an independent negative prognostic factor by multivariate analysis in organ confined disease (Loda M, Febbo P, unpublished). Thus, skp2 may be a suitable therapeutic target in highly proliferative, androgen-independent, prostate cancer.

E-cadherin

The long arm of chromosome 16 (16q22.1) is deleted in both primary and, more frequently, in some metastatic prostate cancer (119). This region contains the *E-cadherin* gene. E-cadherin is found on the membrane of epithelial cells and functions as a Ca^{2+}-dependent epithelial cell adhesion molecule. Its intracellular domain binds directly to *β-catenin*, which links extracellular Wnt signals with transcription factors of the LEF/TCF family. In many carcinomas, cadherins are lost or downregulated. Decreased E-cadherin expression is associated with metastatic progression, while loss of E-cadherin determined by immunohistochemistry is a predictor of poor outcome and overall survival (119). Experimentally, expression of the E-cadherin protein suppresses while loss of expression enhances the invasiveness and motility of epithelial cells. E-cadherin appears to mediate both inhibition of invasion and proliferation via the induction of *p27* (120). These findings link extracellular stimuli to the cell cycle machinery and suggest a role for *E-cadherin* and *p27* in both invasion and metastasis (111).

PTEN

The insulin-like growth factor (IGF) signaling pathway is implicated in both the initiation and progression of prostate cancer. For example, higher plasma IGF-1 levels are associated with prostate cancer risk, while inactivation of *PTEN* is common in prostate cancer cell lines particularly in advanced disease [reviewed in (112)]. Loss of PTEN expression occurs in a subset or in all tumor cells in as many as 80% of prostatic adenocarcinomas as determined by immunohistochemistry. In addition, PTEN loss directly correlates with high Gleason score and advanced stage (121).

The tumor suppressor activity of PTEN is associated with its ability to antagonize phosphoinositide-3 kinase (PI3K) signaling (114). Loss-of-function of PTEN results in deregulated PI3K signaling, and constitutive activation of downstream targets including the Akt/PKB serine/threonine kinase family (Akt), which promotes cell proliferation and survival [reviewed in (115)]. Accordingly, Akt kinase activity is frequently elevated in primary prostate tumors (122).

Androgen Receptor

Androgens with the androgen receptor (*AR*) mediate survival, regeneration, and differentiation processes in the normal prostate (123). In addition, *AR*-mediated transcription appears to be required for prostate cancer survival. In fact, the only effective treatment, albeit temporary, for metastatic prostate cancer is hormonal ablative therapy. However, the duration of response to androgen deprivation therapy is finite. Proposed mechanisms of progression to androgen-independent growth include amplification of the *AR* gene (124), mutations of the *AR* gene [reviewed in (125)], shortened numbers of CAG nucleotide repeat sequences, and recruitment of coactivators (117,126,127). Immunohistochemical studies have demonstrated expression of AR in primary, advanced, and hormone-refractory prostate cancers, suggesting that disease progression is almost never associated with loss of AR expression. There is also considerable heterogeneity of androgen receptor expression in specimens and among patients while the heterogeneity of AR expression increases with increasing Gleason grade (118,128,129).

Clinical trials such as the Prostate Cancer Prevention Trial (PCPT) provided important data on the role of decreasing the amount of available dehydroxytestosterone (DHT), the most active form of testosterone (130). Patients on this trial received long-term administration of the 5-hydroxy reductase inhibitor, finasteride, which lowers levels of circulating DHT. Although finasteride appears to have decreased the incidence of prostate cancer over the course of this trial, the tumors occurring in men having received finasteride were reported as having a higher Gleason grade. However, there is concern that this represents an as yet poorly described morphologic change akin to what is seen in biopsies that follow antiandrogen treatment (131,132). Molecular correlates are being investigated to understand the findings of this important chemopreventive trial.

Using microarray-based profiling of isogenic prostate cancer xenograft models developed from metastatic human prostate tumors in combination with interfering RNA (RNAi), Chen et al. identified that a modest increase in androgen receptor mRNA was the only change consistently associated with the development of resistance to antiandrogen therapy (133). They concluded that the increase in androgen receptor mRNA and protein was both necessary and sufficient to convert prostate cancer growth from a hormone-sensitive to a hormone-refractory stage and was dependent on a functional ligand-binding domain. Moreover, their work demonstrated that androgen receptor antagonists showed agonistic activity in cells with increased androgen receptor levels.

Craft et al. demonstrated that the tyrosine kinase receptor *Her-2/neu* can modulate responses in the setting of low androgen levels by restoring *AR* function, resulting in ligand independent growth and thus clinical progression of the cancer (134). Yeh et al. have shown that Her-2/neu can increase growth rate, PSA level, and AR transactivation in prostate cancer cells via the MAP kinase pathway (135). In addition, Her-2/neu protein expression increases progressively from untreated patients to those subjected preoperatively to androgen ablation to maximal levels in androgen-independent tumors (136). These studies in human tumors strongly support the contention that Her-2/neu overexpression can both superactivate the existing AR pathway and substitute for it to confer androgen-independent tumor cell growth.

c-myc

One of the most frequent genetic changes detected by means of comparative genomic hybridization (CGH) in hormone refractory prostate cancer is the gain of 8q and especially the 8q-qter region (137,138). One potential target at the 8q24 region is the *myc* gene. The c-*myc* gene is an immediate-early response gene that is activated by mitogenic stimuli, resulting in proliferation. Fluorescent *in situ* hybridization analysis has identified high-level amplification of c-*myc* in greater than 20% of recurrent and metastatic prostate cancers (138,139). Amplification of c-*myc* correlates with high level of c-myc protein expression (139). Furthermore, inhibition of c-*myc* expression can mediate tumor regression in a prostate cancer zenograft (140). Also, c-*myc* can cooperate with *ras* to induce prostate cancer in various rat and murine model systems. Evaluation of case-matched prostate cancer biopsies from patients undergoing androgen ablation suggests that levels of c-myc expression increase after castration (141). Bubendorf et al. using FISH on tissue microarrays, showed high-level c-*myc* amplification in 11% of metastases from patients with hormone refractory disease, suggesting a role for c-myc in metastatic progression (142). Importantly, transgenic mice expressing human c-myc in the mouse prostate develop murine prostatic intraepithelial neoplasia followed by invasive adenocarcinoma (143). However, there may be other, currently unknown target genes at the distal 8q locus, whose increased copy number is selected during cancer progression. One such candidate gene is prostate stem cell antigen.

Prostate Stem Cell Antigen

Prostate stem cell antigen (PSCA) may play a role in stem cell/progenitor cell functions such as self-renewal and/or proliferation. PSCA, a prostate-specific cell surface protein, maps distal to c-myc at the 8q24.2 locus. PSCA mRNA is expressed strongly in 80% of primary prostate cancers and is overexpressed in androgen-independent prostate cancer xenografts (144). PSCA protein is overexpressed in cancer compared to normal in 36% of primary tumors and in 100% of bone metastases (145). In addition, *PSCA* is coamplified with c-*myc*, and *PSCA* amplification correlates with overexpression (146). As it localizes to the surface of prostate cancer cells and because of its almost exclusive expression in prostate, PSCA may in addition also represent an important therapeutic target. In fact, anti-PSCA antibodies that recognize PSCA expressed on the surface of live cells are efficiently internalized after antigen recognition and kill tumor cells *in vitro* in an antigen-specific fashion upon conjugation with maytansinoid (147).

Estrogen Receptor Beta

Estrogens, via the interaction with their receptors, play important roles in the control of cellular growth and differentiation. Importantly, estrogens are known to play a role in the development of the male reproductive system (148). The effects of estrogens on prostate epithelium are still largely unknown although estrogens have been used in the treatment of prostate cancer because of their growth-inhibitory effects.

Although it was initially thought that estrogens mediate their action through a single receptor, the estrogen receptor α(ERα), a second ER has been identified and termed ERβ (149). Whereas these two receptors share structural similarities (47% identity) and some functional properties, it is clear that individual characteristics allow them to have distinct biologic functions. The putative diverse biologic function of the two receptors should not only be ascribed to different ligands but, more importantly, to their different tissue distribution. Interestingly, only ERβ and not ERα transcripts were previously detected in rodent prostate epithelial cells. However, no abnormalities in either ERβ or double ERα and ERβ knockouts (ER$\alpha\beta$KO) have been found in the prostate (150–152) [for comprehensive reviews, see (148)]. ERβ mRNA appears to be expressed in both basal and luminal cells (153), although ERβ protein is not expressed in secretory cells and ERα is expressed only in stromal cell nuclei. ERβ transcripts were found to be decreased in both localized and hormone refractory prostate cancers relative to normal prostate tissue, suggesting that loss of ERβ correlated with disease progression (154). However, ERβ protein is widely expressed in androgen-independent, metastatic tumors [(57) and reviewed in (56)].

It is interesting to note that many genes expressed by the basal cells, which do not depend on androgens for survival, such as bcl-2 (155,156), *Her-2-neu* (136), and *PSCA* (144) get "re-expressed" in advanced, androgen-independent cancers. Intriguingly, ERβ seems to follow the same path. Except for the keratin profile and the almost universal expression of the androgen receptor (AR) in these tumors, metastatic, androgen-independent prostate tumors thus seem to display a "basaloid" phenotype. Whether ERβ enhances or suppresses prostate cancer development and/or progression remains to be established.

Alpha-Methylacyl-CoA Racemase

Alpha-methylacyl-CoA racemase (AMACR) is an enzyme that plays an important role in bile acid biosynthesis and β-oxidation of branched-chain fatty acids (157,158). In particular, this enzyme catalyzes the conversion of branched fatty acids from *R* to *S* configuration and allows them to undergo peroxisomal β-oxidation with generation of hydrogen peroxide and potential procarcinogenic oxidative damage (159,160). AMACR is upregulated in prostate cancer and, along with the loss of p63 and high-molecular-weight cytokeratins, is a useful marker of prostatic malignancy in prostate biopsies (54, 161–165). Interestingly, AMACR mRNA and protein expression is downregulated in hormone refractory, metastatic prostate cancer. Thus, AMACR expression appears to be independent of androgen regulation and likely related inversely to tumor differentiation (166).

Fatty Acid Synthase

Fatty acid synthase (FAS) catalyzes the synthesis of palmitate from the condensation of malonyl-CoA and acetyl-CoA, thus playing an important role in energy homeostasis by converting excess carbon intake into fatty acids for storage. Fatty acids synthesis in tumor tissues occurs at very high rates (167). In addition, almost all fatty acids derive from *de novo* synthesis despite adequate nutritional supply (168–170).

Despite its apparently marginal physiologic role under normal conditions, FAS is overexpressed at both protein and mRNA level in prostate carcinoma [reviewed in (150)] (Fig. 6B.2). Its high expression has also been associated with aggressive biologic behavior (151). Interestingly, the highest levels of FAS expression are found in androgen-independent bone metastases (152).

FAS has been shown to play a major role in the synthesis of phospholipids, primary components of cellular membranes (171). Alterations in membrane lipid composition that may occur as a result of FAS overexpression can thus have profound effects on many cellular processes such as signal transduction pathways.

Activation of the phosphatidylinositol 3′-kinase (PI3K) pathway occurs in the late phases of human prostate cancers (121). In turn, PI3K activation increases FAS transcription at least in part through the activation of sterol response element binding proteins (SREBPs) in prostate cancer cell lines (172). Importantly, in breast epithelial cells, Her-2-neu stimulates the FAS promoter through a PI3K-dependent pathway and mediates increased fatty acid synthesis, while pharmacological inhibition of FAS preferentially induces apoptosis of Her-2-overexpressing breast epithelial cells (173). Because expression of Her-2-neu in prostate cancer increases, with progression toward androgen independence (136) being highest, as is the case for FAS, in prostate cancer metastatic to bone, the oncogenic effects of PI3K activation may be mediated, at least in part, via the induction of FAS expression. Finally, overexpression and enhanced activity of FAS would result in a significant improvement in redox balance despite hypoxic conditions (174).

FAS inhibitors, such as C75 and the mycotoxin cerulenin, as well as RNA interference of FAS message, result in apoptosis of cancer cells (175,176) and decrease the size of prostate cancer xenographs that overexpress the enzyme (177). The de-ubiquitinating enzyme USP2a (ubiquitin-specific protease-2a) interacts with and stabilizes FAS, thus providing post-transcriptional regulation. Interfering with USP2a, which is overexpressed in prostate cancer, results in decreased FAS

protein levels and enhanced apoptosis in prostate cancer cells. Thus, the isopeptidase USP2a plays a critical role in prostate cancer cell survival through FAS stabilization and represents a therapeutic target in this disease (178). USP2a interference may circumvent the undesired effects of FAS inhibitors (179).

Hepsin

Hepsin, a cell surface serine protease, was determined to be overexpressed in localized and metastatic prostate cancer when compared to benign prostate or benign prostatic hyperplasia in several expression array experiments (54,88,164,180). As mentioned above, hepsin expression is increased in PIN compared to the nontransformed adjacent cells, suggesting that dysregulation of hepsin is an early event in the development of prostate cancer (54).

Kruppel-like Factor 6

Kruppel-like factor 6 *(KLF6)* is a zinc finger transcription factor of unknown function, which is mutated in a subset of human prostate cancer (181). Loss-of-heterozygosity analysis revealed that one *KLF6* allele is deleted in more than 70% of primary prostate tumors. The retained allele is mutated in more than 70% of these tumors. Functional studies suggest that wild-type KLF6 upregulates p21 (WAF1/CIP1) in a p53-independent manner and reduces cell proliferation, suggesting that *KLF6* is a tumor suppressor gene.

NKX3.1

NKX3.1 is an androgen-regulated homeobox gene located at 8p21, expressed selectively in the prostate with lower levels also seen in the testis (168,182–184). *NKX3.1* is expressed early in mouse embryogenesis, and its targeted disruption in mice gives rise to aberrations in prostate ductal morphogenesis and secretory protein production. Although no mutations have been identified in this gene (182), recent work suggests that decreased expression is associated with prostate cancer progression (183). Given the possible role of NKX3.1 in prostate carcinogenesis, we (Saatcioglu F. and Loda M, unpublished) studied its expression by immunohistochemistry. Our data indicate that NKX3.1 is specifically expressed in the nuclei of luminal cells of the prostate epithelium and that there is no significant change in NKX3.1 expression or distribution during prostate cancer progression. However, NKX3.1 haplo-insufficiency extends the proliferative stage of regenerating luminal cells, leading to epithelial hyperplasia (169). Thus, immunohistochemistry may not be quantitative enough to detect decreased expression occurring as a consequence of haploinsufficiency.

EZH2

EZH2 (Enhancer of zeste homologue 2), a member of the polycomb gene family, is a transcriptional repressor known to be active early in embryogenesis (170,185), showing decreased expression as cells differentiate. Varambally et al. (186), using cDNA microarray analysis, compared the gene expression patterns found in benign prostate tissue, organ-confined tumors, and androgen-independent metastatic prostate tumors and found that the polycomb group (PcG) protein enhancer of zeste homologue *(EZH2)* was among a group of transcripts whose

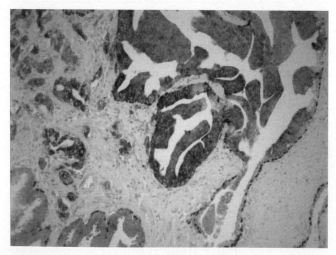

FIGURE 6B.2. Double immunohistochemistry for fatty acid synthase (FAS) and p63 demonstrating overexpression of FAS in both prostate intraepithelial neoplasia (PIN) and invasive carcinoma.

increased expression distinguished metastatic tumors from those localized to the prostate. In addition, RNAi-mediated *EZH2* knockdown leads to growth inhibition in cell culture, and this may be linked to alterations in the cell-cycle profile. These authors showed that the expression of both the EZH2 mRNA and protein progressively increase from benign to organ-confined to metastatic tumors, suggesting that increases in EZH2 precede the development of metastatic foci. These data raise the possibility that EZH2 protein levels might prove useful in predicting patient outcome after prostatectomy. Indeed, immunohistochemical analysis of the EZH2 protein in tissue microarrays predicted outcome independently of Gleason score, presurgical PSA, and stage (187). If validated in larger data sets, these data could provide important additional information useful in patient stratification (188).

Simultaneous Assessment of Multiple Markers: Genetics, Genomics, and Proteomics

Gene Expression Profiling

Several methods of comparative gene expression have been described over the years, such as representational difference analysis (RDA) or serial analysis of gene expression (SAGE), each with its distinct advantages and disadvantages. The first one identifies differences in gene expression in a sequence-independent manner but is not high throughput. The latter yields quantitative expression methods but is labor intensive and restricted in its source of information to a few tumors or cell lines. More recently, gene expression profiling using either cDNA or oligonucleotide microarrays have been successfully applied in the molecular diagnostics of cancer.

The genetic basis of cancer including prostate cancer is indisputable. Although not proven, it is widely accepted that the heterogeneity in clinical behavior is either genetically determined or determined by a complex interaction of genetic and environmental factors. There is also increasing proof that prostate cancer can be genetically classified into different subtypes (54,89,90,164,186,189). The implications of this are that using genetic stratification the clinical behavior of prostate cancer can be predicted.

The expression data obtained by microarray technology must be subjected to complex analytical methods. These include the use of supervised learning techniques for the identification of genes whose expression levels are predictive of rapid relapse after surgical resection, and the use of unsupervised learning methods (clustering) for the identification of previously unrecognized subgroups of tumors. It has been found that a gene expression signature of metastasis exists in a subset of primary tumors (190), and the presence of that signature is predictive of eventual metastatic potential in prostate adenocarcinoma. These findings suggest that contrary to the prevailing model of metastasis development, the metastatic potential of primary tumors is encoded in the bulk of the primary tumor at the time of diagnosis (89). Interestingly, one of the genes in the model was a well-known indicator of poor prognosis when overexpressed (chromogranin A), while another, PDGF receptor beta, represents a potential therapeutic target of Gleevec.

A general approach to cancer classification has been applied to a variety of tumor types including prostate cancer. As a result, efforts to develop a molecular taxonomy of cancer have yielded gene expression correlates of histologic grade and clinical outcome. Because these gene expression signatures are subtle, it is critical to attempt to validate these initial results in independent sets of samples and with different techniques.

Proteomics

Recent achievements in genomics have created an infrastructure of biologic information. The enormous success of genomics promptly induced a subsequent explosion in proteomics technology, the emerging science for systematic study of proteins in complexes, organelles, and cells. Proteomics is developing powerful technologies to identify novel proteins, to quantify the differential expression of proteins under different states, to study aspects of protein–protein interaction and, most importantly, to identify patterns of protein expression in tissues or sera that would predict recurrence or response to therapy. The dynamic nature of protein expression, protein interactions, and protein modifications requires measurement as a function of time and cellular state. These types of studies require many measurements, and thus high-throughput protein identification is essential. The most powerful, currently available technology to study protein expression in cells is mass spectrometry [reviewed in (191)], which allows for the characterization of extremely small samples (e.g., from laser capture microdissected material).

Analysis of tumors with expression array and genomic array technology can be compared and contrasted with the proteomic platform in biopsies and resection specimens, as well as body fluids such as serum. Proteomics applied to serum samples can identify unique profiles that may be used for prognosis and diagnosis of prostate cancer (192). The output of a proteomic platform is a protein profile that can differentiate benign from malignant (192) or provide prognostic/predictive information. One can also image the use of protein or expression array profiles to identify patients at highest risk for developing a disease state (e.g., prostate cancer) or even which patients would benefit from a treatment protocol.

Genome-wide Scanning

The power of comparative genomic hybridization (CGH) has been clearly proved as a tool to characterize chromosomal imbalances in neoplasias. Comparative genomic hybridization and, more recently, array-CGH can detect a number of recurrent regions of amplification or deletion. This has led to the identification of new chromosomal loci involved in the development and progression of tumors. Although mutations in any of the classic oncogenes and tumor suppressor genes are not found in high frequency in primary prostate cancers, a large number of studies have identified nonrandom somatic genome alterations. Using comparative genomic hybridization (CGH) to screen the DNA of prostate cancer, the most common chromosomal alterations in prostate cancer are losses at 1p, 6q, 8p, 10q, 13q, 16q, and 18q and gains at 1q, 2p, 7, 8q, 18q, and Xq (124,138,193, 194). The application of novel SNP informatic platforms (97) to a series of prostate cancer specimens specifically recognized regions of deletion on chromosomes 1p33-34, 3q27, 8p21, 10q23, 15q12, 16q23-24, and 17p13. LOH in prostate cancer localized to 1p, 8p21, 10q23 (the site of the tumor suppressor gene *PTEN*), 16q23 (the site of the tumor suppressor gene *E-cadherin*), and 17p13 (the site of the *p53* gene) had all been previously reported by multiple investigators (98). Thus, when CGH data from different studies are combined, a pattern of nonrandom genetic aberrations appears. As is the case for array CGH, SNP analysis allows investigators to study simultaneously multiple tumors for common regions of genetic loss.

On the basis of these technical developments, we have begun to characterize the prostate cancer genome on the latest SNP arrays. This latest generation of arrays contains probes for 120,000 SNPs. The SNP markers on this array are spaced across the genome with a mean intermarker distance of 9 kb. Thus, these arrays provide the highest resolution of any array-based genome mapping method yet tested.

Samples of androgen-dependent lymph node metastatic prostate cancer, androgen-independent metastatic prostate cancer, prostate cancer xenografts, and prostate cancer cell lines have been analyzed on the 11K platform and preliminary maps of LOH, gene amplficiation, and homozygous deletion have been developed. As shown previously (97), the arrays robustly detect LOH, and we can again define distinct genetic subtypes of prostate cancer by organizing tumors through hierarchical clustering based on LOH. As shown in Figure 6B.3, LOH inferred based on length of homozygous regions robustly separates tumor from normal (normal samples are in the middle and shown little to no inferred LOH). Moreover, two distinct tumor clusters can be seen (a major cluster on the left and one on the right). This clustering appears to be driven, at least in part, by differences on chromosomes 2 and 8.

Homozygous deletion mapping has also been analyzed. Although not as prevalent as LOH, 14 novel regions of homozygous deletion in this initial data set have been detected. Finally, gene amplification events can be detected. As an example, high-level amplification of the androgen-receptor in an androgen-independent prostate cancer xenograft was detected.

The genome-wide information obtained by both the SNP chip and array CGH analysis of pure tumor samples can be merged with expression data obtained from corresponding frozen tumor material. Merging genomic and transcriptome signatures of solid tumors will begin to unravel patterns of activation or silencing of entire pathways essential for tumor initiation or progression. This will accomplish the ultimate goal of classifying tumors not only by traditional clinicopathologic parameters but by molecular genetic means as well. One can speculate that targets will be identified for the subsequent synthesis of chemical compounds aimed at inactivation of pathways. Importantly, simple genomic analysis of paraffin-embedded tumors will eventually

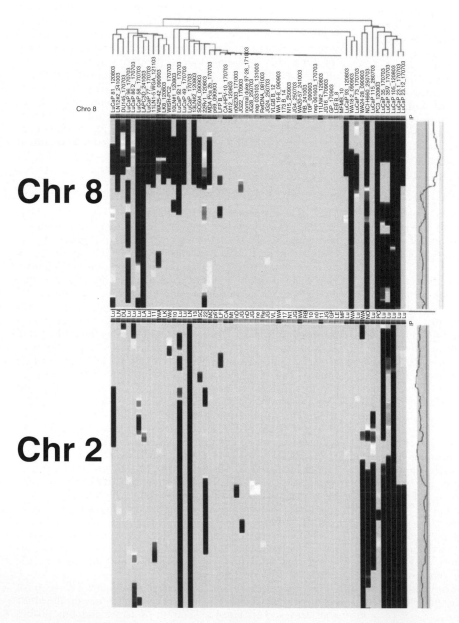

FIGURE 6B.3. Regions of loss of heterozygosity (LOH) in tumors and xenografts compared to normal samples. dChipSNP was used to generate inferred LOH maps, which were then used in hierarchical clustering. The group of samples in the center without LOH are normal germ-line samples. Two distinct tumor clusters can be seen that differ with respect to LOH patterns on chromosomes 2 and 8. (See color insert.)

be indicative of the expression signature of a given tumor (e.g., LOH of the PTEN locus will reflect activation of the PI3 kinase pathway and such a tumor may be targeted with Akt inhibitors).

Chromosomal Instability and Telomeres

Chromosomal instability is an important molecular mechanism during the pathogenesis of malignant transformation in human epithelial tissues (195), yet the molecular mechanisms responsible for chromosome destabilization during carcinogenesis are largely unknown. One route to chromosomal instability is through defective telomeres (196,197). Telomeres, which consist of multiple repeats of a 6-base-pair unit (TTAGGG), complexed with several different binding proteins, protect chromosome ends from fusing with other chromosome ends or other chromosomes containing double-strand breaks (198). However, in the absence of compensatory mechanisms, telomeric DNA is subject to loss due to cell division and possibly oxidative damage. Telomere shortening leads to chromosomal instability that, in mouse models, causes an increased cancer incidence that is likely a result in chromosome fusions, subsequent breakage, and rearrangement (199,200). Telomeres within human carcinomas are often found to be abnormally reduced in length. Telomeres from prostate cancer cells are consistently shorter than those from cells in the adjacent normal prostate tissue (201,202). As outlined above, telomere shortening occurs in the intraepithelial phase of carcinoma (55). Thus, telomere shortening is a prevalent biomarker in human prostate neoplasia occurring early in the process of prostate carcinogenesis.

MOUSE MODELS OF PROSTATE CANCER AS A TOOL FOR BIOMARKER DISCOVERY AND VALIDATION

Mouse models of prostate cancer are an invaluable tool for the understanding of genetic and biochemical pathways relevant to prostate tumorigenesis.

The anterior, dorsolateral, and ventral lobes constitute the three anatomically discrete murine paired lobes. The anterior lobe or coagulating gland plays a role in coagulating seminal fluid. The dorsolateral lobe, roughly corresponding to the human peripheral zone, can be divided into dorsal and lateral lobes based on the anatomic origin of the ducts in the urethra (203). The ventral lobe is the most responsive to androgen action in terms of atrophy and regeneration in castration and testosterone replenishment, respectively. The location of origin of the prostatic ducts in the urethra would appear to represent the best basis for determining homology of prostatic lobes or anatomic regions between mice and man. However, such anatomic homology is no guarantee of functional homology [reviewed in (204)].

In the human prostate gland, the peripheral, central, and transitional zones differ in histologic appearance, point of origin of the prostatic ducts in the urethra, and association with specific disease processes (63). Response to hormones and physiological function differ sometimes substantially in homologous lobes between species [reviewed in (204)].

Although it is beyond the scope of this chapter to give a comprehensive review of all available animal models of prostate cancer, some examples with targeted disruption of tumor suppressor genes or prostate-specific expression of putative

oncogenes, outlined below, provide support for the role of many of the biomarkers described above in human prostate tumorigenesis.

The Transgenic Adenocarcinoma Mouse Prostate Model

The first attempts to generate transgenic models of CaP have used minimal or long rat probasin (rPB) promoter constructs linked to SV40 T antigen (205,206). The TRAMP model has many similarities to human prostate cancer including the development of PIN-like lesions, the development of spontaneous cancer, the development of hormone refractory cancer following androgen withdrawal, and a low incidence of metastatic disease. The TRAMP model has proved to be extremely useful to study prostate cancer. A case in point is the expression by TRAMP tumors of the metabolic oncogene FAS (described above). Pflug et al. have shown that FAS plays a significant role in early tumorigenesis and metastases (187). Importantly, this model provided the setting for preclinical testing of FAS inhibitors.

The hormone refractory TRAMP tumors have a small cell/neuroendocrine appearance and uniformly express neuroendocrine markers (207). Therefore, although this model maintains some features seen in human prostate cancer progression, the morphology does not represent the vast majority of tumors seen after hormone ablation.

NKX3.1

The homeobox gene NKX3.1, one of the biomarkers described above, has emerged as an important regulator of prostate embryonic development. Although NKX3.1 is transiently expressed in several nonurogenital tissues during embryonic and postnatal development, its expression in adults is highly restricted, being expressed only in the prostate (all three lobes in the mouse) and the bulbourethral gland, and not in any adult female tissues (208–210). In the embryonic UGS, NKX3.1 expression is confined to the epithelium and demarcates regions where prostatic buds will arise, predating their emergence by 2 days (208). NKX3.1, along with PSCA and p63, is one of the earliest markers of prostatic epithelium. Importantly, NKX3.1 expression is highly regulated by androgens, with mRNA levels decreasing 10- to 30-fold within 3 days of castration (209,210), and its expression in the human prostate cell line LNCaP is markedly increased upon androgen stimulation (168). AR signaling thus appears to be directly required for maintenance of NKX3.1 expression. Mice with targeted disruption of the NKX3.1 locus exhibited abnormal ductal morphogenesis with fewer prostatic duct tips than wild-type controls, although the overall size and weight of prostatic lobes was normal. In addition, prostatic epithelium exhibited altered production of secretory proteins in adults. These results show that other genes must cooperate with NKX3.1 in specification of the prostate (208).

NKX3.1 itself has also been implicated in prostate tumorigenesis. NKX3.1 loss in the mouse leads to a preneoplastic phenotype of age-dependent prostatic hyperplasia and dysplasia. The human orthologue maps to 8p21, a chromosomal region that undergoes frequent LOH in prostate cancer. Coding region mutations, however, have not yet been identified in human prostate cancers (182), but other mechanisms of gene inactivation may be operating. The locus is haplo-insufficient in the mouse, as NKX3.1 heterozygotes exhibit some degree of age-dependent prostate hyperplasia and dysplasia (208).

Importantly, a majority of *NKX3.1*(+/−); *PTEN*(+/−) mice greater than 1 year of age develop invasive adenocarcinoma, which is frequently accompanied by metastases to lymph nodes (211).

Androgen Receptor Transgenics

Because of the crucial albeit controversial role that the androgen receptor plays in the pathogenesis and progression of prostate cancer, AR was targeted to the prostate with the probasin promoter (212). Although no morphologic changes were seen in young mice, prostate epithelial cells showed an increase in proliferative rates. Interestingly, older mice developed PIN but no invasive cancer.

myc Transgenics

Chromosome 8q gain in prostate cancer is a common event (213), and FISH has demonstrated low-level amplification of c-*myc*, which maps to 8q24, in more than 20% of advanced prostate cancer cases. c-*myc* amplification correlated with overexpression of c-myc protein (139). The cell-surface marker PSCA, originally discovered on the basis of its overexpression in prostate cancer and discussed above, also maps to 8q24. In most cases evaluated by dual-probe FISH, c-*myc* and *PSCA* were c-amplified (146).

The loss of *Mxi1*, an antagonist of the myc oncoprotein, is functionally equivalent to *myc* overexpression. In fact, proliferation and dysplasia of the prostatic epithelium are increased in prostates from *Mxi1* mutant mice compared to wild-type controls, suggesting that the observed PIN lesions may be the result of aberrant growth control due to loss of Mxi1 function (214). In addition, studies in human prostate cancer have identified frequent *MXI1* mutations (215). More recently, transgenic mice expressing human c-*myc* in the prostate were shown to develop prostatic intraepithelial neoplasia followed by invasive adenocarcinoma (143). Interestingly, microarray-based expression profiling identified a myc prostate cancer expression signature, which included the putative human tumor suppressor *NXK3.1*, while human prostate tumor databases revealed that the myc prostate cancer signature includes the Pim-1 kinase, a gene known to cooperate with *myc* in tumorigenesis, and defines a subset of human, "*myc*-like" cancers.

p27/PTEN Knockouts: Akt Transgenics

Targeted gene disruption of *PTEN* results in embryonic lethality in homozygous mice, but heterozygotes develop preneoplastic and frankly malignant lesions at multiple sites, demonstrating that *PTEN* is a potent tumor suppressor. In the prostate, these mice develop epithelial hyperplasia and dysplasia, consistent with a role for PTEN as an important regulator of prostatic epithelial growth *in vivo*. The CDK inhibitor *p27* is frequently downregulated in PIN and prostate cancer and has utility as a prognostic marker (51). Mutations are rare, and downregulation occurs through other mechanisms including ubiquitin-mediated proteolysis. The *p27* chromosomal region 12p12-13 is frequently lost in prostate cancer (216–218) and the mouse *p27* gene is haplo-insufficient for tumor suppression in multiple tissues (219), with heterozygous mice exhibiting hyperplasia in multiple organs, including the prostate (220). The loss of a single allele may thus be sufficient to promote prostate tumorigenesis. Inactivation of both

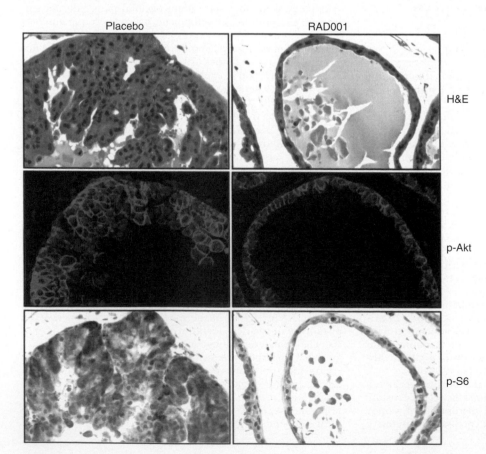

FIGURE 6B.4. Reversal of the prostate intraepithelial neoplasia (PIN) phenotype with mammalian target of rapamycin (mTOR) inhibition. Phospho-Akt is unaffected while phospho-S6 kinase staining is abolished. (See color insert.)

PTEN and p27 are a common occurrence in advanced prostate cancers (121). PTEN activity leads to the induction of p27 expression, which in turn can negatively regulate the transition through the cell cycle. The concomitant inactivation of one PTEN allele and either haplo-insufficiency or knockout of p27 in the mouse results in prostate carcinoma with complete penetrance within 3 months of age. In fact, these cancers recapitulate the natural history and pathological features of human prostate cancer (221).

Loss-of-function mutations in PTEN thus lead to deregulated PI3K signaling, resulting in constitutive activation of downstream targets including the Akt serine/threonine kinase family [reviewed in (115)]. In keeping with these data, Akt kinase activity is frequently elevated in primary prostate tumors (122). Transgenic mice were generated in which expression of activated Akt1 was spatially restricted to the prostate (murine prostate restricted Akt kinase activity transgenic expression model, or MPAKT) (222). Expression of Akt1 in the VP of the MPAKT mice resulted in activation of the $p70^{S6K}$ pathway and the induction of PIN similar in character to that observed in PTEN+/− mice. These mice, while long-lived, die at a 30% frequency due to bladder obstruction. Moreover, expression profiling revealed a novel angiogenic/hypoxia signature in these mice and the identification of an angiogenic plasma factor also found elevated in patients with prostate cancer (222). There is a marked overlap in the phenotype induced by activation of Akt and that resulting from loss of PTEN (223). Importantly, mammalian target of rapamycin (mTOR) inhibition in the MPAKT model induces epithelial cell apoptosis and the complete reversal of a neoplastic phenotype (Fig. 6B.4). Induction of cell death requires the mitochondrial pathway as prostate-specific coexpression of bcl-2 blocks apoptosis. Thus, there is an mTOR-dependent survival signal required downstream of Akt (224).

CONCLUSION

Prostate cancer exhibits a wide range of biological behavior. Preoperative serum PSA, Gleason tumor grade, and stage are the most widely used variables at present in predicting prognosis, relapse, and metastatic potential. As a result of screening, patients increasingly present with organ-confined disease. Yet, a significant percentage of these patients suffer recurrence after prostatectomy. The goal of molecular staging of prostate cancer is to identify genes involved in pathways relevant to prostate cancer pathogenesis and to use them as prognostic and/or predictive markers in both serum- and tissue-based assays. In this chapter, we have discussed the technologies available for the discovery and assessment of biomarkers and many biomarkers that have been found to be relevant in the various stages of prostate cancer progression. The challenge ahead is to conclusively determine the role some of these genes play as prognostic and/or predictive markers using large, retrospective, possibly multi-institutional databases with long-term follow-up. More importantly, such markers need to be applied to needle biopsy specimens, thus guiding therapeutic options. Potential therapeutic targets are also beginning to emerge. This will result in novel and more specific therapeutic modalities for a disease in which the mainstay of treatment, androgen ablation, is only temporarily effective.

ACKNOWLEDGMENTS

This work was supported by grants from the NCI (RO1, PO1, SPORE in prostate cancer), the Gelb Center for Genitourinary Oncology at the Dana Farber Cancer Institute, and a Prostate Cancer Foundation award to M.L.

References

1. Sakr WA, Haas GP, Cassin BF, et al. The frequency of carcinoma and intraepithelial neoplasia of the prostate in young male patients [see Comments]. J Urol 1993;150:379–385.
2. Han M, Partin AW, Zahurak M, et al. Biochemical (prostate specific antigen) recurrence probability following radical prostatectomy for clinically localized prostate cancer. J Urol 2003;169:517–523.
3. Stamey TA, Johnstone IM, McNeal JE, et al. Preoperative serum prostate specific antigen levels between 2 and 22 ng/ml correlate poorly with post-radical prostatectomy cancer morphology: prostate specific antigen cure rates appear constant between 2 and 9 ng/ml. J Urol 2002;167:103–111.
4. Klotz L. Active surveillance: an individualized approach to early prostate cancer. BJU Int 2003;92:657.
5. Barry MJ. Clinical practice. Prostate-specific-antigen testing for early diagnosis of prostate cancer. N Engl J Med 2001;344:1373–1377.
6. Morganti G, Gianferrari L, Cresseri A, et al. Recherches clinico-statistiques et genetiques sur les neoplasies de la prostate. Acta Genet Med Gemellol (Roma) 1956;6:304–305.
7. Lichtenstein P, Holm NV, Verkasalo PK, et al. Environmental and heritable factors in the causation of cancer—analyses of cohorts of twins from Sweden, Denmark, and Finland. N Engl J Med 2000;343:78–85.
8. Rokman A, Ikonen T, Mononen N, et al. ELAC2/HPC2 involvement in hereditary and sporadic prostate cancer. Cancer Res 2001;61:6038–6041.
9. Tavtigian SV, Simard J, Teng DH, et al. A candidate prostate cancer susceptibility gene at chromosome 17p. Nat Genet 2001;27:172–180.
10. Carpten J, Nupponen N, Isaacs S, et al. Germline mutations in the ribonuclease L gene in families showing linkage with HPC1. Nat Genet 2002;30:181–184.
11. Xu J, Zheng SL, Komiya A, et al. Germline mutations and sequence variants of the macrophage scavenger receptor 1 gene are associated with prostate cancer risk. Nat Genet 2002;32:321–325.
12. Rebbeck TR, Walker AH, Zeigler-Johnson C, et al. Association of HPC2/ELAC2 genotypes and prostate cancer. Am J Hum Genet 2000;67:1014–1019.
13. Wang L, McDonnell SK, Elkins DA, et al. Role of HPC2/ELAC2 in hereditary prostate cancer. Cancer Res 2001;61:6494–6499.
14. Suarez BK, Gerhard DS, Lin J, et al. Polymorphisms in the prostate cancer susceptibility gene HPC2/ELAC2 in multiplex families and healthy controls. Cancer Res 2001;61:4982–4984.
15. Xu J, Zheng SL, Carpten JD, et al. Evaluation of linkage and association of HPC2/ELAC2 in patients with familial or sporadic prostate cancer. Am J Hum Genet 2001;68:901–911.
16. Zhou A, Paranjape J, Brown TL, et al. Interferon action and apoptosis are defective in mice devoid of 2′,5′-oligoadenylate-dependent RNase L. EMBO J 1997;16:6355–6363.
17. Kerr IM, Brown RE. pppA2′p5′A2′p5′A: an inhibitor of protein synthesis synthesized with an enzyme fraction from interferon-treated cells. Proc Natl Acad Sci USA 1978;75:256–260.
18. Casey G, Neville PJ, Plummer SJ, et al. RNASEL Arg462Gln variant is implicated in up to 13% of prostate cancer cases. Nat Genet 2002;32:581–583.
19. Rokman A, Ikonen T, Seppala EH, et al. Germline alterations of the RNASEL gene, a candidate HPC1 gene at 1q25, in patients and families with prostate cancer. Am J Hum Genet 2002;70:1299–1304.
20. Rennert H, Bercovich D, Hubert A, et al. A novel founder mutation in the RNASEL gene, 471delAAAG, is associated with prostate cancer in Ashkenazi Jews. Am J Hum Genet 2002;71:981–984.
21. Wang L, McDonnell SK, Elkins DA, et al. Analysis of the RNASEL gene in familial and sporadic prostate cancer. Am J Hum Genet 2002;71:116–123.
22. Silverman RH. Implications for RNase L in prostate cancer biology. Biochemistry 2003;42:1805–1812.
23. DeMarzo AM, Nelson WG, Isaacs WB, et al. Pathological and molecular aspects of prostate cancer. Lancet 2003;361:955–964.
24. Smith JR, Freije D, Carpten JD, et al. Major susceptibility locus for prostate cancer on chromosome 1 suggested by a genome-wide search. Science 1996;274:1371–1374.
25. Berthon P, Valeri A, Cohen-Akenine A, et al. Predisposing gene for early-onset prostate cancer, localized on chromosome 1q42.2-43. Am J Hum Genet 1998;62:1416–1424.
26. Gibbs M, Stanford JL, McIndoe RA, et al. Evidence for a rare prostate cancer-susceptibility locus at chromosome 1p36. Am J Hum Genet 1999;64:776–787.
27. Xu J, Meyers D, Freije D, et al. Evidence for a prostate cancer susceptibility locus on the X chromosome. Nat Genet 1998;20:175–179.
28. Berry R, Schroeder JJ, French AJ, et al. Evidence for a prostate cancer-susceptibility locus on chromosome 20. Am J Hum Genet 2000;67:82–91.

29. Bova GS, Partin AW, Isaacs SD, et al. Biological aggressiveness of hereditary prostate cancer: long-term evaluation following radical prostatectomy. *J Urol* 1998;160:660–663.

30. Ross RK, Pike MC, Coetzee GA, et al. Androgen metabolism and prostate cancer: establishing a model of genetic susceptibility. *Cancer Res* 1998;58: 4497–4504.

31. Huggins C, Hodges CV. Studies on prostatic cancer: I. The effect of castration, of estrogen and of androgen injection on serum phosphatases in metastatic carcinoma of the prostate. 1941. *J Urol* 2002;168:9–12.

32. Isaacs JT. The biology of hormone refractory prostate cancer. Why does it develop? *Urol Clin North Am* 1999;26:263–273.

33. Feldman BJ, Feldman D. The development of androgen-independent prostate cancer. *Nat Rev Cancer* 2001;1:34–45.

34. Rubin MA, Putzi M, Mucci N, et al. Rapid ("warm") autopsy study for procurement of metastatic prostate cancer. *Clin Cancer Res* 2000;6: 1038–1045.

35. Roudier MP, True LD, Higano CS, et al. Phenotypic heterogeneity of end-stage prostate carcinoma metastatic to bone. *Hum Pathol* 2003;34:646–653.

36. Amin MB, Grignon DJ, Humphrey PA, et al. *Gleason grading of prostate cancer: a contemporary approach.* 1st ed. Philadelphia: Lippincott Williams & Wilkins, 2003.

37. Humphrey PA, American Society for Clinical Pathology. *Prostate pathology.* Chicago: American Society for Clinical Pathology, 2003.

38. Cheville JC, Tindall D, Boelter C, et al. Metastatic prostate carcinoma to bone: clinical and pathologic features associated with cancer-specific survival. *Cancer* 2002;95:1028–1036.

39. Hofer MD, Bismar TA, Kuefer R, et al. Determining pathologic risk factors for disease progression in high risk prostate cancer patients treated with radical prostatectomy, 2004 (*submitted*).

40. Aprikian AG, Cordon-Cardo C, Fair WR, et al. Neuroendocrine differentiation in metastatic prostatic adenocarcinoma. *J Urol* 1994;151: 914–919.

41. Mucci NR, Akdas G, Manely S, et al. Neuroendocrine expression in metastatic prostate cancer: evaluation of high throughput tissue microarrays to detect heterogeneous protein expression. *Hum Pathol* 2000;31: 406–414.

42. Bostwick DG, Qian J, Pacelli A, et al. Neuroendocrine expression in node positive prostate cancer: correlation with systemic progression and patient survival. *J Urol* 2002;168:1204–1211.

43. Korenchuk S, Lehr JE, MClean L, et al. VCaP, a cell-based model system of human prostate cancer. *In Vivo* 2001;15:163–168.

44. Lee YG, Korenchuk S, Lehr J, et al. Establishment and characterization of a new human prostatic cancer cell line: DuCaP. *In Vivo* 2001;15: 157–162.

45. True LD, Buhler K, Quinn J, et al. A neuroendocrine/small cell prostate carcinoma xenograft—LuCaP 49. *Am J Pathol* 2002;161:705–715.

46. Gingrich JR, Barrios RJ, Morton RA, et al. Metastatic prostate cancer in a transgenic mouse. *Cancer Res* 1996;56:4096–4102.

47. O'Shaughnessy JA, Kelloff GJ, Gordon GB, et al. Treatment and prevention of intraepithelial neoplasia: an important target for accelerated new agent development. *Clin Cancer Res* 2002;8:314–346.

48. Shih IM, Zhou W, Goodman SN, et al. Evidence that genetic instability occurs at an early stage of colorectal tumorigenesis. *Cancer Res* 2001;61: 818–822.

49. Montironi R, Mazzucchelli R, Scarpelli M. Precancerous lesions and conditions of the prostate: from morphological and biological characterization to chemoprevention. *Ann N Y Acad Sci* 2002;963:169–184.

50. Magi-Galluzzi C, Montironi R, Cangi MG, et al. Mitogen-activated protein kinases and apoptosis in PIN. *Virchows Arch* 1998;432:407–413.

51. Macri E, Loda M. Role of p27 in prostate carcinogenesis. *Cancer Metastasis Rev* 1998;17:337–344.

52. De Marzo AM, Meeker AK, Epstein JI, et al. Prostate stem cell compartments: expression of the cell cycle inhibitor p27Kip1 in normal, hyperplastic, and neoplastic cells. *Am J Pathol* 1998;153:911–919.

53. Downing SR, Russell PJ, Jackson P. Alterations of p53 are common in early stage prostate cancer. *Can J Urol* 2003;10:1924–1933.

54. Dhanasekaran SM, Barrette TR, Ghosh D, et al. Delineation of prognostic biomarkers in prostate cancer. *Nature* 2001;412:822–826.

55. Meeker AK, Gage WR, Hicks JL, et al. Telomere length assessment in human archival tissues: combined telomere fluorescence in situ hybridization and immunostaining. *Am J Pathol* 2002;160:1259–1268.

56. Signoretti S, Loda M. Estrogen receptor beta in prostate cancer: brake pedal or accelerator? *Am J Pathol* 2001;159:13–16.

57. Leav I, Lau KM, Adams JY, et al. Comparative studies of the estrogen receptors beta and alpha and the androgen receptor in normal human prostate glands, dysplasia, and in primary and metastatic carcinoma. *Am J Pathol* 2001;159:79–92.

58. Moore RA. The evolution and involution of the prostate gland. *Am J Pathol* 1936;12:599–624.

59. Rich AR. On the frequency of occurrence of occult carcinoma of the prostate. *J Urol* 1934;33:215–223.

60. Franks LM. Atrophy and hyperplasia in the prostate proper. *J Pathol Bacteriol* 1954;68:617–621.

61. Feneley MR, Young MP, Chinyama C, et al. Ki-67 expression in early prostate cancer and associated pathological lesions. *J Clin Pathol* 1996;49: 741–748.

62. Weinstein RS, Gardner WA. Pathology and pathobiology of the urinary bladder and prostate. *Monographs in pathology*; Vol xi, no 34. Baltimore: Williams & Wilkins, 1992;221.

63. McNeal JE. Normal histology of the prostate. *Am J Surg Pathol* 1988;12: 619–633.

64. De Marzo AM, Marchi VL, Epstein JI, et al. Proliferative inflammatory atrophy of the prostate: implications for prostatic carcinogenesis. *Am J Pathol* 1999;155:1985–1992.

65. Ruska KM, Sauvageot J, Epstein JI. Histology and cellular kinetics of prostatic atrophy. *Am J Surg Pathol* 1998;22:1073–1077.

66. Putzi MJ, De Marzo AM. Morphological transitions between proliferative inflammatory atrophy and high-grade prostatic intraepithelial neoplasia. *Urology* 2000;56:828–832.

67. Liavag I. Atrophy and regeneration in the pathogenesis of prostatic carcinoma. *Acta Pathol Microbiol Scand* 1968;73:338–350.

68. Shah R, Mucci NR, Amin A, et al. Postatrophic hyperplasia of the prostate gland: neoplastic precursor or innocent bystander? *Am J Pathol* 2001;158: 1767–1773.

69. Macoska JA, Trybus TM, Wojno KJ. 8p22 loss concurrent with 8c gain is associated with poor outcome in prostate cancer. *Urology* 2000;55: 776–782.

70. Tsujimoto Y, Takayama H, Nonomura N, et al. Postatrophic hyperplasia of the prostate in Japan: histologic and immunohistochemical features and p53 gene mutation analysis. *Prostate* 2002;52:279–287.

71. Nakayama M, Bennett CJ, Hicks JL, et al. Hypermethylation of the human glutathione S-transferase-pi gene (GSTP1) CpG island is present in a subset of proliferative inflammatory atrophy lesions but not in normal or hyperplastic epithelium of the prostate: a detailed study using laser-capture microdissection. *Am J Pathol* 2003;163:923–933.

72. Lee WH, Morton RA, Epstein JI, et al. Cytidine methylation of regulatory sequences near the pi-class glutathione S-transferase gene accompanies human prostatic carcinogenesis. *Proc Natl Acad Sci U S A* 1994;91:11733–11737.

73. Lin X, Tascilar M, Lee WH, et al. GSTP1 CpG island hypermethylation is responsible for the absence of GSTP1 expression in human prostate cancer cells. *Am J Pathol* 2001;159:1815–1826.

74. Millar DS, Ow KK, Paul CL, et al. Detailed methylation analysis of the glutathione S-transferase pi (GSTP1) gene in prostate cancer. *Oncogene* 1999;18:1313–1324.

75. Zha S, Gage WR, Sauvageot J, et al. Cyclooxygenase-2 is up-regulated in proliferative inflammatory atrophy of the prostate, but not in prostate carcinoma. *Cancer Res* 2001;61:8617–8623.

76. Parsons JK, Nelson CP, Gage WR, et al. GSTA1 expression in normal, preneoplastic, and neoplastic human prostate tissue. *Prostate* 2001;49: 30–37.

77. van Leenders GJ, Gage WR, Hicks JL, et al. Intermediate cells in human prostate epithelium are enriched in proliferative inflammatory atrophy. *Am J Pathol* 2003;162:1529–1537.

78. De Marzo AM, Nelson WG, Meeker AK, et al. Stem cell features of benign and malignant prostate epithelial cells. *J Urol* 1998;160:2381–2392.

79. van Leenders G, Dijkman H, Hulsbergen-van de Kaa C, et al. Demonstration of intermediate cells during human prostate epithelial differentiation in situ and in vitro using triple-staining confocal scanning microscopy. *Lab Invest* 2000;80:1251–1258.

80. Verhagen AP, Ramaekers FC, Aalders TW, et al. Colocalization of basal and luminal cell-type cytokeratins in human prostate cancer. *Cancer Res* 1992;52:6182–6187.

81. Rubin MA. Tech.Sight. Understanding disease cell by cell. *Science* 2002; 296:1329–1330.

82. Lindeman N, Waltregny D, Signoretti S, et al. Gene transcript quantitation by real-time RT-PCR in cells selected by immunohistochemistry-laser capture microdissection. *Diagn Mol Pathol* 2002;11:187–192.

83. Emmert-Buck MR, Bonner RF, Smith PD, et al. Laser capture microdissection. *Science* 1996;274:998–1001.

84. Strausberg RL. The Cancer Genome Anatomy Project: new resources for reading the molecular signatures of cancer. *J Pathol* 2001;195:31–40.

85. Strausberg RL, Greenhut SF, Grouse LH, et al. In silico analysis of cancer through the Cancer Genome Anatomy Project. *Trends Cell Biol* 2001;11: S66–S71.

86. Jordan B. Historical background and anticipated developments. *Ann N Y Acad Sci* 2002;975:24–32.

87. Lipshutz RJ, Fodor SP, Gingeras TR, et al. High density synthetic oligonucleotide arrays. *Nat Genet* 1999;21:20–24.

88. Magee JA, Araki T, Patil S, et al. Expression profiling reveals hepsin overexpression in prostate cancer. *Cancer Res* 2001;61:5692–5696.

89. Singh D, Febbo PG, Ross K, et al. Gene expression correlates of clinical prostate cancer behavior. *Cancer Cell* 2002;1:203–209.

90. Rhodes DR, Barrette TR, Rubin MA, et al. Meta-analysis of microarrays: interstudy validation of gene expression profiles reveals pathway dysregulation in prostate cancer. *Cancer Res* 2002;62:4427–4433.

91. Elkahloun AG, Gaudet J, Robinson GS, et al. In situ gene expression analysis of cancer using laser capture microdissection, microarrays and real time quantitative PCR. *Cancer Biol Ther* 2002;1:354–358.

92. So A, Goldenberg J, Gleave ME. Prostate specific antigen: an updated review. *Can J Urol* 2003;10:2040–2050.

93. Weir EG, Partin AW, Epstein JI. Correlation of serum prostate specific antigen and quantitative immunohistochemistry. *J Urol* 2000;163:1739–1742.

94. Gregorakis AK, Holmes EH, Murphy GP. Prostate-specific membrane antigen: current and future utility. *Semin Urol Oncol* 1998;16:2–12.

95. Griewe GL, Dean RC, Zhang W, et al. p53 immunostaining guided laser capture microdissection (p53-LCM) defines the presence of p53 gene mutations in focal regions of primary prostate cancer positive for p53 protein. *Prostate Cancer Prostatic Dis* 2003;6:281–285.

96. Moul JW. Angiogenesis, p53, bcl-2 and Ki-67 in the progression of prostate cancer after radical prostatectomy. *Eur Urol* 1999;35: 399–407.

97. Lieberfarb ME, Lin M, Lechpammer M, et al. Genome-wide loss of heterozygosity analysis from laser microdissected prostate cancer using single nucleotide polymorphic allele (SNP) arrays and a novel bioinformatics platform dChipSNP. *Cancer Res* 2003;63:4781–4785.

98. Abate-Shen C, Shen MM. Molecular genetics of prostate cancer. *Genes Dev* 2000;14:2410–2434.

99. Ren C, Li L, Yang G, et al. RTVP-1, a tumor suppressor inactivated by methylation in prostate cancer. *Cancer Res* 2004;64:969–976.

100. Fernandez PL, Hernandez L, Farre X, et al. Alterations of cell cycle-regulatory genes in prostate cancer. *Pathobiology* 2002;70:1–10.

101. Zhang Z, Li M, Wang H, et al. Antisense therapy targeting MDM2 oncogene in prostate cancer: effects on proliferation, apoptosis, multiple gene expression, and chemotherapy. *Proc Natl Acad Sci USA* 2003;100: 11636–11641.

102. Cory S, Huang DC, Adams JM. The Bcl-2 family: roles in cell survival and oncogenesis. *Oncogene* 2003;22:8590–8607.

103. Cory S, Adams JM. The Bcl2 family: regulators of the cellular life-or-death switch. *Nat Rev Cancer* 2002;2:647–656.

104. Waltregny D, Leav I, Signoretti S, et al. Androgen-driven prostate epithelial cell proliferation and differentiation in vivo involve the regulation of p27. *Mol Endocrinol* 2001;15:765–782.

105. Tsvetkov LM, Yeh KH, Lee SJ, et al. p27(Kip1) ubiquitination and degradation is regulated by the SCF(Skp2) complex through phosphorylated Thr187 in p27. *Curr Biol* 1999;9:661–664.

106. Gstaiger M, Jordan R, Lim M, et al. Skp2 is oncogenic and overexpressed in human cancers. *Proc Natl Acad Sci USA* 2001;98:5043–5048.

107. Latres E, Chiarle R, Schulman BA, et al. Role of the F-box protein Skp2 in lymphomagenesis. *Proc Natl Acad Sci USA* 2001;98:2515–2520.

108. Hershko D, Bornstein G, Ben-Izhak O, et al. Inverse relation between levels of p27(Kip1) and of its ubiquitin ligase subunit Skp2 in colorectal carcinomas. *Cancer* 2001;91:1745–1751.

109. Haldar S, Basu A, Croce CM. Bcl2 is the guardian of microtubule integrity. *Cancer Res* 1997;57:229–233.

110. Gjertsen BT, Logothetis CJ, McDonnell TJ. Molecular regulation of cell death and therapeutic strategies for cell death induction in prostate carcinoma. *Cancer Metastasis Rev* 1998;17:345–351.

111. Thomas GV, Szigeti K, Murphy M, et al. Down-regulation of p27 is associated with development of colorectal adenocarcinoma metastases. *Am J Pathol* 1998;153:681–687.

112. Paez J, Sellers WR. PI3K/PTEN/AKT pathway. A critical mediator of oncogenic signaling. *Cancer Treat Res* 2003;115:145–167.

113. Slingerland J, Pagano M. Regulation of the CDK inhibitor p27 and its deregulation in cancer. *J Cell Physiol* 2000;183:10–17.

114. Maehama T, Dixon JE. The tumor suppressor, PTEN/MMAC1, dephosphorylates the lipid second messenger, phosphatidylinositol 3,4,5-trisphosphate. *J Biol Chem* 1998;273:13375–13378.

115. Vazquez F, Sellers WR. The PTEN tumor suppressor protein: an antagonist of phosphoinositide 3-kinase signaling. *Biochim Biophys Acta* 2000; 1470:M21–M35.

116. Thomas GV, Schrage MI, Rosenfelt L, et al. Preoperative prostate needle biopsy p27 correlates with subsequent radical prostatectomy p27, Gleason grade and pathological stage. *J Urol* 2000;164:1987–1991.

117. Trapman J, Cleutjens KB. Androgen-regulated gene expression in prostate cancer. *Semin Cancer Biol* 1997;8:29–36.

118. Sadi MV, Barrack ER. Image analysis of androgen receptor immunostaining in metastatic prostate cancer. Heterogeneity as a predictor of response to hormonal therapy. *Cancer* 1993;71:2574–2580.

119. Umbas R, Schalken JA, Aalders TW, et al. Expression of the cellular adhesion molecule E-cadherin is reduced or absent in high-grade prostate cancer. *Cancer Res* 1992;52:5104–5109.

120. St Croix B, Sheehan C, Rak JW, et al. E-Cadherin-dependent growth suppression is mediated by the cyclin-dependent kinase inhibitor p27(KIP1). *J Cell Biol* 1998;142:557–571.

121. McMenamin ME, Soung P, Perera S, et al. Loss of PTEN expression in paraffin-embedded primary prostate cancer correlates with high Gleason score and advanced stage. *Cancer Res* 1999;59:4291–4296.

122. Sun M, Wang G, Paciga JE, et al. AKT1/PKB alpha kinase is frequently elevated in human cancers and its constitutive activation is required for oncogenic transformation in NIH3T3 cells. *Am J Pathol* 2001;159: 431–437.

123. Yong EL, Lim J, Qi W, et al. Molecular basis of androgen receptor diseases. *Ann Med* 2000;32:15–22.

124. Visakorpi T, Kallioniemi AH, Syvanen AC, et al. Genetic changes in primary and recurrent prostate cancer by comparative genomic hybridization. *Cancer Res* 1995;55:342–347.

125. Gelmann EP. Molecular biology of the androgen receptor. *J Clin Oncol* 2002;20:3001–3015.

126. Giovannucci E, Stampfer MJ, Krithivas K, et al. The CAG repeat within the androgen receptor gene and its relationship to prostate cancer. *Proc Natl Acad Sci USA* 1997;94:3320–3323.

127. Schoenberg MP, Hakimi JM, Wang S, et al. Microsatellite mutation (CAG24—>18) in the androgen receptor gene in human prostate cancer. *Biochem Biophys Res Commun* 1994;198:74–80.

128. Sadi MV, Walsh PC, Barrack ER. Immunohistochemical study of androgen receptors in metastatic prostate cancer. Comparison of receptor content and response to hormonal therapy. *Cancer* 1991;67:3057–3064.

129. Magi-Galluzzi C, Xu X, Hlatky L, et al. Heterogeneity of androgen receptor content in advanced prostate cancer. *Mod Pathol* 1997;10:839–845.

130. Thompson IM, Goodman PJ, Tangen CM, et al. The influence of finasteride on the development of prostate cancer. *N Engl J Med* 2003;349:213–222.

131. Rubin MA, Kantoff PW. Effect of finasteride on risk of prostate cancer: how little we really know. *J Cell Biochem* 2004;91:478–482.

132. Rubin MA, Kantoff PW. Prevention of prostate cancer with finasteride. *N Engl J Med* 2003;349:1569–1572; author reply 1569–1572.

133. Chen CD, Welsbie DS, Tran C, et al. Molecular determinants of resistance to antiandrogen therapy. *Nat Med* 2004;10:33–39.

134. Craft N, Shostak Y, Carey M, et al. A mechanism for hormone-independent prostate cancer through modulation of androgen receptor signaling by the HER-2/neu tyrosine kinase. *Nat Med* 1999;5:280–285.

135. Yeh S, Lin HK, Kang HY, et al. From HER2/Neu signal cascade to androgen receptor and its coactivators: a novel pathway by induction of androgen target genes through MAP kinase in prostate cancer cells. *Proc Natl Acad Sci USA* 1999;96:5458–5463.

136. Signoretti S, Montironi R, Manola J, et al. Her-2-neu expression and progression toward androgen independence in human prostate cancer. *J Natl Cancer Inst* 2000;92:1918–1925.

137. Nupponen NN, Visakorpi T. Molecular cytogenetics of prostate cancer. *Microsc Res Tech* 2000;51:456–463.

138. Nupponen NN, Kakkola L, Koivisto P, et al. Genetic alterations in hormone-refractory recurrent prostate carcinomas. *Am J Pathol* 1998;153:141–148.

139. Jenkins RB, Qian J, Lieber MM, et al. Detection of c-myc oncogene amplification and chromosomal anomalies in metastatic prostatic carcinoma by fluorescence in situ hybridization. *Cancer Res* 1997;57:524–531.

140. Steiner MS, Anthony CT, Lu Y, et al. Antisense c-myc retroviral vector suppresses established human prostate cancer. *Hum Gene Ther* 1998;9: 747–755.

141. Thompson TC, Southgate J, Kitchener G, et al. Multistage carcinogenesis induced by ras and myc oncogenes in a reconstituted organ. *Cell* 1989;56: 917–930.

142. Bubendorf L, Kononen J, Koivisto P, et al. Survey of gene amplifications during prostate cancer progression by high-throughout fluorescence in situ hybridization on tissue microarrays. *Cancer Res* 1999;59:803–806.

143. Ellwood-Yen K, Graeber TG, Wongvipat J, et al. Myc-driven murine prostate cancer shares molecular features with human prostate tumors. *Cancer Cell* 2003;4:223–238.

144. Reiter RE, Gu Z, Watabe T, et al. Prostate stem cell antigen: a cell surface marker overexpressed in prostate cancer. *Proc Natl Acad Sci USA* 1998; 95:1735–1740.

145. Gu Z, Thomas G, Yamashiro J, et al. Prostate stem cell antigen (PSCA) expression increases with high Gleason score, advanced stage and bone metastasis in prostate cancer. *Oncogene* 2000;19:1288–1296.

146. Reiter RE, Sato I, Thomas G, et al. Coamplification of prostate stem cell antigen (PSCA) and MYC in locally advanced prostate cancer. *Genes Chromosomes Cancer* 2000;27:95–103.

147. Ross S, Spencer SD, Holcomb I, et al. Prostate stem cell antigen as therapy target: tissue expression and in vivo efficacy of an immunoconjugate. *Cancer Res* 2002;62:2546–2553.

148. Couse JF, Korach KS. Estrogen receptor null mice: what have we learned and where will they lead us? *Endocr Rev* 1999;20:358–417.

149. Kuiper GG, Enmark E, Pelto-Huikko M, et al. Cloning of a novel receptor expressed in rat prostate and ovary. *Proc Natl Acad Sci USA* 1996;93: 5925–5930.

150. Baron A, Migita T, Tang D, et al. Fatty acid synthase: a metabolic oncogene in prostate cancer? *J Cell Biochem* 2004;91:47–53.

151. Epstein JI, Carmichael M, Partin AW. OA-519 (fatty acid synthase) as an independent predictor of pathologic state in adenocarcinoma of the prostate. *Urology* 1995;45:81–86.

152. Rossi S, Graner E, Febbo P, et al. Fatty acid synthase expression defines distinct molecular signatures in prostate cancer. *Mol Cancer Res* 2003;1: 707–715.

153. Shughrue PJ, Lane MV, Scrimo PJ, et al. Comparative distribution of estrogen receptor-alpha (ER-alpha) and beta (ER-beta) mRNA in the rat pituitary, gonad, and reproductive tract. *Steroids* 1998;63:498–504.

154. Latil A, Bieche I, Vidaud D, et al. Evaluation of androgen, estrogen (ER alpha and ER beta), and progesterone receptor expression in human prostate cancer by real-time quantitative reverse transcription-polymerase chain reaction assays. *Cancer Res* 2001;61:1919–1926.

155. McDonnell TJ, Navone NM, Troncoso P, et al. Expression of bcl-2 oncoprotein and p53 protein accumulation in bone marrow metastases of androgen independent prostate cancer. *J Urol* 1997;157:569–574.

156. McDonnell TJ, Troncoso P, Brisbay SM, et al. Expression of the protooncogene bcl-2 in the prostate and its association with emergence of androgen-independent prostate cancer. *Cancer Res* 1992;52:6940–6944.

157. Ferdinandusse S, Denis S, Clayton PT, et al. Mutations in the gene encoding peroxisomal alpha-methylacyl-CoA racemase cause adult-onset sensory motor neuropathy. *Nat Genet* 2000;24:188–191.

158. Kotti TJ, Savolainen K, Helander HM, et al. In mouse alpha-methylacyl-CoA racemase, the same gene product is simultaneously located in mitochondria and peroxisomes. *J Biol Chem* 2000;275:20887–20895.

159. Ockner RK, Kaikaus RM, Bass NM. Fatty-acid metabolism and the pathogenesis of hepatocellular carcinoma: review and hypothesis. *Hepatology* 1993;18:669–676.

160. Tamatani T, Hattori K, Nakashiro K, et al. Neoplastic conversion of human urothelial cells in vitro by overexpression of H$_2$O$_2$-generating peroxisomal fatty acyl CoA oxidase. *Int J Oncol* 1999;15:743–749.

161. Luo J, Zha S, Gage WR, et al. Alpha-methylacyl-CoA racemase: a new molecular marker for prostate cancer. *Cancer Res* 2002;62:2220–2226.

162. Rubin MA, Zhou M, Dhanasekaran SM, et al. alpha-methylacyl coenzyme a racemase as a tissue biomarker for prostate cancer. *JAMA* 2002; 287:1662–1670.

163. Welsh JB, Sapinoso LM, Su AI, et al. Analysis of gene expression identifies candidate markers and pharmacological targets in prostate cancer. *Cancer Res* 2001;61:5974–5978.

164. Luo J, Duggan DJ, Chen Y, et al. Human prostate cancer and benign prostatic hyperplasia: molecular dissection by gene expression profiling. *Cancer Res* 2001;61:4683–4688.

165. Jiang Z, Woda BA, Rock KL, et al. P504S: a new molecular marker for the detection of prostate carcinoma. *Am J Surg Pathol* 2001;25:1397–1404.

166. Kuefer R, Varambally S, Zhou M, et al. alpha-methylacyl-CoA racemase: expression levels of this novel cancer biomarker depend on tumor differentiation. *Am J Pathol* 2002;161:841–848.

167. Medes G, Thomas A, Weinhouse S. Metabolism of neoplastic tissue. IV. A study of lipid synthesis in neoplastic tissue slices in vitro. *Cancer Res* 1953;13:27–29.

168. He WW, Sciavolino PJ, Wing J, et al. A novel human prostate-specific, androgen-regulated homeobox gene (NKX3.1) that maps to 8p21, a region frequently deleted in prostate cancer. *Genomics* 1997;43:69–77.

169. Magee JA, Abdulkadir SA, Milbrandt J. Haploinsufficiency at the Nkx3.1 locus. A paradigm for stochastic, dosage-sensitive gene regulation during tumor initiation. *Cancer Cell* 2003;3:273–283.

170. Francis NJ, Kingston RE. Mechanisms of transcriptional memory. *Nat Rev Mol Cell Biol* 2001;2:409–421.

171. Swinnen JV, Van Veldhoven PP, Timmermans L, et al. Fatty acid synthase drives the synthesis of phospholipids partitioning into detergent-resistant membrane microdomains. *Biochem Biophys Res Commun* 2003;302: 898–903.

172. Van de Sande T, De Schrijver E, Heyns W, et al. Role of the phosphatidylinositol 3'-kinase/PTEN/Akt kinase pathway in the overexpression of fatty acid synthase in LNCaP prostate cancer cells. *Cancer Res* 2002;62:642–646.

173. Kumar-Sinha C, Ignatoski KW, Lippman ME, et al. Transcriptome analysis of HER2 reveals a molecular connection to fatty acid synthesis. *Cancer Res* 2003;63:132–139.

174. Hochachka PW, Rupert JL, Goldenberg L, et al. Going malignant: the hypoxia-cancer connection in the prostate. *Bioessays* 2002;24:749–757.

175. Kuhajda FP, Pizer ES, Li JN, et al. Synthesis and antitumor activity of an inhibitor of fatty acid synthase. *Proc Natl Acad Sci USA* 2000;97:3450–3454.

176. De Schrijver E, Brusselmans K, Heyns W, et al. RNA interference-mediated silencing of the fatty acid synthase gene attenuates growth and induces morphological changes and apoptosis of LNCaP prostate cancer cells. *Cancer Res* 2003;63:3799–3804.

177. Pizer ES, Pflug BR, Bova GS, et al. Increased fatty acid synthase as a therapeutic target in androgen-independent prostate cancer progression. *Prostate* 2001;47:102–110.

178. Graner E, Tang D, Rossi S, et al. The isopeptidase USP2a regulates the stability of fatty acid synthase in prostate cancer. *Cancer Cell* 2004;5: 253–261.

179. Clegg DJ, Wortman MD, Benoit SC, et al. Comparison of central and peripheral administration of C75 on food intake, body weight, and conditioned taste aversion. *Diabetes* 2002;51:3196–3201.

180. Stamey TA, Warrington JA, Caldwell MC, et al. Molecular genetic profiling of Gleason grade 4/5 prostate cancers compared to benign prostatic hyperplasia. *J Urol* 2001;166:2171–2177.

181. Narla G, Heath KE, Reeves HL, et al. KLF6, a candidate tumor suppressor gene mutated in prostate cancer. *Science* 2001;294:2563–2566.

182. Voeller HJ, Augustus M, Madike V, et al. Coding region of NKX3.1, a prostate-specific homeobox gene on 8p21, is not mutated in human prostate cancers. *Cancer Res* 1997;57:4455–4459.

183. Bowen C, Bubendorf L, Voeller HJ, et al. Loss of NKX3.1 expression in human prostate cancers correlates with tumor progression. *Cancer Res* 2000;60:6111–6115.

184. Kim MJ, Bhatia-Gaur R, Banach-Petrosky WA, et al. Nkx3.1 mutant mice recapitulate early stages of prostate carcinogenesis. *Cancer Res* 2002;62: 2999–3004.

185. Mahmoudi T, Verrijzer CP. Chromatin silencing and activation by Polycomb and trithorax group proteins. *Oncogene* 2001;20:3055–3066.

186. Varambally S, Dhanasekaran SM, Zhou M, et al. The Polycomb group protein EZH2 is involved in progression of prostate cancer. *Nature* 2002; 419:624–629.

187. Pflug BR, Pecher SM, Brink AW, et al. Increased fatty acid synthase expression and activity during progression of prostate cancer in the TRAMP model. *Prostate* 2003;57:245–254.

188. Sellers WR, Loda M. The EZH2 Polycomb transcriptional repressor—a marker or mover of metastatic prostate cancer? *Cancer Cell* 2002;2: 349–350.

189. Luo J, Dunn T, Ewing C, et al. Gene expression signature of benign prostatic hyperplasia revealed by cDNA microarray analysis. *Prostate* 2002; 51:189–200.

190. Ramaswamy S, Ross KN, Lander ES, et al. A molecular signature of metastasis in primary solid tumors. *Nat Genet* 2003;33:49–54.

191. Adam BL, Qu Y, Davis JW, et al. Serum protein fingerprinting coupled with a pattern-matching algorithm distinguishes prostate cancer from benign prostate hyperplasia and healthy men. *Cancer Res* 2002;62: 3609–3614.

192. Petricoin EF III, Ornstein DK, Paweletz CP, et al. Serum proteomic patterns for detection of prostate cancer. *J Natl Cancer Inst* 2002;94: 1576–1578.

193. Cher ML, MacGrogan D, Bookstein R, et al. Comparative genomic hybridization, allelic imbalance, and fluorescence in situ hybridization on chromosome 8 in prostate cancer. *Genes Chromosomes Cancer* 1994;11: 153–162.

194. Joos S, Bergerheim US, Pan Y, et al. Mapping of chromosomal gains and losses in prostate cancer by comparative genomic hybridization. *Genes Chromosomes Cancer* 1995;14:267–276.

195. Cahill DP, Kinzler KW, Vogelstein B, et al. Genetic instability and darwinian selection in tumours. *Trends Cell Biol* 1999;9:M57–M60.

196. Hackett JA, Greider CW. Balancing instability: dual roles for telomerase and telomere dysfunction in tumorigenesis. *Oncogene* 2002;21: 619–626.

197. Counter CM, Avilion AA, LeFeuvre CE, et al. Telomere shortening associated with chromosome instability is arrested in immortal cells which express telomerase activity. *EMBO J* 1992;11:1921–1929.

198. McClintock B. The stability of broken ends of chromosomes in Zea mays. *Genetics* 1941;26:234–282.

199. Artandi SE, Chang S, Lee SL, et al. Telomere dysfunction promotes nonreciprocal translocations and epithelial cancers in mice. *Nature* 2000;406: 641–645.

200. Blasco MA, Lee HW, Hande MP, et al. Telomere shortening and tumor formation by mouse cells lacking telomerase RNA. *Cell* 1997;91: 25–34.

201. Donaldson L, Fordyce C, Gilliland F, et al. Association between outcome and telomere DNA content in prostate cancer. *J Urol* 1999;162:1788–1792.

202. Sommerfeld HJ, Meeker AK, Piatyszek MA, et al. Telomerase activity: a prevalent marker of malignant human prostate tissue. *Cancer Res* 1996; 56:218–222.

203. Sugimura Y, Cunha GR, Donjacour AA. Morphogenesis of ductal networks in the mouse prostate. *Biol Reprod* 1986;34:961–971.

204. Castrillon DH, DePinho RA. Modeling prostate cancer in the mouse. *Adv Cancer Res* 2001;82:187–204.

205. Kasper S, Sheppard PC, Yan Y, et al. Development, progression, and androgen-dependence of prostate tumors in probasin-large T antigen transgenic mice: a model for prostate cancer. *Lab Invest* 1998;78:i–xv.

206. Greenberg NM, DeMayo F, Finegold MJ, et al. Prostate cancer in a transgenic mouse. *Proc Natl Acad Sci USA* 1995;92:3439–3443.

207. Kaplan-Lefko PJ, Chen TM, Ittmann MM, et al. Pathobiology of autochthonous prostate cancer in a pre-clinical transgenic mouse model. *Prostate* 2003;55:219–237.

208. Bhatia-Gaur R, Donjacour AA, Sciavolino PJ, et al. Roles for Nkx3.1 in prostate development and cancer. *Genes Dev* 1999;13:966–977.

209. Sciavolino PJ, Abrams EW, Yang L, et al. Tissue-specific expression of murine Nkx3.1 in the male urogenital system. *Dev Dyn* 1997;209: 127–138.

210. Bieberich CJ, Fujita K, He WW, et al. Prostate-specific and androgen-dependent expression of a novel homeobox gene. *J Biol Chem* 1996;271: 31779–31782.

211. Abate-Shen C, Banach-Petrosky WA, Sun X, et al. Nkx3.1; pten mutant mice develop invasive prostate adenocarcinoma and lymph node metastases. *Cancer Res* 2003;63:3886–3890.

212. Stanbrough M, Leav I, Kwan PW, et al. Prostatic intraepithelial neoplasia in mice expressing an androgen receptor transgene in prostate epithelium. *Proc Natl Acad Sci USA* 2001;98:10823–10828.

213. Roylance R, Spurr N, Sheer D. The genetic analysis of prostate carcinoma. *Semin Cancer Biol* 1997;8:37–44.

214. Schreiber-Agus N, Meng Y, Hoang T, et al. Role of Mxi1 in ageing organ systems and the regulation of normal and neoplastic growth. *Nature* 1998;393:483–487.

215. Prochownik EV, Eagle Grove L, Deubler D, et al. Commonly occurring loss and mutation of the MXI1 gene in prostate cancer. *Genes Chromosomes Cancer* 1998;22:295–304.

216. Kibel AS, Christopher M, Faith DA, et al. Methylation and mutational analysis of p27(kip1) in prostate carcinoma. *Prostate* 2001;48:248–253.

217. Kibel AS, Freije D, Isaacs WB, et al. Deletion mapping at 12p12-13 in metastatic prostate cancer. *Genes Chromosomes Cancer* 1999;25: 270–276.

218. Kibel AS, Schutte M, Kern SE, et al. Identification of 12p as a region of frequent deletion in advanced prostate cancer. *Cancer Res* 1998;58:5652–5655.

219. Fero ML, Randel E, Gurley KE, et al. The murine gene p27Kip1 is haploinsufficient for tumour suppression. *Nature* 1998;396:177–180.

220. Cordon-Cardo C, Koff A, Drobnjak M, et al. Distinct altered patterns of p27KIP1 gene expression in benign prostatic hyperplasia and prostatic carcinoma. *J Natl Cancer Inst* 1998;90:1284–1291.

221. Di Cristofano A, De Acetis M, Koff A, et al. Pten and p27KIP1 cooperate in prostate cancer tumor suppression in the mouse. *Nat Genet* 2001;27:222–224.

222. Majumder PK, Yeh JJ, George DJ, et al. Prostate intraepithelial neoplasia induced by prostate restricted Akt activation: the MPAKT model. *Proc Natl Acad Sci U S A* 2003;100:7841–7846.

223. Bernal-Mizrachi E, Wen W, Stahlhut S, et al. Islet beta cell expression of constitutively active Akt1/PKB alpha induces striking hypertrophy, hyperplasia, and hyperinsulinemia. *J Clin Invest* 2001;108:1631–1638.

224. Majumder PK, Febbo PG, Bikoff R, et al. mTOR inhibition reverses Akt-dependent prostate intraepithelial neoplasia via regulation of apoptotic and Hif1-dependent pathways. *Nat Med* 2004 *(in press)*.

CHAPTER 7 ■ PREVENTION OF PROSTATE CANCER

JAVIER HERNANDEZ AND IAN M. THOMPSON JR.

INTRODUCTION

Major advances have been accomplished during the past decade in the diagnosis and treatment of prostate cancer. However, prostate cancer remains a significant health-related problem in our population. Prostate cancer is the most common cancer and the second most common cause of cancer death in men and thus is a significant public health concern in the United States. Prior to the introduction of widespread prostate-specific antigen (PSA) screening for prostate cancer, the disease presented mostly at advanced stages. Since the advent of PSA testing in the 1980s, the detection of localized prostate cancer and nonmetastatic, high-grade disease has increased and the rate of metastatic prostate cancer has decreased (1,2). Approximately 75% of prostate cancers currently diagnosed are identified while the disease is confined to the prostate, in contrast to a 25% rate of organ-confined disease prior to the introduction of PSA screening (3,4). With this early detection of prostate cancer, 5-year cancer-specific survival rates have increased from approximately 70% in the early 1980s to more than 90% a decade later (5). A recent report from the US Centers for Disease Control and Prevention in collaboration with leading cancer organizations noted a 3.4% annual percentage decrease in prostate cancer deaths from 1992 to 2000 (6).

The reason for this decline in mortality in prostate cancer is not completely clear. Possible explanations include widespread PSA screening with attendant early detection and cure, changes in dietary habits (e.g., reduction in dietary fat or increased use of micronutrients), early use of hormonal treatment, or even chemoprevention of prostate cancer by certain agents. The notion that PSA screening may have had an impact on decreased mortality rates is attractive when evaluating outcomes from recent radical prostatectomy series (7,8). PSA screening, however, has major limitations. Concerns about the detection of clinically insignificant disease and the economic implications of widespread screening are only some of the controversial aspects of PSA screening (9–11). Recent data also indicate that approximately 15% of men diagnosed with prostate cancer with a PSA <2.5 ng/dL will have aggressive cancer (12). As a result, there has been a focus on early detection using various PSA derivatives as well as other biomarkers (13–15).

In addition to the unknown impact of screening and treatment prompted by PSA diagnosis on ultimate population mortality from the disease, very serious concerns regarding the cost of this approach have arisen. The stage migration caused by PSA detection has resulted in large numbers of men treated for cure but with modalities that some have argued are more expensive than treatment of late-stage disease (11). Conversely, a study from U.S. military medical centers demonstrated significant costs associated with the treatment of prostate cancer in the last year of life of patients dying from this malignancy (16). Other investigators have estimated the expense and associated survival benefit of treating critically ill cancer patients, demonstrating that limited benefits are usually obtained at a high cost (17). Against this backdrop, strategies designed to prevent prostate cancer may prove beneficial not just in reducing the burden of disease for the individual but also in reducing the cost burden for society.

RATIONALE FOR PREVENTION

Prevention strategies for prostate cancer may have two pragmatic goals. One such goal would be prevention of disease over the lifetime in a man who would otherwise manifest the disease. Another somewhat different approach would be to modulate the risk of progression of premalignant lesions or clinically insignificant cancer into clinically significant disease. Such an approach might be thought of as reduction in risk of progression, rather than prevention. In either case, the ultimate outcome would be beneficial—an individual man would not face the diagnosis of prostate cancer during his lifetime.

Experience with preventive strategies in other malignancies and disease processes have proved to be successful. A recent report described the use of aspirin against secondary prevention of cardiovascular disease as a "best buy" (18). With regard to cancer, a number of malignancies have been clearly linked with environmental factors such as diet and tobacco use, among others. Efforts to increase awareness and reduce risk among the population are underway (19). Chemoprevention has been proved effective in a number of neoplasms as well, including breast and colorectal disease. Tamoxifen and raloxifen are known to reduce the incidence of estrogen-receptor-positive breast cancer in women (20).

As stated previously, preventive strategies could potentially have major economic implications, recognizing that the costs associated with the actual preventive efforts would have to be taken into consideration as well. The impact of prevention of prostate cancer on quality-of-life–related issues would have to be considered as well, just as it is a major consideration with screening and treatment practices (21). One clear-cut advantage of a prevention strategy, compared with treatment for cure, is the lack of treatment-related morbidity such as postprostatectomy incontinence or radiation cystitis.

HORMONAL MANIPULATION

There is strong evidence indicating an association between androgens and the risk of prostate cancer. Testosterone, much of which originates from the Leydig cells, is converted to dihydrotestosterone (DHT) within prostate cells by the enzyme

5α-reductase. DHT, with much greater affinity for the androgen receptor than testosterone, plays a crucial role in the development of the prostate gland. Individuals affected by hereditary 5α-reductase deficiency fail to have adequate levels of DHT to allow proper development of the prostate and external genitalia and present with varying degrees of ambiguous external genitalia (22). These individuals have a rudimentary prostate, undetectable serum PSA levels as adults, no evidence of prostatic epithelium on prostate biopsy, and fail to develop benign prostatic hyperplasia (BPH) or prostate cancer (23). Conversely, some investigators have also suggested that higher levels of testosterone may pose a higher risk for prostate cancer, although these observations have not been uniform (24,25). Observations across different ethnic groups also support a direct role of androgens in the risk for prostate cancer. Androgen levels tend to be higher in African-American and non-Hispanic white men than in lower risk populations such as Japanese men (26). Additionally, Japanese men have lower levels of 5α-reductase activity compared to their higher risk counterparts.

Advances in molecular biology have facilitated identification of various genetic polymorphisms associated with an increased risk for prostate cancer. Many of these genes are directly related to androgen activity. The gene that has been the focus of the most intense molecular studies is the androgen receptor (AR), which binds both testosterone and dihydrotestosterone and transactivates the gene with androgen response elements (27–29). Additional studies have evaluated the role of other genes involved with androgen metabolism (SRD5A2, CYP17, CYP3A4) and the risk of prostate cancer (30–32). Evidence from these studies indicates that genetic alterations directly related to androgen metabolism may have an impact on the risk of prostate cancer and provides a further rationale for hormonal manipulation as a chemopreventive strategy for prostate cancer. A myriad of methods to modulate the androgenic milieu are options for prostate cancer prevention. Among these are antigonadotropins (synthetic estrogens, LHRH agonists), nonsteroidal antiandrogens, steroidal antiandrogens, adrenal androgen inhibitors, steroidal 5α-reductase inhibitors, as well as natural antiandrogens and antiestrogens (33). Because any chemoprevention strategy recommended for otherwise healthy men must place as its paramount goal a virtually nil risk of side effects, many of these agents would be unacceptable for widespread use for chemoprevention due to their unacceptably high risk of toxicity.

Finasteride is a competitive inhibitor of 5α-reductase that blocks the conversion of testosterone to DHT within prostatic cells (34). Extensive evidence from clinical trials has demonstrated a role for 5α-reductase in the treatment of BPH and prevention of BPH-related outcomes. The Proscar Long-Term Efficacy and Safety Study (PLESS) indicated that finasteride reduces the risk of acute urinary retention and the need for BPH-related surgery by approximately 50% (35). A more recent large-scale clinical trial evaluating the role of combination therapy for BPH confirmed a role for finasteride in the prevention of clinical progression of BPH (36). These observations along with the ones previously discussed raised the possibility that 5α-reductase inhibitors might be effective chemopreventive agents against prostate cancer. Preclinical data suggest a chemopreventive role for finasteride against prostate cancer. Tsukamoto conducted a study in F344 rats to evaluate the effect of finasteride on rat prostate carcinogenesis. In this study, finasteride prevented the progression of microscopic prostate carcinoma to macroscopic disease (37). Other clinical observations further support the notion that finasteride might be effective in the prevention of prostate cancer. Men randomized to take finasteride in the PLESS study were less likely to be diagnosed with prostate cancer compared to the placebo group (38). These results did not achieve statistical significance ($P = .7$); however, a relatively small number of patients ($n = 644$) underwent prostate biopsy. Another study suggested that finasteride can delay the progression of prostate cancer in men with a detectable PSA after radical prostatectomy with no clinical or radiographic evidence of metastasis (39).

Most recently, the Southwest Oncology Group (SWOG) supported by the National Cancer Institute (NCI) released the results of the Prostate Cancer Prevention Trial (PCPT) (12). PCPT is the first phase III trial conducted for the prevention of prostate cancer. In this study, 18,882 men 55 years or older who had a normal digital rectal examination (DRE) and a PSA level equal to or less than 3.0 ng/mL were randomized to receive 5 mg of finasteride daily versus placebo after a run-in period of 3 months. Participants remained on the study drug for 7 years. A prostate biopsy was recommended if, during one of the annual visits, participants were found to have a PSA level greater than 4.0 ng/mL after adjusting for the finasteride effect and/or an abnormal digital rectal examination. A prostate biopsy was recommended at the end of the 7-year study period for all participants who had not been found to have prostate cancer. This trial demonstrated an overall 24.8% reduction in the prevalence of prostate cancer over the 7-year period in men who received finasteride. Of concern was the observation of a higher proportion of high-grade tumors (Gleason score 7 or higher) in the finasteride group. Additionally, men on the finasteride arm of the study were more likely to report sexual side effects, although the likelihood of lower urinary tract symptoms and the need for interventions, such as transurethral resection of the prostate, was lower in this group. The latter findings are consistent with those of the PLESS and Medical Therapy of Prostatic Symptoms (MTOPS) trials.

Multiple questions arise from PCPT. Some have cautioned against widespread use of finasteride for the prevention of prostate cancer (40,41). The higher proportion of high-grade tumors among men in the finasteride group can be of concern and warrants further investigation. Some investigators have suggested that high-grade tumors can be induced by finasteride through lowering dihydrotestosterone levels and mechanisms that select for emergence of androgen-independent clones (42). Arguing against this is evidence that response to traditional hormonal therapy is seen in the majority of patients treated with finasteride who subsequently undergo traditional hormonal therapy.

Another explanation for the difference in the rate of high-grade disease in the finasteride arm of the PCPT is that the drug causes histologic and architectural changes that make the tumors appear to be of a higher grade. With recognition of these cytologic and architectural changes, a World Health Organization consensus conference has recommended against assigning a tumor grade using Gleason score in patients who had received previous treatment due to the possible misclassification of grade (43). An observation in the initial PCPT paper argues for this explanation: If finasteride indeed induced the development of high-grade tumors, it should be expected that there would be a growing excess number of high-grade tumors in this group over the 7 years of study. On the other hand, if finasteride led to architectural and cytologic changes that "make tumors look worse," due to the relatively rapid onset of these changes, one would expect high-grade tumors to be more commonly seen in the first years of the study and that there would be no increase in this fraction over time. As was noted by the authors in the original manuscript, the latter observation was noted—more than double the number of high-grade tumors were seen in the first year of the study in the finasteride arm with no increase in the rate of high-grade tumors over time. Important as well was the concept that tumor grade was a secondary end-point of the PCPT and that the study was not designed nor powered for conclusions in this regard.

What, then, is the impact of the PCPT on clinical practice? First, it is clear that a 24.8% reduction in the risk of prostate cancer is a potentially huge public health benefit. The 50,000 men in the United States alone who would not face the diagnosis of prostate cancer on an annual basis is an enormous impact. The additional benefit in symptoms related to BPH [fewer transurethral resections of the prostate (TURP), fewer cases of urinary retention, improved symptoms] must also be considered, especially given the confirmation and extension of these observations in the MTOPS trial. This double-blind clinical trial demonstrated that finasteride led to a 34% risk reduction of overall clinical progression of BPH compared to placebo. When used in combination with doxazosin, the overall risk reduction increased to 66% compared to placebo (36). On the other hand, patients must be counseled regarding the potential and unknown risks of this strategy including the yet-unclear risk of high-grade disease and of sexual toxicity that, while very commonly reported in both groups, was slightly more common in men receiving finasteride. (Importantly, all studies to date suggest that if sexual toxicity is reported by a patient receiving finasteride, this side effect resolves if the drug is discontinued.) Ultimately, it will be the balance of the clear-cut reduction in prostate cancer risk against the potential side effects that will lead to an informed decision by the patient.

CYCLOOXYGENASE-2 INHIBITORS AND NONSTEROIDAL ANTI-INFLAMMATORY DRUGS

Cyclooxygenases (COX-1 and COX-2) are involved in the conversion of arachidonic acid to prostaglandins and other eicosanoids. COX-1 is expressed in almost all tissues throughout the body to include platelets, endothelial cells, gastrointestinal tract, and renal microvasculature. COX-2, on the other hand, is usually undetectable in most tissues except in response to injury or hypoxia when its expression is stimulated by inflammatory cytokines, growth factors, or endotoxins. Prostaglandins and eicosanoids exert their activity by influencing tumor cell proliferation, resistance to apoptosis, enhanced hormonal responsiveness, angiogenesis, and tumor invasion (44).

Interest in the use of COX-2 inhibitors in the prevention of cancer comes from the initial experience with these agents in colon cancer. Prospective clinical trials in patients with familial adenomatous polyposis were begun after early observations of increased COX-2 expression in colon cancer and evidence from animal models (45,46). Steinbach demonstrated a 28% reduction in polyp burden in these patients after a six-month course of celecoxib compared to a 4.5% reduction in the placebo group (47). COX-2 overexpression has been associated with multiple other neoplasms such as bladder, breast, prostate, hepatocellular, endometrial, cervical, ovarian, and pancreatic carcinomas, among others (48). These findings in addition to the extensive experience with COX-2 inhibitors since their introduction in the late 1990s have led to further investigations of these agents for both treatment and prevention regimens for prostate cancer and other genitourinary malignancies.

Growing evidence suggests an association between COX-2 and prostate cancer. O'Neill measured the expression of COX-1 and COX-2 by reverse-transcription polymerase chain reaction (RT-PCR) in multiple tissues and found the highest levels of both forms in the prostate (49). Hsu evaluated the apoptotic activity of the COX-2 inhibitor celecoxib in androgen-responsive LNCaP and androgen-nonresponsive PC-3 cells and demonstrated the induction of apoptosis in both cell lines (50). Other COX-2 inhibitors including rofecoxib, DuP697, and NS398 demonstrated significantly less efficacy in the induction of apoptosis. Additionally, this study concluded that treatment of these cell lines with celecoxib did not affect bcl-2 expression. Unlike the results of other studies that suggested that inhibition of COX-2 induces apoptosis through downregulation of bcl-2, these authors found no effect on bcl-2 expression with celecoxib (51).

The findings that multiple potent COX-2 inhibitors have varying degrees of anticancer activity raise the possibility that the mechanisms of action may be independent of COX-2. This possibility is supported by the findings of Ghosh and Meyers (52). These investigators concluded that the eicosanoid 5-hydroxyeicosatetraenoic acid (5-HETE) was critical for prostate cancer cell survival. They noted dramatic cellular apoptosis in LNCaP and PC3 cell cultures with the addition of an inhibitor of 5-lipoxygenase. Cell survival in the presence of the inhibitor was possible only by the addition of 5-HETE. Conversely, the addition of androgen in the presence of an inhibitor of 5-lipoxygenase did not allow cell survival. Interestingly, this study noted proapoptotic activity in the presence of an inhibitor of 5-lipoxygenase but not with inhibitors of 12-lipoxygenase or cyclooxygenase.

Nonetheless, selective COX-2 inhibitors have been demonstrated to affect PC-3 tumor cell growth through a variety of mechanisms including induction of apoptosis, downregulation of vascular endothelial growth factor (VEGF), and reduced angiogenesis (53). Evidence suggests that COX-2 inhibitors do not suppress growth of normal prostate stromal cells and correlates with the observation that levels of COX-2 mRNA are 3.4-fold higher in prostate cancer than in benign tissue (54,55).

Epidemiologic observations support the potential of nonsteroidal anti-inflammatory drugs (NSAIDs) and COX-2 inhibitors in prostate cancer prevention. Two large case-control studies addressed the relationship between nonsteroidal anti-inflammatory drug use and the risk of prostate cancer. Roberts evaluated 1362 white men between ages 50 and 79 in a longitudinal study of lower urinary tract symptoms. With a median follow-up of 66 months, the odds ratio for prostate cancer was 0.45 [95% confidence interval (CI), 0.28 to 0.73] in NSAID users compared with nonusers (56). A greater reduction in risk was noted in older men, suggesting a dose-response relationship. Another case control study of 417 prostate cancer patients and 420 controls examined the association of prostate cancer and NSAIDs. Regular use of both over-the-counter and/or prescription NSAIDs was associated with a 66% reduction in the risk of prostate cancer (57). In a large multiracial study population, a similar association between prostate cancer and daily aspirin use was noted (58). Another study found no protective effect of NSAIDs against prostate cancer, but concerns with this study's methodology have subsequently been raised (59,60).

Clinical trials in humans evaluating the effectiveness of COX-2 inhibitors for prostate cancer prevention are limited. In a small pilot study, Derksen evaluated the efficacy of celecoxib in patients with biochemical recurrence after definitive treatment and found an inhibitory effect on serum PSA levels in the majority of patients (61). A large-scale trial is currently examining rofecoxib for prostate cancer prevention.

ANTIOXIDANTS

Reactive oxygen species have been implicated as potential agents involved in the onset and progression of various malignancies including prostate cancer. The oxidative damage by these species may be exerted on multiple cellular components including lipids, proteins, and nucleic acids. DNA mutations may lead to altered gene function, potentially contributing to malignant transformation and progression of disease (62). Evidence from clinical trials published in the middle to late portion of the past decade seems to indicate a promising role for vitamin E and selenium as possible chemopreventive agents against prostate cancer potentially through their antioxidant activity (63,64). The Selenium and Vitamin E Cancer Prevention Trial (SELECT) is an ongoing phase III randomized, placebo-controlled trial designed to evaluate the efficacy of each of these agents alone and in combination in the prevention of prostate cancer (65). Background discoveries and rationale leading to the development of this clinical trial are summarized (66).

Selenium

Selenium is a nonmetallic trace mineral found in grains, meat, yeast, and some vegetables. Selenium content in some of these dietary sources may be dependent on the selenium soil content where they are grown. Selenium is an essential component of several extracellular and cellular glutathione peroxidases that protect cells from oxidative damage by catalyzing the reduction of lipid hydroperoxides (67). The usual dietary intake of selenium in the United States ranges between 80 and 120 μg/day, and the recommended dietary allowance is 0.87 μg/kg (68).

A multitude of experimental models have demonstrated the ability of selenium to inhibit tumorigenesis (69–71). The role of selenium in cancer prevention may be through antioxidant, antiproliferative, proapoptotic, cytotoxic, and/or proimmunogenic activities (72). However, most of the recent interest in selenium as a chemopreventive agent comes from observations noted in a large clinical trial evaluating the effectiveness of selenium in the prevention of skin malignancies (64). In this trial, a total of 1312 study participants with a documented prior history of skin cancer were randomized to receive 200 μg per day of elemental selenium versus placebo. The subjects were then followed for a period of 4.5 years to assess the development of skin cancers or other malignancies. The investigators found no difference in the rates of skin cancers in the study groups. However, a two-thirds reduction in the incidence of prostate cancer was noted among men randomized to selenium. Further analysis from a select group of subjects within this trial suggested a greater benefit in prostate cancer reduction among those men 65 years of age or younger, with low baseline selenium serum levels and low serum PSA values (73). Additional epidemiologic evidence on this subject comes from the Health Professionals Follow-Up Study that found a two-thirds reduction in prostate cancer risk among men with the highest quartile of selenium measured in toenail clippings (74). Additional findings from two large, randomized trials conducted in China indicate that selenium may be effective in reducing overall mortality from stomach and esophageal cancers as well (75,76). High levels of selenium have been associated with a one half to two thirds reduction in the risk of advanced prostate cancer (77).

Vitamin E (α-Tocopherol)

Vitamin E includes a group of fat-soluble chemical compounds with antioxidant activity. The most active and most commonly used form of vitamin E supplementation is α-tocopherol (78). However, there is some evidence that γ-tocopherol may have greater activity in preventing prostate cancer than α-tocopherol (79,80). In addition to its antioxidant activity, some of the other mechanisms by which vitamin E is thought to reduce the risk of cancer are through inhibition of prostaglandin synthesis, inhibition of protein kinase C activity, modulation of cell proliferation, and regulation of the cell cycle (81–83). Data from both cell culture and animal prostate cancer models have supported a potential role for vitamin E altering prostate cancer growth and proliferation (84,85).

Early epidemiologic observations suggesting a protective activity for vitamin E against prostate cancer comes from the Alpha-Tocopherol, Beta-Carotene (ATBC) Cancer Prevention Study (86). This study was a randomized, double-blind, placebo-controlled primary intervention trial designed to assess the effectiveness of α-tocopherol, β-carotene, or both administered over 5 to 8 years in preventing lung cancer or other cancers among more than 29,000 male smokers from Finland. On a secondary end-point analysis, study investigators found a 32% decrease (95% confidence interval = −47% to −12%) in the incidence of prostate cancer among subjects receiving α-tocopherol (87). The risk reduction noted was more significant for clinically evident prostate cancer (stages B to D). The study also found a 41% reduction (95% confidence interval = −65% to −1%) in prostate cancer–related deaths among men receiving α-tocopherol. Interestingly, a recent postintervention follow-up study evaluating cancer incidence and cause-specific mortality demonstrated a posttrial relative risk for prostate cancer of 0.88 (95% confidence interval = 0.76 to 1.03) for participants receiving α-tocopherol compared to those not receiving the agent (88). These results suggest that there is no late protective effect of α-tocopherol against prostate cancer once administration of the agent has been discontinued for several years.

Findings from the Health Professional Follow-up Study also demonstrated a protective effect against prostate cancer among men taking vitamin E supplementation (89). In this study, the protective effect of vitamin E was noticed only in smokers. Although vitamin E did not reduce the overall risk of prostate cancer, it was associated with a decreased risk of metastatic or fatal prostate cancer (RR 0.44, 95% confidence interval = 0.18 to 1.07). Another study that followed Swiss men for a 17-year period noted an association between low levels of plasma α-tocopherol in serum and an increased risk for prostate cancer among smokers (90). Taken together, these studies have suggested a role for vitamin E in the prevention of prostate cancer among smokers. However, validation of these findings is needed in the general population.

SELECT AND OTHER CLINICAL TRIALS

The Selenium and Vitamin E for Cancer Prevention Trial (SELECT Trial) is a phase III randomized, double-blind, placebo-controlled trial of selenium (200 μg daily) and vitamin E (400 IU), either agent alone, or placebo only, to determine the efficacy of these agents as chemopreventive interventions against prostate cancer (65). The goal of this study is to accrue more than 32,000 men with a normal DRE and a PSA level <4 ng per mL. Duration of therapy will range between 7 and 12 years depending on the date of randomization for the individual subject. Results of this study are expected in 2012. The primary end-point of this study is the clinical incidence of prostate cancer, determined by current clinical recommendations for prostate cancer screening with DRE and PSA measurements. Contrary to PCPT, the SELECT trial does not require an end-of-study prostate biopsy.

Another SWOG, NCI-sponsored clinical trial is evaluating the effectiveness of selenium in preventing prostate cancer in patients who have high-grade prostatic intraepithelial neoplasia (PIN) (91). The goal of this study is to accrue 1165 men with a diagnosis of high-grade PIN and no evidence of cancer. The participants will be randomized to receive either placebo or selenium. The main objective of this study is to determine the 3-year incidence rate of prostate cancer in this group of patients. Likewise, the National Cancer Institute of Canada is sponsoring a phase II randomized clinical trial to determine if supplementation with soy protein isolate, vitamin E, and selenium can delay the development of prostate cancer in men with a diagnosis of high-grade PIN. In this two-arm study, participants will be randomized to either placebo or a combination of all three study agents.

OTHER DIETARY INTERVENTION

Multiple other dietary interventions/modifications are currently being investigated as possible alternatives to prevent and/or modulate the development of prostate cancer. Dietary fat intake, dietary soy protein, and carotenoids, among others, have all been associated with a risk of prostate cancer. We briefly review some of the epidemiologic data pointing toward some of these agents as potential targets for chemoprevention studies.

Migration studies of Japanese men who moved to Los Angeles County provide strong evidence that environmental factors are significant contributors in the progression of prostate cancer (92). Additionally, epidemiologic studies indicate that incidence of prostate cancer in a given population is associated with levels of per capita fat consumption (93). Data from the Health Professionals Follow-Up Study showed a direct relationship between high fat intake, particularly from animal fat, and the risk of advanced prostate cancer (94). Although the precise mechanism by which dietary fat contributes to the overall risk for prostate cancer is not certain, it is presumed that, in all likelihood, the role of dietary fat in tumorigenesis is a complex process potentially linked to other dietary factors (95).

Increased intake of soy protein has also been considered as a potential contributor to the lower incidence of prostate cancer among men in some Asian countries (96). Genistein and daidzein are two of the most common isoflavonoids found in dietary soy products, and the typical Western diet contains small amounts of these components compared to Asian diets. Various animal model studies have demonstrated the ability of these agents to decrease tumor growth, inhibit metastasis, and prevent prostate-related cancer (97–99).

Carotenoids are another series of compounds that have received considerable attention for cancer prevention. It is important to recognize that, in spite of initial epidemiologic studies showing a cancer-preventive effect of β-carotene, subsequent randomized studies demonstrated an increased incidence and mortality from prostate cancer in men receiving β-carotene supplementation (100). Studies involving lycopene, on the other hand, have been more favorable. Lycopene is another carotenoid that has been studied as a preventive agent for prostate cancer, and it can be found in tomato products, watermelon, and other vegetables. One of the largest studies investigating the association of dietary lycopene intake and the risk of prostate cancer was the Health Professionals Follow-Up Study (101). The investigators found that frequent tomato consumption or lycopene intake was associated with a decreased risk for prostate cancer. The investigators found a stronger association between intake of tomato sauce, the primary source of bioavailable lycopene, and the reduction of prostate cancer risk. Another study found no association between lycopene ingestion and the risk of prostate cancer (102). This latter study, however, did not indicate the type of tomato product ingested.

Although it is extremely tempting to make clinical recommendations based on data from epidemiologic studies, it is best to consider these studies as hypothesis-generating whose findings must be confirmed by appropriately designed and powered clinical trials (Table 7.1).

TABLE 7.1

CURRENT NIH-SPONSORED CLINICAL TRIALS ON CHEMOPREVENTION/COMPLEMENTARY THERAPY FOR PROSTATE CANCER

Phase III Randomized Study of Selenium and Vitamin E for the Prevention of Prostate Cancer (SELECT Trial)

Phase IIB Randomized Chemoprevention Study of Eflornithine (DFMO) in Patients at High Genetic Risk For Prostate Cancer

Randomized Study of Isoflavones in Reducing Risk Factors in Patients with Stage I or II Prostate Cancer

Randomized Pilot Study of Isoflavones versus Lycopene Prior to Radical Prostatectomy in Patients with Localized Prostate Cancer

Phase I Study of Lycopene for the Chemoprevention of Prostate Cancer

Phase III Randomized Study of Selenium as Chemoprevention of Prostate Cancer in Patients with High-Grade Prostatic Intraepithelial Neoplasia

Phase II Randomized Study of Vitamin E, Selenium, and Soy Protein Isolate in Patients with High-Grade Prostatic Intraepithelial Neoplasia

Phase I Randomized Study of Neoadjuvant Celecoxib Followed by Prostatectomy in Patients with Localized Prostate Cancer

Phase II Randomized Study of Doxercalciferol in Patients with Localized Prostate Cancer

Phase II Randomized Study of Toremifene Followed by Radical Prostatectomy in Patients with Stage I or II Adenocarcinoma of the Prostate

Phase II A Chemoprevention Study of an Investigational Drug (GTX-006/Acapodene) in Men with High Grade Prostate Intraepithelial Neoplasia (PIN)

http://clinicaltrials.gov/ct/search?term=chemoprevention+of+prostate+cancer&submit=Search.

CHALLENGES WITH CLINICAL TRIALS

Conducting large-scale clinical trials carries a variety of challenges that ranges from recruitment strategies, assuring compliance, and the use of appropriate end points (103–106). Issues involving cost, size of the study, and the number of volunteers willing or available to participate have a direct impact on the success of the study. Due to these factors, it is often difficult to conduct more than a handful of large-scale prevention trials per decade for a particular disease process.

Successful completion of a prevention clinical trial does not guarantee that the protective effect, if one is found, is durable. As noted earlier, a postintervention evaluation of the ATBC study results demonstrated loss of the protective effects of α-tocopherol against prostate cancer on long-term follow-up. One may also have to consider the possibility that, even when a chemopreventive agent is found to be effective in reducing the incidence of a given disease, the agent may not have an impact in overall and disease-specific survival, reducing the benefit of the chemopreventive intervention.

The record to date suggests that, in the end, a mixed message is almost always the case for large chemoprevention trials. In the case of finasteride and PCPT, the risk of high-grade disease and sexual toxicity must be balanced against a substantial overall decreased risk of prostate cancer (12). The case with tamoxifen and the Breast Cancer Prevention Trial is similar (107). In spite of a 49% reduction in the incidence of breast cancer among women in the tamoxifen arm of the study, there is concern about the increased risk of endometrial cancer and thromboembolic complications among women randomized to tamoxifen. Otherwise healthy patients may be less willing to accept the risks associated with chemopreventive interventions as compared to patients in treatment clinical trials in which there may be a greater acceptance of side effects and toxicities.

References

1. Tarone RE, Chu KC, Brawley OW. Implications of stage-specific survival rates in assessing recent declines in prostate cancer mortality rates. *Epidemiology* 2000;11:167–170.
2. Ries LAG, Eisner MP, Kosary CL, et al., eds. *SEER Cancer Statistics Review, 1973–1998*. Bethesda, MD: National Cancer Institute, 2002.
3. Smith DS, Catalona WJ. The nature of prostate cancer detected through prostate specific antigen based screening. *J Urol* 1994;152:1732–1736.
4. Catalona WJ, Smith DS, Ratliff TL, et al. Detection of organ-confined prostate cancer is increased through prostate-specific antigen-based screening. *JAMA* 1993;270:948–954.
5. Landis SH, Murray T, Bolden S, et al. Cancer statistics, 1999. *CA Cancer J Clin* 1999;49:8–31.
6. Weir HK, Thun MJ, Hankey BF, et al. Annual report to the nation on the status of cancer, 1975–2000, featuring the uses of surveillance data for cancer prevention and control. *J Natl Cancer Inst* 2003;95:1276–1299.
7. Jhaveri FM, Klein EA, Kupelian PA, et al. Declining rates of extracapsular extension after radical prostatectomy: evidence for continued stage migration. *J Clin Oncol* 1999;17:3167–3172.
8. Moul JW, Wu H, Sun L, et al. Epidemiology of radical prostatectomy for localized prostate cancer in the era of prostate-specific antigen: an overview of the Department of Defense Center for Prostate Disease Research national database. *Surgery* 2002;132:213–219.
9. Neal DE, Leung HY, Powell PH, et al. Unanswered questions in screening for prostate cancer. *Eur J Cancer* 2000;36:1316–1321.
10. McNaughton Collins M, Ransohoff DF, et al. Early detection of prostate cancer. Serendipity strikes again. *JAMA* 1997;278:1516–1519.
11. Benoit RM, Naslund MJ. The socioeconomic implications of prostate-specific antigen screening. *Urol Clin North Am* 1997;24:451–458.
12. Thompson IM, Goodman PJ, Tangen CM, et al. The influence of finasteride on the development of prostate cancer. *N Engl J Med* 2003;349:215–224.
13. Ornstein DK, Andriole GL. Screening for prostate cancer in 1999. AUA Office of Education, Houston, TX 1999:Lesson 11–7.
14. Bok RA, Small EJ. Bloodborne biomolecular markers in prostate cancer development and progression. *Nat Rev Cancer* 2002;2:918–926.
15. Banez LL, Prasanna P, Sun L, et al. Diagnostic potential of serum proteomic patterns in prostate cancer. *J Urol* 2003;170(2 Pt 1):442–446.
16. Piper NY, Kusada L, Lance R, et al. Adenocarcinoma of the prostate: An expensive way to die. *Prostate Cancer Prostatic Dis* 2002;5:164–166.
17. Schapira DV, Studnicki J, Bradham DD, et al. Intensive care, survival, and expense of treating critically ill cancer patients. *JAMA* 1993;269:783–786.
18. Probstfield JL. How cost-effective are new preventive strategies for cardiovascular disease?. *Am J Cardiol* 2003;91:22G–27G.
19. Wilby ML. Improving the health profile: decreasing risk for cancer through primary prevention. *Holist Nurs Pract* 1998;12:52–61.
20. Kinsinger LS, Harris R, Woolf SH, et al. Chemoprevention of breast cancer: a summary of the evidence for the U.S. Preventive Services Task Force. *Ann Intern Med* 2002;137:59–69.
21. Miller AB, Madalinska JB, Church T, et al. Health-related quality of life and cost-effectiveness studies in the European randomised study of screening for prostate cancer and the US prostate, lung, colon and ovary trial. *Eur J Cancer* 2001;37:2154–2160.
22. Imperato-McGinley JL, Guerrero L, Gautier T, et al. Steroid 5 alpha-reductase deficiency in men: An inherited form of male pseudohermaphroditism. *Science* 1974;186:1213–1215.
23. Imperato-McGinley J, Gautier T, Zirinsky K, et al. Prostate visualization studies in males homozygous and heterozygous for 5-alpha-reductase deficiency. *J Clin Endocrinol Metab* 1992;75:1022–1026.
24. Barrett Connor E, Garland C, McPhillips JB, et al. A prospective, population-based study of androstenedione, estrogens, and prostatic cancer. *Cancer Res* 1990;50:169–173.
25. Meikle AW, Stanish WM. Familial prostatic cancer risk and low testosterone. *J Clin Endocrinol Metab* 1982;54:1104–1108.
26. Ross RK, Bernstein L, Lobo RA, et al. 5-alpha-reductase activity and risk of prostate cancer among Japanese and US white and black males. *Lancet* 1992;339:887–889.
27. Balic I, Graham ST, Troyer DA, et al. Androgen receptor length polymorphism associated with prostate cancer risk in Hispanic men. *J Urol* 2002;168:2245–2248.
28. Modugno F, Weissfeld JL, Trump DL, et al. Allelic variants of aromatase and the androgen and estrogen receptors: toward a multigenic model of prostate cancer risk. *Clin Cancer Res* 2001;7:3092–3096.
29. Giovannucci E, Stampfer MJ, Krithivas K, et al. The CAG repeat within the androgen receptor gene and its relationship to prostate cancer. *Proc Natl Acad Sci U S A* 1997;94:3320–3323.
30. Kittles RA, Panguluri RK, Chen W, et al. Cyp17 promoter variant associated with prostate cancer aggressiveness in African Americans. *Cancer Epidemiol Biomarkers Prev* 2001;10:943–947.
31. Walker AH, Jaffe JM, Gunasegaram S, et al. Characterization of an allelic variant in the nifedipine-specific element of CYP3A4: ethnic distribution and implications for prostate cancer risk. Mutations in Brief no. 191. Online. *Hum Mutat* 1998;12:289.
32. Makridakis NM, di Salle E, Reichardt JK. Biochemical and pharmacogenetic dissection of human steroid 5α-reductase type II. *Pharmacogenetics* 2000;10:407–413.
33. Lieberman R. Androgen deprivation therapy for prostate cancer chemoprevention: current status and future directions for agent development. *Urology* 2001;58(2 Suppl 1):83–90.
34. Gormley GJ, Stoner E, Rittmaster RS, et al. Effects of finasteride (MK-906), a 5 alpha-reductase inhibitor, on circulating androgens in male volunteers. *J Clin Endocrinol Metab* 1990;70:1136–1141.
35. McConnell JD, Bruskewitz R, Walsh P, et al. The effect of finasteride on the risk of urinary retention and the need for surgical treatment among men with benign prostatic hyperplasia. *N Engl J Med* 1998;338:557–563.
36. McConnell JD, Roehrborn CG, Bautista OM, et al. The long-term effect of doxazosin, finasteride, and combination therapy on the clinical progression of benign prostatic hyperplasia. *N Engl J Med* 2003;349:2387–2398.
37. Tsukamoto S, Akaza H, Onozawa M, et al. A five-alpha reductase inhibitor or an antiandrogen prevents the progression of microscopic prostate carcinoma to macroscopic carcinoma in rats. *Cancer* 1998;82:531–537.
38. Andriole GL, Guess HA, Epstein JI, et al. Treatment with finasteride preserves usefulness of prostate-specific antigen in the detection of prostate cancer: results of a randomized, double-blind, placebo-controlled clinical trial. PLESS study group. Proscar long-term efficacy and safety study. *J Urol* 1998;52:195–201; discussion 201–202.
39. Andriole GL, Lieber M, Smith J, et al. Treatment with finasteride following radical prostatectomy for prostate cancer. *Urology* 1995;45:491–497.
40. Scardino PT. The prevention of prostate cancer—the dilemma continues. *N Engl J Med* 2003;349:297–299.
41. Reynolds T. Prostate cancer prevention trial yields positive results, but with a few cautions. *J Natl Cancer Inst* 2003;95:1030–1031.
42. Cote RJ, Skinner EC, Salem CE, et al. The effect of finasteride on the prostate gland in men with elevated serum prostate-specific antigen levels. *Br J Cancer* 1998;78:413–418.
43. Algaba F, Epstein JI, Aldape HC, et al. Assessment of prostate carcinoma in core needle biopsy—definition of minimal criteria for the diagnosis of cancer in biopsy material. *Cancer* 1996;78:376–381.
44. Smith WL, De Witt DL, Garavito RM. Cyclooxygenases: structural, cellular, and molecular biology. *Annu Rev Biochem* 2000;69:145–182.
45. Koki AT, Leahy KM, Masferrer JL. Potential utility of COX-2 inhibitors in chemoprevention and chemotherapy. *Expert Opin Investig Drugs* 1999;8:1623–1638.
46. Oshima M, Dinchuk JE, Kargman SL, et al. Suppression of intestinal polyposis in Apc Δ716 knockout mice by inhibition of cyclooxygenase 2 (COX-2). *Cell* 1996;87:803–809.
47. Steinbach G, Lynch P, Phillips RKS, et al. The effect of celecoxib, a cyclooxygenase-2 inhibitor, in familial adenomatous polyposis. *N Engl J Med* 2000;342:1946–1952.
48. Subongkot S, Frame D, Leslie W, et al. Selective cyclooxygenase-2 inhibition: a target in cancer prevention and treatment. *Pharmacotherapy* 2003;23:9–28.
49. O'Neill GP, Ford-Hutchinson AW. Expression of mRNA for cyclooxygenase-1 and cyclooxygenase-2 in human tissues. *FEBS Lett* 1993;330:156–160.
50. Hsu AL, Ching TT, Wang DS, et al. The cyclooxygenase-2 inhibitor celecoxib induces apoptosis by blocking Akt activation in human prostate cancer cells independently of Bcl-2. *J Biol Chem* 2000;275:11397–11403.
51. Liu XH, Yau S, Kirshenbaum A, et al. NS-398, a selective cyclooxygenase-2 inhibitor, induces apoptosis and down-regulates bcl-2 expression in LNCaP cells. *Cancer Res* 1998;58:4245–4249.
52. Ghosh J, Myers CE. Inhibition of arachidonate 5-lipoxygenase triggers massive apoptosis in human prostate cancer cells. *Proc Natl Acad Sci U S A* 1998;95:13182–13187.
53. Liu XH, Kirschenbaum A, Yao S, et al. Inhibition of cyclooxygenase-2 suppresses angiogenesis and the growth of prostate cancer in vivo. *J Urol* 2000;164(3 Pt 1):820–825.
54. Kamijo T, Sato T, Nagatomi Y, et al. Induction of apoptosis by cyclooxygenase-2 inhibitors in prostate cancer cell lines. *Int J Urol* 2001;8:S35–S39.
55. Gupta S, Srivastava M, Ahmad N, et al. Over-expression of cyclooxygenase-2 in human prostate adenocarcinoma. *Prostate* 2000;42:73–78.
56. Roberts RO, Jacobson DJ, Girman CJ, et al. A population-based study of daily nonsteroidal anti-inflammatory drug use and prostate cancer. *Mayo Clin Proc* 2002;77:219–225.

57. Nelson JE, Harris RE. Inverse association of prostate cancer and non-steroidal anti-inflammatory drugs (NSAIDs): results of a case-control study. *Oncol Rep* 2000;7:169–170.

58. Habel LA, Zhao W, Stanford JL. Daily aspirin use and prostate cancer risk in a large, multiracial cohort in the US. *Cancer Causes Control* 2002;13:427–434.

59. Irani J, Ravery V, Pariente JL, et al. Effect of nonsteroidal anti-inflammatory agents and finasteride on prostate cancer risk. *J Urol* 2002;168:1985–1988.

60. Pruthi RS, Derksen JE, Gaston K. Re: Effect of nonsteroidal anti-inflammatory agents and finasteride on prostate cancer risk [Comment]. *J Urol* 2003;169:2304.

61. Derksen JE, Pruthi RS. COX-2 inhibitors in PSA recurrent prostate cancer: a pilot study [Abstract]. *J Urol* 2002;167(Suppl 304):1199.

62. Fleshner NE, Kucuk O. Antioxidant dietary supplements: Rationale and current status as chemopreventive agents for prostate cancer. *Urology* 2001;57(4 Suppl 1):90–94.

63. Heinonen OP, Albanes D, Huttunen JK, et al. Prostate cancer and supplementation with alpha-tocopherol and ß-carotene: incidence and mortality in a controlled trial. *J Natl Cancer Inst* 1998;90:440–446.

64. Clark LC, Combs GF Jr, Turnbull BW, et al. Effects of selenium supplementation for cancer prevention in patients with carcinoma of the skin. A randomized controlled trial. Nutritional Prevention of Cancer Study Group. *JAMA* 1996;276:1957–1963.

65. Klein EA, Thompson IM, Lippman SM, et al. SELECT: the next prostate cancer prevention trial. Selenum and Vitamin E Cancer Prevention Trial. *J Urol* 2001;166:1311–1315.

66. Bostwick DG, Alexander EE, Singh A, et al. Antioxidant enzyme expression and reactive oxygen species damage in prostatic intraepithelial neoplasia and cancer. *Cancer* 2000;89(1):123–134.

67. El-Bayoumy K. The role of selenium in cancer prevention. In: Devita VT, Hellman S, Rosenberg S, eds. *Cancer prevention*. Philadelphia: JB Lippincott, 1991:1–15.

68. National Academy of Sciences. *Recommended dietary allowances*, 10th ed. Washington, DC: National Academy Press, 1989:217–224.

69. Redman C, Scott JA, Baines AT, et al. Inhibitory effect of selenomethionine on the growth of three selected human tumor cell lines. *Cancer Lett* 1998;125(1-2):103–110.

70. Webber MM, Perez-Ripoll EA, James GT. Inhibitory effects of selenium on the growth of DU-145 human prostate carcinoma cells in vitro. *Biochem Biophys Res Commun* 1985;130:603–609.

71. Webber MM. Selenium prevents the growth stimulatory effects of cadmium on human prostatic epithelium. *Biochem Biophys Res Commun* 1985;127:871–877.

72. Combs GF Jr, Clark LC. Selenium and cancer. In: Garewal H, ed. *Antioxidants and disease prevention*. New York: CRC Press, 1997.

73. Clark LC, Dalkin B, Krongrad A, et al. Decreased incidence of prostate cancer with selenium supplementation: Results of a double-blind cancer prevention trial. *Br J Urol* 1998;81:730–734.

74. Yoshizawa K, Willett WC, Morris SJ, et al. Study of prediagnostic selenium level in toenails and the risk of advanced prostate cancer. *J Natl Cancer Inst* 1998;90:1219–1224.

75. Blot WJ, Li JY, Taylor PR, et al. Nutrition intervention trials in Linxian, China: Supplementation with specific vitamin/mineral combinations, cancer incidence, and disease-specific mortality in the general population. *J Natl Cancer Inst* 1993;85:1483–1492.

76. Li JY, Taylor PR, Li B, et al. Nutrition intervention trials in Linxian, China: Multiple vitamin/mineral supplementation, cancer incidence, and disease-specific mortality among adults with esophageal dysplasia. *J Natl Cancer Inst* 1993;85:1492–1498.

77. Yoshizawa K, Willett WC, Morris SJ, et al. Study of prediagnostic selenium level in toenails and the risk of advanced prostate cancer. *J Natl Cancer Inst* 1998;90:1219–1224.

78. Pappas AM. Vitamin E. Tocopherols and tocotrienols. In: Pappas AM, ed. *Antioxidant status, diet, nutrition, and health*. Boca Raton, FL: CRC Press, 1998.

79. Moyad MA, Brumfield SK, Pienta KJ. Vitamin E, alpha- and gamma-tocopherol, and prostate cancer. *Semin Urol Oncol* 1999;17:85–90.

80. Helzlsouer KJ, Huang HY, Alberg AJ, et al. Association between alpha-tocopherol, gamma-tocopherol, selenium, and subsequent prostate cancer. *J Natl Cancer Inst* 2000;92:2018–2023.

81. Traber MG, Packer L. Vitamin E: beyond antioxidant function. *Am J Clin Nutr* 1995;62:1501s–1509s.

82. Mahoney CW, Azzi A. Vitamin E inhibits protein kinase C activity. *Biochem Biophys Res Commun* 1988;154:694–697.

83. Venkateswaran V, Fleshner NE, Klotz LH. Modulation of cell proliferation and cell cycle regulators by vitamin E in human prostate carcinoma cell lines. *J Urol* 2002;168(4 Pt 1):1578–1582.

84. Pastori M, Pfander H, Boscoboinik D, et al. Lycopene in association with alpha-tocopherol inhibits at physiological concentrations proliferation of prostate carcinoma cells. *Biochem Biophys Res Commun* 1998;250:582–585.

85. Fleshner N, Fair WR, Huryk R, et al. Vitamin E inhibits the high-fat diet promoted growth of established human prostate LNCaP tumors in nude mice. *J Urol* 1999;161:1651–1654.

86. The Alpha-Tocopherol, Beta Carotene Cancer Prevention Study Group. The effect of vitamin E and beta carotene on the incidence of lung cancer and other cancers in male smokers. *N Engl J Med* 1994;330:1029–1035.

87. Heinonen OP, Albanes D, Virtamo J, et al. Prostate cancer and supplementation with alpha-tocopherol and beta-carotene: incidence and mortality in a controlled trial. *J Natl Cancer Inst* 1998;90:440–446.

88. Virtamo J, Pietinen P, Huttunen JK, et al. Incidence of cancer and mortality following alpha-tocopherol and beta-carotene supplementation: a postintervention follow-up. *JAMA* 2003;290:476–485.

89. Eichholzer M, Stahelin HB, Ludin E, et al. Smoking, plasma vitamins C, E, retinol, and carotene, and fatal prostate cancer: seventeen-year follow-up of the prospective Basel study. *Prostate* 1999;38:189–198.

90. Hsing AW, Comstock GW, Abbey H, et al. Serologic precursors of cancer: retinol, carotenoids, and tocopherol and risk of prostate cancer. *J Natl Cancer Inst* 1990;82:941–946.

91. Southwest Oncology Group, National Cancer Institute (NCI), Eastern Cooperative Oncology Group, Cancer and Leukemia Group B. Selenium in preventing cancer in patients with neoplasia of the prostate. Available at: http://clinicaltrials.gov/ct/show/NCT00030901?order=10. Accessed May 20, 2004.

92. Shimizu H, Ross RK, Bernstein L, et al. Cancers of the prostate and breast among Japanese and white immigrants in Los Angeles County. *Br J Cancer* 1991;63:963–966.

93. Yu H, Harris RE, Gao YT, et al. Comparative epidemiology of cancers of the colon, rectum, prostate and breast in Shanghai, China versus the United States. *Int J Epidemiol* 1991;20:76–81.

94. Giovannucci E, Rimm EB, Colditz GA. et al. A prospective study of dietary fat and risk of prostate cancer. *J Natl Cancer Inst* 1993;85:1571–1579.

95. Kolonel LN, Nomura AM, Cooney RV. Dietary fat and prostate cancer: current status. *J Natl Cancer Inst* 1999;91:414–428.

96. Adlercreutz H. Western diet and western diseases: some hormonal and biochemical mechanisms and associations. *Scand J Clin Lab Invest Suppl* 1990;201:3–23.

97. Aronson WJ, Tymchuk CN, Elashoff RM, et al. Decreased growth of human prostate LNCaP tumors in SCID mice fed a low-fat, soy protein diet with isoflavones. *Nutr Cancer* 1999;35:13013–13016.

98. Zhou JR, Yu L, Zhong Y, et al. Inhibition of orthotopic growth and metastasis of androgen-sensitive human prostate tumors in mice by bioactive soybean components. *Prostate* 2002;53:143–153.

99. Pollard M, Wolter W. Prevention of spontaneous prostate-related cancer in Lobund-Wistar rats by a soy protein isolate/isoflavone diet. *Prostate* 2000;45:101–105.

100. Heinonen OP, Albanes D, Virtamo J. Prostate cancer and supplementation with alpha-tocopherol and beta-carotene: incidence and mortality in a controlled trial. *J Natl Cancer Inst* 1998;90:440–446.

101. Giovannucci E, Rimm EB, Liu Y, et al. A prospective study of tomato products, lycopene, and prostate cancer risk. *J Natl Cancer Inst* 2002;94:391–398.

102. Le Marchand L, Hankin JH, Kolonel LN, et al. Vegetable and fruit consumption in relation to prostate cancer risk in Hawaii: a reevaluation of the effect of dietary beta-carotene. *Am J Epidemiol* 1991;133:215–219.

103. Lieberman R. Prostate cancer chemoprevention: Strategies for designing efficient clinical trials. *Urology* 2001;57(4 Suppl 1):224–229.

104. Thompson IM, Kouril M, Klein EA, et al. The Prostate Cancer Prevention Trial: current status and lessons learned. *Urology* 2001;57(4 Suppl 1):230–234.

105. Pauler DK, Gower KB, Goodman PJ, et al. Biomarker-based methods for determining noncompliance in a prevention trial. *Control Clin Trials* 2002;23:675–685.

106. Moinpour CM, Atkinson JO, Thomas SM, et al. Minority recruitment in the Prostate Cancer Prevention Trial. *Ann Epidemiol* 2000;10(8 Suppl):S85–S91.

107. Wolmark N, Dunn BK. The role of tamoxifen in breast cancer prevention: issues sparked by the NSABP Breast Cancer Prevention Trial (P-1). *Ann N Y Acad Sci* 2001;949:99–108.

CHAPTER 8 ■ SCREENING AND EARLY DETECTION

CHAPTER 8A
Screening and Early Detection of Prostate Cancer: Prostate Specific Antigen and Related Kallikreins

Thomas Steuber, Kevin M. Slawin, and Hans Lilja

INTRODUCTION

Human glandular kallikrein 3 (hK3), commonly known as prostate-specific antigen (PSA), and human glandular kallikrein 2 (hK2) represent the most widely studied and clinically important members of the human glandular kallikrein family. Due to their restricted tissue expression patterns with high abundance in human prostate glands, PSA and hK2 have been thoroughly evaluated as candidate biomarkers for benign and malignant prostatic disease. Since its clinical introduction as a serum marker for the detection and staging of prostate cancer, PSA has had a profound and dramatic impact on the diagnosis and management of prostate cancer and more recently on benign prostatic hyperplasia (BPH). Through intensive study of the molecular biology and biochemistry of PSA, hK2, and related kallikreins, researchers have continued to improve and refine the utility of these markers. Through these efforts, new markers and innovative molecular methods have been developed that promise to improve on the already impressive performance of total PSA testing as a tool in managing prostatic disease, both prostate cancer and BPH.

BIOLOGY OF HUMAN GLANDULAR KALLIKREIN GENE LOCUS PRODUCTS

The Human Kallikrein Gene Family

The human kallikrein gene family was, until recently, thought to consist of only three genes (hKLK 1 to 3) (1). However, since the discovery of new kallikrein genes, it is now evident that the human tissue kallikrein gene family contains 15 functional genes (2,3). The human kallikrein gene locus spans a region of approximately 300 kb on chromosome 19q13.4. It is formed of 15 kallikrein genes (hKLK 1 to 15), localized in tandem, with no intervention from other genes, and is known to comprise the largest cluster of proteases within the human genome (Fig. 8A.1). The length of all human kallikrein genes range from 4 to 10 kp, with most of the differences attributed to variations in intron length.

The close physical linkage of hKLK2, hKLK3, and hKLK4, in conjunction with their primary expression in the prostate gland, indicates that common prostate-specific and androgen regulatory elements may be controlling their expression.

Androgen Regulation of hKLK3 and hKLK2 Transcription

The mode of hormonal regulation has been extensively studied for hKLK3 and hKLK2 (4). The PSA gene represents an androgen-related gene, as evidenced by the increased transcription that occurs in response to the binding of systemic steroid hormones to the androgen receptor (AR). The AR is a receptor that binds as a homodimer to specific DNA sequences, termed androgen-responsive elements (AREs). The hKLK3 gene has been reported to contain three ARE genes: AREI and AREII are situated in the proximal promoter, and AREIII is located 4 kb upstream of the transcription initiation site (5). It has been shown that AREIII mediates the key control over the transcription of hKLK3. Functional androgen response elements have also been described for the promoter of the hKLK2 gene (6). Both AREI and AREIII, but only one of the nonconsensus AREs found in hKLK3, are conserved in hKLK2. AREIII has been shown to be the major control region for hK2 but has been reported to have lower androgenic inducibility than the PSA promoter.

Tissue Expression and Biologic Function of PSA and hK2

Prostate-specific antigen (PSA; hK3 protein) and human glandular kallikrein (hK2 protein) are protein products of human hKLK3 and hKLK2 genes. Due to their remarkable tissue specificity in human males, PSA and hK2 represent the most valuable tissue markers for benign and malignant prostatic disorders identified so far. Recent studies point to evidence that hK4 and hK11, although expressed at lower levels, may also be useful indicators of prostate cancer (7,8).

PSA and hK2 share 86% identity of their nucleotides and 79% homology at the amino acid level. At the protein level, both PSA and hK2 contain a signal peptide (17 amino acids), a propeptide (7 amino acids), and a mature enzyme (237 amino acids). Although the proteins share substantial structural similarity, they differ significantly in their profiles of enzyme activity (1).

Like other serine proteases, PSA is translated as an inactive pre-pro-PSA precursor. During passage through the secretory pathway, the signal peptide is released to yield the pro-PSA. Pro-PSA, the precursor or zymogen form of PSA, is composed

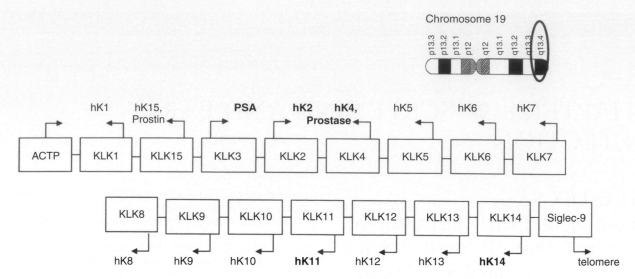

FIGURE 8A.1. Human kallikrein gene locus chromosome 19q13.4, ≈300 kb. (Adapted from Yousef GM, Diamandis EP. The new human tissue kallikrein gene family: structure, function, and association to disease. *Endocr Rev* 2001;22:184–204.)

of 244 amino acid residues, including an amino-terminal propeptide of 7 amino acids. Three studies reported that recombinant hK2 could convert inactive pro-PSA into the mature, enzymatically active, 237-amino acid active single-chain PSA protease, by release of the propeptide *in vitro* (9–11), thus suggesting a possible physiological connection between hK2 and PSA. These findings indicate that one function of hK2 may be the regulation of PSA activity *in vivo*. Furthermore, the activity of PSA is most likely generated by a cascade of events that includes precursor processing and activation of pro-hK2, which can then activate pro-PSA. Pro-hK2 may have autocatalytic activity, which has been demonstrated by its ability to transform independently into enzymatically active hK2 by release of the propeptide (12). The mechanisms that activate pro-kallikreins may be complex and involve several additional enzymes. Both pro-PSA and pro-hK2 have been identified in serum, suggesting that they may also prove to be useful markers for prostate cancer.

PSA manifests chymotrypsin-like proteolytic enzyme activity (13,14), hydrolyzing the peptide bonds of the carboxy-terminal after certain tyrosine and leucine residues (15,16). However, PSA activity is unique in that it is ineffective at hydrolysis of peptide bonds that are most sensitive to the action of native chymotrypsin (16). Contrary to original reports indicating that PSA may also demonstrate some trypsin-like activity (e.g., the ability to hydrolyze peptide bonds of the carboxy-terminal of arginine and lysine residues), PSA has now been shown to be virtually devoid of this type of activity (14). The enzyme action of PSA is believed to be mainly directed against the major gel-forming proteins (semenogelin I and II), and fibronectin in freshly ejaculated semen (17–20). Proteolysis of these proteins induces liquefaction of semen, which results in subsequent release of motile spermatozoa (21,22). *In vitro*, PSA also has been reported to cleave insulin-like growth factor–binding protein-3 (IGF-BP3) (23), thus increasing levels of free IGF-I. However, the identity of several of these reported IGF-BP3 cleavage sites suggest that this proteolytic activity may be the result of contaminants, such as trace amounts of hK2 or trypsin, present within preparations of purified PSA.

Unlike PSA, hK2 displays the trypsin-like specificity common to most members of the tissue kallikrein family of proteases. hK2 is highly selective for arginine residues (12,24)

while PSA cleaves after hydrophobic residues such as tyrosine and leucine (25,26). Using a chromogenic substrate (H-D-ProPhe-Arg-para-nitroanilide) containing an arginine cleavage site, investigators found hK2 enzymatic activity to be 20,000-fold higher than PSA's enzymatic activity on a comparable substrate containing a tyrosine cleavage site (27). hK2 can cleave semenogelin proteins, but with an activity that is comparable only to that of PSA. Since the level of hK2 in seminal fluid is only about 1% of the level of PSA, the physiologic role of hK2 in the cleavage of semenogelin proteins is unclear. Even though hK2 has trypsin-like activity, it does not appear to function primarily as a classical kininogenase. hK2 displays some ability to release kinin in whole serum, as judged by a physiological assay, but this activity is 1,000-fold lower than that of hK1 (28). However, hK2 cannot release lys-bradykinin from a synthetic kininogen substrate (29). Thus, hK2 displays minor physiological kininogenase activity, but the role of this function in the prostate is unknown. Moreover, it is not known whether the enzymatic activity of hK2 contributes to the progression of cancer, or whether its expression is a consequence of neoplastic development, but other active proteases such as urokinase-type plasminogen activator (uPA) and plasmin are known to be involved in cancer invasion and metastasis. hK2 has been shown to activate single chain urokinase-type plasminogen activator (scuPA) to the active double chain form, uPA, which is highly correlated with prostate cancer metastasis (30). More recently, hK2 has been shown to inactivate the major tissue inhibitor of uPA, plasminogen activator inhibitor-1 (PAI-1) (31). Thus, hK2 may influence the progression of prostate cancer by the activation of uPA, and by the inactivation of the primary inhibitor of uPA, PAI-1.

PSA and, presumably, hK2 are produced primarily by prostate ductal and acinar epithelium and are subsequently secreted into the lumina of the prostatic ducts, eventually forming an important component of seminal fluid.

The mean concentration of PSA in seminal plasma roughly exceeds the physiological concentration of PSA in blood by the factor 10^6 (32). The relative level of hK2 in prostate tissue, seminal plasma, and blood is only 1% of the concentration of PSA. However, it has been observed in LNCaP cells that the amount of hK2 transcripts is around 30% of the amount of PSA transcripts (33), which indicates that these closely related proteases differ in regard to the stability of their mRNA. The tight compartmentalization of PSA and hK2 in the normal prostate is altered in prostatic disease. The disintegration of the continuous layer of basal cells, a characteristic early feature of carcinogenesis, results in loss of the normal glandular architecture and allows substantial leakage of various kallikreins into circulation.

The recombinant expression of the cloned glandular kallikreins has provided the critical preconditions for many of the studies aimed at developing a detailed understanding of the structure and function of the human kallikrein family.

PROSTATE-SPECIFIC ANTIGEN AS A SCREENING TOOL FOR EARLY PROSTATE CANCER DETECTION

In the early 1970s, several groups first identified what we now call PSA in human seminal fluid (34,35). In 1979, PSA was purified from prostate tissue (36), but its clinical significance only became evident in the 1980s, when PSA was first reported to be a potentially useful marker for prostate cancer (35,37–39). Subsequently, PSA screening was introduced into clinical practice. With increasing use from 5.1% in all newly diagnosed prostatic carcinomas in 1984 to 60.6% in 1994, PSA screening has since outperformed digital rectal examination (DRE) in early cancer detection (40,41). Not surprisingly, this has resulted in a remarkable increase in the reported incidence of prostate cancer in many countries, and in particular in the United States.

After almost two decades of widespread PSA-based prostate cancer screening, the appropriateness of prostate cancer screening is still a topic of great debate. This includes the diagnostic performance of the screening test, cancer overdetection, and the relationship between PSA screening and the observed decrease in disease-specific mortality. The following chapter introduces the current opinion on screening practices and the estimated effectiveness of screening to reduce prostate cancer mortality based on the evidence to date. In addition, information from ongoing randomized trials is presented.

The Evidence to Date

By now, it is considered indisputable that the widespread use of PSA screening in Western countries has resulted in significantly increased numbers of diagnosed cancer cases, as well as, identification of cancer in its predominantly early stages. Moreover, since 1991, an annual percentage drop of 4.3% in prostate cancer mortality rates has been observed in the United States (42). Simultaneously, a reversal in the prostate cancer mortality rate has been reported for some European countries, with a significant decrease between 1979 and 1997, especially in the age group 40 to 69 years (43). These trends were significantly associated with a parallel decline of locally advanced or metastatic disease. However, a parallel fall in prostate cancer mortality rate was also demonstrated in England and Wales despite a considerably less widespread use of PSA testing in these countries (44). Thus, the beneficial survival effect of PSA screening in prostate cancer remains controversial and has been heavily debated during the last decade.

Several observational studies among entire populations with heterogeneous screening policies have contributed reports about the mortality effect of screening, with conflicting results. Analysis from regional data, published from Canada, consistently could not confirm significant associations with the intensity of PSA screening and subsequent decreases in prostate cancer mortality (45–47). Coldman and associates even observed an inverse relationship between screening intensity and the extent of the mortality reduction among areas with low (5%) medium (53%) and high (71%) screening intensity in British Columbia, Canada (47). High screening coverage was associated with the lowest reduction (14%), whereas the opposite trend in mortality was observed for low screening coverage areas (29% reduction). Another study from the United States compared cancer-related mortality rates from Seattle, defined as an area with high intensity of screening, with Connecticut, where PSA screening is less frequent. Again, reduction of prostate cancer mortality did not show any significant association with the active screening policy in Seattle (48).

In 1993, a mass screening project among all men aged 45 to 75 years using PSA as the only screening test was launched in the Federal State of Tyrol, which is one of nine federal states of the Republic of Austria (49). When PSA testing became freely available, 32.3% of all Tyrolean men underwent PSA screening. Since the beginning of the screening project, a significant migration to lower PSA levels in patients undergoing radical prostatectomy has been observed. In parallel, the rate of organ confined disease in radical prostatectomy increased from 28.7% in 1993 to more than 80% in 2002. Intriguingly, the mortality rate from prostate cancer in Tyrol decreased significantly between 1993 and 2000, in contrast to the modest downward trend in prostate cancer death rates observed in the rest of Austria. This trend coincides from the temporal point of view with the introduction of PSA testing. These findings, however, require careful interpretation. The mean lead-time, defined as the duration of follow-up needed to accrue the same expected number of incident prostate cancer cases in the absence of screening as detected in the initial screening round, was estimated as 5 to 10 years (50,51). Likewise, the mean survival time of prostate cancer was reported to be at least 5 years. Reduced mortality in Austria, however, has emerged at 2 to 3 years after introducing screening, which was also reported for the reduction onset of cancer related mortality in the United States. This suggests that simultaneous improvement of treatment rather than any screening effect may explain the early reduction in prostate cancer mortality. Chu et al. subsequently presented the concept of incidence based mortality (IBM) among the Surveillance, Epidemiology, and End Results (SEER) program, which represents approximately 10% of the US population (52). In this population, age adjusted prostate cancer mortality rates have dropped below the rate in 1986 for participants 50 to 84 years of age. In the white and black populations, this decrease became evident since 1995 and 1997, respectively. IBM by disease stage revealed that the recent declines were caused by decreases in distant disease mortality. This finding is, however, related to a decline in distant disease incidence rather than improved survival of patients with metastatic disease. This data may represent evidence that implicates a potential beneficial outcome of PSA screening.

Ongoing Trials of Prostate Cancer Screening

The outlined studies and their controversial conclusions on the effect of PSA screening on prostate cancer mortality are limited by small size, irregular screening intensity, contamination by opportunistic PSA testing in the control groups, insufficient observation intervals, and their mainly retrospective design. For unambiguous conclusions on PSA screening benefit on prostate cancer mortality, prospective randomized trials in both Europe and North America have been initiated: The European Randomized Study of Screening for Prostate Cancer (ERSPC) started on July 1, 1994 as a cooperation of the Netherlands and Belgium (53). Finland became the third partner a year later after successfully conducting a pilot study. Subsequently, France, Italy, Switzerland, and Sweden joined and completed this multi-institutional project group. During 1995, the ERSPC explored the possibility of cooperation with the Prostate arm of the North American Prostate, Lung, Colorectal, Ovarian, screening program (PLCO), which was initiated by the National Cancer Institute in 1993 (54). Both studies in conjunction may eventually recruit about 260,000 men, randomized between screening and control arms, which has been estimated to increase the power of both studies to demonstrate or exclude a 20% difference in prostate cancer mortality with a power of 90% (55).

Study Design of PLCO and ERSPC

Different legal requirements for running randomized studies among participating countries resulted in two different randomization procedures: ERSPC trials in Belgium, the Netherlands, Spain, and Switzerland are based on participation of invited volunteers, who are eventually required to give their informed consent before randomization. In contrast, trials in the remainder countries of the ERSPC (Italy, France, Finland, Sweden) and the PLCO centers make use of population registers that identify the eligible population by age, who are subsequently randomized to either the screening or the control arm without their consent.

The PLCO study was designed with a strict joint protocol, which is followed by all participating study centers. In contrast, participants in the ERSPC have agreed on a common core protocol, which allows for variability in the target population and screening procedure. The core age group that is targeted by nearly all ERSPC centers includes men 55 to 69 years old.

The PLCO defined their screening protocol as annual screening and 4.0 ng/mL as the PSA cutoff. Based on considerations on lead-time and overdiagnosis, which are inherent in effective screening, a 4-year screening interval was selected in the ERSPC study centers. Moreover, they defined a PSA level ≥4 ng/mL and/or abnormality in transrectal ultrasound and/or DRE as biopsy criteria in the initial round of the trial [except for Sweden, which started with biannual screening intervals in 1995 and defined a PSA cut-point of ≥3 ng/mL as biopsy criterion (56)].

Subsequently, initial experiences with the outlined screening protocol were included in a logistic regression model, to predict the number of cancers for PSA <4 ng/mL if all men were biopsied (predictive index) (57). After an extensive study of various prediction models, the group considered to omit DRE and transrectal ultrasound (TRUS) as screening tests and decreased the biopsy indication to a PSA of ≤3 ng/mL. This screening policy was subsequently substantiated by a model developed with Microsimulation Screening Analysis (MISCAN), which represents tools that are designed to evaluate cancer screening trials (58). The MISCANs were validated with outcome-data from 42,376 men from initial and second screening rounds of the Dutch ERSPC trial, which facilitate prediction of lead-time and overdetection rates associated with different screening programs. The sensitivities for PSA screening estimated with the model were 64.94% and 99% for the localized, regional, and distant cancers, respectively. Simulation of the current ERSPC screening trial including participants 55 to 75 years of age and a 4-year screening interval demonstrated that prostate cancer detection preceded clinical diagnosis by 10 years, with a medium lead time of 10.3 years (range 9.9 to 11.2 years). The corresponding overdetection rate of 54% (range 51% to 59%) implied that half of the detected cancers would have remained undiagnosed in absence of screening for prostate cancer. Lowering the screening interval to annual screening visits did not substantially change the prediction outcome for lead-time (11.6 years) and overdetection (56%), which supports the concept of a screening interval of 4 years.

Preliminary Results of PLCO and ERSPC

Preliminary data from the Finnish, the Dutch, and the Swedish ERSPC section revealed promising data with regard to the impact of screening on stage migration of detected cancers. Significantly lower rates of localized disease in the control group compared to the screening arm (65% to 69% vs. 86% to 94%) were observed. In addition, only 0.6% metastatic cancers were detected in the screened population, which is much lower than the proportion of 25% reported during the prescreening era (59).

De Koning and associates have estimated what impact both ongoing large-scale randomized controlled screenings may have in proving a substantial decline in prostate cancer related mortality (55). They concluded that the current numbers of subjects enrolled so far has sufficient power to detect a significant difference in prostate cancer mortality of at least 25% between the two arms by 2008, if contamination by opportunistic PSA testing in the control arm remains limited.

In conclusion, preliminary experience from the two large ongoing screening trials so far has contributed to a better understanding of screening procedures, predictive factors for a positive biopsy outcome, and screening intervals. Screening, moreover, has demonstrated a favorable impact on stage migration toward localized disease and results in a marked reduction of patients with advanced prostate cancers. These observations, however, stand opposed to the negative side effects of screening. An example of this is a distinct increase of prostate cancer incidence of 60% to 90%, which represents a considerable overdetection of roughly 50% of all diagnosed cancers. Estimates on the effect of prostate cancer screening on disease specific mortality trends await presentation in 2008.

Diagnostic Capacity of PSA for Early Prostate Cancer Detection

Despite its apparently favorable assessed impact on prostate cancer mortality, the application of serum PSA measurement as a screening tool for the early diagnosis of prostate cancer remains controversial. It is widely recognized that in patients with a PSA below 10 ng/mL, PSA has become increasingly limited in its capacity to correctly identify patients with prostate cancer. The complex process that leads to elevated serum PSA levels in patients with prostate cancer as well as various benign prostatic disorders such as inflammatory processes and BPH, often coexistent in the same patients, makes interpretation of an elevated serum PSA level problematic. Results from large scale prostate cancer screening programs, such as those performed under the aegis of Prostate Cancer Awareness Week and a prospective trial of prostate cancer screening performed at six university centers, demonstrated that approximately 10% to 15% of men in their initial year of screening have a serum PSA level above 4 ng/mL (the historically accepted cutoff value thought to identify patients with a higher likelihood of harboring prostate cancer prompting a recommendation for prostate biopsy) (60,61). However, the positive predictive value of biopsy in this setting was only 12%, and 32% when patients also had a nonsuspicious DRE. Surgery in those patients with prostate cancer found tumors to be pathologically organ-confined in a disappointingly small 62% of cases (62). A large number of negative biopsies are performed, associated with costs and some degree of discomfort, yet up to 40% of the cancers detected were more locally advanced than optimal for screening-detected disease.

Furthermore, a patient with a PSA level below 4 ng/mL was earlier assumed to be at low-risk for prostate cancer.

More recent data, especially in cohorts more thoroughly biopsied with more than 10 cores, demonstrated that 19% to 22% of men with a total PSA in the range 2 to 4 ng/mL will have a positive biopsy.

Following radical prostatectomy, organ-confinement was found in 81% to 84% (63,64). Thus, lowering the cutoff value to a PSA of 2 ng/mL would lead to a marked increase in the number of unnecessarily biopsied men. However, if it is not lowered, 20% of significant and potentially curable cancers would remain undiagnosed.

Therefore, alternate approaches are needed to enhance specificity and sensitivity for detection of localized prostate cancer, as cancer control and functional outcomes after local therapy are most favorable when disease is organ confined.

TOTAL PROSTATE-SPECIFIC ANTIGEN DERIVATIVES IMPROVE METHODS FOR CANCER DETECTION

Total PSA derivatives represent permutations of total serum PSA that have been tested in clinical practice to improve the specificity and sensitivity of prostate cancer screening. These derivatives, including age specific PSA, PSA velocity, and PSA density are based on the observed biological characteristics to be highly related to the prevalence of BPH, which is again increasing with age. The clinical relevance of PSA derivatives in the early detection of prostate cancer is described in Chapter 8B.

Age-Specific PSA Ranges

The average annual increase of serum PSA ranges from 0.1 to 0.5 ng/mL in men with benign prostate hyperplasia, and is presumably driven by an average prostate growth rate of 1.8 mL/yr (65). More recent reports, which studied the correlation of PSA and prostate volume in patients with BPH and no evidence of prostate cancer, established an age-dependent log-linear relationship for prostate volume and serum PSA (66). Oesterling and colleagues proposed the use of age-specific serum PSA reference ranges, to improve the sensitivity of prostate cancer detection in patients of younger age, and that might improve specificity by avoiding the detection of insignificant cancers in the elderly population (67–70) (Table 8A.1).

Several studies evaluating the clinical value of age-adjusted PSA have reported conflicting results. When age-related PSA was employed in large study cohorts and screening populations, its application increased the cancer detection rate from 8 to 18% in men <60 years at the expense of a 45% increase over the number of biopsies performed when standard PSA reference ranges were used. In men >60 years, fewer biopsies would have been taken (21% to 22%) if the 4 ng/mL cutoff had been applied, but at the expense of leaving 12% to 22% of localized cancers undetected (71,72). Thus, the net effect on cancer detection rates using age-adjusted PSA applied to all age ranges was a decrease of only 4%. However, a decrease in cancer detection as great as 39% has been reported by other authors, and has been deemed unacceptable for screening prostate cancer (73).

Partin et al. were in favor of using age-specific PSA ranges in younger men, between the ages of 50 and 59, as 81% of the additional cancers detected had favorable pathological parameters compared with 76% in the older group of men. In addition, 95% of the missed T1c cancers in the older men were histologically favorable and were unlikely to become clinically significant (72). Borer et al. in contrast, found unfavorable pathology in 60% of the older patients, screened using age-adjusted PSA parameters (74).

Race-corrected, age-specific PSA ranges take into account reports that describe higher PSA values in black populations than in white or Asian populations, even when studies are controlled for age, Gleason grade, or clinical stage, which has been associated with a larger tumor volume in black than in white men (1.3 to 2.5 times larger). Several investigators have reported that 40% of cancers in a black population would have been missed if traditional age-specific ranges had been used (75,76).

In summary, age-specific PSA ranges are not to be used without careful consideration of the fact that they might lead to missed, significant, and potentially curable cancers in the older population. In addition, application of age-adjusted PSA in men younger than 60 years leads to a marked increase of men requiring further investigation because of an elevated PSA, making it a cost intensive screening tool.

PSA Velocity

The velocity at which PSA increases on an annual basis has been introduced as another PSA derivative used to achieve improved diagnostic accuracy of serial PSA measurements in prostate cancer screening. This concept was first introduced by Carter and associates in their Baltimore Longitudinal Aging Study (BLAS) (77). A PSA velocity exceeding 0.75 ng/mL yr was associated with a higher risk of prostate cancer than was a slower rise in PSA over time, with 72% sensitivity and 95% specificity. These significant differences between PSA velocity associated with BPH and with prostate cancer were detectable up to 9 years before prostate cancer was diagnosed. Following

TABLE 8A.1

AGE-ADJUSTED PSA CUTOFF VALUE IN NORMAL MEN OF DIFFERENT RACES, SUGGESTED BY STUDIES FROM OESTERLING ET AL. (68,69) AND MORGAN ET AL. (70)

Author	n	Race	40–49	50–59	60–69	70–79
Oesterling et al. (68)	422	White	2.5	3.0	4.0	5.5
Oesterling et al. (69)	286	Asian	2.0	3.0	4.0	5.0
Morgan et al. (70)	1673	African-American	2.0	4.0	4.5	5.5

PSA cutoff (ng/mL) adjusted by age (years)

PSA, prostate-specific antigen.

studies that used longitudinal PSA velocity to identify cancer candidates with relatively short-term intervals of less than 2 years, however, were not able to confirm test results from Carter (78). Subsequently, Carter et al. suggested that PSA velocity is useful if a minimum of three tests are taken over a 2-year period, which was most significant in men with a PSA rise from 2.0 ng/mL at baseline to greater than 4 ng/mL (79). Results from the ERSPC screening program (Rotterdam) including 774 men with a PSA below 4 ng/mL, however, demonstrated that, applied in a multivariate analysis, PSA velocity did not prove to be a useful screening tool for the identification of potentially curable prostate cancers in the low PSA range (80).

The limited utility of PSA velocity may be attributable to the fact that PSA is not cancer specific and that it varies significantly from day to day. Additionally, brief episodes of increased serum PSA levels (e.g., due to transient inflammatory processes) interfere with the accurate measurement of the gradual, natural elevation of serum PSA levels over decades (81). Eastham and colleagues recently reported that nearly half of men who had one abnormal PSA value over a 4-year period subsequently had a normal level, suggesting that intraindividual PSA fluctuation may lead to a false positive interpretation (82). Finally, the fact that PSA results are different when measured on different PSA assays may add some degree of imprecision to PSA velocity determination (83,84). Thus, biological variations coupled with differences in assays probably preclude the gathering of useful information from PSA velocity, except with very long intervals between screenings.

More recent studies introduced the concept of annual pretreatment PSA velocity to predict tumor stage, grade, and time to recurrence after radical prostatectomy (85). Intriguingly, D'Amico and associates reported significantly shorter time to PSA relapse and death from prostate cancer in patients with an annual PSA velocity of more than 2.0 ng/mL compared to an annual velocity of 2.0 ng/mL or less among 1054 patients after surgical therapy for localized prostate cancer. This observation might suggest that PSA rises in short time intervals, which have failed to provide reliable information to distinguish cancer patients from subjects without prostate cancer, are present and more pronounced in cancers with less favorable prognosis compared to tumors with favorable treatment outcome. Thus, evaluation of annual PSA velocity prior to diagnosis has been suggested as a promising approach to identify candidates who may not benefit from local therapy on an individual basis. Reports from other institutions, however, have yet to confirm these initial findings.

PSA Density

The third and most intensively investigated PSA derivative for prostate cancer screening is PSA density, which is defined as the ratio of an individual serum PSA and its corresponding prostate volume, assessed by transrectal ultrasound. This concept was first introduced by Benson and colleagues in 1992 to "correct" serum PSA levels for variable association of these levels with benign and malignant prostatic disease (86). Normal prostate epithelium has been reported to contribute an average of 0.1 ng/mL PSA per gram of tissue to the serum PSA level. The corresponding PSA contribution for BPH tissue is 0.3 ng/mL and for cancerous epithelium it is 3.5 ng/mL (87). However, two aspects limit the use of PSA density. First, results depend on the examiner and the different types of ultrasound devices to estimate the prostatic volume correctly. Second, the ratio of stroma to epithelium has been shown to vary considerably between individuals (88). Because only prostatic epithelium produces PSA and the amount of stroma cannot be estimated from transrectal ultrasound, this influences

PSA density to an unforeseeable extent. Therefore, reports of the utility of PSA density have been conflicting. Initial reports indicated that a cutoff of 0.15 ng/mL for PSA density outperformed the 4 ng/mL PSA cutoff in detecting prostate cancer when PSA was below 10 ng/mL (89). Subsequent analyses, however, were not able to reproduce these initial results (90,91). In a prospective multicenter clinical trial of nearly 5000 participants with a PSA between 4.1 and 9.9 ng/mL and normal findings on DRE, Catalona and colleagues concluded that a PSA density cutoff of higher than 0.15 ng/mL for biopsy resulted in half of the tumors being missed (91).

Further studies examined the extent to which PSA density is comparable to other PSA related factors in predicting cancer in men with an ongoing elevated PSA after an initial negative prostate biopsy. Catalona and colleagues achieved 90% sensitivity while avoiding 31% of the repeat biopsies with a modified PSA density cutoff of 0.1 ng/mL. This predictive performance, however, was also obtained by the application of the free to total PSA ratio (92). Further, in a multivariate analysis of 298 consecutive men who presented with suspected cancer for an initial negative biopsy, Fowler and colleagues showed that in the presence of %free PSA, PSA density, and PSA velocity were no longer independent predictors for second biopsy outcome (93). In another study based on secondary analysis of the pivotal trial that led to FDA approval of free PSA, PSA density and the %free PSA ratio performed identically. In that study, a PSA density cut-point of 0.08 was identical to a %free PSA cut-point of 25% in maintaining 95% sensitivity while avoiding 12% unnecessary biopsies in 163 patients with a serum PSA level between 4 and 10 ng/mL and a normal DRE.

The concept of PSA transition zone density (tz density) was introduced by Djavan et al. as a modification of the traditional PSA density (94). It "corrects" serum PSA levels for the volume of the transition zone, since the transition zone in men with nodular hyperplasia-associated BPH produces 10- to 100-fold more PSA per gram than either the peripheral or central zone, which are less significant sources of PSA in the absence of cancer. In a large, prospective study of 820 men, aged 44 to 77 years at risk for prostate cancer with PSA 4 to 10 ng/mL who underwent repeat biopsy, a PSA tz density cutoff of 0.26 ng/mL cc was superior to the conventional volume-adjusted PSA in predicting cancer. However, the best performance was obtained when a 30% cutoff of the free to total PSA ratio (%fPSA) was used (AUC 74.5% for %fPSA vs. 69.1% for PSA tz density) (95).

In summary, although serum PSA levels adjusted to total or transition zone prostate volume have proven to have a greater specificity than serum PSA levels alone, their performance has been gained by the expense of sensitivity for the initially proposed cut-points of 0.1 to 0.15. Although lower cut-points (0.09) appear to maximize sensitivity and specificity, PSA density requires skilled transrectal ultrasonography, an uncomfortable, invasive, and expensive procedure, to accurately measure the prostate volume. With the advent of the free to total PSA ratio as an equally effective screening tool, which requires a simple blood draw to measure, PSA density has waned as a widely used parameter by clinicians.

FREE AND COMPLEXED PROSTATE-SPECIFIC ANTIGEN FOR PROSTATE CANCER DETECTION

The identification of several different molecular forms of PSA in blood in the early 1990s facilitated the development of immunoassays for the PSA subforms with improved cancer specificity (75,77). This section illustrates the use of free and complexed PSA for early detection of prostate cancer, and describes its promising results to date.

PSA in Peripheral Blood: Free and Complexed PSA

After its release into circulation, PSA presumably follows two major metabolic routes: PSA that was catalytically inactivated during passage through the secretory pathway (primarily by internal cleavage) eventually forms a minor proportion of 5% to 40% of total PSA in serum. This enzymatic inactive subfraction is unable to form complexes with antiproteases in the circulation, thus remaining as free (or "unbound") PSA in blood. Free PSA is cleared with a half-life of 12 to 18 hours by renal glomerular filtration (96). The majority (60% to 95%) of PSA that enters the peripheral blood is catalytically active, thus forming stable, covalent complexes with several of the major physiologic protease inhibitors, such as serin protease inhibitors [α_1-antichymotrypsin (ACT), protein C inhibitor (PCI), α_1-antitrypsin (API)] and another class of antiproteases, encompassing α_2-macroglobulin (AMG) and pregnancy-zone protein (PZP) (16). Intact, active PSA reacts preferentially with AMG (about 20 times more rapidly than in the formation of PSA-ACT complexes). However, PSA-AMG is rapidly metabolized by efficient hepatic clearance mechanisms with a half life of only 6.7 minutes. This results in serum concentrations close to or below detection limits (97). Moreover, PSA-AMG is not immunoreactive, since all antigenic epitopes of PSA are encapsuled and thus hidden by the AMG molecule. PSA-ACT complexes are eliminated from the circulation comparatively slowly, with an estimated half life of 3 days, which corresponds to a decrease of PSA-ACT by approximately 1 ng/mL per day (98). Thus, ACT-PSA accumulates in blood and consequently forms the major component of detectable PSA-antiprotease complexes, the minor component being PSA-API (0.5% to 5%). Both complexed forms make up the total of immunoreactive cPSA.

The proportion of free PSA to total PSA has been reported to vary according to disease type: typically a significantly higher percentage of free PSA is found in blood from men with benign gland enlargements, whereas more pronounced elevations of PSA-ACT levels in serum from men with adenocarcinomas contribute to typical findings of a significantly lower percentage of free PSA in these samples.

Clinical Application of Free PSA

Clinically, the most important application of free PSA (fPSA) is in the identification of free PSA-specific antigenic epitope structures that are unavailable when PSA forms complexes with antiproteases such as ACT (16,97). This phenomenon forms the molecular basis for the generation of assays that can accurately measure the ratio of free to total PSA (99). Lilja and associates were first to design an immunoassay specific for the free, non-complexed PSA form (97) and subsequently, Christensson reported that the ratio of free to total PSA was lower in men with carcinoma (99). Currently, at least three fPSA assay systems are approved as adjuncts to PSA-based prostate cancer screening. By simultaneous immunodetection of both free and total PSA, the calculated ratio (%fPSA = 100 × fPSA/PSA) has greatly improved on the simple use of PSA or its derivatives for prostate cancer detection.

Data from the Dutch ERSPC section clearly demonstrated that lower %fPSA levels more accurately predict a higher risk of prostate cancer than higher levels of total PSA (100) (Table 8A.2). When total PSA is 4 ng/mL, the average risk of prostate cancer is 15% to 20% in patients with a normal DRE but varies from only 3% to as high as 50% when the proportion of fPSA is 40% and 5%, respectively. Numerous large, well-controlled studies of defined study populations have reported confirmatory findings (101,102). One of the largest multicenter studies evaluated a total of 773 men with normal DRE over the truncated range of total PSA between 4 and 10 ng/mL (103). Each had a free and total PSA test using the Hybritech Tandem PSA and Tandem free PSA assay, and had a histologically confirmed diagnosis by at least a sextant prostate biopsy. Applying a cut-off value for %fPSA below 25% would have provided detection of 95% of cancers. At the same time, it would have reduced the biopsy rate by 20% in the total PSA range of 4 to 10 ng/mL. On the basis of these results, %fPSA has been established and FDA-approved for clinical use in the 4 to 10 ng/mL PSA range.

Subsequent investigations focused on the lower PSA range of 2 to 4 ng/mL PSA, found in up to 22% of all patients with significant, yet predominantly favorable prostate cancers. In this PSA range, a cutoff for %fPSA of 27% provided detection of 90% of cancers while, at the same time, preventing 18% of biopsies that otherwise would have been performed, supporting the use of %fPSA in this lower range of total PSA as well (64). In addition, Haese and colleagues reported that in the PSA range of 2 to 4 ng/mL, a percent free PSA cutoff of 18% to

---

TABLE 8A.2

PROBABILITY OF FINDING PROSTATE CANCER WITH VARIOUS COMBINATIONS OF FREE AND TOTAL PSA IN MEN WITH NORMAL FINDINGS ON DIGITAL RECTAL EXAMINATION BASED ON DATA FROM THE DUTCH PROSTATE CANCER SCREENING TRIAL (100)

Probability of prostate cancer in biopsy (%)			
Free PSA (%)	Total PSA 4 ng/mL	Total PSA 10 ng/mL	Total PSA 20 ng/mL
40	2	3	5
30	4	7	15
20	12	19	35
15	19	28	49
10	30	42	63
5	52	64	81

PSA, prostate-specific antigen.

20% can be applied to detect prostate cancer and only moderately increase the number of patients biopsied that would be required to detect one significant cancer compared with the PSA range of 4 to 10 ng/mL (biopsy-to-cancer ratio of 3 to 4:1) (104). As discussed earlier, %fPSA also proved to be the most accurate predictor of biopsy outcome after initial negative biopsy in men suspected of having prostate cancer with PSA levels ranging from 4 to 10 ng/mL, thus outperforming simple derivatives of total PSA.

Although %fPSA is cross-validated in numerous clinical trials and is widely used in current clinical practice, its application is not without drawbacks. Investigators in several recent studies comparing prostate markers for early cancer detection were not able to reproduce the diagnostic performance of %fPSA initially reported in the studies of Catalona and colleagues (105,106). The inconsistencies in diagnostic accuracy of %fPSA may find an explanation in any one or a combination of its properties: Because free PSA increases with age and prostate volume, and decreases as the total PSA increases, the composition of any population studied can influence the results of free PSA studies (107). In fact, it has been observed that the discrimination power of %fPSA between BPH and cancer patients is lost when the prostate volume exceeds 40 cm^3 (108).

Second, fPSA immunodetection is highly susceptible to preanalytical and analytical bias. The limited *in vitro* stability of the free PSA, particularly in serum, warrants very careful handling of specimens including very rapid separation of serum/plasma from the blood cells and analysis of serum within 24 hours of collecting the sample (109). Moreover, prostatic manipulation (vigorous DRE), prostate biopsy, and urethral instrumentation have all been shown to increase total PSA concentrations due primarily to an increase in the free PSA component of total PSA (96). Therefore any manipulation of the prostate gland should be avoided for at least 48 to 72 hours prior to the collection of a sample for measurement of free PSA. Probably the most significant problem in comparing diagnostic performance from study to study is that results vary depending on the manufacturer of the assay. The clinical effect of significant interassay variation was clearly demonstrated by Nixon and associates. In their comparative study of three investigational assays for free PSA among 123 consecutively accrued patients, different %fPSA cutpoints of 22%, 34%, and 34% were identified that would ensure a 95% sensitivity cancer detection, and the number of negative biopsies that would have been prevented were 38%, 19%, and 34%, respectively (110).

In conclusion, %fPSA provides a valuable improvement in specificity while maintaining high sensitivity for prostate cancer in men with a total PSA of 2.6 to 10 ng/mL. In clinical practice, the use of a cutoff between 14% and 25% is best, although individual physicians may choose to raise or lower these cutoff points, depending on whether they desire to be more aggressive in detecting cancer at the cost of performing more unnecessary biopsies (e.g., trend to higher sensitivity) or to be more conservative by accepting a lower sensitivity in return for performing fewer biopsies.

Clinical Application of Complexed PSA

Complexed PSA (cPSA) in serum has been reported to be more robust than free PSA both *in vitro* and *in vivo*: (a) It is less likely to be affected by day-to-day variation because of its significantly longer elimination rate (98), (b) it suffers less from significant *in vitro* instability (107), and (c) it is less affected by prostatic manipulation (96).

The only cPSA immunoassay that is approved by the FDA for prostate cancer detection is based on antibody-mediated elimination of all fPSA, followed by measurement of the remaining PSA (Bayer Immuno 1 cPSA Assay, Bayer Diagnostics, Tarrytown, NY). Alternatively, calculated complexed PSA levels can be generated by subtracting total PSA (tPSA) from fPSA. This calculated cPSA has been shown to achieve sensitivity/specificity comparable to that of measured cPSA (111). For clinical use, a 3.2 ng/mL cutoff for cPSA has been estimated to equal the 4 ng/mL total PSA threshold.

A number of retrospective studies have shown that cPSA is better able to detect prostate cancer than total PSA across all PSA ranges (97,112). However, regardless of promising evidence from various small studies suggesting that the diagnostic accuracy of the cPSA assay is comparable to that of %fPSA (113,114), in the largest multicenter study, only the application of cPSA as a ratio to total PSA (%cPSA) performed as well as %fPSA as a screening tool for prostate cancer over the 2 to 10 ng/mL and 4 to 10 ng/mL PSA range. Intriguingly, in men with a PSA below 6 ng/mL, cPSA by itself performed as well as %fPSA (106). Further investigations that focused on cPSA in the lower PSA range were able to reproduce this trend. In a study by Pearson and associates of 205 men with a PSA of 2.6 to 4.0 ng/mL, cPSA provided specificity equal to that of %fPSA for detecting prostate cancer (AUC 0.63 and 0.64, respectively; $P = .58$) (115) (Table 8A.3).

In conclusion, the use of cPSA seems to show enhanced performance in early detection of prostate cancer, and it is likely that this sub-fraction of total serum PSA will be substituted for total PSA by some in the future. However, although it is significantly more stable and much easier to handle while offering comparable sensitivity and specificity, at least in the lower PSA range, its diagnostic superiority over %fPSA is not yet established and warrants further investigation.

RECENTLY IDENTIFIED MOLECULAR ISOFORMS OF FREE PROSTATE-SPECIFIC ANTIGEN FOR THE DIAGNOSIS OF PROSTATE CANCER

Recently performed molecular studies of PSA have reported significant heterogeneity of free PSA in serum, seminal plasma, and hyperplastic and cancerous tissue. Isoforms of PSA that have retained some or all of the propeptide sequence or that have developed internal cleavages have been identified and have been demonstrated remarkable prostate-disease specificity. With this information in hand, an array of new serum markers have been developed and studied in numerous single and even some multi-institutional evaluations.

BPH-Related Isoforms of Free PSA: BPSA and "Nicked PSA"

Initial difficulties in evaluating the actual structure and composition of free PSA in the blood arise from the fact that free PSA makes up only about one tenth to one third of the trace amount of PSA physiologically released in the circulation. Hence, the serum from an individual patient is insufficient for further free PSA characterization. The PSA concentration in seminal plasma and benign prostate tissue, however, exceeds the concentration of PSA in blood by a factor of approximately 10^6, thus making them ideal media for biochemical characterization of free PSA isoforms. A level of 60% to 70% of PSA in seminal plasma is catalytically active, thus mature, uncleaved, and unbound, and only 5% is found in complex with PCI (16). The remainder of the PSA (30% to 40%) demonstrates internal peptide bond

TABLE 8A.3

OVERVIEW OF CURRENT STUDIES FOR COMPARISON OF TOTAL PSA (TPSA), %fPSA, AND COMPLEXED PSA (CPSA) FOR EARLY DETECTION OF PROSTATE CANCER IN THE 2 TO 4 NG/ML, 2 TO 10 NG/ML, AND 4 TO 10 NG/ML TPSA RANGE

	Year	n (Benign/cancer)	PSA range (ng/mL)	Analyte[assay]	Cutoff/specificity at 95% sensitivity	Cutoff/specificity at 90% sensitivity
					(96% sensitive)	(92% sensitive)
Okegawa et al. (114)	2000	116/24	4–10	tPSA[a]	4.5/6%	4.8/14%
				%fPSA	20/12%	18/35%
				cPSA[b]	3.9/18%	2.7/23%
Djavan et al. (105)	2002	237/103	2–10	tPSA[d]	2.8/4.2%	3.3/14.3%
				%fPSA	7.1/7.7%	9/26.9%
				cPSA[e]	2.5/9.1 %	3.1/20.3%
Partin et al. (103)	2003	160/54	2–4	tPSA[c]	2.06/7.0%	2.2/15%
				%fPSA	27.5/7.5%	21/20%
				cPSA[b]	1.6/5.6%	1.9/20%
		210/181	4–10	tPSA[c]	4.0/6.2%	4.2/8.6%
				%fPSA	21.0/11.0%	18.5/21.5%
				cPSA[b]	3.36/6.8%	3.6/13.3%
Parson et al. (115)	2003	234/82	2–4	tPSA[f]	2.7/9.8%	2.7/11.1%
				cPSA[e]	2.3/20.1%	2.4/25.6%

[a]Tandem R.
[b]Bayer Immuno 1.
[c]Access.
[d]AxSYM.
[e]Bayer ACS 180.
[f]Beckman, San Diego.

cleavages at their C-terminal ending, which renders the molecule inactive. Various cleavage sites have been reported, including Ile_1, $Hist_{54}$, $Phen_{157}$, Lys_{145}, and Lys_{182} (116, 117). Mikolajczyk and associates, using a pan-PSA-specific antibody followed by size-exclusion chromatography, demonstrated that most of the internally clipped PSA in BPH tissue is cleaved at Lys_{145} and Lys_{182} (BPSA) (Fig. 8A.2). This group subsequently constructed a research immunoassay specific for individual BPSA detection to measure fPSA that is either clipped only at $Lys_{182(+)}$, or contains a combination of clips behind both Lys_{182} and Lys_{145} as well (117).

In parallel, Nurmikko and associates reported a different method to detect internally cleaved multichain free PSA in serum (118). Their measurements of "nicked" free PSA (fPSA-N) correspond to free PSA subtracted by single-chain free PSA formats measured by the "intact" PSA assay (fPSA-I), constituting multichain fPSA formats that contain the characteristic clip behind Lys_{145} alone, or in combination with cleavage behind Lys_{182}. Hence, measurement of fPSA-N does not include detection of $Lys_{182(+)}$.

Both serum BPSA and fPSA-N have shown highly significant correlation to BPH volume and have proven in univariable

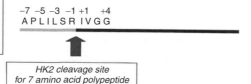

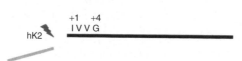

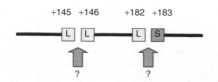

FIGURE 8A.2. Molecular, immunodetectable isoforms of free PSA in the circulation.

TABLE 8A.4

MULTIVARIATE LINEAR REGRESSION ANALYSIS TO
PREDICT TRANSITION ZONE (TZ) VOLUMES
AMONG A COHORT CONSISTING OF CANCER AND
NONCANCER PATIENTS (N = 416)[a]

Variable	P	Model r^2 if variable removed from model
Age	0.1727	0.399
Total PSA	0.0001	0.367
cPSA	0.0004	0.379
Free PSA	<0.0001	0.287
"Intact" fPSA	0.1343	0.408
"Nicked" fPSA	<0.0001	0.322

[a]Full model has r^2 of 0.417. For predicting tz volume, it appears free PSA followed by "nicked" fPSA are the most valuable predictors, as r^2 drops the most when these variables are removed.

(119,120) and multivariable evaluation (121) to be better independent predictors of benign prostatic enlargement than other forms of PSA (Table 8A.4). This indicates the important finding that correlation between prostate volume and free PSA is caused primarily by the contribution of cleaved inactive free PSA.

Furthermore, the capacity of both markers to separate patients with elevated PSA exclusively due to benign prostatic enlargement from those patients who coincidentally have prostate cancer has been studied. Results have been controversial. Neither mean BPSA levels nor mean BPSA/fPSA ratios (mean values of 25% in either the benign or cancer group, $P = .59$) differed in cancer patients from those patients with negative biopsies, although the size of the study cohort was very small (119). On the contrary, in a population-based screening study for prostate cancer, as well as in a referral group of men suspected of having prostate cancer, levels of fPSA-N alone or used with total PSA (PSA-N/T) were significantly higher in noncancer than in cancer patients ($P = .015$ and $P <.0001$, respectively) in the 2 to 10 ng/mL PSA range. Hence, the evaluation of fPSA-N significantly enhanced efforts to distinguish men with prostate cancer from those without the disease (122,123). The outlined structural differences between BPSA and fPSA-N may be one explanation for the differences in their value in separating patients with cancer from those without evidence of prostatic malignancy.

In conclusion, results from different research groups reported in the current literature suggest that the generation and release of cleaved fPSA subforms in blood may be promoted in an environment allowing for more extensive (post translational) proteolytic processing. This could provide substantial insight into benign prostate pathology and the function of the transition zone of patients with pathologic transition zone expansion. Although their clinical role has not yet been established, sensitive assays for the various forms of cleaved fPSA have contributed to knowledge of the mechanism by which %fPSA improves prostate cancer detection.

Cancer-related Free PSA Isoforms: Pro-PSA and "Intact" PSA

To circumvent the problem of limited concentrations of free PSA in serum samples from individuals, PSA eluted from the spent media of prostate cancer cell lines and pooled sera from patients with metastatic spread of prostate cancer have been combined and used to target on free PSA analysis when prostate cancer is present. *In vitro* studies suggested that about 50% of

PSA from androgen-dependent cancer cell lines (LNCaP) was secreted as latent pro-PSA; >40% secreted as mature, single-chain enzyme; and <10% secreted as the N-terminal truncated, single-chain enzyme (124). PSA secreted from LNCaP cells was devoid of internally cleaved multichain forms.

The first two studies of the molecular forms of free PSA in pooled human serum reported conflicting results. Noldus and associates found only inactive mature PSA and cleaved forms of mature PSA (125), while Mikolajczyk et al. using immunoadsorption as the purification method rather than gel filtration, found various zymogen forms of PSA (126). The lack of detection of proPSA in the Noldus study may have resulted from contamination with hK2, which has been shown to cleave proPSA forms to generate mature PSA.

Three conceptually different types of assays have been developed on the basis of the knowledge that single-chain, internally intact forms of free PSA, as opposed to cleaved forms, are associated with prostate cancer. Clinical testing of these has shown significant potential. The first uses an enhanced fluorogenic ELISA to directly measure one or more of the fPSA zymogen forms (127). The second is a functional assay that detects all zymogen forms of PSA by first capturing all free PSA forms and then activating the zymogen forms exclusively by exposing the captured free PSA to hK2 (128). The concentration of proPSA is determined by adding a PSA-specific substrate. The third type of assay uses a fluorogenic ELISA based on antibodies raised against LNCaP-produced free PSA to directly measure the concentration of all non-clipped forms of fPSA, including both the zymogen and the mature inactive molecules (fPSA-I assay) (118). It must be noted that although this assay is said to detect "intact" PSA, it detects both zymogen and mature forms of noncleaved and therefore "intact" enzymatically inactive PSA. There currently is no ELISA assay for the detection of *only* the mature, enzymatically inactive form of free PSA, and its concentration can be calculated only indirectly.

Early studies with assays for proPSA and overall free "intact" PSA (fPSA-I) demonstrated that these PSA isoforms were detectable in patients with PSA below 10 ng/mL. Furthermore, these studies demonstrated that the ratio of noncleaved forms of PSA to free PSA, but not necessarily the absolute concentration of noncleaved forms of free PSA, was higher in patients with prostate cancer than in patients with BPH. The most extensive study (282 patients) of the utility of measuring noncleaved forms of free PSA (fPSA-I) in patients with a PSA between 2 and 10 ng/nL demonstrated that the ratio of fPSA-I/fPSA performed only marginally worse than %fPSA (123). Using fluorogenic ELISAs for the various proPSA forms (−2pPSA, −4pPSA, and combined −5 and −7 pPSA), Catalona et al. demonstrated in a multi-institutional retrospective study of 1091 patients that either 2pPSA or panproPSA (sum of −2, −4, −5, and −7 proPSA) in a ratio with fPSA outperformed either %fPSA or cPSA in patients with a serum PSA in the 2 to 10 ng/mL range (127). In this range, panproPSA/fPSA spared 21% of patients unnecessary biopsies, while %fPSA spared only 13%, and cPSA spared only 9%, of patients unnecessary biopsies ($P <.0001$).

Current literature indicates that proPSA and overall intact PSA (fPSA-I) determination in individual patients provide more consistent cancer discrimination in different patient cohorts than the other forms of PSA. Selective determination of disease-specific free PSA isoforms might provide another piece in the puzzle as we attempt to create a disease-specific marker profile that can correctly distinguish prostate cancer patients from those with an elevated PSA caused by benign prostatic enlargement. However, further evaluation is mandatory and will require more than refinements in detection techniques. Moreover, the exact number and nature of subfractions of free PSA have to be determined.

HUMAN KALLIKREIN-2 IN THE MOLECULAR DIAGNOSIS OF PROSTATE CANCER

Immunohistochemical studies of human prostate glands demonstrated that tissue expression of hK2 differs from that of PSA (129). PSA expression is more pronounced in BPH tissue samples than in tissue containing prostate cancer and diminishes in the process of tumor progression and dedifferentiation. More intensive staining of hK2 in contrast appears in high grade prostate cancer and lymph node metastasis (130) than in low-grade cancer or BPH, thus indicating that hK2 expression is upregulated in the process of carcinogenesis. PSA and hK2 share 79% homology at the amino acid level (131). Further, hk2 concentrations in serum/plasma have been reported to be only as high as 1% to 2% of detectable PSA levels (109). Therefore, the approach to employ hK2 as a serum marker for the early diagnosis of prostate cancer initially was complicated by the need to develop an assay that is devoid of significant immunologic crossreactivity to PSA (<0.01%) and achieves sufficiently low functional detection limits to detect picogram per milliliter concentrations of hK2. The covariance of hK2 and PSA concentrations in blood has been shown to be less than 60%, suggesting an individual and independent contribution of hk2 to PSA. This observation supports its potential as an additional serum marker for prostate cancer detection (132,133).

Clinical Application of hK2 for Prostate Cancer Detection

The first set of studies using clinically useful hK2 assays showed that hK2 by itself did not outperform %fPSA, but suggested that hk2 applied as an algorithm with free PSA (hK2/fPSA) could outperform %fPSA for early cancer detection (134,135). In a large retrospective study, Partin and associates evaluated 937 serum samples of men with prostate cancer or negative biopsy and a total PSA of 2 to 10 ng/mL (136). This evaluation provides preliminary evidence that the hK2/fPSA ratio increases specificity for prostate cancer detection. This increase in specificity is maintained in relatively low PSA ranges (2 to 4 ng/mL) and in %fPSA (10% to 25%) in which additional specificity is most critically needed. Becker and associates reported significant data from their Göteborg study population, including 604 men who underwent prostate biopsy because of a PSA exceeding 3.0 ng/mL or an abnormal DRE (137,138). In their hands, the combination of total PSA, free PSA, and hK2 (hK2 × PSA/fPSA) achieved highest specificity (70%) by correctly identifying 77% of all cancers (sensitivity), which corresponds to a positive predictive value of 45% (Fig. 8A.3).

These results from different institutions, referral cohorts, and screening populations showed that hk2 used as an adjunct to established PSA screening provides significant enhancement to diagnostic capacity for early prostate cancer detection. This implies that there are good reasons to initiate prospective multicenter evaluations that will strive to establish the role of hK2 in the diagnosis of prostate cancer.

The recently suggested research immunoassay that selectively detects the proportion of free hK2 in male human individuals for subsequent generation of the free-to-total hk2 ratio might represent a promising approach to improve the diagnostic ability of hK2 (139). Its clinical evaluation is urgently awaited.

CLINICAL VALUE OF RT-PCR ASSAYS FOR CIRCULATING PSA AND HK2 IN BLOOD

About 20% to 30% of all patients with clinically localized prostate cancer are found to develop locally advanced or metastatic disease after radical surgery. Cancer progression may be attributable to cancer cells in peripheral blood or bone marrow that were not detectable by conventional methods at the time of diagnosis. RT-PCR has been suggested as a highly sensitive marker to detect disseminated cells in blood, other body fluids, or tissue (140). The RT-PCR assay identifies small amounts of mRNA adherent to single cells, and is therefore

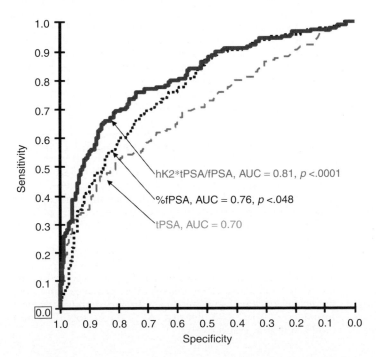

FIGURE 8A.3. ROC (receiver operating characteristics) analysis and area under curve for total PSA, %fPSA, and hK2*tPSA/fPSA in the separation of 460 men with benign prostatic biopsies compared to 144 men with prostate cancer. *P* values illustrate the difference from the area under the curve of tPSA. (From Becker C, Piironen T, Kiviniemi J, et al. Sensitive and specific immunodetection of human glandular kallikrein 2 in serum. *Clin Chem* 2000; 46:198–206, with permission from Elsevier.)

superior to cytology and immunologic approaches in its detection capacity. Highly selective RT-PCR assays for PSA (PSA-mRNA), prostate-specific-membrane antigen (PSMA-mRNA), and hK2 (hK2-mRNA) are available to target prostate cancer cells in the circulation and are currently under clinical evaluation for cancer detection and prediction of progression following local therapy (141–144).

The presence of tumor cells in the circulation, however, does not necessarily indicate that clinically significant metastasis has been established. Melchior and associates reported that up to 65% of patients with organ-confined tumors (pT2) following radical prostatectomy were positive for PSA-mRNA in bone marrow (145). Because this proportion is higher than the percentage of expected recurrence, this would imply that (a) additional factors in the presence of PSA positive cells must promote the establishment of prostate cancer metastasis; and (b) RT-PCR products from prostate cancer cells are not necessarily associated exclusively with the presence of metastatic cancer and may be used as a means to identify clinically significant tumors that require treatment. In a recently published study, Ylikoski and colleagues were able to identify differentially increased copy numbers for hK2 or PSA-mRNA according to prostatic disease (146). Among 70 subjects included in the analysis, blood from 18 of 19 men (95%) with no evidence of prostate cancer did not contain detectable hK2 or PSA-mRNA. In contrast, 70% of the samples from patients with organ-confined and/or clinically localized disease were positive for hK2/PSA-mRNA. Three patients with organ-confined disease at prostatectomy but no detectable hK2/PSA-mRNA were found to have tumors of low pathologic Gleason score. In this study, all of the advanced cancers were above the hK2/PSA-mRNA threshold (>100 mRNA copies). Corey and associates had previously reported similar findings. In peripheral blood obtained prior to radical prostatectomy, the positivity for hK2-mRNA and PSA-mRNA overall was 12.7% and 9%, respectively, but increased up to 30.8% and 46.2%, respectively, in advanced cancer patients (143).

Recent preliminary reports of data may allow for the hypothesis that during the process of progression, initially small tumor lesions are likely to become surrounded by significantly elevated levels of latent or active kallikreins (e.g., of PSA and hK2). At some stage, they are able to establish a link to the systemic circulation from which prostate cells may frequently shed into the blood. If so, circulating levels of hK2 and PSA could become very important signs of clinically significant cancer that requires curative treatment.

MOLECULAR STAGING FOR PROSTATE CANCER

Prediction of pathologic stage prior to local therapy, radiation, or prostatectomy is the essential ingredient for selection of optimal treatment. Cancer control and functional outcomes are most favorable when disease is organ confined. Appropriate selection of treatment requires a trade-off between maximal treatment effectiveness and minimal morbidity. However, serious limitations of conventional oncologic staging using CT, MRI, TRUS, and DRE significantly compromise the accuracy with which prostate cancer can be staged preoperatively. Because extraprostatic extension may be detectable on microscopic evaluation only, it is evident that clinical assessment cannot provide accurate detection of this crucial step in cancer progression. PSA provides biochemical information for staging that is less dependent on the examiner.

PSA in the Local Staging of Prostate Cancer

When PSA was introduced in predicting stage of disease, it outperformed DRE, which showed unsuspected extraprostatic spread in up to 63% (147). Predictive accuracy of serum levels of PSA, however, varies according to observed ranges: When PSA ranges and staging results are analyzed, it can be shown that PSA <4 ng/mL (81% to 84% likelihood of organ-confined cancer) (148) or >10 ng/mL (31% to 55.9% organ confined tumors) (149) correlates reasonably well with extraprostatic tumor expansion. However, in the total PSA range of 4 to 10 ng/mL—the most frequently encountered PSA range—PSA does not provide valuable staging information (53% to 67% organ confinement) (150). Moreover, as PSA production has been shown to be significantly impaired by benign prostatic enlargement, single PSA levels are not sufficiently specific to permit prediction of pathological stage in an individual patient. Multiparameter staging tools (nomograms and predictive algorithms) were developed to improve the accuracy of staging. These are described in a subsequent chapter.

PSA and Distant Staging

PSA has been shown to be a good predictor of a positive bone scan in patients with prostate cancer. The correlation of PSA, tumor grade, and clinical stage revealed that PSA was most accurate in predicting bone scan results. Namely, if PSA was below 20 ng/mL, the negative predictive value was 99.7%. This has resulted in a decrease in the number of bone scans performed in patients with a PSA <20 ng/mL (151).

Free PSA in the Local Staging of Prostate Cancer

Although %fPSA is useful for prostate cancer detection, studies that analyzed %fPSA in predicting stage of prostate cancer have produced conflicting results. While some studies reported that %fPSA provided useful staging information, others failed to demonstrate such findings (152,153). Data from the University of Hamburg reported no difference in %fPSA between patients with organ-confined and non-organ-confined cancers. Nevertheless, a significantly lower %fPSA separated patients who already had seminal vesicle invasion from those who did not (153). Because intrinsic differences such as patient selection, study design, various immunoassays, and %fPSA cutoff values influenced the message of each single study, definitive information can be provided only by a multicenter trial. Therefore, to date the use of %fPSA for the staging of prostate cancer is not established.

Complexed PSA for Staging Prostate Cancer

Several recent studies have evaluated ACT-PSA as a staging tool for prostate cancer, with similar results. cPSA levels have been shown to be higher in patients with extracapsular cancer growth than in patients with organ-confined tumors, and they have been shown to be an independent predictor of extracapsular extension in a multivariate model ($P < 0.05$) (154). The total of cPSA, however, failed to provide more staging information than total PSA (AUC 0.542 to 0.621 and 0.539 to 0.621, respectively) (155). Just as with volume index of total PSA, cPSA density also provides improved prediction of stage, and has been shown to equal the performance of total PSA density (AUC 0.691 to 0.700 and 0.692 to 0.708, respectively).

TABLE 8A.5

SAME MODEL USED TO PREDICT THE AMOUNT OF PROSTATE CANCER TISSUE IN PROSTATECTOMY SPECIMEN OF 172 PATIENTS AFTER RADICAL PROSTATECTOMY[a]

Variable	P	Model r^2 if variable removed from model
DRE	0.507	0.464
Gleason Bx	0.011	0.440
Total PSA	0.049	0.460
cPSA	0.585	0.469
Free PSA	0.008	0.445
"Intact" fPSA	0.059	0.421
"Nicked" fPSA	0.008	0.429
hK2	<0.0001	0.406

DRE, digital rectal examination.
[a]Full model has r^2 of 0.453. Gleason biopsy, total prostate-specific antigen (PSA), free PSA, "nicked" PSA, and hK2 were positively associated with increasing tumor burden. For cancer volume prediction, hK2 appears most valuable given knowledge of all other predictors.

In summary, the current literature indicates that cPSA is equivalent to total PSA in predicting organ confined disease and may be used as a substitute to total PSA in achieving comparable, though not superior, prediction of pathologic stage.

Human Glandular Kallikrein 2 in the Staging of Prostate Cancer

The ability of hK2 to act as a molecular tool for prostate cancer staging was initially evaluated by Haese and associates, with an encouraging outcome (156–158). In their hands, the algorithm hK2*tPSA/fPSA significantly improved the prediction of organ-confined versus non-organ-confined tumors in patients with a total PSA range of up to 66 ng/mL and in the inconclusive range below 10 ng/mL. The process by which hK2 achieves a close association to extraprostatic growth may explain its tight correlation with the individual amount of prostate cancer tissue present, whereas the latter has been shown to be differentially elevated in extraprostatic compared with organ-confined tumors (157). In two correlation analyses, hK2 was the strongest predictor of prostate cancer tissue volume in univariate and multivariate models and independently outperformed various PSA forms and DRE status (Table 8A.5) (121,159). These results encourage further studies to improve staging of prostate cancer. As with the use of hK2 for detection of prostate cancer, potential uncertainties have to be kept in mind when hK2 is analyzed (lack of standardization, different assay principles). Therefore, results from different centers and the performance of different assays—ideally in a multicenter trial—will be required to clarify the role of hK2 as a potential staging tool for prostate cancer.

References

1. Clements JA. The glandular kallikrein family of enzymes: tissue-specific expression and hormonal regulation. *Endocr Rev* 1989;10:393–419.
2. Yousef GM, Luo LY, Diamandis EP. Identification of novel human kallikrein-like genes on chromosome 19q13.3-q13.4. *Anticancer Res* 1999; 19:2843–2852.
3. Yousef GM, Diamandis EP. The expanded human kallikrein gene family: locus characterization and molecular cloning of a new member, KLK-L3 (KLK9). *Genomics* 2000;65:184–194.
4. Cleutjens KB, van Eekelen CC, van der Korput HA, et al. Two androgen response regions cooperate in steroid hormone regulated activity of the prostate-specific antigen promoter. *J Biol Chem* 1996;271:6379–6388.
5. Zhang J, Zhang S, Murtha PE, et al. Identification of two novel cis-elements in the promoter of the prostate-specific antigen gene that are required to enhance androgen receptor-mediated transactivation. *Nucleic Acids Res* 1997;25:3143–3150.
6. Yu DC, Sakamoto GT, Henderson DR. Identification of the transcriptional regulatory sequences of human kallikrein 2 and their use in the construction of calydon virus 764, an attenuated replication competent adenovirus for prostate cancer therapy. *Cancer Res* 1999;59:1498–1504.
7. Xi Z, Klokk TI, Korkmaz K, et al. Kallikrein 4 is a predominantly nuclear protein and is overexpressed in prostate cancer. *Cancer Res* 2004;64: 2365–2370.
8. Nakamura T, Scorilas A, Stephan C, et al. The usefulness of serum human kallikrein 11 for discriminating between prostate cancer and benign prostatic hyperplasia. *Cancer Res* 2003;63:6543–6546.
9. Takayama TKFK, Davie EW. Characterization of the precursor of prostate-specific antigen. Activation by trypsin and by human glandular kallikrein. *J Biol Chem* 1997;272:21582–21588.
10. Lovgren JRK, Karp M, Lundwall A, et al. Activation of the zymogen form of prostate-specific antigen by human glandular kallikrein 2. *Biochem Biophys Res Commun* 1997;238:549–555.
11. Kumar AMS, Goel AS, Millar LS, et al. Expression of pro form of prostate-specific antigen by mammalian cells and its conversion to mature, active form by human kallikrein 2. *Cancer Res* 1997;57:3111–3114.
12. Mikolajczyk SD, Millar LS, Marker KM, et al. Ala217 is important for the catalytic function and autoactivation of prostate-specific human kallikrein 2. *Eur J Biochem* 1997;246:440–446.
13. Lilja H. A kallikrein-like serine protease in prostatic fluid cleaves the predominant seminal vesicle protein. *J Clin Invest* 1985;76:1899–1903.
14. Ban Y, Wang MC, Watt KW, et al. The proteolytic activity of human prostate-specific antigen. *Biochem Biophys Res Commun* 1984;123:482–488
15. Akiyama K, Nakamura T, Iwanaga S, et al. The chymotrypsin-like activity of human prostate-specific antigen, gamma-seminoprotein. *FEBS Lett* 1987;225:168–172.
16. Christensson A, Laurell CB, Lilja H. Enzymatic activity of prostate-specific antigen and its reactions with extracellular serine proteinase inhibitors. *Eur J Biochem* 1990;194:755–763.
17. Lilja H, Abrahamsson PA, Lundwall A. Semenogelin, the predominant protein in human semen. Primary structure and identification of closely related proteins in the male accessory sex glands and on the spermatozoa. *J Biol Chem* 1989;264:1894–1900.
18. Lilja H, Oldbring J, Rannevik G, et al. Seminal vesicle-secreted proteins and their reactions during gelation and liquefaction of human semen. *J Clin Invest* 1987;80:281–285.
19. Lilja H, Lundwall A. Molecular cloning of epididymal and seminal vesicular transcripts encoding a semenogelin-related protein. *Proc Natl Acad Sci U S A* 1992;89:4559–4563.
20. McGee RS, Herr JC. Human seminal vesicle-specific antigen is a substrate for prostate-specific antigen (or P-30). *Biol Reprod* 1988;39:499–510.
21. Lilja H, Laurell CB. Liquefaction of coagulated human semen. *Scand J Clin Lab Invest* 1984;44:447–452.
22. McGee RS, Herr JC. Human seminal vesicle-specific antigen during semen liquefaction. *Biol Reprod* 1987;37:431–439.
23. Cohen P, Graves HC, Peehl DM, et al. Prostate-specific antigen (PSA) is an insulin-like growth factor binding protein-3 protease found in seminal plasma. *J Clin Endocrinol Metab* 1992;75:1046–1053.
24. Frenette G, Deperthes D, Tremblay RR, et al. Purification of enzymatically active kallikrein hK2 from human seminal plasma. *Biochim Biophys Acta* 1997;1334:109–115.
25. Denmeade SR, Lou W, Lovgren J, et al. Specific and efficient peptide substrates for assaying the proteolytic activity of prostate-specific antigen. *Cancer Res* 1997;57:4924–4930.
26. Robert M, Gibbs BF, Jacobson E, et al. Characterization of prostate-specific antigen proteolytic activity on its major physiological substrate, the sperm motility inhibitor precursor/semenogelin I. *Biochemistry* 1997;36: 3811–3819.
27. Mikolajczyk SD, Millar LS, Kumar A, et al. Human glandular kallikrein, hK2, shows arginine-restricted specificity and forms complexes with plasma protease inhibitors. *Prostate* 1998;34:44–50.
28. Deperthes D, Marceau F, Frenette G, et al. Human kallikrein hK2 has low kininogenase activity while prostate-specific antigen (hK3) has none. *Biochim Biophys Acta* 1997;1343:102–106.
29. Bourgeois L, Brillard-Bourdet M, Deperthes D, et al. Serpin-derived peptide substrates for investigating the substrate specificity of human tissue kallikreins hK1 and hK2. *J Biol Chem* 1997;272:29590–29595.
30. Achbarou A, Kaiser S, Tremblay G, et al. Urokinase overproduction results in increased skeletal metastasis by prostate cancer cells in vivo. *Cancer Res* 1994;54:2372–2377.
31. Mikolajczyk SDML, Kumar A, Saedi MS. Human kallikrein 2 (hK2) inactivates and complexes with plasminogen activator inhibitor-1 (PAI-1). *Int J Cancer* 1999;81:438–442.
32. Lilja H, Abrahamsson PA. Three predominant proteins secreted by the human prostate gland. *Prostate* 1988;12:29–38.

33. Ylikoski A, Karp M, Pettersson K, et al. Simultaneous quantification of human glandular kallikrein 2 and prostate-specific antigen mRNAs in peripheral blood from prostate cancer patients. *J Mol Diagn* 2001;3: 111–122.

34. Koyanagi Y, Hara M, Inoue T, et al. Isolation of antigenic component specific for human seminal plasma "-seminoprotein (-Sm)" by electrofocusing. Forensic immunological study of body fluids and secretions. 8. *Nippon Hoigaku Zasshi* 1972;26:78–80.

35. Hara M, Inoue T, Koyanagi Y, et al. Immunoelectrophoretic studies of the protein components in human seminal plasma (especially its specific component). (Forensic immunological study of body fluids and secretions. VI.) *Nippon Hoigaku Zasshi* 1969;23:117–122.

36. Wang MC, Valenzuela LA, Murphy GP, et al. Purification of a human prostate specific antigen. *Invest Urol* 1979;17:159–163.

37. Papsidero LD, Wang MC, Valenzuela LA, et al. A prostate antigen in sera of prostatic cancer patients. *Cancer Res* 1980;40:2428–2432.

38. Wang MC, Papsidero LD, Kuriyama M, et al. Prostate antigen: a new potential marker for prostatic cancer. *Prostate* 1981;2:89–96.

39. Stamey TA, Yang N, Hay AR, et al. Prostate-specific antigen as a serum marker for adenocarcinoma of the prostate. *N Engl J Med* 1987;317: 909–916.

40. Stanford JL, Stephenson RA, Coyle M, et al. *Prostate Cancer Trends 1973-1995, SEER Program.* Bethesda, MD: National Institutes of Health, NIH Publication No. 99–4543;1999;7–15.

41. Jones GW, Mettlin C, Murphy GP, et al. Patterns of care for carcinoma of the prostate gland: results of a national survey of 1984 and 1990. *J Am Coll Surg* 1995;180:545–554.

42. Jemal A, Murray T, Samuels A, et al. Cancer statistics, 2003. *CA Cancer J Clin* 2003;53:5–26.

43. Oliver SE, May MT, Gunnell D. International trends in prostate-cancer mortality in the "PSA ERA." *Int J Cancer* 2001;92:893–898.

44. Oliver SE, Gunnell D, Donovan JL. Comparison of trends in prostate-cancer mortality in England and Wales and the USA. *Lancet* 2000;355: 1788–1789.

45. Labrie F, Candas B, Dupont A, et al. Screening decreases prostate cancer death: first analysis of the 1988 Quebec Prospective Randomized Controlled Trial. *Prostate* 1999;38:83–91.

46. Skarsgard D, Tonita J. Prostate cancer in Saskatchewan Canada, before and during the PSA era. *Cancer Causes Control* 2000;11:79–88.

47. Coldman AJ, Phillips N, Pickles TA. Trends in prostate cancer incidence and mortality: an analysis of mortality change by screening intensity. *CMAJ* 2003;168:31–35.

48. Lu-Yao G, Albertsen PC, Stanford JL, et al. Natural experiment examining impact of aggressive screening and treatment on prostate cancer mortality in two fixed cohorts from Seattle area and Connecticut. *BMJ* 2002;325: 740.

49. Bartsch G, Horninger W, Klocker H, et al. Prostate cancer mortality after introduction of prostate-specific antigen mass screening in the Federal State of Tyrol, Austria. *Urology* 2001;58:417–424.

50. Hugosson J, Aus G, Bergdahl C, et al. Prostate cancer mortality in patients surviving more than 10 years after diagnosis. *J Urol* 1995;154:2115–2117.

51. Stenman UH, Hakama M, Knekt P, et al. Serum concentrations of prostate specific antigen and its complex with alpha 1-antichymotrypsin before diagnosis of prostate cancer. *Lancet* 1994;344:1594–1598.

52. Chu KC, Tarone RE, Freeman HP. Trends in prostate cancer mortality among black men and white men in the United States. *Cancer* 2003;97: 1507–1516.

53. Schroder FH, Denis LJ, Roobol M, et al. The story of the European Randomized Study of Screening for Prostate Cancer. *BJU Int* 2003;92(Suppl 2):1–13.

54. Andriole GL, Reding D, Hayes RB, et al. The Prostate, Lung, Colon, and Ovarian (PLCO) cancer screening trial: status and promise. *Urol Oncol* 2004;22:358–361.

55. de Koning HJ, Liem MK, Baan CA, et al. Prostate cancer mortality reduction by screening: power and time frame with complete enrollment in the European Randomised Screening for Prostate Cancer (ERSPC) trial. *Int J Cancer* 2002;98:268–273.

56. Hugosson J, Aus G, Bergdahl S, et al. Population-based screening for prostate cancer by measuring free and total serum prostate-specific antigen in Sweden. *BJU Int* 2003;92(Suppl 2):39–43.

57. Beemsterboer PM, Kranse R, de Koning HJ, et al. Changing role of 3 screening modalities in the European Randomized Study of Screening for Prostate Cancer (Rotterdam). *Int J Cancer* 1999;84:437–441.

58. Draisma G, Boer R, Otto SJ, et al. Lead times and overdetection due to prostate-specific antigen screening: estimates from the European Randomized Study of Screening for Prostate Cancer. *J Natl Cancer Inst* 2003;95: 868–878.

59. Makinen T, Tammela TL, Hakama M, et al. Tumor characteristics in a population-based prostate cancer screening trial with prostate-specific antigen. *Clin Cancer Res* 2003;9:2435–2439.

60. Catalona WJ, Richie JP, Ahmann FR, et al. Comparison of digital rectal examination and serum prostate specific antigen in the early detection of prostate cancer: results of a multicenter clinical trial of 6,630 men. *J Urol* 1994;151:1283–1290.

61. Crawford ED, Leewansangtong S, Goktas S, et al. Efficiency of prostate-specific antigen and digital rectal examination in screening, using 4.0 ng/ml

62. Partin AW, Kattan MW, Subong EN, et al. Combination of prostate-specific antigen, clinical stage, and Gleason score to predict pathological stage of localized prostate cancer. A multi-institutional update. *JAMA* 1997;277:1445–1451.

63. Lodding P, Aus G, Bergdahl S, et al. Characteristics of screening detected prostate cancer in men 50 to 66 years old with 3 to 4 ng/ml prostate specific antigen. *J Urol* 1998;159:899–903.

64. Catalona WJ, Smith DS, Ornstein DK. Prostate cancer detection in men with serum PSA concentrations of 2.6 to 4.0 ng/mL and benign prostate examination. Enhancement of specificity with free PSA measurements. *JAMA* 1997;277:1452–1455.

65. Bonilla JRC, MC Connel JD. Patterns of prostate growth observed in placebo treated patients in the PLESS trial over four years [Abstract]. *J Urol* 1995;159(Suppl 5):301A.

66. Roehrborn CG, Boyle P, Gould AL, et al. Serum prostate-specific antigen as a predictor of prostate volume in men with benign prostatic hyperplasia. *Urology* 1999;53:581–589.

67. Oesterling JE. Age-specific reference ranges for serum PSA. *N Engl J Med* 1996;335:345–346.

68. Oesterling JE. Age-specific reference ranges for serum prostate-specific antigen. *Can J Urol* 1995;2:23–29.

69. Oesterling JE, Kumamoto Y, Tsukamoto T, et al. Serum prostate-specific antigen in a community-based population of healthy Japanese men: lower values than for similarly aged white men. *Br J Urol* 1995;75:347–353.

70. Morgan TO, Jacobsen SJ, McCarthy WF, et al. Age-specific reference ranges for prostate-specific antigen in black men. *N Engl J Med* 1996;335: 304–310.

71. Catalona WJ, Hudson MA, Scardino PT, et al. Selection of optimal prostate specific antigen cutoffs for early detection of prostate cancer: receiver operating characteristic curves. *J Urol* 1994;152:2037–2042.

72. Partin AW, Criley SR, Subong EN, et al. Standard versus age-specific prostate specific antigen reference ranges among men with clinically localized prostate cancer: a pathological analysis. *J Urol* 1996;155:1336–1339.

73. Bangma CH, Kranse R, Blijenberg BG, et al. The value of screening tests in the detection of prostate cancer. Part II: retrospective analysis of free/total prostate-specific analysis ratio, age-specific reference ranges, and PSA density. *Urology* 1995;46:779–784.

74. Borer JG, Sherman J, Solomon MC, et al. Age specific prostate specific antigen reference ranges: population specific. *J Urol* 1998;159:444–448.

75. Parkin DM, Muir CS. Cancer incidence in five continents. Comparability and quality of data. *IARC Sci Publ* 1992;120:45–173.

76. Oesterling JE, Jacobsen SJ, Chute CG, et al. Serum prostate-specific antigen in a community-based population of healthy men. Establishment of age-specific reference ranges. *JAMA* 1993;270:860–864.

77. Carter HB, Morrell CH, Pearson JD, et al. Estimation of prostatic growth using serial prostate-specific antigen measurements in men with and without prostate disease. *Cancer Res* 1992;52:3323–3328.

78. Brawer MK, Beatie J, Wener MH, et al. Screening for prostatic carcinoma with prostate specific antigen: results of the second year. *J Urol* 1993;150: 106–109.

79. Carter HB, Pearson JD. Prostate-specific antigen testing for early diagnosis of prostate cancer: formulation of guidelines. *Urology* 1999;54:780–786.

80. Roobol MJ, Kranse R, de Koning HJ, et al. Prostate-specific antigen velocity at low prostate-specific antigen levels as screening tool for prostate cancer: results of second screening round of ERSPC (Rotterdam). *Urology* 2004;63:309–313; discussion 313–305.

81. Nadler RB, Humphrey PA, Smith DS, et al. Effect of inflammation and benign prostatic hyperplasia on elevated serum prostate specific antigen levels. *J Urol* 1995;154:407–413.

82. Eastham JA, Riedel E, Scardino PT, et al. Variation of serum prostate-specific antigen levels: an evaluation of year-to-year fluctuations. *JAMA* 2003;289:2695–2700.

83. Link RE, Shariat SF, Nguyen CV, et al. Variation in prostate specific antigen results from 2 different assay platforms: clinical impact on 2304 patients undergoing prostate cancer screening. *J Urol* 2004;171:2234–2238.

84. Semjonow A, De Angelis G, Schmidt HP. In: Brawer MK, ed. *Immunoassays for PSA*, Vol. 1. New York: Dekker; 2001:134.

85. D'Amico AV, Chen MH, Roehl KA, et al. Preoperative PSA velocity and the risk of death from prostate cancer after radical prostatectomy. *N Engl J Med* 2004;351:125–135.

86. Benson MC, Whang IS, Olsson CA, et al. The use of prostate specific antigen density to enhance the predictive value of intermediate levels of serum prostate specific antigen. *J Urol* 1992;147:817–821.

87. Stamey TAYN, Hay AR, McNeal JE, et al. Prostate-specific antigen as a serum marker for adenocarcinoma of the prostate. *N Engl J Med* 1987; 317:909–916.

88. Partin AW, Carter HB, Chan DW, et al. Prostate specific antigen in the staging of localized prostate cancer: influence of tumor differentiation, tumor volume and benign hyperplasia. *J Urol* 1990;143:747–752.

89. Bretton PR, Evans WP, Borden JD, et al. The use of prostate specific antigen density to improve the sensitivity of prostate specific antigen in detecting prostate carcinoma. *Cancer* 1994;74:2991–2995.

90. Cookson MS, Floyd MK, Ball TP Jr, et al. The lack of predictive value of prostate specific antigen density in the detection of prostate cancer in patients

with normal rectal examinations and intermediate prostate specific antigen levels. *J Urol* 1995;154:1070–1073.

91. Catalona WJ, Richie JP, deKernion JB, et al. Comparison of prostate specific antigen concentration versus prostate specific antigen density in the early detection of prostate cancer: receiver operating characteristic curves. *J Urol* 1994;152:2031–2036.

92. Catalona WJ, Beiser JA, Smith DS. Serum free prostate specific antigen and prostate specific antigen density measurements for predicting cancer in men with prior negative prostatic biopsies. *J Urol* 1997;158:2162–2167.

93. Fowler JEBS, Miles D, Yalkut DA Jr. Predictors of first repeat biopsy cancer detection with suspected local stage prostate cancer. *J Urol* 2000;163: 813–818.

94. Djavan B, Zlotta AR, Byttebier G, et al. Prostate specific antigen density of the transition zone for early detection of prostate cancer. *J Urol* 1998;160: 411–418; discussion 418–419.

95. Djavan B, Zlotta A, Remzi M, et al. Optimal predictors of prostate cancer on repeat prostate biopsy: a prospective study of 1,051 men. *J Urol* 2000;163:1144–1148; discussion 1148–1149.

96. Lilja H, Haese A, Bjork T, et al. Significance and metabolism of complexed and noncomplexed prostate specific antigen forms, and human glandular kallikrein 2 in clinically localized prostate cancer before and after radical prostatectomy. *J Urol* 1999;162:2029–2034; discussion 2034–2025.

97. Lilja H, Christensson A, Dahlen U, et al. Prostate-specific antigen in serum occurs predominantly in complex with alpha 1-antichymotrypsin. *Clin Chem* 1991;37:1618–1625.

98. Bjork T, Ljungberg B, Piironen T, et al. Rapid exponential elimination of free prostate-specific antigen contrasts the slow, capacity-limited elimination of PSA complexed to alpha 1-antichymotrypsin from serum. *Urology* 1998;51:57–62.

99. Christensson A, Bjork T, Nilsson O, et al. Serum prostate specific antigen complexed to alpha 1-antichymotrypsin as an indicator of prostate cancer. *J Urol* 1993;150:100–105.

100. Virtanen A, Gomari M, Kranse R, et al. Estimation of prostate cancer probability by logistic regression: free and total prostate-specific antigen, digital rectal examination, and heredity are significant variables. *Clin Chem* 1999;45:987–994.

101. Luderer AA, Chen YT, Soriano TF, et al. Measurement of the proportion of free to total prostate-specific antigen improves diagnostic performance of prostate-specific antigen in the diagnostic gray zone of total prostate-specific antigen. *Urology* 1995;46:187–194.

102. Prestigiacomo AF, Lilja H, Pettersson K, et al. A comparison of the free fraction of serum prostate specific antigen in men with benign and cancerous prostates: the best case scenario. *J Urol* 1996;156:350–354.

103. Catalona WJ, Partin AW, Slawin KM, et al. Use of the percentage of free prostate-specific antigen to enhance differentiation of prostate cancer from benign prostatic disease: a prospective multicenter clinical trial. *JAMA* 1998;279:1542–1547.

104. Haese A, Dworschack RT, Partin AW. Percent free prostate specific antigen in the total prostate specific antigen 2 to 4 ng./ml range does not substantially increase the number of biopsies needed to detect clinically significant prostate cancer compared to the 4 to 10 ng./ml range. *J Urol* 2002;168:504–508.

105. Djavan B, Remzi M, Zlotta AR, et al. Complexed prostate-specific antigen, complexed prostate-specific antigen density of total and transition zone, complexed/total prostate specific antigen ratio, free-to-total prostate-specific antigen ratio, density of total and transition zone prostate-specific antigen: results of the prospective multicenter European trial. *Urology* 2002;60:4–9.

106. Partin AW, Brawer MK, Bartsch G, et al. Complexed prostate specific antigen improves specificity for prostate cancer detection: results of a prospective multicenter clinical trial. *J Urol* 2003;170:1787–1791.

107. Woodrum D, French C, Shamel LB. Stability of free prostate-specific antigen in serum samples under a variety of sample collection and sample storage conditions. *Urology* 1996;48:33–39.

108. Meyer A, Jung K, Lein M, et al. Factors influencing the ratio of free to total prostate-specific antigen in serum. *Int J Cancer* 1997;74:630–636.

109. Piironen T, Pettersson K, Suonpaa M, et al. In vitro stability of free prostate-specific antigen (PSA) and prostate-specific antigen complexed to alpha 1-antichymotrypsin in blood samples. *Urology* 1996; 48(6A Suppl):81–87.

110. Nixon RG, Meyer GE, Blase AB, et al. Comparison of 3 investigational assays for the free form of prostate specific antigen. *J Urol* 1998;160(2): 420–425.

111. Okihara K, Fritsche HA, Ayala A, et al. Can complexed prostate specific antigen and prostatic volume enhance prostate cancer detection in men with total prostate specific antigen between 2.5 and 4.0 ng/ml? *J Urol* 2001;165:1930–1936.

112. Brawer MK, Meyer GE, Letran JL, et al. Measurement of complexed PSA improves specificity for early detection of prostate cancer. *Urology* 1998; 52:372–378.

113. Brawer MK, Cheli CD, Neaman IE. Complexed prostate-specific antigen provides significant enhancement of specificity compared with total prostate specific antigen for detecting prostate cancer. *J Urol* 2000;163:1476–1480.

114. Okegawa T, Noda H, Nutahara K, et al. Comparison of two investigative assays for the complexed prostate-specific antigen in total prostate-specific antigen between 4.1 and 10 ng/ml. *Urology* 2000;55:700–704.

115. Parsons JK, Brawer MK, Cheli CD, et al. Complexed prostate specific antigen (PSA) reduces unnecessary prostate biopsies in the 2.6-4.0 ng/mL range of total PSA. *BJU Int* 2004;94:47–50.

116. Chen Z, Chen H, Stamey TA. Prostate specific antigen in benign prostatic hyperplasia: purification and characterization. *J Urol* 1997;157:2166–2170.

117. Mikolajczyk SD, Millar LS, Marker KM, et al. Seminal plasma contains "BPSA," a molecular form of prostate-specific antigen that is associated with benign prostatic hyperplasia. *Prostate* 2000;45:271–276.

118. Nurmikko P, Vaisanen V, Piironen T, et al. Production and characterization of novel anti-prostate-specific antigen (PSA) monoclonal antibodies that do not detect internally cleaved Lys145-Lys146 inactive PSA. *Clin Chem* 2000;46:1610–1618.

119. Linton HJ, Marks LS, Millar LS, et al. Benign prostate-specific antigen (BPSA) in serum is increased in benign prostate disease. *Clin Chem* 2003; 49:253–259.

120. Canto EI, Singh H, Shariat SF, et al. Serum BPSA outperforms both total PSA and free PSA as a predictor of prostatic enlargement in men without prostate cancer. *Urology* 2004;63:905–910; discussion 910–911.

121. Steuber TNP, Niemela P, Haese A, et al. Association of free-prostate specific antigen subfractions with volume of benign and malignant prostatic tissue. *Prostate* 2005;63(1):13–18.

122. Nurmikko P, Pettersson K, Piironen T, et al. Discrimination of prostate cancer from benign disease by plasma measurement of intact, free prostate-specific antigen lacking an internal cleavage site at Lys145-Lys146. *Clin Chem* 2001;47:1415–1423.

123. Stcuber T, Nurmikko P, Haese A, et al. Discrimination of benign from malignant prostatic disease by selective measurements of single chain, intact free prostate specific antigen. *J Urol* 2002;168:1917–1922.

124. Vaisanen V, Lovgren J, Hellman J, et al. Characterization and processing of prostate specific antigen (hK3) and human glandular kallikrein (hK2) secreted by LNCaP cells. *Prostate Cancer Prostatic Dis* 1999;2:91–97.

125. Noldus J, Chen Z, Stamey TA. Isolation and characterization of free form prostate specific antigen (f-PSA) in sera of men with prostate cancer. *J Urol* 1997;158:1606–1609.

126. Mikolajczyk SD, Grauer LS, Millar LS, et al. A precursor form of PSA (pPSA) is a component of the free PSA in prostate cancer serum. *Urology* 1997;50:710–714.

127. Catalona WJ, Bartsch G, Rittenhouse HG, et al. Serum pro prostate specific antigen improves cancer detection compared to free and complexed prostate specific antigen in men with prostate specific antigen 2 to 4 ng/ml. *J Urol* 2003;170:2181–2185.

128. Niemela P, Lovgren J, Karp M, et al. Sensitive and specific enzymatic assay for the determination of precursor forms of prostate-specific antigen after an activation step. *Clin Chem* 2002;48:1257–1264.

129. Darson MF, Pacelli A, Roche P, et al. Human glandular kallikrein 2 (hK2) expression in prostatic intraepithelial neoplasia and adenocarcinoma: a novel prostate cancer marker. *Urology* 1997;49:857–862.

130. Darson MF, Pacelli A, Roche P, et al. Human glandular kallikrein 2 expression in prostate adenocarcinoma and lymph node metastases. *Urology* 1999;53:939–944.

131. Schedlich LJ, Bennetts BH, Morris BJ. Primary structure of a human glandular kallikrein gene. *DNA* 1987;6:429–437.

132. Becker C, Piironen T, Pettersson K, et al. Clinical value of human glandular kallikrein 2 and free and total prostate-specific antigen in serum from a population of men with prostate-specific antigen levels 3.0 ng/mL or greater. *Urology* 2000;55:694–699.

133. Klee GG, Goodmanson MK, Jacobsen SJ, et al. Highly sensitive automated chemiluminometric assay for measuring free human glandular kallikrein-2. *Clin Chem* 1999;45:800–806.

134. Recker F, Kwiatkowski MK, Piironen T, et al. The importance of human glandular kallikrein and its correlation with different prostate specific antigen serum forms in the detection of prostate carcinoma. *Cancer* 1998; 83:2540–2547.

135. Kwiatkowski MK, Recker F, Piironen T, et al. In prostatism patients the ratio of human glandular kallikrein to free PSA improves the discrimination between prostate cancer and benign hyperplasia within the diagnostic "gray zone" of total PSA 4 to 10 ng/mL. *Urology* 1998;52:360–365.

136. Partin AW, Catalona WJ, Finlay JA, et al. Use of human glandular kallikrein 2 for the detection of prostate cancer: preliminary analysis. *Urology* 1999; 54:839–845.

137. Becker C, Piironen T, Kiviniemi J, et al. Sensitive and specific immunodetection of human glandular kallikrein 2 in serum. *Clin Chem* 2000;46:198–206.

138. Becker C, Piironen T, Pettersson K, et al. Testing in serum for human glandular kallikrein 2, and free and total prostate specific antigen in biannual screening for prostate cancer. *J Urol* 2003;170:1169–1174.

139. Vaisanen V, Eriksson S, Ivaska KK, et al. Development of sensitive immunoassays for free and total human glandular kallikrein 2. *Clin Chem* 2004;50:1607–1617.

140. Ghossein RA, Rosai J, Scher HI, et al. Prognostic significance of detection of prostate-specific antigen transcripts in the peripheral blood of patients with metastatic androgen-independent prostatic carcinoma. *Urology* 1997; 50:100–105.

141. Wood DP, Banerjee M Jr. Presence of circulating prostate cells in the bone marrow of patients undergoing radical prostatectomy is predictive of disease-free survival. *J Clin Oncol* 1997;15:3451–3457.

142. Shariat SF, Gottenger E, Nguyen C, et al. Preoperative blood reverse transcriptase-PCR assays for prostate-specific antigen and human glandular kallikrein for prediction of prostate cancer progression after radical prostatectomy. *Cancer Res* 2002;62:5974–5979.

143. Corey E, Arfman EW, Oswin MM, et al. Detection of circulating prostate cells by reverse transcriptase-polymerase chain reaction of human glandular kallikrein (hK2) and prostate-specific antigen (PSA) messages. *Urology* 1997;50:184–188.

144. Ylikoski A, Sjoroos M, Lundwall A, et al. Quantitative reverse transcription-PCR assay with an internal standard for the detection of prostate-specific antigen mRNA. *Clin Chem* 1999;45:1397–1407.

145. Melchior SW, Corey E, Ellis WJ, et al. Early tumor cell dissemination in patients with clinically localized carcinoma of the prostate. *Clin Cancer Res* 1997;3:249–256.

146. Ylikoski A, Pettersson K, Nurmi J, et al. Simultaneous quantification of prostate-specific antigen and human glandular kallikrein 2 mRNA in blood samples from patients with prostate cancer and benign disease. *Clin Chem* 2002;48:1265–1271.

147. McNeal JE, Villers AA, Redwine EA, et al. Capsular penetration in prostate cancer. Significance for natural history and treatment. *Am J Surg Pathol* 1990;14:240–247.

148. Schroder FH, van der Cruijsen-Koeter I, de Koning HJ, et al. Prostate cancer detection at low prostate specific antigen. *J Urol* 2000;163:806–812.

149. Partin AW, Yoo J, Carter HB, et al. The use of prostate specific antigen, clinical stage and Gleason score to predict pathological stage in men with localized prostate cancer. *J Urol* 1993;150:110–114.

150. Narayan P, Gajendran V, Taylor SP, et al. The role of transrectal ultrasound-guided biopsy-based staging, preoperative serum prostate-specific antigen, and biopsy Gleason score in prediction of final pathologic diagnosis in prostate cancer. *Urology* 1995;46:205–212.

151. Chybowski FM, Keller JJ, Bergstralh EJ, et al. Predicting radionuclide bone scan findings in patients with newly diagnosed, untreated prostate cancer: prostate specific antigen is superior to all other clinical parameters. *J Urol* 1991;145:313–318.

152. Lerner SE, Jacobsen SJ, Lilja H, et al. Free, complexed, and total serum prostate-specific antigen concentrations and their proportions in predicting stage, grade, and deoxyribonucleic acid ploidy in patients with adenocarcinoma of the prostate. *Urology* 1996;48:240–248.

153. Noldus J, Graefen M, Huland E, et al. The value of the ratio of free-to-total prostate specific antigen for staging purposes in previously untreated prostate cancer. *J Urol* 1998;159:2004–2007; discussion 2007–2008.

154. Sokoll LJ, Mangold LA, Partin AW, et al. Complexed prostate-specific antigen as a staging tool for prostate cancer: a prospective study in 420 men. *Urology* 2002;60:18–23.

155. Taneja SS, Hsu EI, Cheli CD, et al. Complexed prostate-specific antigen as a staging tool: results based on a multicenter prospective evaluation of complexed prostate-specific antigen in cancer diagnosis. *Urology* 2002;60:10–17.

156. Haese A, Becker C, Noldus J, et al. Human glandular kallikrein 2: a potential serum marker for predicting the organ confined versus non-organ confined growth of prostate cancer. *J Urol* 2000;163:1491–1497.

157. Haese A, Graefen M, Steuber T, et al. Human glandular kallikrein 2 levels in serum for discrimination of pathologically organ-confined from locally-advanced prostate cancer in total PSA-levels below 10 ng/ml. *Prostate* 2001;49:101–109.

158. Haese A, Graefen M, Becker C, et al. The role of human glandular kallikrein 2 for prediction of pathologically organ confined prostate cancer. *Prostate* 2003;54:181–186.

159. Haese A, Graefen M, Steuber T, et al. Total and Gleason grade 4/5 cancer volumes are major contributors of human kallikrein 2, whereas free prostate specific antigen is largely contributed by benign gland volume in serum from patients with prostate cancer or benign prostatic biopsies. *J Urol* 2003;170:2269–2273.

CHAPTER 8B
Screening for Prostate Cancer

Freddie C. Hamdy, Jenny L. Donovan, and David E. Neal

INTRODUCTION

Prostate cancer screening is one of the most controversial public health issues in urology. The natural aging of the population combined with the continued and widespread use of diagnostic tests, such as serum prostate-specific antigen (PSA), is resulting in an increase in the numbers of men diagnosed with localized prostate cancer. The issue of screening to identify organ-confined prostate cancer has provoked much public and scientific attention, and there is intense debate about its role in improving men's health. The findings from most reviews of the scientific evidence conclude that it is insufficient, at present, to recommend routine population screening because it is unclear whether this would improve either survival or the quality of men's lives. Particular concerns relate to the lack of knowledge about the natural history of screen-detected prostate cancer and the lack of evidence about the effectiveness of treatments. To date, no overall survival advantage has been shown in screen-detected cases for any of the major treatments (radical prostatectomy, radical radiotherapy including brachytherapy, and "watchful waiting," otherwise known as active monitoring or surveillance), and each can result in damaging iatrogenic complications and outcomes, including various levels of incontinence and impotence for radical interventions and anxiety relating to the presence of cancer in watchful waiting. The problem is compounded because many of the published studies contain flawed analyses and unsubstantiated conclusions. Intriguingly, assessment of these same studies has resulted in differing approaches to screening on either side of the Atlantic, and even between states within the United States.

GENERAL CRITERIA FOR ESTABLISHING A SCREENING PROGRAM

In 1968, Wilson and Jungner established key principles that should be satisfied for a disease before introducing screening as a public health policy (1). Despite further refinements, more recent guidelines for screening programs continue to adhere to the merits of Wilson and Jungner's original criteria, the most important of which will be used below as the framework for discussing the issues involved in screening for prostate cancer. The main questions relevant to prostate cancer screening are summarized in Table 8B.1.

THE DISEASE SHOULD BE AN IMPORTANT HEALTH PROBLEM

As the most common male cancer in Europe and the United States and second only to lung cancer in terms of male cancer deaths, there is little doubt that prostate cancer represents a significant public health burden in Western countries (2). In the United States alone, an estimated 220,900 new prostate cancer cases were diagnosed in 2003, with 28,900 deaths attributable to the disease (3).

THERE SHOULD BE A PRECLINICAL STATE MORE AMENABLE TO SUCCESSFUL TREATMENT THAN CLINICAL DISEASE

This remains unclear in prostate cancer. Despite the fact that with increasing age most men will develop microscopic foci of prostate cancer, only a small percentage of these slow-growing tumors will develop into invasive prostate cancer and an even smaller proportion will cause premature death. It is hoped that the epidemiologic investigation of prostate cancer will identify factors—ideally amenable to intervention—that cause the common microscopic form of the disease to progress to invasive disease. However, to date, the etiology of prostate cancer remains virtually unknown and continues to pose a major challenge to epidemiologists. Although both genetics and environment are likely to play a role in the evolution of the disease, the role of genetic factors in prostate cancer susceptibility has stimulated significant interest after a number of genetic linkage analyses based on families that contain several men with prostate cancer, most of whom have early onset disease. Genetic factors will undoubtedly prove important in prostate cancer, although major susceptibility genes account for only 5% to 10% of prostate cancer cases. Whether high-risk genetic mutations or common low-risk genetic polymorphisms (variants) produce familial aggregation remains unclear, although several common polymorphisms are associated with a modest increase in disease risk. Many published studies lack sufficient sample size and statistical power to be conclusive, and even if confirmed, the magnitude of effect would not justify inclusion of genotyping for these polymorphisms within a screening program. The findings for other potential factors such as diet and sexual lifestyle fall short of the evidence required for public health recommendations (4).

THE NATURAL HISTORY OF THE DISEASE SHOULD BE KNOWN

The natural history of prostate cancer in the PSA era is uncertain, because men are far more likely to die with rather than from the disease. The lifetime risk of having microscopic prostate cancer for a man aged 50 years is 42%, although his risk of dying from the disease is about 3% (5). There is little published long-term outcome data for prostate cancer in the PSA era. In clinical practice, it has become customary to state that unless a man has a minimum of 10-year life expectancy, conservative therapy is indicated. This appears to stem from the work by Barnes in the late 1960s who investigated the long-term survival of patients with clinically localized prostate cancer who were treated conservatively (6). Between 1989 and 1997, Johansson et al. carried out a prospective study of the natural history of prostate cancer among 648 men with newly diagnosed prostate cancer from a large county in Sweden (7). The patients were followed up for an average of 14 years, at the end of which the data demonstrated that the higher the stage and grade of the disease, the more likely were the patients to die of prostate cancer, with many men that had well and moderately differentiated, low-volume disease showing a favorable outcome. Johansson et al. concluded that men with early-stage disease were unlikely to benefit from aggressive intervention in the majority of cases. However, further follow-up of this cohort exceeding 15 years was published recently by the same authors, who conclude that although most prostate cancers diagnosed at an early stage have an indolent course, a significant minority of men develop local tumor progression and aggressive metastatic disease may develop in the long term. The authors noted that the risks of prostate cancer mortality increased from 15 per 1000 to 44 per 1000 beyond 15 years from diagnosis (8). These findings would support early radical treatment, notably among patients with an estimated life expectancy exceeding 15 years, with the proviso that those at risk of dying from the disease can be identified at diagnosis. A further multicenter and international analysis by Chodak et al. looked at outcomes in patients receiving no active treatment, and showed similar findings, with poorly differentiated cancers being at particular high risk of death (9). In 1997, Lu-Yao and Yao published data from the Surveillance Epidemiology and End Results (SEER) database, evaluating the outcomes of 59,876 patients diagnosed with prostate cancer over a 10-year period (10). Their results

demonstrated that men with poorly differentiated prostate cancer had a 10-fold greater risk of dying from their disease compared to men with well-differentiated tumors, again confirming previous findings (11). Using the Connecticut Tumor Registry to identify men diagnosed with localized prostate cancer who had been managed conservatively, Albertsen et al. explored the impact men's coexisting medical problems had on their risk of dying from their cancer (12,13). Their analysis concluded that men with well-differentiated disease experienced little if any loss of life, whereas patients with moderately to poorly differentiated disease lost between 4 to 8 years of life compared to age-matched controls. Retrospective analysis reviewing the impact of comorbidity in this same cohort of patients showed that those men whose competing medical problems placed them in the highest risk categories rarely died of prostate cancer.

THERE SHOULD BE AN ACCEPTABLE SCREENING TEST FOR THE DISEASE

The advent of PSA testing in the late 1980s as a simple blood test to indicate the possibility of prostate cancer has revolutionized its diagnosis. Although the triad of PSA, digital rectal examination (DRE), and transrectal ultrasound (TRUS) and biopsies remain important in confirming the diagnosis and staging the disease (14), it is now accepted that neither DRE nor TRUS should be included in a screening context for prostate cancer. In addition, serum PSA concentrations are known to vary in relation to age and prostate gland volume and can be raised after ejaculation, prostate biopsy, surgery, or during prostatitis.

More recently, data from the Prostate Cancer Prevention Trial in the United States, comparing the incidence of prostate cancer diagnosed by end-of-study biopsy between two groups of men receiving either the 5-alpha reductase inhibitor finasteride or placebo, revealed a surprisingly high detection rate (~15%) in men with a low PSA range (<4 ng/ml). This highlights the limitations of serum PSA measurement in the context of prostate cancer screening, and the risk of over-detection and over-treatment of the disease in the general population of asymptomatic men in this age group (15).

THERE SHOULD BE AN ACCEPTED AND EFFECTIVE TREATMENT

Until recently, there was a significant lack of first-degree evidence through large randomized controlled trials that aggressive treatment of localized prostate cancer improves survival and/or quality of life. Outcomes for different treatment options in men with localized prostate cancer are difficult to interpret, because many of the published studies are observational, contain too small numbers, and are otherwise methodologically weak. For example, men treated by watchful waiting may have been selected because they are older, with lower grade tumors, whereas those treated by radiotherapy may have been more likely to have more advanced tumors. Therefore only data from well-conducted large randomized controlled trials can confidently be used to compare treatment options. Such a trial has been performed in Scandinavia (15,16). The trial randomized 695 men with early prostate cancer to either watchful waiting or radical prostatectomy, with a median follow-up of 6.2 years. The most important findings were a 50% reduction in disease-specific mortality following radical prostatectomy, and a 14% increased risk of progression to metastatic disease as well as a 40% increase in local progression in patients receiving watchful waiting. There was no significant difference in overall mortality between the two groups, but morbidity from the surgery was significant, with 49% of patients experiencing varying degrees of urinary leakage, and 100% erectile dysfunction—results that are incompatible with current standard surgical practice in institutions dealing with large numbers of patients (17). Limitations of the study include the following: (a) it essentially preceded the PSA era, as only 5% of cases were detected through screening; (b) more than 50% of men were symptomatic, and 76% had palpable stage T2 tumors—findings which have become unusual in contemporary practice, where most men detected by PSA testing have T1c disease with low PSA levels; (c) the criteria for local progression in the watchful waiting arm were unreliable, defined by the subjective parameters of DRE and symptoms of bladder outflow obstruction, which may have been related to symptomatic benign enlargement of the prostate; and (d) the length of follow-up to date may be insufficient to assess the true impact of the chosen therapy. On the basis of the results from this study alone, therefore, one may conclude that the effectiveness of treatment in screen-detected prostate cancer remains so far unproven. In the United States, the PIVOT (Prostate Cancer Intervention Versus Observation Trial) has been recruiting and randomizing men aged 75 years or lower to a trial of treatment, comparing radical prostatectomy with expectant management, with all-cause mortality as a primary end-point. The trial has closed recently, having recruited 731 men, and the results are awaited (18).

In the United Kingdom, the ProtecT (Prostate testing for cancer and treatment) study is a randomized controlled trial of treatment effectiveness in men with clinically localized prostate cancer that was initiated in 1999 as a feasibility phase, which proved successful (19,20). The main trial started in 2001 and aims to test 130,000 asymptomatic men aged 50 to 70 years over a period of 5 years. Of those, 1800 patients with clinically localized prostate cancer will be randomized to either active monitoring, radical prostatectomy, or radiotherapy. The primary end-point will be survival at 10 years, with a number of secondary end-points including detailed quality of life analyses. The study, funded by the Health Technology Assessment panel of the UK National Health Service (NHS) Research and Development Programme, has been extended recently through further support from Cancer Research UK and the UK Department of Health to include the evaluation of case-finding. This effectively converts the ProtecT study into the intervention arm of a cluster randomized trial of screening. Results will become available within the next decade, at the same time as the other much awaited screening studies in Europe and the United States.

DOES SCREENING FOR PROSTATE CANCER REDUCE MORTALITY FROM THE DISEASE?

Since the introduction of the PSA test, screening for early prostate cancer has become prevalent in the United States, with, as expected, a sharp rise in the incidence of the disease in the early 1990s. This was contrasted by a static incidence rate in countries where screening was not widely practiced, such as the United Kingdom. However, by 1996, the United States started to experience a slow but constant decrease in the prostate cancer mortality rate, which was explained by some as resulting from early aggressive intervention following intensive screening programs. This conclusion can be challenged. First, in view of the protracted natural history of the disease, it is unlikely that early treatment could have caused this reduction in mortality within such a short time period. Second, similar reductions in mortality rates were observed in countries where screening had

not been adopted, such as England and Wales and The Netherlands, suggesting that other factors, including diet and environmental factors yet to be determined, must have been involved in this continuing reduction in mortality from the disease (21,22). A similar trend to that observed in the United States was seen in the Tyrol region of Austria, where in 1993, PSA testing was made freely available to all male inhabitants aged between 45 to 75 years. The effects of this intensive screening and treatment of early disease has been associated with a significant reduction in mortality from prostate cancer between 1993 and 1999, which was in contrast to the modest downward trend in prostate cancer death rates observed throughout the rest of Austria (23). It is clear that current reduction in mortality in Tyrol cannot be attributed to screening alone. More recently, Lu-Yao et al. analyzed mortality data between two areas of the United States with substantially different rates of screening and treatment (24). Using the SEER database, Lu-Yao analyzed data from 94,000 men in Seattle and 120,621 men in Connecticut over an 11-year follow-up period, with the conclusion that in Seattle, intensive PSA screening (5.39-fold compared with Connecticut) and treatment (5.9-fold for radical prostatectomy and 2.3-fold for radiotherapy) did not lead to an improved disease-specific survival rate from prostate cancer, compared with Connecticut practice.

HOW CAN WE STUDY SCREENING?

Screening for prostate cancer can be studied by randomized controlled trials such as the ones currently underway in Europe and the United States. These involve randomizing a population of men at risk of harboring the disease, with good life expectancy, to either an intensive screening program or to no screening. The outcome is measured by analyzing differences in mortality between the two groups, on the assumption that the screened group would have received early aggressive intervention compared with the nonscreened group. The European Randomized Screening for Prostate Cancer (ERSPC) trial and the Prostate, Lung, Colon and Ovary (PLCO) cancer trial in the United States represent such examples (25). The ERSPC trial is a large international cooperative study that was initiated in 1994 involving The Netherlands, Belgium, Finland, Italy, Sweden, Spain, and Switzerland and was planned with a total sample of 190,000 men aged 55 to 74 years. However, over time, targets have changed, and it is now estimated that 120,000 and 140,000 men will be required in each of the intervention and control arms, respectively. These changes were implemented to take into account the variability of countries involved, increased knowledge about compliance within the study, and the increasing rate of contamination (i.e., men in the control arm seeking PSA screening for prostate cancer and potentially receiving subsequent treatment), which now ranges from 10% to 30%. Randomization to the large PLCO study was initiated in 1993. The aim of both studies was originally to detect a 20% mortality reduction in the screened population, with a statistical power of 90%. Data from the prostate arm of the PLCO trial will be merged with ERSPC trial data, and results are expected by approximately 2008. However, treatments are not defined in these studies, and a significant proportion of men may elect 'watchful waiting'. Also, once cancer is diagnosed the treatment is not randomized. It is possible that there may be marked treatment imbalances, compounded by the uncertainty of treatment effectiveness, and ever increasingly sensitive methods of detection, which may not allow the screening studies to show differences sufficient to have an impact on public health policies. Despite these reservations, results are awaited eagerly and will represent a milestone in determining the value of PSA-driven

TABLE 8B.1

STRATEGIC QUESTIONS CONCERNING PROSTATE CANCER SCREENING

Question	Screening worthwhile if:	Screening not supportable if:
Can we identify with sufficient precision those men whose cancers will impinge upon their lives?	The early cellular changes detected through screening are commonly the precursors of later aggressive cancers that would become manifest during the man's lifetime.	There is an uncertain relationship between common microcellular changes and later aggressive cancers that would become manifest.
Is the radical treatment of screen-detected prostate cancer effective and justified?	Radical treatment for localized cancer prolongs life and does not unduly damage quality of life.	Such treatments expose too many men to complications when their prostate cancer would not have become apparent to them during life.
Is there evidence that existing screening programs are effective?	Trends in prostate cancer data support the effectiveness of early radical treatment.	Trends arise largely from a combination of population trends of largely unknown cause.

Frankel S, Smith GD, Donordin J, et al. Screening for prostate cancer. *Lancet* 2003;361(9363):1122–1128.

screening in reducing mortality from prostate cancer, complemented by the UK ProtecT study.

CONCLUSIONS

If screening for prostate cancer were introduced today, men aged between 50 and 70 years would face an uncomfortable burden of uncertainty and potential harm, which have to be weighed against the unknown benefits from intervention. For every 1 million men who agreed to the simple PSA blood test, about 100,000 would have a raised (abnormal) PSA result and face anxiety over possible cancer and the need for biopsy, leading to further anxiety, discomfort, and possible complications. Approximately 20,000 men would then be diagnosed with cancer, and 80,000 would face the anxiety of uncertain future risk. If one-half of those diagnosed with localized disease (10,000) underwent radical prostatectomy, about 10 would die of the operation and, even in the best hands, around 300 would develop urinary incontinence and 4,000 would develop erectile dysfunction. The number whose prostate cancer would eventually have impinged upon their lives is currently unknown, as is the number of deaths that would have been prevented. The dilemmas surrounding the value of screening and treatment in clinically localized prostate cancer thus remain unresolved. Recently published work from Scandinavia sheds some light onto potential benefits of radical prostatectomy in preventing patients from dying from prostate cancer, although aggressive treatment did not improve overall survival compared with watchful waiting. Results from the now-merged ERSPC in Europe and PLCO in the United States, the ProtecT study in the United Kingdom, and the PIVOT study in the United States are awaited eagerly.

Today, the likelihood of harm from prostate cancer screening outweighs the prospect of benefit, leading to the inescapable conclusion that screening remains unjustified outside randomized trials investigating its effects. It is reassuring, however, for the medical community and prostate cancer patients worldwide that these long-standing dilemmas are being resolved through large and robust randomized controlled trials supported by governments and funding institutions in Europe and the United States.

ACKNOWLEDGMENTS

The authors are joint Principal Investigators of the ProtecT Study in the United Kingdom. The ProtecT Study is funded by the Health Technology Assessment panel of the NHS R&D Programme in the UK (ref. 96/20/99).

References

1. Wilson JMG, Junger G. *Principles and practice of screening for disease.* Geneva: World Health Organization, 1968: Public Health Papers, No. 34.
2. Jenson OM, Esteve J, Renhard H. Cancer in the European Community and its member states. *Eur J Cancer* 1990;26:1167–1256.
3. Greenlee RT, Hill-Harmon MB, Murray T, et al. Cancer statistics 2001. *CA Cancer J Clin* 2001;51:15–36.
4. Schaid DJ. The complex genetic epidemiology of prostate cancer. *Hum Mol Genet* 2004;13(Special Issue 1):R103–R121.
5. Whitmore WF Jr. Localised prostate cancer: management and detection issues 1994. *Lancet* 1994;343:1263–1267.
6. Barnes RW. Survival with conservative therapy. *JAMA* 1969;210:331–332.
7. Johansson J, Holmberg L, Johansson S, et al. Fifteen-year survival in prostate cancer: a prospective population based study in Sweden. *JAMA* 1997;227:467–471.
8. Johansson JE, Andren O, Andersson SO, et al. Natural history of early, localized prostate cancer. *JAMA* 2004;291:2757–2758.
9. Chodak GW, Thisted RA, Gerber GS, et al. Results of conservative management of clinically localized prostate cancer. *N Engl J Med* 1994;330:242–248.
10. Lu-Yao GL, Yao SL. Population based study of long-term survival in patients with clinically localised prostate cancer. *Lancet* 1997;349:906–910.
11. Albertsen PC, Frybeck DG, Storer BE, et al. Long-term survival among men with conservatively treated localized prostate cancer. *JAMA* 1995;274:626–631.
12. Albertsen PC, Hanley J, Gleson D, et al. A competing risk analysis of men aged 55-74 years at diagnosis managed conservatively for localized prostate cancer. *JAMA* 1998;280:975–980.
13. Wilkinson BA, Hamdy FC. State-of-the-art staging in prostate cancer. *BJU Int* 2001;87:423–430.
14. Rietbergen J, Kranse R. Evaluation of the digital rectal examination as a screening test for prostate cancer: Rotterdam section of the European Randomized Study of Screening for Prostate Cancer. *J Natl Cancer Inst* 1998;90(23):1817–1823.
15. Donovan JL, Hamdy FC, Neal DE, et al. Prostate testing for cancer and treatment (ProtecT) feasibility study. *Health Technol Assess* 2003;7(14):1–88.
16. Holmberg L, Bill-Axelson A, Helgesen F, et al. A randomised trial comparing radical prostatectomy with watchful waiting in early prostate cancer: Scandinavian Prostatic Cancer Group Study number 4. *N Engl J Med* 2002;347:781–789.
17. Steineck G, Helgesen F, Adolfsson J, et al. Quality of life after radical prostatectomy or watchful waiting. Scandinavian Prostatic Cancer Group Study number 4. *N Engl J Med* 2002;347:790–796.
18. Begg CB, Riedel CR, Bach PB, et al. Variations in morbidity after radical prostatectomy. *N Eng J Med* 2002;346:1138–1144.
19. Wilt TJ, Brawer MK. The Prostate Cancer Intervention Versus Observation Trial (PIVOT). *Oncology (Huntingt)* 1997;11(8):1133–1139.
20. Donovan J, Mills N, Smith M, et al. Improving design and conduct of randomised trials by embedding them in qualitative research: ProtecT (Prostate testing for cancer and treatment) study. *BMJ* 2002;325:766–770.
21. Oliver SE, Gunnell D, Donovan JL. Comparison of trends in prostate cancer mortality in England and Wales and the USA. *Lancet* 2000;355:1788–1789.
22. Schröder FH, Wildhagen MF. Screening for prostate cancer: evidence and perspectives. *BJU Int* 2001;88:811–817.
23. Bartsch G, Horninger W, Klocker H, et al. Prostate cancer mortality after introduction of prostate specific antigen mass screening in the Federal State of Tyrol, Austria. *Urology* 2001;58:417–424.

24. Lu-Yao G, Albertsen PC, Stanford JL, et al. Natural experiment examining impact of aggressive screening and treatment on prostate cancer mortality in two fixed cohorts from Seattle area and Connecticut. *BMJ* 2002;325: 740–745.

25. de Koning HJ, Auvinen A, Berenguer Sanchez A, et al. European Randomized Screening for Prostate Cancer (ERSPC) Trial; International Prostate Cancer Screening Trials Evaluation Group. Large-scale randomised prostate cancer screening trials: program performances in the European Randomized Screening for Prostate Cancer trial and the Prostate, Lung, Colorectal and Ovary Cancer trial. *Int J Cancer* 2002;97:237–244.

26. Frankel S, Smith GD, Donordin J, et al. Screening for prostate cancer. *Lancet* 2003;361(9363):1122–1128.

CHAPTER 8C
Screening for Prostate Cancer: Experience from the Tyrol Study

Wolfgang Horninger, Peter Boyle, and Georg Bartsch

INTRODUCTION

In the early 1990s, a remarkable increase in the incidence of prostate cancer in many countries, particularly in the United States (1), was observed.

This observation can be attributed to the widespread use of prostate-specific antigen (PSA), which was first approved for the detection of recurrent disease in patients with established prostate cancer in 1986. Thereafter, the potential of this test for early diagnosis of prostate cancer was soon recognized. From 1984 until 1994, PSA was increasingly used for diagnostic purposes. In 1984, PSA testing was used in 5.1% and in 1994 in 60.6% of all newly diagnosed prostate carcinomas (2). It has been shown that a great number of cancers detected by PSA testing are clinically significant and potentially curable (3–6).

However, the introduction of PSA testing in prostate cancer screening programs has also led to controversy surrounding several distinct issues, including the sensitivity and specificity of the screening test, treatment of early prostate cancer and, indeed, whether some cancers will do equally well if left untreated, and the side effects of therapy, particularly radical prostatectomy. The two most common cancer screening programs, Papanicolaou smears for cervical cancer and mammographic examination for breast cancer, came into common use and acceptance through widely different mechanisms: the results of randomized trials of mammographic screening for breast cancer and the observation of the decrease in incidence and mortality from cervical cancer after the policy to introduce cervical cancer screening to populations. The current study reports the incidence and mortality rates of prostate cancer in the Federal State of Tyrol, Austria, where regular PSA testing has been made freely available to the population since 1993 and where use of the test has been high. This population is also characterized by being particularly stable. PSA testing was not freely available in the rest of Austria, although it will have been used, probably evolving in a similar manner to the use in many Western countries. A comparison of the mortality rates between Tyrol and the rest of Austria allowed evaluation of the outcome of this natural experiment.

MATERIALS AND METHODS

In 1993, a mass screening project using PSA as the only screening test was launched in the Federal State of Tyrol (one of nine federal states of the Republic of Austria). Previously (1988 to 1992), both PSA and digital rectal examination (DRE) were available and used in the diagnostic workup of symptomatic patients and in a limited way for asymptomatic men. Since 1989, urologists at the Innsbruck University Hospital have promoted the concept of early prostate cancer detection using PSA and DRE. In 1989 to 1992, the number of PSA tests performed in this hospital rose from 2360 to 5878.

Tyrol is an alpine region in Western Austria with, at the 1991 census, 631,410 inhabitants (324,161 women and 307,249 men) in an area of 12,647 km². The region is dominated by the mountains of the Central Alps, and the distances to Innsbruck, the capital, where the central health care unit is located, are not too far (infrequently more than 100 km). This geographic situation, as well as the willingness of the general population to participate in preventive medical programs, caused us to launch a statewide mass screening program with PSA as the only screening test for the early detection of prostate cancer. PSA testing was made freely available by the Social Insurance Company of the Federal State of Tyrol and the University Hospital of Innsbruck to all men aged 45 to 75 years. All men in this age range were advised and encouraged to undergo PSA testing, and information to this effect was distributed to all Tyrolean men by press, radio, and television.

The screening project was performed in collaboration with general practitioners, medical examiners, urologists, medical laboratories, and the Tyrol Blood Bank of the Red Cross. Informed consent was obtained from all volunteers participating in the program. All co-workers were fully informed of the guidelines for withdrawal, storage, and shipping of the blood samples. PSA was assessed immediately on arrival of the blood or serum sample. All volunteers and/or referring physicians were informed about the results. In the case of elevated PSA levels, the volunteers were invited to undergo additional urologic evaluations, and the men with normal PSA levels were invited to have a repeated PSA test 12 months later. More than 80% of all volunteers found to have an elevated PSA level consented to an additional evaluation, which included DRE, transrectal ultrasonography (TRUS), and prostate biopsy. At the time of drawing blood for PSA measurement, no DRE was performed. Several scientific projects (7–11) have been published describing this screening program.

This mass screening program was provided free of charge to men between 45 and 75 years old and to younger men with a family history of prostate cancer. Age-referenced PSA levels (12) in combination with percent free PSA of less than 22%, were initially used as the biopsy criteria. Since October 1995, so-called bisected PSA levels (13) (one-half the age specific reference ranges; Table 8C.1) together with percent free PSA levels of less than 18% were used. Since 2001, complexed PSA was also included in our diagnostic workup. Screened volunteers with a PSA level greater than 10 ng per mL were recommended to undergo biopsy irrespective of their percent free PSA. Since March 1996, PSA transition zone density (11) has been introduced as an additional diagnostic parameter in selecting patients for biopsy to decrease the number of unnecessary

TABLE 8C.1

BISECTED AGE-SPECIFIC REFERENCE RANGES FOR TOTAL PROSTATE-SPECIFIC ANTIGEN

Age (Years)	Normal range (ng/mL)
45–49	0–1.25
50–59	0–1.75
60–69	0–2.25
70–75	0–3.25

biopsies. All men who, according to bisected age-referenced levels and free PSA concentrations, had an elevated PSA concentration were invited to undergo additional urologic evaluation, including DRE and ultrasound-guided biopsies. Urologists performed the DREs and transrectal ultrasound examinations.

Sextant biopsies were initially made using ultrasound guidance with an automatic biopsy gun and an 18-gauge needle; since 1995, 10 systematic biopsies and since 2000, additional contrast-enhanced color Doppler targeted biopsies have been performed.

Patients presenting with organ-confined lesions (T1 and T2) underwent radical prostatectomy or external beam radiotherapy if surgery was not acceptable to them (70.2 Gy, single fraction 1.8 Gy, four-box technique), those with stage T3 lesions underwent external beam radiotherapy (70.2 Gy, single fraction 1.8 Gy, four-box technique), and those with metastatic disease underwent androgen deprivation therapy. Every patient with N1 or M1 disease received hormonal therapy. The policy was such that no patient was treated primarily by surveillance ("watchful waiting").

Data on cancer incidence have been available from the population-based Tyrol Cancer Registry since 1988. Cancer mortality data have been available, independently, from the Austrian Central Statistics Office since 1970. The underlying cause of death was attributed from the death certificates of all deaths in Austria by the Central Statistical Office in Vienna, where they were unaware of the study being performed in Tyrol. The numbers of cases and population estimates are available, annually, in 5-year classes of age. PSA tests were available at no charge for men aged 45 to 75 years, although use among men on either side of these age limits also occurred.

All incidence and mortality rates were calculated for the truncated age range (40 to 79 years) using the world standard population as the reference (14).

The principal hypotheses tested were (a) whether the prostate cancer mortality rates in Tyrol decreased from 1993 and (b) whether the trends in the prostate cancer mortality rates in Tyrol differed from those in the rest of Austria from 1993. The trends in the mortality rates in Tyrol and the rest of Austria were compared within a Poisson regression model:

$$\begin{aligned} \log(\text{rate}) = {} & \beta 0 + \beta 1(\text{year} - 1993) \\ & + \beta 2(\text{year} - 1993)I(\text{year} \supseteq 1993) \\ & + \beta 3 \text{Tyrol} + \beta 4 \text{Tyrol} \\ & \times (\text{year} - 1993) + \beta 5 \text{Tyrol} \\ & \times (\text{year} - 1993)I(\text{year} \supseteq 1993) \end{aligned} \quad (8C.1)$$

This is a "change-point" model in which the term "I(year $\supseteq$ 1993)" is an indicator that permits a different slope from 1993 onward compared with before 1993. The parameter $\beta 0$ gives the estimated log mortality rate in the rest of Austria in 1993; $\beta 3$ represents the difference from this value in Tyrol. A *priori*, no difference was anticipated. The slope of the relationship between the log mortality rates and time was given by $\beta 1$ in the rest of Austria and $\beta 1 + \beta 4$ in Tyrol; thus $\beta 4$ represented the difference in slopes before 1993. The parameter $\beta 2$ gave an estimate of any change in slope from 1993 onward compared with 1992 and before in the rest of Austria. If no change occurred, the estimated value would be about 0; if treatment advances have occurred, a negative estimate would be expected. In Tyrol, the change in the slope from 1993 onward was given by $\beta 2 + \beta 5$. Thus, $\beta 5$ was the crucial parameter in the analysis, as it measured the different slope in Tyrol compared with the rest of Austria from 1993 onward. The goodness of fit of the model was established on the basis of residual plots, and the hypothesis tests were based on changes in the deviance (15). All statistical analysis was carried out using S-plus 2000 (16).

In this analysis we used 1993 as the reference year. This was the beginning of the period at which the practice was different with regard to PSA testing in Tyrol compared with the rest of Austria and so represents the earliest time at which any changes in the trend associated with the mass screening program might theoretically begin. Any other choice of reference year, such as 1995, could be open to criticism on the basis of a post hoc choice, even though one might argue that the earliest time one might begin to see a real benefit from screening would be about 2 years after the introduction. This is because the median survival time for metastatic prostate cancer is about 18 months. If the mass screening program had an effect on the mortality rates, using the earlier date would tend to give conservative results, because no difference in the rates in the two regions should occur for a certain period after the introduction of the mass screening program. The estimated benefit of the mass screening program was calculated by comparing the observed and expected numbers of deaths in Tyrol and by examining the prostate cancer mortality trends in the two regions. The expected numbers of cases and deaths for each year in Tyrol were calculated using the average of the rates from 1986 to 1990 as the reference. The effect of using the data for 1988 to 1990 in the calculation of the expected values should be conservative for incidence and have no influence on mortality.

RESULTS

During 1993, when PSA testing became freely available, 32.3% of all Tyrolean men between 45 and 75 years old underwent PSA screening, and at least 70% of this population were tested at least once during the first 10 years of the study. At the laboratory of the Department of Urology, Innsbruck University, more than 96,000 men were screened at least once. Of these, 10,100 were aged 45 to 49 years and 4900 were aged 40 to 44 years. Thus, a substantial number of men aged 40 to 44 were screened, justifying the inclusion of this age group in the analysis of the incidence and mortality rates.

From 1993 to 2001, 6024 transrectal prostate needle biopsies—as described above—were performed. The overall prostate cancer detection rate was 30.2%. Table 8C.2 shows the major and minor complications of the 6024 transrectal biopsies. The incidence of prostate cancer in men aged 40 to 79 in Tyrol increased between 1988 and 1994 and has remained constant since (Fig. 8C.1). The incidence of organ-confined disease (stages I and II) continued to increase from 1988 until 1998, although the incidence of extraprostatic disease (stage III) declined following a peak in 1994. The incidence of metastatic disease (stage IV) has been declining since 1993 (Fig. 8C.2). The stage reported to the Cancer Registry is a mixture of clinical and pathologic stages.

Since the beginning of the screening project, a significant migration to lower total PSA levels in patients undergoing radical

TABLE 8C.2

COMPLICATIONS OF 6024 TRANSRECTAL NEEDLE PROSTATE BIOPSIES

Complication	Percentage (%)
Gross hematuria >1 day	12.5
Hemospermia	29.8
Significant pain	4.0
Rectal bleeding	0.6
Nausea	0.8
Fever >38.5°C	0.8
Epididymitis	0.7
Sepsis	0.3

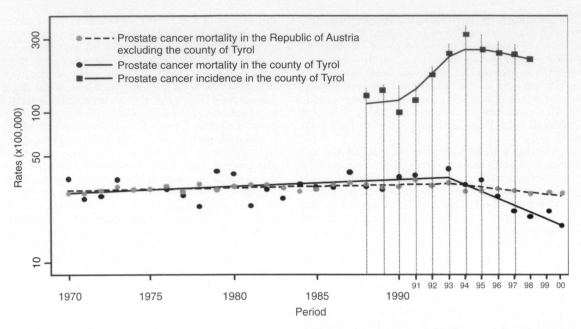

FIGURE 8C.1. Prostate cancer incidence rates in Tyrol and prostate cancer mortality rates in Tyrol and in the rest of Austria.

prostatectomy has been observed. Subsequently, the rate of organ confined diseases in radical prostatectomy increased from 28.7% in 1993 to more than 80% in 2002 (Table 8C.3).

The mortality from prostate cancer in Tyrol decreased significantly between 1993 and 2000, in contrast to the modest downward trend in prostate cancer death rates observed in the rest of Austria (Fig. 8C.1). On the basis of the age-specific prostate cancer mortality rates in Tyrol between 1986 and 1990, 22 fewer prostate cancer deaths in the age range 40 to 79 occurred in 1998 than were expected, 18 fewer deaths than expected occurred in 1999, and 25 fewer deaths than expected occurred in the year 2000 (Table 8C.4).

The fitted values of the model, described above, are shown in Fig. 8C.1. No significant difference was found between the trends in Tyrol and the rest of Austria before 1993 ($\chi^2 = 1.12$,

1 degree of freedom, $P = .29$). The log mortality rates increased at a rate of 0.0113 [standard error (SE) 0.005] per year in Tyrol and 0.0057 (SE 0.0014) in the rest of Austria from 1970 up to and including 1992. No significant difference was found between the estimated rates in 1993 in the two regions of Austria ($P = .13$). A decrease in mortality occurred in Tyrol after 1993 ($\chi^2 = 12.74$, 1 degree of freedom, $P = .0004$), where the log mortality rates decreased at a rate of 0.092 (SE 0.024) per year from 1993 onward. In the rest of Austria, the decrease was 0.0229 (SE 0.0064) per year. From 1993 onward, the trends in the rates show a significant difference between Tyrol and the rest of Austria ($\chi^2 = 7.55$, 1 degree of freedom, $P = .006$). In the analysis, we assumed linear trends between the log mortality rates and year, permitting changes in slopes from 1993 onward in Tyrol and in the rest of Austria. We tested whether the change in

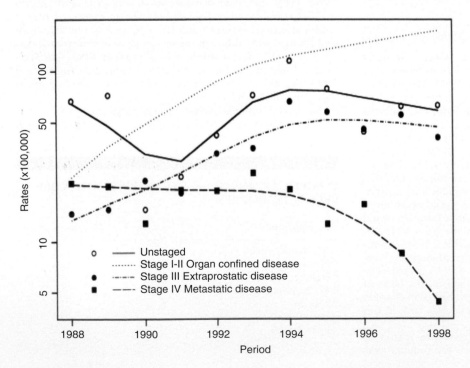

FIGURE 8C.2. Prostate cancer incidence rates in Tyrol by stage in men aged 40 to 79.

TABLE 8C.3

TOTAL PSA AND STAGE MIGRATION IN RADICAL PROSTATECTOMIES SINCE 1993

Year	Mean PSA (ng/mL)	Stage % of organ-confined prostate cancer
1993	14.9	28.7
1994	14.2	27.6
1995	12.7	25.1
1996	9.7	55.8
1997	8.6	65.7
1998	6.3	67.2
1999	6.2	79.1
2000	5.8	82.1
2001	5.3	82.0
2002	4.8	81.0

PSA, prostate-specific antigen.

the slope from 1993 onward was the same in Tyrol as in the rest of Austria. This hypothesis was rejected. Although no statistically significant differences were observed between Tyrol and the rest of Austria before 1993, the fitted value in Tyrol in 1993 was slightly higher than in the rest of Austria (Fig. 8C.1), and this may have some implications for the change in the slope. To investigate the effect of this, we constrained the line before 1993 to be exactly the same in Tyrol as in the rest of Austria. This was achieved by setting $\beta3$ and $\beta4$ both equal to 0 in the model. The rate of increase in the log mortality rate was 0.0061 (SE 0.0013) per year, which was very similar to that for the rest of Austria, as Tyrol is a small part of Austria. In the rest of Austria, the rate of decrease from 1993 onward was 0.0246 (SE 0.0063) per year, and in Tyrol, it was 0.0709 (SE 0.0197) per year. The test statistic for the comparison of the slopes from 1993 onward was $\chi^2 = 5.38$, $P = .02$. Thus, our conclusions were only slightly tempered.

Taking 1995 as the year at which the first change can be reasonably expected yielded a rate of decrease in the rest of Austria from 1995 onward of 0.0309 (SE 0.0104) per year; in Tyrol, it was 0.1505 (SE 0.0410) per year. The latter figure was almost double the corresponding decrease from 1993 and the rate of decrease in the rest of Austria was one third greater. These rates of decrease are significantly different ($\chi^2 = 7.99$, $P = .0047$). Constraining the lines to be identical in Tyrol and the rest of Austria before 1995 yielded very

similar results. In the rest of Austria, the rate of decrease was 0.0328 (SE 0.0103) per year, and in Tyrol, it was significantly greater at 0.1259 (SE 0.0355) per year ($P = .0098$).

Three possibilities could lead to a reduction in the mortality rate from prostate cancer: (a) prevention of the disease, (b) detection of the disease at a stage when it is more likely to be curable, and (c) improvement in the outcome of therapy for metastatic disease. A fourth possibility, that screening would bring forward the time of death in some individuals, is very unlikely to explain the differences observed. Currently, screening for prostate cancer is in a phase of rapid development, with several different approaches used. The general acceptance of prostate cancer screening as a part of public health care programs can only be expected if the benefits in terms of mortality can be demonstrated.

The intermediate end-points of cancer screening include migration to lower cancer stages at the time of diagnosis and lower progression and higher survival rates. The end point of screening programs and the ultimate goal of all cancer research and treatment has to be a reduction in disease-related mortality and improvement in the quality of life. The latter is of particular concern when a screening program could result in more men living longer with cancer and the side effects of the disease and its treatment (17). Screening programs may help control prostate cancer. The term *screening* should only be used if tests suitable for early detection are applied in a clearly defined program (e.g., in the form of population screening). In terms of the costs associated with this type of screening, only primary PSA screening would be acceptable. However, the sensitivity, specificity, and positive predictive value of PSA must be known and must be superior to other diagnostic tools suitable for screening (18,19).

With screening procedures, there is usually a discrepancy between the sensitivity and specificity. In the case of prostate cancer, the cutoff for PSA as a biopsy criterion has to be lowered to improve sensitivity; however, that entails a great number of negative biopsies. Because of its low cost and complete standardization and automation, it would be very attractive to use total PSA as the only biopsy criterion. However, to reduce the number of negative biopsies, additional diagnostic tests such as the assessment of %free PSA and PSA transition zone density should be performed (11). With the help of these two diagnostic tests, approximately 54% of negative biopsies could be avoided (11). In evaluating this program, one should bear in mind that an "aggressive" screening policy has been combined with a complex decision algorithm to maximize prostate cancer detection without unacceptable biopsy rates. Agreement is general that a number of prerequisites have to be fulfilled before a screening program can be introduced as a health policy. These requirements have been described by Wilson and Jungner (20) in a classic paper.

TABLE 8C.4

EXPECTED AND OBSERVED NUMBERS OF PROSTATE CANCER DEATHS IN THE FEDERAL STATE OF TYROL

Year	Deaths expected	Deaths observed	SMR (95% CI) (%)
1991	44	50	114 (84–150)
1992	43	44	101 (74–136)
1993	43	52	121 (90–159)
1994	43	42	97 (70–132)
1995	45	45	101 (74–135)
1996	47	37	79 (56–109)
1997	49	33 (−32%)	67 (46–94)
1998	52	30 (−42%)	58 (39–82)
1999	55	37 (−33%)	
2000	57	32 (−44%)	

SMR, standardized mortality data; CI, confidence interval.

No evidence is yet available from randomized trials that PSA-based screening can decrease prostate cancer mortality rates (21). Nevertheless, the results obtained from the population-based Surveillance, Epidemiology and End Results Program (22–25) show that the incidence of prostate cancer and the mortality rates have declined in recent years. The results of another study (26) suggest that screening for prostate cancer by DRE may be beneficial; screening by DRE was found to be much less common among men who died of histologically confirmed prostate cancer than among age-matched population controls. Currently, two large, prospective studies are underway to examine the impact of PSA-based screening on prostate cancer mortality, but to date, neither has a sufficiently long follow-up to document a reduction in mortality as a direct result of PSA-based screening (27). The results reported here are from a unique natural experiment. The increase in incidence of prostate cancer after the introduction of a uniformly available and free testing program is precisely what is expected if a large proportion of men are screened. The continued increase in local disease incidence, indicating that PSA testing picks up early disease, and the constant decline in the incidence of prostate cancer that has distant spread at diagnosis in the population are encouraging. The fall in prostate cancer mortality rates in Tyrolean men contrasts with the more modest change taking place among all men of the same age in the rest of Austria (Fig. 8C.1) and coincides, from the temporal point of view, with the introduction of PSA testing. The differences we report between the mortality rates in Tyrol and the rest of Austria bear strong similarities to two other phenomena. Mortality rates from cervical cancer in Nordic countries fell after screening became widely available, but not in Norway, where it was not available (28). In addition, the mortality rates from breast cancer in The Netherlands and the United Kingdom have both fallen since the introduction of mammographic screening programs (29), in both cases too quickly to be due to the diagnosis and treatment of clinically undetectable cancers. The absence of a watchful waiting strategy in Tyrol has meant that some patients with stage T3/4 disease will have been treated with hormonal therapy earlier than is usual in the disease course. Recent evidence suggests that earlier hormonal therapy may have a beneficial effect on survival (30). The decline in mortality from prostate cancer seen in the men in the age range for which PSA testing was made available, and where acceptance of testing was high, is the first evidence from a geographically defined population for which screening was available to all its members that the policy of making PSA testing universally available and at no cost may have led to a reduction in death from prostate cancer in that population. Many aspects of prostate cancer screening require better definition by randomized trials, including screening interval, issues relating to lead time, cutoff limits for a PSA test to be considered positive, and estimation of the benefits. Our study was not designed to investigate the important issues relating to economics and psychological impact. Although these necessary data are becoming available, the current demonstration of a decline in mortality from prostate cancer supports, but does not prove, the hypothesis that the policy of making PSA testing available to the population of Tyrol has led to a reduction in prostate cancer death rates. Also, the gap between the absolute numbers of deaths observed and those expected by the pre-PSA testing age-specific mortality rates has been growing in the age range liable to have been screened.

References

1. Stanford JL, Stephenson RA, Coyle M, et al. *Prostate Cancer Trends 1973-1995*, SEER Program. NIH Publication No. 99-4543. Bethesda, MD: National Cancer Institute; 1999:7–15.
2. Jones GW, Mettlin C, Murphy GP, et al. Patterns of care for carcinoma of the prostate gland: results of a national survey of 1984 and 1990. *J Am Coll Surg* 1995;180:545–554.
3. Catalona WJ, Richie JP, Ahmann FR, et al. Comparison of digital rectal examination and serum prostate specific antigen in the early detection of prostate cancer: results of a multicenter clinical trial of 6,630 men. *J Urol* 1994;151:1283–1290.
4. Ohori M, Wheeler TM, Dunn JK, et al. The pathological features and prognosis of prostate cancer detectable with current diagnostic tests. *J Urol* 1994;152:1714–1720.
5. Smith DS, Catalona WJ. The nature of prostate cancer detected through prostate specific antigen based screening. *J Urol* 1994;152:1732–1736.
6. Slawin KM, Ohori M, Dillioglugil O, et al. Screening for prostate cancer: an analysis of the early experience. *CA Cancer J Clin* 1995;45:134–147.
7. Reissigl A, Pointner J, Horninger W, et al. Comparison of different PSA cutpoints for early detection of prostate cancer: results of a large screening study. *Urology* 1995;46:662–665.
8. Reissigl A, Pointner J, Horninger W, et al. PSA based screening for prostate cancer in asymptomatic younger males: pilot study in blood donors. *Prostate* 1997;30:20–25.
9. Reissigl A, Ennemoser O, Klocker H, et al. Frequency and clinical significance of transition zone cancer in prostate cancer screening. *Prostate* 1997;30:130–135.
10. Reissigl A, Klocker H, Horninger W, et al. Usefulness of the ratio free/total PSA in addition to total PSA levels in prostate cancer screening. *Urology* 1996;48:62–66.
11. Horninger W, Reissigl A, Klocker H, et al. Improvement of specificity in PSA based screening by using PSA transition zone density and percent free PSA in addition to total PSA levels. *Prostate* 1998;37:133–137.
12. Oesterling JE, Jacobsen SJ, Chute CG, et al. Serum prostate specific antigen in a community-based population of healthy men: establishment of age specific reference ranges. *JAMA* 1993;270:860–864.
13. Horninger W, Reissigl A, Rogatsch H, et al. Prostate cancer screening in Tyrol, Austria. *Eur J Cancer* 2000;36:1322–1335.
14. Boyle P, Parkin DM. Statistical methods for registries. In: Jensen OM, Parkin DM, McLennan R et al., eds. *Cancer registration: principles and methods*, Vol. 95. Lyon: IARC Scientific Publication; 1995:126–158.
15. McCullagh P, Nelder JA. *Generalized linear models*, 2nd ed. London: Chapman and Hall; 1989.
16. Data Analysis Products Division. *S-plus 2000: User's Guide*. Seattle: Mathsoft; 1999.
17. Boyle P, Severi G. Epidemiology of chemoprevention of prostate cancer. *Eur Urol* 1999;35:370–376.
18. Catalona WJ, Smith DS, Ratliff TL, et al. Measurement of prostate specific antigen in serum as a screening test for prostate cancer. *N Engl J Med* 1991;324:1156–1161.
19. Mettlin C, Murphy GP, Babaian RJ et al., Investigators of the American Cancer Society National Prostate Cancer Detection Project. The results of a five year early prostate cancer detection intervention. *Cancer* 1996;77:150–159.
20. Wilson JMG, Jungner G. *Principles and practice of screening for disease*, Public Health Paper No. 34. Geneva: World Health Organization; 1969.
21. Von Eschenbach A, Ho R, Murphy GP et al., American Cancer Society. Guidelines for the early detection of prostate cancer. *Cancer* 1997;80:1805–1807.
22. Smart CR. The results of prostate carcinoma screening in the U.S. as reflected in the surveillance, epidemiology, and end results program. *Cancer* 1997;80:1835–1844.
23. Hankey BF, Feuer EJ, Clegg LX, et al. Cancer surveillance series: interpreting trends in prostate cancer—Part I: evidence of the effects of screening in recent prostate cancer incidence, mortality and survival rates. *J Natl Cancer Inst* 1999;91:1017–1024.
24. Feuer J, Merrill RM, Hankey BF. Cancer surveillance series: interpreting trends in prostate cancer—Part II: cause of death misclassification and the recent rise and fall in prostate cancer mortality. *J Natl Cancer Inst* 1999;91:1025–1032.
25. Etzioni R, Legler JM, Feuer EJ, et al. Cancer surveillance series: interpreting trends in prostate cancer—Part III: quantifying link between population prostate specific antigen testing and recent declines in prostate cancer mortality. *J Natl Cancer Inst* 1999;91:1033–1039.
26. Jacobsen SJ, Bergstralh EJ, Katusic SK, et al. Screening digital rectal examination and prostate cancer mortality: a population-based case-control study. *Urology* 1998;52:173–179.
27. Boyle P. Prostate specific antigen (PSA) testing as screening for prostate cancer: the current controversy. *Ann Oncol* 1998;9:1263–1264.
28. Laara E, Day NE, Hakama M. Trends in mortality from cervical cancer in the Nordic countries: association with organised screening programs. *Lancet* 1987;1:1247–1249.
29. van den Akker-van Marle E, de Konig H, Boer R, et al. Reduction in breast cancer mortality due to the introduction of mass screening in The Netherlands: comparison with the United Kingdom. *J Med Screen* 1999;6:30–34.
30. Messing EM, Manola J, Sarosdy M, et al. Immediate hormonal therapy compared with observation after radical prostatectomy and pelvic lymphadenectomy in men with nodepositive prostate cancer. *N Engl J Med* 1999;341:1781–1788.

CHAPTER 9 ■ PROSTATE NEEDLE BIOPSY TECHNIQUES AND INTERPRETATION

KATSUTO SHINOHARA, VIRAJ A. MASTER, THOMAS CHI, AND PETER R. CARROLL

INTRODUCTION AND HISTORICAL PERSPECTIVE

Early, appropriate, and efficient detection efforts are likely to lead to improved outcomes of care for men with prostate cancer. Transrectal ultrasound (TRUS) guided needle biopsy of the prostate is the standard method for the early detection of prostate cancer.

Prostate biopsy was first described in 1930 when Ferguson successfully obtained cancer cells by aspirating prostate tissue through a transperineally introduced 18 G needle (1). In 1937, Astraldi described the first transrectal core needle biopsy of the prostate (2). Since then, various instruments have been developed for core needle biopsy. Until the 1980s, a prostate biopsy was commonly done using a large caliber needle, such as a Vim-Silverman or True-cut needle, and was often performed under anesthesia. The biopsy was done either transrectally or transperineally, and was directed to the palpable abnormality using only finger-guidance.

TRUS of the prostate was first reported by Wild and Reid in 1955 and popularized by Watanabe et al. in the early 1970s (3,4). In the late 1980s, TRUS guided prostate biopsy using an 18 G needle loaded in a spring-action device was first introduced (5). Since then, prostate biopsy under ultrasound guidance using an automated device has become a standard procedure. In 1989 Hodge et al. proposed the modern model of performing a biopsy of defined areas of the prostate, namely the "sextant" method of prostate biopsy (para-sagittal biopsy at the apex, mid-gland, and base bilaterally) (6). After the initial introduction of sextant, systematic prostate biopsy, little refinement of the technique was made until, in an editorial, Stamey suggested moving the biopsies more laterally to better sample the anterior horns of the peripheral zone and avoid sampling error (6–8). Such recommendations were supported by the meticulous whole-mount analyses of radical prostatectomy specimens, which helped to further delineate the zonal anatomy of the prostate as well as the spatial origin of prostate cancers (9). Thereafter, technological developments that have improved TRUS and its role in prostate cancer detection include an automated spring-loaded prostate biopsy device, multi-axial planar imaging, and a better understanding of prostate zonal anatomy (10,11).

CURRENT TECHNIQUE

Preparation

Any anticoagulation medications or antiplatelet medications such as aspirin, nonsteroidal antiinflammatory drugs (NSAIDs), and Plavix should be stopped 1 week prior to biopsy. Antibiotics, most commonly fluoroquinolones, are given before biopsy and continued for a total of 48 to 72 hours. Usage of antibiotics significantly reduces the risk of septicemia (12). If a patient is known to have heart valve disease or is susceptible to endocarditis, appropriate antibiotics, usually ampicillin and gentamicin, should be given according to the American Heart Association's recommendation for antibiotic prophylaxis (13). Patients with artificial joints or prostheses need to be appropriately covered with parenteral antibiotics, as well. A Fleets enema may be given approximately 1 hour prior to the procedure. This will not only evacuate rectal contents including gas and fecal matter, which causes interference on ultrasound imaging, but also reduce infection rates in some studies (14).

Transrectal Ultrasonography

Transrectal ultrasonography not only guides the needle into the designated area of the prostate, but also gives information regarding prostate size and shape, tumor localization and stage, and seminal vesicle pathology. Currently either a bi-plane probe or end-fire probe with variable frequency between 5 MHz and 10 MHz is used for transrectal prostate biopsy.

Anesthesia

The administration of anesthetic agents before TRUS biopsy reduces patient discomfort. This may be important, as a study from The Netherlands examining the reasons of men refusing to attend a prostate cancer screening showed that 18% of men felt that the prostate biopsy would be painful (15). Nash et al. at the University of California San Francisco (UCSF) first conducted a randomized, double-blind study of local infiltration of 1% lidocaine around the prostate vascular pedicle in 64 patients (16). Mean pain scores were significantly lower on the side injected with lidocaine as compared to the saline control. The finding that use of anesthetic techniques (topical, injected, or both) is beneficial has been shown by many investigators, although there are a few studies where a benefit has not been shown (17–20). The previously described technique of injecting lidocaine at the vascular pedicle can be associated with systemic circulation of lidocaine, which may result in a bad taste sensation, ear tingling, or vertigo. In addition, this type of nerve block does not completely anesthetize the anterior part of the gland. Currently at UCSF, a 1% lidocaine 10 cc and 7.5% sodium bicarbonate 1 cc solution mixture is used to reduce the burning sensation associated with injection. The solution is injected directly into the prostate at three locations in each lobe by inserting a 22 gauge needle all the way to the anterior capsule at the base, mid-gland, and the apex. As the needle is pulled back, 1 to 2 cc of anesthetic is infiltrated into the prostate parenchyma at each location. This technique allows adequate local anesthesia without a significant risk of systemic absorption of injected lidocaine.

Biopsy Technique

For prostate biopsy, an 18 G needle loaded in a spring-action automated biopsy device is commonly used. When the trigger button of this device is pushed, the inner needle advances 23 mm first, followed by the outer, hollow-core needle. The prostate tissue is caught between the inner and outer needle and is, therefore, automatically disengaged from the prostate gland. This needle biopsy device is designed to obtain approximately 15 through 17 mm of tissue from the tip of the needle before the activation (Fig. 9.1).

Many urologists, both in academic and community practice, utilize an extended sextant biopsy technique, obtaining two specimens from each sextant, which results in a 12 core sample acquisition (21,22). At UCSF, in addition to extended sextant biopsies, a pair of samples along the anterior capsule of the apex/mid gland is routinely taken (Fig. 9.2). Lesion-directed biopsies are routinely performed as well. Using such a scheme, the cancer detection rate at UCSF and most other centers approximates 44%. Biopsy results which are stratified according to serum prostate-specific antigen (PSA) ranges are shown in Table 9.1. Extended-pattern biopsy techniques are associated with improved cancer detection rates compared to the previously standard, sextant (6 core) technique (21).

Repeat Biopsy

With conventional transrectal ultrasound technology, sampling errors are inevitable and a negative biopsy does not rule out malignancy with certainty. The management of the patient with repeatedly negative prostate biopsies and clinical characteristics suggestive of cancer, such as an elevated PSA or abnormal digital rectal exam, remains a challenging problem for physicians and patients. Repeat prostate biopsies will detect cancer in 16–41% of cases in which an initial biopsy was negative (21). At UCSF, Shinohara et al. attempted to identify predictors of positive biopsy in order to be able to avoid unnecessary biopsy procedures in patients at low risk for malignancy, studying 325 men with a history of two or more negative biopsies. The mean age of this patient population was 61 years, and the patients had a mean serum PSA of 13.8. The repeat, positive biopsy rate

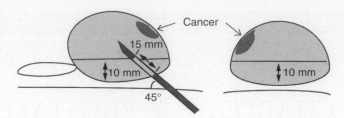

FIGURE 9.2. Illustration of failure to sample the apices of the prostate during needle biopsy. As the biopsy needle is inserted almost 45° from the rectal wall, the commonly performed "apex biopsy" spares significant amount of apico-anterior tissue since apico-anterior tissue is always spared by routine sextant biopsy. It is also critically important to note that because the needle removes only 15 through 17 mm of tissue for analysis, this approach would fail to sample the anterior horn of the prostate.

in these patients was 38%. The percentage of patients with a positive biopsy decreased as the number of previous negative biopsies increased: 40% in patients with two or three prior negative biopsies, 36% in patients with four or five prior negative biopsies, and 17% in patients with six prior negative biopsies. Using a Cox proportional hazards model, predictors of positive biopsy were identified including higher serum PSA, increased age, hypoechoic lesions on an ultrasound, and a smaller prostate. Interestingly, abnormal pathology [prostatic intraepithelial neoplasia (PIN), atypical small acinar proliferation (ASAP)] on previous biopsy, abnormal digital rectal exam, and transition zone volume were not significant predictors of a positive biopsy (unpublished data).

Repeat Biopsy Technique

When performing repeat biopsy, the standard parasagittal loci, lateral mid-prostate and base, anterior apex, and transition zones should be sampled. In addition, additional needle biopsies should be obtained from the site of any initial high-grade prostatic intraepithelial neoplasia (HGPIN) or ASAP, as well as any suspicious lesions seen on ultrasonography. The most common areas missed on initial biopsy are at the apices as well as in the anterior prostate (Fig. 9.2 illustrates missed anterior lesions). Takashima et al. carefully examined radical prostatectomy specimens from 62 T1c cancer patients and reported that T1c cancer is densely located at the apex to the mid-portion in the anterior half of the gland (23). Meng et al. reported that adding anterior apical biopsies to the extended sextant biopsy scheme increased cancer detection, especially in patients with a normal digital rectal examination (24). In those undergoing repeat biopsy, additional biopsies should be directed to areas not previously sampled, such as the very apex, very lateral edges, mid-line, and along the anterior capsule. Recently a series of TRUS guided transperineal template prostate biopsies showed significant apico-anterior cancer detection in patients with a normal digital rectal examination (25). Therefore, a transperineal approach is favored by some for secondary/repeat biopsies.

Strategy for HGPIN and Atypical Small Acinar Proliferation

HGPIN is found on a varying but significant fraction of prostate biopsies (1%–25%), with most modern series having an average of 5% (26). PIN is characterized by architecturally benign prostate acini which are lined by cytologically atypical cells. HGPIN may be a precursor lesion to adenocarcinoma (27,28). The discovery of HGPIN on first prostate biopsy usually

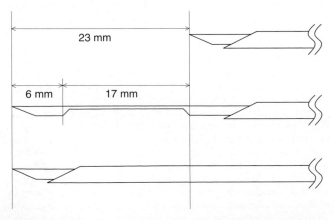

FIGURE 9.1. Diagram of automated 18 G needle for prostate biopsy. After pushing trigger button, inner needle advances 23 mm (**middle**) followed by outer needle advancing the same length (**bottom**). It is designed to take 15 through 17 mm tissue cores from the tip of the needle (**top**).

TABLE 9.1

RECENT BIOPSY RESULTS WITH EXTENDED PLUS 2 ANTERIOR BIOPSY SCHEME AT UCSF

PSA Range (ng/mL)	Total No. Pts.	Pts. with Cancer, No. (%)	Pts. with ASAP[a], No. (%)	Pts. with HGPIN[b], No. (%)
2.5–3.9	60	25 (41.7)	1 (1.7)	2 (3.3)
4.0–9.9	613	254 (41.4)	22 (3.6)	11 (1.8)
10–19.9	263	120 (45.6)	9 (3.4)	7 (2.7)
≥20	96	60 (62.5)	1 (1.0)	1 (1.0)
Total	1032	459 (44.4)	33 (3.2)	21 (2.0)

Pts, patients.
[a]Atypical small acinar proliferation.
[b]High-grade prostatic intraepithelial hyperplasia.

prompts repeat prostate biopsy in 3 to 6 months. Published series of those with HGPIN who undergo repeat biopsies show a cancer detection rate of 30% to 50%. However, Lefkowitz et al. reported that with extended biopsy schemes showing HGPIN, repeat biopsy showed cancer in only 2.3% of cases. They recommended that immediate repeat biopsy is not necessary after 12 core biopsies showing HGPIN.

ASAP, which has also previously been termed atypical adenomatous hyperplasia or atypia, is characterized by the crowding and proliferation of small glands; however, cytologic atypia is minimal (29). This lesion has been less well characterized than HGPIN, but ASAP alone is identified in 5% of patients undergoing needle biopsy. Iczkowski et al. proposed further classification of this lesion into three categories (favor benign, uncertain, and favor malignant) and suggest correlation of each category to subsequent cancer detection (30). Importantly, the association of ASAP with prostate cancer is higher than that of HGPIN. Contemporary biopsy series looking at the influence of ASAP have shown the probability of detecting adenocarcinoma on repeat biopsy is 40% to 50%. Having both HGPIN and atypia together on the first biopsy may increase the rate of cancer detection on the second biopsy to as high as 75% (31). In one study by Park et al. between 1991 and 1998, 45 men with atypia underwent re-biopsy and 23 of the 45 men (51%) were found to have cancer. Ninety-one percent of these patients had a positive biopsy for cancer on their repeat biopsy, while 9% required two or more biopsy sessions (32).

Cancer is more likely to be detected in the sextant where HGPIN or ASAP was found.

Role of Saturation Biopsy

Extensive or "saturation" biopsy has been recommended by some investigators to maximize cancer detection rates in patients with clinical criteria that put them at high risk for prostate cancer despite a previous benign biopsy. This type of biopsy scheme has been performed in the office using periprostatic block, with intravenous sedation, or in the outpatient surgery center with general or spinal anesthetic (33–35). While most of the saturation biopsy protocols are done transrectally, there are also reports of transperineal saturation biopsy (36). Generally, irrespective of the anesthetic used, these saturation biopsy protocols obtain 22 to 24 cores per patient. Borboroglu et al. found 17 of 57 men (30%) of their cohort had adenocarcinoma identified using a 6-region, saturation-biopsy pattern (34). Interestingly, 41% of these men had only one positive biopsy core, while 11% of patients developed urinary retention. Stewart et al. used a radial biopsy

pattern separated by 20° to 30° and found a similar detection rate of 34% in 224 patients. The overall complication rate was 12%, which included 5% of men requiring hospitalization for hematuria (35). Finally, Rabets et al. recently published a 29% overall positive biopsy rate in 116 consecutive patients who underwent 24 core saturation biopsy regimens in the office after previous negative biopsies (37). This 29% to 34% rate of cancer detection is similar to repeat, extended (10 or 12 core) prostate biopsy, which is generally accomplished with less morbidity. As extended pattern biopsy schemes become the standard of care for initial prostate biopsy, the need for secondary biopsies, by any technique, will be reduced.

Complications

Transrectal prostate biopsies can be associated with a number of complications. These include minor complications such as hematuria, hematospermia, and discomfort during the exam, which are frequently seen and generally self-limiting. Rodriguez et al. reported that in 128 patients followed prospectively, 71% experienced immediate hematuria, and in 47%, persistent hematuria, usually quite limited, was seen for up to 3 to 7 days after transrectal prostate biopsy (38). Other published rates of hematuria range between 13% and 58%. In 70% of cases, hematuria resolves within 48 hours of biopsy (39,40). Hematospermia rates range between 9% and 36% and can last up to several months (39,41).

Seeding of prostate cancer via the needle biopsy tract is rare, although it has been reported in the literature. Since its first description in 1953, more than 20 cases of tumor seeding have been published (42–56). Reported incidences based on retrospective studies have ranged from 0.15% (46) to 2% (42). The majority of these cases have been reported as perineal tumor seeding after transperineal needle biopsy, even up to 14 years after biopsy (55). Bastacky et al. reported a 2% rate of tumor seeding, and 6 of 7 cases were secondary to transrectal biopsy needle tracks (42). Similarly, Koppie et al. reported two patients who presented with recurrence of tumor at the rectal wall after transrectal biopsy (57). Hara et al. studied circulating PSA-specific mRNA by reverse transcriptase polymerase chain reaction (RT-PCR) technique before and after prostate biopsy. After biopsy, PSA-specific mRNA was found in 25.8% of cases with a negative biopsy and 45.7% of cases with a positive biopsy. This study indicated that prostate biopsy may disseminate prostate cells into the circulation. However, the risk of developing metastatic disease due to biopsy appears to be small. While the mechanism of such seeding is unknown, it has been proposed that seeding depends on at least three tumor factors: (a) cytokine characteristics, including adhesion, cohesion, and intercellular junction of tumor cells, (b) the "fertility" of the tissue in which tumor cells are seeded, and (c) the number of seeded cells, which in turn depends on needle size and the amount of stromal cells present in the tumor (43). Perineal recurrence is associated with a poor prognosis (54), whereas cases of transrectal needle tract seeding have responded to modalities such as hormone ablation therapy and external beam radiation (57).

Historically, transrectal prostate biopsy has been associated with extremely high rates of infectious complications. In 1982, Thompson et al. reported that without prophylactic antibiotics, 100% of patients develop bacteremia and 87% show laboratory evidence of urinary tract infection (58). The same group showed that bacteria found in the blood and urine following transrectal biopsy covered a broad range of microbes, including aerobic Gram-positive and Gram-negative organisms, as well as anaerobic flora (59). With an enema alone, 44% of patients may develop bacteriuria, and 16% bacteremia (14).

In 1982, Crawford et al. published a randomized control double blind study of 63 patients establishing the effectiveness of prophylactic antibiotics in preventing urinary tract infection and sepsis. Using 2 days of carbenicillin, the study group showed a decrease in positive urine cultures from 36% to 9%. Similarly, fever was reduced from 48% to 17%. Three patients in the placebo group developed Gram-negative sepsis, whereas one patient in the treatment group developed sepsis (12). Similarly, Ruebush et al. performed a double blind comparison of trimethoprim-sulfamethoxazole for prophylaxis after tranrectal prostate biopsy. They found no change in the frequency of fever or bacteremia (18% and 70%, respectively) but they did find a reduction of bacteriuria from 21% to 0% (60). Since that time, the use of prophylactic antibiotics has become the standard of care. Looking at 4303 patients given a 5-day course of prophylactic ciprofloxacin, Berger et al. identified fever (defined at temperature >38.5°C) in only 0.8% (41). Similarly, Desmond et al. reported a fever incidence of 0.6% in 670 patients given 1 to 3 days of ciprofloxacin prophylaxis (61). Rates of urinary tract infection following transrectal prostate biopsy are in the range of 0.7% to 4% (40,62,63).

Rectal bleeding can occur in 2% to 8% of patients (38,41, 64). Mild bleeding may occur more frequently. Most of the time, bleeding is mild and stops spontaneously or responds well to digitally applied perineal or rectal pressure. However, there have been reports of severe bleeding that requires further intervention. Maatman et al. described the effective use of a tampon inserted into the rectum for 30 to 60 minutes, which prevented the need for further intervention in cases of rectal bleeding refractory to digitally applied pressure (65). Brullet et al. described five patients representing 1% of their 550 consecutive patients undergoing TRUS-guided prostate biopsy who presented with rectal bleeding and symptoms of hypovolemia. These patients were effectively treated with emergency colonoscopy and endoscopic injection of epinephrine and polidocanol, which resulted in permanent hemostasis in all 5 cases (66). Only one case of a clinically significant pelvic hematoma has been reported to date (67).

UTILITY OF TRANSRECTAL ULTRASOUND AND PROSTATE BIOPSY IN ACTIVE SURVEILLANCE ("WATCHFUL WAITING") PATIENTS

An emerging cohort of patients are those with a diagnosis of low-grade, low-stage prostate cancer who are being placed on active surveillance regimens with selective, delayed definitive therapy. A small group of studies has reported on different methods for monitoring such patients with serial PSA measurements, but also for performing regular transrectal ultrasound imaging of the prostate and prostate biopsy. Hruby et al. reported on the use of serial semi-annual transrectal ultrasonography in a "watchful waiting" cohort followed at the University of Toronto (68). In this program, 180 men were prospectively enrolled, of whom 136 had 2 or more serial TRUS studies. Changes in gland volume and the number of hypoechoic lesions were examined. In the entire cohort, 28 men were found to have progressive disease. In these 28 patients, TRUS progression was defined as a new or enlarging hypochoic peripheral zone nodule or a documented increase in gland volume of 30% or greater at the time of progression. Only 7 of 28 (25%) patients had progression based on TRUS, and all but one were found to have a growth of an existing nodule or the development of a new nodule. Six of 28 (21%) men were found to have progression on the basis of cancer grade.

PROSTATE BIOPSY AS A PREDICTOR OF OUTCOME FOLLOWING TREATMENT

McNeal first suggested in 1969 that malignant behavior of prostate cancer is tightly correlated with the volume of the primary tumor (69). Clinical understaging is not uncommon (70). Understaging and undergrading are less common with extended pattern biopsies (71–73). Better preoperative assessment of tumor volume and stage would guide more appropriate therapy and, hopefully, better outcomes. Each element of prostate biopsy (such as number of positive cores and volume of cancer in each core) may give important clinical and prognostic information. However, no single method of tumor quantification has emerged as the best predictor of outcome (74).

Number or Percentage of Positive Cores and Treatment Failure

The most commonly used tumor quantification method is the assessment of the number of positive cores, or the percentage of positive cores. Numerous studies have shown a correlation between the number of positive biopsies and tumor characteristics, including extracapsular extension (ECE) of prostate cancer, tumor volume, stage, seminal vesicle invasion, surgical margin status, and lymph node metastases (75–78). Holland et al. found that the number of positive sextant biopsies was a predictor of ECE and positive surgical margins (79). Patients with negative margins had an average of 2.3 positive biopsies, while patients with positive margins had an average of 3.5 biopsies. A correlation between percentage of positive cores and disease recurrence in intermediate- and high-risk patients has been shown. D'Amico et al. studied a cohort of 960 patients with intermediate risk characteristics and sextant biopsies undergoing radical prostatectomy, and first showed that tumors involving 1 or 2 cores (<34% of cores) were associated with a better outcome than those with 4 to 6 cores (>67% of cores) (80). This study, with a mean follow-up time of 46 months, showed men with <34% cores had a 86% biochemical control rate, versus an 11% biochemical control rate for men with >67% cores. UCSF investigators showed that for patients with a high risk of cancer using modified D'Amico risk criteria, the likelihood of disease recurrence 5 years after surgery was 24%, 34%, and 59% for patients with 0% to 33%, 33% to 66%, and >66% positive biopsies, respectively (81).

Grossklaus et al. have reported that the percentage of biopsy tissue with cancer was an excellent predictor of pathologic stage and of tumor volume (82). In this study of 135 men undergoing radical prostatectomy, an increasing percentage of tumor in the biopsy and bilateral positive cores was associated with increased risk of ECE ($P <.01$). Makhlouf et al. examined the effect of sampling more cores on the predictive accuracy of pathologic grade in the final prostate specimen (73). This study looked at 75 consecutive patients undergoing radical prostatectomy who had undergone either traditional sextant or ≥ 8 biopsy core sampling. They found that 58% of the patients who underwent sextant biopsy scores had their final pathologic grade changed after prostatectomy versus 29% of the patients in the ≥ 8 biopsy core group, which was statistically significant. In summary, needle biopsy with an appropriate number of cores does help to predict stage and grade, albeit not with complete certainty.

Utility of Individual Core Samples

Traditionally, many urologists obtain needle biopsies and bunch them as left-side and right-side specimens, without discriminating between the apical, mid, and base regions of the prostate. This is done because submission of needle biopsy specimens in separate containers adds significantly to pathology charges. Nelson et al. have shown that the greatest percentage of a single biopsy core involved by cancer is highly predictive of PSA-free survival (83). Badalament et al. studied the location of positive biopsy cores (apex vs. base) in 210 patients and found significant differences in positive margin rates if the biopsy was positive at the base (6% positive margin) versus at the apex (22% positive margin) (75). However, other groups specifically looking at apical biopsies have concluded that individual core labeling may have a low positive predictive value for a positive apical margin (84,85). At UCSF, our practice pattern is to label cores separately, as the location of a positive biopsy appears to correlate with the risk of ECE at that site (86).

Tumor Length in Core Biopsies/Percentage of Cancer in Each Core

The amount of prostate cancer in each core can be measured with a micrometer along the long axis of each core. There continues to be some disagreement in the literature about the significance of total tumor length. Recently, Naya et al. reviewed 430 patients who underwent radical prostatectomy in the PSA era for whom biopsy information was present (87). In this study, a number of factors predicted for extracapsular extension. A tumor length of 7 mm or greater was the strongest predictor of extraprostatic extension at the neurovascular bundle/posterolateral region on a given side ($P <.0001$), followed by a positive basal core location. If patients with 1 positive biopsy core with a tumor length of 7 mm or greater were excluded, the risk of extraprostatic extension at the ipsilateral neurovascular bundle was only 10%. Again, this does require needle biopsies to be individually analyzed. However, in an earlier cohort of patients, Bruce et al. found that approximately 25% of patients with <2 mm of tumor in the biopsy specimen had extraprostatic disease at the time of radical prostatectomy. It should be noted that the majority of patients in this study had less than six core biopsies, so it is likely the prostate gland was undersampled. Freedland et al. have reported that the percentage of biopsy tissue with cancer was the strongest independent predictor of biochemical recurrence after radical prostatectomy (88). These authors divided percent biopsy tissue with cancer into less than 20%, 20% through 55%, and greater than 55% categories. Interestingly,

patients with intermediate risk profiles based on PSA and biopsy Gleason score, but with cancer involving <20% of core tissue, had biochemical recurrence rates similar to patients who were in the low-risk category on the basis of PSA and Gleason score. Further, patients who were in the intermediate risk group but who had cancer involving >55% of the sample had PSA failure rates similar to patients in the high-risk category. One potential limitation of the study was the short follow-up, with a median of 28 months.

ADJUNCTIVE TECHNIQUES TO INCREASE DETECTION OF PROSTATE CANCER

Color Doppler

Color Doppler was first described in 1993 as a potential means of differentiating malignant tissue from benign growth. It interprets reflected sound as a measure of blood flow in prostatic vessels. This takes advantage of the hypervascular nature of malignant prostatic tissue to visualize vascular flow. Increased angiogenesis in prostate cancer tissue results in higher microvessel density when compared to that of benign tissue (89). Initial studies indicated that color Doppler could be used to identify cancers such as isoechoic, hypervascular tumors that are not visible using conventional gray-scale ultrasound. Prostate cancer can appear isoechoic to benign tissue on gray-scale ultrasound in 40% of cases (90).

However, the data supporting the routine use of color Doppler is not conclusive. Cornud et al. found that in 94 patients with T1c prostate cancer who were treated with radical prostatectomy, ECE and seminal vesicle invasion (SVI) were present more often in tumors identified by color Doppler than in those which were not visualized. However, this study did not compare color Doppler to conventional gray-scale ultrasound for staging purposes (91). Roy et al. evaluated 85 patients with gray-scale and color Doppler, including the use of ultrasound contrast made of galactose-based air microbubbles. The addition of contrast to color Doppler increased the sensitivity and specificity of color Doppler from 54% and 79% to 93% and 87%, respectively (92). Similarly, Frauscher et al. found that the use of contrast in color Doppler increased detection of prostate cancer by 2.6 times when compared to conventional gray-scale, ultrasound-guided biopsy. Other studies have shown that even when predictors of pathologic stage such as Gleason grade are controlled for, color Doppler may detect more prostate cancers (93–95).

Reasons accounting for color Doppler's potential inability to identify some prostate cancers may include the presence of factors such as prostatitis that can increase prostatic blood flow, or the fact that low-grade tumors demonstrate lower blood flows. However, Arger et al. found that pathologic categories of prostate cancer types did not correlate well with different levels of vascularity (96). Interestingly, there may be a future role for color Doppler in predicting behavior and aggressiveness of cancer, Gleason grade and rate of relapse, response to hormone treatment, and invasion of the neurovascular bundle (97–99). Additional studies refining the use of color Doppler are necessary before this technique can be established as a reliable means of staging and identifying prostate cancer (100).

Power Doppler

Power Doppler imaging (PDI) makes use of detecting and amplifying small differences between blood flow in different vessels,

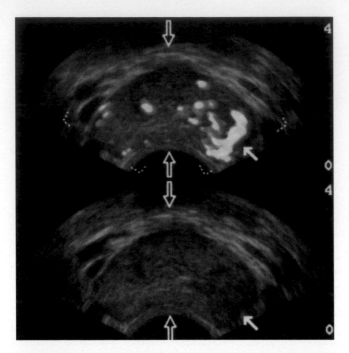

FIGURE 9.3. Comparison of traditional TRUS versus power Doppler ultrasonography of the prostate. The patient is a 63-year-old man with an elevated PSA and abnormal left-side prostate exam. The bottom panel shows traditional gray-scale ultrasonographic image of the prostate and the top panel shows the power Doppler image of the same area. The hypervascular areas corresponded well to geographically directed biopsies, which showed the extent of prostate cancer to be greater than that detected by conventional gray-scale ultrasound. (See color insert.)

allowing imaging of very small tumor vessels (Fig. 9.3) (101). This results in a sensitivity that is three to four times that of color Doppler alone (102). Okihara et al. reported a sensitivity of 98% and a negative predictive value (NPV) of 98%, significantly higher than that of gray-scale ultrasound for visualization of prostate cancer. However, in their study, the positive predictive value (PPV) was 59%, equivalent to that of gray-scale ultrasound (103).

PDI also allows for three-dimensional reconstruction of blood flow, and Sauvain et al. reported about 323 patients where power Doppler with 3-D reconstruction yielded a sensitivity of 92% and a specificity of 72% for detecting prostate cancer, slightly better than the sensitivity and specificity of gray-scale ultrasound, which were 88% and 58%, respectively. In this study, the presence of vasculature crossing the prostate capsule could be identified, and the authors concluded that this may be a means to use power Doppler with 3-D reconstruction for cancer staging (104).

MRI/MRS to Image Cancer and Guide Prostate Biopsy

Magnetic resonance imaging (MRI) can be used to identify prostate cancer both locally and regionally. Endorectal MRI can be performed by placing a magnetic coil in the rectum, which allows improved visualization of prostatic zonal anatomy and an improved delineation of tumor location, volume, and stage. Patients are imaged in a whole-body scanner using a pelvic phased-array coil combined with an inflatable, balloon-covered endorectal surface coil positioned in the rectum. A full evaluation requires the use of both T1- and T2-weighted images. On T1 images, the prostate appears homogenous, and on T2 images, areas of cancer appear as lower-intensity zones

surrounded by normal areas of higher intensity. Additionally, MRI imaging often allows for visualization of the prostate capsule. Postbiopsy hemorrhage can appear as high-intensity areas on T1-weighted images, and this can make the distinction between normal and cancerous tissue more difficult.

Wide ranges of sensitivity and specificity in detecting ECE and SVI have been reported in the literature. For ECE, sensitivity has been reported as ranging between 13% and 95%, and specificity between 49% and 97%. For SVI, sensitivity ranges between 20% and 95%, and specificity ranges between 82% and 98% (105–113). Careful selection of patients may increase the utility of MRI for staging. For example, Cornud et al. found that MRI alone yielded a specificity of 95% and a sensitivity of 50% to 69% for detecting pT3 disease in 336 high-risk patients, as defined by more than three positive cores on sextant biopsy, positive digital rectal examination (DRE), and PSA >10 ng/mL (114). Providing MRI readers with clinical data also likely plays a role in accurate interpretation of images. Dhingsa et al. demonstrated that providing blinded readers with clinical data improved tumor detection from 27% to 37% (115). There are no current data which suggest the routine use of MRI for assessment and staging of prostate cancer, though its use may become more frequent as radiologists become more experienced in its use, and availability and cost improve over time.

Magnetic resonance spectroscopy (MRS) has also been used with MRI to increase the accuracy of radiographic assessment. MRS detects metabolic activity of tissues and can differentiate normal from cancerous tissues based on ratios of creatine, choline, and citrate production and consumption (116). Cancerous tissue has been associated with lower citrate levels and higher levels of choline and creatine when compared to that of tissue containing BPH or normal prostate (117). With refinement in resolution, MRS may help to improve intraobserver variability and increase accuracy of staging (118). The conjunctive use of MRI and MRS may also help to predict for a higher grade of cancer, with early image enhancement potentially being indicative of more aggressive, poorly differentiated tumors (119). There may also be a role for combined MRI/MRS in preoperative selection and treatment planning for patients undergoing brachytherapy (120).

At UCSF, the utility of adjunctive MRI/MRS to predict prostate cancer detection in patients with previous negative prostate biopsies has been recently studied. Fifty-six patients who underwent at least two prior transrectal ultrasound-guided needle biopsy sessions underwent endorectal MRI/MRS. Following that, a repeat TRUS needle biopsy was performed with systemic random biopsy and additional cores taken at abnormal MRI/MRS areas. In this group, 22 of 59 (39%) patients were diagnosed with cancer. When compared to a contemporary cohort of 269 patients with a similar negative biopsy history who did not undergo MRI/MRS, the positive biopsy rate was not statistically different [22 of 56 (39%) vs. 102 of 269 (38%), P = .968]. The sensitivity, specificity, positive predictive value, and negative predictive value of MRI/MRS in this setting were 95%, 18%, 43%, and 86%, respectively. MRI/MRS predicted the correct location of the tumor in 17 of 22 (77%) patients. Similar results have been subsequently reported by others (121). In summary, these data continue to show that men with a history of multiple negative biopsies still have a significant risk for harboring prostate cancer. MRI is sensitive in detecting prostate cancer, but the lack of specificity, along with cost, limits its utility in prostate cancer detection in patients with prior negative biopsies.

D'Amico et al. first reported the use of MR-guided transperineal prostate biopsies on a single patient in 2000 (122,123). In these reports, they were able to use abnormal MRI findings to direct the prostate biopsy and detect cancer. Recently, Coleman et al. from the National Cancer Institute (NCI) reported their limited experience with transrectal MRI directed biopsies in two patients (124). No complications were noted and the targeted tissue of interest was obtained with a core needle biopsy. MR guidance has also been used in conjunction with TRUS (MRI-ultrasound image fusion process) to highlight abnormal regions of the prostate for biopsy (125).

SUMMARY AND THE FUTURE OF PROSTATE BIOPSY

Current biopsy technique, including the use of extended-pattern biopsy schemes, use of antibiotics, and local anesthetic techniques, allows for reasonably efficient and safe detection of prostate cancer as well as providing important prognostic information on which treatment decisions can be made. The roles of more advanced imaging techniques such as MRI/MRSI or power Doppler still needs to be defined. However, the procedure still is not optimally efficient and can be associated with significant costs and side effects. The development and validation of newer imaging techniques and/or serum or tissue-based markers could lead to significant refinements in prostate cancer detection, obviating the need for current biopsy techniques.

ACKNOWLEDGMENTS

This research is supported by NIH 5P50CA089520-02 UCSF Prostate Cancer SPORE (Specialized Program of Research Excellence).

References

1. Ferguson RS. Prostatic neoplasms: their diagnosis by needle puncture and aspiration. *Am J Surg* 1930;9:507–511.
2. Astraldi A. Diagnosis of cancer of the prostate: biopsy by rectal route. *Urol Cutaneous Rev* 1937;41.421.
3. Wild J, Reid J. Fourth Annual Conference in Ultrasound Therapy, 1955.
4. Watanabe H, Kato H, Kato T, et al. Diagnostic application of ultrasonotomography to the prostate. *Nippon Hinyokika Gakkai Zasshi* 1968;59:273–279.
5. Lee F, Torp-Pedersen ST, Carroll JT, et al. Use of transrectal ultrasound and prostate-specific antigen in diagnosis of prostatic intraepithelial neoplasia. *Urology* 1989;34:4–8.
6. Hodge KK, McNeal JE, Terris MK, et al. Random systematic versus directed ultrasound guided transrectal core biopsies of the prostate. *J Urol* 1989;142:71–74; discussion 74–75.
7. Stamey TA. Making the most out of six systematic sextant biopsies. *Urology* 1995;45:2–12.
8. Freedland SJ, Amling CL, Terris MK, et al. Is there a difference in outcome after radical prostatectomy between patients with biopsy Gleason sums 4, 5, and 6? Results from the SEARCH database. *Prostate Cancer Prostatic Dis* 2003;6:261–265.
9. Freiha FS, McNeal JE, Stamey TA. Selection criteria for radical prostatectomy based on morphometric studies in prostate carcinoma. *NCI Monogr* 1988;7:107–108.
10. Torp-Pedersen S, Lee F, Littrup PJ, et al. Transrectal biopsy of the prostate guided with transrectal US: longitudinal and multiplanar scanning. *Radiology* 1989;170:23–27.
11. Lee F, Torp-Pedersen ST, Siders DB, et al. Transrectal ultrasound in the diagnosis and staging of prostatic carcinoma. *Radiology* 1989;170:609–615.
12. Crawford ED, Haynes AL Jr, Story MW, et al. Prevention of urinary tract infection and sepsis following transrectal prostatic biopsy. *J Urol* 1982;127:449–451.
13. Dajani AS, Taubert KA, Wilson W, et al. Prevention of bacterial endocarditis. Recommendations by the American Heart Association. *JAMA* 1997;277:1794–1801.
14. Lindert KA, Kabalin JN, Terris MK. Bacteremia and bacteriuria after transrectal ultrasound guided prostate biopsy. *J Urol* 2000;164:76–80.
15. Nijs HG, Essink-Bot ML, DeKoning HJ, et al. Why do men refuse or attend population-based screening for prostate cancer? *J Public Health Med* 2000;22:312–316.
16. Nash PA, Bruce JE, Indudhara R, et al. Transrectal ultrasound guided prostatic nerve blockade eases systematic needle biopsy of the prostate. *J Urol* 1996;155:607–609.
17. Walsh K, O'Brien T, Salemmi A, et al. A randomised trial of periprostatic local anaesthetic for transrectal biopsy. *Prostate Cancer Prostatic Dis* 2003;6:242–244.
18. Obek C, Ozkan B, Tunc B, et al. Comparison of 3 different methods of anesthesia before transrectal prostate biopsy: a prospective randomized trial. *J Urol* 2004;172:502–505.
19. Haq A, Patel HR, Habib MR, et al. Diclofenac suppository analgesia for transrectal ultrasound guided biopsies of the prostate: a double-blind, randomized controlled trial. *J Urol* 2004;171:1489–1491.
20. Ozveri H, Cevik I, Dillioglugil O, et al. Transrectal periprostatic lidocaine injection anesthesia for transrectal prostate biopsy: a prospective study. *Prostate Cancer Prostatic Dis* 2003;6:311–314.
21. Presti JC Jr. Prostate biopsy: how many cores are enough? *Urol Oncol* 2003;21:135–140.
22. Presti JC Jr, O'Dowd GJ, Miller MC, et al. Extended peripheral zone biopsy schemes increase cancer detection rates and minimize variance in prostate specific antigen and age related cancer rates: results of a community multi-practice study. *J Urol* 2003;169:125–129.
23. Takashima R, Egawa S, Kuwao S, et al. Anterior distribution of Stage T1c nonpalpable tumors in radical prostatectomy specimens. *Urology* 2002;59:692–697.
24. Meng MV, Franks JH, Presti JC Jr, et al. The utility of apical anterior horn biopsies in prostate cancer detection. *Urol Oncol* 2003;21:361–365.
25. Kawakami S, Kihara K, Fujii Y, et al. Transrectal ultrasound-guided transperineal 14-core systematic biopsy detects apico-anterior cancer foci of T1c prostate cancer. *Int J Urol* 2004;11:613–618.
26. Meng MV, Shinohara K, Grossfeld GD. Significance of high-grade prostatic intraepithelial neoplasia on prostate biopsy. *Urol Oncol* 2003;21:145–151.
27. Oyasu R, Bahnson RR, Nowels K, et al. Cytological atypia in the prostate gland: frequency, distribution and possible relevance to carcinoma. *J Urol* 1986;135:959–962.
28. Prange W, Erbersdobler A, Hammerer P, et al. Significance of high grade prostatic intraepithelial neoplasia in needle biopsy specimens. *Urology* 2001;57:486–490.
29. Helpap BG, Bostwick DG, Montironi R. The significance of atypical adenomatous hyperplasia and prostatic intraepithelial neoplasia for the development of prostate carcinoma. An update. *Virchows Arch* 1995;426:425–434.
30. Iczkowski KA, MacLennan GT, Bostwick DG. Atypical small acinar proliferation suspicious for malignancy in prostate needle biopsies: clinical significance in 33 cases. *Am J Surg Pathol* 1997;21:1489–1495.
31. Alsikafi NF, Brendler CB, Gerber GS, et al. High-grade prostatic intraepithelial neoplasia with adjacent atypia is associated with a higher incidence of cancer on subsequent needle biopsy than high-grade prostatic intraepithelial neoplasia alone. *Urology* 2001;57:296–300.
32. Park S, Shinohara K, Grossfeld GD, et al. Prostate cancer detection in men with prior high grade prostatic intraepithelial neoplasia or atypical prostate biopsy. *J Urol* 2001;165:1409–1414.
33. Jones JS, Oder M, Zippe CD. Saturation prostate biopsy with periprostatic block can be performed in office. *J Urol* 2002;168:2108–2110.
34. Borboroglu PG, Comer SW, Riffenburgh RH, et al. Extensive repeat transrectal ultrasound guided prostate biopsy in patients with previous benign sextant biopsies. *J Urol* 2000;163:158–162.
35. Stewart CS, Leibovich BC, Weaver AL, et al. Prostate cancer diagnosis using a saturation needle biopsy technique after previous negative sextant biopsies. *J Urol* 2001;166:86–91; discussion 91–92.
36. Bott SR, Henderson A, McLarty E, et al. A brachytherapy template approach to standardize saturation prostatic biopsy. *BJU Int* 2004;93:629–630.
37. Rabets JC, Jones JS, Patel A, et al. Prostate cancer detection with office based saturation biopsy in a repeat biopsy population. *J Urol* 2004;172:94–97.
38. Rodriguez LV, Terris MK. Risks and complications of transrectal ultrasound guided prostate needle biopsy: a prospective study and review of the literature. *J Urol* 1998;160:2115–2120.
39. Beerlage HP, de Reijke TM, de la, Rosette JJ, et al. Considerations regarding prostate biopsies. *Eur Urol* 1998;34:303–312.
40. Webb JA, Shanmuganathan K, McLean A. Complications of ultrasound-guided transperineal prostate biopsy. A prospective study. *Br J Urol* 1993;72:775–777.
41. Berger AP, Gozzi C, Steiner H, et al. Complication rate of transrectal ultrasound guided prostate biopsy: a comparison among 3 protocols with 6, 10 and 15 cores. *J Urol* 2004;171:1478–1480; discussion 1480–1481.
42. Bastacky SS, Walsh PC, Epstein JI. Needle biopsy associated tumor tracking of adenocarcinoma of the prostate. *J Urol* 1991;145:1003–1007.
43. Haddad FS, Somsin AA. Seeding and perineal implantation of prostatic cancer in the track of the biopsy needle: three case reports and a review of the literature. *J Surg Oncol* 1987;35:184–191.
44. Addonizio JC, Kapoor SN. Perineal seeding of prostatic carcinoma after needle biopsy. *Urology* 1976;8:513–515.
45. Brausi M, Latini A, Palladini PD. Local seeding of anaplastic carcinoma of prostate after needle biopsy. *Urology* 1986;27:63–64.
46. Burkholder GV, Kaufman JJ. Local implantation of carcinoma of the prostate with percutaneous needle biopsy. *J Urol* 1966;95:801–804.

47. Clarke BG, Leadbetter WF, Campbell JS. Implantation of cancer of the prostate in site of perineal needle biopsy: report of a case. *J Urol* 1953;70: 937–939.

48. Desai SG, Woodruff LM. Carcinoma of prostate. Local extension following perineal needle biopsy. *Urology* 1974;3:87–88.

49. Emtage JB, Perez-Marrero R. Extension of carcinoma of prostate along perineal needle biopsy tract. *Urology* 1986;27:548–549.

50. Fortunoff S. Needle biopsy of the prostate: a review of 346 biopsies. *J Urol* 1962;87:159–163.

51. Goldman EJ, Samellas W. Local extension of carcinoma of the prostate following needle biopsy. *J Urol* 1960;84:575–576.

52. Labardini MM, Nesbit RM. Perineal extension of adenocarcinoma of the prostate gland after punch biopsy. *J Urol* 1967;97:891–893.

53. Puigvert A, Elizalde C, Matz JA. Perineal implantation of carcinoma of the prostate following needle biopsy: a case report. *J Urol* 1972;107:821–824.

54. Moul JW, Miles BJ, Skoog SJ, et al. Risk factors for perineal seeding of prostate cancer after needle biopsy. *J Urol* 1989;142:86–88.

55. Moul JW, Bauer JJ, Srivastava S, et al. Perineal seeding of prostate cancer as the only evidence of clinical recurrence 14 years after needle biopsy and radical prostatectomy: molecular correlation. *Urology* 1998;51:158–160.

56. Warden SS, Schellhammer PF, el-Mahdi A. Well differentiated carcinoma of the prostate seeding a perineal needle biopsy tract. *Br J Urol* 1984;56:436.

57. Koppie TM, Grady BP, Shinohara K. Rectal wall recurrence of prostatic adenocarcinoma. *J Urol* 2002;168:2120.

58. Thompson PM, Pryor JP, Williams JP, et al. The problem of infection after prostatic biopsy: the case for the transperineal approach. *Br J Urol* 1982;54:736–740.

59. Thompson PM, Talbot RW, Packham DA, et al. Transrectal biopsy of the prostate and bacteraemia. *Br J Surg* 1980;67:127–128.

60. Ruebush TK, McConville JH, Calia FM II. A double-blind study of trimethoprim-sulfamethoxazole prophylaxis in patients having transrectal needle biopsy of the prostate. *J Urol* 1979;122:492–494.

61. Desmond PM, Clark J, Thompson IM, et al. Morbidity with contemporary prostate biopsy. *J Urol* 1993;150:1425–1426.

62. Aus G, Hermansson CG, Hugosson J, et al. Transrectal ultrasound examination of the prostate: complications and acceptance by patients. *Br J Urol* 1993;71:457–459.

63. Collins GN, Lloyd SN, Hehir M, et al. Multiple transrectal ultrasound-guided prostatic biopsies—true morbidity and patient acceptance. *Br J Urol* 1993;71:460–463.

64. Pearlman CK. Transrectal biopsy of the prostate. *Trans West Sect Am Urol Assoc* 1955;22:125–130; discussion 130–131.

65. Maatman TJ, Bigham D, Stirling B. Simplified management of post-prostate biopsy rectal bleeding. *Urology* 2002;60:508.

66. Brullet E, Guevara MC, Campo R, et al. Massive rectal bleeding following transrectal ultrasound-guided prostate biopsy. *Endoscopy* 2000;32:792–795.

67. Seymour MA, Oesterling JE. Anterior rectal wall hematoma: complication of transrectal ultrasound-guided biopsy of prostate. *Urology* 1992;39: 177–181.

68. Hruby G, Choo R, Klotz L, et al. The role of serial transrectal ultrasonography in a 'watchful waiting' protocol for men with localized prostate cancer. *BJU Int* 2001;87:643–647.

69. McNeal JE. Origin and development of carcinoma in the prostate. *Cancer* 1969;23:24–34.

70. Javidan J, Wood DP. Clinical interpretation of the prostate biopsy. *Urol Oncol* 2003;21:141–144.

71. Grossfeld GD, Chang JJ, Broering JM, et al. Under staging and under grading in a contemporary series of patients undergoing radical prostatectomy: results from the Cancer of the Prostate Strategic Urologic Research Endeavor Database. *J Urol* 2001;165:851–856.

72. Grossklaus DJ, Coffey CS, Shappell SB, et al. Prediction of tumour volume and pathological stage in radical prostatectomy specimens is not improved by taking more prostate needle-biopsy cores. *BJU Int* 2001;88:722–726.

73. Makhlouf AA, Krupski TL, Kunkle D, et al. The effect of sampling more cores on the predictive accuracy of pathological grade and tumour distribution in the prostate biopsy. *BJU Int* 2004;93:271–274.

74. Epstein JI, Potter SR. The pathological interpretation and significance of prostate needle biopsy findings: implications and current controversies. *J Urol* 2001;166:402–410.

75. Badalament RA, Miller MC, Peller PA, et al. An algorithm for predicting nonorgan confined prostate cancer using the results obtained from sextant core biopsies with prostate specific antigen level. *J Urol* 1996;156: 1375–1380.

76. Borirakchanyavat S, Bhargava V, Shinohara K, et al. Systematic sextant biopsies in the prediction of extracapsular extension at radical prostatectomy. *Urology* 1997;50:373–378.

77. Wills ML, Sauvageot J, Partin AW, et al. Ability of sextant biopsies to predict radical prostatectomy stage. *Urology* 1998;51:759–764.

78. Ravery V, Boccon-Gibod LA, Dauge-Geffroy MC, et al. Systematic biopsies accurately predict extracapsular extension of prostate cancer and persistent/recurrent detectable PSA after radical prostatectomy. *Urology* 1994;44:371–376.

79. Huland H, Hammerer P, Henke RP, et al. Preoperative prediction of tumor heterogeneity and recurrence after radical prostatectomy for localized prostatic carcinoma with digital rectal examination, prostate specific antigen and the results of 6 systematic biopsies. *J Urol* 1996;155:1344–1347.

80. D'Amico AV, Whittington R, Malkowicz SB, et al. Clinical utility of the percentage of positive prostate biopsies in defining biochemical outcome after radical prostatectomy for patients with clinically localized prostate cancer. *J Clin Oncol* 2000;18:1164–1172.

81. Grossfeld GD, Latini DM, Lubeck DP, et al. Predicting disease recurrence in intermediate and high-risk patients undergoing radical prostatectomy using percent positive biopsies: results from CaPSURE. *Urology* 2002;59: 560–565.

82. Grossklaus DJ, Coffey CS, Shappell SB, et al. Percent of cancer in the biopsy set predicts pathological findings after prostatectomy. *J Urol* 2002;167: 2032–2035; discussion 2036.

83. Nelson CP, Rubin MA, Strawderman M, et al. Preoperative parameters for predicting early prostate cancer recurrence after radical prostatectomy. *Urology* 2002;59:740–745; discussion 745–746.

84. Taneja SS, Penson DF, Epelbaum A, et al. Does site specific labeling of sextant biopsy cores predict the site of extracapsular extension in radical prostatectomy surgical specimen? *J Urol* 1999;162:1352–1357; discussion 1357–1358.

85. Rogatsch H, Horninger W, Volgger H, et al. Radical prostatectomy: the value of preoperative, individually labeled apical biopsies. *J Urol* 2000; 164:754–757; discussion 757–758.

86. Elliott SP, Shinohara K, Logan SL, et al. Sextant prostate biopsies predict side and sextant site of extracapsular extension of prostate cancer. *J Urol* 2002;168:105–109.

87. Naya Y, Slaton JW, Troncoso P, et al. Tumor length and location of cancer on biopsy predict for side specific extraprostatic cancer extension. *J Urol* 2004;171:1093–1097.

88. Freedland SJ, Csathy GS, Dorey F, et al. Clinical utility of percent prostate needle biopsy tissue with cancer cutpoints to risk stratify patients before radical prostatectomy. *Urology* 2002;60:84–88.

89. Bigler SA, Deering RE, Brawer MK. Comparison of microscopic vascularity in benign and malignant prostate tissue. *Hum Pathol* 1993;24: 220–226.

90. Scardino PT, Shinohara K, Wheeler TM, et al. Staging of prostate cancer. Value of ultrasonography. *Urol Clin North Am* 1989;16:713–734.

91. Cornud F, Hamida K, Flam T, et al. Endorectal color Doppler sonography and endorectal MR imaging features of nonpalpable prostate cancer: correlation with radical prostatectomy findings. *Am J Roentgenol* 2000;175: 1161–1168.

92. Roy C, Buy X, Lang H, et al. Contrast enhanced color Doppler endorectal sonography of prostate: efficiency for detecting peripheral zone tumors and role for biopsy procedure. *J Urol* 2003;170:69–72.

93. Shigeno K, Igawa M, Shiina H, et al. Transrectal colour Doppler ultrasonography for quantifying angiogenesis in prostate cancer. *BJU Int* 2003;91:223–226.

94. Shigeno K, Igawa M, Shiina H, et al. The role of colour Doppler ultrasonography in detecting prostate cancer. *BJU Int* 2000;86:229–233.

95. Newman JS, Bree RL, Rubin JM. Prostate cancer: diagnosis with color Doppler sonography with histologic correlation of each biopsy site. *Radiology* 1995;195:86–90.

96. Arger PH, Malkowicz SB, VanArsdalen KN, et al. Color and power Doppler sonography in the diagnosis of prostate cancer: comparison between vascular density and total vascularity. *J Ultrasound Med* 2004;23: 623–630.

97. Ismail M, Petersen RO, Alexander AA, et al. Color Doppler imaging in predicting the biologic behavior of prostate cancer: correlation with disease-free survival. *Urology* 1997;50:906–912.

98. Okihara K, Watanabe H, Kojima M. Kinetic study of tumor blood flow in prostatic cancer using power Doppler imaging. *Ultrasound Med Biol* 1999;25:89–94.

99. Kravchick S, Cytron S, Peled R, et al. Colour Doppler ultrasonography for detecting perineural invasion (PNI) and the value of PNI in predicting final pathological stage: a prospective study of men with clinically localized prostate cancer. *BJU Int* 2003;92:28–31.

100. Cheng S, Rifkin MD. Color Doppler imaging of the prostate: important adjunct to endorectal ultrasound of the prostate in the diagnosis of prostate cancer. *Ultrasound Q* 2001;17:185–189.

101. Sakarya ME, Arslan H, Unal O, et al. The role of power Doppler ultrasonography in the diagnosis of prostate cancer: a preliminary study. *Br J Urol* 1998;82:386–388.

102. Rubin JM, Bude RO, Carson PL, et al. Power Doppler US: a potentially useful alternative to mean frequency-based color Doppler US. *Radiology* 1994;190:853–856.

103. Okihara K, Kojima M, Nakanouchi T, et al. Transrectal power Doppler imaging in the detection of prostate cancer. *BJU Int* 2000;85: 1053–1057.

104. Sauvain JL, Palascak P, Bourscheid D, et al. Value of power Doppler and 3D vascular sonography as a method for diagnosis and staging of prostate cancer. *Eur Urol* 2003;44:21–30; discussion 30–31.

105. Yu KK, Hricak H, Alagappan R, et al. Detection of extracapsular extension of prostate carcinoma with endorectal and phased-array coil MR imaging: multivariate feature analysis. *Radiology* 1997;202:697–702.

106. Rifkin MD, Zerhouni EA, Gatsonis CA, et al. Comparison of magnetic resonance imaging and ultrasonography in staging early prostate cancer. Results of a multi-institutional cooperative trial. *N Engl J Med* 1990;323: 621–626.

107. Perrotti M, Kaufman RP Jr, Jennings TA, et al. Endo-rectal coil magnetic resonance imaging in clinically localized prostate cancer: is it accurate? *J Urol* 1996;156:106–109.
108. Carroll PR, Presti JC Jr, Small E, et al. Focal therapy for prostate cancer 1996: maximizing outcome. *Urology* 1997;49:84–94.
109. Ikonen S, Karkkainen P, Kivisaari L, et al. Magnetic resonance imaging of clinically localized prostatic cancer. *J Urol* 1998;159:915–919.
110. Maio A, Rifkin MD. Magnetic resonance imaging of prostate cancer: update. *Top Magn Reson Imaging* 1995;7:54–68.
111. Bartolozzi C, Menchi I, Lencioni R, et al. Local staging of prostate carcinoma with endorectal coil MRI: correlation with whole-mount radical prostatectomy specimens. *Eur Radiol* 1996;6:339–345.
112. Deasy NP, Conry BG, Lewis JL, et al. Local staging of prostate cancer with 0.2 T body coil MRI. *Clin Radiol* 1997;52:933–937.
113. Tuzel E, Sevinc M, Obuz F, et al. Is magnetic resonance imaging necessary in the staging of prostate cancer? *Urol Int* 1998;61:227–231.
114. Cornud F, Flam T, Chauveinc L, et al. Extraprostatic spread of clinically localized prostate cancer: factors predictive of pT3 tumor and of positive endorectal MR imaging examination results. *Radiology* 2002;224:203–210.
115. Dhingsa R, Qayyum A, Coakley FV, et al. Prostate cancer localization with endorectal MR imaging and MR spectroscopic imaging: effect of clinical data on reader accuracy. *Radiology* 2004;230:215–220.
116. Purohit RS, Shinohara K, Meng MV, et al. Imaging clinically localized prostate cancer. *Urol Clin North Am* 2003;30:279–293.
117. Koutcher JA, Zakian K, Hricak H. Magnetic resonance spectroscopic studies of the prostate. *Mol Urol* 2000;4:143–152; discussion 153.
118. Yu KK, Scheidler J, Hricak H, et al. Prostate cancer: prediction of extracapsular extension with endorectal MR imaging and three-dimensional proton MR spectroscopic imaging. *Radiology* 1999;213:481–488.
119. Jager GJ, Ruijter ET, van de Kaa CA, et al. Dynamic TurboFLASH subtraction technique for contrast-enhanced MR imaging of the prostate: correlation with histopathologic results. *Radiology* 1997;203:645–652.
120. Clarke DH, Banks SJ, Wiederhorn AR, et al. The role of endorectal coil MRI in patient selection and treatment planning for prostate seed implants. *Int J Radiat Oncol Biol Phys* 2002;52:903–910.
121. Yuen JS, Thng CH, Tan PH, et al. Endorectal magnetic resonance imaging and spectroscopy for the detection of tumor foci in men with prior negative transrectal ultrasound prostate biopsy. *J Urol* 2004;171:1482–1486.
122. D'Amico AV, Tempany CM, Cormack R, et al. Transperineal magnetic resonance image guided prostate biopsy. *J Urol* 2000;164:385–387.
123. Cormack RA, D'Amico AV, Hata N, et al. Feasibility of transperineal prostate biopsy under interventional magnetic resonance guidance. *Urology* 2000;56:663–664.
124. Coleman JA, Susil RC, Krieger A et al., eds. *MRI guided prostate biopsy with biological image acquisition and targeting in a standard 1.5T scanner*. San Francisco, CA: American Urological Association, Annual Meeting, 2004.
125. Kaplan I, Oldenburg NE, Meskell P, et al. Real time MRI-ultrasound image guided stereotactic prostate biopsy. *Magn Reson Imaging* 2002;20:295–299.

CHAPTER 10 ■ STAGING SYSTEMS FOR PROSTATE CANCER

DAVID C. MILLER AND JAMES E. MONTIE

Definition of the extent of a patient's cancer is a prerequisite for designing a plan for successful therapy. Practitioners historically rely on clinical staging, a description of the anatomic extent of disease, to allow selection of therapy, comparison of results of different treatments, and assignment of a prognosis for an individual or a group of patients. Cancer staging is continually evolving through advances in imaging, histopathologic tissue examination, and detection of occult metastases. Moreover, it is increasingly accepted that other factors, in addition to the anatomic extent of disease, may strongly influence an individual patient's prognosis. Indeed, the prognostic limitations of "staging" in the classical sense are illustrated by our increasing recognition that mathematical models, such as nomograms, may offer more precise predictions of a prognosis or therapeutic response than does staging alone. Thus, a clear challenge lies before us to efficiently select the best parameters from a potentially large menu that will improve prediction of outcome, with or without treatment, in an individual patient. It seems likely that, in the future, the term "staging" may become obsolete as we become more sophisticated in our understanding of why a particular treatment works in one patient and not in another, despite an equivalent extent of disease.

GENERAL CONCEPTS

Staging

Care for a cancer patient must address three fundamental issues: (a) establishing diagnosis, (b) defining extent of disease, and (c) administering appropriate treatment. If the cancer poses a threat to the patient and treatment is effective in some but not all patients, assessment of the extent of the disease is a prerequisite for logical pursuit of treatment decisions. Local therapy only, regardless of effectiveness, will not cure a patient with known or unknown metastases. In general, of all prognostic factors, a description of anatomic spread remains the most powerful predictor of patient survival (1). Disease extent has historically been described by stages, with increasing tumor burden or spread designated by a higher stage and associated with a diminished survival. In the 1950s, staging concepts began to include Tumor-Node-Metastasis (TNM) classification. Within each reference of T, N, or M, there are categories based on tumor size or extent, number and/or size of regional nodes containing metastases, and distant metastases, referred to as *TNM variables* (2). Each of these variables is combined by designation of tumor size and involvement (T1 to T4), number of nodes involved (N0 to N3), and distant metastases (M0 to M1). Assignment of a T, N, or M variable is dependent on the quality of data obtained from staging studies, such as digital rectal examination (DRE) or radionuclide bone scan for prostate cancer. A combination of each of these three variables then places the patient into what is known as a "bin." For prostate cancer, there are 32 possible bins based on the different permutations of the TNM variables (4*4*2 = 32) (2).

An advantage of the bin model is that it allows for a precise classification of a patient's cancer into a discrete category. A disadvantage of the bin model is evident with the addition of other variables, because the number of bins increases exponentially with additional variables. For example, adding just one more variable for the histologic grade of prostate cancer (well, moderate, or poorly differentiated) results in the creation of 96 bins (4*4*2*3 = 96). Inclusion of other prognostic variables quickly makes the concept unworkable on a practical basis. In the TNM system, the bins are grouped into stages that have clinical relevance, such as predicting survival as compared to other stages. Stages, based on similar reasoning, were historically developed without the use of the TNM classification. The Whitmore A, B, C, and D stages for prostate cancer are one example. TNM-based stages have gained wider acceptance since 1992. Nonetheless, a clear disadvantage of any staging system is that it puts patients into categories that may be somewhat arbitrary and diminishes the value of retaining data as a continuous variable, such as size of the cancer. Clearly evident in prostate cancer is the arbitrary and likely nonreproducible changes in the categorization of the T stage between the 1992, 1997, and 2002 editions of the staging manual. Even though statistical segregation of the T2 subcategories was evident in retrospective datasets, the choice of a 1.0 cm nodule or one half of the gland involved was arbitrarily chosen. Another disadvantage of any staging classification is that the stage must be changed if new data become available. For example, improvements in imaging technology, more precise histologic evaluation, and better identification of micrometastases have the potential to change the patient population underlying the stages. This "stage migration" of patients, for example, from T2,N0,M0 to T3,N0,M0 or T2,N1,M0 may well change the prediction of survival on which the stage categorization was based and thus undermine the reliability of the stage predictors of outcome (2,3). Stage migration is certainly present in prostate cancer using transrectal ultrasound (TRUS)–guided needle biopsy of seminal vesicles, step-section reconstruction of the entire prostate to identify microscopic capsular penetration, or identification of micrometastases in lymph nodes.

Such limitations in the staging classification do not imply a lack of value in the definition of the extent of disease. As our understanding of the biology of cancer improves, additional information that may also contribute to predicting survival or treatment success must be incorporated into the decision process. Reliance on anatomic staging by itself will ultimately prove insufficient.

121

PROGNOSTIC FACTORS (ANALYTIC CONSIDERATIONS)

A prognostic factor is a marker of disease that increases accuracy in predicting outcome. Prognostic factors may help estimate survival, select therapy, evaluate response to therapy, compare data, act as an intermediate endpoint, and define qualifications for clinical trials. As additional prognostic factors are proposed, the methodology used to evaluate the success of the factors is receiving additional scrutiny and standardization (2–4).

Prognostic factors may also contribute to the description of the natural history of the disease. However, if the natural history of the disease is altered by therapy, the relevance of a factor may change (2). Some factors are prognostic for particular therapies only at a certain stage or only in the context of other factors. The American Joint Committee on Cancer (AJCC) proposes the following criteria for evaluation of putative prognostic factors: They must be (a) significant, (b) independent, and (c) clinically important (2). "Significant" means that the factor rarely occurs by chance. "Independent" means that the factor retains value after controlling for other prognostic factors. "Clinically important" implies that the information obtained through the factor will influence clinical decisions. The guidelines to evaluate prognostic factors in oncology are under development and are only a general overview of some of the methodologic issues discussed here (4). The need for precise and critical evaluation of a proposed prognostic factor is imperative. Inadequate evaluation could have profound negative consequences on treatment decisions and health care costs.

The predictive power of a prognostic factor is evaluated by a statistical model that examines significance and independence. Significance of a prognostic factor can be evaluated by univariate analyses as well as by multivariate models, which provide information on both significance and independence. A commonly applied analysis to show the difference in survival attributable to a particular variable is a Kaplan-Meier survival curve, corresponding to univariate tests. The influence on the variable of interest by another variable known to have significance is not examined in this analysis. To examine the influence of several prognostic factors, a regression model, such as the Cox proportional hazard model, is often used. The stepwise regression model is often used for exploratory studies evaluating a new factor. However, the results may be misleading because the same data set is used to select the model and to establish the regression coefficients. The order of entry of variables can also influence outcome.

Many variables now proposed as prognostic factors are not simply present or absent but are continuous; that is, they are constantly being altered by time and interventions. This can make the construction of levels or cutoff points that define high or low risk problematic. Division of the groups at median values, often used in the past, may not adequately define patient groups. Cutoff points are often determined by computing the significance at multiple cutoff point levels and then choosing the one with the strongest significance level. This selected cutoff point is then used for generation of P-values, survival curves, and regression coefficients involving that factor. These are all biased, however, by preselection of the cutoff point using the same data, and the possibility of false identification of a significant prognostic factor increases substantially. Analysis of a different data set is necessary to confirm the value of the marker. Establishment of the cutoff point before analysis of significance provides an unbiased evaluation of the factor.

Sample size is a common limitation in the evaluation of a prognostic variable. Retrospective studies may allow larger numbers of patients to be evaluated and are easier to conduct than prospective studies. However, bias may be introduced if stored tissue is necessary because of a disproportionate number of larger tumors. If multiple studies must be performed in an individual prospective project, there also may be a selection bias for larger tumors. Precise inclusion and exclusion criteria must be specified in the study design criteria.

Subset analyses can be a source of confusion in studying the relationship between a prognostic variable and a response to treatment. When a subset analysis is found to be significant, unless this interaction was noted at the start of the study, the results should be viewed as providing a hypothesis to be tested on additional data. A noteworthy current example in urologic oncology is the observation that patients with minimal rather than severe metastatic prostate cancer responded most favorably to androgen blockade combined with leuprolide acetate and flutamide, compared to luteinizing hormone-releasing hormone agonist alone (5). This finding was not anticipated at the initiation of the trial, and the subsets included fewer than 15% of all the patients in the trial. Confirmation of the apparent treatment selectivity requires prospective validation using another data set.

BACKGROUND OF STAGING

Credit for categorizing prostate cancer in various stages belongs to Whitmore (6). In 1956, he proposed four groups:

A. Clinically latent prostate cancer
B. Clinically manifest early prostate cancer
C. Clinically manifest locally advanced prostate cancer
D. Clinically manifest advanced prostate cancer with evidence of distant metastases

This classification became the international standard and has withstood the test of time. Proposed modifications also have been accepted in various forms, all attempting to quantify the size of the local lesions.

In the late 1970s, there was increased interest in the oncologic community to shift to a TNM form of anatomic staging to allow for more precise definition of the amount and sites of the cancer. Initial attempts at staging prostate cancer were not widely accepted. In 1986, the Organ Systems Coordinating Center of the National Cancer Institute appointed a blue-ribbon committee, headed by Whitmore and Catalona, and charged it "to develop a simple and reproducible staging system for prostate cancer that would have prognostic and therapeutic relevance" (7). An attempt was made to amalgamate the traditional Whitmore A, B, C, D system with a newer TNM system. Although this approach provided several advantages, the format was cumbersome for the urologic practitioner and was not supported by international oncologic organizations. In 1987, the third revision of the TNM system was published (8). This classification was particularly confusing because of the description of apical disease. This system was widely criticized in Europe and largely ignored in the United States.

In 1992, the fourth TNM system was presented with consensus approval of a large segment of academic urologists, the AJCC, and the International union against cancer (UICC) (9). Although far from ideal and undoubtedly subject to refinement in the future, this categorization appears workable for practitioners caring for prostate cancer patients as well as researchers performing clinical trials (10).

In the development of the 1992 AJCC/UICC system, several concepts were important. The general organization of the Whitmore system remains as follows: Stage A becomes T1, stage B becomes T2, and stage C becomes T3. This organization conforms to general TNM rules categorizing organ-confined tumors as T2 and local extension outside the organ of origin as T3. A T4 category also was added to segregate lesions invading other surrounding organs. The subcategories within each category used in the 1992 system were based on recommendations proposed by the National Cancer Institute committee in 1989 (7). Over the years, many different institutions have proposed different definitions for subcategories within T1(A), T2(B), or T3(C), often empirically derived and not subjected to rigorous testing. An extensive review of the vast array of definitions for proposed subcategories would accomplish little.

The 1992 system was able to accommodate changes in imaging that might define a local lesion better, without the need to change the categories. Historically, DRE exclusively defined the local extent of the disease. Staging was based on observations that an isolated nodule generally implied disease that was confined within the prostate, whereas disease palpable in both lobes had a higher likelihood of extension outside the capsule or into the seminal vesicle. Prognosis from surgical or radiation therapy tended to correlate adequately with local stage as defined by these subcategories.

In the 1997 edition of the system, the general classifications remained constant but some consolidation of subclassifications was undertaken, driven largely by an effort to make clinical staging consistent with pathologic staging (11). For example, the previous T2a (one half-lobe) and T2b (one lobe) were consolidated to T2a (one lobe) to be consistent with the pathology grouping of pT2a (unilateral) versus pT2b (bilateral). There was not universal agreement that this change was wise because of evidence that supported a separate T2a (one half-lobe) category with a similar prognosis to T1c cancers (12). In the 2002 edition, the T-staging reverted again to the 1992 original classification of T2a, T2b, and T2c. Pathologic staging was changed to conform to the clinical staging guidelines (13) (see Table 10.1).

TABLE 10.1

2002 AMERICAN JOINT COMMITTEE ON CANCER/INTERNATIONAL UNION AGAINST CANCER TNM STAGING CLASSIFICATION

Stage	Definition
Primary tumor, clinical (T)	
TX	Primary tumor cannot be assessed
T0	No evidence of primary tumor
T1	Clinically inapparent tumor not palpable or visible by imaging
	T1a: Tumor incidental histologic finding in 5% or less of tissue resected
	T1b: Tumor incidental histologic finding in more than 5% of tissue resected
	T1c: Tumor identified by needle biopsy [e.g., because of elevated prostate-specific antigen (PSA) levels]
T2	Tumor confined within the prostate[a]
	T2a: Tumor involves half of one lobe or less
	T2b: Tumor involves more than half of one lobe but not both
	T2c: Tumor involves both lobes
T3	Tumor extends through the prostate capsule[b]
	T3a: Extracapsular extension (unilateral nor bilateral)
	T3b: Tumor invades seminal vesicle(s)
T4	Tumor is fixed or invades adjacent structures other than the seminal vesicle(s): bladder neck, external sphincter, rectum, levator muscles, pelvic wall, or all the above
Primary tumor, pathologic (pT)	
pT2[c]	Organ confined
	pT2a: Unilateral, involving half of one lobe or less
	pT2b: Unilateral, involving more than half of one lobe but not both lobes
	pT2c: Bilateral
pT3	Extraprostatic extension
	pT3a: Extraprostatic extension
	pT3b: Seminal vesicle invasion
pT4	Invasion of bladder, rectum
Regional lymph nodes (N)	
NX	Regional lymph nodes cannot be assessed
N0	No regional lymph node metastasis
N1	Metastasis in regional lymph node or nodes
Distant metastases[d] (M)	
MX	Distant metastasis cannot be assessed
M0	No distant metastasis
M1	Distant metastasis
	M1a: Nonregional lymph node(s)
	M1b: Bone(s)
	M1c: Other site(s)

[a]Tumor found in one or both lobes by needle biopsy, but not palpable or reliably visible by imaging, is classified as T1c.
[b]Invasion into the prostatic apex or into (but not beyond) the prostatic capsule is classified as T2, not T3.
[c]There is no pathologic T1 classification.
[d]When more than one site of metastasis is present, the most advanced category is used; pM1c is most advanced.
Adapted with permission from Greene FL, Page DL, Fleming ID, et al. *Cancer staging manual*, 6th ed. New York: Springer; 2002.

CLINICAL STAGING

Digital Rectal Examination

Currently, clinical T-stage classification relies primarily on DRE; however, the limitations of DRE in the precise description of the local extent of disease are well known. Indeed, clinicians have long recognized the difficulty in detection of extracapsular disease, especially in cases in which the palpable disease is located near a margin. Many studies have grouped cases together as stage B–C, acknowledging the uncertainty in assigning the appropriate clinical stage. Furthermore, despite its widespread use in quantifying the presence and volume of disease in the prostate, substantial concerns remain about the intra- and/or interobserver variability of DRE. Both Phillips and Thompson (14) and Varenhorst et al. (15) have demonstrated subjectivity in the DRE. Angulo et al. demonstrated that the DRE is only slightly better than chance in interobserver variability for clinical T-stage (1992) subgroups (16). Most extracapsular extension is microscopic, unapparent on DRE, but seen with an alarming frequency with step-sectioning of the entire radical prostatectomy specimen. In surgical series using a pathologic examination that reconstructs the entire prostate, the incidence of penetration through the capsule or seminal vesicle invasion by the cancer ranges from 30% to 60% (17–20). Thus, the sensitivity of DRE to stratify a key factor in T staging (i.e., confinement within the prostate) is disappointingly low.

Transrectal Ultrasound (TRUS)

The introduction of TRUS of the prostate in the early 1980s inspired hope that a substantial improvement in local staging was on the horizon. Unfortunately, further clinical experience tempered this enthusiasm greatly and indicated that TRUS may be only marginally better than DRE at characterizing the extent of the primary tumor (21,22). Furthermore, the performance of TRUS is operator-dependent and must be appreciated in that context. Although TRUS is now routinely used for anatomic guidance during prostate needle biopsy, its ability to reliably define the extent of the intraprostatic disease (i.e., separate T1c from T2 or T2a from T2b) or to identify extraprostatic extension remains inconclusive. In one study, Tiguert et al. found that prostate cancer patients with a normal DRE, but abnormal findings on TRUS, had pathologic and disease-specific survival outcomes that were less favorable than men with normal findings on both DRE and TRUS, but similar to patients with palpable abnormalities on DRE. Therefore, the authors concluded that TRUS has an important role in distinguishing clinical stage T1 and T2 lesions (23). However, such discriminatory capacity has not been consistently confirmed, and the subclassification of impalpable cancers that are visible on TRUS is generally discouraged (24). In selected cases, TRUS can facilitate confirmation of neurovascular bundle or seminal vesicle invasion by directed biopsies. However, these must be interpreted cautiously because the biopsy needle may pass through the prostate and the intraprostatic cancer may be misinterpreted as being outside the gland (25).

It has been suggested that various technical modifications in transrectal ultrasonography may refine its role in prostate cancer staging; however, conclusive data to support this hypothesis remains unavailable. Color Doppler ultrasonography is gaining increasing acceptance but, again, changes in vascular flow may be nonspecific (26). In a study of 47 men with clinically localized prostate cancer, Kravchik et al. evaluated the performance of color Doppler TRUS

(CD-TRUS)–guided neurovascular bundle-adjacent biopsies in predicting the presence of perineural invasion and extraprostatic extension (pT3 disease) in subsequent radical prostatectomy specimens. Although quite accurate in predicting perineural invasion, CD-TRUS–guided biopsies had a low positive predictive value (24%) for extraprostatic disease (27). More recently, using power Doppler sonography, Sauvain et al. reported a significant association between the detection of vessels perforating the posterior prostate capsule and extraprostatic extension (pT3 disease) at the time of radical prostatectomy (28). Finally, computer analysis of sonographic data, as opposed to operator evaluation, has been investigated as a potentially more objective application of this technology (29). Despite this ongoing research, many urologists maintain that the contribution of TRUS imaging to the clinical staging of prostate cancer patients is limited at best (30).

Prostate Biopsy Information

A traditional practice for TRUS-guided biopsy includes sextant biopsies with an 18-gauge core needle of the peripheral zone, in addition to directed biopsies at DRE- or TRUS-identified abnormalities (31–33). Contemporary data support taking a greater number of cores to increase the amount of information obtained and to improve the accuracy of prostate cancer diagnosis (34–37). Indeed, in 2004, the standard of care has shifted away from the traditional sextant biopsy, and it is now generally accepted that at least 8 (and possibly 10) laterally directed, peripheral zone biopsies are necessary for sufficient evaluation (38,39).

With regard to prostate cancer staging, there is a growing body of evidence that supports prostate biopsy tumor volume as a useful surrogate for primary tumor size. As a result, quantification of the amount of tumor on prostate needle biopsy has been proposed as an important adjunct to contemporary staging practices (40–43). In general, multiple studies have demonstrated a consistent association between greater volumes of cancer in the biopsy specimen and various adverse pathologic and survival outcomes (43). Several measures of biopsy tumor volume have been evaluated and applied clinically, including the number or percentage of cores involved with cancer, the percentage of cancer in each core, the total percentage of cancer in the entire biopsy specimen, and the number of (linear) millimeters of carcinoma (40). On the basis of each of these parameters, significant associations have been reported between increased biopsy tumor volume and a greater risk of one or more adverse outcomes, including extraprostatic extension, lymph node involvement, seminal vesicle invasion, and biochemical recurrence following radical prostatectomy (40–44). Unfortunately, there remains no consensus regarding the most feasible, reproducible, and valid method for quantifying biopsy tumor volume data and, prior to the incorporation of such data into routine staging practices, additional study is necessary to establish the most discriminatory biopsy volume cut-point. In the future, prostate biopsy tissue may be used for genomic and/or proteomic analyses that serve to identify subsets of genes or proteins that provide novel and powerful prognostic information that could revolutionize our current approach to clinical and pathologic staging (45).

Bone Scan

The propensity for prostate cancer to metastasize to bone prompts urologists to rely heavily on radionuclide bone scintigraphy as a clinical staging modality among men at risk for distant metastases. Whereas approximately 50% of the marrow must be replaced for the abnormality to be evident on a plain radiograph of the bone, a bone scan may be abnormal if only 10% of the bone is replaced. Historically, all newly diagnosed prostate cancer patients received a bone scan. Currently, many patients have smaller-volume disease, and the rate of patients presenting with metastatic disease is decreasing (46). Some data suggest that the diagnostic yield of bone scintigraphy among men with a PSA level of less than 10 or 20 ng/mL is extremely low. Indeed, Oesterling et al. found no bone scans positive for metastases among men with PSA levels less than 8 ng/mL; if the PSA was less than 20 ng/mL, the yield was less than 2% (47). In a nationwide sample from the National Cancer Database (NCDB), Miller et al. reported similar results, in that only 8% of bone scans were positive among more than 10,000 men with a pretreatment PSA of less than or equal to 10 ng/mL and well- or moderately differentiated cancers (48). Regrettably, despite their potentially low yield, several studies indicate continued, and perhaps unnecessary, utilization of bone scans as an initial staging modality in patients at low risk for distant (M1) disease (48–51). Moreover, despite the recommendations of contemporary practice guidelines, the use of staging bone scans among high-risk patients (e.g., PSA greater than 10) is not universal. In this population, omission of bone scintigraphy from the staging evaluation may lead to problematic underestimations of the extent of disease and result in suboptimal therapeutic planning (48,49,52,53).

In patients with bone scan–documented metastases, the scintigraphic findings are useful not only to characterize the anatomic extent of disease but also to possibly identify patients at risk for early progression. Specifically, scintigraphic findings of disease limited to the axial skeleton and/or a small number of metastatic deposits is associated with more favorable survival outcomes. This is true even among patients with hormonally responsive cancers (54,55). The identification of possible micrometastases of prostate cancer in a bone marrow aspirate is a recent observation, and data suggest a worse prognosis in those men who have PSA-positive cells by reverse transcriptase–polymerase chain reaction (RT-PCR) in the bone marrow at the time of radical prostatectomy (56). However, despite the fact that such identified cells are cytogenetically abnormal, consistent with spread from the primary tumor, many of the 25% to 50% of patients with apparently localized disease and epithelial cells in the bone marrow do not demonstrate relapse with relatively short follow-up (56–58). In this context, refinements in staging practices based on the detection of circulating prostate cancer cells cannot be justified based on current evidence; however, should additional data emerge, a substantial change in the M categorization may be warranted.

Computed Tomography

Computed tomography (CT) of the pelvis has proved to be of limited value in staging of prostate cancer (59). Because most local extension is microscopic, CT understandably fails to detect such extraprostatic disease. In patients with relatively favorable lesions, such as well- or moderately differentiated histology or a PSA of less than 10 ng/mL, the yield of abnormal findings on CT is sufficiently low that its use is not recommended in the initial staging evaluation (52). Indeed, among a nationwide sample of more than 5000 men meeting these low-risk criteria, only 11% of men undergoing staging CT evaluations had findings consistent with metastatic (N1–N3) disease (48). In selected high-risk patients (e.g., PSA greater than 10 or high-grade tumors), CT may provide valuable information on the status of pelvic lymph nodes. In such

a carefully selected patient population, the yield of staging CT studies is appreciably higher (48). Among contemporary patients, however, it should be emphasized that most lymph node metastases are of very small volume and are not reliably identified as abnormal on a CT scan. In cases where gross adenopathy is apparent, confirmatory aspiration biopsy is appropriate to further enhance the precision of the staging work-up (60).

Magnetic Resonance Imaging

Historically, magnetic resonance imaging (MRI) has been unnecessary in most patients with newly diagnosed adenocarcinoma of the prostate (48). In general, MRI with traditional body surface coils provides minimal additional information about the local staging of prostate cancer beyond that provided by DRE or TRUS (61). Moreover, considerable interobserver variability has perennially limited the widespread application of prostate MRI (62). More recently, however, the development and refinement of more specialized imaging techniques have prompted a reassessment of the role of MRI as a prostate cancer staging modality. It is widely recognized that the use of an endorectal surface coil provides superior quality images of the prostate, and several single-institution studies have suggested high levels (i.e., more than 80%) of staging accuracy with this technique (63–66). Endorectal coil MRI may have particular value in detecting previously unrecognized extracapsular extension (resulting in upstaging from clinical stage T2 to clinical stage T3 disease), thereby influencing prognostic counseling and therapeutic decision-making (67,68). However, the optimal application of endorectal coil technology remains controversial, with two recent meta-analyses yielding conflicting results with regard to its impact on the accuracy of clinical staging (69,70). A potentially useful adjunct to endorectal coil MRI is magnetic resonance spectroscopic imaging (MRSI), an emerging technology that provides unique functional information by distinguishing between normal and abnormal tissue metabolism (68). Prostate MRSI has been shown to reliably distinguish between benign and malignant tissue based on characteristic shifts in the metabolic (spectroscopic) peaks of specific molecules (e.g., choline, creatine, and citrate) (68). Moreover, MRSI findings have been shown to correlate directly with tumor biology in that more aggressive tumors (e.g., higher Gleason sum) are associated with greater metabolic abnormalities. Although still in evolution, it has been proposed that the functional information provided by MRSI, combined with the anatomic precision of endorectal coil MRI, may improve the accuracy and reliability of MRI as it relates to prostate cancer staging (68).

In addition to the assessment of prostatic and peri-prostatic anatomy, MRI technology may be particularly valuable for the detection of clinically occult lymph node metastases among men with apparently localized disease (71). In a widely publicized report, Harisinghani et al. demonstrated that the combination of high-resolution MRI with a lymphotropic superparamagnetic nanoparticle imaging agent (monocrystalline iron oxide) was significantly superior to conventional MRI in its ability to identify small and previously unrecognized lymph node metastases. Indeed, among 334 lymph nodes sampled, the positive predictive value for MRI combined with magnetic nanoparticles was 95%, versus 56% for conventional MRI; the overall diagnostic accuracy of this novel technique was also substantially superior, at 97%, versus 76% for MRI alone (71). Although its widespread application is not yet established, high-resolution MRI with magnetic nanoparticles has the potential to transform the clinical staging of newly diagnosed prostate cancer.

Overview of Staging Procedures

Historically, staging defines the anatomic extent of the disease, which happens to be the most important single factor in defining a patient's prognosis. The contribution of staging relies most critically on the judgment of localized versus metastatic disease. In patients with apparent localized disease, now comprising 80% to 90% of patients with newly diagnosed prostate cancer, wide variability exists in the natural history of the disease, the response to surgery or radiation, and the need for salvage therapies after the failure of an initial treatment. Anatomic extent of disease is inadequate to reliably segregate patients with clinically localized disease. Patients rely on their physician for counsel about the potential success of a treatment, and physicians must provide patients with outcome probabilities for their individual cases. Ultimately, symptomatic local recurrence, metastatic disease, or death from prostate cancer are the concern of all. However, we must currently rely on pathologic staging and PSA relapse as harbingers of ultimate failure and surrogate endpoints. Enormous energy has been expended on subclassifying T1 and T2 disease by ultrasonography or other imaging findings, the extent or type of cancer in the biopsy cores, the number of cores involved, and so on. It is unlikely that substantial progress will be forthcoming using only further manipulation of data on the local extent of disease. A good example of such a dilemma is the confusion evident on the contribution of perineural invasion to the prediction of pathologic stage. Conflicting data exist on the association of perineural invasion and extracapsular extension and reliability as a prognostic factor (72,73).

However, grade and PSA level are also independent predictors of outcomes after therapy. Urologic researchers have done a poor job of incorporating the important information provided by PSA level and Gleason score grading into a practical format that allows a clinician to predict treatment outcomes. One impediment to the development of appropriate prediction models is poorly defined outcomes. Because manifestations of ultimate disease progression in prostate cancer are only seen after 10 to 15 years, surrogate endpoints of pathologic stage after radical prostatectomy or rising PSA levels after treatment are commonplace. Each of these endpoints has limitations. Pathologic stage evaluates organ confinement, degree of extracapsular extension, and margin status. The "Partin Tables" are popular nomograms that use clinical stage, PSA level, and Gleason score to predict probability of organ confinement, seminal vesical invasion, or lymph node metastases (74). However, follow-up information with this data set on PSA relapse is not yet available. The value of the Partin Tables in the initial form is limited because most patients who have extracapsular extension, but also have negative seminal vesicles and lymph nodes, are still apparently cured with radical prostatectomy alone, and few patients have positive seminal vesicles or lymph nodes. Margin status emerges as an independent predictor of relapse within pathologic stages and individual Gleason score groups (19,75,76). There is a consensus among pathologists to convey the margin status by a plus sign (e.g., T2b + N0, M0), but such a practice is not yet accepted fully by the AJCC or widely adopted into clinical practice (77).

Efforts to improve the combined prognostic value of the Gleason score, PSA level, and clinical stage are becoming increasingly refined. According to a review by Ross et al. in 2001, 29 published models were available for predicting outcomes of radical prostatectomy using preoperative information (78). D'Amico et al. are leaders in using statistical models to estimate cancer volume and in incorporating multiple variables, including some pathologic findings from the radical prostatectomy specimen (79–84). Kattan et al. at Memorial Sloan-Kettering Cancer Center have developed multiple nomograms to predict the occurrence of numerous and diverse endpoints after radical prostatectomy, external radiation, and brachytherapy, as well as among patients with more advanced disease. Nomograms have been consistently shown to outperform clinical experts in terms of their calibration (e.g., their predictions closely approximate actual outcomes) and discrimination (e.g., their ability to distinguish between patients that will and will not reach a particular endpoint). Furthermore, an important strength of the nomogram methodology has been the validation of these models in multi-institutional datasets (85,86).

In this context, a feasible vision for future urologists will include an easily accessible Internet or personal digital assistant (PDA) tool that efficiently incorporates contemporary prognostic variables to estimate the probability of a successful outcome for a specific treatment in an individual patient. Frequent updating of the model will be necessary because of changes in the character of the disease that are influenced by early detection strategies (87). Staging of anatomic extent of disease will undoubtedly be part of the input data. Ultimately, this information will allow patients to better weigh the risks and benefits of their treatment options. This type of reliable information would be extremely helpful for clinical research to compare different treatments in the absence of randomized trials. Finally, such models would allow testing of new putative prognostic factors, such as molecular biologic data, to see if the additional expense provides truly meaningful information. Such is the future of staging as it evolves into a larger package of prediction of outcome (1).

References

1. Hermanek P, Sobin LH, Fleming ID. What do we need beyond TNM? *Cancer* 1996;77:815–817.
2. Burke HB, Henson DE. Criteria for prognostic factors and for an enhanced prognostic system. *Cancer* 1993;72:3131–3135.
3. Fielding LP, Henson DE. Multiple prognostic factors and outcome analysis in patients with cancer. *Cancer* 1993;71:2426–2429.
4. Simon R, Altman DG. Statistical aspects of prognostic factor studies in oncology. *Br J Cancer* 1994;69:979–985.
5. Crawford DE, Eisenberger MA, McLeod DG, et al. A controlled trial of leuprolide with and without flutamide in prostatic carcinoma. *N Engl J Med* 1989;321:419–424.
6. Whitmore WF Jr. Hormone therapy in prostatic cancer. *Am J Med* 1956; 21:697–713.
7. Catalona WJ, Whitmore WF Jr. New staging systems for prostate cancer. *J Urol* 1989;142:1302–1304.
8. Beahrs OH, Henson DE, Hutter RVP, et al. *Manual for staging of cancer*, 3rd ed. Philadelphia, PA: JB Lippincott Co; 1988.
9. Beahrs OH, Henson DE, Hutter RVP, et al. *Manual for staging of cancer*, 4th ed. Philadelphia, PA: JB Lippincott Co; 1992.
10. Montie JE. 1992 staging system for prostate cancer. *Semin Urol* 1993;11: 10–13.
11. Fleming ID, Cooper JS, Henson DE, et al. *Manual for staging of cancer*, 5th ed. Philadelphia, PA: Lippincott-Raven Publishers; 1997.
12. Stamey TA, Sözen TS, Yemoto CM, et al. Classification of localized untreated prostate cancer based on 791 men treated only with radical prostatectomy: common ground for therapeutic trials and TNM subgroups. *J Urol* 1998; 159:2009–2012.
13. Greene FL, Page DL, Fleming ID, et al. *Cancer staging manual*, 6th ed. New York: Springer; 2002.
14. Phillips TH, Thompson IM. Digital rectal examination and cancer of the prostate. *Urol Clin North Am* 1991;18:459–465.
15. Varenhorst E, Berglund K, Lofman O, et al. Inter-observer variation in assessment of the prostate by digital rectal examination. *Br J Urol* 1993;72: 173–176.
16. Angulo JC, Montie JE, Bukowsky T, et al. Interobserver consistency of digital rectal examination in clinical staging of localized prostatic carcinoma. *Urol Oncol* 1995;1:199–205.
17. Voges GE, McNeal JE, Redwine EA, et al. Morphologic analysis of surgical margins with positive findings in prostatectomy for adenocarcinoma of the prostate. *Cancer* 1992;69:520–526.
18. Humphrey PA, Walther PJ. Adenocarcinoma of the prostate. Part II: tissue prognosticators. *Am J Clin Pathol* 1993;100:356–369.
19. Epstein JI, Pizov G, Walsh PC. Correlation of pathologic findings with progression after radical retropubic prostatectomy. *Cancer* 1993;71:3582–3592.

20. Ohori M, Scardino PT, Lapin SL, et al. The mechanisms and prognostic significance of seminal vesicle involvement by prostate cancer. *Am J Surg Pathol* 1993;17:1252–1261.

21. Scardino PT, Shinohara K, Wheeler TM, et al. Staging of prostate cancer, value of ultrasonography. *Urol Clin North Am* 1989;16:713–734.

22. Rifkin MD, Zerhouni EA, Gatsonis CA, et al. Comparison of magnetic resonance imaging and ultrasonography in staging early prostate cancer. *N Engl J Med* 1990;323:621–626.

23. Tiguert R, Gheiler EL, Grignon DJ, et al. Patients with abnormal ultrasound of the prostate but normal digital rectal examination should be classified as having clinical stage T2 tumors. *J Urol* 2000;163:1486–1490.

24. Augustin H, Graefen M, Palisaar J, et al. Prognostic significance of visible lesions on transrectal ultrasound in impalpable prostate cancers: implications for staging. *J Clin Oncol* 2003;21:2860–2868.

25. Terris MK, McNeal JE, Freiha FS. Efficacy of transrectal ultrasound-guided seminal vesicle biopsies in the detection of seminal vesicle invasion by prostate cancer. *J Urol* 1993;149:1035–1039.

26. Cornud F, Belin X, Piron D, et al. Color Doppler-guided prostate biopsies in 591 patients with an elevated serum PSA level: impact on Gleason score for nonpalpable lesions. *Urology* 1997;49:709–714.

27. Kravchick S, Cytron S, Peled R, et al. Colour Doppler ultrasonography for detecting perineural invasion (PNI) and the value of PNI in predicting final pathological stage: a prospective study of men with clinically localized prostate cancer. *BJU Int* 2003;92:28–31.

28. Sauvain JL, Palascak P, Bourscheid D, et al. Value of power Doppler and 3D vascular sonography as a method for diagnosis and staging of prostate cancer. *Eur Urol* 2003;44:21–30.

29. Giesen RJB, Huynen AL, Aarnink RG, et al. Computer analysis of transrectal ultrasound images of the prostate for the detection of carcinoma: a prospective study in radical prostatectomy specimens. *J Urol* 1995;154: 1397–1400.

30. Werner-Wasik M, Whittington R, Malkowicz SB, et al. Prostate imaging may not be necessary in nonpalpable carcinoma of the prostate. *Urology* 1997;50:385–389.

31. Huland H, Hubner D, Henke RP. Systematic biopsies and digital rectal examination to identify the nerve-sparing side for radical prostatectomy without risk of positive margin in patients with clinical stage T2, N0 prostatic carcinoma. *Urology* 1994;44:211–214.

32. Wills ML, Sauvageot J, Partin AW, et al. Ability of sextant biopsies to predict radical prostatectomy stage. *Urology* 1998;51:759–764.

33. Borirakchanyavat S, Bhargava V, Shinohara K, et al. Systematic sextant biopsies in the prediction of extracapsular extension at radical prostatectomy. *Urology* 1997;50:373–378.

34. Eskew LA, Bare RL, McCullough DL. Systematic 5 region prostate biopsy is superior to sextant method for diagnosing carcinoma of the prostate. *J Urol* 1997;157:199–203.

35. Egevad L, Norberg M, Mattson S, et al. Estimation of prostate cancer volume by multiple core biopsies before radical prostatectomy. *Urology* 1998;52:653–658.

36. Dietrick DD, McNeal JE, Stamey TA. Core cancer length in ultrasound-guided systematic sextant biopsies: a preoperative evaluation of prostate cancer volume. *Urology* 1995;45:987–992.

37. Conrad S, Graefen M, Pichlmeier U, et al. Systematic sextant biopsies improve preoperative prediction of pelvic lymph node metastases in patients with clinically localized prostatic carcinoma. *J Urol* 1998;159: 2023–2029.

38. Presti JC Jr, Chang JJ, Bhargava V, et al. The optimal systematic prostate biopsy scheme should include 8 rather than 6 biopsies: results of a prospective clinical trial. *J Urol* 2000;163:163–166.

39. Gore JL, Shariat SF, Miles BJ, et al. Optimal combinations of systematic sextant and laterally directed biopsies for the detection of prostate cancer. *J Urol* 2001;165:1554–1559.

40. Javidan J, Wood DP. Clinical interpretation of the prostate biopsy. *Urol Oncol* 2003;21:141–144.

41. Freedland SJ, Aronson WJ, Terris MK, et al. The percentage of prostate needle biopsy cores with carcinoma from the more involved side of the biopsy as a predictor of prostate specific antigen recurrence after radical prostatectomy: results from the Shared Equal Access Regional Cancer Hospital (SEARCH) database. *Cancer* 2003;98:2344–2350.

42. Che M, Sakr W, Grignon D. Pathologic features the urologist should expect on a prostate biopsy. *Urol Oncol* 2003;21:153–161.

43. Epstein JI, Potter SR. The pathological interpretation and significance of prostate needle biopsy findings: implications and current controversies. *J Urology* 2001;166:402–410.

44. Nelson CP, Dunn RL, Wei JT, et al. Contemporary preoperative parameters predict cancer-free survival after radical prostatectomy: a tool to facilitate treatment decisions. *Urol Oncol* 2003;21:213–218.

45. Kumar-Sinha C, Chinnaiyan AM. Molecular markers to identify patients at risk for recurrence after primary treatment for prostate cancer. *Urology* 2003;62:19–35.

46. Demers RY, Swanson GM, Weiss KL, et al. Increasing incidence of cancer of the prostate. *Arch Intern Med* 1994;154:1211–1216.

47. Oesterling JE, Martin SK, Bergstralh EJ, et al. The use of prostate-specific antigen in staging patients with newly diagnosed prostate cancer. *JAMA* 1993;269:57–60.

48. Miller DC, Hafez KS, Stewart A, et al. Prostate carcinoma presentation, diagnosis, and staging: an update from the National Cancer Data Base. *Cancer* 2003;98:1169–1178.

49. Cooperberg MR, Lubeck DP, Grossfeld GD, et al. Contemporary trends in imaging test utilization for prostate cancer staging: data from the Cancer of the Prostate Strategic Urologic Research Endeavor. *J Urol* 2002;168: 491–495.

50. Plawker MW, Fleisher JM, Vapnek EM, et al. Current trends in prostate cancer diagnosis and staging among United States urologists. *J Urol* 1997; 158:1853–1858.

51. Kindrick AV, Grossfeld GD, Stier DM, et al. Use of imaging tests for staging newly diagnosed prostate cancer: trends from the CaPSURE database. *J Urol* 1998;160:2102–2106.

52. Carroll P, Coley C, McLeod D, et al. Prostate-specific antigen best practice policy—part II: prostate cancer staging and post-treatment follow-up. *Urology* 2001;57:225–229.

53. Bahnson RR, Hanks GE, Huben RP, et al. National Comprehensive Cancer Network. NCCN Practice Guidelines for Prostate Cancer. *Oncology (Huntington)* 2000;14:111–119.

54. Yamashita K, Denno K, Ueda T, et al. Prognostic significance of bone metastases in patients with metastatic prostate cancer. *Cancer* 1993;71: 1297–1302.

55. Knudson G, Grinis G, Lopez-Majano V, et al. Bone scan as a stratification variable in advanced prostate cancer. *Cancer* 1991;68:316–320.

56. Wood DR, Banerjee M. Presence of circulating prostate cells in the bone marrow of patients undergoing radical prostatectomy is predictive of disease-free survival. *J Clin Oncol* 1997;15:3451–3457.

57. Mueller P, Carrol P, Bowers E, et al. Low frequency epithelial cells in bone marrow aspirates from prostate carcinoma patients are cytogenetically aberrant. *Cancer* 1998;83:538–546.

58. Slovin SF, Scher HI. Detectable tumor cells in the blood and bone marrow: smoke or fire? *Cancer* 1998;83:394–398.

59. Engeler CE, Wasserman NF, Zhang G. Preoperative assessment of prostatic carcinoma by computerized tomography. *Urology* 1992;40:346–350.

60. Van Poppel H, Ameye F, Oyen R, et al. Accuracy of combined computerized tomography and fine needle aspiration cytology in lymph node staging of localized prostate carcinoma. *J Urol* 1993;151:1310–1314.

61. Tempany CMC, Rahmouni AD, Epstein JI, et al. Invasion of the neurovascular bundle by prostate cancer: evaluation with MR imaging. *Radiology* 1991;181:107–112.

62. Schiebler ML, Yankaskas BC, Tempany C, et al. MR imaging in adenocarcinoma of the prostate: inter-observer variation and efficacy for determining stage C disease. *AJR Am J Roentgenol* 1992;158:559–562.

63. Yu KK, Scheidler J, Hricak H, et al. Prostate cancer: prediction of extracapsular extension with endorectal MR imaging and three-dimensional proton MR spectroscopic imaging. *Radiology* 1999;213:481–488.

64. Huch Boni RA, Boner JA, Debatin JF, et al. Optimization of prostate carcinoma staging: comparison of imaging and clinical methods. *Clin Radiol* 1995;50:593–600.

65. Chelsky MJ, Schnall MD, Seidmon JE, et al. Use of endorectal surface coil magnetic resonance imaging for local staging of prostate cancer. *J Urol* 1993;150:391–395.

66. Kier R, Wain S, Troiano R. Fast spin-echo MR images of the pelvis obtained with a phased-array coil: value in localizing and staging prostate carcinoma. *AJR Am J Roentgenol* 1993;161:601–606.

67. D'Amico AV, Schnall M, Whittington R, et al. Endorectal coil magnetic resonance imaging identifies locally advanced prostate cancer in select patients with clinically localized disease. *Urology* 1998;51:449–454.

68. Coakley FV, Qayyum A, Kurhanewicz J. Magnetic resonance imaging and spectroscopic imaging of prostate cancer. *J Urol* 2003;170:69–75.

69. Sonnad SS, Langlotz CP, Schwartz JS. Accuracy of MR imaging for staging prostate cancer: a meta-analysis to examine the effect of technologic change. *Acad Radiol* 2001;8:149–157.

70. Engelbrecht MR, Jager GJ, Laheij RJ, et al. Local staging of prostate cancer using magnetic resonance imaging: a meta-analysis. *Eur Radiol* 2002;12:2294–2302.

71. Harisinghani MG, Barentsz J, Hahn PF, et al. Noninvasive detection of clinically occult lymph-node metastases in prostate cancer. *N Engl J Med* 2003;348:2491–2499.

72. Egan AJM, Bostwick DG. Prediction of extraprostatic extension of prostate cancer based on needle biopsy findings: perineural invasion lacks significance on multivariate analysis. *Am J Surg Pathol* 1997;21: 1496–1500.

73. Stone NN, Stock RG, Parikh D, et al. Perineural invasion and seminal vesicle involvement predict pelvic lymph node metastasis in men with localized carcinoma of the prostate. *J Urol* 1998;160:1722–1726.

74. Partin AW, Kattan MW, Subong ENP, et al. Combination of prostate specific antigen, clinical stage, and Gleason score to predict pathologic stage of localized prostate cancer: a multi-institutional update. *JAMA* 1997; 277:1445–1451.

75. Fesseha T, Sakr W, Grignon D, et al. Prognostic implications of a positive apical margin in radical prostatectomy specimens. *J Urol* 1887;158: 2176–2179.

76. Blute ML, Bostwick DG, Seay TM, et al. Pathologic classification of prostate carcinoma: the impact of margin status. *Cancer* 1998;82:902–908.

77. Sakr WA, Wheeler TM, Blute M, et al. Staging and reporting of prostate cancer—sampling of the radical prostatectomy specimen. *Cancer* 1996; 78:366–368.
78. Ross PL, Scardino PT, Kattan MW. A catalog of prostate cancer nomograms. *J Urol* 2001;165:1562–1568.
79. D'Amico AV, Whittington R, Schultz D, et al. Outcome based staging for clinically localized adenocarcinoma of the prostate. *J Urol* 1997;158: 1422–1426.
80. Renshaw AA, Richie JP, Loughlin KR, et al. The greatest dimension of prostate carcinoma is a simple, inexpensive predictor of prostate specific antigen failure in radical prostatectomy specimens. *Cancer* 1998;83: 748–752.
81. D'Amico AV, Whittington R, Malkowicz SB, et al. The combination of preoperative prostate specific antigen and postoperative pathological findings to predict prostate specific antigen outcome in clinically localized prostate cancer. *J Urol* 1998;160:2096–2101.
82. D'Amico AV, Whittington R, Malkowicz SB, et al. Calculated prostate cancer volume greater than 4.0 cm^3 identifies patients with localized prostate cancer who have a poor prognosis following radical prostatectomy or external-beam radiation therapy. *J Clin Oncol* 1998;16:3094–3100.
83. D'Amico AV, Desjardin A, Chen MH, et al. Analyzing outcome-based staging for clinically localized adenocarcinoma of the prostate. *Cancer* 1998;83:2172–2180.
84. D'Amico AV, Desjardin A, Chung A, et al. Assessment of outcome prediction models for patients with localized prostate carcinoma managed with radical prostatectomy or external beam radiation therapy. *Cancer* 1998; 82:1887–1896.
85. Diblasio CJ, Kattan MW. Use of nomograms to predict the risk of disease recurrence after definitive local therapy for prostate cancer. *Urology* 2003;62:9–18.
86. Graefen M, Karakiewicz PI, Cagiannos I, et al. International validation of a preoperative nomogram for prostate cancer recurrence after radical prostatectomy. *J Clin Oncol* 2002;20:3206–3212.
87. Stamey TA, Donaldson AN, Yemoto CE, et al. Histological and clinical findings in 896 consecutive prostates treated only with radical retropubic prostatectomy: epidemiologic significance of annual changes. *J Urol* 1998;160:2412–2417.

CHAPTER 11 ■ THE UTILITY OF OUTCOME PREDICTION MODELS FOR PROSTATE CANCER THERAPY

ANDREW J. STEPHENSON AND MICHAEL W. KATTAN

INTRODUCTION

The early detection of prostate cancer through the use of widespread prostate-specific antigen (PSA) screening and systematic ultrasound-guided prostate biopsy has resulted in the diagnosis of an increasing number of patients with clinically localized prostate cancer who are candidates for definitive therapy. Radical prostatectomy (RP), external-beam radiotherapy (EBRT), and transperineal interstitial radiotherapy (IRT) are the potential treatment options for these patients, and the reported overall long-term success rates associated with these treatments exceed 65% (1–3). Presently, there are no randomized trials to demonstrate the superiority of one treatment over another, although it is apparent that the success of each of these therapies may vary depending on the characteristics of an individual's cancer. For example, IRT as monotherapy is generally not offered to patients with high-risk features although it may provide equivalent cancer control compared to RP and EBRT for patients with low-risk disease.

Even if one therapy were proven to provide superior oncological results, it may not represent the optimal intervention for an individual patient. Long-term cancer control is not the only goal a patient wishes to pursue when choosing among treatment alternatives. He is also interested in minimizing the impact of therapy on his quality of life. He may be unwilling to accept the treatment option with the highest likelihood of cure if it is also associated with unacceptable morbidity. All the treatment options for prostate cancer impact quality of life to varying degrees. For example, RP is associated with a higher incidence of urinary incontinence, while EBRT and IRT are associated with higher rates of bowel dysfunction and irritative bladder symptoms. Each of these therapies also affects sexual function to varying degrees.

In the absence of evidence demonstrating the superiority of one treatment over another in terms of oncological efficacy and treatment-related morbidity, the patient is best suited to decide which treatment, if any, is best for him by weighing the consequences, both good and bad, for each treatment option under consideration. The relative impact of treatment-related morbidity on quality of life may be highly individualized. Only the patient can gauge how much he is willing to compromise urinary continence, for example, for long-term cancer control. As such, the physician is in a poor position to make treatment decisions for these patients. At the heart of decision making is patient preference, which the physician is also unable to quantify. Some patients may have an aversion to radical surgery while others will be satisfied only if the prostate cancer has been surgically removed. If a patient is not involved in choosing among treatment options for his prostate cancer, he is more likely to regret his treatment choice in the future, especially if he experiences a bad outcome.

Accurate estimations of the likelihood of treatment success, complications, and long-term morbidity are essential to patient counseling and informed decision making. Properly informing the patient of the likelihood of treatment success and morbidity will improve his satisfaction after treatment. This rationale is based on the work in the area of regret, where not consulting multiple specialists is a risk factor for regret of treatment choice (4). If given an overly optimistic likelihood of success (both oncological and functional), a patient is more likely to be surprised and experience more regret when his treatment fails compared to one who is given an accurate estimation of treatment success. Likewise, a patient who is given an overly pessimistic prediction of treatment success will regret the decision not to pursue definitive therapy if he learns later on that he may have had a reasonable chance for a successful outcome. Accurate estimations of risk are essential for the physician if he is to recommend against treatment for a patient with indolent or incurable disease or for the rational application of adjuvant treatment strategies for patients at risk for disease progression after definitive local therapy. Accurate risk estimations are also required for clinical trial design to ensure homogeneous high-risk patient groups for whose members new cancer therapeutics will be investigated.

Traditionally, clinical judgment has formed the basis for risk estimation, patient counseling, and decision making. However, we have difficulty with outcome prediction due to the biases that exist at all stages of the prediction process (5,6). Clinicians do not recall all cases equally; certain cases can stand out and exert an unsuitably large influence when predicting future outcomes. We tend to be inconsistent when processing our mental database and tend to resort to heuristics (i.e., rules of thumb) when processing becomes difficult (7). When it comes to making a prediction, we tend to predict the outcome we prefer rather than the outcome with the highest probability (5). Finally, we have a difficult time learning from our mistakes during the feedback process. Numerous prognostic variables for prostate cancer progression have been identified including serum PSA, clinical stage, biopsy Gleason sum, pathologic stage, prostatectomy specimen Gleason sum, surgical margins, and tumor volume. Likewise, the recovery of potency after RP is influenced by preoperative erectile function, patient age, comorbid medical conditions, cavernous nerve preservation, and individual surgical technique (8). Clinicians have difficulty weighing the relative importance of each of these factors when formulating outcome predictions.

To obtain more accurate predictions, researchers have developed predictive tools based on statistical models (9). In general, these predictive models have been proven to perform as well as or better than clinical judgment when predicting

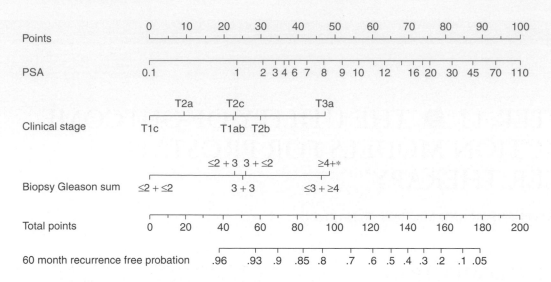

Instructions for Physician: Locate the patient's PSA on the PSA axis. Draw a line straight upward to the Points axis to determine how many points toward recurrence the patient receives for his PSA. Repeat this process for the Clinical Stage and Biopsy Gleason Sum axes, each time drawing straight upward to the Points axis. Sum the points achieved for each predictor and locate this sum on the Total Points axis. Draw a line straight down to find the patient's probability of remaining recurrence free for 60 months assuming he does not die of another cause first.

Note: This nomogram is not applicable to a man who is not otherwise a candidate for radical prostatectomy. You can use this only on a man who has already selected radical prostatectomy as treatment for his prostate cancer.

Instruction to Patient: "Mr. X, if we had 100 men exactly like you, we would expect between (predicted percentage from nomogram – 10%) and (predicted percentage + 10%) to remain free of their disease at 5 years following radical prostatectomy, and recurrence after 5 years is very rare."

FIGURE 11.1. Preoperative nomogram based on 983 patients treated at The Methodist Hospital (Houston, TX) for predicting the 5-year probability of freedom from PSA recurrence after definitive therapy with radical prostatectomy. (From Kattan MW, Eastham JA, Stapleton AM, et al. A preoperative nomogram for disease recurrence following radical prostatectomy for prostate cancer. *J Natl Cancer Inst* 1998;90:766–771, with permission.)

outcome probabilities (10). Statistical models predicting the likelihood of long-term cancer control, urinary continence, and potency will be useful for the individual patient when deciding upon RP as the treatment for his prostate cancer.

A popular approach to developing predictive models is to group patients with similar characteristics, and to make a prediction for each group. For example, D'Amico et al. developed a model that predicts cancer control for patients treated with radical prostatectomy, external-beam radiotherapy, or brachytherapy by placing patients into mutually exclusive risk groups based on clinical stage, biopsy Gleason sum, and pretreatment PSA level (11). While risk grouping is a logical approach, grouping patients is an inefficient use of the data and tends to reduce the predictive accuracy of a prognostic model. When predicting outcome for a subset of patients, the relative importance of prognostic variables in another patient group is ignored. The method of counting risk factors and variables should also be avoided because this assumes that each variable exerts an equal prognostic weight on the outcome, which is unlikely to represent the true relation between variables and prognosis (12). In addition, risk-grouping requires converting continuous variables into categorical variables, which removes information about the actual value.

An alternative method to risk groups is to develop continuous multivariable models called *nomograms*. A nomogram is a graphic representation of a mathematical formula or algorithm that incorporates several predictors modeled as continuous variables to predict a particular endpoint. Nomograms consist of sets of axes; each variable is represented by a scale, with each value of that variable corresponding to a specific number of points according to its prognostic significance. For

example, the nomogram shown in Figure 11.1 assigns each PSA level a unique point value that represents its prognostic significance. In a final pair of axes, the total point value from all the variables is converted to the probability of reaching the endpoint. By using scales, nomograms calculate the *continuous* probability of a particular outcome.

By incorporating all relevant continuous predictive factors for individual patients, nomograms provide more accurate predictions than models based on risk-grouping and they generally surpass clinical experts at predicting outcomes by calculating probabilities in a uniform fashion (5,10,14,15). Several studies have documented the superior performance of nomograms compared to risk-grouping schemata (15–17). This may stem from the fact that risk groups consist of patients with *similar*—albeit not identical—characteristics, resulting in heterogeneity within a risk group that reduces the predictive accuracy (5,18). The heterogeneity inherent in risk groups is illustrated in Figure 11.2, where the 5-year progression-free probability (PFP) after RP was calculated using a continuous, multivariable preoperative nomogram among patients classified as low-, intermediate-, and high-risk using the criteria of D'Amico et al. (11). While low-risk patients uniformly had a high likelihood of being free of progression by the nomogram, a substantial proportion of intermediate- and even high-risk patients had a calculated 5-year PFP of 90% or more. A considerable overlap in the nomogram predictions is also evident among intermediate- and high-risk patients. A risk group is composed of a mixture of patients and is only useful for gauging the prognosis for that group of patients. A patient does not care about the outcome of his (heterogeneous) group; he cares about his individual prognosis. His physician should do the same.

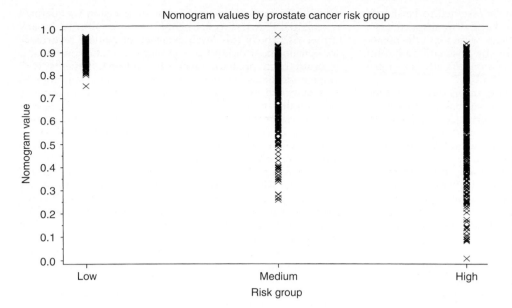

FIGURE 11.2. Five-year progression-free probability after radical prostatectomy calculated by preoperative nomogram (13) for patients classified as low-, intermediate-, and high-risk by D'Amico et al. (From D'Amico AV, Whittington R, Malkowicz SB, et al. Biochemical outcome after radical prostatectomy, external beam radiation therapy, or interstitial radiation therapy for clinically localized prostate cancer. *JAMA* 1998;280:969–974, with permission.)

In contrast to risk groups, a nomogram makes a tailored predicted probability based on the characteristics of the individual patient. While nomograms are more complex than risk groups, this added complexity results in higher predictive accuracy for both patient and physician. Nomograms have been adapted for use on personal digital assistants (PDAs) and personal computers to facilitate their use in the office or for research purposes. These nomograms are available in the public domain for free download from www.nomograms.org.

The superior predictive accuracy of continuous, multivariable nomograms versus risk groups is illustrated by comparing the ability of the Partin Tables to predict the pathologic features of prostate cancer with a suite of nomograms that we have recently developed. The Partin Tables combined serum PSA (four categories), clinical stage (seven categories), and biopsy Gleason sum (five categories) to predict the pathological stage of prostate cancer that is assigned as one of four mutually exclusive groups [organ-confined, established extracapsular extension (ECE), seminal vesicle invasion (SVI) (19), or lymph node involvement (LNI) (20)] (21). These tables underestimate the probability of ECE, for example, because a substantial proportion of patients with lymph node metastases and SVI will also have ECE. Among patients with prostate cancer in our institutional database, the predictive accuracy of the Partin Tables for predicting organ-confined disease, SVI, and LNI was 0.71, 0.72, and 0.74, respectively (19,20,22). In contrast, nomograms incorporating PSA, clinical stage, and Gleason sum modeled as continuous variables had a concordance index for predicting organ-confined disease, SVI, and LNI of 0.74, 0.84, and 0.76, respectively (18,19,21).

Several considerations apply when designing predictive models. A model should accurately predict which patients will and will not reach the endpoint (*discrimination*), generate predictions that closely approximate actual outcomes (*calibration*), and perform consistently when applied to different data sets (*validation*). They should also be based on a sufficient number of cases; specifically, they must incorporate a sufficiently large proportion of cases that reach the endpoint of interest. Predictive models should incorporate an appropriate number of variables, including variables that are statistically insignificant. If the model uses only statistically significant variables, they tend to exert an inappropriately large influence, resulting in falsely narrowed

confidence intervals (CI) that make the nomogram appear more accurate than it is (23,24). Ideally, a predictive model should demonstrate *generalizability*. That is, it should repeatedly perform with similar accuracy when applied to *heterogeneous* novel populations. Prognostic models lose their generalizability when they use small data sets, use data sets with a large proportion of missing information, incorrectly impute or delete missing records, or incorporate an inappropriate number of variables (25). Furthermore, for greatest utility in the clinical setting, nomograms should incorporate parameters that are reliable and routinely employed, and they should be easy to use.

The nomograms developed by Kattan et al. are based on Cox proportional hazards or logistic regression analysis modified by restricted cubic splines (25). Unmodified regression models require variables to assume linear relations, which is not ideal because it assumes that incremental changes represent the same significance across the spectrum of values. For example, a rise in PSA from 2 ng/mL to 4 ng/mL would represent the same impact as a rise from 302 ng/mL to 304 ng/mL. The application of cubic splines imparts flexibility to the nomogram by allowing continuous variables to maintain nonlinear relations. Machine learning modeling methods such as artificial neural networks offer greater flexibility than traditional statistical methods and theoretically may lead to enhanced predictive accuracy if data sets contain highly predictive nonlinear or interactive effects. However, traditional statistical methods appear to perform as well as machine learning methods and offer the added advantage of reproducibility and interpretability through the generation of hazard ratios and tests of significance for the predictors (26).

These nomograms use data in their most elemental forms to extract the maximum amount of useful information. For example, the primary and secondary Gleason grades are used as independent variables, rather than the Gleason sum alone, since several combinations of primary and secondary Gleason grades can result in the same Gleason sum (e.g., 3 + 3 = 6, 2 + 4 = 6, 4 + 2 = 6), but these combinations may reflect quite different disease states with different prognoses (27).

An important approach incorporated into these nomograms is that patients receiving secondary treatment *before* demonstrating disease progression are classified as treatment failures. This approach is used because the secondary treatment was probably prompted by some evidence of recurrence, so the time of secondary treatment is assumed to be shortly before the recurrence would have been demonstrated (24). Censoring (or excluding) these patients would bias the nomogram toward improved outcomes, but by designating adjuvant therapy equivalent to disease progression, the efficacy of primary therapy is better evaluated.

The discrimination of these nomograms is measured using the concordance index (or c-index), rather than the area under the receiver operating characteristic curve (AUC). While the AUC requires binary outcomes (e.g., cure/fail), the c-index functions in the presence of case censoring and is more appropriate for analyzing time-to-event data (28).

Lastly, these nomograms are calibrated and validated to evaluate their accuracy. While external validation represents the gold standard for evaluating accuracy and reproducibility, bootstrapping (29) remains a legitimate alternative that can be used alone or in concert with external validation to assess the nomogram's precision (25).

NOMOGRAMS AVAILABLE FOR PROSTATE CANCER RECURRENCE AFTER DEFINITIVE THERAPY

Many nomograms exist for prostate cancer recurrence after definitive local therapy (9). There is also a critical need for nomograms that estimate the likelihood of treatment-related morbidity (e.g., urinary incontinence and erectile dysfunction). This discussion, however, will be restricted to four contemporary models that predict the continuous risk of disease progression after local definitive therapy with RP (13,30), EBRT (17), or transperineal IRT (31). Each of the pretreatment models predicts the 5-year probability of remaining free from disease progression (i.e., the PFP), based on PSA relapse after definitive therapy. The pretreatment nomograms are useful when deciding upon the definitive treatment options for clinically localized prostate cancer. The postoperative model predicts the 7-year PFP after RP. The postoperative nomogram is useful for deciding upon the need for adjuvant local or systemic therapy after RP.

RADICAL PROSTATECTOMY

Both pretreatment and posttreatment nomograms have been developed to predict the continuous probability of disease progression after RP (13,30).

Pretreatment

Clinical stage, biopsy Gleason score, and pretreatment serum PSA level are known pretreatment variables associated with disease progression after RP (1,32). These factors have been combined by Partin et al. to predict the pathologic stage of the prostatectomy specimen (21). Although this endpoint is useful for surgical planning, it often does not correlate with the risk of disease progression (33). In fact, Hull et al. found 50% of patients with nonorgan-confined disease to be free from disease recurrence at 10 years after RP, confirming that the presence of extraprostatic disease does not imply definite disease progression (1).

Kattan et al. developed a pretreatment nomogram that predicts the 5-year PFP for patients who choose RP based on clinical stage, biopsy-derived primary and secondary Gleason grades, and pretreatment PSA level (13). The model was based on 983 patients with clinically localized prostate cancer

treated by a single surgeon. Disease progression was defined as an initial PSA rise to 0.4 ng/mL or more followed by any further rise above this level, evidence of clinical recurrence (local, regional, or distant), administration of adjuvant therapy, or death from prostate cancer. In addition, patients with lymph node metastasis in whom a prostatectomy was aborted were classified as treatment failures at the time of surgery. The overall 5-year PFP for this cohort was 73%. The nomogram is accurate and discriminating with a concordance index (c-index) of 0.75 when applied to external validation cohort (34). It was also validated in the African-American population with a c-index of 0.74 (35).

The 5-year endpoint is insufficient to predict the likelihood of cure after RP as a substantial number of patients are at risk for disease progression beyond 5 years (36,37). After 10 years, however, recurrence is rare. Among patients treated with RP in our own series, disease progression was observed in 3 of 284 patients who had an undetectable PSA at 10 years or later after RP (38). Thus, the 10-year PFP would appear to be a sufficient endpoint for estimating the likelihood that a man will be cured of his prostate cancer by RP alone.

Several investigators have demonstrated that the results of systematic prostate biopsy provide important preoperative prognostic information for prostate cancer recurrence after radical prostatectomy (39,40). Inclusion of systematic biopsy results in the D'Amico risk groups improved the ability of this model to predict biochemical recurrence after RP (40). We recently developed a new preoperative nomogram incorporating clinical stage, biopsy Gleason grade, PSA, number of positive prostate biopsy cores, and number of negative prostate biopsy cores to predict the 10-year probability of cancer recurrence after RP. However, inclusion of the number of positive and negative cores resulted in only a mild improvement in predictive accuracy over stage, grade and PSA in independent validation (c-index 0.79 vs. 0.78) (41). Similar results were reported by Graefen et al., who demonstrated minimal improvement in the predictive accuracy of stage, grade, and PSA in a predictive model that included the number of positive cores and the number of cores containing high-grade cancer (42).

Posttreatment

Kattan et al. also developed a postoperative nomogram to identify patients at high risk for experiencing disease progression after RP (see Fig. 11.3) (30). This instrument uses the pretreatment PSA level, Gleason sum of the prostatectomy specimen, extracapsular extension, margin status, seminal vesical invasion, and lymph node status to predict the 7-year probability of disease progression. The model was based on 996 men with clinically localized prostate cancer treated by a single surgeon. Treatment failure was defined as an initial PSA rise to 0.4 ng/mL or more, followed by any further rise above this level, clinical evidence of disease progression (local or distant), initiation of adjuvant therapy, or death from prostate cancer. The 7-year progression-free probability for the cohort was 73%. The nomogram had a c-index of 0.80 when applied to an international validation cohort and 0.83 when applied to a cohort of African-Americans (35,43).

The postoperative nomogram was recently updated and enhanced to calculate the 10-year probability of prostate cancer recurrence after RP (38). Given that a patient's prognosis improves with the disease-free interval maintained after RP, we have also enabled the 10-year progression-free probability to be adjusted to reflect this changing prognosis. When applied to two independent validation datasets, the nomogram was demonstrated to be accurate and discriminating (c-index 0.81 and 0.79).

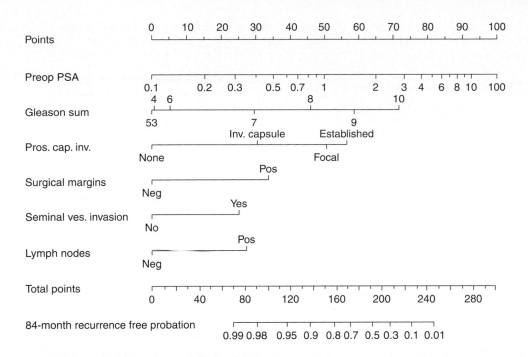

Instructions for Physician: Locate the patient's PSA on the PSA axis. Draw a line straight upward to the Points axis to determine how many points toward recurrence the patient receives for his PSA. Repeat this process for the other axes, each time drawing straight upward to the Point axis. Sum the points achieved for each predictor and locate this sum on the Total Points axis. Draw a line straight down to find the patient's probability of remaining recurrence free for 84 months assuming he does not die of another cause first.

Instruction to Patient: "Mr. X, if we had 100 men exactly like you, we would expect between (predicted percentage from nomogram − 10%) and (predicted percentage + 10%) to remain free of their disease at 7 years following radical prostatectomy, and recurrence after 7 years is very rare."

FIGURE 11.3. Postoperative nomogram based on 996 patients treated at the Methodist Hospital, Houston, TX, for predicting freedom from PSA recurrence after radical prostatectomy. For Prostatic Capsular Invasion (Pros. cap. inv.) "None" refers to L0-L1, "Inv. capsule" refers to L2, "Focal" refers to L3F, and "Established" refers to L3E. Preop, preoperative; ves., vesicle. (From Kattan MW, Wheeler TM, Scardino PT. Postoperative nomogram for disease recurrence after radical prostatectomy for prostate cancer. *J Clin Oncol* 1999;17:1499–1507, with permission.)

EXTERNAL BEAM RADIOTHERAPY

Kattan et al. developed a pretreatment nomogram to predict the 5-year PFP after treatment with three-dimensional conformal EBRT based on clinical stage, biopsy Gleason sum, pretreatment PSA level, use of neoadjuvant androgen deprivation therapy, and radiation dose (see Fig. 11.4) (17). The model was based on 1042 men treated at Memorial Sloan-Kettering Cancer Center (MSKCC) between 1988 and 1998. PSA failure was based on the American Society for Therapeutic Radiology and Oncology (ASTRO) criteria, with failure defined as three cumulative rises of serum PSA level, with the failure date designated as the midpoint in time between the first rise and the PSA level immediately before this rise (44). Bootstrap analysis yielded a *c*-index of 0.73 and external validation with a cohort of 912 men treated at the Cleveland Clinic yielded a *c*-index of 0.76, which was significantly superior to the best risk grouping model available (17).

TRANSPERINEAL INTERSTITIAL PERMANENT BRACHYTHERAPY

Kattan et al. developed a pretreatment nomogram that predicts the 5-year PFP after transperineal IRT with ^{125}I seeds in

the absence of adjuvant hormonal therapy based on pretreatment PSA level, clinical stage, biopsy Gleason sum, and the co-administration of EBRT (see Fig. 11.5) (31). The model was based on 920 men treated for T1-2 prostate cancer at Memorial Sloan-Kettering Cancer Center, with treatment failure defined by a modified version of the ASTRO criteria, the administration of adjuvant hormonal deprivation therapy, clinical evidence of disease progression (local, regional, or distant), or death from prostate cancer. External validation with 1827 men treated at the Seattle Prostate Institute demonstrated a *c*-index of 0.61, and further validation with 765 men treated at Arizona Oncology Services yielded a *c*-index of 0.64.

LIMITATIONS OF NOMOGRAMS

While clinically useful for counseling patients, nomograms are far from perfect and cannot be applied to all men with prostate cancer. In general, nomograms are constructed and validated using patients treated at academic centers, whose outcomes may differ considerably from outcomes of patients treated at community health centers, since the quality and availability of treatments can vary with the location and experience level of the treating physician (45,46). Recently, the preoperative nomogram was validated on a cohort of patients treated at both academic and community centers and was observed to overestimate the likelihood

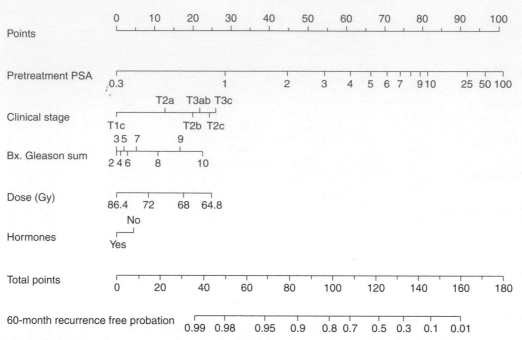

Instructions for Physician: Locate the patient's PSA on the PSA axis. Draw a line straight upward to the Points axis to determine how many points toward recurrence the patient receives for his PSA. Repeat this process for the other axes, each time drawing straight upward to the Points axis. Sum the points achieved for each predictor and locate this sum on the Total Points axis. Draw a line straight down to find the patient's probability of remaining recurrence free for 60 months assuming he does not die of another cause first.

Note: This nomogram is not applicable to a man who is not otherwise a candidate for radiation therapy. You can use this only on a man who has already selected radiation therapy as treatment for his prostate cancer.

Instruction to Patient: "Mr. X, if we had 100 men exactly like you, we would expect between (predicted percentage from nomogram − 10%) and (predicted percentage + 10%) to remain free of their disease at 5 years following conformal radiation therapy, and recurrence after 5 years is very rare."

FIGURE 11.4. Three-dimensional conformal radiation therapy (3D-CRT) nomogram, based on 1042 patients treated at MSKCC, for predicting freedom from PSA recurrence after radiation therapy, Bx. Gleason sum, biopsy Gleason sum. (From Kattan MW, Zelefsky MJ, Kupelian PA, et al. Pretreatment nomogram for predicting the outcome of three-dimensional conformal radiotherapy in prostate cancer. *J Clin Oncol* 2000;18:3352–3359, with permission.)

of cure amongst these patients (particularly for those with probabilities of recurrence of less than 35%) (47). All nomograms were developed in populations of patients treated with RP, EBRT, or transperineal IRT, and thus they are only applicable for patients who otherwise would be candidates for each of these treatments. Since a patient and his physician may exert a selection bias for a particular treatment, it would be most appropriate to apply the nomogram as a last step in the decision-making process after the patient has chosen a particular treatment.

These nomograms use serum PSA relapse as a measure of disease progression. Although PSA universally antedates clinical disease recurrence, it has not been validated as a surrogate endpoint for disease-specific mortality (37,48). However, as a sensitive marker of disease recurrence, PSA recurrence is a valuable endpoint for counseling patients regarding the likelihood of treatment success. However, the probability of developing clinical recurrence and death from prostate cancer are more meaningful endpoints to predict. A nomogram was recently developed that predicts the 5-year probability of distant metastases (with or without the use of salvage androgen-deprivation therapy) among patients treated with EBRT (18). We are currently working to develop nomograms to predict the probability of metastatic progression after RP.

The outcome predictions determined by the nomograms for RP, EBRT, and transperineal IRT should not be used alone to compare treatments. In particular, clinicians and patients should not simply pick the treatment with the highest nomogram prediction of freedom from recurrence. Although all the

nomograms use PSA recurrence as the primary endpoint, the definitions of PSA recurrence are different for each of them. Gretzer et al. applied the ASTRO criteria of recurrence to a series of surgically treated patients and produced an apparent improvement in the 15-year progression-free probability from 68% (based on a single PSA rise of greater than or equal to 0.2 ng/mL) to 90% (49). Even if a similar definition of recurrence is employed for patients treated by RP, EBRT, and transperineal IRT, the PSA outcome may be biased in favor of EBRT and IRT. The reason for this bias is that before a patient who is managed with radiotherapy or brachytherapy can be considered a PSA failure, he must first achieve a PSA nadir, which can take several years (50). Conversely, patients who are managed with RP will reach their PSA nadir within the first few weeks postoperatively. Consequently, among patients who are destined to fail biochemically, the time to failure will be earlier for surgically treated patients (51). It is also apparent that biochemical progression after RP and after EBRT are not equivalent endpoints to compare. In the absence of salvage androgen-deprivation therapy, the reported median interval from biochemical recurrence to metastatic progression has been estimated to be 8 years after RP, compared to only 3 years after EBRT (37,52). Thus, it would appear that patients who experience biochemical recurrence after EBRT are at a considerably higher risk of early metastatic progression than those who recur following RP.

Continuous, multivariable models such as nomograms currently represent the most accurate and discriminating tools for predicting the outcome of patients who undergo definitive

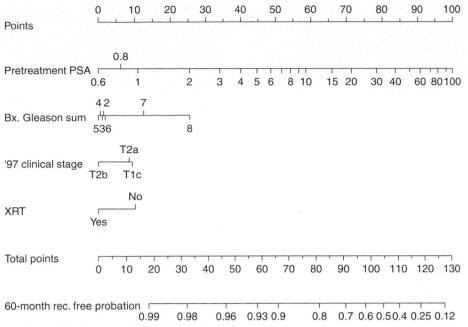

FIGURE 11.5. Nomogram for predicting 5-year freedom from PSA recurrence after permanent prostate brachytherapy without neoadjuvant androgen ablative therapy. XRT, x-ray therapy; Bx. Gleason sum, biopsy Gleason sum. (From Kattan MW, Potters L, Blasko JC, et al. Pretreatment nomogram for predicting freedom from recurrence after permanent prostate brachytherapy in prostate cancer. *Urology* 2001;58:393–399, with permission.)

therapy for localized prostate cancer. When a patient faces the difficult decision of choosing among the treatment options for prostate cancer, the nomograms for prostate cancer recurrence after RP, EBRT, and transperineal IRT provide accurate estimations of treatment success with each of these therapies. Equipped with this information, the patient is more likely to be confident in his treatment decision and less likely to experience regret in the future. However, it should be emphasized that nomogram predictions must be interpreted as such; they do not make treatment recommendations or act as a surrogate for physician-patient interactions, nor do they provide definitive information on symptomatic disease progression or complications associated with treatments. Thus, the current nomogram prediction should serve as the initial basis upon which to further explore these issues when selecting a treatment for prostate cancer. Future nomograms that predict the likelihood of metastatic progression, cancer-specific mortality, and long-term urinary and sexual function are likely to have great utility for the patient and physician as they explore treatment alternatives.

References

1. Hull GW, Rabbani F, Abbas F, et al. Cancer control with radical prostatectomy alone in 1,000 consecutive patients. *J Urol* 2002;167:528–534.
2. Shipley WU, Thames HD, Sandler HM, et al. Radiation therapy for clinically localized prostate cancer: a multi-institutional pooled analysis. *JAMA* 1999;281:1598–1604.
3. Ragde H, Elgamal AA, Snow PB, et al. Ten-year disease free survival after transperineal sonography-guided iodine-125 brachytherapy with or without 45-gray external beam irradiation in the treatment of patients with clinically localized, low to high Gleason grade prostate carcinoma. *Cancer* 1998;83:989–1001.
4. Miles BJ, Giesler B, Kattan MW. Recall and attitudes in patients with prostate cancer. *Urology* 1999;53:169–174.
5. Kattan MW. Expert systems in medicine. In: Smelser NJ, Baltes PB, eds. *International encyclopedia of the social and behavioral sciences.* Oxford: Pergamon; 2001;5135–5139.
6. Hogarth RM. *Judgement and choice: the psychology of decision,* 2nd ed. Chichester: John Wiley and Sons; 1987.
7. Kattan MW. Introduction. *Semin Urol Oncol* 2002;20:79–81.
8. Rabbani F, Stapleton AM, Kattan MW, et al. Factors predicting recovery of erections after radical prostatectomy. *J Urol* 2000;164:1929–1934.
9. Ross PL, Scardino PT, Kattan MW. A catalog of prostate cancer nomograms. *J Urol* 2001;165:1562–1568.
10. Ross PL, Gerigk C, Gonen M, et al. Comparisons of nomograms and urologists' predictions in prostate cancer. *Semin Urol Oncol* 2002;20: 82–88.
11. D'Amico AV, Whittington R, Malkowicz SB, et al. Biochemical outcome after radical prostatectomy, external beam radiation therapy, or interstitial radiation therapy for clinically localized prostate cancer. *JAMA* 1998;280: 969–974.
12. Antman EM, Cohen M, Bernink PJ, et al. The TIMI risk score for unstable angina/non-ST elevation MI: a method for prognostication and therapeutic decision making [see *Comments*]. *JAMA* 2000;284:835–842.
13. Kattan MW, Eastham JA, Stapleton AM, et al. A preoperative nomogram for disease recurrence following radical prostatectomy for prostate cancer. *J Natl Cancer Inst* 1998;90:766–771.
14. Meehl PE. Causes and effects of my disturbing little book. *J Pers Assess* 1986;50:370–375.
15. D'Amico AV, Whittington R, Malkowicz SB, et al. A multivariate analysis of clinical and pathological factors that predict for prostate specific antigen

failure after radical prostatectomy for prostate cancer. *J Urol* 1995; 154:131–138.

16. Kattan MW, Leung DH, Brennan MF. Postoperative nomogram for 12-year sarcoma-specific death. *J Clin Oncol* 2002;20:791–796.

17. Kattan MW, Zelefsky MJ, Kupelian PA, et al. Pretreatment nomogram for predicting the outcome of three-dimensional conformal radiotherapy in prostate cancer. *J Clin Oncol* 2000;18:3352–3359.

18. Kattan MW, Zelefsky MJ, Kupelian PA, et al. Pretreatment nomogram that predicts 5-year probability of metastasis following three-dimensional conformal radiation therapy for localized prostate cancer. *J Clin Oncol* 2003;21:4568–4571.

19. Koh H, Kattan MW, Scardino PT, et al. A nomogram to predict seminal vesicle invasion by the extent and location of cancer in systematic biopsy results. *J Urol* 2003;170:1203–1208.

20. Cagiannos I, Karakiewicz P, Eastham JA, et al. A preoperative nomogram identifying decreased risk of positive pelvic lymph nodes in patients with prostate cancer. *J Urol* 2003;170:1798–1803.

21. Partin AW, Kattan MW, Subong EN, et al. Combination of prostate-specific antigen, clinical stage, and Gleason score to predict pathological stage of localized prostate cancer. A multi-institutional update. *JAMA* 1997; 277:1445–1451.

22. Bianco FJ Jr, Kattan MW, Eastham JA, et al. Prediction and outcomes of men with organ confined prostate cancer after radical prostatectomy. 2004 (*in press*).

23. Harrell FE Jr. Design: S-Plus function for biostatistical/epidemiologic modeling, testing, estimation, validation, graphics, prediction, and typesetting by storing enhanced model design attributes in the fit. 1998.

24. Kattan MW, Scardino P. Prediction of progression: nomograms of clinical utility. *Clin Prostate Cancer* 2002;1:90–96.

25. Harrell FE, Lee KL, Mark DB Jr. Multivariable prognostic models: issues in developing models, evaluating assumptions and adequacy, and measuring and reducing errors. *Stat Med* 1996;15:361–387.

26. Kattan MW. Comparison of Cox regression with other methods for determining prediction models and nomograms. *J Urol* 2003;170:S6–S9; discussion S10.

27. Chan T, Partin A, Walsh P, et al. Prognostic significance of Gleason score 3 + 4 versus Gleason score 4 + 3 tumor at radical prostatectomy. *Mod Pathol* 2000;13:95A.

28. Begg CB, Cramer LD, Venkatraman ES, et al. Comparing tumour staging and grading systems: a case study and a review of the issues, using thymoma as a model. *Stat Med* 2000;19:1997–2014.

29. Efron B, Tibshirani RJ. An introduction to the bootstrap. 1993.

30. Kattan MW, Wheeler TM, Scardino PT. Postoperative nomogram for disease recurrence after radical prostatectomy for prostate cancer. *J Clin Oncol* 1999;17:1499–1507.

31. Kattan MW, Potters L, Blasko JC, et al. Pretreatment nomogram for predicting freedom from recurrence after permanent prostate brachytherapy in prostate cancer. *Urology* 2001;58:393–399.

32. Pound CR, Partin AW, Epstein JI, et al. Prostate-specific antigen after anatomic radical retropubic prostatectomy. Patterns of recurrence and cancer control. *Urol Clin North Am* 1997;24:395–406.

33. Wheeler TM, Dillioglugil O, Kattan MW, et al. Clinical and pathological significance of the level and extent of capsular invasion in clinical stage T1-2 prostate cancer. *Hum Pathol* 1998;29:856–862.

34. Graefen M, Karakiewicz PI, Cagiannos I, et al. International validation of a preoperative nomogram for prostate cancer recurrence after radical prostatectomy. *J Clin Oncol* 2002; 20(15):3206–3212.

35. Bianco FJ Jr, Kattan MW, Scardino PT, et al. Radical prostatectomy nomograms in black American men: accuracy and applicability. *J Urol* 2003; 170:73–76; discussion 76–77.

36. Dillioglugil O, Leibman BD, Kattan MW, et al. Hazard rates for progression after radical prostatectomy for clinically localized prostate cancer. *Urology* 1997;50:93–99.

37. Pound CR, Partin AW, Eisenberger MA, et al. Natural history of progression after PSA elevation following radical prostatectomy. *JAMA* 1999; 281:1591–1597.

38. Stephenson AJ, Scardino PT, Eastham JA, et al. Postoperative nomogram predicting the 10-year probability of prostate cancer recurrence after radical prostatectomy. *J Clin Oncol.* 2005 (*in press*).

39. Freedland SJ, Aronson WJ, Terris MK, et al. Percent of prostate needle biopsy cores with cancer is significant independent predictor of prostate specific antigen recurrence following radical prostatectomy: results from SEARCH database. *J Urol* 2003;169:2136–2141.

40. D'Amico AV, Whittington R, Malkowicz SB, et al. Utilizing predictions of early prostate-specific antigen failure to optimize patient selection for adjuvant systemic therapy trials. *J Clin Oncol* 2000;18:3240–3246.

41. Stephenson AJ, Scardino PT, Eastham JA, et al. Predicting the 10-year probability of prostate cancer recurrence after radical prostatectomy: a new preoperative nomogram. 2005. (*in press*).

42. Graefen M, Ohori M, Karakiewicz PI, et al. Assessment of the enhancement in predictive accuracy provided by systematic biopsy in predicting outcome for clinically localized prostate cancer. *J Urol* 2004;171: 200–203.

43. Graefen M, Karakiewicz PI, Cagiannos I, et al. Validation study of the accuracy of a postoperative nomogram for recurrence after radical prostatectomy for localized prostate cancer. *J Clin Oncol* 2002;20:951–956.

44. American Society for Therapeutic Radiology and Oncology Consensus Panel Consensus statement: guidelines for PSA following radiation therapy. *Int J Radiat Oncol Biol Phys* 1997;37:1035–1041.

45. Hu JC, Gold KF, Pashos CL, et al. Role of surgeon volume in radical prostatectomy outcomes. *J Clin Oncol* 2003;21:401–405.

46. Begg CB, Riedel ER, Bach PB, et al. Variations in morbidity after radical prostatectomy. *N Engl J Med* 2002;346:1138–1144.

47. Greene KL, Meng MV, Elkin EP, et al. Validation of the Kattan preoperative nomogram for prostate cancer recurrence using a community based cohort: results from Cancer of the Prostate Strategic Urological Research Endeavor (capsure). *J Urol* 2004;171:2255–2259.

48. D'Amico AV, Moul JW, Carroll PR, et al. Surrogate end point for prostate cancer-specific mortality after radical prostatectomy or radiation therapy. *J Natl Cancer Inst* 2003;95:1376–1383.

49. Gretzer MB, Trock BJ, Han M, et al. A critical analysis of the interpretation of biochemical failure in surgically treated patients using the American Society for Therapeutic Radiation and Oncology criteria. *J Urol* 2002; 168:1419–1422.

50. Kuban DA, Thames HD, Levy LB, et al. Long-term multi-institutional analysis of stage T1-T2 prostate cancer treated with radiotherapy in the PSA era. *Int J Radiat Oncol Biol Phys* 2003;57:915–928.

51. D'Amico AV. How to compare results after surgery or radiation for localized prostate carcinoma. *Cancer* 2002;95:2041–2043.

52. Lee WR, Hanks GE, Hanlon A. Increasing prostate-specific antigen profile following definitive radiation therapy for localized prostate cancer: clinical observations. *J Clin Oncol* 1997;15:230–238.

CHAPTER 12 ■ IMAGING IN PROSTATE CANCER

MICHAEL MULLERAD, AMITA SHUKLA-DAVE, AND HEDVIG HRICAK

INTRODUCTION

Prostate cancer, a remarkably heterogeneous disease, is the most common malignancy and the second leading cause of cancer death in American men (1). Undiagnosed cases have been found in as many as 64% of autopsies, depending on age (2). The high incidence of indolent prostate cancer and the slow progression of the disease make it difficult to evaluate the benefits of early diagnosis and the need for screening. It is therefore unsurprising that prostate cancer screening has been a controversial issue. Currently, both the American Urological Association (AUA) and the American Cancer Society (ACS) recommend that early detection of prostate cancer be offered to asymptomatic men 50 years of age or older with an estimated life expectancy of more than 10 years. Testing at an earlier age should be limited to men with defined risk factors, such as having a first-degree relative with prostate cancer or being African American (3). The U.S. Preventive Services Task Force (USPSTF) found good evidence that prostate-specific antigen (PSA) screening can detect early-stage prostate cancer, but concluded that evidence was insufficient to determine whether the benefits of prostate screening outweigh the harms (4).

The report published by Holmberg et al. demonstrated for the first time that radical prostatectomy (RP) significantly reduces disease-specific mortality when compared to watchful waiting (median follow-up time of 6.2 years) (5). Partly as a result of these findings, the strategy of watchful waiting could be replaced by new approaches, including disease prevention with a finasteride-based treatment (6) and active surveillance of early prostate cancer (7) that periodically monitors PSA and biopsy features in order to detect disease progression (in terms of the PSA doubling time, and "upgrading" at repeat biopsy). Other treatment options aimed at eradicating the cancer (surgery, radiation, and cryotherapy) are expected to gain strength in light of the findings of Holmberg et al.

All treatment options would benefit from an imaging modality that allowed clear visualization of the primary tumor in every patient. Unfortunately, although much progress has been made, as yet no such modality exists. Current techniques for imaging the primary tumor allow us to gain information only in selective cases. The appropriate use of imaging in evaluating patients with prostate cancer should therefore take into account significant clinical tumor prognostic factors, such as PSA, PSA doubling time, prostate biopsy findings, and, for patients after surgery, the final pathology findings. These prognostic factors have become complementary to prostate cancer imaging and allow the physician to properly assess the patient.

IMAGING FOR PROSTATE CANCER STAGING

Transrectal Ultrasonography (TRUS) and TRUS-guided Biopsy

Indications

Transrectal ultrasonography (TRUS) continues to play an important role in prostate cancer as a tool for guiding biopsy. When prostate cancer is suspected based on an abnormal digital rectal examination (DRE) or an elevated serum PSA level, the essential diagnostic test is a needle biopsy of the prostate. The AUA guidelines for prostate biopsy are a PSA level of 4.0 ng per mL or more, a significant rise in PSA level, or an abnormal DRE (3).

Technique

Patient preparation is not usually required before TRUS, although some physicians recommend a single, self-administered disposable enema before the study. We recommend an enema and antibiotic prophylaxis (e.g., ciprofloxacin 250 mg pre- and postprocedure). However, if after such treatment the patient develops a urinary tract infection, empirical treatment given should consist of second- or third-generation cephalosporin, amikacin, or a carbapenem due to natural selection of resistant bacteria (8). TRUS is well tolerated except in patients with marked prostate enlargement, acute prostatitis, or large hemorrhoids. DRE should be performed before ultrasound probe insertion. The probe is inserted after adequate lubrication, and double condom coverage of the probe is recommended. In patients allergic to latex, use condoms made of a different material. If there is difficulty inserting the endorectal probe, manual relaxation of the sphincter and use of lidocaine gel will help.

The diagnosis of prostate cancer requires a biopsy. The standard of care is the "systematic" sextant biopsy using an 18g needle driven by a spring-loaded, hand-held biopsy "gun." Cores are taken from six areas, or sextants, of the peripheral zone (PZ): left and right each of apex, middle, and base. Cores should also be taken from any suspicious abnormal areas. A single biopsy session has a sensitivity of 70% to 80% for the detection of cancer (9). To minimize the need for repeat biopsy sessions, it is usual to take more cores during the first session. There is growing evidence that 10 or 12 cores taken from the medial and lateral apex, middle, and base of each side increase sensitivity (15% to 30% more cancers detected) (10). Biopsies become increasingly painful after six to eight samples; therefore, many urologists inject local anesthetic (1% lidocaine without epinephrine) (11) around the nerves laterally at the junction of the seminal vesicles and base of the prostate and wait 10 minutes before taking samples. Separate samples of the anterior prostate [or transition zone (TZ)] are usually not taken unless multiple previous biopsy sessions have failed to find a suspected cancer (a high PSA level with an abnormal DRE and multiple negative PZ biopsies) or imaging by TRUS or magnetic resonance imaging (MRI) suggests an anterior cancer.

Findings

After placement of the ultrasound probe in the rectum, the prostate and seminal vesicles are visualized and images are recorded in the transverse and sagittal planes. TRUS can measure with reasonable accuracy (±10%) the size of the prostate gland (12), an important factor in computing "PSA density" (serum PSA in ng/mL divided by the volume of the prostate in cm^3) (13). Tumors, depending on their size, grade, and location, usually appear hypoechoic relative to the normal PZ of the prostate, as shown in Figure 12.1 (14). As a diagnostic test for cancer, ultrasound is as accurate as the DRE and complements the physical examination. Some palpable cancers are not visible on ultrasound and some visible cancers are not palpable (14–16). With the shift toward small, early-stage cancers, most cancers detected today are not visible on ultrasound (low sensitivity) and many hypoechoic areas do not prove to be malignant on biopsy (low specificity). Therefore, TRUS images have limited value in cancer diagnosis, and ultrasound alone should never be used to rule out the presence of a cancer.

TRUS has also been used to evaluate the extent of local disease. The criteria for extracapsular extension (ECE) are bulging or irregularity of the capsule adjacent to a hypoechoic lesion. The length of contact of a visible lesion with the capsule is also associated with the probability of ECE (17). Seminal vesicle invasion (SVI) is heralded by visible extension of a hypoechoic lesion at the base of the prostate into a seminal vesical or by echogenic cancer within the normally fluid-filled seminal vesical (18). Accuracy improved when sonographic findings were interpreted in concert with the DRE and PSA to estimate the likelihood of extraprostatic extension (19). Today, however, tumors are smaller at the time of diagnosis and local extension is uncommon. Modern nomograms based on standard clinical data (i.e., stage, grade, and PSA) more accurately estimate the probability of ECE, SVI, and lymph node metastases (20). Still, these algorithms provide no information about the location of the cancer or of ECE. There has been some enthusiasm for color duplex Doppler ultrasonography to identify cancer in hypervascular areas (21,22), but there is no clear evidence of greater sensitivity, specificity, or staging accuracy (Fig. 12.1B).

TRUS continues to play an important role in therapy. Worldwide, TRUS is the imaging modality of choice for directing brachytherapy seeds into the prostate (23). Cryotherapy of the prostate requires ultrasound guidance (24) as does high-intensity focused ultrasound (HIFU), which, coupled with sonographic targeting, is used for focal ablation of prostate cancers (25). Novel treatment approaches, such as hyperthermia, cryoablation, photodynamic therapy, direct injection of oncolytic viruses, and gene therapy, also depend on TRUS for easy access to prostate cancers (26). Until MRI guidance is widespread and much less expensive than it is now, TRUS will continue to play a major role in the management of prostate cancer patients.

Complications

Major complications are rare and include urosepsis (0.1%) and rectal bleeding that requires intervention (27).

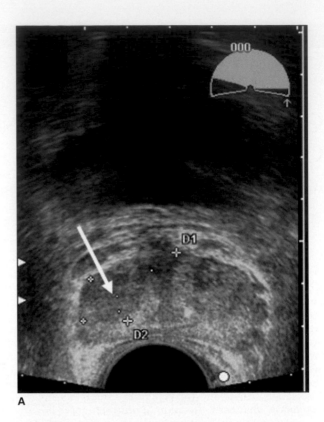

A

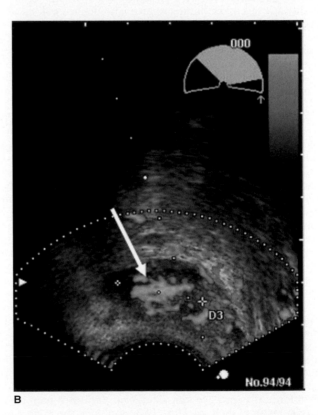

B

FIGURE 12.1. The use of gray-scale and Doppler ultrasound in the detection of prostate cancer: Gray-scale (**A**) and Doppler (**B**) transverse transrectal ultrasound images demonstrate a hypoechoic region (*arrows*) in the right side of the peripheral zone (PZ) suspicious for cancer. Doppler ultrasonography (**B**) identifies hypervascular areas in the lesion, indicating cancer (see color insert). (Courtesy of Dr. Fred Lee, University of Wisconsin.)

Immediate morbidity:

Rectal bleeding (2.1%), mild hematuria (62%), severe hematuria (0.7%), and moderate to severe vasovagal episodes (2.8%) (27).

Delayed morbidity:

Fever (2.9%), hematospermia (9.8%), recurrent mild hematuria (15.9%), persistent dysuria (7.2%), and urinary tract infection (10.9%) (27).

Computed Tomography

The role of computed tomography (CT) in prostate cancer management can be divided into two principal categories: initial staging and posttreatment follow-up.

Indications

In the initial staging of prostate cancer, established nomograms based on clinical data (PSA, Gleason Grade, DRE) provide risk stratification estimates that enable physicians to assess the need for further evaluation, including imaging tests such as CT. The majority of patients with newly diagnosed localized prostate cancer are at low risk for metastases. The diagnostic yield of CT is low in these patients, and false positive results are more common than true positives, leading to inaccurate staging, additional diagnostic work-up, and, sometimes, inappropriate treatment. Decision analysis studies show that nonstratification of patients by prognostic factors is costly and unjustified (28). Cutoff parameters for the appropriate use of CT have been recommended: CT is not recommended for patients with a PSA of less than 20 ng per mL, a Gleason score of less than 7, or a clinical stage of less than T3. However, unusual or discrepant clinical data may call for imaging, even if an individual falls below recommended risk thresholds. According to the AUA guidelines, there is no indication for CT in a patient with a PSA level of less than 25 ng per mL (3).

Technique

CT examination of the pelvis requires careful patient preparation. Complete opacification of the alimentary tract is essential, as unopacified small bowel loops in the pelvis can be misinterpreted as tumor masses. At least 1 hour before the examination, 600 to 1,000 mL of dilute oral contrast material should be given. Opacification of the rectosigmoid colon, however, is rarely needed in a study for prostate cancer. Ideally, the urinary bladder should be distended. A distended bladder will displace small bowel loops out of the pelvis, making it easier to identify other pelvic structures. For the evaluation of prostate cancer, delayed images showing contrast opacification of the bladder are unnecessary unless there is a need to visualize the distal ureters. Dense contrast opacification of the bladder may actually result in imaging artifacts and obscure adjacent structures. The routine use of an intravenous contrast medium is recommended to facilitate differentiation between lymph nodes and blood vessels. Transaxial CT images should extend from below the symphysis pubis up to the aortic bifurcation if only imaging of the pelvis is required. If the patient is being evaluated for advanced disease, imaging of the entire pelvis and abdomen may be required, although retroperitoneal lymphadenopathy is almost never found in the absence of pelvic lymphadenopathy in patients with prostate cancer.

Findings

Due mainly to the lack of soft-tissue contrast, the CT appearance of normal prostate tissue and normal seminal vesicles (Fig. 12.2) is similar to the CT appearance of prostate cancer,

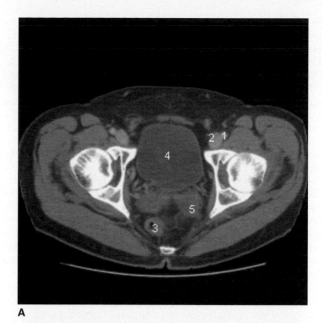

A

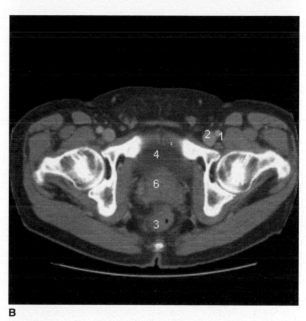

B

FIGURE 12.2. Axial contrast-enhanced computed tomography (CT) images demonstrate normal pelvic anatomy (1-femoral artery, 2-femoral vein, 3-rectum, 4-urinary bladder, 5-seminal vesical, 6-prostate).

even when ECE and SVI are present (29). Consequently, even in high-risk patients, the role of CT in local staging is limited to the assessment of nodal involvement (30). Limited ECE and SVI are better assessed on MRI or TRUS. CT can be useful as a baseline examination in clinically apparent, high-risk patients with grossly advanced local disease (gross ECE, gross SVI, or invasion of surrounding structures including bladder, rectum, levator ani muscles, or pelvic floor). Use of CT will generally be prior to radiation or medical therapy. Such patients will nearly always fall above the cut-off recommendations for the appropriate use of CT imaging based on DRE, PSA and Gleason grade; they will also be at risk for lymph node metastases, which may be assessed concurrently.

In the assessment of metastatic disease, evaluation for lymph node and bone metastases is essential. Nodal disease outside the pelvis as well as liver and lung metastases are features of late-stage prostate cancer. The regional nodes for prostate cancer (designated as N1 in the TNM Staging System) are pelvic nodes, including obturator, iliac [internal, external, or not otherwise specified (NOS)], and sacral [lateral, presacral, promontory (Gerota's)] or NOS sites (Fig. 12.3). The diagnosis of nodal metastases on CT has been based solely on nodal size. The recommended size threshold for diagnosis of lymph node metastases in prostate cancer patients is a short axis diameter of greater than 1.0 cm. However, the correlation between nodal enlargement and metastatic involvement is poor (31). Reports of CT sensitivity for the detection of lymph node metastases vary, but most are in the range of 36% (28). One study reported values of 85% sensitivity and 67% specificity (32), although specificity has occasionally been reported as low as 25% (33). Oyen et al. showed a sensitivity of 78% and specificity of 97% using size criteria of 0.6 cm (34). The same study also reported specificity of 100% for CT combined with CT-guided fine-needle aspiration (FNA) biopsy. The decreased size criteria have not been broadly accepted, nor has the use of FNA been widely adopted.

Metastatic lymph nodes (M1) are any nodes that lie outside the confines of the true pelvis, as outlined earlier. Nodal disease often progresses in stepwise fashion, such that retroperitoneal or mediastinal nodal disease is most often accompanied by pelvic lymphadenopathy (35). If staging by cross-sectional imaging is initially limited to the pelvis, evaluation of the abdominal nodes is warranted whenever enlarged pelvic lymph nodes are identified. Nevertheless, metastases to pelvic lymph nodes are uncommon with early-stage prostate cancer and are found in only 2% to 5% of patients (36,37). These metastases are most often microscopic, too small to be detected on imaging. Neither CT nor MRI can be used to rule out lymph node metastases. Removal of grossly enlarged nodes has not been shown to have therapeutic value in prostate cancer (38). Controversy persists over the therapeutic value of pelvic lymphadenectomy (PLND) performed during radical retropubic prostatectomy (38,39). While the long-term survival for such patients is excellent (85% at 10 years), few remain free of recurrent cancer without additional systemic therapy (40). PLND is not recommended as an independent procedure in patients treated with definitive radiation therapy because metastases often bypass the pelvic lymph nodes.

Bone scan and MRI are superior to CT in diagnosis and follow-up of bone metastases (41,42). Lytic and blastic bone metastases will commonly be visible on CT (Fig. 12.4B,E), however, and should not be overlooked.

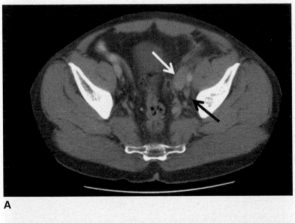

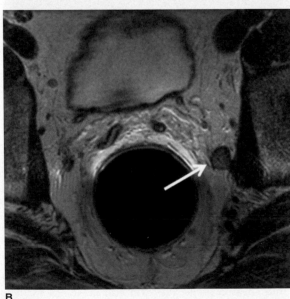

FIGURE 12.3. A: Axial contrast-enhanced computed tomography (CT) image demonstrates enlarged lymph nodes (*black arrow*: obturator node; *white arrow*: external iliac node); B: Axial T2-weighted MR image depicts an enlarged left obturator lymph node (*white arrow*).

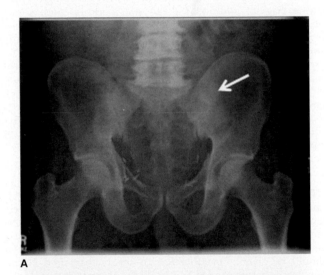

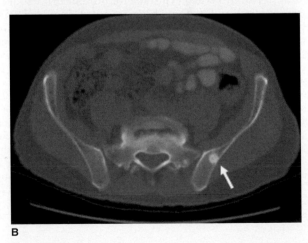

FIGURE 12.4. Iliac bone metastasis demonstrated on (A) plain film (*white arrow*), (B) axial CT scan (*white arrow*), and (C) axial T1-weighted MRI (*white arrow*). Bone metastasis involving the spine vertebra demonstrated on (D) sagittal T1-weighted MRI (*black arrow*) and (E) axial CT scan (*white arrow*).

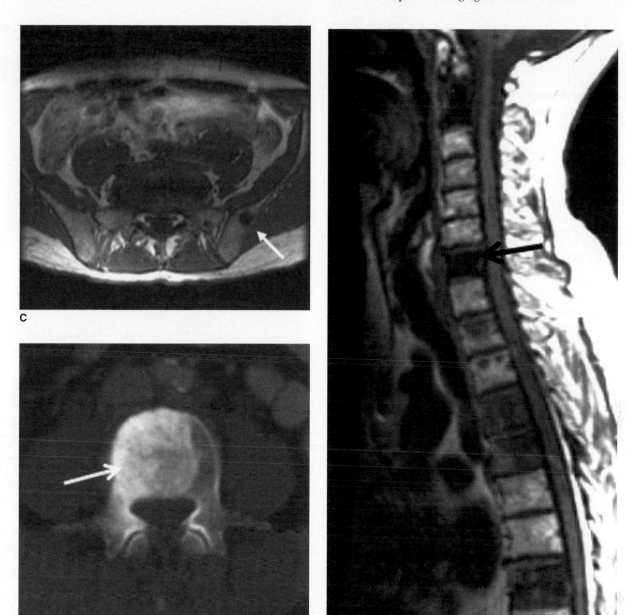

FIGURE 12.4. Continued.

Magnetic Resonance Imaging

Indications

The role of MRI in the pretreatment evaluation of patients with newly diagnosed prostate cancer remains controversial. Of all the imaging techniques available, MRI offers the greatest promise for accurate local staging, but problems of interobserver variability and high examination cost must be resolved before it can be recommended for general clinical use. Although exact patient selection criteria have yet to be worked out, patients for whom MRI is likely to be cost-effective are those at intermediate risk for extraprostatic disease based on established clinical prognostic factors (e.g., patients with 35% to 65% probability of having ECE based on PSA, Gleason score, and DRE). The AUA guidelines find no indication for MRI in a patient with a PSA level of less than 25 ng/mL (3).

Technique

Optimal MR imaging of prostate cancer requires the use of an endorectal coil in conjunction with a pelvic phased-array coil on a 1.5-Tesla or higher strength magnet. Although the patient should be carefully screened before coil placement, tolerance for endorectal coil placement is high. Contraindications for the use of the endorectal coil include a recent history of rectal surgery, inflammatory bowel disease, radiation therapy (RT) to the pelvis within the previous 6 weeks, use of anticoagulant drugs or a history of bleeding tendency, and the known presence of lesions (e.g., fistula or large hemorrhoids) or obstruction of the colon or rectum. To produce T2-weighted images of excellent resolution for local staging, thin slices (3 mm) and a small (14 cm) field of view are required (43).

Adequate evaluation of the pelvis requires both T1- and T2-weighted spin-echo MR images. T1-weighted images should be taken in the axial plane from below the symphysis pubis up to the aortic bifurcation. T2-weighted images (fast spin-echo) should be obtained in the axial plane from below the prostatic apex to above the seminal vesicles. T2-weighted images should be obtained in the coronal or sagittal plane for optimal visualization of the seminal vesicles. A flow-sensitive sequence (e.g., gradient-recalled echo sequence) is indicated when the patency of blood vessels is questioned or when there is a need to differentiate lymph nodes from vascular structures. The use of an intravenous contrast medium is not recommended for evaluation of the prostate gland (44).

Findings

The signal intensity and detection of prostate cancer on MRI depend on the type of imaging sequence used. On T1-weighted images, the prostate demonstrates homogeneous medium signal intensity. On T2-weighted MR images, cancer most commonly demonstrates decreased signal intensity within the high-signal-intensity normal PZ (45) (Fig. 12.5). While MRI has been most effective for detecting prostate cancer in the PZ, it also has great potential for the evaluation of tumors in the TZ, especially when it is combined with magnetic resonance spectroscopic imaging (MRSI) (46). Findings indicative of TZ cancer include: (a) a homogenous low-signal-intensity region in the TZ (especially in the absence of dominant PZ tumor); (b) poorly defined lesion margins; (c) lack of a low-signal-intensity rim (seen commonly in association with benign adenomatous nodules); (d) interruption of the pseudocapsule (TZ/PZ boundary of low signal intensity); and (e) urethral or anterior fibromuscular stromal invasion (47). Tumors in the TZ and those located in the anterior part of the PZ should be carefully sought during MRI interpretation in patients with rising PSA and multiple negative biopsies because these areas often are not routinely sampled or targeted during TRUS-guided biopsy.

Postbiopsy hemorrhage may hamper tumor detection in the prostate, leading to either under- or over-estimation of the tumor presence and local extent. The imaging appearance depends upon the length of time between the biopsy and the MRI, and the MRI should be delayed for at least 3 to 4 weeks after biopsy (48,49). While prostate cancer detection rates as high as 92% have been reported, the results of large multicenter studies were disappointingly low, with only 60% of lesions greater than 5 mm in any one dimension being detected on MRI scans (50).

The use of MRI for prostate cancer staging is gaining acceptance in select centers. On endorectal coil MRI, extracapsular extension can be identified by a contour deformity with a step-off or angulated margin, an irregular bulge or edge retraction, a breech of the capsule with evidence of direct tumor extension, obliteration of the recto-prostatic angle, or asymmetry of the neurovascular bundles (51,52) (Figs. 12.5, 12.6). The criteria for seminal vesicle invasion include contiguous low-signal-intensity tumor extension from the base of the gland into the seminal vesicles; tumor extension along the ejaculatory duct (nonvisualization of the ejaculatory duct); asymmetric decrease in the signal intensity of the seminal vesicles; and decreased conspicuity of the seminal vesicle wall on T2-weighted images (Fig. 12.6). While transaxial planes of section are essential in the evaluation of extracapsular invasion, the addition of coronal plane images facilitates the diagnosis of extracapsular

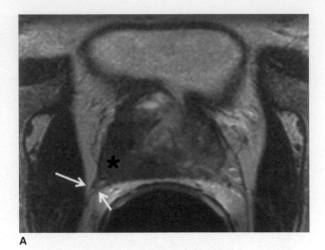

A

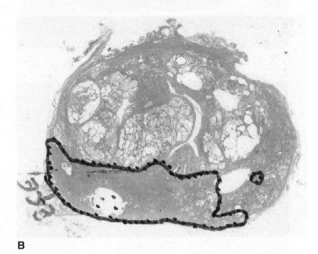

B

FIGURE 12.5. (A) Axial T2-weighted MR image with (B) corresponding step-section pathology. Prostate cancer (*) demonstrates decreased signal intensity within the high-signal-intensity normal PZ. A large tumor in the right side of the PZ demonstrates a focal bulge and tumor envelopment of the neurovascular bundle (*arrows*); both findings indicate extracapsular extension. Corresponding step-section pathology shows tumor (outlined) and site of established extracapsular extension.

extension. Combined axial, coronal, and sagittal planes of section facilitate the assessment of seminal vesical and bladder neck invasion.

The reported accuracy of MRI in staging prostate cancer ranges from 54% to 90% (45,50,51). These results have raised concerns about interobserver variability. During the past few years, however, more encouraging results for endorectal MRI have been obtained. The diagnostic performance of experienced readers has improved, with reported accuracy reaching between 75% and 93% (53–55). These values far exceed those reported for both TRUS and CT. The improved performance of endorectal MRI is likely due to a number of factors: the maturation of MRI technology (e.g., faster imaging sequences, more powerful gradient coils, and postprocessing image correction), better understanding of morphologic criteria used to diagnose ECE or SVI, and greater reader experience.

In the evaluation of lymph node metastases (Fig. 12.3B), efficacy data for MRI and CT are similar, with both modalities having low sensitivity. Promising results have been obtained in the use of highly lymphotropic superparamagnetic iron nanoparticles; these gain access to lymph nodes by means

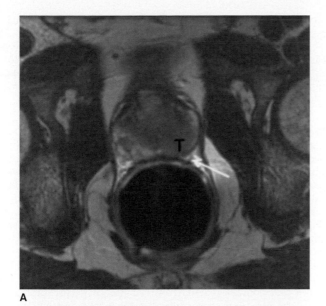

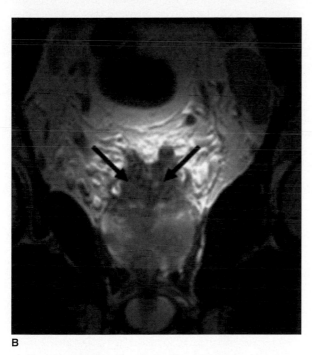

FIGURE 12.6. (A) Axial and (B) coronal T2-weighted MR images demonstrate a large left-side prostate cancer tumor (T) with evidence of bilateral seminal vesicle invasion (*black arrows*) and left-side ECE (*white arrow*).

of interstitial-lymphatic fluid transport and enter lymphatic tissue but not metastatic tissue, providing tissue contrast within in the lymph node and allowing detection of metastases (79). The sensitivity of MRI for metastases may be increased through use of these compounds, which appear to allow detection of metastases in normal-sized nodes (56,57).

MRI has been shown to be both sensitive and specific in the diagnosis of bone metastases; in fact, small metastatic deposits in the bone and those without cortical involvement may be detected earlier on MRI than on bone scans (Fig. 12.4C,D). However, other causes of altered marrow signal (e.g., infection, infarction, trauma) can mimic metastatic disease on MRI, and the examination is therefore limited to answering a specific question raised by other modalities (58). Therefore,

bone scintigraphy continues to be the initial test of choice for assessing bony metastases due to its overall sensitivity and its ability to survey the entire skeleton.

The performance of MRI in the local staging of prostate cancer will almost certainly continue to improve as MR technology, including MRSI, continues to advance.

Proton Magnetic Resonance Spectroscopic Imaging

The combination of MRI and proton MRSI may become an important tool in the detection and staging of prostate cancer (59–62). ^{1}H MRSI of the prostate gland expands the diagnostic assessment of prostate cancer through the detection of cellular metabolites. With 1.5-Tesla clinical MRI, it is possible to obtain a three-dimensional metabolic map of the entire gland with a resolution of 0.24 mL. The major metabolites observed in an MRSI spectrum from the normal prostate PZ are choline-containing compounds [3.21 parts per million (ppm)], creatine (3.02 ppm), and citrate (2.5–2.8 ppm). Citrate is synthesized, stored, and secreted by glandular tissue in the prostate (63–67). The choline peak consists mainly of choline, phosphocholine, and glycerophosphocholine, which are constituents of cell membrane synthesis and degradation pathways and have been shown to be elevated in many malignancies (68–75). The creatine peak is comprised of creatine and phosphocreatine (61).

The MRSI studies performed to date have shown that noninvasive differentiation of cancer from healthy tissue, as predicted by the extract studies, is possible. Choline-containing compounds have been found to be elevated and citrate reduced in *pathology-proven* cancer compared to healthy PZ tissue (61,68,76,77). Representative data from healthy PZ tissue, as well as from prostate gland with Gleason 4 + 3 cancer, are shown in Figures 12.7 and 12.8 with step-section histopathology. On MRSI, the healthier region of the prostate PZ exhibits high levels of citrate, while the region suspicious for cancer shows reduced citrate and elevated choline. Voxels are designated as suspicious for cancer based on the (choline + creatine)/citrate ratio as defined in the literature (61,78).

In a recent study conducted by Zakian et al. MRI/MRSI data from a subset of 123 patients were compared to step-section histopathology. The study demonstrated that tumor detection

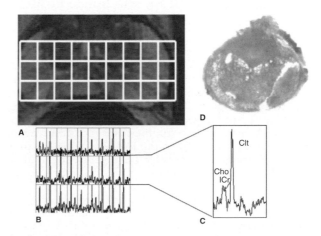

FIGURE 12.7. MRI with spectroscopy (MRSI) for a healthy section of prostate gland: (A) T2-weighted image; (B) spectra corresponding to the grid in (A); (C) normal spectra demonstrating elevated citrate and equivalent choline and creatine; (D) step-section pathology showing no cancerous areas.

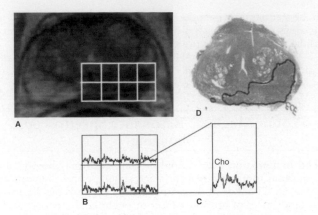

FIGURE 12.8. MRI with spectroscopy of a patient with Gleason 4 + 3 prostate cancer: (**A**) T2-weighted image demonstrates a large tumor volume and evidence of extracapsular extension. The cancer voxels are highlighted and the corresponding spectra are seen in (**B**) and (**C**); spectra demonstrate elevated choline and no citrate; the corresponding step-section tumor map (**D**) shows a Gleason score 4 + 3 cancer (outlined) and ECE.

on MRSI is Gleason-grade dependent. Pathology identified 239 lesions. MRSI overall sensitivity was 56% for tumor detection, increasing from 44% in Gleason pattern 3 + 3 lesions to 89% in lesions with a Gleason pattern greater than or equal to 4 + 4. There was a significant correlation between (choline + creatine)/citrate and Gleason pattern. Tumor volume assessed by MRSI also correlated positively with Gleason grade. Thus, MRSI metabolic and volumetric data correlate with pathologic Gleason grade and may help to noninvasively predict prostate cancer aggressiveness (79). The addition of MRSI to MRI also significantly improves the evaluation of extracapsular extension and decreases interobserver variability, enhancing the overall value of MRI in the evaluation of prostate cancer (59–62,76–78). To date, combined use of MRI and MRSI has been limited to only a few centers. A multicenter American College of Radiology Imaging Network (ACRIN) trial is planned to compare tumor detection using MRI alone to tumor detection using MRI plus MRSI.

Technetium^{99m}-Diphosphonate Bone Scintigraphy (Bone Scan) and Single Positron Emission Tomography

---

Indications

Bone scintigraphy with technetium^{99m}-diphosphonate remains the mainstay for the detection of metastatic prostate cancer spread to skeletal bone. The use of the bone scan has been modified in recent years by the measurement of PSA. If the PSA is less than 10 ng/mL (80), the chances of positive bone scan are less than 1%. When the PSA is between 10 to 50 ng/mL, the incidence of positive bone scan rises to about 10%, and when the PSA is in excess of 50 ng/mL, it rises to about 50%. In our practice, we generally reserve bone scanning for patients with PSA greater than 10 ng/mL. However, the AUA guidelines indicate bone scan for clinically localized prostate cancer patients only if PSA is greater than 20.0 ng/mL or if prostate cancer is poorly differentiated or high grade (3).

After prostatectomy, bone involvement is unlikely, as long as the PSA is below 2 ng/mL. A bone scan is not generally indicated following treatment of prostate cancer unless there is a rising PSA or specific, reproducible "bone" pain (81). There

have been only scattered reports of documented bone metastases with undetectable PSA following RP (82).

In the face of rising PSA, a negative bone scan suggests disease recurrence in the prostatic fossa, which may be treated locally. In contrast, a positive bone scan in the same setting signifies distant metastatic disease requiring systemic therapy.

Findings

Bone scintigraphy with technetium^{99m}-diphosphonate remains the primary means of skeletal imaging after radical retropubic prostatectomy or RT (81,83). The whole-body bone scan is simple to perform and is a sensitive method for detecting osseous metastases. The most common appearance is that of focally increased tracer uptake, usually in the axial skeleton, related to host osteoblastic bone response to tumor invasion (Fig. 12.9). Less often, an area of reduced uptake may be present, which reflects extensive damage to bone with little osteoblastic response. It should be noted that metastatic bone lesions are the result of implantation of metastatic cells within the bone marrow. Ninety percent of lesions are detected in bones that contain red marrow because of its predominant blood supply. Over time, there is progressive destruction of bone from the medullary cavity outward that is driven by biochemical mediators (cytokines) that are released by tumor cells. These mediators activate osteoclasts, which are responsible for the resorption of bone matrix. The osteoblastic response to this process, which is detected on the bone scan, is a secondary phenomenon.

One limitation of bone scans is that they are rarely positive before PSA values are high (around 30 ng per mL) (84). However, bone scans are more reliable than symptoms alone in the evaluation of bony metastatic disease, and as many as 34% of

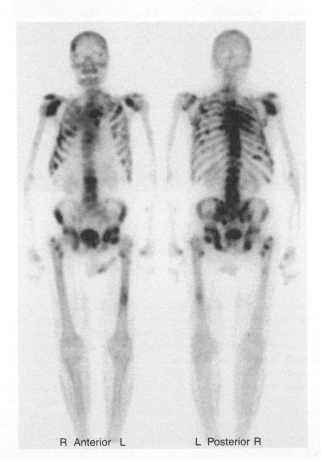

R Anterior L   L Posterior R

FIGURE 12.9. Bone scintigraphy with technetium^{99m}-diphosphonate demonstrating widespread bone metastasis, seen as increased uptake.

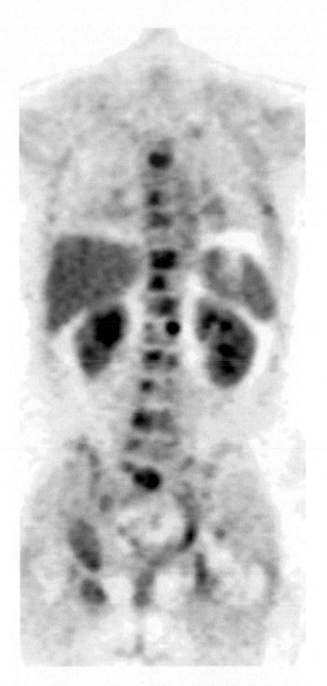

FIGURE 12.10. Bone technetium^{99m}-diphosphonate single photon emission tomography (SPECT), demonstrating prostate cancer metastasis to the vertebra.

asymptomatic patients may have abnormal scans (85). In the evaluation of 1403 patients with prostate cancer, the bone scan was 28% more sensitive than plain radiographs in detecting skeletal metastases (85).

If the bone scan is positive for metastatic disease, imaging assessment is essentially completed. Equivocal findings may warrant further imaging studies; depending on the level of clinical suspicion, these studies may include plain radiographs and positron emission tomography (PET) or, in some instances, MRI—specifically bone marrow MRI.

The long list of reasons for false-positive scans includes Paget disease, degenerative joint disease, previous trauma, and bone-marrow fibrosis—causes that are common in middle-aged and elderly men (86). Some of these conditions can be ruled out

or confirmed by single photon emission tomography (SPECT) imaging of the skeleton (Fig. 12.10). Studies of the skeleton that use SPECT are also more sensitive in the detection of metastatic disease than planar images alone. This technique has particular utility in the evaluation of the spine in patients with lower-back pain indicating possible metastatic disease. For instance, sites of abnormal uptake can be localized to the vertebral body, posterior elements of a vertebra, or to intervertebral joints. On the basis of the location and appearance of the lesion on SPECT images, the finding will be more suspicious for degenerative osteochondrosis, compression fracture, degenerative arthritis of intervertebral joints, or metastasis (87,88). In some cases, these findings may also direct other radiologic studies for more specific diagnosis (89,90).

Efforts have been made to quantify the tumor burden from osseous metastases. One of several proposed methods is the bone scan index (BSI). The BSI was shown to be an independent marker of prognosis in patients with androgen-independent prostate carcinoma (91). Studies investigating the utility of this parameter in monitoring treatment effects are currently underway. The simple quantification of the area of bone involved by metastases has also been shown to be an independent prognostic marker in patients with advanced prostate cancer (92).

Positron Emission Tomography and PET/CT

Most clinical PET studies to date have been performed with the glucose analogue FDG [fluorodeoxyglucose (2-deoxy-2-[18F]fluoro-D-glucose)]. The magnitude of elevated FDG uptake and accumulation within tumors is commonly expressed by the standardized uptake value (SUV), defined by the ratio of the activity per unit mass in the lesion to the administered activity per unit patient mass. Initial results of prostate cancer imaging with FDG were disappointing (93–95). However, many of these negative results might have been related to the use of older image reconstruction algorithms, leading to streak artifacts in the pelvis. In a recent study using iterative image reconstruction and FDG PET, the smallest tumor detectable was a stage T1c prostate carcinoma with a Gleason grade of 6 and a PSA of 8.3 (96). Nevertheless, FDG is not well suited for the detection of all prostate cancers, including instances of local or metastatic disease, especially when the cancer is low grade. FDG imaging is limited by the fact that this agent is excreted by the kidneys and hence accumulates in the urinary bladder. Detection of smaller foci of tracer accumulation in the adjacent prostate bed will therefore remain difficult. It is hoped that combined PET/CT will prove helpful in this regard.

The recent development of combined PET/CT units, where both instruments are housed in a common gantry, permits accurate anatomical localization of lesions with abnormal radiotracer accumulation and therefore more accurately demonstrates bony and pelvic lymph node disease. In the evaluation of bony metastasis, precise location of metastatic disease enables more precise treatment follow-up. New radiotracers for assessing different aspects of tumor biology are being developed, as is the simultaneous use of multiple tracers. Recently, work has been done with ^{11}C-methionine, which traces amino acid transport and protein synthesis (97). Other tracers are choline (labeled to either ^{11}C or ^{18}F) or acetate (labeled to ^{11}C).

The value of PET imaging can vary between patients with androgen-dependent as compared to androgen-independent prostate cancer. It is likely that dedifferentiated tumors (i.e., androgen-independent carcinomas) are metabolically more active and therefore more easily identified with FDG PET. ^{18}F-fluoro-dihydrotestosterone (FDHT) is an F-18 labeled testosterone which binds to androgen receptors on the prostate cancer cell surface. Preliminary studies with this new radio-tracer suggest an inverse relationship between the degree of binding of FDHT on prostate cancer cells and the intensity of FDG uptake in these lesions. That is to say, with increasing dedifferentiation, prostate cancer metastases appear less avid on FDHT imaging but demonstrate an increasing intensity of FDG uptake.

In summary, the concept of using PET with multiple radio-tracers that address different steps and processes of tumor metabolism and differentiation is likely to play an important role in the future of metabolic prostate cancer imaging.

Imaging with Monoclonal Antibodies (^{111}In–capromab Pendetide)

[111]In–capromab pendetide (ProstaScint) is a radiolabeled murine monoclonal immunoglobulin G antibody (7E11-C5.3). The antibody recognizes the intracellular epitope of prostate-specific membrane antigen (PSMA), a 100 kDa transmembrane glycoprotein that is relatively specific for human prostate epithelial cells (98,99). PSMA is expressed by virtually all prostate cancers and its expression is further increased in poorly differentiated, metastatic, and hormone-refractory carcinomas. There is no crossover reaction with PSA and, unlike PSA, PSMA is not down-regulated in undifferentiated or hormonally treated cancer cells (100,101). After initial studies, the U.S. Food and Drug Administration quickly approved imaging for postprostatectomy patients with rising PSA, no clear evidence for metastatic disease in other imaging studies, and a high clinical suspicion of occult metastatic disease. The antibody is fairly specific, but as many as 4 days are required for antibody binding to prostatic cells and clearance for background activity from the blood pool. Therefore, for imaging, the antibody is labeled to [111]indium (with a half-life of approximately 3 days) as a radiotracer, using glycyl-tyrosyl-n-diethylenetriaminepentaacetic acid lysine (GYK-DTPA) as a linker-chelator. The compound is administered intravenously. Planar and SPECT of the pelvis and abdomen is performed at 30 minutes (blood pool) and again 96 to 120 hours later (delayed images). Some institutions also use labeled red cells for imaging of the blood pool. Blood pool activity is then subtracted from [111]in–capromab pendetide images to better identify accumulation of the antibody in tissues. Some studies have found [111]in–capromab pendetide scans to be of little value for the preoperative detection of nodal disease as well as the postoperative detection of extrapelvic disease recurrence (102,103).

ROLE OF IMAGING IN TREATMENT PLANNING AND DELIVERY

Treatment Planning for Surgery

One important use of imaging for surgical treatment planning is assessing the risk of extracapsular extension prior to nerve-sparing RP in patients at intermediate clinical risk for capsular penetration. Such an assessment can help determine the appropriateness of nerve-sparing surgery as well as which neurovascular bundle(s) should be preserved. Because TRUS has not been shown to be more accurate than DRE in diagnosing extracapsular extension, MR imaging is probably the preferred technique for further evaluation of local stage in patients who are at intermediate risk for capsular penetration (50,52,104–106).While multicenter trials have not yet confirmed the value of MRI in this setting, in a study done at a single institution, Wei et al. reported that of 76 patients, 24%

had a more aggressive surgical plan when MRI was reviewed together with the clinical data. In a high-risk group, Bayesian analysis showed that the probability that a neurovascular bundle would have to be resected to avoid a positive margin increased from 39% to 78% with positive MRI findings and decreased from 39% to 19% with negative MRI findings (107). A study by Coakley et al. showed that MRI can help predict intraoperative blood loss, as a direct association was found between increased blood loss and the prominence of the apical periprostatic veins on MRI (108). In a recently published multivariate analysis of risk factors for time to recovery of urinary continence, the length of the membranous urethra on coronal endorectal MRI proved to be an independent predictor (109). Those with longer-than-average (14 mm) membranous urethra lengths experienced a more rapid return to stable continence.

Endorectal coil MRI (erMRI) can contribute still further to surgical planning. Visualization of a large, anterior TZ cancer on the preoperative MRI (Fig. 12.11) leads to more distal transection

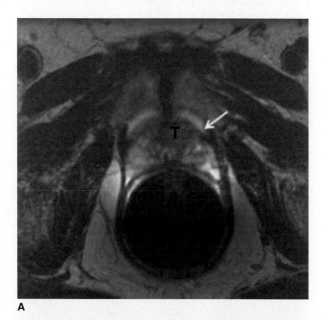

A

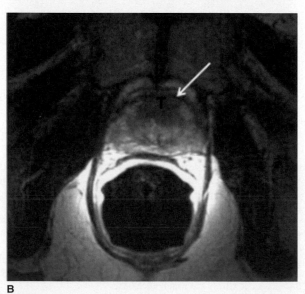

B

FIGURE 12.11. Two axial T2-weighted magnetic resonance (MR) images demonstrate a transitional zone tumor (T) (*arrows*) and direct tumor invasion into the anterior fibromuscular stoma.

of the dorsal vein complex over the urethra. A prominent tumor in the posterior apex warns the surgeon to dissect widely in that difficult area.

While the staging accuracy of MRI has not yet been firmly established in large clinical trials, in our institution the information about the cancer provided by endorectal MRI has led to better patient selection, safer operations, and a lower rate of positive surgical margins.

Treatment Planning for Radiation Therapy

Treatment planning in modern radiation oncology is image-based. Advances in imaging technology and the development of sophisticated radiation dose calculation algorithms have led to remarkable improvements in tumor localization and the generation of dose-distribution plans that conform to the anatomical configuration of tumor targets. The development of image-based computer treatment planning systems during the 1980s allowed CT image data to be incorporated into radiotherapy treatment plans, heralding three-dimensional conformal radiation therapy (3D-CRT) (110,111). The 3D-CRT approach is comprised of a series of procedures to define target and nontarget tissue structures from patient-specific 3D image data sets, the design of treatment portals using beam's-eye view displays, calculation and display of 3D dose distributions, and the analysis and evaluation of structure-specific dose-volume data. The use of conventional radiotherapy dose levels of 65 to 70 Gy, administered with traditional 2D planning and delivery treatment techniques, has had limited success in controlling localized prostate cancer. By improving the conformality of the dose distribution, the 3D-CRT approach has allowed significant increases in the tumor dose to levels beyond those feasible with conventional 2D radiotherapy, but without a concomitant increase in toxicity. Intensity modulated radiotherapy (IMRT) is an advanced mode of conformal radiotherapy that has enabled higher doses of radiation to be delivered to the prostate with greater precision (112–114). Treatment planning is based on inverse planning algorithms and iterative computer-driven optimization that generate treatment fields with varying radiation intensities within each beam. In prostate cancer, IMRT has resulted in reduced rectal toxicity and has permitted tumor dose escalation to previously unattainable levels (up to 86 Gy), with improvements in both local tumor control and disease-free survival.

Recent advances in imaging allow anatomic subregions of the tumor to be defined according to their levels of radiosensitivity or radioresistance. IMRT enables differential dose-painting to selectively increase the dose to specific tumor-bearing regions. It is possible to simultaneously deliver different radiation dose prescriptions to multiple target sites. To be able to dose-paint, one needs to know the tumor location, volume, and extent. Furthermore, information regarding tumor biology (e.g., tumor aggressiveness, angiogenesis, or hypoxia) is becoming essential (115). For example, functional imaging is already capable of identifying foci of hypoxic tumor clones that may require enhanced local doses. Recent data suggest that foci of high Gleason score prostate cancer may require doses of 90 Gy to achieve maximal levels of local control (116). The ability of MRSI to identify high Gleason score (i.e., greater than 8) prostate cancer and the improved tumor localization provided by the combining of MRI and MRSI data has allowed the first IMRT dose-painting clinical trials to be designed. On the basis of such anatomic/metabolic information, patient-specific parametric images have been used to dose-paint during brachytherapy as well (115).

MRI by itself may not be sufficient for treatment planning because it does not provide anatomical information in terms of electron density as needed for dose calculations. Therefore, helical and multidetector CT scanners, which are known to yield consistently high-quality anatomic images devoid of motion artifact, may be of value. With spatial registration of the images from the two modalities, x-ray attenuation data from CT and tissue contrast from MRI can provide a powerful planning tool. Combined CT/MRI images are increasingly used in the treatment planning of prostate cancer. Other information that is becoming essential for treatment planning includes the length of the membranous urethra (easily measured from sagittal or coronal MR images) for determining the caudal margin of the planning target volume and for sparing the penile bulb; the tumor loco-regional stage, including extracapsular extension and seminal vesical involvement (best assessed by MRI); and the presence of nodal metastasis (assessed by either CT or MRI).

Brachytherapy of Prostate Cancer

Technological advances in TRUS and CT have allowed successful development of the transperineal technique for brachytherapy (117). TRUS-guided transperineal radioactive seed implantation allows better distribution of seeds compared with open implants and more effective interstitial radiation. This low-morbidity treatment has the advantage of delivering a high dose of radiation to a confined area while doing relatively little damage to adjacent normal tissue (117). Real-time TRUS guidance allows accurate intraoperative needle placement, and postimplant CT or MRI allows assessment of the distribution of radioactive seeds within the prostate (118). If necessary, adjunctive external beam radiation may be directed to areas not adequately treated by the seed implants.

Cryosurgery of Prostate Cancer

Cryotherapy has reemerged largely because it can be performed percutaneously with real-time ultrasound guidance. The cryosurgical probe is guided into the prostate gland using the transperineal approach. The use of cryosurgery for prostate cancer has remained limited, however, due to a high complication rate and a lack of long-term results documenting the effectiveness of the technique. Shinohara et al. reported that the complication rate (excluding impotence) in their cohort of cryosurgery-treated patients was 51% (119). The most common serious complication was bladder outflow obstruction requiring transurethral resection in 23% of patients. Impotence occurred in 84% of patients (119).

ROLE OF IMAGING IN FOLLOW-UP OF PATIENTS WITH PROSTATE CANCER

The role of imaging after therapy depends on the treatment applied [watchful waiting, radical prostatectomy, radiation therapy, or androgen deprivation therapy (ADT)] and on clinical and laboratory findings. Regardless of the type of treatment, serial measurements of PSA and digital rectal examination (DRE) are the standard tools used in monitoring for tumor recurrence, with rising PSA being the earliest and most common indication of recurrence. When the PSA is elevated, three main categories of prostate cancer recurrence are considered: PSA-only relapse, local recurrence, and distant metastasis (most commonly nodal or bone metastasis). The key clinical consideration in evaluating a patient with suspected recurrence is the differentiation between local and metastatic relapse. Clinical nomograms used to statistically predict whether a recurrence is more likely local or metastatic have been widely studied and their clinical relevance has been determined (120–122). The nomograms are based on clinical parameters such as the tumor stage and grade at the time of diagnosis and the PSA doubling time (120–122). Distant recurrence is suggested by a short PSA doubling time (less than 10 months) in a patient with a high-grade cancer (Gleason sum of 8–10) or a high pathologic stage (SVI or LN metastases). In contrast, local recurrence is typically marked by a prolonged doubling time (more than 10 months) in a patient with a Gleason sum of 2–7, a positive surgical margin, and no involvement of the seminal vesicles or lymph nodes (123).

After potentially curative surgery, PSA should decline to an undetectable level within 21 to 30 days and remain undetectable thereafter (124,125). PSA falls more slowly after definitive radiation therapy than after surgery and may not reach a nadir until 18 to 30 months after treatment (126,127). Assessment for bony metastasis is discussed in the earlier section on MRI and technetium^{99m}-diphosphonate bone scintigraphy.

Assessing Effects of Hormonal Therapy

To date, the accepted use of hormone deprivation therapy has been for the treatment of metastatic prostate cancer. The availability of reversible androgen blockade using luteinizing hormone-releasing hormone (LHRH) agonists has led to a number of situations where LHRH agonists have been used prior to surgery or RT in selected patients. Reports on the efficacy of neoadjuvant antiandrogen therapy prior to RP have indicated a significant reduction in PSA, prostate volume, tumor volume, and a lower rate of positive surgical margins (128). Although there is disagreement over whether neoadjuvant hormones can downstage a cancer, there is no doubt that they reduce prostate volume (128,129). This is an advantage in patients with large prostates (greater than 40 to 50 mL) who are scheduled to undergo brachytherapy, because a smaller prostate gland reduces the number of radioactive seeds that must be placed. TRUS is the least expensive and most common imaging modality used to monitor tumor progression in patients undergoing hormonal therapy, but its value has not been proven (130). Bone scintigraphy can also be used to assess treatment response, as uptake usually decreases following hormone therapy. As a caveat, in prostate as well as breast cancer patients, a "flare" phenomenon may be observed following chemotherapy or hormonal deprivation therapy, whereby uptake increases in known metastatic bone lesions, peaking at 6 weeks after treatment as the healing process accelerates bone turnover (131,132). These changes can last for several months, and care must be taken to avoid misinterpreting the increase in intensity of tracer uptake in known metastasis, or even the appearance of apparently new lesions, as evidence of progression of disease. Awareness of the clinical situation and interaction with the referring physician can help prevent this mistake.

Hormone therapy affects erMRI as well. Apoptosis of prostate glandular cells leads to reduction of T2 signal and difficulties in identifying residual cancer with MRI (129). The effect of hormone therapy on MRSI spectra has been shown to depend on the treatment duration (133,134). Minimal metabolic changes occur with short-term exposure (less than 6 weeks), while medium (7 to 16 weeks) and long-term (more than 16 weeks) therapy dramatically reduce metabolite levels. Citrate levels decline more rapidly than choline levels, and healthy PZ is affected sooner than cancer. After long-term hormone therapy there is a widespread absence of metabolites throughout the gland; however, cancer remains detectable as a persistent choline peak, a feature not seen in treated healthy tissue. After short-to-intermediate hormone therapy, cancer detection is based on an adjusted (choline + creatine)/citrate

cutoff ratio (higher than in untreated gland) for the duration of the treatment, and the sensitivity and specificity of MRI and of combined MRI/MRSI remain the same as in the untreated gland. Combined chemotherapy and hormonal therapy in patients with high-risk, locally advanced prostate cancer has demonstrated a depletion of metabolites after 2 and 4 months of therapy (135).

Recently, PET imaging has been used to assess the metabolic activity of osseous metastases and has proven helpful in differentiating active bony metastasis from osteoblast activity that is merely related to healing bone. This question can be better addressed by PET than by either bone scan or CT (136).

Detecting Prostatic Fossa Recurrence Following Radical Prostatectomy

Imaging has not been widely used for the detection of local recurrence. TRUS, CT, and MRI have been evaluated for detection of local recurrence following prostatectomy. TRUS is the most commonly used imaging study. Leventis et al. (137) showed that TRUS is more sensitive than DRE (76% vs. 44%, respectively), although it is less specific (67% vs. 91%, respectively). The overall TRUS-guided biopsy detection rate was 41%. A tissue diagnosis for local recurrence was more likely to be achieved with TRUS-guided biopsy in patients with a PSA level greater than 4 ng/mL and positive DRE and TRUS findings (137). In a study evaluating CT detection of local recurrence after RP, only 36% of lesions were detected. In all cases in which the recurrence was detected, the tumor size was greater than 2 cm (138). Recent studies have shown that endorectal MRI can detect local recurrence in many patients with a rising PSA but no palpable tumor in the prostatic fossa. Silverman et al. have demonstrated the potential of endorectal MRI in the evaluation of local recurrence following prostatectomy with excellent sensitivity (100%) and specificity (100%) (139). A study by Sella et al. confirmed the high efficacy of MRI (sensitivity for detecting a recurrence was 95%, and specificity was 100%) (140).

MRI can detect local recurrences in the perianastomotic area and retrovesical space (Fig. 12.12), the sites also well identified on TRUS (137). However, 30% of local recurrences, as shown by MRI, can occur elsewhere in the pelvis, at sites of retained seminal vesicles or at the lateral or anterior surgical margins (140). MRI has the potential to direct a transrectal biopsy to these sites and thus may lead to a better diagnostic yield than TRUS. In addition, unlike TRUS, MRI using both an endorectal and a pelvic phased-array coil allows concomitant evaluation of pelvic lymph nodes and osseous structures, permitting the detection of all sites of pelvic relapse in a single examination.

Although studies have shown the value of ^{111}in–capromab pendetide radioimmunoscintigraphy for the detection of local recurrence in the prostate bed when there is rising PSA (141, 142), the prevailing opinion is that ^{111}in–capromab pendetide imaging is not useful for the detection of local recurrence.

In a retrospective study, Seltzer et al. (143) showed that both helical CT and FDG PET detect metastatic disease more accurately than ^{111}in–monoclonal antibody imaging.

As mentioned earlier, FDG imaging is limited by the fact that this agent is excreted by the kidneys and hence accumulates in the urinary bladder. Detection of smaller foci of tracer accumulation in the adjacent prostate bed will therefore remain difficult.

Follow-up After Radiation Therapy

Follow-up after RT is more difficult than after RP because of the potential contribution of residual prostatic tissue to the

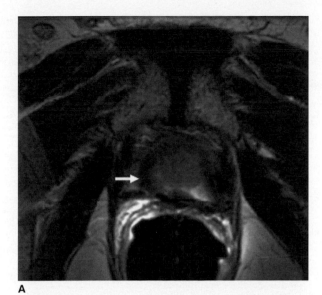

A

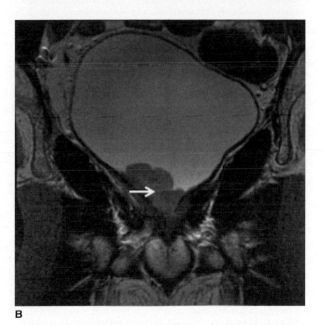

B

FIGURE 12.12. **(A)** Axial and **(B)** coronal T2-weighted magnetic resonance (MR) images of a local recurrence (*white arrows*) at the site of anastomosis.

serum PSA (144). If serum PSA persistently rises above baseline levels, disease progression is suspected and further evaluation is warranted (145). TRUS may be used in the evaluation of disease progression, but its accuracy is limited by loss of the normal zonal anatomy of the prostate after RT. In assessing patients after RT, the most appropriate and helpful use of TRUS may lie not in screening but in guiding biopsies of suspicious areas of the prostate (145).

MRI can also be used after primary RT to detect tumor progression or recurrence. Radiation treatment reduces T2-weighted signal intensity throughout the prostate gland and diminishes contrast between healthy treated tissue and cancer. On T2-weighted images, recurrent tumors appear hypointense compared to the surrounding PZ and hyperintense compared to the levator ani muscles.

Following radiotherapy, MRSI demonstrates an absence of detectable metabolites in most voxels, presumably due to widespread cellular death. However, finding voxels in which choline is the only detectable metabolite should raise a suspicion of cancer.

References

1. Jemal A, Thomas A, Murray T, et al. Cancer statistics, 2002. *CA Cancer J Clin* 2002;52:23–47.
2. Sakr WA, Grignon DJ, Crissman JD, et al. High grade prostatic intraepithelial neoplasia (HGPIN) and prostatic adenocarcinoma between the ages of 20–69: an autopsy study of 249 cases. *In Vivo* 1994;8:439–443.
3. Prostate-specific antigen (PSA) best practice policy. American Urological Association (AUA). *Oncology (Huntingt)* 2000;14:267–272, 277–278, 280 passim.
4. U.S. Preventive Services Task Force. *Guide to Clinical Preventive Services*, 2nd ed. Washington, DC: Office of Disease Prevention and Health Promotion, 1996.
5. Holmberg L, Bill-Axelson A, Helgesen F, et al. A randomized trial comparing radical prostatectomy with watchful waiting in early prostate cancer. *N Engl J Med* 2002;347:781–789.
6. Thompson IM, Goodman PJ, Tangen CM, et al. The influence of finasteride on the development of prostate cancer. *N Engl J Med* 2003;349:215–224.
7. Parker C. Active surveillance: towards a new paradigm in the management of early prostate cancer. *Lancet Oncol* 2004;5:101–106.
8. Tal R, Livne PM, Lask DM, et al. Empirical management of urinary tract infections complicating transrectal ultrasound guided prostate biopsy. *J Urol* 2003;169:1762–1765.
9. Roehl KA, Antenor JA, Catalona WJ. Serial biopsy results in prostate cancer screening study. *J Urol* 2002;167:2435–2439.
10. Gore JL, Shariat SF, Miles BJ, et al. Optimal combinations of systematic sextant and laterally directed biopsies for the detection of prostate cancer. *J Urol* 2001;165:1554–1559.
11. Nash PA, Bruce JE, Indudhara R, et al. Transrectal ultrasound guided prostatic nerve blockade eases systematic needle biopsy of the prostate. *J Urol* 1996;155:607–609.
12. Terris MK, Stamey TA. Determination of prostate volume by transrectal ultrasound. *J Urol* 1991;145:984–987.
13. Benson MC, Whang IS, Pantuck A, et al. Prostate specific antigen density: a means of distinguishing benign prostatic hypertrophy and prostate cancer. *J Urol* 1992;147:815–816.
14. Shinohara K, Wheeler TM, Scardino PT. The appearance of prostate cancer on transrectal ultrasonography: correlation of imaging and pathological examinations. *J Urol* 1989;142:76–82.
15. Ohori M, Wheeler TM, Scardino PT, The New American Joint Committee on Cancer and International Union Against Cancer. TNM classification of prostate cancer. Clinicopathologic correlations. *Cancer* 1994;74:104–114.
16. Ohori M, Kattan MW, Utsunomiya T, et al. Do impalpable stage T1c prostate cancers visible on ultrasound differ from those not visible? *J Urol* 2003;169:964–968.
17. Ukimura O, Troncoso P, Ramirez EI, et al. Prostate cancer staging: correlation between ultrasound determined tumor contact length and pathologically confirmed extraprostatic extension. *J Urol* 1998;159:1251–1259.
18. Ohori M, Shinohara K, Wheeler TM, et al. Ultrasonic detection of nonpalpable seminal vesicle invasion: a clinicopathological study. *Br J Urol* 1993;72:799–808.
19. Ohori M, Egawa S, Shinohara K, et al. Detection of microscopic extracapsular extension prior to radical prostatectomy for clinically localized prostate cancer. *Br J Urol* 1994;74:72–79.
20. Partin AW, Mangold LA, Lamm DM, et al. Contemporary update of prostate cancer staging nomograms (Partin Tables) for the new millennium. *Urology* 2001;58:843–848.
21. Halpern EJ, Frauscher F, Strup SE, et al. Prostate: high-frequency Doppler US imaging for cancer detection. *Radiology* 2002;225:71–77.
22. Kuligowska E, Barish MA, Fenlon HM, et al. Predictors of prostate carcinoma: accuracy of gray-scale and color Doppler US and serum markers. *Radiology* 2001;220:757–764.
23. Zelefsky MJ, Yamada Y, Cohen G, et al. Postimplantation dosimetric analysis of permanent transperineal prostate implantation: improved dose distributions with an intraoperative computer-optimized conformal planning technique. *Int J Radiat Oncol Biol Phys* 2000;48:601–608.
24. De La Taille A, Benson MC, Bagiella E, et al. Cryoablation for clinically localized prostate cancer using an argon-based system: complication rates and biochemical recurrence. *BJU Int* 2000;85:281–286.
25. Chaussy C, Thuroff S. Results and side effects of high-intensity focused ultrasound in localized prostate cancer. *J Endourol* 2001;15:437–440; discussion 447–448.
26. Shalev M, Kadmon D, Teh BS, et al. Suicide gene therapy toxicity after multiple and repeat injections in patients with localized prostate cancer. *J Urol* 2000;163:1747–1750.
27. Djavan B, Waldert M, Zlotta A, et al. Safety and morbidity of first and repeat transrectal ultrasound guided prostate needle biopsies: results of a prospective European prostate cancer detection study. *J Urol* 2001;166:856–860.
28. Wolf JS Jr, Cher M, Dall'era M, et al. The use and accuracy of cross-sectional imaging and fine needle aspiration cytology for detection of pelvic lymph node metastases before radical prostatectomy. *J Urol* 1995;153:993–999.
29. Platt JF, Bree RL, Schwab RE. The accuracy of CT in the staging of carcinoma of the prostate. *Am J Roentgenol* 1987;149:315–318.

30. Engeler CE, Wasserman NF, Zhang G. Preoperative assessment of prostatic carcinoma by computerized tomography. Weaknesses and new perspectives. *Urology* 1992;40:346–350.

31. Tiguert R, Gheiler EL, Tefilli MV, et al. Lymph node size does not correlate with the presence of prostate cancer metastasis. *Urology* 1999;53:367–371.

32. Walsh JW, Amendola MA, Konerding KF, et al. Computed tomographic detection of pelvic and inguinal lymph-node metastases from primary and recurrent pelvic malignant disease. *Radiology* 1980;137:157–166.

33. Rorvik J, Halvorsen OJ, Albrektsen G, et al. Lymphangiography combined with biopsy and computer tomography to detect lymph node metastases in localized prostate cancer. *Scand J Urol Nephrol* 1998;32:116–119.

34. Oyen RH, Van Poppel HP, Ameye FE, et al. Lymph node staging of localized prostatic carcinoma with CT and CT-guided fine-needle aspiration biopsy: prospective study of 285 patients. *Radiology* 1994;190:315–322.

35. Flocks RH, Culp D, Porto R. Lymphatic spread from prostatic cancer. *J Urol* 1959;81:194–196.

36. Soh S, Kattan MW, Berkman S, et al. Has there been a recent shift in the pathological features and prognosis of patients treated with radical prostatectomy? *J Urol* 1997;157:2212–2218.

37. Petros JA, Catalona WJ. Lower incidence of unsuspected lymph node metastases in 521 consecutive patients with clinically localized prostate cancer. *J Urol* 1992;147:1574–1575.

38. Gervasi LA, Mata J, Easley JD, et al. Prognostic significance of lymph nodal metastases in prostate cancer. *J Urol* 1989;142:332–336.

39. Bishoff JT, Reyes A, Thompson IM, et al. Pelvic lymphadenectomy can be omitted in selected patients with carcinoma of the prostate: development of a system of patient selection. *Urology* 1995;45:270–274.

40. Cheng L, Zincke H, Blute ML, et al. Risk of prostate carcinoma death in patients with lymph node metastasis. *Cancer* 2001;91:66–73.

41. Taoka T, Mayr NA, Lee HJ, et al. Factors influencing visualization of vertebral metastases on MR imaging versus bone scintigraphy. *AJR Am J Roentgenol* 2001;176:1525–1530.

42. Traill ZC, Talbot D, Golding S, et al. Magnetic resonance imaging versus radionuclide scintigraphy in screening for bone metastases. *Clin Radiol* 1999;54:448–451.

43. Hricak H, White S, Vigneron D, et al. Carcinoma of the prostate gland: MR imaging with pelvic phased-array coils versus integrated endorectal-pelvic phased-array coils. *Radiology* 1994;193:703–709.

44. Huncharek M, Muscat J. Serum prostate-specific antigen as a predictor of staging abdominal/pelvic computed tomography in newly diagnosed prostate cancer. *Abdom Imaging* 1996;21:364–367.

45. Schnall MD, Pollack HM. Magnetic resonance imaging of the prostate gland. *Urol Radiol* 1990;12:109–114.

46. Zakian KL, Eberhardt S, Hricak H, et al. Transition zone prostate cancer: metabolic characteristics at 1H MR spectroscopic imaging—initial results. *Radiology* 2003;229:241–247.

47. Eberhardt SC, Coakley FV, Schwartz LH, et al. Endorectal MR imaging and spectroscopic imaging of transition zone prostate cancer [Abstract]. *Radiology* 2001;221(P):584.

48. Ikonen S, Kivisaari L, Vehmas T, et al. Optimal timing of post-biopsy MR imaging of the prostate. *Acta Radiol* 2001;42:70–73.

49. White S, Hricak H, Forstner R, et al. Prostate cancer: effect of postbiopsy hemorrhage on interpretation of MR images. *Radiology* 1995;195:385–390.

50. Rifkin MD, Zerhouni EA, Gatsonis CA, et al. Comparison of magnetic resonance imaging and ultrasonography in staging early prostate cancer. Results of a multi-institutional cooperative trial. *N Engl J Med* 1990;323:621–626.

51. Outwater EK, Petersen RO, Siegelman ES, et al. Prostate carcinoma: assessment of diagnostic criteria for capsular penetration on endorectal coil MR images. *Radiology* 1994;193:333–339.

52. Yu KK, Hricak H, Alagappan R, et al. Detection of extracapsular extension of prostate carcinoma with endorectal and phased-array coil MR imaging: multivariate feature analysis. *Radiology* 1997;202:697–702.

53. Bernstein MR, Cangiano T, D'Amico A, et al. Endorectal coil magnetic resonance imaging and clinicopathologic findings in T1c adenocarcinoma of the prostate. *Urol Oncol* 2000;5:104–107.

54. Cornud F, Flam T, Chauveinc L, et al. Extraprostatic spread of clinically localized prostate cancer: factors predictive of pT3 tumor and of positive endorectal MR imaging examination results. *Radiology* 2002;224:203–210.

55. May F, Treumann T, Dettmar P, et al. Limited value of endorectal magnetic resonance imaging and transrectal ultrasonography in the staging of clinically localized prostate cancer. *BJU Int* 2001;87:66–69.

56. Bellin MF, Roy C, Kinkel K, et al. Lymph node metastases: safety and effectiveness of MR imaging with ultrasmall superparamagnetic iron oxide particles—initial clinical experience. *Radiology* 1998;207:799–808.

57. Harisinghani MG, Barentsz J, Hahn PF, et al. Noninvasive detection of clinically occult lymph-node metastases in prostate cancer. *N Engl J Med* 2003;348:2491–2499.

58. Pomeranz SJ, Pretorius HT, Ramsingh PS. Bone scintigraphy and multimodality imaging in bone neoplasia: strategies for imaging in the new health care climate. *Semin Nucl Med* 1994;24:188–207.

59. Coakley FV, Kurhanewicz J, Lu Y, et al. Prostate cancer tumor volume: measurement with endorectal MR and MR spectroscopic imaging. *Radiology* 2002;223:91–97.

60. Heerschap A, Jager GJ, van der Graaf M, et al. Proton MR spectroscopy of the normal human prostate with an endorectal coil and a double spin-echo pulse sequence. *Magn Reson Med* 1997;37:204–213.

61. Kurhanewicz J, Vigneron DB, Hricak H, et al. Three-dimensional H-1 MR spectroscopic imaging of the in situ human prostate with high (0.24–0.7 cm^3) spatial resolution. *Radiology* 1996;198:795–805.

62. Schiebler ML, Schnall MD, Pollack HM, et al. Current role of MR imaging in the the staging of adenocarcinoma of the prostate. *Radiology* 1993;189:339–352.

63. Kurhanewicz J, Vigneron DB, Nelson SJ, et al. Citrate as an in vivo marker to discriminate prostate cancer from benign prostatic hyperplasia and normal prostate peripheral zone: detection via localized proton spectroscopy. *Urology* 1995;45:459–466.

64. Kurhanewicz J, Dahiya R, Macdonald JM, et al. Citrate alterations in primary and metastatic human prostatic adenocarcinomas: ^{1}H magnetic resonance spectroscopy and biochemical study. *Magn Reson Med* 1993;29:149–157.

65. Liney GP, Turnbull LW, Lowry M, et al. In vivo quantification of citrate concentration and water T2 relaxation time of the pathologic prostate gland using 1H MRS and MRI. *Magn Reson Med* 1997;15:1177–1186.

66. Costello LC, Littleton GK, Franklin RB. Regulation of citrate-related metabolism in normal and neoplastic prostate. In: Sharma RK, Criss WE, eds. *Endocrine control in neoplasia*. New York: Raven Press, 1978:303–314.

67. Costello LC, Franklin RB. Citrate metabolism of normal and malignant prostate epithelial cells. *Urology* 1997;50:3–12.

68. Heerschap A, Jager GJ, van der Graaf M, et al. In vivo proton MR spectroscopy reveals altered metabolite content in malignant prostate tissue. *Anticancer Res* 1997;17:1455–1460.

69. Fulham MJ, Bizzi A, Dietz MJ, et al. Mapping of brain tumor metabolites with proton MR spectroscopic imaging: clinical relevance. *Radiology* 1992;185:675–686.

70. Heesters MA, Kamman RL, Mooyaart EL, et al. Localized proton spectroscopy of inoperable brain gliomas. Response to radiation therapy. *J Neurooncol* 1993;17:27–35.

71. Dewhirst MW, Sostman HD, Leopold KA, et al. Soft-tissue sarcomas: MR imaging and MR spectroscopy for prognosis and therapy monitoring. Work in progress. *Radiology* 1990;174:847–853.

72. Koutcher JA, Ballon D, Graham M, et al. P-31 NMR spectra of extremity sarcoma: diversity of metabolic profiles and changes in response to chemotherapy. *Magn Reson Med* 1990;16:19–34.

73. McBride DQ, Miller BL, Nikas DL, et al. Analysis of brain tumors using ^{1}H magnetic resonance spectroscopy. *Surg Neurol* 1995;44:137–144.

74. Sijens PE, Knopp MV, Brunetti A, et al. ^{1}H MR spectroscopy in patients with metastatic brain tumors: a multicenter study. *Magn Reson Med* 1995;33:818–826.

75. Rutter A, Hugenholtz H, Saunders JK, et al. One-dimensional phosphorus-31 chemical shift imaging of human brain tumors. *Invest Radiol* 1995;30:359–366.

76. Scheidler J, Hricak H, Vigneron DB, et al. Prostate cancer: localization with three-dimensional proton MR spectroscopic imaging—clinicopathologic study. *Radiology* 1999;213:473–480.

77. Wefer AE, Hricak H, Vigneron DB, et al. Sextant localization of prostate cancer: comparison of sextant biopsy, magnetic resonance imaging and magnetic resonance spectroscopic imaging with step section histology. *J Urol* 2000;164:400–404.

78. Males R, Vigneron D, Star-Lack J, et al. Clinical application of BASING and spectral/spatial water and lipid suppression pulses for prostate cancer staging and localization by in vivo 3D 1H magnetic resonance spectroscopic imaging. *Magn Reson Med* 2000;43:17–22.

79. Zakian KI, Sircar K, Hricak H, et al. Correlation of proton MR spectroscopic imaging with Gleason score based on step-section pathologic analysis after radical prostatectomy. *Radiology* 2005;234:804–814.

80. Lin K, Szabo Z, Chin BB, et al. The value of a baseline bone scan in patients with newly diagnosed prostate cancer. *Clin Nucl Med* 1999;24:579–582.

81. Terris MK, Klonecke AS, McDougall IR, et al. Utilization of bone scans in conjunction with prostate-specific antigen levels in the surveillance for recurrence of adenocarcinoma after radical prostatectomy. *J Nucl Med* 1991;32:1713–1717.

82. Spencer JA, Golding SJ. Patterns of lymphatic metastases at recurrence of prostate cancer: CT findings. *Clin Radiol* 1994;49:404–407.

83. Algra PR, Bloem JL, Tissing H, et al. Detection of vertebral metastases: comparison between MR imaging and bone scintigraphy. *Radiographics* 1991;11:219–232.

84. Cher ML, Bianco FJ Jr, Lam JS, et al. Limited role of radionuclide bone scintigraphy in patients with prostate specific antigen elevations after radical prostatectomy. *J Urol* 1998;160:1387–1391.

85. Palmer E, Henrikson B, McKusick K, et al. Pain as an indicator of bone metastasis. *Acta Radiol* 1988;29:445–449.

86. Turner JW, Hawes DR, Williams RD. Magnetic resonance imaging for detection of prostate cancer metastatic to bone. *J Urol* 1993;149:1482–1484.

87. Schirrmeister H, Glatting G, Hetzel J, et al. Prospective evaluation of the clinical value of planar bone scans, SPECT, and (18)F-labeled NaF PET in newly diagnosed lung cancer. *J Nucl Med* 2001;42:1800–1804.

88. Savelli G, Maffioli L, Maccauro M, et al. Bone scintigraphy and the added value of SPECT (single photon emission tomography) in detecting skeletal lesions. *Q J Nucl Med* 2001;45:27–37.

89. Delpassand ES, Garcia JR, Bhadkamkar V, et al. Value of SPECT imaging of the thoracolumbar spine in cancer patients. *Clin Nucl Med* 1995;20: 1047–1051.

90. Even-Sapir E, Martin RH, Barnes DC, et al. Role of SPECT in differentiating malignant from benign lesions in the lower thoracic and lumbar vertebrae. *Radiology* 1993;187:193–198.

91. Sabbatini P, Larson SM, Kremer A, et al. Prognostic significance of extent of disease in bone in patients with androgen-independent prostate cancer. *J Clin Oncol* 1999;17:948–957.

92. Noguchi M, Kikuchi H, Ishibashi M, et al. Percentage of the positive area of bone metastasis is an independent predictor of disease death in advanced prostate cancer. *Br J Cancer* 2003;88:195–201.

93. Effert PJ, Bares R, Handt S, et al. Metabolic imaging of untreated prostate cancer by positron emission tomography with 18fluorine-labeled deoxyglucose. *J Urol* 1996;155:994–998.

94. Hofer C, Laubenbacher C, Block T, et al. Fluorine-18-fluorodeoxyglucose positron emission tomography is useless for the detection of local recurrence after radical prostatectomy. *Eur Urol* 1999;36:31–35.

95. Liu IJ, Zafar MB, Lai YH, et al. Fluorodeoxyglucose positron emission tomography studies in diagnosis and staging of clinically organ-confined prostate cancer. *Urology* 2001;57:108–111.

96. Turlakow A, Larson SM, Coakley F, et al. Local detection of prostate cancer by positron emission tomography with 2-fluorodeoxyglucose: comparison of filtered back projection and iterative reconstruction with segmented attenuation correction. *Q J Nucl Med* 2001;45:235–244.

97. Jager PL, Vaalburg W, Pruim J, et al. Radiolabeled amino acids: basic aspects and clinical applications in oncology. *J Nucl Med* 2001;42:432–445.

98. Troyer JK, Beckett ML, Wright GL Jr. Detection and characterization of the prostate-specific membrane antigen (PSMA) in tissue extracts and body fluids. *Int J Cancer* 1995;62:552–558.

99. Troyer JK, Beckett ML, Wright GL Jr. Location of prostate-specific membrane antigen in the LNCaP prostate carcinoma cell line. *Prostate* 1997; 30:232–242.

100. Kahn D, Williams RD, Manyak MJ et al. The ProstaScint Study Group. 111Indium-capromab pendetide in the evaluation of patients with residual or recurrent prostate cancer after radical prostatectomy. *J Urol* 1998; 159:2041–2046; discussion 2046-2047.

101. Kahn D, Williams RD, Seldin DW, et al. Radioimmunoscintigraphy with 111indium labeled CYT-356 for the detection of occult prostate cancer recurrence. *J Urol* 1994;152:1490–1495.

102. Ponsky LE, Cherullo EE, Starkey R, et al. Evaluation of preoperative ProstaScint scans in the prediction of nodal disease. *Prostate Cancer Prostatic Dis* 2002;5:132–135.

103. Thomas CT, Bradshaw PT, Pollock BH, et al. Indium-111-capromab pendetide radioimmunoscintigraphy and prognosis for durable biochemical response to salvage radiation therapy in men after failed prostatectomy. *J Clin Oncol* 2003;21:1715–1721.

104. Smith JA Jr, Scardino PT, Resnick MI, et al. Transrectal ultrasound versus digital rectal examination for the staging of carcinoma of the prostate: results of a prospective, multi-institutional trial. *J Urol* 1997;157:902–906.

105. Sanchez-Chapado M, Angulo JC, Ibarburen C, et al. Comparison of digital rectal examination, transrectal ultrasonography, and multicoil magnetic resonance imaging for preoperative evaluation of prostate cancer. *Eur Urol* 1997;32:140–149.

106. Ikonen S, Karkkainen P, Kivisaari L, et al. Magnetic resonance imaging of clinically localized prostatic cancer. *J Urol* 1998;159:915–919.

107. Wei DC, Coakley FV, Hricak H, et al. Impact of endorectal MRI on preoperative decision of nerve preservation/resection during radical prostatectomy (RP). *J Urol* 2001;165(Suppl. 5):356. Abstract 1461.

108. Coakley FV, Eberhardt S, Wei DC, et al. Blood loss during radical retropubic prostatectomy: relationship to morphologic features on preoperative endorectal magnetic resonance imaging. *Urology* 2002;59:884–888.

109. Coakley FV, Eberhardt S, Kattan MW, et al. Urinary continence after radical retropubic prostatectomy: relationship with membranous urethral length on preoperative endorectal magnetic resonance imaging. *J Urol* 2002;168:1032–1035.

110. Ling CC, Fuks Z. Conformal radiation treatment: a critical appraisal. *Eur J Cancer* 1995;31A:799–803.

111. McShan DL, Fraass BA, Lichter AS. Full integration of the beam's eye view concept into computerized treatment planning. *Int J Radiat Oncol Biol Phys* 1990;18:1485–1494.

112. Burman C, Chui CS, Kutcher G, et al. Planning, delivery, and quality assurance of intensity-modulated radiotherapy using dynamic multileaf collimator: a strategy for large-scale implementation for the treatment of carcinoma of the prostate. *Int J Radiat Oncol Biol Phys* 1997;39:863–873.

113. Intensity Modulated Radiation Therapy Collaborative Working Group. Intensity-modulated radiotherapy: current status and issues of interest. *Int J Radiat Oncol Biol Phys* 2001;51:880–914.

114. Ling CC, Humm J, Larson S, et al. Towards multidimensional radiotherapy (MD-CRT): biological imaging and biological conformality. *Int J Radiat Oncol Biol Phys* 2000;47:551–560.

115. Townsend DW, Cherry SR. Combining anatomy and function: the path to true image fusion. *Eur Radiol* 2001;11:1968–1974.

116. Pickett B, Vigneault E, Kurhanewicz J, et al. Static field intensity modulation to treat a dominant intra-prostatic lesion to 90 Gy compared to seven field 3-dimensional radiotherapy. *Int J Radiat Oncol Biol Phys* 1999;44: 921–929.

117. Porter AT, Blasko JC, Grimm PD, et al. Brachytherapy for prostate cancer. *CA Cancer J Clin* 1995;45:165–178.

118. Dubois DF, Prestidge BR, Hotchkiss LA, et al. Source localization following permanent transperineal prostate interstitial brachytherapy using magnetic resonance imaging. *Int J Radiat Oncol Biol Phys* 1997;39: 1037–1041.

119. Shinohara K, Connolly JA, Presti JC Jr, et al. Cryosurgical treatment of localized prostate cancer (stages T1 to T4): preliminary results. *J Urol* 1996;156:115–120; discussion 120-121.

120. Kattan MW, Wheeler TM, Scardino PT. Postoperative nomogram for disease recurrence after radical prostatectomy for prostate cancer. *J Clin Oncol* 1999;17:1499–1507.

121. D'Amico AV, Whittington R, Malkowicz SB, et al. The combination of preoperative prostate specific antigen and postoperative pathological findings to predict prostate specific antigen outcome in clinically localized prostate cancer. *J Urol* 1998;160:2096–2101.

122. Partin AW, Pearson JD, Landis PK, et al. Evaluation of serum prostate-specific antigen velocity after radical prostatectomy to distinguish local recurrence from distant metastases. *Urology* 1994;43:649–659.

123. Jhaveri FM, Klein EA. How to explore the patient with a rising PSA after radical prostatectomy: defining local versus systemic failure. *Semin Urol Oncol* 1999;17:130–134.

124. Laufer M, Pound CR, Carducci MA, et al. Management of patients with rising prostate-specific antigen after radical prostatectomy. *Urology* 2000; 55:309–315.

125. Partin AW, Oesterling JE. The clinical usefulness of prostate specific antigen: update 1994. *J Urol* 1994;152:1358–1368.

126. Critz FA, Levinson AK, Williams WH, et al. Prostate specific antigen nadir achieved by men apparently cured of prostate cancer by radiotherapy. *J Urol* 1999;161:1199–1203; discussion 1203–1205.

127. Pollack A, Zagars GK, Antolak JA, et al. Prostate biopsy status and PSA nadir level as early surrogates for treatment failure: analysis of a prostate cancer randomized radiation dose escalation trial. *Int J Radiat Oncol Biol Phys* 2002;54:677–685.

128. Soloway MS, Sharifi R, Wajsman Z et al. The Lupron Depot Neoadjuvant Prostate Cancer Study Group. Randomized prospective study comparing radical prostatectomy alone versus radical prostatectomy preceded by androgen blockade in clinical stage B2 (T2bNxM0) prostate cancer. *J Urol* 1995;154:424–428.

129. Chen M, Hricak H, Kalbhen CL, et al. Hormonal ablation of prostatic cancer: effects on prostate morphology, tumor detection, and staging by endorectal coil MR imaging. *Am J Roentgenol* 1996;166: 1157–1163.

130. Pinault S, Tetu B, Gagnon J, et al. Transrectal ultrasound evaluation of local prostate cancer in patients treated with LHRH agonist and in combination with flutamide. *Urology* 1992;39:254–261.

131. Pollen JJ, Witztum KF, Ashburn WL. The flare phenomenon on radionuclide bone scan in metastatic prostate cancer. *Am J Roentgenol* 1984; 142:773–776.

132. Schneider JA, Divgi CR, Scott AM, et al. Flare on bone scintigraphy following taxol chemotherapy for metastatic breast cancer. *J Nucl Med* 1994;35:1748–1752.

133. Mueller-Lisse UG, Vigneron DB, Hricak H, et al. Localized prostate cancer: effect of hormone deprivation therapy measured by using combined three-dimensional 1H MR spectroscopy and MR imaging: clinicopathologic case-controlled study. *Radiology* 2001;221:380–390.

134. Mueller-Lisse UG, Swanson MG, Vigneron DB, et al. Time-dependent effects of hormone-deprivation therapy on prostate metabolism as detected by combined magnetic resonance imaging and 3D magnetic resonance spectroscopic imaging. *Magn Reson Med* 2001;46:49–57.

135. Zakian KL, Dyke J, Kurhanewicz J, et al. Tracking metabolic response to neo-adjuvant chemotherapy in prostate cancer by proton magnetic resonance spectroscopic imaging. *Proceedings of the International Society of Magnetic Resonance in Medicine*, Eighth Scientific Meeting. Denver, 2000:1894.

136. Yeung H, Schoder H, Larson S. Utility of PET/CT for assessing equivocal PET lesions in oncology—initial experience [Abstract]. *J Nucl Med* 2002;43:32P.

137. Leventis AK, Shariat SF, Slawin KM. Local recurrence after radical prostatectomy: correlation of US features with prostatic fossa biopsy findings. *Radiology* 2001;219:432–439.

138. Kramer S, Gorich J, Gottfried HW, et al. Sensitivity of computed tomography in detecting local recurrence of prostatic carcinoma following radical prostatectomy. *Br J Radiol* 1997;70:995–999.

139. Silverman JM, Krebs TL. MR imaging evaluation with a transrectal surface coil of local recurrence of prostatic cancer in men who have undergone radical prostatectomy. *Am J Roentgenol* 1997;168:379–385.

140. Sella T, Schwartz LH, Swindle PW, et al. Suspected local recurrence after radical prostatectomy: endorectal coil MR imaging. *Radiology* 2004;231:379–385.

141. Sodee DB, Malguria N, Faulhaber P et al. The ProstaScint Imaging Centers. Multicenter ProstaScint imaging findings in 2154 patients with prostate cancer. *Urology* 2000;56:988–993.

142. Raj GV, Partin AW, Polascik TJ. Clinical utility of indium 111-capromab pendetide immunoscintigraphy in the detection of early, recurrent prostate carcinoma after radical prostatectomy. *Cancer* 2002;94:987–996.

143. Seltzer MA, Barbaric Z, Belldegrun A, et al. Comparison of helical computerized tomography, positron emission tomography and monoclonal antibody scans for evaluation of lymph node metastases in patients with prostate specific antigen relapse after treatment for localized prostate cancer. *J Urol* 1999;162:1322–1328.

144. Montie JE. Follow-up after radical prostatectomy or radiation therapy for prostate cancer. *Urol Clin North Am* 1994;21:673–676.

145. Ferguson JK, Oesterling JE. Patient evaluation if prostate-specific antigen becomes elevated following radical prostatectomy or radiation therapy. *Urol Clin North Am* 1994;21:677–685.

CHAPTER 13 ■ TREATMENT OF EARLY STAGE PROSTATE CANCER

CHAPTER 13A
Advising Patients with Early Prostatic Cancer on Their Treatment Decision

William U. Shipley, Peter T. Scardino, Donald S. Kaufman, and Michael W. Kattan

Patients diagnosed with early prostate cancer find themselves facing a very difficult treatment decision. Although there are many sources of information readily available to patients and their families, including books written for the informed layperson by physicians, the Internet, popular magazines, newspaper articles, and word-of-mouth, these sources often add to the patient's sense of confusion, and therefore fail in their avowed purpose of enabling the patient to make a reasoned and comfortable decision.

While prostate cancer is unequivocally lethal in some patients, many others don't actually die from their cancer, and the physician's advice, therefore, must take into account the variable natural history of the disease. While the lifetime risk of an American male diagnosed with prostatic cancer is estimated to be about 16%, the risk of his dying of this disease is only about 3.6% (1,2). Appropriate advice regarding the initial treatment of this disease requires an assessment of risk: How likely is an individual's cancer to progress or metastasize over his remaining lifetime? What is the probability of success with treatment for the risk of his cancer? What are the risks of side effects and complications with each type of treatment? In patients with particularly low-risk prostate cancer at diagnosis, as determined by physical examination, Gleason score, and prostate-specific antigen (PSA), it is unclear whether any of the available curative treatments will actually prolong survival, but each treatment has a significant risk of producing short- or long-term dysfunction. Avoiding or deferring treatment is a plausible option for select patients, but inaction in treating a cancer is clearly unacceptable to many individuals, no matter how powerful the arguments in favor of that approach.

TREATMENT CONSIDERATIONS

Advising a patient to be observed or treated for his newly diagnosed prostatic cancer involves balancing risks, benefits, and uncertainties. The most commonly recommended approaches are either active observation ("watchful waiting") or a treatment designed to eradicate the cancer. These options, which include active observation, radical prostatectomy, or radiation therapy, are thoroughly dealt with in Chapters 13B through 13G.

The physician's responsibility in advising a patient at diagnosis is to be certain that the patient understands his treatment options, including the risks of side effects and complications connected with active treatment, and, if possible, to advise him without prejudice which active treatment seems optimal for his particular clinical situation. The historic facts that must be considered in this setting are the life expectancy (e.g., age, comorbidity) of the patient, the probability of metastases and of death from his prostate cancer in the absence of treatment over time, the particular characteristics of the primary tumor (i.e., its prognostic features), the effectiveness of the treatments being considered, the complication rate and side effects of each treatment, and an understanding of the patient's individual concerns for each health state at risk that could be affected by the cancer and its treatment (e.g., living with an untreated cancer, becoming impotent, or being incontinent of urine). Using the clinical stage, serum PSA level, and the biopsy Gleason score of the tumor, individual tumor presentations have been stratified into three major risk groups (Table 13A.1). These stratifications, while imperfect, present the risk of tumor recurrence following therapy, giving a reasonable estimation of the probability of the treatment to achieve its goal, which is the eradication of the cancer. Recently, sophisticated statistical approaches to prognostic risk-group classification have been developed, which have likely added value to the simplified popular system now in use (Table 13A.1). A more accurate risk-classification system may be particularly important for those patients assigned to the intermediate- and high-risk groups, which may contain cohorts of patients who have a more favorable outcome with treatment by surgery or radiation therapy. Methods such as the use of nomograms or recursive partitioning analysis are sophisticated models that rely on continuous risk scales (3–6). It is likely that such newer prognostic models will become more reliable predictors of outcome and thus give us better information, including molecular markers with which to better advise our patients (7). Newer models may also enable doctors to identify patients within the intermediate- and high-risk groups who have a uniquely poor chance of achieving cure with standard treatment approaches and thus may identify such subgroups as being more appropriately treated with combined modality treatments or novel therapy (5).

In each of these cancer-risk strata, it is not possible to state, based on what we know now, that there are significant differences in the cure rate utilizing radical prostatectomy, conformal high-dose radiation therapy, or brachytherapy. Since cancer control is similar with these three modalities, physicians should provide patients with a good understanding of the risk of the side effects of each treatment. This type of assessment has been extensively studied over the last decade (8,9). The selection of treatment should be tailored to avoid the risk of those treatment-related side effects that will particularly trouble an individual patient. A list of the advantages and disadvantages of each of the four methods for managing patients with early prostate

TABLE 13A.1

ESTIMATION OF THE RISK OF TUMOR RECURRENCE FOR CLINICALLY LOCALIZED AND REGIONAL PROSTATE CANCER

Low risk	Intermediate risk	High risk	Very high risk
Clinical T1a–T2a and	Clinical T2b–T2c or	Clinical T3a–T3b or	Clinical T3c–T4 or
Gleason score 2–6 and	Gleason score 7 or	Gleason score 8–10 or	Any T, N1–3
PSA <10 ng/mL	PSA 10–20 ng/mL	PSA >20 ng/mL	

cancer as well as their contraindications are given in Tables 13A.2 to13A.4.

ACTIVE OBSERVATION ("WATCHFUL WAITING")

This management option is also called surveillance or active monitoring. This is a decision to defer active treatment until the PSA rises substantially or until symptoms appear. The rationale behind active observation for patients with early prostate cancer is the consistent observation that most men with small volume, low-grade cancer have an excellent prognosis, such that most will never develop symptoms of the cancer and most will die from causes other than prostate cancer. The advantages of observation are that it avoids the risks of overtreatment, and that it limits the risks of treatment side effects either by eliminating or postponing them (Table 13A.2).

The main disadvantage is the risk that the tumor might progress beyond the possibility of cure and eventually cause severe disability and even death. The delay in treatment may also make subsequent treatment more difficult, with increased side effects for the patient. Some patients may also suffer from anxiety living with an untreated tumor (Tables 13A.3 and 13A.4). There is now Class I evidence from a prospective randomized trial of men mostly with intermediate-risk prostate cancer that watchful waiting leads to a significantly greater risk of metastases (27% compared to 13% after radical prostatectomy), and a greater risk of cancer-related death 8 years later (13% compared to 7%), compared to radical prostatectomy (10). However, these tumors were not PSA-detected but discovered on the basis of a nodule or symptoms requiring transurethral resection of the prostate (TURP). There is considerable evidence that the median time from PSA rise to the development of a clinically recognized disease is around 7 years. Thus, the 8 years of observation in the Swedish study may correspond to 15 years in a US study because of the

TABLE 13A.2

THE ADVANTAGES OF THE MAIN TREATMENT OPTIONS FOR EARLY PROSTATE CANCER

External beam radiation therapy	Radical prostatectomy
• Effective long-term cancer control with high-dose treatments • Very low risk of urinary incontinence • Available for cure of patients over a wide range of ages and in those with significant comorbidity • Combined with hormone therapy treatment, offers an improved chance for a cure in high-risk disease • Treatments can eradicate extensions of tumor beyond the margins of the prostate	• Effective long-term cancer control • Predictions of prognosis can be more precise based on pathologic features in specimen • Pelvic lymph node dissection is possible through the same incision • PSA failure is easy to detect
Brachytherapy • Cancer control rates appear equal to surgery and EBRT for organ-confined tumors • Quicker than EBRT (single treatment) • Risk of incontinence is low in patients without a previous TURP • Available for cure of patients over a wide range of ages and in those with some comorbidity	**Active Observation** • Reduces overtreatment • Avoids or postpones treatment-associated complications • Has no effect on work or social activities

TURP, transurethral resection of the prostate; EBRT, external beam radiation therapy.

TABLE 13A.3

THE DISADVANTAGES OF THE MAIN TREATMENT OPTIONS FOR EARLY PROSTATE CANCER

External beam radiation therapy	Radical prostatectomy
• Significant risk of impotence • Best outcomes require 3-D conformal treatments with doses above 72 Gy • Low risk of later rectal symptoms • Knowledge of possible metastasis to lymph nodes is not available • Up to half of patients have some temporary bladder or bowel symptoms during treatment	• Significant risk of impotence • Risk of operative morbidity • The risk of complications is operator dependent, to some extent • Low risk of long-term incontinence
Brachytherapy	**Active Observation**
• Significant risk of impotence • Successful cancer control is operator dependent, to some extent • Low risk of later rectal symptoms • Knowledge of possible metastasis to lymph nodes is not available • Treatment not appropriate for tumor outside the prostate capsule • Up to half of patients have some temporary bladder or bowel symptoms with treatment	• Tumor may progress beyond the possibility for cure • Later treatment may result in more side effects • Living with untreated cancer may cause anxiety

widespread use of PSA early detection. A modification of the strategy of observation is to defer initial treatment with the stated goal that curative treatment will be given only when it is needed (i.e., when there is clear evidence that the cancer is progressing).

TABLE 13A.4

CONTRAINDICATIONS TO THE MAIN TREATMENT OPTIONS FOR EARLY PROSTATE CANCER

External beam radiation therapy	Radical prostatectomy
• Previous pelvic irradiation • Active inflammatory disease of the rectum • Very low bladder capacity • Chronic moderate or severe diarrhea from any cause	• Higher medical operative risk, including a "medical" age of 70 or greater • Neurogenic bladder • Morbid fear of surgery
Brachytherapy	**Active Observation**
• Previous pelvic irradiation • Prior TURP • Large-volume gland • Marked voiding symptoms • Large or high-grade tumor burdens • Chronic moderate or severe diarrhea • Active inflammatory disease of the rectum	• Patient's preference • High-grade tumors • Expected survival of more than 10 years

TURP, transurethral resection of the prostate; EBRT, external beam radiation therapy.

In such a "deferred-definitive-therapy" approach, the patient is closely followed with periodic physical exams, PSA, and in selected patients a repeat needle biopsy. The cancer is "actively monitored" and definitive treatment—radical prostatectomy, external beam radiation, or brachytherapy—is offered with curative intent upon progression. In a recent study with a PSA-based trigger point, the probability of remaining on active observation was 67% at 2 years and 48% at 4 years after diagnosis (1,11). Some patients, however, did demand treatment in the absence of objective evidence of progression. It is yet unclear what proportion of the patients who underwent deferred treatment were in fact successfully cured. Monitoring with periodic medical evaluation is an appropriate option for well-informed patients who wish to minimize the short-term risks of immediate therapy and who accept the risks of deferred treatment. With a short life expectancy, active monitoring may be appropriate for patients in any stage of cancer in the absence of symptoms or signs of impending morbidity from the disease.

EXTERNAL BEAM RADIATION THERAPY

External beam radiation therapy (EBRT) is described in detail in Chapter 13F. In the last decade, radiation oncologists have refined the technique of EBRT with the development of three-dimensional conformal external beam radiation therapy using many high-energy photon fields and computer software to integrate computed tomography (CT) images of the patient's internal anatomy, which allows the volume receiving the high dose to "conform" more exactly to the shape of the tumor. More recently, further refinements of conformal EBRT have become available using intensity modulation of the radiation treatment fields (IMRT). There is a reduction in side effects of EBRT on urinary and bowel function with conformal ERBT compared to conventional EBRT (12–15). This is shown in

TABLE 13A.5

PATIENT-REPORTED HEALTH-RELATED OUTCOMES AFTER EXTERNAL BEAM RADIATION THERAPY

Symptom	Conventional EBRT (12–14)	3-D conformal EBRT (15)
Wearing absorptive pads for urine leakage	3%–7%	2%
Bowel urgency	35%	22%
Rectal bleeding	10%–20%	8%
Bothered by any bowel dysfunction	8%	4%

Table 13A.5 for patient-reported, health-related outcomes after utilizing these two forms of EBRT. The main complications of conformal ERBT include a significant risk of impotency and a low risk of later rectal symptoms. The main contraindications to ERBT include active inflammatory disease of the rectum, previous pelvic irradiation, a low capacity bladder, or chronic diarrhea (Table 13A.4).

For patients with low-risk prostate cancer, many series utilizing EBRT report 5-year PSA-progression-free outcomes ranging from 70% to 85% (2). There are several series of patients treated with EBRT since 1989 (when the "PSA era" began) with follow-up long enough to report 10-year PSA-failure-free outcomes, which range from 62% to 83% (16–19). As discussed in Chapter 13F, there are both Class I and II evidence that is now compelling that optimal results require high-dose (greater than 72 Gy) conformal treatment. Tables 13A.2 to 13A.4 show the advantages and disadvantages of EBRT as well as the contraindications to EBRT.

BRACHYTHERAPY

Brachytherapy involves placing radioactive sources in the prostate itself. New technology for seed placement and improved radiation dose distribution has shown brachytherapy as monotherapy to be an effective treatment option for men with early clinically organ-confined prostate cancer, as described in Chapter 13G. Cancer control data from the Seattle group yields biochemical disease-free probability of 86% at 7 years for low-risk patients (20). This group has recently published an update of their series with some 13-year actuarial results. For "lower risk" patients, they reported the biochemical disease-free probability at 3, 5, 10, and 13 years of 84%, 79%, 76%, and 74%, respectively (21). No other brachytherapy series has as long a follow-up as this one. Centers of excellence have concluded that brachytherapy is an effective technique with an acceptable safety profile for selected patients with low-risk tumors. Tables 13A.2 to 13A.4 show the advantages and disadvantages of brachytherapy, as well as the contraindications.

RADICAL PROSTATECTOMY

Refinements of the techniques of radical prostatectomy, including nerve-sparing, in the last 20 years have resulted in a low perioperative morbidity and mortality and a high probability of complete tumor eradication (22–24). The advantages of surgery for men with localized tumors are the high likelihood that these patients will live their lives free of prostate cancer and the ease of detecting a treatment recurrence promptly (Table 13A.2). The late complications of radical prostatectomy—urinary incontinence and erectile dysfunction—are less common than before. Radical prostatectomy by the open and the laparoscopic approaches are described in Chapters 13C and 13D. Actuarial progression-free rates after radical retropubic prostatectomy from several recent series range from 47% to 73% for men 10 years after operation for stage T1 and T2 prostate cancer (2). Complications following radical prostatectomy can be divided into those that occur early in the postoperative period and those that are late complications. The risks of perioperative complications reported from several centers of excellence are less than 1% for sepsis, myocardial infarction, rectal injury, or mortality. There is a slightly higher risk of pulmonary embolism, deep vein thrombosis, and wound infection. Late complications include urinary incontinence (defined as leaking more than 2 tablespoons a day with moderate or significant bother for the patient) in 8% of men of all ages after radical prostatectomy (25,26). In centers of excellence the rate of severe incontinence is less than 3%. The major contraindication to radical prostatectomy is in patients with medical comorbidities, such as heart or lung disease, hypertension, or a "medical" age of 70 or greater, that significantly increase operative risks. The advantages and disadvantages of radical prostatectomy are given as well as its contraindications in Tables 13A.2 to 13A.4.

CONCLUSION

How to best advise an individual patient on the choice of the treatment that will be optimal for him is still more an art than a science. Recently the treatment decision-making process has been shown to affect the overall satisfaction of the patient with his treatment choice. Miles et al. surveyed men who were treated following screening-detected, localized prostatic cancer (27,28). Many men were satisfied with their treatment. However, the dissatisfied patients responding to the questionnaire included those who "rushed" into a decision. They concluded that they should have sought a second opinion or perhaps not had any treatment at all. The present state-of-the-art method for the thoughtful well-informed patient is to ensure that the patient is afforded the opportunity to play a significant part in his treatment. This important requirement is enhanced by the patient having the opportunity to consult with a multidisciplinary team consisting of a urologic surgeon, a radiation oncologist, and a medical oncologist. This decision-making process provides an opportunity for patient/physician interactions that represent the best that evidence-based medicine can offer.

References

1. Choo R, Klotz L, Danjoux C, et al. Feasibility study: watchful waiting for localized low to intermediate grade prostate carcinoma with selective delayed intervention based on prostate specific antigen, histological and/or clinical progression. *J Urol* 2002;167:1664.
2. Scardino PF, Abbas F, Adolffson J. Management of localized and regional prostatic cancer. In: Denis L, Bartsch G, Khoury S et al., eds. *Third international consultation on prostate cancer*. Paris: Health Communications Limited, 2003:219–247.

3. Kattan MW, Eastham JA, Stapleton AMF, et al. A preoperative nomogram for disease recurrence following radical prostatectomy for prostate cancer. *J Natl Cancer Inst* 1998;90:766–771.

4. Kattan MW, Zelefsky MJ, Kupelian PA, et al. Pretreatment nomogram for predicting the outcome of 3-dimensional conformal radiotherapy in prostate cancer. *J Clin Oncol* 2000;18:3352–3359.

5. Kattan MW. Nomograms are superior to staging and risk grouping systems for identifying high-risk patients: preoperative application in prostate cancer. *Curr Opin Urol* 2003;13:111–116.

6. Thames HD, Kuban DA, Levy LB, et al. Prognostic risk group stratification for clinical and biochemical failure after external beam radiation of prostate cancer. *T J Radiat Oncol Biol Phys* 2004;60:s231, Abstract 166.

7. Chakravarti A, Heydon K, Wu CL, et al. Loss of p16 expression is of prognostic significance in locally advanced prostate cancer: an analysis from the Radiation Therapy Oncology Group Protocol 86–10. *J Clin Oncol* 2003;21:3328–3334.

8. Clark JA, Inui TS, Skillman RA, et al. Patients' perceptions of quality of life after treatment for early prostate cancer. *J Clin Oncol* 2003;21:3777–3784.

9. Calcotte JA, Clark JA, Stark PC, et al. Long-term treatment related complications of brachytherapy for early prostate cancer: a survey of patients previously treated. *J Urol* 2001;166:494–499.

10. Holmberg L, Bill-Axelson A, Helgesen F, et al. A randomized trial comparing radical prostatectomy with watchful waiting in early prostate cancer. *N Engl J Med* 2002;347:781–789.

11. Zietman AL, Thakral HJ, Wilson L, et al. Conservative management of prostate cancer in the PSA era: the incidence and time course of subsequent therapy. *J Urol* 2001;166:1702–1706.

12. Potosky AL, Legler J, Albertsen PC, et al. Health outcomes after prostatectomy or radiotherapy for prostate cancer: results from the Prostate Cancer Outcomes Study. *J Natl Cancer Inst* 2000;92:1582.

13. Fowler FJ Jr, Barry MJ, Lu-Yao G, et al. Outcomes of external-beam radiation therapy for prostate cancer: a study of Medicare beneficiaries in three surveillance, epidemiology, and end results areas. *J Clin Oncol* 1996;14:2258.

14. Talcott JA, Rieker P, Clark JA, et al. Patient-reported symptoms after primary therapy for early prostate cancer: results of a prospective cohort study. *J Clin Oncol* 1998;16:275.

15. Hanlon AL, Watkins Bruner D, Peter R, et al. Quality of life study in prostate cancer patients treated with three-dimensional conformal radiation therapy: comparing late bowel and bladder quality of life symptoms to that of the normal population. *Int J Radiat Oncol Biol Phys* 2001; 49:51.

16. Symon Z, Griffith KA, McGlaughlin PW, et al. Dose escalation for localized prostate cancer: substantial benefit observed with 3 D conformal therapy. *Int J Radiat Oncol Biol Phys* 2003;57:384–390.

17. Zelefsky M, Fuks Z, Chan H, et al. 10-year results of dose escalation with 3-dimensional conformal radiotherapy for patients with clinically localized prostate cancer. *Int J Radiat Oncol Biol Phys* 2003;57:s749–s750, Abstract 4.

18. Pollack A, Hanlon Al, Horwitz EM, et al. Prostate cancer radiotherapy dose response: an update of the fox chase experience. *J Urol* 2004;171:1132–1136.

19. Zietman AL, Chung CS, Coen JJ, et al. 10-year outcome for men with localized prostate cancer treated with external radiation therapy: results of a cohort study. *J Urol* 2004;171:210–214.

20. Grimm PD, Blasko JC, Sylvester JE, et al. 10-year biochemical (prostate-specific antigen) control of prostate cancer with (125)I brachytherapy. *Int J Radiat Oncol Biol Phys* 2001;51:31.

21. Ragde H, Grado GL, Nadir BS. Brachytherapy for clinically localized prostate cancer: 13-year disease-free survival of 769 consecutive prostate cancer patients treated with permanent implants alone. *Arch Esp Urol* 2001;54:739.

22. Walsh PC. Anatomic radical retropubic prostatectomy. In: Walsh P, Retik A, Vaughan E Jr et al., eds. *Campbell's urology*, Vol. 3. Philadelphia, PA: WB Saunders, 1998:2565.

23. Catalona WJ, Ramos CG, Carvalhal GF. Contemporary results of anatomic radical prostatectomy. *CA Cancer J Clin* 1999;49:282.

24. Eastham JA, Scardino PT. Radical prostatectomy for clinical stage T1 and T2 prostate cancer. In: Vogelzang NJ, Scardino PT, Shipley WU et al., eds. *Comprehensive textbook of genitourinary oncology*, Vol. 2. Philadelphia, PA: Lippincott Williams & Wilkins, 2000:722.

25. Eastham JA, Goad JR, Rogers E, et al. Risk factors for urinary incontinence after radical prostatectomy. *J Urol* 1996;156:1707.

26. Stanford JL, Feng Z, Hamilton AS, et al. Urinary and sexual function after radical prostatectomy for clinically localized prostate cancer. *JAMA* 2000;283:354.

27. Miles BJ, Giesler B, Kattan MW. Recall and attitudes in patients with prostate cancer. *Urology* 1999;53:169–174.

28. Hoffman RM, Hunt WC, Gilliland FD, et al. Satisfaction with treatment decisions for clinically localized prostatic carcinoma. Results from the Prostate Cancer Outcomes Study. *Cancer* 2003;97:1553–1562.

CHAPTER 13B
Active Surveillance for "Good-Risk" Prostate Cancer: Rationale, Method, and Results

Arthur C. Grabowski and Laurence Klotz

INTRODUCTION

The prevalence of histologic prostate cancer in men over 50 years old is 30% to 40% (1–4). A large proportion of this histologic, or "latent," prostate cancer is never destined to progress or affect the lifespan of the patient. The lifetime risk of being diagnosed with prostate cancer has almost doubled, from 9.5% in the pre–prostate-specific antigen (PSA) era to 17.1% currently (5–7). In a recent prostate cancer prevention study, a strategy of routine systematic biopsies of the prostate in each man, regardless of PSA, resulted in 24.4% of patients in the placebo group diagnosed with prostate cancer over a 7-year period (8). Meanwhile, the risk of dying from prostate cancer remains at approximately 3% (7). As the lifetime risk of being diagnosed approaches the known rate of histologic (mostly insignificant) prostate cancer, the risk of overtreatment looms large. At least two studies have tried to model the over-diagnosis rate, suggesting it is between 30% and 84% (9,10). Factors contributing to this are the increasing use of PSA screening and more extensive biopsy strategies employing 8 to 13 cores (11). Additionally, biopsies are often repeated until a cancer diagnosis is made (12). In most patients, prostate cancer progresses slowly. Most patients, particularly with "good-risk" disease, are destined to die of other causes. Clearly, aggressive treatment of all diagnosed cases would represent overtreatment. All treatments carry with them inherent morbidity that can adversely affect quality of life (13–15). Furthermore, current treatments for prostate cancer are not always effective in controlling the malignancy, even when it is localized (15). The central challenge in localized prostate cancer is to identify the minority of patients with aggressive prostate cancer and offer them curative treatment, while sparing the remainder of them the morbidity of unnecessary treatment.

RATIONALE FOR ACTIVE SURVEILLANCE

Since the advent of PSA in 1989, substantial resources have been directed toward the early detection and treatment of prostate cancer. Mortality rates have fallen about 20% during this period (16). Whether this improvement in mortality is due to these efforts or to other causes is the subject of intense controversy. Other factors, including dietary and lifestyle modification, and a trend toward earlier initiation of androgen ablation for recurrent disease, may explain some or all of the fall in mortality. Indeed, Lu-Yao (16) has demonstrated that the fall in prostate cancer patient mortality in Connecticut—where screening is uncommon and the incidence of prostate cancer is correspondingly lower—is equivalent to a similar reduction in Oregon, a highly screened population. Thus, it remains uncertain whether our efforts at early diagnosis and early local treatment have resulted in a decline in prostate cancer mortality.

Prostate cancer is typically slow growing. Work by Sakr (2,17) has indicated that, in the typical patient, the disease develops in his 30s and takes 20 years to become clinically detectable. Studies by Pound (18) demonstrate that in patients who fail radical prostatectomy and go on to die of prostate cancer, a median of 16 years elapses from surgery until death. The "watchful waiting" studies, most of which accrued patients from the pre-PSA era, also demonstrate that disease-related mortality in populations of prostate cancer patients only becomes substantial after 10 years. The lead time afforded by PSA screening likely increases this to 15 years in screened populations. In addition, it is particularly clear that low-grade prostate cancer is associated with low progression rates and high survival rates in the intermediate term.

One indirect piece of evidence supporting the long window of curability can be derived from nomograms predicting the likelihood of biochemical recurrence based on the PSA level, Gleason grade, and clinical stage. The 5-year biochemical disease-free survival (DFS) with radical prostatectomy is 95% using the Kattan nomograms of a patient with clinical stage T1c, Gleason grade 6 prostate cancer, with PSA of 5 ng/mL (19). If intervention is delayed until the PSA reaches 10 ng/mL, the 5-year DFS is still 90%; and with further delay, until the PSA is 15 ng/mL, it is 85%. Thus, following such a patient during a period of PSA doubling or tripling is still associated with a high chance of cure.

Widespread use of PSA testing has also resulted in a profound stage migration (20). Most patients newly diagnosed with prostate cancer have clinically impalpable, stage T1c disease. Additionally, these patients typically have a PSA that is only mildly elevated (<10 ng/mL). These patients usually have slowly growing cancer with a long window of curability. This is also supported by the Albertson data (Table 13B.1) (21).

A meta-analysis of six surveillance series comprising 828 patients reported by Chodak indicated that at 10 years, disease-specific survival was 87% for well- and moderately differentiated cancers, and metastasis-free survival was 81% and 58%, respectively (22). These studies incorporated an "either/or" approach (i.e., either radical treatment or surveillance; surveillance offered no opportunity for delayed radical local therapy) and reflected a prestage migration population. Thus, many patients with favorably prognostic factors, who were diagnosed considerably earlier in their disease process than the average patient in this nonsurveillance population, are likely to have an incredibly long natural history.

EXPECTANT MANAGEMENT APPROACHES

Two basic variants of expectant management have evolved. The first is a noninterventionalist approach, which aims to limit the morbidity of the disease without administering curative treatment. The term "watchful waiting" can be applied to this approach, implying that there is no benefit to radical local therapy. A more recent development is an interventionalist approach called "active surveillance with curative intent." This implies active monitoring of the patient's disease and intervention with curative intent at the first signs of progression. Active surveillance relies on the ability to recognize a biologic change in the cancer that would warrant an intervention and thus separate the clinically insignificant from the life-threatening cancers. Both strategies rely on appropriate patient selection, but active surveillance also relies on rigorous patient monitoring.

The main advantage of expectant management strategies is the avoidance of overtreatment and its consequent morbidities. There are also several potential drawbacks. The most obvious disadvantage stems from incorrect patient selection leading to inappropriate assignment of patients to expectant management or vice versa. This can result from an underestimation of the natural history of the patient's cancer or an overestimation of the patient's comorbidities.

Appropriate patient selection is the crux of expectant management strategies. With the watchful-waiting strategy, it is the most important factor. It involves taking into consideration tumor factors and patient comorbidities, as well as patient wishes and values. With the active surveillance strategy, patient selection is not as critical because further selection can be made during the follow-up period when patients are actively monitored for progression. Other disadvantages are not as obvious; these include the anxiety and decreased quality of life ascribed to living with cancer (13,15). These can be even more pronounced with active surveillance, given that every surveillance visit may initiate a change in treatment course. The costs of watchful waiting and active surveillance protocols have not been examined. Active surveillance is likely to be more costly than watchful waiting alone, given the need for periodic invasive tests such as repeat prostatic biopsies. The efficacy of active surveillance depends on close surveillance, and compliance may be problematic for some patients. Finally, active surveillance is reliant on the presumption that monitoring will be able to detect clinically significant progression with enough lead time that an intervention can still be curative.

Watchful Waiting

The surveillance studies in the published literature are summarized in Table 13B.2 (15,21,24,26,28–34). A number of observations can be made from these studies. Mortality from other causes is common in all cohorts and likely reflects the average age of patients at entry. Cause-specific survival varies substantially, from 30% to 80% at 15 years. This reflects patient selection at study entry. In contrast to the range of outcomes, there are some important similarities between these studies. All reflect natural history from the pre-PSA era. The stage-migration phenomenon of the last decade had not occurred when these studies were carried out, and none offered salvage radical therapy for local progression. Watchful waiting in these series consisted of no active treatment until symptomatic metastases developed, at which point androgen ablation was offered. Additionally, these series are characterized by problems of selection bias to varying degrees. Confounding issues include the use of aspiration cytology for diagnosis, exclusion of higher risk patients, elderly cohorts, and inclusion of T1a patients.

TABLE 13B.1

PROSTATE CANCER MORTALITY IN AN ACTIVE SURVEILLANCE COHORT ACCORDING TO GRADE

Gleason score	Prostate cancer mortality at 15 yr
2–4	4%–7%
5	6%–11%
6	18%–30%
7	42%–70%
8–10	60%–87%

Patients with low grade prostate cancer by and large do not die of their disease. As grade increases, the risk of death also goes up; but for Gleason 6, this remains at only 18 to 30% (21).

TABLE 13B.2

SUMMARY OF WATCHFUL WAITING SERIES

Reference	Stage	Year last patient accrued	N	Survival (%) 5 yr	10 yr	15 yr
Hanash, 1972 (24)	A	1942	50	86	52	22
	B		129	19	4	1
Lerner, 1991 (28)	T1b–T2	1982	279	88	61	
				95 CSS	80 CSS	
Adolfsson, 1992 (30)	T1–T2	1982	122	82	50	
				99 CSS	84 CSS	
Johansson, 1997 (26)	T1–T2	1984	223		41	21
					86 CSS	81 CSS
Albertsen, 1998 (21)	unknown	1984	767			Gl ≤5: 89–96
						Gl 6: 70–82
						Gl 7: 30–58
						Gl 8-10: 13–40
Handley, 1988 (29)		1985	278			
Waaler, 1993 (31)	T2	1985	28	94 CSS		
Whitmore, 1991 (32)	T2	1986	37	95	90	62
George, 1988 (33)	Tx	1986	120	86	66	66
Aus, 1995 (34)	T1–T4	1991	301	80 CSS	50 CSS	30 CSS
Holmberg, 2002 (15)	T1–T2	1999	348	91 CSS		
				82 OS		

CSS, cancer-specific survival; OS, overall survival; Gl, Gleason score.

One striking feature of these studies stands out: Every series contains a large subset of long-term survivors, particularly in the group with favorable clinical parameters. This is a critical observation. In the absence of treatment, a substantial subset of patients with prostate cancer is not destined to die of the disease. The challenge, of course, is to identify that subset accurately.

The first randomized trial comparing radical prostatectomy with watchful waiting recently reported a 50% reduction in prostate cancer deaths, although a significant overall survival benefit has not yet been demonstrated (15). This outcome, while providing strong support for radical prostatectomy for some patients with localized prostate cancer, in no way undermines the case for active surveillance for good-risk patients. Cause-specific survival in the observation group was 91% with a median follow-up of 6.5 years, suggesting that many men don't require therapy. Secondly, the patients in this study were largely accrued in the pre-PSA era. Forty-five percent had a PSA >10 ng/mL, 75% were T2, and 30% had Gleason ≥7. These patients had, in aggregate, significantly more advanced disease than the typical candidate for active surveillance: PSA mildly elevated, T1c, with small volume of low-grade (Gleason <7) cancer. These more advanced patients still benefited from surgical intervention. In this intermediate- to high-risk group, the number of patients needed to treat for each prostate cancer death prevented was 15. This number is likely much higher for good-risk prostate cancer. Thus, the Holmberg study confirms that favorable-risk patients may not require therapy; and if they do, they likely have a long window of curability.

Active Surveillance Studies

Since the prediction of clinically insignificant disease is problematic and inaccurate, an alternative strategy has been developed that allows patient entry into an expectant management protocol with rigorous monitoring and the option of salvage curative therapy, should signs of progression develop. This is referred to as active surveillance (37,38). Two studies have prospectively implemented such active surveillance protocols with curative intent (39,40). Each study has used different eligibility criteria as well as follow-up protocols.

Choo et al. were the first to report on a prospective active surveillance protocol consisting of 206 patients (40,41). Eligibility criteria included untreated biopsy-proven prostate cancer with a PSA of ≤15 ng/mL, Gleason ≤7, and tumor, nodes, and metastases (TNM) stage ≤T2b, N0, M0. All patients with Gleason 7 cancer were over 70 years of age or had significant comorbid conditions. After obtaining informed consent, patients were followed with a PSA and a digital rectal examination (DRE) every 3 months for the first 2 years and every 6 months thereafter, until they met specific criteria defining rapid or clinically significant progression. These criteria are summarized in Table 13B.3.

Eighty percent of the patients in this series fulfilled the criteria for favorable disease (i.e., PSA <10 ng/mL, Gleason ≤6, T ≤2a). The median age was 70 with a range of 49 to 84 years. Eighty percent of patients had Gleason 6 or less, and the same proportion had a PSA <10 ng/mL (with the median being 6.5 ng/mL). With a median follow-up of 45 months, 96 patients (40%) came off watchful observation while 145 have remained on surveillance. Eight percent of patients came off surveillance because of rapid biochemical progression; 10% for clinical progression; 4% for histologic progression; and 16% because of patient preference. Two percent of patients died of other causes.

The distribution of PSA doubling times (PSA DT) is shown in Figure 13B.1. The median PSA DT was 7 years. Only 21% of patients had a PSA DT of <3 years. Forty-two percent had a PSA DT >10 years, suggesting an indolent course of disease in these patients.

Patients were rebiopsied 1.5 to 2 years after being placed on the surveillance protocol. Grade remained stable in 92% of patients; only 8% demonstrated significant rise (Gleason score >2). Whether this represents true grade progression or

TABLE 13B.3

CRITERIA FOR PROGRESSION ON ACTIVE SURVEILLANCE

PSA progression (all 3)
- PSA doubling time <2 years, based on at least three separate measurements over a minimum of 6 months
- Final PSA ≥8 ng/mL
- P value <.05 from a regression analysis of ln (PSA) on time

Clinical progression (any one)
- more than 200% increase in the product of the maximum perpendicular diameters of the primary lesion, as measured digitally
- local progression of prostate cancer requiring TURP
- development of ureteric obstruction
- radiologic and/or clinical evidence of distant metastasis

Histologic progression
- Gleason score ≥8 on re-biopsy of prostate at 12–18 months

TURP, transurethral resection of the prostate.

an initial undersampling is unknown. Regardless, it is a low percentage of patients that is consistent with the recent publication by Epstein and Walsh, demonstrating a 12.9% rate of grade progression over 2 to 3 years (42).

Nine patients (of 206) had a radical prostatectomy after they manifested a PSA doubling time of less than 2 years. All had Gleason score of 5–6, PSA <10 ng/mL, and pT1-2 at study entry. The final pathology was as follows: 3/9 were pT2, five were pT3a-c, and one was N1. For a group of patients with favorable clinical characteristics, this is a high rate of locally advanced disease and it supports the view that a short PSA DT is associated with a more aggressive phenotype. A PSA DT of <2 years in patients with otherwise favorable clinical features portends a high likelihood of advanced disease. Fortunately, this scenario is uncommon. This also suggests that, insofar as cure of the patients with early rapid biochemical progression is a goal, the optimal PSA DT threshold for intervention should be greater than 2 years. The optimal threshold is likely in the range of 3 years. In this series, that represented 22% of patients. One patient died of prostate cancer 6 years after study entry; one has metastatic disease.

Carter et al. also reported their preliminary results of active surveillance in a carefully selected population of 81 men who had been followed for longer than 1 year (with the median being 23 months) (39). Selection criteria are shown in Table 13B.4.

The median age of enrolled patients was 65 years (range, 52 to 73 years). The median PSA was 5 ng/mL (range, 1 to 13 ng/mL). Patients were followed semi-annually with a PSA, a free-to-total PSA ratio, and a digital rectal examination (DRE). A 12-core transrectal ultrasound guided biopsy was performed annually. Progression was defined based on the presence of any of the previously defined adverse pathologic findings (Table 13B.4) on the repeat biopsy.

Twenty-five of the patients (31%) progressed at a median of 14 months from diagnosis (range, 12 to 52 months), with the majority progressing within the first 2 years. Of those who progressed, 13 underwent radical prostatectomy. Final pathology showed organ-confined disease in 11 out of 13 patients, with eight of these 11 having a Gleason score ≤6 and three of these 11 having a Gleason score of 7. Two patients had established extracapsular extension, of which one had a Gleason 9 cancer, and the other had a Gleason 7 cancer. Interestingly, the patient with the Gleason 9 cancer was also on the protocol the longest out of all who progressed. In the evaluation of factors that predicted progression, increasing PSA density and decreasing free-to-total PSA ratio were found to have a statistically significant association with progression. However, because of significant overlap, these factors could not be used to separate the two groups.

Zeitman and Schellhammer recently published a retrospective review of 199 men with T1–T2 prostate cancer and PSA <20 ng/mL, managed with active surveillance (43). Median follow-up was 3.4 years. Overall survival at 5 years and 7 years was 77% and 63%, respectively, and disease-specific survival was 98% and 98%, respectively. At 5 years and 7 years, the proportion of patients who were alive and untreated was 43% and 26%, respectively. Sixty-three patients were treated radically. The median PSA rise, from diagnosis to treatment, was 2.9 ng/mL in the treated cohort, compared with 0.9 ng/mL in the untreated group.

Zeitman and Schellhammer's study raised another concern: Active surveillance may simply be a version of delayed therapy, unless patients die of comorbid illness in the interim. However, the indication for intervention in this series was a mild rise in PSA (<3 ng/mL) over a prolonged period. One wonders whether patients panicked because of the slow rise in PSA. This emphasizes that conservative management in the modern PSA era requires that the patient and the doctor both agree to a course of treatment. This involves an understanding that PSA will likely progress slowly over time, but that slow progression is not a reason for intervention.

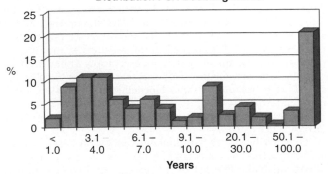

Distribution PSA Doubling Times

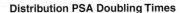

FIGURE 13B.1. Doubling times of PSA in 231 patients on an active surveillance protocol. These data are based on a median follow-up of 55 months. Median PSA doubling time was 7 years. Median number of measurements was 7 (range, 3 to 19). Twenty percent of patients had a PSA DT <3 years.

TABLE 13B.4

ENTRY CRITERIA FOR ACTIVE SURVEILLANCE

TNM stage	T1c
PSA density	<0.15 ng/mL/cm³ (based on TRUS)
Age	>65 regardless of comorbidity
	≤65 with significant comorbidity (unless patient insisted)
Biopsy	minimum 1 sextant
	absence of any one of the following adverse pathologic findings:
	• any Gleason pattern 4 or 5
	• ≥3 cores involved with cancer
	• ≥50% of any one core involved

PSA, prostate-specific antigen; TRUS, transrectal ultrasound; TNM, tumor, node metastasis.

PATIENT SELECTION

In an attempt to define insignificant prostate cancer, Stamey studied prostates obtained from 139 consecutive radical cysto-prostatectomy specimens, of which 55 (40%) had prostate cancer. Given the clinical prevalence of T1b–T4 prostate cancer of 8% at the time, the authors concluded that the tumor volumes in the top 92nd percentile (0.5 to 6.1 mL) were clinically significant. The arbitrary assumption is that 8% is the clinically significant cancer rate. The arbitrariness of this is of concern. If it were set at 4%, then the clinically significant cancer volume would be closer to 1 mL. Conversely, if it were set at 12% then the clinically significant cancer volume would be 0.2 mL (4). The median age of the patients in the study was 65 years; therefore, the applicability of this volume cut point to patients much older or much younger is limited. Epstein et al. (44) utilized the above data with historical radical prostatectomy cohorts from Johns Hopkins School of Medicine (45,46) to codify insignificant cancers as those having the following characteristics: clinical stage T1c; tumor volume <0.2 mL; no Gleason pattern 4 or 5; organ confined and no evidence of seminal vesicle or lymph node invasion. Tumors between 0.2 and 0.5 mL were identified as minimal. Since then other authors have collapsed these two categories into one, despite the propensity of some of the 0.2 to 0.5 mL tumors to display capsular invasion (46–50). Using this definition, many groups have reported on the incidence of insignificant disease. The incidences vary widely, from up to 30% in T1c patients, as reported by the Johns Hopkins group (44,48,51) to values as low as 9% to 12% in other series (49, 52,53). Contemporary radical prostatectomy series report insignificant prostate cancer in 5.8% to 26% of the specimens (4,53–56). Crucially, the designation of "insignificant" disease is based on histologic volume, not natural history. It is likely, in view of the epidemiologic data, that many patients with more substantial volume of disease have insignificant prostate cancer.

Interestingly, Augustin et al. (53) reported a rise in the insignificant cancer rate in the last two years of their series to around 9.5%. This may not be coincidental. As PSA screening becomes established, the initial incidence bump is returning to a new baseline. The initial increased incidence may have included a lot of significant cancers diagnosed earlier because of the added leadtime effect of PSA, as well as many insignificant cancers, which were diluted in that incidence bump. Entrance into this new era of post-incidence bump PSA initiated diagnosis, coupled with more extensive biopsy strategies, will result in insignificant cancers composing a larger proportion of the whole.

Numerous preoperative predictive algorithms have been developed to estimate the risk of having insignificant disease. Table 13B.5 summarizes the variable success of these algorithms in patients with T1c prostate cancer. Recently, Kattan published three predictive nomograms, each with an increasing number of variables that estimated the probability of insignificant disease (50). The area under the receiver operating characteristics curves for these models varied from 0.64 for the basic model to 0.79 for the most complex model, which required knowledge of the pretreatment PSA, clinical stage, primary and secondary biopsy Gleason score, ultrasound prostate volume, and total mm of cancer in the biopsy (50). To reiterate, these nomograms were based on histology, not natural history, and may have underrepresented the true incidence of insignificant disease.

The probability of insignificant disease should not be used in a vacuum and should be adjusted to patient's life expectancy. Dugan et al. attempted to address this issue by building a model to calculate the clinically significant tumor volume at different ages based on theoretical doubling times of cancer growth and Gleason grade (57). Using this model and assuming a doubling time of 6 years, a 50-year-old must have a Gleason score of <5 and a cancer volume of <0.1 mL, a 60-year-old must have a Gleason score of <6 and a cancer volume

TABLE 13B.5

STUDIES AND VARIOUS CRITERIA TO PREDICT INSIGNIFICANT DISEASE IN THE RADICAL PROSTATECTOMY SPECIMEN

Reference	N	Prediction rule		PPV, %	NPV, %
Elgamel et al. (47)	100	• log PSA • <3 mm Ca		88.5[a]	75.0
Goto et al. (49)	170	• PSAD <0.10 • 1 core of ≤2 mm Ca • no Gl pattern 4/5		75.0[b]	94.9
Epstein et al. (44)	157	• <3 cores of Ca • <50% Ca/core • no Gl pattern 4/5 • PSAD <0.10	• <3 mm Ca on 1 core • no Gl pattern 4/5 • PSAD <0.15	79.3	85.9
Carter et al. (51)	240	Same as Epstein (44)		75[c]	75
Epstein et al. (48)	163	• <3 cores of Ca • <50% Ca/core • no Gl pattern 4/5 • f/t PSA ≥0.15		94.4	77.2
Augustin et al. (53)	480	• <1% Ca on biopsy • no Gl pattern 4/5 • PSAD <0.10		45.0[d]	93.3

Gl, gleason score; PPV, positive predictive value; NPV, negative predictive value; PSAD, prostate-specific antigen density; f/t PSA, free to total PSA ratio.
[a]PPV and NPV based on 90 cases.
[b]included patients with T1–T3 disease.
[c]PPV and NPV based on 72 cases.
[d]Based on an undefined subset of 480/1254 patients with Gleason ≤6 (may include T2 patients).
Modified from Epstein JI, Chan DW, Sokoll LJ, et al. Nonpalpable stage T1c prostate cancer: prediction of insignificant disease using free/total prostate specific antigen levels and needle biopsy findings. J Urol 1998;160:2407–2411.

of <2.4 mL, a 70-year-old must have a Gleason score of <7 and a cancer volume of <5.0 mL, and an 80-year-old must have a Gleason score of <8 and a cancer volume of <8.8 mL (57). This study demonstrated that tumor volume needs to be interpreted in the context of the patient's life expectancy. It also showed that relatively large tumor volumes may be insignificant in patients whose life expectancy is short, and insignificant tumors do not necessarily need to be impalpable. Unfortunately, this model has little direct clinical applicability because acceptable Gleason scores were arbitrarily assigned to a decade of life, and life expectancy was based on average life tables without taking individual comorbidities into consideration. Furthermore, although several studies have correlated biopsy parameters (i.e., percentage of cancer, cancer length in mm, number of positive cores) with increasing tumor volume in the radical prostatectomy specimen, a prediction tool to estimate volume remains elusive (58).

Albertsen et al. illustrated another approach to the same problem using competing risk analysis (21). This strategy balances the risk of dying from prostate cancer against the risk of dying from other causes. When the probability of dying from other causes exceeds the probability of dying from prostate cancer, the benefits of radical therapy become less visible and alternative strategies such as expectant management become more attractive. Competing risk analysis involves estimating a patient's life expectancy given the comorbidities that may be present. Krahn et al. has demonstrated that clinicians are able to predict life expectancy with a modest degree of accuracy (59). The average prediction error ranged from 2.4 to 5.2 years. Patients' own assessments of their health status can be useful in predicting their life expectancy as demonstrated by Welch et al. (60). Table 13B.6 displays the life expectancies of patients according to their own assessment of their overall health (60). Using this, one can select patients for expectant management based on their predicted life expectancy and disease-risk category.

The two prospective active surveillance studies had very different eligibility criteria and follow-up protocols. However, certain problems were common to both. Neither of the protocols initially required an extended 10- to 12-core biopsy regimen or a repeat sextant biopsy before enrollment. This may have contributed to the majority of patients in the Johns Hopkins series progressing within 2 years, when the first repeat biopsies would have been done. Progression on rebiopsy may have represented an undersampling of the prostate at study entry. These authors acknowledged this limitation and have since recommended a repeat 12-core transrectal ultrasound (TRUS) biopsy prior to enrollment in the protocol (39,63).

An increased number of biopsies and an increased number of cores may facilitate accurate estimation of cancer volume and extent. Epstein et al. rebiopsied 193 T1c radical prostatectomy specimens in a sextant fashion (64); 30% of these biopsies were negative. Decreased tumor volume, increased gland size, and lower tumor grade of the radical prostatectomy specimen were all independent predictors of a negative biopsy. Patients with "limited cancer" (defined as ≤3 mm of cancer on one core with no Gleason pattern 4 or 5 and PSA <10 ng/mL) on the first biopsy and no cancer on the repeat biopsy had a 62% chance of having pathologically insignificant or minimal disease in the specimen. However, of the patients with minimal cancer on both the first and repeat biopsy, 50% still had moderate tumors in the radical prostatectomy specimen. Moderate cancer was defined as organ confined with volume >0.5 mL; or with focal capsular penetration but Gleason score ≤7; or with established capsular penetration, Gleason score ≤7, and negative margins. Conversely, the finding of significant cancer (i.e., more than limited) on repeat biopsy correlated very well with the finding of moderate to advanced disease in the radical prostatectomy specimen. Furthermore, 26% of patients who initially had limited disease on the first biopsy had significant disease on re-biopsy.

The second issue to consider when using biopsy results to select patients concerns the upgrading of the Gleason score in the radical prostatectomy specimens, which occurs in 35%–38% of patients with a single sextant biopsy (65,66). Fleshner et al. examined this issue and found that repeating the biopsy reduces upgrading by half, to 19% (67). Similarly, Epstein et al. found that grade progression in their active surveillance cohort occurred mostly in the first follow-up biopsy, suggesting undersampling as the cause (42). This demonstrates that a repeat biopsy is useful for excluding patients with moderate to advanced cancer from an expectant management protocol. However, it does not provide a lot of reassurance about the extent of tumor in those who continue to have limited amount or no cancer on rebiopsy.

An alternative strategy to rebiopsy would be to include more cores on the initial biopsy. Multiple studies have demonstrated that increasing the number of cores improves cancer detection (12). It also makes sense that this strategy would be helpful in excluding significant disease in patients where expectant management is being considered. In Kattan's nomogram for the prediction of insignificant cancer, the total number of millimeters of negative biopsy cores is included along with the total number of millimeters of positive cores (50). Makhlouf et al. compared a sextant biopsy with ≥8 cores and found a reduction in the grade discordance between the

---

TABLE 13B.6

LIFE EXPECTANCY ACCORDING TO PATIENT SELF-REPORTED HEALTH STATUS

Age	Average life expectancy (yr)	Life expectancy according to self-reported health status			
		Excellent	Good	Fair	Poor
65	16	21	16	14	11
70	13	18	13	11	8
75	10	14	10	8	6
80	7	11	8	6	5

Light gray = 10–15 years life expectancy.
Dark gray ≤7–8 years life expectancy.
Based on Welch et al. (60), Anderson (61), and National Vital Statistics Report (62).

biopsy and the radical prostatectomy specimen with more cores (68). However, it is unknown whether increasing the number of cores is equivalent to re-biopsy with regard to accuracy of predicting tumor volume and grade. It is not unreasonable to infer from Kattan's nomograms that the more tissue sampled, the more confident one can be in the results. Therefore, unless at least 10 cores were sampled on the initial biopsy, a repeat is warranted (at some point) in patients planning to be followed on an active surveillance protocol.

MONITORING AND FOLLOW-UP

Role of PSA

PSA, DRE, and repeat biopsies were all used in the two prospective active surveillance studies to monitor patients (39,40). However, the triggers for intervention were quite different. PSA seems like a logical marker for cancer progression as it is associated with tumor volume and grade (69,70). In addition, virtually all men with advanced cancer (i.e., bone or soft-tissue metastases) have marked elevation of PSA (71,72). The major drawback to its use is its lack of specificity for prostate cancer in the 2-22 ng/mL range (73). As a result, a number of derivatives of PSA, which include PSA velocity, PSA doubling time, free-to-total PSA ratio, and PSA density have been examined for their utility in monitoring patients in active surveillance protocols.

PSA doubling time has received a lot of attention in this respect. Schmid et al. was one of the first to correlate shortening of PSA DT with increasing cancer volume and stage (70). Since then, others have demonstrated its utility as a prognostic factor for progression after therapy (74,75). Recently, D'Amico has validated it as a surrogate marker for death when measured after PSA recurrence, regardless of previous therapy (76). Choo et al. arbitrarily chose a PSA DT of <2 years as one of the criteria for intervention in their active surveillance cohort (40). This doubling time may be too short, as 6 out of 9 patients thus detected who went on to have a radical prostatectomy had extraprostatic disease. McLaren et al. also examined PSA DT in a watchful waiting cohort and found that a doubling time of <3 years was associated with clinical progression (defined as palpable enlargement in the tumor nodule or increase in T stage) in more than 80% of patients by 18 months from diagnosis. Egawa et al. looked at PSA DT before radical prostatectomy and found that a doubling time ≤3 years was more common with pT3 disease at radical prostatectomy (77). The primary concern with using PSA DT as a trigger

for curative intervention is that it may act as a marker of aggressive disease that has already progressed and is no longer localized. In fact, in Egawa's series, 3/19 patients with a PSA DT ≥6 years had pT3 disease, and two of these had positive margins at radical prostatectomy (77). Others have suggested that prostate cancer doubling time may be underestimated when the calculation is based on serial PSA changes (78,79). Furthermore, PSA DT calculations are subject to the vagaries of the biologic variation of PSA (80,81). The optimal method for PSA doubling time calculation is uncertain. McLaren et al. demonstrated no difference between using the first and last available values compared with using regression analysis (82). A novel way of analyzing serial PSA measurements was described by Vollmer et al. (83). Their analysis suggested that relative PSA velocity and PSA amplitude can be combined to have a more powerful predictive ability for progressors in an active surveillance group than PSA DT alone. Other options include the subtracted PSA DT (subtracting base line PSA, thought to be due to benign prostatic hyperplasia (BPH), from subsequent values); and rolling PSA DT (recalculating the PSA DT every 2 years). The use of PSA DT to predict which patients are destined to progress and which are not is promising but remains investigational. Further work needs to be done to evaluate a safe cut-off value and the best method to calculate it.

Derivatives of PSA such as percent free PSA (%fPSA), PSA velocity, and PSA density have also been examined for their ability to stratify progressors from nonprogressors in an active surveillance protocol. Khan et al. examined these three factors in the John Hopkins active surveillance cohort and found that in different combinations and using various cut-offs they could predict which patients would have progression on repeat biopsy (Table 13B.7) (63). In their study, progression was defined only based on adverse pathologic findings at repeat biopsy, which was performed on an annual basis. At the very least, the analysis could be used to identify patients who could forgo a repeat biopsy.

Do et al. examined the rate of change of %fPSA in the University of Toronto active surveillance cohort (84). They found that the slope of the change in %fPSA was negatively correlated with the doubling time of PSA and initial T stage. Attempts to stratify patients who progressed by the slope of the change in %fPSA dichotomized around the median slope showed a trend that was not statistically significant (log rank $P = .07$). Arguably there may be some interaction in such an analysis as the doubling time of PSA <2 years was one of the criteria for progression. Nevertheless, using the rate of change of %fPSA to predict for aggressive cancers is a concept that has promise and needs further investigation.

TABLE 13B.7

CRITERIA TO PREDICT PROGRESSION AT NEXT BIOPSY

	Findings at initial biopsy to predict progression at first repeat	Findings at first repeat biopsy to predict progression at second repeat	Findings at second repeat biopsy to predict progression at third repeat
N	106	67	36
Criteria	Vol ≤40.5	PSA vel >0.29	%fPSA <20.5
	%fPSA ≤19.5	%fPSA <16.5	Vol >55.5
	or Vol ≥40.5		PSA vel <1.7
	PSA ≥7.95		
Sensitivity	82	71	100
Specificity	83	88	70
Accuracy	83	83	75

PSA vel, PSA velocity.

Role of the Clinical Exam

Intervention criteria that are based solely on changes on a DRE are subjective and prone to error. This is due to the inaccuracy and significant interexaminer variation of the DRE in the detection of prostate cancer and the estimation of its volume (85–87). Furthermore, it would be unusual for a significant change in prostate cancer volume to be detected only on the assessment by the digital rectal exam and not accompanied by changes in the PSA. Despite this, the DRE is an important part of the follow-up protocol as it allows for the potential detection of aggressive cancer that is not secreting PSA. In Choo's study 10/37 patients (27%) that progressed did so on the basis of a change on the DRE (40). At the very least, a change in the DRE can act as a trigger for rebiopsy.

Role of Imaging

Hruby et al. examined the role of TRUS in the follow-up of patients managed in the University of Toronto active surveillance protocol (88). Although TRUS was undertaken prospectively in this cohort, there were no criteria based on TRUS findings for intervention or change in management. The resulting analysis can therefore only address whether TRUS was of value in the clinical decision to intervene once one of the previously established criteria was met. In this subpopulation of 28 patients, a total of 7 (25%) had TRUS changes consistent with progression. Thorough analysis of these changes revealed that TRUS did not aid the clinician with the decision to intervene and could not be recommended as an adjunct investigation once other progression criteria were met (88). Its role as a tool to predict progression is unknown.

The utility of bone scans in patients managed on active surveillance with a PSA ≤15 ng/mL appears to be limited. Yap et al. analyzed the 299 bone scans performed on 244 patients in the University of Toronto active surveillance protocol and found none of them to be positive (89). Bone scans were done routinely on an annual basis for the first 2 years and then biannually thereafter until the PSA was ≥15 ng/mL when annual scans were resumed. Based on the data, the probability of a negative bone scan with a PSA <15 was estimated to be 88% to 100% (95% confidence interval) (89). It must be noted that this protocol was open to patients with favorable prostate cancer (Stage T1b–T2bN0M0, Gleason score ≤7 and PSA ≤15 ng/mL).

Role of Repeat Biopsies

Progression on repeat biopsies has been used in both prospective active surveillance cohorts as an indication for intervention. The biopsy criteria for intervention varied. The John Hopkins group based their criteria solely on the finding of adverse pathologic factors, which were the same as those used to exclude patients from the active surveillance protocol. This required patients to undergo repeat biopsies on an annual basis. While having the advantage of being simple and previously validated to predict for significant disease, this approach carries with it the morbidity and quality of life loss that is attributable to this invasive investigation (48,51). More importantly, such a requirement may increase the noncompliance rate as men refuse follow-up biopsies. In the Johns Hopkins cohort 67 of 78 patients (86%) had the first follow-up biopsy in a cohort that was followed for a minimum of 12 months (63). It is not clear what happened to the 14% of patients not biopsied and whether further decreases in the biopsy rate at year 2 and 3 of follow-up are due to refusal or other reasons. The burden of yearly repeat biopsies is considerable. An ideal follow-up protocol would combine repeat biopsies with less invasive monitoring.

In the Johns Hopkins cohort, the conversion rate to unfavorable pathology was 25.4% at year 1, 16.7% at year 2, and 0 at year 3 (63). Whether these rates would have been lower with more rigorous biopsy strategies at entry is unknown but not unreasonable to speculate. However, the fact that progression does occur beyond the first repeat biopsy suggests the need for more than one repeat biopsy in the protocol.

In the University of Toronto active surveillance protocol, only one follow-up biopsy was planned at 12–18 months post enrollment. The criterion for histological progression was arbitrarily defined as an increase in the Gleason score to 8 or higher, which accounted for 5/37 (13.5%) of those who progressed (40). An additional 4 patients with predominant Gleason 4 pattern on re-biopsy had definitive therapy.

The biopsy criteria for triggering intervention depend on the population being followed. Cancers that are more aggressive may be tolerated in older patients with significant comorbidities and poor life expectancy. In patients who are healthier and younger, assurance of low-volume, low-stage, and low-grade disease is more important. The discrepancy in the criteria between the two prospective studies likely relates to the difference in the life expectancies of their patients. Indirect evidence for this comes from the different median age of the two cohorts, 65 in the Johns Hopkins cohort versus 70 in the University of Toronto cohort.

CURRENT STUDIES

The approach of active surveillance with selective delayed intervention makes sense, but warrants formal evaluation in a prospective comparative trial. In Canada, we have opened a feasibility trial, randomizing good-risk patients between this approach and definitive therapy (e.g., patient's choice of surgery, brachytherapy, or external beam irradiation). This trial will test the willingness of 100 patients to consent to be randomized between these two arms. The intent, if the trial confirms the feasibility of this randomization, will be to enroll this initial cohort of randomized patients into a large-scale randomized trial comparing active surveillance to definitive therapy.

CONCLUSION

Watchful waiting (with palliative intent only) is clearly appropriate for patients who are elderly, have significant comorbidity, and have favorable clinical parameters. The use of comorbidity indices facilitates the identification of patients whose life expectancy is diminished relative to the natural history of their prostate cancer. The likelihood of a prostate cancer death in these patients is low.

Many good-risk patients, however, fall into a gray zone where there may be benefits of curative treatment, particularly if they have a more biologically aggressive disease than average. In these patients, a policy of close monitoring with selective intervention for those who progress rapidly is appealing. This approach is currently the focus of several clinical trials and preliminary analysis of these has demonstrated that it is feasible. Most patients who understand the basis for this approach will remain on observation long term. If patients are selected properly (i.e., good-risk and low-volume disease) and followed carefully (with early intervention for evidence of progression), it is likely that the majority with indolent disease will not suffer from it, and the minority with aggressive disease will still be amenable to cure. Thus, almost all will die of other causes.

References

1. Breslow N, Chan CW, Dhom G, et al. Latent carcinoma of prostate at autopsy in seven areas. The International Agency for Research on Cancer, Lyons, France. *Int J Cancer* 1977;20:680–688.

2. Sakr WA, Haas GP, Cassin BF, et al. The frequency of carcinoma and intraepithelial neoplasia of the prostate in young male patients. *J Urol* 1993;150:379–385.

3. Franks LM. Latent carcinoma of the prostate. *J Pathol Bacteriol* 1954;68:603–616.

4. Stamey TA, Freiha FS, McNeal JE, et al. Localized prostate cancer. Relationship of tumor volume to clinical significance for treatment of prostate cancer. *Cancer* 1993;71:933–938.

5. Seidman H, Mushinski MH, Gelb SK, et al. Probabilities of eventually developing or dying of cancer—United States, 1985. *CA Cancer J Clin* 1985;35:36–56.

6. Boring CC, Squires TS, Tong T. Cancer statistics, 1993. *CA Cancer J Clin* 1993;43:7–26.

7. Jemal A, Tiwari RC, Murray T, et al. Cancer statistics, 2004. *CA Cancer J Clin* 2004;54:8–29.

8. Thompson IM, Goodman PJ, Tangen CM, et al. The influence of finasteride on the development of prostate cancer. *N Engl J Med* 2003;349:215–224.

9. McGregor M, Hanley JA, Boivin JF, et al. Screening for prostate cancer: estimating the magnitude of overdetection. *CMAJ* 1998;159:1368–1372.

10. Etzioni R, Penson DF, Legler JM, et al. Overdiagnosis due to prostate-specific antigen screening: lessons from U.S. prostate cancer incidence trends. *J Natl Cancer Inst* 2002;94:981–990.

11. Singh H, Canto EI, Shariat SF, et al. Improved detection of clinically significant, curable prostate cancer with systematic 12-core biopsy. *J Urol* 2004;171:1089–1092.

12. Presti JC Jr. Prostate biopsy: how many cores are enough? *Urol Oncol* 2003;21:135–140.

13. Penson DF, Feng Z, Kuniyuki A, et al. General quality of life 2 years following treatment for prostate cancer: what influences outcomes? Results from the Prostate Cancer Outcomes Study. *J Clin Oncol* 2003;21:1147–1154.

14. Hoffman RM, Hunt WC, Gilliland FD, et al. Patient satisfaction with treatment decisions for clinically localized prostate carcinoma. Results from the Prostate Cancer Outcomes Study. *Cancer* 2003;97:1653–1662.

15. Steineck G, Helgesen F, Adolfsson J, et al. Quality of life after radical prostatectomy or watchful waiting. *N Engl J Med* 2002;347:790–796.

16. Lu-Yao G, Albertsen PC, Stanford JL, et al. Natural experiment examining impact of aggressive screening and treatment on prostate cancer mortality in two fixed cohorts from Seattle area and Connecticut. *BMJ* 2002;325:740.

17. Sakr WA, Grignon DJ, Haas GP, et al. Age and racial distribution of prostatic intraepithelial neoplasia. *Eur Urol* 1996;30:138–144.

18. Pound C, Partin AW, Eisenberger MA, et al. Natural history of progression after PSA elevation following radical prostatectomy. *JAMA* 1999;281:1591–1597.

19. Kattan M, Zelefsky MJ, Kupelian PA, et al. Pretreatment nomogram for predicting the outcome of three-dimensional conformal radiotherapy in prostate cancer. *J Clin Oncol* 2000;18:3352–3359.

20. Cooperberg MR, Lubeck DP, Mehta SS, et al. Time trends in clinical risk stratification for prostate cancer: implications for outcomes (data from CaPSURE). *J Urol* 2003;170:S21–S25; discussion S26–S27.

21. Albertsen P, Hanley IA, Gleason DF, et al. Competing risk analysis of men aged 55 to 74 years at diagnosis managed conservatively for clinically localized prostate cancer. *JAMA* 1998;280:975–980.

22. Chodak G. The management of localized prostate cancer. *J Urol* 1994; 7th edition, Volume 3:1766.

23. Cook G, Watson FR. Twenty nodules of prostate cancer not treated by total prostatecotmy. *J Urol* 1968;100:672–674.

24. Hanash K, Utz DC, Cook EN. Carcinoma of the prostate: a 15 year followup. *J Urol* 1972;107:450–453.

25. Johansson J, Adami H, Andersson S. High 10 year survival rate in patients with early, untreated prostatic cancer. *JAMA* 1992;267:2191–2196.

26. Johansson J, Holmberg L, Johansson S. Fifteen-year survival in prostate cancer. A prospective, population-based study in Sweden. *JAMA* 1997;277:467–471.

27. Barnes R, Hirst A, Rosenquist R. Early carcinoma of the prostate: comparison of stages A and B. *J Urol* 1976;115:404–405.

28. Lerner S, Seale-Hawkins C, Carlton CE Jr. The risk of dying of prostate cancer in patients with clinically localized disease. *J Urol* 1991;146:1040–1045.

29. Handley R, Carr TW, Travis D. Deferred treatment for prostate cancer. *Br J Urol* 1988;62:249–253.

30. Adolfsson J, Carstensen J, Lowhagen T. Deferred treatment in clinically localized prostate carcinoma. *Br J Urol* 1992;69:183–187.

31. Waaler G, Stenwig AE Prognosis of localised prostatic cancer managed by "watch and wait" policy. *Br J Urol* 1993;72:214–219.

32. Whitmore W, Warner JA, Thompson IM. Expectant management of localized prostatic cancer. *Cancer* 1991;67:1091–1096.

33. George N. Natural history of localised prostatic cancer managed by conservative therapy alone. *Lancet* 1988;1:494–496.

34. Aus G, Hugosson I, Norlen L. Long-term survival and mortality in prostate cancer treated with noncurative intent. *J Urol* 1995;154:460–465.

35. Sandblom G, Dufmats D, Varenhorst E. Long-term survival in a Swedish population-based cohort of men with prostate cancer. *Urology* 2000;56:442–447.

36. Madsen P, Graversen PH, Gasser TC, et al. Treatment of localized prostatic cancer. Radical prostatectomy versus placebo. A 15-year follow-up. *Scand J Urol Nephrol* 1988;110(Suppl.):95–100.

37. Parker C. Active surveillance: towards a new paradigm in the management of early prostate cancer. *Lancet Oncol* 2004;5:101–106.

38. Parker C. Active surveillance: an individualized approach to early prostate cancer. *BJU Int* 2003;92:2–3.

39. Carter HB, Walsh PC, Landis P, et al. Expectant management of nonpalpable prostate cancer with curative intent: preliminary results. *J Urol* 2002;167:1231–1234.

40. Choo R, Klotz L, Danjoux C, et al. Feasibility study: watchful waiting for localized low to intermediate grade prostate carcinoma with selective delayed intervention based on prostate specific antigen, histological and/or clinical progression. *J Urol* 2002;167:1664–1669.

41. Choo R, DeBoer G, Klotz L, et al. PSA doubling time of prostate carcinoma managed with watchful observation alone. *Int J Radiat Oncol Biol Phys* 2001;50:615–620.

42. Epstein JI, Walsh PC, Carter HB. Dedifferentiation of prostate cancer grade with time in men followed expectantly for stage T1c disease. *J Urol* 2001;166:1688–1691.

43. Zietman AL, Thakral H, Wilson L, et al. Conservative management of prostate cancer in the prostate specific antigen era: the incidence and time course of subsequent therapy. *J Urol* 2001;166:1702–1706.

44. Epstein JI, Walsh PC, Carmichael M, et al. Pathologic and clinical findings to predict tumor extent of nonpalpable (stage T1c) prostate cancer. *JAMA* 1994;271:368–374.

45. Epstein JI, Pizov G, Walsh PC. Correlation of pathologic findings with progression after radical retropubic prostatectomy. *Cancer* 1993;71:3582–3593.

46. Epstein JI, Carmichael M, Partin AW, et al. Is tumor volume an independent predictor of progression following radical prostatectomy? A multivariate analysis of 185 clinical stage B adenocarcinomas of the prostate with 5 years of followup. *J Urol* 1993;149:1478–1481.

47. Elgamal AA, Van Poppel HP, Van de Voorde WM, et al. Impalpable invisible stage T1c prostate cancer: characteristics and clinical relevance in 100 radical prostatectomy specimens—a different view. *J Urol* 1997;157:244–250.

48. Epstein JI, Chan DW, Sokoll LJ, et al. Nonpalpable stage T1c prostate cancer: prediction of insignificant disease using free/total prostate specific antigen levels and needle biopsy findings. *J Urol* 1998;160:2407–2411.

49. Goto Y, Ohori M, Arakawa A, et al. Distinguishing clinically important from unimportant prostate cancers before treatment: value of systematic biopsies. *J Urol* 1996;156:1059–1063.

50. Kattan MW, Eastham JA, Wheeler TM et al., eds. Counseling men with prostate cancer: a nomogram for predicting the presence of small, moderately differentiated, confined tumors. *J Urol* 2003;170:1792–1797.

51. Carter HB, Sauvageot J, Walsh PC, et al. Prospective evaluation of men with stage T1c adenocarcinoma of the prostate. *J Urol* 1997;157:2206–2209.

52. Lerner SE, Seay TM, Blute ML, et al. Prostate specific antigen detected prostate cancer (clinical stage T1c): an interim analysis. *J Urol* 1996;155:821–826.

53. Augustin H, Hammerer PG, Graefen M, et al. Insignificant prostate cancer in radical prostatectomy specimens: time trends and preoperative prediction. *Eur Urol* 2003;43:455–460.

54. Noguchi M, Stamey TA, McNeal JE, et al. Relationship between systematic biopsies and histological features of 222 radical prostatectomy specimens: lack of prediction of tumor significance for men with nonpalpable prostate cancer. *J Urol* 2001;166:104–109; discussion 109–110.

55. Soh S, Kattan MW, Berkman S, et al. Has there been a recent shift in the pathological features and prognosis of patients treated with radical prostatectomy? *J Urol* 1997;157:2212–2218.

56. Stamey TA, Donaldson AN, Yemoto CE, et al. Histological and clinical findings in 896 consecutive prostates treated only with radical retropubic prostatectomy: epidemiologic significance of annual changes. *J Urol* 1998;160:2412–2417.

57. Dugan JA, Bostwick DG, Myers RP, et al. The definition and preoperative prediction of clinically insignificant prostate cancer. *JAMA* 1996;275:288–294.

58. Lewis JS Jr, Vollmer RT, Humphrey PA. Carcinoma extent in prostate needle biopsy tissue in the prediction of whole gland tumor volume in a screening population. *Am J Clin Pathol* 2002;118:442–450.

59. Krahn MD, Bremner KE, Asaria J, et al. The ten-year rule revisited: accuracy of clinicians' estimates of life expectancy in patients with localized prostate cancer. *Urology* 2002;60:258–263.

60. Welch HG, Albertsen PC, Nease RF, et al. Estimating treatment benefits for the elderly: the effect of competing risks. *Ann Intern Med* 1996;124:577–584.

61. Anderson RN. United States life tables, 1997. *Natl Vital Stat Rep* 1999;47:1–37.

62. Births, marriages, divorces, and deaths: provisional data for August 1998. *Natl Vital Stat Rep* 1998;47:1–2.

63. Khan MA, Carter HB, Epstein JI, et al. Can prostate specific antigen derivatives and pathological parameters predict significant change in expectant management criteria for prostate cancer? *J Urol* 2003;170:2274–2278.

64. Epstein JI, Walsh PC, Sauvageot J, et al. Use of repeat sextant and transition zone biopsies for assessing extent of prostate cancer. *J Urol* 1997;158: 1886–1890.

65. Steinberg DM, Sauvageot J, Piantadosi S, et al. Correlation of prostate needle biopsy and radical prostatectomy Gleason grade in academic and community settings. *Am J Surg Pathol* 1997;21:566–576.

66. Cookson MS, Fleshner NE, Soloway SM, et al. Correlation between Gleason score of needle biopsy and radical prostatectomy specimen: accuracy and clinical implications. *J Urol* 1997;157:559–562.

67. Fleshner NE, Cookson MS, Soloway SM, et al. Repeat transrectal ultrasound-guided prostate biopsy: a strategy to improve the reliability of needle biopsy grading in patients with well-differentiated prostate cancer. *Urology* 1998;52:659–662.

68. Makhlouf AA, Krupski TL, Kunkle D, et al. The effect of sampling more cores on the predictive accuracy of pathological grade and tumour distribution in the prostate biopsy. *BJU Int* 2004;93:271–274.

69. Stamey TA, Yang N, Hay AR, et al. Prostate-specific antigen as a serum marker for adenocarcinoma of the prostate. *N Engl J Med* 1987;317: 909–916.

70. Schmid HP, McNeal JE, Stamey TA. Observations on the doubling time of prostate cancer. The use of serial prostate-specific antigen in patients with untreated disease as a measure of increasing cancer volume. *Cancer* 1993; 71:2031–2040.

71. Chybowski FM, Keller JJ, Bergstralh EJ, et al. Predicting radionuclide bone scan findings in patients with newly diagnosed, untreated prostate cancer: prostate specific antigen is superior to all other clinical parameters. *J Urol* 1991;145:313–318.

72. Bluestein DL, Bostwick DG, Bergstralh EJ, et al. Eliminating the need for bilateral pelvic lymphadenectomy in select patients with prostate cancer. *J Urol* 1994;151:1315–1320.

73. Stamey TA, Johnstone IM, McNeal JE, et al. Preoperative serum prostate specific antigen levels between 2 and 22 ng./ml. correlate poorly with post-radical prostatectomy cancer morphology: prostate specific antigen cure rates appear constant between 2 and 9 ng./ml. *J Urol* 2002;167:103–111.

74. Hull GW, Rabbani F, Abbas F, et al. Cancer control with radical prostatectomy alone in 1,000 consecutive patients. *J Urol* 2002;167:528–534.

75. Hanks GE, Hanlon AL, Lee WR, et al. Pretreatment prostate-specific antigen doubling times: clinical utility of this predictor of prostate cancer behavior. *Int J Radiat Oncol Biol Phys* 1996;34:549–553.

76. D'Amico AV, Moul JW, Carroll PR, et al. Surrogate end point for prostate cancer-specific mortality after radical prostatectomy or radiation therapy. *J Natl Cancer Inst* 2003;95:1376–1383.

77. Egawa S, Arai Y, Tobisu K, et al. Use of pretreatment prostate-specific antigen doubling time to predict outcome after radical prostatectomy. *Prostate Cancer Prostatic Dis* 2000;3:269–274.

78. Berges RR, Vukanovic J, Epstein JI, et al. Implication of cell kinetic changes during the progression of human prostatic cancer. *Clin Cancer Res* 1995;1:473–480.

79. Egawa S, Matsumoto K, Suyama K, et al. Observations of prostate specific antigen doubling time in Japanese patients with nonmetastatic prostate carcinoma. *Cancer* 1999;86:463–469.

80. Bangma CH, Hop WCJ, Schroder FH. Serial prostate specific antigen measurements and progression in untreated confined (stages T0 to 3NxM0, grades 1 to 3) carcinoma of the prostate. *J Urol* 1995;154:1403–1406.

81. Gerber GS, Gornik HL, Goldfischer ER, et al. Evaluation of changes in prostate specific antigen in clinically localized prostate cancer managed without initial therapy. *J Urol* 1998;159:1243–1246.

82. McLaren DB, McKenzie M, Duncan G, et al. Watchful waiting or watchful progression? Prostate specific antigen doubling times and clinical behavior in patients with early untreated prostate carcinoma. *Cancer* 1998; 82:342–348.

83. Vollmer RT, Egawa S, Kuwao S, et al. The dynamics of prostate specific antigen during watchful waiting of prostate carcinoma: a study of 94 Japanese men. *Cancer* 2002;94:1692–1698.

84. Do V, Choo R, De Boer G, et al. The role of serial free/total prostate-specific antigen ratios in a watchful observation protocol for men with localized prostate cancer. *BJU Int* 2002;89:703–709.

85. Smith DS, Catalona WJ. Interexaminer variability of digital rectal examination in detecting prostate cancer. *Urology* 1995;45:70–74.

86. Stamey TA, McNeal JE, Freiha F, et al. Morphometric and clinical studies on 68 consecutive radical prostatectomies. *J Urol* 1988;139:1235–1241.

87. Spigelman SS, McNeal JE, Freiha FS, et al. Rectal examination in volume determination of carcinoma of the prostate: clinical and anatomical correlations. *J Urol* 1986;136:1228–1230.

88. Hruby G, Choo R, Klotz L, et al. The role of serial transrectal ultrasonography in a 'watchful waiting' protocol for men with localized prostate cancer. *BJU Int* 2001;87:643–647.

89. Yap BK, Choo R, Deboer G, et al. Are serial bone scans useful for the follow-up of clinically localized, low to intermediate grade prostate cancer managed with watchful observation alone? *BJU Int* 2003;91: 613–617.

CHAPTER 13C
Radical Prostatectomy for Clinical Stage T1 and T2 Prostate Cancer

James A. Eastham and Peter T. Scardino

A successful radical prostatectomy is a surgical tour de force. Among the most complex operations performed by urologists, radical prostatectomy challenges surgeons by results that are highly sensitive to fine details in surgical technique. Modern outcomes research has repeatedly documented that the results and complications of this operation vary markedly among surgeons, even among experienced surgeons. The elusive goals of modern radical prostatectomy are complete removal of the cancer with negative surgical margins, minimal blood loss, no serious perioperative complications, and complete recovery of continence and potency. No surgeon achieves such results uniformly. The purpose of this chapter is to provide surgeons with details about our approach to this operation, which we have modified frequently in a continual effort to improve the results. The technique described here is not the only successful approach. Various techniques work as well. We hope readers will discern the important anatomical and surgical principles from ours and other approaches that will allow them to improve their own techniques.

INTRODUCTION

Patients diagnosed with a clinically localized prostate cancer face a daunting variety of management choices, including conservative management (e.g.,"watchful waiting") (see Chapter 13A), brachytherapy and/or external-beam irradiation therapy with or without neoadjuvant hormonal therapy, as well as surgery. As we have learned to characterize the nature of each cancer (see Chapter 6), we can now "risk adjust" treatment decisions (see Chapter 15B). Physicians have long sought to guide patients through these choices based on their best judgment about the threat posed by the cancer, the effectiveness of treatment, and the life expectancy of the patient. Today, many patients wish to participate more actively in decisions about their care, weighing the risks of treatment-related complications as well as the anxiety of living with an untreated or uncontrolled cancer. Patient utilities (see Chapter 11) measure the value patients place on a health state, whether living with cancer or becoming incontinent, allowing quantitative assessments of the risk-benefit ratio of different therapeutic options specific to each patient's preferences as well as the nature of his cancer and life expectancy. Radical prostatectomy remains a mainstay of treatment because it offers patients a high level of confidence that they can live out their life free of cancer recurrence.

For nearly a century, radical prostatectomy has been an effective way to achieve long-term control of clinically localized prostate cancer. The first radical prostatectomy was performed by Billroth in 1867 at the Zurich clinic. A retropubic approach for resection of benign adenomas was introduced by Millin in the 1940s. This approach was modified for radical extirpation of the prostate and seminal vesicles and rapidly adopted by urologists (1–4). Retropubic prostatectomy offers several advantages over the perineal approach. The anatomy is more familiar to urologists, there are fewer rectal injuries, a staging pelvic lymphadenectomy can easily be performed, and the wide exposure offers great flexibility to adapt the operation to each individual's anatomy, permitting more consistent preservation of the neurovascular bundles and a lower rate of positive surgical margins. Radical retropubic prostatectomy therefore has become our standard procedure for removal of the prostate for treatment of localized prostate cancer.

Since the late 1970s, clear definition of periprostatic anatomy has allowed the development of an operation that is more respectful of the intricate anatomy of the periprostatic tissues. Outcomes after radical prostatectomy—cancer control as well as recovery of continence and erectile function—are exquisitely sensitive to fine details in the surgical technique. Surgical margins in radical prostatectomy specimens are measured in millimeters, yet a positive margin (e.g., ink touching cancer at the edge of the specimen) confers a significantly increased risk of recurrence (5–7). Technical refinements have resulted in lower rates of urinary incontinence (8–10), higher rates of recovery of erectile function (9,11,12), less blood loss, fewer transfusions (13–15), shorter hospital stays (16,17), as well as lower rates of positive surgical margins (18–21). A thorough understanding of periprostatic anatomy that emphasizes vascular control permits the safe performance of a radical prostatectomy with reduced morbidity.

This chapter describes the indications for radical retropubic prostatectomy, the preoperative preparation and perioperative management, and the long-term outcomes, including continence and erectile function. We emphasize key aspects of periprostatic anatomy and surgical technique that allow the procedure to be performed safely with minimal complications. Step-by-step details of the surgical technique have been previously published (13,22).

PREOPERATIVE ASSESSMENT

Radical prostatectomy is curative only if the entire tumor is removed. Accurate preoperative characterization of the cancer allows the surgeon to plan an operation tailored to the size, location, and extent of each patient's cancer, as well as the anatomy of each patient's prostate and periprostatic tissues. Today, the probability of successful treatment can be estimated from nomograms that consider the important prognostic factors such as clinical stage, Gleason grade, and serum prostate-specific-antigen (PSA) levels (23). The other element in appropriate selection of alternative treatments is thorough assessment of the physiologic status of the patient and documentation of comorbid conditions. Finally, the risks posed by the surgery (e.g., incontinence, erectile dysfunction, acute surgical morbidity) and the patient's own values must be brought into the decision-making process.

Although radical retropubic prostatectomy results in excellent long-term cancer-specific survival rates (5,7,24,25), the need for active treatment continues to be questioned (26–30). Some argue that the risk posed by localized cancers is low (27) and that decision-analysis models show only a marginal benefit for treatment compared with watchful waiting (26). Chodak and associates (28) analyzed the risk of metastases and of death from cancer with conservative management of clinical stage T1 to T2 cancers. The risk of metastasis at 10 years was 19% for well-differentiated cancers, 42% for moderately differentiated cancers, and 74% for poorly differentiated cancers (Fig. 13C.1). The cancer-specific mortality rate at 10 years was only 13% for well- and moderately differentiated tumors, but 66% for poorly differentiated tumors. Note that in Figure 13C.1, when the primary tumor was not controlled, the risk of developing metastases persists, even accelerates, after 10 years (28). Perhaps the best study to document the impact on mortality was published by Albertsen et al. (30),

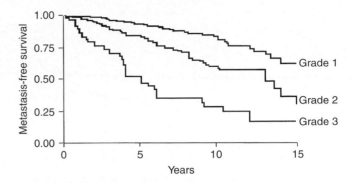

FIGURE 13C.1. Metastasis-free survival rate among conservatively managed patients with localized prostate cancer (cT1-2, NX, M0), according to tumor grade. (From Chodak GW, Thisted RA, Gerber GS, et al. Results of conservative management of clinically localized prostate cancer. *N Engl J Med* 1994;330:242, with permission.)

and it is described in detail in Chapter 13A. In a population-based study, Albertsen et al. documented the 15-year cancer-specific mortality rate by age and Gleason grade in men managed conservatively. Well-differentiated tumors (Gleason sum 2 to 4) seldom caused death within 15 years, but moderately and poorly differentiated cancers proved lethal far more often (Fig. 13A.4), even in elderly men. In a previous study, Albertsen et al. had emphasized that men with well-differentiated cancer (Gleason sum 2 to 4) survived as long as the age-matched controls, but the remaining 91% of patients, who had moderately or poorly differentiated tumors, lost an average of one-third of their remaining life expectancy (29). Perhaps the most compelling evidence that active treatment reduces the risk of mortality from prostate cancer comes from the recently completed Scandinavian trial, which randomized men with localized prostate cancer to either watchful waiting or radical prostatectomy (31). The primary endpoint of this study was death due to prostate cancer. During a median follow-up of 6.2 years, death due to prostate cancer occurred in 31 of 348 of those assigned to watchful waiting and in 16 of 347 of those assigned to radical prostatectomy (relative hazard, 0.5; 95 percent confidence interval, 0.27 to 0.91; $P = 0.02$) (Fig. 13C.2). The men assigned to surgery had a lower relative risk of distant metastases than the men assigned to watchful waiting (relative hazard, .63; 95 percent confidence interval, 0.41 to 0.96). There was no significant difference between surgery and watchful waiting in terms of overall survival.

Although several studies have reported the favorable prognosis of patients with well-differentiated cancers and support watchful waiting for many of these men, poorly differentiated tumors progress rapidly and have a high cancer-specific mortality rate when both managed conservatively (29,31,32) and when treated (5,7). We conducted a study of patients treated with radical prostatectomy for clinically localized prostate cancer to determine if poor results after surgery for high-grade cancers were attributable to the aggressive nature of the cancer itself or to the advanced stage at diagnosis (33). Poorly differentiated cancer, defined as a Gleason score of 7 or more in the biopsy specimen, was present in 298 (30%) of 1,003 patients. Cancers detected solely because of an elevated PSA level (T1c, $n = 335$) were nearly as likely (24%) to be poorly differentiated as cancers detected by digital rectal examination (DRE) (T2 or T3a, $n = 668$), of which 32% were poorly differentiated on biopsy. However, 49% of the poorly differentiated T1c cancers were confined to the prostate, compared with only 28% of the poorly differentiated cancers detected by DRE ($P = .001$) (31). And the prognosis for the

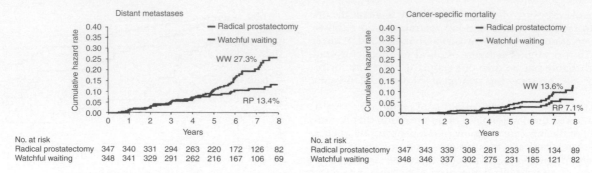

FIGURE 13C.2. Swedish randomized trial comparing radical prostatectomy and watchful waiting. Surgical excision alters the natural history of prostate cancer, reducing metastases and cancer-specific mortality by 50% at 8 years.

poorly differentiated T1c cancers was significantly better (5-year freedom from progression, 69% vs. 55%, P = .047). Although poorly differentiated tumors often extend outside the prostate at the time of diagnosis, a poorly differentiated cancer can be controlled by radical prostatectomy if detected while still confined (5-year freedom from progression was 91%) (33). Therefore, Gleason grade alone should not be used to exclude a patient with a potentially curable prostate cancer.

The extent of capsular penetration is an important prognostic feature in patients with clinically localized prostate cancer (5,7,34). The role of DRE, transrectal ultrasound (TRUS), and magnetic resonance imaging (MRI) to assess the presence and location of extracapsular extension (ECE) has been reviewed (35–37). The accuracy of each of these modalities is limited, unfortunately. The presence of a palpable nodule suggests ECE in 37.4% of patients (35,36), but 18% of patients with no palpable tumor (T1c) have ECE. When the results of DRE and TRUS were combined (if either was positive, the patient was predicted to have ECE), the results were better, with a positive predictive value of 79% and an overall accuracy of 82% (37). Endorectal coil MRI may also add to the accuracy of DRE (36,37).

The results of systematic needle biopsy may also indicate areas suspicious for ECE (38,39). Information about the location of positive biopsies, the length of cancer in each core, the grade of cancer, and the presence of perineural invasion can help characterize the location and extent of cancer within the prostate (38–41). The presence of ECE is not a contraindication to radical prostatectomy because long-term cancer control is possible in more than two thirds of patients with microscopic ECE (Fig. 13C.3). However, knowledge of the presence and location of ECE will allow the surgeon performing radical prostatectomy to modify the operation by performing a wider excision in the involved area so that the tumor can be removed with decreased risk of a positive surgical margin (18,19). Improved imaging studies or other techniques that can detect ECE are urgently needed.

Seminal vesicle involvement (SVI) is well-established as a poor prognostic feature. Patients with SVI not only have an increased incidence of nodal metastasis (43), but also a worse prognosis, even in the absence of lymph node involvement (5,7,44,45). To identify reliable criteria for detecting SVI preoperatively, we compared radical prostatectomy specimens and TRUS (46). Based on our findings, we developed three criteria for SVI: (a) a hypoechoic lesion at the base of the prostate, (b) an "adhesion sign" resulting from loss of the echo reflections from the normal fat plane between the prostate and the seminal vesicle, and (c) "posterior convexity" of the seminal vesicles. These criteria, combined with serum PSA level, allow us to classify patients into those with low risk and those

with high risk of SVI. Sixty-two percent of patients with a PSA level of more than 10 ng/mL and a positive TRUS had SVI. However, only 3% of patients with a PSA level of less than 10 ng/mL and a negative TRUS had SVI (47). MRI has proved superior to TRUS in detecting SVI, especially when the image is enhanced by use of an endorectal coil (48,49). Although SVI may not be an absolute contraindication to radical prostatectomy, its presence has profound implications that could alter treatment recommendations.

STANDARDIZED PATHWAY FOR RADICAL RETROPUBIC PROSTATECTOMY

Because of the increasing emphasis on cost control for medical care, standardized treatment pathways have been developed to control costs without compromising the quality of patient care. These pathways standardize patient care to increase efficiency by identifying factors that contribute to patient costs and eliminating or controlling items deemed unnecessary. Koch et al. (50) reported on the use of a standardized pathway for patients undergoing radical retropubic prostatectomy. This method resulted in a reduction in total hospital stay, operating-room time, material utilization, antibiotic usage, routine laboratory studies, and refinement of postoperative pain management. The standardized pathway reduced hospital charges substantially, with no discernible effect on morbidity rates. We evaluated the treatment of 50 patients at our facilities, with one half treated according to the normal protocol and the other half treated according to the standardized pathway (17). The average hospital stay was reduced by 32%, and the total hospital charges were decreased 34% for those patients on the standardized pathway. This improved cost efficiency occurred without compromising the quality of patient care. All patients undergoing radical retropubic prostatectomy at our facilities are now treated according to a standardized protocol.

SELECTING PATIENTS FOR PELVIC LYMPHADENECTOMY

With stage migration and improved patient selection, the rate of lymph node metastases in patients undergoing radical prostatectomy has declined sharply over the last decade (51,52). As a result, the majority of patients gain no benefit from a pelvic lymph node dissection (PLND). Accurate preoperative prediction of lymph node status could eliminate the need for PLND for patients who have the lowest risk of lymph node

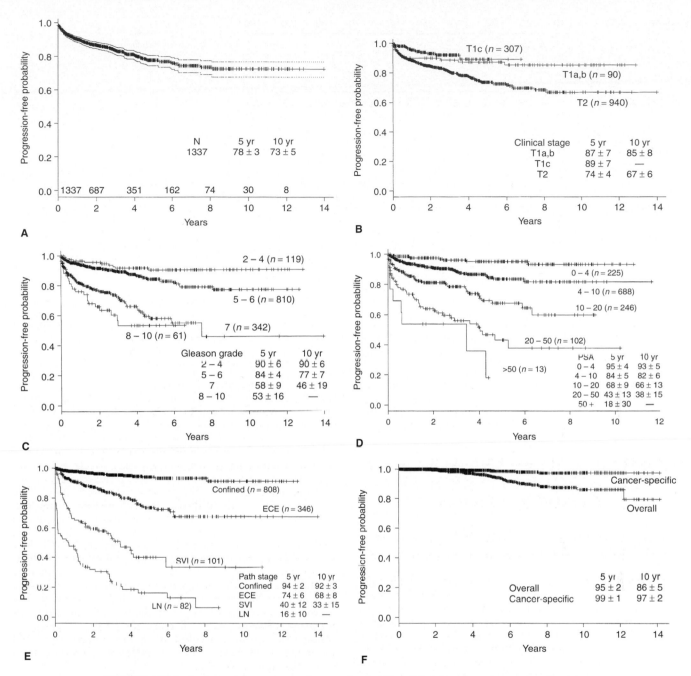

FIGURE 13C.3. A: Actuarial nonprogression rate [probability of freedom from progression by rising prostate-specific-antigen (PSA) level, clinical recurrence, or any other treatment for prostate cancer] for 1,337 consecutive cT1-2 patients managed by intent to treat with radical prostatectomy, 1983–1998. **B:** By clinical stage. **C:** By Gleason grade in the biopsy specimen. **D:** By preoperative PSA level. **E:** By pathologic stage. Patients who had positive nodes found at lymphadenectomy but no radical prostatectomy are included as treatment failures. **F:** Overall and cancer-specific survival rate for these patients. (ECE, extracapsular extension; LN, lymph node; SVI, seminal vesicle involvement) (42).

metastases. Radiographic imaging techniques, however, have low sensitivity for detecting microscopic lymphatic metastases. As a result, several investigators have created algorithms to predict lymph node status. We prospectively collected multi-institutional data on patients with clinically localized prostate cancer treated with radical retropubic prostatectomy (42). We performed a nonrandomized analysis of 7,014 patients treated with radical prostatectomy at six institutions between 1985 and 2000. Exclusion criteria consisted of preoperative androgen ablation therapy, salvage radical prostatectomy, or pretreatment PSA >50 ng/mL. Preoperative predictors of lymph node metastases consisted of pretreatment PSA,

clinical stage (1992 TNM, tumor, node, metastasis), and biopsy Gleason sum. These predictors were used in logistic regression-analysis-based nomograms to predict the probability of lymph node metastases. Overall, 5,510 patients were included and had complete clinical and pathologic information. Lymph node metastases were present in 206 patients (3.7%). Pretreatment serum PSA, biopsy Gleason sum, and clinical stage represented predictors of lymph node status (*P* <.001). Bootstrap corrected predictive accuracy of this three-variable nomogram (i.e., clinical stage, Gleason sum, and PSA) was .76 (Fig. 13C.4). The negative predictive value of our nomogram was .99 when they predicted ≤3% chance of positive lymph

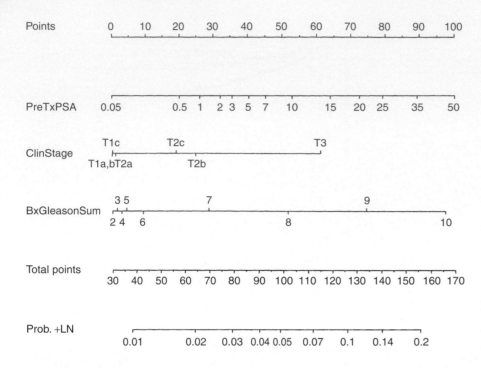

FIGURE 13C.4. Three-variable nomogram (serum PSA level, biopsy Gleason sum, and clinical stage) to predict the probability of positive lymph nodes.

nodes. Using clinical information, we produced a calibrated and validated nomogram, which accurately predicts pathologically negative lymph nodes in men with localized prostate cancer who were candidates for radical prostatectomy (42).

COMPLICATIONS AND SURGICAL TECHNIQUES TO REDUCE COMPLICATIONS

Early Complications: Hemorrhage, Rectal Injury, and Thromboembolism

Hemorrhage is the most common intraoperative complication during radical retropubic prostatectomy. Traditionally, radical prostatectomy has been accompanied by substantial blood loss and the frequent need for transfusions (53,54). A more thorough understanding of the anatomy of the dorsal vein complex and the periprostatic fascia has allowed development of techniques to control these vessels early in the course of the operation (13,53,55). By giving special attention to the major blood supply to the prostate and seminal vesicles, the surgeon can perform the radical retropubic prostatectomy with reduced blood loss. The key steps in this surgical procedure are complete control of the dorsal vein complex and anterior periprostatic veins, identification and control of the small branches from the neurovascular bundles to the prostate posterolaterally, and dissection of the seminal vesicles and vas with control of the many small vessels between the base of the bladder and the seminal vesicles (13). When bleeding is reduced, the surgeon can focus on complete excision of the cancer, selective preservation of the neurovascular bundles responsible for erection, and precise construction of the vesicourethral anastomosis.

Table 13C.1 summarizes the estimated blood loss from several large radical prostatectomy series (14,15,24,56–60). Over the years, we have modified the operative techniques to significantly reduce our blood loss (13). This, together with a more stringent transfusion policy, has reduced the rate of homologous transfusion to less than 10% of patients who did not donate autologous blood.

Other intraoperative complications occur much less frequently. Early complication rates from several large medical centers are summarized in Table 13C.2 (14,60–62). Operative mortality, defined as death within 30 days of surgery, was not reported for the 4,413 men summarized in Table 13C.2. Rectal injury was also uncommon, occurring in less than 1% of patients. Factors that predispose the patient to rectal injury include previous pelvic radiation therapy, rectal surgery, and/or transurethral resection of the prostate (63). Injury most often occurs during the apical dissection, with division of the rectourethralis muscle when the surgeon is unsure of the depth of incision. If a rectal injury occurs, it should not be repaired until after the prostatectomy has been completed. The injury is closed in two inverted layers, and the anal sphincter is dilated. To reduce the potential of fistula formation, omentum may be placed between the rectum and vesicourethral anastomosis, although we have not generally found this necessary. The omentum is mobilized by opening the peritoneum in the rectovesical cul-de-sac and delivering a segment of omentum through the opening. A colostomy is rarely necessary unless the injury is extensive or there is evidence of proctitis from prior radiation treatment.

TABLE 13C.1

ESTIMATED BLOOD LOSS (EBL) IN PATIENTS UNDERGOING RADICAL RETROPUBIC PROSTATECTOMY

Series (ref)	No. patients	Mean EBL (mL)	Range
Rainwater et al. (56)	316	1,020	100–4,320
Zincke et al. (24)	1,728	600	—
Eastham et al. (57)	954	800	150–5,000
Coakley et al. (58)	143	1,626	500–4,400
Goldschlag et al. (59)	221	1,073	—
Lepor et al. (15)	1,000	819	—
Maffezzini et al. (14)	300	600	200–2,200
Augustin et al. (60)	1,243	1,284	—

TABLE 13C.2

PERIOPERATIVE COMPLICATIONS AND MORTALITY OF RADICAL RETROPUBIC PROSTATECTOMY IN CONTEMPORARY SERIES[a]

Complications	Catalona et al. (61) (N = 1,870)		Lerner et al. (62) (N = 1,000)		Maffezzini et al. (14) (N = 300)		Augustin et al. (60) (N = 1,243)		Overall (N = 4,413)	
	N	%	N	%	N	%	N	%	N	%
Mortality	0	0	0	0	0	0	0	0	0/4,413	0
Rectal Injury	1	.1	6	.6	1	.3	3	.2	11/4,413	.3
Colostomy	—	—	0	0	0	0	0	0	0/4,413	0
Ureteral Injury	1	.1	—	—	1	.3	4	.3	6/3,413	.2
Myocardial Infarction	2	.1	7	.7	—	—	1	.1	10/4,113	.2
Pulmonary Embolism	39[b]	2	6	.6	1	.3	2	.2	48/4,413	1.1
Thrombophlebitis/DVT	—	—	14	1.4	1	.3	16	1.3	31/2,543	1.2
Sepsis	—	—	2	.5	—	—	3	.2	5/2,243	.2
Wound Infection or Dehiscence	17	.9	9	.9	3	1	20	1.6	49/4,413	1.1
Lymphocele	—	—	—	—	3	1	37	3	40/1,543	2.6
Prolonged Fluid Leak	7	.4	—	—	—	—	16	1.3	23/3,113	.7
Premature Catheter Loss	1	.1	—	—	—	—	5	.4	6/3,113	.2
Anastomotic Stricture	71	4	87	8.7	2	.7	—	—	160/2,510	5

[a]Notice that complications are not mutually exclusive, that is, one patient may have had more than one complication.
[b]Includes all thromboembolic complications.

Deep venous thrombosis and pulmonary embolism occur in approximately 2% of patients after radical retropubic prostatectomy (Table 13C.2). Cisek and Walsh reported thromboembolic complications in 2% of patients (64), which often occurred after discharge from the hospital. Patients are encouraged to ambulate the morning after the operation and to perform dorsiflexion exercises while in bed to prevent venous stasis.

Methods to Reduce Blood Loss

Dorsal Vein Complex

The prostate is mobilized by incising the endopelvic fascia laterally in the groove between the prostate and the levator ani muscles. This fascial incision is extended sharply toward the pelvis where the fascia condenses into the puboprostatic ligaments. Blunt dissection using the surgeon's finger will divide the remaining fascia posteriorly and mobilize the prostate from the levator ani muscles. The puboprostatic ligaments need not be divided if the apex of the prostate is adequately exposed.

To prevent significant back bleeding, the superficial dorsal vein complex is ligated at the bladder neck, and the deep dorsal vein complex is suture-ligated at the mid-prostate (Fig. 13C.5). The first suture marks the site of division of the bladder neck later in the operation. The suture at the level of the mid- to apical prostate traverses the anterior surface of the gland from one cut edge of endopelvic fascia to the other. This suture should not be carried all the way to the prostatic

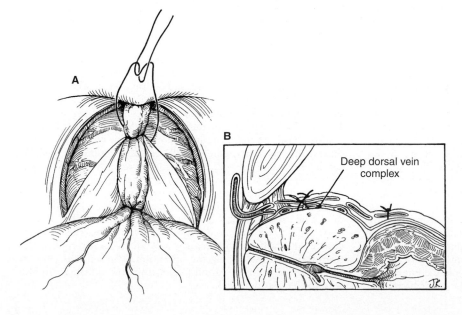

FIGURE 13C.5. The superficial dorsal vein complex is suture-ligated at the bladder neck, approximately 1 cm cephalad to the junction of the prostate and bladder (**A,B**). A deeper suture is placed around the superficial and deep dorsal vein complex midway toward the apex, extending from one cut edge of endopelvic fascia to the other. These sutures limit back bleeding on transection of the dorsal vein complex.

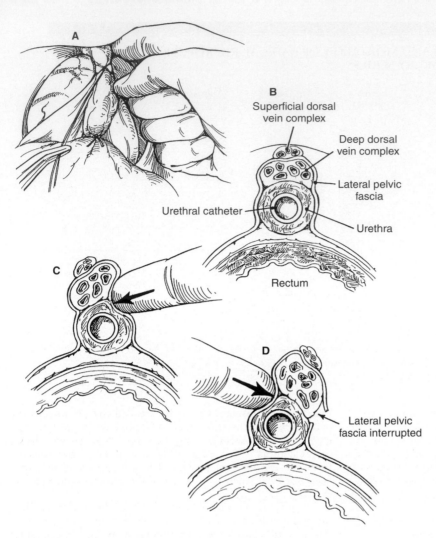

FIGURE 13C.6. Countertraction placed on the hemostatic figure-eight suture around the deep dorsal vein complex at mid-prostate facilitates blunt finger dissection in the plane between the dorsal vein complex and the urethra (**A,B**). The lateral pelvic fascia is weakened with finger dissection applied from both sides (**C,D**).

apex as this may result in displacement of the neurovascular bundles more anteriorly, placing them at risk for damage during their mobilization later in the procedure. This suture is tied and tagged with a large hemostat. Cephalad traction on this ligature will place tension on the lateral pelvic fascia surrounding the dorsal vein complex, allowing the surgeon to weaken this fascia bluntly in the groove between the dorsal vein complex and the urethra just distal to the apex of the prostate (Fig. 13C.6) (55).

A right-angle clamp can then be passed through the weakened fascia beneath the entire dorsal vein complex anterior to the urethra. The clamp is used to grasp an 18-gauge stainless steel wire looped on the end. The wire, which is brought beneath the dorsal vein complex (Fig. 13C.7), serves as a template so that the complex can be transected evenly and sharply with a 15-blade knife. By adjusting the upward tension on the wire and downward traction on the prostate with a sponge stick, the surgeon can divide the dorsal vein complex sufficiently far from the apex to minimize the risk of a positive surgical margin.

Bleeding from the dorsal vein complex is controlled by sewing together the incised edges of the lateral pelvic fascia on either side of the complex, using a continuous 00 polyglactin absorbable suture on a CT-2 needle (Fig. 13C.8). Finally, the suture is sewn through the periosteum of the pubis, compressing the superficial veins between the fascia and the pubic bone.

Lateral Vascular Pedicles and Seminal Vesicles

The thick lateral vascular pedicle supplying the prostate is encountered toward the base of the prostate (Fig. 13C.9). The lateral vascular pedicles are isolated with a right-angle clamp and controlled with clips or ties (Fig. 13C.9 A,B). Full division of the lateral pedicle exposes the lateral edge of the seminal vesicle (Fig. 13C.9C).

Control of bleeding and exposure of the seminal vesicle is improved if the vascular band of tissue between the bladder and the base of the prostate and seminal vesicles is deliberately isolated, clipped, and divided (Fig. 13C.9C). This ensures a wide lateral margin around the base of the prostate. The seminal vesicles can then be bluntly dissected from the bladder base. As the mobilization of the seminal vesicles continues, the vascular pedicle at the tip of the seminal vesicles can be exposed, clipped, and divided (Fig. 13C.10). We usually dissect the seminal vesicles from lateral to medial, ending with the identification and division of the ampulla of the vas. Occasionally, this dissection is easier if the vas is divided first. The artery to the vas must be carefully secured. Meticulous control of the small vessels surrounding the seminal vesicles laterally and anteriorly will substantially reduce the overall blood loss during the operation. The seminal vesicles and vas can then be mobilized, within their fascia, all the way to the bladder neck.

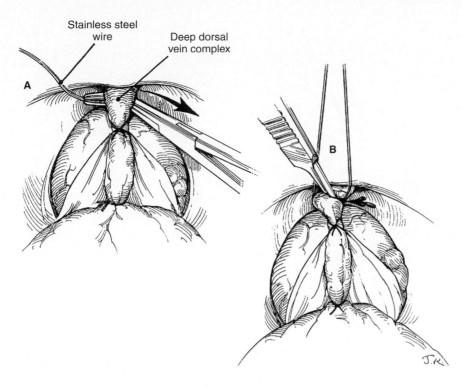

FIGURE 13C.7. A long-nosed, right-angled clamp is passed through the weakened fascia between the urethra and dorsal vein complex and grasps a stainless steel wire that is looped on the end (**A**). The wire serves as a guide to allow a square transection of the dorsal vein complex and its surrounding fascia (**B**). By this maneuver, the dorsal venous complex can be divided close to or far from the apex of the prostate, as the surgeon chooses, with care to avoid a positive surgical margin.

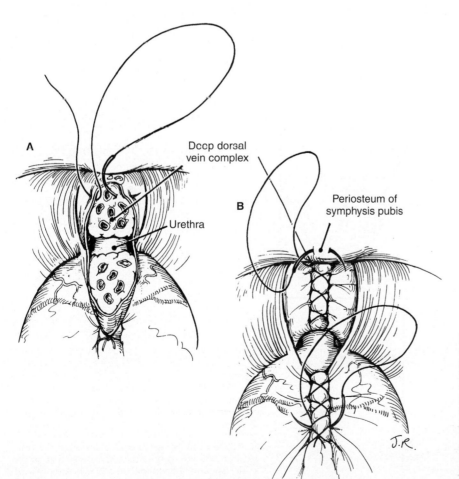

FIGURE 13C.8. Bleeding from the transected dorsal vein complex is controlled by oversewing the cut edges of the lateral pelvic fascia vertically with a continuous suture (**A**), the last pass of which is brought through the periosteum of the pubis (**B**) to compress the superficial venous complex above the lateral pelvic fascia and to fix the fascia to the periosteum, simulating the function of the puboprostatic ligaments. Back bleeding from the ventral prostate is controlled with clips or with a continuous hemostatic suture, taking care not to draw the neurovascular bundles medially (**B**).

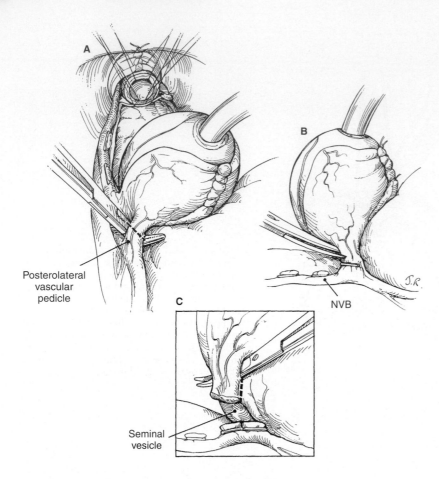

Posterolateral
vascular
pedicle

NVB

Seminal
vesicle

FIGURE 13C.9. Upward traction on the separate catheter placed through the prostate into the bladder allows the lateral vascular pedicles of the prostate to be easily isolated (**A**), controlled with clips (**B**), and divided to expose the lateral aspect of the seminal vesicle. Further exposure is gained by division of the vascular bands between the bladder neck and the seminal vesicles and prostate (**C**). (NVB, neurovascular bundle.)

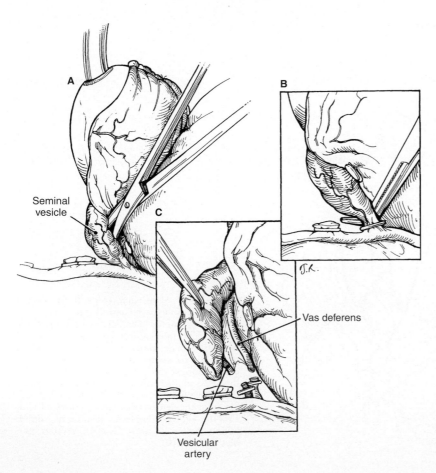

Seminal
vesicle

Vas deferens

Vesicular
artery

FIGURE 13C.10. The seminal vesicles are typically approached laterally and the plane between the vesicles and the bladder developed with scissors and finger dissection. The major blood supply to the seminal vesicles lies anterior and lateral. When these vessels are clipped and divided close to the wall of the vesicle, it is easier to identify the large artery that enters at the apex of the seminal vesicle. The ampulla of the vas are clipped to include the vasal arteries and divided.

THE ROLE OF THE SURGEON IN PATIENT OUTCOMES AFTER RADICAL PROSTATECTOMY: POSITIVE SURGICAL MARGINS

For radical prostatectomy to be successful, the cancer must be completely removed. Cancer present at the margin of resection (a positive surgical margin) after radical prostatectomy (RP) is associated with a 2- to 4-fold increased risk of recurrence even after adjusting for other known risk factors including the pretreatment serum level of PSA, clinical stage, grade, and pathological stage (level of extracapsular extension, seminal vesicle invasion, and status of the pelvic lymph nodes). Of these prognostic factors, only the status of the surgical margins can be influenced by surgical technique. We recently examined variations in the rate of positive surgical margins among 4,629 men treated with radical prostatectomy for clinically localized prostate cancer by 44 individual surgeons after controlling for severity of disease and volume of cases per surgeon (18). Patients were excluded if they previously received androgen deprivation therapy or had radiation therapy to the pelvis. Positive surgical margins were defined as cancer at the inked margin of resection. Other risk factors analyzed were serum PSA level, grade (Gleason sum), level of extracapsular extension (e.g., none, present, invasion into the capsule, focal extracapsular extension, established extracapsular extension), seminal vesicle invasion, pelvic lymph node metastases, surgeon, and volume of cases per surgeon. In multivariable analysis, surgeon was associated with surgical margin status after controlling for all other clinical and pathological variables (Table 13C.3). After further adjustment for surgical volume, individual surgeon remained associated with surgical margin status.

While the clinical and pathologic features of cancer are associated with the risk of a positive margin in radical prostatectomy specimens, the technique used by individual surgeons is also a factor. In a recent review of the literature, the rate of positive surgical margins in major institutions was 25%. This rate can be reduced to less than 10% with deliberate surgical planning. Lower rates of positive surgical margins for high volume surgeons suggest that experience and careful attention to surgical details, adjusted for the characteristics of the cancer being treated, can decrease positive surgical margin rates and improve cancer control with radical prostatectomy.

Late Complications: Bladder Neck Contracture and Incontinence

Bladder neck contracture is usually the result of poor mucosa-to-mucosa apposition at the time of the urethrovesical anastomosis. Eversion of the bladder neck mucosa and proper placement of the urethral sutures under direct vision will help reduce the incidence of this complication. Patients with a bladder neck contracture often note a dribbling urinary stream or symptoms of overflow incontinence. Assessment should include a urinary flow rate, determination of postvoid residual urine, and flexible cystoscopy to evaluate the anastomotic site. Most bladder neck contractures can be managed using a urethral dilating balloon. Severe bladder neck contractures may require cold-knife incision and, if recurrent, may require periodic dilatation to maintain an adequate urine flow (65).

Urinary incontinence is still one of the most troubling side effects occurring after radical retropubic prostatectomy. Although an anatomic approach to radical prostatectomy has resulted in a diminished rate of incontinence, incontinence rates vary widely (8–10,24,61,66–72) (Table 13C.4). Incontinence has been reported in 5% to 23% of postprostatectomy patients by surgeons from large medical centers and from 5% to 32% when reported by patients in response to quality-of-life questionnaires (8–10,24,61,66–72). These variations derive from different definitions of continence, different patient populations, and different times of assessment after the operation. In a multivariate analysis, the factors independently associated with persistence of incontinence are increasing patient age ($P < .001$), surgical technique ($P < .001$), preservation of neurovascular bundles ($P < .01$), and development of an anastomotic stricture ($P < .01$) (Table 13C.5). Over a 13-year period, the rate of urinary stress incontinence was 9% in a Scardino et al. population of 581 patients who were continent before the operation (8). Deliberate changes in surgical technique (Fig. 13C.11), introduced in 1990, however, resulted in a substantial improvement in the continence rate from 82% to 95% at 24 months (8). These specific modifications include less manipulation of the urethra distal to the apex of the prostate, preservation of all periurethral tissue distal to the apex of the prostate, inclusion of a small amount of urethra and a large amount of the oversewn lateral pelvic fascia covering the dorsal venous complex in the anastomotic sutures, and full thickness eversion of the bladder neck to reduce the risk of an anastomotic stricture. The median time to recovery of complete urinary control in this series was 6 weeks, with 92% continent at 12 months and 95% at 24 months (Fig. 13C.11). Less than 1% of patients had leakage severe enough to require an artificial sphincter.

While there is no standard definition for continence following radical prostatectomy, patient questionnaires seem better than physician interviews as a means of assessing recovery of urinary control. A variety of these instruments has been developed and validated. Key aspects of questionnaires include the collection of baseline and long-term follow-up data, the assessments of multiple functions, and an assessment of patient bother. We have instituted a prospective study whereby all patients receiving care for clinically localized prostate cancer complete baseline and follow-up quality-of-life questionnaires using validated instruments. Preliminary results suggest that while differences exist between the various treatment options, patient bother appears to be low (Table 13C.6). Further objective information

TABLE 13C.3

ANALYSIS FOR RISK OF A POSITIVE SURGICAL MARGIN BASED ON CLINICAL AND PATHOLOGICAL PARAMETERS

Variable	P
Serum PSA Level	<.01
Extracapsular Extension	
Capsule Invasion Versus None	<.01
Focal Versus None	<.01
Established Versus None	<.01
Positive Versus None	<.01
Seminal Vesicle Invasion	.86
Lymph Node Involvement	.56
Radical Prostatectomy Gleason Sum	<.01
Surgical Volume	.01
Surgery Date	<.01
Surgeon	.05

From Eastham JA, Kattan MW, Riedel E, et al. Variations among individual surgeons in the rate of positive surgical margins in radical prostatectomy specimens. *J Urol* 2003;170:2292.

TABLE 13C.4

INCIDENCE OF INCONTINENCE AFTER RADICAL PROSTATECTOMY

Series (ref)	n	% Incontinent	Definition of incontinence
Investigator Interview			
Steiner et al. (10)	593	8	Leaks with moderate activity
Zincke et al. (24)	1,728	5	Requires three or more pads per day
Catalona et al. (61)	1,325	8	Any use of pads
Geary et al. (66)	458	20	Requires pads
Eastham et al. (8)	390	5	Leaks with moderate activity
Noh et al. (9)	244	23	Any use of pads
Patient Surveys			
Litwin et al. (67)	98	25	"Bother" score
Murphy et al. (68)	1,796	19	Requires pads
Walsh et al. (69)	62	5	Requires pads
Sebesta et al. (70)	674	32	Any pad use or changing underwear to stay dry
Population Surveys			
Stanford et al. (71)	1,291	8.4	Severe incontinence
		21.6	Requires pads
Fowler et al. (72)	738	31	Pads or clamps

from patient-reported questionnaires is needed to better council patients about quality-of-life outcomes after radical prostatectomy.

Incontinence, however, is only one aspect of urinary quality of life. Irritative symptoms and symptoms of urinary obstruction can also impact overall urinary function. This is nicely illustrated by data from the Scandinavian Prostate Cancer Group Study, which randomized men with clinically localized prostate cancer to either watchful waiting or radical prostatectomy and followed urinary quality of life over the time course of the study (73) (Table 13C.7). While urinary leakage is certainly more problematic following radical prostatectomy and results in significant patient distress, those undergoing watchful waiting have significantly more urinary

TABLE 13C.5

UNIVARIATE AND MULTIVARIATE ANALYSIS OF THE RISK FACTORS FOR INCONTINENCE AFTER RADICAL PROSTATECTOMY

Risk Factor	Parameter Estimate P	
	Univariate analysis	Multivariate analysis
Patient Weight (Continuous)	.002	Not available
Lower Urinary Tract Symptoms (None vs. Requiring Treatment)		
Obstructive	.004	.111
Irritative	.624	.1860
Prostate Size by Transrectal Ultrasound (Continuous)	.441	.250
Transurethral Resection of Prostate (Yes or No)	.001	.349
Clinical Stage (T1a,b/T1c/T2a/ T2b/T2c/T3)	.001	.158
Tumor Palpable at Apex	.289	.707
Operative Blood Loss (Continuous)	.016	.829
Postoperative Bleeding (Presence/ Absence of Clinically Significant Bleeding)	.577	.647
Pathologic Stage (Confined, ECE vs. SVI, +LN)	.310	.733
Nerve Resection (None vs. Unilateral vs. Bilateral)	.001	.015
Anastomotic Stricture (Yes or No)	.001	.015
Patient Age (Continuous)	.001	.0001
Anastomotic Technique (Old or New)	.001	.0001

ECE, extracapsular extension; +LN, positive lymph nodes; SVI, seminal vesicle involvement.
From Eastham JA, Kattan MW, Rogers E, et al. Risk factors for urinary incontinence after radical prostatectomy. *J Urol* 1996;156:1707, with permission.

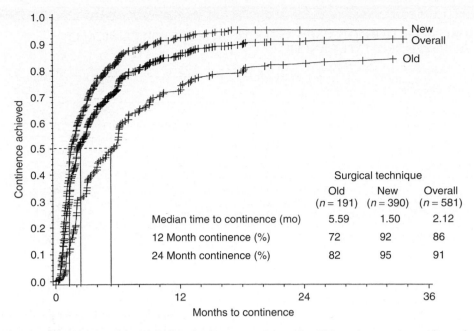

FIGURE 13C.11. Actuarial probability of achieving continence for 581 continent patients who underwent radical prostatectomy for clinically localized (cT1-3,NX,M0) prostate cancer: for the entire group, for the old (191), and new (390) anastomotic techniques. With the new technique, median time to continence was 1.5 months, and 95% of patients were continent at 24 months. (From Eastham JA, Goad JR, Rogers E, et al. Risk factors for urinary incontinence after radical prostatectomy. *J Urol* 1996;156:1707, with permission.)

TABLE 13C.6

QUALITY-OF-LIFE ASSESSMENT OF URINARY CONTINENCE RELATIVE TO BASELINE FOR PATIENTS UNDERGOING TREATMENT FOR CLINICALLY LOCALIZED PROSTATE CANCER

Treatment	Function				Bother			
	3-mo	6-mo	9-mo	12-mo	3-mo	6-mo	9-mo	12-mo
Brachytherapy	.87	.93	.97	.93	.92	.96	1	1
Laparoscopic RP	.64	.75	.88	NA	.87	.95	1.05	NA
Open RP	.67	.81	.86	.84	.88	.97	.99	.96
External Beam RT	.90	.94	.95	.71	.91	.95	1.03	.79
Watchful Waiting	1.04	.96	1.03	1.03	1.14	1.08	1.01	1.16

RP, radical prostatectomy; RT, radiation therapy; NA, not available.
Baseline values are 1.0. Numbers are relative to baseline status.

TABLE 13C.7

ASSESSMENT OF URINARY FUNCTION RELATIVE TO BASELINE FOR MEN TREATED WITH EITHER RADICAL PROSTATECTOMY OR WATCHFUL WAITING FOR CLINICALLY LOCALIZED PROSTATE CANCER

Function	%		Relative risk (95% CI): RP vs. WW
	RP	WW	
Leak Once Per Week or More Often	49	21	2.3 (1.6–3.2)
Distress from Leakage	29	9	3 (1.8–5.2)
Urinary Obstruction	28	44	.6 (.5–.9)
Low/Moderate Urinary Quality of Life	40	45	.9 (.7–1.2)

RP, radical prostatectomy; WW, watchful waiting.
From Steineck G, Helgesen F, Adolfsson J, et al. Scandinavian Prostatic Cancer Group Study Number 4. Quality of life after radical prostatectomy or watchful waiting. *N Engl J Med* 2002;347(11):790–796.

TABLE 13C.8

QUALITY-OF-LIFE OUTCOMES AFTER TREATMENT FOR CLINICALLY
LOCALIZED PROSTATE CANCER

QOL Domain	Brachytherapy $n = 84$	EBRT $n = 147$	Open RP $n = 671$	Control $n = 112$
Incontinence	83%	89%	79%[a]	93%
Irritative Voiding	69%[a]	83%	90%	88%
Bowel Function	78%[a]	85%[a]	93%	92%
Sexual Function	28%[a]	35%[a]	37%[a]	61%
Obstructive Symptoms, AUA-SI	12.6[a]	9	6.1	7

EBRT: External Beam Radiation Therapy; AUA-SI: American Urological Association Symptom Index.
Percent values are in reference to baseline, which is 100%.
[a]Denotes values significantly different from the control population.
Wei JT, Dunn RL, Sandler HM, et al. Comprehensive comparison of health-related quality of life after contemporary therapies for localized prostate cancer. *J Clin Oncol* 2002;20(2):557–566.

obstructive symptoms, such that overall urinary quality of life was similar among the two treatment groups. This is further illustrated by data from the University of Michigan (Table 13C.8) (74). Considering any individual factor in isolation would not reflect global aspects of overall or urinary quality of life.

Urodynamic studies of patients who are incontinent after radical prostatectomy have not elucidated a predominant mechanism of incontinence. Most studies have suggested, however, that the functional length of the urethra is the most important factor in postprostatectomy incontinence (75–78). We believe a "hands-off" approach to the external sphincter tissues beyond the apex of the prostate and fixation of the urethra to the lateral pelvic fascia preserve the maximum amount of functional urethral length within the pelvis and contribute significantly to the maintenance of continence after the procedure (8).

Methods to Reduce Bladder Neck Contracture and Incontinence

After division of the dorsal venous complex and control of bleeding, the levator ani fibers are bluntly and sharply dissected away from the apex of the prostate, exposing the urethra. The operative field should be dry enough to permit precise division of the anterior urethra and placement of the anastomotic sutures under direct vision (Fig. 13C.12). To secure the cut edge of the urethra, we place the anastomotic sutures at this point, rather than attempt to place sutures in the retracted urethral stump later in the procedure. Four 00 monocryl absorbable sutures on a UR-6 needle are placed from inside out, just 3 mm into the urethra, then deeply into the hood of the lateral pelvic fascia. Next, the catheter is withdrawn, exposing the undivided posterior urethra and the firm fibrous layer of Denonvilliers fascia beneath (Fig. 13C.13 A). Two additional posterior sutures are placed through the posterior layer of fascia and through the urethra, from outside in, at the 5 o'clock and 7 o'clock positions. These two sutures must be well away from the previously mobilized neurovascular bundles. Finally, the posterior urethra and rectourethralis muscles is divided, and the prostate is dissected away from the rectum beneath Denonvilliers' fascia (Fig. 13C.13 B).

Once the bladder neck has been divided and the prostate removed, the bladder neck is reconstructed (Fig. 13C.14). The mucosa is everted anteriorly with fine absorbable sutures (Fig. 13C.14 A,B), and the bladder neck is closed posteriorly with a running 00 polyglactin absorbable suture until it is approximately 26 to 30 Fr. in diameter (Fig. 13C.14 C). The

mucosa must be fully everted 360 degrees around the reconstructed bladder neck.

On completion of the bladder neck reconstruction, the previously placed urethral sutures are placed through the reconstructed bladder neck (Fig. 13C.15). All sutures are placed such that the knots are tied on the outside of the lumen. The original Foley catheter (20 Fr., 5-mL balloon) is now passed through the urethra and into the bladder, the balloon is inflated with 15 mL of sterile water, and the sutures are tied.

Late Complications: Erectile Dysfunction

Potency is defined as the ability to obtain an erection that is sufficient for vaginal penetration and sexual intercourse. Current surgical techniques and a more precise understanding of the autonomic innervation of the corpora cavernosa allow preservation of sexual function in many men. Quinlan and associates (79) demonstrated that recovery of potency was quantitatively related to the preservation of nerves. They found that three factors were associated with recovery of potency after radical prostatectomy: age, clinical and pathologic stage, and preservation of the neurovascular bundles (NVB). Approximately 90% of men younger than 50 were potent if either one or both neurovascular bundles were preserved. For men older than 50, return of potency was more likely if both neurovascular bundles were preserved, rather than one. Catalona et al. (61) reported potency in 68% of patients when both nerves were preserved and 47% when one nerve was spared. They also demonstrated a strong correlation between preservation of potency and age.

We have developed a nomogram to predict the return of potency based on a series of 314 previously potent patients treated since 1993 with radical prostatectomy for cT1a to T3a prostate cancer after 1993. Factors significantly associated with recovery of spontaneous erections satisfactory for intercourse included the age of the patient, the quality of erections before the operation, and the degree of preservation of the neurovascular bundles (Table 13C.9) (12). Time after surgery is also an important factor in the recovery of potency. The median time to recovery of an international index of erectile function (IIEF) ≥17 was 24 months, while 42 months was required to reach an IIEF ≥26 (Fig. 13C.16).

The return of postoperative sexual function after radical retropubic prostatectomy is dependent not only on the preservation of the autonomic innervation to the corpora cavernosa (i.e., the neurovascular bundles), but also on the preservation of the vascular branches to the corpora cavernosa (80). Accessory

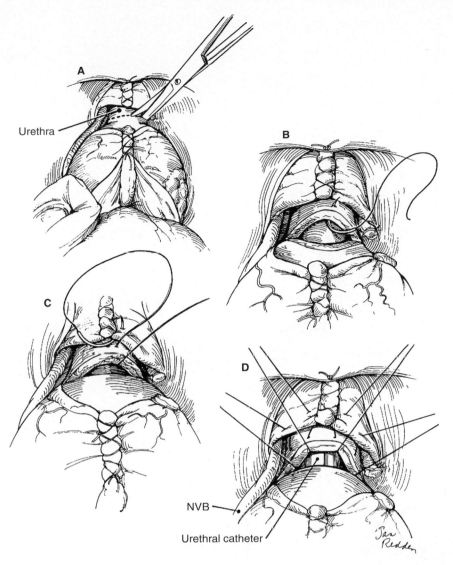

FIGURE 13C.12. Close-up views of urethra at the prostatic apex, illustrating the site of anterior division (**A,B**) and the placement of the anterior anastomotic sutures beneath the mucosa of the urethra and then separately through the thick layer of lateral pelvic fascia (**C,D**) that was oversewn to control the dorsal vein complex. (NVB, neurovascular bundle.)

arterial branches that supply the corpora have been described (81,82). When these branches are preserved, a normal arterial inflow to the penis postoperatively will be maintained. This may enable a patient to remain potent after surgery or, for a patient who is impotent, adequate arterial inflow will ensure an adequate response to medical treatment.

The anatomic approach to radical retropubic prostatectomy has made it possible to completely remove the prostate, with reduced morbidity in the majority of patients with clinically localized prostate cancer. Removal of the cancer and preservation of the nerves responsible for erectile function are often competing goals. Cancers most often penetrate the prostatic capsule posterolaterally, directly over the neurovascular bundles (Fig. 13C.17) (83). In several series, attempts to preserve the neurovascular bundles has increased the rate of positive surgical margins posterolaterally (84). In a review of the literature from centers of excellence, Abbas and Scardino found reported rates of positive margins varied from 14% to 41%, with a mean of 25% (85). In another review, Weider and Soloway noted the remarkable variation in positive margin rates, varying from 0% to 71%, with an overall rate of 28% in radical retropubic prostatectomy series in which no adjuvant hormonal therapy was used before the operation (21). In multivariate analysis, positive margins confer a greater risk of recurrence (5). With deliberate attention to surgical

planning, we reduced our rate of positive margins from 24% before 1987 to 8% in 1993 (85). Consequently, we believe that positive margins are common, that such margins reduce the chances that a cancer will be cured, and that most positive margins can be avoided with careful surgical planning (19,85).

Methods to Reduce Positive Surgical Margins and Preserve Erectile Function

Minimizing the rate of positive surgical margins requires careful dissection in four areas: anteriorly, when the dorsal vein complex is divided; at the apex; posterolaterally, near the neurovascular bundles; and at the bladder neck.

Anterior cancers are difficult to detect preoperatively and difficult to palpate intraoperatively. A recent review of our radical prostatectomy series has suggested that anterior cancers are present in approximately 20% of patients. The dorsal vein complex must be divided sufficiently distal to the anterior prostate to avoid an anterior positive margin. We believe that using a surgical wire during division of the dorsal venous complex facilitates the anterior dissection of the prostate. The wire, which is brought beneath the dorsal vein complex (Fig. 13C.6), serves as a template so that the complex can be

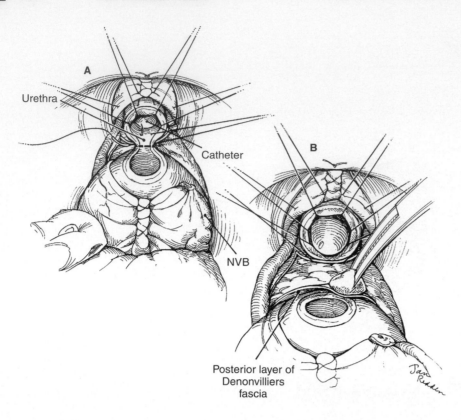

Urethra

Catheter

NVB

Posterior layer of
Denonvilliers
fascia

FIGURE 13C.13. After the nerves have been dissected free (or divided), the remaining urethra and posterior layer of Denonvilliers fascia beneath it are divided (**A**). Two posterior anastomotic sutures are placed at 5 o'clock and 7 o'clock through the fascia and urethra (**A**). The correct plane of dissection adjacent to the rectum is determined with the aid of a Kitner dissector (**B**). (NVB, neurovascular bundle.)

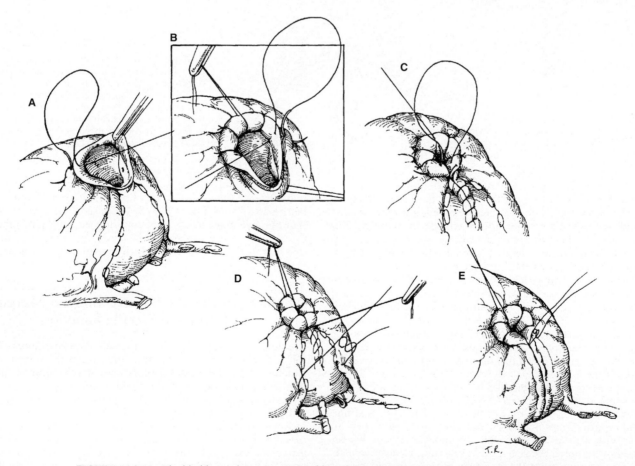

FIGURE 13C.14. The bladder neck is reconstructed by everting the mucosa anteriorly (**A,B**) and closing the bladder posteriorly with a running suture, creating a "tennis-racket" closure (**C**). The suture closest to the trigone should include muscle but little mucosa to avoid tethering the ureteral orifices. In a separate layer, the lateral vascular pedicles of the bladder are brought together in the midline to reinforce the closure and assure hemostasis (**D,E**), creating a cone shape to the reconstructed bladder neck.

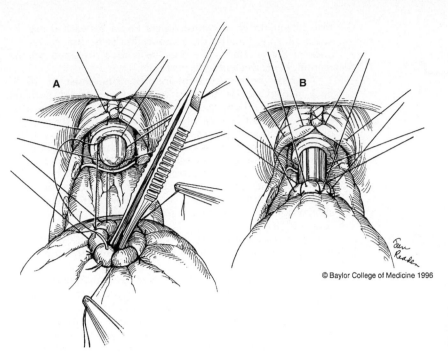

© Baylor College of Medicine 1996

FIGURE 13C.15. The sutures already placed through the urethra are now placed through the bladder neck (**A**) to provide a mucosa-to-mucosa anastomosis (**B**).

transected evenly and sharply with a 15-blade knife. By adjusting the upward tension on the wire and downward traction on the prostate with a sponge stick, the surgeon can divide the dorsal vein complex sufficiently far from the apex to minimize the risk of a positive surgical margin.

A lateral approach to the neurovascular bundles (Fig. 13C.18) allows wide exposure of the apex (Fig. 13C.18C,D) so that the apical tissue can be completely resected. The deep (posterior) layer of Denonvilliers fascia must be deliberately incised, releasing the neurovascular bundle laterally

and allowing a deep plane of dissection along the fat of the anterior rectal wall. The risk of a positive surgical margin will be greatly increased unless this deep layer of fascia is included in the excised specimen. This apical dissection is performed without a catheter in the prostate to give the prostate more mobility. The lateral pelvic fascia over the neurovascular bundle can be incised more medially or laterally to the nerve, depending on the extent or location of the tumor and whether the nerves are to be preserved. A "peanut," or Kitner, dissector is used to gently brush the nerves laterally

TABLE 13C.9

RESULTS OF COX PROPORTIONAL HAZARDS ANALYSIS FOR PREDICTION OF SPONTANEOUS RECOVERY OF ERECTIONS FOR 314 PATIENTS UNDERGOING RADICAL PROSTATECTOMY SINCE 1993 FOR CT1A-T3A PROSTATE CANCER BASED ON PREOPERATIVE AND THE COMBINATION OF PREOPERATIVE AND INTRAOPERATIVE PARAMETERS (12)

	Age		
Probability (%) of recovery of potency by 24 mo (36 mo)	<60 Yr	60–65 Yr	>65 Yr
Preoperative Parameters			
Preoperative Potency			
Full Erection	63 (69)	44 (49)	37 (42)
Full Erection, Recently Diminished	48 (54)	31 (36)	26 (30)
Partial Erection	35 (40)	22 (25)	18 (21)
Preoperative and Intraoperative Parameters			
Bilateral Nerve Sparing			
Full Erection	70 (76)	49 (55)	43 (49)
Full Erection, Recently Diminished	53 (59)	34 (39)	30 (35)
Partial Erection	43 (49)	27 (31)	23 (27)
Unilateral or Bilateral Neurovascular Bundle Damage			
Full Erection	60 (67)	40 (46)	35 (41)
Full Erection, Recently Diminished	44 (50)	28 (32)	24 (28)
Partial Erection	35 (40)	21 (25)	18 (21)
Unilateral Neurovascular Bundle Resection			
Full Erection Recently Diminished	26 (30)	15 (18)	13 (15)
Full Erection	17 (20)	10 (12)	8.5 (10)
Partial Erection	13 (15)	7.5 (8.8)	6.3 (7.5)

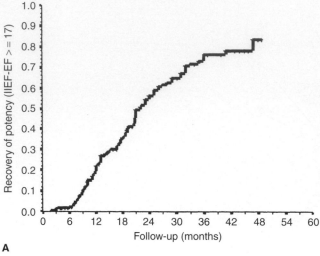

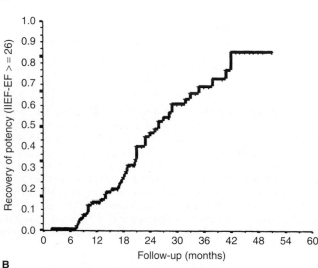

FIGURE 13C.16. Probability of recovery of potency over time after bilateral nerve sparing radical prostatectomy. (**A**). IIEF ≥17. (**B**). IIEF ≥26.

away from the prostate. Small clips placed parallel to the neurovascular bundle are used to control the small vascular bands that are usually present, particularly near the apex of the prostate. Once the posterior anastomotic sutures are placed (Fig. 13C.12), the posterior urethra together with the

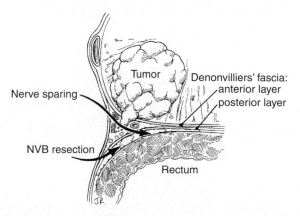

FIGURE 13C.17. The lateral plane of dissection is selected based on preoperative and intraoperative assessment of the extent of the tumor. A wider dissection (i.e., resection of the neurovascular bundle) may be required in an attempt to obtain adequate surgical margins. (NVB, neurovascular bundle.)

firm fibrous layer of Denonvilliers fascia beneath it are divided sharply. Finally, the rectourethralis is divided at the apex of the prostate. The prostate is then dissected off the rectum, beneath Denonvilliers fascia.

We have been successful in preserving most or all of both neurovascular bundles in the majority of patients using this lateral approach, while still allowing a wider dissection around the apex of the prostate, especially posteriorly. Once the apex is completely mobilized, a second catheter is placed through the urethra to facilitate dissection (Fig. 13C.8). Traction on this catheter allows the remaining neurovascular bundles to be dissected away bluntly. The nerves lie close to the prostate, near the base. Dissection too close to the prostate will result in a positive margin in this area, shown to be associated with an increased risk of recurrence (Fig. 13C.8).

When resection of one or both neurovascular bundles is necessary, we use a technique for placing interposition grafts from the sural nerve to one or both neurovascular bundles (Fig. 13C.19) (86,87). Surgeons have performed nerve grafts successfully for decades to replace damaged or transected peripheral sensorimotor nerves. The basis for nerve regeneration, and consequently for nerve grafting, is the ability of axons to produce axon sprouts. Following nerve transection, axon sprouts will invariably grow, forming a neuroma, if they do not come into contact with an environment that channels their growth. The cut end of a nerve sprouts minifascicles that contain axon sprouts, fibroblasts, Schwann cells, and capillaries. The minifascicles grow haphazardly for a limited distance and then form a neuroma. However, if the axons encounter an empty nerve sheath, growth becomes organized and directed, resulting in a new nerve. A nerve graft functions to provide a conduit through which regenerating nerve fibers are directed to meet with the distal end of the transected nerve. These concepts support the hypothesis that cavernous nerve grafts may restore penile autonomic innervation and the ability to achieve spontaneous erections following deliberate neurovascular bundle resection at the time of radical prostatectomy. One third of patients with bilateral nerve resection and placement of bilateral nerve grafts have had spontaneous, medically unassisted erections sufficient for sexual intercourse. The greatest return of function is observed 14 to 18 months after surgery. Having established the ability of nerve grafts to restore natural, spontaneous erectile function after wide resection of both neurovascular bundles, we began to perform unilateral interposition nerve grafts when one neurovascular bundle was resected. Between July 1998 and June 2002, 108 preoperatively potent patients underwent placement of a unilateral interposition cavernous nerve graft. With a median follow-up of 24 months (5 to 52 months), 42% with unilateral nerve resection with a graft and 24% with unilateral nerve resection without a graft were potent. In our experience, nerve grafts provide one solution to a common surgical dilemma. In a patient with a large, high-grade cancer located adjacent to the posterolateral capsule, should we dissect close to the prostate to preserve the nerve or close to the nerve, risking recovery of potency? Over the past 3 years, we have performed nerve grafts in about 15% of all previously untreated patients. The risks were very low: there was only one graft-related complication (cellulitis), and the overall operating-room time, blood loss, and hospital stays were identical in grafted and non-grafted patients. Final proof of the efficacy of nerve grafts must await completion of a prospective randomized trial comparing nerve grafts to no grafts after unilateral NVB resection. Until then, surgeons must use sound judgment and informed consent to decide, along with their patients, whether a nerve graft is indicated when a NVB is damaged or resected during radical prostatectomy.

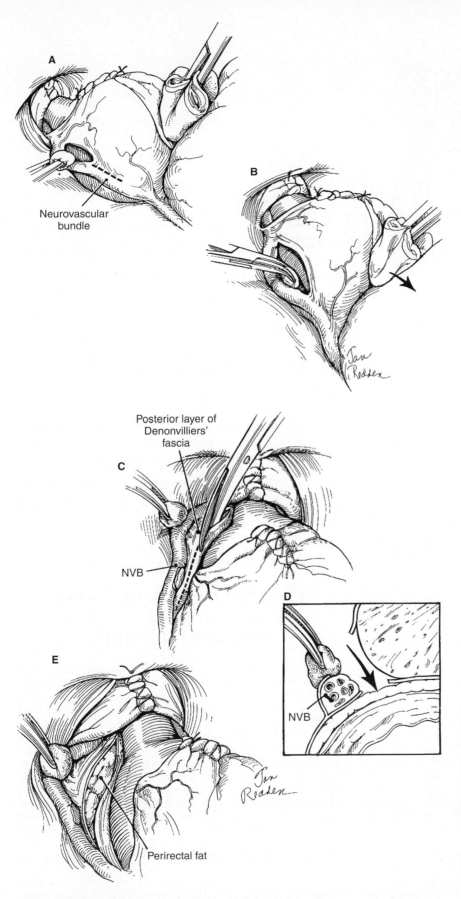

A

Neurovascular
bundle

B

Posterior layer of
Denonvilliers'
fascia

C

NVB

D

NVB

E

Perirectal fat

FIGURE 13C.18. Preservation of left neurovascular bundle (NVB). After the dorsal vein complex has been divided, the prostate is rotated to the right and the levator muscles are bluntly dissected away. The lateral pelvic fascia is then incised in the groove between the prostate and the neurovascular bundle. The neurovascular bundle is most easily dissected away from the apical third of the prostate (**A,B**). The small branches of the vascular pedicle to the apex must be divided. The posterior layer of Denonvilliers fascia is then incised, releasing the NVB from the prostate and urethra (**C–E**) so that the nerves will not be tethered when the urethral anastomotic sutures are tied.

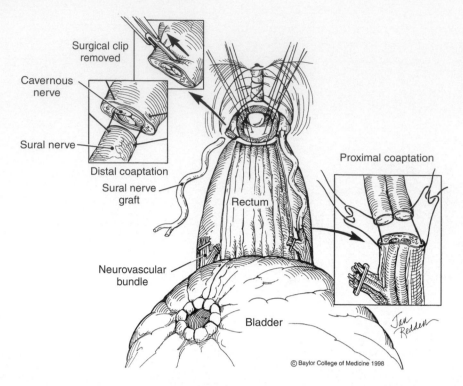

FIGURE 13C.19. Sural nerve grafts can be interposed between severed ends of the cavernous nerves when these nerves must be resected to assure complete excision of the cancer. The nerve graft is reversed, and distal branches are coapted to proximal ends of cavernous nerves near the lateral vascular pedicle. Note the surgical clip across the distal end of the severed right neurovascular bundle. (From Kim ED, Scardino PT, Hampel O, et al. Interposition of sural nerve restores function of cavernous nerves resected during radical prostatectomy. *J Urol* 1999;161:188, with permission.)

Finally, the bladder neck should be divided well away from the prostate. Tapering the bladder neck into the prostatic urethra does not improve the rate of long-term continence but does increase the rate of positive surgical margins (88).

OPTIMIZING OUTCOMES AFTER RADICAL PROSTATECTOMY

The most favorable outcome that can be achieved following radical prostatectomy is complete tumor resection (freedom from clinical recurrence) with full recovery of continence and potency. Risks of individual complications and side effects after this procedure such as erectile dysfunction and incontinence are reasonably well documented in the literature. However, taken in isolation, these risks do not adequately inform patients of the possibility of becoming cancer-free while at the same time returning to their preoperative functional state. We retrospectively reviewed our database from July 1998 through July 2003 and identified 1,133 men who underwent radical prostatectomy for clinical stage T1 to T3a prostate cancer. Patients were excluded if they had received previous radiation to the pelvis or neoadjuvant hormonal therapy, or if they were incontinent or impotent prior to surgery. A total of 862 men met these criteria and were analyzed for biochemical recurrence, and time to recovery of both continence (defined as not having to wear any protective pads/devices) and potency (full erections with/without sildenafil). Mean patient age was 57.8 years (range, 36 to 75 years) while mean pretreatment PSA was 6.73 ng/mL (range, 0.29 to 113.4 ng/mL). Pathologic stage was T0 in five patients, T2 in 30, T2a in 129, T2b in 485, T2c in 20, T3a in 140, T3b in 35, T3c in 3, and T4 in 15 patients. The positive surgical margin rate was 12.5%. There were no perioperative deaths. The attainment of complete cancer resection

(non-detectable postoperative serum PSA level) with full continence and potency (an optimal outcome) was attained in 30% of men at 12 months, 42% at 24 months, 47% at 36 months, and 53% at 48 months (Fig. 13C.20). These retrospective results, based on physician interview of the patient, suggest that an optimal outcome after radical prostatectomy can be achieved in the majority of cases if performed at a center with a large experience. The results also suggest that there is room for improvement for many patients undergoing radical prostatectomy.

CANCER CONTROL AFTER RADICAL RETROPUBIC PROSTATECTOMY

Reports of long-term, cancer-specific survival rates after radical prostatectomy have clearly shown that many such patients live out their lives free of cancer (5,7,24,25). Gibbons et al. (25) reported 82% cancer-specific survival at 15 to 35 years. Zincke et al. (24) reported 90% 10-year and 82% 15-year, cancer-specific survival for 3,170 patients with T1-T2NXM0 cancers treated with radical prostatectomy. Han et al., updating outcomes from Johns Hopkins, reported 96% 10-year and 90% 15-year actuarial, cancer-specific survival for 2,404 men undergoing radical prostatectomy (7). Finally, Bianco et al. reported 5-, 10-, and 15-year cancer-specific survival of 99%, 96%, and 93%, respectively, for 1,700 men treated between 1983 and 2003 with a mean follow-up of 6 years (range, 1 to 20 years). Clearly, radical prostatectomy results in excellent long-term cancer-specific survival.

After a radical prostatectomy, serum PSA levels should become undetectable (89). Although rare cases of disease recurrence after radical prostatectomy with an undetectable serum

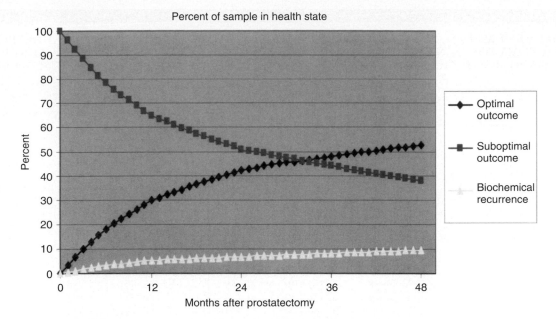

FIGURE 13C.20. Results of Markov model demonstrating the probability of achieving an optimal outcome: complete urinary continence, full erectile function (IIEF ≥ 26), and free of cancer recurrence.
Optimal outcome = potent, continent, recurrence-free.
Suboptimal outcome = impotent and/or incontinent.
Biochemical recurrence = any serum PSA rise of 0.2 ng/mL or greater.

TABLE 13C.10

PROGRESSION-FREE RATE DETERMINED BY PROSTATE SPECIFIC ANTIGEN (PSA), AFTER RADICAL RETROPUBIC PROSTATECTOMY

Group (ref)	No. patients	Clinical stage	Years of RP	PSA nonprogression, %		
				5-yr	10-yr	15-yr
Han et al. (7)	2,404[a]	T1-2NX	1982–1999	84	72	61
Trapasso et al. (96)	425[b]	T1-2NX	1987–1992	69	47	
Zinke et al. (24)	3,170[a]	T1-2NX	1966–1991	70	52	40
Catalona and Smith (97)	1,778[c]	T1-2NX	1983–1993	78	65	
Hull et al. (5)	1,000[b]	T1-2NX	1983–1998	78	75	
Authors' Series	1,700[a]	T1-2NX	1983–2003	84	78	73

[a]Progression defined as a serum PSA >.2 ng/mL.
[b]Progression defined as a serum PSA >.4 ng/mL.
[c]Progression defined as a serum PSA >.3 ng/mL.

PSA level have been documented (90,91), in most men a rising PSA level is the earliest indicator of persistent or recurrent cancer (89,92–95). From several major institutions, we now have remarkably similar 5-year, progression-free probabilities of 69% to 84% in over 8,700 patients treated between 1966 and 1998 (Table 13C.10) (5,7,24,96,97). At 10 years, progression-free probabilities range from 47% to 78% (Table 13C.10).

Progression rates depend on the clinical stage, Gleason grade, and serum PSA level before radical prostatectomy as well as pathologic findings in the radical prostatectomy sspecimen. Up to 15-year outcomes have been reported for anatomic radical prostatectomy based on preoperative and pathologic factors (Table 13C.11) (98). Recently, Scardino calculated the risk of recurrence in his personal series of 1,700 consecutive patients with clinical stage T1-2 N0 or X,

M0 cancer scheduled for radical prostatectomy and followed closely with serum PSA levels for 1 month to 240 months (mean, 72 months) (5). Progression, or treatment failure, was defined as a rising serum PSA greater than 0.2 ng/mL, (i.e., clinical evidence of local or distant recurrence or the initiation of adjuvant radiotherapy or hormonal treatment). At 5 years, 84% were free of progression, at 10 years 78% were; and at 15 years, 73% were free of progression (Table 13C.11; Fig. 13C.21).

Of particular interest are patients with high-grade cancers (Gleason sum 7 to 10). Of patients with Gleason 3 + 4 = 7 cancers in the radical prostatectomy specimen, 68% were free of progression at 15 years. When the tumor was Gleason 4 + 3 = 7, in the radical prostatectomy specimen, 51% were free of progression at 15 years. Even patients with Gleason sum 8 to 10 cancers fared well, with 27% free of progression

TABLE 13C.11

ACTUARIAL (PSA-BASED) 5-, 10-, AND 15-YEAR NONPROGRESSION RATES (%) AFTER RADICAL RETROPUBIC PROSTATECTOMY FOR CLINICALLY LOCALIZED PROSTATE CANCER ACCORDING TO CLINICAL STAGE, GLEASON SCORE IN THE BIOPSY SPECIMEN, PATHOLOGIC STAGE, AND PREOPERATIVE SERUM PSA LEVEL

	John Hopkins University			MSKCC spore prostate cancer database[a]		
	5-Yr	10-Yr	15-Yr	5-Yr	10-Yr	15-Yr
N	2,404	2,404	2,404	4,037	4,037	4,037
BCR	412	412	412	630	630	630
BCR-free	84%	74%	66%	82%	75%	73%
PSA (ng/cc)						
≤4	94 (92–96)	91 (87–93)	67 (34–86)	92 (89–95)	89 (85–93)	86 (80–92)
>4 & <10	89 (86–91)	79 (74–83)	75 (69–80)	87 (85–89)	80 (77–83)	78 (74–81)
≥10 (or 10–20)	73 (68–78)	57 (48–64)	54 (44–63)	75 (72–78)	68 (64–71)	66 (62–70)
≥20	60 (49–69)	48 (36–59)	48 (36–59)	58 (54–62)	52 (47–57)	50 (43–56)
Clinical Stage						
cT1a,b	90 (83–95)	85 (76–91)	75 (58–86)	90 (85–95)	85 (79–92)	83 (76–90)
cT1c	91 (88–93)	76 (48–90)	76 (48–90)	88 (86–90)	79 (73–85)	NA
cT2a	86 (83–88)	75 (71–79)	66 (59–72)	85 (82–88)	77 (81–77)	75 (70–80)
cT2b	75 (70–79)	62 (56–68)	50 (41–58)	74 (70–79)	69 (64–75)	69 (64–75)
cT2c	71 (61–79)	57 (45–68)	57 (45–68)	71 (68–75)	64 (59–68)	62 (57–67)
cT3	60 (45–72)	49 (34–63)	NA	54 (44–64)	51 (40–62)	NA
Specimen Gleason						
2 to 4	100	100	100	100	100	100
5	98 (96–99)	94 (90–96)	86 (78–92)	92 (90–94)	89 (86–92)	88 (84–92)
6	95 (93–97)	88 (83–92)	73 (59–82)	91 (89–93)	83 (80–86)	81 (78–85)
7	73 (69–76)	54 (48–59)	48 (41–56)	77 (75–79)	70 (66–74)	67 (63–72)
3 + 4	81 (77–84)	60 (53–67)	59 (51–65)	82 (79–84)	74 (69–79)	72 (62–82)
4 + 3	53 (44–61)	33 (22–43)	33 (22–43)	60 (50–70)	53 (44–64)	53 (44–64)
8 to 10	44 (36–52)	29 (22–37)	15 (5–28)	41 (35–47)	33 (24–42)	NA
Pathologic Stage						
Organ Confined	97 (95–98)	93 (90–95)	84 (77–90)	93 (92–94)	89 (87–91)	87 (85–89)
EPE+, GS <7, SM−	97 (94–98)	93 (89–96)	84 (70–92)	92 (89–94)	89 (84–94)	86 (79–92)
EPE+, GS <7, SM+	89 (80–94)	73 (61–82)	58 (41–71)	74 (64–84)	65 (54–76)	65 (54–76)
EPE+, GS ≥7, SM−	80 (75–85)	61 (52–68)	59 (50–67)	76 (66–86)	68 (61–75)	65 (56–74)
EPE+, GS ≥7, SM+	58 (49–66)	42 (32–52)	33 (23–44)	60 (53–67)	55 (44–66)	55 (44–66)
SV+, LN−	48 ((38–58)	30 (19–41)	17 (5–35)	44 (38–50)	31 (24–38)	28 (19–37)
LN+	26 (19–35)	10 (5–18)	0	25 (18–32)	15 (5–25)	0
Negative Margins	NR	NR	NR	87 (86–88)	81 (79–83)	79 (76–82)
Positive Margins	NR	NR	NR	66 (63–69)	56 (52–60)	54 (49–59)

BCR, post surgery PSA relapse.

Δ single surgeon series (ref. 98).

[a]Includes 1,092 radical prostatectomies performed by a single surgeon at Baylor College of Medicine.

at 10 years. These progression rates are substantially lower than the 15-year cancer mortality rates reported by Albertsen and his colleagues for patients with Gleason sum 7 to 10 cancers (30).

Once the prostate is removed, the most powerful prognostic factor is the pathologic stage (Table 13C.11; Fig. 13C.21). When the cancer is confined to the prostate (defined as cancer not extending into the periprostatic soft tissue), 91% to 97% of patients remain free of progression at 5 years and 85% to 92% remain free at 10 years (5,34). Focal penetration through the capsule, into the periprostatic soft tissue alone, in the absence of seminal vesicle invasion, results in a 73% 15-year non-progression rate. Established penetration through the prostatitic capsule into the periprostatic soft tissue alone, in the absence of seminal vesicle invasion, results in a 42% 15-year non-progression rate. Even some patients with seminal vesicle invasion (pT3cN0) can be cured with surgery, with 30% being free of disease recurrence at 10 years (Table 13C.11).

CONCLUSION

Radical retropubic prostatectomy reliably eradicates the cancer in most men with clinically localized (cT1a to T3a,NX,M0) prostate cancer. Although technically complex, this operation can generally be performed with a low level of acute and long-term morbidity, but the results are highly sensitive to fine details in surgical technique. Rates of blood loss, positive surgical margins, incontinence, and erectile dysfunction vary widely from surgeon to surgeon. With careful attention to surgical technique, cancer control rates should improve further, and the effect of the operation on quality of life should continue to decrease.

The goal of radical prostatectomy should be to excise the cancer completely, without positive surgical margins and with long-term preservation of urinary and sexual function in all patients. This lofty goal has not yet been achieved in every case by any surgeon, but we should all aspire to this standard.

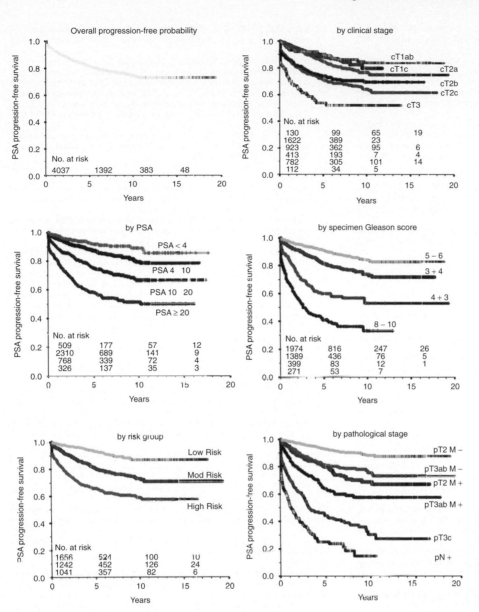

FIGURE 13C.21. Probability of freedom from progression after radical prostatectomy alone. The study population includes 1,700 consecutive patients who agreed to radical prostatectomy, whether or not the operation was actually performed. In 14 patients with positive nodes, the operation was abandoned.

References

1. Kuchler H. Uber prostatavergrosserungh. *Dtsch Klin* 1866;18:458.
2. Millin T. *Retropubic urinary surgery*. Baltimore, MD: Williams & Wilkins, 1947.
3. Ansell JS. Radical transvesical prostatectomy: preliminary report on an approach to surgical excision of localized prostate malignancy. *J Urol* 1959;82:373.
4. Campbell EW. Total prostatectomy with preliminary ligation of the vascular pedicles. *J Urol* 1959;81:464.
5. Hull GW, Rabbani F, Abbas F, et al. Cancer control with radical prostatectomy alone in 1,000 consecutive patients. *J Urol* 2002;167(2 Pt 1):528–534.
6. Kausik SJ, Blute ML, Sebo TJ, et al. Prognostic significance of positive surgical margins in patients with extraprostatic carcinoma after radical prostatectomy. *Cancer* 2002;95(6):1215–1219.
7. Han M, Partin AW, Zahurak M, et al. Biochemical (prostate-specific antigen) recurrence probability following radical prostatectomy for clinically localized prostate cancer. *J Urol* 2003;169(2):517–523.
8. Eastham JA, Kattan MW, Rogers E, et al. Risk factors for urinary incontinence after radical prostatectomy. *J Urol* 1996;156:1707.
9. Noh C, Kshirsagar A, Mohler JL. Outcomes after radical retropubic prostatectomy. *Urology* 2003;61(2):412–416.
10. Steiner MS, Morton RA, Walsh PC. Impact of anatomical radical prostatectomy on urinary continence. *J Urol* 1991;145:512.
11. Walsh PC. Technique of vesicourethral anastomosis may influence recovery of sexual function following radical prostatectomy. *Atlas Urol Clin North Am* 1994;2:59.
12. Rabbani F, Stapleton AM, Kattan MW, et al. Factors predicting recovery of erections after radical prostatectomy. *J Urol* 2000;164(6):1929–1934.
13. Goad JR, Scardino PT. Modifications in the technique of radical retropubic prostatectomy to minimize blood loss. *Atlas Urol Clin North Am* 1994;20:65.
14. Maffezzini M, Seveso M, Taverna G, et al. Evaluation of complications and results in a contemporary series of 300 consecutive radical retropubic prostatectomies with the anatomic approach at a single institution. *Urology* 2003;61(5):982–986.
15. Lepor H, Nieder AM, Ferrandino MN. Intraoperative and postoperative complications of radical retropubic prostatectomy in a consecutive series of 1,000 cases. *J Urol* 2001;166(5):1729–1733.
16. Smith JA, Bray WL, Koch MO. Cost efficient management of the patient with localized prostate cancer. *AUA Update Series* 1997;16:122.
17. Leibman BD, Dillioglugil O, Abbas F, et al. Impact of a clinical pathway for radical retropubic prostatectomy. *Urology* 1998;52:94.
18. Eastham JA, Kattan MW, Riedel E, et al. Variations among individual surgeons in the rate of positive surgical margins in radical prostatectomy specimens. *J Urol* 2003;170:2292.
19. Han M, Partin AW, Chan DY, et al. An evaluation of the decreasing incidence of positive surgical margins in a large retropubic prostatectomy series. *J Urol* 2004;171(1):23–26.
20. Klein EA, Kupelian PA, Tuason L, et al. Initial dissection of the lateral fascia reduces the positive margin rate in radical prostatectomy. *Urology* 1998;51:766.
21. Wieder JA, Soloway MS. Incidence, etiology, location, prevention and treatment of positive surgical margins after radical prostatectomy for prostate cancer. *J Urol* 1998;160:299.

22. Walsh PC. Radical retropubic prostatectomy. In: Walsh PC, Retik AB, Vaughn ED Jr, eds. *Campbell's urology*, 8th ed. Philadelphia, PA: WB Saunders, 2002:3107.

23. Kattan MW, Eastham JA, Stapleton AMF, et al. A preoperative nomogram for disease recurrence following radical prostatectomy for prostate cancer. *J Natl Cancer Inst* 1998;90:766.

24. Zincke H, Oesterling JE, Blute ML, et al. Long-term (15 years) results after radical prostatectomy for clinically localized (stage T2c or lower) prostate cancer. *J Urol* 1994;152:1850.

25. Gibbons RP, Correa RJ Jr, Brannen GE, et al. Total prostatectomy for clinically localized prostate cancer: long-term results. *J Urol* 1989;141:564.

26. Fleming C, Wasson JH, Albertsen PC, et al. A decision analysis of alternative treatment strategies for clinically localized prostate cancer. Prostate Patient Outcomes Research Team. *JAMA* 1993;269:2650.

27. Johansson JE, Adami HO, Anderson SO, et al. High 10-year survival rate in patients with early, untreated prostatic cancer. *JAMA* 1992;267:2191.

28. Chodak GW, Thisted RA, Gerber GS, et al. Results of conservative management of clinically localized prostate cancer. *N Engl J Med* 1994;330:242.

29. Albertsen PC, Fryback DG, Storer BE, et al. Long-term survival among men with conservatively treated localized prostate cancer. *JAMA* 1995;274:626.

30. Albertsen PC, Hanley JA, Gleason DF, et al. Competing risk analysis of men aged 55 to 74 years at diagnosis managed conservatively for clinically localized prostate cancer. *JAMA* 1998;280:975.

31. Holmberg L, Bill-Axelson A, Helgesen F et al. Scandinavian Prostatic Cancer Group Study Number 4. A randomized trial comparing radical prostatectomy with watchful waiting in early prostate cancer. *N Engl J Med* 2002;347(11):781–789.

32. Egawa S, Shoji K, Go M, et al. Long-term impact of conservative management on localized prostate cancer. *Urology* 1993;42:520.

33. Balaji KC, Wheeler TM, Scardino PT. Poorly differentiated prostate cancers (PCa) detected by PSA are more likely to be organ confined than those detected by digital rectal examination. *Proc Am Soc Clin Oncol* 1999;18:318a (abstract 1222).

34. Wheeler TM, Dilliogluil O, Kattan MW, et al. Clinical and pathological significance of the level and extent of capsular invasion in clinical stage T1–2 prostate cancer. *Hum Pathol* 1998;29:856.

35. Ohori M, Egawa S, Shinohara K, et al. Detection of microscopic extracapsular extension prior to radical prostatectomy for clinically localized prostate cancer. *Br J Urol* 1994;74:72.

36. D'Amico AV, Whittington R, Schnall M, et al. The impact of the inclusion of endorectal coil magnetic resonance imaging in a multivariate analysis to predict clinically unsuspected extraprostatic cancer. *Cancer* 1995;75:2368.

37. Coakley FV, Eberhardt S, Kattan MW, et al. Urinary continence after radical retropubic prostatectomy: relationship with membranous urethral length on preoperative endorectal magnetic resonance imaging. *J Urol* 2002;168(3):1032–1035.

38. Epstein JI, Walsh PC, Brendler CB. Radical prostatectomy for impalpable prostate cancer: the Johns Hopkins experience with tumors found on transurethral resection (stages T1A and T1B) and on needle biopsy (stage T1C). *J Urol* 1994;152(Pt. 2):1721.

39. Canto EI, Slawin KM. Early management of prostate cancer: how to respond to an elevated PSA? *Annu Rev Med* 2002;53:355–368.

40. Goto Y, Ohori M, Arakawa A, et al. Distinguishing clinically important from unimportant prostate cancers before treatment: value of systematic biopsies. *J Urol* 1996;156:1059.

41. Bastacky SI, Walsh PC, Epstein JI. Relationship between perineural tumor invasion on needle biopsy and radical prostatectomy capsular penetration in clinical stage B adenocarcinoma of the prostate. *Am J Surg Pathol* 1993;17:336.

42. Cagiannos I, Karakiewicz P, Eastham JA, et al. A pre-operative nomogram identifying prostate cancer patients with decreased risk of positive pelvic lymph nodes. *J Urol* 2003;170:1798.

43. Middleton RG, Smith JA, Melzer RB. Patient survival and local recurrence rate following radical prostatectomy for prostatic carcinoma. *J Urol* 1986;136:422.

44. Epstein JI, Carmichael M, Walsh PC. Adenocarcinoma of the prostate invading the seminal vesicle: definition and relation of tumor volume, grade and margins of resection to prognosis. *J Urol* 1993;149:1040.

45. Ohori M, Scardino PT, Lapin SL, et al. The mechanism and prognostic significance of seminal vesicle involvement by prostate cancer. *Am J Surg Pathol* 1993;17:1252.

46. Ohori M, Shinohara K, Wheeler TM, et al. Ultrasonic detection of nonpalpable seminal vesicle invasion: a clinicopathological study. *Br J Urol* 1993;72:799.

47. Terris MK, McNeal JE, Freiha FS, et al. Efficacy of transrectal ultrasound-guided seminal vesicle biopsies in the detection of seminal vesicle invasion by prostate cancer. *J Urol* 1993;149:1035.

48. D'Amico AV, Schnall M, Whittington R, et al. Endorectal coil magnetic resonance imaging identifies locally advanced prostate cancer in select patients with clinically localized disease. *Urology* 1998;51:449.

49. Rorvik J, Halvorsen OJ, Albrektsen G, et al. MRI with an endorectal coil for staging of clinically localised prostate cancer prior to radical prostatectomy. *Eur Radiol* 1999;9:29.

50. Koch MO, Smith JA Jr, Hodge EM, et al. Prospective development of a cost-efficient program for radical retropubic prostatectomy. *Urology* 1994;44:311.

51. Burkhard FC, Bader P, Schneider E, et al. Reliability of preoperative values to determine the need for lymphadenectomy in patients with prostate cancer and meticulous lymph node dissection. *Eur Urol* 2002;42(2):84–90.

52. Hoenig DM, Chi S, Porter C, et al. Risk of nodal metastases at laparoscopic pelvic lymphadenectomy using PSA, Gleason score, and clinical stage in men with localized prostate cancer. *J Endourol* 1997;11(4):263–265.

53. Reiner WG, Walsh PC. An anatomical approach to the surgical management of the dorsal vein and Santorini's plexus during radical retropubic surgery. *J Urol* 1979;121:198.

54. Peters CA, Walsh PC. Blood transfusions and anesthetic practices in radical retropubic prostatectomy. *J Urol* 1985;134:81.

55. Myers RP. Improving the exposure of the prostate in radical retropubic prostatectomy: longitudinal bunching of the deep venous plexus. *J Urol* 1989;142:1282.

56. Rainwater LM, Segura JW. Technical consideration in radical retropubic prostatectomy: blood loss after ligation of dorsal venous complex. *J Urol* 1990;143:1163.

57. Eastham JA, Scardino PT, Yawn DH, et al. Preoperative autologous blood donation in radical retropubic prostatectomy: a cost-effectiveness analysis. *Int J Technol Manag* 2001;3:322.

58. Coakley FV, Eberhardt S, Wei DC, et al. Blood loss during radical retropubic prostatectomy: relationship to morphologic features on preoperative endorectal magnetic resonance imaging. *Urology* 2002;59(6):884–888.

59. Goldschlag B, Afzal N, Carter HB, et al. Is preoperative donation of autologous blood rational for radical retropubic prostatectomy? *J Urol* 2000;164(6):1968–1972.

60. Augustin H, Hammerer P, Graefen M, et al. Intraoperative and perioperative morbidity of contemporary radical retropubic prostatectomy in a consecutive series of 1243 patients: results of a single center between 1999 and 2002. *Eur Urol* 2003;43(2):113–118.

61. Catalona WJ, Carvalhal GF, Mager DE, et al. Potency, continence and complication rates in 1,870 consecutive radical retropubic prostatectomies. *J Urol* 1999;162(2):433–438.

62. Lerner SE, Blute ML, Lieber MM, et al. Morbidity of contemporary radical retropubic prostatectomy for localized prostate cancer. *Oncology* 1995;9:379.

63. McLaren RH, Barrett DM, Zincke H. Rectal injury occurring at radical retropubic prostatectomy for prostate cancer: etiology and treatment. *Urology* 1993;42:401.

64. Cisek LJ, Walsh PC. Thromboembolic complications following radical retropubic prostatectomy. *Urology* 1993;42:406.

65. Surya BV, Provet J, Johanson KE, et al. Anastomotic strictures following radical prostatectomy: risk factors and management. *J Urol* 1990;143:755.

66. Geary ES, Dendinger TE, Freiha FS, et al. Incontinence and vesical neck strictures following radical retropubic prostatectomy. *Urology* 1995;45:1000.

67. Litwin MS, Hays RD, Fink A, et al. Quality-of-life outcomes in men treated for localized prostate cancer. *JAMA* 1995;273:129.

68. Murphy GP, Mettlin C, Menck H, et al. National patterns of prostate cancer treatment by radical prostatectomy: results of a survey by the American College of Surgeons Committee on Cancer. *J Urol* 1994;152:1817.

69. Walsh PC, Marschke P, Ricker D, et al. Patient-reported urinary continence and sexual function after anatomic radical prostatectomy. *Urology* 2000;55(1):58–61.

70. Sebesta M, Cespedes RD, Luhman E, et al. Questionnaire-based outcomes of urinary incontinence and satisfaction rates after radical prostatectomy in a national study population. *Urology* 2002;60(6):1055–1058.

71. Stanford JL, Feng Z, Hamilton AS, et al. Urinary and sexual function after radical prostatectomy for clinically localized prostate cancer: the Prostate Cancer Outcomes Study [In Process Citation]. *JAMA* 2000;283:354.

72. Fowler FJ Jr, Barry MJ, Lu-Yao G, et al. Patient-reported complications and follow-up treatment after radical prostatectomy. The national Medicare experience: 1988–1990 (updated June 1993). *Urology* 1993;42:622.

73. Steineck G, Helgesen F, Adolfsson J, et al. Scandinavian Prostatic Cancer Group Study Number 4. Quality of life after radical prostatectomy or watchful waiting. *N Engl J Med* 2002;347(11):790–796.

74. Wei JT, Dunn RL, Sandler HM, et al. Comprehensive comparison of health-related quality of life after contemporary therapies for localized prostate cancer. *J Clin Oncol* 2002;20(2):557–566.

75. Presti JC Jr, Schmidt RA, Narayan PA, et al. Pathophysiology of urinary incontinence after radical prostatectomy. *J Urol* 1990;143:975.

76. Hutch JA, Fisher R. Continence after radical prostatectomy. *Br J Urol* 1968;40:62.

77. Rudy DC, Woodside JR, Crawford ED. Urodynamic evaluation of incontinence in patients undergoing modified Campbell radical prostatectomy: a prospective study. *J Urol* 1984;132:708.

78. O'Donnell PD, Finan BF. Continence following nerve sparing radical prostatectomy. *J Urol* 1989;142:1227.

79. Quinlan DM, Epstein JI, Carter BS, et al. Sexual function following radical prostatectomy: influence of preservation of neurovascular bundles. *J Urol* 1991;145:998.

80. Catalona WJ, Bigg SW. Nerve-sparing radical prostatectomy: evaluation of results after 250 patients. *J Urol* 1990;143:538.
81. Bahnson RR, Catalona WJ. Papaverine testing of impotent patients following nerve-sparing radical prostatectomy. *J Urol* 1988;139:773.
82. Breza J, Abuseif SR, Orvis BR, et al. Detailed anatomy of penile neurovascular structures: surgical significance. *J Urol* 1989;141:437.
83. Rosen MA, Goldstone L, Lapin S, et al. Frequency and location of extracapsular extension and positive surgical margins in radical prostatectomy specimens. *J Urol* 1992;148:331.
84. Killeen KP, Libertino JA, Sughayer MA, et al. Pathologic review of consecutive radical prostatectomy specimens. Nerve sparing versus non-nerve sparing. *Urology* 1991;38:212.
85. Abbas F, Scardino PT. Why neoadjuvant androgen deprivation prior to radical prostatectomy is unnecessary. *Urol Clin North Am* 1996;23:587.
86. Kim ED, Scardino PT, Hampel O, et al. Interposition of sural nerve restores function of cavernous nerves resected during radical prostatectomy. *J Urol* 1999;161:188.
87. Kim ED, Nath R, Kadmon D, et al. Bilateral nerve graft during radical retropubic prostatectomy: 1-year followup. *J Urol* 2001;165(6 Pt 1): 1950–1956.
88. Licht MR, Klein EA, Tuason L, et al. Impact of bladder neck preservation during radical prostatectomy on continence and cancer control. *Urology* 1994;44:883.
89. Oesterling JE, Chan DW, Epstein JI, et al. Prostate specific antigen in the preoperative and postoperative evaluation of localized prostate cancer treated with radical prostatectomy. *J Urol* 1988;139:766.
90. Goldrath DE, Messing EM. Prostate specific antigen: not detectable despite tumor progression after radical prostatectomy. *J Urol* 1989;142: 1082.
91. Takayama T, Krieger JN, True LD, et al. Recurrent prostate cancer despite undetectable prostate specific antigen. *J Urol* 1992;148:1541.
92. Lightner DJ, Lange PH, Reddy PK, et al. Prostate specific antigen and local recurrence after radical prostatectomy. *J Urol* 1990;144:921.
93. Stein A, deKernion JB, Dorey F. Prostate specific antigen related to clinical status 1 to 14 years after radical retropubic prostatectomy. *Br J Urol* 1991; 67:626.
94. Amling CL, Bergstralh EJ, Blute ML, et al. Defining prostate specific antigen progression after radical prostatectomy: what is the most appropriate cut point? *J Urol* 2001;165(4):1146–1151.
95. Partin AW, Pound CR, Clemens JQ, et al. Serum PSA after anatomic radical prostatectomy. *Urol Clin North Am* 1993;20:713.
96. Trapasso JG, deKernion JB, Smith RB, et al. The incidence and significance of detectable levels of serum prostate specific antigen after radical prostatectomy. *J Urol* 1994;152:1821.
97. Catalona WJ, Smith DS. Cancer recurrence and survival rates after anatomical radical retropubic prostatectomy for prostate cancer: intermediate results. *J Urol* 1998;160:2428.
98. Han M, Partin AW, Pound CR, et al. Long-term biochemical disease-free and cancer-specific survival following anatomic radical retropubic prostatectomy: the 15-year Johns Hopkins experience. *Urol Clin North Am* 2001;28:555–565.

CHAPTER 13D
Laparoscopic Radical Prostatectomy

*A. Karim Touijer and
Bertrand Guillonneau*

INTRODUCTION

The surgical treatment for localized prostate cancer aims to offer the best cancer control and functional results with the least morbidity. Recent advances during the last two decades have led to a better understanding of the intricate pelvic and periprostatic anatomy and continuous refinements of the radical retropubic prostatectomy technique, resulting in higher cure rates (1–3) and improvement of the morbidity (4–6).

At the same time, laparoscopic surgery emerged as a minimally invasive approach with a low morbidity profile that was gaining popularity in many surgical fields. The first

attempt of the laparoscopic approach to radical prostatectomy occurred in 1991. However, in their publication of the initial series of nine patients, the authors concluded that laparoscopic radical prostatectomy (LRP) was feasible but technically challenging and "not an efficacious surgical alternative to open prostatectomy for malignancy" (7). Surgical teams from France took up the challenge of refining the technique and, with accumulated experience, developed a feasible, reproducible, and teachable operation widely practiced in urologic centers worldwide (8). Today the laparoscopic approach to treatment of clinically localized adenocarcinoma of the prostate is an established technique that respects the same oncologic principles of open surgery and strives to preserve continence and erectile function to the greatest extent possible.

This chapter describes the surgical technique as currently performed at Memorial Sloan-Kettering Cancer Center (MSKCC) with an overview of the oncologic and functional results.

OPERATIVE TECHNIQUE

Possible Difficulties

Laparoscopic radical prostatectomy obeys the same indication and contraindication rules as radical retropubic prostatectomy (RRP). There are no specific contraindications to the laparoscopic approach. However, certain conditions increase the difficulty of the procedure. Certainly, morbid obesity is the most common. Technically, in a patient with a body mass index greater than 35, access to the apex becomes more challenging as the distance from the anterior abdominal wall to the prostate is increased. Bleeding in the operative field is also increased because of the dense fatty tissue obscuring the vision of blood vessels, and the Trendelenburg position is often not as well-tolerated. It may be necessary in morbidly obese patients to place additional trocars and to adapt their position to the specific anatomy of the patient. A large prostate gland generally represents a technical challenge. This can particularly become an issue during the lateral dissection when a nerve-sparing procedure is planned. The presence of a prostatic median lobe adds to the difficulty of the bladder neck dissection. This is due to the close proximity of the ureteral orifices and the risk of entering erroneously the dissection plane of the adenomectomy rather than that of the radical prostatectomy. Previous history of prostate treatment (e.g., transurethral resection or incision of the prostate, suprapubic prostatectomy, external beam radiation therapy, or brachytherapy) does not contraindicate a laparoscopic approach per se but certainly adds to the technical complexity of this procedure. Finally, a previous history of intra-abdominal surgery justifies specific precautions in accessing the abdomen if a laparoscopic route is chosen but may incline the surgeon to prefer a subperitoneal route according to their habits and experience.

Preoperative Care

Prevention of intraoperative and postoperative thromboembolic disease remains an essential element of perioperative care, particularly since the operation adds three risk factors: cancer surgery, pelvic surgery, and elevated intra-abdominal pressure. Compression stockings are mandatory during the surgery and usually during the first postoperative night. Furthermore, our practice is a daily subcutaneous injection of low-molecular-weight heparin adapted to the patient's risk. It must be started 3 hours before the operation and administered daily afterwards until discharged from the hospital. Finally, the third key element to thromboprophylaxis is early postoperative ambulation.

Patients also receive antibiotic prophylaxis with a single preoperative dose of intravenous second generation cephalosporin.

Patient Positioning

Patient positioning is an essential step of the procedure. The surgeon should supervise all the steps of this set-up in order to prevent the perils of positioning for the patient and to ensure an ergonomic set-up for the surgical team.

The patient is positioned in a low lithotomy position with both arms set along the body to avoid brachial plexus injuries. The shoulders are adequately padded with large foam, and the patient is secured to the operating table with surgical tape. Shoulder supports are not appropriate as they carry the risk of postoperative pain from compression; the thoracic wrap by a wide surgical tape is more comfortable for the patient. Particular attention should be paid to the degree of compression around the calves, due to the reported risk of compartment syndrome. The low lithotomy position with the patient's buttocks placed at the end of the table allows, if necessary, intraoperative access to the rectum and perineum (Fig. 13D.1). After usual skin preparation, the abdomen, from the costal margins to the perianal region, is disinfected and the patient is draped. An 18-french Foley catheter is inserted, and the bladder drained.

A right-handed surgeon stands on the patient's left side with his assistant opposite. The scrub nurse stands on the surgeon's left with the instrument table. The monitor is placed between the patient's legs, to the surgeon's eye level. After a radial umbilical incision, a Veress needle is introduced and insufflation is started after the safety maneuvers. Once the intra-abdominal pressure reaches the preset maximum of 12 mm Hg, a 10-mm trocar is inserted through the umbilicus for passage of the 0-degree laparoscope, and the patient is then positioned in a steep Trendelenburg position. Four other 5-mm trocars are inserted: one into the left iliac fossa, one in the midline halfway between the umbilicus and the pubic symphysis, one at the level of the umbilicus in the right pararectal fossa, and one in the right iliac fossa at McBurney's point. The surgeon uses the two ports close to the laparoscope in order to have an ergonomic approach to the surgical field with the instruments in correct triangulation, while the assistant has at his/her disposal the lateral right and the suprapubic ports (Fig. 13D.2).

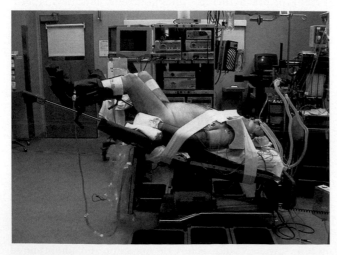

FIGURE 13D.1. Patient positioning.

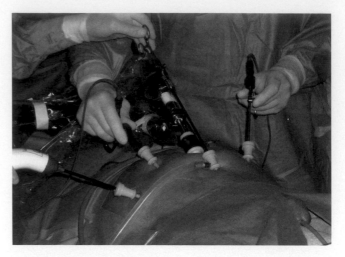

FIGURE 13D.2. Ports placement.

The Pelvic Lymph Node Dissection

Operative Steps

The peritoneal incision is vertical, lateral to the medial umbilical ligaments, starting from the vas deferens and is usually about 5 cm long downwards.

The external iliac vein is easily found; the lymphatic and fatty tissue lateral, medial, and inferior to it should be bluntly dissected. Distally on the vein, the surgeon should be aware of a frequent accessory circumflex vein. The first landmark to be found is Cooper ligament. The lymphatic vessels can be transected safely at its contact, using either surgical clips or bipolar cautery. The dissection of the lymphatic packet should be continued cephalad from the pubic bone to the iliac veins confluence, exposing the obturator nerve and vessels. Small blood vessels from the lateral pelvic wall and posterior to the obturator nerve should be controlled, as they can be a source of unnecessary bleeding, obscuring vision. Finally, the hypogastric part of the lymph node packet is freed after control and transection of the main lymphatic vessels at the level of the iliac venous confluence. The node packet is left in the obturator fossa, and the same node dissection is performed contralaterally. A 5-mm laparoscope is introduced through a lateral port, and the nodes are placed in a laparoscopic bag and extracted through the umbilical incision.

Indications

In our practice, the preoperative prostate cancer nomogram prediction of lymph node invasion dictates whether a bilateral pelvic lymph node dissection will be performed or not prior to prostatectomy (9). We have set, as a high-risk group, patients with a probability of lymph node invasion of 1.5% or greater. Such a cut-off predicts negative lymph node status correctly 99.1% of the time and identifies 94% of all men with positive lymph nodes.

Results

Using the above selection criteria, lymph node dissection was avoided in 58% of the patients. When performed, the average number of nodes removed was 8.8 (range, 0–21) and positive lymph nodes were found in 1.5% of the overall patient population and in 4.2% of the subset with node dissection.

The Radical Prostatectomy

We will describe here the transperitoneal approach with first dissection of the seminal vesicles. Six standardized steps can be outlined (10).

First Step: Posterior Approach to the Seminal Vesicles

Incising the Pouch of Douglas. The sigmoid colon is held gently by the assistant, retracting the rectum cephalad. The surgeon incises the posterior vesical peritoneum transversally approximately 2 cm above the level of the cul de sac of Douglas. The dissection should then follow the inferior peritoneal flap and exposes Denonvilliers fascia. At this level, any dissection into fatty tissue should alert the surgeon of a dissection taken too close to the rectum or the bladder.

Freeing the Seminal Vesicles. Denonvilliers fascia is transversally incised; the vasa deferentia are dissected and coagulated with bipolar forceps then transected. One must be aware and carefully coagulate the deferential artery running along the opposite side. Division of the vasa deferentia allows access to the seminal vesicles. The latter should be dissected along its surface to individualize the two seminal vesicle arteries—one at the tip and the second at the base. These arteries are meticulously and selectively coagulated with the tip of the bipolar forceps facing the surface of the vesicles to avoid any thermal injury to the neural plexus in close proximity (Fig. 13D.3).

At the end of this dissection, the seminal vesicles and vasa deferentia are completely mobilized.

Opening Denonvilliers Fascia. Incision of Denonvilliers fascia allows an easier and safer dissection later in the operation by separating the rectum from the prostatic pedicles. To facilitate the exposure, the assistant retracts the vasa deferentia upward and places Denonvilliers fascia on tension. Denonvilliers fascia is then incised medially and horizontally bringing into view the prerectal fatty tissue (Fig. 13D.4). Further dissection toward the prostatic apex or laterally is ill-advised at this time.

Second Step: Anterior Approach of the Prostate

Entering Retzius' Space. The bladder is filled with approximately 180 mL of saline to help identify its contours and retract it posteriorly. The anterior parietal peritoneum is incised medially from one umbilical ligament to the other. This incision allows clear identification of the urachus that is divided

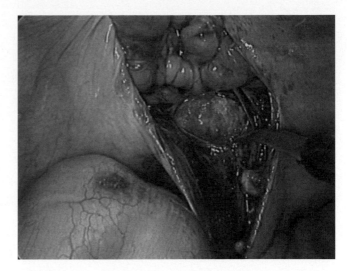

FIGURE 13D.4. Opening of Denonvilliers fascia.

last, minimizing the risk of injury. It is essential to free the bladder wall from its anterior and lateral attachments in order to create a large working space and allow a tension-free vesicourethral anastomosis at the end of the operation. The bladder is emptied with a syringe.

Exposing the Endopelvic Fascia. The fat over the fascia covering the prostate must be swept laterally to expose clearly the endopelvic fascia and the puboprostatic ligaments. The superficial dorsal vein is easily identified and coagulated with bipolar forceps. The endopelvic fascia is identified lateral to the prostate, and incised on its line of reflection, uncovering the levator ani muscle fibers (Fig. 13D.5). Often, muscle fibers and blood vessels extend to the anterolateral aspect of the prostatic apex. The veins, once identified, are coagulated and transected. Sometimes, an artery is identified cephalad to the veins. It should be dissected and preserved, since it does not penetrate the prostate but runs toward the sphincteric complex along the urethra. Incision of the puboprostatic ligaments is done under visual control away from the Santorini venous plexus. The incision can be prolonged toward the fascia that covers the dorsal vein laterally. Although delicate, this step will delineate the anatomy and facilitate further dissection and exposure of the dorsal venous complex and the urethra later during the operation.

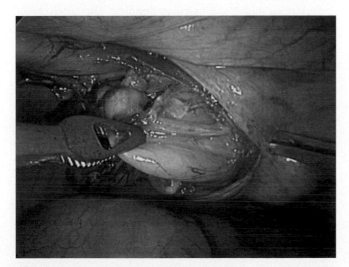

FIGURE 13D.3. Control of seminal vesicle artery.

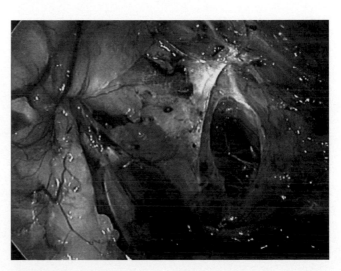

FIGURE 13D.5. Opening of the endopelvic fascia.

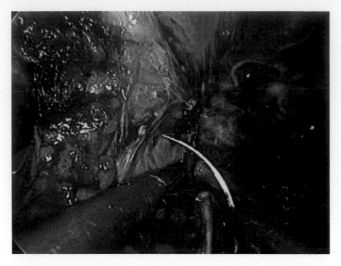

FIGURE 13D.6. Ligation of the dorsal venous complex.

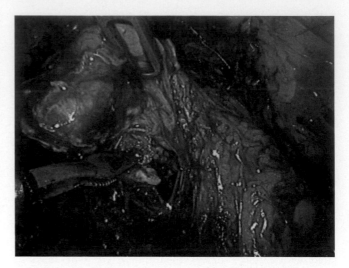

FIGURE 13D.8. Exposure of the prostatic vascular pedicle.

Ligating the Dorsal Venous Complex. The dorsal venous complex is ligated with a 2-0 absorbable suture on an SH needle, passing underneath the venous plexus from one side to the other such that the curve of the needle follows the curve of the pubic symphysis (Fig. 13D.6). Depending on the size of the plexus, a second separate suture or a figure-8 stitch may be placed to make the ligation safer. At this point of the operation, transection of the complex is unnecessary and will be done later. A back-bleeding stitch, ligating the preprostatic venous plexus, is placed.

Third Step: Bladder Neck Dissection

The anatomic landmarks of this step are not well defined. To identify the bladder neck area, the anterior preprostatic fat must be retracted cephalad creating a faint outline of the anterior vesicoprostatic junction. The site where the bladder neck should be dissected is exactly where the fat becomes adherent. This step requires careful hemostasis anteriorly. We have not found that traction on the Foley catheter to pull the balloon to the bladder neck facilitates identification of the correct plane of dissection. The bladder neck is incised transversally, and the tip of the catheter is pulled up by a grasper via the suprapubic port to expose the posterior aspect of the bladder neck (Fig. 13D.7). The surgeon grasps the posterior

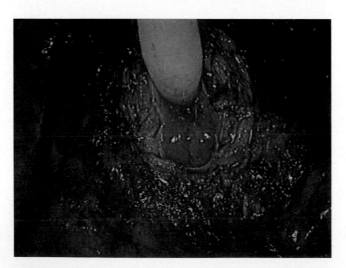

FIGURE 13D.7. Exposure of the posterior aspect of the bladder neck.

bladder neck and separates the bladder from the prostate, reaching the longitudinal muscular fibers between the prostate base and the bladder neck. This layer should be incised in order to gain access to the previously dissected retrovesical space. The vasa deferentia and the seminal vesicles are then simply brought into the operating field by the assistant. This maneuver exposes on both sides the lateral prostatic pedicles (Fig. 13D.8).

Fourth Step: Lateral Dissection of the Prostate

The assistant grasps the vas and the seminal vesicle and retracts them upward. The inferior and medial landmark is easily identified by the posterior layer of Denonvilliers fascia previously dissected during the first step of the procedure. The superior and medial landmark is delineated by incising the periprostatic fascia along the prostate from the base to the apex. The lateral prostatic pedicle is controlled high on the base of the prostate, theoretically at a safe distance from the neurovascular elements of the bundle. The magnification allows a good visualization of the pedicles. However, because of the traction on the seminal vesicles, they appear to rise vertically, which facilitates their exposure but distorts their normal anatomical orientation. It is, therefore, important for the surgeon to re-orient him- or herself constantly during the dissection of the pedicles and be cognizant of the exact location of the neurovascular bundle.

Preserving the Neurovascular Bundles: The Inter-Fascial Technique. Once the pedicle is controlled, the two fascial incisions (superior periprostatic and inferior Denonvilliers fascia) can be joined to develop, with careful and blunt dissection, an avascular interfascial plane, leaving lateral and posterior the neurovascular bundle partially recovered by a fascia. This reduces the possible risk of mechanical injury to the bundle (Fig. 13D.9). It is preferable to continue the apical dissection of the bundle after transecting the dorsal venous plexus, which gives mobility to the gland and facilitates the exposure of the apical and the distal third of the prostate.

Preserving the Neurovascular Bundles: The Extrafascial Technique. With greater risk of extracapsular extension, the interfascial dissection is not recommended as it may increase the likelihood of a positive surgical margin. It is therefore necessary to dissect wider, lateral to the periprostatic fascia and directly into the neurovascular bundle. In this wider dissection, one encounters the adipose tissue and vascular elements within the bundle, which increases the degree of bleeding and requires accurate hemostasis, with fine bipolar forceps or surgical clips.

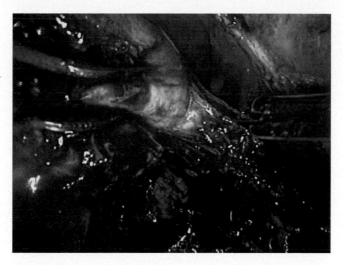

FIGURE 13D.9. Interfascial plane of neurovascular bundle dissection.

Non–nerve-sparing Procedure. If nerve sparing is not considered, the prostatic pedicles are transected far from the prostate and the posterolateral attachments of the prostate are not dissected but simply controlled (using bipolar coagulation or clips) and divided. It is important to remember that the risk of rectal injury becomes higher because the dissection is performed close to the rectum, in the perirectal fat (11).

Fifth Step: Apical Dissection of the Prostate

Division of the Dorsal Venous Complex. The incision of the dorsal venous complex is tangential to the prostate to avoid iatrogenic incision into the anterior aspect of the prostate and the apex. Gradually, the avascular plane of dissection situated between the dorsal venous complex and the urethra is developed to perfectly expose the anterior and lateral urethral walls.

Division of Denonvilliers Fascia. At the apex, the neurovascular bundles are divergent from the prostate but must be followed until their entrance into the pelvic floor, below and lateral to the urethra (Fig. 13D.10). The key element in this dissection is to follow the anatomic contours of the prostate. At the completion of this step, the neurovascular bundles and the rectum are separated away from the prostate. The remainder of Denonvilliers fascia and the rectourethralis muscle fibers are then divided. The only attachment left is the urethra.

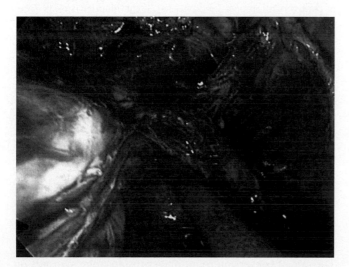

FIGURE 13D.10. Apical dissection of the neurovascular bundle.

Incising the Urethra. The prostate is retracted cephalad and the urethra is sharply incised with laparoscopic scissors. Using the 5-mm laparoscope introduced through a lateral port, the specimen is completely freed and placed in a laparoscopic bag. Through a midline extension of the umbilical incision, the specimen is extracted and macroscopically examined. Frozen sections are obtained if necessary. The umbilical incision is closed around a 10-mm trocar, and the abdomen is reinsufflated. The surgical field is copiously irrigated and hemostasis attained.

Sixth Step: Urethrovesical Anastomosis

It is not necessary to evert the bladder mucosa or to resize the bladder neck. However, in some cases with a large bladder neck, an anterior or posterior tennis-racket reconstruction is required. Throughout this portion of the procedure, the surgeon works with two needle-holders, using a 3-0 resorbable suture with an RB1 needle. All the sutures are tied intracorporeally. The Béniqué helps guide the needle into the urethra. The first three sutures are posterior, placed at the 5, 6, and 7 o'clock positions, going inside-out on the urethra and outside-in on the bladder neck. These sutures are therefore tied intraluminally. Four other sutures are symmetrically placed at 4 and 8 o'clock, then 2 and 10 o'clock, and tied outside the lumen. Three final anterior stitches are placed at the 11, 12 and 1 o'clock positions, going outside-in on the urethra and inside-out on the bladder. Once the sutures are tied, a Foley catheter is inserted. The bladder is filled with 180 mL of saline to ascertain a watertight anastomosis and confirm the correct position of the catheter.

Completing the Operation

The abdominal pressure is lowered to 5 mm Hg, to check for venous bleeding. One or two suction drains are placed, one posterior through the incision of the cul de sac of Douglas, and a second anteriorly in Retzius' space. The 5-mm trocars are removed under visual control and the port sites are checked to exclude any vascular injury, particularly of the epigastric vessels. The incisions are conventionally closed and sterile dressing applied.

Operative Variants

Technical Points

Extraperitoneal Approach. The extraperitoneal approach has been described (12,13) and is currently used by several teams. The theoretical advantages are the absence of peritoneotomy and therefore a decreased risk of bowel injury, peritoneal irritation, and quicker development of Retzius' space. However, the drawbacks are a reduced and less ergonomic working space and a potential for increased tension at the urethrovesical anastomosis due to limited bladder mobilization. Additionally, the extraperitoneal approach does not provide an accurate dissection of the tips of the seminal vesicles, which, given the proximity of the neurovascular bundles, may be relevant if a nerve-sparing approach is planned.

Technique

After an infraumbilical incision, the fascia is incised and the prevesical space is bluntly dissected with a finger. A 10-mm trocar is then inserted; the pressure of the insufflation (12 mm Hg) and the dissecting movements of the tip of the scope complete the development of the space. Once the space is sufficiently opened, the other operative trocars are inserted as previously described.

Other Operative Strategies. Different strategies have been developed. Some start the operation by developing the Retzius' space first, forgoing the posterior dissection of the seminal vesicles (14). Others follow the retrograde retropubic prostatectomy approach (15), mimicking the Walsh technique (16). Laparoscopically, the retrograde approach does not seem to keep the advantage of dissecting in the visual axis.

The Anastomosis. The urethrovesical anastomosis can correctly be done with a running suture (17). A running anastomosis was described with either two hemicircumferential sutures and three intracorporeal knots (17) or with two 6-inch sutures extracorporeally tied together at their ends and running from the 6:30 position to the 12 o'clock position for one and from the 5:30 to the 12 o'clock position for the other. Both sutures are then tied together at the 12 o'clock requiring only one intracorporeal knot (18). There are several pros and cons regarding the different techniques. To summarize, interrupted sutures are theoretically less ischemic, can be done in all situations, do not necessitate the active coordination of the assistant, and are easier to place and tie since the sutures are shorter. On the other hand, during the running anastomosis it is important to maintain proper and constant tension on the suture and to avoid the inadvertent knotting or locking which may jeopardize the quality of the anastomosis. However, only one or three knots are needed. There are no comparative studies evaluating running versus an interrupted anastomosis and the choice of either technique is subject to surgeon's preference and laparoscopic skills.

The Trocars

Other descriptions of laparoscopic radical prostatectomy include a 5-ports technique inserted in a fan array with a 10-mm port at the level of the umbilicus, two 5-mm ports lateral to the right rectus abdominis muscle and a 10-mm and a 12-mm port lateral to the left rectus abdominis muscle (14), or a 6-ports technique inserted in a W-shaped arrangement with a 13-mm port at the level of the umbilicus, a 5-mm port left lateral, 10-mm left medial, 5-mm right lateral, 10-mm right medial, and a 5-mm port right suprapubic (15). In the absence of a robotic arm camera holder, the "fan-shaped" set-up is certainly more adapted, since the assistant holding the camera is not affected by the surgeon's movements. Also, it allows the surgeon to operate seated, using the two trocars in front of him or her. However, this setup is less ergonomic, as the working instruments are not placed in a triangular fashion, which expands the instruments' working range, which is particularly valuable during the urethrovesical anastomosis.

Instrumentation

A variety of instruments can be used during laparoscopic radical prostatectomy. Endovascular staplers can be used to control the prostatic pedicles in a non-nerve sparing procedure (14). Apart from the cost, the major critique is that the rectum can be inadvertently injured.

The use of harmonic scissors has been advocated by some surgeons to theoretically decrease the heat diffusion at the level of the capsular arteries and thus protect the neurovascular bundles from thermal injury. With the same goal, the use of clips to control pedicular vessels has been advocated. No data are presently available to confirm this theoretical advantage over accurate and selective bipolar coagulation. It appears that having an anatomical dissection of all the structures is the best way to avoid possible injury to both nerves and vessels.

The Use of the "Robotics"

Voice-controlled Robotic Arm Camera Holder. The use of a voice-controlled robotic arm camera holder allows the surgeon to control rapidly and safely the optic mobilization (19–21),

and frees the assistant from holding the camera, allowing them to be totally and actively involved in the operation. It is practically impossible to manually hold the camera without any shaking or inadvertent contact with the tissue. Subjectively, there may be less smudging and fogging of the laparoscope. Finally, the robotic arm ensures excellent stability of the image that avoids the stress and tiredness of the surgeon when he or she has to control any involuntary movement of his or her assistant.

Remote-controlled Laparoscopic Surgery. The use of remote device to perform laparoscopic radical prostatectomies has been demonstrated and confirmed by several teams (22–24). The advantages are not yet demonstrated and are still debatable. A sub-chapter in this textbook is dedicated to this topic (See Chapter 13E).

Postoperative Care

Analgesics

The usual analgesic protocol consists of intravenous morphine sulfate or equivalent in the postanesthesia care unit and intravenous ketorolac tromethamine started immediately postoperatively and given on a scheduled basis for the first 24 to 48 hours while the patient is hospitalized. Patients are discharged on oral cyclo-oxygenase-2 inhibitors and oral analgesics for breakthrough pain. Major analgesics are rarely necessary and should raise the suspicion for postoperative complications.

Nutrition

Oral intake is usually resumed the evening of surgery starting with a clear liquid diet and advanced to regular diet on the first postoperative day. Intravenous perfusion is stopped when oral intake is well tolerated, usually between the 12th and the 24th hour after the operation.

Anti-thrombosis Care

It is necessary to emphasize the importance of thromboprophylaxis based on low molecular weight heparin and early ambulation.

Bladder Catheter Removal

There is no set time for catheter removal. The reported mean duration of catheterization in the Montsouris experience was 5.8 days (25). The group from Creteil reported a mean bladder catheterization of 5.7 days and 4 days in another report by Nadu et al. (26,27). In the Heidelberg series, the reported period of catheterization was 13 days (28). If the bladder neck is "preserved," and if the anastomosis is watertight during the operation, the catheter can be removed as early as the third day after surgery. However, this practice is associated with an increased risk of acute urinary retention and anastomotic leakage. Therefore, our practice is to remove the catheter between the fifth and the seventh postoperative day, without cystogram, depending on the surgeon's intraoperative assessment of the quality of the anastomosis as well as the patient's postoperative course. In our last 200 patients, the average duration of catheterization was 7 days. If the quality of the anastomosis is uncertain, the bladder drainage should be prolonged. In this situation, a cystogram is necessary to assess the anastomotic healing status.

TECHNICAL FEASIBILITY

Surgical Conversion

The rate of conversion to an open prostatectomy depends on the surgeon's experience and technical skills. In the published series from Montsouris, 12 of the first 50 and two of the next 50 patients were converted to open surgery, and no conversions occurred in the following 467 patients (25). Many other teams report a similar experience (29,30). The main causes of conversion are either hemorrhage rendering the visualization of the surgical field unsafe or failure to progress.

Intraoperative complications are mainly due to hemorrhage from the Santorini venous plexus. In this event, vascular control should be attempted by compressing the plexus with a clamp or by momentarily increasing the intraperitoneal pressure to 15 or even 20 mm Hg and to place a new ligature. If hemostasis seems impossible and if the decision to convert is made, it is always possible to compress the plexus with a clamp.

Other sources of surgical difficulty include locally advanced prostate cancer, prior hormonal therapy where the prostate is of a reduced size with ill defined surgical borders, and a history of prostatic surgery (e.g., transurethral resection of the prostate or suprapubic prostatectomy). These should be considered preoperatively and a decision regarding the appropriate surgical approach made.

Finally it is important to complete a correct and watertight urethrovesical anastomosis. When this cannot be achieved, a minilaparotomy must be done to perform the anastomosis in the conventional way.

The patient needs to be informed beforehand that there is always a risk for an open surgical conversion, although the conversion rate decreases with experience. There will always be difficult cases for which laparoscopic surgery cannot be completed. One must keep in mind that the surgical benefit is for the patient and that the key word is safety; if this means conversion to a conventional retropubic approach, there must be no hesitation.

Operative Time

LRP requires advanced laparoscopic skills and excellent anatomical knowledge. At the end of the operation, the anastomosis is a critical surgical step, technically demanding, time consuming, and it determines the quality of the postoperative results. Obviously, with experience surgical time decreases. At present, the mean operative time reported by different teams is around 200 minutes, which is more or less comparable to the operative time required for the retropubic procedure (10, 15,31,32).

SPECIFIC COMPLICATIONS

In large series of LRP, the overall incidence of procedure-related complications varies from 17% to 19% and continues to decrease with experience (15,25). In a comprehensive description of the incidence and the severity of complications following 567 consecutive LRP, the Montsouris group reported a total, major, and minor complication rate of 17%, 4%, and 14.6%, respectively.

Hemorrhage

The Dorsal Venous Complex

It is essential to remember that a laparoscopic procedure cannot be continued in case of bleeding, as hemorrhage interferes considerably with vision and makes the operation uncertain and dangerous. A laparoscopic surgeon should pay careful attention to any bleeder before moving to the next step of the operation, as hemostasis and hence visibility is paramount to the progression of a controlled and anatomically safe dissection. The laparoscopic approach provides a dramatic decrease in intraoperative bleeding compared to open surgery. In our recent experience, the mean intraoperative blood loss was 336 mL (range, 100–1100 mL) with a less than 2% transfusion rate. There is no doubt that the pneumoperitoneum, set at 12 mm Hg, helps to collapse small veins, but the dramatic magnification and the visual accessibility to the operative field plays an important role by allowing the surgeon to distinguish anatomical details that are not at the scale of open surgery. In the various series, intraoperative bleeding averages less than 500 mL, and the transfusion rate is less than 5% (29–31,33). The hemorrhagic risk is greatest at the dorsal venous complex and the prostatic pedicles during nerve-sparing procedures.

The Epigastric Vessels Injury

The inferior epigastric vessels are at risk during port placement for LRP, particularly at the pararectus site. Transillumination to locate the epigastric vessels is not helpful, and this complication should always be suspected, leading to a fundamental rule of laparoscopic surgery that all the trocars should be removed under direct vision with a decreased abdominal pressure. Such injury requires surgical hemostasis using resorbable suture, placed either with a Reverdin or a Carter–Thomason needle. This complication often goes unreported and the true incidence is unknown. In our recent experience it occurred in three patients, two of whom required blood transfusion because the injury was unrecognized despite the usual precautions.

Bowel Complications

Rectal Injury

The reported incidence of intraoperative rectal injury in patients undergoing LRP ranges from less than 1% to 2.7% (15,29). In the Montsouris experience of 1000 LRP, rectal injury was noted in 13 patients and repaired primarily in 11; in the remaining two patients, the diagnosis was made postoperatively and required reoperation and temporary colostomy; the majority of rectal injuries occurred during non-nerve sparing prostatectomy (11). In the Creteil experience of 300 LRP, six rectal injuries were reported. One patient developed a rectourethral fistula treated by a diverting colostomy (34). Rassweiller et al. reported three rectal injuries and seven rectal fistulas in a series of 438 LRP. All of the rectal injuries occurred in the first 219 patients (28).

Two types of rectal injuries should be distinguished. The first is a rectal tear, which most commonly occurs during the dissection of the posterior surface of the prostatic apex, often recognized intraoperatively, and the second is diagnosed postoperatively after the patient develops a rectourethral fistula. The latter is secondary to either a microperforation or a thermal or ischemic injury to the anterior rectal wall during a vigorous dissection.

While opinions on early postoperative care (e.g., antibiotics, low-fiber diet, anal dilatation, and cystogram prior to Foley catheter removal) are similar, management of the rectal injury itself remains debatable in regard to interposition of healthy tissue between the rectal repair and the urethrovesical anastomosis and the need for a diverting colostomy. In the absence of gross fecal soiling, it is acceptable to repair the defect with a two-layer primary closure after debridement of any devitalized tissue. While interposition of an omental flap or pararectal fat flap provides extra safety, it is routinely not necessary. However, in face of a large, devitalized rectal laceration or gross soiling, a temporary diverting colostomy is advisable. In difficult cases due to surgeon's inexperience, inflamed prostate, large-volume gland with a narrow pelvis, and during non–nerve sparing LRP, a meticulous dissection and the use of either intrarectal digital manipulation—rectal bougie or balloon—may become indispensable while incising Denonvilliers fascia and dissecting the posterior surface of the prostate.

The incidence of postoperative rectourethral fistulas is unknown. The reported cases of rectourethral fistulas following LRP were successfully treated by a diverting colostomy and prolonged bladder drainage (15), but if primary healing is not achieved, surgical closure should be considered.

Ileus

Postoperative ileus following LRP has been reported in 1% of the cases and managed conservatively. In our experience, prior abdominal surgery, intraoperative or postoperative blood loss, or operative time were not found to be significant risk factors (25). Minimal anastomotic urine leakage is a more likely the cause. Moreover, in face of an ileus, even non-febrile, an unrecognized bowel injury needs to be considered.

Urologic Complications

Bladder Injury

Bladder injury rarely occurs during LRP. When it does occur, it is usually during the division of the urachus and the development of the retropubic space. The reported incidence of bladder injury in the literature is 1.38% (25). All injuries were identified and repaired intraoperatively in a two layer closure, and bladder drainage was maintained for at least 7 days.

Ureter Injury

Ureteral complications are unusual during LRP. The reported incidence is 0.7% (25). They occur either during the dissection of the seminal vesicles by mistakenly identifying the ureter as a vas deferens or by inadvertent thermal injury. Another reported ureteral complication is a postoperative anuria caused by incorporating the ureteral orifices in the urethrovesical anastomotic sutures.

When the injury is not identified intraoperatively, a persistent urine leakage or uroperitoneum with a watertight anastomosis suggests the diagnosis. The treatment consists of a ureteral reimplantation. It is essential to identify the vas deferens based on its relationship with the seminal vesicle, from which it is separated by a large deferential artery. If the identification is difficult, the vas is easily approached more laterally as it crosses the iliac vessels and tracked down to the level of the seminal vesicle.

Urinary Leak

The true incidence of anastomotic leakage is uncertain, as most small leaks remain undiagnosed and resolve spontaneously with bladder drainage. The reported incidence of anastomotic leak following LRP ranges from 1% to 10% (25,30). An increased and prolonged urine output from the pelvic drain suggests the diagnosis. Confirmation by cystogram is often unnecessary. In the majority of the cases, this involves the posterior aspect of the anastomosis and is managed conservatively by prolonging the bladder drainage. After a transperitoneal LRP, severe leak is usually manifested by back pain, uroperitoneum, and ileus with laboratory signs of intraperitoneal urine reabsorption. If the leak persists despite conservative treatment, a ureteral injury should be ruled out. To prevent the leak, posterior approximation of the bladder to the urethra is essential and should be carefully performed.

Anastomotic Stricture

The anastomotic stricture rate after LRP varies from 0% to 3.3% (15,25,32). This lower incidence may be attributed to a tension-free anastomosis achieved by the bladder mobilization during transperitoneal LRP.

Complication Specific to Pelvic Lymph Node Dissection

Obturator Nerve Injury

One patient developed a partial obturator nerve paralysis, probably secondary to a thermal injury. This paralysis resolved spontaneously without any sequel in less than 6 months.

Lymphoceles

Lymphoceles are a common complication of the pelvic lymph node dissection, even after a transperitoneal approach. The incidence of lymphocele after radical prostatectomy is difficult to assess, as most remain asymptomatic and resolve spontaneously. Salomon et al. reported two cases of lymphorrhea treated by prolonged drainage (26). Most of the time lymphoceles are asymptomatic; however, in case of infection or compression to the adjacent organs a percutaneous or laparoscopic drainage is warranted.

ONCOLOGIC RESULTS

Oncologic results are based on pathologic examination of the operative specimen and biological nonprogression. Since there are no prospective randomized, controlled studies comparing LRP to other treatment modalities of prostate cancer, and, overall, the oncologic follow-up is too short, no definitive conclusion about the oncological efficacy of LRP can be made.

Pathologic Evaluation

Oncological efficacy following radical prostatectomy is measured by the rate of positive surgical margins, biochemical recurrence, and cancer-specific survival.

Positive Surgical Margin Rate

A positive surgical margin (PSM) is defined as presence of cancer at the inked margin of resection in the prostatectomy specimen. A PSM results from either an iatrogenic incision into the prostate, a transection through cancer in an area of extracapsular extension, or cancer extending to the edge of the surgical specimen (35). The first type of PSM is related to a technical error rather than the biologic nature of the disease. The prognostic significance of a PSM is a higher risk of biochemical, local, and systemic progression (36,37). The positive surgical margin rate following LRP varies widely among series, depending on the population selected, the experience of the surgeon, and the pathologist. The positive surgical margin rate ranges from 11.4% to 26.4% (31,38). In the series of 1000 consecutive LRP from Montsouris, the PSM rate was 19.2% overall, 15.4% in pT2, and 31% in pT3 (39). In a recent experience of 100 consecutive patients operated on at MSKCC, the PSM rate is 9%, 3.4% for pT2, 21% for pT3, and 66% for pT4 tumors. The number, site, and extent of PSM was shown to adversely impact the prognosis of prostate cancer treated surgically (36,37,40,41). In published LRP series, PSM at the apex predominate (37.8%–58%), followed by the posterolateral site (10.5%–30%). However, in the contemporary series from MSKCC, PSM at the mid- and posterolateral sites predominate, 40% and 45% respectively. The apex was involved in 25% of the cases.

Biochemical Evaluation

Having only been performed within the past 6 years, long-term progression-free probability data after LRP is unavailable. However, in the published short-term follow-up of the first 1000 LRP performed at the Montsouris Institute between 1998 and 2002, the 3-year actuarial progression-free probability was 90.5%, with progression defined as a prostate-specific antigen (PSA) greater than 0.1 ng/mL and a median follow-up period of 12 months. According to the pathological stage, the biochemical progression free survival at 3 years was 91.8% for pT2a N0/Nx, 88% for pT2b N0/Nx, 77% for pT3a N0/Nx, 44% for pT3b N0/Nx, and 50% for pT1-3N1 (P <.001). The importance of the surgical margin status was found in the laparoscopic group with 94% progression-free survival for patients with negative surgical margins and 80% in case of positive margins (P <.001). This analysis indicated that preoperative PSA, pathological stage, surgical margin status, and Gleason score in the radical prostatectomy specimens all had significant impact on cancer recurrence. The data regarding the prognostic factors in the laparoscopic series are similar to those previously published in studying the open retropubic approach. This suggests that the pathologic characteristics of the surgical specimens are comparable, and the chance of definitive cure by the two techniques should be similar. In the author's experience, including the Montsouris and MSKCC patients, the actuarial progression-free probability at 3 years is 88% for pT2 [95% confidence interval (CI), 83%–93%], 73% for pT3a (95% CI, 57%–88%), and 47% for pT3b (95% CI, 36%–62%), with a median follow-up of 12 months (Fig. 13D.11).

Clinical Evaluation

The question of an additional oncological risk related to the laparoscopic route is controversial but needs to be considered. The majority of tumors operated on are intracapsular organ-confined tumors, which are therefore not exposed to the pneumoperitoneum, and which can have little or no risk of

dissemination. The risk of cutaneous tumor seeding is probably very low in view of the number of laparoscopic radical prostatectomies performed for prostate cancer throughout the world and for which no such case has been reported (42).

URINARY FUNCTION

The literature assessing the functional results following radical prostatectomy is marked by a lack of uniformity in the definitions used and the methodology by which the data is gathered and analyzed. The patient, the surgeon, and the assessment tools are all sources of subjectivity and bias. These hindrances are best alleviated by the use of validated questionnaires, administered by a third party (43). In interpreting the published data of laparoscopic radical prostatectomy, two problems emerge: the follow-up is short and the continuous improvements in the technique create a heterogeneous patient population, particularly the first patients in each experience.

Urinary function in 507 patients treated at Montsouris, with a minimum follow-up of 12 months, was assessed by the International Continence Society male questionnaire filled out confidentially by the patients every 6 months following surgery and reviewed by a research specialist. Patients were considered continent when they did not require any protection. Patients who used pad(s) even for only a few drops were considered incontinent. At 12 months after laparoscopic radical prostatectomy, 79% of patients ($n = 401$) recovered complete urinary control and 92% of patients ($n = 466$) were either totally continent or using only one pad per day. Median time to achieve continence was 1.5 months (range, 1–18). Patients younger than 70 years were more likely to achieve total urinary control than older patients (P <.001). Clinical and pathologic tumor stage ($P = .8$ and $P = .7$, respectively), preoperative PSA ($P = .2$), prior surgery for benign prostatic hyperplasia [transurethral prostatectomy (TURP) or suprapubic prostatectomy] ($P = .4$), and the development of an early anastomotic leak ($P = .2$) did not influence the postoperative continence status. Neither surgical technique used, with or without puboprostatic ligaments preservation, nor the quality of neurovascular bundle preservation, affected the continence recovery or time to achieve continence. Difficulty of the surgery was assessed by blood loss, patient body mass index, and specimen weight. Specimen weight was the only significant factor associated with postoperative incontinence ($P = .02$). In a review of the continence rate at 3 months following laparoscopic radical

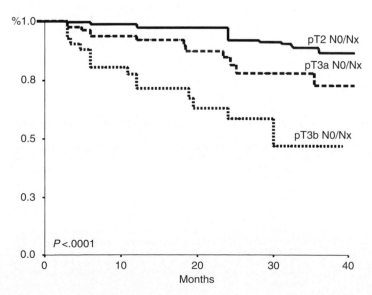

FIGURE 13D.11. Percentage of biochemical progression–free survival (PSA >0.1 ng/mL) according to pathologic stage.

prostatectomy in the patients treated with LRP at MSKCC, 48% were totally continent, and 27% had a mild stress urinary incontinence requiring a pad occasionally or no more than one pad every 24 hours.

SEXUAL FUNCTION

The evaluation of potency is a very difficult task. No evaluation scale is really appropriate to evaluate a function that varies with time and is affected by a variety of factors.

The nerve-sparing technique is now performed in every case where it is functionally important and oncologically feasible without risk for the patient.

Interposition sural nerve grafting during radical prostatectomy provides a potential pathway to restore autonomic innervation and offers men an increased possibility of recovery of spontaneous erections (44). Turk et al. demonstrated the technical feasibility of sural nerve grafting laparoscopically (45). Between 2000 and 2002, 116 patients with a mean age of 59 years (range, 44–70) and with normal preoperative erectile function were selected for nerve sparing procedure and assessed postoperatively with self-questionnaire. The rate of erection obtained without any medical help ranges from 60% to 80%, and the rate of sexual intercourse, achieved eventually with the assistance of oral drugs, ranges from 33% to 74%, for unilateral and bilateral nerve sparing surgery, respectively. Among the 92 patients with bilateral preservation of the vascular bundle, 52% recovered potency in the first 3 months allowing satisfactory intercourse. Some others series confirmed equivalent rates when bilateral nerve sparing was technically successful (26,29).

Since sexual preservation is a critical point, hopefully this rate will improve with time and the quality of erections will allow patients to resume a satisfactory sexual life. Evaluation of potency in the MSKCC experience showed that at 3 months 75% of the patients were having erections and 37.5% were able to have intercourse with or without oral therapy. In the subset of preoperatively fully potent patients with bilateral nerve preservation, 54% are able to have intercourse with or without oral agents versus 33% after unilateral preservation. This experience supports the fact that anatomical and functional nerve-sparing surgery is technically feasible through a laparoscopic approach with satisfactory results.

CONCLUSION

Laparoscopic radical prostatectomy is a treatment modality of clinically localized prostate cancer. It requires advanced laparoscopic skills, knowledge of the prostatic anatomy, and expertise in surgical oncology. Laparoscopy offers the benefit of low perioperative morbidity, short convalescence, and a magnified vision of the surgical field allowing an accurate dissection. These benefits should theoretically translate to an improvement in postoperative quality of life, mainly continence and erectile function. But most importantly, these advantages are supported by equivalent short-term oncological outcomes compared to open retropubic radical prostatectomy. If confirmed on larger well-designed clinical trials, the above benefits would make laparoscopy the approach of choice to perform an effective and less morbid radical prostatectomy.

ACKNOWLEDGMENT

Dr. Karim Touijer is supported by NIH Grant T32-82088.

References

1. Hull GW, Rabbani F, Abbas F, et al. Cancer control with radical prostatectomy alone in 1,000 consecutive patients. *J Urol* 2002;167:528–534.
2. Han M, Partin AW, Piantadosi S, et al. Era specific biochemical recurrence-free survival following radical prostatectomy for clinically localized prostate cancer. *J Urol* 2001;166:416–419.
3. Catalona WJ, Smith DS. Cancer recurrence and survival rates after anatomic radical retropubic prostatectomy for prostate cancer: intermediate-term results. *J Urol* 1998;160:2428–2434.
4. Eastham JA, Kattan MW, Rogers E, et al. Risk factors for urinary incontinence after radical prostatectomy. *J Urol* 1996;156:1707–1713.
5. Goad JR, Eastham JA, Fitzgerald KB, et al. Radical retropubic prostatectomy: limited benefit of autologous blood donation. *J Urol* 1995;154:2103–2109.
6. Steiner MS, Morton RA, Walsh PC. Impact of anatomical radical prostatectomy on urinary continence. *J Urol* 1991;145:512–514; discussion 514-515.
7. Schuessler WW, Schulam PG, Clayman RV, et al. Laparoscopic radical prostatectomy: initial short-term experience. *Urology* 1997;50:854–857.
8. Guillonneau B, Cathelineau X, Barret E, et al. [Laparoscopic radical prostatectomy. Preliminary evaluation after 28 interventions]. *Presse Med* 1998;27:1570–1574.
9. Kattan MW, Eastham JA, Stapleton AM, et al. A preoperative nomogram for disease recurrence following radical prostatectomy for prostate cancer. *J Natl Cancer Inst* 1998;90:766–771.
10. Guillonneau B, Vallancien G. Laparoscopic radical prostatectomy: initial experience and preliminary assessment after 65 operations. *Prostate* 1999;39:71–75.
11. Guillonneau B, Gupta R, El Fettouh H, et al. Laparoscopic [correction of laproscopic] management of rectal injury during laparoscopic [correction of laproscopic] radical prostatectomy. *J Urol* 2003;169:1694–1696.
12. Bollens R, Vanden Bossche M, Roumeguere T, et al. Extraperitoneal laparoscopic radical prostatectomy. Results after 50 cases. *Eur Urol* 2001;40:65–69.
13. Raboy A, Ferzli G, Albert P. Initial experience with extraperitoneal endoscopic radical retropubic prostatectomy. *Urology* 1997;50:849–853.
14. Gill IS, Zippe CD. Laparoscopic radical prostatectomy: technique. *Urol Clin North Am* 2001;28:423–436.
15. Rassweiler J, Sentker L, Seemann O, et al. Laparoscopic radical prostatectomy with the Heilbronn technique: an analysis of the first 180 cases. *J Urol* 2001;166:2101–2108.
16. Walsh PC, Lepor H. The role of radical prostatectomy in the management of prostatic cancer. *Cancer* 1987;60:526–537.
17. Hoznek A, Salomon L, Rabii R, et al. Vesicourethral anastomosis during laparoscopic radical prostatectomy: the running suture method. *J Endourol* 2000;14:749–753.
18. Van Velthoven RF, Ahlering TE, Peltier A, et al. Technique for laparoscopic running urethrovesical anastomosis: the single knot method. *Urology* 2003;61:699–702.
19. Jacobs LK, Shayani V, Sackier JM. Determination of the learning curve of the AESOP robot. *Surg Endosc* 1997;11:54–55.
20. Merola S, Weber P, Wasielewski A, et al. Comparison of laparoscopic colectomy with and without the aid of a robotic camera holder. *Surg Laparosc Endosc Percutan Tech* 2002;12:46–51.
21. Hubens G, Ysebaert D, Vaneerdeweg W, et al. Laparoscopic adrenalectomy with the aid of the AESOP 2000 robot. *Acta Chir Belg* 1999;99:125–127; discussion 127-129.
22. Abbou CC, Hoznek A, Salomon L, et al. Laparoscopic radical prostatectomy with a remote controlled robot. *J Urol* 2001;165:1964–1966.
23. Pasticier G, Rietbergen JB, Guillonneau B, et al. Robotically assisted laparoscopic radical prostatectomy: feasibility study in men. *Eur Urol* 2001;40:70–74.
24. Tewari A, Peabody J, Sarle R, et al. Technique of da Vinci robot-assisted anatomic radical prostatectomy. *Urology* 2002;60:569–572.
25. Guillonneau B, Rozet F, Cathelineau X, et al. Perioperative complications of laparoscopic radical prostatectomy: the Montsouris 3-year experience. *J Urol* 2002;167:51–56.
26. Katz R, Salomon L, Hoznek A, et al. Patient reported sexual function following laparoscopic radical prostatectomy. *J Urol* 2002;168:2078–2082.
27. Nadu A, Salomon L, Hoznek A, et al. Early removal of the catheter after laparoscopic radical prostatectomy. *J Urol* 2001;166:1662–1664.
28. Rassweiler J, Seemann O, Schulze M, et al. Laparoscopic versus open radical prostatectomy: a comparative study at a single institution. *J Urol* 2003;169:1689–1693.
29. Eden CG, Cahill D, Vass JA, et al. Laparoscopic radical prostatectomy: the initial UK series. *BJU Int* 2002;90:876–882.
30. Hoznek A, Salomon L, Olsson LE, et al. Laparoscopic radical prostatectomy. The Creteil experience. *Eur Urol* 2001;40:38–45.
31. Dahl DM, L'Esperance JO, Trainer AF, et al. Laparoscopic radical prostatectomy: initial 70 cases at a U.S. university medical center. *Urology* 2002;60:859–863.
32. Turk I, Deger S, Winkelmann B, et al. Laparoscopic radical prostatectomy. Technical aspects and experience with 125 cases. *Eur Urol* 2001;40:46–52; discussion 53.

33. Guillonneau B, Vallancien G. Laparoscopic radical prostatectomy: the Montsouris technique. *J Urol* 2000;163:1643–1649.
34. Katz R, Borkowski T, Hoznek A, et al. Operative management of rectal injuries during laparoscopic radical prostatectomy. *Urology* 2003;62:310–313.
35. Wieder JA, Soloway MS. Incidence, etiology, location, prevention and treatment of positive surgical margins after radical prostatectomy for prostate cancer. *J Urol* 1998;160:299–315.
36. Sofer M, Hamilton-Nelson KL, Civantos F, et al. Positive surgical margins after radical retropubic prostatectomy: the influence of site and number on progression. *J Urol* 2002;167:2453–2456.
37. Epstein JI, Pizov G, Walsh PC. Correlation of pathologic findings with progression after radical retropubic prostatectomy. *Cancer* 1993;71:3582–3593.
38. Salomon L, Levrel O, de la Taille A, et al. [Localization of positive surgical margins after retropubic, perineal and laparoscopic radical prostatectomy]. *Prog Urol* 2002;12:628–634.
39. Guillonneau B, el-Fettouh H, Baumert H, et al. Laparoscopic radical prostatectomy: oncological evaluation after 1,000 cases at Montsouris Institute. *J Urol* 2003;169:1261–1266.
40. Watson RB, Civantos F, Soloway MS. Positive surgical margins with radical prostatectomy: detailed pathological analysis and prognosis. *Urology* 1996;48:80–90.
41. Blute ML, Bostwick DG, Bergstralh EJ, et al. Anatomic site-specific positive margins in organ-confined prostate cancer and its impact on outcome after radical prostatectomy. *Urology* 1997;50:733–739.
42. Bangma CH, Kirkels WJ, Chadha S, et al. Cutaneous metastasis following laparoscopic pelvic lymphadenectomy for prostatic carcinoma. *J Urol* 1995;153:1635–1636.
43. Sebesta M, Cespedes RD, Luhman E, et al. Questionnaire-based outcomes of urinary incontinence and satisfaction rates after radical prostatectomy in a national study population. *Urology* 2002;60:1055–1058.
44. Kim ED, Nath R, Kadmon D, et al. Bilateral nerve graft during radical retropubic prostatectomy: 1-year followup. *J Urol* 2001;165:1950–1956.
45. Turk IA, Deger S, Morgan WR, et al. Sural nerve graft during laparoscopic radical prostatectomy. Initial experience. *Urol Oncol* 2002;7:191–194.

CHAPTER 13E
Robot-assisted Radical Prostatectomy

Peter N. Wiklund and Stefan Carllson

INTRODUCTION

Radical prostatectomy is an effective treatment for patients with localized prostate cancer. However, many men with untreated prostate cancer do not die from the disease, but if operated on, they may suffer from a loss of potency and/or incontinence due to the surgical procedure. The fact that several patients are subjected to surgery without benefit in survival is in itself a challenge. This challenge is enhanced, however, by the morbidity caused by the radical prostatectomy. There will be a need to find treatments with less morbidity for patients with localized prostate cancer. The search for less morbidity has led to the development of minimally invasive surgical procedures such as laparoscopic and robot-assisted prostatectomy. Several centers have published relatively large series on the use of laparoscopic prostatectomy in the treatment of localized prostate cancer, whereas only limited experience is at hand regarding robot-assisted prostatectomy. There is still a controversy on whether the patients will benefit from these minimally invasive procedures compared with open surgery (1). Laparoscopic radical prostatectomy is a demanding procedure that requires a long learning curve and vast laparoscopic experience. In the original series described by Schuessler et al. (2) the long operative times and the associated complications reported were a limit of the technique until 1999, when the

technical improvements allowed shorter operating times and fewer complications (3,4).

Recently, robots have been introduced to assist in the development of minimally invasive prostate cancer surgery. The term "robot-assisted surgery" in prostate cancer treatment usually refers to the use of the da Vinci robot (Fig. 13E.1) from Intuitive Surgical, Inc. in Sunnyvale, CA. However, a true robot is an enslaved device under human control that accomplishes its assignment without human assistance. This is not the case for the use of the da Vinci robot because it requires the surgeon to guide every movement performed by the robot. Nevertheless, the terms "robotic" and "robot-assisted surgery" are used in this chapter to describe when surgeons perform radical prostatectomy with computer-enhanced master-slave telemanipulators (5). This master-slave system offers three-dimensional (3-D) visualization, wristed instrumentation, intuitive finger-controlled movements, and ergonomic seating position for the surgeon. These features have been suggested to translate into a more easily learned prostatectomy than the laparoscopic approach (6). Our experience at Karolinska Hospital, Stockholm, Sweden, would agree with this notion. We started a robot-assisted prostatectomy program in January 2002. Two urologists with extensive experience in open retropubic prostatectomy, but without any laparoscopic experience, were started on a training program. The first robot-assisted prostatectomy was completed in less than 5 hours, suggesting that the use of the robot system greatly improved the learning curve compared to conventional laparoscopy (Fig. 13E.2). The operating time can be lowered to around 2 hours, allowing for 2 to 3 procedures during a normal working day if theater turnover can be kept to less than 1.5 hours (7).

SURGICAL TECHNIQUE

There is no need for a modification of the surgical approach with the robotic technique compared to conventional laparoscopy. However, the wristed (Endowrist) instruments enable the surgeon to dissect with ease around corners and angles, allowing better preservation of the neurovascular bundles and a more precise dissection than with straight laparoscopy or with open surgery. The 3-D and 10x magnification visualization system and the good eye-hand coordination enabled by the robotic system are also important advantages for the surgeon who is learning the technique of minimally invasive prostatectomy. It seems clear that surgeons with extensive experience in open radical prostatectomy surgery will benefit from these features. A potential disadvantage of robot technology is the lack of tactile sensation, but the 3-D visualization allows the surgeon to compensate for this drawback. Both the transperitoneal and the extraperitoneal approach can be used. The extraperitoneal route may decrease the number of intestinal complications, whereas the intraperitoneal approach may decrease the intraoperative bleeding. However, the complication rate is low regardless of the route used, and the most familiar approach for the surgeon should probably be used. As for all laparoscopic operations, optimal preparations are necessary when robot-assisted surgery is scheduled. Thus, training of the team, patient selection, set up of the robot, patient positioning, port placements, instrument choice, and surgical technique must all be considered. The operating surgeon is seated at the console and does not scrub (Fig. 13E.1). One of the robotic arms controls the binocular endoscope, and the other arms control the robotic instruments (Fig. 13E.1). Two finger-controlled handles (called "masters") control the robotic arms and camera. Manipulation of the masters is transmitted to a computer that filters, scales, and relays the surgeon's movements to the robotic

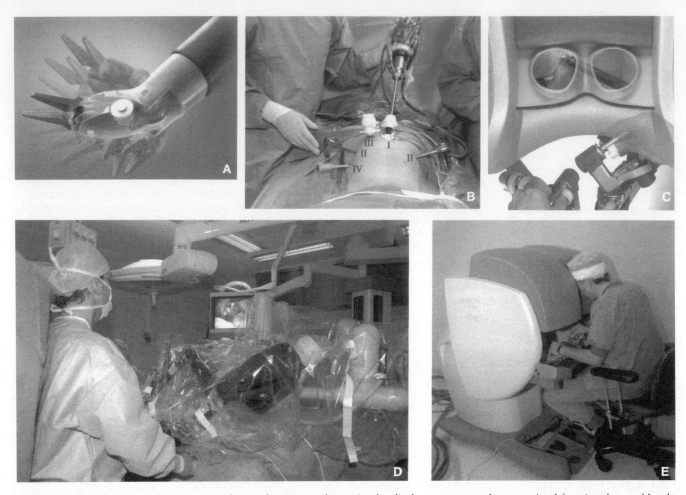

FIGURE 13E.1. The robotic instruments used in performing a robot-assisted radical prostatectomy have a wristed function that enables the surgeon to dissect with ease around corners and angles (**A**). Positioning of the five ports used during robot-assisted prostatectomy (**B**). Finger-controlled handles (masters), which control the robotic arms and camera (**C**). The assistant surgeon and the cart with surgical arms holding the camera and instruments (**D**). Surgeon's console (**E**).

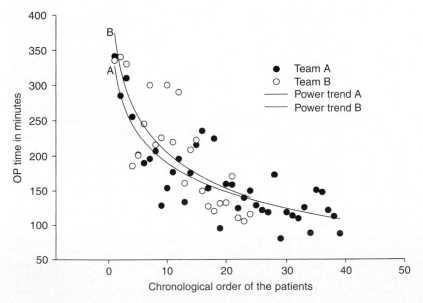

FIGURE 13E.2. Operative times for two surgeons performing robot-assisted prostatectomy at the Karolinska Hospital, Stockholm, Sweden. Note that the learning curve is almost horizontal after only 20 procedures, indicating a procedure that is relatively easy to learn.

arms and instruments. This scaling allows for finer and more precise execution of the operation, and tremor is eliminated.

The patient is placed in a Trendelenburg position with adequate padding of the pressure points by use of gel pads. At our hospital, 5 ports are placed for this operation. A 12-mm port is placed at the umbilicus for introduction of the binocular scope. The remaining ports are placed under camera control to visualize the abdominal wall. Two 8-mm ports are used for the robotic instrument arms, placed 9–10 cm on both sides of the midline on a line joining the anterosuperior iliac spine to the umbilicus. Two additional ports are introduced in the right side for use by the assistant surgeon. The lateral one is a 5-mm port, and the medial one is a 10-mm port. It takes approximately 30 minutes from introduction of the first port to the actual beginning of surgery at our institution. Conventional laparoscopic instruments are used by the assistant surgeon and include an atraumatic grasper, scissors, intracorporeal clips, and suction. We perform the dissection using two robotic instruments: bipolar forceps (left hand) and round-tip scissors (right hand). A needle driver is used during the anastomosis. A detailed description of the technique of da Vinci robot-assisted prostatectomy has been presented (8).

CLINICAL OUTCOME

It is clear that robot-assisted prostatectomy reduces bleeding and postoperative pain compared with open retropubic prostatectomy (Table 13E.1). This may translate into earlier discharge from the hospital. In Menon's series, 95% of the patients were discharged within 24 hours (7). We have similar data from our institution; most patients were discharged the day after surgery. In a majority of conventional laparoscopic prostatectomy series, the patients have been hospitalized for several days after surgery. This difference may be due in part to the fact that in straight laparoscopy, the surgical procedure is longer lasting, but it could also be related to other factors such as an insurance system that does not give financial incentives toward discharging patients early, or the patients wish to remain in the hospital until the catheter is removed (9).

CANCER CONTROL

Several studies have shown good results regarding cancer control when conventional laparoscopy has been used (11–14). However, the number of patients with positive margins is likely a combination of the pathologic tumor stage and the surgical technique. The more pT3 patients, the more positive margins are found in the laparoscopy series, which is not different as compared to open prostatectomy series. Menon et al. have published excellent results on cancer control in their series on robot-assisted prostatectomy (10). However, the status regarding positive margins is controversial in this study because a different approach has been used in the detection of positive margins compared with open surgery (Table 13E.1). Positive margins were assessed by intraoperative distal biopsies in the apical region. In our series, 24% of the patients showed positive margins; most of these were detected dorsolaterally, in the area of the neurovascular bundle. It is unclear if the 3-D and 10x magnification visual system and the improved eye-hand coordination enabled by the robot system will improve cancer control, but the results do not appear inferior to open surgery (Table 13E.1).

URINARY CONTROL

The risk of incontinence following open retropubic radical prostatectomy varies widely, from 5% to 10% when reported by surgeons from large series and from 20% to 30% when patients were evaluated by questionnaire (15). Menon's group are reporting excellent results on continence rate and found that patients achieved continence much quicker after robot-assisted prostatectomy than after open surgery (10). In our series at

TABLE 13E.1

PUBLISHED EXPERIENCE ON ROBOT-ASSISTED PROSTATECTOMY COMPARED TO RETROPUBIC RADICAL PROSTATECTOMY AND LAPAROSCOPIC RADICAL PROSTATECTOMY

	LRP	RARP	KHRAP	RRP	VIP
No. patients	40	40	30	100	200
Mean preoperative PSA (ng/mL)	6.9	5.7	7.7	7.3	6.4
Mean operating time	258	274	191	163	160
Estimated blood loss	391	256	217	910	153
No. discharge home less than 24 hr (%)	26 (65)	32 (80)	15 (50)	0	186 (93)
No. Pathological Stage (%)					
pT2	92.5	82.5	75	93	87
pT3	7.5	17.5	25	7	13
Mean postoperative gleason score	6.8	6.8	6.1	6.6	6.9
Pos. margins (%)					
Focal	12.5	12.5	7	15	5
Extensive	12.5	5	17	8	1
Totals	25	17.5	24	23	6

LRP, Laparoscopic radical prostatectomy; RARP, Robot-assisted radical prostatectomy; RRP, Retropubic radical prostatectomy; VIP, Vattikuti Institute Prostatectomy.
From Menon M, Shrivastava A, Tewari A, et al. Laparoscopic and robot assisted radical prostatectomy: establishment of a structured program and preliminary analysis of outcomes. *J Urol* 2002;168:945–949; First 40 patients at Henry Ford Hospital, Detroit, Mich. *Robot-assisted radical prostatectomy, Karolinska Hospital, Stockholm (KHRAP), Sweden; first 30 patients*; Robot-assisted prostatectomy (VIP) 200 patients; Tewari A, Srivasatava A, Menon M, et al. A prospective comparison of radical retropubic and robot-assisted prostatectomy: experience in one institution. *BJU International* 2003;92:205–210, with permission.

the Karolinska Hospital, we evaluated continence by use of a questionnaire. None of the patients used more than one pad per 24 hours in our series (75 patients). The continence rate after conventional laparoscopy is very high, ranging from 85% to 97% in published series (12,13,16,17). It is clear that the anastomosis between the urethra and bladder neck, and the dissection of the apex, is easier to perform due to the improved vision and wristed instruments enabled by the use of robotics. However, whether this will translate into better results regarding continence remains to be seen.

SEXUAL FUNCTION

One of the most important factors in reducing the morbidity of radical prostatectomy is to increase the number of patients that recover their sexual function after surgery. Menon's group has reported that robot-assisted prostatectomy enhances the return of erections and the ability to have intercourse compared to open surgery (10). In our study, the International Index of Erectile Function (IIEF) score was 15.6 before surgery. After bilateral or unilateral nerve-sparing, the score was 9.1 for both groups of patients. After 6 to 12 months follow-up, 41% and 44% of the patients were able to have unassisted intercourse, respectively. Thus, we had similar results regardless of whether unilateral or bilateral nerve-sparing was attempted, which was unexpected. Longer follow-up is needed to evaluate if robot-assisted prostatectomy will show better results regarding sexual side effects compared with open surgery and conventional laparoscopy.

CONVERSION RATE

A conversion rate of <5% is reported in most series of laparoscopic prostatectomies. In our experience at the Karolinska Hospital, the conversion rate for robot-assisted prostatectomies is 1%. In the initial series by Bentas et al. (9), a conversion rate of 5% was reported, whereas Tewari et al. (10) reported no conversions in their series. After mastering of the technique of conventional laparoscopy as well as robot-assisted prostatectomy, the conversion rate is negligible.

COMPLICATIONS

There are several large series reporting the complications of laparoscopic radical prostatectomy (11–13,18), whereas only limited reports on robot-assisted prostatectomy have been published (9,10). After conventional laparoscopy, anastomotic leakage is a common problem (12–14,16). We have not encountered this problem in any of our patients; neither has Menon's group (10). This could be attributed to the 3-D visualizing system and the fine-wristed instruments, enabling a more refined surgical technique in creation of the anastomosis to the urethra. However, in the series from Bentas et al. (9), prolonged anastomotic leak was noted in 10% of the patients. Other complications observed include pulmonary embolism, deep vein thrombosis, obturator nerve injury, trocar injury to epigastric artery, venous plexus bleeding, and urinary tract infection. In our series of 75 patients, one patient had a bowel perforation that led to a reoperation, and one patient had ureteric stenosis at the level of the iliac vessels. No patient required intraoperative transfusion at our institution. Similar results have been reported from Menon's group, whereas Bentas et al. (9) reported 500 mL bleeding requiring 7 intraoperative and 6 postoperative transfusions (32%). The high incidence of bleeding complications was probably due to

a different surgical approach with ascending preparation of the dorsal aspect of the prostate.

In general, the complication rate seems similar between conventional laparoscopic and robot-assisted procedures. However, the learning curve and the operating time appear to favor robot-assisted prostatectomy and may translate to earlier discharge, reduced postoperative pain score, and less bleeding (7).

THE COST

The da Vinci surgical system costs $1.2 million, with a maintenance fee of $100,000/year after the first year. The average cost of disposables is $1,500 in the United States (7), and $2,000 at the Karolinska Hospital in Stockholm. These costs are at least in part balanced by cost savings of decreased hospital stay, fewer blood transfusions, and lower complication rate. The robotic system may appear expensive; however, taking into account the cost for magnetic resonance imaging (MRI) cameras and computed tomography (CT) scans, the cost for a robot is less impressive. It has been suggested that the cost for robotic surgery is an average of $150 more than for open surgery in the United States (7). If the data are further established on tumor-free margins, and less incontinence and impotence, the cost of the procedure will be of lesser importance. At our institution, the overall cost for the robot-assisted prostatectomy is approximately $1,000 more than conventional surgery. It is notoriously difficult to calculate hospital costs; however, the shorter rehabilitation is of benefit for both the patient and the health insurance system.

FUTURE ASPECTS OF ROBOT-ASSISTED SURGERY

It is unclear if the next generation of robots will further improve the surgical results. They will likely be less expensive compared to the current systems, and new instruments allowing more precise dissection are likely to be developed. This may enhance the possibility to perform nerve-sparing surgery and reduce the morbidity inflicted by prostate cancer surgery. Another possibility lies in the development of less nerve-damaging instruments using ultrasound, cautery, or laser technique. The option of performing remote surgery with robots is another future challenge. Whether this will be of interest is unclear. In theory, it will be possible to be operated on by leading surgeons even in smaller institutions with less experience. However, in case of a need for conversion, experienced surgeons will have to be present.

CONCLUSION

Unlike laparoscopic prostatectomy, which is difficult and time-consuming to learn (6), robot-assisted prostatectomy can be learned more easily by surgeons skilled in open prostatectomy. The availability of surgical robots with 3-D vision and wristed instruments with greater degrees of freedom than rigid laparoscopic instruments will possibly facilitate the performance of laparoscopic radical prostatectomy in the future. It remains to be scientifically evaluated whether these features will translate into better results regarding continence rate, erectile function, and cancer control. However, it seems clear that the patient will benefit in less postoperative pain, decreased bleeding, and shorter hospital stay compared to open surgery.

References

1. Artibani W, Grosso G, Novara G, et al. Is laparoscopic radical prostatectomy better than traditional retropubic radical prostatectomy? An analysis of peri-operative morbidity in two contemporary series in Italy. *Eur Urol* 2003;44:401–406.
2. Guillonneau B, Cathelineau X, Barret E, et al. Laparoscopic radical prostatectomy: technical and early oncological assessment of 40 operations. *Eur Urol* 1999;36:14–20.
3. Schuessler WW, Schulam PG, Clayman RV, et al. Laparoscopic radical prostatectomy: initial short–term experience. *Urology* 1997;50:854–857.
4. Abbou CC, Salomon L, Hoznek A, et al. Laparoscopic radical prostatectomy: preliminary results. *Urology* 2000;55:630–634.
5. Guillonneau B. What robotics in urology? A current point of view. *Eur Urol* 2003;43:103–105.
6. Menon M, Shrivastava A, Tewari A, et al. Laparoscopic and robot assisted radical prostatectomy: establishment of a structured program and preliminary analysis of outcomes. *J Urol* 2002;168:945–949.
7. Menon M. Robotic radical retropubic prostatectomy. *BJU International* 2003;91:175–176.
8. Tewari A, Peabody J, Sarle R, et al. Technique of da Vinci robot-assisted anatomic radical prostatectomy. *Urology* 2002;60:569–572.
9. Bentas W, Wolfram M, Jones J, et al. Robotic technology and the translation of open radical prostatectomy to laparoscopy: the early Frankfurt experience with robotic radical prostatectomy and one year follow-up. *Eur Urol* 2003;44:175–181.
10. Tewari A, Srivasatava A, Menon M, et al. A prospective comparison of radical retropubic and robot-assisted prostatectomy: experience in one institution. *BJU International* 2003;92:205–210.
11. Guillonneau B, Rozet F, Cathelineau X, et al. Perioperative complications of laparoscopic radical prostatectomy: the Montsouris 3-year experience. *J Urol* 2002;167:51–56.
12. Rassweiler J, Sentker L, Seemann O, et al. Laparoscopic radical prostatectomy with the Heilbronn technique: an analysis of the first 180 cases. *J Urol* 2001;166:2101–2108.
13. Türk I, Deger S, Winkelmann B, et al. Laparoscopic radical prostatectomy: technical aspects and experience with 125 cases. *Eur Urol* 2001;40:46–53.
14. Dahl DM, L'Esperance JO, Trainer AF, et al. Laparoscopic radical prostatectomy: initial 70 cases at a U.S. university medical center. *Urology* 2002;60:859–863.
15. Noldus J, Palisaar J, Huland H. Treatment of prostate cancer: the clinical use of radical prostatectomy. *EAU Update Series* 2003;1:16–22.
16. Hoznek A, Salomon L, Olsson LE, et al. Laparoscopic radical prostatectomy: the Créteil experience. *Eur Urol* 2001;40:38–45.
17. Eden CG, Cahill D, Vass TH, et al. Laparoscopic radical prostatectomy: the initial UK series. *BJU International* 2002;90:876–882.
18. Gregori A, Simonato A, Lissiani A, et al. Laparoscopic radial prostatectomy: perioperative complications in an initial and consecutive series of 80 cases. *Eur Urol* 2003;44:190–194.

CHAPTER 13F
3D Conformal Radiotherapy for Localized Prostate Cancer

Howard M. Sandler and
Jeff Michalski

INTRODUCTION

External beam radiation therapy techniques for prostate cancer have evolved dramatically from the early 1990s to the present. Previously, traditional or conventional radiation therapy approaches often have employed a four-field "box" treatment arrangement that encompassed the pelvic lymph nodes, seminal vesicles, and the prostate gland. By necessity, the volumes irradiated were large, to assure coverage of the target tissue that could harbor subclinical, microscopic, or gross disease. The boost treatment to the prostate, with or without the seminal vesicles, would be done with either a similar four-field method or with rotational fields that treated the large target volumes, along with adjacent organs at risk, to cumulative radiation doses in the range of 64 Gy to 70 Gy. The high-dose volumes would inherently be box-shaped or cylindrical and would not resemble the actual irregular shape of the anatomical targets they were intended to treat. As a result, the upper limit of radiation dose was constrained to 70 Gy due to the large amounts of bowel and bladder that would be coincidentally irradiated. Exceeding that radiation dose in the pre–three-dimensional (3D) era was associated with a significant risk of morbidity (1).

The availability of powerful computers and workstations has changed the manner in which modern radiation therapy is planned and delivered. Dedicated radiation oncology computed tomography (CT) scanners allow the capture of complete volumetric anatomical information from which a 3D radiation therapy treatment plan is created. Radiation-dose distributions can be shaped using customized beam apertures that shield the nearby organs at risk from receiving high doses of radiation therapy. Three-dimensional treatment planning includes the volumetric calculation of radiation dose to the target volume of each organ at risk, including unspecified tissues. The dose distributions and anatomical structures are then viewed on a 3D rendered volumetric display or in multiple reconstructions in axial, sagittal, and coronal planes. Finally, graphic analytical tools, such as dose-volume histograms (DVH) are computed to facilitate plan review and approval.

Conformal radiation therapy takes many forms. In this chapter we will focus on 3D conformal radiation therapy (3D-CRT) planning and delivery. Intensity-modulated radiation therapy (IMRT), proton-beam radiation therapy, and even high-dose-rate (HDR) brachytherapy can also be considered conformal radiation therapy (CRT) methods, but they are so unique in their physical characteristics that they are addressed in other chapters. The process of treatment planning without volumetric dose calculation has been described as "two-and-one-half" dimensional (2.5-D) treatment planning or virtual simulation without volumetric dose calculation. True 3D planning requires the volumetric dose calculation, display, recording, and reporting of DVHs and dose statistics. This data is then used to review and score plans for conformality and to choose a plan that optimally treats a target volume while protecting normal tissues. Virtual simulation or 2.5-D planning describes the use of CT data for structure display on digitally reconstructed radiographs for beam orientation and aperture design. While radiation dose might be calculated on single or multiple axial planes, the full volumetric dosimetry information for treatment plan review and scoring is not available with virtual simulation only.

CONFORMAL RADIATION THERAPY SIMULATION AND TREATMENT PLANNING

The process of 3D-CRT planning entails patient positioning and immobilization followed by acquisition of a treatment-planning CT dataset. Image segmentation is the process of defining target volumes and organs at risk by contouring anatomy on a slice-by-slice basis. Radiation beams are created with a virtual simulation software tool that is analogous to the operation of a conventional fluoroscopic isocentric radiation therapy simulator. The radiation beams or apertures are shaped using a beam's eye view (BEV) display, and the contributing dose from each beam is entered into the treatment-planning software. Finally, the plan is reviewed using a variety of dose display and analysis tools.

Patient Immobilization and Positioning

Patient immobilization devices are more frequently used in 3D CRT compared to traditional treatment planning. Some investigators have reported improved treatment setup accuracy with these devices, whereas others have reported no significant advantage with their use (2,3). In a randomized study, Kneebone demonstrated that the average simulation-to-treatment deviation of the isocenter position was 8.5 mm in a control group and 6.2 mm in an immobilized group (P <.001). The use of immobilization devices reduced isocenter deviations exceeding 10 mm from 30.9% to 10.6% in the immobilized arm (P <.001). The average deviations in the anteroposterior, right-left, and superior-inferior directions were reduced to 2.9 mm, 2.1 mm, and 3.9 mm respectively for the immobilized group (4).

Each radiation therapy center is advised to study and review the treatment setup variations with either method and choose the one that gives the best reproducibility.

There is significant debate regarding the appropriate positioning for patients who have localized prostate carcinoma. Some groups advocate a prone position, which minimizes prostate positional uncertainty and decreases the volume of rectum irradiated with conformal radiation therapy when the seminal vesicles are irradiated (5). More recent data suggest that a prone position is associated with greater prostate motion accompanying normal ventilation. The increased intra-abdominal pressure associated with breathing in a supine position results in significant movement of the prostate and seminal vesicles. Dawson et al. (6) evaluated the impact of breathing on the position of the prostate gland in four patients treated in four different positions on whom radiopaque markers were implanted in the periphery of the prostate using transrectal ultrasound guidance. Fluoroscopy was performed in four different positions: prone in a foam cast cradle, prone in a thermoplastic mold, supine on a flat table, and supine with a false table under the buttocks. During normal breathing, maximum movement of prostate markers seen in the prone position (cranial-caudal) ranged from 0.9 to 5.1 mm and anterior-posterior ranged up to 3.5 mm. In the supine position, prostate movements during normal breathing were less than 1 mm in all directions; however, deep breathing resulted in movements of 3.8 to 10.5 mm in the cranial-caudal direction in the prone position (with and without thermoplastic mold). This range was reduced to 2.7 mm in the supine position and to 0.5 to 2.1 mm with the use of the false table top. Deep breathing resulted in anterior-posterior skeletal movements of 2.7 to 13.1 mm in the prone position, whereas in the supine position these variations were negligible.

Malone et al. (7) also characterized inaccuracies in prostatic gland location due to respiration observed fluoroscopically in 28 patients on whom three gold fiducial markers were implanted under ultrasound guidance at the apex, posterior wall, and base of prostate. Patients were immobilized on a customized thermoplastic shell placed on a rigid pelvic board. A second group of 20 patients were evaluated both prone (with or without thermoplastic shell) and supine (without immobilization shell). When the patients were immobilized prone in the thermoplastic shell, the prostate moved synchronously with respiration of a mean distance of 3.3 ± 1.8 mm (range, 1–10 mm). In 9 of 40 observations (23%) the displacements were 4 mm or greater. The respiratory-associated prostate movement decreased significantly when the thermoplastic shells were removed. Prostate movement with respiration was significantly less in the patients placed in the supine position without shells (6–12).

Target Volume Definition

After the acquisition of the treatment-planning CT scan, the image data needs to be segmented in order for the treatment-planning computer to render 3D images and compute dose to the various targets and normal organs. Segmentation refers to the assignment of CT visualized grayscale structures to logical anatomic labels. This target and normal organ definition can be done with a computer-pointing device, such as a mouse and a drawing utility in the treatment-planning program. Organs with high contrast relative to adjacent tissues (e.g., skin, bone, and lung) can be segmented using automatic grayscale image threshold identification utilities.

The identification of target volumes and normal organs at risk is the critical element of 3D-CRT planning. The International Commission for Radiation Units (ICRU) has encouraged the use of common terminology to describe these volumes and report prescription and dosimetric data. The ICRU No. 50 and ICRU No. 62 bulletins established guidelines for defining both targets and organs at risk (13,14). The gross tumor volume (GTV) represents any disease that can be identified by imaging modalities or physical examination. Because prostate cancer is often found to be multifocal at the time of radical prostatectomy, the entire gland is commonly considered the GTV for radiation treatment planning purposes. The clinical target volume (CTV) encompasses the GTV and may add margin for microscopic extension of disease. The CTV may expand the GTV to account for direct extension or the CTV can be extended to encompass adjacent organs or regions of spread. In prostate cancer, the CTV may encompass the seminal vesicles and possibly the regional pelvic lymph nodes. In selected patients, it is necessary to outline the seminal vesicles, which in most patients are well demonstrated on the cross-section CT scans of the pelvis, superior, lateral, and posterior to the base of the prostate. Nomograms have been developed by Partin et al. (15), Pisansky et al. (16) and Roach et al. (17), who constructed mathematical formulas to determine the probability of seminal vesicle or pelvic lymph node involvement in patients with carcinoma of the prostate using prostate-specific antigen (PSA), clinical stage, pretreatment PSA, and Gleason score.

Kestin et al. (18) published an analysis of 344 radical prostatectomy specimens in which they measured the length of seminal vesicles, length of involvement, and percentage of seminal vesicle involved. They found an excellent correlation between the various prognostic parameters and the probability of seminal vesicle involvement. Also, in 81 patients with positive seminal vesicle involvement, the median length of tumor presence was 1 cm, and in the entire population only 7% of patients had seminal vesicle involvement beyond 1 cm. They concluded that in selected patients seminal vesicles need to be treated, and only 2.5 cm (approximately 60% of the seminal vesicle) should be included within the CTV, unless there is radiographic evidence of involvement.

When there is evidence of extraprostatic extension on either physical examination or imaging modalities such as magnetic resonance imaging (MRI) (clinical stage T3), we routinely include the seminal vesicles for the total radiation dose prescription. In cases where the disease is confined to the gland (clinical stages T1-2) and the risk of seminal vesicle invasion exceeds 15%, we will commonly define two clinical target volumes. The first encompasses the prostate and the seminal vesicles, and the second boost target volume will be the prostate alone. In these cases, a radiation dose that controls subclinical disease will be prescribed to the first target volume, and a higher dose will be intended for the prostate itself.

Involvement of the pelvic lymph nodes in carcinoma of the prostate also is closely related to clinical tumor stage, pretreatment PSA, and Gleason score, and the above-mentioned Partin nomograms (15,16) or the Roach formulas (19) provide the means to determine the risk of pelvic lymph node involvement. Kestin et al. (18) noted that only 1% of low-risk patients (PSA <10 ng/mL, Gleason score ≤6, and clinical stage

≤T2a) had lymph node involvement compared with 27% in patients with higher risk factors.

To aid in the identification of the prostatic apex, a retrograde urethrogram can be performed using 25% iodinated contrast material. The prostatic apex is 3 to 13 mm above the most proximal aspect of the urogenital diaphragm as defined by the urethrogram (20,21). Care should be taken not to overinflate the urethra with iodinated contrast as this may distend or move the prostate from its relaxed position (7). An MRI study done by Mah did not demonstrate significant deviation of the prostate when urethral contrast was injected for urethrography (22). A rubber catheter or hollow tube to deflate flatus in the rectum helps avoid the introduction of systematic errors in organ and target definition due to rectal distension (23). An enema prior to simulation will empty the rectum and allow the prostate to move to its most posterior position. This allows use of a tighter uncertainty margin posteriorly.

Some authors feel that MRI may be more accurate in delineating the prostate and seminal vesicles (24). Several publications have shown some discrepancy (.5 to 1 cm) in defining the location of the apex of the prostate using CT scanning or MRI (25–27). Parker et al. (28) studied coregistration of CT and MR images in the radiation treatment planning of six patients with localized prostate cancer to assist with GTV delineation and identification of prostate position during radiation therapy. The overall magnitude of contoured GTV was similar for MRI and CT; however, there were spatial discrepancies in contouring between the two modalities. The greatest systematic discrepancy was at the posterior apical prostate border, which was 3.6 mm more posterior on MR- than CT-defined contouring.

The planning target volume (PTV) envelops the CTV with a margin to account for uncertainties in treatment delivery. The uncertainties may be related to setup variations or internal organ motion. Variations in patient anatomy and position, and internal target or normal organ motion during treatment, need to be carefully identified and addressed during the treatment-planning process and in the delivery of radiation therapy. These uncertainties will influence the actual absorbed dose of irradiation delivered to the target volume when compared with initial treatment-planning dose distribution (29). Two important scenarios are an insufficient dose delivered to the tumor volume and excessive irradiation doses given to normal tissues. The possible errors that may be encountered have been defined as systematic or random and interfraction or intrafraction. Motion of the target volume is taken into consideration when the margins for PTV are defined according to ICRU reports 50 and 62 (13,14). More problematic and challenging is the unpredictable internal motion of the target of the normal tissues related to physiologic processes, such as filling of the bladder or the rectum during and between treatments.

The magnitude of the PTV margin depends on several treatment-related factors. A technologist's inability to precisely reproduce a patient's position on a daily basis is one contributing factor. Some patients may move while on the treatment table because of fatigue or discomfort. Internal organs, including the prostate gland, can shift because of variable filling of the bladder and rectum. The shifts can be anisotropic with most movement occurring in the anterior and posterior directions. Table 13F.1 summarizes several studies of treatment uncertainty in prostate cancer patients (29). These studies investigated both internal organ motions and setup errors to determine an appropriate margin for the planning target volume. Increasing the size of the PTV margin increases the probability of encompassing the CTV by the prescribed isodose from a complete course of radiation therapy. In order to assure that an adequate radiation dose is encompassing all areas at risk of harboring disease, the radiation oncologist needs to include an appropriate PTV margin. There is a trade-off between assuring nearly 100% coverage during each treatment and the volume of adjacent organs irradiated unnecessarily. The PTV margin does not account for radiation beam penumbra. When defining beam aperture or field shape, additional margin needs to be added to account for this dosimetric falloff near the edge of the beam.

Antolak et al. (40), in a study of 17 patients with prostate cancer who underwent CT scanning for treatment planning and three subsequent CT scans obtained at approximately 2-week intervals during external beam fractionated irradiation, observed CTV motion of 0.09 cm (left to right), 0.36 cm (cranial-caudal), and 0.41 cm (anterior-posterior). Prostate mobility was not significantly correlated with bladder volume, but both prostate and seminal vesicle positions were significantly influenced by rectal volume. From this study, the authors concluded that margins between the CTV and PTV necessary to enclose 95% of the PTV were 7 mm in the lateral and cranial-caudal directions and 11 mm in the anterior-posterior direction. They felt that more consistent methods for reproducing prostate position, for instance, emptying the rectum, and more sophisticated beam aperture optimization are needed to guarantee consistent coverage of the CTV while avoiding additional irradiation to organs at risk.

Zelefsky et al. (43) evaluated prostate and seminal vesicle motion in 50 patients treated in the prone position using CT scans for initial treatment planning and three scans obtained throughout the course of radiation therapy. Before the initial CT scans, patients had an enema and were given 250 mL of bowel contrast by mouth. Patients had an empty bladder and 10 mL of air was inserted into the rectum via rectal catheter. Prior to all CT scans, patients voided, and no additional procedures were performed. Relative to the initial planning CT, mean displacements of the prostate were -1.2 ± 2.9 mm in the anterior-posterior (AP), -0.5 ± 3.3 mm in the superior-inferior, and -0.6 ± 0.8 mm in the lateral directions. The seminal vesicle displacements were -1.4 ± 4.9 mm, 1.3 ± 5.5 mm, and -0.8 ± 3.1 mm in the AP, superior-inferior (SI), and lateral directions, respectively (negative values indicated displacements to the posterior, inferior, and left directions). A combination of rectal volume larger than 60 mL or a bladder volume larger than 40 mL was found to be predictive for systematic deviations of the prostate and seminal vesicles of more than 3 mm. Based on the data and the prescription of irradiation dose to achieve at least 93% coverage of the CTV, Zelefsky et al. calculated the margins to be added to the CTV for defining the PTV. Based on these reports, it is apparent that beyond the CTV, additional margins of 5 to 8 mm are necessary to provide adequate coverage of the prostate and 6 to 11 mm for adequate coverage of the seminal vesicles when there is no organ distension that would result in a systematic error.

In a study of 11 patients with repeating CT scans during a course of radiation therapy for prostate cancer, van Herk et al. (33) showed that the largest deviation in prostate position was 2.7 mm in the anterior-posterior direction with a rotation about the left-right axis of 4 degrees. They found that the apex of the prostate does not move, and the majority of any motion is rotation around the apex. Melian et al. (38), in a study of 13 patients with carcinoma of the prostate on whom they superimposed the PTV on serial CT scans, noted that one standard deviation displacement of the PTV center mass with respect to the planning scan center of mass was 1.2 mm in the lateral, 4 mm in the anterior-posterior, and 3.1 mm in the superior-inferior directions. Movement was significantly larger in the superior part of the PTV above the base of the bladder compared with the distal portion. There was a significant correlation between bladder volume and changes in PTV position, particularly in the anterior-posterior and superior-inferior directions. Also, there was a correlation between the rectal volume and the position of the PTV in the anterior-posterior direction, with

TABLE 13F.1

SUMMARY OF PROSTATE MOTION STUDIES

Study, First Author	N	Comments	Displacement (mm)	Maximum (mm)
Ten Haken (30)	50	$+30$–$50\ cm^3$ of contrast in R	62% >5	20
Schild (31)	18	$60 \rightarrow 180\ cm^3$ of contrast in R	17% >5	17
	11	$60 \rightarrow 180\ cm^3$ of contrast in B	9% >5	8
Balter (32)	10	ROM, full B, weekly portals relative to a reference portal image	Max. exp. ($P = .05$)	
			AP: 4.5	7.5
			Lat: 1.7	2
			SI: 3.7	5
Van Herk (33)	11	3-4 CT, biweekly, full B, displacement between 2 CT	AP: SD = 2.7	
			Lat: SD = .9	
			Si: SD = 1.7	
Roeske (34)	10	Weekly CT, full B, relative to initial CT	AP: mean = −.4, SD = 3.9	5.3 (mean)
			Lat: mean = −.6, SD = .7	
			SI: mean = −.2, SD = 3.2	6.3 (mean)
Crook (27)	55	Gold seeds, full B, initial and second film before boost	Post: mean = 5.6, SD = 4.1	
			Inf: mean = 5.9, SD = 4.5	
Beard (35)	30	2 CT, 4 weeks apart, empty B	AP: 40% >5	Post: 13
			Inf: 7% >5	Inf: 8
Althof (36)	9	^{125}I seed implants, 6 sets of x-rays, relative to first x-rays	AP: SD = 1.5	7
			Lat: SD = .8	3
			SI: SD = 1.7	4
Rudat (37)	28	Weekly CT, empty B and R, relative to mean position	AP: SD = 3.7	13
			Lat: SD = 1.9	7
Melian (38)	13	4 CT scans, prone, relative to init. CT Lat: mean = .3, SD = 1.2	AP: mean = −.7, SD = 4.0	
			SI: mean = .4, SD = 3.1	
Roach (17)	10	Biweekly CT scans, full B, relative to first CT	Ant: 23%, post: 27% >5	14
			Lat: 0% >5	4.5
			Sup: 20%, inf: 3% >5	8
Vigneault (39)	11	ROM, EPI over course of treatment, relative to init. EPI	AP: mean = .5, SD = 3.5	10.8
			Lat: mean = .3, SD = 1.9	8.8
			SI: mean = .7, SD = 3.6	9.9
Tinger (23)	8	Weekly CT, full B, relative to init. CT	AP: mean = .5, SD = 2.6	
			Lat: mean = 0, SD = .9	
			SI: mean = 1.5, SD = 3.9	
Antolak (40)	17	4 CT, biweekly, full B, relative to init. CT	AP: SD = 3.6	
			Lat: SD = .7	
			SI: SD = 3.6	
Dawson (6)	6	Weekly CT, empty B, relative to init. CT		AP: 7.1
				SI: 9.3
Stroom (41)	15	TPCT + 3 CT scans, supine	AP: SD = 2.8	
			SI: SD = 2.8	
Stroom (42)	15	TPCT + 3 CT scans, prone	AP: SD = 2.1	
			SI: SD = 1.7	
Zelefsky (43)	50	TPCT + CT scans, empty B, prone, relative to TPCT	AP: mean = −1.2, SD = 2.9	
			Lat: mean = −.6, SD = .8	
			SI: mean = −.5, SD = 3.3	

R, rectum; B, bladder; ROM, radio-opaque marker; Max. exp., maximum expected; lat, lateral; SD, standard deviation; init., initial; post, posterior; inf, inferior; ant, anterior; sup, supine; EPI, electronic portal imaging; TPCT, treatment planning CT; AP, anterior-posterior; SI, superior-inferior.
From Langen KM, Jones DTL. Organ motion and its management. *Int J Radiat Oncol Biol Phys* 2001;50:265–278, with permission.

larger rectal volume associated with anterior displacement of the PTV. Analysis of DVHs showed that these displacements in the prostate position had an impact on the dose received by the PTV as well as by the adjacent bladder and rectal walls. By requiring patients to void prior to the scan procedures, changes in bladder volume were decreased but not completely eliminated.

Strategies to reduce the uncertainty in daily treatment delivery and therefore reduce the magnitude of the PTV margin have been successfully introduced. Each of these methods employs daily imaging of the prostate with the patient in the treatment position on the linear accelerator treatment table. Some institutions have employed radiopaque implanted fiducial markers that are subsequently imaged with electronic portal imaging devices. Crook et al. (27) evaluated prostate motion in 55 patients in whom gold seeds were implanted at the base of the gland. Initial simulation was obtained in a supine position with a full bladder and repeated after patients received 40 Gy. The location of the seeds relative to bony landmarks was recorded on plain radiographs. A urethrogram was performed at the initial simulation and 10 to 15 mL of barium were inserted in the rectum. No contrast material was used during the second simulation. Prostate motion was observed in the posterior direction (5.6 mm ± 4.1 mm) and in the inferior direction (5.9 mm ± 4.5 mm). In 30% of the patients the base of the prostate was displaced posteriorly and 11% in the inferior direction by more than 10 mm. Vigneault et al. (39) investigated inter- and intrafraction daily motion of the prostatic apex relative to pelvic bony structures in 11 patients using radiopaque markers implanted under ultrasound guidance near the prostatic apex. Patients were treated with a four-field box technique using 23 MV photons. Over 900 digital portal images were obtained throughout the radiation therapy course. After the completion of treatment, a transrectal ultrasound was performed in 8 of 11 patients to verify that the position of the radiopaque markers had not shifted. Marker displacements up to 1.6 cm were measured between 2 consecutive days of treatment on portal images. The marker displacement relative to the center of the irradiation field was sensitive to both setup variations and internal prostate motion. The authors performed treatment movies (6 consecutive electronic portal images during the same treatment fraction) and observed no visible intratreatment displacement of the markers.

Transabdominal ultrasound has been used to localize the prostate for treatment planning and during daily radiation therapy delivery with an accuracy parallel to that of CT scanning of the pelvis (Fig. 13F.1). Lattanzi et al. (44) studied 23 patients with CT simulations on whom prostate-only fields based on CT scans were created with no planning target volume (PTV) margin. Ten of the patients also had prostate localization with a transabdominal ultrasound system. The absolute magnitude difference in CT and ultrasound was small (AP mean 3 mm ± 1.8 mm, lateral mean 2.4 mm ± 1.8 mm, superior-inferior mean 4.6 mm ± 2.8 mm). The authors felt the transabominal ultrasound was simple and expeditious and improved their ability to localize the position of the prostate with the patient at the treatment machine for daily irradiation. Functionally, it was found to be equivalent to CT scanning. Lattanzi et al. (45) then performed daily CT scan and transabdominal ultrasound prostate localization during a course of radiation therapy in 35 patients. A 3D comparison of prostate position was determined in 69 daily CT and ultrasound studies. The magnitude of difference between the CT and ultrasound localization ranged from 0 to 7 mm in the anterior-posterior, 0 to 6.4 mm in the lateral, and 0 to 6.7 mm in the superior-inferior dimensions. The corresponding directed average disagreements were extremely small (less than 1 mm in all dimensions).

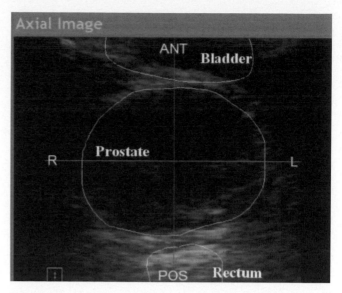

FIGURE 13F.1. Transabdominal ultrasound taken at the linear accelerator just prior to treatment. Contours from the planning CT scan of the prostate, bladder, and rectum are superimposed on the ultrasound images (*white lines*) to allow alignment of the isocenter (*green and red line intersection*) to the treatment plan. (See color insert.)

Huang et al. (46) evaluated intrafraction motion using a transabdominal ultrasound system in 20 patients during 200 IMRT treatments for prostate cancer. The mean magnitude shifts were 0.1 ± 0.4 mm in the left to right, 0.2 ± 1.3 mm in the anterior, and 0.1 ± 1 mm in the superior directions. Maximum range of motion occurred in the AP dimension, from 6.8 mm anteriorly to 4.6 mm posteriorly. The percentage of treatments during which prostate motion was judged to be 5 mm or less was 100%, 99%, and 99.5% in the right-to-left, AP, and superior-inferior directions, respectively. The degree of intrafraction motion was significantly smaller than interfraction motion. There was no correlation between the two types of movement.

Yan et al. (47) have developed a strategy of adaptive radiation therapy. Patients undergo daily CT imaging during the first week of radiation therapy. A patient-specific PTV is then calculated and the patients are re-planned. A patient-specific margin allows reduction of the PTV that is otherwise calculated based on population averages. This strategy does mean some patients will be treated to larger PTVs if their CTV error is larger than average. Those patients may require other strategies to account for organ motion if dose escalation is necessary.

Organs at risk need to be defined for the treatment-planning process. In the treatment of prostate cancer, the organs at risk include the bladder, rectum, femoral heads, and occasionally the small bowel. There can be considerable variation in the definition of these organs from physician to physician. When comparing dosimetric constraints and clinical outcomes from various series, a consistent definition of these structures is important. The Radiation Therapy Oncology Group (RTOG) has described their method for normal organ definition (48). The femoral heads are contoured from the level of the ischial tuberosities to their proximal joint at the pelvis. The rectum and bladder are both defined as solid organs. Inferiorly, the rectum is defined from the level of the ischial tuberosities. It extends superiorly until the colon moves anteriorly toward the sigmoid. The bladder is contoured inferiorly from the prostate base to the dome. Radiation to the penile bulb tissue of the corpora spongiosa inferior to the prostatic apex and urogenital diaphragm appears to play a role in the development of radiation induced erectile dysfunction (49, 50). MR images may allow more accurate definition of the prostate apex, urogenital diaphragm, and penile bulb (51).

It has been argued that the bladder and rectum, being hollow organs, should have the inner contents subtracted from volumetric dose information. The remaining volume then represents the volume of the organ wall. Unfortunately, the calculation of wall volume is not a trivial task and either requires the added work of contouring both the inner and rectal walls or additional software that is not available on many 3D-SCRT computer-planning systems. As a result, most institutions and cooperative groups report dosimetry data to the whole organ volume. Early clinical outcomes suggest that wall volume may indeed be a more important parameter with respect to 3D dosimetry than the whole organ volume (52–54).

Beam Selection and Shaping

The process of beam selection and shaping with 3D-CRT is analogous to the same process with conventional simulation. 3D-CRT planning systems display a "virtual patient" reconstructed from the CT image data and the segmented structures. Radiation beams can be added and displayed from the perspective of a subject in the treatment room ("room view" or "physician's eye view") and from the perspective of the linear accelerator radiation source ("beam's eye view" or

BEV). The beam's eye view display allows a physicist or dosimetrist to set collimator positions and shape the field to encompass the projected PTV. The field shaping can be designated with freehand shapes for cerrobend blocks or with multileaf collimation. Alternatively, blocks can be automatically generated to fit the contours of the PTV as displayed in the BEV (Fig. 13F.2). The advantage that the BEV display offers over conventional simulation is the ability to actually see the spatial relationships of the target volume and organs at risk. The 3D renderings of the targets and adjacent organs can be adjusted with transparency or color controls to allow visualization of overlaps between them.

A critical enhancement of the BEV is the digitally reconstructed radiograph (DRR). The DRR is a projected plane x-ray image that is computed from the CT data. The DRR is helpful in the planning process and aids in treatment verification. In treatment planning, the DRR is used with the BEV to assist the physician or dosimetrist to define the treatment aperture. If all nearby anatomical structures have not been contoured, the DRR helps identify possible unintentional irradiation of those regions. The DRR also serves as a prescription image that can be used to confirm patient setup and desired localization of the target volume by comparing it to verification port films or electronic portal images taken at the treatment machine.

A variety of treatment techniques have been described for 3D conformal radiation therapy for prostate cancer. One of the first methods simply applies traditional orthogonal four-field beam orientation but employs BEV shaping

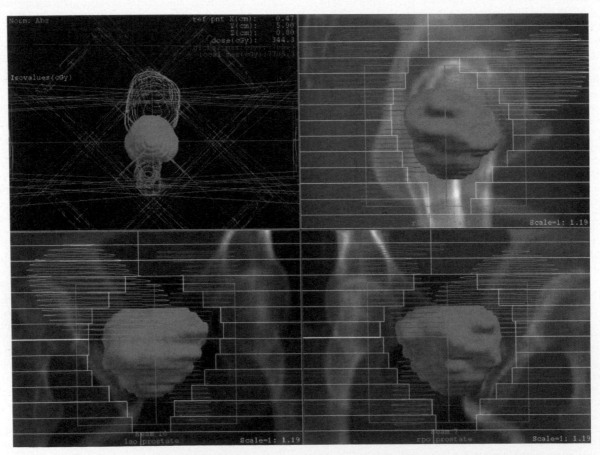

FIGURE 13F.2. Beam's eye view displays on lateral (*upper right panel*) and two obliquely-oriented (lower panels) digital reconstructed radiographs. Graphic representations of multileaf collimator leaves demonstrate beam shaping relative to the contour of the PTV (*solid light blue*) and shielding of the rectum (*brown wire cage*) and bladder (*yellow wire cage*). The left upper panel displays a six-field 3D conformal beam arrangement viewed along the superior-inferior axis. (See color insert.)

(55,56). A four-field 3D-CRT technique confers a significant advantage over a conventional four-field "box" or bilateral 120 degree arc technique (30,57). A four-field 3D-CRT technique shields significant portions of the bladder and rectum from the primary beam in the lateral projections. This leads to significant sparing of these organs from a high radiation dose.

A six-field technique has been favored by many institutions. This technique employs parallel opposed anterior and posterior oblique fields in addition to the traditional lateral fields. Typically the oblique fields are angled 45 degrees from the lateral, although they can be at shallower angles to the organs at risk. Compared to a four-field conformal technique employing prescription doses of 70 to74 Gy, the six-field technique does not appear to confer a clear dosimetric advantage. However, institutions that have delivered radiation doses in excess of 74 Gy have preferred a six-field technique, as it may reduce dose for the bladder, rectum, and the bilateral femoral heads (30,57,58). We commonly use unevenly weighted beams in the six-field technique with 40% of the dose contribution coming from the lateral fields and the other 60% of the dose divided evenly between the anterior and posterior oblique fields. The lateral beams are weighted more heavily in our six-field technique because this direction allows maximum shielding of the bladder and rectum. Beam's eye view treatment planning with a six-field technique significantly improves PTV coverage and provides better bladder and rectum sparing compared to traditional bilateral arcs (Table 13F.2). Perez compared 174 patients planned with either 3D conformal radiation therapy or standard radiation therapy and demonstrated that when field sizes were adjusted to adequately encompass the planning target volumes, there was a significant reduction in the volumes of bladder and rectum irradiated with conformal technique (58).

A noncoplanar technique has been described and used at the University of Michigan since 1992. This technique employs two lateral fields paired with noncoplanar anterior inferior oblique fields. The direction of the anterior inferior obliques is selected on a patient-by-patient basis using angles that optimally exclude the maximum amount of bladder and rectum. This technique has been demonstrated to effectively reduce the volume of the bladder and rectal walls that receive significant radiation dose (59).

A technique employing blocked arc fields has been used at the University of California, San Francisco. This technique has been used in patients treated for the prostate without the seminal vesicles. Bilateral 120 degree arc fields are blocked in the corners with a 2 cm margin on the PTV. This technique results in a lower dose to the rectum and a tighter dosimetric margin around the prostate compared to either a six-field or four-field fixed beam 3D-CRT technique (60,61).

The choice of technique for any given institution may depend as much on the availability of technical resources as any dosimetric advantage that the various techniques may or may not have. For example, the noncoplanar method may not be possible on all linear accelerators due to the presence of a beam stop or limited clearance of the gantry and collimator to the patient. In some busy clinics, the longer treatment times with six fields compared to four fields may not be justified if doses less than 74 Gy are utilized.

Because 3D-CRT employs more shaped fields than conventional radiation therapy, automatic beam-shaping devices are necessary to make the treatment process more efficient. If customized cerrobend metal alloy blocks are used for each field, a therapist much enter the treatment room before each of six or seven fields to manually change the block aperture. Multileaf collimators allow for automatic and remote field shaping adjustment. This enhances operational efficiency of the accelerator and reduces treatment times from more than 20 minutes to 12 minutes.

Plan Optimization and Review

Following the application of multiple radiation beams and shaping with BEV tools, the treatment-planning computer will calculate the radiation distribution based upon the characteristics of the treatment machine's x-ray output. The radiation dose distribution can be displayed on the segmented patient CT data with color-wash or wire-frame contours (Fig. 13F.3). Room view displays with interactive, real-time image-manipulation tools help review the adequacy of the dose distribution. Areas of radiation under-dosage to a target or over-dosage to an organ at risk can be identified.

Review of multiple dose levels is difficult with room-view displays because of overlap and crowding of objects on the computer screen. Planar two-dimensional (2-D) displays of

TABLE 13F.2

COMPARISON OF MEAN DOSIMETRIC PARAMETERS FOR THREE-DIMENSIONAL (3D) CONFORMAL OR STANDARD BILATERAL ARC ROTATION IN CARCINOMA OF PROSTATE

Parameter	Prostate irradiation only	
	3D conformal therapy	Standard therapy
Number of observations	87	87
Percent PTV receiving ≥ prescribed dose	92.9 ± 13.9	92.9 ± 10.8
ICRU dose (Gy)	69.1 ± 2.6	69.2 ± 2.6
Minimum tumor dose (Gy)	66.3 ± 5.3	63.5 ± 8.6
Mean tumor dose (Gy)	69.8 ± 2.6	69.7 ± 2.8
Maximum dose (Gy)	71.7 ± 2.4	71.3 ± 2.8
Percent volume rectum ≥65 Gy	33.7 ± 15	62.7 ± 21
Percent volume rectum ≥70 Gy	8.5 ± 11.8	28.8 ± 28.9
Percent volume bladder ≥65 Gy	22.3 ± 12.5	50.5 ± 22.8
Percent volume bladder ≥70 Gy	6.3 ± 8.4	19.4 ± 24.4

PTV, planning target volume; ICRU, international commission on radiation units and measurements.
From Perez CA, Michalski J, Ballard S, et al. Cost benefit of emerging technology in localized carcinoma of the prostate. *Int J Radiat Oncol Biol Phys* 1997,39:875–883.

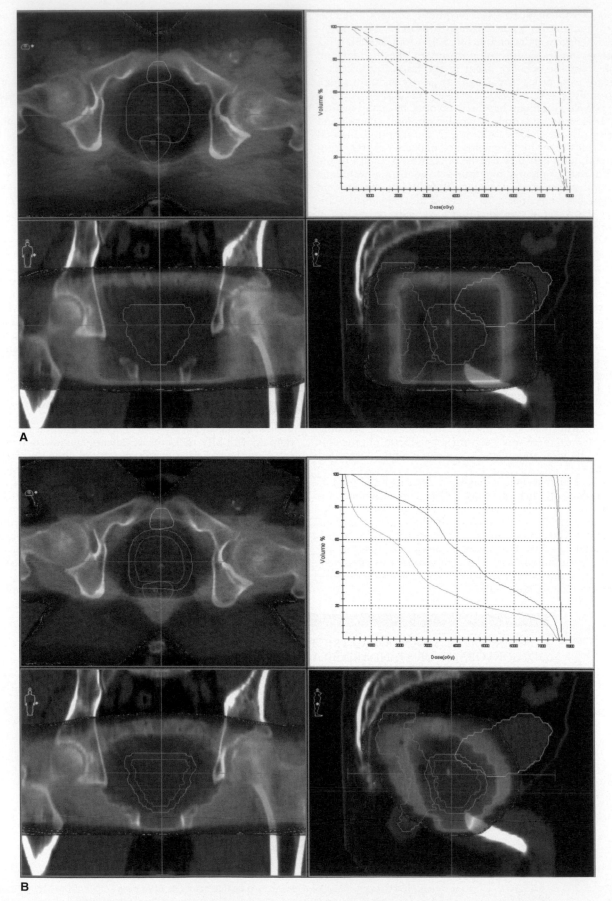

FIGURE 13F.3. Radiation dose distribution is represented by a color-wash display on axial, sagittal, and coronal CT reconstructions for (**A**) 2-D "arc" plan and (**B**) 3D six field conformal plan. The upper-right panel in each group is a DVH of the bladder, rectum, and PTV. (See color insert.)

cross-sectional axial or reconstructed sagittal and coronal CT scans facilitate review of multiple dose levels.

Both the room view and 2-D image reconstructions limit the radiation oncologist to a few dose levels reviewed at one time. In order to take advantage of the complete dosimetric data available for plan interpretation, dose volume histograms (DVHs) are calculated. DVHs summarize the complete dose distribution to a target or organ at risk in a linear graph model. On the horizontal axis, the radiation dose can be represented in Gray (Gy) or as a percent of the prescribed dose. The vertical axis represents the organ volume in cubic centimeters or as a percent of the whole organ. A differential DVH is a plot of equally spaced dose bins. A cumulative, or integral, DVH is a plot of the volume of a structure receiving certain dose or higher, against dose. The cumulative DVH is generally more helpful for plan interpretation and review (Fig. 13F.4).

The DVH facilitates identification that either an underdosed region of a target or an overdosed region of an organ at risk exists. The DVH can be displayed with dose statistics, such as minimum, maximum, or mean dose to the volume. The DVH's most significant shortcoming is the lack of spatial information provided. The DVH may reveal that an unacceptable dose distribution is present, but it does not illustrate its location. For this reason, the DVH, room view, and 2-D reconstructions are complementary.

The radiation therapy planning process is iterative. The plan is created by a dosimetrist and then reviewed by the radiation oncologist and physicist. It is common for the plan to be redone with modifications in field shaping or with a change in the relative dose contribution per field to optimize the dose distribution.

TUMOR CONTROL WITH 3D CONFORMAL RADIOTHERAPY

Before beginning a detailed discussion of the results of 3D conformal radiotherapy (3D-CRT), one must review how tumor-control outcomes are commonly assessed. Determining the success of treatment following 3D-CRT is more complex than treatment appraisal following radical prostatectomy because radiotherapy, by its nature, is a relatively tumor-specific therapy and can eliminate neoplastic cells while sparing normal prostatic epithelium, the result of which, in contrast to radical prostatectomy, can be a patient cured of prostate cancer who also has a detectable PSA. Studies of patients following radiotherapy (RT) generally use either a PSA defined endpoint (sometimes called biochemical control or biochemical failure), a biopsy-determined pathologic endpoint, or a clinical endpoint, such as time to distant metastases, death from prostate cancer, or overall survival. Given the long time interval between biochemical failure and death from prostate cancer, many studies have focused on biochemical failure, recognizing that the link between biochemical failure and prostate cancer death has yet to be completely forged.

Many different definitions of biochemical failure following RT have been devised. In order to standardize the definition, a consensus conference was sponsored by the American Society of Therapeutic Radiology and Oncology (ASTRO), and a definition was designed that took into account the fluctuating nature of serial PSA values over time following RT. Thus, the consensus definition stated that "three consecutive increases in PSA is a reasonable definition of biochemical failure after radiation therapy...the date of failure should be the midpoint between the postirradiation nadir PSA and the first of the three consecutive rises" (62). This definition, generally known as "the ASTRO definition," has become widely used, although its use was cautioned against for patients who received combined androgen suppression therapy (AST) and RT. After its adoption, the definition has been criticized primarily for the backdating of failure to the midpoint between the postirradiation nadir and the first rise in PSA. This backdating results in discrepancy of outcome reporting with varying lengths of clinical follow-up.

More recently, there have been proposed definitions that seem to offer better sensitivity and specificity in identifying patients who are at risk for clinical consequences subsequent to biochemical failure. These definitions rely on a fixed magnitude rise (of 2 or 3 ng/mL) in PSA above the lowest value observed following treatment and are sometimes known as "the Houston definition," after work performed by statisticians at the M.D. Anderson Cancer Center in Houston (63–65). Advantages of this type of definition include greater specificity and potentially the ability to use this definition for both patients treated with RT alone and for patients treated with RT combined with AST (66). Recent attempts to improve upon the ASTRO definition have also been challenged to create a definition that crosses all treatment modalities, including radical prostatectomy and brachytherapy. However, since surgery and brachytherapy are intrinsically more ablative than

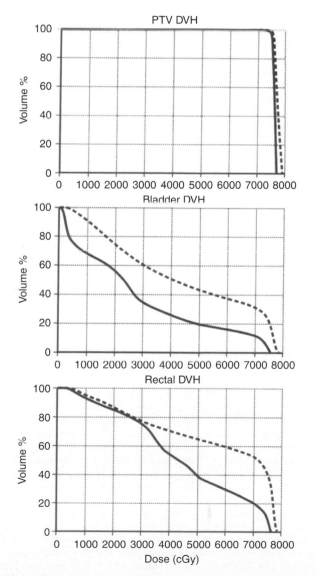

FIGURE 13F.4. Cumulative DVHs demonstrate coverage of the PTV and a reduction in dose to the bladder and rectum using 3D-CRT (*solid*) compared to a 2-D plan with bilateral 120 degree arcs (*dash*).

RT, there does not seem to be a definition that can be applied across all modalities.

Besides biochemically-defined definitions, such as the ASTRO definition, prostate biopsies following RT have been used to define treatment success. The potential advantage for biopsy-defined success or failure compared with biochemical failure is that biopsy can confirm local failure, while biochemical failure can be due to local or distant disease. The largest post-RT prostate biopsy experience consisted of nearly 500 patients who were prospectively biopsied several times following conventional radiotherapy (67). Significantly, this trial confirmed the finding that the time to pathologically confirmed complete response following RT can be prolonged. That is, of patients who showed residual cancer on their first posttreatment biopsy done 12 to18 months following RT, 30% of these converted to negative biopsies upon subsequent evaluation. The time to reach nadir PSA for this group of patients was 26 months. Thus, the conventional wisdom of discounting the significance of a positive post-RT biopsy for the first 2 to 3 years was confirmed. Also, this study using conventional RT showed approximately 30% local failure, indicating suboptimal tumor eradication with conventional dose therapy. Further, this study also established that biopsy-determined locally recurrent disease at 36 months was prognostically important and perhaps should be employed in studies assessing new RT strategies where local efficacy assessment is the primary endpoint. The importance of ensuring local disease eradication with RT should not be underestimated, since studies suggest that the failure to obtain local control may result in a late wave of distant metastases that might have been prevented if local control had been achieved at the outset (68).

Finally, along the lines of assessing outcome of treatment, dynamic indices of PSA following RT may be important. PSA values that are rising rapidly following RT are probably an indication of distant metastases (69) and are more likely to result in prostate-cancer-specific death. D'Amico analyzed two large databases to assess PSA doubling time following primary RT or surgery and found that PSA doubling times of 3 months or less were associated with prostate-specific deaths, while more slowly rising PSA patterns following treatment could not be associated with prostate cancer mortality, given the competing causes of death in this patient population of mostly older men (70). Similarly, using a complex model taking into account baseline factors, Taylor has shown that clinical failure is most strongly associated with the slope of log-transformed PSA values, (i.e., PSA doubling time) (71). One potential criticism of dynamic constructs of PSA following treatment is that calculation of the doubling time or using a statistical model may hamper clinical implementation, compared with either the ASTRO- or a Houston-styled definition of treatment failure.

As previously noted in this chapter, 3D-CRT has allowed the safe delivery of higher doses of radiotherapy in an attempt to intensify the local application of RT and to result in more local tumor control and, hopefully, more cures. As 3D-CRT became more widespread, the radiotherapy community first tested the application of higher doses for tolerability (72) and then for efficacy. It was recognized relatively early in the modern radiotherapy era that higher doses of external beam therapy could not be safely delivered with conventional techniques; an upper limit of 70 Gy was often considered to be the maximum safe dose. So, any discussion of the efficacy of 3D-CRT can be translated into a discussion of higher doses, since higher doses can only be applied with 3D-CRT techniques (or other focused radiotherapy technologies such as IMRT or proton beam).

Higher doses of external RT have been shown to improve biochemical disease control, usually using the ASTRO definition, and, in at least one study so far, have been shown to improve survival. Early adopters of 3D-CRT technology have the longest follow-up information, and in a study with more than 5 years of follow-up data, both pre-radiotherapy PSA and radiotherapy dose were powerfully and significantly associated with biochemical control (ASTRO), especially for those patients whose pre-RT PSA is between 10 to 20 ng/mL. For example, among patients with PSA 10 to 20 ng/mL, the PSA control was 79% when doses ≥76 Gy were used and only 24% when doses <72 Gy were used (73). The decreased ability to observe dose-related effects for patients presenting with higher PSA (>20 ng/mL) and lower PSA (<10 ng/mL) can be interpreted as showing that lower doses are acceptable for the lowest risk patient since they generally have smaller volumes of cancer, and that local control is less meaningful for higher risk patients who are less common and statistically harder to evaluate and also may have distant metastatic disease not influenced by more intensive local treatment. Another study showed that for intermediate-risk patients (primarily PSA 10–20 ng/mL or Gleason 7 patients), the dose-control relationship was quite steep with a hazard ratio of .92 per Gy of additional radiotherapy, indicating that each additional Gy of 3D-CRT reduced the biochemical failure rate by 8% (74). In order to evaluate higher risk patients further, one study pooled data from three centers to accumulate more information on high Gleason score patients, and 180 Gleason 8 to 10 patients treated with 3D-CRT were analyzed. In addition to T-stage and pretreatment PSA, the treatment dose was significant in predicting freedom from biochemical relapse (ASTRO definition), especially in the T1-T2 patients, indicating at least some effect of dose for patients who might be expected to harbor subclinical metastatic disease. Additionally, the data seemed to be superior to biochemical control data from contemporary reports of surgically treated patients (75).

Another approach to evaluating the effect of dose—and thus 3D-CRT—on outcome has been to use a nomogram approach (76). This has been used successfully for several clinical prostate cancer scenarios, including the development and validation of a pretreatment 3D-CRT nomogram that uses ASTRO-defined biochemical relapse at 5 years as the primary endpoint. This nomogram assigns a number of points to various prognostic factors, including PSA, T-stage, and Gleason score, but also incorporates the delivered conformal radiotherapy dose. The nomogram assigns the most points (where more points predicts a worse outcome) for higher pretreatment PSA values, which confirms the generally held belief that an elevated PSA is the strongest factor in predicting PSA-determined relapse. Of note, though, is that the number of points assigned as a function of dose is as strong at affecting outcome as the well known prognostic factors of Gleason score and T-stage.

The ideal method of assessing the benefit of 3D-CRT or higher treatment doses is through randomized clinical trials. One relatively large trial has been reported showing a benefit of higher doses of 3D-CRT (77). Patients with T1-T3 prostate cancer (301) were randomized to either conventionally delivered RT of 70 Gy or conformally boosted RT to 78 Gy. Patients with any Gleason score and any PSA were eligible, and AST was not used. The primary endpoint was ASTRO-defined biochemical freedom from failure. With a 60-month median follow-up, the trial showed an overall benefit to the use of higher dose 3D-CRT. The 6-year freedom from failure for all patients was improved from 64% to 70% ($P = .03$). But in line with a smaller effect observed for lower risk patients, this study also showed no benefit for patients with a pretreatment PSA lesser than or equal to 10 ng/mL and a larger benefit for those with higher volume cancer and a PSA greater than 10 ng/mL. For the higher PSA patients, the 5-year freedom from relapse was improved from approximately 44% to 72%. This study, while large enough to detect differences in biochemical relapse, may not be large enough to observe differences in

TABLE 13F.3

RESULTS OF CONFORMAL THERAPY FOR INTERMEDIATE RISK PROSTATE CANCER PATIENTS

	Dose (Gy)	5-Yr bNED (%)	Patients
Fox Chase Cancer Center (73)	<72	24	PSA 10-20 ng/mL
	72–76	65	Any Gleason
	76+	79	Any T-stage
MSKCC nomogram estimate (76)	70	51	PSA <15 ng/mL
	75	66	Gleason 7
	80	70	T2a
M. D. Anderson Cancer Center	70	44	PSA >10 ng/mL
Randomized Trial (77)	78	72	Any Gleason
			T1-T3

bNED, biochemical non-evidence.

prostate-cancer-specific mortality or overall survival. So following a large phase I, dose-escalation clinical trial directed by the Radiation Therapy Oncology Group (RTOG), the group has initiated a definitive phase III dose comparison trial (RTOG P-0126) using 3D-CRT (or IMRT) to deliver either 70.2 Gy or 79.2 Gy. This study will enroll 1,520 patients and is designed to detect an overall survival advantage to higher dose 3D-CRT, if such an advantage exists.

For a summary of data regarding dose and biochemical control for intermediate-risk patients treated with 3D-CRT (see Table 13F.3).

Given the data presented in Table 13F.3 showing a benefit in biochemical control with 3D-CRT, are there data suggesting a reduction in prostate cancer death or an improvement in overall survival? One might need to wait until large trials, such as RTOG P-0126 are completed, but there are some indications from previous studies. Older phase III RTOG studies from the 1970s have some built-in dose variability, and this variability was examined (78) to see if higher protocol doses yielded better survival. For patients who received protocol doses greater than 66 Gy, overall and prostate-cancer-specific survival was better than for patients who received protocol-compliant doses of less than 66 Gy, although the observed benefit was restricted to patients with Gleason scores of 8 to 10. The randomized trial from M.D. Anderson Cancer Center (77) was designed to observe differences in biochemical

freedom from relapse, but also showed an interesting reduction in the incidence of observed distant metastases in the higher dose arm (2% vs. 12%, $P = .056$) for patients with pretreatment PSA >10 ng/mL, strengthening the supposition that improved local control results in fewer distant metastases. This reduction in distant metastases with higher doses has also been observed in a single institution study of 3D-CRT (79) but not in a nomogram analysis, although it is postulated that the dose range is narrow and the follow-up interval is relatively short in the datasets used to derive the nomogram (80).

High dose 3D-CRT has also been compared with other treatment modalities, albeit not in a randomized phase III manner. However, large datasets of T1-T2 prostate cancer patients from two centers were pooled and biochemical control outcome was assessed for patients treated with high dose (>72 Gy) conformal external beam (EB) RT brachytherapy with a permanent implant (PI) alone, for brachytherapy combined with external beam treatment (COMB), and for radical prostatectomy (RP). The outcome data extend beyond 5 years and show no difference when all patients are considered or when the patients are broken into favorable and unfavorable subsets (Fig. 13F.5) (81). This modern data seems to validate strongly the role of high dose 3D-CRT and affirms its role in the treatment of localized prostate cancer. Given the long natural history of prostate cancer, one might question whether the durability of the biochemical control rate—usually noted

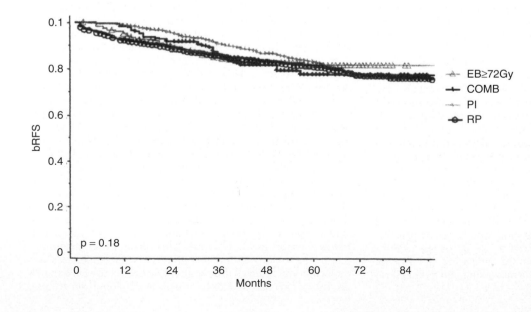

FIGURE 13F.5. Biochemical relapse-free results by treatment modality. EB, external beam, COMB, combined permanent seed implant and EB, PI, permanent seed implant, RP, radical prostatectomy, bRFS, biochemical relapse-free survival. (Reprinted with permission from Kupelian PA. Radical prostatectomy, external beam radiotherapy <72 Gy, external beam radiotherapy ≥72 Gy, permanent seed implantation, or combined seeds external beam radiotherapy for stage T1-T2 prostate cancer. *Int J Radiation Oncology Biol Phys* 2004;58:25.)

at 5 or 6 years—is adequate following 3D-CRT. However, some data suggest that biochemical freedom from recurrence at 5 years is relatively durable and that recurrences beyond this point are uncommon. In the large dataset used to generate the 3D-CRT nomogram, there were no recurrences beyond 63 months and there were 649 patient-months of follow-up beyond 60 months (76). For patients without biochemical failure, even those mainly treated with conventional RT (82), if the PSA is less than 2 ng/mL 5 years after completing RT, the risk of biochemical failure when followed an additional 5 to 10 years later seems to be only about 20% and is comparable to the failure rate observed beyond 5 years for those patients treated with radical prostatectomy.

Although it is much more common for younger men to undergo radical prostatectomy in the US (83), especially those who are diagnosed at age 60 or younger where the ratio of surgery to radiotherapy is approximately 8:1, there is no outcome data to suggest that radiotherapy is less effective when used in younger patients nor that the durability of disease control is worse among those irradiated. In a large review of patients treated with 3D-CRT to higher doses, disease control was no different at 7 years after therapy for those younger than 60 years old compared with those older than 60 (84). This series also showed that lower doses were associated with a higher failure rate, but this effect was independent of the age at the time of treatment. Apparently, in the age of high-dose 3D-CRT, radiation treatments can be delivered to younger men without regard to undue concerns about the long term efficacy.

TOLERANCE OF 3D CONFORMAL RADIOTHERAPY

It seems clear that organ toxicity following RT is related to the RT dose delivered to the structure at risk for toxicity. In general, the relationship between dose and toxicity is complex and mostly follows a sigmoid-type relationship, with no or little toxicity for lower dose exposures followed as the dose increases by a dose range associated with rapidly increasing observed toxicities with small increases in dose, until nearly everyone exposed above a certain dose level has some toxicity. This relationship can be modified by poorly understood, patient-specific issues (i.e., diabetes, collagen-vascular diseases, inflammatory bowel disease, previous transurethral resection of the prostate) and ultimately should be measured using patient-reported, validated quality-of-life measurements. Since tumor control, like toxicity, is also dose-related, radiation therapy dose prescriptions are often pushed to the edge of the steep part of the dose-toxicity curve in order to maximize the probability of tumor elimination.

How has 3D-CRT and dose escalation affected the toxicity profile of external beam radiotherapy? Doses have increased from 70 Gy or below for even the largest DRE-detected prostate cancers treated in the 1980s to up near 80 Gy for relatively small volume, PSA-detected cancers treated today. It was observed early in the CT-guided treatment era that higher toxicity was associated with higher doses, unless careful attention was paid to reducing the exposure of normal structures. For prostate cancer external beam treatment, the organs at risk include bowel—especially rectal-related toxicity, which is considered the most common dose-limiting structure; bladder, which is more resistant to the effects of RT; and structures associated with sexual function. In a 1990 study using CT-guided but nonconformal RT, the risk of moderate-to-severe proctitis rose from 20% for patients treated to 70 Gy or less to 60% for patients treated to 75 Gy or more, indicating that dose escalation could not be safely performed using conventional radiotherapy delivery techniques (1).

Most analyses of RT toxicities have used a physician-determined scale to quantify toxicity, where grade 1 to 2 toxicity indicates mild or moderate toxicity, perhaps requiring medical management, while grade 3 to 4 toxicity is more severe and involves surgical procedures such as endoscopic ablation of regions of mucosal rectal bleeding or bowel diversion or prolonged hospitalization for treatment. Grade 5 toxicity is fatal and very rare following RT. Various centers have reviewed detailed 3D dosimetric information and devised relationships that quantify the association between rectal toxicity and dose among patients treated with 3D-CRT. For example, investigators at Memorial Sloan-Kettering Cancer Center (MSKCC) observed an overall dose-response for grade $\geq$2 rectal toxicity (54). More specifically, treatment-related factors associated with this level of toxicity include: enclosure of the entire rectum by 50% isodose line on the center of the treated volume and a higher maximum dose to the rectal wall. Compared to the 60% moderate-to-severe proctitis with conventional treatment of 75 Gy or more, the MSKCC data show only 15% grade $\geq$2 rectal toxicity with doses as high as 81 Gy when using 3D-CRT. Others have found that the maximum dose to a rectal volume of at least 10 cm^3 is important and still others have shown similar dose-volume relationships (85–87). The significance of these studies is the understanding that treatment-related parameters can have a direct effect upon observed toxicities, and more important, that reducing the exposure of normal organs may reduce the observed toxicity, further encouraging technological improvements in radiotherapy dose delivery. Patient-related factors associated with more toxicity include older age, diabetes, hemorrhoids, previous transurethral resection of the prostate (TURP), use of aspirin or warfarin, and inflammatory bowel disease.

Some of the best studied 3D-CRT prostate cancer patients are those treated on the large, prospective, phase I study of 3D-CRT dose escalation managed by RTOG, called RTOG 9406. This trial enrolled patients serially through five sequential dose levels: 68.4 Gy, 73.8 Gy, 79.2 Gy, all in 1.8 Gy daily increments; then 74 Gy and 78 Gy in 2.0 Gy daily fractions. Toxicity assessed with a physician-reported late (>120 days) toxicity scoring regimen was compared to historical data from previous RTOG trials. Approximately 1,000 patients were enrolled, making this perhaps the largest oncology phase I study, and toxicity data are available for the first four dose levels (88). Of 255 patients treated to dose-level four, 74 Gy in 2.0 Gy daily fractions, there were only 7 patients (3%) who had grade 3 toxicity of any type (5 bladder, 2 bowel)—although sexual function was not prospectively assessed—and there were no grade 4 or 5 toxicities. There were 20% grade 2 toxicities, which are generally considered mild. Based upon historical RTOG data using non-3D-CRT techniques to doses greater than or equal to 70 Gy, 37 grade 3 or greater events would have been expected, indicating that 3D-CRT allows for higher doses with less toxicity than conventionally delivered RT.

In a randomized study comparing conventional to 3D-CRT with all patients treated to what today would be considered relatively low doses of 64 Gy in daily fractions of 2 Gy, 225 men were treated and followed for late bowel or bladder toxicity (89). For bowel toxicity, there were 5% with grade 2 toxicities in the 3D-CRT arm and 14% grade 2 (plus 1% grade 4) in the conventional arm (P = .006). For bladder toxicity, there were 20% grade 2 or greater in the conformal arm and 23% grade 2 or greater in the conventional arm (P = .34). The time course to toxicity in this study was similar to other toxicity studies; most events occurred within the first 2 to 3 years, with few new events beyond 3 years. These data are similar in nature to the toxicity data observed in the M.D. Anderson Cancer Center randomized dose trial. In this study, however, the 78 Gy arm, which had a better biochemical freedom from relapse, had an increased risk of greater than or equal to grade 2 bowel toxicity than the 70 Gy arm (26% vs. 12% at 5 years), with no statistically significant increase in greater than or equal to grade 2 bladder toxicity (8% vs. 13%) (90).

Although physician-reported outcome data are important, patient-reported quality-of-life (QOL) data may be more significant, as physicians tend to underreport some events (91). A large cross-sectional study reviewed the health-related QOL outcome of 1,014 subjects including age-matched controls without prostate cancer and patients treated for prostate cancer with 3D-CRT (with or without AST) and other modalities (92). QOL was measure with the Expanded Prostate Cancer Index Composite (EPIC) instrument. With a median time since therapy of 29 months, the 3D-CRT patients did not differ from control men in the overall urinary function and bother measures, while differences in bowel, sexual, and hormonal scales were noted. The sexual and hormonal differences were aggravated by the use of AST (93). Of interest, there was no difference in QOL as a function of 3D-CRT parameters, such as dose or treatment volume, perhaps indicating that with conformal therapy, such treatment parameters are less important than patient-specific issues, which have been harder to quantify (94). Others have found similar information, indicating that patients who receive 3D-CRT have bladder function no different than aged-matched control men, but increased bowel complaints, albeit generally mild (95).

There have been reports of increased bowel toxicity when conventional RT is combined with AST (96), but this relationship was not confirmed when a population treated only with 3D-CRT was studied (97). Sexual dysfunction occurs as a late effect up to 2 years after 3D-CRT and has a frequency of approximately 30% to 40% (98). Higher doses to the neurovascular structures surrounding the prostate may influence long-term potency (50) and represent another area in which improvements in dose conformality may result in less morbidity (99). Sildenafil seems to be effective in helping ameliorate impotence when it occurs following external beam therapy (100).

3D CONFORMAL RADIOTHERAPY AND BRACHYTHERAPY

Brachytherapy, usually performed with permanent implantation of radioactive seeds, is widely used for prostate cancer, although it has never been—and likely never will be—compared to RT in a randomized trial. Nevertheless, the results of brachytherapy when used as monotherapy to doses of approximately 144 Gy are apparently excellent in low-risk patients but perhaps less good in more advanced disease situations (101). For higher risk patients, combined external beam therapy of 40 to 50 Gy and a lower dose of brachytherapy (approximately 108 Gy) is an alternative that may result in as excellent a disease control as 3D-CRT, albeit with the potential of higher toxicity, although data are currently conflicting (102–104). The treatment volume for patients who received external radiotherapy in combination is usually the prostate and seminal vesicles with a 1 to 2 cm margin. Thus, the benefit of the combination approach may be to treat subclinical disease just outside the prostate capsule, a region that may be underdosed during brachytherapy performed as monotherapy to the prostate gland alone. A randomized trial, RTOG 0232 (http://www.rtog.org/summaries/gu.html) is underway to compare the survival, quality of life, and economic impact of brachytherapy alone versus brachytherapy in combination with external beam for low- and intermediate-risk prostate cancer patients.

FUTURE DIRECTION FOR 3D-CRT

3D-CRT has led to substantial improvements in prostate cancer disease control compared with conventional radiotherapy techniques, primarily by allowing safe dose escalation from under 70 Gy to near 80 Gy. This dose escalation has occurred in a steep part of the dose-response curve and the influence on prostate cancer disease control has been large. To a great extent, the ability to implement this intensified therapy safely has been a result of improvements in imaging, primarily computed tomography, and in computing power and daily imaging of the prostate target volume. New changes in 3D-CRT will also take advantage of enhancements in daily imaging and computing. In the foreseeable future, one can expect that MR imaging will become widely used in radiotherapy planning to more accurately define the prostate gland (105) and to define within the gland itself abnormal regions that could benefit from partial gland dose augmentation (106). Advances in computing capability will allow for more accurate dose calculation algorithms involving Monte Carlo calculations (107) that can take into account the subtle but perhaps still important dosimetric inhomogeneities that occur because of the increased density of skeletal structures in the pelvis and decreased density of bowel gases.

References

1. Smit WG, Helle PA, van Putten WL, et al. Late radiation damage in prostate cancer patients treated by high dose external radiotherapy in relation to rectal dose. *Int J Radiat Oncol Biol Phys* 1990;18:23–29.
2. Nutting CM, Khoo VS, Walker V, et al. A randomized study of the use of a customized immobilization system in the treatment of prostate cancer with conformal radiotherapy. *Radiother Oncol* 2000;54:1–9.
3. Rosenthal SA, Roach M III, Goldsmith BJ, et al. Immobilization improves the reproducibility of patient positioning during six-field conformal radiation therapy for prostate carcinoma. *Int J Radiat Oncol Biol Phys* 1993; 27:921–926.
4. Kneebone A, Gebski V, Hogendoorn N, et al. A randomized trial evaluating rigid immobilization for pelvic irradiation. *Int J Radiat Oncol Biol Phys* 2003;56:1105–1111.
5. Zelefsky MJ, Happersett L, Leibel SA, et al. The effect of treatment positioning on normal tissue dose in patients with prostate cancer treated with three-dimensional conformal radiotherapy. *Int J Radiat Oncol Biol Phys* 1997;37:13–19.
6. Dawson LA, Litzenberg DW, Brock KK, et al. A comparison of ventilatory prostate movement in four treatment positions. *Int J Radiat Oncol Biol Phys* 2000;48:319–323.
7. Malone S, Crook JM, Kendal WS, et al. Respiratory-induced prostate motion: quantification and characterization. *Int J Radiat Oncol Biol Phys* 2000; 48:105–109.
8. Weber DC, Nouet P, Rouzaud M, et al. Patient positioning in prostate radiotherapy: is prone better than supine? *Int J Radiat Oncol Biol Phys* 2000;47:365–371.
9. Kitamura K, Shirato H, Seppenwoolde Y, et al. Three-dimensional intrafractional movement of prostate measured during real-time tumor-tracking radiotherapy in supine and prone treatment positions. *Int J Radiat Oncol Biol Phys* 2002;53:1117–1123.
10. Bayley AJ, Catton CN, Haycocks T, et al. A randomized trial of supine vs prone positioning in patients undergoing escalated dose conformal radiotherapy for prostate cancer. *Radiother Oncol* 2004;70:37–44.
11. McLaughlin PW, Wygoda A, Sahijdak W, et al. The effect of patient position and treatment technique in conformal treatment of prostate cancer. *Int J Radiat Oncol Biol Phys* 1999;45:407–413.
12. Litzenberg D, Dawson LA, Sandler H, et al. Daily prostate targeting using implanted radiopaque markers. *Int J Radiat Oncol Biol Phys* 2002;52: 699–703.
13. Prescribing, Recording, and Reporting Photon Beam Therapy (Supplement to ICRU Report No. 50), Report No. 62, International Commission on Radiation Units and Measurements, Washington, DC, 1999.
14. Prescribing, Recording, and Reporting Photon Beam Therapy, Report No. 50, International Commission on Radiation Units and Measurements, Washington, DC, 1993.
15. Partin AW, Yoo J, Carter HB, et al. The use of prostate specific antigen, clinical stage and Gleason score to predict pathological stage in men with localized prostate cancer. *J Urol* 1993;150:110–114.

16. Pisansky TM, Blute ML, Suman VJ, et al. Correlation of pretherapy prostate cancer characteristics with seminal vesicle invasion in radical prostatectomy specimens. *Int J Radiat Oncol Biol Phys* 1996;36:585–591.

17. Roach M, Faillace-Akazawa P, Malfatti C III. Prostate volumes and organ movement defined by serial computerized tomographic scans during three-dimensional conformal radiotherapy. *Radiat Oncol Investig* 1997;5:187–194.

18. Kestin L, Goldstein N, Vicini F, et al. Treatment of prostate cancer with radiotherapy: should the entire seminal vesicles be included in the clinical target volume? *Int J Radiat Oncol Biol Phys* 2002;54:686–697.

19. Roach M III, Marquez C, Yuo HS, et al. Predicting the risk of lymph node involvement using the pre-treatment prostate specific antigen and Gleason score in men with clinically localized prostate cancer [see Comments]. *Int J Radiat Oncol Biol Phys* 1994;28:33–37.

20. Wilder RB, Fone PD, Rademacher DE, et al. Localization of the prostatic apex for radiotherapy treatment planning using urethroscopy. *Int J Radiat Oncol Biol Phys* 1997;38:737–741.

21. Rasch C, Barillot I, Remeijer P, et al. Definition of the prostate in CT and MRI: a multi-observer study. *Int J Radiat Oncol Biol Phys* 1999;43:57–66.

22. Mah D, Freedman G, Movsas B, et al. To move or not to move: measurements of prostate motion by urethrography using MRI. *Int J Radiat Oncol Biol Phys* 2001;50:947–951.

23. Tinger A, Michalski JM, Cheng A, et al. A critical evaluation of the planning target volume for 3-D conformal radiotherapy of prostate cancer. *Int J Radiat Oncol Biol Phys* 1998;42:213–221.

24. Perrotti M, Kaufman RP Jr, Jennings TA, et al. Endo-rectal coil magnetic resonance imaging in clinically localized prostate cancer: is it accurate? *J Urol* 1996;156:106–109.

25. Algan O, Hanks GE, Shaer AH. Localization of the prostatic apex for radiation treatment planning. *Int J Radiat Oncol Biol Phys* 1995;33:925–930.

26. Cox JA, Zagoria RJ, Raben M. Prostate cancer: comparison of retrograde urethrography and computed tomography in radiotherapy planning. *Int J Radiat Oncol Biol Phys* 1994;29:1119–1123.

27. Crook JM, Raymond Y, Salhani D, et al. Prostate motion during standard radiotherapy as assessed by fiducial markers. *Radiother Oncol* 1995;37:35–42.

28. Parker CC, Damyanovich A, Haycocks T, et al. Magnetic resonance imaging in the radiation treatment planning of localized prostate cancer using intra-prostatic fiducial markers for computed tomography co-registration. *Radiother Oncol* 2003;66:217–224.

29. Langen KM, Jones DT. Organ motion and its management. *Int J Radiat Oncol Biol Phys* 2001;50:265–278.

30. Ten Haken RK, Perez-Tamayo C, Tesser RJ, et al. Boost treatment of the prostate using shaped, fixed fields. *Int J Radiat Oncol Biol Phys* 1989;16:193–200.

31. Schild SE, Casale HE, Bellefontaine LP. Movements of the prostate due to rectal and bladder distension: implications for radiotherapy. *Med Dosim* 1993;18:13–15.

32. Balter JM, Sandler HM, Lam K, et al. Measurement of prostate movement over the course of routine radiotherapy using implanted markers. *Int J Radiat Oncol Biol Phys* 1995;31:113–118.

33. van Herk M, Bruce A, Kroes AP, et al. Quantification of organ motion during conformal radiotherapy of the prostate by three dimensional image registration. *Int J Radiat Oncol Biol Phys* 1995;33:1311–1320.

34. Roeske JC, Forman JD, Mesina CF, et al. Evaluation of changes in the size and location of the prostate, seminal vesicles, bladder, and rectum during a course of external beam radiation therapy. *Int J Radiat Oncol Biol Phys* 1995;33:1321–1329.

35. Beard CJ, Kijewski P, Bussiere M, et al. Analysis of prostate and seminal vesicle motion: implications for treatment planning. *Int J Radiat Oncol Biol Phys* 1996;34:451–458.

36. Althof VG, Hoekstra CJ, te Loo HJ. Variation in prostate position relative to adjacent bony anatomy. *Int J Radiat Oncol Biol Phys* 1996;34:709–715.

37. Rudat V, Schraube P, Oetzel D, et al. Combined error of patient positioning variability and prostate motion uncertainty in 3D conformal radiotherapy of localized prostate cancer. *Int J Radiat Oncol Biol Phys* 1996;35:1027–1034.

38. Melian E, Mageras GS, Fuks Z, et al. Variation in prostate position quantitation and implications for three-dimensional conformal treatment planning. *Int J Radiat Oncol Biol Phys* 1997;38:73–81.

39. Vigneault E, Pouliot J, Laverdiere J, et al. Electronic portal imaging device detection of radioopaque markers for the evaluation of prostate position during megavoltage irradiation: a clinical study. *Int J Radiat Oncol Biol Phys* 1997;37:205–212.

40. Antolak JA, Rosen II, Childress CH, et al. Prostate target volume variations during a course of radiotherapy. *Int J Radiat Oncol Biol Phys* 1998;42:661–672.

41. Stroom JC, Koper PC, Korevaar GA, et al. Internal organ motion in prostate cancer patients treated in prone and supine treatment position. *Radiother Oncol* 1999;51:237–248.

42. Stroom JC, Kroonwijk M, Pasma KL, et al. Detection of internal organ movement in prostate cancer patients using portal images. *Med Phys* 2000;27:452–461.

43. Zelefsky MJ, Crean D, Mageras GS, et al. Quantification and predictors of prostate position variability in 50 patients evaluated with multiple CT scans during conformal radiotherapy. *Radiother Oncol* 1999;50:225–234.

44. Lattanzi J, McNeeley S, Pinover W, et al. A comparison of daily CT localization to a daily ultrasound-based system in prostate cancer. *Int J Radiat Oncol Biol Phys* 1999;43:719–725.

45. Lattanzi J, McNeeley S, Hanlon A, et al. Ultrasound-based stereotactic guidance of precision conformal external beam radiation therapy in clinically localized prostate cancer. *Urology* 2000;55:73–78.

46. Huang E, Dong L, Chandra A, et al. Intrafraction prostate motion during IMRT for prostate cancer. *Int J Radiat Oncol Biol Phys* 2002;53:261–268.

47. Yan D, Lockman D, Brabbins D, et al. An off-line strategy for constructing a patient-specific planning target volume in adaptive treatment process for prostate cancer. *Int J Radiat Oncol Biol Phys* 2000;48:289–302.

48. Michalski JM, Purdy JA, Winter K, et al. Preliminary report of toxicity following 3D radiation therapy for prostate cancer on 3DOG/RTOG 9406. *Int J Radiat Oncol Biol Phys* 2000;46:391–402.

49. Merrick GS, Wallner K, Butler WM, et al. A comparison of radiation dose to the bulb of the penis in men with and without prostate brachytherapy-induced erectile dysfunction. *Int J Radiat Oncol Biol Phys* 2001;50:597–604.

50. Fisch BM, Pickett B, Weinberg V, et al. Dose of radiation received by the bulb of the penis correlates with risk of impotence after three-dimensional conformal radiotherapy for prostate cancer. *Urology* 2001;57:955–959.

51. Steenbakkers RJ, Deurloo KE, Nowak PJ, et al. Reduction of dose delivered to the rectum and bulb of the penis using MRI delineation for radiotherapy of the prostate. *Int J Radiat Oncol Biol Phys* 2003;57:1269–1279.

52. Koper PC, Heemsbergen WD, Hoogeman MS, et al. Impact of volume and location of irradiated rectum wall on rectal blood loss after radiotherapy of prostate cancer. *Int J Radiat Oncol Biol Phys* 2004;58:1072–1082.

53. Boersma LJ, van den Brink M, Bruce AM, et al. Estimation of the incidence of late bladder and rectum complications after high-dose (70–78 GY) conformal radiotherapy for prostate cancer, using dose-volume histograms. *Int J Radiat Oncol Biol Phys* 1998;41:83–92.

54. Skwarchuk MW, Jackson A, Zelefsky MJ, et al. Late rectal toxicity after conformal radiotherapy of prostate cancer (I): multivariate analysis and dose-response. *Int J Radiat Oncol Biol Phys* 2000;47:103–113.

55. Soffen EM, Hanks GE, Hwang CC, et al. Conformal static field therapy for low volume low grade prostate cancer with rigid immobilization. *Int J Radiat Oncol Biol Phys* 1991;20:141–146.

56. Fiorino C, Reni M, Cattaneo GM, et al. Comparing 3-, 4- and 6-fields techniques for conformal irradiation of prostate and seminal vesicles using dose-volume histograms. *Radiother Oncol* 1997;44:251–257.

57. Magrini SM, Cellai E, Rossi F, et al. Comparison of the conventional 'box technique' with two different 'conformal' beam arrangements for prostate cancer treatment. *Cancer Radiother* 1999;3:215–220.

58. Perez CA, Michalski J, Ballard S, et al. Cost benefit of emerging technology in localized carcinoma of the prostate. *Int J Radiat Oncol Biol Phys* 1997;39:875–883.

59. Marsh LH, Ten Haken RK, Sandler HM. A customized non-axial external beam technique for treatment of prostate carcinomas. *Med Dosim* 1992;17:123–127.

60. Akazawa PF, Roach M III, Pickett B, et al. Three dimensional comparison of blocked arcs vs four and six field conformal treatment of the prostate. *Radiother Oncol* 1996;41:83–88.

61. Roach M III, Akazawa PF, Pickett B, et al. Bilateral arcs using "averaged beam's eye views": a simplified technique for delivering 3-D based conformal radiotherapy. *Med Dosim* 1994;19:159–168.

62. Consensus statement: guidelines for PSA following radiation therapy. American Society for Therapeutic Radiology and Oncology Consensus Panel. *Int J Radiat Oncol Biol Phys.* 1997;37:1035–1041.

63. Horwitz EM, Thames HD, Kuban DA, et al. Definitions of biochemical failure that best predict clinical failure in prostate cancer patients treated with external beam radiation alone—a multi-institutional pooled analysis. *Int J Radiat Oncol Biol Phys* 2003;57:S147.

64. Kuban DA, Thames HD, Levy LB, et al. Failure definition-dependent differences in outcome following radiation for localized prostate cancer. Can one size fit all? *Int J Radiat Oncol Biol Phys* 2003;57:S146–S147.

65. Thames H, Kuban D, Levy L, et al. Comparison of alternative biochemical failure definitions based on clinical outcome in 4839 prostate cancer patients treated by external beam radiotherapy between 1986 and 1995. *Int J Radiat Oncol Biol Phys* 2003;57:929–943.

66. Pickles T, Kim-Sing C, Morris WJ, et al. Evaluation of the Houston biochemical relapse definition in men treated with prolonged neoadjuvant and adjuvant androgen ablation and assessment of follow-up lead-time bias. *Int J Radiat Oncol Biol Phys* 2003;57:11–18.

67. Crook J, Malone S, Perry G, et al. Postradiotherapy prostate biopsies: what do they really mean? Results for 498 patients. *Int J Radiat Oncol Biol Phys* 2000;48:355–367.

68. Coen JJ, Zietman AL, Thakral H, et al. Radical radiation for localized prostate cancer: local persistence of disease results in a late wave of metastases. *J Clin Oncol* 2002;20:3199–3205.

69. Sartor CI, Strawderman MH, Lin XH, et al. Rate of PSA rise predicts metastatic versus local recurrence after definitive radiotherapy. *Int J Radiat Oncol Biol Phys* 1997;38:941–947.

70. D'Amico AV, Moul JW, Carroll PR, et al. Surrogate end point for prostate cancer-specific mortality after radical prostatectomy or radiation therapy. *J Natl Cancer Inst* 2003;95:1376–1383.

71. Taylor JMG, Yu M, Sandler HM. Individualized predictions of disease progression following radiation therapy for prostate cancer. *J Clin Oncol* 2005;23:816–825.

72. Sandler HM, Perez-Tamayo C, Ten Haken RK, et al. Dose escalation for stage C (T3) prostate cancer: minimal rectal toxicity observed using conformal therapy. *Radiother Oncol* 1992;23:53–54.

73. Pollack A, Hanlon AL, Horwitz EM, et al. Prostate cancer radiotherapy dose response: an update of the fox chase experience. *J Urol* 2004;171: 1132–1136.

74. Symon Z, Griffith KA, McLaughlin PW, et al. Dose escalation for localized prostate cancer: substantial benefit observed with 3D conformal therapy. *Int J Radiat Oncol Biol Phys* 2003;57:384–390.

75. Fiveash JB, Hanks G, Roach M, et al. 3D conformal radiation therapy (3DCRT) for high grade prostate cancer: a multi-institutional review. *Int J Radiat Oncol Biol Phys* 2000;47:335–342.

76. Kattan MW, Zelefsky MJ, Kupelian PA, et al. Pretreatment nomogram for predicting the outcome of three-dimensional conformal radiotherapy in prostate cancer. *J Clin Oncol* 2000;18:3352–3359.

77. Pollack A, Zagars GK, Starkschall G, et al. Prostate cancer radiation dose response: results of the M. D. Anderson phase III randomized trial. *Int J Radiat Oncol Biol Phys* 2002;53:1097–1105.

78. Valicenti R, Lu J, Pilepich M, et al. Survival advantage from higher-dose radiation therapy for clinically localized prostate cancer treated on the Radiation Therapy Oncology Group trials. *J Clin Oncol* 2000;18:2740–2746.

79. Jacob R, Hanlon AL, Horwitz EM, et al. The relationship of increasing radiotherapy dose to reduced distant metastases and mortality in men with prostate cancer. *Cancer* 2004;100:538–543.

80. Kattan MW, Zelefsky MJ, Kupelian PA, et al. Pretreatment nomogram that predicts 5-year probability of metastasis following three-dimensional conformal radiation therapy for localized prostate cancer. *J Clin Oncol* 2003;21:4568–4571.

81. Kupelian PA, Potters L, Khuntia D, et al. Radical prostatectomy, external beam radiotherapy <72 Gy, external beam radiotherapy > or = 72 Gy, permanent seed implantation, or combined seeds/external beam radiotherapy for stage T1-T2 prostate cancer. *Int J Radiat Oncol Biol Phys* 2004;58:25–33.

82. Yock TI, Zietman AL, Shipley WU, et al. Long-term durability of PSA failure-free survival after radiotherapy for localized prostate cancer. *Int J Radiat Oncol Biol Phys* 2002;54:420–426.

83. Harlan LC, Potosky A, Gilliland FD, et al. Factors associated with initial therapy for clinically localized prostate cancer: prostate cancer outcomes study. *J Natl Cancer Inst* 2001;93:1864–1871.

84. Zelefsky MJ, Marion C, Fuks Z, et al. Improved biochemical disease-free survival of men younger than 60 years with prostate cancer treated with high dose conformal external beam radiotherapy. *J Urol* 2003;170:1828–1832.

85. Huang EH, Pollack A, Levy L, et al. Late rectal toxicity: dose-volume effects of conformal radiotherapy for prostate cancer. *Int J Radiat Oncol Biol Phys* 2002;54:1314–1321.

86. Dale E, Olsen DR, Fossa SD. Normal tissue complication probabilities correlated with late effects in the rectum after prostate conformal radiotherapy. *Int J Radiat Oncol Biol Phys* 1999;43:385–391.

87. Wachter S, Gerstner N, Goldner G, et al. Rectal sequelae after conformal radiotherapy of prostate cancer: dose-volume histograms as predictive factors. *Radiother Oncol* 2001;59:65–70.

88. Michalski JM, Winter K, Purdy JA, et al. Toxicity after three-dimensional radiotherapy for prostate cancer with RTOG 9406 dose level IV. *Int J Radiat Oncol Biol Phys* 2004;58:735–742.

89. Dearnaley DP, Khoo VS, Norman AR, et al. Comparison of radiation side-effects of conformal and conventional radiotherapy in prostate cancer: a randomised trial. *Lancet* 1999;353:267–272.

90. Kuban D, Pollack A, Huang E, et al. Hazards of dose escalation in prostate cancer radiotherapy. *Int J Radiat Oncol Biol Phys* 2003;57:1260–1268.

91. Talcott JA, Rieker P, Clark JA, et al. Patient-reported symptoms after primary therapy for early prostate cancer: results of a prospective cohort study. *J Clin Oncol* 1998;16:275–283.

92. Wei JT, Dunn RL, Sandler HM, et al. Comprehensive comparison of health-related quality of life after contemporary therapies for localized prostate cancer. *J Clin Oncol* 2002;20:557–566.

93. Hollenbeck BK, Wei JT, Sanda MG, et al. Neoadjuvant hormonal therapy impairs sexual outcome among younger men who undergo external beam radiotherapy for localized prostate cancer. *Urology* 2004;63:946–950.

94. Sandler HM, Dunn RL, Wei JT, et al. Health related quality of life following 3D conformal external beam radiotherapy: treatment factors influence patient-reported outcome. *Int J Radiat Oncol Biol Phys* 2000;48:249.

95. Hanlon AL, Bruner DW, Peter R, et al. Quality of life study in prostate cancer patients treated with three-dimensional conformal radiation therapy: comparing late bowel and bladder quality of life symptoms to that of the normal population. *Int J Radiat Oncol Biol Phys* 2001;49:51–59.

96. Hanks GE, Pajak TF, Porter A, et al. Phase III trial of long-term adjuvant androgen deprivation after neoadjuvant hormonal cytoreduction and radiotherapy in locally advanced carcinoma of the prostate: the Radiation Therapy Oncology Group protocol 92-02. *J Clin Oncol* 2003;21:3972–3978.

97. Valicenti RK, Winter K, Cox JD, et al. RTOG 94-06: is the addition of neoadjuvant hormonal therapy to dose-escalated 3D conformal radiation therapy for prostate cancer associated with treatment toxicity? *Int J Radiat Oncol Biol Phys* 2003;57:614–620.

98. Chinn DM, Holland J, Crownover RL, et al. Potency following high-dose three-dimensional conformal radiotherapy and the impact of prior major urologic surgical procedures in patients treated for prostate cancer. *Int J Radiat Oncol Biol Phys* 1995;33:15–22.

99. Kao J, Turian J, Meyers A, et al. Sparing of the penile bulb and proximal penile structures with intensity-modulated radiation therapy for prostate cancer. *Br J Radiol* 2004;77:129–136.

100. Incrocci L, Hop WC, Slob AK. Efficacy of sildenafil in an open-label study as a continuation of a double-blind study in the treatment of erectile dysfunction after radiotherapy for prostate cancer. *Urology* 2003;62:116–120.

101. D'Amico AV, Whittington R, Malkowicz SB, et al. Biochemical outcome after radical prostatectomy, external beam radiation therapy, or interstitial radiation therapy for clinically localized prostate cancer [see Comments]. *JAMA* 1998;280:969–974.

102. Sarosdy MF. Urinary and rectal complications of contemporary permanent transperineal brachytherapy for prostate carcinoma with or without external beam radiation therapy. *Cancer* 2004;101:754–760.

103. Merrick GS, Butler WM, Wallner KE, et al. Long-term urinary quality of life after permanent prostate brachytherapy. *Int J Radiat Oncol Biol Phys* 2003;56:454–461.

104. Ghaly M, Wallner K, Merrick G, et al. The effect of supplemental beam radiation on prostate brachytherapy-related morbidity: morbidity outcomes from two prospective randomized multicenter trials. *Int J Radiat Oncol Biol Phys* 2003;55:1288–1293.

105. Meirovitz A, Troyer S, Evans V, et al. Rectum and prostate separation by MRI vs CT in external beam and post-implant patients. *Int J Radiat Oncol Biol Phys* 2003;57:S334.

106. Pickett B, Vigneault E, Kurhanewicz J, et al. Static field intensity modulation to treat a dominant intra-prostatic lesion to 90 Gy compared to seven field 3-dimensional radiotherapy. *Int J Radiat Oncol Biol Phys* 1999;44:921–929.

107. Demarco JJ, Chetty IJ, Solberg TD. A Monte Carlo tutorial and the application for radiotherapy treatment planning. *Med Dosim* 2002;27:43–50.

CHAPTER 13G
Intensity Modulated Radiotherapy and Proton Beam Therapy for the Treatment of Prostate Cancer

Steven A. Leibel, Zvi Fuks, and Anthony Zietman

Since the late 1980s, early detection strategies have resulted in prostate cancer being routinely discovered at a stage when, in all likelihood, it is still locally confined. As a result, the efficacy of any local treatment is of paramount importance because therapy is potentially curative (1). The relative inability of conventional radiotherapy to control localized prostate cancer results from resistance of subpopulations of tumor clonogens to dose levels of 65 to 70 Gy, the maximum feasible with traditional two-dimensional treatment planning and delivery techniques. Efforts to improve the outcome of localized prostate cancer have greatly accelerated during the past two decades, following the development and implementation of three-dimensional conformal radiation therapy (3D-CRT). Three-dimensional treatment planning systems combine advanced imaging technology with sophisticated radiation dose calculation algorithms to generate dose distributions that ensure that the prescribed dose conforms to the anatomical boundaries of the prostatic target volume. At the same time, a rapid decrease in the dose delivered to the normal tissues adjacent to the targeted tumor permits effective exclusion of the rectum and the urinary bladder from the volume carried to high-dose levels. Accordingly, 3D-CRT has allowed increases in the tumor dose to levels beyond those feasible with conventional 2D radiotherapy (2). Evidence indicates that radiation-induced morbidity is reduced with 3D conformal techniques and that the outcome is improved when higher dose levels are administered (2–9). In a prospective trial conducted by Pollack et al. (9) patients were randomized to receive either 70 Gy or 78 Gy. The overall 6-year freedom-from-failure rates (clinical and PSA relapse-free survival) were 70% for patients who received 78 Gy and 64% for those treated to 70 Gy ($P = .03$). It is important to note that in this trial the 6-year rate of grade 2 or higher rectal complications increased from 12% for patients treated to 70 Gy to 26% for those treated to 78 Gy ($P = .001$) (9). Thus, although higher dose levels appear to be essential for enhancing the local cure of prostate cancer patients, improved techniques that more tightly confine the high-dose distribution to the planning target volume (PTV) are necessary to decrease the risk of rectal toxicity and improve the therapeutic ratio when high doses are administered.

Experimental and clinical evidence indicate that the biologic effects of radiation on both tumors and normal tissue structures are dose dependent, and the resultant dose-response curves when plotted graphically are sigmoidal in shape (10). Tumor dose-response curves are typically described in terms of the dose that controls the tumors in 50% of the patients treated, the TCD_{50}, and the γ_{50}, representing the change in tumor control probability (in percent) with a 1% change in dose about the TCD_{50}. Based on data from prostate biopsy specimens obtained at 2.5 years or more (median 3.3 years) after treatment, Levegrün et al. (11) showed that the population average TCD_{50} for fractionated radiotherapy in prostate cancer was 70.5 Gy and that the γ_{50} was 2.9. Similar findings have been generated based on prostate-specific antigen (PSA) outcome. For example, Fowler et al. (12), using published data from several institutions, found that for intermediate risk patients the TCD_{50} was 65.6 Gy and the γ_{50} was 2. TCD_{50} and γ_{50} parameters vary with definition of risk group and length of follow-up. As shown in Table 13G.1, the Memorial Sloan-Kettering Cancer Center (MSKCC) tumor control probability (TCP) modeling data demonstrated that the TCD_{50} values for low-, intermediate-, and high-risk patients were 68.3, 72.8, and 77.3 Gy, respectively. The corresponding γ_{50} values were 4.6, 4.9, and 5.2, indicating that the dose-response curves for each risk group (representing subpopulations of patients with more homogeneous phenotypic features) are steeper than the more heterogeneous population average curve. From these data, the calculated TCD_{50} values for low-, intermediate-, and high-risk patients were approximately 78, 83, and 88 Gy, respectively (11). These findings are consistent with PSA outcome data of patients treated with escalating dose levels at MSKCC (2) and indicate that prostate tumors with more aggressive biologic phenotypes are more radioresistant. However, the data also show that even for more favorable phenotypes, conventional doses of 65 to 70 Gy appear insufficient and that dose levels of 81 Gy or higher are necessary for a maximal local cure. Because it is not possible at the present time to identify the more resistant phenotypes that require higher dose levels, it appears necessary to provide the maximal feasible therapeutic doses to all eligible patients.

To reduce the likelihood of radiation induced toxicity, the delivery of ultra high-dose radiation, defined as levels greater than 78 Gy, requires advanced radiotherapeutic techniques such as intensity-modulated radiotherapy (IMRT) or proton beam radiotherapy. These approaches share the common attribute of precisely targeting the high radiation dose to the prostate while excluding, to the greatest level possible, the surrounding normal tissues. Computer-based 3D construction of anatomy is routinely performed, allowing greater anatomical definition and the ability to distinguish between the prostate and normal tissues. This chapter describes the IMRT and proton beam approaches to the treatment of localized prostate cancer. The toxicity observed and biochemical outcomes achieved with these treatment modalities are also summarized.

INTENSITY-MODULATED RADIOTHERAPY

IMRT is an advanced form of 3D-CRT that applies highly specialized treatment planning and delivery systems to produce improved dose distributions that conform to the tumor target with significantly enhanced precision (2,13–15). Several techniques of IMRT have been implemented in clinical practice, and their approaches to treatment planning and delivery are quite different. The MSKCC simulation and treatment planning techniques for patients with localized prostate cancer have previously been described in detail (2,16,17). The methods used for patient set-up, immobilization, anatomical image acquisition, and delineation of the target volume and critical organs are similar to those used in 3D-CRT. Because the daily filling states of the bladder and rectum can lead to variations in prostate location and geometry, the simulation and each treatment session at MSKCC are performed after the patient empties his bladder to decrease prostate and seminal vesicle positional variability. The bowel is also emptied before simulation.

At MSKCC, the PTV is delineated on each relevant computed tomography (CT) slice by encompassing the prostate and seminal vesicles with a 1 cm margin. The margin at the interface with the rectum is reduced to 0.6 cm. The walls of the rectum and bladder, the pelvic bones, and the skin surface are also identified on each CT slice. Portions of the small bowel and/or sigmoid colon when adjacent to the PTV are also contoured and taken into consideration, if necessary, in designing the treatment plan.

Treatment Planning and Delivery of IMRT

Computer-automated Optimization of Treatment Planning

IMRT uses the inverse treatment planning technique and computer-aided optimization to generate intensity-modulated beam profiles. Inverse treatment planning is distinct in its basic approach from forward planning used in 3D-CRT. Forward planning begins with an arbitrary selection of a set of beam specifications (e.g., directions, weights, shapes, wedges) and calculation of the resulting dose distribution. Field parameters are then adjusted by trial and error until a satisfactory dose distribution is derived. In contrast, a mathematical approach is used in inverse planning to translate a desired dose distribution to the target volume and normal organs into a clinically applicable treatment plan. A computer-aided optimization algorithm modifies the intensity profile of each radiation beam in an iterative fashion until a dose distribution is produced that matches as nearly as possible the predefined dose specifications for the tumor and normal tissue structures (18). The result is a series of radiation beams with changing intensities across the treatment field. Multiple intensity-modulated beams with different profiles are used to achieve a composite homogeneous dose distribution within the PTV.

TABLE 13G.1

CHARACTERISTICS OF DOSE-RESPONSE CURVES BASED ON BIOPSY OUTCOME IN 103 PATIENTS WITH T1C TO T3 PROSTATE CANCER TREATED WITH THREE-DIMENSIONAL CONFORMAL RADIATION THERAPY

Patient subgroup	Number of patients	TCD_{50} (Gy)	γ_{50}
All patients	103	70.5	2.9
Low risk	43	68.3	4.6
Intermediate risk	37	72.8	4.9
High risk	22	77.3	5.2

TABLE 13G.2

MSKCC IMRT TEMPLATE FOR 81 GY PROSTATE TREATMENT PLAN[a]

Structure	Optimization parameters			Treatment plan criteria		
	Max dose/penalty	Min dose/penalty	Volume	Structure	Dose	Volume
PTV (excluding rectal overlap)	82.5 Gy/50	79.5 Gy/50		PTV	max 90 Gy	$V_{95} > 90\%$
PTV (rectal overlap)	78 Gy/20	75.5 Gy/10				
Rectum	77 Gy/20			Rectal wall	75.6 Gy	30%
Rectum	32.5 Gy		30%	Rectal wall	47 Gy	53%
Bladder	79.5 Gy/35					
Bladder	32.5 Gy		30%	Bladder wall	47 Gy	53%

Max, maximum; Min, minimum; V_{95}, volume receiving 95% of dose; PTV, planning target volume.

[a]The IMRT template defines the parameters that are used as a starting point for optimization and the criteria are used to evaluate the plan. From Leibel SA, Fuks Z, Zelefsky MJ, et al. Technological advances in external beam radiation therapy for the treatment of localized prostate cancer. *Semin Oncol* 2003;30:596–615, with permission.

The MSKCC inverse algorithm makes use of a least-squares objective function and conjugate gradient minimization methods to find an optimum solution consistent with a set of predefined constraints. These include minimum and maximum dose constraints for the tumor target and dose as well as dose-volume constraints for normal tissue structures. The constraints can be violated with a cost or penalty. The penalties specified for the tumor and the normal tissues define the relative importance of each constraint in meeting the goals of the plan. The optimization parameters and treatment plan criteria for prostate cancer patients treated with IMRT at MSKCC to 81 Gy and 86.4 Gy are shown in Tables 13G.2 and 13G.3, respectively (2). Since structure definition plays such a fundamental part of IMRT planning, an important feature of the MSKCC system is the ability to define substructures, such as partially overlapping target and normal tissue structures, and to specify dose constraints for them. For example, the intersection of the PTV and rectum is defined as a distinct structure, and the maximum dose to this region is constrained to a lower value than other portions of the PTV. Because of the strict dose constraint placed on the rectal wall, the entire PTV does not receive the full prescription dose. Thus, an IMRT plan for prostate treatments typically delivers at least 95% of the prescription dose to at least 90% of the PTV (2).

Once the number and orientation of the beams are selected, and the dose constraints and penalties specified, the optimization algorithm divides each radiation field into a series of pencil beams or rays and alters the weights of each ray in an iterative manner until the composite 3D dose distribution conforms to the specified objectives. The treatment fields derived by this method vary in their intensity, and when the fields are combined, the dose distribution conforms tightly to the PTV and exhibits a steep fall-off of the dose within the adjacent normal tissue. It is important to note that the field shapes are not prespecified with the inverse planning approach. Instead, the optimization process determines the field apertures as well as the intensity patterns.

Delivery of Intensity-modulated Beams

Delivery of intensity-modulated beams requires multileaf collimators (MLC), operated in either the dynamic (19) or multisegment static (step-and-shoot) modes (20). The MSKCC system for IMRT delivery uses MLC in a dynamic mode. With

TABLE 13G.3

MSKCC IMRT TEMPLATE FOR 86.4 GY PROSTATE TREATMENT PLAN[a]

Structure	Optimization parameters			Treatment plan criteria		
	Max dose/penalty	Min dose/penalty	Volume	Structure	Dose	Volume
PTV (excluding rectal overlap)	88 Gy/50	84.5 Gy/50		PTV	max 90 Gy	CTV V_{100} >85%; PTV $V_{95} > 85\%$
PTV (rectal overlap)	73.5 Gy/20	72 Gy/10				
Mid PTV (urethral region)	85.5 Gy/10	83.5 Gy/10		Mid PTV	max 89 Gy	
Rectum	73.5 Gy/20			Rectal wall	75.6 Gy	30%
Rectum	26 Gy		30%	Rectal wall	47 Gy	53%
Bladder	76 Gy/35					
Bladder	26 Gy		30%	Bladder wall	47 Gy	53%

Max, maximum; Min, minimum; V_{95}, volume receiving 95% of dose; PTV, planning target volume; CTV, clinical target volume.

[a]The IMRT template defines the parameters used as a starting point for optimization, and the criteria are used to evaluate the plan. From Leibel SA, Fuks Z, Zelefsky MJ, et al. Technological advances in external beam radiation therapy for the treatment of localized prostate cancer. *Semin Oncol* 2003;30:596–615, with permission.

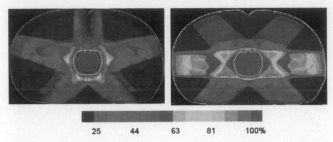

FIGURE 13G.1. Left: Midplane axial color wash dose distribution display of a five-field coplanar prostate IMRT plan for 15 MV x-rays, consisting of fields placed at angles of 0°, 75°, 135°, 225°, and 285°. **Right:** Midplane axial color wash dose distribution display of a six-field coplanar prostate 3D-CRT plan for 15 MV x-rays, consisting of one pair of lateral and two pairs of oblique fields. In these displays a band of the color spectrum corresponds to a range of doses. The prescription dose is normalized to 100%. The red region corresponds to the prescription isodose distribution (100% to 105%). The PTV contour is yellow, the clinical target volume is green, and the rectum is magenta. (From Leibel SA, Fuks Z, Zelefsky MJ, et al. Technological advances in external beam radiation therapy for the treatment of localized prostate cancer. *Semin Oncol* 2003;30:596–615, with permission.) (See color nsert.)

this approach, each pair of opposing leaves forms an individual "sliding window" that travels across the targeted tissue under computer control as the radiation is delivered. The width of the window and the speed of the leaves are continuously adjusted, according to a preplanned scheme, to generate the necessary intensity pattern. A computer program, called the "leaf sequencer," converts the intensity profiles of each intensity-modulated beam into leaf positions, stored as a function of monitor units in a dynamic multileaf collimation (DMLC) file. This information is transferred to the MLC control computer of the treatment machine, which guides the function of the MLC during treatment.

At MSKCC, a coplanar five-field IMRT technique is used to treat patients to dose levels of 81 Gy or higher (21). The maximum dose limit within the PTV is 110%. The dose distribution of this treatment plan is shown in Figure 13G.1. Compared to a typical 3D-CRT plan, also shown in Figure 13G.1, the high-dose volume in the IMRT conforms better to the shape of the PTV and sculpts around instead of transecting the adjacent rectum.

Dose Escalation with 3D-CRT/IMRT

The concept of dose escalation with 3D-CRT and IMRT in prostate cancer was tested in a study at MSKCC, beginning in October 1988, and 1,684 patients were treated through July 2001 (2,8,17,22,23). The dose was increased from 64.8 to 86.4 Gy by increments of 5.4 Gy in consecutive groups of patients. A total of 907 patients received 64.8 to 81 Gy with 3D-CRT and 777 received 81 to 86.4 Gy with IMRT. The treatment volume included the entire prostate and seminal vesicles but did not encompass the regional pelvic lymph nodes. A three-month course of neoadjuvant androgen deprivation therapy was administered to 746 patients (44%) with large-volume prostate glands to decrease the target volume for irradiation and to reduce the risk of treatment-related complications (24). Androgen deprivation was discontinued at the completion of radiotherapy in all such cases. In other patients, androgen deprivation therapy was given only when indicated for relapsing disease.

In the patients treated with 3D-CRT, a decrease in grade 3 to 4 rectal and bladder toxicity was observed from 6.9% in patients treated historically to more than 70 Gy using conventional techniques (25) to 2.2% for those treated to 75.6 to 81 Gy with 3D-CRT (8). However, the 5-year actuarial rate of grade 2 rectal bleeding for patients receiving 75.6 to 81 Gy

was 17%, compared with 5% for those treated to 64.8 to 70.2 Gy (P <.001) (8). Thus, although 3D-CRT reduced the risk of severe toxicity, grade 2 rectal bleeding continued to be a clinical concern. IMRT was introduced to overcome this difficulty and enhance the potential for dose escalation.

Toxicity levels in 171 patients treated to 81 Gy with IMRT were subsequently compared with the toxicity observed in 61 patients treated to the same dose level with 3D-CRT. The acute and late urinary toxicity for the IMRT and 3D-CRT techniques was not significantly different. However, the combined rates of acute grade 1 and 2 rectal toxicities and the incidence of late grade 2 rectal bleeding were significantly lower (P = .05 and P = .0001, respectively) in the IMRT patients. Notably, the 3-year actuarial rate of late grade 2 to 3 rectal bleeding was 3% for IMRT compared with 15% for 3D-CRT (P <.001). Only one case of grade 3 rectal bleeding was observed in each treatment group (21). At 7 years the actuarial rate of grade 2 rectal bleeding in the 171 patients treated with IMRT remains 3% (Zelefsky M, unpublished data, 2004).

The rates of late rectal and urinary toxicity observed in 772 patients treated with IMRT are shown in Table 13G.4. A total of 698 patients received 81 Gy and 74 were treated to 86.4 Gy. With median follow-up time of 36 months (range 6 to 76 months), only 11 patients (1.4%) have developed grade 2 rectal bleeding, and six (0.8%) have experienced grade 3 toxicity. Overall, the 3-year actuarial rate of late grade 2 to 3 rectal toxicity was 2.6%. The rate for patients treated to 86.4 Gy was significantly greater than for those treated to 81 Gy (8% vs. 1%, P = .008) (2,23). These findings demonstrate that the improved conformality and reduction of irradiated rectal tissue with IMRT resulted in a decrease in rectal toxicity as compared to 3D-CRT, permitting a safe escalation of dose to 86.4 Gy.

Outcome of High-dose Radiotherapy

Dose escalation had a significant impact on PSA relapse-free survival. Biochemical failure was defined as three successive increases in the PSA value after a posttreatment nadir level was achieved with date of failure being the midpoint in time between the last nonrising and the first rising PSA value (26). Patients were categorized into three prognostic groups. Those with T1 to T2 tumors, Gleason scores of 6 or less, and pretreatment PSA levels of 10 ng/mL or less were classified as a favorable prognosis group. An increase in any one of the three variables classified patients into an intermediate group, whereas those with an increase in two or more variables comprised an unfavorable prognosis group (2,22).

As shown in Figure 13G.2, the biochemical outcome in each prognostic group was directly related to dose. The 5-year actuarial PSA relapse-free survival rate for patients in the favorable prognosis group who received 81 to 86.4 Gy was 96% compared to 86% for those treated to 75.6 Gy and 65% for patients receiving conventional dose levels of 64.8 to 70.2 Gy (81

TABLE 13G.4

INCIDENCE OF LATE RECTAL AND URINARY TOXICITY IN 772 PROSTATE CANCER PATIENTS TREATED WITH IMRT TO 81 AND 86.4 GY

Toxicity grade	Rectal	Urinary
None	658 (85.2%)	478 (62%)
1	97 (12.6%)	200 (25.9%)
2	11 (1.4%)	89 (11.5%)
3	6 (0.8%)	5 (0.6%)
4	0	0

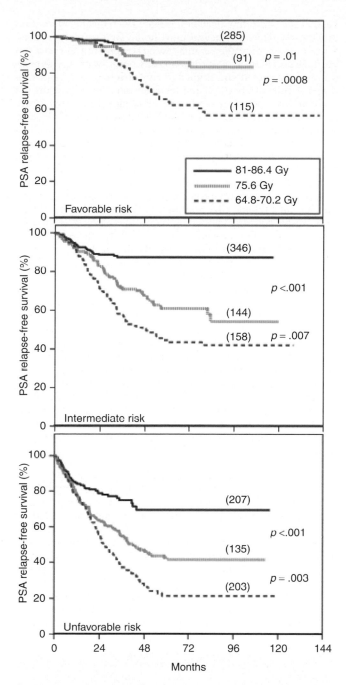

FIGURE 13G.2. Actuarial PSA relapse-free survival according to dose for patients in the favorable (**top**), intermediate (**middle**), and unfavorable (**bottom**) prognostic groups. The values in parentheses indicate number of patients per subgroup. (From Leibel SA, Fuks Z, Zelefsky MJ, et al. Technological advances in external beam radiation therapy for the treatment of localized prostate cancer. *Semin Oncol* 2003;30:596–615, with permission.)

survival with increasing dose might be attributed to improved local control. To examine this concept, sextant prostate biopsies were performed at 2.5 years or more after 3D-CRT or IMRT in 304 patients. Of the patients receiving 81 Gy, 88% (64/73) had negative biopsies indicating local tumor control, compared with 77% (105/137) after 75.6 Gy, (45/69) 65% after 70.2 Gy, and 44% (11/25) after 64.8 Gy (81 Gy vs. 75.6 Gy, $P = .05$; 81 Gy vs. 70.2 Gy, $P = .001$) (2). Patients at MSKCC with intermediate and unfavorable prognostic features are now being treated to 86.4 Gy. Whether this or higher dose levels will incrementally improve local tumor control requires further investigation. Nonetheless, it is clear that such high dose levels can only be delivered with advanced IMRT techniques.

DOSE PAINTING WITH IMRT

The MSKCC TCP modeling studies described above suggested that eradication of high Gleason score tumors may require dose levels on the order of 90 Gy (11). However, escalation of the prostate dose to 91.8 Gy, using the MSKCC IMRT approach, is limited by the ability to produce treatment plans that would deliver acceptable dose levels to the PTV with sufficient sparing of the urethra and rectum. On the other hand, IMRT can be used to increase the dose to selected tumor-bearing regions within the prostate. Such areas can now be identified using new molecular-based imaging methods, providing the potential for localizing tumor foci with specified phenotypic expressions of varying radiosensitivities. For example, magnetic resonance spectroscopic imaging (MRSI) can identify intraprostatic foci of prostate cancer, and their phenotypic features can be categorized according to the spectroscopic characteristics (27–29). Prostate cancer is distinguished by an increase in the ratio of choline and creatine to citrate, and a direct relationship has been demonstrated between the magnitude of the ratio and the Gleason score (30). Higher Gleason scores have been found to correlate with MRSI-defined voxels having a choline + creatine:citrate ratio of 2 or more and voxels in which choline is the only detectable metabolite. As shown in Figure 13G.3, radiation distributions can be produced with IMRT that permit the simultaneous delivery of different dose prescriptions to multiple target sites (called dose painting), providing a technique for differential dose painting to

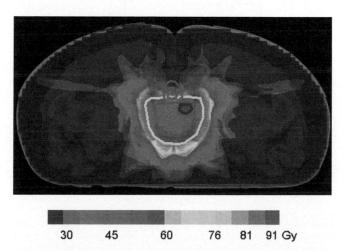

FIGURE 13G.3. Midplane axial color wash dose distribution display of a 9-field coplanar prostate IMRT plan for 15 MV x-rays with dose painting. In this plan the planning target volume (*contour in yellow*) is treated to a dose of 81 Gy and the image-detected target volume (*contour in blue*) simultaneously receives 91 Gy. (See color insert.)

to 86.4 Gy vs. 75.6 Gy, $P = .01$; 75.6 Gy vs. 64.8 to 70.2 Gy, $P = .008$). The corresponding rates for patients with intermediate prognosis were 87% compared to 61% and 44%, respectively (81 to 86.4 Gy vs. 75.6 Gy, $P < .001$; 75.6 Gy vs. 64.8 to 70.2 Gy, $P = .007$). For those in the unfavorable prognostic group, the 5-year actuarial PSA relapse-free survival rate for 81 to 86.4 Gy was 69% compared to 43% for 75.6 Gy and only 22% for 64.8 to 70.2 Gy (81 to 86.4 Gy vs. 75.6 Gy, $P < .001$; 75.6 Gy vs. 64.8 to 70.2 Gy, $P = .003$) (2).

Because radiation was limited to the prostate alone, it is reasonable to assume that the improvement in PSA relapse-free

selectively increase the dose to specific image-defined regions within the prostate (27,31,32). This departure from traditional treatment planning philosophy represents a new paradigm in the management of prostate cancer with IMRT.

PROTON BEAM THERAPY

X-rays (now more correctly but confusingly known as photons) generated by linear accelerators are fundamentally constrained by an inherent property, their "depth-dose profile." This term describes the deposition of radiation within tissue along the path of the penetrating beam. Regardless of beam energy or intensity, the intrinsic shape of this profile is the same with a maximal dose relatively close to the skin and an exponential decrease in dose beyond this point (Fig. 13G.4). The latter property ensures that radiation will always stream beyond the target like a tail. By contrast, the dose deposited by a beam of monoenergetic protons *increases* slowly with depth but reaches a sharp maximum near the end of the particles' range (the Bragg peak). The dose falls to zero after the Bragg

peak at the end of the particles' range (33). This means that no radiation is deposited beyond this point. By using attenuating filters in the path of the beam between the generating cyclotron (particle accelerator) and the skin, this point of energy deposition may be spread and shaped to conform with the shape of a target within the body. If the location of a tumor within the body and the densities of the surrounding normal tissues are accurately determined, it is possible to design exquisitely conformed treatments for deep-seated tumors. Hypothetically, this approach should deliver lower integral radiation doses (doses to nontarget tissues) than can be achieved with photons (34). On average this "dose bath" is about half that of x-rays. The great attraction of the proton beam comes from these physical properties. Though the physical properties of protons are distinctive, the biologic effects on tissue are not. The proton beam does not have greater cell-killing power than conventional photon radiation. The dose deposited by a proton beam is expressed as Cobalt Gray Equivalent (CGE), and this term may be used interchangeably with the unit Gray that's used in conventional photon treatment.

In the early days of proton therapy treatment there were few facilities, beam energies were low, and planning was laborious. Commercially developed cyclotrons now produce 150 to 250 MeV beams, which are of greater interest to the clinician (Fig. 13G.5). These energies correspond to a range in tissue of 15 to 30 cm, sufficient to reach most human tumors and in particular the prostate. Two dedicated hospital-based cyclotron facilities now exist in the United States with three more currently in the planning or construction stages. Randomized trials are underway for tumors in several sites, and the hypotheses of dose escalation and reduced normal tissue injury upon which all conformal radiation strategies are predicated are now being put to the test.

Proton Therapy for Prostate Cancer at MGH

The earliest clinical trial of proton beam in prostate cancer was the phase I/II study reported by Shipley et al. (35) in 1979. Seventeen patients with locally advanced tumors were treated at the Harvard Cyclotron/Massachusetts General Hospital (MGH) with pelvic fields administered with photon beams to a dose of 50.4 Gy and a perineal proton boost to a total of 75.6 CGE. The perineal approach was necessitated by the range limitation imposed by the Harvard Cyclotron's 16 MeV-proton beam. The morbidity profile was favorable with

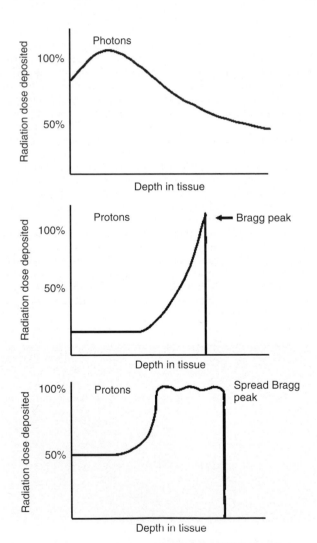

FIGURE 13G.4. The deposition of radiation within tissue. **Top:** Photon (conventional x-ray) beam: note the high dose beneath the skin slowing and exponentially tailing off. **Middle:** Proton beam: rising to the Bragg peak at depth with no subsequent deposition of radiation. **Bottom:** Proton beam with a spread Bragg peak: this effect is produced by modulating filters within the beam in air and spreads and sculpts the beam to conform to the shape of a target deep within the tissue.

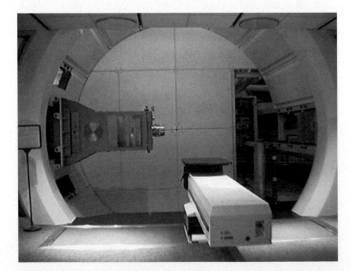

FIGURE 13G.5. Gantry and treatment couch for the delivery of proton beam therapy at the Massachusetts General Hospital. (See color insert.)

only 2 urethral strictures, both in patients who had had prior transurethral prostatic resections (TURPs), and no severe late rectal complications.

In a subsequent study using the same beam configuration, 202 men with T3-4 tumors were randomized in a phase III trial (36). All patients received 50.4 Gy delivered with conventional photons using a 4-field box beam arrangement. Half were randomized to receive a boost to 67.2 Gy using conventional photons through lateral portals, and the other half were boosted to a total dose of 77.2 CGE with a perineal proton beam (Fig. 13G.6). The endpoints were clinical local failure based on a digital rectal examination, a positive post-treatment TURP specimen, or a positive rebiopsy. After 1989 PSA was used in follow-up allowing for a biochemical evaluation of outcome. There was a trend towards an improvement in local control at 8 years, but this did not reach statistical significance (73% high dose vs. 59% low dose, $P = .09$). There was, however, a statistically significant improvement in local disease control at 5 and 8 years for the subset with Gleason score 7-10 tumors treated in the high-dose arm (94% and 84% vs. 64% and 19%). The percentage of positive rebiopsies was also lower for this subset in the high-dose arm although biases will have been introduced here because not all men with negative digital rectal examinations consented to rebiopsy. This significant gain in local control was not seen in men with lower Gleason grade tumors. The improved local outcome for men did not translate into a gain in terms of disease-free survival (biochemical or clinical) or overall survival. With regards to toxicity, an actuarial incidence of urethral stricture was seen in 19% of those in the high-dose arm and only 8% in the low-dose arm ($P = .07$). This was usually relieved by urologic intervention such that it was only a persistent problem in 2% of patients in each arm. Corresponding figures for late hematuria were 14% and 8%, respectively. The actuarial rates of rectal bleeding were higher in the high-dose arm (32% vs. 12%) but in only one patient did this represent a grade 4 complication (37). Among the 78 patients fully potent prior to irradiation who had not had endocrine therapy for a relapse, the risk of subsequent impotence was equal at 60% and 62% (36).

To gain greater insight into the relationship between dose and rectal bleeding, an analysis was performed relating the dose delivered and the proportion of the rectum receiving it to the incidence of rectal bleeding (38). Patients receiving at least 76.5 CGE to at least 40% of their anterior rectal wall had an 81% actuarial risk of rectal bleeding, as compared with 25% who received this dose to less than 40%. This analysis has provided important information that is currently being used to define dose constraints in many active 3D-CRT trials.

Proton Therapy for Prostate Cancer at Loma Linda University Medical Center

In 1991 a program of proton beam therapy for patients with prostate cancer began at the dedicated hospital-based facility at the Loma Linda University Medical Center (LLUMC) in California. Depending upon their estimated risk of nodal disease, patients were either treated with a combination of pelvic photon fields and a proton boost to their prostate or with protons to the prostate alone. All proton treatments were given using opposed lateral 225 to 250 MeV beams which, together with the regular use of a water-filled rectal balloon, reduced the volume of the rectum that was irradiated. The total prostate dose was usually 74 to 75 CGE in 37 to 40 daily fractions. Between 1991 and 1997, 1,255 men were treated. The median follow-up time was 63 months. Using three successive rises in PSA as a surrogate endpoint, the investigators reported 5-year PSA relapse-free survival rates of 90%, 84%, 65%, and 48% for men with pretreatment PSA values of less than 4, 4 to 10, 10.1 to 20, and more than 20 ng/mL, respectively. Late grade 3 morbidity was seen in 16 patients (1%) and grade 4 in 2 patients (0.2%) Gastrointestinal toxicity included grade 3 rectal bleeding and pain in 2 patients and a bowel obstruction requiring a colostomy in 1 patient. Of the 14 patients with grade 3 urinary toxicity, 8 developed urethral strictures, 4 had hematuria, and 1 experienced dysuria. Overall, the 5- and 10-year actuarial rates for freedom from grade 3 and 4 gastrointestinal and urinary toxicity were all 99%, supporting the hypothesis that modest dose escalation may be safely achieved using conformal proton beam therapy (39).

New Protocols

In 1995 the MGH and LLUMC jointly initiated a trial randomizing 390 men with T1-2N0-XM0 adenocarcinoma of the prostate and a pretreatment PSA of less than 15 ng/mL to receive either a 19.8 or a 28.8 CGE proton boost to the prostate followed without interruption by 50.4 Gy using 3D conformal photons to the prostate and seminal vesicles. Although accrual is now complete, the results in terms of freedom from local failure (by planned rebiopsy) or biochemical failure are still many years off. It is of note that 97% of men in both arms completed protocol treatment, suggesting that even high doses of radiation were acutely tolerable. In the first analysis of toxicity 3 years after the first patient was accrued, 242 patients were evaluable. Combined grade 3 urinary and rectal toxicity was observed in 6.6% of those randomized to 70.2 CGE and 2.5% of those randomized to 79.2 CGE (39). Only one grade 4 toxicity was seen, a case of temporary urinary retention in a man in the high-dose arm. Currently, a new phase I/II study is being activated by this group in which men with early stage prostate cancer will be treated using protons alone to 82 CGE. If this dose level is found to be tolerable, it will be tested in a randomized fashion against 75.6 CGE, a dose midway between the two arms of the first trial.

CONCLUSION

Several dramatic technologic advances made over the past two decades have enhanced the precision and improved the outcome of external beam irradiation in the treatment of localized prostate cancer. IMRT has greatly facilitated the ability to deliver higher dose levels to the prostate. The results of the MSKCC dose-escalation study confirm the validity of the 3D-CRT/IMRT paradigm both in terms of reducing late radiation-induced morbidity and improving local tumor

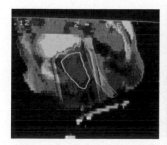
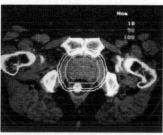

FIGURE 13G.6. Left: Sagittal CT reconstruction showing a perineal proton boost. The patient is in the lithotomy position. Note the rectal probe displacing the posterior rectal wall from the path of the proton beam. **Right:** Transverse CT slice showing the tightly conformal proton radiation isodose distribution encircling the prostate gland. (See color insert.)

control and disease-free survival. The safety of 86.4 Gy has now been demonstrated. Whether the outcome will be further improved at this dose level, especially for patients with unfavorable prognosis disease, remains to be established. Dose escalation can also be achieved with proton beam therapy and dose-escalation studies are now being conducted at MGH and LLUMC. Intensity-modulated proton beam technology is being developed, and its potential in the treatment of prostate cancer has been demonstrated (40). As data from dose-escalation studies using IMRT and proton therapy mature, a randomized trial would be important in determining which approach leads to the highest benefit-to-risk ratio.

References

1. Zietman AL. Radiation therapy or prostatectomy: an old conflict revisited in the PSA era. *Semin Radiat Oncol* 1998;8:81–86.
2. Leibel SA, Fuks Z, Zelefsky MJ, et al. Technological advances in external beam radiation therapy for the treatment of localized prostate cancer. *Semin Oncol* 2003;30:596–615.
3. Dearnaley DP, Khoo VS, Norman AR, et al. Comparison of radiation side-effects of conformal and conventional radiotherapy in prostate cancer: a randomized trial. *Lancet* 1999;353:267–273.
4. Pollack A, Hanlon AL, Horwitz EM, et al. Prostate cancer radiotherapy dose response: an update of the fox chase experience. *J Urol* 2004;171:1132–1136.
5. Lyons JA, Kupelian PA, Mohan DA, et al. Importance of high radiation doses (72 or greater) in the treatment of stage T1-T3 adenocarcinoma of the prostate. *Urology* 2000;55:85–90.
6. Perez CA, Michalski JM, Purdy JA, et al. Three-dimensional conformal or standard irradiation in localized carcinoma of prostate: preliminary results of a nonrandomized comparison. *Int J Radiat Oncol Biol Phys* 2000;47:629–637.
7. Fiveash JB, Hanks G, Roach M III, et al. 3D conformal radiation therapy (3DCRT) for high grade prostate cancer: a multi-institutional review. *Int J Radiat Oncol Biol Phys* 2000;47:335–342.
8. Zelefsky MJ, Fuks Z, Hunt M, et al. High-dose radiation delivered by intensity modulated radiation therapy (IMRT) improves the outcome of localized prostate cancer. *J Urol* 2001;166:876–881.
9. Pollack A, Zagars GK, Starkschall G, et al. Prostate cancer radiation dose response: results of the M.D. Anderson phase III randomized trial. *Int J Radiat Oncol Biol Phys* 2002;53:1097–1105.
10. Munro TR, Gilbert CW. The relation between tumour lethal doses and the radiosensitivity of tumour cells. *Br J Radiol* 1961;34:246–259.
11. Levegrün S, Jackson A, Zelefsky MJ, et al. Risk group dependence of dose-response for biopsy outcome after three-dimensional conformal radiation therapy for prostate cancer. *Radiother Oncol* 2002;63:11–26.
12. Fowler JF, Ritter MA, Chappell RJ, et al. What hypofractionation scheme should be tested for prostate cancer? *Int J Radiat Oncol Biol Phys* 2003;56:1093–1104.
13. Leibel SA, Fuks Z, Zelefsky MJ, et al. Intensity-modulated radiotherapy. *Cancer J* 2002;8:164–176.
14. Ling CC, Burman CM, Chui CS, et al. Conformal radiation treatment of prostate cancer using inversely planned intensity-modulated photon beams produced with dynamic multileaf collimation. *Int J Radiat Oncol Biol Phys* 1996;35:721–730.
15. Burman CM, Chui CS, Kutcher GJ, et al. Planning, delivery, and quality assurance of intensity-modulated radiotherapy using dynamic multileaf collimator: a strategy for large-scale implementation for the treatment of carcinoma of the prostate. *Int J Radiat Oncol Biol Phys* 1997;39:863–873.
16. Fuks Z, Leibel SA, Kutcher GE, et al. Three dimensional conformal treatment: a new frontier in radiation therapy. In: DeVita VT Jr, Hellman S, Rosenberg SA, eds. *Important advances in oncology*. Philadelphia, PA: JB Lippincott Co, 1991:151–172.
17. Leibel SA, Zelefsky MJ, Kutcher GJ, et al. Three-dimensional conformal radiation therapy in localized carcinoma of the prostate: interim report of a phase I dose-escalation study. *J Urol* 1994;152:1792–1798.
18. Spirou SV, Chui C-S. A gradient inverse planning algorithm with dose-volume constraints. *Med Phys* 1998;25:321–333.
19. Spirou SV, Chui C-S. Generation of arbitrary fluence profiles by dynamic jaws or multileaf collimators. *Med Phys* 1994;21:1031–1041.
20. Fraas BA, Kessler ML, McShan DL, et al. Optimization and clinical use of multisegment intensity-modulated radiation therapy for high dose conformal therapy. *Semin Radiat Oncol* 1999;9:60–77.
21. Zelefsky MJ, Fuks Z, Happersett L, et al. Clinical experience with intensity modulated radiation therapy (IMRT) in prostate cancer. *Radiother Oncol* 2000;55:241–249.
22. Zelefsky MJ, Leibel SA, Gaudin PB, et al. Dose escalation with three-dimensional conformal radiation therapy affects the outcome in prostate cancer. *Int J Radiat Oncol Biol Phys* 1998;41:491–500.
23. Zelefsky MJ, Fuks Z, Hunt M, et al. High-dose intensity modulated radiotherapy for prostate cancer: early toxicity and biochemical outcome in 772 patients. *Int J Radiat Oncol Biol Phys* 2002;53:1111–1116.
24. Zelefsky MJ, Leibel SA, Burman CM, et al. Neoadjuvant hormonal therapy improves the therapeutic ratio in patients with bulky prostatic cancer treated with three-dimensional conformal radiation therapy. *Int J Radiat Oncol Biol Phys* 1994;29:755–761.
25. Leibel SA, Hanks GE, Kramer S. Patterns of care outcomes studies: results of the national practice in adenocarcinoma of the prostate. *Int J Radiat Oncol Biol Phys* 1984;10:401–409.
26. American Society for Therapeutic Radiology and Oncology Consensus Panel. Consensus statement: guidelines for PSA following radiation therapy. *Int J Radiat Oncol Biol Phys* 1997;37:1035–1041.
27. Ling CC, Humm J, Larson S, et al. Towards multidimensional radiotherapy (MD-CRT): biological imaging and biological conformality. *Int J Radiat Oncol Biol Phys* 2000;47:551–556.
28. Kurhanewicz J, Vigneron DB, Hricak H, et al. Three-dimensional H-1 MR spectroscopic imaging of the in situ human prostate with high (0.24–0.7-cm^3) spatial resolution. *Radiology* 1996;198:795–805.
29. Wefer AE, Hricak H, Vigneron DB, et al. Sextant localization of prostate cancer: comparison of sextant biopsy, magnetic resonance imaging and magnetic resonance spectroscopic imaging with step section histology. *J Urol* 2000;164:400–404.
30. Zakian KL, Sircar K, Kleinman S, et al. Correlation of proton MR spectroscopic imaging with Gleason score based on step section radical prostatectomy. *Radiology* 2002;225(Suppl.):628 (Abstract).
31. Pickett B, Vigneault E, Kurhanewicz J, et al. Static field intensity modulation to treat a dominant intra-prostatic lesion to 90 Gy compared to seven field 3-dimensional radiotherapy. *Int J Radiat Oncol Biol Phys* 1999;43:921–929.
32. Xia P, Pickett B, Vigneault E, et al. Forward or inversely planned segmental multileaf collimator IMRT and sequential tomotherapy to treat multiple dominant intraprostatic lesions of prostate cancer to 90 Gy. *Int J Radiat Oncol Biol Phys* 2001;51:244–254.
33. Archambeau J, Bennett G, Levine G. Proton radiation therapy. *Radiology* 1974;110:445–447.
34. Suit HD, Urie M. Proton beams in radiation therapy. *J Natl Cancer Inst* 1992;84:155–164.
35. Shipley WU, Tepper JE, Prout GR, et al. Proton radiation as boost therapy for localized prostatic carcinoma. *JAMA* 1979;241:1912–1915.
36. Shipley WU, Verhey LJ, Munzenrider JE, et al. Advanced prostate cancer: the results of a randomized comparative trial of high dose irradiation boosting with conformal protons compared with conventional dose irradiation using photons alone. *Int J Radiat Oncol Biol Phys* 1995;32:3–12.
37. Benk V, Adams J, Shipley WU, et al. Late rectal bleeding following combined x-ray and proton high dose irradiation for patients with stages T3-4 prostate carcinoma. *Int J Radiat Oncol Biol Phys* 1996;26:551–557.
38. Hartford AC, Niemierko A, Adams JA, et al. Conformal irradiation of the prostate: estimating long-term rectal bleeding risk using dose-volume histograms. *Int J Radiat Oncol Biol Phys* 1996;36:721–730.
39. Slater JD, Rossi CJ, Yonemoto LT, et al. Proton therapy for prostate cancer: the initial Loma Linda University experience. *Int J Radiat Oncol Biol Phys* 2004;59:348–352.
40. Cella L, Lomax A, Miralbell R. Potential role of intensity modulated proton beams in prostate cancer radiotherapy. *Int J Radiat Oncol Biol Phys* 2001;49:217–223.

CHAPTER 13H
Brachytherapy
Michael J. Zelefsky and W. Robert Lee

MODERN TRANSPERINEAL IMPLANTATION TECHNIQUES

Improved outcomes and reduced treatment-related complications after prostate brachytherapy depend to a large extent on the quality of the implant and dose distribution. A meticulous approach, attention to detail in the operating room, close collaboration of the radiation oncologist with the medical physicist in the design of the preplan or intraoperative treatment plan, and attention to quality assurance are critical ingredients for a successful outcome.

Preplanned Technique

Transrectal ultrasound imaging is obtained several days to weeks before the planned procedure to assess the prostate volume. A computerized plan is generated from the transverse ultrasound images, which will in turn demonstrate the ideal location of seeds within the gland to deliver the prescription dose to the prostate. Several days to weeks later, the implantation procedure is performed, and needles are placed through a perineal template according to the coordinates determined by the preplan. Needle placement is performed under ultrasound-guidance, and the radioactive seeds are individually deposited within the needle with the aid of an applicator or with pre-loaded seeds on a semi-rigid strand containing the preplanned number of seeds. In the latter case, this is accomplished by stabilizing the needle obturator that holds the seed column in a fixed position while the needle is withdrawn slowly while depositing a row or series of seeds within the gland. In the initial phases of the Seattle experience, seeds were homogenously distributed throughout the prostate gland, which resulted in an increased central (urethral) dose and higher incidence of grade 3–4 urinary complications. In order to decrease the risk of severe urinary toxicity, a modified peripheral-based needle placement and seed-loading schema was implemented (1,2). The average seed activity used ranges from 0.3 to 0.6 mCi, and the median number of needles used is approximately 30 (2 4).

Intraoperative Treatment Planning

While an intraoperative treatment planning implantation technique has been associated with excellent clinical outcomes, there are limitations to this approach. These include the technical difficulties associated with simulating or matching the exact configurations of the prostate, rectum, and bladder of the preplan obtained in the un-anesthetized patient compared with the patient's anatomy during the operative procedure. Consequently, intraoperative adjustments of seed and needle placements are frequently required, and the actual postimplantation dose distribution will not always resemble the idealized preplan. In addition, intraprostatic needle placement causes distortion and edema of the gland, which could lead to significant discrepancies between the preplan anatomic geometry and actual anatomic conditions during the procedure (5,6). At the same time, such deviations may lead to unintentional increased doses delivered to normal tissue structures such as the urethra and rectum, increasing the risks of treatment-related morbidity.

Others have described a treatment planning technique using an ultrasound-based transperineal approach, which eliminates the need for preplanning and rather relies upon the intraoperative determination of the prostate volume and the calculation of the cumulative seed activity necessary to deliver the prescription dose to the target volume based on the Anderson I-125 nomogram (7). The revised nomogram represented an approximate 25% increase in the required activity compared with the original nomogram. In general 75% of the necessary activity would be placed at the periphery of the gland, and the remaining 25% of the seeds would be placed centrally. Others have described "hybrid interactive planning" where intraoperative determination of seed placement was made using Manchester source placement principles (2). While these intraoperative approaches were initially neither computer-based nor optimized treatment plans (which could have more easily accounted for the three-dimensional configuration in the target and normal tissue structures), these techniques attempt to address some of the above-mentioned limitations of the preplanning approach.

At Memorial Sloan-Kettering Cancer Center (MSKCC), an intraoperative conformal optimization and planning system for ultrasound-based implantation has been used since 1996 that obviates the need for preplanning (8). This technique involves an inverse-planning conformal optimization system that incorporates acceptable dose ranges allowed within the target volume as well as dose constraints for the rectal wall and urethra. An ultrasound probe is positioned in the rectum, and the prostate and normal anatomy are identified. Needles are inserted through the perineal template and positioned at the periphery of the prostate. The prostate is subsequently scanned from apex to base, and these 0.5-cm images are transferred to the treatment planning system using a PC-based video capture system. On the computer monitor, the prostate contours and the urethra are digitized on each axial image with a 5-mm margin. Needle positions are identified on each image, and their coordinates are incorporated into a genetic algorithm optimization program (9,10). After the optimization program identifies the optimal seed-loading pattern and the dose calculations are completed, isodose displays are superimposed on each transverse ultrasound image and carefully evaluated (Fig. 13H.1). Dose volume histograms for the target volume, rectum, and urethra are also carefully assessed. If portions of the target volume are found to be under-dosed or higher urethral doses on selected images are observed, appropriate adjustments are made with the deletion of a seed or insertion of a new needle position, and revised isodose distributions are immediately generated. The entire planning process from the contouring of images to the generation of the seed-loading pattern requires approximately 10 minutes. Seeds are then loaded with a standard applicator. The prescribed dose delivered to the entire prostate is 144 Gy. The median seed strength is 0.3 to 0.4 mCi, and the median number of needles required is 20.

Advocates of preplanning approaches have raised concerns about additional operating room time required for intraoperative planning, but with the availability of commercial software programs, the additional time requirements are only 7 to 20 minutes. Intraoperative planning and, in particular, computer-based and conformal optimized treatment planning will more consistently achieve excellent target coverage and reduced doses to surrounding normal tissue structures, although excellent dosimetric and biochemical outcomes have been achieved with preplanning methods. Several comparative analyses comparing a preplan approach with intraoperative planning are summarized in Table 13H.1 (8,11,12). Nevertheless, it should be noted that a well executed preplanned implant from an experienced practitioner will result in an excellent outcome with quality comparable to an intraoperative-based implant.

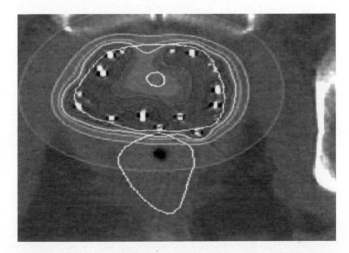

FIGURE 13H.1. Dose distribution of a low dose rate (LDR) implant using intraoperative conformal treatment planning.

TABLE 13H.1

COMPARISON OF DOSIMETRIC OUTCOMES BETWEEN INTRAOPERATIVE PLANNING AND PREPLANNING APPROACHES

Series (ref)	$V_{100}{}^a$	$D_{90}{}^a$	$V_{150}{}^a$
Memorial Sloan-Kettering Cancer Center (8)	96% vs. 86%	116% vs. 88%	71% vs. 66%
Cleveland Clinic Foundation (11)	85% vs. 76%	136% vs. 120%	34% vs. 27%
Tel Aviv University (12)	95% vs. 58%	113% vs. 53%	45% vs. 21%

^{a}Intraoperative vs. preplanned outcome.

Isotope Considerations for Prostate Brachytherapy

In the retropubic implant era, 160 Gy with I-125 was prescribed to a median peripheral dose (MPD), which assumed the target was in the configuration of a perfect ellipsoid. A reanalysis of the dosimetry of I-125 performed by AAPM Task Group 43 revealed that the actual dose delivered for a 160-Gy implant was approximately 10% lower (13). At the present time, the commonly used dose for an I-125 interstitial implantation is 144 Gy, prescribed to the isodose surface, which completely encompasses the prostate as contoured from imaging studies. The recommended prescription dose for palladium-103 (Pd-103) based upon a consensus from the National Institute of Standards and Technology (NIST 1999) is 125 Gy (14). There are important physical differences between these two isotopes. The half-life of I-125 is 60 days with a mean photon energy of 27 KeV and an initial dose rate of 7 cGy per hour. In contrast, the half-life of Pd-103 is 17 days with a mean photon energy of 21 KeV and an initial dose rate of 19 cGy per hour. Based upon radiobiologic considerations, because of its initial lower dose rate, I-125 may be more appropriate for low-grade tumors with a slower proliferating tumor cell population, whereas Pd-103 may be the more appropriate isotope for more rapidly proliferating tumor clones, given its higher initial dose rate (ie, higher Gleason scores) (15). Dosimetric analyses of treatment plans performed with either isotope have not revealed significant differences between these isotopes (16). One retrospective report (17) failed to demonstrate any benefit in terms of local tumor control or long-term complications for either isotope.

Recently, Wallner et al. (18) reported the preliminary results of an ongoing Phase III prospective trial comparing I-125 and Pd-103 for low-risk prostate cancer. In this report, 110 patients of a total planned 380 were randomized to implantation alone with I-125 (144 Gy) and Pd-103 (125 Gy). Six months after implantation, 41% of patients treated with Pd-103 required alpha blockers for urinary symptoms, compared with 44% of patients treated with I-125. American Urologic Association (AUA) scores peaked in both groups at one month after the implant and then gradually declined. While a difference was noted for AUA scores between these groups at 6 months from the procedure, fewer to no differences were noted between the AUA scores of the treatment groups at 9 and 12 months after the procedure. At the present time it appears there are no dramatic differences between the treatment groups. Completion of the trial and appropriate follow-up will be necessary to clarify if any differences exist in the acute and long-term morbidities between the treatment groups.

Post-implantation Evaluation and Quality Assurance for Prostate Brachytherapy

As part of maintaining quality assurance for prostate brachytherapy, the American Brachytherapy Society has recommended that routine evaluation of the implant procedure must be performed with imaging studies of the prostate, such as computed tomography (CT) scanning, and subsequently contouring the implanted prostate (19). Commercial software is routinely available to determine the coverage of the prostate and dose to critical normal tissue structures. Isodose curves and dose-volume histograms produce a detailed analysis of the radiation dose distribution relative to the prostate and surrounding normal tissues. Dosimetric parameters recommended for this evaluation include V_{100} for the target (volume of the prostate receiving 100% of the prescription dose), D_{90} of the target (dose delivered to 90% of the prostate), and the average and maximum rectal and urethral doses. Post-implantation evaluation is performed on the day of the procedure or 30 days after the procedure. The latter time point may be preferable where prostate edema is less significant after the implant and would less likely underestimate the prostate coverage with the prescription dose.

The percentage of the target covered with the prescription dose observed after prostate brachytherapy using standard preplanning techniques varies widely. Several authors have attempted to define acceptable levels of dose coverage of the prostate after transperineal implantation (TPI). Based on early data from patients implanted with the preplanned CT technique at MSKCC, Willins and Wallner concluded that 80% coverage of the prostate with the prescription dose was adequate (20). Bice et al. (21) examined multiple dosimetric parameters obtained from 50 prostate implants performed in five institutions using preplanning techniques. In that analysis the average V_{100} (percent volume of the prostate exposed to the prescription dose) for the respective five centers in ascending order was 77.5%, 84.3%, 87%, 88.4%, and 94.5%. Average maximal rectal doses calculated for each of the centers were 195 Gy, 263 Gy, 271 Gy, 292 Gy, and 354 Gy. No data were reported regarding urethral doses, although it was suggested that implants performed at centers that achieved higher percentages of target coverage with the prescription dose noted a concomitant increase in the central urethral dose (reflected in a greater percentage of the target volume receiving >150% of the prescription dose).

Zelefsky et al. reported dosimetric outcomes for intraoperative planning (8). The median V_{100}, V_{90}, and D_{90} values for the intraoperative technique were 96%, 98%, and 116%, respectively. In contrast, the V_{100}, V_{90}, and D_{90} values for a CT preplan and ultrasound manual approaches were 86%, 89%, and 88%, respectively, and 88%, 92%, and 94%, respectively (intraoperative optimization versus other techniques: $P < .001$). A multivariate analysis determined that the intraoperative technique (compared with other techniques) was an independent predictor of improved target coverage for each dosimetric parameter analyzed ($P < .001$). Maximum and average urethral doses were significantly reduced when the intraoperative technique was introduced as shown in Figure 13H.2 (22). Others have also demonstrated improved dosimetric outcomes with intraoperative planning techniques (11,23-26). A summary of published dosimetric outcomes after TPI based on post-implantation CT-based analyses is shown in Table 13H.2.

INDICATIONS AND CONTRAINDICATIONS FOR TPI

The ideal candidates for permanent interstitial implantation are those with favorable risk prognostic features who have a high

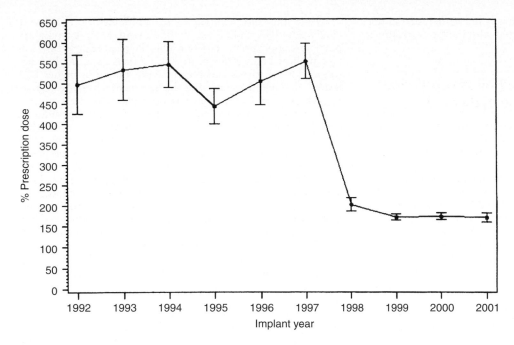

FIGURE 13H.2. Maximal urethral dose expressed as a percentage of the prescription dose (PD) depicted over time. A significant decrease of the urethral dose was observed in 1998 with the introduction of the intraoperative conformal technique.

likelihood of organ-confined disease. This group includes those with prostate-specific antigen (PSA) levels <10 ng/mL with Gleason scores <7. The pretreatment work-up should include a magnetic resonance imaging (MRI) of the prostate with endorectal coil to assess the integrity of the prostatic capsule as well as the geometry of the gland. Such information is invaluable in the planning aspects of TPI as well as in determining whether a patient is a candidate for the procedure. The prostate gland size should preferably be <60 mL. With larger gland sizes, the pubic arch may interfere with needle placement to the antero-lateral portions of the gland resulting in inadequate coverage of the target volume. In addition, larger glands require more seeds and activity to achieve coverage of the gland with the prescription dose, resulting in a concomitant increase in the central urethral doses and potentially increasing the risk of urinary morbidity. One report indicated that patients with median lobe hyperplasia have a higher incidence of acute urinary symptoms after prostate brachytherapy (27). The size of the prostate can usually be effectively reduced with combined androgen blockade therapy. An approximate 30% volume reduction is often observed after 3 months of androgen deprivation.

A prior transurethral resection (TURP) increases the risks of urinary morbidity after TPI (28,29). In these patients implantation should be performed with caution. Using a uniform loading seed pattern, Blasko et al. (29) reported an increased incidence of incontinence and superficial urethral necrosis after TPI among patients with a prior history of a TURP. Wallner et al. (30) observed in 11 patients who underwent TURP prior to TPI a 3-year actuarial incidence of incontinence of 6%. Stone et al. (31) reported on 43 patients treated with TPI using a modified peripheral seed-loading technique. While the authors observed no cases of urinary incontinence, the 4-year incidence of superficial urethral necrosis was 16%. As noted above, patients with pre-existing significant urinary obstructive symptoms are more likely to experience acute urinary morbidity after TPI, and this would represent a relative contraindication to brachytherapy.

Patients who possess relative contraindications for external beam radiotherapy may be more suitable for TPI. These include patients with bilateral hip replacements where CT-based treatment planning is technically difficult due to the substantial artifact created by the prostheses precluding adequate visualization of the target volume. Ultrasound-based TPI would be an appropriate alternative for such patients. In most cases, patients with hip prosthesis are able to tolerate extended dorsal lithotomy position for adequate perineal exposure during TPI. Patients with their small bowel in close proximity to the prostate volume are not ideal candidates for high-dose, three-dimensional conformal

TABLE 13H.2

OUTCOME OF LDR BRACHYTHERAPY ACCORDING TO PROGNOSTIC RISK GROUPINGS

Series (ref.)	Treatment	Follow-up, mo	Outcome, % (*n*) Low risk	Intermediate risk	High risk
Merrick et al. (3)	I-125/Pd-103 IERT	38	96 (90)	98 (121)	79 (61)
Kollmeier et al. (40)	I-125/Pd-103[a]	75	88 (75)	81 (70)	65 (98)
Blasko et al. (37)	I-125	41.5	94 (103)	82 (107)	65 (20)
Zelefsky et al. (39)	I-125	48	88 (112)	77 (92)	38 (22)
Sylvester et al. (41)	I-125/Pd-103	63	85 (63)	77 (92)	45 (77)
Kwok et al. (42)	I-125	94	85 (41)	63 (33)	24 (20)
Potters et al. (43)	I-125/Pd-105	82	89 (451)	78 (554)	63 (418)

[a]60% with neoadjuvant ADT.

radiation therapy (3D-CRT) and are better suited for TPI due to lower doses to the bowel expected with the latter treatment intervention.

PSA Fluctuations in the Follow-up Period after Prostate Brachytherapy

It is important for clinicians to recognize that natural oscillations of PSA levels are often observed after prostate radiotherapy. Similar to what has been observed after external beam radiotherapy, PSA levels can spontaneously increase or "bounce" after prostate brachytherapy. The etiology of PSA bounces has not been elucidated, but it has been suggested that it could represent radiation-induced prostatitis (32,33). Several series have reported the occurrence of this phenomenon, ranging from 24% to 35% of treated patients (32–34). The median time for these fluctuations to manifest has been reported to be 1.5 to 2 years after implantation. The average magnitude of the PSA elevations has been noted to be in the range of 1.0 ng/mL. Merrick et al. (34) reported that factors predictive of such fluctuations include a higher clinical stage, lower V_{150} levels, lower initial PSA levels post-implantation, and lower PSA nadir levels. These temporary fluctuations appear to carry no long-term prognostic significance for the patient.

BIOCHEMICAL AND DISEASE CONTROL OUTCOMES WITH LOW DOSE RATE (LDR) BRACHYTHERAPY

Similar to the predictors of biochemical outcome after external beam radiotherapy for prostate cancer, PSA relapse-free survival after transperineal implantation depends on several prognostic variables including the pretreatment PSA, Gleason score, clinical stage, and implant dose delivered to the target volume. Because of the variability in the definitions of relapse used by various investigators when reporting biochemical outcome after implantation, it is difficult to compare published studies.

While some have defined a PSA failure based on achieving an absolute PSA nadir level of <0.2 ng/mL (35), it would appear more appropriate to define a biochemical relapsed state as an established rising PSA profile rather than a specific PSA absolute value. Patients can present with stable but higher PSA levels (>0.5 ng/mL) years after therapy, yet remain disease free. In addition, similar to what has been reported after external beam radiotherapy, PSA levels can fluctuate after implantation, and in 30% of patients, transient PSA rises have been described that subsequently resolve spontaneously without treatment interventions (32–34). Using the American Society of Therapeutic Radiation Oncology (ASTRO) Consensus Statement definition, three consecutive rising PSA values from nadir point would be a reasonable definition to utilize for the definition of biochemical relapse. A working group has been established to develop a multi-institution data set to explore optimal definitions of biochemical relapse after prostate brachytherapy that would most closely and reliably correlate with long-term outcome.

Grimm et al. (36) reported the outcome of 125 patients treated between 1988 and 1990 with TPI using I-125 and followed for a median of 81 months. A PSA relapse in that report was defined as three consecutive PSA elevations above the nadir PSA level. Among patients defined as having low-risk disease (PSA <10, Gleason <7, and clinical stage <T2b), the 10-year PSA relapse-free survival outcome was 87%. Improved long-term outcomes were noted for both favorable- and intermediate-risk patients who were treated after their initial learning curve was achieved, compared with the initial patients treated at their center (Fig. 13H.3) (36). Blasko et al. (37) reported the outcome of 230 patients treated with a median follow-up of 41 months with Pd-103. Most patients in this report had favorable risk features, whereas only approximately 30% and 20%, respectively, of the patients had Gleason scores >6 and PSA levels >10 ng/mL. The 7-year PSA relapse-free survival (RFS), with relapse defined as two consecutive rising PSA values, was 83%. Post-implantation biopsies were performed on 201 patients. The incidence of negative, indeterminate, and positive post-implant biopsies were 80%, 17%, and 3%, respectively (37).

Brachman et al. (38) reported on 695 patients treated with brachytherapy alone (I-125 or Pd-103) and followed for a

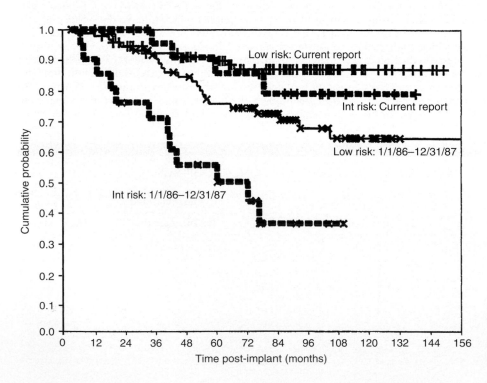

FIGURE 13H.3. Comparison of freedom from prostate-specific antigen (PSA) progression by interval implanted and risk stratum according to the Seattle Prostate Institute experience.

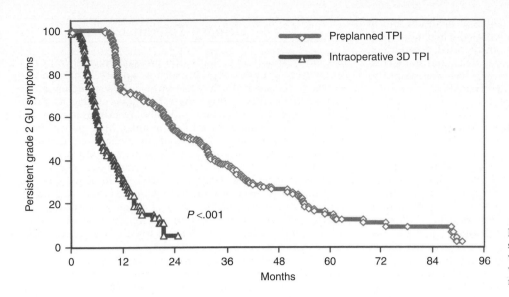

FIGURE 13H.4. Resolution of urinary side effects comparing patients treated with a preplanned implant technique versus an intraoperative real-time planning technique at MSKCC.

median of 51 months. The 5-year actuarial PSA relapse-free survival outcomes for patients with pretreatment PSA levels of 0 to 4, >4 to 10, and >10 ng/mL were 87%, 74%, and 48%, respectively. In an update of the 5-year outcome of CT-based preplanned TPI alone at MSKCC (39), patients were characterized as having favorable risk disease if their pretreatment PSA level was ≤10.0 ng/mL and Gleason score ≤6; those with one and two adverse prognostic features (PSA >10 ng/mL and Gleason score >6) were classified as having intermediate and unfavorable risk disease, respectively. The median follow-up in that report was 48 months (range: 12–126 months) and PSA relapse was defined according to the ASTRO Consensus Statement. The overall 5-year PSA RFS rate was 71%. The 5-year PSA RFS rates for favorable-risk ($n = 146$), intermediate-risk ($n = 85$), and unfavorable-risk ($n = 17$) patients were 88%, 77%, and 38%, respectively ($P <.001$) (Fig. 13H.4). Multivariate analysis identified pretreatment PSA >10 ng/mL and Gleason score >6 as independent predictors for biochemical outcome after TPI.

Investigators from the Mount Sinai School of Medicine reported 8-year outcomes of I-125 implantation for 243 patients with a minimum follow-up of 5 years (40). The 8-year PSA RFS outcome for patients with low-risk disease (stage T2a or less, Gleason score <7, PSA <10) was 88%. Among patients with intermediate-risk features (stage T2b or Gleason score 7 or initial PSA levels 10 to 20) and unfavorable-risk characteristics (two or more adverse features, Gleason 8 or higher and PSA >20), the 8-year biochemical outcomes were 81% and 65%, respectively. In a subset analysis, among patients with low-risk disease who had an optimal dose based on retrospective post-implantation dosimetry evaluation delivered with the implant (D_{90} >140 Gy; $n = 49$) the PSA RFS at 8 years was 94%, compared with 75% for patients ($n = 23$) who received suboptimal dose levels with the implant ($P = .02$). Table 13H.2 summarizes the published biochemical outcomes after low-dose rate interstitial seed implantation according to prognostic risk groups (41,42).

COMPARISON OF OUTCOME TO OTHER TREATMENT INTERVENTIONS

In the absence of randomized trials and the different patient populations selected for specific local therapy, it is difficult to retrospectively compare the biochemical outcome of TPI with other local treatment interventions for patients with localized prostatic cancer. Nevertheless, several reports have made efforts to compare similar patients based on prognostic risk groups treated at single institutions with TPI, external beam radiotherapy, and radical prostatectomy (RP) (44–46).

Zelefsky et al. (45) compared the outcome of favorable risk patients treated at MSKCC with either 3D-CRT (median dose 70.2 Gy) or preplanned I-125 transperineal brachytherapy. Patients with favorable-risk prostate cancer were defined as having a pretreatment PSA <10.0 ng/mL, Gleason score <6, and stage <T2b. Between 1989 and 1996, 137 patients were treated with 3D-CRT and 145 with TPI. The median ages of the 3D-CRT and TPI groups were 68 years and 64 years, respectively. The median dose of 3D-CRT was 70.2 Gy, and the median implant dose was 150 Gy. The median follow-up times for the 3D-CRT and TPI groups were 36 and 24 months, respectively. Eleven patients (8%) in the 3D-CRT group and 12 patients (8%) in the TPI group developed a biochemical relapse. The 5-year PSA RFS rates for the 3D-CRT and the TPI groups were similar (88% and 82%, respectively; $P = .09$).

In a recent analysis of the MSKCC experience using intraoperative conformal treatment planning for permanent implantation, the biochemical outcomes for favorable-risk patients were compared with similar patients treated with intensity modulated radiotherapy (IMRT) treated to 81 Gy. With a median follow-up of 4 years in each group, the biochemical outcomes for the brachytherapy group and high-dose IMRT patients were 95% and 90%, respectively (unpublished data). D'Amico et al. (47) recently compared the outcome of low-risk patients treated between 1997 and 2002 with radical prostatectomy ($n = 322$) and MRI-guided I-125 implantation ($n = 196$). With a median follow-up of 4 years, the 5-year PSA RFS for patients treated with surgery and brachytherapy were 93% and 95%, respectively.

Sequelae of LDR Brachytherapy; Acute and Late Toxicity

Transient urinary morbidity related to radiation-induced urethritis or prostatitis represents the most common side effects after TPI. Symptoms include urinary frequency, urgency, and dysuria. Because of the varying definitions of toxicity reported in the literature, it is difficult to quantify the likelihoods of treatment-related toxicities after TPI. Many reports have not described toxicity outcomes using actuarial methods, and in some studies, only severe toxicity is reported while more moderate complications (grade 2) were not reported. In addition, various implantation techniques, seed activity, and source distribution patterns used by different centers have contributed to the wide range of morbidities reported after TPI.

Acute Urinary Retention

Acute urinary retention (AUR) is a known risk that can occur immediately after prostate brachytherapy, and the incidence varies in the literature as shown in Table 13H.3 (4,48–51). Locke et al. (48) reported the experience from Seattle in 62 consecutive patients followed after prostate brachytherapy. In that prospective study all patients were evaluated with baseline AUA scores, uroflowimetry, and prostate volume assessments. Patients were contacted at monthly intervals to obtain accurate follow-up information. Catheterization was required in 42% (26 of 62) of the patients. The incidence of urinary retention was observed in 34% at 1 week, 29% at 1 month, and 18% at 3 months from completion of the procedure. Among many variables analyzed, a prostate volume >33 mL was an independent predictor of AUR. Other reports in the literature have indicated much lower incidence of AUR after prostate brachytherapy. Crook et al. (49) studied 150 patients treated between 1999 and 2001 with prostate brachytherapy. In this group 13% developed AUR ($n = 20$). Of these 20 patients, 55% received prior neoadjuvant androgen deprivation (NAAD) to decrease the size of the prostate prior to the procedure compared with 27% among patients who were not pretreated with NAAD. A multivariate analysis revealed that larger prostate volumes and prior hormone therapy were each independent predictors of AUR.

Terk et al. (52) reported on 251 patients treated with TPI; 137 were implanted with I-125, and 114 patients were treated with Pd-103. Overall, urinary retention requiring catheterization in more than 48 hours developed in 5.5% of patients. Among patients with pre-implantation International Prostate Symptom Score (IPSS) >20, 10 to 20, and <10, the rates of acute urinary retention after TPI were 29%, 11%, and 2%, respectively. One recent report (53) demonstrated an association between the volume of the transitional zone (TZ) noted on MRI and the incidence of AUR. Among patients with MRI-defined TZ volumes of <50 mL, 50 to 60 mL, and >60 mL the incidence of AUR was 0% (0/40), 33% (1/3), and 71% (5/7), respectively. In a multivariate analysis, Crook et al. (54) observed that only the baseline urinary function and IPSS score were predictors of AUR, while transitional zone index was not a significant predictor of this endpoint. These data in combination with the lack of correlation of AUR with dose delivered to the urethra or prostate suggest that the etiology of AUR is most likely related acute trauma to the prostate gland during the implant procedure.

Urinary Tolerance

In general, almost all patients after prostate brachytherapy develop acute urinary symptoms such as urinary frequency, urgency, and occasional urge incontinence. Depending upon the isotope used, these symptoms often peak at one to three months after the procedure and subsequently gradually decline over the ensuing three to six months. Most patients significantly benefit with the use of an alpha-blocker, which ameliorates such symptoms in 60% to 70% of patients.

Grimm et al. (1) summarized the tolerance outcome in 310 patients who received I-125 or Pd-103 for localized disease. Approximately 90% of patients experienced grade 1–2 acute urinary symptoms, which included urinary frequency, urgency, and obstructive symptoms during the first 12 months after the procedure. Grade 3 acute toxicity was observed in 8% of patients, and 1.5% suffered a grade 4 toxicity. Late grade 3 and 4 toxicities were observed in 7% and 1%, respectively. These authors also reported urinary incontinence rates ranging from 6% to 48% among patients with a prior history of a TURP. Among those patients without a history of TURP and with modest gland volumes, the incidence of chronic urethritis and incontinence was found to be <3%.

The 5-year tolerance outcome of CT-preplanned implantation at MSKCC was reported by Zelefsky et al. (39). One hundred thirty-five patients (55%) developed acute grade 2 urinary symptoms after TPI. These symptoms included urinary frequency and urgency, which were generally treated with alpha-blocker medications. Patients were characterized as having late grade 2 urinary toxicity if acute symptoms persisted for more than 1 year after TPI or had become clinically manifest at that time. One hundred patients (40%) developed late grade 2 urinary toxicity, and the 5-year actuarial likelihood of grade 2 urinary toxicity was 41%. These symptoms often persisted in these patients during the first year after TPI and were effectively managed with alpha-blocker therapy. The actuarial likelihoods of grade 2 urinary symptom resolution at 1, 2, and 3 years after TPI were 19%, 50%, and 70%, respectively. Twenty-three patients (9%) developed urethral strictures after TPI (grade 3 urinary toxicity). The 5-year likelihood of stricture development was 10% and the median time to development was 18 months. One grade 4 late urinary toxicity (0.4%) was observed early in this experience, requiring urinary diversion and a colostomy.

Brown et al. (55) reported on 87 patients who underwent TPI, and urinary symptoms were carefully assessed after the procedure. Urinary effects such as frequency, nocturia, and dysuria generally developed two to three weeks post-implantation and peaked three to four months after the procedure. A gradual decline of the severity of symptoms was noted in approximately 75% of patients during the first 12 months. In this series, 41% of patients experienced acute grade 2–3 urinary morbidity with 6% having acute grade 3 urinary morbidity.

TABLE 13H.3

INCIDENCE OF ACUTE URINARY RETENTION AFTER LDR BRACHYTHERAPY

Series	n	Treatment	% AUR	Predictors for AUR
Princess Margaret Hospital (48)	150	I-125	13	Prostate volume and prior hormone usage
Brigham & Women's Hospital (49)	50	I-125	12	TZ volume (BPH)
Seattle (47)	62	I-125/Pd-103	34	TZ volume >50 mL
Columbia (4)	91	I-125/Pd-103	12	60% AUR
Marseilles (50)	60	I-125	13	Number of needles used >33
Pending	251	I-125	5.5	Prostate volume >35 mL

AUR, acute urinary retention; BPH, benign prostatic hyperplasia; TZ, transrtional zone.

After 12 months 22% of patients experienced persistent urinary morbidity. Of this latter group, approximately 70% of these patients were characterized as having persistent grade 1 and 30% as having persistent grade 2–3 symptoms.

From the above published reports, when compared with conformal radiotherapy, there appears to be a higher incidence of grade 2 genitourinary (GU) acute symptoms with standard implantation techniques. The increased likelihood of such symptoms is related to the higher doses inevitably delivered to the urethra, which generally averages 1.5 to 2 times more than the prescription dose. The uniform source and needle placement initially used by the Seattle group was associated with central doses that were in excess of 200% of the prescription dose (37). This prompted these investigators to use a modified peripheral seed loading approach to minimize the urethra dose to 150% or less of the prescription dose (37). Several reports have demonstrated that acute urinary symptoms and late urinary morbidity after TPI correlate with the central target doses and the proximity of seed placement to the urethra. Stokes et al. (56) demonstrated a reduction in grade 2 symptoms (from 42% to 19%) when the central dose was reduced by placement of half-strength radioactive seeds in the periurethral area. Wallner et al. (57) have previously demonstrated a correlation of late urethral toxicity with the urethral dose from TPI. In that study the average maximal urethral dose among patients with late grade 2 and 3 urinary toxicities was 592 Gy, compared with 447 Gy for those who had minimal (grade 1) or no late urinary toxicity (P = .03).

With the introduction of intraoperative conformal planning for ultrasound-based implantation in 1996 at MSKCC, a significant reduction in the average and maximal urethral doses achieved with this approach translated into an improved urinary tolerance profile and quality of life for treated patients. Zelefsky et al. (58) reported reduced incidence of grade 2 acute urinary symptoms and more rapid resolution of symptomatology with this technique compared with a preplanned technique previously used at the institution. These data highlight the important relationship between the urethral dose and urinary symptoms after prostate brachytherapy. Careful attention to this parameter during intraoperative planning is important for achieving an optimal outcome, and a modified peripherally loaded implant not in conjunction with computer-generated optimization and planning will not necessarily consistently achieve lower urethral doses.

Rectal Tolerance

Reports of grade 2 rectal toxicity after prostate brachytherapy ranges in the literature from 2% to 12%. The incidence of grade 3 or 4 rectal toxicity is unusual (<2%). Grimm et al. (1) reported grade 2 late proctitis in 2% to 12% of patients treated at the Seattle Prostate Institute, but no grade 3 or 4 GI complications were reported. The actuarial incidence of late grade 2 rectal bleeding was 9%. In general, such symptoms were treated with conservative measures and resolved in all cases. One patient (0.4%) developed a grade 4 rectal complication.

Erectile Function

Although reports have noted relatively low rates of impotence after prostate implantation (59,60), this endpoint was only evaluated at 2 years after implantation. There is a paucity of long-term data available critically examining this issue. Stock et al. (61) also reported gradual declining erectile function with continued follow-up after brachytherapy in 89 patients. However, the median follow-up in that report was only 15 months. It appears that impotence rates after TPI are likely underestimated in the literature. With longer follow-up observations, Zelefsky et al. (8) reported that whereas the incidence of impotence at 2 years after implantation was 21%, the rate increased to 42% at 5 years after the procedure.

Excellent responses have been observed with sildenafil citrate in the treatment of post-treatment impotence after brachytherapy. In one report, 80% of patients responded well to the medication (62). These results are consistent with similar responses reported with this medication for prostate cancer patients with erectile dysfunction after external beam radiotherapy (63). In one study (64), the addition of neoadjuvant androgen deprivation had a significant impact on the potency preservation rate after prostate brachytherapy. Among patients treated with brachytherapy alone who developed impotence after implantation, 30 of 37 (81%) responded to sildenafil, compared with a response rate of 22 of 48 (46%) for patients who received neoadjuvant androgen deprivation therapy in combination with brachytherapy (P = .04).

COMBINATION EXTERNAL BEAM RADIOTHERAPY AND LDR BRACHYTHERAPY

While excellent PSA relapse free survival rates have been achieved for patients with favorable-risk disease using brachytherapy alone, results are generally suboptimal for patients with adverse prognostic features treated with this approach. The likely explanation for the inferior outcome with implantation alone in this group may be related to an insufficient radiation dose or dose rate to overcome radioresistant tumor clonogens. In addition, brachytherapy alone may not deliver adequate dosage to the periprostatic tissues in patients with higher risks of extra-prostatic disease involvement. The rationale for incorporating external beam radiotherapy with brachytherapy for patients with adverse prognostic risk factors is related to the need to deliver escalated radiation doses to this cohort of patients. Combining external beam radiotherapy with a brachytherapy boost (in the form of interstitial permanent implantation or temporary implantation with afterloading catheters, ie, high-dose-rate brachytherapy) represents equally effective approaches for delivering higher radiation doses necessary for optimal tumor control.

When a combined modality approach is chosen for a patient, various treatment schemes have been used to integrate the brachytherapy with the external beam radiotherapy. In general, 45 to 50 Gy of external beam radiotherapy is delivered using conventional or conformal-based techniques to the prostate and peri-prostatic tissues. If a low-dose-rate boost is used, the brachytherapy prescription dose has been 90 Gy for palladium-103 implants and 110 Gy for I-125 implants. In the absence of clinical trials comparing various approaches—high-dose-rate brachytherapy boosts versus low-dose-rate boosts; the optimal sequence of therapy (brachytherapy boost preceding the external beam radiotherapy or vice versa); and the optimal isotope to be used for combined modality therapy—there is no definitive evidence at the present time demonstrating the superiority of a particular treatment strategy over another.

Outcome of Combination External Beam Radiotherapy and LDR Brachytherapy

Blasko et al. (65) reported on the outcome of 231 patients treated with 45 Gy of conventionally planned external beam radiotherapy followed 2 to 4 weeks later by a boost with I-125 (110 Gy) or Pd-103 (90 Gy). The mean PSA in this group of patients was 15.6 ng/mL, and 35% presented with a Gleason score >7. The median follow-up period was 58 months. The 8-year PSA RFS for favorable-, intermediate-, and unfavorable-risk features treated with this combination regimen was 87%, 85%, and 62%, respectively. These results were similar to the biochemical outcomes observed for patients in similar risk groups, treated at their center with permanent implantation without supplemental external beam radiotherapy. Singh et al. (66) reported on 65 patients treated at MSKCC with intermediate- or unfavorable-risk prostate cancer treated with 3D-CRT and Pd-103 who were followed for a median of 2 years. The 3-year PSA RFS was 87%, with a median PSA value at last follow-up of 0.25 ng/mL. The PSA relapse-free survival rate was 90% for patients who had an initial PSA <10 ng/mL and 80% for those who had an initial PSA >10 ng/mL. Merrick et al. (67) reported a 97% 6-year PSA relapse-free survival outcome among intermediate-risk hormone naïve patients who were treated with a combination regimen. Critz et al. (68) reported on 689 patients with early-stage prostate cancer treated with transperineal ultrasound-guided implantation using I-125 followed 3 weeks later by the delivery of 45 Gy of conventional external beam radiotherapy. The pretreatment PSA levels were <10 ng/mL and Gleason scores <7 in 73% and 76% of patients, respectively. No patients received neoadjuvant or adjuvant hormonal therapy. PSA relapse was defined as a PSA nadir level >0.2 ng/mL or a subsequent rising PSA above this level. The median follow-up in that report was 4 years. The actuarial 5-year PSA relapse-free survival rates for patients with pretreatment PSA levels 0 to 4 ng/mL ($n = 50$), 4 to 10 ng/mL ($n = 451$), >10 to 20 ng/mL ($n = 144$), and >20 ng/mL ($n = 44$) were 94%, 93%, 75%, and 69%, respectively.

In the absence of randomized prospective trials, it is difficult to define clearly the clinical indications and benefits of combined external beam radiotherapy and brachytherapy. Specifically, further studies are needed to determine if the combined approach achieves significantly superior biochemical outcomes for patients with adverse prognostic features compared with brachytherapy alone. It also remains unclear whether the combined approach is necessary for patients with favorable-risk disease where the results of monotherapy alone have been excellent. In recent retrospective comparisons, no differences in biochemical outcome have been observed for patients with favorable-risk prognostic features treated with brachytherapy alone when compared with combined external beam radiotherapy and brachytherapy. At the present time, combined external beam radiotherapy and brachytherapy should be reserved as a treatment option for selected patients with intermediate- or high-risk prognostic features, whereas monotherapy appears to be sufficient for those with favorable-risk features.

Sequelae of Combination External Beam Radiotherapy and LDR Brachytherapy

There is a paucity of information regarding the long-term tolerance of combined external beam radiotherapy and brachytherapy for patients with localized prostate cancer. Critz et al. (35) reported grade >2 rectal toxicities in 23% and grade >2 urinary toxicities in 20% of treated patients using this approach. The higher toxicity rates in this report may be attributed to their use of the retropubic open technique in some of these patients rather than a transperineal, ultrasound-guided technique. The tolerance profile for patients treated with combined external beam radiotherapy and TPI at MSKCC was reported by Singh et al. (66). Four patients (6%) with acute urinary retention required Foley catheterization within 48 hours of the implant procedure. The catheter remained in place for median of 5 days. Twenty-three patients (42%) developed grade 2 urinary symptoms after completion of therapy requiring alpha-blocker medications. Three patients (4%) noted rare stress incontinence, and no patient described urge incontinence. Of the 65 patients treated, 45 (68%) reported at their last follow-up that their urinary symptoms had returned to their pretreatment level. Eight patients (13%) developed grade 2 rectal bleeding within 6 months from the completion of therapy. No grade 3 or 4 rectal toxicities have been observed. Five patients (8%) reported increased frequency of bowel movements that were managed with conservative measures. Forty-four of the patients (66%) were potent prior to the initiation of treatment. Of these, 17 (26%) developed erectile dysfunction. Merrick et al. (67) have reported higher rates of erectile dysfunction with combination of brachytherapy and external beam radiotherapy compared with brachytherapy alone (Fig. 13H.5).

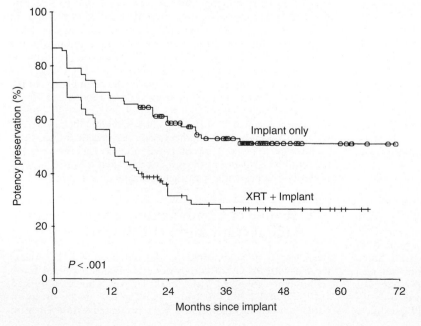

FIGURE 13H.5. Data from Merrick et al. (66) demonstrating Kaplan-Meier potency preservation curves for men treated with external beam radiation therapy (EBRT) with a brachytherapy boost ($n = 91$, plus symbols) and with implant only ($n = 90$, open circles).

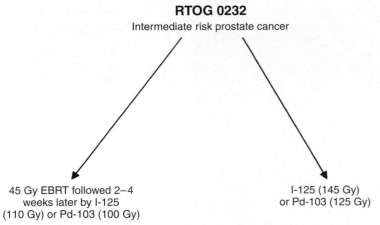

RTOG 0232

Intermediate risk prostate cancer

45 Gy EBRT followed 2–4
weeks later by I-125
(110 Gy) or Pd-103 (100 Gy)

I-125 (145 Gy)
or Pd-103 (125 Gy)

Stratification by stage (T1c vs T2a-T2b); Gleason score (≤6 vs 7); PSA
(<10 vs >10–20); and neoadjuvant hormonal therapy.

FIGURE 13H.6. RTOG protocol schema.

Single institution experiences have documented somewhat increased morbidity following combined treatment using conventional brachytherapy and external beam radiation therapy (EBRT) techniques (68). The Radiation Therapy Oncology Group conducted a phase II study (RTOG P-0019) to assess the acute and late toxicity for patients with intermediate-risk clinically localized prostate cancer. Between January 2001 and November 2001, 138 patients from 20 institutions were entered on this study. Acute toxicity information was available in 131 patients, and 127 patients were analyzable for late toxicity. All patients were treated with external beam radiation therapy (45 Gy/25 fractions) followed 2 to 6 weeks later by an interstitial implant using I-125 to deliver an additional 108 Gy. Thirty-five patients (27%) had preradiotherapy androgen deprivation. The median follow-up was 20 months. The most commonly reported acute toxicity was urinary frequency and dysuria. Acute grade 3 toxicity was documented in 10/131 (7.6%) patients. No grade 4–5 acute toxicity has been observed. Late grade 3 toxicity has been observed in six men (five urinary, one bowel). The 18-month estimate of late grade 3 genitourinary/gastrointestinal (GU/GI) toxicity is 3.3% [95% confidence interval (CI): 0.1–6.5]. No late grade 4–5 toxicity has been observed. In the 61 men who reported no impotence at baseline and received no androgen deprivation, the 18-month rate of grade 2–3 impotence was 45.5% (95% CI, 32.6–58.5%). These data suggest that compared with brachytherapy alone, the acute and late morbidity observed in this multi-institutional, cooperative group study is somewhat increased consistent with previous reports from single institutions.

A phase III trial, RTOG 0232, has recently been activated that compares permanent source brachytherapy as monotherapy with the combination of external beam treatment followed by brachytherapy for patients with intermediate-risk prostate cancer (Fig. 13H.6). The primary endpoint of this study is survival outcome and secondary endpoints include PSA relapse-free survival, distant metastases-free survival, and quality-of-life endpoints. The required number of patients for this study is 1,250. Eligibility criteria for this study include: clinical stage T1c-T2b, Gleason <7 with PSA 10 to 20 ng/mL or Gleason 7 with a PSA <10 ng/mL. The AUA voiding symptom score should be <15 and prostate volume <60 grams. The combined regimen is similar to what was employed for RTOG P-0019. Quality assurance for this cooperative group study will mandate that there will be a central review of the pathology. Each participating institution will require credentialing status by the Radiologic Physics Center for prostate brachytherapy. In addition, electronically transferred external beam and post-implantation data will be sent to the Image Guided Therapy Center in St Louis, Missouri.

HIGH-DOSE-RATE BRACHYTHERAPY

Modern temporary prostate brachytherapy relies on high-dose rate (HDR) afterloading machines. These devices contain a single high-intensity Ir-192 source (5 to 10 Ci) that is replaced every 3 months. The source is attached to the end of a wire that is controlled by the afterloading machine. The machine can position the source precisely for a specified period of time (usually measured in seconds). The source can thus be moved within needles to a number of locations allowing the treating physician to create a dose distribution of virtually any shape or size.

Most HDR prostate brachytherapy techniques utilize transrectal ultrasound to guide the needles into place within and around the prostate (69). A variety of perineal templates have been devised to assist needle placement. In some centers, ultrasound-based treatment planning allows treatment to be delivered at the time of the needle placement (70). Most sites, however, use CT images for the treatment planning process. The HDR needles are identified and the prostate gland is contoured on the CT images. Nearby structures (ie, urethra, rectum) are identified and a dose plan is created that delivers the desired dose to the prostate while limiting the dose to the urethra and rectum (Fig. 13H.7A,7B).

Outcome of HDR Temporary Prostate Brachytherapy

Most reports of HDR brachytherapy combined with external beam radiotherapy (EBRT) to date have focused on men with T1–3 tumors with intermediate- or high-risk features (>T2b, Gleason >6, and pretreatment PSA >10). The number of men with favorable risk factors for favorable disease included in these reports is small. The biochemical relapse-free survival (BRFS) results of several series are summarized in Table 13H.4 (69,71–75). For centers that have reported their results on multiple occasions, only the most recent update is discussed.

Mate et al. reported one of the early experiences from the United States using HDR brachytherapy combined with EBRT (69). These authors from the Seattle Prostate Institute treated 104 men between 1989 and 1995. All men were treated with HDR brachytherapy (12 to 16 Gy in 4 fractions) followed by EBRT (50.4 Gy/28 fractions). The median follow-up was 45 months (range 10–89 months). Biochemical recurrence was defined as three consecutive rises in PSA following treatment.

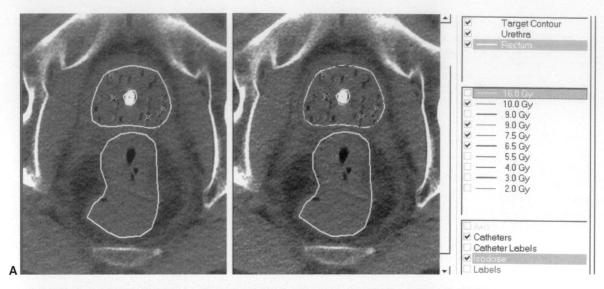

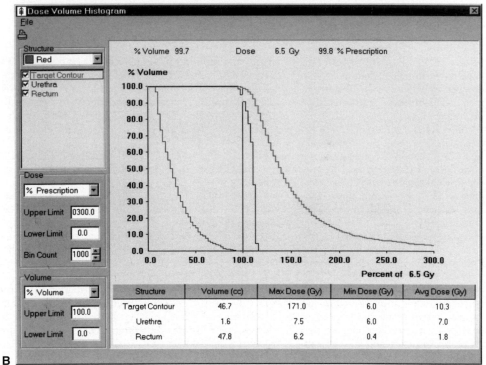

FIGURE 13H.7. A: HDR dose distribution. **B:** Dose volume histogram illustrating dose to target urethra and rectum. (See color nsert.)

TABLE 13H.4

BIOCHEMICAL RELAPSE-FREE SURVIVAL FOLLOWING HDR BRACHYTHERAPY AND EBRT

Author (ref)	n	%T1–2	Med F/U	Implant dose, Gy	# Fractions	EBRT dose, Gy	BRFS, % (yr)
Borghede (72)	50	76	45 mo	20	2	50	84[c]
Dinges (73)	82	26	24 mo	18–20	2	45	53 (2)
Mate (69)	104	90	45 mo	12–16	4	50.4	84 (5)[c]
Galalae (74)	144	68	8 yr	30[b]	2	50	73 (5)
Martinez (75)	207	91	4.7 yr	16.5–23	2–3	46	74 (5)

EBRT, external beam radiation therapy; PSA, prostate-specific antigen; BRFS, biochemical relapse-free survival.
[a]18-month crude rate.
[b]Prescription dose to the peripheral zone.
[c]For patients with pretreatment PSA <20 ng/mL.

At 5 years, in those men with a pretreatment PSA below 20 ng/mL, the BRFS was estimated to be 84%.

The Kiel group has updated its results with 144 men treated between 1986 and 1992 (74). The treatment schedule included 50 Gy EBRT to the pelvic lymph nodes (40 Gy to the prostate) and an additional 30 Gy delivered to the prostate by HDR in two separate fractions. Fifty-four men (37.5%) received adjuvant androgen deprivation. This series has the most mature follow-up of any reported with a median follow-up of 8 years (range 60–171 months). Biochemical recurrence was defined as a rising PSA on three consecutive determinations, all above 1.0 ng/mL. The five-year estimate of BRFS was 73% for all patients.

Martinez has updated his experience treating 207 men with HDR and EBRT between 1991 and 2000 on a prospective dose-escalation study (75). Patients were treated with EBRT to 46 Gy in 23 fractions and HDR was delivered in 2 to 3 fractions of 5.5 to 11.5 Gy. No patients received hormonal therapy prior to recurrence. The ASTRO consensus definition of biochemical recurrence was used. The mean follow-up is 4.7 years. The 5-year estimate of BRFS was 74%.

Conclusive statements about the efficacy of HDR are difficult to make for a variety of reasons: (a) the patients included in these series are very heterogeneous (some series include a majority of men with T1–2 disease while in others most men have extracapsular disease); (b) BRFS is defined very differently with some series using an absolute PSA level to define cure and others relying on a rising PSA to define recurrent disease, still others use the ACD to calculate BRFS; (c) in some series pretreatment or adjuvant androgen deprivation therapy is administered. From the recent results with EBRT, it is clear that increasing radiation dose leads to an improvement in BRFS; whether HDR is a superior method to achieve an increased prostate dose awaits further prospective trials.

Morbidity of HDR Temporary Prostate Brachytherapy

The acute and late morbidity reported following HDR is summarized in Table 13H.5 (69,72–75). Most of the data are crude percentages; one report includes actuarial numbers. All of these reports rely on physician assessment and to date no patient-reported results have been published.

The most common late GU morbidity is the development of urethral stricture. Most series have observed that urethral strictures are more common in men with a history of previous TURP. In most cases the strictures can be managed with dilation in the office or in the outpatient surgical setting. Late GI morbidity can take the form of rectal bleeding, rectal ulcer, or (in rare cases) prostato-rectal fistulas.

PATTERNS OF PRACTICE OF BRACHYTHERAPY IN THE UNITED STATES

It is estimated that 20,000 to 40,000 patients are treated with brachytherapy in the management of their localized prostate cancer. Recently Lee et al. (76) reported the results of the Patterns of Care Survey for Brachytherapy Practice. A random survey was conducted in the United States of 59 facilities treating prostate cancer patients in 1999. A weighted sample size of 13,293 patients (36%; unweighted sample size = 162) was treated with prostate brachytherapy (PB). Brachytherapy was used in 36% of men treated with radiation therapy nationally. The mean age of the men treated with brachytherapy was younger than the population of men treated with EBRT alone. Nearly one-half of men receiving brachytherapy also received EBRT. Supplemental EBRT was used more frequently in men with higher-risk disease. Androgen deprivation therapy (ADT) was used in 40% of PB patients.

In this survey it was observed that the vast majority of men treated with brachytherapy received low-dose-rate permanent sources (89%). Fifty-four percent of men received PB monotherapy (PBM), and the remaining 46% were treated with EB in addition to PB (EBPB). The mean age of men treated with PBM was greater than men treated with EBPB (68.92 vs 66.15; $P = .0223$). The mean pretreatment PSA for the PBM group was lower than the EBPB group (7.06 vs. 13.19; $P = .0008$). The Gleason score was lower in men treated with PBM compared with men treated with EBPB ($P = .003$). The prognostic groupings were more favorable in patients treated with PBM compared with the EBPB group ($P = .0037$). The use of ADT did not differ according to treatment with PBM or EBPB ($P = .2502$).

Ultrasound was used for treatment planning and intraoperative guidance in the vast majority of cases (implant procedure = 85% or preplanning = 82%). Of the men treated with low-dose rate PB, 59% were treated with I-125, and 41% were treated with Pd-103. Iodine-125 was used more frequently in men treated with PBM and Pd-103 was used more frequently in men treated with EBPB. Post-implant dosimetry was documented in 61% of cases treated with low-dose rate PB; 47% of cases used CT imaging as part of this quality assessment.

TABLE 13H.5

ACUTE AND LATE MORBIDITY FOLLOWING HDR BRACHYTHERAPY

Author (ref.)	n	Med F/U	Acute Gr3+,%	Late Gr3+ GI,%	Late Gr3+ GU,%
Borghede (72)	50	45 mo	8	0	6
Dinges (73)	82	24 mo	7	4[a]	16
Mate (69)	104	45 mo	ND	0	7
Galalae (74)	144	8 yr	ND	4	2
Martinez (75)	207	4.7 yr	ND	1	8

GI, gastrointestinal; GU, genitourinary.
[a]Three patients with prostato-rectal fistulas.

HEATH-RELATED QUALITY OF LIFE FOLLOWING PROSTATE BRACHYTHERAPY

In one of the first analyses of Health-Related Quality of Life (HRQOL) in men treated with PB, Brandeis compared generic and disease-specific HRQOL in men treated with PB (with and without EBRT) to men treated with radical prostatectomy (RP) and age-matched healthy controls (77). The study incorporated the Short Form (SF)-36 and the University of California Los Angeles Prostate Cancer Index (UCLA PCI) questionnaires in a cross-sectional design. The men with prostate cancer completed the various questionnaires 3 to 17 months (median 7.5) following treatment. The PB group included 48 men treated with PB (14 received EBRT in addition to PB and 34 did not), and the RP group included 74 men. There were 134 men in the control group. Compared with men in the RP group, men treated with PB were older, less healthy, and had less formal education. Generic HRQOL did not differ greatly among the three groups. In fact, the only generic HRQOL domain in the SF-36 that differed was physical function, with RP patients scoring higher than the PB or control groups. Disease-specific HRQOL measures were very different between the groups. Urinary function (leakage) was worse in the PB group than in controls, but better than in the RP group. The PB group had worse bowel function than controls and the RP group. Sexual function and bother were worse in the PB group than controls, but no different from the RP group. The authors also divided the PB group according to whether EBRT was also given and found that men who received both EBRT and PB scored worse in all disease-specific HRQOL domains compared with those men treated with PB alone.

Davis and colleagues from Eastern Virginia Medical School have reported on HRQOL in men treated with PB alone, EBRT, and RP for clinically localized prostate cancer (78). These investigators mailed the SF-36, the UCLA PCI, and the IPSS questionnaire to more than 600 men following definitive treatment. The response rate was greater than 80% in all groups. Important demographic differences between the treatment groups were identified. Men treated with RP tended to be younger, healthier, and less likely to receive neoadjuvant androgen deprivation therapy, compared with men treated with PB. The median time from treatment to survey completion was longer in the men treated with RP compared with the men treated with PB (37.9 months versus 22.4 months, $P > .05$). The raw and adjusted SF-36 scores were not significantly different between men treated with RP and those treated with PB. Examination of the urinary, bowel, and sexual domains of the PCI indicated that men treated with PB had better sexual and urinary function than men treated with RP. Men treated with PB also reported less sexual bother than men treated with RP.

Bacon et al. have analyzed a subset of men being followed in the Health Professionals Follow-up Study (79). The authors reported on 842 men that had been diagnosed with clinically localized prostate cancer between 1993 and 1998. The study population had completed the SF-36 and UCLA PCI questionnaires. These men received various treatments, including radical prostatectomy ($n = 421$), external beam radiation therapy ($n = 221$), brachytherapy ($n = 69$), hormonal treatment ($n = 33$), watchful waiting ($n = 31$), and other ($n = 67$). The authors provide no information as to whether some men included in the PB group also received EBRT. In addition, no information was provided concerning the use of ADT in combination with PB, RP, or EBRT. Age-adjusted generic HRQOL scores showed very small differences according to treatment group with the RP group having the highest scores.

Significant differences were observed in sexual, urinary, and bowel HRQOL according to treatment group. Men treated with PB and EBRT reported higher sexual and urinary function as well as less sexual bother compared with men treated with RP. The men treated with PB or EBRT, however, also reported significantly worse bowel function, bowel bother, and urinary bother (in the case of PB) than men treated with RP.

In a recent report from investigators at the University of Michigan, Wei et al. have provided a cross-sectional analysis of more than 1,000 men treated with RP, PB, or EBRT between 1995 and 1999 (80). The PB group included an unreported percentage of men treated with a combination of EBRT and PB, and the PB group was more likely to be treated with ADT. The PB group had the shortest time between treatment and completion of the HRQOL questionnaires (median 21 months, range 4–52 months). These authors used a number of validated questionnaires including the Expanded Prostate cancer Index Composite (EPIC) instrument and compared the HRQOL in each group with a group of age-matched controls. The EPIC instrument was constructed by modifying the UCLA PCI instrument and adding items that address irritative urinary symptoms, irritative bowel symptoms, symptoms related to androgen deprivation, and items expanding the assessment of function-specific bother in each of these new domains. Measures of generic HRQOL [SF-36 and Functional Assessment of Cancer Therapy-General (FACT-G)] did not differ between controls and treatment groups. Using the EPIC instrument, however, the PB group was found to have significantly worse urinary, bowel, and sexual HRQOL compared with controls. A comparison of HRQOL scores in men at least one year from completion of therapy found that the PB group had significantly worse urinary irritative, bowel, and sexual symptoms than the RP or EBRT groups. By excluding the patients that received EBRT from the PB group, sexual HRQOL was similar to the EBRT group and superior to the RP group.

When all these cross-sectional studies are considered together, several statements can be offered. First, when HRQOL is measured with a generic instrument (SF-36, for instance), there do not appear to be any large differences between men treated for prostate cancer and similarly aged men without cancer or those with cancer who have yet to receive definitive treatment. Second, when HRQOL is measured with a symptom-specific instrument, there are often differences between men treated for prostate cancer and similarly aged men without cancer. Third, it appears that there are treatment specific changes in HRQOL within the urinary, bowel, and sexual domains. Specifically, it appears that men treated with RP have more difficulty within the sexual and certain urinary domains compared with men treated with PB or EBRT. On the other hand, PB and EBRT are associated with more bowel dysfunction than RP, and PB is associated with more urinary bother than EBRT or RP. The strength of these conclusions is tempered by the cross-sectional nature of these reports. Prospective data collection, including baseline values, is required to examine the net effect of any treatment on various HRQOL domains.

Lee and colleagues have reported a prospective study examining HRQOL in a group of men treated with PB (81). In a pilot study reported in 2000, the authors studied 31 men who had completed the Fact Assessment of Cancer Therapy—Prostate (FACT-P) questionnaire prior to PB and at several times (1, 3, 6, and 12 months) following PB. All men were treated with PB alone; no EBRT was utilized. Clinically meaningful decreases in the FACT-P scores (indicating decreased HRQOL) were noted 1 month following PB with a return to baseline by 12 months. An examination of the domains of the FACT-P demonstrated that the HRQOL decreases occurred in the Functional Well-Being (FWB), Physical Well-Being (PWB), and Prostate Cancer Symptom (PCS) subscales.

In a later report from the same group at Wake Forest University, Lee compared changes in HRQOL as measured by FACT-P in men treated with PB, RP, or EBRT (82). Ninety men were included (PB = 44, RP = 23, EBRT = 23). The study design did not use randomization: treatment was chosen based on the recommendation of the treating physicians and the wishes of the patient. The authors compared the HRQOL profiles in each of the treatment groups. After adjusting for baseline HRQOL, there were significant differences in HRQOL at 1 month according to treatment group. Men treated with PB or RP experienced larger declines in HRQOL at 1 month following treatment than men treated with EBRT. Importantly, however, by 1 year there were no significant differences in HRQOL according to treatment group. In fact, the HRQOL scores for all groups at 12 months were not significantly different than baseline scores for any of the treatment groups.

Prospective results from the Cancer of the Prostate Strategic Urologic Research Endeavor (CaPSURE) database have been published very recently (83). Downs et al. studied 419 men treated with PB alone ($n = 92$) or RP ($n = 327$). The authors used the SF-36 and the UCLA PCI instruments to measure generic and prostate cancer specific HRQOL prior to therapy and at 6-month intervals following treatment. Early functional impairment in most generic domains was observed with a return to baseline scores by 18 to 24 months. Following treatment, generic HRQOL did not differ between the men treated with RP or those treated with PB. There were differences between the groups in disease-specific domains. Patients treated with PB had significantly higher urinary function scores 6 months following treatment when compared with men treated with RP. Urinary bother scores were not different between the groups. Sexual function decreased and sexual bother increased in both groups, but to a lesser degree in men treated with PB, despite the fact that men treated with RP had higher sexual function scores prior to treatment.

In some of the reports above, the PB groups contained men treated with PB alone and men treated with a combination of PB and EBRT. The best way to determine whether the addition of EBRT to PB is associated with a decrease in HRQOL compared with treatment with PB alone is by way of a randomized trial. The RTOG has recently opened such a trial (RTOG P-0232, Bradley Prestidge, P.I.). For the time being, there is at least a suggestion that the addition of EBRT may decrease HRQOL.

In conclusion, these reports generally indicate that prostate brachytherapy and external beam radiotherapy are associated with significantly less incontinence but more urinary obstructive symptoms compared with radical prostatectomy. Compared with surgery, brachytherapy and external beam radiotherapy are associated with significantly more rectal symptoms but somewhat less sexual dysfunction.

References

1. Grimm PD, Blasko JC, Ragde H, et al. Does brachytherapy have a role in the treatment of prostate cancer? *Hematol Oncol Clin North Am* 1996;10:653.
2. Shanahan TG, Nanavati PJ, Mueller PW, et al. A comparison of permanent prostate brachytherapy techniques: pre-plan vs. hybrid interactive planning with postimplant analysis. *Int J Radiat Oncol Biol Phys* 2002;53:490.
3. Merrick GS, Butler WM, Galbreath RW, et al. Five-year biochemical outcome following permanent interstitial brachytherapy for clinical T1-T3 prostate cancer. *Int J Radiat Oncol Biol Phys* 2001;51:41.
4. Lee N, Wuu CS, Brody R, et al. Factors predicting for post-implantation retention after permanent prostate brachytherapy. *Int J Radiat Oncol Biol Phys* 2000;48:1457.
5. Bealieu L, Aubin S, Taschereau R, et al. Dosimetric impact of the variation of the prostate volume and shape between pre-treatment planning and treatment procedure. *Int J Radiat Oncol Biol Phys* 2002;53:215.
6. Stone NN, Roy J, Hong S, et al. Prostate gland motion and deformation caused by needle placement during brachytherapy. *Brachytherapy* 2002;1:154.
7. Stock RG, Stone NN, Wesson MF, et al. A modified technique allowing ultrasound-guided three dimensional transperineal prostate implantation. *Int J Radiat Oncol Biol Phys* 1995;32:219.
8. Zelefsky MJ, Yamada Y, Cohen G, et al. Postimplantation dosimetric analysis of permanent transperineal prostate implantation: improved dose distributions with an intraoperative computer-optimized conformal planning technique. *Int J Radiat Oncol Biol Phys* 2000;48:601.
9. Yu Y, Zhang JBY, Brasacchio RA, et al. Automated treatment planning engine for prostate seed implant brachytherapy. *Int J Radiat Oncol Biol Phys* 1999;43:647.
10. Lee EK, Gallagher RJ, Silvern D, et al. Treatment planning for brachytherapy: an integer programming model, two computational approaches and experiments with permanent prostate implant planning. *Phys Med Biol* 1999;44:145.
11. Wilkinson DA, Lee EJ, Ciezki JP, et al. Dosimetric comparison of pre-planned and OR-planned prostate seed brachytherapy. *Int J Radiat Oncol Biol Phys* 2000;48:1241.
12. Matzkin H, Kaver I, Bramante-Schreiber L, et al. Comparison between two iodine-125 brachytherapy implant techniques: pre-planning and intraoperative by various dosimetry quality indicators. *Radiother Oncol* 2003;68:289.
13. Nath R, Anderson LL, Luxton G, et al. Dosimetry of interstitial brachytherapy sources: recommendations of the AAPM Radiation Committee Task Group No. 43. *Med Phys* 1995;22:209.
14. Beyer D, Nath R, Butler W, et al. American Brachytherapy Society recommendations for clinical implementation of NIST-1999 standards for (103) palladium brachytherapy. *Int J Radiat Oncol Biol Phys* 2000;47:273.
15. Ling CC. Permanent implants using Au-198, Pd-103 and I-125: radiobiological considerations based on the linear quadratic model. *Int J Radiat Oncol Biol Phys* 1992;23:81.
16. Dicker AP, Lin CC, Leeper DB, et al. Isotope selection for permanent prostate implants? An evaluation of 103Pd versus 125I based on radiobiological effectiveness and dosimetry. *Semin Urol Oncol* 2000;18:152.
17. Cha CM, Potters L, Ashley R, et al. Isotope selection for patients undergoing prostate brachytherapy. *Int J Radiat Oncol Biol Phys* 1999;45:391.
18. Wallner K, Merrick G, True L, et al. 125I versus 103Pd for low risk prostate cancer: morbidity outcomes from a prospective randomized trial. *Cancer J* 2002;8:67.
19. Nag S, Bice W, DeWyngaert K, et al. The American Brachytherapy Society recommendations for permanent prostate brachytherapy post-implant dosimetric analysis. *Int J Radiat Oncol Biol Phys* 2000;46:221.
20. Willins J, Wallner K. CT-based dosimetry for transperineal I-125 prostate brachytherapy. *Int J Radiat Oncol Biol Phys* 1997;39:347.
21. Bice WS Jr, Prestidge BR, Grimm PD, et al. Centralized multiinstitutional postimplant analysis for interstitial prostate brachytherapy. *Int J Radiat Oncol Biol Phys* 1998;41:921.
22. Zelefsky MJ, Yamada Y, Marion C, et al. Improved conformality and decreased toxicity with intraoperative computer-optimized transperineal ultrasound-guided prostate brachytherapy. *Int J Radiat Oncol Biol Phys* 2003;55:956.
23. D'Amico AV, Cormack R, Tempany CM, et al. Real time magnetic resonance image guided interstitial brachytherapy in the treatment of select patients with clinically localized prostate cancer. *Int J Radiat Oncol Biol Phys* 1998;42:507.
24. Messing EM, Zhang JB, Rubens DJ, et al. Intraoperative optimized inverse planning for prostate brachytherapy: early experience. *Int J Radiat Oncol Biol Phys* 1999;44:810.
25. Stock RG, Stone NN, Lo YC. Intraoperative dosimetric representation of the real-time ultrasound implant. *Tech Urol* 2000;6:95.
26. Beyer DC, Shapiro RH, Puente F. Real-time optimized intraoperative dosimetry for prostate brachytherapy: a pilot study. *Int J Radiat Oncol Biol Phys* 2000;48:1483.
27. Nguyen J, Wallner K, Han B, et al. Urinary morbidity in brachytherapy patients with median lobe hyperplasia. *Brachytherapy* 2002;1:42.
28. Zelefsky MJ, Whitmore WF, Leibel SA, et al. Impact of transurethral resection on the long-term outcome of patients with prostatic carcinoma. *J Urol* 1993;150:1860.
29. Blasko JC, Ragde H, Grimm PD. Transperineal ultrasound-guided implantation of the prostate: morbidity and complications. *Scand J Urol Nephrol* 1991;137:113.
30. Wallner K, Lee H, Wasserman S, et al. Low risk of urinary incontinence following prostate brachytherapy in patients with a prior transurethral prostate resection. *Int J Radiat Oncol Biol Phys* 1997;37:565.
31. Stone NN, Ratnow ER, Stock RG, et al. Prior transurethral resection does not increase morbidity following real time ultrasound-guided prostate seed implantation. *Tech Urol* 2000;6:123.
32. Cavanagh W, Blasko JC, Grimm PD, et al. Transient elevation of serum prostate-specific antigen following I-125/Pd-103 brachytherapy for localized prostate cancer. *Semin Urol Oncol* 2000;18:160.
33. Critz FA, Williams WH, Benton JB, et al. Prostate specific antigen bounce after radioactive seed implantation followed by external beam radiation for prostate cancer. *J Urol* 2000;163:1085.

34. Merrick GS, Butler WM, Wallner KE, et al. Prostate-specific antigen spikes after permanent prostate brachytherapy. *Int J Radiat Oncol Biol Phys* 2002;54:450.

35. Critz FA, Williams WH, Levinson KA, et al. Simultaneous irradiation for prostate cancer: intermediate results with modern techniques. *J Urol* 2000;164:738.

36. Grimm PD, Blasko JC, Sylvester JE, et al. 10-year biochemical (prostate-specific antigen) control of prostate cancer with I-125 brachytherapy. *Int J Radiat Oncol Biol Phys* 2001;51:31.

37. Blasko JC, Grimm PD, Sylvester JE, et al. Palladium 103 brachytherapy for prostate carcinoma. *Int J Radiat Oncol Biol Phys* 2000;46:839.

38. Brachman DG, Thomas T, Hilbe J, et al. Failure-free survival following brachytherapy alone or external beam irradiation alone for T1-T2 prostate tumors in 2222 patients: results from a single practice. *Int J Radiat Oncol Biol Phys* 2000;48:111.

39. Zelefsky MJ, Hollister T, Raben A, et al. Five year biochemical outcome and toxicity with transperineal CT-planned permanent I-125 prostate implantation for patients with localized prostate cancer. *Int J Radiat Oncol Biol Phys* 2000;47:1261.

40. Kollmeier MA, Stock RG, Stone N. Biochemical outcomes after prostate brachytherapy with 5-year minimal follow-up: importance of patient selection and implant quality. *Int J Radiat Oncol Biol Phys* 2003;57:645.

41. Sylvester JE, Blasko JC, Grimm PD, et al. Ten-year biochemical relapse-free survival after external beam radiation and brachytherapy for localized prostate cancer: the Seattle experience. *Int J Radiat Oncol Biol Phys* 2003;57:944.

42. Kwok Y, DiBiase SJ, Amin PP, et al. Risk group stratification in patients undergoing permanent (125) I prostate brachytherapy as monotherapy. *Int J Radiat Oncol Biol Phys* 2002;53:588.

43. Potters L, Huang D, Caluguru E, et al. Importance of implant dosimetry for patients undergoing prostate brachytherapy. *Urology* 2003;62:1073.

44. D'Amico AV, Whittington R, Malkowicz SB, et al. Biochemical outcome after radical prostatectomy, external beam radiation therapy, or interstitial radiation therapy for clinically localized prostate cancer. *JAMA* 1998;280:969.

45. Zelefsky MJ, Wallner KE, Ling CC, et al. Comparison of the 5-year outcome and morbidity of three-dimensional conformal radiotherapy versus transperineal permanent iodine-125 implantation for early-stage prostatic cancer. *J Clin Oncol* 1999;17:517.

46. Stokes SH. Comparison of biochemical disease-free survival of patients with localized carcinoma of the prostate undergoing radical prostatectomy, transperineal ultrasound-guided radioactive seed implantation or definitive external beam irradiation. *Int J Radiat Oncol Biol Phys* 2000;47:129.

47. D'Amico AV, Tempany CM, Schultz D, et al. Comparing PSA outcome after radical prostatectomy or magnetic resonance imaging-guided partial prostatic irradiation in select patients with clinically localized adenocarcinoma of the prostate. *Urology* 2003;62:1062.

48. Locke J, Ellis W, Wallner K, et al. Risk factors for acute urinary retention requiring temporary intermittent catheterization after prostate brachytherapy: a prospective study. *Int J Radiat Oncol Biol Phys* 2002;52:712.

49. Crook J, McLean M, Catton C, et al. Factors influencing risk of acute urinary retention after TRUS-guided permanent prostate seed implantation. *Int J Radiat Oncol Biol Phys* 2002;52:453.

50. Thomas MD, Cormack R, Tempany CM, et al. Identifying the predictors of acute urinary retention following magnetic resonance-guided prostate brachytherapy. *Int J Radiat Oncol Biol Phys* 2000;47:905.

51. Salem N, Simonian-Sauve M, Rosello R, et al. Predictive factors of acute urinary morbidity after iodine-125 brachytherapy for localised prostate cancer: a phase 2 study. *Radiother Oncol* 2003;66:159.

52. Terk MD, Stock RG, Stone NN. Identification of patients at increased risk for prolonged urinary retention following radioactive seed implantation of the prostate. *J Urol* 1998;160:1379.

53. Merrick GS, Butler WM, Galbreath RW, et al. Relationships between the transition zone index of the prostate gland and urinary morbidity after brachytherapy. *Urology* 2001;57:524.

54. Crook J, Toi A, McLean M, et al. The utility of transition zone index in predicting acute urinary morbidity after 125-I prostate brachytherapy. *Brachytherapy* 2002;1:131.

55. Brown D, Colonias A, Miller R, et al. Urinary morbidity with a modified peripheral loading technique of transperineal (125) I prostate implantation. *Int J Radiat Oncol Biol Phys* 2000;47:353.

56. Stokes SH, Real JD, Adams PW, et al. Transperineal ultrasound-guided radioactive seed implantation for organ confined carcinoma of the prostate. *Int J Radiat Oncol Biol Phys* 1997;37:337.

57. Wallner KE, Roy J, Harrison L, et al. Dosimetry guidelines to minimize urethral and rectal morbidity following transperineal I-125 prostate brachytherapy. *Int J Radiat Oncol Biol Phys* 1995;32:465.

58. Zelefsky MJ, Yamada Y, Marion C, et al. Improved conformality and decreased toxicity with intraoperative computer-optimized transperineal ultrasound-guided prostate brachytherapy. *Int J Radiat Oncol Biol Phys* 2003;55:956.

59. Sharkey J, Chovnick SD, Behar RJ, et al. Minimally invasive treatment for localized adenocarcinoma of the prostate: review of 1048 patients treated with ultrasound-guided palladium-103 brachytherapy. *J Endourol* 2000;14:343.

60. Benoit RM, Naslund MJ, Cohen JK. Comparison of complications between ultrasound-guided prostate brachytherapy and open prostate brachytherapy. *Int J Radiat Oncol Biol Phys* 2000;47:909.

61. Stock RG, Stone NN, Iannuzzi C. Sexual potency following interactive ultrasound-guided brachytherapy for prostate cancer. *Int J Radiat Oncol Biol Phys* 1996;35:267.

62. Merrick GS, Butler WM, Lief JH, et al. Efficacy of sildenafil citrate in prostate brachytherapy patients with erectile dysfunction. *Urology* 1999;53:1112.

63. Zelefsky MJ, McKee AB, Lee H, et al. Efficacy of oral sildenafil in patients with erectile dysfunction after radiotherapy for carcinoma of the prostate. *Urology* 1999;53:775.

64. Potters L, Torre T, Fearn PA, et al. Potency after permanent prostate brachytherapy for localized prostate cancer. *Int J Radiat Oncol Biol Phys* 2001;50:1235.

65. Blasko JC, Grimm PD, Sylvester JE, et al. The role of external beam radiotherapy with I-125/Pd-103 brachytherapy for prostate carcinoma. *Radiother Oncol* 2000;57:273.

66. Singh A, Zelefsky MJ, Raben A, et al. Combined 3-dimensional conformal radiotherapy and transperineal Pd-103 permanent implantation for patients with intermediate and unfavorable risk prostate cancer. *Int J Cancer* 2000;90:275.

67. Merrick GS, Butler WM, Lief JH, et al. Biochemical outcome for hormone naïve intermediate risk prostate cancer managed with permanent interstitial brachytherapy and supplemental external beam radiation. *Brachytherapy* 2002;1:95.

68. Critz FA, Williams WH, Levinson AK, et al. Simultaneous irradiation for prostate cancer: intermediate results with modern techniques. *J Urol* 2000;164:738.

69. Mate TP, Gottesman JE, Hatton J, et al. High dose-rate afterloading ^{192}iridium prostate brachytherapy: feasibility report. *Int J Radiat Oncol Biol Phys* 1998;41:525.

70. Martinez AA, Kestin LL, Stromberg JS, et al. Interim report of image-guided conformal high-dose-rate brachytherapy for patients with unfavorable prostate cancer: the William Beaumont Phase II Dose-escalating Trial. *Int J Radiat Oncol Biol Phys* 2000;47:343.

71. Puthawala AA, Syed AM, Austin PA, et al. Long-term results of treatment for prostate carcinoma by staging pelvic lymph node dissection and definitive irradiation using low-dose rate temporary iridium-192 interstitial implant and external beam radiotherapy. *Cancer* 2001;92:2084.

72. Borghede G, Hedelin H, Holmang S, et al. Combined treatment with temporary short-term high dose rate iridium-192 brachytherapy and external beam radiotherapy for irradiation of localized prostatic carcinoma. *Radiother Oncol* 1997;44:237.

73. Dinges S, Deger S, Koswig S, et al. High-dose rate interstitial with external beam irradiation for localized prostate cancer—results of a prospective trial. *Radiother Oncol* 1998;48:197.

74. Galalae RM, Kovacs G, Schultze J, et al. Long-term outcome after elective irradiation of the pelvic lymphatics and local dose escalation using high-dose-rate brachytherapy for locally advanced prostate cancer. *Int J Radiat Oncol Biol Phys* 2002;52:81.

75. Martinez AA, Gustafson G, Gonzalez J, et al. Dose escalation using conformal high-dose-rate brachytherapy improves outcome in unfavorable prostate cancer. *Int J Radiat Oncol Biol Phys* 2002;53:316.

76. Lee WR, Moughan J, Owen JB, et al. The 1999 patterns of care study of radiotherapy in localized prostate carcinoma: a comprehensive survey of prostate brachytherapy in the United States. *Cancer* 2003;98:1987.

77. Brandeis JM, Litwin MS, Burnison CM, et al. Quality of life outcomes after brachytherapy for early stage prostate cancer. *J Urol* 2000;163:851.

78. Davis JW, Kuban DA, Lynch DF, et al. Quality of life after treatment for localized prostate cancer: differences based on treatment modality. *J Urol* 2001;166:947.

79. Bacon CG, Giovannucci E, Testa M, et al. The impact of cancer treatment on quality of life outcomes for patients with localized prostate cancer. *J Urol* 2001;166:1804.

80. Wei JT, Dunn RL, Sandler HM, et al. Comprehensive comparison of health-related quality of life after contemporary therapies for localized prostate cancer. *J Clin Oncol* 2002;20:557.

81. Lee WR, McQuellon RP, Case LD, et al. Early quality of life assessment in men treated with permanent source interstitial brachytherapy for clinically localized prostate cancer. *J Urol* 1999;162:403.

82. Lee WR, McQuellon RP, Harris-Henderson K, et al. A preliminary analysis of health-related quality of life in the first year after permanent source interstitial brachytherapy (PIB) for clinically localized prostate cancer. *Int J Radiat Oncol Biol Phys* 2000;46:77.

83. Downs TM, Sadetsky N, Pasta DJ, et al. Health related quality of life patterns in patients treated with interstitial prostate brachytherapy for localized prostate cancer—data from CaPSURE. *J Urol* 2003;170:1822.

CHAPTER 14 ■ MANAGEMENT OF HIGH RISK PROSTATE CANCER

CHAPTER 14A
Combined Hormone Therapy and Modern Radiation Therapy for High-Risk Prostate Cancer

Michel Bolla and Mack Roach, III

First introduced by Huggins in 1941 (1), androgen deprivation as a therapeutic intervention is based on the apparent dependence of prostatic epithelial and adenocarcinoma cells on androgenic hormones. This dependency explains the fact that after primary treatment with orchiectomy or estrogens more than 80% of patients with locally advanced prostate cancer (LadCaP) respond favorably. Unfortunately, hormonal manipulation is generally not curative and has side effects (2). Estrogen and castration have been largely abandoned and replaced by luteinizing hormone-releasing hormone (LHRH) analogues because of similar efficacy, reversibility, and less toxicity (3).

During the 1970s external beam irradiation (EBRT) became the treatment of choice for the treatment of LadCaP in the radiotherapy community. EBRT could effectively encompass the prostate, the seminal vesicles, and the tissues surrounding the prostate within the high-dose volume. However, when given alone the long-term results with EBRT were associated with a relatively high risk of local relapse, distant metastasis, and a poor long-term survival (4–6).

There has been a substantial decline in the incidence of LadCaP-T3-4 N0 M0 and any T N1-3 M0 (2002 TNM classification) due to mass screening (7,8). Contemporary patients with high-risk prostate cancer (HriCaP) include the occasional patients with LadCaP, but more frequently patients with lower clinical stages (T1-2) and with poor prognostic factors, namely, Gleason 8 to 10 or PSA >20 ng/mL. Such patients have a significant risk of relapse within and outside the irradiated volume. The challenge was, and still is, to improve local control by innovative techniques of irradiation *and* to address the risk of systemic as well as regional disease. The importance of the first goal as a major endpoint is supported by the evidence that the 20-year metastasis-free survival rate of pN0 patients is 70% versus 13% for patients in whom local control is not achieved ($P <.00001$) (9). The second goal is achieved in part by achieving local control (thus eliminating the nidus for metastatic disease) and by suppressing micrometastatic disease by combining androgen deprivation as it has been done for locally advanced breast carcinomas with tamoxifen (10). More recently the importance of controlling regional disease has come to light.

RATIONALE FOR COMBINING ANDROGEN DEPRIVATION WITH RADIATION

The theoretical basis for combining hormonal therapy with radiotherapy was not well elucidated at the very start of these trials. Since completion of these trials, it is now clear that there are several potential benefits of combining these two modalities, including:

(a) decreasing the volume of the prostate with hormonal therapy thus decreasing the volume of the treatment fields, particularly when three-dimensional conformal radiation therapy (3D-CRT) is used;
(b) inhibiting repopulation during irradiation, thereby reducing the risk of local relapse within the irradiated volume;
(c) suppressing sub-clinical distant metastases.

The dosimetric benefits resulting from the downstaging (or downsizing) induced by neoadjuvant hormonal treatment has been shown by using dose-volume-histogram (DVH) analyses. Zelefsky and Harrison reported on the experience at the Memorial Sloan-Kettering Cancer Center: 45 patients were prospectively studied and the DVH of the prostate, bladder, and rectum were compared before and after hormonal therapy. The median reduction in the volumes of the bladder and rectum receiving 95% of the dose were 46% and 18%, respectively (11). On the basis of these findings, it was postulated that such a dramatic reduction in the volume of normal tissues irradiated might have a potential impact of late toxicity, particularly if higher doses of radiation were prescribed. Unfortunately, the clinical experiences thus far have not verified the theoretical advantages associated with the volume reductions resulting from hormonal therapy (12,13). To date, a large phase I-II dose-escalation study demonstrated an increased level of urinary (GU) morbidity, a large phase III trial demonstrated an increase in gastrointestinal (GI) morbidity, and at least one retrospective study demonstrated worse GU and GI morbidity associated with the use of neoadjuvant hormonal therapy (NHT) (14). We are not aware of any prospective or retrospective studies showing a reduction in morbidity with the use of NHT. Thus, until proven otherwise this theoretical clinical benefit due to improved DVH should be considered questionable at best.

Another rationale for combining hormones and radiation is to improve the effectiveness of radiation. To test the relative effect of neoadjuvant and adjuvant deprivation on the radiation response of a transplantable androgen-dependent tumor, Zietman et al. (15) used the transplantable androgen-dependent

Shionogi tumor, a spontaneous murine mammary carcinoma. This tumor was grown as allografts in the hind limbs of athymic nude mice. Tumors were treated by radiation alone, once the average diameter was 6 mm; radiation was preceded 12 days earlier by orchiectomy (neoadjuvant therapy); radiation was followed by orchiectomy (adjuvant therapy) or by orchiectomy with radiation given once the tumors had regrown in an androgen-unresponsive mode. The endpoint was the TCD 50 dose necessary to locally control 50% of tumors. In this experiment, it was observed that the TCD 50 was: 85.7 Gy for radiotherapy alone, 43.4 Gy (neoadjuvant androgen deprivation), 69.0 Gy (radiation followed one day after by adjuvant androgen deprivation), and 74.9 Gy (radiation followed 12 days after by adjuvant androgen deprivation). Thus, although the radiation response was significantly enhanced by both modalities, neoadjuvant androgen deprivation provided the greatest effect.

Joon et al. (16) used Dunning R3327-G rat prostate tumors, grown in the flanks of Copenhagen rats up to a volume of 1 mL, to test the hypothesis that there is a supra-additive interaction between androgen ablation and radiation through modulation of apoptosis. Androgen ablation was realized by castration, and androgen restoration was achieved with silastic tube implants containing testosterone. A histochemical assay was set up to identify apoptotic cells and quantify the apoptotic index, determined by dividing the number of apoptotic cells by the number of tumor cells. Tumors from intact and castrated irradiated control rats had average apoptotic indices of 0.4% and 1%, respectively. Irradiation of intact rats to 7 Gy resulted in a peak apoptotic response at 6 hours of 2.3%. A supra-additive apoptotic response was obtained when castration was initiated 3 days prior to 7 Gy radiation, with peak levels of about 10.1%. When the radiation was administered at increasing times beyond 3 days after castration, the apoptotic response gradually decreased to the level obtained in intact rats 28 days after castration. All these results are consistent with the better results obtained by neoadjuvant hormonal manipulation with respect to the adjuvant setting, but are not conclusive proof. Nevertheless, they are obtained from animal models under experimental conditions that do not allow hormonal treatment during and after irradiation to be delivered in a more protracted way.

Not all animal studies support supra-additive interactions between radiation and hormonal therapy, however (17). Pollack et al. investigated in LNCaP cells grown in vitro, and apoptosis was measured with a terminal deoxynucleotidyl transferase-mediated dUTP-biotin nick end labeling (TUNEL) assay. Clonogenic survival was used to determine overall cell death, and the results were corrected for differences in plating efficiency from the various growth conditions. There was a consistent supra-additive increase in apoptosis in cells exposed to androgen deprivation and radiotherapy, as compared to either treatment given individually. In contrast, significant radiosensitization by androgen deprivation was not observed by clonogenic survival even when the conditions of androgen deprivation varied. They concluded: "In LNCaP prostate tumor cells supra-additive apoptosis did not translate into radiosensitization by clonogenic survival." They also concluded: "Because clonogenic survival is a measure of overall cell death, either the level of apoptosis is too small a component of overall cell death or the increases in apoptosis occurred in a subpopulation that would have been killed by other mechanisms." Their findings appear to demonstrate that androgen deprivation does not sensitize prostate cancer cells to radiotherapy. The findings of RTOG 9413 (discussed below) may provide important insights into the clinical relevance of these animal studies.

RESULTS OF THE PHASE III TRIALS

The earliest trials incorporating hormonal therapy and radiotherapy were launched prior to the LHRH era with patients managed using estrogen or surgical castration (see Table 14A.1). The first trial was conducted at the MD Anderson Cancer Center (18), including a small cohort of 78 T3 tumors treated by pelvic radiotherapy alone or combined with DES (5 mg). The long-term follow-up demonstrated a striking difference in disease-free survival persisting at 10 and 15 years, but no improvement in overall survival (19). The Medical Research Council multicentric trial (20) focused on the treatment of 277 cases of T2–4 NX M0 prostate cancer by castration ($n = 90$), radiotherapy ($n = 88$), or combined treatment ($n = 99$). The specific details of irradiation were left to the discretion of each treatment center. With a median follow-up of 4 to 4.5 years, the use of orchiectomy was associated with a delay in the onset of distant metastases, but radiotherapy and orchiectomy proved equally effective in controlling local disease. The major trials demonstrating a survival benefit were launched by the Radiation Therapy Oncology Group (RTOG) and the European Organisation on Research and Treatment on Cancer (EORTC), all using goserelin acetate (Zoladex), a LHRH analogue. The schema for these five phase III trials are shown in Figure 14A.1.

CONCOMITANT AND ADJUVANT HORMONAL TREATMENT

The EORTC study 22863 (Fig. 14.A) recruited 415 patients with cT1-2 grade 3, cT3-4 N0 M0 to compare radiotherapy and adjuvant hormone therapy to radiotherapy alone, with hormone therapy in case of relapse. Eighty-two percent of these patients were T3, 10% T4, and 89% N0. The hormone treatment was oral cyproterone acetate 50 mg 3 times daily for 1 month, beginning 1 week before the start of radiotherapy, and subcutaneous injection of goserelin (Zoladex) 3.6 mg every 4 weeks for 3 years starting on the first day of radiotherapy. The pelvic target volume received 50 Gy and the prostatic target volume 20 Gy. With a median follow-up of 66 months, there was a significant difference in survival—78% in favor of the combination versus 62% for radiotherapy alone ($P = .001$) and survival without clinical relapse: 78% versus 40%, respectively ($P <.001$) (25). The 5-year cumulative incidence of locoregional failure was 1.7% versus 16.4% in the radiotherapy alone arm ($P <.0001$) and survival without clinical or biological failure (nadir of 1.5 ng/mL) was 81% versus 43% ($P <.001$). These results confirm those of 1997 (21). Three risk categories—low, intermediate, and high—were formed according to prognostic index with respect to disease-free survival. The hazard-ratio for combined treatment versus radiotherapy alone was 0.12 (0.01–1.01; $P = .05$) in the low-risk category, 0.28 (0.18–0.46; $P = .0001$) in the intermediate-risk category, and 0.39 (0.24–0.63; $P = .0001$) in the high-risk category, indicating that each risk category benefits from concomitant and adjuvant HT.

ADJUVANT HORMONAL TREATMENT

The RTOG trial 85-31 was designed to evaluate the effectiveness of indefinite goserelin alone after radiotherapy; 977 patients with stages T3-T4 M0 with or without lymph node involvement, or pT3 after radical prostatectomy in the event of capsule invasion, positive margins, or seminal

TABLE 14A.1

SUMMARY OF MAJOR PROSPECTIVE TRIALS USING HORMONAL THERAPY AND RADIOTHERAPY

First author (Institution), yr (ref)	Study design (n)	Sequencing of hormonal therapy	Conclusions
Neglia (M.D. Anderson) 1977 (18)	EBRT +/− Estrogen (78)	Adjuvant?	Improved disease-free survival
Fellows (MRC) 1992 (20)	EBRT vs. Castration vs. both (277)	Adjuvant?	Delayed onset of distant metastasis
Bolla (EORTC) 1997 (21)	EBRT +/− CAB × 1 wk prior to RT and the LHRH × 3 yr (415)	Concomitant and Adjuvant	Survival advantage
Pilepich (RTOG) 2003 (22)	EBRT +/− LHRH for life after completing radiotherapy (977)	Adjuvant for life (RTOG 8531)	Survival advantage[a]
Pilepich (RTOG) 2001 (23)	EBRT +/− CAB starting 2 mo before and during EBRT (471)	Neoadjuvant (RTOG 8610)	Survival advantage[b]
Hanks (RTOG) 2003 (13)	EBRT + CAB starting 2 mo before and during EBRT +/− 2 yr of Adjuvant LHRH (1554)	Neoadjuvant vs. Neoad Neoadjuvant + Adjuvant	Survival advantage[c]
Roach (RTOG) 2003 (24)	Four arms: 1 and 2 CAB starting 2 months before and during EBRT and arms 3 and 4 CAB × 4 mo starting immediately after completing EBRT (1323)	Short Term Neoadjuvant vs. Short term Adjuvant	Progression-free survival advantage[d]

EBRT, external beam radiation therapy; CAB, combined androgen blockade.
[a]Updated analysis.
[b]limited to Gleason 2-6 tumors only.
[c]limited to Gleason 8-10 tumors only.
[d]Follow-up too early to expect survival endpoint.

vesicle involvement were included. Monthly administration of goserelin was started either during the last week of radiation therapy and was continued indefinitely or until relapse (Arm 1) or started at relapse (Arm 2). In fact, nearly a third of the patients took it for less than 2 years, one-third for 2 to 5 years, and only one-third received it more than 5 years (26). Of note, even after adjustment for early failures, the best survivals were seen for patients treated with >5 years of hormonal therapy. Antiandrogen therapy was not given at the very start of goserelin in order to inhibit the initial rise of LH and then of testosterone. Fifteen percent of patients had undergone radical prostatectomy in group 1 and 14% in group 2, and 29% and 26% had lymph node involvement, respectively. The pelvic target volume received 45 Gy and the prostate target volume 65 Gy to 70 Gy. Patients with a pT3 tumor received 60 Gy to 65 Gy to the postoperative target volume.

In the initial analysis, with a median follow-up of 5.6 years, the eight-year local failure rate was 23% vs. 37% ($P < .0001$). Distant metastasis was likewise favorably affected with the immediate use of hormone manipulation, with a distant metastasis rate of 27% and 37% ($P < .0001$). Disease-free survival and NED survival with PSA of 1.5 ng/mL or less were both statistically significant in favor of Arm 1 ($P < .0001$). But in this initial report, overall survival was not statistically significant: 49% vs. 47% ($P = .36$). Interestingly, subset analysis by Gleason score revealed a statistically significant overall survival ($P = .036$) and cause-specific survival ($P = .019$) in favor of the adjuvant HT arm for centrally reviewed Gleason 8-10 patients who had not previously undergone prostatectomy (27). With a median follow-up time of 7.3 years for all 977 randomized patients, a statistical significance was reached on this most recent update for 5-year and 10-year overall survival in

favor of the adjuvant HT arm, with 76% vs. 71% and 53% vs. 38% alive at those time points, respectively. However, the improvement in survival appears preferentially in patients with Gleason scores 7-10 (22).

Of note in RTOG 8531, 173 patients had biopsy-proven pN1 lymph nodes, and 98 of these received RT plus adjuvant HT. For those patients, there was a significant improvement in 5 year progression-free survival with PSA <1.5 ng ($P = .0001$) and metastatic-free survival ($P = .02$) with a median follow-up of 4.9 years (28). These data are in keeping with those of Gransfors et al. (29) who compared the combination of orchiectomy and radiotherapy ($n = 45$) to radiotherapy alone and androgen ablation at clinical disease progression ($n = 46$) for T1–4 pN0-3 M0 disease. Unfortunately, this study was closed prematurely due to insufficient accrual. Despite the small numbers, after a median follow-up of 9.3 years there was a significant difference in overall survival ($P = .02$) and progression-free survival ($P = .005$) in favor of the combined arm. This difference was mainly caused by lymph node-positive tumors.

SHORT-TERM NEOADJUVANT AND CONCOMITANT

The RTOG trial 8610 was designed to test the potential value of combined androgen blockade (CAB) with goserelin and flutamide, prior (2 months) and during radiation therapy (2 months) with respect to radiotherapy alone (23). A total of 471 patients with stage T2b-c (tumors measuring at least 5×5 cm at rectal examination); T3 and T4 M0 prostate cancers were included. Patients with regional lymph nodes

RTOG 8531 Schema

Stratify		Randomize	
Histologic differentiation			Radiation therapy[a] plus goserelin acetate[b]
2–5			
6–7			
8–10			
Nodal status			
None			vs.
Below common iliacs			
Common iliacs			
Para-aortics			Radiation therapy[a] alone
Acid phosphatase status			
Not elevated			
Elevated			
Prior radical prostatectomy			
No			
Yes			

[a]Radiation therapy: 44–46 Gy to the regional lymphatics, then 2–25 Gy boost to the prostate.
[b]Goserelin acetate: 3.6 mg q4wk. Patients started during last week of radiotherapy and continued indefinitely or until sign of disease progression.

Eligibility
T1–T2,N1,M0
T3,N0–N1,M0
pT3,N0–N1,M0

RTOG 8610 Schema

Stratify		Randomize	
Clinical stage			Radiation therapy[a] plus goserelin acetate[b] and flutamide[c]
B2, C			
T3–T4			
Differentiation			
Moderate			vs.
Poor			
			Radiation therapy[a] alone

[a]Radiation therapy: 44–46 Gy to the regional lymphatics, then 20–25 Gy boost to the prostate.
[b]Goserelin acetate: 3.6 mg q4wk. Patients started 2 months before the start of radiotherapy and stopped at the completion of radiotherapy.
[c]Flutamide: 250 mg orally three times per day. Patients started 2 months before start of radiotherapy and stopped at the completion of radiotherapy.

Eligibility
Bulky (≥25 cm² palpable tumor dimensions) clinical stage B2 and C

FIGURE 14A.1. Treatment schema for the Radiation Therapy Oncology Group (RTOG) 8531 and RTOG 8610 randomized prospective trials of radiation therapy and adjuvant hormone therapy.

EORTC Schema

Stratify		Randomize	
Clinical stage			Radiation therapy[a] plus goserelin acetate[b]
T1–T2			
T3–T4			
Extraperitoneal pelvic lymph node biopsy			
Negative			vs.
Positive			
Irradiation technique			Radiation therapy[a] alone
4 field boost			
2 field boost			
Institution			

[a]Radiation therapy: 50 Gy to the regional lymphatics, then 20 Gy boost to the prostate.
[b]Goserelin acetate: Patients started during first day of radiotherapy and continued monthly for 3 years. 150 mg of cyproterone acetate (steroidal antiandrogen) was given orally for 1 month starting 1 week before the goserelin acetate.

Eligibility
T1–T2,N0–N1,M0
T3–T4,N0–N1,M0

RTOG 9202 Schema

Stratify		Randomize	
Clinical stage			Radiation therapy[a] plus goserelin acetate[b] and flutamide[c]
T2c			
T3			
T4			
PSA			
≤30			vs.
>30			
Grade			
Well			Radiation therapy[a] plus goserelin acetate[b] and flutamide[c] plus goserelin acetate[d]
Moderate			
Poor or undifferentiated			
Nodal status (pathologic)			
Negative			
Positive			
Not done			

[a]Radiation therapy: 50 Gy to the regional lymphatics, then 20 Gy boost to the prostate.
[b]Goserelin acetate: 3.6 mg q4wk. Patients started 2 months before start of radiotherapy and stopped at the completion of radiotherapy.
[c]Flutamide: 250 mg orally three times per day. Patients started 2 months before start of radiotherapy and stopped at the completion of radiotherapy.
[d]Goserelin acetate: 3.6 mg q4wk. Patients started during last week of radiotherapy and continued for 2 years.

Eligibility
T2c–T4,N0–N1,M0

FIGURE 14A.2. Treatment schema for the European Organization for Research and Treatment of Cancer (EORTC) and Radiation Therapy Oncology Group (RTOG) 9202 randomized prospective trials of radiation therapy and adjuvant hormonal therapy. (PSA, prostate-specific antigen.)

were eligible, provided the involved nodes were below the common iliac chain and 7% had a positive nodal status in the combined treatment arm versus 9% in the radiotherapy-alone arm. Thirty percent of patients had a T2 tumor, 70% T3–4, and 91% of tumors were node negative. Hormonal treatment consisted of oral flutamide (250 mg 3× day) and a subcutaneous injection of goserelin, 3.6 mg every 4 weeks. The pelvis received 45 Gy and the prostate target volume 65 Gy to 70 Gy. With a median follow-up of 6.7 years, at 8 years, androgen ablation has been associated with an improvement in local control (42% vs. 30%, $P = .016$); a reduction in the incidence of distant metastases (34% vs. 45%, $P = .04$), an improvement

of disease-free survival (33% vs. 21%, $P = .004$), biochemical disease-free survival with a PSA nadir of 1.5 ng/mL (24% vs. 10%, $P = .0001$), and cause-specific mortality (23% vs. 31%, $P = .05$) was also noted. Subset analysis demonstrated that a significant enhancement in overall survival was seen in patients with Gleason score 2-6: 70% versus 52%, $P = .015$ (23). Of note, however, it is of interest that in a meta-analysis of RTOG trials, a benefit to T1-2 Gleason score = 7 with Nx disease was suggested (26).

RTOG 9413 Schema

Stratify

Stage
T1c, T2a
T1b, T2b
T2c–T4
PSA
≥30
<30
Gleason score
<7
7–10

Randomize

Radiation therapy[a] plus
goserelin acetate or
leuprolide acetate and
flutamide[c]
vs.
Radiation therapy[b] plus
goserelin acetate or
leuprolide acetate and
flutamide[c]
vs.
Radiation therapy[a] plus
goserelin acetate or
leuprolide acetate and
flutamide[d]
vs.
Radiation therapy[b] plus
goserelin acetate or
leuprolide acetate and
flutamide[d]

[a]Radiation therapy: 50.4 Gy to the regional lymphatics, then 19.8 Gy boost to the prostate.
[b]Radiation therapy: 70.2 Gy to the prostate only.
[c]Total androgen suppression: flutamide 250 mg orally twice per day and goserelin acetate or leuprolide acetate 3.6 q4wk. Patients started 2 months before start of radiotherapy and stopped at the completion of radiotherapy.
[d]Total androgen suppression: flutamide 250 mg orally twice per day and goserelin acetate or leuprolide acetate 3.6 q4wk. Patients started 2 months after completion of radiotherapy.

Eligibility
T1–T4,N0–NX,M0
Estimated risk of lymph node involvement >15%

FIGURE 14A.3. Treatment schema for the Radiation Therapy Oncology Group and RTOG 9413 randomized prospective trials of radiation therapy and adjuvant hormonal therapy. (PSA, prostate-specific antigen.)

SHORT-TERM NEOADJUVANT AND CONCOMITANT VERSUS SHORT-TERM ADJUVANT COMBINED ANDROGEN SUPPRESSION WITH WHOLE PELVIS OR PROSTATE-ONLY RADIOTHERAPY

The RTOG 9413 study (Fig. 14A.3) is a four-arm trial devoted to patients T1c–4 N0 M0 PSA <100 ng with an estimated risk of lymph node involvement of >15%. It randomized patients between neoadjuvant concurrent hormone therapy (NCHT) 2 months before and 2 months during RT (as on RTOG 8610) and adjuvant hormone therapy (AHT), for 4 months beginning immediately after the completion of RT. This study also included a second randomization between whole pelvis radiotherapy (WPRT) followed by a boost to the prostate or prostate-only radiotherapy (PORT). A total of 1,323 patients were accrued. With a median follow-up of 59.5 months, WPRT plus NCHT improved the 4-year freedom from progression (61%) compared with PORT + NCHT (45%), PORT + AHT (49%) and WPRT + AHT (47%) ($P = .008$) (24). These investigators noted that, based on the findings of

RTOG 8610, longer follow-up is required to determine whether the improved progression-free survival will translate into a difference in specific and overall survival.

The findings of RTOG 9413 both support and disprove elements of what was commonly believed about the interactions of neoadjuvant hormonal therapy and radiotherapy. For example, it is not surprising that there is an enhanced biologic interaction when HT is given short term before and during WPRT (Arm 1) compared to WPRT and AHT (Arm 3). However, NCHT, delivered with PORT (Arm 2), failed to render a better outcome than PO and AHT (Arm 4). Taken together, these findings suggest that the benefits of neoadjuvant short-term radiotherapy are manifested in pelvic lymph nodes (24).

The findings of RTOG 9413 contradict conventional thinking by failing to show benefit to PORT. This finding is consistent with a number of trials incorporating neoadjuvant hormonal therapy prior to radical prostatectomy (30–33). Despite the fact that they consistently demonstrate a reduction of the rate of positive margins and extracapsular extension, to date no difference in outcome has been shown (34). This suggests that the favorable histologic changes are in some sense an artifact, because they are not associated with a corresponding improvement in clinical outcome. Similar findings were noted by Laverdiere et al. who observed that, although the positive biopsy rate was reduced with longer-duration hormonal therapy, the biochemical control rate was unchanged (35). A preliminary analysis of a trial reported by Crook et al. also supports the notion that, although longer-induction hormonal therapy can result in more dramatic histological response in the prostate, it may not translate into an improved outcome (36). These findings, when taken together, imply that the apparent benefit of improved local control based on RTOG 8610 may, in fact, be an artifact similar to the surgical series as well as the biopsy results from the studies reported by Laverdiere et al. and Crook et al.

NEOADJUVANT AND CONCOMITANT +/– ADJUVANT LONG-TERM HORMONAL TREATMENT

The aim of RTOG protocol 9202 (Fig. 14A.2), devoted to patients classified T2c–4 N0, was to assess the value of a long-term adjuvant suppression (LTAD) after a short-term androgen suppression (STAD) according to the one used in protocol 86-10. All patients received 2 months of CAB with goserelin and flutamide before radiotherapy, followed during radiotherapy. A radiation dose of 65–70 Gy was given to the prostate. Then patients were randomly assigned to receive no additional therapy or 24 months of goserelin. This trial, activated in 1992, was closed in April 1995 after accruing 1,554 cases, a sufficient number of patients to show a 6% potential survival advantage. With a median follow-up time of 5.8 years, the LTAD arm showed significant improvement in all efficacy endpoints except 5-year overall survival: 80% versus 78.5 % ($P = .73$) compared with the STAD. In a subset of patients as part of the original study design to confirm the early findings of RTOG 8531, patients with tumor Gleason scores 8-10, treated on the LTAD arm, had significantly better overall survival: 81% vs. 70.7% ($P = .04$) (13).

UNSOLVED QUESTIONS

- *Is combined androgen suppression during 4 or 6 months of value as compared with LHRH analogue alone?*
  The rationale of using an antiandrogen in association with an LHRH agonist or castration is to block the androgens of adrenal origin, which are left free to continue

to stimulate prostate cancer (37). A meta-analysis of 27 randomized trials devoted to advanced prostate cancer has shown that the addition of an antiandrogen to androgen suppression, by surgery or drug controls, improved the 5-year survival by about 2% or 3%, with a range of uncertainty between 0% and 5% (38). In a more recent analysis, a larger effect is suggested if steroidal anti-androgens are excluded (39). In RTOG trials 8610, 9202, and 9413, 4 months of antiandrogen are used, and one month when combined with LHRH therapy in EORTC trial 22961. We do not know the optimal duration of combined androgen blockade, but we do know that antiandrogens inhibit the transient rise of LH and subsequently block the clinical effects of testosterone, which may have a potential harmful effect when LHRH analogues are prescribed alone (3,40,41).

- *Is neo-adjuvant HT of value before RT?*

We have no definitive answer in the absence of a randomized trial comparing a neoadjuvant and concomitant AD with concomitant AD, and a STAD with a survival endpoint. In daily practice, starting AD with a first shot 2 months before radiotherapy may be useful to decrease the tumor volume of HriCaP and improve DVH, while treating the patient immediately instead of awaiting the onset of irradiation. The serial studies reported by Laverdiere et al. shed some light on this question (35). Between 1990 and 1999, they entered 481 patients into two successive, prospective, randomized studies, including 161 in Study 1 and 325 in Study 2. Eligible patients had clinical stages T2-T3 prostate cancer. In the first study, patients were randomly allocated to EBRT alone (group 1), EBRT preceded by 3 months of NHT (group 2), and NHT concomitant and AHT for a total of 10 months (group 3). In the second study, they compared NCHT for a total of 5 months to NCHT and short-term AHT (total 10 months) with EBRT. In Study 1, at a median follow-up of 5 years, the 7-year biochemical-free survival rates were 42%, 66%, and 69% in groups 1 to 3, respectively, and significantly different between groups 1 and 2 ($P = .009$) and between groups 1 and 3 ($P = .003$) but not between groups 2 and 3 ($P = .6$). In Study 2, biochemical-free survival rates at 4 years were 65%. There was no significant difference between the two arms, and these investigators concluded that adding a short course of AHT after NHT provided no advantage.

- *Is STAD as effective as LTAD?*

STAD may certainly be beneficial for some HriCaP as shown by RTOG 8610. However, based on RTOG 8531, 9202, and EORTC trials, LTAD is recommended for the highest risk patients. The aim of EORTC equivalence trial 22961, initiated in 1997 and closed in 2001, was to compare surveillance to hormone therapy with an LHRH analogue (triptorelin) for 30 months, after external irradiation and CAB for 6 months, to determine the best adjuvant hormonal scheme to be associated with external irradiation (42). The findings of RTOG 9202 suggest that not all patients fare better with the use of LTAD, supporting the findings of the meta-analysis of RTOG trials (26).

- *Is LTAD alone as effective as LTAD plus RT?*

This is the standing controversy. Merit is due to the National Cancer Institute in Canada, which launched a randomized trial (43) comparing CAB (a SQ injection of 3.6 mg of goserelin every 4 weeks and flutamide at a dose of 750 mg/day or orchiectomy) plus radiation therapy 65 Gy to 69 Gy in 35 to 37 fractions associated with the same hormonal treatment, in stages T3–4 N0 M0 disease. This study started in 1996, has to accrue at least

650 patients, and will determine whether the combined approach is more effective than hormonal therapy alone. However, if the findings from RTOG 9202 hold up regarding equivalence of 4 months of combined hormonal therapy and radiotherapy to the same plus LTAD, it could prove a moot point, because few men would chose life-long castration over 4 months. Furthermore, the proof of a biologic interaction between hormonal therapy and radiotherapy from RTOG 9413 provides a clear rationale for an improved outcome with a combined approach.

- *What is the value of escalating dose and does it obviate the need for androgen deprivation?*

In RTOG and EORTC trials, the specified dose ranged between 65 Gy and 70 Gy without the benefits of escalating the dose of radiation delivered. Numerous studies evaluating escalating doses have shown a dose-response relationship for biochemical control (44–46), and a retrospective case-matched study has shown an advantage in cause-specific death for high-dose versus low-dose RT in the absence of HT (47). The intermediate results of the randomized study of the M.D. Anderson Cancer Center comparing 78 Gy 3D-CRT to a 70 Gy conventional radiotherapy show a significant increase in survival without biochemical relapse at 4 years in patients with cT1–2, PSA >10 ng/mL: 90% versus 60% ($P = .003$) (48). Clearly, higher-dose EBRT (>70–72 Gy) appears to be better than lower doses and capable of rendering results very similar to those associated with radical prostatectomy and brachytherapy; but can androgen deprivation be omitted (49)? There has not been a definitive study addressing this question. However, RTOG 9413 suggests that patients with a risk of lymph node involvement >15% benefit from irradiation of pelvic lymph nodes, and there is no reason to think that would change simply because a higher dose of radiation is delivered to the prostate.

MORBIDITY AND QUALITY OF LIFE

AD is known to adversely affect quality of life, leading to increased fatigue, hot flashes, limitations in daily activities, erectile difficulties, diarrhea, and breast swelling with antiandrogen therapy. Such side effects can be best assessed by a self-administered questionnaire (50). Treatment-related side effects and sexual dysfunction may gradually disappear once the hormonal treatment has stopped, depending on its duration. Patients who receive a short-term androgen suppression will recuperate earlier from the side effects, which may have a positive impact on the overall quality of life. The possible gains in terms of length of life will have to be balanced against a prolonged burden of treatment. In EORTC trial 22863, hot flashes were present among patients taking adjuvant hormonal treatment in 62% of the cases, but only 34% of the patients were suffering from more than three hot flushes per day. The figures pertaining to change in erectile potency are likely to be grossly underestimated due to patient and physician concerns about privacy. In RTOG trial 9202, there was a small but significant increase in the frequency of 5-year late radiation grades 3, 4, and 5 gastrointestinal toxicity ascribed to the LTAD arm (2.6% vs. 1.2% $P = .037$), the cause of which was not clear.

CONCLUSIONS

Androgen ablative therapy prescribed with external irradiation increases clinical and biochemical relapse-free survival in patients

TABLE 14A.2

GUIDELINES REGARDING SEQUENCING OF HORMONAL THERAPY ACCORDING TO RISK GROUPS (2002 TNM CLASSIFICATION)

Risk	EBRT	Neoadjuvant/ Concomitant	Adjuvant +/– Concomitant
Low			
T1c-2a, Gleason ≤6, PSA ≤10 ng/mL	+	–	–
Intermediate			
T2b, or 10 <PSA <20, or Gleason 7	+ᵃ	+	–
High			
(T2c, PSA >20)ᵇ, Gleason >7	+	+ᶜ	+
Very high			
T3–4, N1	+	+ᶜ	+

ᵃConsider high dose >72 Gy as alternative to hormonal therapy.
ᵇThere are no data yet published that demonstrate that patients with clinical stage T2c, or PSA >20 ng/mL, benefit from long-term adjuvant hormonal therapy.
ᶜRTOG 9202 starts with neoadjuvant hormonal therapy followed by concomitant and adjuvant.

with locally advanced prostate cancer T2c–4 N0–1 M0. According to Gleason score and modalities of administration, a significant improvement in overall survival has been shown. There appears to be a survival advantage for patients with poorly differentiated tumors, with either LHRH analog being prescribed alone after the last week of irradiation and continued until relapse ($P = .03$) compared to EBRT alone (RTOG trial 8531), or CAB given before and during irradiation and followed by 2 years of LHRH analogue ($P = .04$) (RTOG Trial 9202). There is also a survival advantage for patients with Gleason score 2-6 ($P = .015$) with a CAB prescribed 2 months before and during radiation therapy (RTOG trial 8610). There appears to be a survival advantage whatever the histologic grade with LHRH analogue administered during and after irradiation for a total duration of 3 years ($P = .001$) (EORTC trial 22863) or longer (update of 8531) compared to EBRT alone. The choice has to be made taking into account the patient's feeling regarding quality of life. In the near future, randomized trials will enable us to better define the optimal chronology and duration of hormonal therapy, the value of combined androgen blockade versus LHRH alone, the role of using an androgen deprivation alone, and the potential of chemotherapy to enhance the results of hormonal radiotherapy. On the basis of these data, Table 14A.2 proposes guidelines.

References

1. Huggins C, Stevens RE, Hodges CV. The effects of castration on advanced carcinoma of the prostate gland. *Arch Surg* 1941;43:207–211.
2. Schroder FH. What is new in endocrine therapy of prostatic cancer? *Prog Clin Biol Res* 1990;357:45–52.
3. Parmar H, Phillips RH, Lightman SL, et al. Randomised controlled study of orchidectomy vs. long-acting D-Trp-6-LHRH microcapsules in advanced prostatic carcinoma. *Lancet* 1985;2:1201–1205.
4. Bagshaw MA, Cox RS, Ray GR. Status of prostate cancer at Stanford University. *NCI Monogr* 1988;7:47–60.
5. Hanks GE, Corn BW, Lee WR, et al. External beam irradiation of prostate cancer: conformal treatment techniques and outcomes for the 1990s. *Cancer* 1995;75:1972–1977.
6. Roach M III, Lu J, Pilepich MV, et al. Long-term survival after radiotherapy alone: Radiation Therapy Oncology Group prostate cancer trials. *J Urol* 1999;161:864–868.
7. Bolla M, Bartelink H, Gibbons R, et al. Treatment of regional disease. Prostate cancer. In: Murphy G, Denis L, Chatelain C, et al. ed. *First international consultation on prostate cancer, Monaco,* June 20-21-22 1996. Monaco: Scientific Communication International Ltd, 1997;259–266.
8. Cooperberg MR, Broering JM, Litwin MS, et al. The contemporary management of prostate cancer in the United States: lessons from the Cancer of the Postate Strategic Urologic Research Endeavor (CapSURE), a national disease registry. *J Urol* 2004;171:1393–1401.
9. Leibel SA, Fuks Z, Zelefsky MJ, et al. The effects of local and regional treatment on the metastatic outcome in prostatic carcinoma with pelvic lymph node involvement. *Int J Radiat Oncol Biol Phys* 1994;28:7–16.
10. Overgaard M, Jensen MB, Overgaard J, et al. Postoperative radiotherapy in high-risk postmenopausal breast-cancer patients given adjuvant tamoxifen: Danish Breast Cancer Cooperative Group DBCG 82c randomised trial. *Lancet* 1999;353:1641–1648.
11. Zelefsky MJ, Harrison A. Neoadjuvant androgen ablation prior to radiotherapy for prostate cancer: reducing the potential morbidity of therapy. *Urology* 1997;49:38–45.
12. Michalski JM, Purdy JA, Winter K, et al. Preliminary report of toxicity following 3D radiation therapy for prostate cancer on 3DOG/RTOG 9406. *Int J Radiat Oncol Biol Phys* 2000;46:391–402.
13. Hanks GE, Pajak TF, Porter A, et al. Phase III trial of long-term adjuvant androgen deprivation after neoadjuvant hormonal cytoreduction and radiotherapy in locally advanced carcinoma of the prostate: the Radiation Therapy Oncology Group Protocol 92-02. *J Clin Oncol* 2003;21:3972–3978.
14. Schultheiss TE, Lee WR, Hunt MA, et al. Late GI and GU complications in the treatment of prostate cancer. *Int J Radiat Oncol Biol Phys* 1997;37:3–11.
15. Zietman AL, Prince EA, Nakfoor BM, et al. Androgen deprivation and radiation therapy: sequencing studies using the Shionogi in vivo tumor system. *Int J Radiat Oncol Biol Phys* 1997;38:1067–1070.
16. Joon DL, Hasegawa M, Sikes C, et al. Supraadditive apoptotic response of R3327-G rat prostate tumors to androgen ablation and radiation. *Int J Radiat Oncol Biol Phys* 1997;38:1071–1077.
17. Pollack A, Salem N, Ashoori F, et al. Lack of prostate cancer radiosensitization by androgen deprivation. *Int J Radiat Oncol Biol Phys* 2001;51:1002–1007.
18. Neglia WJ, Hussey DH, Johnson DE. Megavoltage radiation therapy for carcinoma of the prostate. *Int J Radiat Oncol Biol Phys* 1977;2:873–883.
19. Zagars GK, Johnson DE, von Eschenbach AC, et al. Adjuvant estrogen following radiation therapy for stage C adenocarcinoma of the prostate: long-term results of a prospective randomized study. *Int J Radiat Oncol Biol Phys* 1988;14:1085–1091.
20. Fellows GJ, Clark PB, Beynon LL, et al. A Medical Research Council Study Treatment of advanced localized prostatic cancer by orchiectomy, radiotherapy, or combined treatment. *Br J Urol* 1992;70:304–309.
21. Bolla M, Gonzalez D, Warde P, et al. Improved survival in patients with locally advanced prostate cancer treated with radiotherapy and goserelin. *N Engl J Med* 1997;337:295–300.
22. Pilepich MV, Winter K, Lawton C, et al. Androgen suppression adjuvant to radiotherapy in carcinoma of the prostate. Long-term results of phase III RTOG study 85-31. *Int J Radiat Oncol Biol Phys* 2003;2003:S172–S173.
23. Pilepich MV, Winter K, John MJ, et al. Phase III Radiation Therapy Oncology Group (RTOG) trial 86-10 of androgen deprivation adjuvant to definitive radiotherapy in locally advanced carcinoma of the prostate. *Int J Radiat Oncol Biol Phys* 2001;50:1243–1252.
24. Roach M III, DeSilvio M, Lawton C, et al. Phase III trial comparing whole-pelvic versus prostate-only radiotherapy and neoadjuvant versus adjuvant combined androgen suppression: Radiation Therapy Oncology Group 9413. *J Clin Oncol* 2003;21:1904–1911.

25. Bolla M, Collette L, Blank L, et al. Long-term results with immediate androgen suppression and external irradiation in patients with locally advanced prostate cancer (an EORTC study): a phase III randomised trial. *Lancet* 2002;360:103–106.

26. Roach M, Lu J, Pilepich MV, et al. Predicting long term survival, and the need for hormonal therapy: a meta-analysis of RTOG prostate cancer trials. *Int J Radiat Oncol Biol Phys* 2000;47:617–627.

27. Lawton CA, Winter K, Murray K, et al. Updated results of the phase III Radiation Therapy Oncology Group (RTOG) trial 85-31 evaluating the potential benefit of androgen suppression following standard radiation therapy for unfavorable prognosis carcinoma of the prostate. *Int J Radiat Oncol Biol Phys* 2001;49:937–946.

28. Lawton CA, Winter K, Byhardt R, et al. Radiation Therapy Oncology Group. Androgen suppression plus radiation versus radiation alone for patients with D1 (pN+) adenocarcinoma of the prostate (results based on a national prospective randomized trial, RTOG 85-31). *Int J Radiat Oncol Biol Phys* 1997;38:931–939.

29. Granfors T, Modig H, Damber JE, et al. Combined orchiectomy and external radiotherapy versus radiotherapy alone for nonmetastatic prostate cancer with or without pelvic lymph node involvement: a prospective randomized study. *J Urol* 1998;159:2030–2034.

30. VanPoppel H, Ridder DD, Elgamal AA, et al. Neoadjuvant hormonal therapy before radical prostatectomy decreases the number of positive surgical margins in stage T2 prostate cancer: interim results of a prospective randomized trial. *J Urol* 1995;154:429–434.

31. Pedersen KV, Lundberg S, Hugosson J, et al. Neoadjuvant hormonal treatment with triptorelin versus no treatment prior to radical prostatectomy: a prospective randomized multicenter study. *Am Urol Assoc* 1995;153:391A.

32. Fair WR, Israeli RS, Wang Y, et al. Neoadjuvant androgen-deprivation therapy (ADT) prior to radical prostatectomy results in a significantly decreased incidence of residual micrometastatic disease as detected by nested RT-PCR with primers. *Int J Radiat Oncol Biol Phys* 1995;153:391A.

33. Gleave ME, Goldenberg SL, Jones EC, et al. Maximal biochemical and pathological downstaging requires 8 months of neoadjuvant hormonal therapy prior to radical prostatectomy. *J Urol* 1995;153:392A.

34. Soloway MS, Pareek K, Sharifi R, et al. Neoadjuvant androgen ablation before radical prostatectomy in cT2bNxM0 prostate cancer: 5-year results. *J Urol* 2002;167:112–116.

35. Laverdiere J, Nabid A, De Bedoya LD, et al. The efficacy and sequencing of a short course of androgen suppression on freedom from biochemical failure when administered with radiation therapy for T2-T3 prostate cancer. *J Urol* 2004;171:1137–1140.

36. Crook JM, Ludgate C, Lim J, et al. Preliminary report of a multi center Canadian phase III randomized trial of 3 months vs 8 months neoadjuvant androgen ablation prior to standard dose radiotherapy for clinically localized prostate cancer. In: Cox, ed. *Proceedings of American Society for Therapeutic Radiology and Oncology 44th annual meeting,* October 6-10, 2002. New Orleans: Elsevier Science, 2002:134.

37. Labrie F, Belanger A, Simard J, et al. Combination therapy for prostate cancer. Endocrine and biologic basis of its choice as new standard first-line therapy. *Cancer* 1993;71:1059–1067.

38. Prostate Cancer Trialists' Collaborative Group. Maximum androgen blockade in advanced prostate cancer: an overview of the randomised trials. *Lancet* 2000;355:1491–1498.

39. Klotz L. Combined androgen blockade in prostate cancer: meta-analyses and associated issues. *BJU Int* 2001;87:806–813.

40. Noguchi K, Uemura H, Harada M, et al. Inhibition of PSA flare in prostate cancer patients by administration of flutamide for 2 weeks before initiation of treatment with slow-releasing LH-RH agonist. *Int J Clin Oncol* 2001;6:29–33.

41. Bubley GJ. Is the flare phenomenon clinically significant? *Urology* 2001;58:5–9.

42. Bolla M, de Reijke Th, et al. Long term adjuvant hormonal treatment with LHRH analogue versus no further treatment in locally advanced prostatic carcinoma treated by external irradiation and a six months combined androgen blockade. A phase III study. EORTC trial 22961. Brussels: EORTC Data Center, 1997.

43. Warde P, Kostashuk E, Bell D, et al. Intergroup (NCIC CTG, CUOG, ECOG, CALGB, SWOG) Phase III randomized trial comparing total androgen blockade versus total androgen blockade plus pelvic irradiation in clinical stage T3-4, N0, M0 adenocarcinoma of the prostate. 1995.

44. Hanks GE, Lee WR, Hanlon AL, et al. Conformal technique dose escalation for prostate cancer: biochemical evidence of improved cancer control with higher doses in patients with pretreatment prostate-specific antigen > or = 10 ng/ml [see Comments]. *Int J Radiat Oncol Biol Phys* 1996;35:861–868.

45. Roach M, Meehan S, Kroll S, et al. Radiotherapy (XRT) for high-grade (HG) clinically localized adenocarcinoma of the prostate (CAP). *J Urol* 1996;156:1719–1723.

46. Pollack A, Zagars GK. External beam radiotherapy dose response of prostate cancer. *Int J Radiat Oncol Biol Phys* 1997;39:1011–1018.

47. Hanks GE, Hanlon AL, Pinover WH, et al. Dose selection for prostate cancer patients based on dose comparison and dose response studies. *Int J Radiat Oncol Biol Phys* 2000;46:823–832.

48. Pollack A, Zagars GK, Smith LG, et al. Preliminary results of a randomized radiotherapy dose-escalation study comparing 70 Gy with 78 Gy for prostate cancer. *J Clin Oncol* 2000;18:3904–3911.

49. Kupelian PA, Potters L, Khuntia D, et al. Radical prostatectomy, external beam radiotherapy <72 Gy, external beam radiotherapy > or = 72 Gy, permanent seed implantation, or combined seeds/external beam radiotherapy for stage T1-T2 prostate cancer. *Int J Radiat Oncol Biol Phys* 2004;58:25–33.

50. Potosky AL, Knopf K, Clegg LX, et al. Quality-of-life outcomes after primary androgen deprivation therapy: results from the Prostate Cancer Outcomes Study. *J Clin Oncol* 2001;19:3750–3757.

CHAPTER 14B
Surgical Management of Clinical T3 (cT3) and Node Positive (pN+) Adenocarcinoma of the Prostate

Gregory S. Schenk, Michael L. Blute, and Horst Zincke

INTRODUCTION

The management of clinical stage T3 adenocarcinoma of the prostate has remained controversial for many years. Risk stratification has led to a better understanding of which patients are at greatest risk of mortality from their cancer (1). The use of hormonal therapy (HT) and advances in surgical technique have provided a therapeutic regimen that improves survival while minimizing treatment-associated morbidity. However, the problem of locally advanced disease remains substantial despite the stage migration, which has been witnessed during the prostate specific antigen (PSA) era (from 1987 onward) (2). Prostate cancer is now the most common malignancy diagnosed in American men and the second leading cause of cancer-specific death after lung cancer (3). In 2003, approximately 220,900 men will be diagnosed with prostate cancer and 28,900 will die from this disease in the United States (3). An increased awareness of prostate cancer by the public has induced more men to have routine digital rectal examination (DRE) and PSA testing. This has led to unprecedented changes in prostate cancer presentation. While dramatic shifts have been observed in the numbers of patients presenting with metastatic (decreased) and clinically localized disease (increased), cT3 disease has remained relatively stable for the past 20 years (4). The National Cancer Data Base (NCDB), which records clinical stage, and the population-based Surveillance, Epidemiology, and End Result (SEER) registry, which records most accurate stage, both confirm these findings (5,6). Analysis from the NCDB regarding 51,459 patients diagnosed during 1998 reveals that 10.5% were American Joint Committee on Cancer (AJCC) stage III [T3, N0, M0, any Gleason score (2–10)] (6). Previously, cT3 has accounted for 3% to 37% of patients in various treatment series (7). Currently, about 23,000 patients with locally advanced prostate cancer are diagnosed each year in the United States. The surgical management and outcomes of these patients and those found to have node-positive (pN+) disease after radical prostatectomy (RP) are reviewed in this chapter.

STAGING

The AJCC defines clinical stage T3a as unilateral or bilateral extracapsular extension and cT3b as extension into the seminal vesicle (8). The proper management of patients with locally advanced prostate cancer, defined as extending beyond the confines of the prostatic capsule (palpable induration that extends into the lateral sulci or cephalad and into the seminal vesicles without evidence for metastatic disease), is widely debated. Historical arguments against RP need to be examined in light of contemporary data that show minimal morbidity along with a new multimodality therapy paradigm of treatment for advanced disease (9). Furthermore, the number of patients currently presenting for surgical management of their cT3 prostate cancer has steadily decreased over the last two decades. In 1987, 25% of prostatectomies performed at the Mayo Clinic were for men with clinically assessed T3 disease (Fig. 14B.1). Since 1995, the percentage with cT3 cancer has ranged between 3% to 5%, and in 2002, patients with cT3 cancer accounted for only 5% of all prostatectomies performed at the Mayo Clinic, where aggressive surgical management has been advocated for over 20 years (2,10). This significant decrease (25% vs. 5%, P <.001) may be explained by stage migration; however, current category one recommendations for radiation treatment (RT) with androgen ablation for cT3 disease (despite its only moderate outcome) may also have contributed to fewer patients presenting to a tertiary referral center for surgery (11). For the youngest men with stages C (palpable with clinical evidence of extension beyond the prostate) and D (lymph node involvement or distant metastasis) prostate cancer, prostatectomy rates are only 19% and 8%, respectively, while the radiation treatment rate for clinical stage C disease is 54% (12). Thus, in spite of only moderate results, albeit inferior as compared to RP, the majority of men with clinically staged T3 disease are treated with RT.

GOALS OF TREATMENT AND INITIAL EVALUATION

Most investigators would agree that the treatment goals for cT3 disease are as follows: (a) eliminate local tumor, (b) prevent progressive disease dissemination of tumor cells, (c) prolong survival, and (d) maintain quality of life. Patients, many of whom present with obstructive symptoms, are considered candidates for surgery when they have biopsy-proven disease, 10 years or more of life expectancy, low or no co-morbidities, no extension to the pelvic side walls or vesical neck (cystoscopically assessed), and no regional or systemic disease

as assessed by computed tomographic (CT) imaging of the pelvis and abdomen and by bone scintigraphy. Magnetic resonance imaging (MRI) is obtained if CT or bone scan are positive in only one area. In a young patient with no significant adenopathy, lesser than or equal to 2 cm pelvic nodes, and no significant comorbidities, RP would be offered as a treatment option possibly in conjunction with adjuvant hormonal or radiation therapy, depending on the pathological staging. If preoperative evaluation revealed that the patient had enlarged nodes along the greater vessels, surgery would not be offered. In addition, preoperative serum PSA levels are of questionable value when determining the appropriateness of a cT3 prostate cancer patient for surgery. We recently reviewed 173 patients who presented to our institution with a serum PSA greater than or equal to 50 ng/mL and who subsequently underwent radical retropubic prostatectomy. Among these patients, 43% had node positive disease and began adjuvant HT (AHT) immediately following surgery. Even within this elevated PSA range, 16% of these patients had pathologically confirmed, organ-confined disease. The 10-year cause-specific survival for this group is 87%, and 80% of these patients are free from metastasis at 10 years (manuscript in preparation, Mayo Data). Therefore, the extent of the preoperative evaluation is similar to that performed for patients with localized disease except a thorough attempt is made to determine the patients' M (metastasis) status prior to surgery.

The DRE is inaccurate in predicting pathologic stage on radical prostatectomy specimens (Table 14B.1) (7,13). Other avenues of staging continue to be investigated. MRI, particularly endorectal MRI for staging of prostate cancer, is being vigorously studied (14). However, the ability of MRI alone to predict stage is variable (15); therefore, MRI is currently only used in clinical research studies. Our patients with limited cT3 are still offered a surgical component to manage their disease regardless of locally advanced disease on MRI.

TREATMENT OPTIONS

While frequently employed to treat clinically localized disease, RP has not been widely accepted to treat cT3, probably because of the perceived notion that surgery is technically not feasible, morbidity is high, and pN+ disease is present. Therapeutic options include expectant management, conservative surgery (i.e., transurethral resection of the prostate, TURP), external beam radiotherapy (EBRT), interstitial seed implantation, and combined EBRT and interstitial brachytherapy as well as primary excision, all with or without HT.

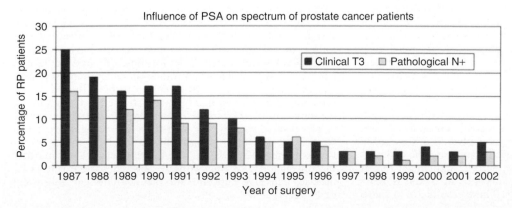

FIGURE 14B.1. Influence of PSA on clinical presentation and pathologic outcome of patients treated with radical prostatectomy (RP).

Nonsurgical Management

Conservative Management

While the natural history of clinical T3 prostate cancer is difficult to ascertain because the majority of patients are treated upon diagnosis, some studies do report expectant management and provide some insight. Patients with stage T3 disease have an average survival of two to three years (16–18). More recently, Adolfsson et al. (19) updated their cohort of 50 men with locally advanced prostate cancer (cT3) with a follow-up to at least 12 years or until death. Though cancer-specific survival at 12 years was 70%, two-thirds of patients eventually received definitive treatment (HT, EBRT, or RP) and of the 10 patients with 12- to 14-year-survival, all had started HT early in the course of their disease. Only 4% of these expectantly managed patients had poorly differentiated tumors on fine-needle aspiration biopsy. This is in stark contrast to the majority of series reporting on cT3 prostate cancer, where usually high grade, high volume, and aggressive tumor activity are noted. For example, the control arm of the Medical Research Council (MRC) study (20), which delayed therapy until systemic progression, studied patients with locally advanced disease or asymptomatic metastasis and reported 5-year cause-specific survival and overall survival rates of 46% and 40%, respectively. The immediately treated group was less likely to require TURP, less likely to develop major complications, and had a significant survival benefit in the M0 group. While this was the first demonstration of a survival benefit for early HT in locally advanced prostate cancer, it also revealed that 60% of untreated patients died of metastatic prostate cancer.

TURP with or without adjuvant treatment has also been employed to manage cT3 disease. Tomlinson et al. compared two similar groups, treated by either RP or TURP. In the patients treated with TURP, the likelihood of long-term survival was low, and there was symptomatic local recurrence in 75% of patients; in contrast, the patients treated with RP had a local recurrence of only 8% (21). In general, the role of TURP should be limited to those patients who are unsuitable candidates for surgery or radiation and are in need of symptomatic relief after failing hormonal management (22,23). A recent review of the morbidity associated with TURP in locally advanced prostate cancer revealed the International Prostate Symptom Score improved from 21.1 to 11 ($P = .002$); however, a 29% reoperation rate was also noted (24).

Androgen Deprivation Monotherapy

HT alone is infrequently used to manage locally advanced prostate cancer. The timing of endocrine monotherapy was evaluated in a randomized fashion by the MRC trials (20); both overall and disease-specific survivals were significantly longer in patients who received early endocrine treatment. Disease-specific survival at 5 years in the deferred-treatment arm was 46% compared with 60% in the immediate-treatment arm. Furthermore, the immediately treated patients were less likely to develop major complications, such as spinal cord compression or pathologic fractures, and fewer immediately treated patients needed TURP. The MRC trial was the first trial to demonstrate a clear survival benefit for immediate HT in locally advanced prostate cancer.

Recently, Fowler et al. studied 208 men with locally advanced prostate cancer who were treated with gonadal androgen ablation or gonadal androgen ablation plus an antiandrogen (25). The actuarial 5-year and 8-year, cause-specific survivals were 92% and 80%, respectively, with 22 patients at risk at 8 years; the actuarial all-cause survivals at 5 and 8 years were 59% and 41%, respectively. These results are in sharp contrast to earlier hormonal monotherapy reports. For example, the European Organization for Research and Treatment of Cancer (EORTC) reported that 34% of patients treated with hormonal monotherapy progressed to metastatic disease within 2 years and that 22% died of disease within 2 years of initiating treatment (18).

Recent studies evaluating the role of high-dose bicalutamide have shown similar survival outcomes to those observed with castration; the 5-year overall survival for both treatment groups was approximately 50% (26). Seretta et al. reported an actuarial 5-year overall survival of 40% in 25 patients with T3-T4 N0 M0 prostate carcinoma treated with flutamide, 250 mg, 3 times daily (27). These two reports also investigated whether the treatments would preserve sexual function without losing efficacy compared to orchiectomy. Antiandrogen monotherapy in patients with locally advanced disease has a similar survival outcome to orchiectomy with improved quality of life benefits with regard to sexual interest, physical capacity, and bone mineral density (28). However, in the phase III studies of 150 mg bicalutamide monotherapy for patients with M0 disease, the incidence of gynecomastia and breast tenderness was 49.4% and 40.1%, respectively, in the antiandrogen group, and 4.4% and 1.9% in the orchiectomy group (26). In addition, neither treatment compares favorably with modern radiation or surgical series reports. For example, the updated overall survival rate in the largest surgical series is 53% at 15 years, and cause-specific survivals are 87% and 78% at 10 and 15 years, respectively (29). This contrasts with 50% overall survival at 5 years in the above mentioned androgen monotherapy series.

Radiotherapy (RT)

External beam radiation has been the most commonly employed treatment for cT3 disease, with 54% of newly diagnosed patients receiving RT (12). After definitive treatment, the local recurrence rate is the most accurate measure of the treatment's ability to control the primary tumor (30,31). A report of 120 patients who were randomized to receive RT only, neoadjuvant hormonal therapy (NHT) plus RT, or NHT plus RT plus AHT, and subsequently underwent prostate biopsies, revealed positive biopsy rates of 65%, 28%, and 5%, respectively, at 2 years (32). Unfortunately, RT alone has serious limitations in cT3 patients, especially regarding local disease control. Establishing control of the primary tumor eliminates a source of continued tumor dissemination and reduces morbidity from local progression. Zagars et al. reported that without local control the 10-year incidence of freedom from metastatic disease was only 41% compared to 64% with local control (33). Finally, interstitial radiotherapy as a single modality is not used for locally advanced disease.

In an attempt to improve patient survival, hormonal manipulation in conjunction with RT has been employed (34–36). Bolla et al. showed that RT and concomitant HT continued for 3 years provided a significant improvement in both 5-year disease-free (74% vs. 40%, $P = .0001$) and cancer-specific survival (94% vs. 79%, $P = .0001$). Although the follow-up was short, this and similar reports have made HT with RT the standard treatment for those cT3 patients receiving RT (37–40). Advances in radiation technology have also allowed increasing doses of radiation to be delivered to the prostate, and this too has been investigated (41). While the combination of HT plus RT has been shown to be effective in prospective studies, the long-term effect might be due to continuing androgen depression, particularly in regard to PSA outcome (42). Overall, the 10-year data are not mature. In contrast, RP, in the properly selected patient with cT3 disease, can give superior survival with longer follow-up (≥15 years) (43).

Primary Surgical Management

For more than 20 years, surgical management has been advocated at the Mayo Clinic in the treatment of locally advanced disease (44). Multiple Mayo Clinic publications report the effectiveness of this therapeutic regimen in men with locally advanced disease (9,29). The advantages to surgical removal of the prostate gland include accurate pathologic staging, allowing judicious use of adjuvant therapy in those patients at highest risk for disease progression and death from prostate cancer. Extirpation also identifies the 27% of patients who are clinically overstaged (i.e., upon pathologic review, have organ-confined tumors) and who are potentially curable (Table 14B.1).

When performed by an experienced surgeon, RP can lead to excellent functional recovery. This eliminates the substantial risk of increased morbidity from local progression and, as noted, provides superior local control and improves overall outcome. In those patients found to have node-positive disease, RP provides accurate staging and identification of patients who would likely benefit from adjuvant hormonal therapy. In the only randomized prospective study comparing immediate HT to observation after RP and pelvic lymph node dissection in men with node-positive disease, Messing et al. validated the Mayo Clinic's longstanding practice by showing significant improvements in both overall- and cause-specific survival for the patient cohort receiving immediate HT (45).

Surgical Technique

The success of RP for locally advanced disease relies on the presence of an intact barrier overlying the tumor and on the removal of all tumor-bearing tissue. Precise knowledge of the location and frequency of residual tumor, extracapsular extension, and positive margins may indicate patients in whom improved surgical techniques are needed for complete tumor excision. About 70% to 80% of clinically palpable prostate cancers originate in the peripheral zone, or PZ (46). As these tumors grow, they are more likely to extend into the posterolateral and rectal periprostatic soft tissue (47,48). Villers et al. demonstrated that capsular penetration occurs preferentially through perineural spaces (49). These spaces represent relatively weak areas in the anatomic capsule that facilitate the spread of cancer. The importance of the wide en bloc excision of the prostate and surrounding lateral prostatic (pelvic) fascia, which contain the neurovascular bundles, is emphasized by the fact that 60% of RP specimens with positive posterolateral margins contained tumor in the ipsilateral resected neurovascular bundle (50). There is generally no role for nerve-sparing procedures when RP is performed for clinical T3 disease. Many of these patients may need AHT.

About 20% to 25% of patients with palpable (PZ) tumors have a positive surgical margin posteriorly on the rectal surface of the prostate (47,51). An iatrogenic positive surgical margin may be avoided by precisely entering the plane posterior to Denonvilliers' fascia, anterior to the smooth muscle layer

of the rectal wall, and inferior to the rectal fascia. In this way, both layers of Denonvilliers' fascia are removed en bloc with the prostate gland (51). Posterior dissection of the prostate is initiated at the apices of the seminal vesicles; anterior/posterior Denonvilliers' fascia is not entered proximally. Step-sectioning of the carcinomatous prostates demonstrated extension of the carcinoma to within 8 mm of the apical margin in 80% of the specimens (52), and, in whole mounts of clinically localized disease, cancer was present in the apical section of 74% of specimens (53). A complete understanding of the complex apical anatomy facilitates complete tumor removal (54,55). Frozen section analysis is crucial and can guide the extent of the apical dissection. In the presence of a positive margin, a wider excision, if prudent and possible, can be performed. In the event of a proximal positive margin or gross but limited tumor invasion of the bladder neck, the circular smooth muscle fibers of the bladder neck are resected with care to preserve the ureteral orifices. The bladder neck is reconstructed using the visceral bladder fascia for closure at the 6 o'clock position of the vesical neck (56).

The prognostic implications of positive surgical margins (especially gross residual disease) have been demonstrated (57–59). Multivariate analysis has demonstrated that positive surgical margins were a significant predictor of clinical disease recurrence and biochemical failure ($P = .0017$, RR 1.55, CI 1.18–2.04) (48). The natural biologic behavior (tumor grade and volume) of the tumor may be more influential with regard to disease outcome than minute local residual tumor; however, the immediate goal of any cancer operation is surgical margins that are clear of tumor (60). Therefore, the following procedures related to key anatomic points potentially improve cancer removal and thus local control: (a) wide excision of the neurovascular bundles (Fig. 14B.2), (b) en bloc removal of both layers of Denonvilliers' fascia and both ampullae of the vas deferens and seminal vesicles from the tips of the seminal vesicles distally to the vesicle neck proximally (Fig. 14B.3),

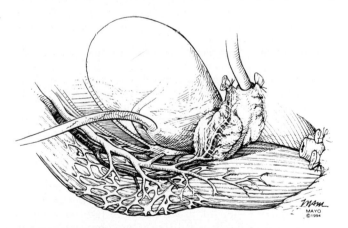

FIGURE 14B.2. After the urethra is divided, the neurovascular bundle is transected. The lateral pelvic fascia and neurovascular bundles are widely excised en bloc with the prostate.

TABLE 14B.1

STAGING ERRORS FOR PATIENTS UNDERGOING RADICAL PROSTATECTOMY FOR CLINICAL T3 PROSTATE CANCER

cT3	pT2a	pT2b	pT3a	pT3b	pT4	pT2–pT4 N+	Margin+
1,236[a](%)	140 (11)	200 (16)	265 (21)	280 (23)	13 (1)	336 (27)	613 (50)

[a]Pathologic staging was unavailable for two patients.

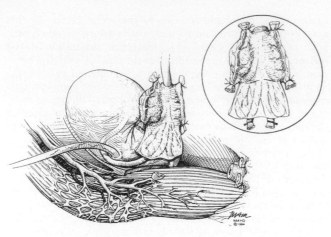

FIGURE 14B.3. En bloc removal of both layers of Denonvilliers fascia and both ampullae of the vas deferens and seminal vesicles from the tips of the seminal vesicles distally to the vesicle neck proximally. Inset: Radical prostatectomy specimen after wide excision of the lateral pelvic fascia, neurovascular bundles, and both layers of Denonvilliers' fascia en bloc with the prostate.

(c) precise apical dissection guided by intraoperative frozen section analysis of the margins, and (d) wider excision of the circular smooth muscle fibers of the bladder neck with reconstruction in the event that a positive margin is found on intraoperative frozen section analysis or gross but limited invasion of the bladder neck is noted.

Morbidity

Modern radical prostatectomy is well tolerated, and the morbidity associated with the procedure in men with locally advanced disease is not different from that seen in patients with clinically localized disease (7,9). Higher clinical stage does not appear to predispose patients to higher operative morbidity or longer hospitalization (9).

A recent analysis describes the 15-year results of RP in cT3 disease among patients treated during the PSA era exclusively (61). The complications and continence rates following RP in cT3 patients mirrored those observed following surgery in cT2 disease. During this period, over 93% of patients in both groups achieved complete urinary control within 1 year following surgery. These improved outcomes refute the notion that the surgical morbidity associated with cT3 disease is greater than cT2; thus, surgical management should not be withheld secondary to this concern.

Another advantage of RP over nonsurgical therapies is that RP prevents the local morbidities associated with the extension and invasion of prostate cancer into surrounding pelvic structures. As discussed above, the complications related to local cancer progression, such as bladder outlet obstruction, ureteral obstruction, infection, and gross hematuria, are significantly reduced in patients treated with radical prostatectomy when compared to patients not receiving radical prostatectomy (21). Because any one treatment may not completely eradicate all cancer from every patient presenting with cT3 disease, maintenance of a high quality of life is important. Preventing localized cancer progression minimizes the loss to quality of life (33,62,63). Radical prostatectomy also imparts improved survival benefits over nonextirpating therapies (64).

Staging

Clinical staging is inaccurate; indeed, many patients who are diagnosed with clinically localized disease are found to have pT3

disease on final pathologic examination (65). The percentage of patients found to have been clinically understaged in localized disease has decreased during the PSA era (2). Furthermore, clinical overstaging is also a well-documented observation in a substantial number of patients (Table 14B.1). A recent review of the experience at the Mayo Clinic with 841 patients, who presented during the PSA era (1987–1997) with cT3 prostate cancer and who subsequently underwent radical retropubic prostatectomy, reveals clinical overstaging in 27% of these patients (61). Therefore, an aggressive surgical approach to these cT3/pT2 patients provides an opportunity for a prolonged disease-free period or even cure after monotherapy.

Clinical Results

Between 1967 and 2002, 13,612 US patients underwent radical retropubic prostatectomy and bilateral pelvic lymphadenectomy at the Mayo Clinic. Of these patients, 1,236 (9%) had locally advanced disease (cT3) and were candidates for surgery, as described earlier. All patients had palpable induration extending beyond the gland and a negative workup for distant metastases. Mean patient age was 64 years (median 65, range 41–79). Follow-up ranged between 0.1 and 33.4 years (median 10.6, mean 10). Tumor grade was established using the Gleason grading system. In general, patients were followed every 3 to 6 months for 2 years postoperatively, every 6 months for the next 3 years, and then annually. DRE and serum PSA (since 1987) were performed at each follow-up visit. Radionuclide bone scans and abdominal-pelvic CT scans were performed if there was any evidence of cancer progression. Palpable local recurrence was confirmed by transrectal needle biopsy. Systemic progression was diagnosed on the basis of a positive bone scan, CT scan, and plain films. PSA progression was considered to be a value greater than 0.4 ng/mL (66). Overall survival rates in the Mayo Clinic cT3 series (1967–2002) at 5, 10, 15, and 20 years were 90%, 74%, 53%, and 32%, respectively; cancer-specific survival rates were 94%, 87%, 78%, and 66%, respectively (Fig. 14B.4). Rates for survival free of local progression, free of systemic progression, and free of local and systemic progression with a PSA level greater than 0.4 ng/mL are displayed in Figure 14B.5. Of these 1,236 patients, 571 patients (46%) received postoperative adjuvant treatment: 489 (40%) received HT, 154 (12%) received RT, and of these patients, 72 received both HT and RT.

Of the patients with cT3 prostate cancer who were treated at the Mayo Clinic during the PSA era (1987–1997), 841 patients underwent RP. The 5-year, 10-year and 15-year freedom from local or distant disease recurrence rates were 85%, 73%, and 63%, respectively. When a detectable serum PSA ≥0.4 ng/mL is included among the defining criteria for cancer recurrence, approximately half of the patients (60% at 5 years, 44% at 10 years) remained disease free without AHT. Cause specific survival (CSS) at 15 years was 79% (61).

Adjuvant Hormonal Therapy

Early hormonal therapy following local control by RP has been shown to improve overall survival in patients with locally advanced disease (67–69). Zincke et al. first reported on the effects of immediate AHT after RP in patients with stage C and D1 tumors (10,68–70). A combined modality approach to patients with cT3 disease or poor prognostic indicators (PSA >10 ng/mL, Gleason score ≥7, DNA aneuploidy, seminal vesical involvement, PSA doubling time less than one year) can reduce not only the incidence of PSA and systemic progression, but may improve the cause-specific survival for these patients (67). While RP effectively controls local progression, those with pT3/N+ cancer or high-risk features frequently have distant relapse (65).

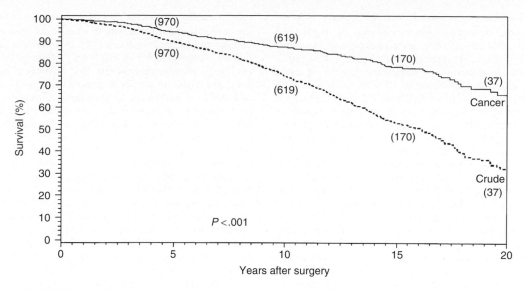

FIGURE 14B.4. Crude and cause-specific survival rates after radical prostatectomy for patients with clinical stage T3 prostate cancer. Numbers in parentheses represent number of living patients in each category at 5, 10, 15, and 20 years after surgery.

Overall, adjunctive systemic therapy combined with effective local treatment is required to achieve the best possible control (67).

The frequency of pN+ disease among patients undergoing RP at Mayo Clinic decreased from 16% in 1987 to 3% in 2002 (Fig. 14B.1). Within the 1,236 patients (1967–2002) who had RP for cT3 disease, 27.2% were found to be pN+ on final analysis (Table 14B.1). A prospective randomized surgical trial recently showed the benefit of AHT in patients with pN+ disease (45). As noted above, Messing and associates showed both overall survival (P = .02) and cause-specific survival (P = .001) to be significantly improved for those patients receiving immediate AHT after RP in node-positive disease (45).

A recent retrospective analysis by Myers et al. of 289 patients who had pN+ disease after RP (1966–1988) updated a previously reported cohort and eliminated from analysis those

patients who received NAHT (71,72). All patients were followed yearly, with 125 alive at last follow-up and a mean follow-up of 15.3 years. A total of 231 patients received AHT (within 90 days of RP), and 58 received no AHT. The AHT group had significantly worse pathological features, including percentage with margin positive (P < .001), extraprostatic extension (P = .015), tumor volume (P = .008), and pathologic grade (P = .006). In univariate analysis, AHT patients had significantly better progression-free survival with regard to systemic or local recurrence end points (P < .001). In addition, AHT patients had significantly better cause-specific survival than patients not treated with HT (P = .015). Actual cause-specific survival for patients with AHT at 15 and 20 years was 75% and 72%, respectively, compared with 58% and 51% survival in patients not treated with HT. Using the Cox model, the relative risk (95% confidence interval) associated with the use of HT was .54 (.33–.89). After adjusting for grade, stage,

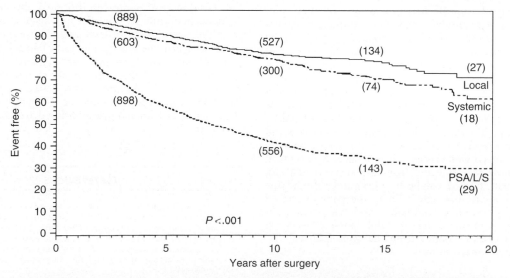

FIGURE 14B.5. Survival free of progression after radical prostatectomy for patients with clinical stage T3 prostate cancer. Numbers in parentheses represent number of patients in each category at 5, 10, 15, and 20 years after surgery. (PSA, prostate-specific antigen, >0.4 ng/mL.)

age, ploidy, extraprostatic extension, margin status, tumor dimension, and positive nodes (one versus two or more), the relative risk of .38 (.21–.69) for early androgen-deprivation therapy remains statistically significant ($P = .002$). This retrospective analysis demonstrates a significant benefit of early AHT in terms of cause-specific survival. While a benefit was not demonstrated in terms of overall survival, the importance of not dying from prostate cancer as an endpoint should be emphasized. It should also be noted that the patients who received AHT had significantly worse pathological features and were at increased risk of dying from prostate cancer.

The question of whether prostatectomy has a benefit in node-positive patients has produced equivocal results (73,74). To address the effect of local treatment (i.e., RP), Ghavamian et al. reported in a retrospective matched comparison analysis of pN+ patients that those patients treated with RP plus orchiectomy had significant improvements in overall and cause-specific survival when compared to orchiectomy alone, refuting the notion that RP may not be beneficial (74). One criticism of the report was that within the group treated after 1987, when PSA testing was available, the effect of RP on cause-specific survival at 5 years was less pronounced and not significant (RP plus orchiectomy $79 \pm 8\%$, orchiectomy $63 \pm 9\%$, risk ratio .42, 95% CI .08–2.25, $P = .19$). Analysis of these 34 pairs from the PSA era (now with 10-year follow-up) reveals that the cause-specific survival at 10 years was significant (RP plus orchiectomy $79 \pm 7\%$, orchiectomy $29 \pm 8\%$, risk ratio 0.26, 95% CI 0.10–0.71, $P = .008$). This confirms previous reports that the beneficial effect of AHT in regard to cause-specific survival is not apparent before nine years (75). The addition of radical prostatectomy to orchiectomy in this matched cohort reduces the risk of dying from prostate cancer by 74% and effectively prevents local recurrence.

Adjuvant Radiotherapy

Several studies have investigated the efficacy of radical prostatectomy with or without adjuvant radiotherapy (76). Two reports in the early 1990s studied men with pathologic stage C cancer who were treated with radical prostatectomy and who received adjuvant irradiation (55–60 Gy) (77,78). Disease-free outcomes were improved in the patients who received both surgery and adjuvant irradiation compared to similar patients who were treated with surgery only and no irradiation. In 1996, Schild et al. compared a large series of prostate cancer patients treated with surgery and adjuvant RT versus surgery alone (79). Those patients receiving adjuvant RT had an improved freedom from failure (defined as a serum PSA ≤ 0.3 ng/mL and no clinical evidence of disease recurrence) (57% vs. 40%, $P = .049$). In the same report, the majority of failures were distant in both treatment arms. Therefore, while adjuvant RT may decrease new seeding of cancer cells from unresected areas, all patients required systemic therapy for their disease. A subset analysis in patients whose tumors extended directly beyond the capsule showed that radiotherapy after surgery improved their freedom from progression. In contrast, radiotherapy after surgery did not improve disease-free survival in patients whose seminal vesicles were involved with cancer. When patients with seminal vesicle invasion were eliminated from the survival analysis, 81% of the patients treated with both surgery and radiotherapy were free from failure, but only 50% of the patients treated with surgery only were free from failure at 5 years. Thus, patients with locally advanced disease, while possibly receiving some beneficial disease control from adjuvant RT, will frequently develop distant metastasis.

Neoadjuvant Hormonal Therapy

Another potential adjunct to radical prostatectomy in patients with locally advanced cancer is hormonal therapy before radical prostatectomy. Hormone therapy, which uses reversible luteinizing hormone releasing agents, markedly decreases both prostatic volume and serum PSA levels (80). Preoperative hormone therapy was investigated for its effect on pathologic downstaging, reducing the positive margin rate, and possibly allowing complete surgical excision of locally advanced cancers (81–84). The effect of NAHT on pathologic downstaging in patients with cT3 disease was minimal compared to the effects of NAHT in patients with clinically organ-confined disease. In one study, 15 patients received LHRH agonist plus flutamide therapy before prostatectomy for cT3 prostate cancer (85). Although prostatic volume in these patients decreased 40% to 50%, less than one-third of the patients were clinically downstaged. A recent report from the European Study Group on Neoadjuvant Treatment of Prostate Cancer compared the 4-year outcomes of 182 men with cT3 cancer who were randomly assigned to treatment with immediate prostatectomy or with 3 months of NAHT and prostatectomy (86). NAHT did not show statistically significant benefits in pathologic downstaging (25% NAHT, 13% immediate prostatectomy, $P = .18$) or in PSA progression (>1 ng/mL) (37% NAHT, 44% immediate prostatectomy, $P = .50$). In 72 patients with cT3 prostate cancer at the Mayo Clinic, NAHT did not improve progression-free survival rates at five years (48% NAHT, 62% immediate prostatectomy, $P = .08$) nor did it improve disease-specific survival rates (89% NAHT, 97% immediate prostatectomy, $P = .052$) (87). Overall, while NAHT is conceptually appealing, careful controlled studies do not show improvement in progression-free survival and show little improvement in organ-confinement rates.

CONCLUSION

No prospective randomized studies comparing RP and RT in cT3 patients have been reported; therefore, the management of locally advanced prostate cancer continues to be controversial. The clinical scenario is common as approximately 20,000 patients are diagnosed each year with locally advanced disease in the US. Clinical staging errors continue to be a problem. The most recent analysis shows that 27% of cT3 patients are overstaged and may be cured upon confirmation of organ-confined disease. For those patients found to be clinically understaged, AHT improves survival and provides excellent control of the local tumor. Thus, an aggressive surgical approach toward cT3 patients permits pathologic staging and directs subsequent treatment, if needed. Overall, the morbidity associated with RP for cT3 has been shown to approximate that seen in RP for localized disease. Presently, there is no consensus in the management of cT3 patients, and the majority of patients are treated with RT and HT, and not surgery. Suitable candidates for surgery should be offered RP, as this treatment is associated with better survival rates (64). The long-term clinical results for RP combined with AT, in those patients who require additional treatment, have been excellent.

References

1. Blute ML, Bergstralh EJ, Iocca A, et al. Use of Gleason score, prostate specific antigen, seminal vesicle and margin status to predict biochemical failure after radical prostatectomy. *J Urol* 2001;165:119–125.
2. Amling CL, Blute ML, Lerner SE, et al. Influence of prostate-specific antigen testing on the spectrum of patients with prostate cancer undergoing radical prostatectomy at a large referral practice. *Mayo Clin Proc* 1998; 73:401–406.
3. Jemal A, Murray T, Samuels A, et al. Cancer statistics 2003. *CA Cancer J Clin* 2003;53:5–26.
4. Ries LA, Eisner MP, Kosary CL et al., eds. *SEER cancer statistics review, 1973–1999.* Bethesda, MD: National Cancer Institute, 2002.

5. Stephenson RA. Prostate cancer trends in the era of prostate-specific antigen. An update of incidence, mortality, and clinical factors from the SEER database. *Urol Clin North Am* 2002;29:173–181.

6. Miller DC, Hafez KS, Stewart A, et al. Prostate carcinoma presentation, diagnosis, and staging: an update from the National Cancer Data Base. *Cancer* 2003;98:1169–1178.

7. Iocca A, Zincke H. Management of clinical T3 prostate cancer. *AUA Updat* 1999;18:250–255.

8. Greene FL, Page DL, Fleming ID et al., eds. *AJCC (American Joint Committee on Cancer) cancer staging manual*, 6th ed. New York: Springer-Verlag, 2002:309–313.

9. Lerner SE, Blute ML, Zincke H. Extended experience with radical prostatectomy for clinical stage T3 prostate cancer: outcome and contemporary morbidity. *J Urol* 1995;154:1447–1452.

10. Zincke H, Fleming TR, Furlow WL, et al. Radical retropubic prostatectomy and pelvic lymphadenectomy for high-stage cancer of the prostate. *Cancer* 1981;47:1901–1910.

11. Bahnson RR, Hanks GE, Huben RP, et al. NCCN practice guidelines for prostate cancer. *Oncology (Huntingt)* 2000;14:111–119.

12. Meltzer D, Egleston B, Abdalla I. Patterns of prostate cancer treatment by clinical stage and age. *Am J Public Health* 2001;91:126–128.

13. Ravery V, Boccon-Gibod L. T3 prostate cancer: how reliable is clinical staging? *Semin Urol Oncol* 1997;15:202–206.

14. Coakley FV, Qayyum A, Kurhanewicz J. Magnetic resonance imaging and spectroscopic imaging of prostate cancer. *J Urol* 2003;170:S69–S75; discussion S75–S76.

15. Purohit RS, Shinohara K, Meng MV, et al. Imaging clinically localized prostate cancer. *Urol Clin North Am* 2003;30:279–293.

16. Whitmore WF Jr. Hormone therapy in prostatic cancer. *Am J Med* 1956;21(5):697–713.

17. Nesbit RM, Baum WC. Endocrine control of prostatic carcinoma: clinical and statistical survey of 1,818 cases. *JAMA* 1950;143:1317–1320.

18. Pavone-Macaluso M, de Voogt HJ, Viggiano G, et al. Comparison of diethylstilbestrol, cyproterone acetate and medroxyprogesterone acetate in the treatment of advanced prostatic cancer: final analysis of a randomized phase III trial of the European Organization for Research on Treatment of Cancer Urological Group. *J Urol* 1986;136:624–631.

19. Adolfsson J, Steineck G, Hedlund PO. Deferred treatment of locally advanced nonmetastatic prostate cancer: a long-term follow-up. *J Urol* 1999;161:505–508.

20. The Medical Research Council Prostate Cancer Working Party Investigators Group. Immediate versus deferred treatment for advanced prostatic cancer: initial results of the Medical Research Council Trial. *Br J Urol* 1997;79:235–246.

21. Tomlinson RL, Currie DP, Boyce WH. Radical prostatectomy: palliation for stage C carcinoma of the prostate. *J Urol* 1977;117:85–87.

22. Fleischmann JD, Catalona WJ. Endocrine therapy for bladder outlet obstruction from carcinoma of the prostate. *J Urol* 1985;134:498–500.

23. Gee WT, Cole JR. Symptomatic stage C carcinoma of prostate. Traditional therapy. *Urology* 1980;15:335–337.

24. Crain DS, Amling CL, Kane CJ. Palliative transurethral prostate resection for bladder outlet obstruction in patients with locally advanced prostate cancer. *J Urol* 2004;171:668–671.

25. Fowler JE Jr, Bigler SA, White PC, et al. Hormone therapy for locally advanced prostate cancer. *J Urol* 2002;168:546–549.

26. Iversen P, Tyrrell CJ, Kaisary AV, et al. Bicalutamide monotherapy compared with castration in patients with nonmetastatic locally advanced prostate cancer: 6.3 years of follow-up. *J Urol* 2000;164:1579–1582.

27. Serretta V, Daricello G, Dispensa N, et al. Long-term outcome of antiandrogen monotherapy in advanced prostate carcinoma: 12-year results of a phase II study. *BJU Int* 2003;92:545–549; discussion 549–550.

28. Iversen P. Bicalutamide monotherapy for early stage prostate cancer: an update. *J Urol* 2003;170:S48–S52; discussion 552–54.

29. Amling CL, Leibovich BC, Lerner SE, et al. Primary surgical therapy for clinical stage T3 adenocarcinoma of the prostate. *Semin Urol Oncol* 1997;15:215–221.

30. Scardino PT, Wheeler TM. Local control of prostate cancer with radiotherapy: frequency and prognostic significance of positive results of postirradiation prostate biopsy. *NCI Monogr* 1988;7:95–103.

31. Egawa S, Wheeler TM, Greene DR, et al. Detection of residual prostate cancer after radiotherapy by sonographically guided needle biopsy. *Urology* 1992;39:358–363.

32. Laverdiere J, Gomez JL, Cusan L, et al. Beneficial effect of combination hormonal therapy administered prior and following external beam radiation therapy in localized prostate cancer. *Int J Radiat Oncol Biol Phys* 1997;37:247–252.

33. Zagars GK, von Eschenbach AC, Ayala AG, et al. The influence of local control on metastatic dissemination of prostate cancer treated by external beam megavoltage radiation therapy. *Cancer* 1991;68:2370–2377.

34. Bolla M, Gonzalez D, Warde P, et al. Improved survival in patients with locally advanced prostate cancer treated with radiotherapy and goserelin. *N Engl J Med* 1997;337:295–300.

35. Bolla M, Collette L, Blank L, et al. Long-term results with immediate androgen suppression and external irradiation in patients with locally advanced prostate cancer (an EORTC study): a phase III randomised trial. *Lancet* 2002;360:103–106.

36. Laverdiere J, Nabid A, De Bedoya LD, et al. The efficacy and sequencing of a short course of androgen suppression on freedom from biochemical failure when administered with radiation therapy for T2-T3 prostate cancer. *J Urol* 2004;171:1137–1140.

37. Pilepich MV, Winter K, John MJ, et al. Phase III Radiation Therapy Oncology Group (RTOG) trial 86-10 of androgen deprivation adjuvant to definitive radiotherapy in locally advanced carcinoma of the prostate. *Int J Radiat Oncol Biol Phys* 2001;50:1243–1252.

38. Hanks GE, Pajak TF, Porter A, et al. Phase III trial of long-term adjuvant androgen deprivation after neoadjuvant hormonal cytoreduction and radiotherapy in locally advanced carcinoma of the prostate: the Radiation Therapy Oncology Group protocol 92-02. *J Clin Oncol* 2003;21:3972–3978.

39. Lawton CA, Winter K, Murray K, et al. Updated results of the phase III Radiation Therapy Oncology Group (RTOG) trial 85-31 evaluating the potential benefit of androgen suppression following standard radiation therapy for unfavorable prognosis carcinoma of the prostate. *Int J Radiat Oncol Biol Phys* 2001;49:937–946.

40. Granfors T, Modig H, Damber JE, et al. Combined orchiectomy and external radiotherapy versus radiotherapy alone for nonmetastatic prostate cancer with or without pelvic lymph node involvement: a prospective randomized study. *J Urol* 1998;159:2030–2034.

41. Leibel SA, Fuks Z, Zelefsky MJ, et al. Technological advances in external-beam radiation therapy for the treatment of localized prostate cancer. *Semin Oncol* 2003;30:596–615.

42. Padula GD, Zelefsky MJ, Venkatraman ES, et al. Normalization of serum testosterone levels in patients treated with neoadjuvant hormonal therapy and three-dimensional conformal radiotherapy for prostate cancer. *Int J Radiat Oncol Biol Phys* 2002;52:439–443.

43. Ward JF, Zincke H. Radical prostatectomy for the patient with locally advanced prostate cancer. *Curr Urol Rep* 2003;4:196–204.

44. Zincke H, Utz DC, Taylor WF. Bilateral pelvic lymphadenectomy and radical prostatectomy for clinical stage C prostatic cancer: role of adjuvant treatment for residual cancer and in disease progression. *J Urol* 1986;135:1199–1205.

45. Messing EM, Manola J, Sarosdy M, et al. Immediate hormonal therapy compared with observation after radical prostatectomy and pelvic lymphadenectomy in men with node-positive prostate cancer. *N Engl J Med* 1999;341:1781–1788.

46. McNeal JE, Redwine EA, Freiha FS, et al. Zonal distribution of prostatic adenocarcinoma. Correlation with histologic pattern and direction of spread. *Am J Surg Pathol* 1988;12:897–906.

47. Rosen MA, Goldstone L, Lapin S, et al. Frequency and location of extracapsular extension and positive surgical margins in radical prostatectomy specimens. *J Urol* 1992;148:331–337.

48. Kausik SJ, Blute ML, Sebo TJ, et al. Prognostic significance of positive surgical margins in patients with extraprostatic carcinoma after radical prostatectomy. *Cancer* 2002;95:1215–1219.

49. Villers A, McNeal JE, Redwine EA, et al. The role of perineural space invasion in the local spread of prostatic adenocarcinoma. *J Urol* 1989;142:763–768.

50. Epstein JI. Evaluation of radical prostatectomy capsular margins of resection. The significance of margins designated as negative, closely approaching, and positive. *Am J Surg Pathol* 1990;14:626–632.

51. Stamey TA, Villers AA, McNeal JE, et al. Positive surgical margins at radical prostatectomy: importance of the apical dissection. *J Urol* 1990;143:1166–1172; discussion 1172–1173.

52. Byar DP, Mostofi FK. Carcinoma of the prostate: prognostic evaluation of certain pathologic features in 208 radical prostatectomies examined by the step-section technique. *Cancer* 1972;30:5–13.

53. Leibovich BC, Blute ML, Bostwick DG, et al. Proximity of prostate cancer to the urethra: implications for minimally invasive ablative therapies. *Urology* 2000;56:726–729.

54. Myers RP, Goellner JR, Cahill DR. Prostate shape, external striated urethral sphincter and radical prostatectomy: the apical dissection. *J Urol* 1987;138:543–550.

55. Myers RP. Practical surgical anatomy for radical prostatectomy. *Urol Clin North Am* 2001;28:473–490.

56. Ghavamian R, Zincke H. An updated simplified approach to nerve-sparing radical retropubic prostatectomy. *BJU Int* 1999;84:160–163.

57. Paulson DF, Moul JW, Walther PJ. Radical prostatectomy for clinical stage T1-2N0M0 prostatic adenocarcinoma: long-term results. *J Urol* 1990;144:1180–1184.

58. Cheng WS, Frydenberg M, Bergstralh EJ, et al. Radical prostatectomy for pathologic stage C prostate cancer: influence of pathologic variables and adjuvant treatment on disease outcome. *Urology* 1993;42:283–291.

59. van den Ouden D, Bentvelsen FM, Boeve ER, et al. Positive margins after radical prostatectomy: correlation with local recurrence and distant progression. *Br J Urol* 1993;72:489–494.

60. Lerner SE, Blute ML, Bergstralh EJ, et al. Analysis of risk factors for progression in patients with pathologically confined prostate cancers after radical retropubic prostatectomy. *J Urol* 1996;156:137–143.

61. Ward JF, Slezak JM, Blute ML, et al. Radical prostatectomy for clinically advanced (cT3) prostate cancer since the advent of prostate-specific antigen testing: 15-year outcome. *BJU Int* 2005;95:751–756.

62. Kaplan ID, Prestidge BR, Bagshaw MA, et al. The importance of local control in the treatment of prostatic cancer. *J Urol* 1992;147:917–921.

63. Fuks Z, Leibel SA, Wallner KE, et al. The effect of local control on metastatic dissemination in carcinoma of the prostate: long-term results in patients treated with 125I implantation. *Int J Radiat Oncol Biol Phys* 1991;21:537–547.

64. Barry MJ, Albertsen PC, Bagshaw MA, et al. Outcomes for men with clinically nonmetastatic prostate carcinoma managed with radical prostatectomy, external beam radiotherapy, or expectant management: a retrospective analysis. *Cancer* 2001;91:2302–2314.

65. Zincke H, Oesterling JE, Blute ML, et al. Long-term (15 years) results after radical prostatectomy for clinically localized (stage T2c or lower) prostate cancer. *J Urol* 1994;152:1850–1857.

66. Amling CL, Bergstralh EJ, Blute ML, et al. Defining prostate specific antigen progression after radical prostatectomy: what is the most appropriate cut point? *J Urol* 2001;165:1146–1151.

67. Zincke H, Lau W, Bergstralh E, et al. Role of early adjuvant hormonal therapy after radical prostatectomy for prostate cancer. *J Urol* 2001;166: 2208–2215.

68. Zincke H. Combined surgery and immediate adjuvant hormonal treatment for stage D1 adenocarcinoma of the prostate: Mayo Clinic experience. *Semin Urol* 1990;8:175–183.

69. Zincke H, Utz DC, Thule PM, et al. Treatment options for patients with stage D1 (T0-3,N1-2,M0) adenocarcinoma of prostate. *Urology* 1987;30: 307–315.

70. Zincke H, Utz DC, Myers RP, et al. Bilateral pelvic lymphadenectomy and radical retropubic prostatectomy for adenocarcinoma of prostate with regional lymph node involvement. *Urology* 1982;19:238–247.

71. Zincke H, Bergstralh EJ, Larson-Keller JJ, et al. Stage D1 prostate cancer treated by radical prostatectomy and adjuvant hormonal treatment. Evidence for favorable survival in patients with DNA diploid tumors. *Cancer* 1992;70:311–323.

72. Myers RB, Slezak EJ, Farrow JM, et al. Use of adjuvant hormonal therapy with radical prostatectomy in lymph node-positive disease: rationale and contribution to outcome. In: Bangma ChH, Newling DWW, ed. *Prostate and renal cancer, benign prostatic hyperplasia, erectile dysfunction and basic research: an update*. Boca Raton, FL: Parthenon Publishing Group, 2003:390–399.

73. Cadeddu JA, Partin AW, Epstein JI, et al. Stage D1 (T1-3, N1-3, M0) prostate cancer: a case-controlled comparison of conservative treatment versus radical prostatectomy. *Urology* 1997;50:251–255.

74. Ghavamian R, Bergstralh EJ, Blute ML, et al. Radical retropubic prostatectomy plus orchiectomy versus orchiectomy alone for pTxN+ prostate cancer: a matched comparison. *J Urol* 1999;161:1223–1227; discussion 1227–1228.

75. Seay TM, Blute ML, Zincke H. Long-term outcome in patients with pTxN+ adenocarcinoma of prostate treated with radical prostatectomy and early androgen ablation. *J Urol* 1998;159:357–364.

76. Petrovich Z, Lieskovsky G, Stein JP, et al. Comparison of surgery alone with surgery and adjuvant radiotherapy for pT3N0 prostate cancer. *BJU Int* 2002;89:604–611.

77. Morgan WR, Zincke H, Rainwater LM, et al. Prostate specific antigen values after radical retropubic prostatectomy for adenocarcinoma of the prostate: impact of adjuvant treatment (hormonal and radiation). *J Urol* 1991;145:319–323.

78. Stein A, deKernion JB, Dorey F, et al. Adjuvant radiotherapy in patients post-radical prostatectomy with tumor extending through capsule or positive seminal vesicles. *Urology* 1992;39:59–62.

79. Schild SE, Wong WW, Grado GL, et al. The result of radical retropubic prostatectomy and adjuvant therapy for pathologic stage C prostate cancer. *Int J Radiat Oncol Biol Phys* 1996;34:535–541.

80. Oesterling JE, Andrews PE, Suman VJ, et al. Preoperative androgen deprivation therapy: artificial lowering of serum prostate specific antigen without downstaging the tumor. *J Urol* 1993;149:779–782.

81. Van Poppel H, De Ridder D, Elgamal AA et al., The Belgian Uro-Oncological Study Group. Neoadjuvant hormonal therapy before radical prostatectomy decreases the number of positive surgical margins in stage T2 prostate cancer: interim results of a prospective randomized trial. *J Urol* 1995;154:429–434.

82. Andros EA, Daneshgari F, Crawford ED. Neoadjuvant hormonal therapy in stage C adenocarcinoma of the prostate. *Clin Invest Med* 1993;16: 510–515.

83. Aprikian AG, Fair WR, Reuter VE, et al. Experience with neoadjuvant diethylstilboestrol and radical prostatectomy in patients with locally advanced prostate cancer. *Br J Urol* 1994;74:630–636.

84. Armas OA, Aprikian AG, Melamed J, et al. Clinical and pathobiological effects of neoadjuvant total androgen ablation therapy on clinically localized prostatic adenocarcinoma. *Am J Surg Pathol* 1994;18:979–991.

85. Sassine AM, Schulman CC. Neoadjuvant hormonal deprivation before radical prostatectomy. *Eur Urol* 1993;24:46–50.

86. Schulman CC, Debruyne FM, Forster G et al., European Study Group on Neoadjuvant Treatment of Prostate Cancer. 4-year follow-up results of a European prospective randomized study on neoadjuvant hormonal therapy prior to radical prostatectomy in T2-3N0M0 prostate cancer. *Eur Urol* 2000;38:706–713.

87. Amling CL, Blute ML, Bergstralh EJ, et al. Preoperative androgen-deprivation therapy for clinical stage T3 prostate cancer. *Semin Urol Oncol* 1997;15:222–229.

CHAPTER 14C
The Role of Hormonal Therapy Combined with Surgery in the Management of Prostate Cancer

Alan So and S. Larry Goldenberg

THE MULTIMODALITY APPROACH TO CANCER TREATMENT

The goal of curative cancer therapy requires elimination of all tumor cells from both the primary site and all distant metastases. The concept of multimodality therapy involves the utilization of two or more therapies, usually with different mechanisms of action, to remove as many cancerous cells from the body as possible. For example, surgery and radiation therapy may be effective for loco-regional treatment but when combined with chemotherapy and/or endocrine therapy, the overall outcome improves for both local and distant sites of disease. Traditionally, systemic treatments applied after primary local therapy, known as adjuvant therapy (AT), are intended to remove obvious or nonobvious spread of disease that cannot be completely eradicated by targeted therapy alone. This type of therapy has been effective in the management of breast (1), colon (2), bladder (3), and ovarian cancers (4). Neoadjuvant therapy (NT) attempts to maximize the benefits of surgery or radiation by applying chemotherapy or endocrine treatment *prior* to loco-regional treatment. NT has been shown to improve survival in advanced breast (5), lung (6), nasopharyngeal (7), esophageal (8), and bladder cancers (9). This chapter will focus on the hypothesis of and current experience with combined use of hormonal therapy and radical prostatectomy, administered either adjuvantly or neoadjuvantly, to maximize cancer cure in men with prostate cancer.

The Potential Benefits of Neoadjuvant Therapy

The concept of NT and prostate cancer remains theoretical—a hypothesis to be proven. Tumor regression or "debulking" may facilitate loco-regional management by allowing for a smaller, and thus more focused, radiation treatment field or a more complete surgical resection. Downstaging will decrease physiologic damage to surrounding organs, allow for possible organ or function-sparing surgery, and, most importantly, provide better loco-regional cancer control by reducing positive surgical margin rates. Some examples are neoadjuvant chemotherapy (NC) administered in locally advanced gastric tumors to attempt curative resection (10), and maximal organ preservation during radical surgery of soft tissue sarcomas (11), laryngeal cancers (12), breast cancers (13), and Ewing's sarcomas (14).

Beginning with the pioneering work of Huggins and Hodges, prostate cancer research has revealed a multifaceted and interwoven relationship between cancer and androgen with different signaling cascades and protein coactivators (15). Following castration, the hormone resistant phenotype develops because of a complex process that involves both selection and outgrowth of preexisting clones of androgen-independent cells (clonal selection) and adaptive up-regulation of genes that help the cancer cells survive and grow after androgen ablation (adaptation). It has been shown that the number of androgen-resistant clones in hormone naive prostate cancers is actually very low, in the order of 1 in 10^5–10^6 (16). This important fact suggests that the maximal effect of androgen-induced apoptosis in prostate cancer (i.e., maximal percentage of cells affected) would occur when androgen deprivation is started at an earlier stage of tumor growth (17,18).

By applying systemic therapy earlier in the course of disease and prior to definitive loco-regional therapy, the effectiveness of distant tumor control may be optimized. Experimental animal models and early clinical trial data suggest that administration of systemic therapy is most likely to affect cure when tumor burden is low (19) and when the theoretical number of resistant clones against that particular therapy is at a minimum. Furthermore, the delivery of chemotherapeutics should be optimal prior to surgical or radiation damage to the tumor's inherent vasculature that would limit drug delivery to target cells.

Neoadjuvant therapy may also provide important prognostic information about a particular tumor. Pathologic assessment of a neoadjuvantly treated specimen can reflect on the effectiveness of the administered therapy and predicts for later sensitivity of recurrent/persistent cancer as has been described in the treatment of osteosarcoma (20) and breast cancer (13). Also, the primary tumor response to neoadjuvant therapy has been shown to correlate with overall survival in soft-tissue sarcomas and head and neck cancers (20,21), and in a recent study of 100 patients treated with neoadjuvant hormonal therapy (NHT) and radical prostatectomy, Kitigawa et al. showed that the amount of histopathological change after initiation of NHT correlated with the overall biochemical recurrence-free rates (22).

In surgical science, the NT paradigm also provides a unique opportunity to study tumor biology in the living host. The bioprofile of excised tissue specimens after NT treatment may provide information about the biologic effect of a novel therapeutic, and provide valuable information concerning tumor behavior and pathophysiology.

Animal Model Studies

In the Shionogi tumor model, androgen withdrawal actively induces apoptosis and tumor regression in a highly reproducible manner with up to a 2-log cell kill; however, androgen-independent tumors invariably recur 1 month after castration (23). Using this tumor model, Gleave et al. found that neoadjuvant castration decreased local recurrence rates after tumor excision by 50%. The tumor-free survival in mice treated with primary excision plus castration at time of recurrence ("delayed hormone therapy") was 20%, less than half that of mice treated with neoadjuvant castration and excision of the regressed tumor (despite both groups starting with similar initial tumor volumes and having complete wide excision of tumor) (24).

Using this same tumor model, So et al. have recently shown that maximal apoptosis-induced effects of hormonal therapy occur when castration is performed early in the course of disease, when tumor burden is at its lowest (17). Mice that were castrated earliest ultimately had tumor recurrence later, and progressed slower than those mice undergoing delayed castration. Although this model cannot address the issue of the effect of NHT on subclinical metastases, it does support the hypothesis that early application of hormonal therapy before radical prostatectomy may reduce not only the positive margin rates but also the subsequent risk of local and distant recurrence.

Preoperative Risk Assessment and Neoadjuvant Therapy

Although higher tumor stage, grade, and pre-operative serum PSA levels correlate with higher pathologic stage, no single preoperative prognostic variable exists that can be applied independently and individually to predict pathologic stage (25). Up to two-thirds of clinically localized tumors are understaged with positive margin rates as high as 30% being reported following radical prostatectomy (26–28). These are the high risk patients who could theoretically benefit most from NHT. NHT is less likely to alter outcome in low-risk tumors (PSA <10 ng/mL, Gleason score = 6, stage T1c), since most of these patients do well with surgery alone.

Postoperative Risk Assessment and Adjuvant Therapy

Multiple studies have confirmed that pathological grading is the most accurate means of predicting long-term disease-specific and biochemical survival (29,30). Khan et al. showed that in their cohort of 1,955 men treated with radical prostatectomy, clinico-pathologic information including pathologic stage, Gleason score, and surgical margin status could stratify patients into various risk categories (31). Similar studies have confined the significance of pathologic Gleason score, margin status, and pathologic stage in predicting progression after surgery (32–34).

Pathologic stage also predicts survival. Epstein et al. showed that patients with pT3 disease had between 58% to 68% progression-free rates while those with organ-confined disease (pT2) had 85% progression-free survival rates (32). The amount of capsular penetration ("focal" vs. "established") and the surgical margin status have also been shown to predict for postoperative failure. Positive margins are associated with a 45% chance of PSA recurrence failure compared to only 21% in patients with negative margins (35,36). In Babaian's cohort of 265 men, a positive margin of >3 mm, seminal vesicle invasion (pT3b), and amount of tumor involvement at the margins were significant clinico-pathological variables in a multivariate analysis (37). Similarly, Kattan studied 990 patients postradical prostatectomy and found that seminal vesicle involvement and nodal status (N+) were two independent variables most associated with a poor prognosis (38).

Pathological assessment of prostatectomy specimens is an invaluable tool to predict high-risk patients. Ultimately, these patients with high-risk features are most likely to benefit from any type of adjuvant or neoadjuvant therapy, including radiation therapy or hormonal therapy, to consolidate local therapies.

REVERSIBLE ANDROGEN SUPPRESSION THERAPY

The availability of several classes of potent, well-tolerated, and reversible agents for androgen withdrawal therapy provides the means for offering NHT prior to radical prostatectomy. Several classes of drugs induce castrate levels of testosterone through suppression of luteinizing hormone (LH) release from the pituitary gland (39–41). In a majority of patients, serum testosterone returns to baseline levels by three months.

Pickles et al. showed that in their group of 666 men treated with hormonal therapy for three to six months prior to radiation therapy, 97% recovered to normal levels (42).

Further, Lamb et al. showed that in a cohort of 818 men with prostate cancer treated with radiation treatment and either 3 or 6 months of NHT, short term androgen blockade was well tolerated and no difference in sexual recovery was found between those receiving hormonal therapy or radiation alone (43).

Gleave et al. have shown that longer androgen suppression results in longer time to testosterone recovery. In a randomized Canadian Uro-Oncology Group (CUOG) trial comparing 3 versus 8 months of NHT, at 3 months after surgery, mean testosterone levels had recovered in the 3-month group, but they remained at about 50% of baseline in the 8-month group. At 12 months, 17% of the 3-month group and 34% of the 8-month group continued to have subnormal levels of testosterone. The suppression of testosterone occurred in association with a low level of serum LH. As LH recovered, testosterone increased, suggesting an ongoing hypothalamic suppression of pituitary LH secretion as an explanation for the continued suppression of androgen (44). Although longer androgen suppression may delay recovery, this study has shown that a majority of patients recover to normal testosterone levels.

Availability of PSA as a Marker of Tumor Regression

PSA gene expression is androgen regulated (45,46). After institution of androgen ablation therapy, serum PSA levels decrease rapidly and dramatically for two reasons: down-regulation of androgen-regulated PSA gene expression and apoptosis. Patterns of PSA response reflect intrinsic biologic characteristics of tumors. For example, although significant downsizing occurs after 3 months of therapy, serum PSA does not reach undetectable levels after 3 months in most patients. This suggests that optimal duration of NHT may be longer than 3 months presumably because maximal tumor regression occurs when PSA reaches its nadir level.

Pathological Changes Following Hormone Therapy

Size and Volume

NHT studies have offered the opportunity to investigate the pathological effects of androgen deprivation on benign and malignant prostate tissue. Grossly, NHT significantly reduces the size of both hyperplastic nodules and prostate cancers. After three months of androgen deprivation, total prostate size decreased 25% to 37% (18,47). Gleave et al. found that prostate size continued to decrease with ongoing treatment, up to an additional 13% if continued for 8 months. Lilleby has shown that total prostate size reduced 33%, 35%, 45%, and 46% at 3, 6, 9, and 12 months, respectively (48). Similarly, cancer volume is also reduced after three months of NHT. Armas et al. showed that cancers were grossly visible in only 15% of patients receiving NHT versus 60% in case-matched controls (49). In a randomized study, Vailancourt et al. estimated tumor volume based on relative tumor area on pathological slides (50). They showed that average volume was reduced by 55%, from 4.66 cm^3 to 2.11 cm^3.

In most published series, a percentage of patients was found to be pathologically T0, that is, tumor cannot be found in the microscopic analysis. The pT0 rates range from 4% to 17% (50–52) in patients treated with 3 months of NHT. In the Canadian study, pT0 was found in 5.1% after 3 months of

NHT and 8.3% after 8 months (53). Though it is possible that all cancer cells were eradicated, the high rates of pT0 in these studies may also be explained by: (a) incomplete examination of the gland, (b) lack of familiarity with hormone-related effects, (c) microscopic foci of tumor that are too small to be seen (51,54).

Histology

The histologic changes in the prostate that are induced by NHT have been well described. Apoptosis, or programmed cell death, occurs in normal, benign hyperplastic, and malignant prostatic epithelial cells following hormonal ablation (17). Apoptotic cell death appears to be a "genetic suicide" process that requires activation of a series of genes and is characterized morphologically by shrunken cells with condensed and fragmented nuclei (apoptotic bodies). Initiation of apoptosis may, in part, be cell-cycle specific or regulated by epigenetic factors and begin at different times in different populations of cells.

Both Vailancourt et al. and Bullock et al. showed that NHT-treated prostate cancers had increased cellular vacuolization with small nucleoli, decreased intraluminal crystalloids, and higher Gleason score because of a reduction in cytoplasm causing an apparent reduction of gland diameter and thereby gland density (50,55). Atrophy occurs to the greatest extent in the peripheral zone of the gland, with the least effect in the central zone (55) (Fig. 14C.1).

Does NHT also eliminate prostatic epithelial neoplasia (PIN) (55)? Androgen therapy results in nuclear pyknosis, a lack of prominent nucleoli, and an overall flattening of the epithelial proliferation of high-grade PIN (HPIN), with less pronounced cellular tufting (56). These changes are interpreted as an increase in the frequency of flat HPIN versus the more common micropapillary and tufting forms noted in nontreated cases (57). Thus, it may be possible that hormonal therapy induces regression of PIN (49,50,54) but there is no concrete evidence to support this theory (55).

NHT Effect on Tumor Grading

With the profound histopathological changes described above, grading of tumors becomes challenging, prompting some authors (50) to recommend that Gleason scoring not be performed on specimens after NHT. Many studies have shown an upward shift of Gleason score in the hormonally treated radical prostatectomy (RP) specimens compared with the baseline biopsy grade

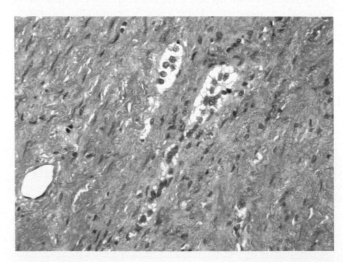

FIGURE 14C.1. H & E stained prostate specimen (40× magnification) after 6 months of neoadjuvant hormone therapy. Tumor is atrophic with significant vacuolization.

(49,50,58–60) well beyond what would be predicted from undergrading in needle biopsies (61). Bullock et al. have shown that the higher scores were the result of an increase in the frequency of Gleason 5 as either the primary or, more commonly, the secondary grade (55), due not to the emergence of a more aggressive, possibly androgen-resistant clone of cells, but rather to artifact introduced by the Gleason grading system itself.

That this is artifact is supported by studies showing a lower rate of proliferative activity in treated cases (Ki-67 immunohistochemical stains) (49,56) and a predominance of diploid DNA content (49,62). The presence of pronounced therapy-induced alterations likely indicates that the tumor is responding favorably to treatment; in fact, Kitigawa showed that higher response to NHT is correlated to longer biochemical recurrence-free survival postprostatectomy (22).

Recently, chemoprevention studies have focused on the histopathologic changes associated with the use of alpha-1 reductase inhibitors such as finasteride (type II inhibitor) and dutasteride (type I and II inhibitor) (63). Although not as profound, these agents cause similar changes in prostate cancer and thus affect the "apparent" Gleason score (64).

Clinical Studies Using Neoadjuvant Hormone Therapy

The hypotheses of NHT in prostate cancer as based on the above rationale are as follows: (a) Preoperative reversible androgen withdrawal should decrease tumor burden/downstage tumors so that the tumor is fully resectable, minimize surgical trauma to surrounding organs, and reduce positive surgical margins and capsular penetration rates. (b) NHT should decrease local and systemic recurrence. (c) Ultimately, NHT plus radical prostatectomy should improve overall survival. The first two hypotheses have been tested in trials of both short-term and long-term NHT.

Nonrandomized Clinical Studies of 3 Months of NHT

Most nonrandomized trials noted impressive decreases in serum PSA, prostatic volume, and positive margin rates following 3 months of NHT (Table 14C.1). Soloman et al. (65) published a large phase II series of 156 patients with T2/T3 tumors

treated with between 3 and 6 months of an LHRH agonist plus flutamide. Positive margin rates were 11.5% compared to 35% in historical controls. Powell et al. showed in the SWOG 9109 phase II study that patients with clinical T3 and T4 tumors treated with four months of NHT and radical prostatectomy had a positive margin rate of 30% and surprising 5-year progression-free and overall survival rate of 70% and 90%, respectively (66).

Investigators at Memorial Sloan-Kettering Cancer Center have conducted a series of studies on NHT. Aprikian et al. (73) reported that most patients with locally advanced cT3 tumors did not benefit from between 2 and 8 months of neoadjuvant DES. A subsequent phase II study of 141 patients with cT1 or cT2 tumors found significant decreases in serum PSA (>98%) and a 38% decrease in prostatic volume after 3 months of LHRH agonist with flutamide (67). Pathologic staging revealed increased organ-confined rates (74% vs. 49%) and decreased positive margin rates (10% vs. 33%) when compared to a group of 72 concurrent controls that did not receive NHT. However, at 48 months follow-up, no differences in PSA recurrence rates were apparent in a post hoc analysis (77). Smaller nonrandomized studies by Sassine and Schulman (69,78) and by Haggman et al. (70) also reported 40 to 50% decreases in positive margin rates in patients pretreated with 3 months of NHT when compared to historical controls. Curiously, two reports on small cohorts of patients with cT2 or cT3 tumors by McFarlane et al. (71) and Oesterling et al. (72) suggested no improvement in pathologic outcome following short-term NHT, and Witjes et al. (79) found no statistical benefit in the reduction of positive margins in stage T3 patients (59% vs. 43%, P = .14). These conflicting results of nonrandomized studies illustrate that outcome (pathologic stage, positive margin rates, and risk of PSA recurrence) depends on many factors, including the proportion of patients with T3 tumors, the level of preoperative serum PSA, the length of postoperative follow up, and the time period during which the study accrued (stage migration toward earlier diagnosis began in the early 1990s). Conclusions from such discordant studies are drawn with caution, but taken together the results suggest that 3 months of NHT resulted in encouraging pathologic downsizing/downstaging and set the stage for prospective randomized clinical trials to further test the hypothesis.

Randomized Clinical Studies of 3 Months of NHT

To date, eight phase III randomized studies comparing 0 versus 3 months of NHT have been published (68,74,79–84).

TABLE 14C.1

NONRANDOMIZED CLINICAL TRIALS OF NHT WITH RADICAL PROSTATECTOMY

Investigator	Sample size	Clinical stage	Serum PSA	Duration of NHT	Positive margin %	Follow up
Fair, 1993, 1997 (67,68)	74	T2	8.7 (median)	3 month	10	18%/48 months
Solomon, 1993 (65)	156	T2/T3	NA	3–6 months	11.5	NA
Schulman, 1994 (69)	40	T2/T3	NA	3 months (mean)	32	NA
Haggman, 1993 (70)	40	T2/T3	NA	3 months	31	15%/3 months
McFarlane, 1993 (71)	22	T2b/T3	14.8	3 months	32	NA
Oesterling, 1993 (72)	22	T2b/T3	30	1.5 months	68	NA
Aprikian, 1994 (73)	55	T2b/T3	20.4 (median)	3 months (median)	33	62%/26 months
Soloway, 1995 (74)	37	T2b–3	NA	3–16 months	41	Mean—38.4 months
Gleave, 1996, 2000 (75,76)	156	T1c–3	11.5 (mean)	8 months	6	None
Meyer, 1999 (52)	680	T1–3	NA	3 months	24.8	Mean—38 months
Powell, 2002 (66)	55	T3–4	NA	4 months	30	6.1 years (median)

TABLE 14C.2

RANDOMIZED CLINICAL TRIALS OF NHT WITH RADICAL PROSTATECTOMY

Investigator	Sample size	Clinical stage	Change in PSA	Duration of NHT	Positive margin %	Type	Change in TRUS
Labrie, 1995 (80)	161	T2–3	NA	3 months	8 vs. 34	L + F	NA
Soloway, 1995, 2002 (74,85)	303	T2b	14.3 to <0.5 in 70	3 months	18 vs. 48 (stat. sig. only in T2)	L + F	44–35 cm³
Van Poppel, 1995 (81)	130	T2b–3	14 to 1.0 μg/L	6 weeks	20 vs. 46	EP	43–29 cm³
Goldenberg, 1996 (82)	213	T1–2	13 to 1.1 μg/L	3 months	28 vs. 65	CPA	43–33 cm³
Hugosson and Aus 1996, 2002 (83,86)	111	T1–3a	NA	3 months	23.6 vs. 45.5	T + C	NA
Witjes, 1997 (79)	354	T2–3	20 to 0.8 μg/L	3 months	27 vs. 46	G + F	38–27 cm³
Fair, 1997 (68)	148	T2b/T3	NA	3 months	18 vs. 37	G + F	NA
Selli and Bono, 2002 (87,88)	393	T2a–3b	NA	3–6 months	25.9 at 12 weeks, 19.7% after 24 weeks vs. 46.5%	G + B	NA
Gleave, 2003 (89)	549	T1–2	NA	3–8 months	12% at 8 months, 23% at 3 months	L + F	NA
Prezioso, 2004 (84)	167	T1–2	NA	0 vs. 3 months	60% vs. 39%	L + CPA	NA

The primary endpoint in all of these trials was pathologic staging and positive margin rates. All studies (Table 14C.2) demonstrated significant decreases in positive surgical margins after 3 months of NHT, ranging from 21% to 26% (80,84). Soloway et al. (74,85) published the results of a multicenter randomized study comparing 0 versus 3 months of leuprolide and flutamide prior to radical prostatectomy. Positive margin rates decreased from 48% in the control group to 18% in the NHT group. Organ-confined disease (pT2) was reported twice as frequently in the NHT group (53%) compared to the surgery alone group (22%). A randomized multicenter trial by the CUOG using 3 months of cyproterone acetate also reported a 50% reduction in positive margin rates (65% vs. 28%) and doubling of the organ-confined rate (20% vs. 42%) (82). The greatest reduction occurred in apical margin rates, likely related to the decrease in gland size which facilitated surgical removal.

Fair and Kava (68) reported results of a randomized trial comparing 0 versus 3 months of NHT (LHRH plus flutamide) in 148 patients with clinically confined prostate cancer. Overall, the incidence of positive margins decreased from 37% to 18% (P <.05). The decrease in positive margins was greatest in high-risk patients with pretreatment PSA levels >10 ng/mL (63% vs. 18%), suggesting that these men may be the most likely to benefit from NHT.

The randomized studies of 3 months of NHT (Table 14C.2) consistently reported 90% decreases in serum PSA levels, 30% decreases in prostatic volume, 50% decreases in positive margin rates in cT1 or cT2 (but not cT3) disease, and higher organ-confined rates, but no differences in incidence of seminal vesicle involvement or positive lymph nodes. Soloway et al. (85) reported 5-year follow-up data on 265 evaluable patients in the U.S. Intergroup Study and found that 35.4% of the NHT group compared to 32.4% of the surgery alone group had PSA levels >0.4 ng/mL (P = .663). The CUOG study did not demonstrate any statistical differences in PSA failure at 36 months follow-up, with recurrence rates of 35% and 40% in the control and NHT arms, respectively (90). These studies did not reveal biochemical recurrence free-advantages in patients with high Gleason scores or high PSA prior to treatment, but caution is warranted in interpreting these trials since they were not designed methodologically to detect differences in survival.

Clinical Studies of Longer-term NHT (Greater than 3 Months Duration)

Although a degree of downsizing occurs after 3 months of NHT, maximum volume reduction and serum PSA does not reach undetectable levels in most patients within this period of time. Serum PSA levels decreasing during the first 2 months are due to rapid down-regulation in gene expression (91). Further decreases after the second month of androgen withdrawal reflect ongoing imbalances between apoptotic prostate epithelial cell death and decreased tumor cell proliferation, resulting in a reduction in the number of PSA-producing cells. These observations suggest that optimal duration of NHT exceeds 3 months.

A prospective phase II trial was carried out to study the biochemical and pathologic effects of 8 months of NHT prior to surgery in 156 men (75). Different mechanisms for PSA decline after institution of therapy produced two distinct slopes: a precipitous drop during the first month and a more gradual subsequent decrease that continued into the eighth month of therapy. Serum PSA decreased to undetectable or nadir levels in 22% of patients after 3 months, 42% after 5 months, and 84% after 8 months. After 8 months of NHT, serum PSA levels were <0.5 ng/mL in 18% of patients, <0.4 ng/mL in 82% of patients, <0.3 ng/mL in 76% of patients, and <0.2 ng/mL in 66%. Most patients in this study had organ-confined, stage pT2 tumors (79%), and half of these had only microfoci or small volume tumors occupying less than 5% of the prostate. The positive margin rate was 5.8%, lower than that reported after 3 months of NHT in similar cohorts of patients (68,83,85). No cancer was identified in the radical prostatectomy specimen (pT0) in 13% of cases. Microscopic extension through prostatic capsule with negative margins (pT3M–) was reported in 13% of the patients. The pathologic stage and risk of positive margins increased with higher clinical T-stage, grade, and pretreatment serum PSA levels. None of 65 patients with T1c or T2a tumors had positive margins compared to 7.5% of 79 with T2b and 25% of 12 patients with

T3a disease. Positive margins were identified in 2% of patients with Gleason scores of 4, 5% with scores of 5 or 6, and 11% with Gleason scores of ≥7. None of 99 patients with PSA levels <10 ng/mL had positive margins, compared to 15% of 57 with PSA levels ≥10 ng/mL.

Although patients with organ-confined tumors tended to have lower mean PSA nadir levels, the nadir PSA value was not predictive of pathologic stage in individual patients. After a mean of 52 months postoperative follow-up, biochemical recurrences occurred in 19 patients (12.2%), most within the first 2 years of surgery. Risk of biochemical recurrence after 8 months of NHT remained proportional to known risk factors for recurrence, including pretreatment serum PSA, Gleason score, and pathologic stage.

In another study, Meyer et al. (52) reported on 680 men who were followed for 38 months after NHT and radical prostatectomy. They reported an overall PSA failure rate of 33% at 5 years. Patients who received neoadjuvant androgen ablation for longer than 3 months (mean 5 months) had a significantly lower risk of PSA failure than those treated by radical prostatectomy alone (hazard ratio = 0.52, 95% CI 0.29 to 0.93).

Apparent improvement in recurrence rates in uncontrolled studies must be interpreted with caution. Any potential benefit of longer-term NHT is best confirmed by phase III studies, of which two are currently published. The PROSIT study examined 393 patients who were randomly selected to have no NHT (131 patients), 3 months of NHT (131 patients) using goserelin depot and bicalutamide, or 6 months of NHT (131 patients) (87). Patients treated with 6 months of NHT had significantly lower positive margin rates (18.7% of stage B, 35.5% of stage C) versus 3 months NHT (25.9% of stage B, 34.3% of stage C) or RP-only group (46.5% of stage B, 75.9% of stage C). The positive margin rate was not different between the 3-month NHT and 6-month NHT groups in those patients with stage C disease; however, in this group NHT provided the largest difference in margin-positive rates when compared to radical prostatectomy alone. Furthermore, 6 months of NHT had the highest proportion of pathologic stage B tumors compared to the other two groups, supporting the concept that pathologic changes still occur after 3 months of androgen ablation.

Another phase III study examining the long-term effects of NHT was initiated by the CUOG (53). CUOG-P95A randomized 547 men with clinically confined prostate cancer to either 3 months or 8 months of leuprolide acetate and flutamide prior to radical prostatectomy. The study was powered to detect a 25% decrease in PSA recurrence, assuming a 30% recurrence in the 3-month arm after 3 years. Groups were balanced for clinical stage, Gleason grade, and serum PSA. Analysis of biochemical and pathologic changes demonstrated significant differences between groups. Mean serum PSA decreased 89% to 0.12 ng/mL after 3 months, with a further 53% reduction to 0.056 ng/mL from 3 months to 8 months. Presurgery PSA nadir levels were <0.1 ng/mL in 35% versus 73%, and ≥0.3 ng/mL in 37% versus 10% after 3 months versus 8 months, respectively. TRUS-determined prostatic volume decreased 37% from a mean of 40.5 cm³ to 25.7 cm³ after 3 months of NHT (P <.0001) and a further 11% to 22.8 cm³ after 8 months (P <.03). Positive margin rates were 23% and 12% in the 3-month and 8-month groups, respectively (P <.01). This phase III study confirms that there is ongoing biochemical and pathological regression of prostate tumors between 3 and 8 months of NHT, in keeping with data from the PROSIT trial that showed improved downstaging in stage C tumors after 6 months of NHT versus 3 months and in support of the hypothesis generated by phase II studies that optimal duration of NHT is indeed longer than 3 months.

Data of the 3-year PSA recurrence rates in the CUOG-P95A trial have been recently presented (89). Although Kaplan-Meier analysis showed a trend toward delay in time to biochemical recurrence in the 8-month group (Log Rank, P = .051), there was no overall statistical significance between the 3-month and 8-month arms. Within the 3-month group, overall PSA recurrence was 25.4% versus 23.6% in the 8-month group. The number of events still remains small and longer follow-up is still required to assess whether a statistical benefit will be seen. Interestingly, however, in the subgroup analysis a statistical difference between the 3-month and 8-month arms was found in the intermediate risk group (one of: Gleason grade 7, serum PSA ≥10 ng/mL, >3 positive biopsies or cT3 disease) of patients when treated in a high volume center (>100 RPs/year).

Questions and Challenges of Neoadjuvant Therapy

Does NHT Result in Artifactual Pathological Understaging?

Following NHT, residual foci of atrophic glands can be difficult to identify with hematoxylin and eosin (H&E) staining, raising the possibility that pT0 staging or low-positive margin rates may report an artifact of histology, that is, downsizing occurring without downstaging (71,72,92). However, there is much evidence that the NHT-induced decrease in positive margin rates is a real, rather than an artifactual, phenomenon. First, all randomized studies which used a single, central, and experienced pathologist reported similar (50%) decreases in positive margin rates. Second, repeat staging of prostatectomy specimens for prostatic acid phosphatase (PAP) and cytokeratin did not increase positive margin rates (75,93). Third, animal model studies (see above) demonstrated 50% reduction in local recurrence and positive margin rates (24). Finally, pathologic stage remained proportional to pretreatment risk factors (serum PSA, T-stage, and Gleason grade), and was an important prognostic predictor for biochemical relapse (76,82,83).

Does NHT Increase Surgical Morbidity?

Concerns have been raised that NHT makes surgery more difficult by increasing periprostatic adhesions. Soloway stated that surgeons noted surgical dissection, particularly seminal vesicle adherence in T2b patients, possibly due to desmoplastic fibrosis (74).

However, there is no objective evidence that NHT adversely affects radical prostatectomy. Randomized series that have documented surgical difficulty, blood loss, length of procedure, and postoperative complications found no significant difference in these parameters between NHT-treated and untreated groups (74,82). Furthermore, apoptosis initiated by androgen withdrawal is a controlled cellular event that is not associated with acute inflammation or scarring.

One technical point is noteworthy: after 8 months of NHT, the prostate can decrease to a small, fusiform swelling of the urethra, which can make it more challenging to palpate the prostatic apex and decide where to divide the urethra. With care, however, this can be done without increasing positive margins, compromising urinary control, or damaging the neurovascular bundles.

Does Tumor Progression Occur During Prolonged NHT?

To study the possible risk of progression and outgrowth of androgen-independent clones during prolonged NHT, proliferation markers and oncoproteins have been assessed in the RP specimens (75,94). The proliferation marker Ki-67 staining remained suppressed in most patients after 8 months of NHT (52,75). Staining for the cyclin-dependent kinase inhibitor, p27, increased in prostate cancer specimens after NHT ranging between 3 and 8 months (95), suggesting that cell cycle arrest is induced by androgen withdrawal in the cancer cells that survive. Levels of the antiapoptotic oncoprotein, Bcl-2, increase during the first 3 months of NHT, and remain elevated after 8 months of therapy (94), consistent with its role in prevention of castration-induced apoptosis (96,97). Taken together, ongoing decreases in serum PSA, ongoing reduction of tumor size, the high percentage of organ-confined and small-volume tumors, and the absence of increased Ki-67 immunostaining suggest that progression from the growth of androgen-independent clones during 8 months of NHT is unlikely.

Are Recurrence Rates Altered by Neoadjuvant Therapy?

With the exception of breast, lung, nasopharyngeal, esophageal, bladder cancers, and Wilm tumors, there is limited survival data to support the use of neoadjuvant therapies for most solid tumors. Indeed, it remains possible that the delay in definitive local therapy by neoadjuvant treatments may actually be detrimental. In prostate cancer, phase III studies do not suggest that recurrence rates are altered; but, these studies were designed with sample sizes based on detecting differences in positive margin rates and not biochemical recurrence rates. At this point in time, longer-term NHT may be beneficial to certain subgroups of intermediate- or high-risk patients but should still be considered investigational and further studied in the context of controlled clinical studies.

Adjuvant Hormonal Therapy

An alternative multimodality approach to the high-risk prostate cancer patient would involve hormone withdrawal following surgery adjuvant hormone therapy (AHT). This would be particularly logical in an individual who has pathologic staging consistent with a high risk for recurrence.

Nonrandomized Studies Using AHT

A number of nonrandomized studies utilizing AHT after radical prostatectomy in high-risk patients have been published (98–105). Seay et al. retrospectively reviewed 790 N+ patients (101) in whom 88% (694 pts) received adjuvant hormonal therapy. Progression-free survival at 5 and 10 years was 94% and 84% in the adjuvantly treated group compared to 56% and 19% in the nontreated historical control group. However, after 10 years, a significant overall cause-specific survival advantage was found only in patients with DNA diploid tumors ($P < .002$). Other retrospective studies have shown the survival benefits of AHT in N+ patients (101,104).

More recently, Zincke et al. reported on the effects of AHT in the setting of pT3b (seminal vesicle involvement) disease (105). In this retrospective analysis of 707 patients, 157 received hormonal therapy within 90 days of surgery. Those patients given adjuvant treatment had better biochemical progression-free survival (67% vs. 23% at 10 years, $P < .001$), better systemic progression-free survival (95% vs. 87%, $P < .001$) and better cause-specific survival (95% vs. 78%, $P < .001$).

Randomized Studies of Adjuvant Hormone Therapy

Currently, there are four randomized, prospective controlled studies assessing radical prostatectomy with AHT (Table 14C.3) (106–109). The largest of these studies is the international Early Prostate Cancer (EPC) study, addressing whether 150 mg of bicalutamide is beneficial when given as monotherapy following radical prostatectomy or radiotherapy (106). A total of 8,113 men with T1b–4 NxM0 enrolled in the study, with 55% (4,454 men) undergoing radical prostatectomy. Endpoints of this study were "objective progression and survival" including PSA recurrence and development of bone metastasis. Patients receiving hormone therapy had a lower overall objective progression (5.1% vs. 7.7%, $P = .0001$). Predictably, those patients with high-risk features (locally advanced, high Gleason score, high pretherapy PSA) had the most significant benefit. The five-year follow-up of EPC trials 24 and 25 revealed that in localized (i.e., low-risk) patients, the overall survival was worse in the Casodex arm (196; 25.2%) deaths versus 174 (20.5%) deaths (hazard ratio = 1.23) (110).

An Eastern Cooperative Oncology Group (ECOG) study assessed the role of AHT after radical prostatectomy in N+ patients. In this study of 98 men, the 47 who were treated with hormonal therapy had better overall, prostate-cancer specific, and progression-free survival ($P < .001$) when compared to those observed in the observation arm (107). Although the

TABLE 14C.3

RANDOMIZED CONTROL TRIALS—RADICAL PROSTATECTOMY AND AHT

Author	Patients	Stage	Type of androgen blockade	Benefits?	Follow-up
See et al. (106)	4454 (2236 treated)	Any pT, N0–/+	Bicalutamide 150 mg	Progression free survival, PSA progression	3 years (median)
Messing (107)	98 (47 treated)	Any pT, N+	Goserelin 3.6 mg monthly or bilateral orchiectomy	Overall survival, prostate-specific survival, progression free survival	7.1 years
Wirth et al. (108)	309 (152 treated)	pT3, N0	Flutamide 250 mg tid	Recurrence-free survival NO survival advantage	6.1 years (median)
Prayer-Galetti et al. (109)	201	pT3	Goserelin	Cancer-specific survival	5 years

number of patients in this trial is small, the benefits of early treatment are comparable to those found in the EPC trial.

A study by Wirth et al. did not show any survival benefits of early AT in patients with N0 disease (108). In this European trial of 352 men with pT3N0, 152 (43%) patients were given adjuvant flutamide with a median follow-up time of 6.1 years. Recurrence-free survival was better in the flutamide group (P = .0041), but there was no difference in overall survival. Limitations of this study include its numbers and, more importantly, the exclusion of 12% of patients from the initial enrollment (43% due to drug toxicity). This study points out the importance of careful postoperative clinicopathological assessment in determining which patients will benefit most from AT.

Taken together, these studies suggest that AHT may be most beneficial in those patients with either metastatic (N+) or locally advanced tumors; however, many questions remain unanswered. For example, the ideal length of time of hormonal therapy has not been established. This is important since many of these men will be of younger age and the long-term side effects with hormonal therapy are not insignificant, including cardiovascular toxicity, anemia, and osteoporosis. An interesting area of further study will be the application of intermittent or "interrupted" androgen blockade instead of continual hormone withdrawal as a protocol for the administration of AT (111).

SUMMARY

Ultimately, the effects of AHT and/or NHT on the quality of life need to be balanced against the potential survival gains of treatment. Other questions yet to be answered include: should NHT continue until PSA reaches nadir in a particular patient (as opposed to all men receiving the same duration of treatment)? Does NHT-induced decrease of positive margins lower local recurrence rates and diminish the need for adjuvant or salvage radiation therapy? Can NHT preselect patients who should be treated with early adjuvant therapies? What is the impact of testosterone recovery rates and patterns on PSA recurrence? What are the phenotypic and genotypic changes induced by NHT? These questions will need to be answered before adjuvant or neoadjuvant therapy is recommended as "standard of care" addition to radical prostatectomy.

There has been a tremendous amount of research to discover methods to maximize the benefits of radical prostatectomy in the management of prostate cancer. Hormone withdrawal, either applied before surgery or early afterward, is a systemic treatment intended to prolong overall survival. Although there are many theoretical benefits of adjuvant or neoadjuvant hormonal therapy, further study is needed to establish overall survival benefits and the effects on quality of life.

The hypothesis of NHT was initially tested in animal models and phase II clinical trials. Large phase III studies reveal interesting data but the null hypothesis, at least regarding biochemical-free recurrence, has not yet been confirmed. The NHT model is a superb opportunity for urologic surgeons to test proof of principle in the human system, evaluating biological markers in the radical prostatectomy specimen.

References

1. Hayward RL, Dixon JM. Current limits of knowledge in adjuvant and neoadjuvant endocrine therapy of breast cancer: the need for more clinical research. *Surg Oncol* 2003;12:289–304.
2. Chawla AK, Kachnic LA, Clark JW, et al. Combined modality therapy for rectal and colon cancer. *Semin Oncol* 2003;30:101–112.
3. Hussain SA, James ND. The systemic treatment of advanced and metastatic bladder cancer. *Lancet Oncol* 2003;4:489–497.
4. Trimbos JB, Timmers P. Chemotherapy for early ovarian cancer. *Curr Opin Obstet Gynecol* 2004;16:43–48.
5. Esserman L. Neoadjuvant chemotherapy for primary breast cancer: lessons learned and opportunities to optimize therapy. *Ann Surg Oncol* 2004;11:3S–8S.
6. Eberhardt WE, Albain KS, Pass H, et al. Induction treatment before surgery for non-small cell lung cancer. *Lung Cancer* 2003;42(Suppl 1): S9–S14.
7. Teo PM, Chan AT. Treatment strategy and clinical experience. *Semin Cancer Biol* 2002;12:497–504.
8. Lordick F, Stein HJ, Peschel C, et al. Neoadjuvant therapy for oesophagogastric cancer. *Br J Surg* 2004;91:540–551.
9. Grossman HB, Natale RB, Tangen CM, et al. Neoadjuvant chemotherapy plus cystectomy compared with cystectomy alone for locally advanced bladder cancer. *N Engl J Med* 2003;349:859–866.
10. Yao JC, Mansfield PF, Pisters PW, et al. Combined-modality therapy for gastric cancer. *Semin Surg Oncol* 2003;21:223–227.
11. Ottaiano A, De Chiara A, Fazioli F, et al. Neoadjuvant chemotherapy for intermediate/high-grade soft tissue sarcomas: five-year results with epirubicin and ifosfamide. *Anticancer Res* 2002;22:3555–3559.
12. The Department of Veterans Affairs Laryngeal Cancer Study Group. Induction chemotherapy plus radiation compared with radiation in patients with advanced laryngeal cancer. *N Engl J Med* 1991;324: 1685–1690.
13. Wolmark N, Wang J, Mamounas E, et al. Preoperative chemotherapy in patients with operable breast cancer: nine-year results from National Surgical Adjuvant Breast and Bowel Project B-18. *J Natl Cancer Inst Monogr* 2001;30:96–102.
14. Shamberger RC, LaQuaglia MP, Gebhardt MC, et al. Ewing sarcoma/primitive neuroectodermal tumor of the chest wall: impact of initial versus delayed resection on tumor margins, survival, and use of radiation therapy. *Ann Surg* 2003;238:563–567; discussion 567–568.
15. So AI, Hurtado-Coll A, Gleave ME. Androgens and prostate cancer. *World J Urol* 2003;21:325–337.
16. Craft N, Chhor C, Tran C, et al. Evidence for clonal outgrowth of androgen-independent prostate cancer cells from androgen-dependent tumors through a two-step process. *Cancer Res* 1999;59:5030–5036.
17. So AI, Bowden M, Gleave M. Effect of time of castration and tumour volume on time to androgen-independent recurrence in Shionogi tumours. *BJU Int* 2004;93:845–850.
18. Gleave ME, La Bianca S, Goldenberg SL. Neoadjuvant hormonal therapy prior to radical prostatectomy: promises and pitfalls. *Prostate Cancer Prostatic Dis* 2000;3:136–144.
19. Skipper HE, Schabel FM Jr, Wilcox WS. Experimental evaluation of potential anticancer agents. XIII. On the criteria and kinetics associated with "curability" of experimental leukemia. *Cancer Chemother Rep* 1964;35:1–111.
20. Bielack SS, Machatschek JN, Flege S, et al. Delaying surgery with chemotherapy for osteosarcoma of the extremities. *Expert Opin Pharmacother* 2004; 5:1243–1256.
21. Phan A, Patel S. Advances in neoadjuvant chemotherapy in soft tissue sarcomas. *Curr Treat Options Oncol* 2003;4:433–439.
22. Kitagawa Y, Koshida K, Mizokami A, et al. Pathological effects of neoadjuvant hormonal therapy help predict progression of prostate cancer after radical prostatectomy. *Int J Urol* 2003;10:377–382.
23. Bruchovsky N, Rennie PS, Coldman AJ, et al. Effects of androgen withdrawal on the stem cell composition of the Shionogi carcinoma. *Cancer Res* 1990;50:2275–2282.
24. Gleave ME, Sato N, Goldenberg SL, et al. Neoadjuvant androgen withdrawal therapy decreases local recurrence rates following tumor excision in the Shionogi tumor model. *J Urol* 1997;157:1727–1730.
25. Partin AW, Yoo J, Carter HB, et al. The use of prostate specific antigen, clinical stage and Gleason score to predict pathological stage in men with localized prostate cancer. *J Urol* 1993;150:110–114.
26. Rosen MA, Goldstone L, Lapin S, et al. Frequency and location of extracapsular extension and positive surgical margins in radical prostatectomy specimens. *J Urol* 1992;148:331–337.
27. Jones EC. Resection margin status in radical retropubic prostatectomy specimens: relationship to type of operation, tumor size, tumor grade and local tumor extension. *J Urol* 1990;144:89–93.
28. Trapasso JG, deKernion JB, Smith RB, et al. The incidence and significance of detectable levels of serum prostate specific antigen after radical prostatectomy. *J Urol* 1994;152:1821–1825.
29. Frazier HA, Robertson JE, Humphrey PA, et al. Is prostate specific antigen of clinical importance in evaluating outcome after radical prostatectomy? *J Urol* 1993;149:516–518.
30. Dillioglugil O, Leibman BD, Kattan MW, et al. Hazard rates for progression after radical prostatectomy for clinically localized prostate cancer. *Urology* 1997;50:93–99.
31. Khan MA, Partin AW, Mangold LA, et al. Probability of biochemical recurrence by analysis of pathologic stage, Gleason score, and margin status for localized prostate cancer. *Urology* 2003;62:866–871.
32. Epstein JI, Partin AW, Potter SR, et al. Adenocarcinoma of the prostate invading the seminal vesicle: prognostic stratification based on pathologic parameters. *Urology* 2000;56:283–288.

33. Tefilli MV, Gheiler EL, Tiguert R, et al. Prognostic indicators in patients with seminal vesicle involvement following radical prostatectomy for clinically localized prostate cancer. *J Urol* 1998;160:802–806.

34. Pound CR, Partin AW, Epstein JI, et al. Prostate-specific antigen after anatomic radical retropubic prostatectomy. Patterns of recurrence and cancer control. *Urol Clin North Am* 1997;24:395–406.

35. Humphrey PA, Frazier HA, Vollmer RT, et al. Stratification of pathologic features in radical prostatectomy specimens that are predictive of elevated initial postoperative serum prostate-specific antigen levels. *Cancer* 1993; 71:1821–1827.

36. Fesseha T, Sakr W, Grignon D, et al. Prognostic implications of a positive apical margin in radical prostatectomy specimens. *J Urol* 1997;158: 2176–2179.

37. Babaian RJ, Troncoso P, Bhadkamkar VA, et al. Analysis of clinicopathologic factors predicting outcome after radical prostatectomy. *Cancer* 2001; 91:1414–1422.

38. Kattan MW, Wheeler TM, Scardino PT. Postoperative nomogram for disease recurrence after radical prostatectomy for prostate cancer. *J Clin Oncol* 1999;17:1499–1507.

39. Cox RL, Crawford ED. Estrogens in the treatment of prostate cancer. *J Urol* 1995;154:1991–1998.

40. The Leuprolide Study Group. Leuprolide versus diethylstilbestrol for metastatic prostate cancer. *N Engl J Med* 1984;311:1281–1286.

41. Mahler C. Is disease flare a problem? *Cancer* 1993;72:3799–3802.

42. Pickles T, Agranovich A, Berthelet E, et al. Testosterone recovery following prolonged adjuvant androgen ablation for prostate carcinoma. *Cancer* 2002;94:362–367.

43. Lamb DS, Denham JW, Mameghan H, et al. Acceptability of short term neoadjuvant androgen deprivation in patients with locally advanced prostate cancer. *Radiother Oncol* 2003;68:255–267.

44. Hurtado-Coll A, Goldenberg SL, Klotz L, et al. Preoperative neoadjuvant androgen withdrawal therapy in prostate cancer: the Canadian experience. *Urology* 2002;60:45–51; discussion 51.

45. Gleave ME, Hsieh JT, Wu HC, et al. Serum prostate specific antigen levels in mice bearing human prostate LNCaP tumors are determined by tumor volume and endocrine and growth factors. *Cancer Res* 1992;52: 1598–1605.

46. Stamey TA, Kabalin JN, Ferrari M, et al. Prostate specific antigen in the diagnosis and treatment of adenocarcinoma of the prostate. IV. Anti-androgen treated patients. *J Urol* 1989;141:1088–1090.

47. Blank KR, Whittington R, Arjomandy B, et al. Neoadjuvant androgen deprivation prior to transperineal prostate brachytherapy: smaller volumes, less morbidity. *Cancer J Sci Am* 1999;5:370–373.

48. Lilleby W, Fossa SD, Knutsen BH, et al. Computed tomography/magnetic resonance based volume changes of the primary tumour in patients with prostate cancer with or without androgen deprivation. *Radiother Oncol* 2000;57:195–200.

49. Armas OA, Aprikian AG, Melamed J, et al. Clinical and pathobiological effects of neoadjuvant total androgen ablation therapy on clinically localized prostatic adenocarcinoma. *Am J Surg Pathol* 1994;18:979–991.

50. Vailancourt L, Ttu B, Fradet Y, et al. Effect of neoadjuvant endocrine therapy (combined androgen blockade) on normal prostate and prostatic carcinoma. A randomized study. *Am J Surg Pathol* 1996;20:86–93.

51. Labrie F, Cusan L, Gomez JL, et al. Neoadjuvant hormonal therapy: the Canadian experience. *Urology* 1997;49:56–64.

52. Meyer F, Moore L, Bairati I, et al. Neoadjuvant hormonal therapy before radical prostatectomy and risk of prostate specific antigen failure. *J Urol* 1999;162:2024–2028.

53. Gleave ME, Goldenberg SL, Chin JL, et al. Randomized comparative study of 3 versus 8-month neoadjuvant hormonal therapy before radical prostatectomy: biochemical and pathological effects. *J Urol* 2001;166: 500–506; discussion 506–507.

54. Tetu B, Srigley JR, Boivin JC, et al. Effect of combination endocrine therapy (LHRH agonist and flutamide) on normal prostate and prostatic adenocarcinoma. A histopathologic and immunohistochemical study. *Am J Surg Pathol* 1991;15:111–120.

55. Bullock MJ, Srigley JR, Klotz LH, et al. Pathologic effects of neoadjuvant cyproterone acetate on nonneoplastic prostate, prostatic intraepithelial neoplasia, and adenocarcinoma: a detailed analysis of radical prostatectomy specimens from a randomized trial. *Am J Surg Pathol* 2002;26: 1400–1413.

56. Tetu B, van der Kwast T, Fradet Y, et al. Morphologic effects of neoadjuvant hormone therapy on prostate cancer. *Mol Urol* 1998;2:103–107.

57. van der Kwast TH, Labrie F, Tetu B. Persistence of high-grade prostatic intra-epithelial neoplasia under combined androgen blockade therapy. *Hum Pathol* 1999;30:1503–1507.

58. Montironi R, Magi-Galluzzi C, Muzzonigro G, et al. Effects of combination endocrine treatment on normal prostate, prostatic intraepithelial neoplasia, and prostatic adenocarcinoma. *J Clin Pathol* 1994;47:906–913.

59. Murphy WM, Soloway MS, Barrows GH. Pathologic changes associated with androgen deprivation therapy for prostate cancer. *Cancer* 1991;68: 821–828.

60. Reuter VE. Pathological changes in benign and malignant prostatic tissue following androgen deprivation therapy. *Urology* 1997;49:16–22.

61. Bostwick DG. Gleason grading of prostatic needle biopsies. Correlation with grade in 316 matched prostatectomies. *Am J Surg Pathol* 1994;18:796–803.

62. Hellstrom M, Wester K, Haggman M, et al. DNA ploidy patterns in androgen-deprived localized prostate cancer. *Eur Urol* 1996;29:420–424.

63. Thompson IM, Goodman PJ, Tangen CM, et al. The influence of finasteride on the development of prostate cancer. *N Engl J Med* 2003;349: 215–224.

64. Civantos F, Soloway MS, Pinto JE. Histopathological effects of androgen deprivation in prostatic cancer. *Semin Urol Oncol* 1996;14:22–31.

65. Soloman MH, McHugh TA, Dorr RP, et al. Hormone ablation treatments as neoadjuvant hormone therapy prior to radical prostatectomy. *Clin Invest Med* 1993;16:532–538.

66. Powell IJ, Tangen CM, Miller GJ, et al. Neoadjuvant therapy before radical prostatectomy for clinical T3/T4 carcinoma of the prostate: 5-year followup, phase II Southwest Oncology Group Study 9109. *J Urol* 2002;168: 2016–2019.

67. Fair WR, Aprikian A, Sogani P, et al. The role of neoadjuvant hormonal manipulation in localized prostatic cancer. *Cancer* 1993;71:1031–1038.

68. Fair WR, Scher HI. Neoadjuvant hormonal therapy plus surgery for prostate cancer. The MSKCC experience. *Surg Oncol Clin N Am* 1997;6: 831–846.

69. Schulman CC. Neoadjuvant androgen blockade prior to prostatectomy: a retrospective study and critical review. *Prostate Suppl* 1994;5:9–14.

70. Haggman M, Hellstrom M, Aus G, et al. Neoadjuvant GnRH-agonist treatment (triptorelin and cyproterone acetate for flare protection) and total prostatectomy. *Eur Urol* 1993;24:456–460.

71. Macfarlane MT, Abi-Aad A, Stein A, et al. Neoadjuvant hormonal deprivation in patients with locally advanced prostate cancer. *J Urol* 1993;150: 132–134.

72. Oesterling JE, Andrews PE, Suman VJ, et al. Preoperative androgen deprivation therapy: artificial lowering of serum prostate specific antigen without downstaging the tumor. *J Urol* 1993;149:779–782.

73. Aprikian AG, Fair WR, Reuter VE, et al. Experience with neoadjuvant diethylstilboestrol and radical prostatectomy in patients with locally advanced prostate cancer. *Br J Urol* 1994;74:630–636.

74. Soloway MS, Sharifi R, Wajsman Z et al. The Lupron Depot Neoadjuvant Prostate Cancer Study Group. Randomized prospective study comparing radical prostatectomy alone versus radical prostatectomy preceded by androgen blockade in clinical stage B2 (T2bNxM0) prostate cancer. *J Urol* 1995;154:424–428.

75. Gleave ME, Goldenberg SL, Jones EC, et al. Biochemical and pathological effects of 8 months of neoadjuvant androgen withdrawal therapy before radical prostatectomy in patients with clinically confined prostate cancer. *J Urol* 1996;155:213–219.

76. Gleave ME, La Bianca SE, Goldenberg SL, et al. Long-term neoadjuvant hormone therapy prior to radical prostatectomy: evaluation of risk for biochemical recurrence at 5-year follow-up. *Urology* 2000;56: 289–294.

77. Kava BR. Interim follow-up of patients receiving neoadjuvant hormonal therapy prior to radical prostatectomy at Memorial Sloan-Kettering Cancer Center: tumor designation as organ-confined and specimen-confined does not appear to result from pathologic understating. *Mol Urol* 1997;1: 141–148.

78. Sassine AM, Schulman CC. Neoadjuvant hormonal deprivation before radical prostatectomy. *Eur Urol* 1993;24(Suppl 2):46–50.

79. Witjes WP, Schulman CC, Debruyne FM, The European Study Group on Neoadjuvant Treatment of Prostate Cancer. Preliminary results of a prospective randomized study comparing radical prostatectomy versus radical prostatectomy associated with neoadjuvant hormonal combination therapy in T2-3 N0 M0 prostatic carcinoma. *Urology* 1997;49:65–69.

80. Labrie F, Cusan L, Gomez JL, et al. Down-staging of early stage prostate cancer: the first randomized trial of neoadjuvant combination therapy with flutamide and a LHRH agonist. *Urology* 1995;44:29.

81. Van Poppel H, De Ridder D, Elgamal AA et al. The Belgian Uro-Oncological Study Group. Neoadjuvant hormonal therapy before radical prostatectomy decreases the number of positive surgical margins in stage T2 prostate cancer: interim results of a prospective randomized trial. *J Urol* 1995;154:429–434.

82. Goldenberg SL, Klotz LH, Srigley J et al. Canadian Urologic Oncology Group. Randomized, prospective, controlled study comparing radical prostatectomy alone and neoadjuvant androgen withdrawal in the treatment of localized prostate cancer. *J Urol* 1996;156:873–877.

83. Hugosson J, Abrahamsson PA, Ahlgren G, et al. The risk of malignancy in the surgical margin at radical prostatectomy reduced almost three-fold in patients given neo-adjuvant hormone treatment. *Eur Urol* 1996;29: 413–419.

84. Prezioso D, Lotti T, Polito M, et al. Neoadjuvant hormone treatment with leuprolide acetate depot 3.75 mg and cyproterone acetate, before radical prostatectomy: a randomized study. *Urol Int* 2004;72:189–195.

85. Soloway MS, Pareek K, Sharifi R, et al. Neoadjuvant androgen ablation before radical prostatectomy in cT2bNxMo prostate cancer: 5-year results. *J Urol* 2002;167:112–116.

86. Aus G, Abrahamsson PA, Ahlgren G, et al. Three-month neoadjuvant hormonal therapy before radical prostatectomy: a 7-year follow-up of a randomized controlled trial. *BJU Int* 2002;90:561–566.

87. Selli C, Montironi R, Bono A, et al. Effects of complete androgen blockade for 12 and 24 weeks on the pathological stage and resection margin status of prostate cancer. *J Clin Pathol* 2002;55:508–513.

88. Bono AV, Pagano F, Montironi R, et al. Effect of complete androgen block-ade on pathologic stage and resection margin status of prostate cancer: progress pathology report of the Italian PROSIT study. *Urology* 2001;57: 117–121.

89. Gleave Mea. Randomized comparative study of 3 vs 8 months of neoadjuvant hormonal therapy prior to radical prostatectomy: 3 year PSA recurrence rates. AUA 2003 meeting, Abstract 2003, ID: 690.

90. Klotz LH, Goldenberg SL, Jewett M et al., Canadian Urologic Oncology Group. CUOG randomized trial of neoadjuvant androgen ablation before radical prostatectomy: 36-month post-treatment PSA results. *Urology* 1999;53:757–763.

91. Sato N, Gleave ME, Bruchovsky N, et al. Intermittent androgen suppression delays progression to androgen-independent regulation of prostate-specific antigen gene in the LNCaP prostate tumour model. *J Steroid Biochem Mol Biol* 1996;58:139–146.

92. Paulson DF. Neoadjuvant androgen-deprivation therapy prior to radical prostatectomy: con. *Urology* 1996;48:539–540.

93. Bazinet M, Zheng W, Begin LR, et al. Morphologic changes induced by neoadjuvant androgen ablation may result in underdetection of positive surgical margins and capsular involvement by prostatic adenocarcinoma. *Urology* 1997;49:721–725.

94. Paterson RF, Gleave ME, Jones EC, et al. Immunohistochemical analysis of radical prostatectomy specimens after 8 months of neoadjuvant hormonal therapy. *Mol Urol* 1999;3:277–286.

95. Tsihlias J, Kapusta LR, DeBoer G, et al. Loss of cyclin-dependent kinase inhibitor p27Kip1 is a novel prognostic factor in localized human prostate adenocarcinoma. *Cancer Res* 1998;58:542–548.

96. McDonnell TJ, Navone NM, Troncoso P, et al. Expression of bcl-2 onco-protein and p53 protein accumulation in bone marrow metastases of androgen independent prostate cancer. *J Urol* 1997;157:569–574.

97. Reed JC. Bcl-2 and the regulation of programmed cell death. *J Cell Biol* 1994;124:1–6.

98. Stein A, deKernion JB. Adjuvant endocrine therapy after radical prostatectomy for stage D1 prostate carcinoma. *Semin Urol* 1990;8:184–189.

99. Zincke H. Combined surgery and immediate adjuvant hormonal treatment for stage D1 adenocarcinoma of the prostate: Mayo Clinic experience. *Semin Urol* 1990;8:175–183.

100. Zincke H, Bergstralh EJ, Larson-Keller JJ, et al. Stage D1 prostate cancer treated by radical prostatectomy and adjuvant hormonal treatment. Evidence for favorable survival in patients with DNA diploid tumors. *Cancer* 1992;70:311–323.

101. Seay TM, Blute MC, Zincke H. Radical prostatectomy and early adjuvant hormonal therapy for pTxN+ adenocarcinoma of the prostate. *Urology* 1997;50:833–837.

102. Cheng WS, Bergstralh EJ, Frydenberg M, et al. Prostate-specific antigen levels after radical prostatectomy and immediate adjuvant hormonal treatment for stage D1 prostate cancer are predictive of early disease outcome. *Eur Urol* 1994;25:189–193.

103. Cheng WS, Frydenberg M, Bergstralh EJ, et al. Radical prostatectomy for pathologic stage C prostate cancer: influence of pathologic variables and adjuvant treatment on disease outcome. *Urology* 1993;42:283–291.

104. Ghavamian R, Bergstralh EJ, Blute ML, et al. Radical retropubic prostatectomy plus orchiectomy versus orchiectomy alone for pTxN+ prostate cancer: a matched comparison. *J Urol* 1999;161:1223–1227; discussion 1227–1228.

105. Zincke H, Lau W, Bergstralh E, et al. Role of early adjuvant hormonal therapy after radical prostatectomy for prostate cancer. *J Urol* 2001;166: 2208–2215.

106. See W, Iversen P, Wirth M, et al. Immediate treatment with bicalutamide 150mg as adjuvant therapy significantly reduces the risk of PSA progression in early prostate cancer. *Eur Urol* 2003;44:512–517; discussion 517–518.

107. Messing EM, Manola J, Sarosdy M, et al. Immediate hormonal therapy compared with observation after radical prostatectomy and pelvic lymphadenectomy in men with node-positive prostate cancer. *N Engl J Med* 1999;341:1781–1788.

108. Wirth MP, Weissbach L, Marx FJ, et al. Prospective randomized trial comparing flutamide as adjuvant treatment versus observation after radical prostatectomy for locally advanced, lymph node-negative prostate cancer. *Eur Urol* 2004;45:267–270; discussion 270.

109. Prayer-Galetti TZF, Capizzi F. Disease-free survival in patients with pathologic "C stage" prostate cancer at radical prostatectomy submitted to adjuvant hormonal treatment. *Eur Urol* 2000;38:504, Abstract 48.

110. See WA, Iversen P, McLeod D, et al. Bicalutamide 150mg alone or as adjuvant to standard care significantly improves progression-free survival in patients with early, non-metastatic prostate cancer. *J Urol* 2004;171:214, Abstract 1061.

111. Pether M, Goldenberg SL. Intermittent androgen suppression. *BJU Int* 2004;93:258–61.

CHAPTER 14D
Integrating Chemotherapy into Multidisciplinary Treatments for Prostate Cancer

Kenneth J. Pienta

Many phase II trials have been published suggesting that multiple drugs and regimens have activity in advanced prostate cancer (1–3). Multiple phase III trials are underway to test the ability of these agents to increase survival of patients in the hormone refractory setting (4,5). Because of the apparent activity of these regimens, many have been moved to earlier disease settings to determine if combining them with standard therapies increases disease-free and overall survival (Fig. 14D.1).

DEFINING THE HIGH-RISK PATIENT UNDERGOING DEFINITIVE LOCAL THERAPY

Many methods have been published to identify patients at risk for recurrence of their disease after surgery or radiation for cure (6). Pretreatment PSA, clinical stage, pathologic stage, and Gleason score have all been demonstrated to give prognostic information, and many nomograms and algorithms have been developed to predict relapse (7–13). Currently, patients at low risk for recurrence are those with T1-T2a disease, PSA <10 ng/mL, and Gleason <6 disease (7) (Table 14D.1). Patients with an intermediate risk of recurrence, i.e., a 30% to 60% chance of relapse, include those with T2b-T3a, PSA 10–20 ng/mL, and a Gleason score of 7. Patients with T3b, PSA >20 ng/mL, and Gleason scores of 8 to 10 are at high risk for recurrence. In analyzing the data from neoadjuvant and adjuvant trials, it is very important to take into consideration the proportions of patients from the various risk groups who were treated as those may have dramatic impacts on the relapse rate.

CHEMOTHERAPY AND PROSTATECTOMY FOR HIGH-RISK LOCALIZED PROSTATE CANCER

Neoadjuvant Therapy and Radical Prostatectomy

The use of NHT (androgen deprivation therapy or ADT) with radical prostatectomy (RP) has been well studied. Results suggest that men undergoing radical prostatectomy with T2b disease have approximately a 40% to 50% chance of having a positive surgical margin. Neoadjuvant hormonal therapy of 3 to 8 months results in positive surgical margins in the 10% to 20% range. However, this decrease in positive surgical margins does not correlate with an increase in disease-free survival as reflected by the recurrence of a measurable PSA. Aus et al. randomized 126 patients with T1b-T3a Nx XM0 disease to 3 months of neoadjuvant hormonal therapy prior to radical prostatectomy versus radical prostatectomy alone and presented results with a median follow-up of 7 years (14). The incidence of positive surgical

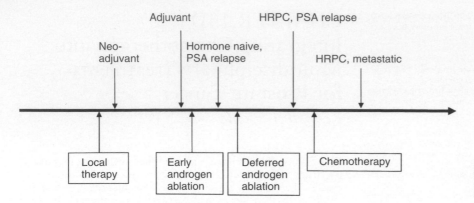

FIGURE 14D.1. Integrating chemotherapy and hormonal therapy into multidisciplinary treatments for prostate cancer.

margins decreased from 45.5% to 23.6% with ADT. However, there was no difference in PSA progression-free survival: 51.5% for patients undergoing RP, and 49.8% for those who received combined treatment. Soloway et al. randomized 282 patients with cT2b Nx M0 disease to treatment with 3 months of neoadjuvant hormonal therapy using leuprolide and flutamide plus radical prostatectomy versus prostatectomy alone (15). Forty-eight percent of patients treated with radical prostatectomy alone had positive surgical margins whereas 18% of patients treated with the neoadjuvant ADT had positive surgical margins. At 5 years, there was no difference in the PSA progression-free survival; 67.6% in the RP alone group, and 64.8% in the combined treatment group. Gleave et al. randomized 547 men with organ-confined prostate cancer to 3 versus 8 months of ADT (16). The positive surgical margin rates were 23% in the 3-month group and 12% in the 8-month group. No difference in progression-free survival has yet been reported. Recently, it has been demonstrated that patients receiving the nonsteroidal antiandrogen bicalutamide in the adjuvant setting after surgery had less risk of objective clinical progression in patients as compared to control patients (hazards ratio 0.58, 95% confidence interval 0.51–0.66, $P <.0001$) (17). However, more time is needed to determine whether this difference will lead to a survival advantage.

Taken together, these data suggest that ADT decreases the positive surgical margin rate from 40% to 50% to 10% to 20% (Table 14D.2). To date, it does not appear that this correlates with an increase in disease-free survival. Several small phase II studies have been undertaken to determine if the addition of chemotherapy in the neoadjuvant setting is beneficial. Pettaway et al. gave 18 men with T3 disease and 15 patients with T2b-T2c, Gleason 7, PSA greater than 10 disease ADT plus 12 weeks of ketoconazole–adriamycin alternating with vinblastine–estramustine (KAVE) chemotherapy (18).

Overall, 17% of the men had a positive surgical margin. Sixty-nine percent of the men were progression-free at a median follow-up of 13 months. Clark et al. treated 18 men with T1c-T3a disease with estramustine and etoposide prior to prostatectomy (19). Thirty-one percent of men had a pT2 disease at the time of surgery. Hussain et al. treated 10 patients (≤T2b, PSA >15, and/or Gleason 8–10 disease) prior to RP with docetaxel and estramustine (20). There was a 30% positive surgical margin rate and no patients achieved a pathologic complete response.

All of these trials combine chemotherapy with ADT therapy in some form. Estramustine lowers testosterone levels to castrate quickly because it is essentially an estradiol molecule with a nonfunctional nitrogen mustard attached. In addition to its hormonal effects, estramustine causes venous thromboses in 5% to 25% of patients on clinical trials (1). Consequently, there has been interest in investigating the effects of chemotherapy agents without hormone therapy in the neoadjuvant setting. Trials that investigate neoadjuvant chemotherapy agents that do not affect circulating testosterone are underway.

Adjuvant Chemotherapy and Radical Prostatectomy

In 1978, the National Prostate Cancer Project initiated two protocols evaluating adjuvant chemotherapy (Protocol 900) or radiation (Protocol 1000) for patients at high risk for relapse (21). There were 170 evaluable patients on Protocol 900 who were randomized to cyclophosphamide 1 g/m^2 every 3 weeks intravenously for 2 years, estramustine 600 mg/m^2 orally daily for 2 years, or observation. Twenty-nine percent of men on Protocol 900 had positive lymph nodes. There was no benefit of adjuvant chemotherapy (cyclophosphamide) or hormonal therapy (estramustine) as measured by overall survival (21). The Eastern Cooperative Oncology Group (ECOG) randomized 98 men with T1-T2 disease and nodal metastases to receive ADT or observation. At a median follow-up of 7.1 years, ADT reduced disease progression from 77% to 18% and overall survival increased from 65% to 85% (22). Currently, the SouthWest Oncology Group (SWOG) is testing the hypothesis that adjuvant chemo-hormonal therapy will improve survival in men with high-risk prostate cancer compared to hormonal therapy alone (SWOG 9921) (5). This trial randomizes men with T3b, T4 or N1 or Gleason greater than or equal to 8, or T3a, +margin, and Gleason 7 disease to 24 months of ADT with combined hormonal blockade versus 24 months of ADT plus mitoxantrone 12 mg/m^2 d1 + prednisone 5 mg B.I.D. d1–21 every 3 weeks for 6 cycles (Fig. 14D.2). It is designed to detect a 30% difference in survival at 10 to 15 years.

TABLE 14D.1

PROSTATE CANCER RECURRENCE RISK BY CRITERIA

Risk for recurrence	Risk criteria
Low	Staged T1-T2a disease
	PSA <10 ng/mL
	Gleason score <6
Intermediate	Staged T2b-T3a
	PSA 10–20 ng/mL
	Gleason score of 7
High	Staged T3b
	PSA >20 ng/mL
	Gleason score of 8–10

TABLE 14D.2

THE USE OF NEOADJUVANT HORMONAL THERAPY WITH RADICAL PROSTATECTOMY

Study	Stage	N	Treatment	Path result	PSA prog
Soloway (15)	T2b	282	None	48% +SM	67.6% @ 5 y.
			3 mo ADT	18% +SM	64.8% @ 5 y.
Gleave (13)		547	3 mo ADT	23% +SM, 5.1% pT0	
			8 mo ADT	12% +SM, 9.3% pT0	
Selli	cT3	393	None	10.4% pT2	
			3 mo ADT	31.4% pT2	
			6 mo ADT	61.2% pT2	
Clark (24)	T1c-T3a	18	Estramustine Etoposide	31% pT2	
Hussain (25)	T2b ≥ PSA >15 and/or Gl 8–10	10	Estramustine Docetaxel	30% +SM	
Pettaway (23)	T2b-T2c, Gl 7	15	Ketoconazole Adriamycin Vinblastine Estramustine	33% pT2	64% DFS @ 13 mo
	PSA >10 T3	18		17% +margin	

ADT, androgen-deprivation therapy; Gl, gleason score.

CHEMOTHERAPY AND RADIOTHERAPY FOR HIGH-RISK LOCALIZED PROSTATE CANCER

Chemotherapy and Concurrent Radiation Therapy

It has been demonstrated that many chemotherapy agents, including estramustine and the taxanes, can function as radiosensitizers (23,24). Due to these radiosensitization effects, chemotherapy has been studied when given in conjunction with radiation, rather than in a pure neoadjuvant setting. A series of phase II trials have been performed to examine the efficacy and toxicity of chemotherapy and radiation. Zelefsky et al. performed a phase II trial administering three 8-week cycles of estramustine–vinblastine (6 weeks of treatment, 2 weeks of rest) in combination with 65 cGy to 70 cGy of conformal three-dimensional (3D) external beam radiation therapy to patients at high risk of recurrence (25). These patients were defined as Gleason 8 to10, PSA greater than 10 or Gleason greater than or equal to 7, PSA greater than 20 or cT3N0M0, PSA greater than 20 or T4N0M0, or TxN1M0. The 2-year progression-free survival rate was 60%, suggesting efficacy as compared to

historical controls. In this trial the vinblastine was given in a dose of 6 mg/m^2/week and gastrointestinal and genitourinary toxicities were acceptable. Khil et al. utilized a vinblastine dose of 3 mg/m^2/week in conjunction with oral estramustine to treat 60 patients with T2-T4 disease in conjunction with 65 cGy to 70 cGy of radiation (26). Toxicity was tolerable and again there appeared to be efficacy in high-risk patients as compared to historical controls with a PSA relapse-free survival of 52% at 5 years. Ben-Josef et al. treated 18 patients with T3-T4 disease or T1-T2 disease, PSA greater than 15, Gleason greater than 7 with a neoadjuvant regimen of oral estramustine or oral etoposide followed by estramustine during external beam radiation (27). Progression-free survival in this small group of patients at 3 years was 73%. More trials are currently underway to determine if chemotherapy alone or in combination with hormonal therapy will boost progression-free survival rates (28). Oh et al. recently studied three patients with T3 disease and 4 patients with T2b disease, PSA greater than 40 ng/mL or endorectal MRI demonstrating nonorgan confined disease (28). Patients were treated with 2 cycles of liposomal doxorubicin at 50 mg/m^2 every 28 days and then treated with ADT plus RT. None of the patients demonstrated a significant response to neoadjuvant doxorubicin as measured by PSA, digital rectal examination (DRE), or endorectal MRI.

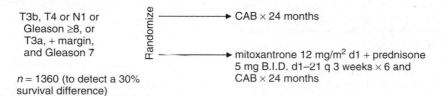

FIGURE 14D.2. SWOG 9921: Phase III Study of Adjuvant Chemotherapy in High-Risk Prostate Cancer. This trial will establish the efficacy of six cycles of adjuvant mitoxantrone chemotherapy plus two years of hormonal therapy versus hormonal therapy alone in high-risk surgical patients. Total accrual is set at 1,360 patients to detect a 30% survival difference.

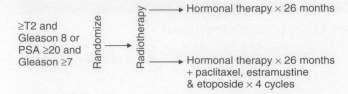

FIGURE 14D.3. RTOG 0521 Phase III Study of AHT with Radiation Therapy. This trial will establish the efficacy of four cycles of adjuvant hormonal therapy plus four cycles of chemotherapy with docetaxel and prednisone versus hormonal therapy alone in high-risk radiation patients. Total accrual is set at 600 patients to detect a 7% survival difference at 4 years.

Adjuvant Chemotherapy and Radiation Therapy

Based on the studies of Bolla et al. and the Radiation Therapy Oncology Group (RTOG), ADT given with radiation therapy and then in the adjuvant setting for patients at high risk for recurrence is now the standard of care (29–32). Recently, it has been demonstrated that in patients undergoing radiation therapy, 5-year progression-free survival was 40% in patients treated with RT alone and 74% in patients receiving RT plus 3 years of ADT (29). Overall survival was 62% in the RT group and 78% in the combined treatment group (29). Overall survival in a high-risk group of patients, those with T3-T4 disease, had survival rates of 60% and 78%, respectively. RTOG 05212 is a phase III protocol which examines the benefit of adding chemotherapy to hormone therapy in the adjuvant setting (Fig. 14D.3) (33). Node-negative patients with Gleason 7 to 10, PSA 20 to 100 or ≥T2, Gleason 8 to 10, PSA ≤100 are randomized to radiation therapy (RT) + ADT for 24 months versus RT + ADT + four cycles of chemotherapy with docetaxel and prednisone given after the radiation. All patients are treated with 8 weeks of ADT prior to starting RT. This trial is powered to detect an increase in survival of 7% at 4 years.

CHEMOTHERAPY AND HORMONAL THERAPY IN PATIENTS WITH A RISING PSA AFTER FAILURE OF LOCAL TREATMENT

A man with a rising PSA after definitive local therapy for cure is considered to have failed primary treatment. If the PSA is low (generally ≤2 ng/mL) and there is no evidence of systemic disease, the patient can be considered for local salvage therapy. If the patient fails salvage therapy, or already has a high PSA, other treatment options must be considered (34). The only standard of care in the treatment of men with a rising PSA after local treatment failure is ADT. A patient with symptoms from metastatic progression should absolutely be treated, but many patients fall into the categories of either PSA-only disease or patients with known metastatic disease (positive radiology studies) that are asymptomatic. Given the data from the adjuvant treatment studies, there is a growing trend to treat patients earlier in their disease course, but there is no right or wrong answers as to timing at this time. Given that this population has minimal disease, it is a popular group of patients on which to try to utilize experimental strategies to eradicate cancer in this setting. Multiple trials using vaccines and other experimental strategies are underway.

CHEMOTHERAPY AND HORMONAL THERAPY FOR HORMONE REFRACTORY PROSTATE CANCER WITH A RISING PSA

Men on hormonal therapy for metastatic prostate cancer invariably fail ADT and become hormone refractory. In the PSA era, often the only sign of hormone failure is a rising PSA. Most traditional chemotherapy trials target men with positive radiographic studies or symptoms. Although docetaxel is an approved therapy in this setting, multiple phase II studies are underway utilizing strategies that offer patients less toxicity. These include vaccine and anti-angiogenesis strategies.

FUTURE DIRECTIONS

The current phase III trials will take place over the next 5 to 10 years and will define the role of chemotherapy in the adjuvant setting as well as in the setting of patients with a rising PSA in the hormone-naïve and hormone-refractory settings. Additional phase I and II trials are underway to define the role of established and new chemotherapeutic agents in the neoadjuvant surgery and radiation settings.

References

1. Lawton CA, Winter K, Murray K, et al. Updated results of the phase III Radiation Therapy Oncology Group (RTOG) trial 85-31 evaluating the potential benefit of androgen suppression following standard radiation therapy for unfavorable prognosis carcinoma of the prostate. *Int J Radiat Oncol Biol Phys* 2001;49:937–946.
2. Hellerstedt BA, Pienta KJ. The current state of hormonal therapy for prostate cancer. *CA Cancer J Clin* 2002;52:154–179.
3. Pilepich MV, Winter K, John MJ, et al. Phase III Radiation Therapy Oncology Group (RTOG) trial 86-10 of androgen deprivation adjuvant to definitive radiotherapy in locally advanced carcinoma of the prostate. *Int J Radiat Oncol Biol Phys* 2001;50:1243–1252.
4. D'Amico AV, Cote K, Loffredo M, et al. Pretreatment predictors of time to cancer specific death after prostate specific antigen failure. *J Urol* 2003; 169:1320–1324.
5. Vaishampayan U, Hussain M. The evolving role of systemic therapy in high risk prostate cancer: strategies for cure in the 21st century. *Crit Rev Oncol Hematol* 2002;42:179–188.
6. Partin AW, Mangold LA, Lamm DM, et al. Contemporary update of prostate cancer staging nomograms (Partin Tables) for the new millennium. *Urology* 2001;58:843–848.
7. Nelson CP, Dunn RL, Wei JT, et al. Contemporary preoperative parameters predict cancer-free survival after radical prostatectomy: a tool to facilitate treatment decisions. *Urol Oncol* 2003;21:213–218.
8. Graefen M, Karakiewicz PI, Cagiannos I, et al. A validation of two preoperative nomograms predicting recurrence following radical prostatectomy in a cohort of European men. *Urol Oncol* 2002;7:141–146.
9. D'Amico AV, Cote K, Loffredo M, et al. Determinants of prostate cancer-specific survival after radiation therapy for patients with clinically localized prostate cancer. *J Clin Oncol* 2002;20:4567–4573.
10. Yossepowitch O, Trabulsi EJ, Kattan MW, et al. Predictive factors in prostate cancer: implications for decision making. *Cancer Invest* 2003;21: 465–480.
11. Aus G, Abrahamsson P-A, Ahlgren G, et al. Three month neoadjuvant hormonal therapy before radical prostatectomy: a 7 year follow-up of a randomized controlled trial. *BJU Int* 2002;90:561–566.
12. Soloway MS, Pareek K, Sharifi R, et al. Neoadjuvant androgen ablation before radical prostatectomy in cT2bNxM0 prostate cancer: 5-year results. *J Urol* 2002;167:112–116.
13. Gleave ME, Goldenberg SL, Chin JL, et al. Randomized comparative study of 3 versus 8 month neoadjuvant hormonal therapy before radical prostatectomy: biochemical and pathologic effects. *J Urol* 2001;166: 500–506.
14. Kelly WK, Curley T, Slovin S, et al. Paclitaxel, estramustine phosphate, and carboplatin in patients with advanced prostate cancer. *J Clin Oncol* 2001;19:44–53.

15. Petrylak DP, Macarthur RB, O'Connor J, et al. Phase I trial of docetaxel with estramustine in androgen-independent prostate cancer. *J Clin Oncol* 1999;17:958–967.
16. Smith DC, Esper P, Strawderman M, et al. Phase II trial of oral estramustine, oral etoposide, and intravenous paclitaxel in hormone-refractory prostate cancer. *J Clin Oncol* 1999;17:1664–1671.
17. Roach M III, Lu J, Pilepich MV, et al. Predicting long-term survival, and the need for hormonal therapy: a meta-analysis of RTOG prostate cancer trials. *Int J Radiat Oncol Biol Phys* 2000;47:617–627.
18. Sandler HM, Narayan S, Smith DC. Combined modality treatment for prostate cancer: role of chemotherapy. *Semin Oncol* 2003;30:95–100.
19. Kent EC, Hussain MH. The rationale for adjuvant chemotherapy for high-risk prostate cancer. *Curr Opin Urol* 2003;13:123–131.
20. Syed S, Petrylak DP, Thompson IM. Management of high-risk localized prostate cancer: the integration of local and systemic therapy approaches. *Urologic Oncology* 2003;21:235–243.
21. Carrol PR, Lee KL, Fuks ZY, et al. Cancer of the prostate. In: DeVita, VT, Hellman, S, Rosenberg, SA, eds. *Cancer principles and practice of oncology.* 6th ed. Philadelphia, PA: Lippincott Williams & Wilkins 2001:1418–1476.
22. Wirth MP, Froehner M. Adjuvant hormonal treatment for prostate cancer: the bicalutamide early prostate cancer program. *Oncology* 2003;65 (Suppl. 1):1–4.
23. Pettaway CA, Pisters LL, Troncoso P, et al. Neoadjuvant chemotherapy and hormonal therapy followed by radical prostatectomy: feasibility and preliminary results. *J Clin Oncol* 2000;18:1050–1057.
24. Clark PE, Peereboom DM, Dreicer R, et al. Phase II trial of neoadjuvant estramustine and etoposide plus radical prostatectomy for locally advanced prostate cancer. *Urology* 2001;57:281–285.
25. Hussain M, Smith DC, El-Rayes BF, et al. Neoadjuvant docetaxel and estramustine chemotherapy in high risk/locally advanced prostate cancer. *Urology* 2003;61:774–780.
26. Schmidt JD, Gibbons RP, Murphy GP, et al. Adjuvant therapy for clinical localized prostate cancer treated with surgery or radiation. *Eur Urol* 1996;29:425–433.
27. Messing ED, Manola J, Sarosdy M, et al. Immediate hormonal therapy compared with observation after radical prostatectomy and pelvic lymphadenectomy in men with node-positive prostate cancer. *N Engl J Med* 1999;341:1781–1788.
28. Bolla M, Collette L, Blank L, et al. Long-term results with immediate androgen suppression and external irradiation in patients with locally advanced prostate cancer (an EORTC study): a phase III randomised trial. *Lancet* 2002;360:103–106.
29. Milas L, Milas MM, Mason KA. Combination of taxanes with radiation: preclinical studies. *Semin Radiat Oncol* 1999;9:12–26.
30. Zelefsky MJ, Kelly WK, Scher HI, et al. Results of a phase II study using estramustine phosphate and vinblastine in combination with high-dose three-dimensional conformal radiotherapy for patients with locally advanced prostate cancer. *J Clin Oncol* 2000;18:1936–1941.
31. Khil MS, Kim JH, Bricker LJ, et al. Tumor control of locally advanced prostate cancer following combined estramustine, vinblastine, and radiation therapy. *Cancer J Sci Am* 1997;3:289–296.
32. Ben-Josef F, Porter AT, Han S, et al. Neoadjuvant estramustine and etoposide followed by concurrent estramustine and definitive radiotherapy for locally advanced prostate cancer: feasibility and preliminary results. *Int J Radiat Oncol Biol Phys* 2001;49:699–703.
33. Oh WK, Kaplan ID, Febbo P, et al. Neoadjuvant doxil chemotherapy prior to androgen ablation plus radiotherapy for high-risk localized prostate cancer. *Am J Clin Oncol* 2003;26:312–316.
34. Ryu S, Gabel M, Khil MS, et al. Estramustine: a novel radiation enhancer in human carcinoma cells. *Int J Radiat Oncol Biol Phys* 1994;30:99–104.

CHAPTER 14E
Quality of Life after Treatment for Localized Prostate Cancer

Mark S. Litwin and Arnold L. Potosky

BACKGROUND AND DEFINITION

The central goal in the care of patients with urological malignancies has traditionally been to maximize survival. Recent advances in chemotherapy regimens, surgical techniques, and radiation delivery have refined the treatment of urologic malignancies so that patients are now living longer with their cancers. This is particularly true in prostate cancer, where patients often live for many years after diagnosis and treatment. Historically, evaluation of the success of cancer therapies has focused on disease-free survival and other clinical parameters, but the advent of the medical outcomes movement has generated greater interest in patient-reported endpoints, such as health-related quality of life and patient satisfaction with health care.

Health-related quality of life (HRQOL) is one of several variables commonly studied in the field of medical outcomes research. HRQOL encompasses a wide range of human experience, including the daily necessities of life, such as food and shelter, intrapersonal and interpersonal responses to illness, and activities associated with professional fulfillment and personal happiness (1). Contemporary interpretations of HRQOL are based on the World Health Organization's longstanding definition of health as a "state of complete physical, mental, and social well-being and not merely the absence of disease" (2). Since cancer affects both quantity and quality of life, all the constituents of well-being must be addressed when treating patients with cancer. Perhaps most importantly, HRQOL involves patients' own perceptions of their health and ability to function in life. Indeed, patient perceptions of physical function have prognostic value in predicting survival (3).

While *quantity* of life is relatively easy to assess in terms of survival, the measurement of *quality* of life presents more challenges, primarily because it is less familiar to most clinicians (4). To quantify these qualitative phenomena, the principles of psychometric test theory are applied. This discipline provides the theoretical underpinnings for the science of survey research. Data are collected with HRQOL surveys, called instruments. Instruments typically contain questions, or items, that are organized into scales. Each scale measures a different aspect, or domain, of HRQOL. Some scales comprise dozens of items, while others may include only one or two items. HRQOL instruments may be general or disease specific. General HRQOL domains address the components of overall well-being, and disease-specific domains focus on the impact of particular organic dysfunctions that may affect HRQOL. General HRQOL instruments typically address general health perceptions, sense of overall well-being, and function in the physical, emotional, and social domains. Disease-specific HRQOL instruments for cancer patients focus on more clinically relevant domains, such as anxiety about cancer recurrence, nausea from chemotherapy, urinary incontinence, impotence, or bowel dysfunction (5).

Psychometric Validation of HRQOL Instruments

The development and validation of new instruments and scales is a long and arduous process. It is not undertaken lightly. Simply drawing up a list of questions that seem appropriate is fraught with potential traps and pitfalls. For this reason, it is always preferable to use established, validated HRQOL instruments (6).

When scales and instruments are developed, they are first pilot tested to ensure that the target population can understand and complete them with ease. Pilot testing is usually preceded by the conduct of focus groups to refine the wording of items and to ensure comprehensive coverage of concepts and domains deemed important by respondents. The initial part of pilot testing an instrument should involve formal cognitive testing. This process is usually led by cognitive psychologists or other behavioral scientists who specialize in developing and assessing the wording and ordering of questionnaire items to ensure that they can be easily understood by respondents, and that the answers that respondents provide are what investigators hope to learn from their study. Cognitive testing is usually performed on a very small number of respondents, usually 5 to 10 volunteers, who are asked to "think aloud" during the process of the interview. Following one or even two rounds of cognitive tests, a larger pilot test is then performed on a somewhat larger sample, using the exact same planned enrollment procedures and materials that are intended for the full study. Pilot testing can reveal problems that might otherwise go unrecognized by researchers. For example, many terms that are commonly used by medical professionals are poorly understood by patients. This may result in missing data if patients leave questions blank. Furthermore, since many patients with urologic malignancy are older and may have poor eyesight, pilot testing often identifies easily corrected visual barriers, such as type size and page layout. In addition, self-administered instruments with complicated skip patterns (e.g., "If you answered yes to item 16b, continue with item 16c; if you answered no to item 16b, skip to item 19a") may be too confusing for even the most competent patients to follow. This, too, can result in missing data and introduce difficulties in the analysis. Pilot testing is a necessary and valuable part of instrument development. It serves as a reality check on those developing the scales. Scales and instruments are also evaluated for two fundamental statistical properties, reliability and validity. These properties should, ideally, be reported immediately after pilot testing if enough respondents participate in the pilot phase.

Reliability refers to how free the scale is of measurement error, that is, what proportion of a patient's test score is true and what proportion is due to chance variation. Two of the most commonly used metrics are test-retest and internal consistency reliability. *Test-retest reliability* is assessed by correlating scale scores measured at two separate time points. *Internal consistency reliability* is a measure of the similarity of an individual's responses across several items, indicating the homogeneity of a scale (7). The statistic most often used to quantify this unidimensionality or internal consistency of a scale is called Cronbach's coefficient alpha (8). The internal consistency can be reported for any scale with more than one item, while test-retest reliability requires the scale to be administered to some patients twice within a short interval, preferably less than 1 month.

Validity refers to how well the scale or instrument measures the attribute it is intended to measure. Validity provides evidence to support drawing inferences about quality of life from the scale scores. Three types of validity usually are evaluated in new scales and instruments. *Content validity*, sometimes referred to as face validity, involves a nonquantitative assessment of the scope and completeness of a proposed scale. It is useful in the early stages of instrument development to seek such an assessment from clinicians and social scientists who are not directly part of the study, and from respondents via focus groups or formal cognitive tests, to improve face validity. *Criterion validity* is a more quantitative approach to assessing the performance of scales and instruments. It requires the correlation of scales scores with future measurable outcomes (predictive validity) and with results from other established tests (concurrent validity). For example, the predictive validity of a new quality of life scale for physical function might be correlated with the number of subsequent physician visits or hospitalizations. Likewise, the concurrent validity of a new sexual function scale might be correlated with objective performance on infusion cavernosometry. A new emotional quality of life scale might be correlated with an established mental health index.

In addition, instruments that are adopted as outcome measures must be responsive to change (9,10). That is, the score must increase or decrease over time in association with progressive improvement or impairment in the domain being measured. It is also useful to establish the minimally important difference (11), or the point difference thought to represent meaningful change or difference among treatment groups. Responsiveness and minimally important difference may be ascertained by correlation with a self-administered global response assessment that measures change on a Likert scale such as markedly, moderately, or minimally worse, unchanged, or minimally, moderately, or markedly better.

Other Considerations When Collecting HRQOL Data

Due to the effort and expertise required to develop and evaluate new scales for the purpose of measuring HRQOL, we recommend using existing instruments to assess general and disease-related HRQOL for men diagnosed with prostate cancer. Fortunately, several instruments have been developed to assess issues unique to men with this disease. Nevertheless, it may be necessary for an investigator to develop new items or scales or adapt existing scales when new questions arise, for example, due to the introduction of newer forms of therapies or other changes in practice. It is also possible that existing instruments or scales may not be sufficiently comprehensive to capture all domains of interest, or lack sufficient sensitivity to detect hypothesized differences in patient outcome across different patient sub-groups or over time since initial therapy. If an existing instrument cannot be found to suit the conditions and questions of a study, we recommend that any new items or scales that are developed be subjected to focus groups and cognitive evaluation at minimum, and further psychometric evaluations via pilot testing whenever possible. Such evaluations should be conducted before the administration of new scales or items in actual study subjects.

Furthermore, quality of life data should not be collected from cancer patients directly by the operating surgeon or treating oncologist or radiotherapist. The main reason for this is that there is evidence that patient and physicians' reports of prostate cancer-specific outcomes differ (12,13). Physician-based reports of urinary and sexual function in their patients, therefore, would not be considered valid if one assumes that the patient report is the "gold standard." Patients have an unconscious desire to produce responses that their physicians want to hear (12), and this introduces measurement error. No matter how objective the treating physician may claim to be, it is impossible to collect statistically meaningful outcomes data through direct questioning. Variations in phrasing, inflection, eye contact, rapport, mood, and other factors are difficult or impossible to eliminate.

Surveys may be administered person-to-person, over the telephone, or can be self-administered via postal mail, e-mail, or the Internet (14). Each mode has different limitations and advantages. Mailed surveys can be simpler and less costly to administer, but often lead to more missing data and can require calling respondents back to complete missing items. Phone or in-person surveys are usually more expensive since they require trained interviewers, but allow for more complex surveys to be administered with more skip patterns, and tend to have fewer missing data than mailed surveys. Web-based data collection has gained popularity in recent years, especially for longitudinal follow-up of enrolled patients who may indicate a preference to be contacted via email. It is convenient for patients, minimizes missing data, avoids data entry errors, and has minimal marginal cost once a secure system has been built. A mixed-mode approach may utilize some combination of web-based, mailed, or emailed surveys followed by telephone follow-up for nonresponders.

HEALTH-RELATED QUALITY OF LIFE INSTRUMENTS

There are numerous validated HRQOL instruments for the study of patients with many different diseases (15). An abundance of literature exists on general HRQOL, and a significant body of work has been published on HRQOL in cancer patients. One of the earliest predecessors to modern quality of life studies is the Karnofsky performance status scale (16). Popularized over 50 years ago, this instrument is actually a measure of physical function, not general HRQOL. Scores are determined by clinicians and not by patients. This work laid an important foundation for the HRQOL movement, although it captures only one part of HRQOL. It is reliable and fairly easy to apply, but it does not present a complete picture of HRQOL, nor is it based on patient self-report. Recently, the National Cancer Institute convened a Cancer Outcomes Measurement Working Group, which conducted a thorough review of HRQOL instruments and includes a detailed chapter on instruments commonly used in men with prostate cancer (17).

HRQOL is often confused with functional status. Although functional status is one important dimension of HRQOL, it is now widely recognized by social scientists that HRQOL is a multidimensional construct consisting of physical function, role function, mental health, vitality, pain, and psychosocial interactions. HRQOL also encompasses the overall sense of satisfaction that an individual experiences in life (18).

General HRQOL Instruments

General quality of life instruments have been extensively researched and validated in many types of patients. Examples include the RAND Medical Outcomes Study 36-Item Health Survey (also known as the SF-36) (19,20), the Quality of Well-Being scale (QWB) (21–25), the Sickness Impact Profile (SIP) (21,26–28), and the Nottingham Health Profile (NHP) (21,29–31). Each assesses various components of HRQOL, including physical and emotional functioning, social functioning, and symptoms. Each has been thoroughly validated and tested.

The most commonly used instrument for measuring general HRQOL among prostate cancer patients is the RAND 36-Item Health Survey, which was developed for the Medical Outcomes Study, which examined a variety of different types of patients (32,33). It is a 36-item, self-administered instrument that takes less than 10 minutes to complete and quantifies HRQOL in eight multi-item scales that address different health concepts: physical function, social function, bodily pain, emotional well-being, energy/fatigue, general health perceptions, role limitation due to physical problems, and role limitation due to emotional problems. The SF-36 can be interviewer-administered or self-administered. Another advantage of the SF-36 is that scale scores in prostate cancer patients can be compared with population norms or with other disease cohorts. A potential limitation of the SF-36 in prostate cancer patients is that the scales may not be sufficiently sensitive to detect subgroup differences, nor to measure changes in general HRQOL over time due to disease-specific decrements in function.

The Profile of Moods States (POMS) (34) and Hospital Anxiety and Depression Scale (HADS) (35) have also been used, though far less frequently than the SF-36, as generic measures focusing on mental health status in prostate cancer patients.

Cancer-targeted HRQOL Instruments

Because of the well-documented association of cancer with psychological stress and emotional anxiety, as well as the deficits in activities of daily living that affect patients living with malignancy, cancer-specific quality of life instruments have become more commonly applied in studies of prostate cancer patients. Several instruments have been developed and tested that measure the special impact of cancer on patients' routine activities. Examples include the European Organization for the Research and Treatment of Cancer Quality of Life Questionnaire (EORTC QLQ-C30) (36), the Functional Assessment of Cancer Therapy (FACT) (37,38), the Cancer Evaluation Rehabilitation System (CARES) (39,40), and the CARES Short Form (41). Each has been validated and tested in patients with various types of cancer.

The EORTC QLQ-C30 was designed to measure cancer-specific HRQOL in patients with a variety of malignancies, and has been used mostly in cancer clinical trials in Europe (36). The EORTC QLQ-C30 was designed as a core instrument for a modular approach to measuring HRQOL for various malignancies; therefore, its 30 items address domains that are common to all cancer patients. The questionnaire includes five general scales (physical, role, emotional, cognitive, and social functioning), a global health scale, three symptom scales (fatigue, nausea/vomiting, and pain), and six single items concerning dyspnea, insomnia, appetite loss, constipation, diarrhea, and financial difficulties due to disease. It is responsive to change, but much more so in patients with metastatic prostate cancer who have more frequently been the subjects of clinical trials than patients with localized disease.

The Functional Assessment of Cancer Therapy-General (FACT-G) is also a modular system focusing on cancer HRQOL, with modules for specific cancers (42). The FACT-G domains include well-being in five main areas: physical, social/family, relationship with doctor, emotional, and functional. The FACT-G includes 28 items and is easily self-administered. The CARES Short Form (CARES-SF) is a 59-item, self-administered instrument that measures cancer-related quality of life with five multi-item scales: physical, psychosocial, medical interaction, marital interaction, and sexual function. A large and valuable database of patients with many different tumors, including urologic tumors, has been collected by the developers of the CARES. These data are helpful when comparing the experience of prostate cancer patients with that of patients with other types of cancer.

Other scales have been used to assess cancer-related HRQOL in prostate cancer patients, including the Functional Living Index for Cancer (FLIC) (43,44), the Quality of Life Index (QL-Index) (45), and the Rotterdam Symptom Checklist (RSCL) (46).

Prostate Cancer-targeted HRQOL Instruments

In the past decade, several instruments specific to prostate cancer have been developed focusing on the urinary, bowel, and sexual domains that are of most frequent concern to prostate cancer survivors. The UCLA Prostate Cancer Index (PCI) was developed to measure disease-targeted HRQOL in men treated for early stage prostate cancer (47). The PCI is a self-administered, 20-item questionnaire that quantifies prostate cancer–specific HRQOL in six separate domains: urinary function, urinary bother, sexual function, sexual bother, bowel function, and bowel bother. The six scales are scored from 0 to 100, with higher scores representing better outcomes. The PCI has been shown to be both reliable and valid with test-retest reliability coefficients of 0.77 in five of six scales and internal consistency alpha coefficients of 0.65 to 0.93 in populations of older men with and without prostate cancer (47). Validated, cross-cultural translations of the PCI are available in Spanish (48), French (49), Dutch (50), and Japanese (51). A validated short form (PCI-SF) is also available (52).

The Expanded Prostate Cancer Index Composite (EPIC) added new items not available on the PCI assessing painful or difficult urination and rectal or urinary bleeding (53). The EPIC also includes a domain on hormonal symptoms, due to the increasing number of asymptomatic patients receiving hormonal ablation therapy.

The FACT-P is a supplemental prostate-targeted module that is used with the FACT-G. It is a 12-item scale that addresses weight loss, appetite, and urinary and erectile difficulties (54). The Prostate Cancer Treatment Outcome Questionnaire (PCTO-Q) (55) was also designed to supplement the FACT-G as a self-administered instrument relevant to prostate cancer patients. The PCTO-Q provides scores in the sexual, urinary, and bowel domains, but it is much longer than the FACT-P.

Another HRQOL disease-specific instrument is the prostate cancer module of the EORTC QLQ-C30. Researchers developed this module to be used in conjunction with the EORTC QLQ-C30 as a measure of disease-specific HRQOL in prostate cancer. Its 20 items include bowel, urinary, and sexuality symptom scales and are reliable and valid in men with localized (56,57) or metastatic (58) prostate cancer. Its scales are scored from 0 to 100 with higher scores representing worse outcomes.

Several other instruments assessing disease-specific symptoms have been evaluated or used for specific study settings, but have not been commonly adopted (59–63).

HEALTH-RELATED QUALITY OF LIFE IN PATIENTS WITH PROSTATE CANCER

In recent years, quality of life research has expanded rapidly in all areas of urologic oncology, including bladder (64), testicular (65), renal (66), and prostate cancer. HRQOL has been reported in numerous observational studies of clinical practice and has more often been incorporated in clinical trials to help enhance the relevance of results to clinical decision making. A recent review of 24 clinical trials of prostate cancer therapies that included HRQOL assessments revealed that 74% of these studies showed some difference in terms of HRQOL outcomes (67). Space limitations prevent a full review of all randomized and observational studies that have examined HRQOL in prostate cancer patients, but prostate cancer will be explored in some depth as an example of how our understanding of patients' experience with urologic cancer treatment can be augmented with HRQOL research.

Metastatic Prostate Cancer

Cancer-specific quality of life has been studied in patients with metastatic prostate cancer by Cassileth et al. (68,69), who used established psychometric instruments to show changes in HRQOL after treatment. Her work suggests that these men are interested in considering quality of life outcomes when selecting specific hormonal therapy. Herr et al. (70) also compared patients receiving hormonal therapy versus observation for metastatic prostate cancer. Their research documented better quality of life scores among patients who elected to defer

treatment over those who underwent early intervention. Litwin et al. (71) followed men with metastatic prostate cancer longitudinally after the initiation of androgen ablation. No differences were found in any of the HRQOL domains between men receiving combined androgen blockade or those undergoing bilateral orchiectomy, even when patients were followed for as long as 24 months. When patients were followed over time, significant improvements were seen in most HRQOL domains during the first year after diagnosis and treatment. Similar findings were also shown in a European trial of men treated with androgen ablation for newly diagnosed metastatic disease (72). Tannock et al. (73) adapted a series of linear analog items from an instrument validated in breast cancer patients and applied it along with the established McGill-Melzack pain questionnaire (74) to measure qualitative response to prednisone in patients with symptomatic bone metastases from prostate cancer. Although Tannock et al. did not develop new scales, they did measure outcomes, such as fatigue, appetite, and anxiety, all of which have been shown to contribute to quality of life in cancer patients. In a study of men with prostate cancer, Ganz et al. (39) used the CARES to discriminate among various clinical stages of the disease. They also demonstrated that among prostate, lung, and colorectal cancer patients, this instrument can be used to document the progressive worsening of quality of life as the cancer advances. These findings were confirmed by Kornblith (75), who used the EORTC Prostate Cancer Quality of Life Questionnaire to survey patients and spouses, demonstrating that as disease progresses, steady declines in HRQOL among patients are paralleled by increasing psychological distress among their spouses. Fossa (76) used an instrument adapted from the EORTC Prostate Cancer Quality of Life Questionnaire to compare doctors' and patients' perceptions of HRQOL following chemotherapy for hormone-resistant prostate cancer and showed that physicians tend to underestimate the effects of metastatic prostate cancer on patients' quality of life. Clark et al. found that regret was substantial among 201 men treated for metastatic prostate cancer two years later, and that it was adversely associated with HRQOL (77). Men with advanced disease were uncertain about the progress of their disease and their decision making. Potosky et al. compared surgical and medical hormonal therapy in 431 men with all stages within 1 year of initial diagnosis, and found little difference in sexual outcomes or general HRQOL between men with early versus advanced disease (78). Siston et al., studying 140 veterans with prostate cancer, found that general HRQOL improved more quickly in men initially diagnosed with distant disease compared with men diagnosed with localized disease (79).

Localized Prostate Cancer

Assessments of HRQOL in men with clinically localized prostate cancer have increased dramatically in the past 15 years, motivated in part by the dramatically increasing incidence of prostate cancer since 1990, and the expectation that most men with this condition will live many years with side effects of therapy.

Two comprehensive literature reviews have been performed describing the effects of prostate cancer on both general and disease-specific HRQOL (80,81). These reviews found that HRQOL can be assessed using scientifically sound methods from the field of psychometric test theory, and that there is a substantial literature on this topic that can be used to guide men and their clinicians in decision making. Here, we provide a brief synopsis of the literature.

Most studies that have compared HRQOL according to initial therapy for early stage prostate cancer have been observational, and thus subject to selection bias. One notable exception was a comparison of radical prostatectomy (RP) versus watchful waiting in a randomized trial (82), which found that erectile dysfunction and incontinence were more common, while urinary obstruction was less common, in the RP group. Bowel problems and general HRQOL were similar in the two arms. These results can be helpful in guiding men who are contemplating surgery versus watchful waiting.

Other common limitations on the utility of observational studies for informing decisions, besides selection bias, include cross-sectional rather than longitudinal measurements, lack of adjustment or stratification on key clinical and socio-demographic baseline variables, and the use of samples drawn from selected institutions or health plans. Most studies lack a control group, which is useful in understanding the unique impact of prostate cancer on HRQOL. Nevertheless, such observational studies are the most commonly available source of information available about HRQOL following prostate cancer treatment, so it is useful to describe briefly several studies having the strongest designs and greatest generalizability, despite the limitations noted.

Some often-cited studies using case series from major academic institutions have reported fairly low rates of incontinence and impotence following radical prostatectomy (83–85). Other single institution reports have shown higher rates of side effects after surgery or beam radiotherapy (86–88). One cross-sectional study of 214 patients from a large HMO plan revealed no differences in general HRQOL when comparing patients who had undergone surgery or radiation or observation alone for clinically localized prostate cancer, or when comparing cases to a group of age-matched control subjects without prostate cancer (89). Another single institution study reported that age, nerve-sparing technique, and prostate size were key predictors of post-prostatectomy impotence (90). Studies from single institutions, tertiary referral centers, or health plans may be limited in their generalizability to community clinical practice due to both patient and health care provider selection.

To avoid this limitation, Fowler et al. surveyed a large national Medicare sample of men diagnosed with prostate cancer (91) and found that sexual and urinary dysfunctions are much more common after radical prostatectomy than previously reported. The same authors also compared 367 patients who had undergone radical prostatectomy with 621 men from the National Cancer Institute's Surveillance, Epidemiology, and End Results (SEER) program who received radiotherapy (92). They found that those who underwent radiotherapy were more likely to worry about their disease than those who underwent prostatectomy. In a later study, Fowler et al. noted significant decrements in body image, mental health, general health, physical activity, worries about cancer and dying, and treatment impact among men receiving ADT after radical prostatectomy (93). These studies of the Medicare population were cross-sectional and did not include adjustments for key clinical prognostic factors.

Talcott et al. (94,95) conducted one of the first truly prospective cohort studies in which patients were assessed with validated HRQOL instruments before treatment and at three and twelve months afterward. Initially, radiotherapy patients had more irritative bowel and bladder symptoms, while surgery patients had more impotence and incontinence (95). Over time, sexual function declined in the radiotherapy group and improved in the surgery group, suggesting that with longer follow-up, treatment group differences in sexual function would continue to narrow. In another study, by the same authors, of 417 patients with longer follow-up, pretreatment baseline differences were found according to socio-demographic, prognostic, and symptom variables (96). Urinary incontinence increased after RP, bowel dysfunction and urinary obstruction increased after beam radiotherapy or brachytherapy (BT), and

sexual function declined in all treatment groups. However, samples for these studies' patients were drawn from two major referral centers and thus may not be generalizable. Another prospective study was performed in the Netherlands within the context of a large, randomized screening trial (97). RP patients reported significantly higher posttreatment incidences of urinary incontinence and erectile dysfunction than beam radiotherapy patients, while the latter experienced more bowel dysfunction.

The Prostate Cancer Outcomes Study (PCOS), initiated in 1994 by researchers at the National Cancer Institute (NCI) and the SEER Program, measured HRQOL outcomes over two years following different therapies using a population-based sample of approximately 3,500 community patients treated in six regions of the US (98). Findings from PCOS have confirmed earlier studies documenting decrements in urinary and sexual function in RP relative to external beam radiotherapy (EBRT) treated patients (99–101). Another PCOS study reported that androgen deprivation therapy (ADT) was commonly used in clinical practice as primary therapy for clinically localized disease, particularly among men with worse prognostic factors, and that such therapy resulted in decrements in sexual function and some aspects of general physical well-being within one year of diagnosis (102). While the strength of PCOS is its generalizability and repeated measures over time, it is not truly prospective, relying on 6-month post-diagnostic recall of pretreatment urinary, bowel, and sexual function. However, a PCOS validation study of posttreatment recall found reasonably high agreement between baseline and 6-month estimates of prediagnostic function, and between prospective and retrospective measures of change over 6 months (103).

Another large, comprehensive study of HRQOL in men with prostate cancer is a national observational cohort known as the Cancer of the Prostate Strategic Urologic Research Endeavor (CaPSURE) (104,105). The study includes over 10,000 men with all stages of biopsy-proven prostate cancer, drawn from more than three dozen community and academic settings. Subjects are assessed with biannual surveys that include validated measures of HRQOL. Among the many important observations made from this disease registry are three longitudinal HRQOL assessments comparing sexual, urinary, and bowel outcomes following surgery or radiation (106–108). In general, postoperative outcomes improve and postradiation outcomes decline over time. Data from CaPSURE have also demonstrated racial differences in HRQOL domains. Compared with white men, African-American men have worse scores in the general domains of physical function and role limitations due to emotional health problems. African-American men report better sexual function but worse sexual bother than white men (109). Cooperberg et al. provided a thorough review of CaPSURE's principal HRQOL findings (110). A valuable resource in describing outcomes and treatment patterns in men with prostate cancer, CaPSURE is limited by its observational nature and patient self-selection.

The recent dissemination of brachytherapy has led to a shift toward assessment of this therapy relative to more commonly established therapies. In a study of 256 men with clinically localized prostate cancer, men treated with BT reported the fewest problems with sexual function compared with men treated with either RP or EBRT (111). In a cross-sectional study of nearly 1,000 men with prostate cancer (and 112 controls) treated in a single institution, HRQOL after BT ($n = 84$) was not beneficial relative to RP or EBRT, and was worse in some domains of HRQOL, notably urinary obstruction and irritation (112). In another study that included 80 BT patients treated in two academically affiliated centers, BT was associated with increased rates of urinary obstruction/irritation and sexual dysfunction, though sexual function was still poorer in surgically treated patients after 24 months (96). In a cross-sectional study of 122 men undergoing BT or RP prostatectomy, the former were more likely to report irritative urinary symptoms and bowel impairment, especially if they had also received EBRT (113). Significant urinary, bowel, and sexual side effects were also reported in a series of French men undergoing BT (114). The HRQOL changes observed following BT appear to persist for at least several years (115,116).

Impact of Disease-specific Function on General HRQOL

While many studies have carefully documented disease-specific dysfunction, more attention has been given to assessing the impact of disease-specific complications on general HRQOL. One study found only temporal changes (117), while another noted declines in general HRQOL relative to controls (118). However, some differences in mental health at 15 months have been found for surgery versus radiotherapy patients, with surgery patients having somewhat better outcomes (119). Another investigation using PCOS data reported that the use of surgery versus radiotherapy had no effect on general HRQOL as measured by the SF-36, but that men who were bothered by their incontinence or impotence were more likely to report worse HRQOL than men not bothered by their dysfunction. It also showed that among men treated with surgery or radiation for localized prostate cancer, urinary dysfunction diminished HRQOL much more than did sexual dysfunction (120). The lack of differences when comparing treatment groups on general HRQOL can obscure important issues with respect to diminished body image, masculinity, and intimacy which are correlated with decrements in sexual function (121).

APPROACHES TO MEASUREMENT OF HRQOL

The Southwest Oncology Group (SWOG) has defined five principles (as cited in Table 14E.1) for HRQOL research in cancer trials (122). It is recommended that investigators start with these guidelines when selecting instruments to assess HRQOL in longitudinal or cross-sectional studies of patients with urologic malignancy. Ideally, instruments should also have demonstrated properties of responsiveness and sensitivity to change in longitudinal studies. Data should be collected at baseline before treatment (if possible) and tracked longitudinally to assess changes related to the disease or its treatments. Important social (e.g., education, income), demographic (e.g., age, race), and clinical (e.g., stage, grade, comorbidity) variables should also be measured at baseline in order to correct for case mix in subsequent predictive modeling. This approach reduces bias in group comparisons. Instruments that may be used to measure comorbidity in men with prostate cancer include the Index of Co-Existent Disease (ICED) (123), the Charlson Index (124), the Deyo Index (125), The Kaplan-Feinstein Index (126), and others (127).

The various components of HRQOL should be measured with different scales to ensure that each receives adequate attention. Many quality of life researchers believe that instruments should always be self-administered by patients independent of interviewers. Others prefer a mixed-mode approach, in which some data are collected by interviewers. Self-assessment of HRQOL frees patient responses from any interviewer bias. Although many instruments use visual analog scales, most quality of life researchers believe that items with specific Likert-type response sets provide more accurate information. Longer instruments may yield richer data sets, but they also increase respondent burden and decrease the reliability and validity of the information. Hence, short instruments are generally preferable when obtaining HRQOL measurements. When collecting HRQOL data with published instruments, the researcher can compare the results to other populations with various chronic diseases, including different types of cancer.

It can be useful to assess the public health impact of prostate cancer by comparing results for prostate cancer patients with individuals of the same age without known disease (128). For example, when measuring sexual function after treatment for prostate cancer, it is more helpful to compare outcomes with age-matched control subjects than with a hypothetical state of perfect sexual function. Since sexual function varies with age, it is critical to maintain the appropriate context of the variable under investigation. This principle holds true with other HRQOL domains as well. However, comparisons of patients with controls has more limited value for guiding newly diagnosed men who must choose among alternative treatments with different profiles of outcomes.

Directions for Future Research in HRQOL

Specific research questions begin with the need for basic descriptive analysis of quality of life in patients treated for urologic cancers. Depiction of the fundamental elements in quality of life for these individuals requires study of their health perceptions and how their daily activities are affected by both their general health and their cancer. Physical and emotional well-being form the cornerstone of this approach, but research must also extend to other issues that can affect a cancer patient's quality of life and satisfaction, such as eating and sleeping habits, anxiety and fatigue, depression, rapport with the physician, presence of a spouse or partner, and social interactions. Characterization of all domains must address not only the actual functions but also the relative importance of these issues to patients.

Beyond simple descriptive analysis, HRQOL outcomes must be compared between patients undergoing different modes of therapy. General and disease-specific HRQOL must be measured to facilitate comparison with patients treated for diabetes, heart disease, arthritis, and other common chronic conditions. Quality of life outcomes may be correlated with medical variables, such as comorbidity, or socio-demographic variables, such as age, race, education, income, insurance status, geographic region, and access to health care. In this context, HRQOL may be linked with many factors other than the traditional medical ones. All clinical trials and observational cohort studies in patients with urologic malignancies should include an HRQOL component.

With better information on quality of life, clinical outcomes, and duration of survival, we will be better able to evaluate new treatment modalities, educate patients, and counsel them individually on what to do when they are diagnosed with urologic malignancies.

Ultimately, research into quality of life following the diagnosis and treatment of men with prostate cancer must be translated into results that are useful for patients facing difficult clinical choices. This informs medical decision-making in a manner that is beneficial for patients, their families, and their physicians. Because uncertainty is well documented in the literature surrounding the management of men with early and advanced prostate cancer, quality of life considerations have assumed a position of paramount importance. Among the most important challenges facing the field of quality of life research in prostate cancer is determining how clinicians can better incorporate quality of life tools and results into practice in order to help patients make decisions that suit their own idiosyncratic preferences.

TABLE 14E.1

SWOG GUIDELINES FOR QUALITY OF LIFE ASSESSMENT IN CANCER TRIALS

- Always measure physical functioning, emotional functioning, symptoms, and global quality of life separately
- Include measures of social functioning and additional protocol-specific measures if resources permit
- Use patient-based questionnaires
- Select brief questionnaires, not interviews
- Select HRQOL measures with published psychometric properties

References

1. Patrick DL, Erickson P. Assessing health-related quality of life for clinical decision-making. In: Walker SR, Rosser RM, eds. *Quality of life assessment: key issues in the 1990's.* Dordrecht: Kluwer Academic Publishers, 1993:11–64.
2. World Health Organization. *Constitution of the World Health Organization, basic documents.* Geneva: WHO, 1948.
3. Fossa SD. Quality of life after palliative radiotherapy in patients with hormone-resistant prostate cancer: single institution experience. *Br J Urol* 1994;74:345–351.
4. Litwin MS. Measuring health related quality of life in men with prostate cancer. *J Urol* 1994;152:1882–1887.
5. Patrick DL, Deyo RA. Generic and disease-specific measures in assessing health status and quality of life. *Med Care* 1989;27:S217–S232.
6. Guyatt GH, Kirshner B, Jaeschke R. Measuring health status: what are the necessary measurement properties? *J Clin Epidemiol* 1992;45:1341–1345.
7. Tulsky DS. An introduction to test theory. *Oncology (Huntingt)* 1990;4: 43–48.
8. Cronbach LJ. Coefficient alpha and the internal structure of tests. *Psychometrika* 1951;16:297–334.
9. Deyo RA, Diehr P, Patrick DL. Reproducibility and responsiveness of health status measures. Statistics and strategies for evaluation. *Control Clin Trials* 1991;12:142S–158S.
10. Stockler MR, Osoba D, Goodwin P et al. European Organization for Research and Treatment of Cancer. Responsiveness to change in health-related quality of life in a randomized clinical trial: a comparison of the prostate cancer specific quality of life instrument (PROSQOLI) with analogous scales from the EORTC QLQ-C30 and a trial specific module. *J Clin Epidemiol* 1998;51:137–145.
11. Sloan JA, Cella D, Frost M, et al. Assessing clinical significance in measuring oncology patient quality of life: introduction to the symposium content overview, and definition of terms. *Mayo Clin Proc* 2002;77:367–370.
12. Litwin MS, Lubeck DP, Henning JM. Differences in urologist and patient assessments of health related quality of life in men with prostate cancer: results of the CaPSURE database. *J Urol* 1998;159:1988–1992.
13. Wei JT, Montie JE. Comparison of patients' and physicians' rating of urinary incontinence following radical prostatectomy. *Semin Urol Oncol* 2000;18:76–80.
14. Lallas CD, Preminger GM, Pearle MS, et al. Internet based multi-institutional clinical research: a convenient and secure option. *J Urol* 2004;171: 1880–1885.
15. Gill TM, Feinstein AR. A critical appraisal of the quality of quality of life measurements. *JAMA* 1994;272:619–626.
16. Karnofsky DA, Buchenal JH. The clinical evaluation of chemotherapeutic agents in cancer. In: MacLeod CM, ed. *Evaluation of chemotherapeutic agents.* New York: Columbia University Press, 1949.
17. Litwin MS, Talcott JA. Measuring quality of life in prostate cancer: progress and challenges. In: Lipscomb J, Gotay CC, Snyder C, eds. *Outcomes assessment in cancer.* Cambridge: Cambridge University Press, 2004.
18. Osoba D. Measuring the effect of cancer on quality of life. In: Osoba D, ed. *Effect of cancer on quality of life,* Chap. 31. Boca Raton, FL: CRC Press, 1991.
19. Stewart AL, Hays RD, Ware JE Jr. The MOS short-form general health survey. Reliability and validity in a patient population. *Med Care* 1988; 26:724–735.
20. Ware JE, Sherbourne CD Jr. The MOS 36-item short-form health survey (SF-36). I. Conceptual framework and item selection. *Med Care* 1992;30: 473–483.
21. McDowell I, Ewell C. *Measuring health: a guide to rating scales and questionnaires.* New York: Oxford University Press, 1987.
22. Kaplan RM, Anderson JP. A general health policy model: update and applications. *Health Serv Res* 1988;23:203–235.
23. Kaplan RM, Ganiats TG, Sieber WJ, et al. The quality of well-being scale: critical similarities and differences with SF-36. *Int J Qual Health Care* 1998;10:509–520.
24. Kaplan RM, Bush JW, Berry CC. Health status: types of validity and the index of well-being. *Health Serv Res* 1976;11:478–507.
25. Kaplan RM, Bush JW. Health-related quality of life measurement for evaluation research and policy analysis. *Health Psychol* 1982;1:61–80.
26. Bergner M, Bobbitt RA, Carter WB, et al. The sickness impact profile: development and final revision of a health status measure. *Med Care* 1981; 19:787–805.
27. Bergner M, Bobbitt RA, Pollard WE, et al. The sickness impact profile: validation of a health status measure. *Med Care* 1976;14:57–67.
28. Pollard WE, Bobbitt RA, Bergner M, et al. The sickness impact profile: reliability of a health status measure. *Med Care* 1976;14:146–155.
29. Hunt SM, McEwen J, McKenna SP. Measuring health status: a new tool for clinicians and epidemiologists. *J R Coll Gen Pract* 1985;35: 185–188.
30. McDowell IW, Martini CJ, Waugh W. A method for self-assessment of disability before and after hip replacement operations. *Br Med J* 1978;2: 857–859.
31. Martini CJ, McDowell I. Health status: patient and physician judgments. *Health Serv Res* 1976;11:508–515.
32. Tarlov AR, Ware JE, Jr., Greenfield S, et al. The Medical Outcomes Study. An application of methods for monitoring the results of medical care. *JAMA* 1989;262:925–930.
33. Stewart AL, Greenfield S, Hays RD, et al. Results from the Medical Outcomes Study. Functional status and well-being of patients with chronic conditions. *JAMA* 1989; 262:907–913.
34. McNair DM, Lorr M, Droppleman LF. *Profile of mood states,* 2nd ed. San Diego, CA: Educational and Industrial Testing Service, 1981.
35. Zigmond AS, Snaith RP. The hospital anxiety and depression scale. *Acta Psychiatr Scand* 1983;67:361–370.
36. Aaronson NK, Ahmedzal S, Bergman B, et al. The European Organization for Research and Treatment of Cancer QLQ-C30: a quality-of-life instrument for use in international clinical trials in oncology. *J Natl Cancer Inst* 1993;85:365–376.
37. Cella DF, Bonomi AE, Lloyd SR, et al. Reliability and validity of the Functional Assessment of Cancer Therapy-Lung (FACT-L) quality of life instrument. *Lung Cancer* 1995;12:199–220.
38. Cella DF, Tulsky DS. Measuring quality of life today: methodological aspects. *Oncology (Huntingt)* 1990;4:29–38.
39. Ganz PA, Schag CA, Lee JJ, et al. The CARES: a generic measure of health-related quality of life for patients with cancer. *Qual Life Res* 1992; 1:19–29.
40. Schag CA, Heinrich RL. Development of a comprehensive quality of life measurement tool: CARES. *Oncology (Huntingt)* 1990;4:135–138.
41. Schag CA, Ganz PA, Heinrich RL. Cancer Rehabilitation Evaluation System—short form (CARES-SF). A cancer specific rehabilitation and quality of life instrument. *Cancer* 1991;68:1406–1413.
42. Cella DF, Tulsky DS, Gray G, et al. The Functional Assessment of Cancer Therapy scale: development and validation of the general measure. *J Clin Oncol* 1993;11:570–579.
43. Schipper H, Clinch J, McMurray A, et al. Measuring the quality of life of cancer patients: the Functional Living Index-Cancer: development and validation. *J Clin Oncol* 1984;2:472–483.
44. Finkelstein DM, Cassileth BR, Bonomi PD, et al. An Eastern Cooperative Oncology Group Study. A pilot study of the Functional Living Index-Cancer (FLIC) scale for the assessment of quality of life for metastatic lung cancer patients. *Am J Clin Oncol* 1988;11:630–633.
45. Spitzer WO, Dobson AJ, Hall J, et al. Measuring the quality of life of cancer patients: a concise QL-index for use by physicians. *J Chronic Dis* 1981;34:585–597.
46. de Haes JC, van Knippenberg FC, Neijt JP. Measuring psychological and physical distress in cancer patients: structure and application of the Rotterdam Symptom Checklist. *Br J Cancer* 1990;62:1034–1038.
47. Litwin MS, Hays RD, Fink A, et al. The UCLA Prostate Cancer Index: development, reliability, and validity of a health-related quality of life measure. *Med Care* 1998; 36:1002–1012.
48. Krongrad A, Perczek RE, Burke MA, et al. Reliability of Spanish translations of select urological quality of life instruments. *J Urol* 1997;158: 493–496.
49. Karakiewicz PI, Kattan MW, Tanguay S, et al. Cross-cultural validation of the UCLA prostate cancer index. *Urology* 2003;61:302–307.
50. Korfage IJ, Essink-Bot ML, Madalinska JB, et al. Measuring disease specific quality of life in localized prostate cancer: the Dutch experience. *Qual Life Res* 2003;12:459–464.
51. Kakehi Y, Kamoto T, Ogawa O, et al. Development of Japanese version of the UCLA Prostate Cancer Index: a pilot validation study. *Int J Clin Oncol* 2002;7:306–311.
52. Litwin MS, McGuigan KA. Accuracy of recall in health-related quality-of-life assessment among men treated for prostate cancer. *J Clin Oncol* 1999; 17:2882–2888.
53. Wei JT, Dunn RL, Litwin MS, et al. Development and validation of the Expanded Prostate Cancer Index Composite (EPIC) for comprehensive assessment of health-related quality of life in men with prostate cancer. *Urology* 2000;56:899–905.
54. Esper P, Mo F, Chodak G, et al. Measuring quality of life in men with prostate cancer using the Functional Assessment of Cancer Therapy-Prostate instrument. *Urology* 1997;50:920–928.

55. Shrader-Bogen CL, Kjellberg JL, McPherson CP, et al. Quality of life and treatment outcomes: prostate carcinoma patients' perspectives after prostatectomy or radiation therapy. *Cancer* 1997;79:1977–1986.

56. Borghede G, Karlsson J, Sullivan M. Quality of life in patients with prostatic cancer: results from a Swedish population study. *J Urol* 1997;158:1477–1485.

57. Borghede G, Sullivan M. Measurement of quality of life in localized prostatic cancer patients treated with radiotherapy. Development of a prostate cancer-specific module supplementing the EORTC QLQ-C30. *Qual Life Res* 1996;5:212–222.

58. Albertsen PC, Aaronson NK, Muller MJ, et al. Health-related quality of life among patients with metastatic prostate cancer. *Urology* 1997;49:207–216.

59. Stockler MR, Osoba D, Corey P, et al. European Organization for Research and Treatment of Cancer. Core Quality of Life Questionnaire. Convergent discriminative and predictive validity of the Prostate Cancer Specific Quality of Life Instrument (PROSQOLI) assessment and comparison with analogous scales from the EORTC QLQ-C30 and a trial-specific module. *J Clin Epidemiol* 1999;52:653–666.

60. Dale W, Campbell T, Ignacio L, et al. Self-assessed health-related quality of life in men being treated for prostate cancer with radiotherapy: instrument validation and its relation to patient-assessed bother of symptoms. *Urology* 1999;53:359–366.

61. Clark JA, Talcott JA. Symptom indexes to assess outcomes of treatment for early prostate cancer. *Med Care* 2001;39:1118–1130.

62. Giesler RB, Miles BJ, Cowen ME, et al. Assessing quality of life in men with clinically localized prostate cancer: development of a new instrument for use in multiple settings. *Qual Life Res* 2000;9:645–665.

63. Clark JA, Bokhour BG, Inul TS, et al. Measuring patients' perceptions of the outcomes of treatment for early prostate cancer. *Med Care* 2003;41:923–936.

64. Fossa SD, Reitan JB, Ous S, et al. Life with an ileal conduit in cystectomized bladder cancer patients: expectations and experience. *Scand J Urol Nephrol* 1987;21:97–101.

65. Fossa SD, Aass N, Ous S, et al. Long-term morbidity and quality of life in testicular cancer patients. *Scand J Urol Nephrol Suppl* 1991;138:241–246.

66. Litwin MS, Fine JT, Dorey F, et al. Health related quality of life outcomes in patients treated for metastatic kidney cancer: a pilot study. *J Urol* 1997;157:1608–1612.

67. Efficace F, Bottomley A, Van Andle G, et al. Beyond the development of health-related-quality-of-life (HRQOL) measures: a checklist for evaluating HRQOL outcomes in cancer clinical trials—does HRQOL evaluation in prostate cancer research inform clinical decision-making? *J Clin Oncol* 2003;21:3502–3511.

68. Cassileth BR, Soloway MS, Vogelzang NJ, et al. Zoladex Prostate Cancer Study Group. Quality of life and psychosocial status in stage D prostate cancer. *Qual Life Res* 1992;1:323–329.

69. Cassileth BR, Soloway MS, Vogelzang NJ, et al. Patients' choice of treatment in stage D prostate cancer. *Urology* 1989;3:57–62.

70. Herr HW, Kornblith AB, Ofman U. A comparison of the quality of life of patients with metastatic prostate cancer who received or did not receive hormonal therapy. *Cancer* 1993;71:1143–1150.

71. Litwin MS, Shpall AI, Dorey F, et al. Quality-of-life outcomes in long-term survivors of advanced prostate cancer. *Am J Clin Oncol* 1998;21:327–332.

72. da Silva FC, Fossa SD, Aaronson NK, et al. The quality of life of patients with newly diagnosed M1 prostate cancer: experience with EORTC clinical trial 30853. *Eur J Cancer* 1996;32A:72–77.

73. Tannock I, Gospodarowicz M, Meakin W, et al. Treatment of metastatic prostatic cancer with low-dose prednisone: evaluation of pain and quality of life as pragmatic indices of response. *J Clin Oncol* 1989;7:590–597.

74. Melzack R. The McGill pain questionnaire: major properties and scoring methods. *Pain* 1975;1:277–299.

75. Kornblith AB, Herr HW, Ofman US, et al. Quality of life of patients with prostate cancer and their spouses: the value of a data base in clinical care. *Cancer* 1994;73:2791–2802.

76. Fossa SD, Aaronson NK, Newling D, et al. The EORTC Genito-Urinary Group. Quality of life and treatment of hormone resistant metastatic prostatic cancer. *Eur J Cancer* 1990;26:1133–1136.

77. Clark JA, Wray NP, Ashton CM. Living with treatment decisions: regrets and quality of life among men treated for metastatic prostate cancer. *J Clin Oncol* 2001;19:72–80.

78. Potosky AL, Knopf K, Clegg LX, et al. Quality-of-life outcomes after primary androgen deprivation therapy: results from the Prostate Cancer Outcomes Study. *J Clin Oncol* 2001;19:3750–3757.

79. Siston AK, Knight SJ, Slimack NP, et al. Quality of life after a diagnosis of prostate cancer among men of lower socioeconomic status: results from the Veterans Affairs Cancer of the Prostate Outcomes Study. *Urology* 2003;61:172–178.

80. Penson DF, Litwin MS. Quality of life after treatment for prostate cancer. *Curr Urol Rep* 2003;4:185–195.

81. Eton DT, Lepore SJ. Prostate cancer and health-related quality of life: a review of the literature. *Psychooncology* 2002;11:307–326.

82. Steineck G, Helgesen F, Adolfsson J, et al. Quality of life after radical prostatectomy or watchful waiting. *N Engl J Med* 2002;347:790–796.

83. Walsh PC, Marschke P, Ricker D, et al. Patient-reported urinary continence and sexual function after anatomic radical prostatectomy. *Urology* 2000;55:58–61.

84. Catalona WJ, Basler JW. Return of erections and urinary continence following nerve sparing radical retropubic prostatectomy. *J Urol* 1993;150:905–907.

85. Gralnek D, Wessells H, Cui H, et al. Differences in sexual function and quality of life after nerve sparing and nonnerve sparing radical retropubic prostatectomy. *J Urol* 2000;163:1166–1169; discussion 1169–1170.

86. Schover LR, Fouladi RT, Warneke CL, et al. The use of treatments for erectile dysfunction among survivors of prostate carcinoma. *Cancer* 2002;95:2397–2407.

87. Yarbro CH, Ferrans CE. Quality of life of patients with prostate treated with surgery or radiation therapy. *Oncol Nurs Forum* 1998;25:685–693.

88. Lim AJ, Brandon AH, Fiedler J, et al. Quality of life: radical prostatectomy versus radiation therapy for prostate cancer. *J Urol* 1995;154:1420–1425.

89. Litwin MS, Hays RD, Fink A, et al. Quality-of-life outcomes in men treated for localized prostate cancer. *JAMA* 1995;273:129–135.

90. Hollenbeck BK, Dunn RL, Wei JT, et al. Determinants of long-term sexual health outcome after radical prostatectomy measured by a validated instrument. *J Urol* 2003;169:1453–1457.

91. Fowler FJ, Barry MJ, Lu-Yao G, et al. Patient-reported complications and follow-up treatment after radical prostatectomy. The National Medicare Experience: 1988-1990. *Urology* 1993;42:622–629.

92. Fowler FJ Jr, Barry MJ, Lu-Yao GL, et al. Outcomes of external-beam radiation therapy for prostate cancer: a study of Medicare beneficiaries in three surveillance, epidemiology, and end results areas. *J Clin Oncol* 1996;14:2258–2265.

93. Fowler FJ Jr, McNaughton Collins M, Walker Corkery E, et al. The impact of androgen deprivation on quality of life after radical prostatectomy for prostate carcinoma. *Cancer* 2002;95:287–295.

94. Talcott JA, Rieker P, Propert KJ, et al. Patient-reported impotence and incontinence after nerve-sparing radical prostatectomy. *J Natl Cancer Inst* 1997;89:1117–1123.

95. Talcott JA, Rieker P, Clark JA, et al. Patient-reported symptoms after primary therapy for early prostate cancer: results of a prospective cohort study. *J Clin Oncol* 1998;16:275–283.

96. Talcott JA, Manola J, Clark JA, et al. Time course and predictors of symptoms after primary prostate cancer therapy. *J Clin Oncol* 2003;21:3979–3986.

97. Madalinska JB, Essink-Bot ML, de Koning HJ, et al. Health-related quality-of-life effects of radical prostatectomy and primary radiotherapy for screen-detected or clinically diagnosed localized prostate cancer. *J Clin Oncol* 2001;19:1619–1628.

98. Potosky AL, Harlan LC, Stanford JL, et al. Prostate cancer practice patterns and quality of life: the Prostate Cancer Outcomes Study. *J Natl Cancer Inst* 1999;91:1719–1724.

99. Potosky AL, Legeler J, Albertsen PC, et al. Health outcomes after prostatectomy or radiotherapy for prostate cancer: results from the Prostate Cancer Outcomes Study. *J Natl Cancer Inst* 2000;92:1582–1592.

100. Stanford JL, Feng Z, Hamilton AS, et al. Urinary and sexual function after radical prostatectomy for clinically localized prostate cancer: the Prostate Cancer Outcomes Study. *JAMA* 2000;283:354–360.

101. Hamilton AS, Stanford JL, Gilliland FD, et al. Health outcomes after external-beam radiation therapy for clinically localized prostate cancer: results from the Prostate Cancer Outcomes Study. *J Clin Oncol* 2001;19:2517–2526.

102. Potosky AL, Reeve BB, Clegg LX, et al. Quality of life following localized prostate cancer treated initially with androgen deprivation therapy or no therapy. *J Natl Cancer Inst* 2002;94:430–437.

103. Legler J, Potosky AL, Gilliland FD, et al. Validation study of retrospective recall of disease-targeted function: results from the Prostate Cancer Outcomes Study. *Med Care* 2000;38:847–857.

104. Lubeck DP, Litwin MS, Henning JM, et al. The CaPSURE database: a methodology for clinical practice and research in prostate cancer. CaPSURE Research Panel. Cancer of the Prostate Strategic Urologic Research Endeavor. *Urology* 1996;48:773–777.

105. Lubeck DP, Litwin MS, Henning JM, et al. Measurement of health-related quality of life in men with prostate cancer: the CaPSURE database. *Qual Life Res* 1997;6:385–392.

106. Litwin MS, Flanders SC, Pasta DJ, et al. Sexual function and bother after radical prostatectomy or radiation for prostate cancer: multivariate quality-of-life analysis from CaPSURE. Cancer of the Prostate Strategic Urologic Research Endeavor. *Urology* 1999;54:503–508.

107. Litwin MS, Pasta DJ, Yu J, et al. Urinary function and bother after radical prostatectomy or radiation for prostate cancer: a longitudinal, multivariate quality of life analysis from the Cancer of the Prostate Strategic Urologic Research Endeavor (In Process Citation). *J Urol* 2000;164:1973–1977.

108. Litwin MS, Sadetsky N, Pasta DJ, et al. Bowel function and bother after treatment for early stage prostate cancer: a longitudinal quality of life analysis from CaPSURE. *J Urol* 2004;171(2):515-519 (in press).

109. Lubeck DP, Kim H, Grossfeld G, et al. Health related quality of life differences between black and white men with prostate cancer: data from the Cancer of the Prostate Strategic Urologic Research Endeavor. *J Urol* 2001;166:2281–2285.

110. Cooperberg MR, Broering JM, Litwin MS, et al. The contemporary management of prostate cancer in the United States: lessons from the Cancer of the Prostate Strategic Urologic Research Endeavor (CapSURE), a national disease registry. *J Urol* 2004;171:1393–1401.

111. Eton DT, Lepore SJ, Helgeson VS. Early quality of life in patients with localized prostate carcinoma: an examination of treatment-related, demographic, and psychosocial factors. *Cancer* 2001;92:1451–1459.

112. Wei JT, Dunn RL, Sandler HM, et al. Comprehensive comparison of health-related quality of life after contemporary therapies for localized prostate cancer. *J Clin Oncol* 2002;20:557–566.

113. Brandeis JM, Litwin MS, Burnison CM, et al. Quality of life outcomes after brachytherapy for early stage prostate cancer. *J Urol* 2000;163:851–857.

114. Joly F, Brune D, Couette JE, et al. Health-related quality of life and sequelae in patients treated with brachytherapy and external beam irradiation for localized prostate cancer. *Ann Oncol* 1998;9:751–757.

115. de Reijke TM, Laguna MP. Long-term complications of brachytherapy in local prostate cancer. *BJU Int* 2003;92:869–873.

116. Henderson A, Laing RW, Langley SE. Quality of life following treatment for early prostate cancer: does low dose rate (LDR) brachytherapy offer a better outcome? A review. *Eur Urol* 2004;45:134–141.

117. Litwin MS, McGuigan KA, Shpall AI, et al. Recovery of health related quality of life in the year after radical prostatectomy: early experience. *J Urol* 1999;161:515–519.

118. Bacon CG, Giovannucci E, Testa M, et al. The association of treatment-related symptoms with quality-of-life outcomes for localized prostate carcinoma patients. *Cancer* 2002;94:862–871.

119. Litwin MS, Lubeck DP, Spitalny GM, et al. Mental health in men treated for early stage prostate carcinoma: a posttreatment, longitudinal quality of life analysis from the Cancer of the Prostate Strategic Urologic Research Endeavor. *Cancer* 2002;95:54–60.

120. Penson DF, Feng Z, Kuniyuki A, et al. Results from the Prostate Cancer Outcomes Study. General quality of life 2 years following treatment for prostate cancer: what influences outcomes? *J Clin Oncol* 2003;21:1147–1154.

121. Clark JA, Inui TS, Silliman RA, et al. Patients' perceptions of quality of life after treatment for early prostate cancer. *J Clin Oncol* 2003;21:3777–3784.

122. Moinpour CM, Hayden KA, Thompson IM, et al. Quality of life assessment in Southwest Oncology Group trials. *Oncology (Huntingt)* 1990;4:79–84, 89; discussion 104.

123. Greenfield S, Apolone G, McNeil BJ, et al. The importance of co-existent disease in the occurrence of postoperative complications and one-year recovery in patients undergoing total hip replacement. Comorbidity and outcomes after hip replacement. *Med Care* 1993;31:141–154.

124. Charlson ME, Pompei P, Ales KL, et al. A new method of classifying prognostic comorbidity in longitudinal studies: development and validation. *J Chronic Dis* 1987;40:373–383.

125. Deyo RA, Cherkin DC, Ciol MA. Adapting a clinical comorbidity index for use with ICD-9-CM administrative databases. *J Clin Epidemiol* 1992;45:613–619.

126. Kaplan MH, Feinstein AR. The importance of classifying initial co-morbidity in evaluating the outcome of diabetes mellitus. *J Chronic Dis* 1974;27:387–404.

127. Albertsen PC, Fryback DG, Storer BE, et al. The impact of co-morbidity on life expectancy among men with localized prostate cancer. *J Urol* 1996;156:127–132.

128. Litwin MS. Health related quality of life in older men without prostate cancer. *J Urol* 1999;161:1180–1184.

CHAPTER 15 ■ TREATMENT OF LOCALLY RECURRENT PROSTATE CANCER

CHAPTER 15A
Definition of Failure Recurrence after Primary Therapy—Radical Prostatectomy and Radiation Therapy

Christopher L. Amling and Anthony Zietman

DEFINING FAILURE AFTER RADICAL PROSTATECTOMY FOR PROSTATE CANCER

The ultimate goal of radical prostatectomy in the treatment of prostate cancer is the eradication of disease by complete removal of all prostatic tissue. Unfortunately, in many cases this does not occur, either because local disease is left behind by incomplete resection or because systemic disease was already present at the time of surgery. Before the advent and widespread use of prostate-specific antigen (PSA) testing, recurrence after prostatectomy was usually defined by the postoperative development of a palpable mass in the prostatic fossa or by evidence of metastatic disease on postoperative imaging studies. These recurrences were often associated with bone pain and/or local symptoms. With postoperative PSA monitoring, and particularly with the use of ultrasensitive PSA assays, "biochemical" recurrence can now be detected many years before the development of clinically evident disease. Although there have been case reports of the development of metastatic disease with an undetectable PSA in the post radical prostatectomy setting (1,2), a detectable and increasing PSA level almost always precedes progression to clinically evident metastases. As such, while the clinical significance of a PSA-detected recurrence can vary significantly, its presence is currently the best and most sensitive determinate of therapeutic failure or recurrence after surgical therapy.

Defining the Ideal PSA Cut Point

To date, there has been no general consensus on what represents the best definition of PSA recurrence after radical prostatectomy. While some radical prostatectomy series use any detectable PSA level as evidence of treatment failure, most define recurrence as occurring at some selected PSA threshold. A PSA cut point of $\geq$0.2 ng/mL has been used by several institutions, while others have used two values of $\geq$0.2 ng/mL, or single values of $\geq$0.3 to 0.5 ng/mL (3–10). One series has used a definition that requires a PSA of $\geq$0.4 ng/mL, but also requires

two values that are rising so that a stable PSA of 0.4 ng/mL would not meet the definition of failure (11). Recent investigations have shown that biochemical outcomes reported after prostatectomy are dependent to some degree on the PSA threshold used to define failure (12,13). In a large surgical series from the Mayo Clinic, the impact of varying definitions of recurrence on outcome reporting was investigated (12). Comparing a PSA cut point of $\geq$0.2 ng/mL to $\geq$0.4 ng/mL, a 14% and 16% improvement in PSA progression-free survival at 5 and 10 years, respectively, was seen, favoring the higher PSA cut point. A definition that required two values (consecutive or not) above a given PSA threshold also has a significant effect on failure rates. Comparing a definition requiring a single PSA value of $\geq$0.4 ng/mL to that requiring two such values revealed a 7% and 18% difference in outcome at 5 and 10 years, respectively, with the better-reported outcomes occurring when two abnormal values were required. Because it takes longer for two PSA values above a given threshold to occur, progression is delayed and outcomes are improved using these kinds of definitions. In addition, if the date of failure is backdated to the first of these two PSA values, a further bias is created. A definition that requires that the failure event be backdated to a time before occurrence of the final PSA required to define recurrence can give the impression that late recurrence does not occur.

The American Society for Therapeutic Radiation and Oncology (ASTRO) definition of biochemical recurrence after radiation therapy for prostate cancer requires three consecutive rises in PSA and backdates the time of failure to a point between the nadir and the first of the rising PSA levels (14). To investigate how the ASTRO definition might affect reported biochemical recurrence rates when applied to radical prostatectomy patients, this definition was applied to such patients in two large surgical series (12,15). The requirement for consecutive PSA increases was shown to delay the event time significantly, and backdating made late recurrence much less likely. Comparing the ASTRO definition to a failure definition of 0.4 ng/mL in the Mayo Clinic series showed a 19% advantage in 10-year recurrence rate with the ASTRO definition (12). In the Johns Hopkins radical prostatectomy series, censoring patients with fewer than three consecutive PSA increases yielded biochemical recurrence rates that were superior to the standard actuarial surgical definition rate by nearly 20% at 15 years (15). Backdating the event time to between the nadir and the first of these rising PSA levels produced an apparent increase in survival from 68% to 80% at 15 years. When both the requirement for three consecutive rising PSA values and backdating were combined, biochemical failure was eliminated after 5 years. This comparison illustrates how differences in the definition of biochemical failure between radical prostatectomy and radiation series make it difficult to compare biochemical outcome between these groups. Recurrence estimates after radical prostatectomy can also be significantly affected by relatively minor changes in the definition used.

What then is the most appropriate PSA cut point at which to define recurrence after radical prostatectomy? While it is generally assumed that any detectable PSA level after radical prostatectomy represents persistent or progressive disease, this generalization may not always be true. Some men develop detectable but stable PSA levels that do not appear to progress further. In a large series of patients who under went radical prostatectomy between 1987 and 1993 at the Mayo Clinic, Amling et al. investigated the ability of various PSA cut points to predict continual upward progression of PSA levels over the subsequent 3-year period (12). It was assumed in this series that recurrent disease would be best represented by a PSA that continues to rise once a detectable PSA is attained, and that a low but stable PSA level may not necessarily represent recurrent disease. Surprisingly, only 49% of patients who reached a PSA threshold of 0.2 ng/mL progressed to a higher PSA value within a 3-year period. It wasn't until the PSA reached 0.4 ng/mL that the vast majority of patients demonstrated a subsequent PSA increase. Based on this data it was proposed that a cut point of greater than or equal to 0.4 ng/mL would be the most appropriate PSA level at which to define failure. In a smaller but very similar study, Freedland et al. investigated 358 men undergoing radical prostatectomy at the West Los Angeles Veterans Medical Center between 1991 and 2001 (13). In this series, a PSA cut point of 0.2 ng/mL was associated with a 100% risk of an increasing PSA over the subsequent 3-year period. These investigators suggested that a cut point of 0.2 ng/mL was the most appropriate for use in defining PSA recurrence. Unfortunately, the results of these two investigations do not answer definitely which is the best cut point to use. However, both suggest that some men develop a low but stable serum PSA level after radical prostatectomy that fails to demonstrate a continual upward trend.

Benign Versus Malignant Sources of Detectable PSA

Although the reason for these low detectable but stable PSA levels after radical prostatectomy is unknown, there are several potential explanations (16,17). One possibility is that an elevated PSA after surgery may be due to residual benign tissue left behind at surgery, particularly at the bladder neck or prostatic apex. Several series have shown that capsular incisions during radical prostatectomy can expose benign prostatic tissue to the margin of resection (16–19). In one series this was found in 37% to 90% of specimens, depending on the surgical approach, retropubic or perineal (18). In a series of 300 consecutive radical prostatectomy specimens submitted to wholemount pathologic analysis, 26% of specimens were found to have benign glandular tissue at the surgical resection margins (19). In the absence of cancer at the surgical margins, some of these patients were observed to develop low but detectable PSA levels in the 0.1 to 0.3 ng/mL range that remain stable, possibly a result of retained benign glands (17). When anastomotic biopsies are performed in men with detectable PSA levels after a radical prostatectomy, 15% to 19% are found to have benign disease in the biopsy specimens (20,21). While it is likely that cancerous tissue coexists with benign tissue in many of these men, these studies demonstrate that it is not uncommon for benign tissue to be left behind at the time of radical prostatectomy.

Persistence of benign glands after radical prostatectomy may be related to surgical technique. Bladder neck preservation is a commonly practiced surgical technique during radical prostatectomy in which the circular bladder neck fibers are preserved by peeling the prostate from its bladder neck attachments. This technique may increase the probability of leaving benign prostate tissue behind at this location (22,23). In one

series, 38% of men had some elements of benign prostatic tissue at the bladder neck margin after radical retropubic prostatectomy (23). Incomplete apical dissection might also result in persistent benign tissue left in an apical location. In a prospective study of 95 consecutive men undergoing radical prostatectomy, a separate 2-mm to 3-mm circumferential biopsy was obtained from around the urethral stump at the apical soft tissue margin after the prostate specimen had been completely removed (24). Benign tissue was found in 54% of these apical soft tissue biopsies. In another report, Ponthieu et al. reported that 43% of apical margin biopsies had some elements of benign prostatic tissue (25). These studies show that persistent benign tissue, left behind at either the bladder neck or prostatic apex, is not uncommon after radical prostatectomy.

The persistence of PSA in the urine of men who have undergone radical prostatectomy may also originate from retained benign tissue, although some have suggested that this PSA is derived from periurethral glands. In a study investigating urinary PSA levels as a potential marker of response to prostate cancer therapy, deVere White collected voided urine samples from 57 patients who had undergone radical prostatectomy, 43 of whom had no evidence of recurrence (26). Considering both margin-positive and margin-negative cases, 77% were found to have elevated urinary PSA levels, which was more than twice as common as finding elevated serum PSA levels (>0.6 ng/mL). They concluded that urinary PSA levels reflect some remaining prostate tissue. In an attempt to localize the source of urinary PSA to prostatic or urethral secretions, Iwakiri compared the first 1 to 5 cc of voided urine to a midstream urine sample, finding consistently higher levels of PSA on the first voided sample (27). They noted that the PSA level in the first voided urine samples did not decrease to undetectable levels in the manner that the serum PSA did, even in the patients who had organ-confined tumors. Moreover, these urinary PSA levels were surprisingly high, with a mean urinary PSA level of 40.2 ng/mL. Takayama found urinary PSA levels that ranged from 0 ng/mL to 19.2 ng/mL in 39 patients after radical prostatectomy with higher levels again seen in the initial portion of the voided urine (28). It was thought that the urinary PSA in these cases originated from periurethral glands.

It is clear from these studies that low levels of PSA are detectable in the urine of men who have undergone radical prostatectomy, although the degree to which these PSA levels contribute to serum PSA levels after radical prostatectomy is unknown.

Use of Ultrasensitive PSA Assays

With increasing use of ultrasensitive PSA assays that detect PSA at levels much lower than standard assays, further questions have arisen regarding the most appropriate PSA level at which to define failure after surgical therapy (29–33). The most important potential utility of ultrasensitive PSA assays is the identification of recurrent disease earlier in its course. Using a PSA assay with a biological detection limit for serum PSA of 0.07 ng/mL, Stamey et al. studied serum samples from 22 patients after radical prostatectomy who later developed recurrent cancer as evidenced by a detectable PSA level of >0.3 ng/mL (29). Recurrence was detected a mean of 310 days earlier using the ultrasensitive assay. In another study using an ultrasensitive assay with a 0.08 ng/mL level of detectability, it was calculated that recurrent disease could be identified with a lead time of 22 months over conventional PSA assays (30). Other studies have shown similar ability to predict biochemical recurrence much earlier than standard assays (31–33). An important clinical question, however, is whether identification of biochemical recurrence at an earlier point in time, yet within the undetectable level of standard assays, provides any benefit with regard to the efficacy of further treatment. While it is accepted that radiation to the prostatic fossa for local recurrence after radical prostatectomy is most beneficial when the PSA is low, there is no current evidence that this therapy is more effective when disease is detected at ultrasensitive PSA levels.

Similar to standard PSA assays, it remains uncertain which PSA threshold detected by ultrasensitive assays truly represents recurrent disease. Using an ultrasensitive assay with a biological detection limit of 0.07 ng/mL, Stamey et al. referred to a "residual cancer detection limit," which was defined in this study as a PSA level of 0.1 ng/mL (29). On screening 187 radical prostatectomy patients without evidence of cancer by a standard assay with a detection limit of 0.3 ng/mL, 11% were found to have evidence of residual cancer as defined by a PSA level of ≥0.1 ng/mL. In another study, an ultrasensitive assay was used to measure serum PSA levels in post-prostatectomy males compared to PSA measurements in hospitalized and healthy females (34). Of the post-prostatectomy patients, 50% had measurable PSA levels (≥0.01 ng/mL) and 21% had levels of ≥0.05 ng/mL. For the female patients tested, 15% had PSA levels between 0.01 ng/mL and 0.05 ng/mL, 2.5% had PSA levels of ≥0.05 ng/mL, and 1.5% had PSA levels of >0.10 ng/mL. The finding of low PSA levels in women raises the possibility that PSA may be produced and released by nonprostatic tissue. Ellis et al. suggested that the circulating nonprostatic source of PSA should be <0.008 ng/mL since most patients after cystoprostatectomy exhibit these levels (30).

Doherty and associates suggested that a PSA of ≤0.01 ng/mL should be the goal after radical prostatectomy (35). With biochemical relapse defined as three consecutive rises in PSA above the nadir PSA reached, the 2-year biochemical disease-free survival rate was significantly lower for patients who reached this undetectable range compared to those with detectable PSA levels of <0.1 ng/mL. However, most studies using ultrasensitive assays have identified small subsets of patients who have detectable but stable PSA levels many years after prostatectomy. Shinghal identified a group of patients with biochemical recurrence after a radical prostatectomy as defined by a PSA of >0.07 ng/mL who had no evidence of progressive disease (36). This group comprised 8.8% of men with biochemical recurrence in their series. Witherspoon and Lapeyrolerie identified 11 of 127 patients after radical prostatectomy who had a slowly increasing PSA of >0.01 ng/mL but <0.02 ng/mL at an average at 36 months postoperatively (31). Ellis et al. identified a small number of patients in their series who had low but detectable PSA levels upon initial testing that in later evaluations could not be detected, and another small group with stable or slowly rising PSA levels between 0.04 ng/mL and 0.08 ng/mL who were more than 7 years after radical prostatectomy without evidence of failure (30).

Proponents of ultrasensitive PSA assays in the postprostatectomy setting suggest that clinically significant recurrences can be detected earlier. While this is undoubtedly true, the serum PSA level that represents a clinically significant recurrence using ultrasensitive assays is uncertain and it remains possible that these assays may overestimate disease recurrence. Thus, a higher PSA threshold may be more appropriate to define treatment failure, particularly when it is to be used in considering additional treatment.

Conclusions Regarding Radical Prostatectomy

Although recurrence after radical prostatectomy is readily detected with the use of both standard and ultrasensitive PSA assays, the most appropriate cut point at which to define failure continues to be uncertain. While ultrasensitive PSA assays can identify biochemical recurrence much earlier in its course than standard assays, the clinical significance of these very low PSA levels is uncertain. Furthermore, it is not known whether the use of additional treatment for recurrence, when PSA is at ultrasensitive levels, will be any more effective than if given when a higher, standard assay threshold is reached. In addition, there are clearly some patients who develop biochemical recurrence that have an indolent course. These patients can often be identified by considering the initial tumor pathology, the timing of PSA recurrence, and the kinetics of PSA rise after biochemical progression has occurred (4,5,37–40). At the same time, there are patients who harbor a more malignant tumor type that is destined upon PSA recurrence to progress to distant metastatic disease. It has been difficult to devise a definition of biochemical failure that encompasses all of these considerations. Consensus on the definition of biochemical failure after surgery would be important to allow consistent outcome comparisons between surgical series and varied patient populations. Unfortunately, at this point in time, the most appropriate definition of biochemical recurrence after radical prostatectomy continues to be debated.

DEFINING FAILURE AFTER RADIATION THERAPY FOR PROSTATE CANCER

PSA Definitions

Prior to the late 1980s the success or failure of curative treatment for prostate cancer was determined using clinical endpoints such as local control, and disease-free or metastasis-free survival. When PSA was first introduced as a surrogate endpoint it led to confusion as it appeared to unearth a considerable amount of previously unsuspected failure (41,42). Men were found who had detectable or rising PSA after radiation but who were clinically disease free and may indeed have lived out their lives never knowing that their cancer had not been eradicated. It was not clear whether or not these men had truly failed. Stamey et al. was the first to apply a strict biochemical definition of failure to radiation-treated patients and asserted that less than 20% had been cured by therapy (43). The evidence was that 80% had a detectable or rising postradiation PSA. Radiation oncologists used the evidence of residual secretory function after radiation of other glands such as the pituitary or thyroid to counterclaim that a certain level of serum PSA was to be expected. The exact serum level compatible with a disease-free state was, however, unclear. Willett et al. showed that 10-year survivors of radiation therapy for prostate cancer had low PSA values, with a median of 0.5 ng/mL. Eighty percent had PSA values below 1.0 ng/mL (44) (Fig. 15A.1). Men without prostate cancer who received incidental radiation to their prostates during treatment for bladder or rectal cancer had median values of 0.5 ng/mL. Other studies showed that after prostate radiation the PSA rarely rose, raising the possibility that a rising PSA could be used as an endpoint (Fig. 15A.2) (45). It was, however, not immediately obvious what size rise or how many sequential rises constituted true failure. As a result of these uncertainties radiation series reported in the literature between 1992 and 1997 used a chaotic range of PSA endpoints: target PSAs of <4.0 ng/mL, <1.5 ng/mL, <1.0 ng/mL, <0.5 ng/mL; two successive rises, three successive rises, rises of >0.2 ng/mL, rises of >1.5 ng/mL. It was also unclear how to deal with patients who had a high but falling PSA in the first few years after radiation as the median time to nadir is around 18 months, or those who had a bouncing PSA. Should they be included? Should they be censored? By 1996 it was evident that series

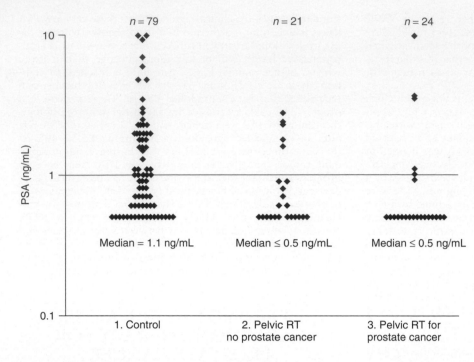

FIGURE 15A.1. Range of serum PSA values in three different groups of men (44):

1. Men who do not have known prostate cancer.
2. Men who do not have known prostate cancer and who have had their prostates irradiated incidentally as part of the treatment of bladder or rectal cancer.
3. Men who are long-term disease-free survivors following radiation therapy for prostate cancer.

The median PSA for groups 2 and 3 was significantly lower than for group 1 (44).

were being reported in so many different ways that they had become incomparable. As the number of differing therapies began to proliferate, it was evident that the playing field needed to be leveled to allow meaningful comparison between them, not to mention between radiation and surgery.

In 1996 The American Society for Therapeutic Radiology and Oncology (ASTRO) sponsored a consensus conference (14) which evaluated the available data and came up with the following guidelines:

1. Biochemical failure is not justification per se to initiate additional treatment.
2. Three consecutive rises in PSA is reasonable definition of biochemical failure after external beam radiotherapy.
3. No definition of failure has, as yet, been shown to be a surrogate for clinical progression or survival.
4. Nadir PSA is a strong prognostic factor but no absolute level is a valid cut point for separating successful and unsuccessful treatment.

These criteria were not recommended for use when radiation is given with androgen deprivation (AD). No comment

was made regarding their use after brachytherapy. The following additional recommendations were made to authors submitting studies for publication:

1. Minimum period of observation should be 24 months.
2. PSA should be measured at 3-month to 4-month intervals for the first 2 years after radiation and every 6 months thereafter.
3. Patients who have one or two rises in PSA but not three be reported separately in the final results.

These recommendations set a new standard which was closely followed in almost all published work for the subsequent 5 years. They unified reporting and ended the chaos. Subsequent studies have shown that, given sufficient follow-up, the ASTRO definition of failure at 5 years strongly correlates with cancer-specific survival at 15 years (46,47). This seemed to confirm the relevance of this biochemical surrogate of failure.

Despite its merits and widespread adoption, a number of problems with the ASTRO definition has subsequently surfaced. It has been argued that the ASTRO definition of biochemical

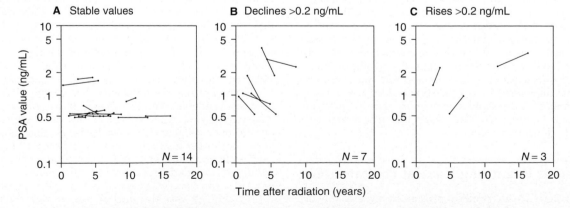

FIGURE 15A.2. Serial PSA values from 24 men without prostate cancer but who received radiation therapy to their prostates as part of the treatment of other pelvic malignancies. In only three of these men was a subsequent PSA rise of >0.2 ng/mL seen to imply that the production of PSA by normal prostatic tissue rarely recovers after radiation (45).

failure, which relies upon a rising PSA, may underestimate true failure because of two principal biases. The first is the issue of the sensitivity of the definition to the length of available follow-up, and the second is that of backdating failure. In addition, the definition needed modification to account for erratic PSA behavior seen after androgen deprivation or brachytherapy.

1. **ASTRO definition is "time sensitive".** Despite the routine use of radiation for over 20 years, the published data have been characterized by relatively short follow-up. This is partly the result of an elderly patient pool with many competing morbidities who are often lost to follow-up as they die, migrate to other locations when they retire, or enter nursing homes. It is a problem compounded by the routine inclusion of men treated recently who contribute little to the value of the data set but greatly shorten the median follow-up. Most modern major series have few patients still in the analysis by 8 years, but actuarial projections of outcome to that time and beyond are common.

Short follow-up is a troubling source of bias as the ASTRO consensus definition of failure is based upon a rising PSA. At least two years of follow-up are necessary for the PSA to decline, then some further period of time during which the patient is in remission, and finally the length of time it takes to witness three rises which will depend upon the frequency of office visits. It therefore usually takes a minimum of 4 to 5 years of follow-up of any treated population to begin to witness failure. Incorporating patients with less follow-up, results in a great deal of data censoring. This in turn leads to over-optimistic projections of outcome.

The important role that length of follow-up plays in determining outcome has been well demonstrated by Vicini et al. (48). They took a group of patients with relatively long follow-up and serially truncated the follow-up in 1-year increments. The less follow-up that was available, the worse the ASTRO method fared at detecting failure (Fig 15A.3). This was particularly pronounced once follow-up fell below 6 years, when the analysis is within the major hazard period for failure. Thus two groups of patients treated by different techniques, and in truth faring equally well, may appear to have different outcomes if the follow-up is shorter for one group than another. This bias alone may explain many of the assertions in the literature that one form of radiation is superior to another.

2. **Backdating appeared to inflate long-term outcome.** The follow-up bias may be compounded by the use of backdating of failure to a point half-way between the last nonrising PSA and the first rise. This was originally contrived in order that the failure event would be recorded at a time close to when it first occurred and at a time that would be comparable to surgical series. In an actuarial analysis the failure rate calculated in any given time interval is based on the number of patients whose failure occurs in the interval divided by the number with no biochemical evidence of failure at the start of the interval. The number of patients at the start of each time interval (the denominator of the rate) decreases with time due to censoring and so the impact of each individual failure is larger for failures that occur later than those that occur earlier. Backdating as required in the ASTRO definition causes failures occurring late to be backdated into an earlier time with a larger denominator and thus the consequence of each failure event is reduced. This has the tendency to reduce the ultimate failure rate and to flatten the actuarial survival curves over their last few years. The latter is an artifact caused by the fact that there are no subsequent failures beyond the time of observation to backdate into the final period of observation. Gretzer et al. using a surgical population to test the ASTRO definition, found that the longer the definition was stretched beyond the median of follow-up the less realistic the outcome (15). One way around this would be to maximize follow-up thus minimizing early censoring and the dilution effect. Zietman et al. reported on a cohort of patients with near complete follow-up out to 10 years in whom censoring had been minimized (though that occurring through death in this elderly population is unavoidable) (50). When the ASTRO definition was compared with a definition which reduces these biases by eliminating all backdating there was remarkably little difference in outcome at 10 years (49% vs. 42%) (Fig. 15A.4). Long follow-up would, therefore, seem to be the best way to minimize the differences in outcome otherwise revealed by these differing definitions.

3. **The ASTRO definition could not manage erratic PSA behavior.** Examples of this are seen in the following situations: small, benign "PSA bounces" seen after external beam radiation; the large and frequent PSA bounces in the second and

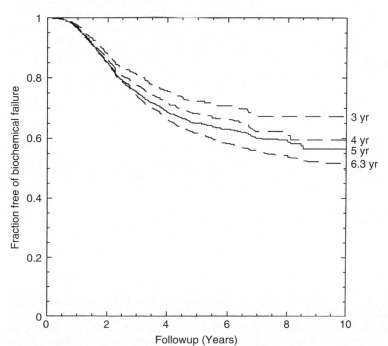

FIGURE 15A.3. A study of 4,839 men treated by conventional dose external beam radiation therapy (EBRT). Biochemical outcome was determined using the ASTRO definition of failure (three successive rises in PSA with the failure date backdated to a midpoint between the nadir and the first rise). In this figure each curve represents the same patients but with serial truncation of follow-up data from full follow-up (median 6.3 years) to just 3 years. This demonstrates the sensitivity of the ASTRO definition to length of follow-up (49).

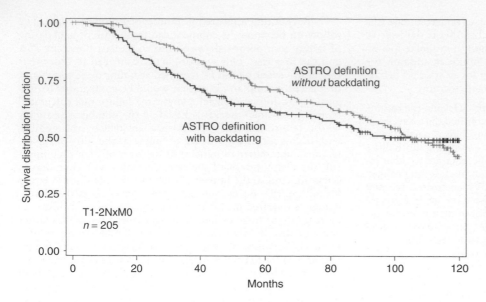

FIGURE 15A.4. A cohort of 205 men treated at the Massachusetts General Hospital from 1991 to 1993 in whom follow-up was maximized (median 9.5 years). If backdating of failure does not take place, then the curve continues a downward descent out to 10 years and the ultimate incidence of failure is higher than when the ASTRO definition is used with backdating (50).

third years after prostate brachytherapy; and the rebound in PSA seen after a short course of neoadjuvant androgen deprivation. The latter two are particularly troublesome as recent Patterns of Care studies show that brachytherapy was a component of treatment in 28% of radiation-treated cases in 1998 and is likely to be currently much higher (51). The same study also showed that androgen deprivation is used together with external radiation with great and increasing frequency. In 1993 it was 9% but by 1998 it was up to 50%. It was being used in 30% of those with favorable disease, 54% of those with intermediate prognosis disease, and 81% of those with unfavorable prognosis. Any definition of failure that cannot cope with such a large proportion of the patients treated by external beam is an unsuitable definition.

At the Massachusetts General Hospital, we have used our dataset to estimate the impact of rebound bounces caused when a man is released from neoadjuvant androgen deprivation if the ASTRO definition is used. PSA bounces were seen 31% of the time and are usually small, with a median of only 0.6 ng/mL. They tend to occur in the second or third year after treatment but may occasionally occur later. If these bounces had occurred in conjunction with regular 3-month follow-up, the ASTRO definition would have scored false failures in 18% of the cases. At its extreme the ASTRO definition could call a failure if the PSA rises on three successive occasions from <0.2 ng/mL (the lower limit of detectability at our laboratory), to 0.2 ng/mL, to 0.3 ng/mL, to 0.4 ng/mL over 9 months. While 18% is a relatively small proportion of the total it is still sufficiently large to vindicate the decision of the original consensus conference to avoid the use of the ASTRO definition in the setting of androgen deprivation. It likely occurs because of the recovery of serum testosterone after discontinuation of AD.

A further concern about any use of the ASTRO definition of failure after short-course androgen deprivation stems from the very early occurrence of the PSA nadir. Indeed it has often occurred by the time the radiation starts. Thus, if backdating is used, one of two confounding effects occur. Firstly, failure rates may be exaggerated over the first few treatment years because backdating pulls the Kaplan-Meier curves several years to the left. Secondly, and in conflict with the first, the impact of each individual failure event will be greatly underestimated because of extended backdating into a time when far more patients are present on the curve.

Redefining PSA Failure After Radiation

In an attempt to grapple with this problem the databases from nine major radiation centers were pooled to provide a dataset of 4,839 patients with long median follow-up (6.3 years) in which alternative definitions could be tested. Thames et al. examined 68 different definitions (49). They confirmed that any definition that relied upon backdating is very sensitive to follow-up time. There was a tendency to worsen outcome in the short term but improve it in the long term due to an artificial flattening of the curve. They suggested an alternative definition based on a rise of 2 ng/mL over the nadir without backdating. This displayed an even higher level of specificity and sensitivity for ultimate clinical failure. The absence of backdating eliminated the follow-up bias. It was able to cope with halting rises because it doesn't specify any number of successive rises. It could also cope with benign bounces seen after brachytherapy or androgen deprivation which rarely exceed 2 ng/mL.

Pickles and Coen have tested this new definition using different datasets and reached similar conclusions. They confirm that it does ultimately detect more failure and that the hazard of failure continues beyond 5 years though at a slightly lower pace (52,53).

It has another advantage over the ASTRO definition. Not only can be it be used to compare different radiation modalities (brachytherapy or external beam), and series with differing follow-up, but it can also be used to compare radiation with surgical series.

It is not currently clear whether this new definition will be universally adopted. It certainly seems to have much merit but more debate is required. It is likely that results will be quoted both ways during the period of transition.

Should a Target PSA Be Reconsidered for High-dose Radiation Therapy?

Concerns also exist about a definition of failure after radiation based upon a rising PSA rather than a target PSA. The use of the latter is possible after surgery as the source of all PSA, the prostate, has been extirpated and a clear target of zero is appropriate. It is well recognized that after radiation some PSA may be produced by surviving prostatic epithelium. There is, however, no agreement as to what constitutes a "normal" postradiation level. It has been argued that the PSA must fall to and remain at ablative levels after radiation in order to assert a disease-free state (54). In a recent study the median PSA for men biochemically disease-free 10 years after conventional dose radiation was 1.0 ng/mL (50). These men are likely truly disease-free by virtue of the stability of their PSA levels and the sheer length of uneventful time that has elapsed since treatment. These data seem to indicate that external radiation at the doses given in the early 1990s was "organ sparing." Thus, cancer has been eradicated while preserving some degree of prostatic secretory function. It does, however, appear that lower PSA levels are currently being achieved by high-dose conformal radiation and by brachytherapy suggesting a greater potential for organ ablation by these modalities (55,56). It would be premature, however, to extrapolate and argue they are more likely to cure or that an ablative PSA (<0.2 ng/mL) is a prerequisite for cure. Partial prostate brachytherapy is now being explored with unknown consequences on the ultimate level of PSA.

A BIOCHEMICAL FAILURE DEFINITION COMMON TO RADIATION AND SURGICALLY TREATED PATIENTS

It is clear that the behavior of PSA after radiation and surgery varies greatly and thus the use of a single definition of biochemical failure is hazardous. The surgical definition of an undetectable PSA cannot apply because radiation, at least at traditional doses, has not been an ablative therapy and thus a residue of "background" PSA production often exists. Equally the ASTRO definition could not work for surgically treated patients because failure would have to be backdated a long way to a point midway between the nadir shortly after prostatectomy and the first rise. This leads to a double and conflicting bias with the calling of failure unreasonably early and to a minimizing of the consequence of each failure event due to the previously mentioned denominator effect (vide supra). It is generally agreed that large and sequential rises in PSA constitute failure. Allowing a 2 ng/mL rise and avoiding backdating will likely identify most failures after any treatment and with high specificity and sensitivity (49). This endpoint, which has so far only been tested in radiation-treated patients, might become a common endpoint for comparative studies between the modalities. A potential problem arises because prostatectomy patients often receive salvage treatment before the PSA reaches 2 ng/mL. If this were the case, then the date of salvage treatment would become the date of failure. This would create a small bias bringing forward surgical failure when compared with radiation but it would likely be of trivial consequence if the series has sufficient follow-up.

DEFINING LOCAL CONTROL AFTER RADIATION BY PROSTATE REBIOPSY

Any local therapy is best judged by an accurate measure of local control. A rising PSA indicates failure but it does not tell its location. Waiting for clinical evidence of a local failure will overestimate the local efficacy of radiation because many patients will die with impalpable disease and many will have clinical evidence of a local failure suppressed by androgen deprivation given for co-existing metastatic disease. Post-radiotherapy prostate biopsies should provide a definitive measure of the success or failure

of local treatment but this is unfortunately not the case (57–59). Radiation kill of prostate tumor cells is primarily a postmitotic event. Prostate tumor cells may have long doubling times and thus histologic resolution may take 2 to 3 years. Biopsies done prior to this time are difficult to interpret because it is not clear whether any tumor elements found are regressing or regrowing. Cancer persistence may therefore be overcalled. Sampling error is another confounding factor. However, it works in the opposite direction to undercall failure. A further large subcategory is those with "indeterminate" rebiopsies.

A prospective study from Ottawa, Canada, has highlighted the problems with prostate rebiopsies and also the best way to obtain data (60). From 1987 to 1996, 498 patients treated with conventional dose external beam radiation were enrolled onto a protocol that mandated rebiopsies starting 12 to 18 months after therapy. If there was residual tumor but a further decline in PSA, biopsies were repeated every 6 to 12 months. Patients with negative rebiopsies were rebiopsied at 36 months. Median follow-up was 54 months, and 978 rebiopsies were ultimately performed.

Several important observations were made:

1. Of patients showing residual tumor on their first rebiopsy at a median of 13 months, 30% showed delayed tumor regression with eventual conversion to negative biopsies at a mean of 30 months. The time to nadir PSA for this group was 26 months.
2. The proportion of indeterminate biopsies decreases with time: 33% at 13 months, 24% at 28 months, 18% at 36 months, and 7% at 44 months. Thirty percent of indeterminate biopsies eventually cleared by a median of 31 months, 34% remained as biopsy failures but without progression to overt local or clear biochemical failure over the period of this study, and 18% progressed to local failure at a median of 38 months. The absence of radiation effect within the prostate made it more likely that subsequent biopsies would move from the indeterminate to the positive category.
3. Proliferation markers such as PCNA and Mib-1 (which show good concordance) were useful in predicting those with positive or indeterminate biopsies who would ultimately go on to overt clinical failure.
4. Nineteen percent of patients who achieved a negative postradiation rebiopsy went on to subsequently biopsy positive at a later time (median of 43 months).
5. Those who achieve low nadir PSAs are the most likely to rebiopsy negative. The median nadir and current PSA values for those who remained without any evidence of disease were 0.4 ng/mL and 0.5 ng/mL, respectively. Dugan et al. have shown that the likelihood of a positive prostate rebiopsy is substantially greater when the PSA is greater than 1 ng/mL than when it is less (60% vs. 9%) (61).

The above observations support the notion that 3 to 4 years should pass following radiation before rebiopsies are performed in order to minimize both false positives and false negatives. The majority of patients treated with conventional-dose radiation who have a rising PSA have a component of local failure.

Because of these limitations postradiation prostate rebiopsy does not form part of routine clinical practice. Rebiopsy would be performed if consideration was being given to a radical salvage therapy such as prostatectomy. Rebiopsy is more commonly used as an endpoint of local control in prospective clinical studies.

References

1. Leibman BD, Dillioglugil O, Wheeler TM, et al. Distant metastasis after radical prostatectomy in patients without an elevated serum prostate specific antigen level. *Cancer* 1995;76:2530–2534.

2. Oefelein MG, Smith N, Carter M, et al. The incidence of prostate cancer progression with undetectable serum prostate specific antigen in a series of 394 radical prostatectomies. *J Urol* 1995;154:2128–2131.

3. Hull GW, Rabbani F, Abbas F, et al. Cancer control with radical prostatectomy alone in 1,000 consecutive patients. *J Urol* 2002;167:528–534.

4. Pound CR, Partin AW, Eisenberger MA, et al. Natural history of progression after PSA elevation following radical prostatectomy. *JAMA* 1999;281:1591–1597.

5. Roberts SG, Blute ML, Bergstralh EJ, et al. PSA doubling time as a predictor of clinical progression after biochemical failure following radical prostatectomy for prostate cancer. *Mayo Clin Proc* 2001;76(6):576–581.

6. Zincke H, Oesterling JE, Blute ML, et al. Long-term (15 years) results after radical prostatectomy for clinically localized (stage T2c or lower) prostate cancer. *J Urol* 1994;152:1850–1857.

7. Catalona WJ, Smith DS. Cancer recurrence and survival rates after anatomic radical retropubic prostatectomy for prostate cancer: intermediate-term results. *J Urol* 1998;160:2428–2434.

8. Han M, Partin AW, Zahurak M, et al. Biochemical (prostate specific antigen) recurrence probability following radical prostatectomy for clinically localized prostate cancer. *J Urol* 2003;169:517–523.

9. Trapasso JG, de Kernion JB, Smith RB, et al. The incidence and significance of detectable levels of serum prostate specific antigen after radical prostatectomy. *J Urol* 1994;152:1821–1825.

10. Moul JW, Douglas TH, McCarthy WF, et al. Black race is an adverse prognostic factor for prostate cancer recurrence following radical prostatectomy in an equal access health care setting. *J Urol* 1996;155:1667–1673.

11. Kattan MW, Wheeler TM, Scardino PT. Postoperative nomogram for disease recurrence after radical prostatectomy for prostate cancer. *J Clin Oncol* 1999;17:1499–1507.

12. Amling CL, Bergstralh EJ, Blute ML, et al. Defining prostate specific antigen progression after radical prostatectomy: what is the most appropriate cut point? *J Urol* 2001;165:1146–1151.

13. Freedland SJ, Sutter ME, Dorey F, et al. Defining the ideal cut point for determining PSA recurrence after radical prostatectomy. *Urology* 2003;61:365–369.

14. American Society for Therapeutic Radiology and Oncology Consensus Panel. Consensus statement: guidelines for PSA following radiation therapy. *Int J Radiat Oncol Biol Phys* 1997;37:1035–1041.

15. Gretzer MB, Trock BJ, Han M, et al. A critical analysis of the interpretation of biochemical failure in surgically treated patients using the American Society for Therapeutic Radiation and Oncology criteria. *J Urol* 2002;168:1419–1422.

16. Ravery V. The significance of recurrent PSA after radical prostatectomy: benign versus malignant sources. *Semin Urol Oncol* 1999;17:127–129.

17. Moul JW. Variables in predicting survival based on treating "PSA-only" relapse. *Urol Oncol* 2003;21:292–304.

18. Boccon-Gibod L, Ravery V, Vordos D, et al. Radical prostatectomy for prostate cancer. The perineal approach increases the risk of surgically induced positive margins and capsular incisions. *J Urol* 1998;160:1383–1385.

19. Mostofi FK, Sesterhenn IA, Davis CJ, et al. Benign prostatic glands in the surgical margin in radical retropubic prostatectomies. *J Urol* 1998;159 (Suppl. 5):297 (#1147A).

20. Fowler JE Jr, Brooks J, Pandey P, et al. Variable histology of anastomotic biopsies with detectable prostate specific antigen after radical prostatectomy. *J Urol* 1995;153:1011–1014.

21. Foster LS, Jajodia P, Fournier G Jr, et al. The value of prostate specific antigen and transrectal ultrasound guided biopsy in detecting prostatic fossa recurrences following radical prostatectomy. *J Urol* 1993;149:1024–1028.

22. Wood DP, Peretsman SJ, Seay TM. Incidence of benign and malignant prostate tissue in biopsies of the bladder neck after radical prostatectomy. *J Urol* 1995;154:1443–1446.

23. Lepor H, Chan S, Melamed J. The role of bladder neck biopsy in men undergoing radical retropubic prostatectomy with preservation of the bladder neck. *J Urol* 1998;160:2435–2439.

24. Shah O, Melamed J, Lepor H. Analysis of apical soft tissue margins during radical retropubic prostatectomy. *J Urol* 2001;165:1943–1949.

25. Ponthieu A, Delgrande J, Ivaldi A. Perioperative biopsy of the sub-apical urethra during prostatectomy for cancer. *Prog Urol* 1996;6:250–255.

26. deVere White RW, Meyers FJ, Soares SE, et al. Urinary prostate specific antigen levels: role in monitoring the response of prostate cancer to therapy. *J Urol* 1992;147:947–951.

27. Iwakiri J, Granbois K, Wehner N, et al. An analysis of urinary prostate specific antigen before and after radical prostatectomy: evidence for secretion of prostate specific antigen by the periurethral glands. *J Urol* 1993;149:783–786.

28. Takayama TK, Vessella RL, Brawer MK, et al. Urinary prostate specific antigen levels after radical prostatectomy. *J Urol* 1994;151:82–87.

29. Stamey TA, Graves HCB, Wehner N, et al. Early detection of residual prostate cancer after radical prostatectomy by an ultrasensitive assay for prostate specific antigen. *J Urol* 1993;149:787–792.

30. Ellis WJ, Vessella RL, Noteboom JL, et al. Early detection of recurrent prostate cancer with an ultrasensitive chemiluminescent prostate-specific antigen assay. *Urology* 1997;50(4):573–579.

31. Witherspoon LR, Lapeyrolerie T. Sensitive prostate specific antigen measurements identify men with long disease free intervals and differentiate aggressive from indolent cancer recurrences within 2 years after radical prostatectomy. *J Urol* 1997;157:1322–1328.

32. Haese A, Huland E, Graefen M, et al. Ultrasensitive detection of prostate specific antigen in the follow-up of 422 patients after radical prostatectomy. *J Urol* 1999;161:1206–1211.

33. Yu H, Diamandis EP, Wong PY, et al. Detection of prostate cancer relapse with prostate specific antigen monitoring at levels of 0.001 to 0.1 microG./L. *J Urol* 1997;157:913–918.

34. Yu H, Diamandis EP. Measurement of serum prostate specific antigen levels in women and in prostatectomized men with an ultrasensitive immunoassay technique. *J Urol* 1995;153:1004–1008.

35. Doherty AP, Bower M, Smith GL, et al. Undetectable ultrasensitive PSA after radical prostatectomy for prostate cancer predicts relapse-free survival. *Br J Cancer* 2000;83(11):1432–1436.

36. Shinghal R, Yemoto C, McNeal JE, et al. Biochemical recurrence without PSA progression characterizes a subset of patients after radical prostatectomy. *Urology* 2003;61(2):380–385.

37. Partin AW, Pearson JD, Landis PK, et al. Evaluation of serum prostate specific antigen velocity after radical prostatectomy to distinguish local recurrence from distant metastasis. *Urology* 1994;43:649–659.

38. Patel A, Dorey F, Franklin J, et al. Recurrence patterns after radical retropubic prostatectomy: clinical usefulness of prostate specific antigen doubling times and log slope prostate specific antigen. *J Urol* 1997;158:1441–1445.

39. Koch MO, Foster RS, Bell B, et al. Characterization and predictors of prostate specific antigen progression rates after radical retropubic prostatectomy. *J Urol* 2000;164:749–753.

40. Pruthi RS, Johnstone I, Tu IP, et al. Prostate-specific antigen doubling times in patients who have failed radical prostatectomy: correlation with histologic characteristics of the primary cancer. *Urology* 1997;49(5):737–742.

41. Kaplan ID, Cox RS, Bagshaw MA. Prostate specific antigen after external beam radiotherapy for prostate cancer. *J Urol* 1993;149:415–419.

42. Zietman AL, Coen JJ, Shipley WU, et al. Radical radiation therapy in the management of prostatic adenocarcinoma: the initial PSA value as a predictor of treatment outcome. *J Urol* 1994;151:640–645.

43. Stamey TA, Ferrari MK, Schmid H-P. The value of serial PSA determinations 5 years after radiotherapy. Steeply increasing values characterize 80% of patients. *J Urol* 1993;150:1856–1859.

44. Willett CG, Zietman AL, Shipley WU, et al. The effect of pelvic radiation therapy on the production of prostatic specific antigen. *J Urol* 1994;151:1579–1581.

45. Zietman AL, Zehr EM, Shipley WU. The production of prostate specific antigen by benign prostatic tissue: the long-term effects of external radiation. *Int J Radiat Oncol Biol Phys* 1999;43:715–718.

46. Pollack A, Hanlon AL, Movsas B, et al. Biochemical failure as a determinant of distant metastasis and death in prostate cancer treated with radiotherapy. *Int J Radiat Oncol Biol Phys* 2003;57:19–23.

47. Kupelian PA, Buchsbaum JC, Patel C. Impact of biochemical failure on overall survival after radiation therapy for localized prostate cancer in the PSA era. *Int J Radiat Oncol Biol Phys* 2002;52:704–711.

48. Vicini FA, Kestin LL, Martinez AA. The importance of adequate follow-up in defining treatment success after external beam irradiation for prostate cancer. *Int J Radiat Oncol Biol Phys* 1999;45:553–561.

49. Thames H, Kuban D, Levy L, et al. A comparison of alternative biochemical failure definitions based on clinical outcome in 4839 prostate cancer patients treated by external beam radiotherapy between 1986 and 1995. *Int J Radiat Oncol Biol Phys* 2003;57:929–943.

50. Zietman AL, Chung CS, Coen JJ, et al. 10-year outcome for men with localized prostate cancer treated with external radiation therapy: results of a cohort study. *J Urol* 2004;171:210–214.

51. Zietman AL, Moughan J, Owen J, et al. The Patterns of Care survey of radiation therapy in localized prostate cancer: similarities between the practice nationally and in minority-rich areas. *Int J Radiat Oncol Biol Phys* 2001;50:75–80.

52. Pickles T, Kim-Sing C, Morris WJ, et al. Evaluation of the Houston biochemical relapse definition in men treated with prolonged neoadjuvant and adjuvant androgen ablation and assessment of follow-up lead-time bias. *Int J Radiat Oncol Biol Phys* 2003;57:11–18.

53. Coen JJ, Chung CS, Shipley WU, et al. The influence of follow-up bias on PSA failure after external radiation for localized prostate cancer: results from a 10 year cohort analysis. *Int J Radiat Oncol Biol Phys* 2003;57:621–628.

54. Critz FA, Williams WH, Holladay CT, et al. Post-treatment PSA ≤0.2 ng/mL defines disease freedom after radiotherapy for prostate cancer using modern techniques. *Urology* 1999;54:968–971.

55. Pollack A, Zagars GK, Smith LG, et al. Preliminary results of a randomized radiotherapy dose-escalation study comparing 70Gy with 78Gy for prostate cancer. *J Clin Oncol* 2000;18:3904–3911.

56. Ragde H, Elgamal AA, Snow PB, et al. Ten-year disease free survival after transperineal sonography-guided iodine-125 brachytherapy with or without 45-gray external beam irradiation in the treatment of patients with clinically localized, low to high Gleason grade prostate carcinoma. *Cancer* 1998;83(5):989–1001.

57. Scardino PT, Wheeler TM. Local control of prostate cancer with radiotherapy: frequency and prognostic significance of positive results of postirradiation prostate biopsy. *NCI Monogr* 1988;7:95–103.

58. Kuban DA, El-Mahdi AM, Schellhammer PF. The significance of postirradiation prostate biopsy with long-term follow-up. *Int J Radiat Oncol Biol Phys* 1992;24:409–414.

59. Babaian RJ, Kojima M, Saitoh M, et al. Detection of residual prostate cancer after external radiotherapy. *Cancer* 1995;75:2153–2158.
60. Crook J, Malone S, Perry G, et al. Postradiotherapy prostate biopsies: what do they really mean? Results for 498 patients. *Int J Radiat Oncol Biol Phys* 2000;48:355–367.
61. Dugan TC, Shipley WU, Young RH, et al. Biopsy after external beam radiation therapy for adenocarcinoma of the prostate: correlation with original histologic grade and current prostatic specific antigen levels. *J Urol* 1991;146:1313–1316.

CHAPTER 15B
Management of Rising Prostate-specific Antigen Following Surgery or Radiation Therapy

Anthony V. D'Amico

INTRODUCTION

Although generally found in an asymptomatic patient with prostate cancer, prostate-specific antigen (PSA)–defined disease recurrence after initial therapy with radical prostatectomy or external beam radiation therapy (EBRT) is considered treatment failure (1) and often triggers the start of secondary therapy (2). However, it remains unknown whether PSA-defined recurrence given time will translate into prostate cancer–specific mortality (PCSM), particularly for men with competing causes of mortality (3).

To identify patients for whom a PSA-defined recurrence is likely to translate into death from prostate cancer, investigators have tried to identify prognostic factors associated with the time to documentation of distant disease recurrence (i.e., positive bone scan) after PSA-defined recurrence. From these investigations (4–8), one posttreatment clinical parameter, a short posttreatment PSA doubling time (PSA-DT), was consistently found to be statistically significantly associated with the time to distant recurrence after PSA-defined recurrence.

Factors were then determined that were associated with the time to PCSM after PSA-defined recurrence. Specifically, D'Amico et al. (9) studied potential candidate determinants of time to PCSM after PSA-defined recurrence in patients treated with radiation therapy and found that, after a PSA-defined recurrence, patients with a short posttreatment PSA-DT had an estimated PCSM and an estimated all-cause mortality that were nearly identical. These results confirmed the findings of Sandler et al. (10) on the prognostic significance of a short posttreatment PSA-DT. Thus, a short posttreatment PSA-DT appears to identify patients with PSA-defined recurrence after radiation therapy that were at high risk for PCSM.

SURROGATE ENDPOINT FOR PROSTATE CANCER-SPECIFIC MORTALITY

In a recent study (11), baseline, treatment, and follow-up data on 8,669 patients with clinical stage T1b-4, NX or N0, M0 adenocarcinoma of the prostate treated with radical prostatectomy or radiation therapy at 44 institutions throughout the United States (12,13) were used to assess whether a short posttreatment PSA-DT after radical prostatectomy or radiation therapy could serve as its surrogate endpoint. Utilizing Cox regression analyses (14), Prentice's criteria (15) were employed to see if a surrogate for prostate cancer-specific mortality could be determined. In the process of the analysis in order to be certain that the magnitude of the PSA-DT would be the same for patients treated surgically and with radiation therapy who experienced the same absolute elevations in PSA level, the nadir PSA level was subtracted from the PSA level after radiation therapy and then the PSA-DT was calculated. This normalization decreased the calculated PSA-DT in the radiation-managed patients.

The results indicated that the posttreatment PSA-DT was statistically significantly associated with time to PCSM and with time to all-cause mortality (all $P_{Cox} < .001$). However, the treatment received was not statistically significantly associated with time to PCSM after PSA-defined disease recurrence for patients with a PSA-DT of less than 3 months ($P_{Cox} = .90$) and for patients with a PSA-DT of 3 months or greater ($P_{Cox} = .28$) when controlling for the specific value of the PSA-DT consistent with the requirements for Prentice's criteria for surrogacy. In that study, among the patients who had a PSA-defined recurrence, including 611 patients treated surgically and 840 patients treated with radiation therapy, 12% (95% CI: 9% to 15%) and 20% (95% CI: 18% to 23%) respectively, had a PSA-DT of <3 months. Furthermore, after a PSA-defined recurrence, a PSA-DT of less than 3 months was significantly associated with time to PCSM (median time: 6 years; hazard ratio = 19.6, 95% confidence interval = 12.5 to 30.9).

Management of the Patient with a Short PSA-DT (<3 months)

Given the median cancer-specific and overall survival after PSA-defined recurrence in patients with a PSA-DT <3 months of only 6 years, as shown in Figures 15B.1 and 15B.2, respectively, and the hazard ratio for cancer-specific mortality following a PSA-defined recurrence of 19.6 suggests these patients already harbor occult micrometastatic prostate cancer. Specifically, the median survival of 1,387 newly diagnosed patients with minimal metastatic prostate cancer has been reported to range from 4.25 to 4.33 years following either orchiectomy or combined hormonal blockade, respectively, from a large randomized trial (16), supporting the hypothesis that patients with a PSA-DT <3 months have occult micrometastatic disease that is likely to be documented on bone scan in relatively short order following PSA failure. In addition, given that a short PSA-DT has been shown to be associated with a short time to bone metastases recurrence after PSA-defined recurrence (4–8), these men are at very high risk for developing metastatic bone disease and subsequent pathologic fracture and spinal cord compression in a relatively short time after PSA-defined recurrence. Therefore, these are the men who are most likely to benefit from an extended relatively symptom-free interval provided by the early salvage hormonal therapy. Consequently, patients with a PSA-DT of <3 months should be given the opportunity to begin androgen-suppression therapy. These patients should also be referred for entry into clinical trials that are examining new forms of systemic therapy, which may further benefit them. One such active trial is Radiation Therapy Oncology Group (RTOG) P-0014, a phase III randomized study of patients with high-risk, hormone-naïve prostate cancer who have failed therapy for localized disease and have a rising PSA with a short PSA-DT. Patients are randomized to either androgen blockade with cycles of immediate chemotherapy or androgen blockade with delayed chemotherapy. The goal is to assess whether chemotherapy known to be effective in hormone-refractory prostate cancer may help address the presence of subclinical metastatic disease known to exist in patients with a rapidly rising PSA.

While a survival benefit is not expected to prompt initiation of salvage hormonal therapy at the time of PSA failure for

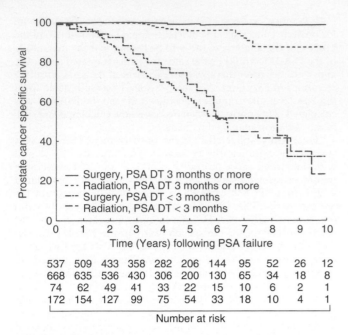

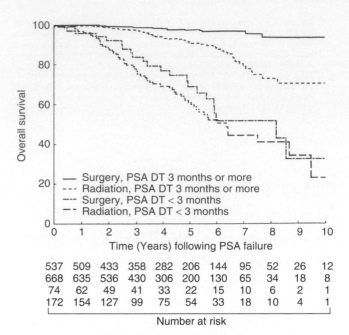

537	509	433	358	282	206	144	95	52	26	12
668	635	536	430	306	200	130	65	34	18	8
74	62	49	41	33	22	15	10	6	2	1
172	154	127	99	75	54	33	18	10	4	1

Number at risk

FIGURE 15B.1. Prostate cancer–specific survival after prostate-specific antigen (PSA)–defined recurrence stratified by treatment received and the value of the posttreatment PSA doubling time (DT). Pairwise two-sided log-rank test was used.
P values are as follows: for a PSA-DT of <3 months (PSA-DT <3 months; surgery vs. radiation), $P = .38$; for PSA-DT of ≥3 months (PSA-DT ≥3 months; surgery vs. radiation), $P < .001$; for PSA-DT of <3 months vs. PSA-DT ≥ 3 months (surgery), $P < .001$; for PSA-DT of <3 months versus PSA-DT ≥ 3 months (radiation), $P < .001$.
PSA-DT ≥3 months (surgery), 3 years: 99.8 [95% CI: 99.4, 100]; 5 years: 99.4 [95% CI: 98.6, 100]; 8 years: 98.9 [95% CI: 97.6, 100]
PSA-DT ≥3 months (radiation), 3 years: 99.6 [95% CI: 99.1, 100]; 5 years: 96.1 [95% CI: 94, 98.2]; 8 years: 87.6 [95% CI: 81.2, 94]
PSA-DT <3 months (surgery), 3 years: 84.1 [95% CI: 74.4, 93.8]; 5 years: 68.8 [95% CI: 55, 82.6]; 8 years: 51.5 [95% CI: 34.8, 68.3]
PSA-DT <3 months (radiation), 3 years: 79.1 [95% CI: 72.5, 85.8]; 5 years: 61.6 [95% CI: 53, 70.4]; 8 years: 41.6 [95% CI: 29.8, 53.4]

FIGURE 15B.2. Overall survival after prostate-specific antigen (PSA)–defined recurrence stratified by treatment received and the value of the posttreatment PSA doubling time (DT). Pairwise two-sided log-rank test was used.
P values are as follows: for PSA-DT of <3 months (PSA-DT < 3 months; surgery vs. radiation), $P = .34$; for PSA-DT of ≥3 months (PSA-DT ≥3 months; surgery vs. radiation), $P < .001$; for PSA-DT <3 months vs. PSA-DT ≥3 months (surgery), $P < .001$; for PSA-DT <3 months vs. PSA-DT ≥3 months (radiation), $P < .001$.
PSA-DT ≥3 months (surgery), 3 years: 99.1 [95% CI: 98.2, 100]; 5 years: 97.6 [95% CI: 95.9, 99.3]; 8 years: 93.9 [95% CI: 89.7, 98.1]
PSA DT ≥3 months (radiation), 3 years: 97.7 [95% CI: 96.4, 98.9]; 5 years: 91.7 [95% CI: 88.9, 94.6]; 8 years: 73 [95% CI: 64.8, 81.4]
PSA-DT <3 months (surgery), 3 years: 84.1 [95% CI: 74.4, 93.8]; 5 years: 68.8 [95% CI: 55, 82.6]; 8 years: 51.5 [95% CI: 34.8, 68.3]
PSA-DT <3 months (radiation), 3 years: 78.5 [95% CI: 71.8, 85.3]; 5 years: 61 [95% CI: 52.1, 69.8]; 8 years: 41 [95% CI: 29.1, 52.8]

patients with a PSA-DT of <3 months, the possibility exists that a survival benefit may exist in patients with larger values of PSA-DT. To that end, a randomized study which enrolled patients with clinically localized prostate cancer and a rising PSA following surgery or radiation therapy and randomized them to immediate versus deferred hormonal therapy has been completed by the European Organization for Research and Treatment of Cancer (EORTC 30943). A definitive answer regarding the impact of the timing of salvage hormonal therapy on survival will be forthcoming from this study.

setting with significant comorbid illness, observation is a reasonable approach given that clinical progression during the relatively short life expectancy is unlikely. Randomized studies that have completed accrual and await follow-up and that have addressed the issue of adjuvant post-prostatectomy radiation therapy in patients with pathologic T3N0 disease include the Southwest Oncology Group (SWOG) Protocol 8794 and the EORTC Protocol 22911. To date, there are no randomized studies that have evaluated postprostatectomy salvage radiation therapy versus observation for patients with a rising PSA.

Management of the Patient with a Long PSA-DT (>1 year)

The long median-time interval (>10 years) from PSA failure to PCSM in patients with a PSA-DT in excess of 1 year (11) makes the presence of occult micrometastatic disease much less likely. Therefore, a second opportunity for long-term cancer control may exist in otherwise healthy patients with prolonged PSA-DT. Specifically, salvage local therapy such as EBRT in the postoperative setting or salvage brachytherapy, cyrosurgery, or prostatectomy in the postradiation setting may be attempted if a radiologic work-up with bone scan and pelvic imaging (CT or MRI) do not disclose metastatic or nodal disease and a biopsy-proven local recurrence is found. However, for patients in this

Management of the Patient with an Intermediate PSA-DT (3–12 months)

The optimal management for the patient whose PSA-DT is intermediate remains unanswered. The current recommendation for patients in this setting who are otherwise healthy is to enroll them in a clinical trial. However, if this is not possible, offering salvage local therapy with or without androgen-suppression therapy is a reasonable approach. The RTOG has conducted a randomized study (9601) of EBRT with or without 2 years of high-dose bicalutamide (Casodex 150 mg) for patients with pathologic (p) stage T3 N0 or pT2 N0 with a positive inked resection margin or positive prostate/fossa anastamosis biopsy and a serum PSA level of at least 0.2 ng/mL but not more than 4.0 ng/mL. This study will provide insight on the role of combined modality as opposed to monotherapy for the patient with a rising PSA in the postoperative setting.

References

1. Moul JW. Prostate specific antigen only progression of prostate cancer. *J Urol* 2000;163:1632–1642.
2. Grossfeld GD, Stier DM, Flanders SC, et al. Use of second treatment following definitive local therapy for prostate cancer. Data from the CaPSURE database. *J Urol* 1998;160:1398–1404.
3. D'Amico AV. Predicting prostate-specific antigen recurrence established: now, who will survive? *J Clin Oncol* 2002;20:3188–3190.
4. Pound CR, Partin AW, Eisenberger MA, et al. Natural history of progression after PSA elevation following radical prostatectomy. *JAMA* 1999; 281:1591–1596.
5. Patel A, Dorey F, Franklin J, et al. Recurrence patterns after radical retropubic prostatectomy: clinical usefulness of prostate specific antigen doubling times and log slope prostate specific antigen. *J Urol* 1997;158: 1441–1445.
6. Roberts SG, Blute ML, Bergstralh EJ, et al. PSA doubling time as a predictor of clinical progression after biochemical failure following radical prostatectomy for prostate cancer. *Mayo Clin Proc* 2001;76:576–581.
7. Lee WR, Hanks GE, Hanlon A. Increasing prostate-specific antigen profile following definitive radiation therapy for localized prostate cancer: clinical observations. *J Clin Oncol* 1997;15:230–238.
8. Sartor CI, Strawderman MH, Lin XH, et al. Rate of PSA rise predicts metastatic versus local recurrence after definitive radiotherapy. *Int J Radiat Oncol Biol Phys* 1997;38:941–947.
9. D'Amico AV, Cote K, Loffredo M, et al. Determinants of prostate cancer specific survival following radiation therapy for patients with clinically localized prostate cancer. *J Clin Oncol* 2002;20:4567–4573.
10. Sandler HM, Dunn RL, McLaughlin PW, et al. Overall survival after prostate-specific-antigen detected recurrence following conformal radiation therapy. *Int J Radiat Oncol Biol Phys* 2000;48:629–633.
11. D'Amico AV, Moul J, Carroll P, et al. Surrogate marker for prostate cancer specific mortality following radical prostatectomy or radiation therapy. *J Natl Cancer Inst* 2003;85:1376–1383.
12. Lubeck DP, Litwin MS, Henning JM, et al. The CaPSURE database: a methodology for clinical practice and research in prostate cancer. CaPSURE Research Panel: Cancer of the Prostate Strategic Urologic Research Endeavor. *Urology* 1996;48:773–777.
13. Sun L, Gancarczyk K, Paquette EL, et al. Introduction to the Department of Defense Center for Prostate Disease Research Multicenter National Prostate Cancer Database, and analysis of changes in the PSA-era. *Urol Oncol* 2001;6:203–209.
14. Neter J, Wasserman W, Kutner M, eds. Simultaneous inferences and other topics in regression analysis—1. In: *Applied linear regression models.* Homewood, IL: Richard D Irwin Inc; 1983:150–153.
15. Prentice RL. Surrogate endpoints in clinical trials: definition and operational criteria. *Stat Med* 1989;8:431–440.
16. Eisenberger MA, Blumenstein BA, Crawford ED, et al. Bilateral orchiectomy with or without flutamide for metastatic prostate cancer. *N Engl J Med* 1998;339:1036–1042.

CHAPTER 15C
Management of Rising Prostate-specific Antigen after Local Surgical Therapy

J. Kellogg Parsons and Alan W. Partin

INTRODUCTION

The advent of prostate-specific antigen (PSA) testing precipitated a profound stage migration in prostate cancer (1). By 1996, 75% of patients were presenting with localized disease (2). The increased proportion of low-stage tumors led to greater numbers of men seeking definitive therapy with radiotherapy or surgery. Surveillance, Epidemiology and End Results (SEER) data indicate that, during the late 1980s and early 1990s, the rate of men undergoing radical prostatectomy more than tripled: from 17.4 per 100,000 in 1988 to 54.6 per 100,000 in 1992 (3). It is now estimated that 40% of men with prostate cancer undergo radical prostatectomy, and that 75,000 radical prostatectomies are performed annually in the United States (4).

Of men who undergo radical prostatectomy as primary treatment for prostate cancer, 15% to 46% will manifest an isolated rise in postoperative PSA within 15 years of follow-up. This phenomenon is referred to as biochemical recurrence. Due to the burgeoning population of postprostatectomy patients, biochemical recurrence now poses a health care issue of considerable magnitude, with thousands of new cases identified each year in the United States (5).

In this chapter, we review the definition, natural history, diagnosis, and treatment of biochemical recurrence after definitive surgical therapy for localized prostate cancer. Throughout our discussion, we emphasize practical considerations in the management of these patients.

DEFINITION OF BIOCHEMICAL RECURRENCE

Appropriate PSA Assays

Currently, there are three commercially available PSA assays applicable to clinical urology, each recognizing different isoforms of PSA: total PSA, free PSA, and complexed PSA. The oldest, most ubiquitous assay is the total PSA assay, which measures all immunoreactive forms of PSA present in serum. The literature on biochemical recurrence is uniformly based on measurements of total PSA, and this assay remains the most appropriate test for postsurgical biochemical surveillance. Ultrasensitive assays for total PSA, capable of detection thresholds of .001 to .01 ng/mL, are not recommended for routine surveillance since they are of unproven clinical value (6), may detect minute amounts of PSA originating from nonmalignant extraprostatic sources (7), and may generate problems with false positive results since there is no definitive management for biochemical recurrence (8).

The free PSA assay increases specificity for prostate cancer diagnosis when used in conjunction with total PSA (9). Since its utility for detecting biochemical recurrence has not been assessed, the free PSA assay should not be applied to postoperative surveillance. The complexed PSA assay also enhances prostate cancer detection by increasing specificity (10). Although preliminary data suggest that complexed PSA may be useful for longitudinally monitoring prostate cancer patients after definitive treatment (11), further studies are warranted before its routine use in this setting may be advocated.

Thus, measurement of total PSA currently remains the gold standard for determining biochemical recurrence after surgery. Hereafter, subsequent statements regarding PSA in this chapter are made in reference only to total PSA.

Timing of Postoperative PSA Surveillance

The oncologic goal of any radical prostatectomy—retropubic, perineal, or laparoscopic—is surgical extirpation of all prostatic tissue. The half-life of PSA is 3.15 days (12). Accordingly, serum PSA should fall to undetectable levels within 21 to 30 days after successful surgery (13). There are no uniform guidelines for postoperative PSA surveillance, and practice patterns vary considerably (14). PSA is typically drawn every 3 months during the first year, every 6 months during the second through fifth years, and every 12 months thereafter unless there is clinical or laboratory evidence of recurrent disease (14,15).

There are no uniform standards governing the required duration of follow-up for patients with a persistently undetectable PSA. Kattan et al. have asserted that biochemical recurrence after 7 years is rare (16). Other data suggest that biochemical recurrence may occur in a substantial number of patients well after 7 years. Among patients with biochemical recurrence in the Johns Hopkins series, 19% first developed detectable PSA levels 6 to 9 years after surgery and 4% developed it 10 years after surgery (17). Similarly, approximately 4% of patients in a series from the Mayo Clinic first experienced biochemical recurrence $8^{1}/_{2}$ or more years after surgery (18). These data imply a need for continued biochemical surveillance for at least 10 years following prostatectomy.

Definition of Recurrence: PSA Level

There has been considerable debate as to what level of PSA constitutes true biochemical failure. Recommendations for cut point range from 0.2 ng/mL to 0.5 ng/mL (16,17,19–21). Much of this disagreement arises from uncertainty over how to classify those men who never achieve undetectable levels of PSA but maintain stable levels in the 0.2 ng/mL to 0.3 ng/mL range. If PSA does not become undetectable within 6 weeks after successful surgery there are two potential explanations: (a) the presence of systemic, micrometastatic disease or (b) the presence of residual benign prostate tissue. Previously, persistent detectable PSA was thought to be caused by occult systemic disease (22).

More recent data, however, suggest that men with a PSA in the early postoperative period that is *detectable but stable* often do not progress. In a recent analysis of 2,782 men who underwent radical prostatectomy for localized disease, Amling et al. noted that 50% of patients with postoperative PSAs in the 0.20 ng/mL to 0.29 ng/mL range and 35% of patients in the 0.3 ng/mL to 0.39 ng/mL range within 3 years of surgery did not subsequently progress (23). In addition, Moul et al. recently observed that as many as 26% of radical prostatectomy specimens may have benign glandular tissue at the margins of surgical resection, which could account for stable postoperative PSA levels of up to 0.3 ng/mL (3).

Misinterpretation as systemic disease of persistent, low levels of serum PSA caused by the presence of unresected benign glands could potentially lead to unnecessarily aggressive adjuvant treatment in these patients. Based on these observations, therefore, several recent publications have cited a level of 0.4 ng/mL as an acceptable cutoff for the definitive diagnosis of biochemical recurrence (3,6,18,23).

Thus, if PSA fails to reach undetectable levels after surgery but remains stable at levels less than 0.4 ng/mL for up to 3 years following surgery (a relatively rare occurrence), recent data suggest that it is reasonable to consider retained benign tissue as a potential source of detectable PSA. In this case, expectant management with serial PSAs is acceptable. However, if a detectable PSA rises above 0.4 ng/mL within 3 years after surgery or never falls below 0.4 ng/mL, the presence of systemic disease should be strongly considered.

NATURAL HISTORY OF BIOCHEMICAL RECURRENCE

Incidence of Biochemical Recurrence

Projected incidences of biochemical recurrence after definitive surgical therapy for localized prostate cancer are derived primarily from large institutional series of patients undergoing radical retropubic prostatectomy. Overall, biochemical failure will eventually occur in about one third of these patients, with 15-year PSA-free actuarial survival rates ranging from 54% to 85% (8,16,17,20,24–26). Rates will vary depending upon pathologic stage of tumor, grade, and margin status. Data on the incidence of biochemical failure after perineal prostatectomy are considerably less extensive, but appear to be similar when compared by equivalent stage, grade, and margin status (27,28). Data on the outcomes from laparoscopic radical prostatectomy are not yet mature, but an early report from the Mountsoris Institute indicates an overall 3-year biochemical failure rate of 10%, which is comparable to the 3-year rates observed in retropubic series (29).

Prediction of Biochemical Recurrence

Several instruments—including formulas, graphs, and tables—have been developed to predict which patients are likely to develop biochemical recurrence. Ross et al. applied the broad term "nomogram" to describe instruments that use a set of input data (such as PSA and tumor grade) to predict outcomes (30). The clinical goal of nomograms is to improve the delivery of care by providing clinicians and patients with additional information on which to base treatment decisions. In the case of biochemical recurrence, stratifying patients by risk identifies those patients who would potentially benefit from adjuvant treatment *before* biochemical recurrence occurs. The rationale is to delay or prevent biochemical recurrence in those patients most likely to develop it, thereby altering disease course and potentially improving cancer specific survival.

In 1995, Partin et al. developed a validated equation for predicting early biochemical recurrence in patients with T2 disease after radical retropubic prostatectomy based on Gleason sum, specimen confinement status, and a sigmoidally transformed PSA value (31). Termed "R_w," or the weighted risk of recurrence, the model was updated in 2001 to account for patients with T1c disease (32). More recently, Khan et al. expanded the Partin tables (originally designed to predict pathologic stage prior to radical prostatectomy) to estimate biochemical disease-free survival (33).

At least 12 other nomograms specifically designed to predict the likelihood of biochemical recurrence after radical prostatectomy have been reported (Table 15C.1) (16,34–44). Consistently, the most important variables in these nomograms are preoperative PSA, Gleason grade, specimen confinement status, and seminal vesicle or lymph node involvement (3). Other variables that correlate with biochemical recurrence include DNA ploidy, angiogenesis, p53, p27, bcl-2, Ki67, and E-cadherin coupled with enhancer of zeste homolog 2 status (43,45). As Kattan has noted, however, it is not yet clear whether these individual markers add anything to current predictive models (46).

Although not specifically designed for predicting biochemical recurrence after radical prostatectomy, nomograms have also been constructed for patients in various stages of clinical disease and treatment. At the discretion of the clinician, they may be applied in the post-radical prostatectomy setting (3,30). Detailed descriptions of these nomograms lie beyond the scope of this chapter; suffice it to say that more than 30 now exist (30). No consensus has been reached as to how each should be applied to clinical practice.

Moreover, there are no data to support the hypothesis that aggressive adjuvant treatment of patients likely to experience biochemical recurrence delays its onset, prevents metastatic progression, or improves cancer specific survival. Nevertheless, we and other institutions (3,16) recommend the use of appropriate, validated nomograms in counseling patients after

TABLE 15C.1

MODELS FOR PREDICTION OF BIOCHEMICAL RECURRENCE AFTER RADICAL RETROPUBIC PROSTATECTOMY

Reference	Yr	Number of patients	Prediction instrument	Prediction variables	Validated?
Partin et al. (31)	1995	216	Equation categorizing men into low-, intermediate-, and high-risk groups	PSA, Specimen Gleason sum, Specimen confinement status	Yes
Bauer et al. (34)	1997	132	Equation categorizing men into low-, intermediate-, and high-risk groups	bcl-2 status, p53 status, PSA, Race, Specimen confinement status	No
Bauer et al. (35)	1998	378	Equation categorizing men into low-, intermediate-, and high-risk groups	PSA, Race, Specimen confinement status, Specimen Gleason sum	Yes
D'Amico et al. (36)	1998	862	Probability graph	Pathological stage, PSA, Specimen Gleason sum, Surgical margin status	No
Kattan et al. (37)	1998	983	Probability nomogram	Biopsy Gleason grade, Clinical stage, PSA	Yes
D'Amico et al. (38)	1999	892	Probability nomogram	Biopsy Gleason grade, Clinical stage, PSA	Yes
Graefen et al. (39)	1999	318	Quantitative analysis of high-grade cancer categorizing men into low- and high-risk groups	Biopsy Gleason grade, Number of positive biopsy cores, Pathological stage, PSA, Specimen Gleason grade	No
Kattan et al. (16)	1999	996	Probability nomogram	Lymph node invasion, PSA, Seminal vesicle invasion, Specimen confinement status, Specimen Gleason sum	Yes
Potter et al. (40)	1999	214	Neural network	DNA ploidy, Patient age, Quantified nuclear grade, Specimen confinement status, Specimen Gleason sum	Yes
D'Amico et al. (41)	2000	823	Percentage of positive biopsy cores categorizing men into risk groups	Biopsy Gleason grade, Clinical stage, Percentage of positive biopsy cores, PSA	Yes
Stamey et al. (42)	2000	326	Equation for probability of biochemical failure	Gleason grade, Lymph node invasion, Percent of intraductal cancer, Prostate weight, PSA, Tumor volume, Vascular invasion	Yes
Blute et al. (44)	2001	2,518	Equation categorizing men into low- and high-risk groups	Adjuvant therapy, Gleason sum, PSA, Seminal vesicle invasion, Surgical margin status	Yes
Moul et al. (43)	2001	1,012	Equation categorizing men into four different risk groups	PSA, Race, Specimen confinement status, Specimen Gleason sum	Yes
Roberts et al. (32)	2001	904	Equation categorizing men into low- and high-risk groups	Gleason sum, Lymph node invasion, Seminal vesicle invasion, Surgical margin status	Yes
Khan et al. (33)	2003	1,955	Probability nomogram	Gleason sum, Pathological stage, Surgical margin status	No

surgery in order to direct those at risk into appropriate clinical trials and/or more rigorous programs of surveillance.

Prediction of Time to Metastases and Death

The natural history of progression to clinically significant metastatic disease and death once biochemical recurrence has occurred is variable but is generally prolonged. Pound et al. reported that in a cohort of 304 patients with biochemical recurrence followed for up to 15 years, only 34% progressed to metastases over a median period of 8 years. Of those who progressed, median time to cancer-specific death after documented metastases was 5 years (17). Similarly, recent combined data on 5,918 radical prostatectomy patients showed a cancer-specific death rate among patients with biochemical recurrence ($n = 611$) of only 4% at a median follow-up of 7 years (47). And in another series from the Cleveland Clinic, overall 5-year survival among patients with biochemical recurrence who did not receive salvage therapy was 94% (96% among patients who received salvage therapy) (48).

Since a majority of men will progress slowly once biochemical recurrence has occurred, efforts have been directed toward identifying the minority of men who will progress more rapidly. As we alluded to previously, time to biochemical recurrence has emerged in many analyses as an important indicator of more aggressive disease. In the Johns Hopkins series, men who recurred within 2 years of surgery developed frank

TABLE 15C.2

ESTIMATION OF METASTASIS-FREE SURVIVAL FOLLOWING BIOCHEMICAL RECURRENCE AFTER RADICAL PROSTATECTOMY

			% with metastasis free survival (95% confidence interval)		
			3 Yr	5 Yr	7 Yr
All patients			78 (73 to 84)	63 (56 to 70)	52 (44 to 60)
Gleason sum 5 to 7	Recurrence >2 yr	PSA-DT >10 mo	95 (83 to 96)	86 (74 to 92)	82 (69 to 90)
		PSA-DT ≤10 mo	82 (54 to 94)	69 (40 to 86)	60 (32 to 80)
	Recurrence ≤2 yr	PSA-DT >10 mo	79 (65 to 88)	76 (61 to 86)	59 (40 to 73)
		PSA-DT ≤10 mo	81 (57 to 93)	35 (16 to 56)	15 (4 to 33)
Gleason sum 8 to 10	Recurrence >2 yr		77 (55 to 89)	60 (33 to 79)	47 (17 to 72)
	Recurrence ≤2 yr		53 (39 to 66)	31 (17 to 45)	21 (9 to 35)

From Pound CR, Partin AW, Eisenberger MA, et al. Natural history of progression after PSA elevation following radical prostatectomy. *JAMA* 1999;281(17):1591–1597; and Laufer M, Pound CR, Carducci MA, et al. Management of patients with rising prostate-specific antigen after radical prostatectomy. *Urology* 2000;55(3):309–315, with permission.

metastases earlier then men who did not (17,49). Amling et al. confirmed this observation in two separate analyses showing that patients who experienced rapid biochemical progression within 1 to 3 years of surgery progressed more quickly to metastases and death (23,50).

Still, a significant number of men who experience biochemical progression many years after surgery will nevertheless progress rapidly (18,50). Because of this, the study of PSA kinetics (measures of PSA changes) has proven valuable in evaluating these patients. Partin et al. showed that PSA velocity (PSAV), the change in PSA per unit time, at one year after surgery correlated with worse outcomes, such that a velocity greater than or equal to 0.75 ng/mL/year was associated with an increased likelihood of early metastases (12).

An even more useful parameter is PSA doubling time (PSA-DT). First described by Patel et al. (51), many studies have subsequently confirmed the accuracy of PSA-DT in estimating the aggressiveness of disease (17,50,52). Conceptually, PSA doubling time represents the amount of time it takes for serum PSA levels to double. It is calculated by: (a) log-transforming longitudinal PSA levels to create a linear relationship between serum PSA level and time; (b) determining the slope of this log-transformed curve; and (c) multiplying the slope of the log-transformed curve by the inverse of the natural log (ln) of 2 (51).

Shorter PSA-DTs are associated with worse prognoses (17,51,52). D'Amico et al. recently reported that PSA-DT accurately predicts prostate cancer-specific mortality, suggesting its potential use as a surrogate for cancer-specific death after surgery or radiation (47). The advantage of PSA-DT over time to recurrence or one year PSAV is that it predicts metastatic progression independent of how many years have elapsed since surgery (18,51). Cut point values for stratifying patients into low-risk and high-risk groups for progression to distant metastases range from 6 (51,52) to 10 months (17). The Johns Hopkins group combined PSA-DT with Gleason sum and time to biochemical recurrence to construct a table predicting those patients less likely to enjoy metastasis-free survival at 3, 5, and 7 years (Table 15C.2) (8,17). As we discuss shortly, combining PSA kinetics with pathologic features in this manner currently represents the most effective means with which to distinguish between local and distant disease.

DIAGNOSIS OF BIOCHEMICAL RECURRENCE: LOCAL VERSUS SYSTEMIC DISEASE

One of the most problematic aspects of evaluating patients with biochemical recurrence is determining the source of the rising PSA; that is, establishing whether it is caused by local or systemic disease. As we previously noted, a PSA ≥0.4 ng/mL within 3 years of surgery in a patient who never achieved undetectable levels likely represents occult systemic disease. But a rising PSA in a patient with a previously undetectable PSA represents a more challenging scenario: should therapy be directed toward the prostatic fossa (i.e., radiotherapy), or systemically with the intent of eradicating distant metastases (i.e., androgen ablation)? Estimates for the incidence of isolated local recurrence vary widely, between 4% and 53%, reflective of the difficulty in establishing this diagnosis (8,15,53–55).

Current diagnostic modalities for distinguishing between local and systemic disease remain limited. Available options (summarized in Tables 15C.3 and 15C.4) are as follows.

TABLE 15C.3

PSA AND PATHOLOGIC VARIABLES FOR DISTINGUISHING BETWEEN LOCAL AND SYSTEMIC DISEASE IN PATIENTS WITH BIOCHEMICAL RECURRENCE AFTER RADICAL PROSTATECTOMY

Variable	Local recurrence	Systemic recurrence
Gleason sum (49)	≤7	>7
Lymph node invasion (49)	no	yes
PSA-DT (17,51,52)	>6 to 10 mo	≤6 to 10 mo
PSA velocity at one year (12,49)	<0.75 ng/mL/yr	≥0.75 ng/mL/yr
Seminal vesicle invasion (49)	no	yes
Time to PSA recurrence (12,50,51,56)	<1 to 2 yr	<1 to 2 yr

TABLE 15C.4

DIAGNOSTIC MODALITIES FOR DISTINGUISHING BETWEEN LOCAL AND SYSTEMIC DISEASE IN PATIENTS WITH BIOCHEMICAL RECURRENCE AFTER RADICAL PROSTATECTOMY

Diagnostic modality	Clinical usefulness for distinguishing between local and systemic recurrence
Digital rectal examination (DRE)	Marginal
Ultrasound-guided biopsy	Marginal
Computed tomography (CT)	Marginal, particularly at low PSA
Magnetic resonance imaging (MRI)	Not defined
Bone scan	Marginal at PSA <10 to 50 ng/mL
Radiolabeled antibody to prostate-specific membrane antigen (PSMA)	Potentially useful—further trials needed in setting of biochemical recurrence
Positron emission tomography (PET)	Not defined

PSA Kinetics and Tumor Pathology

PSA kinetics and tumor pathology are the most useful parameters for estimating the likelihood that isolated local disease is present (6). As mentioned in the preceding section, there are three PSA measurements that suggest the presence of systemic disease: (a) time to biochemical recurrence less than 1 to 2 years (12,50,51,56), (b) PSAV at 1 year greater than or equal to 0.75 ng/mL/year (12), and (c) PSA-DT <6 to 10 months (17, 51,52). All may be used in determining whether an isolated PSA recurrence likely represents local or systemic disease.

In making this determination, PSA kinetics may be combined with tumor pathology. Partin el al. designed a nomogram stratifying patients into low-risk and high-risk groups for distant metastases based on 1-year PSAV, pathologic stage, and Gleason sum (49). The usefulness of using PSA kinetics and tumor pathology in selecting potential patients for radiotherapy was demonstrated by Cadeddu et al., who showed that patients with a time to biochemical recurrence of less than 1 year, Gleason sum greater than 8, or positive seminal vesicles or lymph nodes rarely respond to radiotherapy (57). A summary of PSA and pathologic variables that correlate with an increased likelihood of distant disease is presented in Table 15C.3.

Digital Rectal Examination

Digital rectal examination (DRE) should be performed with the recognition that its diagnostic utility is limited. The postoperative contour of the prostatic fossa is highly variable and correlates poorly to the presence of local recurrence (58). In published series, 23% to 50% of patients with biopsy-proven localized recurrence had no palpable abnormalities (53,59, 60). Management decisions, therefore, should not be based on examination findings alone.

Ultrasound-guided Biopsy

Biopsy directed toward the vesicourethral anastomosis or an ultrasound-detected lesion would seem a straightforward method for either establishing or ruling out local recurrence. Indeed, sensitivities of 76% to 96%, specificities of 26% to 67%, and positive predictive values of up to 95% have been documented with biopsies of ultrasound-identified lesions (53,54,61).

In practice, however, the clinical utility of postprostatectomy biopsy has been the subject of much controversy. There are at least four substantial problems with employing ultrasound-guided biopsy as a diagnostic tool for guiding therapy. First, the true sensitivity of ultrasound in detecting local recurrence is not known. Second, since the true false-negative rate is not known (5,6), negative biopsy does not preclude the presence of local disease. Third, distant disease may exist concomitantly with local disease (6,56), which would render a positive biopsy result irrelevant if one could not be certain that metastatic disease was not also present. Fourth, and perhaps most importantly, postbiopsy salvage radiation therapy to the prostatic bed has produced similar results regardless of whether the biopsy was positive or negative (57,62). Therefore, the role of biopsy in the evaluation of postprostatectomy biochemical recurrence is minimal.

Computed Tomography

Computed tomography (CT) of the abdomen and pelvis has poor yield for identifying local or metastatic disease after radical prostatectomy (63,64). Seltzer et al. suggested that the yield of CT is particularly low for biochemical recurrence patients with lower PSA and PSA velocity (65). Although this analysis included patients who had undergone radiation therapy and cryosurgery as well as radical prostatectomy for primary therapy, a more recent review by Kane et al. of 132 patients with PSA recurrence after radical prostatectomy produced similar results. In this study, only 14% of patients had positive CT scans within 3 years of biochemical recurrence. The mean PSA in this group was 27 ng/mL and the PSA velocity was 1.8 ng/mL/mo—both significantly higher than in the group with negative CT scans (5 ng/mL and 0.7 ng/mL/mo, respectively) (66). As such, performance of CT scan in patients with low PSA and/or low PSA velocity may be considered for obtaining a baseline study, but should not be used to direct local versus systemic care.

Magnetic Resonance Imaging

Since its efficacy in identifying local recurrence is currently unclear, the primary role for endorectal magnetic resonance imaging (MRI) has been to rule out osseous metastases after an equivocal bone scan (6). Several studies are ongoing as to whether new MRI modalities may be useful for identifying soft-tissue and nodal disease. The use of ferromagnetic materials to detect lymph node lesions (67) may prove useful, but at this time MRI should be considered an investigational modality.

Bone Scan

A 1998 survey found that 68% of urologists recommended obtaining a bone scan on patients with biochemical recurrence more than 1 year after surgery, regardless of PSA level (68). Like CT scan, however, bone scan has limited clinical utility in asymptomatic men with biochemical recurrence and low PSA. Among 127 patients who had a bone scan within 3 years of documented biochemical recurrence, only 9.4% were positive, with a mean PSA among those testing positive of 61.3 ng/mL (66). In other studies, the probabilities of a positive bone scan in patients with a PSA less than 40 ng/mL and less than 10 ng/mL were 5% and 1%, respectively (69,70).

On the basis of these data, recent publications have recommended bone scans only for those patients with serum PSA greater than 10 to 50 ng/mL and/or with suspicious PSA kinetics (3,6,69). If serum PSA is less than 10 ng/mL, performance of bone scan may be considered to obtain a baseline study.

Radiolabeled Antibody to Prostate-specific Membrane Antigen

Prostate-specific membrane antigen (PMSA) is a prostate-restricted cell-surface antigen expressed by all prostate cancers. Expression tends to be increased in poorly differentiated, metastatic, and hormone refractory cancers. Antibodies to PSMA tagged with radioactive particles have been developed to identify areas of tumor cell activity to use as information for diagnostic and therapeutic purposes. In 1997, the FDA approved use of a monoclonal, radiolabeled anti-PSMA antibody—capromab pendetide, or ProstaScint (from Cytogen Corporation, Princeton, NJ)—for imaging of soft tissue metastases. Its use in the diagnosis of osseous metastases has not as of yet been approved because the antibody targets the intracytoplasmic portion of the protein, although a more recent incarnation employing a different polyclonal antibody may circumvent this problem (71).

Sensitivities for capromab pendetide range from 62% to 75% (72,73). Many of these results are from early trials performed in patients with significant tumor burden. A more recent trial suggests that capromab pendetide may also be a promising test for discerning local from systemic disease in patients with serum PSA as low as 0.5 ng/mL (74). More prospective trials are needed to fully evaluate capromab pendetide in the setting of biochemical recurrence.

Positron Emission Tomography

Positron emission tomography (PET) scanning, which utilizes a radiolabeled glucose analog to identify areas of increased tumor activity, has had only a limited role in the evaluation of biochemical recurrence, primarily because initial results were disappointing (75,76). Newer radiotracers have since been developed, and studies are ongoing (77). PET scanning should therefore be considered an investigational modality.

MANAGEMENT OF BIOCHEMICAL RECURRENCE

Any discussion of the management of biochemical recurrence after radical surgery merits contemplation of this important caveat: currently, there are no data as to whether treatment of biochemical recurrence prevents or delays the onset of metastatic disease or cancer-specific death. While many current treatment modalities are effective at returning serum PSA to undetectable levels, it is unclear as to whether or not this alters the natural history of the disease.

Expectant Management

Since there is no definitive evidence that treatment of biochemical recurrence will slow progression to metastases and/or death, and since Pound et al. demonstrated that the median time for the onset of metastases in untreated patients after an initial rise in PSA was 8 years (17), expectant management may be an appropriate treatment option in select older patients, particularly those with significant comorbidity and/or a lower probability of disease progression. These patients may be followed closely, with treatment reserved for those with increased PSA doubling times (<6–10 months) or evidence of clinical progression.

Salvage Radiotherapy

Salvage radiotherapy should be considered if PSA kinetics, tumor pathology, and radiologic imaging suggest an isolated local recurrence. "Salvage radiotherapy" is the term for radiation applied to the prostatic bed with curative intent for postoperative biochemical recurrence (78). The efficacy of salvage radiotherapy remains unproven. With little data on cancer-specific survival, response to therapy has been documented with respect to PSA changes. Although 60% to 90% of patients may initially achieve an undetectable PSA after radiation, only 10% to 45% remain free of PSA recurrence 5 years later (78–80).

The single most important prognostic factor in predicting objective response to salvage radiotherapy is pretreatment PSA, with a lower PSA portending a greater likelihood of response. In 1999, the American Society for Therapeutic Radiology and Oncology (ASTRO) consensus panel recommended a PSA treatment threshold of 1.5 ng/mL, citing evidence that salvage radiotherapy administered to men with serum PSA at or below this level resulted in superior efficacy (78). Since then, other studies have substantiated the concept that early salvage radiotherapy achieves a more durable response (80–83). The recommended minimum dose needed to exert a therapeutic effect is 64 Gy to 65 Gy (78).

The benefit of adjuvant hormonal therapy with salvage radiotherapy is unproven. A large, randomized, placebo-controlled trial recently demonstrated that bicalutamide at the time of primary radiotherapy confers a significant survival benefit in patients with high-grade or locally advanced disease (84). One small, retrospective study suggested that hormonal therapy may also be useful at the time of salvage radiotherapy (85). However, there are no prospective data. In order to assess the efficacy of hormonal therapy at the time of salvage radiation, the Radiation Therapy Oncology Group is currently performing a study (RTOG 96-01) randomizing patients with isolated PSA increases after radical prostatectomy to radiotherapy alone versus radiotherapy plus bicalutamide 150 mg each day (80).

In summary, salvage radiotherapy is effective at lowering PSA. It should be considered for patients in whom isolated local recurrence is suspected. Treatment while PSA is still low (<1.5 ng/mL) maximizes the potential response. Studies are ongoing as to whether adjuvant hormonal therapy will improve outcomes.

Hormonal Therapy

Androgen ablation for the treatment of advanced prostate cancer may be achieved with bilateral simple orchiectomy, gonadotropin releasing hormone (GnRh) agonist or antagonist therapy, or oral estrogens. The rationale for using androgen ablation for biochemical recurrence is that, in the absence of an isolated local recurrence, biochemical recurrence corresponds to systemic, micrometastatic disease. Debate as to the appropriate timing of androgen ablation for advanced prostate cancer (early vs. late) has continued for many years. Androgen ablation for isolated biochemical recurrence represents early therapy; androgen ablation after a postprostatectomy patient develops clinical evidence of metastases represents late therapy.

While there are no prospective data on whether the use of early androgen ablation for postprostatectomy biochemical recurrence improves outcomes in this patient group, there are prospective data suggesting that early androgen ablation may be efficacious in prolonging survival in select groups of men with advanced or aggressive disease. Data from the United Kingdom Medical Research Council Study demonstrated that early hormonal ablation delayed progression and improved survival in men with locally advanced or asymptomatic metastatic disease (86). Likewise, Messing et al. determined that early hormonal treatment of radical prostatectomy patients with nodal disease significantly improved cancer specific survival at 7 years (87). It is not known, however, whether these results may be applied to men at risk for biochemical recurrence.

Still, Moul et al. recently reported preliminary, retrospective data from the Department of Defense Center for Prostate Disease Research registry that suggest that men who receive early hormonal therapy for biochemical recurrence have a median PSA progression-free survival of >10 years. In a further analysis of 4,430 patients, men with Gleason sum of >7 or PSA-DT of <12 months who received early hormonal therapy experienced increased time to the onset of frank metastases relative to men who did not. However, no survival benefit was noted (3). Further prospective analyses are needed before determining whether early hormonal therapy at the time of biochemical recurrence will improve survival.

Other means by which the androgen axis may be manipulated include maximum androgen blockade, which combines androgen ablation with an oral anti-androgen such as bicalutamide, oral antiandrogens alone, and 5-alpha reductase inhibitors such as finasteride. There are no conclusive data on the use of any of these modalities for the long-term treatment of biochemical recurrence.

In conclusion, there are no definitive data on whether early or delayed hormonal therapy will alter the natural history of biochemical recurrence, delay the onset of metastases, or improve cancer-specific survival.

Future Approaches to Systemic Therapy

Novel investigational agents with potential applications to men with biochemical recurrence include taxane-based combinations of chemotherapy, including docetaxel (77,88); anti-angiogenic agents, including matrix metalloproteinase inhibitors (which inhibit enzymes believed to play a role in prostate cancer tumor invasion and dissemination) (8); and immune-directed agents, including gene-delivery techniques and therapy (77,89).

SUMMARY

The large number of low-stage prostate cancers being diagnosed as a result of PSA screening has driven an increase in the number of men undergoing radical prostatectomy for clinically localized disease. This in turn has led to a growing population of patients with biochemical recurrence.

The most appropriate assay for diagnosing biochemical recurrence is serum total PSA, which should be checked at 3 months after surgery and at least every 12 months thereafter for a minimum of 10 years. Although some investigators advocate a cut-off of ≥0.4 ng/mL for the diagnosis of biochemical recurrence, a cutoff currently acceptable to all investigators is ≥0.2 ng/mL. Persistent, stable levels below 0.2 ng/mL to 0.4 ng/mL for up to 3 years following surgery may be followed expectantly.

Fifteen-year PSA-free actuarial survival rates vary from 54% to 85%. Several validated nomograms exist to stratify patients by risk for biochemical recurrence, and should be used to counsel patients postoperatively. Disease progression following biochemical recurrence is generally indolent. Time to recurrence, PSAV at 1 year, PSA-DT, and tumor features all correlate with risk of progression to metastases and death.

In distinguishing between patients with local and systemic recurrence, PSA kinetics and tumor features remain the most valuable clinical parameters. Digital rectal examination should be performed, but its usefulness at planning therapy is limited. Ultrasound-guided biopsy of the prostatic fossa is not recommended. CT and bone scan have marginal clinical utility at low PSA levels, but may be considered for baseline studies or in the setting of a rapidly rising PSA. MRI, capromab pendetide, and PET scanning are investigational modalities at this time.

Expectant management should be considered in patients with late recurrence, low PSA-DT, and no evidence of clinical disease. Salvage radiotherapy is efficacious at lowering serum PSA in men suspected of having isolated local recurrence, especially with PSA <1.5 ng/mL. However, it is unclear whether it improves survival. Early hormonal therapy for suspected systemic disease will also lower PSA, but there are no prospective data as to whether it will improve cancer-specific survival.

References

1. Hankey BF, Feuer EJ, Clegg LX, et al. Cancer surveillance series: interpreting trends in prostate cancer—part I: evidence of the effects of screening in recent prostate cancer incidence, mortality, and survival rates. *J Natl Cancer Inst* 1999;91(12):1017–1024.
2. Moul JW. Rising PSA after local therapy failure: immediate vs. deferred treatment. *Oncology (Huntingt)* 1999;13(7):985–990, 993; discussion 985–993, 999.
3. Moul JW. Variables in predicting survival based on treating "PSA-only" relapse. *Urol Oncol* 2003;21(4):292–304.
4. Burkhardt JH, Litwin MS, Rose CM, et al. Comparing the costs of radiation therapy and radical prostatectomy for the initial treatment of early-stage prostate cancer. *J Clin Oncol* 2002;20(12):2869–2875.
5. Moul JW. Prostate specific antigen only progression of prostate cancer. *J Urol* 2000;163(6):1632–1642.
6. Swindle PW, Kattan MW, Scardino PT. Markers and meaning of primary treatment failure. *Urol Clin North Am* 2003;30(2):377–401.
7. Diamandis EP, Yu H. Nonprostatic sources of prostate-specific antigen. *Urol Clin North Am* 1997;24(2):275–282.
8. Lauter M, Pound CR, Carducci MA, et al. Management of patients with rising prostate-specific antigen after radical prostatectomy. *Urology* 2000; 55(3):309–315.
9. Catalona WJ, Partin AW, Slawin KM, et al. Use of the percentage of free prostate-specific antigen to enhance differentiation of prostate cancer from benign prostatic disease: a prospective multicenter clinical trial. *JAMA* 1998; 279(19):1542–1547.
10. Parsons JK, Partin AW. Applying complexed PSA to clinical practice. *Urology* 2004;63:27–32.
11. Allard WJ, Cheli CD, Morris DL, et al. Multicenter evaluation of the performance and clinical utility in longitudinal monitoring of the Bayer Immuno 1 complexed PSA assay. *Int J Biol Markers* 1999;14(2):73–83.
12. Partin AW, Oesterling JE. The clinical usefulness of prostate specific antigen: update 1994. *J Urol* 1994;152(5 Pt 1):1358–1368.
13. Oesterling JE, Chan DW, Epstein JI, et al. Prostate specific antigen in the preoperative and postoperative evaluation of localized prostate cancer treated with radical prostatectomy. *J Urol* 1988;139(4):766–772.
14. Oh J, Colberg JW, Ornstein DK, et al. Current followup strategies after radical prostatectomy: a survey of American Urological Association urologists. *J Urol* 1999;161(2):520–523.
15. Han M, Partin AW, Pound CR, et al. Long-term biochemical disease-free and cancer-specific survival following anatomic radical retropubic prostatectomy. The 15-year Johns Hopkins experience. *Urol Clin North Am* 2001; 28(3):555–565.
16. Kattan MW, Wheeler TM, Scardino PT. Postoperative nomogram for disease recurrence after radical prostatectomy for prostate cancer. *J Clin Oncol* 1999;17(5):1499–1507.
17. Pound CR, Partin AW, Eisenberger MA, et al. Natural history of progression after PSA elevation following radical prostatectomy. *JAMA* 1999; 281(17):1591–1597.
18. Ward JF, Blute ML, Slezak J, et al. The long-term clinical impact of biochemical recurrence of prostate cancer 5 or more years after radical prostatectomy. *J Urol* 2003;170(5):1872–1876.
19. Moul JW, Douglas TH, McCarthy WF, et al. Black race is an adverse prognostic factor for prostate cancer recurrence following radical prostatectomy in an equal access health care setting. *J Urol* 1996;155(5):1667–1673.

20. Zincke H, Oesterling JE, Blute ML, et al. Long-term (15 years) results after radical prostatectomy for clinically localized (stage T2c or lower) prostate cancer. *J Urol* 1994;152(5 Pt 2):1850–1857.

21. Freedland SJ, Sutter ME, Dorey F, et al. Defining the ideal cutpoint for determining PSA recurrence after radical prostatectomy. Prostate-specific antigen. *Urology* 2003;61(2):365–369.

22. Ravery V. The significance of recurrent PSA after radical prostatectomy: benign versus malignant sources. *Semin Urol Oncol* 1999;17(3):127–129.

23. Amling CL, Bergstralh EJ, Blute ML, et al. Defining prostate specific antigen progression after radical prostatectomy: what is the most appropriate cut point? *J Urol* 2001;165(4):1146–1151.

24. Catalona WJ, Smith DS. 5-year tumor recurrence rates after anatomical radical retropubic prostatectomy for prostate cancer. *J Urol* 1994;152(5 Pt 2):1837–1842.

25. Khan MA, Han M, Partin AW, et al. Long-term cancer control of radical prostatectomy in men younger than 50 years of age: update 2003. *Urology* 2003;62(1):86–91; discussion 82–91.

26. Trapasso JG, deKernion JB, Smith RB, et al. The incidence and significance of detectable levels of serum prostate specific antigen after radical prostatectomy. *J Urol* 1994;152(5 Pt 2):1821–1825.

27. Iselin CE, Robertson JE, Paulson DF. Radical perineal prostatectomy: oncological outcome during a 20-year period. *J Urol* 1999;161(1):163–168.

28. Harris MJ. Radical perineal prostatectomy: cost efficient, outcome effective, minimally invasive prostate cancer management. *Eur Urol* 2003;44(3):303–308; discussion 308.

29. Guillonneau B, el-Fettouh H, Baumert H, et al. Laparoscopic radical prostatectomy: oncological evaluation after 1,000 cases at Montsouris Institute. *J Urol* 2003;169(4):1261–1266.

30. Ross PL, Scardino PT, Kattan MW. A catalog of prostate cancer nomograms. *J Urol* 2001;165(5):1562–1568.

31. Partin AW, Piantadosi S, Sanda MG, et al. Selection of men at high risk for disease recurrence for experimental adjuvant therapy following radical prostatectomy. *Urology* 1995;45(5):831–838.

32. Roberts WW, Bergstralh EJ, Blute ML, et al. Contemporary identification of patients at high risk of early prostate cancer recurrence after radical retropubic prostatectomy. *Urology* 2001;57(6):1033–1037.

33. Khan MA, Partin AW, Mangold LA, et al. Probability of biochemical recurrence by analysis of pathologic stage, Gleason score, and margin status for localized prostate cancer. *Urology* 2003;62(5):866–871.

34. Bauer JJ, Connelly RR, Sesterhenn IA, et al. Biostatistical modeling using traditional variables and genetic biomarkers for predicting the risk of prostate carcinoma recurrence after radical prostatectomy. *Cancer* 1997;79(5):952–962.

35. Bauer JJ, Connelly RR, Seterhenn IA, et al. Biostatistical modeling using traditional preoperative and pathological prognostic variables in the selection of men at high risk for disease recurrence after radical prostatectomy for prostate cancer. *J Urol* 1998;159(3):929–933.

36. D'Amico AV, Whittington R, Malkowicz SB, et al. The combination of preoperative prostate specific antigen and postoperative pathological findings to predict prostate specific antigen outcome in clinically localized prostate cancer. *J Urol* 1998;160(6 Pt 1):2096–2101.

37. Kattan MW, Eastham JA, Stapleton AM, et al. A preoperative nomogram for disease recurrence following radical prostatectomy for prostate cancer. *J Natl Cancer Inst* 1998;90(10):766–771.

38. D'Amico AV, Whittington R, Malkowicz SB, et al. Pretreatment nomogram for prostate-specific antigen recurrence after radical prostatectomy or external-beam radiation therapy for clinically localized prostate cancer. *J Clin Oncol* 1999;17(1):168–172.

39. Graefen M, Noldus J, Pichlmeier U, et al. Early prostate-specific antigen relapse after radical retropubic prostatectomy: prediction on the basis of preoperative and postoperative tumor characteristics. *Eur Urol* 1999;36(1):21–30.

40. Potter SR, Miller MC, Mangold LA, et al. Genetically engineered neural networks for predicting prostate cancer progression after radical prostatectomy. *Urology* 1999;54(5):791–795.

41. D'Amico AV, Whittington R, Malkowicz SB, et al. Clinical utility of the percentage of positive prostate biopsies in defining biochemical outcome after radical prostatectomy for patients with clinically localized prostate cancer. *J Clin Oncol* 2000;18(6):1164–1172.

42. Stamey TA, Yemoto CM, McNeal JE, et al. Prostate cancer is highly predictable: a prognostic equation based on all morphological variables in radical prostatectomy specimens. *J Urol* 2000;163(4):1155–1160.

43. Moul JW, Connelly RR, Lubeck DP, et al. Predicting risk of prostate specific antigen recurrence after radical prostatectomy with the Center for Prostate Disease Research and Cancer of the Prostate Strategic Urologic Research Endeavor databases. *J Urol* 2001;166(4):1322–1327.

44. Blute ML, Bergstralh EJ, Iocca A, et al. Use of Gleason score, prostate specific antigen, seminal vesicle and margin status to predict biochemical failure after radical prostatectomy. *J Urol* 2001;165(1):119–125.

45. Rhodes DR, Sanda MG, Otte AP, et al. Multiplex biomarker approach for determining risk of prostate-specific antigen-defined recurrence of prostate cancer. *J Natl Cancer Inst* 2003;95(9):661–668.

46. Kattan MW. Judging new markers by their ability to improve predictive accuracy. *J Natl Cancer Inst* 2003;95(9):634–635.

47. D'Amico AV, Moul JW, Carroll PR, et al. Surrogate end point for prostate cancer-specific mortality after radical prostatectomy or radiation therapy. *J Natl Cancer Inst* 2003;95(18):1376–1383.

48. Jhaveri FM, Zippe CD, Klein EA, et al. Biochemical failure does not predict overall survival after radical prostatectomy for localized prostate cancer: 10-year results. *Urology* 1999;54(5):884–890.

49. Partin AW, Pearson JD, Landis PK, et al. Evaluation of serum prostate-specific antigen velocity after radical prostatectomy to distinguish local recurrence from distant metastases. *Urology* 1994;43(5):649–659.

50. Amling CL, Blute ML, Bergstralh EJ, et al. Long-term hazard of progression after radical prostatectomy for clinically localized prostate cancer: continued risk of biochemical failure after 5 years. *J Urol* 2000;164(1):101–105.

51. Patel A, Dorey F, Franklin J, et al. Recurrence patterns after radical retropubic prostatectomy: clinical usefulness of prostate specific antigen doubling times and log slope prostate specific antigen. *J Urol* 1997;158(4):1441–1445.

52. Roberts SG, Blute ML, Bergstralh EJ, et al. PSA doubling time as a predictor of clinical progression after biochemical failure following radical prostatectomy for prostate cancer. *Mayo Clin Proc* 2001;76(6):576–581.

53. Foster LS, Jajodia P, Fournier G Jr, et al. The value of prostate specific antigen and transrectal ultrasound guided biopsy in detecting prostatic fossa recurrences following radical prostatectomy. *J Urol* 1993;149(5):1024–1028.

54. Connolly JA, Shinohara K, Presti JC, Jr, et al. Local recurrence after radical prostatectomy: characteristics in size, location, and relationship to prostate-specific antigen and surgical margins. *Urology* 1996;47(2):225–231.

55. Zietman AL, Shipley WU, Willett CG. Residual disease after radical surgery or radiation therapy for prostate cancer. Clinical significance and therapeutic implications. *Cancer* 1993;71(Suppl. 3):959–969.

56. Pound CR, Partin AW, Epstein JI, et al. Prostate-specific antigen after anatomic radical retropubic prostatectomy. Patterns of recurrence and cancer control. *Urol Clin North Am* 1997;24(2):395–406.

57. Cadeddu JA, Partin AW, DeWeese TL, et al. Long-term results of radiation therapy for prostate cancer recurrence following radical prostatectomy. *J Urol* 1998;159(1):173–177; discussion 177–178.

58. Lightner DJ, Lange PH, Reddy PK, et al. Prostate specific antigen and local recurrence after radical prostatectomy. *J Urol* 1990;144(4):921–926.

59. Saleem MD, Sanders H, Abu El Naser M, et al. Factors predicting cancer detection in biopsy of the prostatic fossa after radical prostatectomy. *Urology* 1998;51(2):283–286.

60. Fowler JE Jr, Brooks J, Pandey P, et al. Variable histology of anastomotic biopsies with detectable prostate specific antigen after radical prostatectomy. *J Urol* 1995;153(3 Pt 2):1011–1014.

61. Leventis AK, Shariat SF, Slawin KM. Local recurrence after radical prostatectomy: correlation of US features with prostatic fossa biopsy findings. *Radiology* 2001;219(2):432–439.

62. Koppie TM, Grossfeld GD, Nudell DM, et al. Is anastomotic biopsy necessary before radiotherapy after radical prostatectomy? *J Urol* 2001;166(1):111–115.

63. Kramer S, Gorich J, Gottfried HW, et al. Sensitivity of computed tomography in detecting local recurrence of prostatic carcinoma following radical prostatectomy. *Br J Radiol* 1997;70(838):995–999.

64. Johnson PAS. Yield of imaging and scintigraphy assessing bNED failure in prostate cancer patients. *Urol Oncol* 1997;70:995.

65. Seltzer MA, Barbaric Z, Belldegrun A, et al. Comparison of helical computerized tomography, positron emission tomography and monoclonal antibody scans for evaluation of lymph node metastases in patients with prostate specific antigen relapse after treatment for localized prostate cancer. *J Urol* 1999;162(4):1322–1328.

66. Kane CJ, Amling CL, Johnstone PA, et al. Limited value of bone scintigraphy and computed tomography in assessing biochemical failure after radical prostatectomy. *Urology* 2003;61(3):607–611.

67. Harisinghani MG, Barentsz J, Hahn PF, et al. Noninvasive detection of clinically occult lymph-node metastases in prostate cancer. *N Engl J Med* 2003;348(25):2491–2499.

68. Ornstein DK, Colberg JW, Virgo KS, et al. Evaluation and management of men whose radical prostatectomies failed: results of an international survey. *Urology* 1998;52(6):1047–1054.

69. Cher ML, Bianco FJ Jr, Lam JS, et al. Limited role of radionuclide bone scintigraphy in patients with prostate specific antigen elevations after radical prostatectomy. *J Urol* 1998;160(4):1387–1391.

70. Lee CT, Oesterling JE. Using prostate-specific antigen to eliminate the staging radionuclide bone scan. *Urol Clin North Am* 1997;24(2):389–394.

71. Bander NH, Trabulsi EJ, Kostakoglu L, et al. Targeting metastatic prostate cancer with radiolabeled monoclonal antibody J591 to the extracellular domain of prostate specific membrane antigen. *J Urol* 2003;170(5):1717–1721.

72. Quintana JC, Blend MJ. The dual-isotope ProstaScint imaging procedure: clinical experience and staging results in 145 patients. *Clin Nucl Med* 2000;25(1):33–40.

73. Hinkle GH, Burgers JK, Neal CE, et al. Multicenter radioimmunoscintigraphic evaluation of patients with prostate carcinoma using indium-111 capromab pendetide. *Cancer* 1998;83(4):739–747.

74. Raj GV, Partin AW, Polascik TJ. Clinical utility of indium 111-capromab pendetide immunoscintigraphy in the detection of early, recurrent prostate carcinoma after radical prostatectomy. *Cancer* 2002;94(4):987–996.

75. Hofer C, Laubenbacher C, Block T, et al. Fluorine-18-fluorodeoxyglucose positron emission tomography is useless for the detection of local recurrence after radical prostatectomy. *Eur Urol* 1999;36(1):31–35.

76. Effert PJ, Bares R, Handt S, et al. Metabolic imaging of untreated prostate cancer by positron emission tomography with 18fluorine-labeled deoxyglucose. *J Urol* 1996;155(3):994–998.

77. Hricak H, Schoder H, Pucar D, et al. Advances in imaging in the postoperative patient with a rising prostate-specific antigen level. *Semin Oncol* 2003;30(5):616–634.

78. Cox JD, Gallagher MJ, Hammond EH, et al. Consensus statements on radiation therapy of prostate cancer: guidelines for prostate re-biopsy after radiation and for radiation therapy with rising prostate-specific antigen levels after radical prostatectomy. American Society for Therapeutic Radiology and Oncology Consensus Panel. *J Clin Oncol* 1999;17(4):1155.

79. Forman JD, Velasco J. Therapeutic radiation in patients with a rising post-prostatectomy PSA level. *Oncology (Huntingt)* 1998;12(1):33–39; discussion 39, 43–44, 47.

80. Macdonald OK, Schild SE, Vora SA, et al. Radiotherapy for men with isolated increase in serum prostate specific antigen after radical prostatectomy. *J Urol* 2003;170(5):1833–1837.

81. Anscher MS, Clough R, Dodge R. Radiotherapy for a rising prostate-specific antigen after radical prostatectomy: the first 10 years. *Int J Radiat Oncol Biol Phys* 2000;48(2):369–375.

82. Song DY, Thompson TL, Ramakrishnan V, et al. Salvage radiotherapy for rising or persistent PSA after radical prostatectomy. *Urology* 2002;60(2):281–287.

83. Liauw SL, Webster WS, Pistenmaa DA, et al. Salvage radiotherapy for biochemical failure of radical prostatectomy: a single-institution experience. *Urology* 2003;61(6):1204–1210.

84. Bolla M, Collette L, Blank L, et al. Long-term results with immediate androgen suppression and external irradiation in patients with locally advanced prostate cancer (an EORTC Study): a phase III randomised trial. *Lancet* 2002;360(9327):103–106.

85. Eulau SM, Tate DJ, Stamey TA, et al. Effect of combined transient androgen deprivation and irradiation following radical prostatectomy for prostatic cancer. *Int J Radiat Oncol Biol Phys* 1998;41(4):735–740.

86. The Medical Research Council Prostate Cancer Working Party Investigators Group. Immediate versus deferred treatment for advanced prostatic cancer: initial results of the Medical Research Council trial. *Br J Urol* 1997; 79(2):235–246.

87. Messing EM, Manola J, Sarosdy M, et al. Immediate hormonal therapy compared with observation after radical prostatectomy and pelvic lymphadenectomy in men with node-positive prostate cancer. *N Engl J Med* 1999;341(24):1781–1788.

88. Khan MA, Carducci MA, Partin AW. The evolving role of docetaxel in the management of androgen independent prostate cancer. *J Urol* 2003; 170(5):1709–1716.

89. Harrington KJ, Spitzweg C, Bateman AR, et al. Gene therapy for prostate cancer: current status and future prospects. *J Urol* 2001;166(4):1220–1233.

CHAPTER 15D
Adjuvant and Salvage Radiotherapy, Postprostatectomy

Alan Pollack

RATIONALE FOR ADJUVANT AND SALVAGE TREATMENT

Radiotherapy is given after prostatectomy in three main scenarios: (a) adjuvant radiotherapy (ART) in men with an undetectable or just barely detectable prostate-specific antigen (PSA) (a PSA of <0.2 ng/mL is considered adjuvant by most investigators), but with high-risk pathologic features; (b) salvage radiotherapy (SRT) for a delayed rise in PSA (DR-PSA) after the PSA has been undetectable for a period of time; and (c) SRT for a persistently detectable PSA (PD-PSA) after surgery. The rationale for separating adjuvant from salvage is that the overall prognoses after radiotherapy, dose of radiotherapy, and prognostic factors differ to a degree. The salvage patients have been divided into those with a DR-PSA or PD-PSA because the initial considerations in evaluation are different and there may be a distinction in prognosis. The discussions that follow focus on men with no obvious evidence of lymph node involvement pathologically, unless otherwise specified.

Adjuvant Radiotherapy

The judgment to administer ART is based on the recognition of high-risk findings pathologically in the prostatectomy specimen (Table 15D.1) (1–15). The key high-risk features are prostate margin positivity (prostate cancer at the margin of resection), extracapsular extension (ECE), seminal vesicle involvement (SVI), and lymph node involvement (LNI). Table 15D.1 shows that the frequency of ECE is about 40%, margin positivity is 25%, SVI is 10%, and LNI is 5%. Another reason to administer postoperative radiotherapy (RT) includes evidence that some normal prostate was present at the inked margin (a cut-through), even without conclusive evidence that tumor was left behind, and even when the PSA is undetectable. Other pathologic factors, such as perineural invasion, have not consistently been associated with an increased risk of failure biochemically (a postprostatectomy PSA ≥ 0.2 ng/mL) (16–22).

Of the key factors listed, margin positivity has been most conclusively established as a predictor of biochemical and local failure. Approximately 40% to 50% of those with a positive surgical margin will experience a rise in PSA to detectable levels within 5 to 10 years (Table 15D.2) (3,5,23–29). Since it appears that not all patients with positive margins will experience biochemical failure, the extent of extraprostatic extension and the positive margin (focal vs. extensive) (25,26,29–33) should be considered, along with the Gleason score and SVI. A single focal positive margin in the absence of other unfavorable pathologic features has been described as less of an indication; in this setting, extensive extraprostatic extension or Gleason score ≥ 7 disease imparts a greater risk of biochemical failure and a stronger rationale for ART. Likewise the presence of a small amount of ECE as an isolated adverse pathologic finding is not associated with much of an increased risk of biochemical failure, unless the Gleason score is ≥ 7. The enhanced risk of biochemical failure under these conditions is due to both local and distant progression.

Even in "negative margin" cases, when there is a rising PSA later, complete biochemical responses to salvage RT occur, suggesting local residual disease. While a rising PSA after a negative margin has been associated with a worse prognosis in some prostatectomy series and a recent pooled analysis (34,35), not every micron of tissue is pathologically assessed. Obvious ECE with Gleason score ≥ 7 (especially with a major portion or bilateral involvement of the prostate) and negative margins probably has a substantial risk of local persistence on a microscopic level and ART should be considered.

Local persistence of disease is more prevalent following prostatectomy than is generally recognized (see section on endpoints). An autopsy series (36) and reports on aggressive prostatic fossa/urethrovesical anastomosis biopsies (37–40) have documented residual disease in about 50% of prostatectomy cases. Even though men with a focal positive margin and otherwise favorable features have a low biochemical failure rate, long follow-up may be required for failure to manifest, and it may be worthwhile to administer ART in younger men with a long life expectancy. Support for this comes from surgical data that demonstrate a meaningful, continuous risk of biochemical failure between 5 to 10 years, with a yearly relative risk of 2% to 3% on average (6,41–43). Late failures after radical prostatectomy are not insignificant and provide a strong rationale for ART.

Lymph node involvement connotes a very poor prognosis, with a high rate of distant failure. Although there is emerging data that radical prostatectomy or RT should be used along with androgen deprivation when LNI is identified (44), there are few reports on combining prostatectomy with ART in cases of LNI or other high-risk features (45). There is

TABLE 15D.1

INCIDENCE OF ADVERSE PATHOLOGIC FEATURES IN PROSTATECTOMY SPECIMENS FROM CT1-T2 PATIENTS

First author (yr)	Institution	n	ECE	SV+	LN+	Margin+
Ohori (1995)	Baylor	478	43%	12%	5%	16%
Kupelian (1996)	Cleveland Clinic	337	61%	18%	8%	43%
Epstein (1996)	Johns Hopkins	721	58%	7%	8%	23%
Lowe (1997)	OHS	583	35%	4%	3%	15%
Dillioglugil (1997)	Baylor	611	39%	11%	6%	—
Pound (1997)	Johns Hopkins	1,623	52%	6%	7%	—
Bauer (1998)	Walter Reed	378	57%	—	–	—
Ramos (1999)[a]	Wash U	1,620	32%	7%	1%	24%
Gilliland (1999)	USC	1,395	47%	7%	3%	33%
Jhaveri (1999)	Cleveland Clinic	731	54%	—	—	–
Cheng (2000)	Indiana	339	35%	14%	6%	24%
Blute (2000)	Mayo Clinic	2,475	32%	15%	7%	—
Shah (2003)	NYU	535	20%	—	—	11%
Khan (2003)	Johns Hopkins	1,955	35%	4%	4%	10%
Cagiannos (2003)	Pooled	3,903	37%	11%	4%	30.2%

OHS, Oregon Health Sciences University.
[a]T1-T2b (T2c excluded).

no well-established benefit from combining prostatectomy with ART and androgen deprivation in such cases. However, ART might be of some value when there is evidence of an appreciable local/regional tumor burden, such as when there is an extensive positive margin.

Salvage Radiotherapy When There Is a Delayed Rise in PSA (DR-PSA)

In the case of the patient who has manifested biochemical failure without obvious local recurrence (palpable nodule in the prostatic fossa), the choice for SRT is predicated on whether there is a reasonable chance that such treatment will render the patient free of disease. In the setting of a DR-PSA, prostatectomy Gleason score, SVI, time to biochemical failure, pre-RT PSA level, and postprostatectomy (Pre-RT) PSA-DT are considered the dominant factors that should be used to differentiate between local and distant failure

(46–50). Pound et al. (47) have reported that when the Gleason score is ≥8, time to biochemical failure is <2 years and PSA doubling time is <10 months, the probability of distant metastasis is >65% at 5 years. In a recent multi-institutional pooled analysis of over 500 men treated with SRT, Stephenson et al. (35) confirmed that Gleason score ≥8 and PSA doubling time <10 months, along with pre-RT PSA level >2 ng/mL, SVI, and margin negativity, were significantly related to biochemical failure in Cox proportional hazards multivariate analysis. Ideally, none of these factors should be present. However, it is these DR-PSA patients with very favorable characteristics that have a relatively low chance (<20%) of developing distant metastasis within 7 years. Therein is the dilemma. The rationale for RT is to reduce the risk of local progression such that the development of distant metastasis and death from prostate cancer are avoided. One must balance the goal of preventing progression to distant metastasis, the side effects from treatment, and the chance of death due to intercurrent disease; a >10-year life expectancy is an important consideration.

TABLE 15D.2

RELATIONSHIP OF EXTRACAPSULAR EXTENSION AND MARGIN POSITIVITY TO FREEDOM FROM BIOCHEMICAL FAILURE

First author (Yr)	%, 5 yr		%, 10 yr	
	ECE	Margin+	ECE	Margin+
Paulson (1994)	—	42	—	38
Zietman (1994)	27	26	—	—
Watson (1996)	—	66	—	—
Epstein (1996)	78[a,b]	64	68	55
Dillioglugil (1997)	79	–	79	—
Kupelian (1997)	~43	~35	—	—
Grossfeld (2000)	—	52	—	—
Kausik (2002)	—	64	—	55[c]

[a]Established ECE.
[b]4 yr rate.
[c]7 yr rate, all had T3 disease.

Salvage Radiotherapy When There Is a Persistently Detectable PSA (PD-PSA)

In the setting of a PD-PSA, a rationale for local persistence of disease and, therefore, the administration of RT should be apparent. A recent metastatic work-up should have been done, either before or after prostatectomy. The prostatectomy pathologic findings should be reviewed carefully. The finding of a positive margin, especially an extensive margin with high-grade disease, a cut through the prostate (some may be considered a partial prostatectomy when there is palpable or imaging evidence of prostate remaining), or incomplete removal of the seminal vesicles in the setting of T3 disease (especially with ECE at the base or with SVI) offer sound justification for the administration of SRT. If very few lymph nodes were identified in the pathologic review of the lymph node dissection or if palpable residual tissue suggestive of a partial prostatectomy was found on digital rectal examination (DRE), a pre-SRT CT of abdomen and pelvis should be performed. If the PSA is rising sharply (doubling time of <6 months) in the background of a PD-PSA, then the probability of metastasis is high (46–50) and SRT is discouraged.

ENDPOINT CONSIDERATIONS

There has been debate about a clinically relevant definition of biochemical failure and what it demonstrates. Biochemical failure is usually defined as a PSA $\geq$0.2 ng/mL (47,51), although higher values have been recommended (52). A PSA $\geq$0.2 ng/mL is a harbinger of clinical disease relapse and has become the primary early endpoint on which the justification of SRT has been based. A key question is whether the development of a detectable, rising PSA is more reflective of local or distant progression. There are several lines of evidence that a delayed rise in PSA (DR-PSA) represents local progression as a component of failure more often than distant progression alone. First, an autopsy study has shown that residual prostate cancer cells are found in the prostate bed in about 50% of cases (36). Second, aggressive biopsies of the urethrovesical junction and prostatic bed reveal adenocarcinoma in about 50% of cases with a rising PSA, with or without an abnormality on DRE (37–40). Third, when SRT is given, in over 80% the PSA falls significantly in response to RT (53–57). Local persistence of disease appears to be a main contributor to the rising PSA profile in the majority.

Pre-adjuvant Radiotherapy Work-up

Since by definition the PSA is undetectable or just barely detectable ($<$0.2 ng/mL) by most standard assays in this group, and appropriate work-up had been done prior to prostatectomy, there is usually no need for further imaging studies.

Adjuvant Radiotherapy Results and Prognostic Factors

Several series, mostly from the pre-PSA era, have documented a reduction in local and/or clinical recurrence from ART in men who were considered to be at a high risk pathologically

after radical prostatectomy (58–64). Anscher et al. (61) found the 10-year local-control rates to be 92% after ART and 60% after radical prostatectomy alone. Long follow-up was required to demonstrate this difference in clinically palpable recurrence in the prostatic fossa. Improvement in local control from ART has not until recently been associated with a significant reduction in distant metastasis or survival. Do et al. (64) found that in univariate, but not multivariate, analysis, local recurrence was related significantly to distant metastasis. They also reported that the distant metastasis rate was lower in men who received ART compared with radical prostatectomy alone. It should be noted that the studies in which the frequency of distant metastasis has been measured after ART were generally underpowered. Men with biochemical relapse after prostatectomy often received androgen deprivation, which delays the onset of distant metastasis. Death due to intercurrent disease also contributes to the inadequate power; larger patient numbers and longer follow-up are needed to demonstrate that ART reduces distant metastasis and mortality. There is a well-established association between local failure and distant metastasis in men treated primarily with radiotherapy for prostate cancer (65–67), and it is very likely that ART will eventually be shown to have an impact on these other endpoints.

Table 15D.3 displays a summary of several representative series on the relationship of ART to freedom from biochemical failure (FFBF). The range of 5-year rates is most likely related to variations in the patient prognostic characteristics, radiation technique, RT dose, and length of follow-up. When a positive margin was present and the RT dose was $\geq$60 Gy, the FFBF results were usually over 80% (Table 15D.3) (53,63,64,68–75). Many of the retrospective series listed evaluated small numbers of patients. The largest series is from the University of Southern California (USC) (76), with 423 patients treated to doses usually below 50 Gy. In the M.D. Anderson Cancer Center (MDACC) series, the median dose was 60 Gy, and FFBF was higher (88% vs. 69% at 5-year). The differences observed here and between other series could be related to the dose used (77), the use of androgen deprivation in some patients (78–81), an unequal balance of adverse factors (e.g., Gleason score 8–10, SVI or LNI) or how biochemical failure was defined [e.g., PSA $<$0.05 ng/mL, PSA $<$0.1 ng/mL, or 3 rises per the American

TABLE 15D.3

FREEDOM FROM BIOCHEMICAL FAILURE AFTER ADJUVANT RADIOTHERAPY

First author (yr)	n	pStage	Margin+, %	F/U, mo	Dose, Gy	FFBF, %
Schild (1996)	60	T3N0	82	32	62	57 (5 yr)
Coetzee (1996)	30	T2-T3c	100	33	66-70	50 (4 yr)[c]
Morris (1997)	40	T3N0	85	31	60-62	88 (3 yr)
Valicenti (1998)	15	T3cN0	20	~38	64.8	86 (3 yr)[c]
Valicenti (1999)	52	T3N0	83	39	64.8	82 (5 yr)[c]
Vicini (1999)	38	T2c-T4	–	49	59.4	67 (5 yr)[c]
Nudell (1999)	36	T2-T3	97	~23	68	~58 (5 yr)[c]
Leibovich (2000)	76	T2N0	100[a]	29	63	88 (5 yr)[c]
Catton (2001)	54	T2-3N0	96	37	50–62	81 (5 yr)[c]
Mayer (2002)	29	T2-T4	~70	35	60–70	85 (5 yr)[b]
Do (2002)	58	T2-3N0-1	100	78	65	88 (10 yr)[d]
Petrovich (2002)	423	T3N0	—	84	48	69 (5 yr)[c]
Kalapurakal (2002)	35	—	—	36	60-65	86 (5 yr)[c]
Taylor (2003)	75	T2-T3N0	96	68	60	88 (5 yr)[c]
Tsien (2003)	38	T3-T4	89	116	59-69	50 (5 yr)[b]

[a]Single positive margin.
[b]ASTRO or modified rising PSA definition.
[c]detectable PSA >0.05 to 0.2 ng/mL.
[d]PSA >0.5 ng/mL.

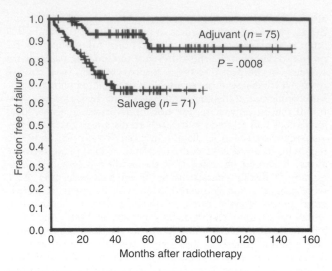

FIGURE 15D.1. Kaplan-Meier FFBF survival curves for patients treated after radical prostatectomy with adjuvant radiotherapy (ART) or salvage radiotherapy (SRT). Biochemical failure was defined as a detectable prostate-specific antigen (PSA) level after radiotherapy (RT). The log-rank test was used to compare outcome. (Reproduced from Taylor N, Kelly JF, Kuban DA, et al. Adjuvant and salvage radiotherapy after radical prostatectomy for prostate cancer. *Int J Radiat Oncol Biol Phys* 2003;56:755–763, with permission.)

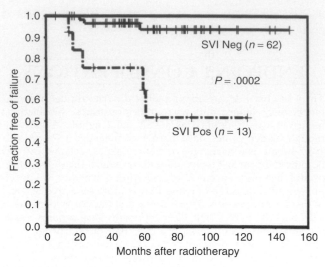

FIGURE 15D.2. Kaplan-Meier FFBF survival curves for patients treated after radical prostatectomy with adjuvant radiotherapy (ART), subdivided by whether seminal vesicle involvement (SVI) was present or not. The log-rank test was used to compare outcome. (Reproduced from Taylor N, Kelly JF, Kuban DA, et al. Adjuvant and salvage radiotherapy after radical prostatectomy for prostate cancer. *Int J Radiat Oncol Biol Phys* 2003;56:755–763, with permission.)

Society of Therapeutic Radiation Oncologists (ASTRO) definition]. In the MD Anderson Cancer Center (MDACC) series (82), there were no biochemical failures beyond 5 years (Fig. 15D.1) using an undetectable PSA as the endpoint. The flatness of the curve after 5 years suggests that these patients have been cured.

A consistent observation in patients treated with ART is that SVI is a highly significant correlate of reduced FFBF (82–84), although other factors such as Gleason score may also be important. Figure 15D.2 illustrates the significance of SVI in patients treated at MDACC (82). The FFBF rates at 5 years were 94% and 65% ($P = .0002$) for those with and without SVI, respectively.

Androgen deprivation has been used sparingly in patients who have an undetectable PSA after radical prostatectomy

(75,82). Because of small patient numbers, it is not possible to ascribe a benefit from applying the combination of ART+AD. However, men treated with ART for SVI have a poor prognosis in terms of FFBF, and in this situation it is worth considering AD (82).

Adjuvant Radiotherapy Versus Radical Prostatectomy Alone

Table 15D.4 summarizes recent retrospective series that have compared radical prostatectomy alone with radical prostatectomy plus ART (63,64,71,83,85,86). In all but the USC series

---

TABLE 15D.4

ADJUVANT RADIOTHERAPY VERSUS RADICAL PROSTATECTOMY ALONE: RECENT COMPARATIVE STUDIES

First author (yr)	*n*	Dose, Gy	FFBF, %	*P*
Schild (1998)	~228	None	40 (5 yr)	.0003
	~60	60–67	90 (5 yr)	
Valicenti (1998)[b]	20	None	48 (3 yr)	.01
	15	64.8	86 (3 yr)	
Valicenti (1999, 2003)[a]	36	None	55 (5 yr)	<.01
	36	64.8	88 (5 yr)	
Leibovich (2000)[a]	76	None	59 (5 yr)	.005
	76	63	88 (5 yr)	
Do (2002)	45	None	25 (5 yr)	.0048
	30	60-68	88 (5 yr)	
Petrovich (2002)	199	None	69 (5 yr)	NS
	423	48	71 (5 yr)	
Bolla (2004)[c]	503	None	52 (5 yr)	<.0001
	502	60	72 (5 yr)	

NS, not significant.
[a]Matched pair analysis.
[b]pT3bN0 (SVI) patients.
[c]EORTC 22911 randomized trial.

(83), ART was found to result in a significant improvement in FFBF. As previously described, the patients at USC were typically treated to doses under 50 Gy, while doses of 60 Gy and higher were used at the other institutions. The USC authors noted that there was an imbalance in prognostic factors, with the patients in the ART group having more high-risk features than those treated with radical prostatectomy alone. In two of the series shown in Table 15D.4, matched-pair analyses were performed (63,87), and in each an obvious gain in FFBF with ART was seen. The cumulative results indicate that the addition of ART reduces the probability of biochemical failure by 40% to 50%. There are two major randomized trials evaluating the efficacy of ART pending—one run by SWOG and one run by the EORTC (88). Recently, the preliminary results of the EORTC trial were presented at American Society of Clinical Oncology (ASCO) (89). There were 1,005 patients with high-risk pathologic features randomized between ART (60 Gy) and no ART. Like the retrospective studies, the use of ART improved FFBF from 52% to 72% (P < .0001). No difference in distant metastasis or survival was observed.

A main consideration with ART is whether it would be better to wait after prostatectomy in high-risk patients until relapse is evidenced and then treat with SRT (90). Since over 50% of men with high-risk pathologic findings at radical prostatectomy develop a rising PSA later, the approach of watchful waiting dooms these men to failure and gives any residual disease in the prostatic bed an opportunity to spread. There are few situations in oncology in which the failure rate is so high where ART would not be applied. However, one must consider that the risk of biochemical failure does not always mean progression to distant metastasis and death due to prostate cancer. The progression of prostate cancer may be very slow and the risk of death due to intercurrent illness may be an overriding consideration. These and other factors relevant to the quandary of comparing ART to SRT are described in detail below.

Adjuvant Radiotherapy Dose and Technique

There is little sound information on the appropriate dose to use for ART after radical prostatectomy. Valicenti et al. (77) reported 3-year FFBF rates of 90% (n = 14) and 64% (n = 38; P = .015) for doses above and below 61.2 Gy in men with pT3N0 prostate cancer treated at Thomas Jefferson University. They did not perform a multivariate analysis, so these values were not adjusted for possible inequity in the distribution of other prognostic factors. In the recent analysis by Taylor et al. (82) from MDACC, a median dose of 60 Gy was used with excellent results (Table 15D.3 and Fig. 15D.1). Petrovich and colleagues (83,91) at USC have the largest ART experience reported. A median dose of 48 Gy was used and FFBF rates of 69% at 5-year and 51% at 10-year were observed. Although FFBF was at the lower end of the values from ART (Table 15D.3), some of the other series in which higher ART doses were used also reported FFBF rates in the same range. The difference might be attributable to the prognostic characteristics of the groups. The recommendations from an ASTRO consensus conference held in 1997 (92) were that ≥64 Gy be used in the treatment of men with a rising PSA after prostatectomy. A slightly lower dose for ART seems reasonable, but doses below 50 Gy may be too low.

Based on the above evidence, the recommended ART dose is 60–64.8 Gy. In many of the prior studies, the dose was prescribed to the isocenter, but now with the more widespread use of 3-D conformal radiotherapy (3D-CRT) (93) and intensity-modulated radiotherapy (IMRT) (94,95), the designation is more appropriately to a planning target volume (PTV). Figure 15D.3 displays the four-field 3D-CRT arrangement used at MDACC for several years. The clinical target volume (CTV) included the bladder neck, which is pulled down into the prostatic fossa and the periprostatic bed clips. There are typically some clips located in the central-lower aspect of the prostatic bed (from the level of the top of the pubic symphysis inferiorly), with sometimes an abundance of clips in the upper region of the surgical bed (superior to the pubic symphysis and posterior to the bladder) where the seminal vesicles were located (Fig. 15D.3). Moreover, in a surprising number of cases, remnants of the seminal vesicles may be seen, and these should also be treated. The anterior-posterior fields were about 10 × 10 cm with the inferior border at the ischial tuberosities. The lateral fields split the rectum posteriorly and extended to the anterior aspect of the pubic symphysis. A block was placed over the anterior-inferior soft tissue below the symphysis and superiorly to shield a portion of the bladder above the prostatic bed.

The use of IMRT in postoperative treatment requires more detailed definition of the CTV and the margin required to account for uncertainties of set-up and target motion. The potential

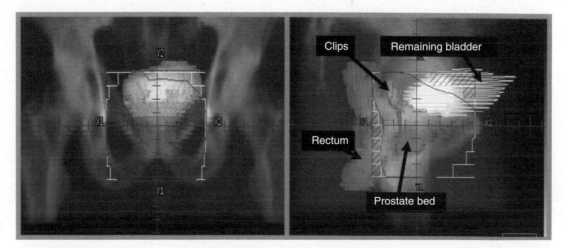

FIGURE 15D.3. The fields used at M.D. Anderson Cancer Center (MDACC) (82) were typically 10 × 10 cm anterior-posterior fields with the inferior border at the ischial tuberosities. This would place the inferior extent usually below the bulb of the penis. The rectum was split posteriorly, and some of the bladder above the prostatic bed was blocked anteriorly. The prostate bed is shown in tomato, the rest of the bladder in yellow, surgical clips in blue (*green when overlaying yellow*), and the rectum in green. Left, anterior-posterior; right, right lateral. (See color insert.)

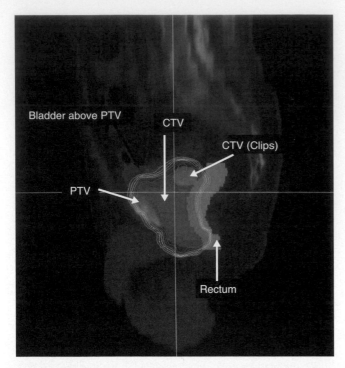

FIGURE 15D.4. An example of a patient planned using intensity-modulated radiotherapy (IMRT). A sagittal image is shown. An 8 mm planning target volume (PTV) was placed around the clinical target volumes (CTVs). (See color insert.)

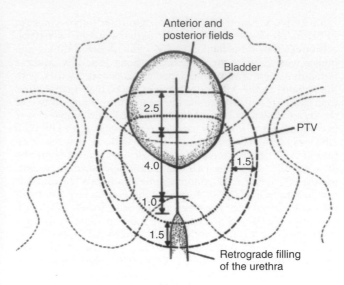

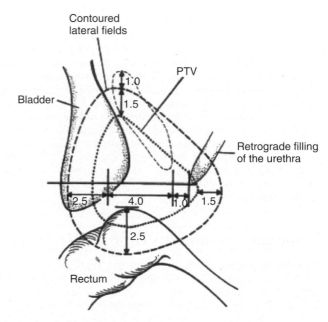

FIGURE 15D.5. Schematic of the radiotherapy fields recommended for RTOG 96-01. A retrograde urethrogram was recommended to define the inferior extent of the field. The urethrogram "beak," delineating the lower aspect of the urogenital diaphragm, is shown. The fields are designed for a patient who had an approximately 4 cm prostate in the superior-inferior dimensions. The size of the prostate should be approximated from any imaging studies done prior to prostatectomy. The fields as depicted are very generous. The posterior margin on the rectum may be too generous if the rectum is empty.

advantage of IMRT is that the dose fall-off is more abrupt and the dose distribution may be more precisely shaped to conform to the CTV; nearby normal structures should consequently be spared to a greater degree. The technique requires attention to many details and probably should not be broadly adopted until more data are published on efficacy and side effects. The Fox Chase Cancer Center (FCCC) method illustrates some of the details that should be considered (Fig. 15D.4). The bladder neck and soft tissue below the bladder neck are outlined from the bulb of the penis to the just above the pubic symphysis. The bladder neck fills the prostatic fossa, the space between the obturator internus muscles laterally, the pubic symphysis anteriorly, and the rectum posteriorly. An 8 mm planning target volume (PTV) is then added around this CTV. One problem with this method is that the bladder is very distensible and changes in volume may distort the CTV, contributing to the uncertainty of containing the CTV in the PTV daily. The patient is simulated with a somewhat full bladder, so that the volume treated is maximal. Another problem is that the anatomy shifts considerably from day to day. Because there is no prostate to localize on, interfraction adjustments using ultrasound may be inaccurate. Although Chinnaiyan et al. (96) have proposed using ultrasound to correct for interfraction motion postprostatectomy, our experience is that without referencing the ultrasound to CT (interfraction correction made with CT and then a reference ultrasound performed), daily ultrasound does not result in the alignment accuracy needed. The recommendation here is that 3D-CRT or conventional techniques (e.g., the methods used in Radiation Therapy Oncology Group (79) protocol 96-01, Fig. 15D.5) be used until research more adequately defines the advantages and drawbacks of IMRT.

Timing of Radiotherapy and Side Effects

Adjuvant RT should be delayed until urinary continence has returned. Some have advocated starting RT within 3 months

(63,83) of prostatectomy. In many cases, it will take longer than 6 months to realize the maximal return of urinary continence. Taylor et al. (82) observed that the timing of RT had little effect on outcome, even when patients were started more than 6 months after prostatectomy; however, patient numbers were small and if a patient developed a detectable PSA prior to RT, they would have then been classified as having received SRT.

Side effects from postprostatectomy radiotherapy are most often relatively mild to moderate, but severe reactions are possible. Since the bladder neck is pulled down into the prostatic fossa, a substantial portion of the bladder is treated. One would expect that acute and late genitourinary (GU) effects would, therefore be quite significant. However, the acute effects appear to be less than when the prostate is in place (76,93,97). In primary treatment of prostate cancer with RT, there is prostatic inflammation and probable acute urethral narrowing that causes increased urinary obstructive symptoms (e.g., frequency, nocturia). Although there are usually some urinary symptoms in the postprostatectomy setting, they are typically less pronounced.

Severe side effects from postoperative RT have been reported (98), but the incidence, when considering all of the available data, is low. Patients who present with a postprostatectomy history of urethral stricture requiring dilatation are at a particularly high risk of developing urinary obstructive problems during RT, as well as later. After ART, the rates of incontinence requiring a pad are similar to when ART is not administered (99,100). The incidence of new onset post-RT urinary incontinence requiring a pad and/or dilatation is <5% (56,88,97,99). Rectal irritation is common but rarely severe. Rectal bleeding appears to be about the same as that for those treated primarily for prostate cancer, with about a 10% to 20% risk of mild intermittent spotting and <5% requiring intervention (e.g., laser coagulation) (56,88,97,99). From these data, the absolute increase over prostatectomy alone in major urinary incontinence is <1%, hematuria (usually transient) is <5%, major rectal bleeding (usually transient) is 2% to 6%, and bowel urgency/incontinence is <5%. There appears to be an absolute increase in impotence from postoperative RT of about 30% compared to prostatectomy alone, but data are limited (62,100).

TABLE 15D.5

SALVAGE RADIOTHERAPY: SELECTED SERIES ILLUSTRATING THE RELATIONSHIP OF POTENTIAL PROGNOSTIC FACTORS TO FREEDOM FROM BIOCHEMICAL FAILURE

First author (yr)	Dose, Gy median (Range)	N	Overall FFBF, % (Time of analysis)	Factor (n)	SubGroup FFBF, % (Time of analysis)	P
McCarthy (1994)	NA (60–65)	37	46 (crude)	PD-PSA (15)	33 (crude)	NA
				DR-PSA (22)	68 (crude)	
Zelefsky (1997)	65 (38–70)	42	53 (2 yr)	PD-PSA (11)	26 (2 yr)	.008
				DR-PSA (31)	66 (2 yr)	
Garg (1998)	66 (54–74)	78	~62 (3 yr)	PD-PSA (37)	60 (3 yr)	.6
				DR-PSA (41)	65 (3 yr)	
Nuddell (1999)	66 (60–74)	69	~45 (4 yr)	PSA failure alone (35)	~55 (4 yr)	NS
	69 (64–74)			Biopsy proven (34)	~35 (4 yr)	
Anscher (2000)	66 (55–70)	89	50 (4 yr)	≤65 Gy (36)	0 yr (Median)	<.0001
				>65 Gy (53)	2.2 yr (Median)	
Pisansky (2000)	64 (54–72)	166	46 (5 yr)	Grade 2 (57)	~63 (5 yr)	<.001
				Grade 3–4 (106)	~37 (5 yr)	
Catton (2001)	62 (54–65)	59	~10 (5 yr)	PD-PSA (21)	16 (5 yr)	<.0001
				DR-PSA (22)	19 (5 yr)	
				Palpable mass (16)	0 (5 yr)	
Leventis (2001)	66 (60–76)	95	24 (5 yr)	<11.8 mo PSADT (23)	16 (5 yr)	.036
				≥11.8 mo PSADT (23)	27 (5 yr)	
Choo (2002)	NA (60–66)	98	~20 (5 yr)	PD-PSA (36)	26 (4 yr)	NA
				DR-PSA (26)	39 (4 yr)	
				Palpable mass (36)	14 (4 yr)	
Chawla (2002)	65 (NA)	54	35 (5 yr)	PD-PSA (NA)	27 (5 yr)	.05
				DR-PSA (NA)	52 (5 yr)	
Song (2002)	67 (61–70)	61	39 (4 yr)	PD-PSA (25)	~18 (4 yr)	.018
				DR-PSA (36)	~45 (4 yr)	
Mosbacher (2002)	61 (60–68)	62	~23 (4 yr)	Gleason ≤7 (43)	~32 (4 yr)	.0032
				Gleason >7 (19)	~7 (4 yr)	
Taylor (2003)	70 (60–78)	71	66 (5 yr)	PD-PSA (27)	43 (5 yr)	.01
				DR-PSA (44)	78 (5 yr)	
Liauw (2003)	66 (61–72)	51	16 (5 yr)	No SVI (37)	~68 (3 yr)	.013
				SVI (14)	~20 (3 yr)	
Macdonald (2003)	65 (61–68)	60	43 (5 yr)	≤64.8 Gy (22)	28 (5 yr)	.026
				>64.8 Gy (38)	59 (5 yr)	
Katz (2003)	67 (38–76)	115	46 (4 yr)	RP Margin Close/Neg (38)	RR 1.42	.02
				RP Margin Pos (54)		

N, overall number of patients treated for salvage; n, number per sub group; NA, not available; NS, not stated; RR, relative risk.

SALVAGE RADIOTHERAPY

Pre-salvage Radiotherapy Work-up

The DRE and imaging studies, such as bone, computed tomography (CT), magnetic resonance imaging (MRI), fluorodeoxyglucose positron emission tomography (FDG-PET), and capromab pendetide (ProstaScint) scans, are not very sensitive indicators of local persistence of disease (101–106). ProstaScint scans may be useful in identifying disease inside or outside the prostatic bed, although variable results have been reported (103,107–111). Novel PET markers may emerge that are more valuable in imaging the surgical bed and elsewhere after prostatectomy when PSA is elevated. Some potential candidate markers are F18-fluorocholine, carbon-11 choline, or carbon-11 acetate (106,112–115). The role of MRI spectroscopy is undefined but may also aid in identifying disease in the prostatic fossa, possibly augmenting CT planning of the radiotherapy clinical target volume (116). Even though biopsies of the prostatic fossa may detect disease about 50% of the time (37–40), there does not appear to be a significant difference in prognosis when prostatic fossa biopsies are positive (55,117).

Despite the insensitivity of imaging, the preprostatectomy work-up for a PD-PSA should be complete, including a bone scan and CT scans of the abdomen and pelvis. If such imaging was not done preprostatectomy, it should be completed pre-RT to ensure that there are no obvious metastases present. Even when bone scan, CT-abdomen, and pelvis have been done preprostatectomy, there may be indications (e.g., a rapidly rising PSA) to repeat the scans prior to SRT. For a DR-PSA, a bone scan, CT-abdomen, and pelvis should be ordered prior to SRT.

Salvage Radiotherapy Results and Prognostic Factors

In general, the results of SRT have been relatively poor, with FFBF rates ranging from 10% to 66% (Table 15D.5) (34,48, 55–57,73,74,82,93,118–123). Several factors predictive of FFBF have been identified. When patients with a persistently detectable PSA (PD-PSA) after radical prostatectomy have been segregated from those with a delayed rise in PSA (DR-PSA), the outcome has usually been worse in univariate analysis for the former group (56,57,82,93,118,120,121,124) (Table 15D.5).

TABLE 15D.6

SALVAGE RADIOTHERAPY: IMPORTANCE OF THE PRE-RADIOTHERAPY PSA LEVEL

First author (yr)	Dose, Gy median (Range)	N	Pre-RT PSA, ng/mL Cut-point (n)	Biochemical non-evidence of disease, % (yr of analysis)	P
Wu (1995)	61 (55–66)	53	<2.5 (27) ≥2.5 (26)	52 (crude) 8 (crude)	.001
Schild (1996)	64 (60–67)	46	≤1.1 (NA) >1.1 (NA)	76 (3 yr) 26 (3 yr)	.02
Morris (1997)	NA (60–64)	48	≤1.7 (24) >1.7 (24)	66 (3 yr) 29 (3 yr)	.03
Forman (1997)	66 (50–74)	47	≤2 (29) >2 (18)	44 (4 yr) 13 (4 yr)	.005
Zelefsky (1997)	65 (38–70)	28	≤1.0 (25)[b] >1.0 (13)	75 (2 yr) 26 (2 yr)	.008
Rogers (1998)[a]	70 (61–70)	34	≤4 (NA) >4 (NA)	60 (3.5yr) 0 (3.5 yr)	.03
Nuddell (1999)	~67 (60–74)	69	≤1.0 (35) >1.0 (34)	57 (4 yr) ~35 (4 yr)	NS
Anscher (2000)	66 (55–70)	89	<2.5 (NA) ≥2.5 (NA)	4.8 yr (median) 1.5 yr (median)	.03
Pisansky (2000)	64 (54–72)	166	≤1.0 (96) >1.0 (70)	53 (5 yr) 38 (5 yr)	.08
Catton (2001)	62 (54–65)	56	≤2.0 (30) >2.0 (26)	29 (5 yr) 4 (5 yr)	<.0001
Leventis (2001)	66 (60–76)	49	<2.1 (24) ≥2.1 (25)	62 (5 yr) 10 (5 yr)	.01
Chawla (2003)	65 (NA)	54	≤1.2 (43) >1.2 (26)	43 (5 yr) 26 (5 yr)	.07
Taylor (2003)	70 (60–78)	71	≤1.0 (46) >1.0 (25)	67 (5 yr) 65 (5 yr)	.87
Macdonald (2003)	65 (61–68)	60	<0.69 (28) ≥0.69 (32)	63 (5 yr) 27 (5 yr)	.016
Stephenson (2004)	65 (38–76)	501	≤1.0 (NA) 1.1-2.0 (NA) >2.0 (NA)	53 (4 yr) 49 (NA) 21 (NA)	<.001

N, overall number of patients treated for salvage; n, number per PSA cut-point group; NA, not available; NS, not stated.
[a]All had confirmed local recurrence by biopsy.
[b]Includes some patients treated adjuvantly.

Yet, in many of these series, the difference in FFBF between patients with a PD-PSA and DR-PSA has been minimal or not seen on multivariate analysis (35,93,119,122–125). Some of those with a PD-PSA will have occult distant metastasis, but the majority of patients probably have regional or residual local disease. In many reports, the numbers of patients treated with SRT are small, and the patients treated for a DR-PSA are not segregated from those with a PD-PSA. If the doubling time is <6 months, occult metastatic disease is likely (35,46–50), whether the treatment is for a DR-PSA or a PD-PSA, and postoperative radiotherapy is not recommended.

In addition to the status of the postoperative PSA (PD-PSA vs DR-PSA), some of the other factors associated with FFBF include a Gleason score of ≥7, SVI, negative prostatectomy margins, palpable prostatic fossa mass, short PSA doubling time, high pre-RT PSA (>1 to >2.5 ng/mL), and RT dose <64–65 Gy. Table 15D.5 displays the results of representative series for most of these factors, with the exception of the pre-RT PSA. The pre-RT PSA level is the most consistent variable related to FFBF in univariate and multivariate analyses. Some examples of the strength of this parameter are shown in Table 15D.6 (35,48,53,57,69,73,74,82,120,123,124,126,127). A standard pre-RT PSA cut-point has not been established, but the evidence demonstrates that the lower the pre-RT PSA, the higher the FFBF will be. The best results have been seen when the pre-RT PSA was ≤1 ng/mL. A significant decline in FFBF is typical when going from a pre-RT PSA ≤1 ng/mL to 1.1–2, to >2 ng/mL. For these reasons, androgen deprivation has been applied in some reports to patients with a high pre-RT PSA and other high-risk features. With these results in mind, Radiation Therapy Oncology Group (RTOG) protocol 96-10 tested radiotherapy alone versus radiotherapy plus 2 years of Casodex® (AstraZeneca) at 150 mg per day; the study is now closed and the results pending follow-up.

Salvage Radiotherapy Dose and Technique

The technique for SRT mirrors that for ART, although doses have traditionally been higher. No class I data apply to the issue of dose, although retrospective studies provide a rationale for delivering 64–68 Gy to the prostatic fossa. Anscher et al. (120) found significantly better results in multivariate analysis when doses above 65 Gy were used (Table 15D.5). Forman and Velasco (54), Valicenti et al. (77), and Macdonald et al. (123) have advocated similar doses. The recommendation of the ASTRO (92) consensus conference was 64 Gy. Along these lines, 64.8 Gy was used in RTOG protocol 96-01. Figure 15D.5 illustrates the four-field conventional RT fields used in RTOG protocol 96-01.

ADJUVANT VERSUS SALVAGE RADIOTHERAPY

The optimal timing of ART versus SRT for patients with high-risk pathologic features is controversial. Schild et al. (90) and Forman et al. (54) have supported the use of a watchful waiting initially and the use of SRT as needed. They reason that 50% of men will be treated unnecessarily and that salvage rates are high, especially when the pre-RT PSA is low (≤1.0 ng/mL is the safest value). In addition, the progression to distant metastasis after prostatectomy once biochemical failure is manifest may be prolonged (47). Although their interpretation of the available data seems reasonable, other factors should be considered.

In absolute terms, there is plainly an advantage to the use of ART (see Table 15D.7). ART improves the 5-year FFBF rate from about 50% to about 80% (>80% when the seminal vesicles are

TABLE 15D.7

ADJUVANT VERSUS SALVAGE RADIOTHERAPY

Author (yr)	N	ART vs. SRT (n)	Dose, Gy median (Range)	Biochemical non-evidence of disease % (yr of analysis)	P
McCarthy (1994)	64	ART (27)	NS (<60–65)	66 (3 yr)	.008
		SRT (22)	NS (<60–65)	68 (3 yr)	
		SRT (15)[a]	NS (<60–65)	32 (3 yr)	
Coetzee (1996)	45	ART (30)	NS (66–70)	50 (5 yr)	NS
		SRT (15)[a]	NS (66–70)	0 (5 yr)	
Morris (1997)	88	ART (40)	NS (60–64)	81 (3 yr)	.0006
		SRT (48)	NS (60–64)	48 (3 yr)	
Valicenti (1998)	79	ART (52)	65 (55–70)	93 (3 yr)	<.0001
		SRT (27)	65 (55–70)	44 (3 yr)	
Schild (1998)	NS	ART (NS)	62 (57–68)	90 (5 yr)	NS
		SRT (55)	64 (60–68)	49 (5 yr)	
Vicini (1999)	61	ART (38)	59.4 (50–61)	67 (5 yr)	<.001
		SRT (23)	61 (59–68)	16 (5 yr)	
Do (2002)	148	ART (58)	65 (59–68)	88 (10 yr)	.07
		SRT (90)	65 (59–68)	45 (10 yr)	
Kalapurakal (2002)	76	ART (35)	60 (60–65)	86 (5 yr)	.02
		SRT (41)	65 (60–70)	57 (5 yr)	
Taylor (2003)	75	ART (75)	60 (51–70)	88 (5 yr)	.0008
		SRT (71)	70 (60–78)	66 (5 yr)	

ART, adjuvant radiotherapy; SRT, salvage radiotherapy; N, overall number of patients treated for salvage; n, number per PSA cut-point group; NS, not stated.
20 patients had a detectable PSA after surgery.
[a]Persistently elevated PSA.

not involved) in the more recent series (Table 15D.3). In contrast, SRT on average results in a FFBF rate of 30% to 40% (Table 15D.5). ART would seem to be preferable to SRT on these grounds. However, the selection of patients for ART and SRT is noteworthy and confounds any attempt to fairly contrast these strategies. For example, the referral of patients with ART may be weighted toward those with very high-risk features such as SVI, Gleason ≥8, or extensive ECE, while men with more favorable features, even with a positive margin, are not referred. Likewise, those with a slowly rising PSA might not be referred for SRT. The reverse is also probable—that men with a very short PSA doubling time would not be referred for SRT. Without an in-depth understanding of the referral patterns and selection practices, it is not possible to cogently attribute a benefit of ART over SRT or vice versa. These considerations aside, the fact that ART is efficacious and that about 50% of men with high-risk pathologic features in the radical prostatectomy specimen will ultimately fail without such treatment makes ART a more attractive approach, particularly when margins are positive.

RECOMMENDATIONS

Both ART and SRT are effective at eradicating locally persistent disease after prostatectomy, and the morbidity of treatment is relatively low. ART results in an approximately 80% and SRT an approximately 35% chance of maintaining an undetectable PSA long term. Radiotherapy doses of 60–64 Gy should be used for ART and 64–68 Gy for SRT. There are well-established prognostic factors that should be used to appropriately select patients for treatment.

References

1. Ohori M, Wheeler TM, Kattan MW, et al. Prognostic significance of positive surgical margins in radical prostatectomy specimens. *Int J Radiat Oncol Biol Phys* 1995;154:1818–1824.
2. Kupelian P, Katcher J, Levin H, et al. Correlation of clinical and pathologic factors with rising prostate-specific antigen profiles after radical prostatectomy alone for clinically localized prostate cancer. *Urology* 1996;48:249–260.
3. Epstein JI, Partin AW, Sauvageot J, et al. Prediction of progression following radical prostatectomy. A multivariate analysis of 721 men with long-term follow-up. *Am J Surg Pathol* 1996;20:286–292.
4. Lowe BA, Lieberman SF. Disease recurrence and progression in untreated pathologic stage T3 prostate cancer: selecting the patient for adjuvant therapy. *J Urol* 1997;158:1452–1456.
5. Dillioglugil O, Leibman B, Kattan M, et al. Hazard rates for progression after radical prostatectomy for clinically localized prostate cancer. *Urology* 1997;50:93–99.
6. Pound CR, Partin AW, Epstein JI, et al. Prostate-specific antigen after anatomic radical retropubic prostatectomy. *Urol Clin North Am* 1997;24:395–406.
7. Bauer JJ, Connelly RR, Seterhenn IA, et al. Biostatistical modeling using traditional preoperative and pathological prognostic variables in the selection of men at high risk for disease recurrence after radical prostatectomy for prostate cancer. *J Urol* 1998;159:929–933.
8. Ramos C, Carvalhal G, Smith D, et al. Clinical and pathological characteristics, and recurrence rates of stage T1C versus T2A or T2B prostate cancer. *J Urol* 1999;161:1525–1529.
9. Gilliland FD, Hoffman RM, Hamilton A, et al. Predicting extracapsular extension of prostate cancer in men treated with radical prostatectomy: results from the Population Based Prostate Cancer Outcomes study. *J Urol* 1999;162:1341–1345.
10. Jhaveri FM, Klein EA, Kupelian PA, et al. Declining rates of extracapsular extension after radical prostatectomy: evidence for continued stage migration. *J Clin Oncol* 1999;17:3167–3172.
11. Cheng L, Slezak J, Bergstralh EJ, et al. Preoperative prediction of surgical margin status in patients with prostate cancer treated by radical prostatectomy. *J Clin Oncol* 2000;18:2862–2868.
12. Blute ML, Bergstralh EJ, Partin AW, et al. Validation of Partin tables for predicting pathological stage of clinically localized prostate cancer. *J Urol* 2000;164:1591–1595.
13. Shah O, Robbins DA, Melamed J, et al. The New York University nerve sparing algorithm decreases the rate of positive surgical margins following radical retropubic prostatectomy. *J Urol* 2003;169:2147–2152.
14. Khan MA, Partin AW, Mangold LA, et al. Probability of biochemical recurrence by analysis of pathologic stage, Gleason score, and margin status for localized prostate cancer. *Urology* 2003;62:866–871.
15. Cagiannos I, Karakiewicz P, Eastham JA, et al. A preoperative nomogram identifying decreased risk of positive pelvic lymph nodes in patients with prostate cancer. *J Urol* 2003;170:1798–1803.
16. de la Taille A, Katz A, Bagiella E, et al. Perineural invasion on prostate needle biopsy: an independent predictor of final pathologic stage. *Urology* 1999;54:1039–1043.
17. Endrizzi J, Seay T. The relationship between early biochemical failure and perineural invasion in pathological T2 prostate cancer. *BJU Int* 2000;85:696–698.
18. D'Amico AV, Wu Y, Chen MH, et al. Perineural invasion as a predictor of biochemical outcome following radical prostatectomy for select men with clinically localized prostate cancer. *J Urol* 2001;165:126–129.
19. Maru N, Ohori M, Kattan MW, et al. Prognostic significance of the diameter of perineural invasion in radical prostatectomy specimens. *Hum Pathol* 2001;32:828–833.
20. O'Malley KJ, Pound CR, Walsh PC, et al. Influence of biopsy perineural invasion on long-term biochemical disease-free survival after radical prostatectomy. *Urology* 2002;59:85–90.
21. Bismar TA, Lewis JS Jr, Vollmer RT, et al. Multiple measures of carcinoma extent versus perineural invasion in prostate needle biopsy tissue in prediction of pathologic stage in a screening population. *Am J Surg Pathol* 2003;27:432–440.
22. Quinn DI, Henshall SM, Brenner PC, et al. Prognostic significance of preoperative factors in localized prostate carcinoma treated with radical prostatectomy: importance of percentage of biopsies that contain tumor and the presence of biopsy perineural invasion. *Cancer* 2003;97:1884–1893.
23. Paulson DF. Impact of radical prostatectomy in the management of clinically localized disease. *J Urol* 1994;152:1826–1830.
24. Zietman AL, Edelstein RA, Coen JJ, et al. Radical prostatectomy for adenocarcinoma of the prostate: the influence of preoperative and pathologic findings on biochemical disease-free outcome. *Urology* 1994;43:828–833.
25. Watson RB, Civantos F, Soloway MS. Positive surgical margins with radical prostatectomy: detailed pathological analysis and prognosis. *Urology* 1996;48:80–90.
26. Epstein JI. Incidence and significance of positive margins in radical prostatectomy specimens. *Urol Clin North Am* 1996;23:651–663.
27. Kupelian PA, Katcher J, Levin HS, et al. Stage T1-2 prostate cancer: a multivariate analysis of factors affecting biochemical and clinical failures after radical prostatectomy. *Int J Radiat Oncol Biol Phys* 1997;37:1043–1052.
28. Grossfeld GD, Tigrani VS, Nudell D, et al. Management of a positive surgical margin after radical prostatectomy: decision analysis. *J Urol* 2000;164:93–99; discussion 100.
29. Kausik SJ, Blute ML, Sebo TJ, et al. Prognostic significance of positive surgical margins in patients with extraprostatic carcinoma after radical prostatectomy. *Cancer* 2002;95:1215–1219.
30. Jones EC. Resection margin status in radical retropubic prostatectomy specimens: relationship to type of operation, tumor size, tumor grade and local tumor extension. *J Urol* 1990;144:89–93.
31. Epstein JI, Pizov G, Walsh PC. Correlation of pathologic findings with progression after radical retropubic prostatectomy. *Cancer* 1993;71:3582–3593.
32. Epstein JI, Pound CR, Partin AW, et al. Disease progression following radical prostatectomy in men with Gleason score 7 tumor. *J Urol* 1998;160:97–100; discussion 101.
33. D'Amico AV, Whittington R, Malkowicz SB, et al. Prostate specific antigen outcome based on the extent of extracapsular extension and margin status in patients with seminal vesicle negative prostate carcinoma of Gleason score < or = 7. *Cancer* 2000;88:2110–2115.
34. Katz MS, Zelefsky MJ, Venkatraman ES, et al. Predictors of biochemical outcome with salvage conformal radiotherapy after radical prostatectomy for prostate cancer. *J Clin Oncol* 2003;21:483–489.
35. Stephenson AJ, Shariat SF, Zelefsky MJ, et al. Salvage radiotherapy for recurrent prostate cancer after radical prostatectomy. *JAMA* 2004;291:1325–1332.
36. Oesterling JE, Epstein JI, Walsh PC. Long-term autopsy findings following radical prostatectomy. *Urology* 1987;29:584–588.
37. Scattoni V, Roscigno M, Raber M, et al. Multiple vesico-urethral biopsies following radical prostatectomy: the predictive roles of TRUS, DRE, PSA and the pathological stage. *Eur Urol* 2003;44:407–414.
38. Leventis AK, Shariat SF, Slawin KM. Local recurrence after radical prostatectomy: correlation of US features with prostatic fossa biopsy findings. *Radiology* 2001;219:432–439.
39. Saleem MD, Sanders H, Abu El Naser M, et al. Factors predicting cancer detection in biopsy of the prostatic fossa after radical prostatectomy. *Urology* 1998;51:283–286.
40. Foster LS, Jajodia P, Fournier G Jr, et al. The value of prostate specific antigen and transrectal ultrasound guided biopsy in detecting prostatic fossa recurrences following radical prostatectomy. *J Urol* 1993;149:1024–1028.
41. Trapasso JG, de Kernion JB, Smith RB, et al. The incidence and significance of detectable levels of serum prostate specific antigen after radical prostatectomy. *J Urol* 1994;152:1821–1825.
42. Catalona W, Smith D. Cancer recurrence and survival rates after anatomic radical retropubic prostatectomy for prostate cancer: intermediate-term results. *J Urol* 1998;160:2428–2434.

43. Amling CL, Blute ML, Bergstralh EJ, et al. Long-term hazard of progression after radical prostatectomy for clinically localized prostate cancer: continued risk of biochemical failure after 5 years. *J Urol* 2000;164:101–105.

44. Pollack A, Horwitz EM, Movsas B. Treatment of prostate cancer with regional lymph node (N1) metastasis. *Semin Radiat Oncol* 2003;13:121–129.

45. Wiegel T, Bressel M. Influence of the extent of nodal involvement on the outcome in stage D1 prostate cancer. *Radiat Oncol Investig* 1994;2:144–151.

46. Patel A, Dorey F, Franklin J, et al. Recurrence patterns after radical retropubic prostatectomy: clinical usefulness of prostate specific antigen doubling times and log slope prostate specific antigen. *J Urol* 1997;158:1441–1445.

47. Pound C, Partin A, Eisenberger M, et al. Natural history of progression after PSA elevation following radical prostatectomy. *JAMA* 1999;281:1591–1597.

48. Leventis AK, Shariat SF, Kattan MW, et al. Prediction of response to salvage radiation therapy in patients with prostate cancer recurrence after radical prostatectomy. *J Clin Oncol* 2001;19:1030–1039.

49. Roberts SG, Blute ML, Bergstralh EJ, et al. PSA doubling time as a predictor of clinical progression after biochemical failure following radical prostatectomy for prostate cancer. *Mayo Clin Proc* 2001;76:576–581.

50. D'Amico AV, Moul JW, Carroll PR, et al. Surrogate end point for prostate cancer-specific mortality after radical prostatectomy or radiation therapy. *J Natl Cancer Inst* 2003;95:1376–1383.

51. Freedland SJ, Sutter ME, Dorey F, et al. Defining the ideal cutpoint for determining PSA recurrence after radical prostatectomy. *Urology* 2003;61:365–369.

52. Amling CL, Bergstralh EJ, Blute ML, et al. Defining prostate specific antigen progression after radical prostatectomy: what is the most appropriate cut point? *J Urol* 2001;165:1146–1151.

53. Schild SE, Buskirk SJ, Wong WW, et al. The use of radiotherapy for patients with isolated elevation of serum prostate specific antigen following radical prostatectomy. *J Urol* 1996;156:1725–1729.

54. Forman JD, Velasco J. Therapeutic radiation in patients with a rising postprostatectomy PSA level. *Oncology (Huntingt)* 1998;12:33–39; discussion 39, 43–44, 47.

55. Mosbacher MR, Schiff PB, Otoole KM, et al. Postprostatectomy salvage radiation therapy for prostate cancer: impact of pathological and biochemical variables and prostate fossa biopsy. *Cancer J* 2002;8:242–246.

56. Choo R, Hruby G, Hong J, et al. (IN)-efficacy of salvage radiotherapy for rising PSA or clinically isolated local recurrence after radical prostatectomy. *Int J Radiat Oncol Biol Phys* 2002;53:269–276.

57. Chawla AK, Thakral HK, Zietman AL, et al. Salvage radiotherapy after radical prostatectomy for prostate adenocarcinoma: analysis of efficacy and prognostic factors. *Urology* 2002;59:726–731.

58. Gibbons RP, Cole BS, Richardson RG, et al. Adjuvant radiotherapy following radiation prostatectomy: results and complications. *J Urol* 1986;135:65–68.

59. Meier R, Mark R, St. Royal I, et al. Postoperative radiation therapy after radical prostatectomy for prostate carcinoma. *Cancer* 1992;70:1960–1966.

60. Cheng WS, Frydenberg M, Bergstralh EJ, et al. Radical prostatectomy for pathologic stage C prostate cancer: influence of pathologic variables and adjuvant treatment on disease outcome. *Urology* 1993;42:283–291.

61. Anscher MS, Robertson CN, Prosnitz R. Adjuvant radiotherapy for pathologic stage T3/4 adenocarcinoma of the prostate: ten-year update. *Int J Radiat Oncol Biol Phys* 1995;33:37–43.

62. Syndikus I, Pickles T, Kostashuk E, et al. Postoperative radiotherapy for stage pT3 carcinoma of the prostate: improved local control. *J Urol* 1996;155:1983–1986.

63. Leibovich BC, Engen DE, Patterson DE, et al. Benefit of adjuvant radiation therapy for localized prostate cancer with a positive surgical margin. *J Urol* 2000;163:1178–1182.

64. Do LV, Do TM, Smith R, et al. Postoperative radiotherapy for carcinoma of the prostate: impact on both local control and distant disease-free survival. *Am J Clin Oncol* 2002;25:1–8.

65. Kuban DA, el-Mahdi AM, Schellhammer PF. Effect of local tumor control on distant metastasis and survival in prostatic adenocarcinoma. *Urology* 1987;30:420–426.

66. Zagars GK, von Eschenbach AC, Ayala AG, et al. The influence of local control on metastatic dissemination of prostate cancer treated by external beam megavoltage radiation therapy. *Cancer* 1991;68:2370–2377.

67. Fuks Z, Leibel SA, Wallner KE, et al. The effect of local control on metastatic dissemination in carcinoma of the prostate: long term results in patients treated with I-125 implantation. *Int J Radiat Oncol Biol Phys* 1991;21:537–547.

68. Coetzee LJ, Hars V, Paulson DF. Postoperative prostate-specific antigen as a prognostic indicator in patients with margin-positive prostate cancer, undergoing adjuvant radiotherapy after radical prostatectomy. *Urology* 1996;47:232–235.

69. Morris MM, Dallow KC, Zietman AL, et al. Adjuvant and salvage irradiation following radical prostatectomy for prostate cancer. *Int J Radiat Oncol Biol Phys* 1997;38:731–736.

70. Valicenti RK, Gomella LG, Ismail M, et al. Durable efficacy of early postoperative radiation therapy for high-risk pT3N0 prostate cancer: the importance of radiation dose. *Urology* 1998;52:1034–1040.

71. Valicenti RK, Gomella LG, Ismail M, et al. The efficacy of early adjuvant radiation therapy for pT3N0 prostate cancer: a matched-pair analysis. *Int J Radiat Oncol Biol Phys* 1999;45:53–58.

72. Vicini FA, Ziaja EL, Kestin LL, et al. Treatment outcome with adjuvant and salvage irradiation after radical prostatectomy for prostate cancer. *Urology* 1999;54:111–117.

73. Nudell DM, Grossfeld GD, Weinberg VK, et al. Radiotherapy after radical prostatectomy: treatment outcomes and failure patterns. *Urology* 1999;54:1049–1057.

74. Catton C, Gospodarowicz M, Warde P, et al. Adjuvant and salvage radiation therapy after radical prostatectomy for adenocarcinoma of the prostate. *Radiother Oncol* 2001;59:51–60.

75. Mayer R, Pummer K, Quehenberger F, et al. Postprostatectomy radiotherapy for high-risk prostate cancer. *Urology* 2002;59:732–739.

76. Petrovich Z, Lieskovsky G, Langholz B, et al. Postoperative radiotherapy in 423 patients with pT3N0 prostate cancer. *Int J Radiat Oncol Biol Phys* 2002;53:600–609.

77. Valicenti RK, Gomella LG, Ismail M, et al. Effect of higher radiation dose on biochemical control after radical prostatectomy for PT3N0 prostate cancer. *Int J Radiat Oncol Biol Phys* 1998;42:501–506.

78. Eulau SM, Tate DJ, Stamey TA, et al. Effect of combined transient androgen deprivation and irradiation following radical prostatectomy for prostatic cancer. *Int J Radiat Oncol Biol Phys* 1998;41:735–740.

79. Corn BW, Winter K, Pilepich MV. Does androgen suppression enhance the efficacy of postoperative irradiation? A secondary analysis of RTOG 85-31. Radiation Therapy Oncology Group. *Urology* 1999;54:495–502.

80. Allison RR, Schulsinger A. Multimodality salvage for patients with persistently elevated postprostatectomy PSA. *Int J Cancer* 2000;90:331–335.

81. Tiguert R, Rigaud J, Lacombe L, et al. Neoadjuvant hormone therapy before salvage radiotherapy for an increasing post-radical prostatectomy serum prostate specific antigen level. *J Urol* 2003;170:447–450.

82. Taylor N, Kelly JF, Kuban DA, et al. Adjuvant and salvage radiotherapy after radical prostatectomy for prostate cancer. *Int J Radiat Oncol Biol Phys* 2003;56:755–763.

83. Petrovich Z, Lieskovsky G, Stein JP, et al. Comparison of surgery alone with surgery and adjuvant radiotherapy for pT3N0 prostate cancer. *BJU Int* 2002;89:604–611.

84. Kalapurakal JA, Huang CF, Neriamparampil MM, et al. Biochemical disease-free survival following adjuvant and salvage irradiation after radical prostatectomy. *Int J Radiat Oncol Biol Phys* 2002;54:1047–1054.

85. Schild SE. Radiation therapy after prostatectomy: now or later? *Semin Radiat Oncol* 1998;8:132–139.

86. Valicenti RK, Gomella LG, Ismail M, et al. Pathologic seminal vesicle invasion after radical prostatectomy for patients with prostate carcinoma: effect of early adjuvant radiation therapy on biochemical control. *Cancer* 1998;82:1909–1914.

87. Valicenti RK, Gomella LG, Perez CA. Radiation therapy after radical prostatectomy: a review of the issues and options. *Semin Radiat Oncol* 2003;13:130–140.

88. Bolla M, van Poppel H, van Cangh PJ, et al. Acute and late toxicity of post-operative external irradiation in pT3N0 prostate cancer patients treated within EORTC trial 22911. *Int J Radiat Oncol Biol Phys* 2002;54 (Suppl. 1):62–63.

89. Bolla M, van Poppel H, Van Cangh P, et al. Does post-operative radiotherapy (P-XRT) after radical prostatectomy (Px) improve progression-free survival (PFS) in pT3N0 prostate cancer (PC)? EORTC 22911. *Annu Meet Proc ASCO* 2004;23:382.

90. Schild SE. Radiation therapy (RT) after prostatectomy: the case for salvage therapy as opposed to adjuvant therapy. *Int J Cancer* 2001;96:94–98.

91. Petrovich Z, Lieskovsky G, Langholz B, et al. Nonrandomized comparison of surgery with and without adjuvant pelvic irradiation for patients with pT3N0 adenocarcinoma of the prostate. *Am J Clin Oncol* 2001;24:537–546.

92. Cox J, Gallagher M, Hammond E et al. American Society for Therapeutic Radiology and Oncology Consensus Panel. Consensus statements on radiation therapy of prostate cancer: guidelines for prostate re-biopsy after radiation and for radiation therapy with rising prostate-specific antigen levels and radical prostatectomy. *J Clin Oncol* 1999;17:1155.

93. Zelefsky MJ, Aschkenasy E, Kelsen S, et al. Tolerance and early outcome results of postprostatectomy three-dimensional conformal radiotherapy. *Int J Radiat Oncol Biol Phys* 1997;39:327–333.

94. Bastasch MD, Teh BS, Mai WY, et al. Post-nerve-sparing prostatectomy, dose-escalated intensity-modulated radiotherapy: effect on erectile function. *Int J Radiat Oncol Biol Phys* 2002;54:101–106.

95. Teh BS, Mai WY, Augspurger ME, et al. Intensity modulated radiation therapy (IMRT) following prostatectomy: more favorable acute genitourinary toxicity profile compared to primary IMRT for prostate cancer. *Int J Radiat Oncol Biol Phys* 2001;49:465–472.

96. Chinnaiyan P, Tomee W, Patel R, et al. 3D-ultrasound guided radiation therapy in the post-prostatectomy setting. *Technol Cancer Res Treat* 2003;2:455–458.

97. Duchesne GM, Dowling C, Frydenberg M, et al. Outcome, morbidity, and prognostic factors in post-prostatectomy radiotherapy: an Australian multicenter study. *Urology* 2003;61:179–183.

98. Edgren M, Lennernas B, Haggman M, et al. Postoperative radiotherapy after prostatectomy can be associated with severe side effects. *Anticancer Res* 2001;21:2231–2235.

99. Van Cangh PJ, Richard F, Lorge F, et al. Adjuvant radiation therapy does not cause urinary incontinence after radical prostatectomy: results of a prospective randomized study. *J Urol* 1998;159:164–166.

100. Formenti SC, Lieskovsky G, Skinner D, et al. Update on impact of moderate dose of adjuvant radiation on urinary continence and sexual potency in prostate cancer patients treated with nerve-sparing prostatectomy. *Urology* 2000;56:453–458.

101. Hofer C, Laubenbacher C, Block T, et al. Fluorine-18-fluorodeoxyglucose positron emission tomography is useless for the detection of local recurrence after radical prostatectomy. *Eur Urol* 1999;36:31–35.

102. Cher ML, Bianco FJ Jr, Lam JS, et al. Limited role of radionuclide bone scintigraphy in patients with prostate specific antigen elevations after radical prostatectomy. *J Urol* 1998;160:1387–1391.

103. Seltzer MA, Barbaric Z, Belldegrun A, et al. Comparison of helical computerized tomography, positron emission tomography and monoclonal antibody scans for evaluation of lymph node metastases in patients with prostate specific antigen relapse after treatment for localized prostate cancer. *J Urol* 1999;162:1322–1328.

104. Lattouf JB, Saad F. Digital rectal exam following prostatectomy: is it still necessary with the use of PSA? *Eur Urol* 2003;43:333–336.

105. Kane CJ, Amling CL, Johnstone PA, et al. Limited value of bone scintigraphy and computed tomography in assessing biochemical failure after radical prostatectomy. *Urology* 2003;61:607–611.

106. de Jong IJ, Pruim J, Elsinga PH, et al. 11C-choline positron emission tomography for the evaluation after treatment of localized prostate cancer. *Eur Urol* 2003;44:32–38; discussion 38–39.

107. Kahn D, Williams R, Haseman M, et al. Radioimmunoscintigraphy with IN-111-labeled capromab pendetide predicts prostate cancer response to salvage radiotherapy after failed radical prostatectomy. *J Clin Oncol* 1998; 16:284–289.

108. Murphy GP, Elgamal AA, Troychak MJ, et al. Follow-up ProstaScint scans verify detection of occult soft-tissue recurrence after failure of primary prostate cancer therapy. *Prostate* 2000;42:315–317.

109. Raj GV, Partin AW, Polascik TJ. Clinical utility of indium 111-capromab pendetide immunoscintigraphy in the detection of early, recurrent prostate carcinoma after radical prostatectomy. *Cancer* 2002;94:987–996.

110. Ponsky LE, Cherullo EE, Starkey R, et al. Evaluation of preoperative ProstaScint scans in the prediction of nodal disease. *Prostate Cancer Prostatic Dis* 2002;5:132–135.

111. Thomas CT, Bradshaw PT, Pollock BH, et al. Indium-111-capromab pendetide radioimmunoscintigraphy and prognosis for durable biochemical response to salvage radiation therapy in men after failed prostatectomy. *J Clin Oncol* 2003;21:1715–1721.

112. Price DT, Coleman RE, Liao RP, et al. Comparison of [18 F]fluorocholine and [18 F]fluorodeoxyglucose for positron emission tomography of androgen dependent and androgen independent prostate cancer. *J Urol* 2002; 168:273–280.

113. Picchio M, Landoni C, Messa C, et al. Positive [11C]choline and negative [18F]FDG with positron emission tomography in recurrence of prostate cancer. *AJR Am J Roentgenol* 2002;179:482–484.

114. Kotzerke J, Volkmer BG, Neumaier B, et al. Carbon-11 acetate positron emission tomography can detect local recurrence of prostate cancer. *Eur J Nucl Med Mol Imaging* 2002;29:1380–1384.

115. Oyama N, Miller TR, Dehdashti F, et al. 11C-acetate PET imaging of prostate cancer: detection of recurrent disease at PSA relapse. *J Nucl Med* 2003;44:549–555.

116. Hricak H, Schoder H, Pucar D, et al. Advances in imaging in the postoperative patient with a rising prostate-specific antigen level. *Semin Oncol* 2003;30:616–634.

117. Koppie TM, Grossfeld GD, Nudell DM, et al. Is anastomotic biopsy necessary before radiotherapy after radical prostatectomy? *J Urol* 2001;166: 111–115.

118. McCarthy JF, Catalona WJ, Hudson MA. Effect of radiation therapy on detectable serum prostate specific antigen levels following radical prostatectomy: early versus delayed treatment. *J Urol* 1994;151:1575–1578.

119. Garg MK, Tekyi-Mensah S, Bolton S, et al. Impact of postprostatectomy prostate-specific antigen nadir on outcomes following salvage radiotherapy. *Urology* 1998;51:998–1002.

120. Anscher MS, Clough R, Dodge R. Radiotherapy for a rising prostate-specific antigen after radical prostatectomy: the first 10 years. *Int J Radiat Oncol Biol Phys* 2000;48:369–375.

121. Song DY, Thompson TL, Ramakrishnan V, et al. Salvage radiotherapy for rising or persistent PSA after radical prostatectomy. *Urology* 2002;60: 281–287.

122. Liauw SL, Webster WS, Pistenmaa DA, et al. Salvage radiotherapy for biochemical failure of radical prostatectomy: a single-institution experience. *Urology* 2003;61:1204–1210.

123. Macdonald OK, Schild SE, Vora SA, et al. Radiotherapy for men with isolated increase in serum prostate specific antigen after radical prostatectomy. *J Urol* 2003;170:1833–1837.

124. Wu JJ, King SC, Montana GS, et al. The efficacy of postprostatectomy radiotherapy in patients with an isolated elevation of serum prostate-specific antigen. *Int J Radiat Oncol Biol Phys* 1995;32:317–323.

125. Peyromaure M, Allouch M, Eschwege F, et al. Salvage radiotherapy for biochemical recurrence after radical prostatectomy: a study of 62 patients. *Urology* 2003;62:503–507.

126. Forman JD, Meetze K, Pontes E, et al. Therapeutic irradiation for patients with an elevated post-prostatectomy prostate specific antigen level. *J Urol* 1997;158:1436–1439; discussion 1439–1440.

127. Rogers R, Grossfeld GD, Roach M III, et al. Radiation therapy for the management of biopsy proved local recurrence after radical prostatectomy. *J Urol* 1998;160:1748–1753.

CHAPTER 15E
Salvage Radical Prostatectomy for Recurrence of Prostate Cancer after Radiation Therapy

James A. Eastham and Peter T. Scardino

INTRODUCTION

One of the most perplexing problems faced by urologists and oncologists is the management of patients with a rising serum prostate-specific antigen (PSA) level after definitive local therapy (1). The initial challenge is to determine whether the PSA originates from local persistence (i.e., recurrence) of cancer, from distant metastases, or both. If the recurrence is local, an opportunity remains for cure by additional treatment at the primary site. While patients with relapsing disease after radiation therapy differ in their risk of death from prostate cancer, many will develop local progression, metastasis, and death (2). The recognition that local recurrence after radiation therapy portends a poor prognosis has led to the development of improved methods for early detection of recurrence, as well as the development of alternative treatment strategies for radio-resistant cancers. Unfortunately, by the time relapse becomes clinically evident, the cancer has usually progressed beyond the point where salvage therapy might be effective. The challenge to the clinician, therefore, is to detect local recurrences while the cancer is still amenable to salvage therapy. At the same time, diagnostic tests must be both sensitive and specific; that is, they need to identify the majority of clinically threatening cancers, while excluding patients with metastatic disease and those with relapse that is not likely to be life-threatening.

Further treatment options for men with local recurrence of prostate cancer after radiation therapy include expectant management; immediate, continuous, or intermittent hormonal therapy; or further local therapy with radio-frequency thermal ablation, high-intensity focused ultrasonography, cryoablation, or salvage radical prostatectomy. Only salvage surgery has been shown to eradicate the cancer for 10 years or more. Candidates for salvage prostatectomy should be otherwise healthy with a life expectancy greater than 10 years, have a cancer that was initially and is now potentially curable with radical prostatectomy, and have no evidence of severe radiation cystitis or proctitis. If an initial pelvic lymph node dissection was performed, it must have been negative.

The major problem today with salvage prostatectomy is that the cancer is already advanced by the time most patients and their physicians will accept the operation. While stage-for-stage outcomes after salvage radical prostatectomy resemble results of standard radical prostatectomy, the majority of patients undergoing salvage radical prostatectomy have a pathologically advanced cancer [seminal vesicle invasion (SVI) and/or lymph node metastases]. Salvage prostatectomy, while technically challenging, provides excellent local control of radio-recurrent cancer and can eradicate the disease in a high proportion of patients treated when the cancer is confined to the prostate or immediate periprostatic tissue. As for standard prostatectomy, patient selection is of utmost importance.

DEFINING PROGRESSION AFTER RADIATION THERAPY FOR PROSTATE CANCER: CLINICAL VERSUS BIOCHEMICAL RECURRENCE

The goal of radiation therapy in men with localized prostate cancer is to cure the patient of his disease. Despite improved methods of delivery (ultrasound-guided brachytherapy, 3-D conformal techniques, and intensity-modulated radiation therapy) that have permitted giving higher radiation doses with fewer side effects, up to one third of men treated with radiation therapy will have evidence of treatment failure by 5 years (3).

Clinical Local Recurrence

Clinical local recurrence, defined as relapse, detectable on physical examination and characterized by signs and symptoms such as urinary outlet obstruction, has been a critical measure of the efficacy of radiation therapy. Clinical recurrence both predicts and ultimately causes disease dissemination (2,4). Kaplan et al. demonstrated that patients with clinical relapse had a shorter disease-specific survival rate than those with clinically normal prostates 10 years after external-beam radiation therapy (2). Fuks et al. calculated that the relative risk of metastatic spread was fourfold higher in patients with clinical local relapse than in patients with apparent local control (4). At 15 years, 77% of patients who had local recurrence developed metastatic disease compared with 24% of patients without relapse. These investigators correlated the presence or absence of local relapse with the time of onset of metastatic disease. Patients with local recurrence developed metastases sooner than those without local failure, implying that the latter group of patients developed metastatic disease secondary to their local recurrence and not because of preexisting micrometastases.

The true incidence of clinical local recurrence after radiation therapy has been a matter of much debate. The slow growth rate of prostate cancer mandates that long-term follow-up is necessary for accurate data. Diagnosis of recurrence by digital rectal examination (DRE) is difficult in an irradiated field. In addition, interpretation of data has often been confounded by hormonal therapy, which can mask the true rate of clinical local recurrence. Kaplan et al. reported 15-year clinical recurrence rates of 17%, 22%, 35%, and 39% for Stanford stages T1a, T1b–T1d, T2, and T3 tumors, respectively (2). However, their study did not remove patients receiving hormonal treatment from analysis. In contrast, Holzman et al. reported a 53% clinical local recurrence rate for patients with clinical T3 lesions a mean of 8 years after treatment with gold seeds and external-beam radiation therapy (5). Ninety percent of such patients required surgical intervention for complications from their local recurrence. Likewise, Schellhammer and El-Mahdi reviewed their experience with patients who did not receive elective hormonal therapy (6). Clinical local failure occurred in 4.6%, 19%, and 28% of patients with clinical stage T1, T2, and T3 tumors, respectively, only 5 to 10 years after external-beam radiotherapy. Despite the paucity of unambiguous long-term data, there is overall agreement that higher rates of clinical relapse occur with tumors of higher initial stage and grade treated by radiation therapy.

Biochemical Recurrence

The vast majority of men with recurrence after radiation therapy for localized prostate cancer are found to have an elevated and rising serum PSA level (1). In 1997, the American Society for Therapeutic Radiology and Oncology (ASTRO) defined guidelines for PSA recurrence after radiation therapy (7). While the panel agreed that biochemical failure did not necessarily predict clinical progression, they did consider biochemical failure an appropriate endpoint for clinical trials. The ASTRO definition of biochemical failure after radiation therapy is three consecutive increases in serum PSA levels at least 6 months apart. The date of biochemical failure is the midpoint between postirradiation serum PSA nadir and the first of three consecutive serum PSA increases (7). The panel also concluded that while serum PSA nadir is an important prognostic variable, no absolute value was defined to separate successful from unsuccessful treatments. While this definition has high specificity, meaning that most men with three consecutive rises in serum PSA level over an 18-month period do indeed have cancer recurrence and persistence, it lacks sensitivity, in that many men with prostate cancer who have not been cured with local radiation therapy will not manifest three consecutive rises in serum PSA levels until the cancer has advanced beyond the point were additional local therapy might still be curative. In addition, the concept of "PSA-bounce," a temporary rise in serum PSA levels within the first 2 to 3 years after radiation therapy (which may occur in up to 15% of patients), and the difficulty of interpreting the expected rise in serum PSA levels in men who receive temporary neoadjuvant or adjuvant androgen deprivation therapy can make interpretation of serum PSA levels after radiation therapy even more difficult. Improved methods of identifying patients with radio-resistant prostate cancer are needed if we are to improve patient selection and outcomes after local salvage therapies.

Using the ASTRO definition of disease recurrence, Shipley et al. examined 1,765 men with clinically localized prostate cancer (clinical stage T1–T2) treated with radiation therapy between 1988 and 1995 to determine 5-year and 7-year PSA recurrence-free rates (3). For men with a pretreatment serum PSA level <10 ng/mL, the PSA recurrence-free rates at 5 and 7 years were 77.8% and 72.9%, respectively. In those with pretreatment serum PSA levels of 10–20, 20–30, or >30 ng/mL, the 5-year PSA recurrence-free rates were 68%, 51%, and 31%, respectively. These investigators also determined that serum PSA nadir was a prognostic factor. Men with a serum PSA nadir of ≤0.5 ng/mL had a 5-year PSA recurrence-free survival of 83% compared to men with a serum PSA nadir of 0.6 to 0.9, 1 to 1.9, and ≥2 ng/mL who had a 5-year PSA recurrence-free survival of 68%, 56%, and 28%, respectively (3).

POSTRADIATION PROSTATE BIOPSY

Because of the importance of complete local tumor eradication to overall survival and because of the difficulties inherent in appreciating local recurrence clinically, a number of investigators have performed postradiation prostatic biopsies in an attempt to detect patients who have failed radiation therapy early. The hypothesis has been that microscopic recurrence precedes and is more frequent than clinical recurrence. The incidence of microscopic cancer might better estimate the success of radiation therapy, and early detection might improve the success of salvage therapies, such as radical prostatectomy.

Despite the rationale for postradiation biopsies, a number of investigators have questioned whether microscopic prostate cancer is equivalent to clinical recurrence. First, because the rate of positive biopsies may decrease with time, the significance of any given biopsy has been questioned. Cox and Stoffel biopsied patients at 6-month intervals after radiation therapy and found that the rate of positive biopsies decreased from 60% at 6 months to 19% at 30 months (8). Second, some have reported a lack of correlation between positive postradiation biopsies and disease progression. In the series reported by Cox and Stoffel, recurrence and survival rates did not differ among patients with positive and negative biopsies (8). Similar results were reported by others (9,10).

Recent work by multiple groups, however, has failed to support the contention that microscopic local cancer is not a poor prognostic indicator. In a report by Kiesling et al., only one of 38 patients with a positive biopsy converted to a negative biopsy 12 months after radiation therapy (11). Unlike Cox and Stoffel, these investigators only included in their report patients who had not received hormonal therapy. The use of hormonal therapy likely explains the divergent results between these two studies because hormonal therapy can promote local tumor regression, alter the course of localized and metastatic prostate cancer, and cause false-negative biopsies.

Long-term follow-up of patients who did not receive hormonal therapy has likewise demonstrated that positive biopsies do predict ultimate clinical local and distant recurrence. Scardino et al. reported that 66% of patients with normal DRE and positive biopsies developed clinical recurrences 5 years after treatment with gold seeds and external-beam radiation (12,13). Among those with negative biopsies and clinically benign prostates, only 29% relapsed. Freiha and Bagshaw biopsied 64 patients at least 18 months after external-beam radiation therapy (14). Forty-seven percent of patients with positive biopsies and negative lymph nodes developed metastatic disease, compared with only 10% with negative biopsies and negative lymph nodes. Seven of 28 patients with positive biopsies had clinically benign prostates. Kuban et al. selectively biopsied patients with clinically negative prostate glands and reported similar findings (15). Although only 18% of patients had microscopic local disease, 53% of these patients developed clinical local failure, a rate three times higher than those without microscopic disease.

Nevertheless, some patients with positive biopsies do not develop clinical recurrence, at least not during the intervals reported in the literature. Eighteen percent of patients with positive biopsies in the series of Scardino et al. (12) did not have clinical evidence of recurrence 10 years after treatment. In the report by Kuban et al. (16), 19% of patients had no evidence of disease 10 years after radiation therapy. Although it is possible that some patients have not been followed sufficiently long for recurrence to become manifest, it is conceivable that some biopsies may have detected clinically latent cancers. Equally important is the fact that a significant percentage of patients with negative biopsies develop local and distant recurrences. Thirty-two percent of patients with negative biopsies ultimately failed radiation therapy in the study by Scardino et al. (12). Kuban et al. reported that false-negative biopsies occurred in 24% of patients treated with ^{125}I and in 9% of those treated with external-beam therapy (17,18). Although some of these patients probably had micrometastatic disease at presentation, it is clear that biopsies failed to detect many local recurrences. The best explanation for this lack of sensitivity is that sampling errors occurred when the biopsies were taken. This is especially likely when one considers the variation in biopsy techniques used in each study. Some investigators did single transperineal biopsies, whereas others performed multiple, random transrectal biopsies.

DIAGNOSIS OF LOCAL RECURRENCE

It is clear that local recurrences, whether microscopic or macroscopic, predict and lead to prostate cancer progression. Unfortunately, by the time relapse becomes clinically evident, the tumor has generally progressed beyond the point at which salvage therapy might be effective. The challenge to the clinician, therefore, is to detect local relapses before they cease to be amenable to salvage therapy. At the same time, diagnostic tests of microscopic or subclinical local recurrence must be both sensitive and specific (i.e., they need to identify the majority of clinically threatening cancers).

DEFINING LOCAL RECURRENCE AFTER RADIATION THERAPY

Defining the site or sites of disease recurrence in men with a rising serum PSA level after radiation therapy can be difficult. While digital rectal examination (DRE) is a routine part of clinical staging, a normal DRE is not evidence for lack of local recurrence. Similarly, induration on DRE is not proof of local recurrence and may represent scar tissue. Transrectal ultrasonography (TRUS), computed tomography (CT) scan, and endorectal magnetic resonance imaging (MRI) have not proven helpful in determining the site of recurrence, but TRUS is useful for biopsy guidance and is performed at the time of systematic prostate biopsy. In most cases imaging studies to detect metastatic disease are negative (1,16).

Local recurrence after radiation therapy is defined as a rising PSA level in conjunction with a positive needle biopsy of the prostate at least 18 to 24 months after completion of irradiation. A biopsy taken earlier is not reliable, as the cancer may be regressing (19). Care must be taken in evaluating postradiation prostate biopsies because radiation induced atypia may be difficult to distinguish from residual cancer with severe radiation changes. Bostwick et al. have defined strict criteria by which prostate cancer can be histologically differentiated from postradiation atypia (20).

For men with local recurrence after radiation therapy for clinically localized prostate cancer, options for further treatment of local recurrence include expectant management, immediate continuous or intermittent hormonal therapy, or further local therapy with radio frequency thermal ablation, high-intensity focused ultrasonography, cryoablation, or salvage radical prostatectomy (21) (Fig. 15E.1). Only salvage surgery has been shown to help long-term cancer control (22).

SALVAGE RADICAL PROSTATECTOMY

The ultimate goal of early detection of local prostate cancer recurrence after radiation therapy is to improve the efficacy of salvage therapy, with the hypothesis that early recurrences will more likely be organ-confined and therefore amenable to salvage strategies. Radical prostatectomy has been used successfully to eradicate locally recurrent cancer after definitive radiotherapy, but complications are common (22–26). From these studies, several generalizations can be made. First, the procedure is usually reserved for patients in excellent health with a life expectancy of at least 10 years. Second, patients must have no evidence of metastatic disease; if an initial pelvic lymph node dissection was performed, it must have been negative. Third, salvage surgery should be offered only to those for whom both initial cancer and recurrent cancer are clinically

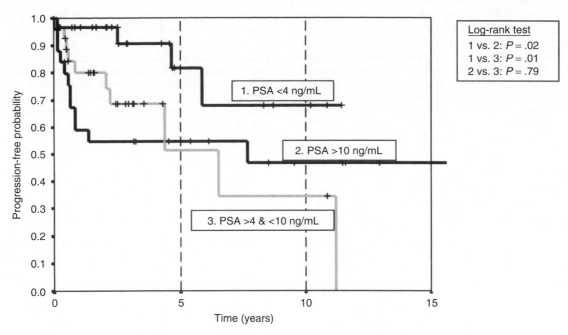

FIGURE 15E.1. Risk of recurrence after salvage radical prostatectomy according to pre-operative serum PSA level. Men with a serum PSA level <4 ng/mL were more likely to remain cancer-free than men with higher pre-operative serum PSA levels.

organ-confined and potentially curable with radical prostatec-tomy. Patients should have no evidence of severe radiation cystitis or proctitis. In all of these studies, candidates for salvage surgery were highly motivated individuals who accepted the higher morbidity associated with this approach.

Salvage radical prostatectomy is technically challenging. Short-term and long-term complication rates have been reported to exceed those of standard radical prostatectomies. Patients who consider salvage prostatectomy must be highly motivated and understand and accept the attendant morbidities. Table 15E.1 lists the rate of complications in existing salvage prostatectomy series. Overall, mean estimated blood loss and operative time do not differ significantly from estimated blood loss and operative time for standard radical prostatectomy.

However, approximately 5% to 15% of patients in these series had rectal injuries, and as many as 25% will have some other early complication of surgery, such as ureteral transection, prolonged anastomotic leakage, and pulmonary embolism. Rectal and other intraoperative injuries are especially common in those patients who had prior staging pelvic lymphadenectomy or open-seed implantation, both of which are associated with extensive fibrosis between the bladder, iliac vessels, prostate, and rectum; the former is now infrequently performed and the latter has been abandoned. Thirty-one percent of patients who had previously undergone pelvic surgery in the series from Baylor University had a surgical complication, compared with only 9% of patients who received radiation alone (22).

TABLE 15E.1

COMPLICATIONS OF SALVAGE RADICAL PROSTATECTOMY

				%			Incontinence (%)[a]	
Author	Yr	N	EBL, mL	Strictures	Rectal injuries	Other[b]	Mild	Severe
Thompson et al. (26)	1988	5	—	0	0	20	20	60
Link et al. (27)	1991	14	1,000	7	0	—	3.6	—
Moul and Paulson (28)	1991	4	800	—	—	100	0	—
Ahlering et al. (29)	1992	11	—	—	0	—	64	—
Pontes et al. (30)	1992	35	—	11.5	6	9	28	17
Stein et al. (31)	1992	11	1,100	18	0	27	64	—
Zincke et al. (32)	1992	32	—	19	6.3	25	26.7	—
Brenner et al. (33)	1994	10	1,650	10	0	20	10	10
Rogers et al. (22)	1995	40	910	27.5	15	20	58	—
Gheiler et al. (25)	1998	30	1,100	13	7	17	23	26

EBL, estimated blood loss.
[a]Severe incontinence implies >2 pads per day, and mild incontinence indicates stress incontinence requiring <2 pads per day.
[b]Other major operative complications including postoperative hemorrhage, ureteral injury, prolonged anastomotic leakage.

We have performed over 100 salvage radical prostatectomies. Salvage surgery can be safely performed after failed external beam radiotherapy, brachytherapy (open or ultrasound-guided) or combinations of these techniques. Most of our patients (89%) were treated with a retropubic approach, although selected patients (11%) following open brachytherapy underwent a combined abdominoperineal approach. Early in our series (prior to 1993), the mean estimated blood loss, transfusion requirements, and average hospital stay were greater than that for standard radical prostatectomy, but in the past 10 years the morbidity of the operation has changed substantially. Rectal injuries occurred in 15% of patients treated prior to 1993, but are now rare (Table 15E.2). With full bowel preparation before the operation, rectal injuries can be repaired primarily without altering postoperative recovery. The re-operation rate was significantly less for patients treated since 1993 (3% vs 15%, $P = .05$). There were no perioperative deaths in our series. Using current surgical techniques, salvage radical prostatectomy is technically feasible, with immediate intraoperative and postoperative outcomes similar to men undergoing standard radical prostatectomy.

Long-term complications, however, remain high. The development of an anastomotic stricture has continued to be problematic. The overall anastomotic stricture rate was 30% and did not change significantly over time. Twelve patients required multiple interventions for strictures. In multivariable analysis of factors associated with postoperative strictures, an antegrade or abdominoperineal approach (used in patients who had undergone prior pelvic surgery) and a poor quality anastomosis as judged by the surgeon were significant predictors (Table 15E.3). Careful attention to surgical detail, with a mucosa-to-mucosa anastomosis, is critical to preventing an anastomotic stricture (34). We have recently changed our anastomotic technique at the time of salvage radical prostatectomy in the hopes of reducing the incidence of stricture. Following removal of the prostate, the 'original' bladder-neck opening is closed in two layers and a new 26 to 30 French opening is made anteriorly away from the field of radiation. Further follow-up is needed to evaluate whether this technical modification will reduce the anastomotic stricture rate.

In addition, the risk of urinary incontinence remains high. For our entire series of 100 patients undergoing salvage radical prostatectomy, the overall (95% confidence limits) recovery of urinary control was 62% (49%–74%). For the period prior to 1993, 45% (26%–64%) recovered urinary control while after 1993 the rate of recovery improved to 66% (49%–84%). This likely reflects not only an improvement in

TABLE 15E.2

INTRAOPERATIVE FINDINGS AND POSTOPERATIVE COURSE IN 100 PATIENTS UNDERGOING SALVAGE RADICAL RETROPUBIC PROSTATECTOMY

	1984–1992 Early group ($n = 40$)	1993–2002 contemporary group ($n = 60$)
Mean operative time, hours (Range)	**4.4 (2.8–7)**	**3.7 (2.2–6.3)**
Operative Approach		
Standard Retropubic	19 (48%)	56 (93%)
Antegrade Retropubic	10 (25%)	4 (7%)
Abdominoperineal	11 (28%)	0
Blood Loss		
Median Amount, mL (Range)	1,000 (100–2400)	1,000 (350–4,000)
Patients Transfused (%)	13 (39)	17 (29)
Intraoperative Complication		
Rectal Injury (%)	6 (15)	1 (1.6)
Diverting Colostomy (%)	2 (5)	0
Ureteral Injury (%)	2 (5)	3 (5)
Obturator Nerve Injury (%)	0	1 (1.6)
Median Length of Stay, Days (Range)	10 (6–16)	3 (2–7)
Hospital Readmission (%)	5 (13)	8 (13)
Postoperative Complications		
Lymphocele (%)	0	2 (3.3)
Urinary Tract Infection (%)	1 (2.5)	2 (3.3)
Re-Explore for Bleeding (%)	2 (5)	0
UVJ Stricture (%)	1 (2.5)	1 (1.6)
Vesicourethral/Perineal Fistula (%)	1 (2.5)	1 (1.6)
Septic Shock (%)	1 (2.5)	0
Thrombophlebitis (%)	1 (2.5)	0
Additional Major Procedure		
Colostomy Closure (%)	2 (5)	0
Ureteral Reimplantation (%)	1 (2.5)	1 (1.6)
Delayed Cystectomy (%)	1 (2.5)[a]	1 (1.6)[a]

UVJ, ureterovesical junction.
[a]14 mo after salvage radical prostatectomy.

TABLE 15E.3

FACTORS ASSOCIATED WITH THE DEVELOPMENT OF AN ANASTOMOTIC STRICTURE

	Univariate			Multivariable		
	HR	95% CI	P	HR	95% CI	P
Non-standard Approach	5.0	1.7–15.2	.004	23.0	3.6–151	.001
Poor Anastomosis	2.2	0.7–6.8	.16	5.8	1.4–23.0	.01
External-beam Radiotherapy	4.8	1.1–20.7	.04	5.1	0.9–29.1	.06
Pre-radiotherapy PLND	0.4	0.1–1.9	.28	0.3	0.1–2.3	.24
TRUS Size >25 mL	2.1	0.8–5.6	.13	0.6	0.2–1.7	.30

HR, hazard ratio; CI, confidence interval; TRUS, transrectal ultrasound; PLND, pelvic lymph node dissection

surgical technique, but better-targeted radiation therapies leading to better preservation of the sphincteric mechanism. Twenty-three patients with persistent, severe urinary incontinence were dry after insertion of an artificial urinary sphincter and only one patient has required sphincter revision. The artificial sphincter insertion rate did not improve over time. Smaller prostate size and nerve-sparing radical prostatectomy were associated with recovery of continence (Table 15E.4).

Erectile dysfunction has been considered almost inevitable after salvage radical prostatectomy, but in selected cases, one or both neurovascular bundles may be preserved. While overall postsurgical potency is low 16% (95% CI, 4%–28%), many men have erectile dysfunction prior to salvage prostatectomy. The 5-year recovery was 45% (95% CI, 16%–75%) for men who were potent preoperatively. Of 7 patients who underwent bilateral nerve sparing procedures, 5 (71%) have recovered functional erections. Importantly, in men undergoing neurovascular bundle preservation we have not had a positive surgical margin in the area where the nerve bundle was preserved. In addition, we have recently used nerve grafts (35) to replace the cavernous nerves in patients potent before the operation who require either unilateral or bilateral neurovascular bundle resection. While follow-up is short, in selected patients potency can be maintained even in the salvage setting. Additional follow-up is required to determine the success of nerve-grafting in this patient population, especially those men receiving bilateral nerve grafts.

The major problem today with salvage radical prostatectomy is that the cancer is already advanced by the time most patients and their physicians will accept the operation. In the initial series of Scardino and colleagues, 54% had pathologically advanced cancer, defined as SVI and/or lymph node metastases (Table 15E.5) (22). Preoperative serum PSA levels, but not clinical stage or biopsy grade, had a positive correlation with pathologic stage (22). In this initial study, if the preoperative PSA was less than 10 ng/mL, only 15% of the patients had advanced pathologic features, compared to 86% if the PSA level was greater than 10 ng/mL (22). With increasing experience, however, we have determined that the lower the serum PSA level is at the time of salvage surgery (preferably <4.0 ng/mL), the more likely the opportunity for cure (Fig. 15E.1). This further highlights the need for alternative methods of defining cancer persistence and recurrence following radiation therapy rather than the ASTRO definition (7).

Data for cancer control outcomes from several salvage radical prostatectomy series are summarized in Table 15E.6. Cancer-specific survival in each of these series is greater than 90%. When serum PSA levels are used to detect recurrence following salvage prostatectomy, the actuarial non-progression rates in our series at 5 and 10 years are 57% and 38%, respectively (Table 15E.6; Fig. 15E.2). The 5-year actuarial non-progression rate was 86% for patients with organ-confined cancer (pT2N0), 61% for those with extracapsular extension, and 48% for those with SVI. Stage for stage, these results resembled those of standard radical prostatectomy (17) (Table 15E.7).

TABLE 15E.4

PREDICTORS OF URINARY CONTINENCE RECOVERY AFTER SALVAGE RADICAL PROSTATECTOMY

	5-year continence recovery (95% CI)			Multivariable Analysis		
	Present	Absent	P	HR	95% CI	P
TRUS Size <25 cc	84% (70–99)	40% (20–59)	.001	4.4	1.9–10	.0005
Nerve-sparing RP[a]	65% (46–100)	58% (43–75)	.27	2.1	1.1–4.1	.03
Positive Surgical Margins	79% (57–100)	58% (44–73)	.02	2.1	.9–4.6	.07
Clinical Stage T1-T2a	81% (60–100)	52% (36–68)	.23	1.3	.6–2.5	.49
No SVI or LNI	61% (46–77)	63% (41–85)	.74	1.2	.6–2.5	.56
PSA <10 ng/mL	63% (47–78)	50% (22–78)	.11	1.2	.4–3.2	.76
Patient Age <65 yr	69% (52–86)	54% (37–71)	.3	1.1	.5–2.1	.94

CI, confidence interval; HR, hazard ratio; TRUS, transrectal ultrasound; RP, radical prostatectomy; SVI, seminal vesicle invasion; LNI, lymph node involvement.
[a]Includes patients who had bilateral nerve-sparing and unilateral nerve-sparing, with or without nerve graft.

TABLE 15E.5

PATHOLOGICAL OUTCOMES IN 100 MEN UNDERGOING SALVAGE RADICAL PROSTATECTOMY BETWEEN 1984 AND 2003

	Overall (n = 100)	1984–1994 (n = 48)	1995–2003 (n = 52)	P
Organ-confined	32%	17%	46%	.002
Extraprostatic	45%	67%	25%	.005
Seminal Vesicle Invasion	38%	50%	27%	.003
Positive Surgical Margin	29%	31%	8%	.004
Positive Lymph Nodes	9%	4%	14%	.02

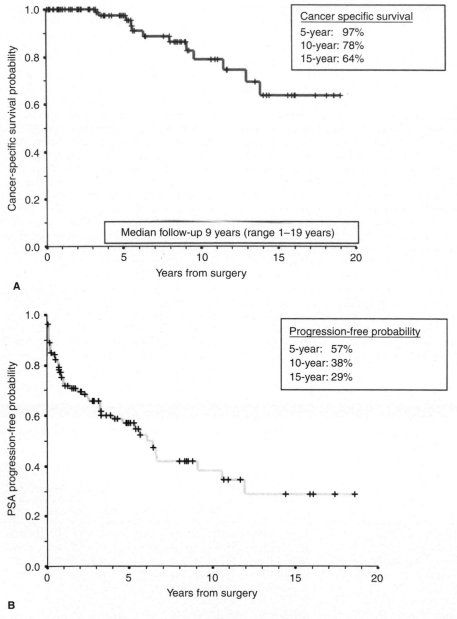

FIGURE 15E.2. Kaplan-Meier estimates for outcomes after salvage radical prostatectomy for 100 patients in our series. None received adjuvant treatment before relapse. **A:** Cancer-specific survival. **B:** Progression-free probability. Progression was defined as either a serum prostate-specific antigen (PSA) level of ≥0.2 ng/mL and/or clinical recurrence. Median time to serum PSA failure after surgery was 6.1 years. **C:** Progression-free probability according to pathologic stage of disease.

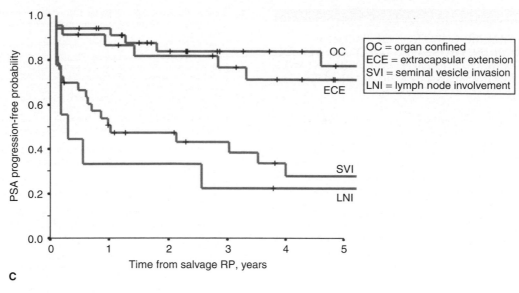

c

FIGURE 15E.2. Continued.

SALVAGE LAPAROSCOPIC RADICAL PROSTATECTOMY

Salvage surgery has been described using the laparoscopic approach. The largest series to date is from Vallancien et al. who reported their results from 7 patients treated between 2000 and 2002 who had failed either external beam radiation therapy (5 patients) or brachytherapy (2 patients) (38). Average operating time was 190 minutes (range 170–210 minutes). None of the patients had preservation of the neurovascular bundles. There were no intraoperative complications or transfusions. Pathologic examination of the resected specimens included three with extraprostatic extension (pT3a), three with SVI (pT3b), and one with invasion of the bladder neck (pT4a). The positive surgical margin rate was 28%. With follow-up ranging from four to 21 months, two have failed biochemically. Five of seven (71%) were continent and none had developed an anastomotic stricture. While these functional results (continence and anastomotic strictures) are excellent compared to open salvage radical

prostatectomy, the positive surgical margin rate was much higher (28% vs 8%) even though no attempts were made to preserve the neurovascular bundles. Whether or not this translates into a higher rate of failure awaits further follow-up.

CONCLUSION

Salvage prostatectomy, while technically challenging, provides excellent local control of radiorecurrent cancer, and it can eradicate the disease in a high proportion of patients treated when the cancer is confined to the prostate or immediate periprostatic tissue. As with standard prostatectomy, patient selection is of utmost importance. Patients should be in good health with a life expectancy greater than 10 years, have a local tumor proven by biopsy, and have no evidence of metastatic disease. As outcomes continue to improve, patients may be more willing to accept this treatment option after failure of definitive radiation therapy. Continuing surgical challenges include the high rate of urinary incontinence and anastomotic strictures. While these outcomes appear better

---

TABLE 15E.6

OUTCOMES AFTER SALVAGE RADICAL PROSTATECTOMY IN SELECTED SERIES OF PATIENTS

Authors	N	Clinical stage	Non-progression rate, % 5 Yr	Non-progression rate, % 10 Yr	Clinical non-progression rate, % 5 Yr	Clinical non-progression rate, % 10 Yr	Cancer-specific survival rate, % 5 Yr	Cancer-specific survival rate, % 10 Yr
Rogers et al. (22)	38	T1-3 N0NX	55	33	83	67	95	87
Amling et al. (36)	108	T1b-N+	70	44	—	42	90	60
Gheiler et al. (25)	40	T2-3N0	47.4	—	87.5	—	—	—
Current series[a]	100	T1-3 N0NX	57	38	90	81	97	78

[a]Includes the patients detailed in reference (22).

TABLE 15E.7

LONG-TERM CANCER CONTROL OUTCOMES: STANDARD RADICAL PROSTATECTOMY (RP) VERSUS SALVAGE RADICAL PROSTATECTOMY; PERCENTAGES REPRESENT PROGRESSION-FREE PROBABILITIES; DATA SUMMARIZED FROM REFERENCE (37)

Pathology	Standard RP N = 1,000		Salvage RP N = 100	
	5 Yr	10 Yr	5 Yr	10 Yr
Organ-confined	94.9%	92.2%	86.0%	86.0%
Extraprostatic Extension	76.3%	71.4%	61.6%	41.0 %
Seminal Vesicle Invasion	37.4%	37.4%	47.6%	32.6%
Positive Lymph Nodes	18.5%	7.4%	60.0%	—

with a laparoscopic approach, this must be balanced against the higher rate of positive surgical margins. Improved methods to identify radio recurrent prostate cancer while it is still confined to the prostate are also needed to enhance patient outcomes. Our data suggests that the serum PSA level should be <4 ng/mL prior to salvage prostatectomy in order to have a realistic chance of cure. Improved methods of defining failure, rather than reliance on the ASTRO definition, are needed.

References

1. Djavan B, Moul JW, Zlotta A, et al. PSA progression following radical prostatectomy and radiation therapy: new standards in the new millennium. *Eur Urol* 2003;43:12–27.
2. Kaplan ID, Prestidge BR, Bagshaw MA, et al. The importance of local control in the treatment of prostatic cancer. *J Urol* 1992;147:917–921.
3. Shipley WU, Thames HD, Sandler HM, et al. Radiation therapy for clinically localized prostate cancer: a multi-institutional pooled analysis. *JAMA* 1999;281(17):1598–1604.
4. Fuks Z, Leibel S, Wallner K, et al. The effect of local control on metastatic dissemination in carcinoma of the prostate: long-term results in patients treated with I-125 implantation. *Int J Radiat Oncol Biol Phys* 1991;21:537.
5. Holzman M, Carlton CE Jr, Scardino PT. The frequency and morbidity of local tumor recurrence after definitive radiotherapy. *J Urol* 1991;146:1578.
6. Schellhammer PF, El-Mahdi AM. Local failure and related complications after definitive treatment of carcinoma of the prostate by irradiation or surgery. *Urol Clin North Am* 1990;17:835.
7. American Society for Therapeutic Radiology and Oncology Consensus Panel. Consensus statement: guidelines for PSA following radiation therapy. *Int J Radiat Oncol Biol Phys* 1997;37:1035–1041.
8. Cox JD, Stoffel TJ. The significance of needle biopsy after irradiation for stage C adenocarcinoma of the prostate. *Cancer* 1977;40:156.
9. Leach GE, Cooper JF, Kagan AR, et al. Radiotherapy for prostatic carcinoma: postirradiation prostatic biopsy and recurrence patterns with long-term follow-up. *J Urol* 1982;128:505.
10. Kagan AR, Steckel RJ. Surveillance of patients with prostate cancer after treatment: the roles of serologic and imaging studies. *Med Pediatr Oncol* 1993;21:327.
11. Kiesling VJ, McAninch JW, Goebel JL, et al. External beam radiotherapy for adenocarcinoma of the prostate: a clinical follow-up. *J Urol* 1980;124:851.
12. Scardino PT, Frankel JM, Wheeler TM, et al. The prognostic significance of postirradiation biopsy results in patients with prostatic cancer. *J Urol* 1986;135:510.
13. Scardino PT, Wheeler TM. Local control of prostate cancer with radiotherapy: the frequency and prognostic significance of positive postirradiation prostate biopsy results. *Natl Cancer Inst Monogr* 1988;7:95.
14. Freiha FS, Bagshaw MA. Carcinoma of the prostate: results of postirradiation biopsy. *Prostate* 1984;5:19.
15. Kuban D, El-Mahdi A, Schellhammer P. Prognostic significance of post-irradiation biopsies. *Oncology* 1993;7:29.
16. Epstein JI, Pizov G, Walsh PC. Correlation of pathologic findings with progression after radical retropubic prostatectomy. *Cancer* 1993;71:3582–3593.
17. Kuban DA, El-Mahdi AM, Schellhammer PF. I-125 interstitial implantation for prostatic cancer. What have we learned 10 years later? *Cancer* 1989;63:2415.
18. Kuban DA, El-Mahdi AM, Schellhammer PF. The significance of postirradiation prostate biopsy with long-term follow-up. *Int J Radiat Oncol Biol Phys* 1992;24:409.
19. Crook JM, Perry GA, Robertson S, et al. Routine prostate biopsies following radiotherapy for prostate cancer: results for 226 patients. *Urology* 1995;45:624–631.
20. Bostwick DG, Egbert BM, Fijardo LF. Radiation injury of the normal and neoplastic prostate. *Am J Surg Pathol* 1982;6:541.
21. Miles BJ, Herman JR, Reiter RE, et al. Salvage radical prostatectomy for local recurrence of prostate cancer after radiotherapy. In: Vogelzang NJ, Scardino PT, Shipley WU et al., eds. *Comprehensive textbook of genitourinary oncology*, 2nd ed. Philadelphia, PA: Lippincott Williams & Wilkins, 2000:813.
22. Rogers E, Ohori M, Kassabian VS, et al. Salvage radical prostatectomy: outcome measured by serum prostate specific antigen levels. *J Urol* 1995;153:104–110.
23. Cheng L, Sebo TJ, Slezak J, et al. Predictors of survival for prostate carcinoma in patients treated with salvage radical prostatectomy after radiation therapy. *Cancer* 1998;83:2164–2171.
24. Tefilli MV, Gheiler EL, Tiguert R, et al. Salvage surgery or salvage radiotherapy for locally recurrent prostate cancer. *Urology* 1998;52:224–229.
25. Gheiler EL, Tefilli MV, Tiguert R, et al. Predictors for maximal outcome in patients undergoing salvage surgery for radiorecurrent prostate cancer. *Urology* 1998;51:789–795.
26. Thompson IM, Rounder JB, Spence CR, et al. Salvage radical prostatectomy for adenocarcinoma of the prostate. *Cancer* 1988;61:1464.
27. Link P, Freiha FS. Radical prostatectomy after definitive radiation therapy for prostate cancer. *Urology* 1991;37:189.
28. Moul JW, Paulson DF. The role of radical surgery in the management of radiation recurrent and large volume prostate cancer. *Cancer* 1991;68:1265.
29. Ahlering TE, Lieskovsky G, Skinner DG. Salvage surgery plus androgen deprivation for radioresistant prostatic adenocarcinoma. *J Urol* 1992;147:900.
30. Pontes JE, Montie J, Klein E, et al. Salvage surgery for radiation failure in prostate cancer. *Cancer* 1992;71:976.
31. Stein A, Smith RB, DeKernion JB. Salvage radical prostatectomy after failure of curative radiotherapy for adenocarcinoma of prostate. *Urology* 1992;40:197.
32. Zincke H. Radical prostatectomy and exenterative procedures for local failure after radiotherapy with curative intent: comparison of outcomes. *J Urol* 1992;147:894.
33. Brenner PC, Russo P, Wood DP, et al. Salvage radical prostatectomy in the management of locally recurrent prostate cancer after 125I implantation. *Br J Urol* 1995;75:44.
34. Eastham JA, Kattan MW, Rogers E, et al. Risk factors for urinary incontinence after radical retropubic prostatectomy. *J Urol* 1996;156:1707–1712.
35. Kim ED, Scardino PT, Hampel O, et al. Interposition of sural nerve restores function of cavernous nerves resected during radical prostatectomy. *J Urol* 1999;161:188–192.
36. Amling CL, Blute ML, Lerner SE, et al. Influence of prostate-specific antigen testing on the spectrum of patients with prostate cancer undergoing radical prostatectomy at a large referral practice [see Comments]. *Mayo Clin Proc* 1998;73:401–406.
37. Hull GW, Rabbani F, Abbas F, et al. Cancer control with radical prostatectomy alone in 1,000 consecutive patients. *J Urol* 2002;167:528–534.
38. Vallancien G, Gupta R, Cathelineau X, et al. Initial results of salvage laparoscopic radical prostatectomy after radiation failure. *J Urol* 2003;170:1838–1840.

CHAPTER 16 ■ ADVANCED PROSTATE CANCER

CHAPTER 16A
Initial Management of Metastatic Prostate Cancer

Paul D. Maroni, J. Brantley Thrasher, and E. David Crawford

INTRODUCTION

Despite tremendous research effort, few areas of urologic oncology contain as much uncertainty and controversy about appropriate therapy as the hormonal manipulation of advanced prostate cancer. In 1941, Huggins and Hodges (1) provided evidence widely accepted that patients with symptomatic metastatic disease benefit from some form of testosterone suppression. Most trials in the late 20th century expanded to treating patients with symptomatic and asymptomatic/radiographic metastatic disease. More recently, a wave of enthusiasm has spread over the growing population of men with prostate-specific antigen (PSA) relapse after local therapy for prostate carcinoma thus clouding further the exact definition of what constitutes "metastatic" disease in a given individual. Certainly, the presence of cancer cells inside the organism yet outside the boundaries of the organ of origin would provide biological proof of metastasis, but the investigational focus until lately has been primarily on patients with extensive, measurable disease. This is largely due to the relatively recent availability of PSA, a serum marker that is mostly accepted as a surrogate of disease. This marker has the means of detecting subclinical disease, thus creating a paradigm in the management of malignancy that is not available for most other solid-organ tumors. An even more recent entry into the population of men likely to benefit from hormonal therapy are "candidates" for advanced disease or men with high-risk features based on clinical, laboratory, and pathologic parameters.

Another realm of controversy in the management of patients with advanced disease is the utility of surgical and medical therapies and combinations thereof. Bilateral surgical orchiectomy, luteinizing-hormone-releasing hormone analogs (LHRHa), and estrogens all provide patients with castrate levels of testosterone, but small amounts of androgens are released by the adrenal glands. Surgical adventures into the removal of the adrenal glands have largely been abandoned for the many medications available that block the activity of adrenal androgens, namely, steroidal and nonsteroidal antiandrogens, and addition of one of these components to medical or surgical castration is considered combined/complete androgen blockade or maximum androgen blockade (CAB/MAB). The monotherapy versus CAB debate continues despite a wealth of studies largely due to the incalculable value physicians and patients place on different outcomes. When clear

and meaningful expansion of life is in doubt, patient benefit must be found in other areas and quality of life issues will be addressed when possible. In this chapter, we present a brief history of hormonal manipulation, an overview of methods of castration, a contemporary review of the literature on clinical trials comparing CAB with monotherapy, the optimum timing of treatment, and newer hormonal manipulations such as intermittent androgen deprivation (IAD).

EARLY HISTORY OF HORMONAL THERAPY FOR PROSTATE CANCER

The first scientific observation of the relationship of castration to prostate size was made in 1786 by the father of scientific surgery, John Hunter (2). The discovery of prostate cancer metastasizing to the bone occurred about 30 years after the first description of prostate cancer in 1818 by George Langstaff (3). While castration was being used to remedy urinary retention in the late 1800s (4, 5), another half century passed before Huggins discovered the relationship between testosterone and prostate cancer and refined castration therapies for advanced disease (1). Serum improvements in the acid and alkaline phosphatases were associated with cancer-related symptom relief. These findings would later earn him the Nobel Prize for physiology and medicine, and Huggins remarked that "this will benefit man forever.... A thousand years from now people will be taking this treatment" (6). Likely due to the absence of other therapies, hormonal manipulation became a mainstay of treatment for symptomatic metastatic disease. Some authors have suggested that hormone treatment of prostate cancer potentially cures patients, but the typical expectation is that a patient enjoys a variable period of tumor shrinkage or suspension followed ultimately by progressive expansion or development of clones stimulated by nonandrogenic growth factors, such as IL-6 (7–9). While the hypothesis that androgen deprivation lengthens life expectancy has never been tested in a randomized fashion, Nesbit and Baum's (10) retrospective review of 417 patients demonstrated increased survival in patients who received hormonal manipulation (Fig. 16A.1).

Castrate levels of testosterone are achievable in most patients treated with estrogens, LHRH analogs, or orchiectomy, but roughly 20% of patients do not respond to treatment and those that do often have clinical progression to hormone refractory disease at 18 to 24 months (11). Many patients with castrate levels of testosterone continue to have measurable levels of dihydrotestosterone (DHT) in the prostate thought secondary to nontesticular sources of androgen (12). Huggins et al. attempted to eliminate the contribution of adrenal androgens by performing bilateral adrenalectomy in patients with progressing prostate cancer, but three of four patients died in the early postoperative period from mineralocorticoid deficiency, curbing any enthusiasm for this mode of therapy (13).

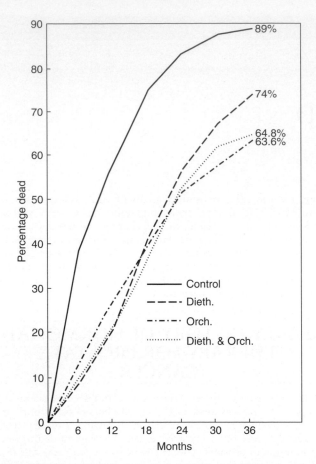

FIGURE 16A.1. Three-year survival in patients with metastasis at presentation with hormonal therapy compared to previously untreated cohort (From Nesbit RM, Baum WC. Endocrine control of prostatic carcinoma: clinical and statistical survey of 1818 cases. *JAMA* 1950; 143:1317.)

Through the 1950s, mild interest in adrenalectomy returned with the availability of exogenous cortisol, and subjective improvement in pain was noted in 73% of patients with a 6.6% objective response rate (14–23). Ultimately this procedure was largely abandoned as a therapy for prostate cancer due to the poor objective response rates and the tremendous morbidity associated with the surgery and cortisol replacement. Similarly, medical blockade of adrenocortical function using aminoglutethimide or spironolactone resulted in the majority of patients experiencing subjective relief of pain, but objective responses were rare and short-lived (24–26). Side effects were substantial, with most patients experiencing lassitude, anorexia, and depression, with some episodes of hypotension, nausea, and vomiting. Therefore, interest in CAB waned until improved methods of medical castration became available.

Discoveries in the late 1960s and 1970s contributed to advances in medical therapies for the treatment of metastatic prostate cancer. Up through this time, synthetic estrogens were the primary means of medical castration, but the Veterans Administration Cooperative Urological Research Group (VACURG) studies raised serious concerns regarding cardiac events in patients receiving diethylstilbestrol (DES), in particular the 5 mg/day dosage. Schally and Guillemin received the Nobel Prize for physiology and medicine in 1977 for independently isolating and synthesizing naturally occurring LHRH (27,28). Since then, numerous synthetic analogs have been developed that have a greater potency than the naturally occurring compound due to increased receptor affinity and reduced susceptibility to enzymatic degradation (29). Administration of these

analogs results in release and depletion of pituitary LH, followed by a down-regulation of LHRH receptors. As a result, the pituitary becomes refractory to further stimulation by LHRH, resulting in castrate levels of testosterone. These compounds usually cause an early increase, or flare, in serum testosterone within days and castrate levels are attained by 4 weeks (30). Multiple LHRH analogs are available and include goserelin (Zoladex), leuprolide (Lupron, Eligard, Viadur), buserelin (Suprefact), and triptorelin (Decapeptyl, Trelstar). These compounds are available in a variety of formulations, but are commonly given as intramuscular or subcutaneous depots that last between 1 and 4 months with longer acting implants/depots available or being developed (Table 16A.1). The advantages of LHRHa therapy are tolerance and reversibility; however, these compounds have high repeating costs and result in a loss of libido, impotence, and hot flashes. Also of concern is the increase in the level of testosterone after the initial administration of LHRH analogs. This flare phenomenon may cause an increase in pain and result in serious side effects such as ureteric obstruction and paralysis in patients with extensive spinal column metastases (31). Investigations into antiandrogenic compounds in the late 1960s/early 1970s led to the availability of several agents that inhibited or blocked the testosterone receptor with few or minor side effects (32, 33). The addition of these antiandrogens before initiating LHRH analog therapy has been found to block flare side effects (34). Antiandrogens finally allowed a less morbid method for addressing adrenal androgens and led into the modern era of investigation of the role of hormonal manipulation in advanced prostate cancer. These agents can be classified into steroidal and nonsteroidal antiandrogens, with the distinctions being the molecular chemical structure and the physiologic progestational effects of steroidal compounds, namely impotence and loss of libido.

The nonsteroidal antiandrogens act only at the androgenic receptors and do not have progestational side effects. This local effect results in increased LH and serum testosterone, which preserves libido and potency in 80% of patients (35). The nonsteroidal antiandrogens currently available include flutamide (Eulexin), nilutamide (Anandron), and bicalutamide (Casodex) (Fig. 16A.2). Flutamide has a short half-life (6 to 8 hours) with 3-times daily dosing (250 mg), but daily dosing (500 mg) has also been shown to be safe and effective at lower cost (36). The most frequently reported side effects include gynecomastia, nausea, vomiting, diarrhea, and liver dysfunction. Hepatotoxicity has been reported in approximately three per 100,000 flutamide users and is thought to be the result of metabolites formed via the cytochrome P-450 system (37). The package insert addendum from 1999 recommends pretreatment evaluation of serum transaminases and monthly checks for the first 4 months on treatment with periodic checks thereafter. Nilutamide has a longer half-life (45 hours) than flutamide, which allows for a single oral dose of 300 mg daily. Its side effects include hot flashes, nausea, visual disturbances, alcohol intolerance, and interstitial pneumonitis (38). Bicalutamide is a newer nonsteroidal antiandrogen that has a half-life of 7 to 10 days, which allows for administration of a single daily dose. It possesses a fourfold higher affinity for the rat androgen receptor than 2-hydroxyflutamide, the active metabolite of flutamide (39). Currently, a dosage of 50 mg orally once daily has been recommended for the use as a component of CAB while 150 mg once daily has been investigated as single-agent therapy (40,41). Bicalutamide has a dose-dependent incidence of gynecomastia and breast pain that can be as high as 74% lending to high dropout rates in certain studies (42). This antiandrogen is considered the standard for use in current combination regimens.

Steroidal antiandrogens include cyproterone acetate (CPA), megestrol acetate, and medroxyprogesterone acetate. CPA has been widely used across the world as a combined-therapy and

TABLE 16A.1

AVAILABLE LUTEINIZING-HORMONE-RELEASING HORMONE ANALOGS

Compound	Trade name (Manufacturer)	Dose	Route
Buserelin acetate	Suprefact (Aventis)	0.5 mg–TID × 7 days, then 0.2 mg QD	SQ
		6.3 mg–2 mo	
		9.45 mg–3 mo	
		0.4 mg TID	Intranasal
Goserelin acetate	Zoladex (Astrazeneca)	3.6 mg–1 mo	SQ
		10.8 mg–3 mo	
Leuprolide acetate	Lupron (TAP)	7.5 mg–1 mo	IM
		22.5 mg–3 mo	
		30 mg–4 mo	
	Eligard (Sanofi-Synthelabo)	7.5 mg–1 mo	SQ
		22.5 mg–3 mo	
	Viadur (Bayer)	72 mg–12 mo	SQ implant
Triptorelin pamoate	Trelstar (Pharmacia/Upjohn) Decapaptyl SR (Ipsen)	3.75 mg–1 mo	IM

monotherapy agent. One advantage of CPA is the amelioration of hot flashes induced by medical and surgical castration (43). Megestrol and medroxyprogesterone acetate have been used as second-line agents in hormone refractory prostate cancer with disappointing results (44), but have perhaps found greatest use in the treatment of intolerable hot flashes from hormone ablation therapy (45). Worrisome for both steroidal and non steroidal compounds is the concept that mutant clones may potentially be stimulated by exposure to these agents as has been demonstrated in certain prostate cancer cell lines (46,47).

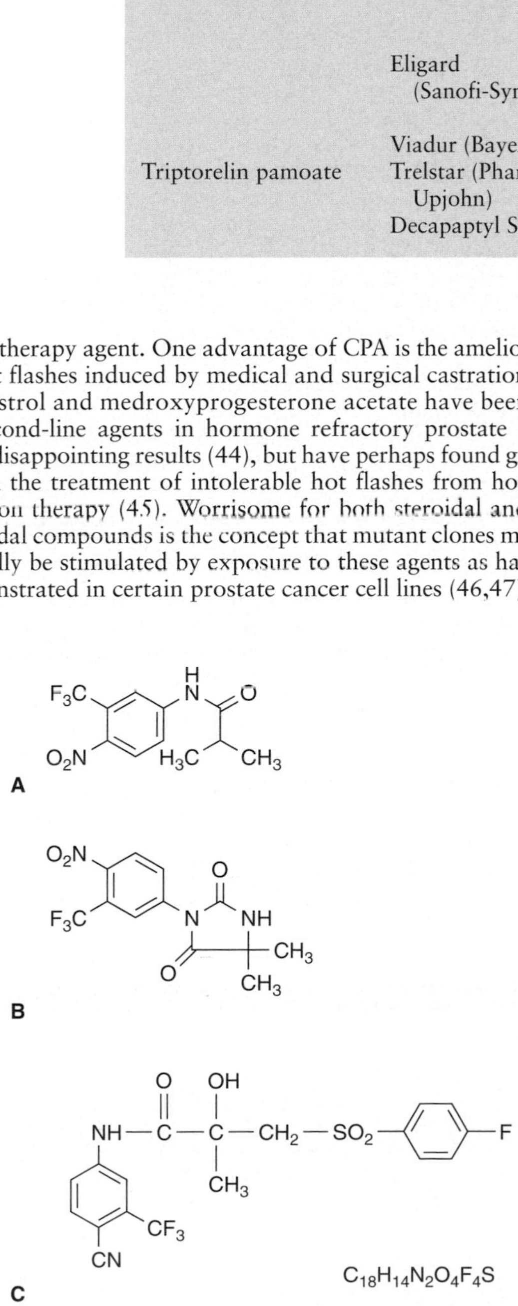

FIGURE 16A.2. Molecular structure of nonsteroidal antiandrogens. **A:** Flutamide. **B:** Nilutamide. **C:** Bicalutamide. (From *Physicians' Desk Reference,* 52nd ed. Montvale, NJ: Medical Economics Company, 1998;1222, 2023, 3152, with permission.)

MAXIMUM ANDROGEN BLOCKADE

The studies of Geller et al. (48) suggested a significant contribution toward continued androgenic stimulation of prostate cancer cells from adrenal androgens in men who had undergone medical or surgical castration. These authors noted that in castrated men, the concentration of DHT in prostate tissue remained at up to 40% of the level detected in untreated men. They also noted that extremely small levels of DHT resulted in an increase in prostatic protein synthesis. Labrie has spent tremendous basic science effort in forwarding the benefit of inhibition with antiandrogens (49). Conversely, an animal study by Trachtenberg suggested a testosterone threshold (50). He used the Dunning prostate-cancer model in castrated rats implanted with testosterone pellets of variable concentration and noted that tumor volume did not increase over castrate control until serum concentration was well above castrate levels. He also hypothesized that more men might sustain erectile function with adequate cancer control if higher levels of testosterone were tolerated. The idea of a critical threshold for prostatic cell growth has also been supported by others (51, 52). While combined therapy has synergistic effects on nondiseased prostate growth in the rat, the Dunning prostate-cancer model has not shown a tumor growth or survival benefit of combined androgen blockade with either cyproterone acetate or flutamide (Fig. 16A.3) (49,53,54). Despite mixed basic scientific data suggesting benefit of combined androgen blockade in the treatment of prostate cancer, numerous small scale trials proceeded largely due to the poor prognosis of individuals with metastatic prostate cancer and the lack of other effective therapeutic options.

The major catalyst for the rejuvenation of clinical interest in using an antiandrogen in combination with testicular androgen ablation was a study by Labrie et al. (55). Thirty-seven patients with stage-C and stage-D prostate cancer received buserelin and nilutamide. None of the patients had received prior hormonal therapy. A positive objective response was reported in 97% of the patients, with a median follow-up of only 4.2 months. None of the patients had measurable lesions,

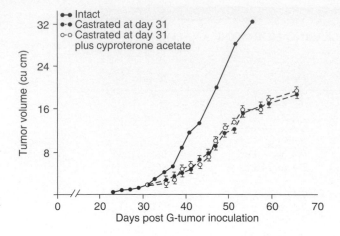

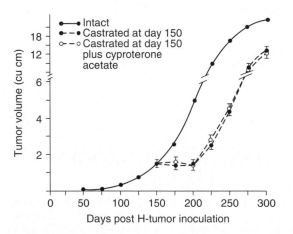

FIGURE 16A.3. Castration and cyproterone acetate do not affect Dunning R-3327-implanted prostate cancer growth more than castration alone. [From Ellis WJ, Isaacs JT. Effectiveness of complete versus partial androgen withdrawal therapy for the treatment of prostatic cancer as studied in the Dunning R-3327 system of rat prostatic adenocarcinoma. *Cancer Res* 1985;45(12 pt 1):6041.]

bringing into question the ability to accurately assess objective response. However, the authors suggested that first-line CAB produced response rates 25% to 30% higher than conventional testicular androgen ablation. Labrie et al. recommended CAB as an "initial therapy" based on the theory that some cancer cells are "hypersensitive" to androgens (56). Castration eradicates the clones of cancer cells that require the largest amounts of DHT but not the clones that grow with

lower DHT concentrations. These clones require adrenal androgen blockade. Labrie et al. also suggested that monotherapy resulted in persistent levels of cellular androgens, which ultimately result in the development of androgen-hypersensitive tumors, which are more resistant to antihormonal therapy (57,58). Therefore, their early clinical trials and animal experiments rejuvenated the concept of early CAB, suggesting response rates that were much higher than historical controls.

Review of Randomized Trials

Supporting Maximum Androgen Blockade

The excellent results reported by Labrie et al. (55) had neither a large patient population nor a randomized design. Therefore, their results were met with considerable skepticism. A large number of controlled studies have been initiated to test the hypothesis that CAB is superior to conventional monotherapy. The study designs have varied, and a variety of LHRH agonists or orchiectomy have been used for castration in combination with three different antiandrogens—flutamide, nilutamide, and CPA. Three independent randomized studies have shown significant benefits for CAB over castration alone in either time to progression or survival (59–62). These studies are summarized in Table 16A.2.

The study conducted by the Southwest Oncology Group (SWOG; INT 0036) randomized 603 patients with previously untreated stage-D2 carcinoma of the prostate to leuprolide-plus-placebo versus leuprolide-plus-flutamide (59). The National Prostatic Cancer Project criteria were used to evaluate response. A significantly longer progression-free survival rate (16.5 vs. 13.9 months, P = .039) and overall survival rate (35.6 vs. 28.3 months, P = .035) were noted in the group that received CAB. Patients with minimal disease and good performance status enjoyed a more significant benefit. The difference in overall survival rate was 19 months (48 months for CAB, and 19 months for single-agent leuprolide) in favor of patients with minimal disease. However, this subgroup consisted of only 41 patients in each arm. The only adverse event reported significantly more often in the CAB group was diarrhea (13.6% vs. 4.9%, P ≤.001). The conclusion of the INT 0036 study was that leuprolide combined with flutamide was superior to leuprolide alone and thus the extrapolation that CAB was superior to monotherapy. However, there were questions raised about compliance in the control arm and whether or not the flare phenomenon contributed to the worse outcome seen in the control group.

The European Organization of Research and Treatment of Cancer (EORTC) conducted a phase III randomized study (EORTC 30853) that compared CAB (goserelin acetate, 3.6 mg

TABLE 16A.2

TRIALS THAT SUPPORT THE EFFICACY OF COMBINED ANDROGEN BLOCKADE

Primary author	*n*	Treatment	Follow-up	Response rate	Progression-free survival	Survival
Crawford 1989 (SWOG; INT 0036)	603	Leuprolide + placebo vs. leuprolide + flutamide	48 mo	36.1% vs. 42.8%	13.9 mo vs. 16.5 mo	22.3 mo vs. 35.6 mo (P = .035)
Denis 1993 (EORTC 30853)	310	Orchiectomy + placebo vs. goserelin + flutamide	5 yr	59% vs. 58%	46 wk vs. 71 wk	27.1 mo vs. 34.4 mo (P = .02)
Dijkman 1997	423	Orchiectomy + placebo vs. orchiectomy + nilutamide	8.5 yr	24% vs. 41%	14.7 mo vs. 21.2 mo	29.8 mo vs. 37 mo (P = .013)

every 4 weeks subcutaneously, plus flutamide, 250 mg 3 times a day orally) with bilateral orchiectomy in 310 patients (60). The initial report (interim analysis) showed no differences in terms of progression and survival (62); however, the subsequent review of the data at 5 years of follow-up demonstrated a statistical difference in favor of CAB. With a mean follow-up of 5 years, there was a 25-week increase in time to progression (71 weeks vs. 46 weeks) and a 7-month increase in overall survival (34.4 months vs. 27.1 months) noted in the CAB group. This statistically significant difference closely approximated that found in the INT 0036 (59). Additionally, CAB provided the most benefit to those patients with minimal disease. The most frequent side effects reported in both treatment arms were hot flashes and gynecomastia, both of which were more common in the combination arm. Hot flushes were reported for 58% of patients who underwent orchiectomy and 68% of patients treated with CAB. The corresponding differences with respect to gynecomastia were 8% and 19%, respectively.

The International Anandron Study Group compared the combination of bilateral orchiectomy alone versus bilateral orchiectomy plus 300 mg per day of nilutamide in 457 patients (61). With 8.5 years of follow-up, a 7-month increase was found in the CAB arm in both time to progression (21.2 months vs. 14.7 months) and survival rate (37 months vs. 29.8 months). The overall response rate of 41% was significantly higher than the 24% response rate with orchiectomy alone. Also, more patients in the CAB group than in the orchiectomy group had a decrease in pain (74% vs. 68%, $P = .046$) and normalization of PSA and prostatic acid phosphatase levels (51% vs. 32%, $P = .027$) at 1 month. Early normalization of PSA was shown to predict an improved long-term response to hormonal therapy in terms of interval to disease progression and death. A total of 15.5% of the patients in the nilutamide group and 9% in the placebo group were withdrawn from the study prematurely because of adverse or intercurrent events. Respiratory disorders, visual disturbances (difficulty with light-to-dark adaptation or blurred vision), and transient increases in liver enzyme levels were reported more commonly in the nilutamide group.

Refuting Maximal Androgen Blockade

Although several large and well-designed studies have supported the superiority of CAB, 22 studies refute these findings or showed trends that did not achieve statistical significance (63–84). Comprehensive analysis of the survival data from these studies has been published by the Prostate Cancer Trialists' Collaborative Group (85). A few of these studies will be highlighted as follows. The Danish Prostatic Cancer Group randomized 262 patients to either orchiectomy plus placebo or to CAB consisting of goserelin acetate depot, 3.6 mg subcutaneously once every 4 weeks, plus flutamide, 250 mg by mouth 3 times a day (71). Neither the interim analysis (median follow-up of 39 months) nor the final analysis (median follow-up of 57 months) found significant differences between treatment groups for time to progression of disease (16.5 months vs. 16.8 months) and survival rate (22.7 months vs. 27.6 months). Advantages to CAB were seen in the subgroup of patients with minimal metastatic disease in terms of time to progression and survival, but they were not significant.

Iversen et al. attempted to perform combined analysis of the EORTC 30853 and the Danish Prostatic Cancer Group 86 study because of the almost identical design of the protocols (84). A combined analysis of 591 patients from the two studies revealed a significantly longer time to objective progression of disease in the combination group ($P = .04$). However, the time from objective progression to death was longer in the orchiectomy group, and no differences in overall survival were noted between the treatment groups.

Numerous studies that compared CAB using flutamide with monotherapy refute the benefits of CAB (68–77). Fourcade et al. (71) performed a double-blind, placebo-controlled, randomized study in 245 patients comparing goserelin acetate depot, 3.6 mg subcutaneously injected every 4 weeks, with goserelin acetate depot in the same dose plus flutamide, 250 mg by mouth 3 times daily. Complete and partial responses were noted in 77.9% of patients in the combination group and in 80.8% of those in the monotherapy group. At 4 years median follow-up, no significant difference in time to disease progression or overall survival was found.

Reporting for the International Prostate Cancer Study Group, Tyrell et al. used a similar study design with identical drug dosages (69). They evaluated 586 patients and reported no statistically significant difference between treatment groups in the rate of objective response, interval to progression, and overall median survival. When these parameters were subcategorized to evaluate those with locally advanced disease and those with metastatic disease separately, no significant differences could be ascertained.

Eisenberger et al. have reported the results of a large randomized study (SWOG INT-0105) that compared bilateral orchiectomy alone and orchiectomy plus flutamide (76). This study is the largest trial to date and enrolled almost 1,400 patients. This study also failed to demonstrate the superiority of CAB versus monotherapy in terms of time to progression (20.4 months vs. 18.6 months, respectively) and overall survival (33.5 months vs. 29.9 months, respectively) (Fig. 16A.4 and 16A.5). It also failed to demonstrate an advantage of CAB in patients with minimal disease with respect to overall survival and progression-free survival (Table 16A.3). It did show a statistically significant difference in the normalization of serum PSA (81% vs. 69%) in favor of the combination arm. However, this decrease in PSA levels did not correlate into a survival advantage and questions the validity of PSA level as a prognostic marker in advanced disease. This study is thought to be the definitive study in evaluating the usefulness of CAB because of its size, the fact that the flare phenomenon is avoided, and it is constructed to prospectively evaluate the relative benefits in patients with good performance status and minimal disease. The study was constructed to detect a 25% improvement in survival, so the fact that there was not a statistically significant improvement does not mean that there was no benefit to CAB, just that it was less than projected.

SWOG INT-0105 has been the only study to also enroll patients in a quality of life (QOL) protocol (86). Patients completed a comprehensive battery of QOL questions at assignment

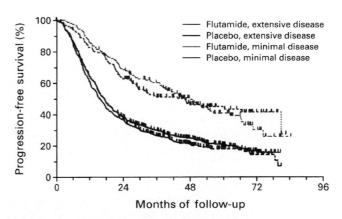

FIGURE 16A.4. Progression-free survival among eligible patients with follow-up, according to treatment assignment and extent of disease. (From Eisenberger MA, Blumenstein BA, Crawford ED, et al. Bilateral orchiectomy with or without flutamide for metastatic prostate cancer. *N Engl J Med* 1998;339:1036, with permission.)

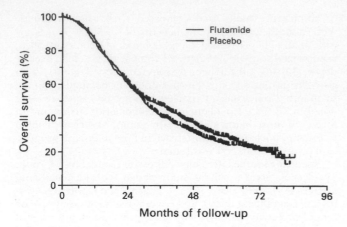

FIGURE 16A.5. Overall survival among eligible patients with follow-up, according to treatment assignment. (From Eisenberger MA, Blumenstein BA, Crawford ED, et al. Bilateral orchiectomy with or without flutamide for metastatic prostate cancer. *N Engl J Med* 1998; 339:1036, with permission.)

and then at 1, 3, and 6 months after initiating treatment. Most patients showed improvement, but those in the flutamide arm showed statistically more significant episodes of diarrhea and worse overall emotional functioning. Those receiving flutamide also discontinued the treatment more often and showed less overall improvement in most QOL dimensions, suggesting that the addition of flutamide might actually detract from the palliative benefits of bilateral orchiectomy.

META-ANALYSIS OF CONTROLLED STUDIES

Most meta-analyses have reported slightly in favor of CAB for reasons ranging from slightly decreased rates of progression or slightly increased survival. Bertagna et al. performed a meta-analysis of seven randomized, placebo-controlled studies that compared orchiectomy plus nilutamide with orchiectomy plus placebo in 1,056 eligible patients with metastatic prostate cancer and demonstrated a 16% ($P = .05$) reduction in risk of disease progression (87). The response rate in the combination arm was 50%, compared with 33% in the monotherapy group. Statistically significant differences also were found in favor of CAB with regard to improvement in bone pain and normalization of tumor markers. However, the 10% decrease in risk of death in the CAB group did not reach statistical significance. Denis and Murphy reported on a meta-analysis of 22 international studies involving 5,425 patients with advanced prostate cancer treated with either testicular androgen deprivation or CAB (88). At 5 years, 55.8% of the patients in the CAB group and 58.1% in the testicular androgen-deprivation group were dead, which led to the conclusion that CAB resulted in a relative 7% better 5-year survival rate than testicular androgen deprivation. However, the authors cautioned that because of a standard deviation of 4% and the greater cost and side effects associated with CAB, the gap between the two groups was modest.

The Prostate Cancer Trialists' Collaborative Group (85) updated an overview of 27 randomized trials with 5,932 deaths (72%) in 8,275 patients. The 5-year survival rate was 23.6%

TABLE 16A.3

OVERALL SURVIVAL AND PROGRESSION-FREE SURVIVAL IN THE SOUTHWEST ONCOLOGY GROUP INT-0105

Variable	Placebo group	Flutamide group	Risk ratio (90% CI)	P value
Eligible patients with follow-up—total no. (no. who died)	685 (480)	697 (468)		
Minimal disease	146 (71)	141 (76)		
Extensive disease	539 (409)	556 (392)		
Median follow-up—mo	49.2	50.1		
Survival—median no. of months (95% CI)[a]				
Overall, not stratified	29.9 (28.5–32.1)	33.5 (28.9–38.1)		0.16
Stratified			0.91 (0.81–1.01)[b]	0.14
Minimal disease	51.0 (40.0–?)	52.1 (48.1–63.8)		
Extensive disease	27.5 (24.6–29.9)	28.5 (25.7–31.4)		
Progression-free survival—median no. of months (95% CI)				
Overall, not stratified	18.6 (17.2–21.0)	20.4 (18.2–22.7)		0.26
Stratified				0.21
Minimal disease	46.2 (29.1–?)	48.1 (37.8–56.5)		
Extensive disease	16.0 (14.7–17.7)	17.5 (15.6–19.0)		

[a]The planned primary statistical test was the stratified log-rank test for survival. A question mark indicates cases in which the upper limit of the 95%-confidence interval (CI) could not be estimated.
[b]The risk ratio in this analysis was the hazard ratio for death in the flutamide group as compared with the placebo group.

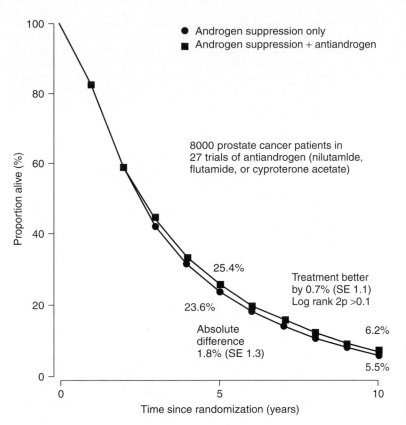

FIGURE 16A.6. Survival in 27 randomized prostate cancer trials: maximum androgen blockade versus castration alone. 8,275 patients, 5,932 deaths. (From Prostate Cancer Trialists' Collaborative Group. Maximum androgen blockade in advanced prostate cancer: an overview of the randomized trials. *Lancet* 2000;355:1491, with permission.)

and 25.4% in the monotherapy and combined-therapy groups, respectively (Fig. 16A.6). This study subcategorized the results to evaluate different types of antiandrogens and castration. It appears that CAB using CPA is no more effective than castration alone and is slightly unfavorable in terms of benefit, while studies including only nilutamide and flutamide appear to be slightly favorable. This improvement has been estimated to be as high as 5% in a meta-analysis of 20 randomized trials using nonsteroidal antiandrogens (89). This final analysis from the PCTCG concluded that the addition of an antiandrogen was likely to confer approximately 2% to 3% survival advantage at 5 years. A surprising secondary finding from this study was the suggestion that MAB was not of more benefit in 1,000 men with no evidence of metastasis (M0). The Blue Cross/Blue Shield meta-analysis similarly concluded that men with good prognostic factors are not helped by MAB, but a subgroup analysis by the Anandron/Nilutamide Study Group suggested that patients with good prognostic indicators benefit more (90,91). An extensive, but strongly recommended, review from the Department of Health and Human Services Evidence Reports/Technology Assessment also found the benefit of CAB to be modest (92). This well-referenced review by many of the authors from the Blue Cross/Blue Shield meta-analysis group encompasses all issues surrounding androgen therapy for prostate cancer.

The meta-analyses have been criticized for several reasons. Many of the studies included in analyses were immature when analyzed or contained too few patients to reach statistical significance. These points are highlighted in an article by Blumenstein, who demonstrated the weakness of using a meta-analysis to compare the trials involving CAB (93). Also, three different antiandrogens have different endocrinologic effects and therefore may not be comparable treatments. Although only a small advantage was seen in favor of CAB, this was only with respect to survival and does not address the benefits of the decrease in pain, normalization of markers, and the length of symptom-free survival. Quality of life has been

partially assessed in only one trial suggesting higher morbidity with CAB.

Currently, no clear consensus about the advantage of CAB as first-line therapy for metastatic prostate cancer over castration alone exists. After reviewing the current literature, it can be concluded that the original observations made by Labrie concerning the significant advantage of CAB have not been confirmed to the extent hoped. Also, in most studies a higher incidence of adverse events in the CAB groups was found, which can be attributed to the addition of the antiandrogens. It is important to note that there are no large trials evaluating an LHRH agonist with or without bicalutamide. At best, with CAB our patients should expect very modest returns in life expectancy (months) with potential for some delay in objective progression at the risk of incurring a degree of troublesome side effects.

COMPARISON OF MEDICAL AND SURGICAL CASTRATION

While DES and castration were the initially available therapies for palliative treatment of metastatic prostate cancer, the arrival of other androgenic manipulators raised the question of relative effectiveness. Over 30 years of randomized trials have progressed beginning with the VACURG studies in the late 1960s (94–97). Invariably, comparison of methods of castration between studies during this period is difficult due to numerous updates and/or changes in staging and grading techniques. With the exception of the testosterone flare as previously described, numerous authors have demonstrated comparative reduction in serum testosterone and response to treatment between the available methods of castration (98–100). Two trials have compared bilateral orchiectomy to DES (1 and 5 mg) without demonstrable difference in survival outcome at up to 10 years

(78,94,95). Nine randomized trials have compared LHRH analogs to DES (3 mg) or surgical castration also without any arm showing survival or time to progression benefit (100–108). The 28-day dosage of goserelin and intranasal buserelin have been the most extensively investigated with one study addressing leuprolide. Triptorelin is biochemically comparable to leuprolide in terms of PSA response and response to treatment, but no other head-to-head or survival studies have been reported for this class of medications (109).

Perhaps indicative of the investigative era, none of these studies included quality of life assessments. Cassileth et al. surveyed 115 men on goserelin and 32 men who had surgical castration and found improvements over the course of the study in the Functional Living Index in the group treated with LHRH analog while the orchiectomy group remained unchanged (110). Litwin et al. have used validated quality of life questionnaires in a small group of patients with either surgical or medical castration and showed that measured indices were equivalent in either group (111). The cost of care has been analyzed, and understandably DES and surgical castration are markedly less expensive than treatment with LHRHa and CAB (92).

DATA ON OTHER COMBINATIONS

With the availability of four formulations of LHRH analog and numerous steroidal and nonsteroidal antiandrogens, questions about the optimal medication or combinations remain. The Casodex Combination Study Group had the ambitious goal of comparing LHRHa plus bicalutamide versus LHRHa plus flutamide (112). In their final analysis of 813 mostly stage D2 patients with a median follow-up of 160 weeks, bicalutamide therapy met the predetermined definitions of equivalence with flutamide (Fig. 16A.7). Dropout rates were 10% with bicalutamide and 16% with flutamide, with diarrhea being significantly worse in the flutamide arm. Of interest, the

investigators on this study generated a treatment scheme where patients were also randomized to receive either goserelin or leuprolide in a 2-to-1 ratio (113). Time to progression, survival, and tolerability were similar in both groups. For reasons not easily explained, the best performing combination was leuprolide plus bicalutamide while the worst was leuprolide plus flutamide; goserelin in combination with antiandrogens distributed between these two treatment groups.

ANTIANDROGEN MONOTHERAPY

The sole use of antiandrogens for initial hormonal therapy has a potential role in the treatment of advanced or metastatic prostate cancer as a means of satisfactorily controlling disease and limiting impairment of quality of life. Direct inhibition of the testosterone receptor would allow for some hormonal effects of circulating testosterone, namely, the maintenance of sexual interest and function. Initial comparisons of low-dose bicalutamide (50 mg) versus castration postponed enthusiasm for this approach as response and survival parameters proved the superiority of medical and surgical castration despite improved quality of life in antiandrogen monotherapy groups (114–117). Large-scale randomized trials with higher doses of bicalutamide have provided mixed results in patients with metastatic and locally advanced T3/4 disease (41, 118). Tyrrell et al. used optimal-dose estimation arms and demonstrated improved PSA response at a dose of 150 mg (vs. 100 mg), thus the higher dose was used for the remainder of the study. With over 800 patients enrolled with metastatic disease, the study was stopped after the 2-year follow-up review due to a 6-week median survival benefit to castration. Patients in the bicalutamide monotherapy arm had better overall sexual interest and physical capacity with fewer hot flushes, but significantly more breast tenderness that did not lend to withdrawal from therapy (Table 16A.4). The authors concluded that bicalutamide monotherapy may still be an option in a well-counseled patient

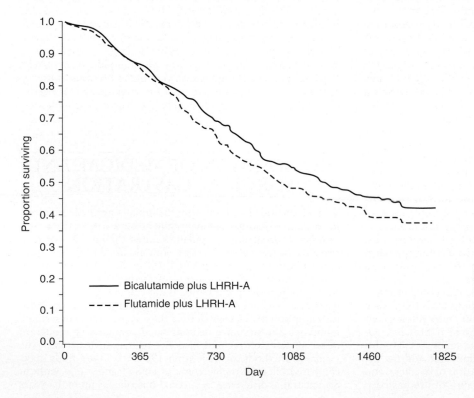

FIGURE 16A.7. Survival with CAB with bicalutamide versus flutamide from the Casodex Combination Study Group. [From Schellhammer PF, Sharifi R, Block NL, et al. Clinical benefits of bicalutamide compared with flutamide in combined androgen blockade for patients with advanced prostatic carcinoma: final report of a double-blind, randomized, multicenter trial. Casodex Combination Study Group. *Urology* 1997;50(3):330, with permission.]

TABLE 16A.4

SIDE EFFECTS OF BICALUTAMIDE 150 MG AND CAB

Adverse event	No. 150 mg Bicalutamide (%)	No. castration (%)
Gynecomastia	155 (49.4)	7 (4.4)
Breast pain	126 (40.1)	3 (1.9)
Pain	60 (19.1)	37 (23.1)
Constipation	43 (13.7)	23 (14.4)
Aggravation reaction	42 (13.4)	31 (19.4)
Infection	42 (13.4)	23 (14.4)
Hot flashes	41 (13.1)	80 (50.0)
Back pain	40 (12.7)	26 (16.3)
Hematuria	39 (12.4)	13 (8.1)
Pelvic pain	36 (11.5)	16 (10.0)
Asthenia	36 (11.5)	12 (7.5)
Urinary tract infection	33 (10.5)	24 (15.0)
Abdominal pain	33 (10.5)	9 (5.6)
Urinary retention	31 (9.9)	18 (11.3)
Diarrhea	20 (6.4)	20 (12.5)

with metastatic disease who wishes to avoid certain side effects of castration. A secondary analysis of this data showed that patients with PSA less than 400 ng/mL or less than 6 metastatic sites had equivalent outcomes with castration or antiandrogen monotherapy (119). A surplus of androgen receptors in patients with extensive disease might reconcile the poorer results in this population. Despite early termination in the group of patients with metastatic disease, the trial continued in the M0 patients. Iversen et al. (120) reported on the 6.3-year median follow-up that time to progression and survival were similar in this patient cohort (Fig. 16A.8). The Italian Prostate Cancer Project also evaluated bicalutamide at a dose of 150 mg against MAB with goserelin and flutamide and found no difference in survival in a group of 220 patients, many of whom did not have metastatic disease (118). Similarly, Fourcade et al. randomized 235 men predominantly with metastatic disease to bicalutamide versus castration plus nilutamide. Objective response rates and disease progression were not different between groups while bicalutamide significantly delayed time to treatment failure (121).

Conclusions regarding flutamide as monotherapy are somewhat more difficult to make. Flutamide has been randomized against MAB, orchiectomy, and diethylstilbestrol in 319, 104, and 92 patients, respectively (122–124). Survival time in the DES

study was much shorter in the flutamide group (43.2 months vs. 28.5 months) while survival was equivalent in the other two studies. The remaining antiandrogen nilutamide has not been reported as a sole agent. Thorpe et al. examined CPA acetate monotherapy in a three-armed study of 525 patients comparing monotherapy-with-CPA versus goserelin versus combined therapy (82). CPA performed slightly worse than LHRHa in time to progression. Two other trials with a total of 175 patients have examined CPA against DES (3 mg) and orchiectomy and found no difference in overall survival at up to 5 years (125,126).

The Early Prostate Cancer trials represent some of the most ambitious programs in hormonal therapy (127–129). Over 8,100 patients have been enrolled on several continents and started on bicalutamide 150 mg daily after receiving local therapy [radical prostatectomy (RP) and external beam radiation therapy (XRT)] or be considered candidates for watchful waiting. These three trials have an interesting design based partially on local/national treatment trends. The studies are well-powered to detect differences and have shown that the treatment arms have delay in objective and PSA progression-free survival, in particular in patients with high-risk clinical features, i.e., pretreatment PSA greater than 10, Gleason 7 to 10, positive lymph nodes. However, critics of this study cite that the differences are of dubious clinical utility, for example, treat between 20 (XRT group) and 40 (RP group) patients for 3 years to avoid one patient with objective progression, and note the extraordinary rate of adverse events in the treatment arm, in particular breast pain and gynecomastia, which led to withdrawal in almost 30% of patients. The hope for this study lies in the risk stratification as undoubtedly certain groups will receive increased benefit.

INITIAL VERSUS DELAYED HORMONE THERAPY

Androgen-withdrawal therapy, since its description by Huggins and Hodges in 1941, has been the standard therapy for metastatic prostate cancer (1). It has well-accepted benefits in palliating painful bone metastases and urinary tract obstruction. However, androgen-withdrawal therapy is not curative and the response to therapy is temporary, with most patients progressing within 2 years (130). Since the introduction of androgen-withdrawal therapy, controversy has existed over its optimum timing. Many have advocated initiating treatment at the time of diagnosis in hopes of delaying disease progression and possibly prolonging survival. Others have argued that survival is not prolonged and that the treatment may be deferred until symptoms develop.

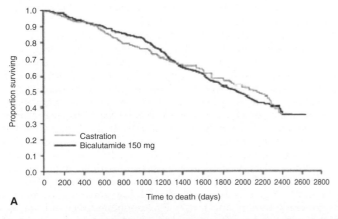
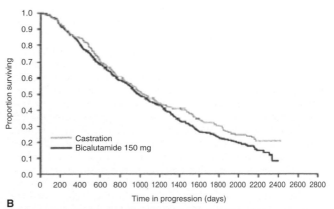

FIGURE 16A.8. Overall and progression-free survival of bicalutamide at 150 mg vs. CAB. [From Iversen P, Tyrrell CJ, Kaisary AV, et al. Bicalutamide monotherapy compared with castration in patients with non-metastatic locally advanced prostate cancer: 6.3 years of followup. *J Urol* 2000;164(5):1579, with permission.]

Early evidence to support the immediate treatment of advanced prostate cancer came from the work of Nesbitt and Baum (10). They compared patients who were treated with orchiectomy, DES, or both, and then compared them with untreated historical controls. The treated group showed a 5-year survival rate of 34% vs. 11% in the untreated group. This and other similar studies provided the basis for the early treatment of advanced prostate cancer. However, these studies have been criticized for their retrospective and nonrandomized design. It was the results of the Veterans Administration Cooperative Urological Research Group study that demonstrated that delaying hormonal therapy did not compromise overall survival (94–97). These results demonstrated that many of the patients died of other causes and that only 41% died from prostate cancer. As a result, the pendulum shifted toward advocating delayed treatment for those with advanced prostate cancer.

With the increasing interest in the biology of prostate cancer, several studies have provided important observations regarding the biologic mechanisms of advanced prostate cancer and the timing of androgen-withdrawal therapy. Using the Dunning R3327 rat prostatic adenocarcinoma model, investigators have been able to show increased regression and survival after castration if the tumor volume was relatively small as opposed to when the tumor was allowed to grow larger (131). Using this same model, Coffey and Isaacs were able to show that the mechanism responsible for the emergence of androgen resistance was the intrinsic heterogeneity of the tumor and not castration (132). They also demonstrated that poorly differentiated, fast-growing androgen-sensitive tumors respond less to androgen withdrawal later in their lifespan. These laboratory studies add support to the theory that early androgen ablation may delay progression.

In addition to laboratory data, clinical data support the early treatment of advanced prostate cancer. A stringent reanalysis of the Veterans Administration Cooperative Urological Research Group data showed that younger patients with high-grade tumors and those with stage D2 disease derive a survival benefit from the early initiation of androgen withdrawal therapy (96). Kramolowsky performed a retrospective review of 68 patients with stage D1 disease, 38 of whom underwent immediate androgen deprivation and 30 who underwent delayed treatment until the onset of bone metastasis (133). With a follow-up of 5 years, the median interval to the appearance of bone metastasis was 43 months in the delayed-treatment group and 100 months in the early-treatment group, a statistically significant advantage. The results of the NCI INT 0036 and the EORTC 30846 also have supported androgen elimination at the time of diagnosis (59, 60).

Two studies provide convincing clinical evidence supporting the early treatment of advanced prostate cancer: the randomized trial reported by the Medical Research Council (134) and the ECOG Stage D1 study (135). The MRC study randomized 934 patients with locally advanced prostate cancer or asymptomatic metastasis to either immediate treatment (orchiectomy or LHRH analog) or the same treatment deferred until an indication occurred. This study showed that there was a more rapid local and distant disease progression in the deferred group as seen by the fact that there was an earlier onset of pain and an increased need for transurethral resection of the prostate in the deferred group. There was also a twofold increase in serious complications, such as pathologic fractures, spinal cord compression, and extraskeletal metastasis, in the deferred group compared with those who received immediate treatment. These results are summarized in Table 16A.5. The need for treatment in the deferred group arose after a median of 9 months. Overall, 67% of the patients died from prostate cancer in the deferred-treatment group, with 5% dying before treatment being initiated and 11% dying of unrelated causes.

TABLE 16A.5

SUMMARY OF THE RESULTS FROM THE MEDICAL RESEARCH COUNCIL PROSTATE CANCER WORKING PARTY INVESTIGATORS GROUP TRIAL

Complication	Treatment group	
	Immediate ($n = 469$)	Deferred ($n = 465$)
Pain from metastasis	121	211
Need for transurethral resection of the prostate	65	141
Pathologic fracture	11	21
Cord compression	9	23
Ureteric obstruction	33	55
Extraskeletal metastasis	37	55
Death from prostate cancer	203	257

From The Medical Research Council Prostate Cancer Working Party Investigators Group. Immediate versus deferred treatment for advanced prostatic cancer: initial results of the Medical Research Council Trial. *Br J Urol* 1997;79:235, with permission.

The overall survival was significantly longer in the patients treated immediately, and this benefit appeared to be greatest in those with M0 disease (Fig. 16A.9). Unfortunately, the survival advantage may have disappeared in the early treatment arm according to an unpublished presentation of this trial in 2000 (136). The Eastern Cooperative Oncology Group trial randomized 98 patients with pathologically positive lymph nodes after radical prostatectomy with lymphadenectomy to immediate or delayed hormonal therapy with goserelin or orchiectomy (135). Survival in the delayed therapy and immediate therapy arms was 65% and 85% respectively at a median of over 7 years of follow-up. Patients receiving immediate therapy were 75% less likely to progress and die of prostate cancer.

The Cochrane databases compiled a meta-analysis of data from four randomized controlled trials in 2001 (137). The trials included are VACURG-I, -II, the MRC trial, and the ECOG trial. The authors concluded that early hormonal therapy definitively reduces disease progression and the subsequent complications with a small improvement (6%) in overall survival at 10 years, but not at earlier time points. Of note, 97% of the patients included in the 10-year analysis were extracted from the VACURG-I data, which makes this result sensitive to the weaknesses of that trial.

Some experimental and clinical evidence supports the early treatment of prostate cancer. Early treatment can delay progression of the disease and improve QOL, in addition to prolonging survival (133). It appears that younger patients with high-grade tumors and those with minimal metastatic disease will derive the most benefit. Moul et al. performed an observational analysis on PSA-only recurrence following radical prostatectomy by extracting data from the Department of Defense Prostate Research Database (138). They found that hormonal therapy initiated prior to a PSA of 5 ng/mL and 10 ng/mL delayed clinical metastasis in patients with Gleason scores 8 to 10 or a PSA doubling time of greater than 12 months (Fig. 16A.10). Patients with low-grade and/or moderate-grade tumors and longer PSA doubling times did not appreciate this benefit. It should be kept in mind that much of the evidence supporting the early treatment of metastatic prostate cancer does not specifically address early therapy with CAB.

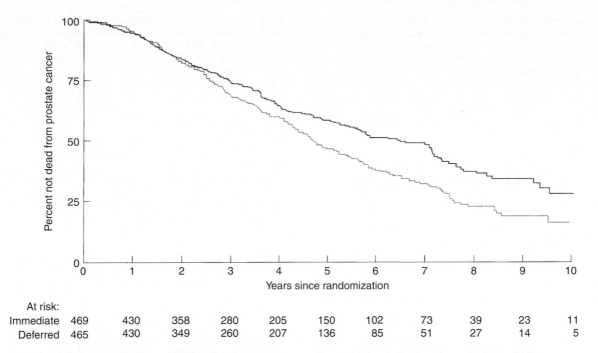

FIGURE 16A.9. Time until death from prostate cancer: all patients, by randomization group (203 of 469 immediate and 257 of 465 deferred treatment). (From The Medical Research Council Prostate Cancer Working Party Investigators Group. Immediate versus deferred treatment for advanced prostatic cancer: initial results of the Medical Research Council Trial. *Br J Urol* 1997;79:235, with permission.)

The appropriate time to initiate hormonal therapy for prostate cancer remains a contentious issue. Certainly, a patient with painful metastasis can expect symptomatic relief from castration. The commonly encountered scenario of the patient with asymptomatic metastasis also should expect a delay in progression and the avoidance of sequelae of progression, if not a measurable increase in survival (137). D1 (lymph node-positive) patients after prostatectomy and patients with advanced disease undergoing external beam radiation therapy have solid evidence that hormonal therapy delays progression and extends survival (135,139). What to do with M0 and locally advanced patients is a little more slippery, but based on the last published results of the MRC trial these patients will benefit from early initiation of androgen deprivation (134). Patients with PSA only recurrence after local therapy present another group with debatable treatment options. Historically, these patients have been started on hormonal therapy if further local therapy is not indicated despite a lack of direct data

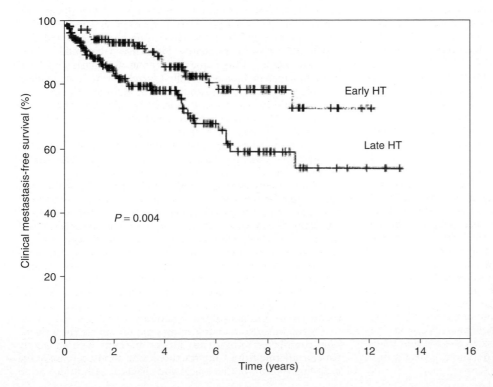

FIGURE 16A.10. Clinical metastasis-free survival in patients with immediate vs. deferred therapy with Gleason score greater than 7 and PSA-DT less than 12 months. [From Moul JW, Wu H, Sun L, et al. Early versus delayed hormonal therapy for prostate specific antigen only recurrence of prostate cancer after radical prostatectomy. *J Urol* 2004;171(3):1141.]

supporting this broad approach likely driven by patient anxiety and supplier-induced demand. Based on the results of Moul et al. starting hormonal therapy before PSA rises to 5 ng/mL or 10 ng/mL in postprostatectomy patients with Gleason scores of greater than 7 or PSA-DT of less than 12 months will have delay to clinical metastasis (138). A rising PSA after local therapy and adjuvant short-term hormonal/chemotherapy in high-risk patients are the subjects of numerous ongoing clinical trials that should have results in the next few years.

INTERMITTENT VERSUS CONTINUOUS HORMONE THERAPY

Unfortunately, most patients with metastatic prostate cancer treated with androgen-withdrawal therapy eventually succumb to the uncontrolled growth of hormone-independent prostate cancer. With a growing knowledge of tumor biology and apoptosis (programmed cell death), there is a better understanding of the mechanisms responsible for the progression to hormone-independent cancer. Bruchovsky et al. (140), using the androgen-dependent Shionogi mammary cancer line, demonstrated that androgen withdrawal altered the ratio of stem cells in the tumor population. There was a 20-fold increase in the proportion of total stem cells and a 500-fold increase in the androgen-independent stem cell population. The investigators hypothesized that progression to hormone independence is associated with the activation of previously androgen-repressed genes, some of which may code for autocrine or paracrine growth factors that substitute for androgens in maintaining the viability of the surviving tumorigenic stem cells. Replacing androgens early and before the initiation of progression should allow for the development of androgen-dependent tumor cells, which should be susceptible to retreatment with androgen withdrawal (131). Using the Shionogi mammary cancer cell line, the interval to androgen independence was increased threefold using intermittent androgen therapy as compared with continuous androgen withdrawal (140). Using the human prostate xenograft LNCaP model, intermittent androgen suppression led to the delayed development of androgen-independent regulation of PSA expression, but not survival (141). These experimental models, which demonstrate the recovery of androgen dependence and apoptotic potential, provide the rationale for intermittent androgen-deprivation treatment.

Since Klotz et al. (142) reported on 20 patients with metastatic prostate cancer treated with intermittent androgen deprivation (DES) and were able to demonstrate satisfactory palliation, at least 14 other clinical studies with almost 650 patients have supported the feasibility of this approach (143–156). Although these studies examined different populations ranging from localized cancer to PSA relapse after local therapy to metastatic disease, several conclusions can be drawn. Patients spend 40% to 60% of the time off treatment and this percentage tends to decrease with time (154). The response of serum PSA level to treatment was found to be predictive of a patient's long-term prognosis. It appears that 32 weeks of treatment was necessary to bring the serum PSA level into the normal range. The failure of serum PSA level to decrease to normal during induction was usually a sign of early progression to androgen independence and portended a poor prognosis. Another observation was that, although patients were off therapy for approximately 3 months, they experienced an increased sense of well-being, and many described a return of libido as well as decrease in frequency of hot flashes (143). Also, it has been noted that up to 8% to 50% of patients can have delayed or no recovery of testosterone. Risk factors for poor testosterone recovery appear to be age and duration of treatment of greater than 2 years (153).

One randomized trial has been published to date. De Laval et al. examined 68 patients with advanced or relapsing prostate cancer and randomized these patients to continuous or intermittent androgen deprivation with the primary outcome as time to androgen independence (157). The 3-year progression rate was 39% in the CAD group and 7% in the IAD group. Although promising, IAD should still be considered investigational therapy or may be used in a well-counseled patient. A large multicenter NCI/SWOG trial is underway in patients with metastatic disease that should definitively answer this question in this population. Other randomized trials are ongoing in Europe, where IAD is currently more popularly received. Several issues will hopefully be addressed in future IAD protocols: (a) appropriate populations, (b) type of therapy (monotherapy vs. MAB), (c) optimal point of cessation and reinitiation of therapy, and (d) cost/quality of life analyses.

HOW TO FOLLOW PATIENTS ON HORMONAL THERAPY

The follow-up arrangements and testing for patients with advanced prostate cancer depend on the patient's goals of therapy and the individual biology of the carcinoma. During office evaluations, an emphasis should also be placed on preventing side effects of disease or treatment that at times can be catastrophic. While patients with localized or regional metastatic disease are prescribed hormonal therapy by their physician, the determination of high recurrence risk groups in these circumstances is poorly defined. As a guideline, patients with clinical factors suggestive of high-risk disease (i.e., PSA >20, clinical stage equal or greater to T2b, Gleason 8 to 10), might benefit from more frequent examinations. Data from SWOG trials of patients receiving treatment for metastatic prostate cancer have defined groups at high risk of recurrence; the factors lending to early failure/death were appendicular skeletal disease, poor performance status, PSA greater than 65 ng/mL, and Gleason score 8 to 10 (158). Messing and Thompson have suggested an algorithm based on these parameters using PSA nadir as the second clinical dividing point recommending high-risk patients having clinic visits every 3 months and all others biannually at first (159). Patients with a PSA nadir of >2 ng/mL may also be categorized as high recurrence risk and should be seen more frequently. The office visit should include questions centered on sequelae of bone metastasis and local growth, which include new bone or neuropathic pain, changes in urinary or fecal habits, and weakness/fatigue. The physical exam should focus on areas indicated by the patient as problematic (orthopedic, neurologic, and rectal exams), a breast examination if on antiandrogens, and general observations for manifestations of osteoporosis. Laboratory evaluations should be directed by clinical judgment, but should include regular PSA measurement. The early detection of anemia and azotemia could potentially avoid morbid complications. Liver function tests should be checked regularly the first few months on nonsteroidal antiandrogen therapy and occasionally thereafter. Clinically directed use of bone scans and plain films might aid in directing palliative intervention with radiotherapy or surgical fixation. All patients with bone metastasis should be cautioned to watch for signs of spinal cord compression including extremity weakness, sudden or insidious onset of urinary and/or fecal incontinence, or other radicular symptoms. Urgent or emergent intervention in such cases can prevent further decrement in neurologic function.

Osteoporosis from androgen deprivation can also be a significant contributor to morbidity and/or mortality with an elderly patient suffering from a hip fracture losing almost 6 years of life expectancy (160). Both surgical and chemical castration lead to

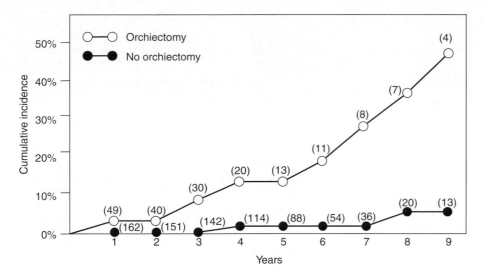

FIGURE 16A.11. Incidence of osteoporotic fracture in men after orchiectomy versus control. [From Daniell HW. Osteoporosis after orchiectomy for prostate cancer. *J Urol* 1997;157(2):439–444.]

approximately 6% to 10% diminution in bone mineral density over the first 2 years with an additional 1% to 2% loss for each additional year on continuous androgen deprivation therapy (161). The incidence of osteoporotic fractures follows this loss in bone with up to 50% of patients suffering fractures after 9 years of therapy (Fig. 16A.11). The trend toward earlier initiation of therapy lends to more men achieving osteoporosis-related complications. While systematic evaluations of the timing of bone mineral density evaluations have not been performed, baseline, annual, and semiannual radiologic studies have been recommended (161). Intravenous pamidronate (60 mg q3 months) and zoledronic acid (4 mg q3 months) have been found to respectively prevent bone loss and increase bone mineral density in men on androgen-deprivation therapy (162). Alternative hormone manipulations such as estrogens and bicalutamide monotherapy have also been found to maintain bone mass (162). To be prudent, men on androgen-deprivation therapy should be counseled to perform regular physical exercise and consider taking calcium (1500 mg) and Vitamin D (600 IU) supplements.

References

1. Huggins C, Hodges CU. Studies on prostate cancer. I. The effect of castration, of estrogen and of androgen injection on serum phosphatases in metastatic carcinoma of the prostate. *Cancer Res* 1941;1:293.
2. Hunter J. Observations on certain parts of the animal oeconomy. In: Palmer JF, ed. *The complete works of John Hunter*, Vol. 4. Philadelphia, PA: Haswell, Barrington, & Haswell, 1841:68.
3. Shelley HS. The enlarged prostate. A brief history of its treatment. *J Hist Med Allied Sci* 1969;24:452.
4. White JW. The results of double castration in hypertrophy of the prostate. *Ann Surg* 1895;22:1.
5. Cabot AT. The question of castration for enlarged prostate. *Ann Surg* 1896;24:265.
6. Marks LS. Androgen Deprivation Treatment: Part I. History. Urological Sciences Research Foundation Website, 2001: www.usrf.org/news/010308-androgen_deprivation.html.
7. Labrie F, Candas B, Gomez J-L, et al. Can combined androgen blockade provide long-term control or possible cure of localized prostate cancer? *Urology* 2002;60(1):115.
8. Kent EC, Hussain MH. The patient with hormone refractory prostate cancer: determining who, when and how to treat. *Urology* 2003;62(Suppl. 6B):134.
9. Culig Z, Klocker H, Bartsch G, et al. Androgen receptors in prostate cancer. *J Urol* 2003;170(Pt 1):1363.
10. Nesbit RM, Baum WC. Endocrine control of prostatic carcinoma: clinical and statistical survey of 1818 cases. *JAMA* 1950;143:1317.
11. Schellhammer PF. Combined androgen blockade for the treatment of metastatic cancer of the prostate. *Urology* 1996;47:622.
12. Geller J, De La Vega DJ, Albert JD, et al. Tissue dihyrotestosterone levels and clinical responses to hormonal therapy in patients with advanced prostate cancer. *J Clin Endocrinol Metab* 1984;58:36.
13. Huggins C, Scott WW. Bilateral adrenalectomy in prostatic cancer. *Ann Surg* 1945;122:1031.
14. Bhanalaph T, Varkarakis MJ, Murphy GP. Current status of bilateral adrenalectomy for advanced prostatic carcinoma. *Ann Surg* 1974;179:17.
15. Huggins C, Bergenstal DM. Effect of bilateral adrenalectomy on certain human tumors. *Proc Natl Acad Sci U S A* 1952;38:73.
16. Baker WJ. Bilateral adrenalectomy for carcinoma of the prostate gland: preliminary report. *J Urol* 1953;70:275.
17. Scardino PL, Prince CL, McGoldrick TA. Bilateral adrenalectomy for prostate cancer. *J Urol* 1953;70:100.
18. Taylor SG III, Li MC, Eckles N, et al. Effect of surgical Addison's disease on advanced carcinoma of the breast and prostate. *Cancer* 1953;6:997.
19. Whitmore WF Jr, Randall HT, Pearson OH, et al. Adrenalectomy in the treatment of prostate cancer. *Geriatrics* 1954;9:62.
20. Fergusson JD. Total adrenalectomy for malignant disease of the prostate and breast. *Proc R Soc Med* 1954;47:1007.
21. Pyrah LN. Bilateral adrenalectomy in the treatment of mammary and prostatic cancer. *Proc R Soc Med* 1954;47:1002.
22. Morales PA, Brendler H, Hotchkiss RS. The role of the adrenal cortex in prostatic cancer. *J Urol* 1955;73:399.
23. MacFarlane DA, Thomas LP, Harrison JH. A survey of total adrenalectomy in cancer of the prostate. *Am J Surg* 1960;99:562.
24. Robinson MRG, Thomas BS. Effect of hormonal therapy on plasma testosterone levels in prostatic carcinoma. *BMJ* 1971;4:391.
25. Worgul TJ, Santen RJ, Samoglik E, et al. Clinical and biochemical effect of aminoglutethimide in the treatment of advanced prostatic carcinoma. *J Urol* 1983;129:51.
26. Walsh PC, Siiteri PK. Suppression of plasma androgens by spironolactone in castrated men with carcinoma of the prostate. *J Urol* 1975;114:254.
27. Matsuo H, Baba Y, Nair RM, et al. Structure of porcine LH- and FSH-releasing hormone. I. The proposed amino acid sequence. *Biochem Biophys Res Commun* 1971;43(6):1334.
28. Yen SS, Rebar R, Van den Berg G, et al. Synthetic luteinizing hormone-releasing factor. A potent stimulator of gonadotropin release in man. *J Clin Endocrinol Metab* 1972;34(6):1108.
29. Schally AV, Coy DH, Arimura A. LHRH agonists and antagonists. *Int J Gynecol Obstet* 1980;18:318.
30. The Leuprolide Study Group. Leuprolide versus diethylstilbesterol for metastatic prostate cancer. *N Engl J Med* 1984;311:1281.
31. Koutsilieris M, Favre N, Tolis G, et al. Objective response and disease outcome in 59 patients with stage D2 prostatic cancer treated with either buserelin or orchiectomy. Disease aggressivity and its association with response and outcome. *Urology* 1986;27:221.
32. Markewitz M, Veenema RJ, Fingerhut B, et al. Cyproterone acetate (SH 714) effect on histology and nucleic acid synthesis in the testes of patients with prostatic carcinoma. A preliminary report. *Invest Urol* 1969;6(6):638.
33. Neri R, Florance K, Koziol P, et al. A biological profile of a nonsteroidal antiandrogen, SCH 13521 (4'-nitro-3'trifluoromethylisobutyranilide). *Endocrinology* 1972;91(2):427.
34. Schroeder FH, Lock TM, Chadha DR, et al. Metastatic cancer of the prostate managed with buserelin versus buserelin plus cyproterone acetate. *J Urol* 1987;137:912.
35. Labrie F, Dupont A, Belanger A, et al. Flutamide eliminates the risk of disease flare in prostatic cancer patients treated with luteinizing hormone-releasing hormone agonist. *J Urol* 1987;138:804.
36. Thrasher JB, Deeths J, Bennett C, et al. Comparative study of the clinical efficacy of two dosing regimens of flutamide. *Mol Urol* 2000;4(3):259.
37. Wysowski DK, Freiman JP, Tourtelot JB, et al. Fatal and nonfatal hepatotoxicity associated with flutamide. *Ann Intern Med* 1993;118:860.

38. Gomez JL, Dupont A, Cusan L, et al. Simultaneous liver and lung toxicity related to the nonsteroidal antiandrogen nilutamide (Anandron): case report. *Am J Med* 1992;92:563.

39. Blackledge GRP. Clinical progress with a new antiandrogen, Casodex (bicalutamide). *Eur Urol* 1996;29(Suppl. 2):96.

40. Blackledge GRP, Cockshott ID, Furr BJA. Casodex (bicalutamide): overview of a new antiandrogen developed for treatment of prostate cancer. *Eur Urol* 1997;31(Suppl. 2):30.

41. Tyrrell CJ, Kaisary AV, Iversen P, et al. A randomised comparison of 'Casodex' (bicalutamide) 150 mg monotherapy versus castration in the treatment of metastatic and locally advanced prostate cancer. *Eur Urol* 1998; 33(5):447.

42. Tyrrell CJ. Immediate treatment with bicalutamide, 150mg/d, following radiotherapy in localized or locally advanced prostate cancer. *Rev Urol* 2004;6(Suppl. 2):S29.

43. de Voogt HJ. The position of cyproterone acetate (CPA), a steroidal antiandrogen, in the treatment of prostate cancer. *Prostate Suppl* 1992;4: 91–95.

44. Dawson NA, Conaway M, Halabi S, et al. A randomized study comparing standard versus moderately high dose megestrol acetate for patients with advanced prostate carcinoma: Cancer and Leukemia Group B study 9181. *Cancer* 2000;88(4):825.

45. Kouriefs C, Georgiou M, Ravi R. Hot flushes and prostate cancer: pathogenesis and treatment. *BJU Int* 2002;89(4):379.

46. Hara T, Miyazaki J, Araki H, et al. Novel mutations of androgen receptor: a possible mechanism of bicalutamide withdrawal syndrome. *Cancer Res* 2003;63(1):149.

47. Godoy-Tundidor S, Hobisch A, Pfeil K, et al. Acquisition of agonistic properties of nonsteroidal antiandrogens after treatment with oncostatin M in prostate cancer cells. *Clin Cancer Res* 2002;8(7):2356.

48. Geller J, Albert J, Vik A. Advantages of total androgen blockade in the treatment of advanced prostate cancer. *Semin Oncol* 1988;15(2 Suppl. 1):53.

49. Labrie F. Mechanism of action and pure antiandrogenic properties of flutamide. *Cancer* 1993;72(Suppl. 12):3816.

50. Trachtenberg J. Optimal testosterone concentration for the treatment of prostatic cancer. *J Urol* 1985;133(5):888.

51. Kyprianou N, Isaacs JT. Quantal relationship between prostatic dihydrotestosterone and prostatic cell content: critical threshold concept. *Prostate* 1987;11(1):41.

52. Van Weerden WM, van Kreuningen A, Moering EP, et al. Pharmacia Award 1990. The biological significance of low testosterone levels and adrenal androgens in the transplantable prostate cancer lines. *Urol Res* 1991; 19(1):1.

53. Ellis WJ, Isaacs JT. Effectiveness of complete versus partial androgen withdrawal therapy for the treatment of prostatic cancer as studied in the Dunning R-3327 system of rat prostatic adenocarcinoma. *Cancer Res* 1985; 45(12 Pt 1):6041.

54. Redding TW, Schally AV. Investigation of the combination of agonist D-Trp-6-LH-RH and the antiandrogen flutamide in the treatment of Dunning R-3327H prostate cancer model. *Prostate* 1985;6(3):219.

55. Labrie F, Dupont A, Belanger A, et al. New approach in the treatment of prostate cancer: complete instead of partial withdrawal of androgens. *Prostate* 1983;4(6):579.

56. Labrie F, Dupont A, Belanger A, et al. New hormonal treatment in cancer of the prostate: combined administration of an LHRH agonist and an antiandrogen. *J Steroid Biochem* 1983;19:999.

57. Labrie F, Belanger A, Simard J, et al. Combination therapy for prostate cancer. Endocrine and biologic basis of its choice as new standard first line therapy. *Cancer* 1993;71(Suppl. 3):1059.

58. Labrie F, Veilleux R, Fournier A. Low androgen levels induce the development of androgen hypersensitive cell clones in Shionogi mouse mammary carcinoma cells in culture. *J Natl Cancer Inst* 1988;80:1138.

59. Crawford ED, Eisenberger MA, McLeod DG, et al. A controlled trial of leuprolide with and without flutamide in prostatic carcinoma. *N Engl J Med* 1989;321:419.

60. Denis LJ, Keuppens F, Smith PH, et al. Maximal androgen blockade: final analysis of EORTC phase III trial 30853. *Eur Urol* 1998;33:144.

61. Dijkman GA, Janknegt RA, De Reijke TM et al. International Anandron Study Group. Long-term efficacy and safety of nilutamide plus castration in advanced prostate cancer, and the significance of early prostate specific antigen normalization. *J Urol* 1997;158:160.

62. Denis LJ, Carneiro de Moura JL, Bono A, et al. EORTC Genitourinary Group and EORTC Data Center. Goserelin acetate and flutamide versus bilateral orchidectomy: a phase III EORTC trial (30853). *Urology* 1993;42:119.

63. Navratil H. Double-blind study of anandron versus placebo in stage D2 prostate cancer patients receiving buserelin. *Prog Clin Biol Res* 1987; 243A: 401.

64. Beland G, Elhilali M, Fradet Y, et al. A controlled trial of castration with and without nilutamide in metastatic prostatic carcinoma. *Cancer* 1990; 66(Suppl. 5):1074.

65. Namer M, Toubol J, Caty A, et al. A randomized double-blind study evaluating Anandron associated with orchiectomy in stage D prostate cancer. *J Steroid Biochem Mol Biol* 1990;37:909.

66. Knonagel H, Bolle JF, Hering F, et al. [Therapy of metastatic prostatic cancer by orchiectomy plus Anandron versus orchiectomy plus placebo. Initial results of a randomized multicenter study]. *Helv Chir Acta* 1989;56:343.

67. Crawford ED, Kasimis BS, Gandara D, et al. A randomized, controlled trial of leuprolide and Anandron versus leuprolide and placebo for advanced prostate cancer. *Proc Am Soc Clin Onc* 1990;9:A523.

68. Schulze H, Kaldenhoff H, Senge T. Evaluation of total versus partial androgen blockade in the treatment of advanced prostatic cancer. *Urol Int* 1988;43:193.

69. Tyrrell CJ, Altwein JE, Klippel F et al. International Prostate Cancer Study Group. Multicenter randomized trial comparing Zoladex with Zoladex plus flutamide in the treatment of advanced prostate cancer. Survival update. *Cancer* 1993;72(Suppl. 12):3878.

70. Iversen P, Rasmussen F, Klarskov P, et al. Long-term results of Danish Prostatic Cancer Group trial 86. Goserelin acetate plus flutamide versus orchiectomy in advanced prostate cancer. *Cancer* 1993;72(Suppl. 12):3851.

71. Fourcade RO, Colombel P, Mangin M. Zoladex plus flutamide versus Zoladex plus placebo in advanced prostatic carcinoma: extended follow-up of the French multicentre study. In: Murphy G, Khoury S, Chatelain C et al., eds. *Proceedings of the 3rd International Symposium on Recent Advances in Urological Cancer: diagnosis and treatment*, June 1992. Paris: Scientific Communication International Ltd., 1993:102.

72. Zalcberg JR, Raghaven D, Marshall V, et al. Bilateral orchidectomy and flutamide versus orchidectomy alone in newly diagnosed patients with metastatic carcinoma of the prostate—an Australian multicentre trial. *Br J Urol* 1996;77:865.

73. Delaere KP, Boccon-Gibod L, Corrado F, et al. Randomized, double-blind, parallel group study of flutamide and orchiectomy versus placebo and orchiectomy in men with D2 adenocarcinoma of the prostate [Abstract]. *Proc ECCO-4* 1987:68.

74. Boccardo F, Pace M, Rubagotti A et al. The Italian Prostatic Cancer Project (PONCAP) Study Group. Goserelin acetate with or without flutamide in the treatment of patients with locally advanced or metastatic prostate cancer. *Eur J Cancer* 1993;29A:1088.

75. Ferrari P, Castagnetti G, Ferrari G, et al. Combination treatment versus LHRH alone in advanced prostatic cancer. *Urol Int* 1996;56(Suppl. 1):13.

76. Eisenberger MA, Blumenstein BA, Crawford ED, et al. Bilateral orchiectomy with or without flutamide for metastatic prostate cancer. *N Engl J Med* 1998;339:1036.

77. Bono AV, DiSilverio F, Robustelli della Cuna G et al. Italian Leuprorelin Group. Complete androgen blockade versus chemical castration in advanced prostatic cancer: analysis of an Italian multicentre study. *Urol Int* 1998;60(Suppl. 1):18.

78. Robinson MR, Smith PH, Richards B, et al. The final analysis of the EORTC Genito-Urinary Tract Cancer Co Operative Group phase III clinical trial (protocol 30805) comparing orchidectomy, orchidectomy plus cyproterone acetate and low dose stilboestrol in the management of metastatic carcinoma of the prostate. *Eur Urol* 1995;28(4):273.

79. Di Silverio F, Serio M, D'Eramo G, et al. Zoladex vs. Zoladex plus cyproterone acetate in the treatment of advanced prostatic cancer: a multicenter Italian study. *Eur Urol* 1990;18(Suppl. 3):54.

80. De Voogt HJ, Studer U, Schroder FH et al. European Organization for Research and Treatment of Cancer (EROTC) Genito-Urinary Tract Cancer Cooperative Group. Maximum androgen blockade using LHRH agonist buserelin in combination with short-term (two weeks) or long-term (continuous) cyproterone acetate is not superior to standard androgen deprivation in the treatment of advanced prostate cancer. Final analysis of EORTC GU Group Trial 30843. *Eur Urol* 1998;33:152.

81. Jorgensen T, Tveter KJ, Jorgensen LH. Total androgen suppression: experience from the Scandinavian Prostatic Cancer Group Study No. 2. *Eur Urol* 1993;24:466.

82. Thorpe SC, Azmatullah S, Fellows GJ, et al. A prospective, randomised study to compare goserelin acetate (Zoladex) versus cyproterone acetate (Cyprostat) versus a combination of the two in the treatment of metastatic prostatic carcinoma. *Eur Urol* 1996;29:47.

83. Theib M, Wirth M, Tunn U, et al. Triptorelin-Cyproteronacetat versus Triptorelin-Placebo: Multizentrische Phase III-Studie an 222 Patienten mit fortgeschrittenem Prostata-Karzinom [Abstract]. *Urologe A* 1996:S41.

84. Iversen P, Suciu S, Sylvester R, et al. Zoladex and flutamide versus orchiectomy in the treatment of advanced prostatic cancer. A combined analysis of two European studies, EORTC 30853 and DAPROCA 86. *Cancer* 1990;66:1067.

85. Prostate Cancer Trialists' Collaborative Group. Maximum androgen blockade in advanced prostate cancer: an overview of the randomized trials. *Lancet* 2000;355:1491.

86. Moinpour CM, Savage MJ, Troxel A, et al. Quality of life in advanced prostate cancer: results of a randomized therapeutic trial. *J Natl Cancer Inst* 1998;90(20):1537.

87. Bertagna C, De Gery A, Hucher M, et al. Efficacy of the combination of nilutamide plus orchidectomy in patients with metastatic prostatic cancer. A meta-analysis of seven randomised double-blind trials (1,056 patients). *Br J Urol* 1994;73:396.

88. Denis L, Murphy GP. Overview of phase III trials on combined androgen treatment in patients with metastatic prostatic cancer. *Cancer* 1993;72:3888.

89. Schmitt B, Wilt TJ, Schellhammer PF, et al. Combined androgen blockade with nonsteroidal antiandrogens for advanced prostate cancer: a systematic review. *Urology* 2001;57(4):727.

90. Samson DJ, Seidenfeld J, Schmitt B, et al. Systematic review and meta-analysis of monotherapy compared with combined androgen blockade for patients with advanced prostate carcinoma. *Cancer* 2002;95(2):361.

91. de Reijke T, Derobert E, Anandron/Nilutamide Study Group. Prognostic factor analysis in patients with advanced prostate cancer treated by castration plus Anandron or placebo: a final update. *Eur Urol* 2002;42:139.

92. Seidenfeld J, Samson DJ, Aronson N, et al. Relative effectiveness and cost-effectiveness of methods of androgen suppression in the treatment of advanced prostate cancer. *Evidence report/technology assessment No. 4*, AHCPR Publication No. 99-E0012. Rockville, MD: Agency for Health Care Policy and Research, May 1999.

93. Blumenstein BA. Some statistical considerations for the interpretation of trials of combined androgen therapy. *Cancer* 1993;72:834.

94. Blackard CE, Byar DP, Jordan WP Jr. Orchiectomy for advanced prostatic carcinoma. A reevaluation. *Urology* 1973;1(6):553.

95. Veterans Administration Cooperative Urological Research Group. Treatment and survival of patients with cancer of the prostate. *Surg Gynecol Obstet* 1967;124(5):1011.

96. Byar DP, Corle DK. Hormone therapy for prostate cancer: results of the Veterans Administration Cooperative Urologic Research Group studies. *Natl Cancer Inst Monogr* 1988;7:165.

97. Christensen MM, Aagaard J, Madsen PO. Reasons for delay of endocrine treatment in cancer of the prostate (until symptomatic metastases occur). *Prog Clin Biol Res* 1990;359:7.

98. Tolis G, Koutsilieris M, Herrera R, et al. Advanced prostatic adenocarcinoma: biological aspects and effects of androgen deprivation achieved by castration or agonistic analogues of LHRH. *Med Oncol Tumor Pharmacother* 1984;1(2):129.

99. Turkes AO, Peeling WB, Griffiths K. Treatment of patients with advanced cancer of the prostate: phase III trial, Zoladex against castration; a study of the British Prostate Group. *J Steroid Biochem* 1987;27(1–3):543.

100. Vogelzang NJ, Chodak GW, Soloway MS et al. Zoladex Prostate Study Group. Goserelin versus orchiectomy in the treatment of advanced prostate cancer: final results of a randomized trial. *Urology* 1995;46(2):220.

101. Kaisary AV, Tyrrell CJ, Peeling WB, et al. Comparison of LHRH analogue (Zoladex) with orchiectomy in patients with metastatic prostatic carcinoma. *Br J Urol* 1991;67(5):502.

102. de Voogt HJ, Klijn JG, Studer U, et al. Orchidectomy versus buserelin in combination with cyproterone acetate, for 2 weeks or continuously, in the treatment of metastatic prostatic cancer. Preliminary results of EORTC-trial 30843. *J Steroid Biochem Mol Biol* 1990;37(6):965.

103. Bruun E, Frimodt-Moller C, Danish Buserelin Study Group. The effect of buserelin versus conventional antiandrogenic treatment in patients with T2-4NXM1 prostatic cancer: a prospective, randomized multicentre phase III trial. *Scand J Urol Nephrol* 1996;30(4):291.

104. Koutsilieris M, Tolis G. Long-term follow-up of patients with advanced prostatic carcinoma treated with either buserelin (HOE 766) or orchiectomy: classification of variables associated with disease outcome. *Prostate* 1985;7(1):31.

105. The Leuprolide Study Group. Leuprolide versus diethylstilbestrol for metastatic prostate cancer. *N Engl J Med* 1984;311(20):1281.

106. Waymont B, Lynch TH, Dunn JA, et al. Phase III randomised study of Zoladex versus stilboestrol in the treatment of advanced prostate cancer. *Br J Urol* 1992;69(6):614.

107. Citrin DL, Resnick MI, Guinan P, et al. A comparison of Zoladex and DES in the treatment of advanced prostate cancer: results of a randomized, multicenter trial. *Prostate* 1991;18(2):139.

108. Huben RP, Murphy GP. A comparison of diethylstilbestrol or orchiectomy with buserelin and with methotrexate plus diethylstilbestrol or orchiectomy in newly diagnosed patients with clinical stage D2 cancer of the prostate. *Cancer* 1988;62(9):1881.

109. Heyns CF, Simonin MP, Grosgurin P et al. South African Triptorelin Study Group. Comparative efficacy of triptorelin pamoate and leuprolide acetate in men with advanced prostate cancer. *BJU Int* 2003;92:226.

110. Cassileth BR, Soloway MS, Vogelzang NJ et al. Zoladex Prostate Cancer Study Group. Quality of life and psychosocial status in stage D prostate cancer. *Qual Life Res* 1992;1(5):323.

111. Litwin MS, Shpall AI, Dorey F, et al. Quality-of-life outcomes in long-term survivors of advanced prostate cancer. *Am J Clin Oncol* 1998;21(4):327.

112. Schellhammer PF, Sharifi R, Block NL et al. Casodex Combination Study Group. Clinical benefits of bicalutamide compared with flutamide in combined androgen blockade for patients with advanced prostatic carcinoma: final report of a double-blind, randomized, multicenter trial. *Urology* 1997;50(3):330.

113. Sarosdy MF, Schellhammer PF, Sharifi R, et al. Comparison of goserelin and leuprolide in combined androgen blockade therapy. *Urology* 1998;52(1):82.

114. Kaisary AV, Tyrrell CJ, Beacock C et al. Casodex Study Group. A randomised comparison of monotherapy with Casodex 50 mg daily and castration in the treatment of metastatic prostate carcinoma. *Eur Urol* 1995;28(3):215.

115. Chodak G, Sharifi R, Kasimis B, et al. Single-agent therapy with bicalutamide: a comparison with medical or surgical castration in the treatment of advanced prostatic carcinoma. *Urology* 1995;46(6):849.

116. Bales GT, Chodak GW. A controlled trial of bicalutamide versus castration in patients with advanced prostate cancer. *Urology* 1996;47(Suppl. 1A):38.

117. Iversen P, Tveter K, Varenhorst E, The Scandinavian Casodex Cooperative Group. Randomised study of Casodex 50 mg monotherapy vs. orchidectomy in the treatment of metastatic prostate cancer. *Scand J Urol Nephrol* 1996;30(2):93.

118. Boccardo F, Barichello M, Battaglia M et al. Italian Prostate Cancer Group. Bicalutamide monotherapy versus flutamide plus goserelin in prostate cancer: updated results of a multicentric trial. *Eur Urol* 2002;42(5):481.

119. Kolvenbag G, Iversen P, Newling D. Antiandrogen monotherapy: a new form of treatment for patients with prostate cancer. *Urology* 2001;58(Suppl. 2A):16.

120. Iversen P, Tyrrell CJ, Kaisary AV, et al. Bicalutamide monotherapy compared with castration in patients with nonmetastatic locally advanced prostate cancer: 6.3 years of followup. *J Urol* 2000;164(5):1579.

121. Fourcade RO, Chatelain C, Poterre M. An open multicentre study to compare the effect and safety of Casodex (bicalutamide) 150 mg monotherapy with castration plus nilutamide in metastatic prostate cancer [Abstract]. *Eur Urol* 1998;33(Suppl. 1):88.

122. Pavone-Macaluso M. Flutamide monotherapy vs. combined androgen blockade in advanced prostate cancer [Abstract]. Interim Report of an Italian Multicenter, Randomized Study. *Proceedings of the 23rd Congress of the Societe Internationale d'Urologie*, Sydney, Australia 1994,

123. Boccon-Gibod L, Fournier G, Bottet P, et al. Flutamide versus orchidectomy in the treatment of metastatic prostate carcinoma. *Eur Urol* 1997;32(4):391.

124. Chang A, Yeap B, Davis T, et al. Double-blind, randomized study of primary hormonal treatment of stage D2 prostate carcinoma: flutamide versus diethylstilbestrol. *J Clin Oncol* 1996;14(8):2250.

125. Pavone-Macaluso M, de Voogt HJ, Viggiano G, et al. Comparison of diethylstilbestrol, cyproterone acetate and medroxyprogesterone acetate in the treatment of advanced prostatic cancer: final analysis of a randomized phase III trial of the European Organization for Research on Treatment of Cancer Urological Group. *J Urol* 1986;136(3):624.

126. Ostri P, Bonnesen T, Nilsson T, et al. Treatment of symptomatic metastatic prostatic cancer with cyproterone acetate versus orchiectomy: a prospective randomized trial. *Urol Int* 1991;46(2):167.

127. See W, Iversen P, Wirth M, et al. Immediate treatment with bicalutamide 150 mg as adjuvant therapy significantly reduces the risk of PSA progression in early prostate cancer. *Eur Urol* 2003;44(5):512.

128. Wirth M, Tyrrell C, Wallace M, et al. Bicalutamide (Casodex) 150 mg as immediate therapy in patients with localized or locally advanced prostate cancer significantly reduces the risk of disease progression. *Urology* 2001;58(2):146.

129. Iversen P, Tammela TL, Vaage S et al. Scandinavian Prostatic Cancer Group (SPCG). A randomised comparison of bicalutamide ('Casodex') 150 mg versus placebo as immediate therapy either alone or as adjuvant to standard care for early non-metastatic prostate cancer. First report from the Scandinavian Prostatic Cancer Group study no. 6. *Eur Urol* 2002;42(3):204.

130. Beynon LL, Chisholm GD. The stable state is not an objective response in hormone-escaped carcinoma of the prostate. *Br J Urol* 1984;56:702.

131. Isaacs JT. The timing of androgen ablation therapy and/or chemotherapy in the treatment of prostatic cancer. *Prostate* 1984,5:1.

132. Isaacs JT, Coffey DS. Adaptation versus selection as the mechanism responsible for the relapse of prostate cancer to androgen ablation therapy as studied in the Dunning R-3327-H adenocarcinoma. *Cancer Res* 1981;41:5070.

133. Kramolowsky EV. The value of testosterone deprivation in stage D1 carcinoma of the prostate. *J Urol* 1988;139:1242.

134. The Medical Research Council Prostate Cancer Working Party Investigators Group. Immediate versus deferred treatment for advanced prostatic cancer: initial results of the Medical Research Council Trial. *Br J Urol* 1997;79:235.

135. Messing EM, Manola J, Sarosdy M, et al. Immediate hormonal therapy compared with observation after radical prostatectomy and pelvic lymphadenectomy in men with node-positive prostate cancer. *N Engl J Med* 1999;341(24):1781.

136. Newling D. Early versus late androgen deprivation therapy in metastatic disease. *Urology* 2001;58(Suppl. 2A):50.

137. Wilt T, Nair B, MacDonald R, et al. Early versus deferred androgen suppression in the treatment of advanced prostate cancer (Cochrane Review). *The Cochrane Library*, Issue 2. Chichester: John Wiley and Sons, 2004.

138. Moul JW, Wu H, Sun L, et al. Early versus delayed hormonal therapy for prostate specific antigen only recurrence of prostate cancer after radical prostatectomy. *J Urol* 2004;171(3):1141.

139. Bolla M, Collette L, Blank L, et al. Long-term results with immediate androgen suppression and external irradiation in patients with locally advanced prostate cancer (an EORTC study): a phase III randomised trial. *Lancet* 2002;360(9327):103.

140. Bruchovsky N, Rennie PS, Coldman AJ, et al. Effects of androgen withdrawal on the stem cell composition of the Shionogi carcinoma. *Cancer Res* 1990;50:2275.

141. Gleave M, Bruchovsky N, Bowden M, et al. Intermittent androgen suppression prolongs time to androgen-independent progression in the LnCAP prostate tumor model. *J Urol* 1994;151:457A [Abstract].

142. Klotz LH, Herr HW, Morse MJ, et al. Intermittent endocrine therapy for advanced prostate cancer. *Cancer* 1986;58:2546.

143. Goldenberg SL, Bruchovsky N, Gleave ME, et al. Intermittent androgen suppression in the treatment of prostate cancer: a preliminary report. *Urology* 1995;45:839.

144. Higano CS, Ellis W, Russell K, et al. Intermittent androgen suppression with leuprolide and flutamide for prostate cancer: a pilot study. *Urology* 1996;48:800.

145. Oliver RT, Williams G, Paris AM, et al. Intermittent androgen deprivation after PSA-complete response as a strategy to reduce induction of hormone-resistant prostate cancer. *Urology* 1997;49(1):79.

146. Theyer G, Hamilton G. Current status of intermittent androgen suppression in the treatment of prostate cancer. *Urology* 1998;52(3):353.

147. Gleave M, Bruchovsky N, Goldenberg SL, et al. Intermittent androgen suppression for prostate cancer: rationale and clinical experience. *Eur Urol* 1998;34(Suppl. 3):37.

148. Horwich A, Huddart RA, Gadd J, et al. A pilot study of intermittent androgen deprivation in advanced prostate cancer. *Br J Urol* 1998;81(1):96.

149. Crook JM, Szumacher E, Malone S, et al. Intermittent androgen suppression in the management of prostate cancer. *Urology* 1999;53(3):530.

150. Kurek R, Renneberg H, Lubben G, et al. Intermittent complete androgen blockade in PSA relapse after radical prostatectomy and incidental prostate cancer. *Eur Urol* 1999;35(Suppl. 1):27.

151. Hruby G, Gurnry H, Turner S, et al. Long-term follow-up of patients treated with intermittent hormone therapy for advanced prostate cancer. *Prostate J* 1999;1:138.

152. Tunn UW. Intermittent endocrine therapy of prostate cancer. *Eur Urol* 1996;30(Suppl. 1):22.

153. Strum SB, Scholz MC, McDermed JE. Intermittent androgen deprivation in prostate cancer patients: factors predictive of prolonged time off therapy. *Oncologist* 2000;5(1):45.

154. Grossfeld GD, Chaudhary UB, Reese DM, et al. Intermittent androgen deprivation: update of cycling characteristics in patients without clinically apparent metastatic prostate cancer. *Urology* 2001;58(2):240.

155. Bouchot O, Lenormand L, Karam G, et al. Intermittent androgen suppression in the treatment of metastatic prostate cancer. *Eur Urol* 2000; 38(5): 543.

156. Leibowitz RL, Tucker SJ. Treatment of localized prostate cancer with intermittent triple androgen blockade: preliminary results in 110 consecutive patients. *Oncologist* 2001;6(2):177.

157. de Leval J, Boca P, Yousef E, et al. Intermittent versus continuous total androgen blockade in the treatment of patients with advanced hormone-naive prostate cancer: results of a prospective randomized multicenter trial. *Clin Prostate Cancer* 2002;1(3):163.

158. Glass TR, Tangen CM, Crawford ED, et al. Metastatic carcinoma of the prostate: identifying prognostic groups using recursive partitioning. *J Urol* 2003;169(1):164.

159. Messing EM, Thompson I Jr. Follow-up of conservatively managed prostate cancer: watchful waiting and primary hormonal therapy. *Urol Clin North Am* 2003;30(4):687.

160. Trombetti A, Herrmann F, Hoffmeyer P, et al. Survival and potential years of life lost after hip fracture in men and age-matched women. *Osteoporos Int* 2002;13(9):731.

161. Daniell HW. Osteoporosis due to androgen deprivation therapy in men with prostate cancer. *Urology* 2001;58(2 Suppl. 1):101.

162. Smith MR. Management of treatment-related osteoporosis in men with prostate cancer. *Cancer Treat Rev* 2003;29(3):211.

CHAPTER 16B
Beyond First-Line Hormones: Options for Treatment of Castration-resistant Disease

Kathleen Beekman, Wayne D. Tilley, Grant Buchanan, and Howard I. Scher

The standard treatment for patients with systemic prostate cancer, regardless of whether prior local therapy has been applied, is to ablate the action of androgens by medical or surgical means (1). The clinical outcomes are well documented: a decline in prostate-specific antigen (PSA), a regression in soft-tissue disease, improvement in osseous disease if present by imaging studies, as well as palliation of disease-related symptoms. After a variable period of time, a rise in PSA is observed, followed in turn by other manifestations of progressing cancer including new metastases on imaging studies and later, disease-related symptoms. Placed in a clinical-state model of prostate cancer that characterizes the disease from prediagnosis to death, we separate patients who have failed androgen-ablative therapies

on the basis of the measured testosterone concentrations in the blood as either noncastrate or castrate (2). This simple, practical, and straightforward approach provides the framework to consider patients with castration-resistant disease as individuals or as a group, using information such as the prior prostate cancer history, previous systemic therapies, and the current disease extent to formulate specific treatment recommendations (Figure 16.B1).

Most important is that many progressive castrate prostate cancers remain sensitive to further hormonal manipulations, including steroidal and nonsteroidal hormone withdrawal (3,4), antiandrogens, estrogens, progestational agents, glucocorticoids, and enzymatic inhibitors of the adrenal androgen synthetic pathway (5). Consistent with the clinical findings are molecular studies showing that despite castrate levels of testosterone, signaling through the androgen receptor is maintained or increased. As such, to classify these tumors as "hormone-refractory" is a misnomer, and this classification should be abandoned. In our view, a more clinically relevant scheme shifts the focus toward the mechanisms associated with continued signaling through the receptor, rather than on the ligand itself (6). Prior therapy must also be considered when formulating management decisions, as it is now recognized that the specific treatment itself can influence the biology of the relapsing tumor, a concept termed "therapy-mediated selection pressure" (7,8). In this section we will focus first on the biology of the relapsing tumor, and then discuss a framework for management decisions based on the prognosis of the individual and the antecedent treatment history.

BIOLOGY OF PROGRESSIVE CASTRATION-RESISTANT PROSTATE CANCER

Androgens are the primary regulators of prostate cancer growth and proliferation. Testosterone, the main circulating androgen, enters the prostate cell where it is converted primarily to dihydrotestosterone (DHT) by the enzyme 5-alpha reductase. DHT then binds to the androgen receptor, a dimerization ensues, and the complex is transported to the nucleus where it binds to androgen response elements in the promoter regions of target genes, including PSA, resulting in an increase or decrease in transcription (9). When androgens are ablated or withdrawn by orchiectomy, a proportion of cells undergoes apoptosis, while those that survive arrest in G1 (10).

Paradoxically, the failure of androgen-ablation therapy in a clinical setting is accompanied by rising serum levels of the androgen-regulated protein, PSA. This observation provides a clear impetus to examine the androgen-signaling pathway in prostate cancer. However, to understand the mechanisms associated with progression despite castrate levels of testosterone requires the direct study of the progressing tumor. This has been limited in part because the performance of a repeat biopsy to characterize the progression of tumors directly is not a part of routine clinical management. Even when a biopsy is considered, the primary manifestations of progression, such as a rising PSA or spread to an osseous site, do not lend themselves to easy acquisition and analysis. Consequently, the overall number of specimens analyzed has been limited, and in particular, there are few reports focused on matched pairs of tumors obtained from the time of diagnosis, and at the time of relapse in the same patient. Despite this, the available reports permit a classification scheme based on: (A) the levels of wild-type receptors, (B) the levels of ligand within the tumor itself, (C) activating mutations in the receptor that affect structure and function, (D) changes in coregulatory molecules including coactivators and corepressors, and (E) factors that lead to activation of the receptor independent of the level of ligand or receptor allowing cross-talk with other signaling pathways (11,12) (Figure 16.B2).

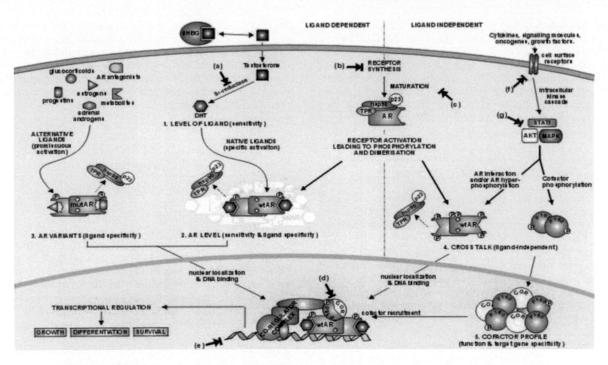

FIGURE 16B.1. Signaling in progressive castration resistant prostate cancer showing points of therapeutic attacks. (Modified from Scher HI, Buchanan G, Gerald W, et al. Targeting the androgen receptor: improving outcomes for castration resistant prostate cancer. *Endocr Relat Cancer* 2004;11:459–476.)

Androgen Receptor Expression

Many studies have addressed the role of androgen receptor (AR) in prostate cancer using xenograft mouse models of the human disease. Analogous to the clinical setting, prostate cancer xenograft lines typically grow only in an androgen-dependent state and are sensitive to androgen ablation, but frequently regrow in a low-androgen environment following castration and continue to secrete PSA. In support of the hypothesis that AR continues to play an important role in growth of castrate-resistant prostate cancer, several studies have demonstrated an increase in the level of AR and/or AR-regulated genes in xenograft tumors following castration in comparison to untreated tumors (13–16). In particular, comprehensive gene expression profiling determined that the AR was the only gene upregulated in the progression from androgen sensitive to castration-resistant growth in all seven human prostate cancer xenograft models analyzed (15). In clinical disease, recent studies have demonstrated an increase in both AR mRNA and protein levels during progression from localized disease to metastatic castrate-resistant prostate cancer (6). Moreover, increased AR levels in clinically localized disease have been associated with relapse following radical prostatectomy, suggesting that the AR is a determinant of metastatic spread (17,18).

Several mechanisms have been proposed to contribute to increased AR levels in castrate-resistant tumors, including increased expression of the AR and AR gene amplification, the latter being demonstrated in up to 29% of castrate-resistant tumors along with a concomitant increase in androgen-regulated genes (19–22). Increased stability and reduced degradation of the AR protein have more recently been identified in prostate cancer (23), which may result from altered posttranslational modifications to the receptor (24–26). There are at least two mechanisms by which increased AR levels may facilitate prostate cancer progression in a castrate environment: (a) hypersensitizing the receptor for activation by low concentrations of ligand (23), and (b) permitting AR antagonists, such as bicalutamide, to act as receptor agonists (15,27).

Level of Ligand

A recent study using laser capture mass spectrometry demonstrated that the level of testosterone in recurrent prostate cancers following androgen ablation was similar to that in untreated benign prostatic disease (28). While the level of dihydrotestosterone, dehydroepiandrosterone, and androstenedione were significantly lower in the recurrent prostate cancer cells in that study, the level of DHT (1.45 nM) was sufficient to

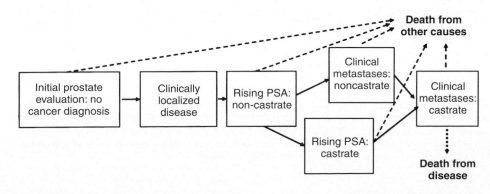

FIGURE 16B.2. Prostrate cancer clinical states. (Modified from Scher HI, Heller G. Clinical states in prostate cancer: towards a dynamic model of disease progression. *Urology* 2000;55:323–327.)

maintain AR signaling and expression of PSA (28). Moreover, it has recently been shown that genes involved in steroid biosynthesis are overexpressed in recurrent human prostate tumors and CWR22 xenografts, suggesting that tumors may be able to compensate locally for systemic androgen deprivation (16,22). Alternatively, sequestration of androgens by steroid hormone-binding globulin, which is synthesized and secreted by prostatic epithelial and stromal cells (29), may allow tumor cells to accumulate androgens.

Androgen Receptor Structure

The AR has a modular structure, consisting primarily of a large amino-terminal transactivation domain (NTD), a centrally located DNA-binding domain (DBD), and a carboxy-terminal ligand-binding domain (LBD) that confers high affinity and specificity for androgen binding. AR gene mutations have been reported in prostate cancer at a frequency of 5% to 50%, with a higher frequency reported in more advanced disease and following androgen-ablation therapy (30). In contrast to the inherited syndrome of androgen insensitivity, where AR gene mutations result in a loss of receptor function, those detected in prostate cancer occur in distinctly different regions of the receptor, and generally confer promiscuity or increased sensitivity for receptor activation by other steroid hormones and/or by the specific antiandrogen used in clinical management of the disease (6,8,31). These observations led to the concept of therapy-mediated selection pressure, which is exemplified by the detection of AR gene mutations which confer enhanced receptor activity in response to flutamide but not to other antiandrogens in tumors from patients treated with hydroxyflutamide plus orchiectomy or Luteinizing-hormone releasing hormone (LHRH) agonists/antagonists, as part of a combined androgen blockade strategy (32,33). Clinically, patients who progress during treatment with one antiandrogen often respond to another (34,35). The phenomenon of therapy-mediated selection pressure has been observed clinically for many antiandrogens, where a paradoxical decline in PSA levels is observed following discontinuation of specific antiandrogen therapy (36,37). In vitro culture of LNCaP cells with bicalutamide resulted in outgrowth of a subline containing a mutation at codon 741, which conferred increased cell growth and PSA secretion in response to bicalutamide but not flutamide (38). These findings suggest that antiandrogens may elicit different mechanisms leading to a withdrawal response, consistent with clinical observations that second-line therapy with antiandrogens often results in tumor regression. Studies of the autochthonous TRAMP model of prostate cancer (39,40) demonstrate that therapy-mediated selection of AR mutations is not limited to antiandrogen treatment. Whereas noncastrate mice develop mutations in the AR-LBD, mice castrated at 12 weeks of age developed mutations in the NTD (41). Enforced expression of the AR-NTD variant, E231G, in the mouse prostate confers rapid development of prostatic intra-epithelial neoplasia that progresses to invasive and metastatic disease in 100% of mice (42). In contrast, the wild-type AR and the LNCaP AR-LBD variant, which is responsive to other steroid hormones, had minimal effect on the mouse prostate (42). This finding suggests that the AR can also act in an appropriate environment as a proto-oncogene to promote tumor formation. Collectively, the above clinical and animal studies imply that selection of mutations in the AR-LBD most likely occurs during the course of the disease to facilitate progression in response to an available ligand (i.e., estradiol, glucocorticoids, or antiandrogens), whereas mutations in the NTD occurring earlier in disease etiology may alter AR function, per se, to promote tumor formation (43). Although mutations in the AR have not been detected in all patients with castrate-resistant disease, which may reflect technical issues, differences in patient populations, stage of disease, tumor burden, timing of antiandrogen therapy, and prior hormonal manipulations (6,44), it has now been clearly established that mutations are one important mechanism contributing to prostate tumorigenesis, progression following androgen ablation, antiandrogen agonist activity, and withdrawal responses.

Coregulators

Extended culture of LNCaP human prostate cancer cells in androgen-depleted media resulted in sensitization of the AR to 10-fold lower concentrations of androgens and the ability to respond to bicalutamide, without changes in AR structure or level (45). These effects may be explained by changes in the level or function of proteins that orchestrate specific aspects of AR signaling. For example, the transcriptional activity of the AR is mediated, in part, by the recruitment of coregulator proteins that enhance (coactivators) or repress (corepressors) receptor function. An increase in coactivator levels has been shown in prostate cancer compared to benign prostate tissues, and during the development of castrate-resistant disease (23,46–49). These coactivator proteins can selectively enhance the activity of the AR upon binding of alternative ligands, such as estradiol and hydroxyflutamide, sensitize the AR to lower concentrations of native and nonnative ligands, or promote different modes of AR activation by altering conformational changes and homodimerization following ligand binding (41,50–53). Conversely, decreased expression of corepressors such as NCoR and SMRT, which mediate, in part, the antagonist action of bicalutamide, flutamide, and mifepristone, would facilitate increased agonist activity of these agents (54,55). However, while more than 120 AR-interacting proteins have been described, it is not currently known how the majority of these influence receptor function, or which are expressed in the prostate and have altered expression during disease etiology.

Cross-talk with Other Signaling Pathways

Tyrosine kinase receptors, growth factors, and cytokines are able to activate the AR, possibly negating the requirement for ligand, or at least sensitizing the AR to low concentrations of available native or nonnative steroids (56–63). Activation of the AR by these factors in the absence of ligand results in the activation of AR-responsive genes, proliferation of prostate cancer cells, and increased apoptosis resistance during androgen deprivation (59,64).

Increased expression of HER-2/neu has been detected in a proportion of prostate cancers at all stages of disease (65–67). Significantly, a recent retrospective study of aggressively treated, clinically organ-confined prostate cancer demonstrated that 90% of patients who developed extensive metastatic disease requiring androgen ablation already expressed high levels of both HER-2/neu and AR in the primary tumor (Dr. Camela Ricciardelli, University of Adelaide; personal communication). HER-2/neu is thought to promote DNA binding and AR stability through activation of MAPK and Akt, the latter being able to bind directly to the receptor (25,64). Mechanisms that directly activate MAPK and Akt can elicit an analogous effect (64). Importantly, nongenomic effects of hydroxyflutamide appear to enhance the effect of MAPK on the AR, possibly by promoting rapid phosphorylation of the kinase via RAS/RAF association (68), implicating antiandrogens as direct promoters of tumor progression.

Implications for Clinical Management

The evolving evidence that the AR is one of the key critical mediators of continued prostate cancer growth following hormone ablation makes a compelling argument for the development of new strategies that directly target the receptor (6). Such new therapies are necessary for significant advances in the management of patients with advanced prostate cancer who will ultimately fail androgen ablation. Several approaches to achieve this goal have been documented. Reducing the level of AR and suppression of human prostate cancer cell growth *in vitro* and *in vivo* have been achieved with double-stranded RNA interference, antisense oligonucleotides, hammerhead ribozymes, and analogues of the ansamycin antibiotics such as 17-allylamino-17-demethoxygeldanamycin (69–76). Inhibition of AR function has been achieved with dominant negative AR inhibitors, microinjection of AR antibodies, "decoy" double-stranded DNA fragments containing specific AR response elements, and histone deacetylase inhibitors suberoylanilide including hydroxamic acid and phenylbutyrate (74,77–80). Providing issues such as the mode of delivery and the potential for disruption of multiple signaling pathways can be circumvented, these newer approaches that directly target the AR provide considerable promise as therapeutic options for castrate-resistant prostate cancer.

THERAPEUTIC CONSIDERATIONS

Understanding the biology of castration-resistant disease can help place therapeutic options for patients into perspective. The clinical spectrum of patients with prostate cancer who progress despite castrate levels of testosterone includes individuals with tumor burdens ranging from minimal to extensive, who have shown varying degrees and a range of durations of response to primary androgen deprivation therapy. The clinical manifestations may be restricted to a rising PSA alone, a rising PSA with osseous and/or soft-tissue spread, while some show a predominantly visceral disease pattern with PSA levels that are disproportionately low relative to tumor burden. This latter group includes tumors with a predominantly neuroendocrine phenotype, and have a distinctly poor prognosis.

PROGNOSIS

It is often stated that the duration of response to primary androgen deprivation is on the order of 12 to 18 months; however, where the data supporting this conclusion came from is not entirely clear. A critical analysis of outcomes reported with androgen ablation shows that response durations range from months to years, varying as a function of the grade of the tumor and on the initial extent of disease. In a Southwest Oncology Group (SWOG) study evaluating the role of combined androgen blockade, the prognosis of patients with disease limited to the axial skeleton differed significantly from those with disease in the axial and appendicular skeleton (82). Others have demonstrated that prognoses can be defined based on the extent of disease evident on a bone scan (83). Pretherapy PSA doubling times may also be predictive as recent studies have shown that the duration of response, and subsequent prostate cancer specific mortality, is inversely related to PSA doubling times (84). This consideration is important when trying to identify patients at risk of dying of their illness for whom more aggressive approaches may be more appropriate.

The nadir PSA following treatment is also important (85, 86). Figure 16B.3 illustrates serial changes in PSA after androgen deprivation. Noteworthy is that the PSA nadir did not reach undetectable levels, and using a stringent definition of treatment failure, two consecutive rises in PSA, the overall duration of response was less than 6 months. This, too, has prognostic significance, as patients who achieve an undetectable posttherapy nadir have a significantly better prognosis than those who do not (87).

That patients have a range of prognoses is illustrated further using a nomogram for survival of patients with progressive castration-resistant disease treated with a range of therapies (Figure 16B.4). Illustrated are two individuals. The first has a good performance status, no significant comorbidities, and an extent of disease that has not produced significant alterations in alkaline phosphatase, reflecting osseous spread, or lactate dehydrogenase, and a hemoglobin within the normal range. The second is compromised functionally from his disease, with an increased alkaline phosphatase and lactate dehydrogenase, and a significantly lower hemoglobin. The range in the predicted 1-year and 2-year survivals, 90% vs. 20%, and 65% vs. essentially zero, is illustrated. Whether the approaches to these two individuals should be the same is uncertain.

The results with second-line and third-line hormonal manipulations that will be discussed below must be considered in this context, as none have been proven to prolong life. This issue has been complicated further by the results of SWOG 9916 and TAX 327, American Society for Clinical Oncology (ASCO) (88,89). These studies both demonstrated a survival advantage in castrate metastatic prostate cancer with docetaxel-based chemotherapy given on an every-3-week schedule. It is unknown

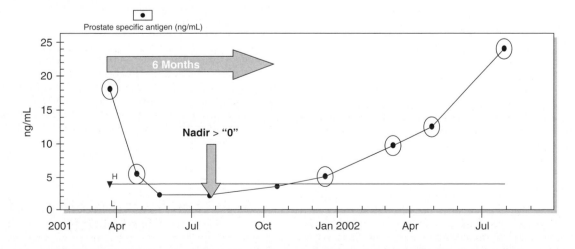

FIGURE 16B.3. Serial changes in PSA following Androgen ablation showing a nadir value above "0".

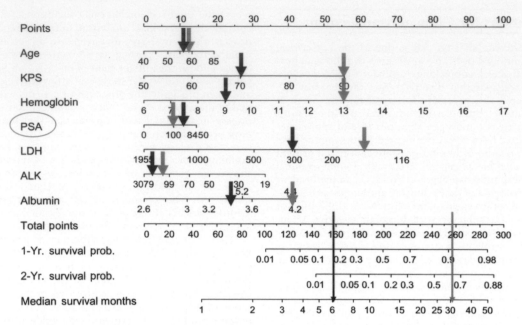

FIGURE 16B.4. Nomogram for survival of patients with progressive castration resistant disease showing two patients with markedly different prognosis (From, Smaletz O, Scher HI, Small EJ, et al. Nomogram for overall survival of patients with progressive metastatic prostate cancer after castration. *J Clin Oncol* 2002;20:3972–3982.)

whether this survival advantage is affected by the timing and sequence of treatments. A current phase III trial conducted by the Eastern Cooperative Oncology Group (ECOG, trial 1899) is testing whether chemotherapy with docetaxel and estramustine is superior to ketoconazole and hydrocortisone in patients with progression after initial hormonal therapy. Until the results of that trial are mature, it is reasonable to approach each patient individually.

Once disease progression occurs on primary hormonal therapy, patients have several options for treatment, including secondary hormonal manipulations, chemotherapy, or experimental approaches. A period of observation may also be appropriate. Indeed, prognostic models have shown that certain key factors such as performance status, PSA, and baseline laboratory values may be utilized to predict the likelihood of continued progression and survival (90,91). These models may be a useful aid to determine which second-line therapy approach is appropriate.

CASTRATION STATUS

One consideration at the outset is the castration status of the patient. This is assessed easily by measuring the level of testosterone in the blood. Those with elevated levels typically include patients who have been treated with antiandrogen monotherapy or a combination of an antiandrogen and the 5-alpha reductase inhibitor finasteride. These patients should be treated first with an approach designed to lower testosterone levels such as a gonadotropin-releasing hormone analog or surgical orchiectomy. The response to such crossover therapies is not well characterized, however, and in one study it was only 30% (92).

An additional question is whether medical therapies to maintain castrate levels of testosterone should be continued when a patient progresses. This is not an issue for patients who have undergone surgical orchiectomy, and while most physicians do maintain treatment, the data justifying this approach is limited. In a retrospective analysis of 341 patients treated in a

series of clinical trials conducted by ECOG, medical castration was discontinued in 16% (n = 55) of patients. These patients had decreased survival compared with those whose castration was continued (10). Although a similar analysis conducted by the Southwest Oncology Group did not show an inferior outcome with discontinuation of castration, the fact that exogenous testosterone administration can induce disease flares argues for maintenance of castrate states. However, only a small number of patients had discontinuation of medical castration (16% of 205 patients) in this series. Long recognized is that the administration of exogenous androgens may result in a clinical flare of the disease. This is another example of the continued hormone sensitivity of the disease, which may be manifest by an increase in pain, urinary obstruction, or spinal cord compression (93). In one series, exogenous testosterone was utilized as a means to increase sensitivity to cytotoxic drugs. The approach was not only unsuccessful, but resulted in a shortened survival for those receiving testosterone relative to those who did not (94). Whether the same "shortened" survival would result if endogenous testosterone levels were allowed to rise by discontinuing medical therapies designed to maintain castrate levels of testosterone is uncertain. Recognizing the concentration of dihydrotestosterone required for growth stimulation of recurrent prostate cancer cell lines was 4 orders of magnitude lower than that required for androgen-dependent LNCaP cells (53), and that in human studies, 15 (28%) of 54 castrate metastatic tumor specimens demonstrated androgen-receptor gene amplification compared with none of the 26 paired primary specimens (95), the increase in enzymes associated with androgen synthesis, along with previous cited studies showing the significance of low levels of intratumoral androgens, argue for continued medical suppression.

ANTIANDROGEN SELECTION PRESSURE

There is emerging evidence that the mechanisms contributing to continued signaling through the androgen receptor within a tumor may depend on the specific therapy to which a tumor has been exposed during treatment of the disease. We have termed this "therapy-mediated selection pressure." The development of specific AR mutations in response to particular therapies is an example of how therapy-mediated selection pressure can affect a patient's disease at the level of the tumor. Clinically, this has been demonstrated as a higher frequency of responses to bicalutamide in patients previously treated with flutamide compared to patients who have not been exposed to flutamide (34). Another example of therapy-mediated selection pressure is the antiandrogen withdrawal response. One cannot have a withdrawal response in the absence of treatment with the specific agent (96).

Up to 40% of patients with progressive castrate prostate cancer will have a clinical benefit after the withdrawal of an antiandrogen. This phenomenon was first observed after the selective discontinuation of flutamide while maintaining treatment with a gonodotropin releasing harmone (GN_{RH}) analog (3). Nonsteroidal and steroid hormone withdrawal responses are characterized by decreasing levels of PSA and tumor regressions when an agent, previously shown to induce regression as therapy, is selectively discontinued at the time of disease progression. Such responses have been reported with nonsteroidal antiandrogens (i.e., flutamide, nilutamide, and bicalutamide), estrogens (diethylstilbestrol), or progestational agents (megestrol acetate) (36,37,97–105). In most series, the overall frequency of response, reported on the basis of posttherapy changes in PSA, are in the range of 25% to 30%, lasting a median duration of 3 to 4 months. In a summary of 132 patients evaluated for a response to withdrawal of "any" antiandrogen, a lower response rate of 10% was observed. Despite the modest frequency, some are quite significant and include regressions of established epidural lesions and hepatic disease.

The antiandrogen withdrawal phenomenon seems to be due to a selection of androgen receptor mutations that yield a promiscuous receptor allowing for stimulation of the receptor with the antiandrogen agent. For example, in 5 of 16 patients treated with the antiandrogen flutamide, a mutation in codon 877 resulting in the substitution of an alanine for a threonine (T877A) was found (33). Functional analysis of this mutation has demonstrated that the substitution allows hydroxyflutamide, the active metabolite of flutamide, to become a strong agonist of the receptor (32). These findings further support the importance of continued androgen receptor signaling with progressive prostate cancer. The exact mechanisms associated with this effect have not been fully elucidated.

THERAPEUTIC OPTIONS

Antiandrogens as Second-line Therapy

Antiandrogens function to block the binding of dihydrotestosterone to the androgen receptor, preventing the translocation of the DHT-androgen receptor complex to the nucleus. There are two general classes, steroidal and non-steroidal. The former includes cyproterone acetate and megestrol acetate, both of which have progestational effects as well, while of the nonsteroidal, three are in general clinical use, including flutamide, bicalutamide, and nilutamide. All function at the level of ligand and do not alter the level of receptor. The nonsteroidal agents in particular agents differ in their affinity for the AR, elimination half-life as well as the exact site of binding as evidenced by the effectiveness of these agents in the second-line and third-line setting.

Interpreting literature reports of second-line and third-line hormonal treatments is limited by differences in reporting, and in particular, that many trials were conducted prior to the acceptance of PSA-based standards of reporting (106). Such is the case despite the controversies surrounding how to interpret PSA-based endpoints in relation to true clinical benefit to the patient. This severely limits comparisons between studies. It should be reported at the outset that to date, no prospectively designed randomized comparative trial has shown a survival benefit for any second-line treatment. This is not surprising given that results of first trials showing a definitive benefit for a cytotoxic agent were not published until 2004, even though response proportions in excess of 50% have been reported for over a decade. Overall, most responses to second-line therapies are short, with a median duration in the range of 3 to 4 months, with selected patients showing more prolonged benefit. Uncertain is whether a patient who responds to one is more likely to respond to a second and third hormonal intervention, which may result in a longer period of "net clinical benefit" for that individual. Such questions can only be addressed through prospectively designed trials that factor in prior treatments in the outcomes analysis.

Flutamide

Flutamide is a nonsteroidal pure antiandrogen that inhibits the binding of DHT to the androgen receptor. It has a shorter half-life and a lower binding affinity for the androgen receptor than bicalutamide. However, flutamide has been the most widely studied in the second-line setting. In one study of 209 patients with progressive disease following either orchiectomy, DES, or a gonadotropin-releasing hormone agonist, flutamide was administered with a response rate of 34.5% (107). The European Organization for Research and Treatment of Cancer reported a similar response rate of 45% ($n = 45$ of 100) following medical or surgical castration (108). Large trials of flutamide following other antiandrogens have not been performed. However, Kojima et al. reported a response rate of 50% ($n = 5$ of 10) based on PSA criteria in patients treated with flutamide after progression on combined androgen blockade with a GnRH agonist and bicalutamide (109). Side effects of flutamide include diarrhea and biochemical hepatitis, which mandates monitoring of liver function while on treatment.

Bicalutamide

Bicalutamide is a nonsteroidal pure antiandrogen with a longer half-life allowing once-a-day dosing and improved patient tolerance relative to flutamide, which it has largely replaced in clinical practice (110). Additional side effects include fatigue and gynecomastia. Standard-dose bicalutamide (50 mg) has not been studied in the castrate metastatic state, although doses of 150 mg daily have shown activity. One study, which analyzed outcomes in relation to prior hormone therapy, showed an overall PSA response rate of 31% (12 of 39) (92). The proportion ranged from 22% (7 of 31) in those not exposed to flutamide to 38% (10 of 26) in those who were. Similar results were observed in a second trial: 22% for those with no prior flutamide exposure versus 43% in those who were (34). This is another example of therapy-mediated selection pressure.

Nilutamide

Nilutamide is an additional nonsteroidal antiandrogen that is given on a daily basis. It is well tolerated with a side effect profile similar to other antiandrogens with some additional effects that are unique to the drug. These include impaired visual adaptation to darkness and interstitial pneumonitis reported in 8% and 2% of patients, respectively (111). Patients should also be advised to avoid alcohol consumption because of the possibility of a disulfiram reaction. A retrospective analysis of patients treated with nilutamide after progression on another antiandrogen demonstrated that 48% (12 of 28) of patients had a PSA decline of greater than 50% (35). A similar report from the University of Chicago demonstrated that 50% of patients treated with nilutamide following treatment with at least one antiandrogen had a PSA response (112). No prospective studies have been reported.

Estrogens

Estrogens have long been included in the therapeutic milieu of progressive prostate cancer although the precise mechanism by which they exert their effects is unknown. They inhibit testicular production of testosterone by inhibiting LHRH from the hypothalamus and subsequent LH by the pituitary gland. They also likely compete for the androgen receptor at higher concentrations. The most commonly studied estrogen agent is diethylstilbesterol (DES). The earliest studies were conducted by the Veterans Administration Cooperation Urological Research Group (VACURG) in the 1960s using 5 mg of DES. These studies demonstrated that DES was as effective as orchiectomy but carried with it significant cardiovascular toxicity. A more recent phase II study of 1 mg oral DES in castrate metastatic patients performed at the University of Michigan demonstrated that 43% (9 of 21) of patients had a decline in PSA of greater than or equal to 50% (113).

PC-SPES is a mixture of Chinese herbs with known estrogenic effects with seeming activity in castration-resistant disease. Administered as monotherapy, side effects included gynecomastic and thromboembolic events similar to those reported with estrogens alone. Serum testosterone levels have also been documented to decline. To evaluate the relative efficacy of the herbal mixture to DES alone, a prospective trial of PC-SPES and DES 3 mg daily was initiated. A PSA decline of greater than or equal to 50% was observed in 24% (10 of 42) of patients in the DES group and 40% (17 of 43) of the PC-SPES-treated patients (114). It should be noted that measurable levels of DES were detected in all lots of the PC-SPES used for this study, although in varying amounts, and the trial was not designed to detect superiority of one agent.

Adrenal Suppression

Approximately 90% of testosterone is removed following medical or surgical castration. The remaining androgens are produced by the adrenal glands, primarily dehydroepiandrosterone (DHEA) and dehydroepiandrosterone sulfate (DHEAS). DHEA and DHEAS have little androgenic activity alone; however, both are converted in peripheral tissues to androstenedione and testosterone. As stated earlier, mechanisms for continued prostate cancer growth following androgen ablation with orchiectomy or a GNRH is the increased sensitivity of the androgen receptor to these circulating androgens as well as an increase in the level of receptor. Such hypersensivity has been demonstrated in prostate cancer cell lines derived from tumors that have progressed despite androgen ablation (23). This is supported by clinical studies that have shown benefit with adrenal suppression in men with progressive androgen-independent prostate cancer. This paradigm once again demonstrates that our terminology for progressive prostate cancer is inadequate and the term "progressive castrate prostate cancer" is more accurate.

Corticosteroids

Glucocorticoids suppress the production of adrenal androgens via negative feedback inhibition of corticotropin-releasing hormone production from the hypothalamus and ACTH production from the pituitary. An early study by Tannock et al. reported that quality of life measurements were improved with prednisone 7.5 mg to 10 mg daily in 38% of patients (14 of 37), doses which are slightly higher than the physiologic replacement dose (115). Most of the more recent data on glucocorticoids comes from control arms of randomized trials testing other agents. For example, in a study comparing prednisone 20 mg daily with flutamide 250 mg three times daily for patients with progressive castrate metastatic prostate cancer, the EORTC reported that 21% (21 of 101) of patients receiving prednisone had a greater than 50% decline in PSA compared with 23% (23 of 100) of the patients receiving flutamide (108). Similar results have been reported with hydrocortisone. The CALGB reported a PSA response of 14.3% (13 of 91) in patients treated with 40 mg of hydrocortisone compared with 18.7% (18 of 96) of patients treated with 40 mg of hydrocortisone and mitoxantrone (116). There has not been a randomized trial to determine which glucocorticoid is more effective, but it appears that inhibiting even low levels of circulating androgens appears to be effective in a sizable proportion of patients.

Understanding the benefits of corticosteroids alone has improved our ability to analyze new agents being tested. Initial reports of suramin, a polysulphonated naphthylurea, demonstrated seemingly high response proportions in patients with progressive castration-resistant disease (117), which appeared to be confirmed in follow-up studies (118,119). Unrecognized at the time was the potential contribution of the glucocorticoids themselves or the role of steroid hormone withdrawal responses on outcome. A prospective, double-blind, randomized comparative trial which controlled for these factors showed no survival benefit relative to hydrocortisone alone (120). This study shows the importance of controlling for patient entry factors that can affect outcomes, and the contribution of responses to hormonal maneuvers as opposed to the test agent itself.

Ketoconazole

Ketoconazole is an azole antifungal which was discovered to produce gynecomastia in men during its initial use. This prompted exploration of its effects on androgen biosynthesis (121). It is now known that ketoconazole exerts its effect through inhibition of cytochrome P-450a-demethylase, a catalyst for the conversion of lanosterol to cholesterol. It results in a significant decline in serum testosterone as a result from both adrenal and testicular production. An initial pilot trial reported a significant need for analgesic use and a decrease in prostatic acid phosphatase levels with 400 mg of ketoconazole given 3 times daily (122). When studied after combined androgen blockade with flutamide and subsequent antiandrogen withdrawal, this dosage of ketoconazole yielded a PSA response of 62.5% (30 of 48) (5). Uncertain at this point is whether similar responses would be observed to low-dose hydrocortisone alone or whether higher doses are necessary, and the relative contribution of hydrocortisone.

In a more recent study from the CALGB, 32% (35 of 108) of patients experienced a decline in PSA with 400 mg of ketoconazole given 3 times daily and replacement hydrocortisone of 40 mg daily (123). In this trial objective regressions were observed in 20% versus 2%, although there was no survival benefit. The study included the measurement of adrenal androgen levels and showed that on aggregate, androstenedione levels were increased at the start of therapy and relatively decreased following treatment. This suggested a correlation between androstenedione levels and the probabililty of response. The median levels in responding patients were 880 mcg/mL versus 530 mcg/mL for nonresponders, with an association between baseline level and survival (hazard ratio 1.6; $p = .034$), although serial levels in individual patients were not reported.

Ketoconazole is associated with significant toxicities including adrenal suppression, and when used with higher doses necessitates coadministration of hydrocortisone. When given with hydrocortisone, nausea and vomiting are reported in approximately 10% of patients. Fatigue, rash, and hepatotoxicity are also reported in 5% to 10% of patients (124). Ketoconazole requires an acidic environment for absorption and avoidance of medications that increase gastric pH such as H2-blockers.

FUTURE DIRECTIONS

Reducing AR Levels

Current evidence shows the importance of continued signaling through the androgen receptor on the growth of castration-resistant prostate cancers. This supports the development of androgen receptor-targeted treatments as a viable therapeutic strategy. This approach could be alone or in combination with strategies directed at the level of ligand, including inhibitors of adrenal synthetic enzymes and novel antiandrogens that interact with the receptor itself or that inhibit receptor function by inhibiting coactivators or activating repressors. The challenge is to eliminate the receptor selectively in the tumor without affecting other androgen-target tissues. Recognizing that each of these approaches is likely to have multiple effects on AR signaling, the strategies under development include those designed to reduce AR levels with double-stranded RNA interference (73) and antisense oligonucleotides (72,74,76). Ansamycin antibiotics induce the degradation of steroid hormone receptors and a number of mutated oncogenes by interfering with Hsp90 binding and preventing protein refolding (69–71,125). These agents, now in clinical testing, reduce the levels of AR and inhibit prostate cancer cell growth *in vivo* in a dose-dependent manner (125). Other Hsp90 substrates affected by this agent include HER2/neu and phosphor-AKT, both of which are expressed at a higher frequency in castration-resistant tumors and opposed to castration-naive tumors.

Histone deacetylase inhibitor, such as suberoylanilide hydroxamic acid and phenylbutyrate, which inhibit chromatin remodeling enzymes recruited by NCoR and SMRT (80), also inhibit prostate cancer cells growth *in vitro* and *in vivo* (78,126). Both are under study against a range of solid tumors including prostate cancer (127,128).

LIGAND-INDEPENDENT ACTIVATION

The family of epidermal growth-factor receptors (EGFr) have been shown to be important in the progression of castrate prostate cancer (129,130). HER2/neu, a member of the EGFr family of receptor tyrosine kinases, is consistently overexpressed in castrate prostate cancer cell lines (58), and inhibition of HER2/neu with trastuzumab, a monoclonal antibody against HER2/neu, has shown antiproliferative activity against prostate cancer cell lines (131). A phase II study of trastuzumab in men with progressive castrate and noncastrate prostate cancer demonstrated no PSA declines in 23 patients. Only six patients had HER2 overexpression as confirmed by IHC with $\geq 2+$ staining using the Hercptest™ (132). The investigators also reported that of the nine matched primary prostate and metastatic samples, three were HER2 positive in the metastatic setting but not in the primary setting, suggesting that HER2 expression varies by clinical state. In a separate phase II trial in

which HER2 positive patients were to be treated with trastuzumab followed by combination therapy with docetaxel at progression, only 7% (7 of 100) of patients screened had HER2/neu overexpression by IHC (133). Thus, the trial was closed. It is important to note that these samples were all from the primary tumors and, based on the data from the previous phase II experience, it is likely that some patients with HER2 overexpression in metastatic disease were overlooked.

Many investigators have begun to take advantage of what is known about "outlaw pathways" that may stimulate the androgen receptor through means other than circulating androgens. These novel, targeted approaches may prove to be the future of treatment for men with progressive castrate metastatic prostate cancer and will help us to further understand the mechanisms by which prostate cancers continue to grow despite androgen ablation.

Calcitriol

Calcitriol (1,25-dihhydroxyvitamin D_3) is also a steroid hormone best known for its activity in regulating calcium and bone metabolism. Epidemiologic studies have demonstrated an association between vitamin D_3 deficiency and the risk of prostate cancer (134). The exact antitumor mechanism through which vitamin D_3 exerts its effects is still unknown, although it is likely a combination of cell-cycle arrest and apoptosis. Vitamin D_3 binds to Vitamin D receptor (VDR), which then complexes with the retinoic-acid receptor. This complex binds to a specific DNA-sequence motif called the vitamin D-response element, which ultimately regulates the transcription of genes involved in apoptosis, differentiation, and cell-cycle arrest.

Unfortunately, clinical trials to date have been disappointing. A phase II trial in men with progressive castrate prostate cancer reported by Osborn et al. demonstrated no responses in 14 patients at a dose of 1.0 to 1.5 mcg daily (135). Therapy was limited by hypercalcemia, so subsequent trials have been aimed at trying to limit the amount of hypercalcemia. Smith and colleagues demonstrated that hypercalcemia can be ameliorated by administration of calcitriol on an every-other day schedule and that substantially higher doses of calcitriol can be well tolerated when using a pulsatile-dosing schedule (136). A recent phase I trial reported from Memorial Sloan-Kettering Cancer Center combined high-dose calcitriol with zoledronic acid. Patients could also receive dexamethasone at disease progression. Doses were escalated to 30 mcg given 3 times per week. Once again, minimal antitumor effects were seen (137). Based on these data, the authors concluded that further phase II trials of calcitriol administered in this manner are not warranted.

Proteosome Inhibition

The ubiquitin-proteosome pathway plays an important role in regulating the cell cycle, neoplastic growth, and metastasis (138). The ordered degradation of these key cell-cycle regulators is required for the cell to progress through the cell cycle and undergo mitosis. The ubiquitin-proteosome pathway is also required for transcriptional regulation. Nuclear factor-κB (NF-κB) is a transcription factor that promotes cell survival, angiogenesis, and metastasis. Its activation is regulated by proteosome-mediated degradation of the inhibitor protein I kappa B alpha-associated protein kinase ($I_K B_\alpha$) (139). Inhibiting the proteosome results in stabilization of the inhibitor protein and thus downregulation of NF-κB and enhanced apoptosis. A recent phase I trial of bortezomib, a specific and reversible inhibitor of the proteosome, was reported by Papandreou et al. in which the dose-limiting toxicities of diarrhea and hypotension were observed at 2.0 mg/m^2. Two (4%) of 47 patients with progressive castrate prostate cancer experienced a PSA decline of greater than or equal to 50% and nine (19%) experienced a stabilization of PSA. Interestingly, a greater than or equal to 50% PSA decline was seen only in the subgroup of patients with a decline in elevated pretreatment serum IL-6 levels, a marker for NF-κB activation (140). A phase II trial of bortezomib is currently underway (Moms et al. Memorial Hospital Clinical Protocol (MSKCC) IRB#02-070) (141).

Endothelin Receptor Antagonists

Endothelin-1 is a potent vasoconstrictor found in normal seminal fluid and found to be elevated in men with castrate prostate cancer (142). It has been shown to inhibit apoptosis in prostate cancer cells when induced by a variety of stimuli, including paclitaxel, and to act as a nociceptive mediator in animal models. Initial results from phase I and phase II trials with an endothelin receptor antagonist, Atrasentan (ABT-627), were promising and demonstrated tolerability of the agent as well as antitumor activity. Sixty-eight percent of men (15 of 22) treated on two separate phase I trials experienced a decline in PSA, ranging from 4% to 89%, and 70% experienced decreased pain as measured on visual analog scales (143). A randomized double-blind phase II trial was performed in men with progressive castrate prostate cancer with three treatment arms, including placebo, 2.5 mg of Atrasentan, and 10 mg of Atrasentan. The primary endpoint of the study was time to disease progression as defined by development of new lesions in the bone or soft tissue, the requirement of palliative treatment with an opioid analgesic for new disease-related pain, a new disease-related symptom that required intervention or was deemed by the investigator to represent progression, or death occurring while the patient was receiving the drug in the study. The investigators reported no significant difference in time to progression in any of the arms (183 days vs. 178 days vs. 137 days, $P = .13$ and $P = .29$). A longer time to PSA progression in the Atrasentan arms compared with the placebo arm (155 vs. 141 vs. 71 days, $P = .002$ and $P = .055$) was identified (144,145).

The results of two phase III trials comparing 10 mg of Atrasentan with placebo were reported at ASCO in 2004. Again, the primary endpoint was time to progression using a combination of clinical and radiographic criteria. In a meta-analysis using data pooled from the two studies, there was a significant delay in time to progression with 10 mg of Atrasentan (HR 1.19, $P = .13$) (146).

COOPERATIVE ALTERATIONS IN SIGNALING PATHWAYS

Although inhibition at the level of the HER2 receptor has not proven to be promising, there is much interest in other aspects of the EGFr pathway. Using the androgen-dependent CWR22 prostate xenograft model, daily oral administration of gefitinib given at the maximal tolerated dose (MTD) (150 mg/kg) resulted in a 54% growth inhibition. When tested in a variant cell line with a decreased dependence on androgen (CWR22LD1), growth was inhibited by 76% (147). Unfortunately, in a phase II trial of 51 patients with androgen-independent prostate cancer treated with gefitinib, only one PSA response occurred and eight had stable disease (148).

Understanding why the antiproliferative effects of EGFr inhibition can be overcome with upregulation of important targets through other means has led to further investigation into

this pathway. One example of this is demonstrated in tumor cell lines that are phosphate and tensin homologue deleted on chromosome 10 (PTEN)-deficient. PTEN is a phosphatase which converts PIP3 into an inactive PIP2. Loss of PTEN leads to a constitutively active PI3-kinase pathway with increased phosphorylation of AKT, a downstream protein of PIP3. Cell lines which are deficient in PTEN, MDA-468, are resistant to treatment with EGFr inhibitors. Reconstitution of PTEN via retroviral infection of the MDA-468 cells resulted in sensitivity to inhibition of EGFr (149,150). In other words, restoring PTEN activity allows for the cell to become dependent upon EGFR and thus become sensitive to inhibition of that target. This effect of PTEN on the EGFr pathway is of particular interest in prostate cancer because of the high rate of PTEN deletion in prostate cancer. PTEN mutations have been observed in up to 80% of prostate cancers and correlate with higher Gleason scores and more advanced disease. Loss of PTEN leads to increased activation of AKT and subsequent activation of a downstream protein important for cell growth, mTOR, which serves as a molecular sensor that regulates protein synthesis. Because of this data, trials are currently underway looking at single-agent and combination therapy targeted at this pathway. It will be important for us to continue to understand both the negative and positive results of any future trials aimed at this pathway. Critical to this study is the inclusion of pharmacodynamic measures to optimize the dose of the study drug based on changes in S6kinase in lymphocytes, and based on the observation that increase in signaling through mTOR increases HIFalpha and in turn angiogenesis, we are monitoring patients with serial FDG PET scans under the hypothesis that decreases in HIFalpha will decrease GLUT1 and in turn decrease FDG accumulation in tumor. Direct tumor biopsies will also be obtained to further characterize this axis.

CONCLUSION

Despite the commonly used descriptors "hormone refractory" or "androgen independent," it is likely that prostate cancer remains dependent upon the hormonal milieu of its environment and the actions of the androgen receptor on targets of cell growth and proliferation. As our knowledge of the androgen receptor and parallel pathways that affect it grows, so will our therapeutic armamentarium. It is crucial to encourage our patients to enroll in clinical trials and for us to critically evaluate both positive and negative results from these trials. A continued interaction between the bench, the bedside, and back again will be essential for the advancement of treatment for these patients.

ACKNOWLEDGMENTS

Support: WT (National Health and Medical Research Council of Australia ID#299048); GB (United States Department of Defense W81XWH-04-1-0017); MS: MSKCC SPORE in prostate cancer.

References

1. Huggins C, Hodges CV. Studies on prostatic cancer I. The effect of castration, of estrogen and of androgen injection on serum phosphatases in metastatic carcinoma of the prostate. *Cancer Res* 1941;1:193–197.
2. Scher HI, Heller G. Clinical states in prostate cancer: towards a dynamic model of disease progression. *Urology* 2000;55:323–327.
3. Kelly WK, Scher HI. Prostate specific antigen decline after antiandrogen withdrawal: the flutamide withdrawal syndrome. *J Urol* 1993;149:607–609.

4. Wirth MP, Froschermaier SE. The antiandrogen withdrawal syndrome. *Urol Res* 1997;25(Suppl. 2):S67–S71.

5. Small EJ, Baron AD, Fippin L, et al. Ketoconazole retains activity in advanced prostate cancer patients with progression despite flutamide withdrawal. *J Urol* 1997;157:1204–1207.

6. Scher HI, Buchanan G, Gerald W, et al. Targeting the androgen receptor: improving outcomes for castration-resistant prostate cancer. *Endocr Relat Cancer* 2004;11:459–476.

7. Buchanan G, Irvine RA, Coetzee GA, et al. Contribution of the androgen receptor to prostate cancer predisposition and progression. *Cancer Metastasis Rev* 2001;20:207–223.

8. Buchanan G, Greenberg NM, Scher HI, et al. Collocation of androgen receptor gene mutations in prostate cancer. *Clin Cancer Res* 2001;7:1273–1281.

9. Brinkmann AO, Jenster G, Kuiper GGJM, et al. The human androgen receptor: structure/function relationship in normal and pathological situations. *J Steroid Biochem Mol Biol* 1992;41:361.

10. Taylor CD, Elson P, Trump DL. Importance of continued testicular suppression in hormone-refractory prostate cancer. *J Clin Oncol* 1993;11:2167–2172.

11. Tilley WD, Buchanan G, Coetzee GA. Androgen receptor signaling in prostate cancer. In: Henderson BE, Ponder BA, Ross RK, eds. *Hormones, genes and cancer.* New York: Oxford University Press, 2003:288–315.

12. Feldman BJ, Feldman D. The development of androgen independent prostate cancer. *Nature Rev Cancer* 2001;1:34–45.

13. Gregory CW, Hamil KG, Kim D, et al. Androgen receptor expression in androgen-independent prostate cancer is associated with increased expression of androgen-regulated genes. *Cancer Res* 1998;58:5718–5724.

14. Presnell SC, Werdin ES, Maygarden S, et al. Establishment of short-term primary human prostate xenografts for the study of prostate biology and cancer. *Am J Pathol* 2001;159:855–860.

15. Chen CD, Welsbie DS, Tran C, et al. Molecular determinants of resistance to antiandrogen therapy. *Nat Med* 2004;10:33–39.

16. Sirotnak FM, She Y, Khokhar NZ, et al. Microarray analysis of prostate cancer progression to reduced androgen dependence: studies in unique models contrasts early and late molecular events. *Mol Carcinog* 2004;41:150–163.

17. Henshall SM, Quinn DI, Lee CS, et al. Altered expression of androgen receptor in the malignant epithelium and adjacent stroma is associated with early relapse in prostate cancer. *Cancer Res* 2001;61:423–427.

18. Ricciardelli C, Choong CS, Buchanan G, et al. Androgen receptor levels in prostate cancer epithelial and peritumoral stromal cells identify non-organ confined disease. *Prostate* 2005;63:19–28.

19. Koivisto P, Kononen J, Palmberg C, et al. Androgen receptor gene amplification: a possible molecular mechanism for androgen deprivation failure in prostate cancer. *Cancer Res* 1997;57:314–319.

20. Bubendorf L, Kononen J, Koivisto P, et al. Survey of gene amplifications during prostate cancer progression by high-throughout fluorescence in situ hybridization on tissue microarrays. *Cancer Res* 1999;59:803–806.

21. Koivisto PA, Helin HJ. Androgen receptor gene amplification increases tissue PSA protein expression in hormone-refractory prostate carcinoma. *J Pathol* 1999;189:219–223.

22. Holzbeierlein J, Lal P, LaTulippe E, et al. Gene expression analysis of human prostate carcinoma during hormonal therapy identifies androgen-responsive genes and mechanisms of therapy resistance. *Am J Pathol* 2004;164:217–227.

23. Gregory CW, Johnson RT, Mohler JL, et al. Androgen receptor stabilization in recurrent prostate cancer is associated with hypersensitivity to low androgen. *Cancer Res* 2001;61:2892–2898.

24. Lin HK, Wang L, Hu YC, et al. Phosphorylation-dependent ubiquitylation and degradation of androgen receptor by AKT require Mdm2 E3 ligase. *EMBO J* 2002;21:4037–4048.

25. Mellinghoff IK, Vivanco I, Kwon A, et al. HER2/neu kinase-dependent modulation of androgen receptor function through effects on DNA binding and stability. *Cancer Cell* 2004;6:517–527.

26. Gaughan L, Logan IR, Neal DE, et al. Regulation of androgen receptor and histone deacetylase 1 by Mdm2-mediated ubiquitylation. *Nucleic Acids Res* 2005;33:13–26.

27. Hara T, Nakamura K, Araki H, et al. Enhanced androgen receptor signaling correlates with the androgen-refractory growth in a newly established MDA PCa 2b-hr human prostate cancer cell subline. *Cancer Res* 2003;63:5622–5628.

28. Mohler JL, Gregory CW, Ford OH III, et al. The androgen axis in recurrent prostate cancer. *Clin Cancer Res* 2004;10:440–448.

29. Hryb DJ, Nakhla AM, Kahn SM, et al. Sex hormone-binding globulin in the human prostate is locally synthesized and may act as an autocrine/paracrine effector. *J Biol Chem* 2002;277:26618–26622.

30. Scher HI, Eisenberger M, D'Amico AV, et al. Eligibility and outcomes reporting guidelines for clinical trials for patients in the state of a rising PSA: recommendations from the Prostate-Specific Antigen Working Group. *J Clin Oncol* 2004;22:537–556.

31. Buchanan G, Yang M, Nahm SJ, et al. Mutations at the boundary of the hinge and ligand binding domain of the androgen receptor confer increased transactivation function. *Mol Endocrinol* 2000;15:46–56.

32. Fenton MA, Shuster TD, Fertig AM, et al. Functional characterization of mutant androgen receptors from androgen-independent prostate cancer. *Clin Cancer Res* 1997;8:1383–1388.

33. Taplin ME, Bubley GJ, Ko YJ, et al. Selection for androgen receptor mutations in prostate cancers treated with androgen antagonist. *Cancer Res* 1999;59:2511–2515.

34. Joyce R, Fenton MA, Rode P, et al. High dose bicalutamide for androgen independent prostate cancer: effect of prior hormonal therapy. *J Urol* 1998;159:149–153.

35. Kassouf W, Tanguay S, Aprikian AG. Nilutamide as second line hormone therapy for prostate cancer after androgen ablation fails. *J Urol* 2003;169:1742–1744.

36. Nieh PT. Withdrawal phenomenon with the antiandrogen Casodex. *J Urol* 1995;153:1070–1072.

37. Akakura K, Akimoto S, Furuya Y, et al. Incidence and characteristics of antiandrogen withdrawal syndrome in prostate cancer after treatment with chlormadinone acetate. *Eur Urol* 1998;33:567–571.

38. Hara T, Miyazaki J, Araki H, et al. Novel mutations of androgen receptor: a possible mechanism of bicalutamide withdrawal syndrome. *Cancer Res* 2003;63:149–153.

39. Greenberg NM, DeMayo F, Finegold MJ, et al. Prostate cancer in a transgenic mouse. *Proc Natl Acad Sci U S A* 1995;92:3459–3443.

40. Gingrich JR, Barrios RJ, Kattan MW, et al. Androgen-independent prostate cancer progression in the TRAMP model. *Cancer Res* 1997;57:4687–4691.

41. Han G, Foster BA, Mistry S, et al. Hormone status selects for spontaneous somatic androgen receptor variants that demonstrate specific ligand and cofactor dependent activities in autochthonous prostate cancer. *J Biol Chem* 2001;276:11204–11213.

42. Han G, Buchanan G, Ittmann M, et al. Mutation of the androgen receptor causes oncogenic transformation of the prostate. *Proc Natl Acad Sci U S A* 2005;102:1151–1156.

43. Buchanan G, Yang M, Cheong A, et al. Structural and functional consequences of glutamine tract variation in the androgen receptor. *Hum Mol Genet* 2004;13:1677–1692.

44. Taplin ME, Rajeshkumar B, Halabi S, et al. Androgen receptor mutations in androgen-independent prostate cancer: Cancer and Leukemia Group B Study 9663. *J Clin Oncol* 2003;21:2673–2678.

45. Culig Z, Hoffmann J, Erdel M, et al. Switch from antagonist to agonist of the androgen receptor bicalutamide is associated with prostate tumour progression in a new model system. *Br J Cancer* 1999;81:242–251.

46. Fujimoto N, Yeh S, Kang HY, et al. Cloning and characterization of androgen receptor coactivator, ARA55, in human prostate. *J Biol Chem* 1999;274:8316–8321.

47. Debes JD, Tindall DJ. The role of androgens and the androgen receptor in prostate cancer. *Cancer Lett* 2002;187:1–7.

48. Debes JD, Sebo TJ, Lohse CM, et al. p300 in prostate cancer proliferation and progression. *Cancer Res* 2003;63:7638–7640.

49. Ngan ES, Hashimoto Y, Ma ZQ, et al. Overexpression of Cdc25B, an androgen receptor coactivator, in prostate cancer. *Oncogene* 2003;22:734–739.

50. Yeh S, Miyamoto H, Shima H, et al. From estrogen to androgen receptor: a new pathway for sex hormones in prostate. *Proc Natl Acad Sci U S A* 1998;95:5527–5532.

51. Yeh S, Kang HY, Miyamoto H, et al. Differential induction of androgen receptor transactivation by different androgen receptor coactivators in human prostate cancer DU145 cells. *Endocrine* 1999;11:195–202.

52. He B, Bowen NT, Minges JT, et al. Androgen-induced NH2- and COOH-terminal interaction inhibits p160 coactivator recruitment by activation function 2. *J Biol Chem* 2001;276:42293–42301.

53. Gregory CW, He B, Johnson RT, et al. A mechanism for androgen receptor-mediated prostate cancer recurrence after androgen deprivation therapy. *Cancer Res* 2001;61:4315–4319.

54. Berrevoets CA, Umar A, Trapman J, et al. Differential modulation of androgen receptor transcriptional activity by the nuclear receptor corepressor (N-CoR). *Biochem J* 2004;379:1147–1154.

55. Hodgson MC, Astapova I, Cheng S, et al. The androgen receptor recruits nuclear receptor CoRepressor (N-CoR) in the presence of mifepristone via its N and C termini revealing a novel molecular mechanism for androgen receptor antagonists. *J Biol Chem* 2005;280:6511–6519.

56. Culig Z, Hobisch A, Cronauer MV, et al. Androgen receptor activation in prostatic tumor cell lines by insulin-like growth factor-I, keratinocyte growth factor, and epidermal growth factor. *Cancer Res* 1994;54:5474–5478.

57. Nazareth LV, Weigel NL. Activation of the human androgen receptor through a protein kinase: a signaling pathway. *J Biol Chem* 1996;271:19900–19907.

58. Craft N, Shostak Y, Carey M, et al. A mechanism for hormone-independent prostate cancer through modulation of androgen receptor signaling by the HER-2/neu tyrosine kinase. *Nat Med* 1999;5:280–285.

59. Yeh S, Lin HK, Kang HY, et al. From HER2/Neu signal cascade to androgen receptor and its coactivators: a novel pathway by induction of androgen target genes through MAP kinase in prostate cancer cells. *Proc Natl Acad Sci U S A* 1999;96:5458–5463.

60. Grossmann ME, Huang H, Tindall DJ. Androgen receptor signaling in androgen-refractory prostate cancer. *J Natl Cancer Inst* 2001;93:1687–1697.

61. Ueda T, Mawji NR, Bruchovsky N, et al. Ligand-independent activation of the androgen receptor by interleukin-6 and the role of steroid receptor coactivator-1 in prostate cancer cells. *J Biol Chem* 2002;277:38087–38094.

62. Ueda T, Bruchovsky N, Sadar MD. Activation of the androgen receptor N-terminal domain by interleukin-6 via MAPK and STAT3 signal transduction pathways. *J Biol Chem* 2002;277:7076–7085.

63. Gregory CW, Fei X, Ponguta LA, et al. Epidermal growth factor increases coactivation of the androgen receptor in recurrent prostate cancer. *J Biol Chem* 2004;279:7119–7130.

64. Wen Y, Hu MC, Makino K, et al. HER-2/neu promotes androgen-independent survival and growth of prostate cancer cells through the AKT pathway. *Cancer Res* 2000;60:6841–6845.

65. Shi Y, Brands FH, Chatterjee S, et al. Her-2/neu expression in prostate cancer: high level of expression associated with exposure to hormone therapy and androgen independent disease. *J Urol* 2001;166:1514–1519.

66. Reese DM, Small EJ, Magrane G, et al. HER2 protein expression and gene amplification in androgen-independent prostate cancer. *Am J Clin Pathol* 2001;116:234–239.

67. Lara PN Jr, Meyers FJ, Gray CR, et al. HER-2/neu is overexpressed infrequently in patients with prostate carcinoma. Results from the California Cancer Consortium Screening Trial. *Cancer* 2002;94:2584–2589.

68. Lee YF, Lin WJ, Huang J, et al. Activation of mitogen-activated protein kinase pathway by the antiandrogen hydroxyflutamide in androgen receptor-negative prostate cancer cells. *Cancer Res* 2002;62:6039–6044.

69. Grenert J, Sullivan W, Fadden P, et al. The amino-terminal domain of heat shock protein (hsp90) that binds geldanamycin is an ATP/ADP switch that regulates hsp90 conformation. *J Biol Chem* 1997;272:23843–23850.

70. Prodromou C, Roe SM, O'Brien R, et al. Identification and structural characterization of the ATP/ADP-binding site in the Hsp90 molecular chaperone. *Cell* 1997;90:65–75.

71. Stebbins CE, Russo AA, Schneider C, et al. Crystal structure of an Hsp90-geldanamycin complex: targeting of a protein chaperone by an antitumor agent. *Cell* 1997;89:239–250.

72. Eder IE, Culig Z, Ramoner R, et al. Inhibition of LncaP prostate cancer cells by means of androgen receptor antisense oligonucleotides (In Process Citation). *Cancer Gene Ther* 2000;7:997–1007.

73. Caplen NJ, Taylor JP, Statham VS, et al. Rescue of polyglutamine-mediated cytotoxicity by double-stranded RNA-mediated RNA interference. *Hum Mol Genet* 2002;11:175–184.

74. Zegarra-Moro OL, Schmidt LJ, Huang H, et al. Disruption of androgen receptor function inhibits proliferation of androgen-refractory prostate cancer cells. *Cancer Res* 2002;62:1008–1013.

75. Solit DB, Zheng FF, Drobnjak M, et al. 17-Allylamino-17-demethoxygeldanamycin induces the degradation of androgen receptor and HER-2/neu and inhibits the growth of prostate cancer xenografts. *Clin Cancer Res* 2002;8:986–993.

76. Eder IE, Hoffmann J, Rogatsch H, et al. Inhibition of LNCaP prostate tumor growth in vivo by an antisense oligonucleotide directed against the human androgen receptor. *Cancer Gene Ther* 2002;9:117–125.

77. Palvimo JJ, Kallio PJ, Ikonen T, et al. Dominant negative regulation of trans-activation by the rat androgen receptor: roles of the N-terminal domain and heterodimer formation. *Mol Endocrinol* 1993;7:1399–1407.

78. Butler LM, Agus DB, Scher HI, et al. Suberoylanilide hydroxamic acid, an inhibitor of histone deacetylase, suppresses the growth of prostate cancer cells in vitro and in vivo. *Cancer Res* 2000;60:5165–5170.

79. Bramlett KS, Dits NF, Sui X, et al. Repression of androgen-regulated gene expression by dominant negative androgen receptors. *Mol Cell Endocrinol* 2001;183:19–28.

80. Marks P, Rifkind RA, Richon VM, et al. Histone deacetylases and cancer: causes and therapies. *Nat Rev Cancer* 2001;1:194–202.

81. Bianco F, Dotan Z, Kattan MW, et al. Fifteen-year cancer-specific and PSA progression-free probabilities after radical prostatectomy. *J Urol* 2004;171:926.

82. Eisenberger MA, Crawford ED, Wolf M, et al. Prognostic factors in stage D2 prostate cancer; important implications for future trials: results of a cooperative intergroup study (INT 0036). *Semin Oncol* 1994;21:613–619.

83. Soloway MS, Ishikawa S, van der Zwaag R, et al. Prognostic factors in patients with advanced prostate cancer. *Urology* 1989;33:53–56.

84. D'Amico AV, Moul JW, Carroll PR, et al. Intermediate end point for prostate cancer-specific mortality following salvage hormonal therapy for prostate-specific antigen failure. *J Natl Cancer Inst* 2004;96:509–515.

85. Beekman KW, Heller G, Wilton A, et al. Defining a new threshold for PSA outcomes in untreated prostate cancer [Abstract 4587]. *Proc ASCO* 2004;23:402.

86. Morote J, Trilla E, Esquena S, et al. Nadir prostate-specific antigen best predicts the progression to androgen-independent prostate cancer. *Int J Cancer* 2004;108:877–881.

87. Stewart A, Scher H, Chen H et al. The clinical significance of a PSA nadir >0.2 to patients with a rising post-operative or post-radiation PSA treated with androgen deprivation. *Proc ASCO* 23:389s(2005).

88. Tannock IF, de Wit R, Berry WR, et al. Docetaxel plus prednisone or mitoxantrone plus prednisone for advanced prostate cancer. *N Engl J Med* 2004;351:1502–1512.

89. Petrylak DP, Tangen CM, Hussain MH, et al. Docetaxel and estramustine compared with mitoxantrone and prednisone for advanced refractory prostate cancer. *N Engl J Med* 2004;351:1513–1520.

90. Smaletz O, Scher HI, Small EJ, et al. Nomogram for overall survival of patients with progressive metastatic prostate cancer after castration. *J Clin Oncol* 2002;20:3972–3982.

91. Smaletz O, Scher HI. Outcome predictions for patients with metastatic prostate cancer. *Semin Urol Oncol* 2002;20:155–163.

92. Scher HI, Liebertz C, Kelly WK, et al. Bicalutamide for advanced prostate cancer: the natural vs. treated history of disease. *J Clin Oncol* 1997;15:2928–2938.

93. Fowler JE Jr, Whitmore WF Jr. The response of metastatic adenocarcinoma of the prostate to exogenous testosterone. *J Urol* 1981;126:372–375.

94. Manni A, Santen RJ, Boucher AE, et al. Androgen depletion and repletion as a means of potentiating the effect of cytotoxic chemotherapy in advanced prostate cancer. *J Steroid Biochem* 1987;27:551–556.

95. Koivisto P, Kononen J, Palmberg C, et al. Androgen receptor gene amplification: a possible molecular mechnaism for androgen deprivation therapy failure in prostate cancer. *Cancer Res* 1997;57:314–319.

96. Scher HI, Kolvenbag GJ. The antiandrogen withdrawal syndrome in relapsed prostate cancer. *Eur Urol* 1997;31(Suppl. 2):3–7; discussion 7–24.

97. Scher HI, Kelly WK. The flutamide withdrawal syndrome: its impact on clinical trials in hormone-refractory prostatic cancer. *J Clin Oncol* 1993;11:1566–1572.

98. Scher H, Kelly WK, Cohen L, et al. Flutamide withdrawal response in patients with metastatic prostate cancer (PC) progressing on hormonal therapy. *Proc Am Soc Clin Oncol* 1993;12:723.

99. Kelly WK, Slovin S, Scher HI. Steroid hormone withdrawal syndromes: pathophysiology and clinical significance. *Urol Clin North Am* 1997;24:421–433.

100. Small EJ, Carroll PR. Prostate-specific antigen decline after Casodex withdrawal: evidence for an antiandrogen withdrawal sydrome. *Cancer* 1995;43:408–410.

101. Small EJ, Srinivas S. The antiandrogen withdrawal syndrome: experience in a large cohort of unselected patients with advanced prostate cancer. *Cancer* 1995;76:1428–1434.

102. Huan SD, Gerridzen RG, Yau JC, et al. Antiandrogen withdrawal syndrome with nilutamide. *Urology* 1997;49:632–634.

103. Bissada NK, Kaczmarek AT. Complete remission of hormone refractory adenocarcinoma of the prostate in response to withdrawal of diethylstilbesterol. *J Urol* 1995;153:1944–1945.

104. Kelly WK. Endocrine withdrawal syndrome and its relevance to the managment of hormone refractory prostate cancer. *Eur Urol* 1998;34(Suppl. 3):18–23.

105. Schellhammer PF, Sharifi R, Block N, et al. A controlled trial of bicalutamide versus flutamide, each in combination with luteinizing hormone-releasing hormone analogue therapy, in patients with advanced prostate cancer. *Urology* 1995;45:745–752.

106. Bubley GJ, Carducci M, Dahut W, et al. Eligibility and response guidelines for phase II clinical trials in androgen-independent prostate cancer: recommendations from the PSA Working Group. *J Clin Oncol* 1999;17:3461–3467.

107. Labrie F, Dupont A, Giguere M, et al. Benefits of combination therapy with flutamide in patients relapsing after castration. *Br J Urol* 1988;61: 341–346.

108. Fossa SD, Slee PH, Brausi M, et al. Flutamide versus prednisone in patients with prostate cancer symptomatically progressing after androgen-ablative therapy: a phase iii study of the European Organization for Research and Treatment of Cancer Genitourinary Group. *J Clin Oncol* 2001; 19:62–71.

109. Kojima S, Suzuki H, Akakura K, et al. Alternative antiandrogens to treat prostate cancer relapse after initial hormone therapy. *J Urol* 2004;171:679–683.

110. Schellhammer PF, Sharifi R, Block NL, et al. A controlled trial of bicalutamide versus flutamide, each in combination with luteinizing hormone-releasing hormone analogue therapy, in patients with advanced prostate carcinoma. *Cancer* 1996;78:2164–2169.

111. Schasfoort EM, Van De Beek C, Newling DW. Safety and efficacy of a non-steroidal anti-androgen, based on results of a post marketing surveillance of nilutamide. *Prostate Cancer Prostatic Dis* 2001;4:112–117.

112. Desai A, Stadler WM, Vogelzang NJ. Nilutamide: possible utility as a second-line hormonal agent. *Urology* 2001;58:1016–1020.

113. Smith DC, Dunn RL, Strawderman MS, et al. Change in serum prostate-specific antigen as a marker of response to cytotoxic therapy for hormone-refractory prostate cancer. *J Clin Oncol* 1998;16:1835–1843.

114. Oh WK, Kantoff PW, Weinberg V, et al. Prospective, multicenter, randomized phase II trial of the herbal supplement, PC-SPES, and diethylstilbestrol in patients with androgen-independent prostate cancer. *J Clin Oncol* 2004;22:3705–3712.

115. Tannock I, Gospodarowicz M, Meakin W, et al. Treatment of metastatic prostatic cancer with low-dose prednisone: evaluation of pain and quality of life as pragmatic indices of response. *J Clin Oncol* 1989;7:590–597.

116. Kantoff PW, Halabi S, Conaway M, et al. Hydrocortisone with or without mitoxantrone in men with hormone-refractory prostate cancer: results of the Cancer and Leukemia Group B 9182 study. *J Clin Oncol* 1999;18:2506–2513.

117. Myers CE, Stein C, LaRocca R, et al. Suramin: an antagonist of heparin-binding tumor growth factors with activity against a broad spectrum of human tumors. *Proc Am Soc Clin Oncol* 1989;8:66.

118. Kobayashi K, Vokes EE, Janisch L, et al. Suramin (SUR) is safe and active in prostate cancer without adaptive control: evidence for a dose-response. *Proc Am Soc Clin Oncol* 1994;13:140.

119. Eisenberger MA, Reyno LM, Jodrell DI, et al. Suramin, an active drug for prostate cancer: interim observations in a phase I trial. *J Natl Cancer Inst* 1993;85:611–621.

120. Small EJ, Meyer M, Marshall ME, et al. Suramin therapy for patients with symptomatic hormone-refractory prostate cancer: results of a randomized phase III trial comparing suramin plus hydrocortisone to placebo plus hydrocortisone. *J Clin Oncol* 2000;18:1440–1450.

121. Pont A, Williams PL, Loose DS, et al. Ketoconazole blocks adrenal steroid synthesis. *Ann Intern Med* 1982;97:370–372.

122. Trachtenberg J, Pont A. Ketoconazole therapy for advanced prostate cancer. *Lancet* 1984;2:433–435.

123. Small EJ, Halabi S, Dawson NA, et al. Antiandrogen withdrawal alone or in combination with ketoconazole in androgen-independent prostate cancer patients: a phase III trial (CALGB 9583). *J Clin Oncol* 2004;22:1025–1033.

124. Small EJ, Baron A, Apodaca D. Simultaneous anti-androgen withdrawal (AAWD) and treatment with ketoconazole (KETO)/hydrocortisone (HD) in patients with advanced "hormone-refractory" prostate cancer (HRPC). *Proc Am Soc Clin Oncol* 1997;16:313a.

125. Solit DB, Scher HI, Rosen N. Hsp90 as a therapeutic target in prostate cancer. *Semin Oncol* 2003;30:709–716.

126. Gore SD, Carducci MA. Modifying histones to tame cancer: clinical development of sodium phenylbutyrate and other histone deacetylase inhibitors. *Expert Opin Investig Drugs* 2000;9:2923–2934.

127. Carducci MA, Gilbert J, Bowling MK, et al. A phase I clinical and pharmacological evaluation of sodium phenylbutyrate on a 120-h infusion schedule. *Clin Cancer Res* 2001;7:3047–3055.

128. Kelly WK, Richon VM, O'Connor O, et al. Phase I clinical trial of histone deactylase inhibitor: suberylanilide hydroxamic acid (SAHA) administered intravenously. *Clin Cancer Res* 2003;9:3578–3588.

129. Scher HI, Sarkis A, Reuter V, et al. Changing pattern of expression of the epidermal growth factor receptor and transforming growth factor-a in the progression of prostatic neoplams. *Clin Cancer Res* 1995;1:545–550.

130. Prewett M, Rockwell P, Rockwell RF, et al. The biologic effects of C225, a chimeric monoclonal antibody to the EGFR, on human prostate carcinoma. *J Immunother Emphasis Tumor Immunol* 1996;19:419–427.

131. Agus DB, Scher HI, Higgins B, et al. Response of prostate cancer to anti-her2/neu antibody in androgen-dependent and -independent human xenograft models. *Clin Cancer Res* 1999;59:4761–4764.

132. Morris MJ, Reuter VE, Kelly WK, et al. HER-2 profiling and targeting in prostate carcinoma. *Cancer* 2002;94:980–986.

133. Lara PN Jr, Chee KG, Longmate J, et al. Trastuzumab plus docetaxel in HER-2/neu-positive prostate carcinoma: final results from the California Cancer Consortium Screening and Phase II Trial. *Cancer* 2004;100:2125–2131.

134. Ahonen MH, Tenkanen L, Teppo L, et al. Prostate cancer risk and predi agnostic serum 25-hydroxyvitamin D levels (Finland). *Cancer Causes Control* 2000;11:847–852.

135. Osborn JL, Schwartz GG, Smith DC, et al. Phase II trial of oral 1,25-dihydroxyvitamin D (calcitriol) in hormone refractory prostate cancer. *Urol Oncol* 1995;1:195 198.

136. Smith DC, Johnson CS, Freeman CC, et al. A phase I trial of calcitriol (1,25 dihydroxycholecalciferol) in patients with advanced malignancy. *Clin Cancer Res* 1999;5:1339–1345.

137. Morris MJ, Smaletz O, Solit D, et al. High-dose calcitriol, zoledronate, and dexamethasone for the treatment of progressive prostate carcinoma. *Cancer* 2004;100:1868–1875.

138. Hideshima T, Richardson P, Chauhan D, et al. The proteasome inhibitor PS-341 inhibits growth, induces apoptosis, and overcomes drug resistance in human multiple myeloma cells. *Cancer Res* 2001;61:3071–3076.

139. Palombella VJ, Rando OJ, Goldberg AL, et al. The ubiquitin-proteasome pathway is required for processing the NF-kappa B1 precursor protein and the activation of NF-kappa B. *Cell* 1994;78:773–785.

140. Papandreou CN, Daliani DD, Nix D, et al. Phase I trial of the proteasome inhibitor bortezomib in patients with advanced solid tumors with observations in androgen-independent prostate cancer. *J Clin Oncol* 2004;22:2108–2121.

141. Morris MS, Beckman KW, Kelly WIC et al., Phase II study of bortezamib for castrate metastatic prostate cancer (A), *Proc ASCO* 23(165):Abstract 4633:2005.

142. Nelson JB, Hedican SP, George DJ, et al. Identification of endothelin-1 in the pathophysiology of metastatic adenocarcinoma of the prostate. *Nat Med* 1995;1:944–949.

143. Carducci MA, Nelson JB, Bowling MK, et al. Atrasentan, an endothelin-receptor antagonist for refractory adenocarcinomas: safety and pharmacokinetics. *J Clin Oncol* 2002;20:2171–2180.

144. Carducci MA, Padley RJ, Breul J, et al., Effect of endothelin-A receptor blockade with Atrasentan on tumor progression in men with hormone-refractory prostate cancer: a randomized, phase II, placebo-controlled trial. *J Clin Oncol* 2003;21:679–689.

145. Carducci MA, Padley RJ, Breul J, et al. Effect of endothelin-a receptor blockade with Atrasentan on tumor progression in men with hormone-refractory prostate cancer: a randomized, phase II, placebo-controlled trial. *J Clin Oncol* 2003;21:679–689.

146. Carducci M, Nelson BJ, Saad F, et al. Effects of Atrasentan on disease progression and biological markers in men with metastatic hormone-refractory prostate cancer: phase 3 study Abstract 4058. *Proc Am Soc Clin Oncol* 2004;23:383.

147. Sirotnak FM, She Y, Lee F, et al. Studies with CWR22 xenografts in nude mice suggest that ZD1839 may have a role in the treatment of both androgen-dependent and androgen-independent human prostate cancer. *Clin Cancer Res* 2002;8:3870–3876.

148. Rosenthal M, Toner GC, Gurney H, et al. Inhibition of the epidermal growth factor receptor (EGFR) in hormone refractory prostate cancer (HRPC): initial results of a phase II trial of gefitinib. *Proc ASCO* 2003;22:416. [Abstract #1671]

149. She QB, Solit D, Basso A, et al. Resistance to gefitinib in PTEN-null HER-overexpressing tumor cells can be overcome through restoration of PTEN function or pharmacologic modulation of constitutive phosphatidylinositol 3'-kinase/AKT pathway signaling. *Clin Cancer Res* 2003;9:4340–4346.

150. Bianco R, Shin I, Ritter CA, et al. Loss of PTEN/MMAC1/TEP in EGF receptor-expressing tumor cells counteracts the antitumor action of EGFR tyrosine kinase inhibitors. *Oncogene* 2003;22:2812–2822.

CHAPTER 16C
Management of Hormone Refractory Prostate Cancer

Miah-Hiang Tay, Mari Nakabayashi, and William K. Oh

INTRODUCTION

Although androgen-deprivation therapy remains the most effective treatment for metastatic prostate cancer, the majority of patients demonstrate evidence of progressive disease after a median duration of 18 to 24 months. Upon disease progression, further secondary hormonal manipulation may lead to additional cancer control, but generally for a shorter duration before the tumor eventually becomes truly refractory to further hormonal manipulation. The median survival of men with hormone refractory prostate cancer (HRPC) has historically been approximately 1 year (1). As therapies for HRPC have not until recently been associated with a survival benefit, the general aim of treatment of HRPC has included palliation of symptoms, if possible by slowing the progression of disease. Previously, such goals were achieved with conservative medical care, since chemotherapy was considered to be relatively ineffective in HRPC until only the recent past (2,3). Such perceptions of the role of chemotherapy are now shifting, as emerging data support the fact that prostate cancer is a chemosensitive disease. Furthermore, newer systemic therapies are exploiting a growing understanding of the biology of HRPC and are targeted against putative pathways of cancer growth in this stage of disease.

Prostate-specific antigen (PSA) has become a primary tool for measuring the disease burden and response to therapy for prostate cancer, including in the patient with HRPC (4). Although its use as a surrogate marker of response is controversial, changes in serum level of PSA have correlated with both objective disease responses and survival (5–11). The first report of this phenomenon by Kelly et al. (12) demonstrated that median survival was nearly twice as long for men with HRPC who experienced a decline in PSA in excess of 50% at 8 weeks after treatment compared to those with a lesser or no decline (23.6 months vs. 12.5 months). This finding has been confirmed by others (5,9,13). In 1999, the Prostate-Specific Antigen Working Group suggested uniform guidelines for reporting PSA changes in phase II studies, specifically a decrease of 50% or more from the baseline PSA, occurring in the absence of clinical or radiographic evidence of disease progression, and confirmed with another measurement 4 weeks later (14). Also, patient quality of life (QOL) measurements and pain scales represent recognized and validated parameters that can determine the efficacy of treatment in patients with symptomatic

HRPC. In fact, the approval of mitoxantrone for the management of HRPC (5,6) by the U.S. Food and Drug Administration (FDA) was based primarily on its beneficial impact on pain and QOL measures (15,16).

This chapter will review the efficacy of cytotoxic chemotherapy, supportive therapies, and promising new systemic treatments in the management of HRPC.

CYTOTOXIC CHEMOTHERAPY

First-generation Drugs and Combinations

The earliest trials from the 1970s to 1980s demonstrated, at best, objective response rates with traditional chemotherapeutic drugs in the range of 10% to 20%, without any evidence of an improvement in overall survival. In part, this was due to the ineffectiveness of the drugs themselves, but also because of difficulty in defining objective responses in a disease such as metastatic prostate cancer, which is dominated by bony involvement. In the era prior to the availability of PSA as a serum marker of drug efficacy, two comprehensive reviews of clinical trials performed in the 1980s and early 1990s confirmed the poor activity of most chemotherapy agents in advanced prostate cancer. In 1985, Eisenberger et al. reported a total response rate of 4.5% in a review of 17 studies, and in 1993 Yagoda and Petrylak reported only a slightly higher response rate of 8.7% in a review of 26 trials. There was no evidence for a survival benefit with any agent (2,17).

Over the past decade, many additional cytotoxic drugs have been investigated. In recent clinical trials, the following chemotherapy drugs have been investigated and show minimal to no activity in HRPC: melphalan (18), ifosfamide (19), temozolamide (20), etoposide (21), idarubicin (22), gemcitabine (23), irinotecan (24), trimetrexate (25), floxuridine (26), and 5-fluorouracil (27). Most of these studies reported overall response rates less than 10%, using either PSA and/or measurable endpoints. Phase II studies of other cytotoxic agents, including cyclophosphamide, doxorubicin, and platinum-based agents, have shown modest improvements in activity. For instance, objective response rates of 30% were reported with single-agent oral cyclophosphamide (28). These response rates are improved when cyclophosphamide is combined with other drugs including doxorubicin, etoposide, estramustine, and vincristine (11,29–31) (Table 16C.1). As single agents, doxorubicin and epirubicin also appear to have some activity. For instance, in two small studies of single-agent doxorubicin, objective response rates were 5% and 33%, respectively (32,33). PSA response rates of 20% to 30% were seen in three studies of epirubicin (34–36). In addition, various combination studies have included doxorubicin, though results have been disappointing. In one phase III trial from the "prePSA" era, the overall objective response rate with the combination of cyclophosphamide, doxorubicin, and methotrexate was only 6%, compared to a 2% with cyclophosphamide alone and no difference in overall survival (37).

The first important contemporary milestone for cytotoxic chemotherapy in the management of HRPC was achieved in 1996 with a Canadian multi-institutional phase III trial restricted to symptomatic HRPC patients (6). In this trial, 161 men with symptomatic HRPC were randomized to either mitoxantrone (12 mg/m^2) given every 3 weeks plus prednisone 10 mg daily versus prednisone alone (Table 16C.2). The primary endpoint of the trial was a palliative response as indicated by at least a 2-point reduction in pain, assessed by a 6-point validated pain questionnaire. Secondary endpoints included a 50% reduction in the total amount of pain medication without an increase in pain, duration of response, and survival. QOL was also evaluated. Although no survival benefit was found, there was a significant decrease in pain (29% vs. 12%) as well as a significant prolongation in the duration of pain relief (43 weeks vs. 18 weeks) in the chemotherapy arm. Palliation was also significantly more likely in men with a PSA response than without (50% vs. 29%). Toxicity was primarily

---

TABLE 16C.1

NONTAXANE COMBINATION CHEMOTHERAPY IN HRPC

Chemotherapy	No.	≥50% PSA response (%)	Measurable response (%)	References (first author)
Doxorubicin + cyclophosphamide	35	16/35(46)	5/15(33)	Small (11)
Doxorubicin + ketoconazole	39	21/38(55)	7/12(58)	Sella (38)
Epirubicin + 5-FU + cisplatin	24	8/20(40)	3/8(38)	Chao (39)
Cyclophosphamide + etoposide	20	2/8(25)	7/20(35)	Maulard-Durdux (29)
Estramustine + vinblastine	25	13/24(54)	2/5(40)	Seidman (40)
	36	22/36(61)	1/7(14)	Hudes (41)
	22	(50)	(43)	Amato (42)
KAVE	46	12/16(75)	31/46(67)	Ellerhorst (43)
Estramustine + etoposide	62	24/62(39)	8/15(53)	Pienta (44)
Estramustine + doxorubicin	31	18/31(58)	5/11(45)	Culine (45)
Estramustine + etoposide + vinorelbine	25	11/22(56)	2/3(67)	Colleoni (46)

KAVE: doxorubicin and ketoconazole alternating with vinblastine + estramustine.

TABLE 16C.2

LANDMARK PHASE III CHEMOTHERAPY TRIALS IN HRPC

Treatment arms	No.	≥50% PSA response (%)	Measurable response (%)	Clinical response (%)	Overall Survival (mo)	Progression free survival (mo)	References (first author)
Mitoxantrone + prednisone vs. prednisone	80	NR	NR	29	NR	43 (wk)	Tannock (6)
				P = .01		P <.0001	
	81			12		18 (wk)	
Mitoxantrone + hydrocortisone vs. hydrocortisone	119	33	7		12.3	3.7	Kantoff (5)
		P = .008		–4.34[a]		P = .25	
	123	22	4		12.6	2.3	
Docetaxel + estramustine q3 wk vs. mitoxantrone + prednisone	386	50	17		18	6	Petrylak (47)
		P <.0001	P = .15	NR	P = .01	P <.0001	
	384	27	11		16	3	
Docetaxel + prednisone q3 wk vs. docetaxel weekly + prednisone vs. mitoxantrone + prednisone	335	45	12	22	18.9	NR	Eisenberger (48)
		[b]P = .0005	[b]P = .1	[b]P = .009	[b]P = .009		
	334	48	8	23	17.3		
		[b]P <.0001	[b]P = .5	[b]P = .005	[b]P = .3		
	337	32	7	13	16.4		

NR, not received.

[a]Quality of life coefficient indicator of treatment effect: 1 for mitoxantrone + hydrocortisone, 0 for hydrocortisone. Negative values favor mitoxantrone and hydrocortisone; positive values are in favor of the hydrocortisone-only group.

[b](vs. mitoxantrone).

hematologic with a 45% event rate of grade-3 or grade-4 toxicity in all treatment courses, though only 1% developed neutropenic fever. In addition, cardiac toxicity was rare and occurred predominantly with cumulative doses greater than 100 mg/m^2. The Cancer and Leukemia Group B (CALGB) reported in 1999 a comparable phase III trial of 242 men with HRPC randomized to mitoxantrone (14 mg/m^2) every 3 weeks plus hydrocortisone 40 mg daily versus hydrocortisone alone (5) (Table 16C.2). This study included both symptomatic and asymptomatic patients, with a primary endpoint of overall survival. Secondary endpoints included time to disease progression, time to treatment failure, objective and PSA response rates, and QOL. As in the Canadian study, median survival durations were similar between the two arms (12.3 months vs. 12.6 months) though time to disease progression and time to treatment failure each favored the combination arm (3.7 months vs. 2.3 months, $P = .25$). In a post-hoc analysis, patients in the combination arm who had a 50% or greater reduction in PSA had a longer median survival duration than those who did not (20 months vs. 10 months). Based on these two randomized studies, mitoxantrone was approved for the palliative treatment of HRPC.

Second-generation Drugs and Combinations

Estramustine phosphate consists of estradiol attached to a nitrogen mustard moiety (49). Although it was first thought that the cytotoxic effect was mediated through an alkylating effect following facilitation of uptake by the estradiol component, it was later determined that the binding of the estramustine and its metabolites to microtubule-associated proteins accounted for its antineoplastic activity. In addition, this mechanism appeared distinct from other antimicrotubule agents such as the vinca alkaloids and taxanes, which bind to the spindles themselves (50). As a single agent, estramustine has variable but generally modest levels of reported activity in HRPC, with objective response rates of 14% to 48% and subjective improvements in pain and performance status (51,52). However, in therapeutic doses, estramustine significantly increases the risk of serious thromboembolic events, with incidence rates of 10% to 20% reported in various trials. Although prophylactic anticoagulation with warfarin or aspirin has been proposed to reduce this toxicity, anticoagulation has not been proven to be effective (53,54).

In vitro studies suggested a synergistic effect when estramustine was combined with other antimicrotubule-directed agents (55–57). When this hypothesis was tested in clinical trials, promising activity was seen (Table 16C.1). For instance, the combination of estramustine and vinblastine yielded a mean PSA response of 42% and objective response of 31% in three phase II studies and one phase III trial (40–42,58). However, in none of these trials did patients experience a median survival greater than 12 months. In the phase III trial, Hudes et al. compared the combination of estramustine and vinblastine to vinblastine alone (58). In this study, the combination of estramustine (600 mg/m^2 on days 1–42 repeated every 8 weeks) and vinblastine (4 mg/m^2 weekly for 6 of 8 weeks) was associated with a significantly longer median survival (12.5 months vs. 9.4 months), time to progression (3.7 months vs. 2.2 months), and 50% PSA response rate (25% vs. 3%) compared with vinblastine alone. The combination of estramustine and vinorelbine also has activity in HRPC with PSA response rates ranging from 24% to 71% and objective response rates of 0% to 13% (59,60).

Although single-agent oral etoposide has minimal activity in HRPC (21), Pienta et al. showed that the combination of etoposide and estramustine had significant activity in a study of 42 patients with HRPC. In this trial, 54% of patients had ≥50% PSA decline and 50% of patients with measurable disease had an objective response (61). However, this combination was difficult to tolerate, requiring reductions in etoposide dose in 25% of the patients as a result of grade-3 or grade-4 leukopenia, five patients developing neutropenic fever, one dying from bone marrow failure, and 2 patients stopping therapy because of nausea and vomiting. Similar efficacy was noted with a lower incidence of toxicity when the duration of etoposide was reduced from 21 days to 14 days (44). Based on the promising results of estramustine and vinblastine, etoposide or vinorelbine, a triple-drug combination using estramustine, etoposide, and vinorelbine was studied by Colleoni et al. in 25 patients. Fifty-six percent of patients had a 50% or greater PSA decline and an objective response was seen in 32% (46). In addition, toxicity with this combination was more moderate, with only 12% developing grade-3 or grade-4 neutropenia, likely due to a shorter duration of etoposide.

Combinations of estramustine with epirubicin or doxorubicin have also been studied. Although significant PSA response rates of 45% to 54% and objective responses as high as 45% have been reported, both combinations demonstrated significant rates of hematologic and cardiovascular toxicity (45,62). Another chemotherapy regimen combined estramustine and vinblastine alternating weekly with doxorubixcin and ketoconazole. In a phase II trial, 31 of 46 patients (67%) had a 50% or greater decline in PSA and 12 of 16 (75%) had a measurable disease response (43). Median response duration was 8.4 months (1.8 months to 14.9 months) and the combination had moderate toxicity, including peripheral edema (49%), deep vein thrombosis (19%), and cardiac events (4%).

Third-generation Drugs and Combinations

Taxanes are among the most active chemotherapy drugs in HRPC (Table 16C.3). Though single-agent paclitaxel has been reported to have response rates using PSA endpoints ranging from only 0% to 34%, paclitaxel plus estramustine demonstrated promising synergy in a clinical trial reported by Hudes et al. (63–65). Estramustine, when combined with paclitaxel administered as a 96-hour infusion, resulted in PSA declines of ≥50% in 53% of patients and objective responses in 45%. Hematologic toxicity, nausea, vomiting, fluid retention, and fatigue were the major toxicities. In order to minimize the hematologic toxicity, later studies administered paclitaxel over shorter durations and in different schedules. For instance, weekly paclitaxel (doses ranging from 60 mg/m^2 to 150 mg/m^2) and estramustine combinations have demonstrated PSA declines of ≥50% in 42% to 62% of patients and objective response in 15% to 39% (66–69). The durations of response range from 5 to 11.5 months and median survivals extend to approximately 17 months. With 1-hour paclitaxel infusions and weekly administration, the toxicity of these regimens is significantly improved and leukopenia, thrombocytopenia, and peripheral neuropathy were not commonly noted. The extent of toxicity generally correlated with the dose of each drug. At higher doses of paclitaxel, higher rates of hematologic and neurologic toxicity were seen, and with higher doses of estramustine, an increased risk of thromboembolism and nausea was seen.

Docetaxel is a semisynthetic taxane with significant single-agent activity (70,72,81,82). Administered every 3 weeks, PSA declines of 50% or greater are seen in 46% to 50%, while weekly docetaxel monotherapy is associated with 41% to 46% rates of PSA decline. Improvements in QOL were demonstrated in a phase II study, with 47% of the patients meeting the criteria for palliative response and 37% achieving significant pain relief (70). In combination with estramustine,

TABLE 16C.3

TAXANE-BASED CHEMOTHERAPY IN HRPC

Taxane schedule	No.	≥50% PSA response (%)	Measurable response (%)	References (first author)
		Docetaxel, single agent		
Weekly	23	9/19(47)	NR	Beer (70)
	64	41/64(64)	2/12(17)	Ferrero (71)
Every 3 weeks	35	16/35(46)	7/25(28)	Picus (72)
		Docetaxel and estramustine		
Weekly	30	23/30(76)	7/12(58)	Sitka Copur (73)
Every 3 weeks	42	18/40(45)	4/20(20)	Sinibaldi (53)
	47	30/44(68)	24/46(50)	Savarese (74)
	17	14/17(82)	1/6(17)	Kreis (8)
	34	20/32(63)	5/18(28%)	Petrylak (7)
		Paclitaxel, single agent		
Every 3 weeks	23	0/23(0)	1/23(4)	Roth (63)
Weekly	18	7/18(34)	4/8(50)	Trivedi (64)
	84	21/84(25)	NR	Berry (68)
		Paclitaxel and estramustine		
Every 3 weeks	34	17/32(53)	4/9(44)	Hudes (75)
	18	9/18(50)	NR	Ferrari (66)
	24	9/24(38)	6/13(46)	Haas (76)
		Other taxane combinations		
TEC	56	36/54(67)	15/33(45)	Kelly (77)
EDC	40	23/34(68)	11/21(52)	Oh (54)
DV	21	11/19(58)	3/5(60)	Koletsky (78)
DCal	37	30/37(81)	8/15(53)	Beer (79)
DThal	36	19/36(53)	NR	Figg (80)

TEC, paclitaxel, estramustine, carboplatin; EDC, estramustine, docetaxel, carboplatin; DV, docetaxel, vinorelbine; DCal, docetaxel, high-dose calcitriol; DThal, docetaxel, thalidomide; NR, not received.

two phase I studies of docetaxel administered every 3 weeks and combined with intermittent estramustine reported PSA declines of ≥50% in 63% to 82% (8,83). Subsequent phase II studies of this combination produced similar response rates of 41% to 70% by PSA criteria and 21% to 55% by conventional measurable disease criteria (53,73,74,84). Though initial trials of this combination used long durations of estramustine, subsequent studies have decreased both the dose and duration of estramustine to minimize toxicity while continuing to exploit a possible synergy between the two drugs.

Two landmark randomized phase III studies comparing docetaxel-containing regimens to mitoxantrone were recently published (47,48) (Table 16C.2). In an intergroup study led by the Southwest Oncology Group (SWOG 9916), 770 men with HRPC were randomized to receive either docetaxel 60 mg/m^2 to 70 mg/m^2 every 3 weeks and estramustine 280 mg 3 times a day for 5 days every 21 days or mitoxantrone 12 mg/m^2 to 14 mg/m^2 plus prednisone 5 mg twice daily. Median survival was increased by 20% in the docetaxel arm (18 months vs. 16 months; $P = .01$). Also, the median duration of response (6 months vs. 3 months; $P < .0001$) and the rate of PSA declines of 50% or greater (50% vs. 27%; $P < .0061$) were significantly longer in the docetaxel arm. Objective measurable response rates, however, were similar (17% vs. 11%; $P = .15$). Although there were more adverse effects, such as pain, fatigue, metabolic disturbances, nausea, and vomiting, in the experimental arm, importantly, this did not translate into increased

toxic death or study discontinuation. In a second phase III study (TAX327), 1,006 patients were randomized to docetaxel 75 mg/m^2 every 3 weeks, docetaxel 30 mg/m^2 weekly for 5 of every 6 weeks, or mitoxantrone 12 mg/m^2. All patients also received prednisone 10 mg daily (48). At a median follow up of 20.7 months, median survival was significantly longer in the docetaxel group compared to mitoxantrone (18.3 months vs. 16.5 months; $P = .04$). In addition, PSA decline rates of ≥50% (47% vs. 32%; $P < .0001$) and pain response (33% vs. 22%; $P = .01$) were both significantly better with docetaxel compared with mitoxantrone. Based on these results, docetaxel every 3 weeks with prednisone was approved by the FDA on May 19, 2004, for the management of HRPC and has become the new standard of care for the management for this disease.

The epothilones are a new class of cytotoxic nontaxane tubulin polymerization agents obtained from the fermentation broth of the myxobacterium *Sorangium cellulosum* (85), and have shown activity in taxane-resistant cell lines (86). A multi-institutional randomized phase II trial of epothilone B analogue (BMS-247550) +/− estramustine phosphate (EMP) was conducted in 92 chemotherapy-naïve patients with progressive castrate-metastatic prostate cancer (87). BMS-247550, alone or in combination with EMP, has significant activity. The combination arm showed >50% decline in PSA in 69%, and 56% in the BMS-247550-alone arm. A higher partial response rate was observed in the combination arm compared with BMS-247550 alone (46% vs.

23%). The regimen was well tolerated but peripheral neuropathy was a prominent side effect, though manageable with longer infusion rates. Phase III studies are ongoing to determine its relative benefit in second-line therapy after taxane failure.

Remaining Questions and Conclusions

One strategy to improve the efficacy of chemotherapy is to increase the number of active agents, often on a taxane +/− estramustine "backbone." For instance, several groups have added carboplatin to the combination of estramustine and either docetaxel or paclitaxel. While these combinations are clearly active, the addition of carboplatin increases toxicity and randomized trials are needed to determine whether there is any additive or synergistic benefit (54,77,88–91). Another strategy is to combine chemotherapy with other so-called targeted systemic therapies, discussed further below.

Another goal of treatment is to continue to maximize QOL. In this regard, the role of estramustine remains unclear. Though some patients tolerate this agent with minimal toxicity, others experience nausea, thrombosis, and other unpleasant side effects. Despite efforts to reduce the dose of estramustine, the randomized trials noted above have suggested that a comparable survival benefit with a generally improved toxicity profile can be achieved by substituting prednisone for estramustine in the first-line treatment of HRPC. It is possible that estramustine may continue to play a role in second-line chemotherapy combinations and in selected clinical trials, but its primary role in combination with docetaxel is in doubt.

In summary, chemotherapeutic options for the management of HRPC have undergone significant evolution over the past decade. The concept that prostate cancer is resistant to chemotherapy—predominant in the 1980s—has been contradicted by a series of phase II and III trials that demonstrated improvements in pain control, QOL, time to disease progression, and survival in men with HRPC. The standard of care for patients with symptomatic HRPC prostate cancer now clearly includes the use of cytotoxic chemotherapy, with docetaxel every 3 weeks and daily prednisone representing the favored first-line chemotherapy regimen in patients with metastatic HRPC. Ongoing clinical trials are investigating whether the earlier use of chemotherapy (e.g., nonmetastatic HRPC, rising PSA and hormone-naïve, adjuvant and neoadjuvant) may have an enhanced effect on survival.

RADIATION THERAPY FOR HRPC

Radiopharmaceuticals

Over 80% of men with metastatic prostate cancer have radiographic evidence of bone involvement, which may lead to complications including pain, skeletal fractures, neurologic impairment, and bone marrow suppression (92). Effective palliative treatment is important in these patients to improve their quality of life. Various radiopharmaceutical drugs have demonstrated efficacy in the palliative management of pain secondary to bone metastases (93). These agents are calcium analog β-particle emitters and localize to osteoblastic metastases. There are three FDA-approved radiopharmaceuticals: strontium-89 chloride (^{89}Sr), samarium-153 lexidronam (^{153}Sm), and sodium phosphorus-32 (^{32}P). ^{32}P is rarely used for bone-pain palliation because of excessive myelosuppression. ^{153}Sm, which has the lowest beta energy emission of the three available agents, has a more favorable toxicity profile

and is an appropriate choice in patients for whom myelosuppression is a particular concern. Randomized trials have demonstrated pain response rates of 60% to 80% with single-agent radiopharmaceuticals in the palliation of bone pain, though the duration of response is generally limited to several months (93).

Little data are available on the efficacy and toxicity of radiopharmaceutical agents after the use of cytotoxic chemotherapy. One small study found that 57% of patients experienced improved pain control with a median response duration of 56 days after ^{89}Sr therapy in 14 patients with prostate cancer resistant to chemotherapy (94). Unfortunately, hematologic toxicity was significant, including transfusion-requiring anemia and prolonged thrombocytopenia. In addition, no PSA declines were noted. Another group conducted a randomized phase III trial comparing ^{89}Sr with palliative local radiation therapy (RT) in 203 patients with symptomatic metastatic prostate cancer (95). Subjective responses were seen in 35% versus 33% and PSA declines greater than 50% were observed in 10% versus 13% of ^{89}Sr and RT arms, respectively. No difference in toxicity and time to progression was noted.

In addition to their ability to relieve pain, bone-targeted radiopharmaceuticals have recently been evaluated in combination with chemotherapy (96,97). Possible synergistic effects of radiopharmaceuticals and chemotherapy on alleviating bone pain and improving bone disease progression have been compared to either radiopharmaceuticals or chemotherapy alone. A randomized phase II trial was conducted to evaluate the efficacy of bone-targeted consolidation therapy consisting of ^{89}Sr and doxorubicin given to patients with stable or responding disease after systemic induction chemotherapy (96). Of an evaluable 103 patients, median survival was 27.7 months in the ^{89}Sr-plus-doxorubicin arm compared with 16.8 months in the doxorubicin-alone arm. The hazard ratio between the two groups was 2.76 (95% CI, 1.44 to 5.29). This intriguing study implied that the combination of a radiopharmaceutical and chemotherapy might have had a sustained antitumor effect in bone that allowed for improved survival. This question is being addressed in an ongoing randomized trial.

A randomized phase III trial of 70 patients treated with low-dose cisplatin plus ^{89}Sr versus ^{89}Sr alone demonstrated that the addition of cisplatin to ^{89}Sr treatment resulted in a significant improvement in pain palliation (98). These regimens were tolerated with only mild adverse effects. Effect on survival needs to be determined by larger randomized phase III trials that are ongoing. Proper selection of patients is key for using radiopharmaceutical drugs. Patients with painful bone metastases, poor analgesic control, and adequate bone marrow function are appropriate candidates for radiopharmaceuticals, though care must be taken in relation to timing of chemotherapy use (99).

The Role of External Beam Radiation Therapy

Local-field external beam radiotherapy is extremely effective in the palliation of symptomatic bony metastases. A standard course of radiation for palliating pain from bony metastases has been a 2-week course with 10 treatments given to a total dose of 3,000 cGy, with higher doses sometimes used. Following such treatment 50% to 80% of patients experience reduction in their pain and complete pain relief is reported in 20% to 50% of patients (100). Until 5 or 10 years ago, patients with painful bony metastases had more widespread disease at the time they underwent palliative radiation than at present because of the more effective secondary hormonal manipulations used at an earlier stage as well as the use of more effective systemic cytotoxic chemotherapy regimens and better pain control management programs now. Recently randomized studies have evaluated the palliative efficacy of standard local-field radiation therapy as described above compared to a single-fraction radiation treatment (101). An RTOG phase III trial comparing whether 8 Gy in a single fraction provides equivalent pain relief to the standard dose of 30 Gy in 10 fractions has also recently been reported (102). Both pain relief and quality of life issues were evaluated by patient self-assessment inventories. Hartsell et al. concluded from this 879-patient randomized study that localized radiation therapy of either form is effective in palliating pain from bony metastases in this modern patient population with complete or partial reduction in pain seen in 66% of the patients. At 3 months of follow-up there was no reported difference in the 30 Gy in 10 fractions compared to the 8 Gy in a single fraction in terms of pain relief or in terms of reduction in narcotic requirements or in frequency of pathologic fractures. Although prior meta-analysis and reviews of comparing retrospective studies of single-fraction versus multiple-fraction palliative regimens have come to differing conclusions supporting or not the equal efficacy of single fractionation (103–105), it now seems clear that single-fraction radiation therapy should be one standard option for many clinical presentations (101,102). There are exceptions to the use of the single-fraction approach—for instance, unfavorable lesions in the long bones that require prophylactic orthopedic internal fixation prior to radiation. Internal fixation of favorable lesions will provide more and rapid pain relief. This facilitates nursing care for these patients and prevents complications which can arise from prolonged immobilization. Postoperative radiation therapy given by local field should be by the fractionated approach and will reduce the risk of further tumor growth and bone disruption (106). Other clinical presentations that may not be appropriate for single-fraction 8 Gy localized field of radiation include those lesions in areas in which adjacent normal tissue may be unduly sensitive to a high single dose of radiation such as the spinal cord, the intestines, or the lungs.

Patients who present with pain as well as spinal cord compression from their bony metastatic disease to the vertebrae, often with extra osseous extension, present a special clinical problem. Magnetic resonance imaging and a thorough neurologic examination as well as the early initiation of steroids are all essential to a favorable outcome from palliation with radiation therapy. There has been a long controversy as to whether treatment for these men does or does not require initial surgical decompression and when possible resection of epidural disease (107). If the patient at presentation with cord compression has not had hormonal therapy, then immediate androgen-deprivation and localized field-radiation is usually appropriate (108). However, as is now most commonly seen, patients with cord compression who are hormonally resistant may have better palliative benefit from decompressive surgical resection followed by radiation. A recently reported randomized trial compared surgery within 24 hours after a study entry followed by 30 Gy and 10 fractions 14 days following surgery with radiation alone with 30 Gy in 10 fractions (109). This study was limited to patients with a single site of spinal cord compression who were not totally paraplegic for more than 48 hours prior to entry. Patients with particularly radiation-sensitive tumors, including lymphoma, leukemia, and germ cell tumors, were excluded. The remainder included a significant percentage with prostate cancer but also included breast and lung cancer patients in substantial numbers. In this phase III study, 101 patients were evaluated. Immediate decompressive surgery plus postoperative radiation therapy, compared to radiation therapy alone, allowed patients to regain and maintain their ability to walk better. This study reported in this patient population that decompressive surgery works best when given as the initial treatment for

cord compression giving significantly better overall results with regard to ambulation, their status with urinary continence, and their cord function as well as fewer steroid and narcotic requirements. This phase III data would suggest that in this patient population very serious attention should be directed toward considering immediate decompressive surgery in patients who have solitary sites of spinal cord compression, who have no contraindications to surgery, and who have an expected longevity of 3 months or more.

In previous decades when there were not so many active second-line hormonally therapeutic regimens or active cytotoxic chemotherapy regimens, wide-field radiation and, in fact, hemibody radiation were often used for palliation. However, this is being used with much less frequency in order to preserve bone marrow function, allowing patients to receive newer chemotherapy regimens that in many instances (see above) have achieved very gratifying remissions and improvement in both the quality of life as well as the duration in responding patients. Finally, there has recently been data supporting the use of low dose prophylactic breast radiation to decrease the risk of antiandrogen inducing symptomatic gynecomastia and breast tenderness, which can improve patient quality of life (110).

NEW SYSTEMIC APPROACHES

New treatment approaches toward HRPC are exploiting molecular pathways that appear to be critical to the growth and survival of prostate cancer cells in the androgen-deprived environment. The most promising agents are targeting cell-signaling pathways, angiogenesis, inflammatory pathways, and the immune system (Table 16C.4).

Targeting Cell-signaling Pathways

An increased understanding of the molecular and cellular mechanisms of prostate tumorigenesis has identified new targets for therapy. The mechanism(s) by which prostate cancers become hormone refractory has not been fully elucidated to date, but it is clear that aberrant androgen receptor (AR) signaling plays a central role in HRPC. It has been postulated that prostate cancer represents a heterogeneous mixture of cells that vary in their dependence on androgen for growth and survival. It has been hypothesized that treatment with androgen deprivation and/or antiandrogen therapy provides selective pressure and may increase the number of cells which are androgen-independent (111). *In vitro* studies indicate that in the castrate state, AR adapts by mutation, amplification, and modulation of coregulatory proteins to become "superactive" in the face of the low amounts of testosterone and dihydrotestosterone in androgen-independent prostate cancer (112–117). Recently, Chen et al. have presented one possible mechanism of resistance to antiandrogen therapy by using prostate cancer xenograft models (118). In their model, the only change consistently associated with the development of resistance to antiandrogens was an increase in AR mRNA and protein levels that were both necessary and sufficient to convert prostate cancer cells to an androgen-independent state, possibly through recruitment of coactivators and corepressors. They concluded that the most important therapeutic implication of this work was that new antiandrogens were needed. Along these lines, a phase II study is evaluating a unique AR antagonist, mifepristone (RU-486). Mifepristone was originally developed as a progesterone and glucocorticoid receptor antagonist that could also inhibit AR. Mechanistically, mifepristone triggers the conformational change in AR by inducing strong interaction between AR and nuclear receptor corepressor (NCoR), which

TABLE 16C.4

INVESTIGATIONAL APPROACHES

Targeted pathways	Examples of agents	Clinical trial (phase)
RTK cell signaling	Imatinib mesylate (Gleevec™)	III
	ZD1839 (Gefinitib)	II
	Trastuzumab (Herceptin™)	II
	CCI-779	II
Angiogenesis	Thalidomide	II
	ABT-627 (Atrasentan™)	III
	MMP inhibitor (BMS275291)	II
	Bevacizumab (Avastin™)	I/II
	PTK787/ZK222584	I
Tumor-specific immune responses	APC8015 (Provenge™)	III
	TRICOM™	II
Apoptosis	Bcl-2 antisense oligonucleotide (G3139)	II
Differentiation	Troglitazone	III
	Vitamin D analogs	II
Proteasome inhibition	Bortezomib (PS-341, Velcade™)	I/II
Osteogenesis	ABT-627 (Atrasentan™)	II
Others	Selenium, vitamin E	III

results in the conversion of AR from a transcriptional activator to a strong transcriptional repressor. The repression is more potent than the AR inhibition by bicalutamide and flutamide. The primary point of this study is to determine its efficacy as second-line hormonal therapy (119).

Recent data have shown that signaling pathways downstream of growth factor receptor tyrosine kinases may also have a significant role in the progression of prostate cancer to a hormone-resistant phenotype (120). Consequently, identifying tyrosine kinase inhibitors (TKIs) targeting receptors or secondary signaling molecules has been an active area of drug development (121). Overexpression of epidermal growth factor receptor (EGFR) has been observed in various types of cancer including prostate cancer (122). Gefitinib (ZD1839) is a selective EGFR TKI approved for the treatment of patients with advanced non-small-cell lung cancer (123). A double-blind, randomized, placebo-controlled phase II trial suggested possible biologic activity of gefitinib in HRPC. Fifty-eight patients were randomized to drug or placebo and their PSA slopes compared (124). PSA doubling time was longer in the gefitinib group compared to placebo (5.0 months vs. 3.9 months) although the difference was not statistically significant ($P = .25$). Preclinical data in prostate cancer cell lines suggests that gefitinib may enhance the cytotoxicity of chemotherapy (125). Ongoing pilot studies also have investigated the efficacy of gefitinib in combination with mitoxantrone plus prednisone or docetaxel plus estramustine. PSA declines and pain responses were observed in 41% and 48% of patients, respectively, though relative additive benefits of gefitinib could not be determined in this small nonrandomized trial (125). However, gefitinib in combination with chemotherapy is feasible and well tolerated.

HER-2/neu, a member of the EGFR family, has also been found to be overexpressed in some prostate cancers, correlating with a poorer prognosis (126,127). Furthermore, expression of HER-2/neu appears to increase with progression to androgen independence (128). Trastuzumab is a humanized monoclonal antibody directed against the extracellular domain of HER-2/neu and shows evidence of antitumor activity in breast cancer cells (129). In patients with HER-2/neu-positive metastatic breast cancer, trastuzumab enhances survival when given with chemotherapy (130). In HRPC, Lara et al. screened for patients

who were HER-2/neu-positive for a phase II trial of trastuzumab plus docetaxel (131). Unfortunately, they reported that 1,000 patients would be needed to accrue to a typical 40-patient phase II efficacy trial, as HER-2/neu overexpression was infrequent in their study, thus the trial could not be completed.

Imatinib mesylate (STI571) is a specific inhibitor of several tyrosine kinases including BCR-Abl, c-KIT, and platelet-derived growth-factor receptor (PDGF-R). The efficacy and safety of imatinib mesylate has been confirmed in patients with chronic myelogenous leukemia and gastrointestinal stromal tumor (132,133), but because of high rates of expression of PDGF-R in prostate cancer, studies with imatinib mesylate are ongoing in prostate cancer. A multicenter, randomized phase III clinical trial comparing imatinib mesylate plus docetaxel to placebo plus docetaxel alone in HRPC is currently underway (134).

Phosphoinositide 3-kinase (PI3-K) signaling is a major signaling component downstream of growth-factor receptors and also a target for the treatment of cancer. In many types of cancers, including prostate cancer, aberrant activation of this pathway has been implicated (135). The PI3-K-Akt signaling pathway is a key regulator of many normal cellular processes including cell proliferation, survival, growth, and motility through multiple downstream targets (136). Hyperactivation of the PI3-K-Akt pathway due to loss of PTEN or increased Akt activity results in hyperproliferation and decreased apoptotis, both hallmarks of tumorigenesis.

Recently, attention has been focused on targeting a signaling molecule called the mammalian target of rapamycin (mTOR). mTOR was originally identified as the target of the macrolide antibiotic, rapamycin, and serves as a pivotal molecule for control of translation of proteins. Specifically, mTOR controls proteins required for G1-phase cell-cycle progression (137). Rapamycin and its analogs (including CCI-779 and RAD001), which inhibit mTOR, have been shown to cause G1-phase cell-cycle arrest. These agents inhibit growth of prostate cancer cell lines *in vitro* and prostate cancer xenograft models (138,139). Several of these agents are in phase II trials in prostate cancer (140).

The success of the cell-signaling target therapy depends on developing specific TKIs that are able to distinguish tumors sensitive to the TKIs from normal tissues (141). In addition, screening genetic information of RTKs may contribute to the effective use of TKIs. It has been found that a certain point mutation in its kinase domain on EGFRs in lung cancer patients confers profound sensitivity to gefitinib therapy (142).

Inhibiting Angiogenesis

Targeting angiogenesis has become an attractive area of cancer therapeutics. Angiogenesis is controlled by a balance between angiogenic factors, such as vascular endothelial growth factor (VEGF), and antiangiogenic factors, such as thrombospondin-1 (143). It is likely that angiogenesis plays a pivotal role in the initiation and propagation of prostate cancer. Thus, inhibiting angiogenesis has been proposed as a cancer treatment strategy. Thalidomide decreases angiogenesis by inhibiting VEGF (144) and has been shown to have activity in HRPC both as a single agent and in combination with chemotherapy in phase II trials (80,145). In addition to thalidomide, current ongoing angiogenesis-targeted phase I/II trials include the monoclonal VEGF antibody bevacizumab and the small molecule TKI PTK787/ZK222584 (146). In a multicenter phase II study (CALGB 90006), 79 patients with progressive, metastatic HRPC were treated with bevacizumab in combination with docetaxel and estramustine. 53 percent (nine out of 17 evaluable patients with measurable disease) showed a partial response, and 65% of patients with evaluable PSA data showed >50% PSA decline (147). A phase III clinical trial is planned to compare docetaxel with or without bevacizumab.

Other angiogenesis inhibitors being tested include VEGF receptor tyrosine kinase inhibitor ZD6474. ZD6474 has additional activity against EGFR, and is currently being tested in phase II trials in solid tumors (148,149). AZD2171 is now in phase I trials (150).

Targeting the Immune System

Immunotherapy intends to induce a tumor-specific immune response in the host. Improved understanding of immune recognition may lead to more effective immunotherapy for prostate cancer (151). Potential targets include PSA, prostatic acid phosphatase (PAP), and prostate-specific membrane antigen (PSMA). Recent immunotherapy trials have included patients with either minimally symptomatic, metastatic HRPC, or hormone-naïve patients whose disease is manifested solely by a rising PSA. Recent approaches include the *ex vivo* stimulation of antigen-specific cytotoxic T-lymphocytes directed at tumor-specific antigens (152). APC8015 consists of autologous dendritic cells loaded with a recombinant fusion protein consisting of PAP linked to granulocyte macrophage colony stimulating factor (GM-CSF) (153). A phase III study of APC8015 demonstrated a significant improvement in time to progression in the subset of patients with Gleason score 7 or less. The regimen was well tolerated with minimal toxicity (154).

Other active strategies enhance the immunogenicity of the tumor through gene modification or costimulatory molecules in the tumor cell vaccines (152). The Eastern Cooperative Oncology Group (ECOG) conducted the phase II randomized study to evaluate the feasibility and tolerability of a prime/boost vaccine strategy using vaccinia virus and fowlpox virus expressing human PSA in 64 eligible patients with biochemical progression after local therapy failure (155). After 19 months of follow-up, a significant proportion of men remained free of PSA progression (45.3%) and clinical progression (78.1%), and nearly half demonstrated an increase in PSA-specific T-cell response. The regimen was well tolerated with few adverse events.

A novel viral vaccine approach incorporates TRICOM, which is a product of recombinant vaccinia and fowlpox viruses which contain genes encoding PSA, intercellular adhesion molecule-1 (ICAM-1), leukocyte function-associated antigen-3 (LFA-3) and B7.1, and is designed in order to enhance antigen presentation and T–cell immunity by introducing more antigens. A recent phase I study demonstrated the safety of a prime/boost schedule with the addition of TRICOM in patients with advanced prostate cancer (156). Phase III studies of APC8015 and TRICOM are currently accruing.

A recent pilot study also demonstrated that vaccine therapy increased T-cell responses even when combined with docetaxel (157).

Targeting Bone-tumor Interaction

Given the fact that prostate cancer is the only malignancy to form predominantly osteoblastic metastases (158,159) and more than 80% of men with metastatic HRPC have radiographic evidence of bone involvement, it is crucial to investigate the agents capable of interfering with bone-tumor interaction. Prostate cancer cells produce growth factors that promote osteoblast growth including endothelin(ET)-1 (160). The ET family has been identified as contributing to the pathophysiology of prostate cancer (161). They are paracrine/autocrine peptides that modulate vasomotor tone, nociception, hormone production, and cell proliferation (160). Endothelin-1 (ET-1) is the predominant circulating endothelin and is uniformly produced by endothelial cells and prostate epithelium, and acts through the ET_A receptor signaling. Higher circulating levels of ET-1 have been observed in men with HRPC compared with those with clinically localized disease or healthy individuals (161). Atrasentan (ABT-627) is a selective ET_A receptor antagonist that blocks or reverses the biologic effects of ET-1 (162). A double-blind, randomized, placebo-controlled phase II study with a 2.5-mg arm and a 10-mg arm was conducted in 288 patients with either asymptomatic or metastatic HRPC in the United States and Europe (163). Time to progression was longer in the 10-mg Atrasentan arm compared with the placebo (183 days vs. 137 days; $P = .13$), and median time to progression was significantly prolonged in the 10-mg Atrasentan arm compared with placebo arm (196 days vs. 129 days; $P = .021$). In the 10-mg Atrasentan arm median time to PSA progression was twice that of the placebo arm (155 days vs. 71 days; $P = .002$). No difference was observed in survival among the groups. The regimen was well tolerated with mild toxicity. A randomized, double-blind, placebo-controlled phase III study of 10 mg Atrasentan investigated the effects on bone alkaline phosphatase (BAP), and survival in 474 patients with metastatic HRPC (164). The data demonstrated that high-baseline BAP is predictive of early disease progression (168 days vs. 85 days; $P < .0001$) and reduced survival (741 days vs. 461 days; $P < .0001$). Another study demonstrated the QOL benefit of Atrasentan by assessing the Functional Assessment of Cancer Therapy-Prostate (FACT-P) quality of life (QOL) instrument and FACT Advanced Prostate Symptom Index (FAPSI) derived from FACT-P ($P < .003$) (165). Atrasentan represents a promising new therapeutic option in targeting bone metastases in advanced prostate cancer.

Inducing Apoptosis

Preclinical studies showed that expression of the *bcl-2* gene and its antiapoptotic protein bcl-2 is elevated in HRPC (166,167). This antiapoptotic effect in prostate cancer cells can be suppressed by bcl-2 antisense oligonucleotide (G3139), which decreases the expression level of bcl-2. In a phase II study of G3139 in combination with docetaxel, a PSA >50% reduction rate was 48% (15 out of 31 patients) and this regimen was well tolerated (168). Whether an enhancement of apoptosis was present beyond docetaxel alone is unclear without a randomized trial, which is planned. Based on observations that retinoids and interferon reduce Bcl-2 expression (169), ECOG conducted a randomized phase II study to investigate the efficacy of 13-cis retinoic acid and interferon-α in combination with paclitaxel (170). This regimen was well tolerated; however, the outcome was insufficient to gain significant support for a phase III trial.

Inducing Differentiation

This category of drugs suppresses tumors by changing their genetic program, thereby altering growth characteristics. Targets of differentiation therapy include the vitamin D pathway. An active metabolite of vitamin D, 1,25-dehydroxyvitamin D (calcitriol), has antineoplastic activity and can induce cell cycle arrest and cellular differentiation of prostate cancer cells, which results in induction of apoptosis (171). A phase II trial of weekly docetaxel plus high-dose calcitriol was reported in patients with metastatic HRPC (79). Eighty-one percent of patients achieved at least a 50% reduction in PSA while 53% of those with measurable disease had a partial response. The combination regimen was well tolerated and demonstrated promising activity compared with trials of docetaxel alone. In addition, significant palliative activity of this regimen has been reported (172). A randomized phase II trial comparing docetaxel to docetaxel plus a high-dose calcitriol formulation recently completed accrual of 232 patients and will be useful to assess the additive benefit of vitamin D to docetaxel chemotherapy. Other differentiation agents being studied include histone deacetylase inhibitors, such as suberoylanilide hydroxamine acid (SAHA) (86).

Targeting the Proteosome

The ubiquitin-proteosome pathway plays a crucial role in cellular homeostasis by degrading proteins in an orderly fashion. Therefore, the pathway controls critical cellular functions, including cell cycle regulation and apoptosis, by controlling the availability of key molecules. Therefore, proteosome inhibition is an attractive target for disrupting cell cycle regulation and causing apoptosis of cancer cells. Proteosome inhibitors cause cancer cell death in part by inhibiting activation of nuclear factor kappa B (NF-κB). NF-κB contributes to various aspects of tumorigenesis including cell growth and proliferation, antiapoptosis, and angiogenesis, and its constitutive activation has been demonstrated in prostate cancer (173). Also, proteosome inhibitors stall the degradation process of many proteins necessary for the progression through the cell cycle (174). A phase I/II trial is currently ongoing to evaluate the effect of the proteosome inhibitor, bortezomib (PS-341), in combination with docetaxel in patients with advanced HRPC (175). A preliminary report of 22 evaluable patients showed that 36% had a >50% decline in PSA, and 17% with measurable disease achieved a partial response. The regimen was well tolerated.

CONCLUSION

With the continual advancement in understanding the molecular basis of cancer, "noncytotoxic" pharmacologic agents targeting specific cellular pathways are currently being tested in HRPC. There are several requirements in order to successfully combine such noncytotoxic agents with the standard chemotherapy drugs such as docetaxel, and improve survival and QOL for HPRC patients. First, the drug must be specific for the target molecule. Second, the target must be differentially expressed in HRPC cells. Third, there should be evidence that the drug can be effectively delivered to the tumor. Fourth, the new agent must have an acceptable safety profile. Finally, the agent should not interfere with the activity of chemotherapy in phase I and II trials. Further research is needed to define the key targets, develop the optimal drugs to interfere with these targets, and ultimately deliver on the promise of improved survival and QOL for prostate cancer patients.

References

1. Smaletz O, Scher HI, Small EJ, et al. Nomogram for overall survival of patients with progressive metastatic prostate cancer after castration. *J Clin Oncol* 2002;20(19):3972–3982.
2. Eisenberger MA, Simon R, O'Dwyer PJ, et al. A reevaluation of nonhormonal cytotoxic chemotherapy in the treatment of prostatic carcinoma. *J Clin Oncol* 1985;3(6):827–841.
3. Yagoda A, Petrylak D, Thompson S. Cytotoxic chemotherapy for advanced renal cell carcinoma. *Urol Clin North Am* 1993;20(2):303–321.
4. Ban Y, Wang MC, Chu TM. Immunologic markers and the diagnosis of prostatic cancer. *Urol Clin North Am* 1984;11(2):269–276.
5. Kantoff PW, Halabi S, Conaway M, et al. Hydrocortisone with or without mitoxantrone in men with hormone-refractory prostate cancer: results of the Cancer and Leukemia Group B 9182 study. *J Clin Oncol* 1999;17(8): 2506–2513.
6. Tannock IF, Osaba D, Stackler MR, et al. Chemotherapy with mitoxantrone plus prednisone or prednisone alone for symptomatic hormone-resistant prostate cancer: a Canadian randomized trial with palliative end points. *J Clin Oncol* 1996;14(6):1756–1764.
7. Petrylak DP, Macarthur R, O'Connor J, et al. Phase I/II studies of docetaxel (Taxotere) combined with estramustine in men with hormone-refractory prostate cancer. *Semin Oncol* 1999;26(5 Suppl. 17):28–33.
8. Kreis W, Budman DR, Fetten J, et al. Phase I trial of the combination of daily estramustine phosphate and intermittent docetaxel in patients with metastatic hormone refractory prostate carcinoma. *Ann Oncol* 1999; 10(1):33–38.
9. Savarese D, Taplin ME, Halabi S, et al. A phase II study of docetaxel (taxotere), estramustine, and low-dose hydrocortisone in men with hormone-refractory prostate cancer: preliminary results of cancer and leukemia group B trial 9780. *Semin Oncol* 1999;26(5 Suppl. 17):39–44.
10. Sinibaldi VJ, Carducci MA, Laufer M, et al. Preliminary evaluation of a short course of estramustine phosphate and docetaxel (taxotere) in the treatment of hormone-refractory prostate cancer. *Semin Oncol* 1999;26(5 Suppl. 17):45–48.
11. Small EJ, Srinivas S, Egan B, et al. Doxorubicin and dose-escalated cyclophosphamide with granulocyte colony-stimulating factor for the treatment of hormone-resistant prostate cancer. *J Clin Oncol* 1996;14(5): 1617–1625.
12. Kelly WK, Scher HI, Mazumdar M, et al. Prostate-specific antigen as a measure of disease outcome in metastatic hormone-refractory prostate cancer. *J Clin Oncol* 1993;11(4):607–615.
13. Scher HI, Kelly WM, Zhang ZF, et al. Post-therapy serum prostate-specific antigen level and survival in patients with androgen-independent prostate cancer. *J Natl Cancer Inst* 1999;91(3):244–251.
14. Bubley GJ, Carducci M, Dahut W, et al. Eligibility and response guidelines for phase II clinical trials in androgen-independent prostate cancer: recommendations from the Prostate-Specific Antigen Working Group. *J Clin Oncol* 1999;17(11):3461–3467.
15. Esper P, Mo F, Chodak G, et al. Measuring quality of life in men with prostate cancer using the functional assessment of cancer therapy-prostate instrument. *Urology* 1997;50(6):920–928.
16. Kornblith AB, Herndon JE II, Zuckerman E, et al. The impact of docetaxel, estramustine, and low dose hydrocortisone on the quality of life of men with hormone refractory prostate cancer and their partners: a feasibility study. *Ann Oncol* 2001;12(5):633–641.
17. Yagoda A, Petrylak D. Cytotoxic chemotherapy for advanced hormone-resistant prostate cancer. *Cancer* 1993;71(Suppl. 3):1098–1109.
18. Smith DC, Jodrell DI, Egorin MJ, et al. Phase II trial and pharmacokinetic assessment of intravenous melphalan in patients with advanced prostate cancer. *Cancer Chemother Pharmacol* 1993;31(5):363–368.
19. Williamson SK, Wolf MK, Eisenberger MA et al, A Southwest Oncology Group study. Phase II evaluation of ifosfamide/Mesna in metastatic prostate cancer. *Am J Clin Oncol* 1996;19(4):368–370.
20. van Brussel JP, Busstra MB, Lang MS, et al. A phase II study of temozolomide in hormone-refractory prostate cancer. *Cancer Chemother Pharmacol* 2000;45(6):509–512.

21. Hussain MH, Pienta KJ, Redman BG, et al. Oral etoposide in the treatment of hormone-refractory prostate cancer. *Cancer* 1994;74(1):100–103.

22. Schmid HP, Maibach R, Bernhard J et al, Swiss Group for Clinical Cancer Research, Berne, Switzerland. A phase II study of oral idarubicin as a treatment for metastatic hormone-refractory prostate carcinoma with special focus on prostate specific antigen doubling time. *Cancer* 1997;79(9): 1703–1709.

23. Morant R, Bernhard J, Maibach R et al, Swiss Group for Clinical Cancer Research (SAKK) Response and palliation in a phase II trial of gemcitabine in hormone-refractory metastatic prostatic carcinoma. *Ann Oncol* 2000;11(2):183–188.

24. Reese DM, Tchekmedyian S, Chapman Y, et al. A phase II trial of irinotecan in hormone-refractory prostate cancer. *Invest New Drugs* 1998;16(4): 353–359.

25. Witte RS, Yeap BY, Trump DL. Trimetrexate in advanced hormone-refractory prostate cancer. An ECOG phase II trial. *Invest New Drugs* 1994; 12(3):255–258.

26. Rajagopalan K, Peereboom D, Budd GT, et al. Phase II trial of circadian infusion floxuridine (FUDR) in hormone refractory metastatic prostate cancer. *Invest New Drugs* 1998;16(3):255–258.

27. Atkins JN, Muss HB, Case LD, et al. Leucovorin and high-dose fluorouracil in metastatic prostate cancer. A phase II trial of the Piedmont Oncology Association. *Am J Clin Oncol* 1996;19(1):23–25.

28. Raghavan D, Cox K, Pearson BS, et al. Oral cyclophosphamide for the management of hormone-refractory prostate cancer. *Br J Urol* 1993;72(5 Pt 1):625–628.

29. Maulard-Durdux C, Dufour B, Hennequin C, et al. Phase II study of the oral cyclophosphamide and oral etoposide combination in hormone-refractory prostate carcinoma patients. *Cancer* 1996;77(6):1144–1148.

30. Bracarda S, Tonato M, Rosi P, et al. Oral estramustine and cyclophosphamide in patients with metastatic hormone refractory prostate carcinoma: a phase II study. *Cancer* 2000;88(6):1438–1444.

31. Daliani DD, Assikis V, Tu SM, et al. Phase II trial of cyclophosphamide, vincristine, and dexamethasone in the treatment of androgen-independent prostate carcinoma. *Cancer* 2003;97(3):561–567.

32. Torti FM, Aston D, Lum BL, et al. Weekly doxorubicin in endocrine-refractory carcinoma of the prostate. *J Clin Oncol* 1983;1(8):477–482.

33. Scher H, Yagoda A, Serber M, et al. Phase II trial of doxorubicin in bidimensionally measurable prostatic adenocarcinoma. *J Urol* 1984;131(6): 1099–1102.

34. van Andel G, Kurth KH, Rietbroek RL, et al. Quality of life assessment in patients with hormone-resistant prostate cancer treated with epirubicin or with epirubicin plus medroxy progesterone acetate—is it feasible? *Eur Urol* 2000;38(3):259–264.

35. Petrioli R, Fiaschi AI, Pozzessere D, et al. Weekly epirubicin in patients with hormone-resistant prostate cancer. *Br J Cancer* 2002;87(7):720–725.

36. Magarotto R, Recaldin E, Molon A, et al. Continuous infusion of epirubicin in metastatic hormone refractory prostate cancer [Abstract]. *Proc Am Soc Clin Oncol* 2001;20:163b.

37. Saxman S, Ansari R, Drasga R et al. A Hoosier Oncology Group Study. Phase III trial of cyclophosphamide versus cyclophosphamide, doxorubicin, and methotrexate in hormone-refractory prostatic cancer. *Cancer* 1992;70(10):2488–2492.

38. Sella A, Kilbourn R, Amato R, et al. Phase II study of ketoconazole combined with weekly doxorubicin in patients with androgen-independent prostate cancer. *J Clin Oncol* 1994;12(4):683–688.

39. Chao D, von Schlippe M, Harland SJ. A phase II study of continuous infusion 5-fluorouracil (5-FU) with epirubicin and cisplatin in metastatic, hormone-refractory prostate cancer: an active new regimen. *Eur J Cancer* 1997;33(8):1230–1233.

40. Seidman AD, Scher HI, Petrylak D, et al. Estramustine and vinblastine: use of prostate specific antigen as a clinical trial end point for hormone refractory prostatic cancer. *J Urol* 1992;147(3 Pt 2):931–934.

41. Hudes GR, Greenberg R, Krigel RL, et al. Phase II study of estramustine and vinblastine, two microtubule inhibitors, in hormone-refractory prostate cancer. *J Clin Oncol* 1992;10(11):1754–1761.

42. Amato RJ, Bui C, Logothetis CJ. Estramustine in combination with vinblastine and mitomycin-C for patients with progressive androgen independent adenocarcinoma of the prostate. *Prostate Cancer Prostatic Dis* 1999;2(2):83–87.

43. Ellerhorst JA, Tu S-M, Amato RJ, et al. Phase II trial of alternating weekly chemohormonal therapy for patients with androgen-independent prostate cancer. *Clin Cancer Res* 1997;3(12 Pt 1):2371–2376.

44. Pienta KJ, Redman BG, Bandekar R, et al. A phase II trial of oral estramustine and oral etoposide in hormone refractory prostate cancer. *Urology* 1997;50(3):401–406; discussion 406-407.

45. Culine S, Kattan J, Zanetta S, et al. Evaluation of estramustine phosphate combined with weekly doxorubicin in patients with androgen-independent prostate cancer. *Am J Clin Oncol* 1998;21(5):470–474.

46. Colleoni M, Graiff C, Vicario G, et al. Phase II study of estramustine, oral etoposide, and vinorelbine in hormone-refractory prostate cancer. *Am J Clin Oncol* 1997;20(4):383–386.

47. Petrylak DP, Tangen C, Hussein M, et al. SWOG 99-16: randomized phase III trial of docetaxel (D)/estramustine (E) versus mitoxantrone (M)/prednisone (P) in men with androgen-independent prostate cancer (AIPCA). [Abstract]. *Proc Am Soc Clin Oncol* 2004;23:3.

48. Eisenberger MA, De Wit R, Berry W, et al. A multicenter phase III comparison of docetaxel (D) + prednisone (P) and mitoxantrone (MTZ) + P in patients with hormone-refractory prostate cancer (HRPC). *Proc Am Soc Clin Oncol* 2004;23:4.

49. Perry CM, McTavish D. Estramustine phosphate sodium. A review of its pharmacodynamic and pharmacokinetic properties, and therapeutic efficacy in prostate cancer. *Drugs Aging* 1995;7(1):49–74.

50. Speicher LA, Barone L, Tew KD. Combined antimicrotubule activity of estramustine and taxol in human prostatic carcinoma cell lines. *Cancer Res* 1992;52(16):4433–4440.

51. Yagoda A, Smith JA Jr, Soloway MS, et al. Phase II study of estramustine phosphate in advanced hormone refractory prostate cancer with increasing prostate specific antigen levels [Abstract]. *J Urol* 1991;145: 384a.

52. Iversen P, Rasmussen F, Asmussen C et al. Danish Prostatic Cancer Group. Estramustine phosphate versus placebo as second line treatment after orchiectomy in patients with metastatic prostate cancer: DAPROCA study 9002. *J Urol* 1997;157(3):929–934.

53. Sinibaldi VJ, Carducci MA, Moore-Cooper S, et al. Phase II evaluation of docetaxel plus one-day oral estramustine phosphate in the treatment of patients with androgen independent prostate carcinoma. *Cancer* 2002; 94(5):1457–1465.

54. Oh WK, Halabi S, Kelly WK, et al. A phase II study of estramustine, docetaxel, and carboplatin with granulocyte-colony-stimulating factor support in patients with hormone-refractory prostate carcinoma: Cancer and Leukemia Group B 99813. *Cancer* 2003;98(12):2592–2598.

55. Hartley-Asp B. Estramustine-induced mitotic arrest in two human prostatic carcinoma cell lines DU 145 and PC-3. *Prostate* 1984;5(1):93–100.

56. Mareel MM, Storme GA, Dragonetti CH, et al. Antiinvasive activity of estramustine on malignant MO4 mouse cells and on DU-145 human prostate carcinoma cells in vitro. *Cancer Res* 1988;48(7):1842–1849.

57. Hartley-Asp B, Kruse E. Nuclear protein matrix as a target for estramustine-induced cell death. *Prostate* 1986;9(4):387–395.

58. Hudes G, Einhorn L, Ross E, et al. Vinblastine versus vinblastine plus oral estramustine phosphate for patients with hormone-refractory prostate cancer: a Hoosier Oncology Group and Fox Chase Network phase III trial. *J Clin Oncol* 1999;17(10):3160–3166.

59. Sweeney CJ, Monaco FJ, Jung SH, et al. A phase II Hoosier Oncology Group study of vinorelbine and estramustine phosphate in hormone-refractory prostate cancer. *Ann Oncol* 2002;13(3):435–440.

60. Smith MR, Kaufman D, Oh W, et al. Vinorelbine and estramustine in androgen-independent metastatic prostate cancer: a phase II study. *Cancer* 2000;89(8):1824–1828.

61. Pienta KJ, Redman B, Hussain M, et al. Phase II evaluation of oral estramustine and oral etoposide in hormone-refractory adenocarcinoma of the prostate. *J Clin Oncol* 1994;12(10):2005–2012.

62. Hemes EH, Fossa SD, Vaage S, et al. Epirubicin combined with estramustine phosphate in hormone-resistant prostate cancer: a phase II study. *Br J Cancer* 1997;76(1):93–99.

63. Roth BJ, Yeap BY, Wilding G, et al. Taxol in advanced, hormone-refractory carcinoma of the prostate. A phase II trial of the Eastern Cooperative Oncology Group. *Cancer* 1993;72(8):2457–2460.

64. Trivedi C, Redman B, Flaherty LE, et al. Weekly 1-hour infusion of paclitaxel. Clinical feasibility and efficacy in patients with hormone-refractory prostate carcinoma. *Cancer* 2000;89(2):431–436.

65. Berry W, Gregurich M, Dakhil S, et al. Phase II randomized trial of weekly paclitaxel (Taxol) with or without estramustine phosphate in patients with symptomatic, hormone-refractory, metastatic carcinoma of the prostate (HRMCP). *Proc Am Soc Clin Oncol* 2001;20(175a):696; [Abstract]

66. Ferrari AC, Chachoua A, Singh H, et al. A Phase I/II study of weekly paclitaxel and 3 days of high dose oral estramustine in patients with hormone-refractory prostate carcinoma. *Cancer* 2001;91(11):2039–2045.

67. Vaishampayan U, Fontana J, Du W, et al. An active regimen of weekly paclitaxel and estramustine in metastatic androgen-independent prostate cancer. *Urology* 2002;60(6):1050–1054.

68. Berry W, Gregurich M, Dakhil S, et al. Phase II randomized trial of weekly paclitaxel with or without estramustine phosphate in patients with symptomatic, hormone-refractory metastatic carcinoma of the prostate. [Abstract]. *Proc Am Soc Clin Oncol* 2001;20:175a.

69. Vaughn DJ, Brown AW Jr, Harker WG, et al. Multicenter phase II study of estramustine phosphate plus weekly paclitaxel in patients with androgen-independent prostate carcinoma. *Cancer* 2004;100(4):746–750.

70. Beer TM, Pierce WC, Lowe BA, et al. Phase II study of weekly docetaxel in symptomatic androgen-independent prostate cancer. *Ann Oncol* 2001; 12(9):1273–1279.

71. Ferrero JM, Foa C, Thezenas S, et al. A weekly schedule of docetaxel for metastatic hormone-refractory prostate cancer. *Oncology* 2004;66(4): 281–287.

72. Picus J, Schultz M. Docetaxel (Taxotere) as monotherapy in the treatment of hormone-refractory prostate cancer: preliminary results. *Semin Oncol* 1999;26(5 Suppl. 17):14–18.

73. Sitka Copur M, Ledakis P, Lynch J, et al. Weekly docetaxel and estramustine in patients with hormone-refractory prostate cancer. *Semin Oncol* 2001;28(4 Suppl. 15):16–21.

74. Savarese DM, Halabi S, Hars V et al. Cancer and Leukemia Group B. Phase II study of docetaxel, estramustine, and low-dose hydrocortisone in

men with hormone-refractory prostate cancer: a final report of CALGB 9780. *J Clin Oncol* 2001;19(9):2509–2516.

75. Hudes GR, Nathan F, Khater C, et al. Phase II trial of 96-hour paclitaxel plus oral estramustine phosphate in metastatic hormone-refractory prostate cancer. *J Clin Oncol* 1997;15(9):3156–3163.

76. Haas N, Roth B, Garay C, et al. Phase I trial of weekly paclitaxel plus oral estramustine phosphate in patients with hormone-refractory prostate cancer. *Urology* 2001;58(1):59–64.

77. Kelly WK, Curley T, Slovin S, et al. Paclitaxel, estramustine phosphate, and carboplatin in patients with advanced prostate cancer. *J Clin Oncol* 2001;19(1):44–53.

78. Koletsky AJ, Guerra ML, Kronish L. Phase II study of vinorelbine and low-dose docetaxel in chemotherapy-naive patients with hormone-refractory prostate cancer. *Cancer J* 2003;9(4):286–292.

79. Beer TM, Eilers KM, Garzotte M, et al. Weekly high-dose calcitriol and docetaxel in metastatic androgen-independent prostate cancer. *J Clin Oncol* 2003;21(1):123–128.

80. Figg WD, Arlen P, Gulley J, et al. A randomized phase II trial of docetaxel (Taxotere) plus thalidomide in androgen-independent prostate cancer. *Semin Oncol* 2001;28(4 Suppl. 15):62–66.

81. Friedland D, Cohen J, Miller R Jr, et al. A phase II trial of docetaxel (Taxotere) in hormone-refractory prostate cancer: correlation of antitumor effect to phosphorylation of Bcl-2. *Semin Oncol* 1999;26(5 Suppl. 17):19–23.

82. Gravis G, Bladou F, Salem N, et al. Weekly administration of docetaxel for symptomatic metastatic hormone-refractory prostate carcinoma. *Cancer* 2003;98(8):1627–1634.

83. Petrylak DP, Macarthur RB, O'Connor J, et al. Phase I trial of docetaxel with estramustine in androgen-independent prostate cancer. *J Clin Oncol* 1999;17(3):958–967.

84. Petrylak D, Shelton GB, England-Owen C, et al. Response and preliminary survival results of a phase II study of docetaxel + estramustine in patients with androgen-independent prostate cancer [Abstract]. *Proc Am Soc Clin Oncol* 2000;19:334a.

85. Gerth K, Bedorf N, Hofle G, et al. Epothilons A and B: antifungal and cytotoxic compounds from *Sorangium cellulosum* (Myxobacteria). Production, physico-chemical and biological properties. *J Antibiot (Tokyo)* 1996;49(6):560–563.

86. Galsky M, Kelly WK. The development of differentiation agents for the treatment of prostate cancer. *Semin Oncol* 2003;30(6):689–697.

87. Kelly WK, Galsky MD, Small EJ, et al. Multi-institutional trial of the epothilone B analogue BMS-247550 with or without estramustine phosphate (EMP) in patients with progressive castrate-metastatic prostate cancer (PCMPC); updated results. *Proc Am Soc Clin Oncol* 2004;23:383; Abstract 4509.

88. Eisenberger MA, DeWit R, Berry W, et al. A multicenter phase III comparison of docetaxel (D) + prednisone (P) and mitoxantrone (MTZ) + P in patients with hormone-refractory prostate cancer (HRPC). *Proc Am Soc Clin Oncol* 2004;22(14S):4.

89. Urakami S, Igawa M, Kikuno N, et al. Combination chemotherapy with paclitaxel, estramustine and carboplatin for hormone refractory prostate cancer. *J Urol* 2002;168(6):2444–2450.

90. Smith DC, Esper P, Strawderman M, et al. Phase II trial of oral estramustine, oral etoposide, and intravenous paclitaxel in hormone-refractory prostate cancer. *J Clin Oncol* 1999;17(6):1664–1671.

91. Smith DC, Chay CH, Dunn RL, et al. Phase II trial of paclitaxel, estramustine, etoposide, and carboplatin in the treatment of patients with hormone-refractory prostate carcinoma. *Cancer* 2003;98(2):269–276.

92. Smith MR. Bisphosphonates to prevent skeletal complications in men with metastatic prostate cancer. *J Urol* 2003;170(6 Pt 2):S55–S57; discussion S57–S58.

93. Serafini AN. Therapy of metastatic bone pain. *J Nucl Med* 2001;42(6):895–906.

94. Gunawardana DH, Lichtenstein M, Better N, et al. Results of strontium-89 therapy in patients with prostate cancer resistant to chemotherapy. *Clin Nucl Med* 2004;29(2):81–85.

95. Oosterhof GO, Roberts JT, de Reijke TM, et al. Strontium(89) chloride versus palliative local field radiotherapy in patients with hormonal escaped prostate cancer: a phase III study of the European Organisation for Research and Treatment of Cancer, Genitourinary Group. *Eur Urol* 2003; 44(5):519–526.

96. Tu SM, Millikan RE, Mengistu B, et al. Bone-targeted therapy for advanced androgen-independent carcinoma of the prostate: a randomised phase II trial. *Lancet* 2001;357(9253):336–341.

97. Mertens WC, Porter AT, Reid RH, et al. Strontium-89 and low-dose infusion cisplatin for patients with hormone refractory prostate carcinoma metastatic to bone: a preliminary report. *J Nucl Med* 1992;33(8):1437–1443.

98. Sciuto R, Festa A, Rea S, et al. Effects of low-dose cisplatin on 89Sr therapy for painful bone metastases from prostate cancer: a randomized clinical trial. *J Nucl Med* 2002;43(1):79–86.

99. Sartor O. Radioisotopic treatment of bone pain from metastatic prostate cancer. *Curr Oncol Rep* 2003;5(3):258–262.

100. Bates T. A review of local radiotherapy in the treatment of bone metastases and cord compression. *Int J Radiat Oncol Biol Phys* 1992;23(1):217–221.

101. Nielsen OS, Bentzen SM, Sandberg E, et al. Randomized trial of single dose versus fractionated palliative radiotherapy of bone metastases. *Radiother Oncol* 1998;47(3):233–240.

102. Hartsell WF, Scott C, Brunner DW, et al. A phase III randomized trial of 8 Gy in one fraction vs. 30 Gy in 10 fractions for palliation of painful bone metastases: preliminary results of RTOG 97-04. *Int J Radiat Oncol Biol Phys* 2003;57(Suppl. 2) (presented at the American Society of Radiation Therapeutic Oncology 45th annual meeting):S124; Abstract 1.

103. Zelefsky MJ, Scher HI, Forman JD, et al. Palliative hemiskeletal irradiation for widespread metastatic prostate cancer: a comparison of single dose and fractionated regimens. *Int J Radiat Oncol Biol Phys* 1989;17(6):1281–1285.

104. Ratanatharathorn V, Powers W, Moss W, et al. Bone metastasis: review and critical analysis of random allocation trials of local field treatment. *Int J Radiat Oncol Biol Phys* 1999;44(1):1–18.

105. Wu JS, Wong R, Johnston M, et al. Meta-analysis of dose-fractionation radiotherapy trials for the palliation of painful bone metastases. *Int J Radiat Oncol Biol Phys* 2003;55(3):594–605.

106. Yazawa Y, Frassica FJ, Chao EY, et al. Metastatic bone disease. A study of the surgical treatment of 166 pathologic humeral and femoral fractures. *Clin Orthop* 1990;(251):213–219.

107. Zelefsky MJ, Scher HI, Krol G, et al. Spinal epidural tumor in patients with prostate cancer. Clinical and radiographic predictors of response to radiation therapy. *Cancer* 1992;70(9):2319–2325.

108. Flynn DF, Shipley WU. Management of spinal cord compression secondary to metastatic prostatic carcinoma. *Urol Clin North Am* 1991;18(1): 145–152.

109. Regine WF, Tibbs PA, Young A. Metastatic spinal cord compression: a randomized trial of direct decompressive surgical resection plus radiation therapy vs. radiotherapy alone. *Int J Radiat Oncol Biol Phys* 2003;57 (Suppl. 2)(presented at the American Society of Radiation Therapeutic Oncology 45th annual meeting:) S125; Abstract 3.

110. Dicker AP. The safety and tolerability of low-dose irradiation for the management of gynaecomastia caused by antiandrogen monotherapy. *Lancet Oncol* 2003;4(1):30–36.

111. Craft N, Chhor C, Tran C, et al. Evidence for clonal outgrowth of androgen-independent prostate cancer cells from androgen-dependent tumors through a two-step process. *Cancer Res* 1999;59(19):5030–5036.

112. Taplin ME, Bubley GJ, Shuster TD, et al. Mutation of the androgen-receptor gene in metastatic androgen-independent prostate cancer. *N Engl J Med* 1995;332(21):1393–1398.

113. Visakorpi T, Hyytinen E, Koivisto P, et al. In vivo amplification of the androgen receptor gene and progression of human prostate cancer. *Nat Genet* 1995;9(4):401–406.

114. Taplin ME, Bubley GJ, Ko YJ, et al. Selection for androgen receptor mutations in prostate cancers treated with androgen antagonist. *Cancer Res* 1999;59(11):2511–2515.

115. Koivisto PA, Helin HJ. Androgen receptor gene amplification increases tissue PSA protein expression in hormone-refractory prostate carcinoma. *J Pathol* 1999;189(2):219–223.

116. Marcelli M, Ittmann M, Mariani S, et al. Androgen receptor mutations in prostate cancer. *Cancer Res* 2000;60(4):944–949.

117. Feldman BJ, Feldman D. The development of androgen-independent prostate cancer. *Nat Rev Cancer* 2001;1(1):34–45.

118. Chen CD, Welsbie DS, Tran C, et al. Molecular determinants of resistance to antiandrogen therapy. *Nat Med* 2004;10(1):33–39.

119. Song LN, Coghlan M, Gelmann EP, et al. Antiandrogen effects of mifepristone on coactivator and corepressor interactions with the androgen receptor. *Mol Endocrinol* 2004;18(1):70–85.

120. Blackledge G. Growth factor receptor tyrosine kinase inhibitors; clinical development and potential for prostate cancer therapy. *J Urol* 2003;170(6 Pt 2):S77–S83; discussion S83.

121. Shawver LK, Slamon D, Ullrich A. Smart drugs: tyrosine kinase inhibitors in cancer therapy. *Cancer Cell* 2002;1(2):117–123.

122. Salomon DS, Brandt R, Ciardiello F, et al. Epidermal growth factor-related peptides and their receptors in human malignancies. *Crit Rev Oncol Hematol* 1995;19(3):183–232.

123. Natale RB. Effects of ZD1839 (Iressa, gefitinib) treatment on symptoms and quality of life in patients with advanced non-small cell lung cancer. *Semin Oncol* 2004;31(3 Suppl 9):23–30.

124. Schroder FH, Wildhagen MF. ZD1839 (gefinitib) and hormone resistant (HR) prostate cancer—final results of a double blind randomized placebo-controlled phase II study. *Proc Am Soc Clin Oncol* 2004;22(14S): Abstract 4698.

125. Trump DL, Wilding G, Small E, et al. Pilot trials of ZD1839 ('Iressa') an orally active selective epidermal growth factor receptor tyrosine kinase inhibitor, in combination with mitoxantrone/prednisone or docetaxel/estramustine in patients with hormone-refractory prostate cancer. *AUA* 2003;169(4):Abstract 105239.

126. Ross JS, Sheehan CE, Hayner-Buchan AM, et al. Prognostic significance of HER-2/neu gene amplification status by fluorescence in situ hybridization of prostate carcinoma. *Cancer* 1997;79(11):2162–2170.

127. Sadasivan R, Morgan R, Jennings S, et al. Overexpression of Her-2/neu may be an indicator of poor prognosis in prostate cancer. *J Urol* 1993; 150(1):126–131.

128. Signoretti S, Montironi R, Manola J, et al. Her-2-neu expression and progression toward androgen independence in human prostate cancer. *J Natl Cancer Inst* 2000;92(23):1918–1925.

129. Slamon DJ, Clark GM, Wong SG, et al. Human breast cancer: correlation of relapse and survival with amplification of the HER-2/neu oncogene. *Science* 1987;235(4785):177–182.

130. Slamon DJ, Leyland-Jones B, Shak S, et al. Use of chemotherapy plus a monoclonal antibody against HER2 for metastatic breast cancer that overexpresses HER2. *N Engl J Med* 2001;344(11):783–792.

131. Lara PN Jr, Chee KG, Longmate J, et al. Trastuzumab plus docetaxel in HER-2/neu-positive prostate carcinoma: final results from the California Cancer Consortium Screening and Phase II Trial. *Cancer* 2004;100(10): 2125–2131.

132. Druker BJ, Talpaz M, Resta DJ, et al. Efficacy and safety of a specific inhibitor of the BCR-ABL tyrosine kinase in chronic myeloid leukemia. *N Engl J Med* 2001;344(14):1031–1037.

133. Druker BJ, Sawyers CL, Kantarjian H, et al. Activity of a specific inhibitor of the BCR-ABL tyrosine kinase in the blast crisis of chronic myeloid leukemia and acute lymphoblastic leukemia with the Philadelphia chromosome. *N Engl J Med* 2001;344(14):1038–1042.

134. Mathew P, Fidler IJ, Logothetis CJ. Combination docetaxel and platelet-derived growth factor receptor inhibition with imatinib mesylate in prostate cancer. *Semin Oncol* 2004;31(2 Suppl. 6):24–29.

135. Vivanco I, Sawyers CL. The phosphatidylinositol 3-kinase AKT pathway in human cancer. *Nat Rev Cancer* 2002;2(7):489–501.

136. Cantley LC. The phosphoinositide 3-kinase pathway. *Science* 2002;296 (5573):1655–1657.

137. Fingar DC, Richardson CJ, Tee AR, et al. mTOR controls cell cycle progression through its cell growth effectors S6K1 and 4E-BP1/eukaryotic translation initiation factor 4E. *Mol Cell Biol* 2004;24(1):200–216.

138. Neshat MS, Mellinghoff IK, Tran C, et al. Enhanced sensitivity of PTEN-deficient tumors to inhibition of FRAP/mTOR. *Proc Natl Acad Sci U S A* 2001;98(18):10314–10319.

139. Dudkin L, Dilling MB, Cheshire PJ, et al. Biochemical correlates of mTOR inhibition by the rapamycin ester CCI-779 and tumor growth inhibition. *Clin Cancer Res* 2001;7(6):1758–1764.

140. Peralba JM, DeGraffenried L, Friedrichs W, et al. Pharmacodynamic evaluation of CCI-779, an inhibitor of mTOR, in cancer patients. *Clin Cancer Res* 2003;9(8):2887–2892.

141. Luo J, Manning BD, Cantley LC. Targeting the PI3K-Akt pathway in human cancer: rationale and promise. *Cancer Cell* 2003;4(4):257–262.

142. Paez JG, Janne PA, Lee JC, et al. EGFR mutations in lung cancer: correlation with clinical response to gefitinib therapy. *Science* 2004;304(5676): 1497–1500.

143. Hanahan D, Folkman J. Patterns and emerging mechanisms of the angiogenic switch during tumorigenesis. *Cell* 1996;86(3):353–364.

144. D'Amato RJ, Loughnan MS, Flynn E, et al. Thalidomide is an inhibitor of angiogenesis. *Proc Natl Acad Sci U S A* 1994;91(9):4082–4085.

145. Figg WD, Dahut W, Duray P, et al. A randomized phase II trial of thalidomide, an angiogenesis inhibitor, in patients with androgen-independent prostate cancer. *Clin Cancer Res* 2001;7(7):1888–1893.

146. George D, Oh W, Gilligan T, et al. Phase I study of the novel, oral angiogenesis inhibitor PTK787/ZK 222584 (PTK/ZK): evaluation of the pharmacokinetic effect of high-fat meal in patients with hormone-refractory prostate cancer (HRPC). *Proc Am Soc Clin Oncol* 2004;22(14S):4689.

147. Picus J, Halabi S, Rini B, et al. The use of bevacizumab (B) with docetaxel (D) and estramustine (E) in hormone refractory prostate cancer (HRPC): initial results of CALGB 90006. *Proc Am Soc Clin Oncol* 2003;22:393; Abstract 1578.

148. Wedge SR, Ogilvie DJ, Dukes M, et al. ZD6474 inhibits vascular endothelial growth factor signaling, angiogenesis, and tumor growth following oral administration. *Cancer Res* 2002;62(16):4645–4655.

149. Heymach JV, Dong RP, Dimery I, et al. ZD6474, a novel antiangiogenic agent, in combination with docetaxel in patients with NSCLC: results of the run-in phase of a two-part, randomized phase II study. *Proc Am Soc Clin Oncol* 2004;22(14S):3051.

150. Medinger M, Mross K, Zirrgiebel U, et al. Phase I dose-escalation study of the highly potent VEGF receptor kinase inhibitor, AZD2171, in patients with advanced cancers wtih liver metastases. *Proc Am Soc Clin Oncol* 2004;22(14S):3055.

151. Fong L, Small EJ. Immunotherapy for prostate cancer. *Semin Oncol* 2003; 30(5):649–658.

152. Kantoff PW, Carroll PR, D'Amico AV eds., et al. Prostate cancer: principles and practice. In: Kantoff PW, Scher HI, ed. (1st ed.) Philadelphia: Lippincott Williams & Wilkins, 2002:708–720.

153. Small EJ, Fratesi P, Reese DM, et al. Immunotherapy of hormone-refractory prostate cancer with antigen-loaded dendritic cells. *J Clin Oncol* 2000; 18(23):3894–3903.

154. Small EJ, Rini B, Higano C, et al. A randomized, placebo-controlled phase III trial of APC8015 in patients with androgen-independent prostate cancer (AiPCa). *Proc Am Soc Clin Oncol* 2003;22(14S): Abstract 1534.

155. Kaufman HL, Wang W, Manola J, et al. Phase II randomized study of vaccine treatment of advanced prostate cancer (E7897): a trial of the Eastern Cooperative Oncology Group. *J Clin Oncol* 2004;22(11):2122–2132.

156. DiPaola RS, Plante M, Petrylak D, et al. A phase I trial of PROSTAVAC-VF/TRICOM vaccination in patients with prostate cancer. *AACR* 2004;45:1035; Abstract 4485.

157. Arlen PM, Gulley J, Dahut W, et al. A phase I study of sequential vaccinations with recombinant Fowlpox-PSA (L155)-TRICOM (rF) alone, or in combination with recombinant vaccinia-PSA (L155)-TRICOM (rV), and the role of GM-CSF, in patients (Pts) with prostate cancer. *Proc Am Soc Clin Oncol* 2004;22(14S): Abstract 2522.

158. Zetter BR. The cellular basis of site-specific tumor metastasis. *N Engl J Med* 1990;322(9):605–612.

159. Jacobs SC. Spread of prostatic cancer to bone. *Urology* 1983;21(4): 337–344.

160. Battistini B, Chailler P, D'Orleans-Juste P, et al. Growth regulatory properties of endothelins. *Peptides* 1993;14(2):385–399.

161. Nelson JB, Hedican SP, George DJ, et al. Identification of endothelin-1 in the pathophysiology of metastatic adenocarcinoma of the prostate. *Nat Med* 1995;1(9):944–949.

162. Opgenorth TJ, Adler AL, Calzadilla SV, et al. Pharmacological characterization of A-127722: an orally active and highly potent ETA-selective receptor antagonist. *J Pharmacol Exp Ther* 1996;276(2):473–481.

163. Carducci MA, Padley RJ, Breul J, et al. Effect of endothelin-A receptor blockade with Atrasentan on tumor progression in men with hormone-refractory prostate cancer: a randomized, phase II, placebo-controlled trial. *J Clin Oncol* 2003;21(4):679–689.

164. Lipton A, Sleep DJ, Hulting SM, et al. Benefit of Atrasentan in men with hormone refractory prostate cancer metastatic to bone. *Proc Am Soc Clin Oncol* 2004;22 (14S): Abstract 4687.

165. Yount S, Cella D, Mulani P, et al. Impact of Atrasentan on prostate-specific outcomes with hormone refractory prostate cancer patients. *Proc Am Soc Clin Oncol* 2004;22(14S): Abstract 4582.

166. Raffo AJ, Perlman H, Chen MW, et al. Overexpression of bcl-2 protects prostate cancer cells from apoptosis in vitro and confers resistance to androgen depletion in vivo. *Cancer Res* 1995;55(19):4438–4445.

167. McDonnell TJ, Troncoso P, Brisbay SM, et al. Expression of the protooncogene bcl-2 in the prostate and its association with emergence of androgen-independent prostate cancer. *Cancer Res* 1992;52(24):6940–6944.

168. Chi KN, Murray RN, Gleave ME, et al. A phase II study of oblimersen sodium (G3139) and docetaxel (D) in patients (pts) with metastatic hormone-refractory prostate cancer (HRPC). *Proc Am Soc Clin Oncol* 2003; 22:393; Abstract 1580.

169. DiPaola RS, Rafi MM, Vyas V, et al. Phase I clinical and pharmacologic study of 13-cis-retinoic acid, interferon alfa, and paclitaxel in patients with prostate cancer and other advanced malignancies. *J Clin Oncol* 1999; 17(7):2213–2218.

170. DiPaola RS, Manola J, Li S, et al. A randomized phase II trial of mitoxantrone, estramustine and vinorelbine or 13-cis retinoic acid, interferon and paclitaxel in patients with metastatic hormone refractory prostate cancer: results of ECOG 3899. 2004 ASCO Meeting 2004;22(14S): Abstract 4594.

171. Beer TM, Myrthue A. Calcitriol in cancer treatment: from the lab to the clinic. *Mol Cancer Ther* 2004;3(3):373–381.

172. Beer TM, Eilers KM, Garzotto M, et al. Quality of life and pain relief during treatment with calcitriol and docetaxel in symptomatic metastatic androgen-independent prostate carcinoma. *Cancer* 2004;100(4):758–763.

173. Suh J, Rabson AB. NF-kappaB activation in human prostate cancer: important mediator or epiphenomenon? *J Cell Biochem* 2004;91(1):100–117.

174. Voorhees PM, Dees EC, O'Neil B, et al. The proteasome as a target for cancer therapy. *Clin Cancer Res* 2003;9(17):6316–6325.

175. Dreicer R, Roth B, Petrylak D, et al. Phase I/II trial of bortezomib plus docetaxel in patients with advanced androgen-independent prostate cancer. *Proc Am Soc Clin Oncol* 2004;22(14S):4654; Abstract.

CHAPTER 17 ■ CLINICAL SIGNS AND SYMPTOMS OF BLADDER CANCER

NIALL M. HENEY

GROSS HEMATURIA

The vast majority of bladder cancers are diagnosed as a result of evaluating a patient for hematuria (1). Total gross painless hematuria (TGPH) is a symptom that mandates further evaluation. In total hematuria, blood is present in the urine throughout micturition, rather than initial or terminal hematuria, in which blood is seen only at the beginning or end of micturition, respectively. The significance of total hematuria is that the blood has originated from the bladder or upper tracts. Bleeding from the bladder neck region or trigone may result in terminal hematuria; bleeding from the prostate or urethra causes initial hematuria. Pain in association with hematuria suggests an inflammatory component and should trigger a search for infection or calculus formation. Of 95 patients with TGPH at a hematuria diagnostic unit, 12 were found to have bladder carcinoma (2). In a similar study of 1,000 consecutive patients with TGPH, 15% had bladder carcinoma (3). Upper-tract bleeding may cause ureteral colic, especially if clots form. Upper-tract clots may be vermiform or spaghetti-like, whereas bladder clots are shapeless.

Hematuria associated with irritative symptoms, such as frequency, dysuria, and urgency, should not lull the physician into assuming that the bleeding has a nonneoplastic origin. Any bleeding in the urine should be a cause for concern, and evaluation should be aimed at ruling out a life-threatening cause. Urine may be turned red by eating beets. Runners' hematuria is a benign condition and occurs after running (4).

MICROSCOPIC HEMATURIA

Microscopic hematuria, or microhematuria, may be symptomatic or asymptomatic. Asymptomatic microhematuria can occur in 13% of the general population, although in a population-based study in Minnesota, urothelial neoplasia was found in only 0.4% of patients (5). Few of these patients underwent full evaluation initially, but they were followed for three or more years without significant additional concerns arising. On the other hand, a study of 246 patients with asymptomatic microhematuria referred for urologic evaluation showed that 14% had a highly significant cause for their bleeding and 16 (6.5%) had bladder cancer (6).

Although the indications for urologic evaluation may seem clear-cut in patients with TGPH or asymptomatic microhematuria, the clinical picture may often be ambiguous. Patients, especially those with carcinoma in situ (CIS) or invasive disease, often have urinary frequency, urgency, burning dysuria, or combinations of the three. In addition, there may be microscopic hematuria. Studies that have quantitated the amount of microhematuria have shown poor correlation between the number of red blood cells (RBCs) per high-power field and the probability of significant disease (5). Although the high prevalence (13%) of microhematuria in the general population argues against full evaluation of all patients in whose urine a few RBCs are found, the repetition of this finding should be cause for concern. If urine is found to be dipstick-positive, it is wise to study the voided urine under the microscope to confirm the presence of RBCs. It may be helpful to do a three-glass test, wherein the spun sediment of the initial, midstream, and terminal urine is examined microscopically to identify the source of the bleeding. RBCs in the initial specimen and not in the midstream or terminal specimens suggest a urethral source, whereas blood cells in similar numbers in all three specimens suggest bladder or upper-tract bleeding.

Evaluation for renal parenchymal disease and urinary tract infection should be performed. In the absence of infection or bladder outlet obstruction, the possibility of neurogenic bladder, vesical calculus, neoplasm, or CIS should be considered, in which case ultrasound of the kidneys and bladder and/or excretion urography with tomography or I+ and I− computed tomography (CT) and urinary cytology should be performed, as they provide additional critical information. Patients with urinary calculi usually shed RBCs in the urine, and urinary cytology is more difficult to interpret in the presence of calculi. Nevertheless, a negative cytologic study is a reassuring finding, although it is not conclusive because well-differentiated and moderately differentiated transitional cell tumors have a high false-negative rate. High-grade transitional cell carcinoma has a false-negative rate of approximately 20%. Flow cytometry has automated the technology of cytologic evaluation, but it is bedeviled by the same limitations as standard cytology. The probability of missing a bladder tumor through cytologic testing is reduced by combining cytologic testing with bladder washings (7), which involves irrigating the bladder with 50 mL of normal saline through a cystoscope or catheter.

The detection of various bladder tumor markers in urine has enhanced our ability to diagnose bladder cancer noninvasively. Nuclear matrix protein (NMP22) and bladder tumor antigen (BTA-stat) are now in routine clinical use (8,9). Fluorescence in situ hybridization assay (FISH) offers greater sensitivity than NMP22, BTA-stat, or voided urine cytology. FISH specificity is less than cytology but better than NMP22 or BTA-stat (10,11).

The sensitivity and specificity of NMP22 was 67% and 84%, compared with 40% and 99% for urine cytology (8). The overall sensitivity of BTA was 40%, versus 16% for cytology, and the specificity of BTA ranged from 82% to 96% for various urologic conditions and normal subjects (9). Sarsody reported the sensitivity for FISH versus BTA and cytology was 71%, 50%, and 26% respectively (10), with FISH specificity of 94.5% (10). Bladder tumor marker assays may be best used in combination with urine cytology.

Patients with unexplained hematuria usually require intravenous urography or retrograde pyelography to evaluate the bladder and upper tracts. Some centers have replaced excretion urography with computed tomography using IV contrast. This provides the most detailed information about the kidneys, ureters, and bladder, with reformatting providing additional perspectives.

Occasionally, a patient harboring a bladder cancer will observe pain or irritative or obstructive symptoms. If such symptoms are associated with hematuria, a full evaluation is required. CIS of the bladder may be difficult to diagnose and may masquerade as interstitial cystitis (12) or prostatitis. The clinician must consider CIS or other forms of bladder cancer if irritative symptoms are persistent or recurrent. Patients who are heavy smokers, who are exposed to known industrial carcinogens or cyclophosphamide, and who have indwelling catheters for many years should be considered at risk for bladder cancer.

Bladder cancer may cause symptoms of bladder outlet obstruction, retention, pelvic fullness, suprapubic discomfort or pressure, or suprapubic mass. Rarely, evidence of metastatic disease may be present, with systemic symptoms of anorexia, weight loss, or pelvic pain or weakness.

Physical Examination

The physical examination usually is unremarkable in patients with bladder cancer. Rarely is a solid pelvic mass felt, and when it is, the condition is usually advanced. If the bladder cancer involves the prostate substance, induration of that organ may be felt on digital rectal examination (DRE). DRE should not be an assessment of the prostate only. An attempt should be made to palpate the base and lateral walls of the bladder, with the physician seeking induration, thickening, or fixation. The rectal wall should be carefully palpated. In women, a careful bimanual examination should be performed and include the vagina and the rectum, although a negative examination does not rule out bladder cancer. The vast majority of bladder cancers are not palpable, as they involve only the urothelium and lamina propria. Tumors that invade muscle may not be palpable, even under anesthesia. Large, widely infiltrating tumors that have invaded deeply into or through the bladder wall may be palpable, however, especially if they are fixed to the pelvic side wall or vagina. Physical examination should include careful palpation of the urethra and the vagina. Inguinal adenopathy may be found. Nodularity in the periumbilical region may be seen in advanced urachal tumors.

CYTOSCOPY

Modern flexible cystoscopes permit almost painless inspections of the urinary bladder. Under intraurethral lidocaine anesthesia, the urethra and bladder can be inspected. This test is diagnostic if a tumor is found. Unfortunately, the converse is not true. Rarely, patient discomfort or bleeding may compromise the study. If so, cystoscopy under either spinal or general anesthesia should be scheduled. In women, the rigid 15.5 Fr. cystoscope provides excellent visualization of the bladder interior. Bladder barbotage may be performed using 50 mL of saline to obtain fluid for cytology or flow cytometry.

Occasionally, office cystoscopy is unnecessary, especially if the urine cytology has been shown to be positive for malignant cells or if intravenous pyelogram, ultrasound, or CT has shown a constant filling defect in the bladder. Under these circumstances, cystourethroscopy should be performed under anesthesia. At this time, a bimanual examination can be performed with the bladder empty. Cystoscopic urine or bladder washings or both can be obtained. Careful inspection of the urethra, including the prostatic urethra, can be performed, and the bladder can be inspected using 30-degree, 70-degree, and 120-degree lenses. A bladder diagram should be completed during or immediately after cystoscopy. The entire bladder interior should be visualized. Papillary or nodular tumor is usually evident. Tumor proximity to ureters and the bladder neck should be particularly noted and recorded. A careful search should be made for flat, velvety erythematous areas, which might harbor CIS, especially in patients with irritative symptoms. Cold-cup biopsies of suspicious areas should be obtained, in addition to selected mucosal biopsy specimens from areas that may not seem very abnormal (13). Biopsies of tumors and prostatic urethra should be performed.

After biopsy specimens have been obtained, transurethral resection (TUR) of all visible tumor should be performed (if possible). The resectionist should obtain underlying muscle for staging purposes. If muscle is not included, the patient's disease cannot be fully staged. While performing the tumor resection, the surgeon has a unique opportunity to assess the depth and extent of tumor invasion. The surgeon often can determine transmural invasion if yellow fat is seen and can formulate an opinion as to the completeness of the resection. If the ureteral orifices are involved, they should be resected. Subsequent stenosis of the ureter is very unlikely.

After completing the resection, the urologist should diagram the location of residual disease and should repeat bimanual examination if it was positive before resection. Transurethral laser ablation of bladder cancer is an option but is more appropriate for recurrent, low-grade superficial tumors not requiring biopsy for histologic evaluation.

References

1. Varkarakis MJ, Gaeta J, Moore RH, et al. Superficial bladder tumor. Aspect of clinical progression. *Urology* 1974;4:414.
2. Turner AG, Hendry WF, Williams GB, et al. Haematuria diagnostic service. *BMJ* 1977;2:29.
3. Lee LW, Davis E Jr. Gross urinary hemorrhage: a symptom, not a disease. *JAMA* 1953;153:782.
4. Siegal AJ, Hennekens CH, Solomon HS, et al. Exercise-related hematuria. *JAMA* 1979;241:391.
5. Mohr DN, Offord KP, Owen RA, et al. Asymptomatic microhematuria and urologic disease. A population-based study. *JAMA* 1986;256:224.
6. Golin AL, Howard RS. Asymptomatic microscopic hematuria. *J Urol* 1980;124:389.
7. Zein T, Wajsman Z, Englander LS, et al. Evaluation of bladder washings and urine cytology in the diagnosis of bladder cancer and its correlation with selected biopsies of the bladder mucosa. *J Urol* 1984;132:670.
8. Stampfer DS, Carpinito GA, Rodruguez-Villanueva J, et al. Evaluation of NMP22 in the detection of transitional cell carcinoma of the bladder. *J Urol* 1998;159:394.
9. Sarosdy MF, deVere White RW, Soloway MS, et al. Results of multicenter trial using the BTA test to monitor for and diagnose recurrent bladder cancer. *J Urol* 1995;154:379.
10. Sarosdy MF, Schellhammer P, Bokinsky G, et al. Clinical evaluation of a multi-target fluorescent in situ hybridization assay for detection of bladder cancer. *J Urol* 2002;168(5):1950.
11. Friedrich MG, Toma MI, Hellstern A, et al. Comparison of multitarget fluorescence in situ hybridization in urine with other noninvasive tests for detecting bladder cancer. *BJU Int* 2003;92(9):911.
12. Utz DC, Hanash KA, Farrow GM. Plight of patient with carcinoma in situ of bladder. *J Urol* 1970;103:160.
13. Heney NM, Szfelbein W, Daly JJ, et al. Positive urinary cytology in patients without evident tumor. *J Urol* 1977;177:223.

CHAPTER 18 ■ THE EPIDEMIOLOGY OF BLADDER CANCER

RONALD K. ROSS, MIMI C. YU, AND JIAN-MIN YUAN

INTRODUCTION AND OVERVIEW

One of the earliest established etiologic, exposure–cancer relationships was between exposures encountered during the manufacturing of synthetic dyes and subsequent bladder cancer development. There were hints of such a relationship by the late 1800s, strong anecdotal evidence by the early 20th century, supportive experimental evidence by the 1930s (that began to pinpoint the carcinogenic chemical exposure to specific arylamines), and strong systematic epidemiologic evidence by the early 1950s (1,2). Also in the 1950s, the first convincing epidemiologic evidence was published that cigarette smoking was by far the most important exposure contributing to bladder cancer development on a population basis (3,4). This smoking and bladder cancer relationship was over time shown to be a highly reproducible finding that extended across genders and many populations worldwide, with estimates from many recent studies indicating that smoking alone could explain half of all bladder cancer occurrence in most Western populations (5–7). This recognition, combined with a series of largely nonproductive major epidemiologic studies in the 1970s to establish other exposures as major contributors to bladder cancer development, such as artificial sweetener use and coffee drinking, has led to substantial neglect by epidemiologists in recent decades in developing any additional hypotheses or in conducting additional major studies to further understand the epidemiology and etiology of this important disease.

The epidemiology of bladder cancer is not, as one might predict, that of a disease whose main established risk factors are cigarette smoking and occupational exposure to arylamines. Although men are at substantially greater risk than women, as predicted from the epidemiology of cigarette smoking, white men have substantially higher rates than African–American men (or for that matter higher than any other racial–ethnic group), which is not as predicted, nor is the strong positive relationship between socioeconomic status and risk. Moreover, there exist many populations around the world with high smoking rates, and consistent with these, high lung cancer rates, yet relatively low bladder cancer rates. These patterns of occurrence strongly suggest that there are still important additional, but as yet unidentified, risk factors, protective factors, or environmental- or genetic-risk modifiers that contribute to bladder cancer susceptibility.

The reason that cigarettes cause bladder cancer has not been definitively established, but it is generally believed that this association is due to small amounts of the same arylamines in cigarette smoke known to cause bladder cancer in occupational settings. Recent evidence suggests that use of permanent hair dyes might also be both an additional substantial population source of arylamines, as well as a substantial contributor to bladder cancer risk, especially among women.

Recent work looking at probable important biomarkers of bladder cancer risk (i.e., arylamine adducts to hemoglobin) strongly suggests that there are additional important arylamines that predict bladder cancer risk, but the main source of exposure remains unknown. Even for established carcinogenic arylamines to the bladder, such as 4-aminobiphenyl hemoglobin adduct, data suggest that major additional unknown sources of exposure exist. Data suggest that genetically determined modification of arylamine metabolism can affect individual bladder cancer risk, no matter what the underlying source of arylamine exposure.

In this chapter, we begin by reviewing the unique demographic patterns of bladder cancer, focusing especially on racial–ethnic variation in risk, socioeconomic characteristics, and bladder cancer risk patterns, and time trends in bladder cancer incidence over the past several decades. While we focus on patterns in a large urban area of the United States, the observed patterns are generally representative of national patterns, and we also provide some international rates for comparative purposes. Bladder cancer, at least in endemic areas, occurs in two major histopathologic subgroups: superficial, papillary transitional-cell bladder cancer with a highly favorable prognosis but with a tendency to occur with multiple lesions and to recur after surgical treatment, and invasive transitional cell bladder cancer with a substantially poorer average survival. We provide comparisons on demographic characteristics for these two major subgroups as well. We then review in detail the epidemiologic and related evidence for the well-established bladder cancer risk or protective factors. We also review and summarize the epidemiologic evidence for some potential bladder cancer risk factors, which have been extensively studied but largely dismissed as significant contributors to bladder cancer occurrence. Finally we discuss areas where there is clearly a need for additional research, including the current status of biomarker research and genetically determined risk modification.

DEMOGRAPHICS

Bladder cancer shows an almost 20-fold international variation in incidence. High-risk populations include non-Latino whites in the United States and most Western Europeans with age-standardized rates (per world population) in men close to 40 per 100,000 population per year. Asians (including Chinese, Japanese, and Indians) are at low risk for bladder cancer, with annual age-standardized rates in men of around 3 to 7 per 100,000 (8).

Age, Sex, and Race

Bladder cancer currently ranks 4th in incidence among all cancers in American men, whereas it ranks only 11th among cancers

357

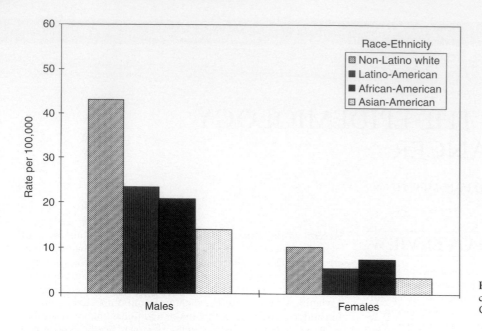

FIGURE 18.1. Incidence rates of bladder cancer by race ethnicity in Los Angeles County, California, 1990–1999.

in women (8). The disease is rare prior to age 35, and two-thirds of cases occur in people aged 65 or older. The huge excess in men is among the most prominent epidemiologic features of bladder cancer. Men overall have a fourfold excess of bladder cancer compared with women, and the male excess is observed to a somewhat comparable degree across all major racial–ethnic groups.

Bladder cancer is a disease for which non-Latino whites are at very high risk relative to other racial groups. In Los Angeles from 1990 to 1999, for example, the age-adjusted incidence rate of bladder cancer in non-Latino white men was approximately twice as high as that in African-American or Latino men. Asian-American men had rates which were lower still, roughly one-third that of non-Latino white men, although there is some variation in rates among the major Asian-American ethnic groups. Women showed a somewhat comparable pattern by race ethnicity, albeit at substantially lower absolute-risk levels (Fig. 18.1).

Social Class

Some population-based cancer registries classify cancer patients according to social class characteristics based on their places of residence. Specifically, census information on income and/or educational levels of residents in the neighborhoods where cancer patients reside is used to rank cancer cases (e.g., in Los Angeles, patients are placed into one of five social-class groupings). Figure 18.2 shows that, in general, high social class individuals, whether white or black or either sex, have a higher risk of bladder cancer.

Time Trends

In the United States, the incidence of bladder cancer in both men and women has been relatively stable during the past

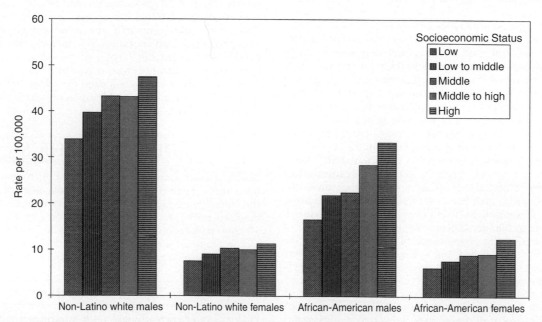

FIGURE 18.2. Incidence rates of bladder cancer by socioeconomic status in non-Latino whites and African-Americans in Los Angeles County, California, 1990–1999.

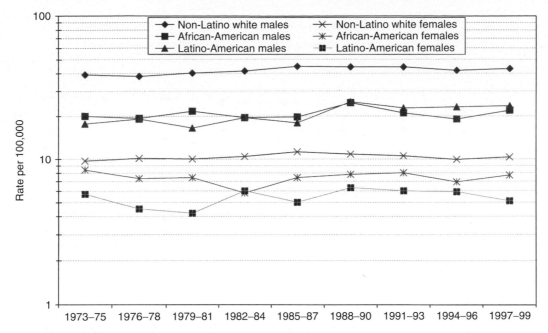

FIGURE 18.3. Secular trends in incidence rates of bladder cancer by sex and major racial–ethnic group in Los Angeles County, California, 1973–1999.

30 years. In Los Angeles, there is no clear indication of declining or increasing incidence among non-Latino whites, African-Americans, or Latinos of either sex (Fig. 18.3).

Histopathology

The uroepithelial cells lining the human bladder can become transformed to tumor cells with different histopathologies. Approximately 93% of tumors of the urinary bladder in the United States are of transitional cell type. The remaining 7% include primarily squamous, glandular, or undifferentiated cell type tumors. In contrast, in Egypt and parts of the Middle East where infection with *Schistosoma haematobium* is endemic, squamous cell carcinoma of the bladder constitutes 55% to 80% of all bladder cancer diagnoses.

Transitional cell carcinoma occurs in two distinct morphologic forms, which have different natural histories and prognoses. Almost two-thirds of transitional cell bladder cancers diagnosed in the Western world are papillary noninfiltrating morphology (i.e., superficial cancer). The remaining transitional cell carcinomas invade the underlying stroma of the bladder (i.e., invasive cancer).

Superficial Versus Invasive Bladder Cancer

Demographic characteristics of superficial and invasive cancers are considerably different. The excess rate of superficial bladder cancer for men over women is somewhat greater than that of invasive bladder cancer. In men, the incidence rate of superficial bladder cancer in non-Latino whites is more than twice that of Latinos or African-Americans, and more than three times that of Asian-Americans. The differences in invasive bladder cancer incidence across racial–ethnic groups, although showing a similar pattern, are smaller than those for superficial bladder cancer. Similar patterns of incidence rates for superficial versus invasive bladder cancer in women are also observed (Table 18.1). Within each race–ethnicity, superficial bladder cancer is twice as common as invasive cancer in non-Latino

white women, while these two histopathologic types of bladder cancer, although at lower absolute risk, are roughly equally distributed in Latino, African-Americans, and Asian-Americans (Table 18.1). By socioeconomic status, although both types show a clear gradient, the difference in superficial cancer incidence between low and high socioeconomic status is greater than that in invasive cancer in both males and females (Table 18.1).

Figure 18.4 shows secular trends of superficial and invasive bladder cancer incidence rates in non-Latino whites in Los Angeles from 1976 to 1999. Incidence rates of superficial

TABLE 18.1

AGE-ADJUSTED INCIDENCE RATES OF SUPERFICIAL AND INVASIVE BLADDER CANCER BY SEX, RACE–ETHNICITY, AND SOCIOECONOMIC STATUS IN LOS ANGELES COUNTY, CALIFORNIA, 1990–1999

	Superficial cancer		Invasive cancer	
	Men	Women	Men	Women
Total	22.5	5.0	11.9	3.4
Race–Ethnicity				
Non-Latino Whites	28.9	6.4	14.2	3.9
Latino-Americans	14.3	2.9	9.2	2.7
African-Americans	11.3	3.7	9.5	3.9
Asian-Americans	8.8	1.9	5.2	1.6
Socioeconomic Status				
Low	11.2	2.4	8.3	2.7
Low to Middle	16.6	3.9	10.1	3.0
Middle	23.1	5.2	11.6	3.5
Middle to High	26.3	5.4	12.2	3.6
High	29.2	6.9	14.8	3.6

Age-adjustment according to the 2000 US population.

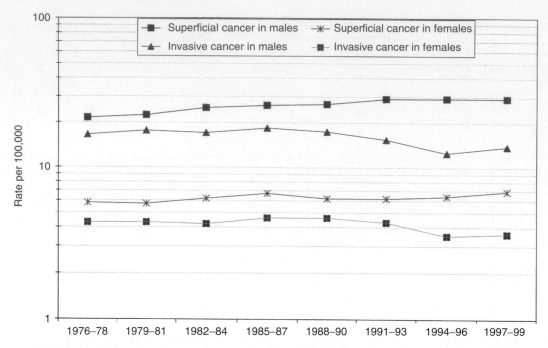

FIGURE 18.4. Secular trends in incidence rates of superficial and invasive bladder cancer in non-Latino whites by gender in Los Angeles County, California, 1976–1999.

bladder cancer have increased while those of invasive bladder cancer have decreased during the past 25 years. The secular trends in men are somewhat stronger than in women.

CIGARETTE SMOKING

The earliest epidemiologic studies on cigarette smoking and bladder cancer were conducted in the 1950s (3,4). Scores of such studies have provided data on this relationship subsequently, although not all were designed specifically for that purpose. Although epidemiologic methods and statistical analytic strategies have improved dramatically since those original studies and much more detail is now known about this relationship, the general conclusion of these first studies was correct: Cigarette smokers, overall, increase their bladder cancer risk some twofold to threefold compared to lifelong nonsmokers. This approximate increase in risk seems to extend across many populations around the world, including multiple racial–ethnic groups. We, and others, have reviewed the individual studies contributing to our understanding of these relationships, and we will not repeat that review here (9). Nonetheless, some additional generalizations can be made about this relationship. Risk of bladder cancer increases with increasing number of cigarettes smoked on a daily basis and with increasing duration of smoking, although it is unclear if this relationship is strictly linear. Risk among ex-smokers is intermediate between current and past smokers, after adjusting for duration and number of cigarettes smoked daily. There is no indication that risk among ex-smokers returns to that of a lifetime nonsmoker even many years after cessation (9). Although cigarette smoking clearly increases bladder cancer risk among both men and women, relative risk appears to be higher in women for a given dose and duration of smoking (10), a finding which is supported by biomarker data on smoking-related carcinogens (11). If inhalation patterns, tar content of cigarettes, or filters modify bladder cancer risk among smokers, the impact of these effects must be very modest as they are not easily detectable by epidemiologic methods. Finally the impact of pipe and cigar smoking on

bladder cancer risk appears to be substantially less than among cigarette smokers. Smokeless tobacco use does not appear to affect risk at all, and environmental tobacco smoke exposure ("passive" smoking) is not yet very well studied in relationship to bladder cancer risk (9).

Although the reason that cigarette smoking causes bladder cancer is unproven, it very likely is due to the presence of carcinogenic arylamines in cigarette smoke including especially 2-naphthylamine and 4-aminobiphenyl (4-ABP) (11). One of the most fascinating features of bladder cancer epidemiology is that, despite the clear importance of cigarette smoking in bladder cancer development as noted above, there exist a number of populations worldwide with high smoking rates and high lung cancer rates in conjunction with these, but relatively low bladder cancer rates (9). In fact, even among different racial–ethnic groups with comparable smoking habits living in the same geographic area, there can be substantial variation in bladder cancer risk, as in Los Angeles.

OCCUPATIONAL EXPOSURES

Although various industries and occupations have been linked to bladder cancer in individual epidemiologic studies, by far the most important, at least historically, is the synthetic dye industry. The historical sequence of events leading to our understanding of this relationship and of the specific etiologic agents involved has been the subject of previous reviews (9). The first synthetic dye, aniline purple, made from aniline, an arylamine present in coal tars, was accidentally formulated in the 1860s. By the late 1800s, synthetic textile dye production was a major industry. The first anecdotal reports of bladder cancer occurring among employees in these chemical dye works were published in 1895, and many others in the United States and Europe followed. Experimental evidence that oral ingestion of 2-naphthylamine, an arylamine extensively used in the manufacturing of industrial dyes, could cause bladder cancer in dogs fueled further interest in a possible etiologic association (12).

Nonetheless, the first systematic epidemiologic evidence that arylamine-exposed chemical dye workers had a large and unequivocal increase in bladder cancer risk was not published until 1954 in London, by Case et al. (2). They observed approximately a 20-fold increase in bladder cancer risk in such workers compared to the general population and concurrently showed that rubber workers, another occupational group with extensive exposure to 2-napthylamine and to benzidene, a chemically related compound, also had substantial elevation in bladder cancer risk.

Other industries and occupations that appear to be at high risk of bladder cancer based on observations from multiple epidemiologic studies include the leather industry, commercial painters, hair dressers, truck drivers, and aluminum workers (13). In fact, many of these associations can be linked to workers in these occupations or industries with exposure to the same arylamines, which have been proven to be human bladder carcinogens in other settings.

ARYLAMINE METABOLISM

The arylamines present in cigarette smoke or in the workplace require metabolic activation to transform into their carcinogenic, reactive metabolites. Hepatic N-hydroxylation, catalyzed by the cytochrome P450 1A2 isoenzyme (CYP1A2), is a critical first step (14). There is some evidence that bioactivation also may take place in extrahepatic tissues, catalyzed by the cyclooxygenases, COX-1 and COX-2 (15). The hydroxylamines are electrophilic and, in circulation, can form adducts with hemoglobin, or can circulate as free or glucuronidated compounds eventually excreted through the kidney. These latter compounds are hydrolyzed in the acidic environment of the bladder lumen, and with or without further local bioactivation by N-acetyltransferase 1 (NAT1) can covalently bind to urothelial DNA. Misrepair of the damage to DNA induced by these adducts can lead to mutations in proto-oncogenes and/or tumor-suppressor genes, a critical step in the process of transforming a normal cell to its malignant phenotype.

Hepatic N-acetylation, catalyzed primarily by NAT2, is a recognized major detoxification pathway for arylamines. There are two distinct phenotypes of NAT2 in humans, commonly labeled as rapid and slow acetylators, respectively, which can be assessed using urine-based bioassays employing caffeine as the metabolic probe (16,17). There is strong epidemiological evidence that NAT2 slow acetylators experience a 30% to 50% increase in risk for bladder cancer relative to NAT2 rapid acetylators (18).

Glutathione S-transferase M1 (GSTM1) is part of a family of enzymes that detoxify reactive chemical entities by promoting their conjugation to glutathione. GSTM1 is polymorphic in humans; about half of the US non-Latino white population lack both copies of the gene and hence exhibit no GSTM1 enzymatic activity. Metabolites of several polycyclic aromatic hydrocarbons present in cigarette smoke are known substrates for GSTM1. There is some human evidence that GSTM1 also detoxifies arylamine metabolites (19). There is strong epidemiological evidence that GSTM1-null individuals experience a 30% to 50% increase in risk for bladder cancer compared to those with one or two copies of the gene (20).

HAIR DYES

Hair dyes represent another substantial source of arylamine exposure in humans. In developed countries, including North America, Europe, and Japan, up to 40% of adult women use hair dyes on a regular basis. There are three major types of hair dyes: permanent dyes, semipermanent dyes, and temporary rinses. Permanent dyes are the most common, accounting for roughly three fourths of all hair dye use. Many commercial brands of hair dyes are mutagenic and some are known to contain recognized animal carcinogens (21).

Early studies of bladder cancer risk in hair dye users, conducted in the 1970s and 1980s, reported largely null results. Few of these studies differentiated among the three major types of hair dyes (permanent, semipermanent, or temporary rinses). In the recent Los Angeles study, personal use of hair dyes was assessed according to the types of hair dyes normally used. Women who reported regular and sustained use of permanent hair dyes were found to experience an increased risk of bladder cancer comparable in level to women who smoked. Risk increased with increasing frequency of hair dye applications and with increasing duration of use (22). Among women who were smokers as well as permanent hair dye users, the level of increased bladder cancer risk was approximately the sum of the individual effects from smoking and use of permanent hair dyes (23). This latter statistical observation is compatible with the notion of a common etiologic pathway (i.e., arylamine exposure) linking these two seemingly distinct environmental exposures to bladder cancer development.

If the arylamines in hair dyes are the etiologic agents responsible for bladder cancer development in users, one would predict a stronger hair dye/cancer association in NAT2 slow versus rapid acetylators. Indeed, in the Los Angeles study, women exhibiting the NAT2 slow acetylation phenotype showed a considerably stronger permanent hair-dye/cancer association than those possessing the NAT2 rapid acetylation phenotype (24).

4-aminobiphenyl (4-ABP) is a potent human bladder carcinogen, which may exist as a contaminant in commercially produced 1,4-phenylenediamine, a key component of many permanent hair dyes. A recent study detected the presence of 4-ABP (in parts per billion) in 8 of 11 commercial brands of hair dyes in the United States, and found nursing mothers who were current users of hair dyes to exhibit significantly elevated levels of 4-ABP DNA adducts in epithelial cells from breast milk relative to nursing mothers who were not currently using hair dyes (25).

BLADDER CANCER IN NONSMOKERS

At the most, only 50% of the bladder cancer burden in a given population can be attributed to tobacco smoking. The search for nonsmoking causes of bladder cancer was the goal of numerous studies launched in the last 30 years, and no credible hypothesis has emerged until recently. Using hemoglobin adducts of selected arylamines as biomarkers of exposure, the Los Angeles study demonstrates that among lifelong nonsmokers, bladder cancer risk increases with increasing exposure to 4-ABP (a potent human bladder carcinogen), presumably from diffuse, as-yet-unidentified sources in the environment (26). Even more interesting is the finding that lifelong nonsmokers who develop bladder cancer are also exposed to higher levels of selected anilines that hitherto had not been linked to human bladder cancer (27).

NONSTEROIDAL ANTI-INFLAMMATORY AGENTS

Nonsteroidal anti-inflammatory agents (NSAIDs) are recognized chemopreventive agents for colon cancer, presumably due to their inhibitory actions on the expression of COX-2, an inducible enzyme whose overexpression has been linked to most major forms of cancer, including bladder cancer. There are consistent experimental data indicating NSAIDs as inhibitors of carcinogen-induced bladder cancer in animals (28). Epidemiologic evidence shows regular and sustained users of NSAIDs to possess a lower risk of bladder cancer (29). The degree of protection seems to vary by class of chemical formulation, in general agreement with experimental findings in animals (29).

DIETARY ANTIOXIDANTS

Carotenoids have been shown to prevent carcinogen-induced bladder cancer in animals. Recent human data strongly suggest that dietary carotenoids protect against bladder cancer in smokers, especially current smokers. Moreover, smokers ingesting high levels of carotenoids have lower hemoglobin adduct levels of 3- and 4-ABP (both of which are contained in tobacco smoke) than comparable smokers with lower intake of dietary carotenoids (30).

Nitrosamines are chemicals that can produce bladder cancer in animals. Humans are exposed to nitrosamines or their precursors via tobacco smoke or diet, including cured meats such as hot dogs and salami. Nitrosamines can be formed *in vivo* from ingested nitrates and secondary amines by nitrate-reducing bacteria in the human bladder, and vitamin C can block this *in vivo* nitrosamine formation (31). In addition to dietary carotenoids, recent work also finds vitamin C intake to be protective against bladder cancer in smokers. Smokers consuming high levels of vitamin C also have lower levels of arylamine hemoglobin adducts than comparable smokers with lower intake of vitamin C (30). It should be noted that the usual close correlation between intake of vitamin C and carotenoids precludes any firm conclusions regarding the separate effects of dietary vitamin C and carotenoids on bladder cancer protection. In other words, it is unclear if the observed dietary protective effect is due to carotenoids alone, vitamin C alone, or both.

OTHER RISK/PROTECTIVE FACTORS

Although our understanding of bladder cancer epidemiology and etiology focuses around the important contribution of exposure from various sources to carcinogenic arylamines, a number of other potential risk or protective factors have also been extensively explored over the past several decades in relationship to bladder cancer occurrence.

For example, a large series of epidemiologic studies were conducted, primarily in the 1970s, on the possible relationship between artificial sweetener use and bladder cancer risk (32). Interest in this relationship was stimulated by a series of experimental studies showing that at least two artificial sweeteners, cyclamate and saccharin, could induce bladder tumors in rats, both independently and as enhancers of the effects of other carcinogens (33). Despite the extensive attention given to this topic by epidemiologists, the overall evidence does not support the use of artificial sweeteners as a risk factor for bladder cancer in doses that humans routinely consume (34).

Similarly, the possible role of caffeine-containing beverages in bladder cancer development was the topic of a large series of epidemiologic studies over several decades (35,36). Interest in this relationship was also stimulated initially by laboratory data indicating that caffeine is mutagenic and could enhance the transforming potential of cell lines exposed to established chemical carcinogens (37,38). Although the literature is highly inconsistent, there are a number of "positive" studies on this

relationship (i.e., suggesting that coffee drinkers have a modest increase in risk). One difficulty in establishing this relationship with certainty is that coffee drinking and cigarette smoking are often correlated on a population basis. Although there have been few statistically powerful studies to test this hypothesis in nonsmokers, there have been a few reports supporting this modest association, while others have proven largely negative (39). If caffeine increases risk, the level of increased risk is quite small, probably at the limit of detectability by epidemiologic methods.

Although not a problem in the United States, it is clear that chronic infection with *Schistosoma haemotobium* substantially increases bladder cancer risk (40). The histologic type of bladder cancer linked to schistosomiasis is squamous cell, however, rather than transitional cell, which comprises the vast majority of cases in the United States and Western Europe. As the mechanism to explain this relationship most likely relates to chronic inflammation, it is not surprising that other types of recurrent urinary tract infections are also associated with bladder cancer, again, especially the usually uncommon squamous histologic subtype (41).

Finally, there are weak but reproducible relationships between ionizing radiation exposure and bladder cancer occurrence (42), and between arsenic exposure from drinking water and bladder cancer, as demonstrated particularly in an area of northeastern Taiwan where the triad of chronic arsenic toxicity, skin cancer, and blackfoot disease is accompanied by an apparent excess in bladder cancer (43). However, these two exposures contribute little to the population risk of bladder cancer in the United States or around the world.

In addition to a series of environmental factors that increase risk, there are also several that appear to reduce risk. The relationships between analgesics and certain dietary protective factors are reviewed previously. Not surprisingly, total fluid intake also appears to be associated with reduced risk, presumably by diluting carcinogens in urine and/or by reducing contact time between urine carcinogens and bladder epithelium, by increasing frequency of micturition (44).

References

1. Case RA, Hosker ME. Tumour of the urinary bladder as an occupational disease in the rubber industry in England and Wales. *Br J Prev Soc Med* 1954;8:39–50.
2. Case RA, Hosker ME, Mc DD, et al. Tumours of the urinary bladder in workmen engaged in the manufacture and use of certain dyestuff intermediates in the British chemical industry. I. The role of aniline, benzidine, alpha-naphthylamine, and beta-naphthylamine. *Br J Ind Med* 1954;11:75–104.
3. Lilienfeld AM, Levin ML, Moore GE. The association of smoking with cancer of the urinary bladder in humans. *AMA Arch Intern Med* 1956;98:129–135.
4. Hammond EC, Horn D. Smoking and death rates; report on forty-four months of follow-up of 187,783 men. II. Death rates by cause. *J Am Med Assoc* 1958;166:1294–1308.
5. Doll R, Peto R. The causes of cancer: quantitative estimates of avoidable risks of cancer in the United States today. *J Natl Cancer Inst* 1981;66:1191–1308.
6. Brennan P, Bogillot O, Cordier S, et al. Cigarette smoking and bladder cancer in men: a pooled analysis of 11 case-control studies. *Int J Cancer* 2000;86:289–294.
7. Brennan P, Bogillot O, Greiser E, et al. The contribution of cigarette smoking to bladder cancer in women (pooled European data). *Cancer Causes Control* 2001;12:411–417.
8. Parkin DM, Whelan SL, Ferlay J et al., eds. *Cancer incidence in five continents*, Vol. VIII. Lyon: International Agency for Research on Cancer, 2002.
9. Ross RK, Jones PA, Yu MC. Bladder cancer epidemiology and pathogenesis. *Semin Oncol* 1996;23:536–545.
10. Castelao JE, Yuan JM, Skipper PL, et al. Gender- and smoking-related bladder cancer risk. *J Natl Cancer Inst* 2001;93:538–545.
11. Partrianakos C, Hoffman D. On the analysis of aromatic amines in cigarette smoke. *J Anal Toxicol* 1979;3:150–154.
12. Hueper WC, Wiley FH, Wolfe HD. Experimental production of bladder tumor in dogs by administration of beta-naphthylamine. *J Ind Hyg Toxicol* 1938;20:46–84.

13. Silverman DT, Levin LI, Hoover RN, et al. Occupational risks of bladder cancer in the United States: I. White men. *J Natl Cancer Inst* 1989;81: 1472–1480.

14. Butler MA, Iwasaki M, Guengerich FP, et al. Human cytochrome P-450PA (P-450IA2), the phenacetin O-deethylase, is primarily responsible for the hepatic 3-demethylation of caffeine and N-oxidation of carcinogenic aryl-amines. *Proc Natl Acad Sci U S A* 1989;86:7696–7700.

15. Wiese FW, Thompson PA, Kadlubar FF. Carcinogen substrate specificity of human COX-1 and COX-2. *Carcinogenesis* 2001;22:5–10.

16. Tang BK, Kadar D, Qian L, et al. Caffeine as a metabolic probe: validation of its use for acetylator phenotyping. *Clin Pharmacol Ther* 1991;49: 648–657.

17. Butler MA, Lang NP, Young JF, et al. Determination of CYP1A2 and NAT2 phenotypes in human populations by analysis of caffeine urinary metabolites. *Pharmacogenetics* 1992;2:116–127.

18. Marcus PM, Vineis P, Rothman N. NAT2 slow acetylation and bladder cancer risk: a meta-analysis of 22 case-control studies conducted in the general population. *Pharmacogenetics* 2000;10:115–122.

19. Yu MC, Ross RK, Chan KK, et al. Glutathione S-transferase M1 genotype affects aminobiphenyl-hemoglobin adduct levels in white, black and Asian smokers and nonsmokers. *Cancer Epidemiol Biomarkers Prev* 1995;4: 861–864.

20. Engel LS, Taioli E, Pfeiffer R, et al. Pooled analysis and meta-analysis of glutathione S-transferase M1 and bladder cancer: a HuGE review. *Am J Epidemiol* 2002;156:95–109.

21. IARC Monographs on the Evaluation of Carcinogenic Risk to Humans. *Occupational exposures of hairdressers and barbers and personal use of hair colourants; some hair dyes, cosmetic colourants, industrial dyestuffs and aromatic amines*, Vol. 57. Lyon: International Agency for Research on Cancer, 1993.

22. Gago-Dominguez M, Castelao JE, Yuan JM, et al. Use of permanent hair dyes and bladder-cancer risk. *Int J Cancer* 2001;91:575–579.

23. Gago-Dominguez M, Chan KK, Ross RK, et al. Permanent hair dyes and bladder-cancer risk. *Int J Cancer* 2001;94:905–906.

24. Gago-Dominguez M, Bell DA, Watson MA, et al. Permanent hair dyes and bladder cancer: risk modification by cytochrome P4501A2 and N-acetyltransferases 1 and 2. *Carcinogenesis* 2003;24:483–489.

25. Turesky RJ, Freeman JP, Holland RD, et al. Identification of aminobiphenyl derivatives in commercial hair dyes. *Chem Res Toxicol* 2003;16:1162–1173.

26. Skipper PL, Tannenbaum SR, Ross RK, et al. Nonsmoking-related aryl-amine exposure and bladder cancer risk. *Cancer Epidemiol Biomarkers Prev* 2003;12:503–507.

27. Gan J, Skipper PL, Gago-Dominguez M, et al. Alkylaniline-hemoglobin adducts and risk of nonsmoking-related bladder cancer. *J Natl Cancer Inst* 2004;96:1425–1431.

28. Rao KV, Detrisac CJ, Steele VE, et al. Differential activity of aspirin, keto-profen and sulindac as cancer chemopreventive agents in the mouse urinary bladder. *Carcinogenesis* 1996;17:1435–1438.

29. Castelao JE, Yuan JM, Gago-Dominguez M, et al. Non-steroidal anti-inflammatory drugs and bladder cancer prevention. *Br J Cancer* 2000;82: 1364–1369.

30. Castelao JE, Yuan JM, Gago-Dominguez M, et al. Carotenoids/vitamin C and smoking-related bladder cancer. *Int J Cancer* 2004;110:417–423.

31. Bartsch H, Pignatelli B, Calmels S, et al. Inhibition of nitrosation. *Basic Life Sci* 1993;61:27–44.

32. Ross RK, Paganini-Hill A, Henderson BE. Epidemiology of bladder cancer. In: Skinner D, Lieskovsky G, eds. *Diagnosis and management of genitourinary cancer*. Philadelphia, PA: WB Saunders, 1988:23–31.

33. Hicks RM, Wakefield JS, Chowaniec J. Letter: co-carcinogenic action of saccharin in the chemical induction of bladder cancer. *Nature* 1973;243: 347–349.

34. Elcock M, Morgan RW. Update on artificial sweeteners and bladder cancer. *Regul Toxicol Pharmacol* 1993;17:35–43.

35. Simon D, Yen S, Cole P. Coffee drinking and cancer of the lower urinary tract. *J Natl Cancer Inst* 1975;54:587–591.

36. Wynder EL, Goldsmith R. The epidemiology of bladder cancer: a second look. *Cancer* 1977;40:1246–1268.

37. Donovan PJ, DiPaolo JA. Caffeine enhancement of chemical carcinogen-induced transformation of cultured Syrian hamster cells. *Cancer Res* 1974; 34:2720–2727.

38. Kuhlmann W, Fromme HG, Heege EM, et al. The mutagenic action of caffeine in higher organisms. *Cancer Res* 1968;28:2375–2389.

39. Viscoli CM, Lachs MS, Horwitz RI. Bladder cancer and coffee drinking: a summary of case-control research. *Lancet* 1993;341:1432–1437.

40. Badawi AF, Mostafa MH, Probert A, et al. Role of schistosomiasis in human bladder cancer: evidence of association, aetiological factors, and basic mechanisms of carcinogenesis. *Eur J Cancer Prev* 1995;4:45–59.

41. Tawfik HN. Carcinoma of the urinary bladder associated with schistosomiasis in Egypt: the possible causal relationship. In: Miller RW, Watanabe S, Fraumeni JF et al., eds. *Unusual occurrences as clues to cancer etiology*. Tokyo: Japan Scientific Societies Press, 1988:197–209.

42. Romanenko A, Morimura K, Wanibuchi H, et al. Urinary bladder lesions induced by persistent chronic low-dose ionizing radiation. *Cancer Sci* 2003; 94:328–333.

43. Chiou HY, Chiou ST, Hsu YH, et al. Incidence of transitional cell carcinoma and arsenic in drinking water: a follow-up study of 8,102 residents in an arseniasis-endemic area in northeastern Taiwan. *Am J Epidemiol* 2001; 153:411–418.

44. Michaud DS, Spiegelman D, Clinton SK, et al. Fluid intake and the risk of bladder cancer in men. *N Engl J Med* 1999;340:1390–1397.

CHAPTER 19 ■ CYTOLOGY AND PATHOLOGY OF CARCINOMAS OF THE URINARY TRACT

ROBERT H. YOUNG AND GRACE T. MCKEE

CYTOLOGY

Cytologic examination of urine is a widely accepted test which is the first step in the investigation of symptoms relating to the urinary tract. It is both diagnostic as it can reveal malignant cells from a transitional cell carcinoma as well as a monitoring test for patients with a history of bladder cancer. Urinary cytology is especially useful in diagnosing carcinoma *in situ* of the bladder as cystoscopy is often negative in these cases. Cytologic examination of urine detects disease not only in the bladder, but in other areas of the urinary tract including the kidneys, ureters, and urethra. Urine cytology is now firmly established as part of the routine workup of patients with urinary tract symptoms with some of the earliest reports of its efficacy dating back to Sanders (1) and Papanicolaou (2). It plays a very important role in the diagnosis of high-grade transitional cell carcinomas as these tumors tend to shed many obviously malignant cells into the urine. However, low-grade transitional cell carcinomas are much more difficult to diagnose cytologically as these tumors are composed of relatively bland cells (3). Although its major role is in the detection of cancer, cytological examination of urine is also useful in the detection of polyoma virus in patients with kidney transplants, a possible of sign of damage to the transplanted kidney (4), and in diagnosing renal allograft rejection (5). In certain centers urine cytology is used for industrial screening of patients exposed to carcinogens such as aniline dyes. Urine cytology is a useful test to monitor patients with transitional cell carcinomas who have been treated surgically, including those with ileal conduits, as well as those who have chemotherapy or intravesical treatment with Bacillus Calmette-Guerin (BCG), for example. Urine cytology also has a place in the workup of certain renal diseases, such as acute interstitial nephritis and glomerular hematuria (6–8), but is not successful in the detection of renal neoplasms. Another use is in the diagnosis of uncommon infections (9). The sensitivity and specificity of urine cytology is high (10), but marked variability in cytologic diagnosis between pathologists has been demonstrated (11).

Epithelium of the Urinary Tract

Urine is produced in the kidneys, passes from the renal calyces to the renal pelves, then through the ureters into the urinary bladder. The tubules within the kidney are lined by a single layer of renal tubular cells. The other channels are lined by multilayered epithelium known as transitional epithelium or urothelium. The number of cell layers varies from two to three in the calyces to five to seven in the bladder mucosa. In the distended state the bladder epithelium appears to be thinned and composed of fewer layers than in the nondistended bladder. The cells comprising the deeper layers of urothelium are small with round nuclei and a small amount of cytoplasm. The superficial layer is composed of larger cells, each of which may overlap several deeper-layer cells, hence they are referred to as "umbrella" cells. These superficial cells have abundant cytoplasm and more than one nucleus, often just two but occasionally even more.

The bladder trigone in women, particularly in the reproductive age group, is usually lined by squamous, rather than transitional, epithelium. Another type of epithelial cell found in the bladder as a result of the frequent presence of the benign metaplasia lesion, cystitis glandularis, is a columnar cell which has the ability to secrete mucin. Thus, in addition to deep and superficial transitional cells, normal urine may contain squamous cells and columnar glandular cells. Squamous cells in urine of women are often vaginal contaminants and reflect the hormonal changes (and sometimes the dysplastic changes) seen in cervicovaginal smears. In men, squamous cells may derive from the urethra.

Types of Urinary Specimens

Freshly voided midmorning or random urine samples are best for cytologic examination as the cells are usually well preserved. With early morning specimens the cells are degenerated, having been lying in urine for some hours. Three urine samples taken on consecutive days produce the best results, with two samples being better than a single one in the sensitivity for detecting bladder carcinoma (12,13).

Cystoscopy urine. Catheterized urine often contains lubricant, which obscures cellular detail. In addition, cell clusters are usually present, a feature which is abnormal in voided specimens. Hence, it is of the utmost importance that clinicians label urine specimens according to the method of collection to prevent overcalling an instrumented sample.

Bladder washings. This type of specimen is obtained by lavaging the bladder with fluid, usually saline, and retrieving the washings for cytologic examination. Bladder and ureteral wash samples are usually very cellular and contain sheets of epithelial cells that apparently have been sheared off during the procedure. This method of collection has been found to be superior to voided urine (14,15).

Ureteral washings. Each ureter can be lavaged separately to determine whether there is evidence of neoplasia. Ureteral washes, like bladder washes, are usually cellular with large clusters of transitional cells, including both superficial and deeper-layer cells.

Laboratory Processing

Aliquots of urine are centrifuged to concentrate the cells, because urine normally contains few cells. In some laboratories filters are still used to prepare the smear before staining. This produces a rather thick, though cellular, smear with a dark background, often difficult to interpret. A few laboratories use cytospin preparations for urine cytology but many laboratories have converted to processing ThinPrep (Cytyc Corporation, Boxborough, MA). With this method the cells are collected on a filter during processing, and then transferred to the glass slide before staining. The stain used for urine cytology is the Papanicolaou stain, in which the cytoplasm of transitional cells stains a greenish-blue and the nuclei are purple. With ThinPrep the background of the smear is clear and bright, the cells are within the demarcated circle on the glass slide, are clearly visible, and are found in larger numbers than with the Millipore filter preparation (16).

Cytology of Normal Urine

Normal urine contains few cells, comprising both deeper-layer and superficial cells with their characteristic features as mentioned earlier. Small nucleoli are also occasionally present (Fig. 19.1). Deeper-layer transitional cells are smaller and have a higher nuclear/cytoplasmic ratio (Fig. 19.2), bearing some resemblance to metaplastic squamous cells in a cervical (Pap) smear. When transitional cells degenerate, the nuclei become smaller and pyknotic, and the cytoplasm becomes vacuolated and contains lipofuschin pigment in the form of reddish-orange globules of varying size. Benign superficial and intermediate squamous cells are also often noted, particularly in women in whom these cells are vaginal contaminants. In men squamous cells are usually derived from the urethra. Other benign cells that are noted in normal urine are renal tubular cells. These cells are much smaller than transitional cells and are always degenerate, with small pyknotic nuclei and granular cytoplasm. Spermatozoa are occasionally seen in urine samples, and may be accompanied by seminal vesicle cells. The latter are hyperchromatic cells which can look abnormal but are recognized by their cytoplasmic pigment. Rarely, benign columnar cells may be noted in urine specimens. Corpora amylacea, rounded laminated structures derived from the prostate gland, are not uncommon in urine specimens from men.

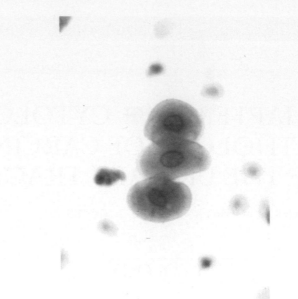

FIGURE 19.2. The three epithelial cells seen in this field are deeper-layer transitional cells. They are smaller than superficial cells and each has only one nucleus. The nuclear/cytoplasmic ratio is higher than that of superficial cells. The cytoplasm is dense.

Crystals can be seen in urine samples. These are of various types: matrix protein crystals, triple phosphate, or cholesterol crystals. Casts also are frequently seen in urine cytology. They may be granular, composed of degenerated renal tubular cells, or hyaline. Large numbers of casts may signify renal disease. They are often associated with calculi of either the kidney or bladder. Catheterized samples and bladder and ureteral washings are much more cellular than normal urine. In addition to single urothelial cells, clusters and sheets are noted, even in benign samples. These groups usually have smooth borders and no cytological features of malignancy (17).

Infections

In the presence of cystitis the preparation shows abundant neutrophils and histiocytes with reactive transitional cells (Fig. 19.3). This is usually due to bacterial infections but other organisms such as *Candida* species may be responsible. Inflammatory cells are also present after radiation and chemotherapy. Carcinoma *in situ* of the bladder, residual tumors, and nonresponding tumors are treated with immunotherapy using intravesical BCG (18,19). Instillation of BCG induces a granulomatous response characterized by epithelioid histiocytes and multinucleated giant cells (20,21) (Fig. 19.4). Both urine cytology and bladder mucosal biopsy are used in patients treated with BCG to assess recurrence (22,23).

Polyoma virus changes are not uncommon in normal urine, but are more often associated with immunosuppression and acute renal allograft complications (24). The cytopathic changes of polyoma virus include single cells with a plasmacytoid appearance as the nucleus is eccentrically placed. There is nuclear enlargement, the nuclear margin is seldom intact, and the chromatin shows degenerative changes, either ground glass in appearance or in the form of a network (Fig. 19.5). At low magnification these cells appear abnormal and can mimic transitional cell carcinoma, hence they have been referred to as decoy cells (25). Large numbers of infected cells are associated with acute renal allograft dysfunction. Other viruses that

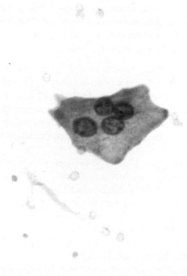

FIGURE 19.1. Superficial transitional (urothelial) cell, also referred to as an umbrella cell. There are four nuclei of relatively uniform size.

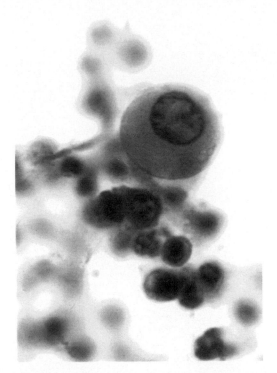

FIGURE 19.3. The deeper-layer transitional cell seen here shows reactive changes in the form of margination of the chromatin as well as a somewhat enlarged nucleus. In the background there are many acute inflammatory cells.

may affect the urinary tract include herpes simplex virus, human papilloma virus, and cytomegalovirus, especially in immunosuppressed patients.

Hematuria

Hematuria may be associated with either renal or other upper- or lower-tract causes. Renal hematuria is accompanied by the

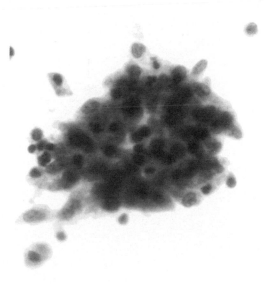

FIGURE 19.4. Urine from patient who had transitional cell carcinoma and was treated with BCG. The cluster of cells in the center of the field represents a granuloma, consisting of epithelioid histiocytes and some lymphocytes.

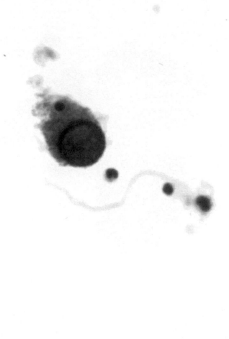

FIGURE 19.5. The cell shown here appears atypical because of the large nucleus. It is a transitional cell showing the cytopathic effects of polyoma virus. These include an eccentrically placed large nucleus which gives the cell a plasmacytoid appearance, and abnormal chromatin, either ground glass as seen here or in the form of a degenerating network.

presence of casts in the urine, both renal tubular and granular types. Red blood cells are lysed by ThinPrep processing and may be difficult to detect. The lysed cells form small clumps of reddish-brown granular material. In addition, 'ghost' or empty red cells are sometimes seen, devoid of hemoglobin. Hematuria associated with urinary tract lesions shows additional features depending on the cause. With cystitis, abundant inflammatory cells are also present. In the presence of bladder calculi, crystals are also seen.

Red blood cells in the urine that originate in the kidney are described as dysmorphic and can be detected by phase-contrast microscopy (26–28), immunocytochemical or immunofluorescent staining (29), or scanning electron microscopy (30).

Urinary Tract Calculi

The cytologic picture includes inflammatory cells, red blood cells that are either ghost cells or lysed, crystalline material, debris, and clusters of transitional cells. The individual cells may show reactive changes in the form of slight nuclear enlargement and small nucleoli. The clusters are usually smooth-bordered (Fig. 19.6) but rarely have irregular borders, mimicking transitional cell carcinoma. However, single cells are not as frequent with calculi as they are in malignant urine. On the other hand, low-grade transitional cell carcinoma can look much less atypical than the cells in patients with calculi (31). Cystoscopy and imaging are necessary to confirm the cytologic diagnosis if carcinoma is suspected.

Malakoplakia

Malakoplakia occurs in the bladder and is more common in women. Michaelis-Gutmann bodies composed of incompletely digested bacteria covered by iron and phosphates are a diagnostic feature (32).

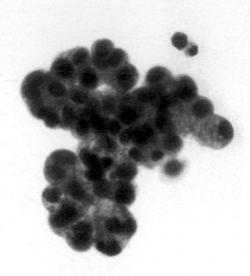

FIGURE 19.6. Clusters of transitional cells in voided urine from a patient with bladder calculi. The cluster has smooth borders and the cells show no atypical features.

Neoplasms of the Urinary Tract

Papillomas

These benign neoplasms, whether of the typical (33) or inverted (34) types, show no specific characteristics on urine cytology.

Grade I Transitional Cell Carcinoma

Only 30% to 60% of grade I carcinomas exfoliate carcinoma cells (35), and only 30% are detected by cytology (36,37). These are difficult to diagnose as malignant in voided urine samples as the cells closely resemble normal urothelial cells. Many single cells are present (Fig. 19.7). These may be columnar or spindled in appearance. Clusters, composed of cells that may appear to be bland or mildly pleomorphic and sometimes spindled, are also noted (Fig. 19.8). Although the cellularity is often increased, the background is clean and inflammatory cells are rare. The cellular changes can be difficult to distinguish from those of calculi as they are often bland with vesicular or finely granular chromatin and inconspicuous nucleoli. These lesions are usually reported either as benign or atypical as there are no features of malignancy. The detection rate for grade I transitional cell carcinomas is notoriously low, so urine cytology is not a reliable screening test for this tumor.

Grade II Transitional Cell Carcinoma

Grade II urothelial carcinomas are composed of cells with appreciable pleomorphism and are more easily detected by urine cytology. Approximately 50% are diagnosed using this method (36,37). Increased cellularity with single malignant cells as well as clusters of tumor cells (Fig. 19.9) are noted in urine. These cells show abnormal, irregular nuclei and granular chromatin. A feature that is often noted is pyknotic, inky-black nuclei in the single neoplastic cells. Tumor cells often appear to be degenerate in cytology samples. Although a definitive diagnosis cannot be made on degenerated cells, there are usually enough viable cells present for a confident interpretation.

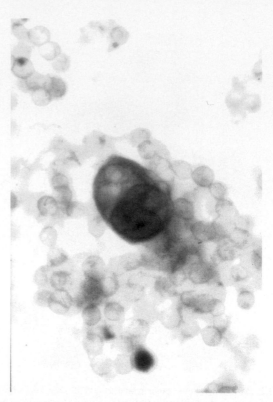

FIGURE 19.7. Single atypical transitional cell surrounded by red blood cells from a grade I transitional cell carcinoma. It looks deceptively bland.

Grade III Transitional Cell Carcinoma

Grade III carcinomas are easily detectable in urine samples. The cellularity is marked with a mixture of single tumor cells, clusters of malignant cells, degenerated cells, and inflammatory cells in a "dirty" background (Fig. 19.10). The neoplastic

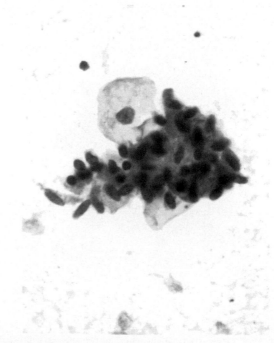

FIGURE 19.8. Cluster of cells from grade I transitional cell carcinoma. Here the cells are small and spindled and there is a superficial cell adjacent for size comparison.

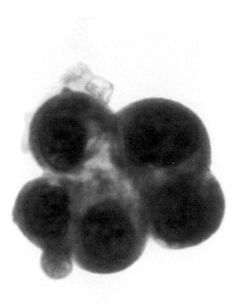

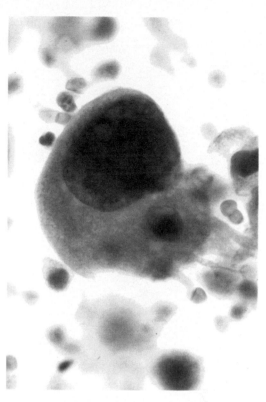

FIGURE 19.9. Cluster of neoplastic cells from a grade II transitional cell carcinoma. There is a high nuclear/cytoplasmic ratio and hyperchromatic nuclei.

FIGURE 19.11. Highly magnified view of a grade III carcinoma cell with an enlarged nucleus and abnormally clumped chromatin.

cells are pleomorphic, varying from round to spindle-shaped, with large, hyperchromatic nuclei and clumped and cleared chromatin (Fig. 19.11). Malignant cells are not always hyperchromatic and sometimes have pale abnormal nuclei. Large nucleoli are frequently seen. When squamous differentiation is present, keratinized malignant cells are noted (Fig. 19.12).

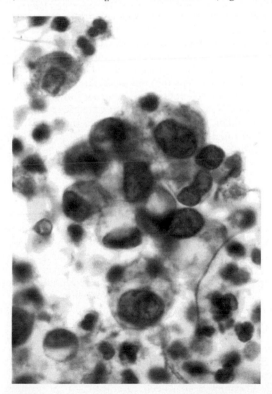

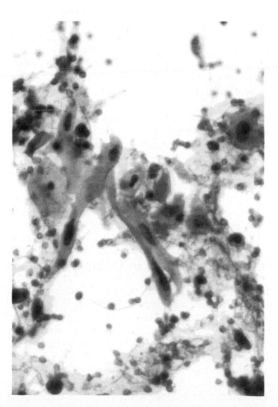

FIGURE 19.10. Cluster of high-grade tumor cells, some vacuolated, accompanied by neutrophil polymorphs and red blood cells.

FIGURE 19.12. Transitional cell carcinoma shows signs of squamous differentiation in the form of keratinized spindled cells with abundant cytoplasm accompanying the smaller neoplastic transitional cells.

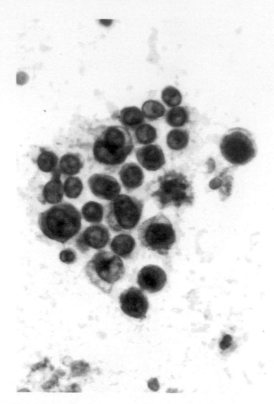

FIGURE 19.13. Abnormal transitional cells are seen in a fairly clean background showing a few red blood cells. The cells vary in size and show an abnormal chromatin pattern. These high-grade cells are from a carcinoma *in situ* that was not visible on cystoscopy.

Carcinoma *In Situ*

Cytology is an important method of detecting this lesion as it is not always visible on cystoscopy. Urine cytology shows abnormal transitional cells, singly (Fig. 19.13) and in clusters. Typically, these samples show a clean background unlike the dirty, inflammatory background of grade III carcinoma. The tumor cells are, however, markedly pleomorphic, resembling high-grade carcinoma cells. Carcinoma *in situ* is diagnosed as a grade III transitional cell carcinoma in 50% of cases (38).

There are occasions when cytology shows evidence of transitional cell carcinoma, either *in situ* or invasive, while cystoscopy and random biopsies are negative. In such cases it may take months before the cytologic diagnosis of carcinoma is verified clinically (39). Urinary cytology is useful in detecting recurrent bladder carcinoma after surgery, chemotherapy, or immunotherapy. Malignant transitional cells in urine originate in sites other than the bladder in 5% to 8% of all transitional cell carcinomas (40,41).

Diagnostic Pitfalls in Urinary Cytology

False-positive cytology is often related to overcalling the atypia seen with cystitis and bladder calculi, especially with the cellular clusters seen in the latter condition. Polyoma virus changes can also mimic malignancy, especially when the infected cells are present in large numbers. Intravesical chemotherapy can produce markedly atypical but degenerate cells that may be mistaken for viable carcinoma cells. Chemotherapy for other cancers necessitating the use of cyclophosphamide, busulphan, and cyclosporin can produce abnormal changes in transitional cells. These changes may be seen 13 to 20 days after starting treatment (42) and include cellular and nuclear enlargement and degeneration without prominent nucleoli or mitoses (Fig. 19.14),

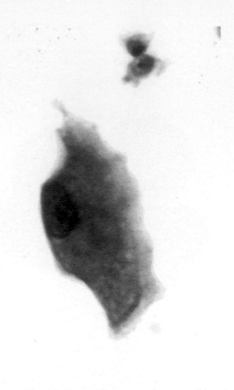

FIGURE 19.14. Atypical transitional cell with abundant cytoplasm. The patient had undergone chemotherapy a few months previously.

but with much background debris (43). However, urothelial carcinoma developed in 5% of cases of hemorrhagic cystitis following cyclophosphamide therapy in one series (44). Postlaser bladder wash specimens contain spindle cells that resemble the spindle cells sometimes seen in low-grade papillary carcinomas (45). Radiation changes noted in voided urine include cellular and nuclear enlargement with multinucleation, hyperchromasia, and prominent nucleoli. The nuclear/cytoplasmic ratio is low and the changes tend to be present in all cells.

False-negative cytologic diagnoses are common with grade I transitional cell carcinomas as they are composed of bland, sometimes columnar, epithelial cells. The presence of abundant inflammatory cells may mask carcinoma cells, also leading to a false-negative report. Three urine samples collected on consecutive days are more likely to detect carcinoma than a single specimen. If a specimen contains malignant cells and this is confirmed on review, normal cystoscopy and biopsy do not exclude a tumor that may have arisen at another site in the urinary tract.

Other Neoplasms

In cases of the uncommon pure squamous cell carcinoma, the cytological features typically consist of malignant cells with keratinized cytoplasm and large hyperchromatic nuclei, but poorly differentiated tumors do not keratinize. Similar features may be seen in cases of the more common transitional cell carcinoma with squamous differentiation.

About 1% of bladder tumors are primary adenocarcinomas arising from cystitis glandularis of intestinal type, urachal remnants, or, rarely, in bladders with extrophy. Gland differentiation is relatively common in cancers that are fundamentally of transitional cell type. Glandular cells have delicate cytoplasm, are often in clusters (Fig. 19.15), and may produce mucin.

The uncommon small-cell carcinoma of the urinary tract may be detectable in some cases (46–48) and should be diagnosed using the criteria applicable in the respiratory tract.

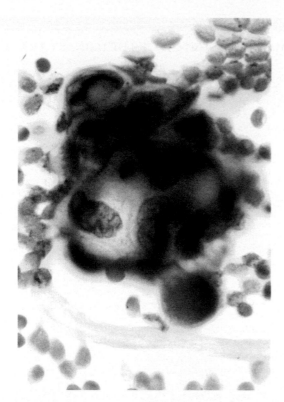

FIGURE 19.15. Cluster of malignant glandular cells in urine. There is vacuolated cytoplasm and nuclei are pushed to the periphery of the cluster. Immunocytochemical staining may be helpful in determining the site of origin of the tumor.

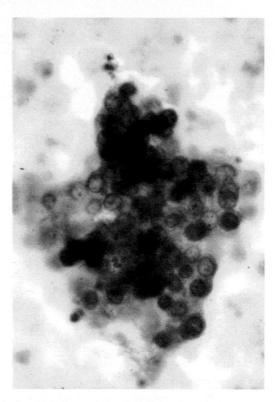

FIGURE 19.16. Group of small adenocarcinoma cells with prominent nucleoli, representing spread from adenocarcinoma of the prostate.

Secondary tumors in the bladder include most commonly squamous cell carcinoma from a cervical carcinoma in women, and, in men, adenocarcinoma from the prostate (Fig. 19.16), but diverse other tumors that metastasize to bladder include breast carcinoma, malignant melanoma, and ovarian carcinoma (49). Cells of a renal cell carcinoma are very rarely found in urine specimens and only seen when there is invasion of the renal pelvis by the tumor.

Ileal Conduit Urine Cytology

Ileal conduits and rectosigmoid segments that function as bladders are constructed following total cystectomy, and regular cytological examination of urine obtained from the new reservoir is used to monitor recurrence of transitional cell carcinoma. This type of specimen contains inflammatory cells, glandular cells from the lining mucosa (Fig. 19.17), mucin, bacteria, and much cellular debris. Recurrent tumors are generally of high grade (41,50). Reported complications following this procedure include stenosis (51,52), the development of adenomas, and adenocarcinomas at or close to the anastomosis site in rectosigmoid bladders (53–55), and squamous cell carcinoma (54).

New Techniques that Complement Urine Cytology

Immunocytochemical Techniques

Carcinoembryonic antigen is detectable in most urothelial neoplasms as is cytokeratin 20 (56) and these tests have been suggested as being of use in diagnosing low-grade transitional cell carcinomas. Other authors claim that a panel of three antibodies

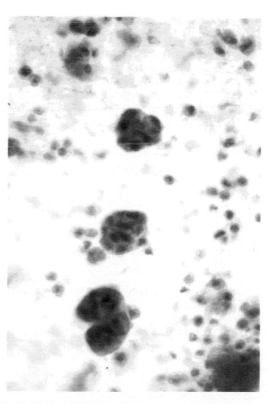

FIGURE 19.17. Small clusters of degenerated glandular cells and inflammatory cells are seen in this specimen of ileal conduit urine.

including cytokeratin 20, p53, and CD44 is more useful (57). Immunocyt is a highly sensitive test which detects cellular markers specific for transitional cell carcinoma in urine (58).

Urine Detection of Survivin

Survivin is a member of the inhibitor-of-apoptosis gene family, and correlates with unfavorable disease and shortened overall survival. It has been found in 78% of bladder cancers but not in normal urothelial cells (59). Its presence in urine samples is detected by a new detection system, confirmed by Western blot and a reverse transcriptase polymerase chain reaction (60).

The BTA (Bladder Tumor Antigen)

This test is useful for the detection of low-grade transitional cell carcinomas but has a high false-positive rate so should be used in conjunction with urine cytology (61,62), but is as informative on its own as in combination with urine cytology according to other authors (63).

NMP22 Immunoassay

The NMP22 (nuclear matrix protein) test is an enzyme immunoassay for nuclear mitotic apparatus protein in voided urine and has a sensitivity of 67% or possibly higher for the high-grade bladder carcinomas (64,65).

ELISA-like Assays

These have been used to measure urinary hyaluronic acid and hyaluronidase markers that are said to be highly sensitive and specific for bladder carcinoma cells (66). The telemoric repeat amplification protocol (TRAP) assay is not as sensitive as urine cytology (67).

Flow Cytometry

Flow cytometry can be used for the detection of bladder cancer and for monitoring treatment (68). The detection rate for bladder cancers is 90% to 94% when combined with cytology (69) especially after intravesical therapy (70). Bladder wash flow cytometry is more sensitive than urine flow cytometry (71–73). Microfluorometry is another new technique which has a very high false-positive rate (74).

Fluorescence *In Situ* Hybridization (FISH)

FISH is more sensitive than cytology for urine specimens but not for bladder washings (75).

Although many new tests have been developed recently urine cytology is still the most economical and simplest test available for the detection of transitional carcinoma, with the caveat that low-grade tumors may be missed using this technique (76).

PATHOLOGY

Transitional Cell Carcinoma

Transitional cell carcinoma (urothelial carcinoma) is conventionally divided into two types, the papillary and nonpapillary (flat-sessile) types. The former, which account for approximately 25% of primary transitional cell tumors of the bladder (77), and for the majority of tumors of the upper tract, is discussed first here. This is followed by a consideration of invasive transitional cell carcinoma, some of its special variants, and, finally, other forms of primary carcinoma (Table 19.1). These tumors are morphologically fundamentally the same wherever they are encountered in the urinary tract (78–83)

TABLE 19.1

PRIMARY CARCINOMAS OF THE URINARY TRACT

1. *Transitional cell carcinoma*
   Papillary
   Nonpapillary
   (i) Transitional cell carcinoma *in situ*
   (ii) Invasive transitional cell carcinoma
   Variants
   With squamous differentiation and/or glandular
       differentiation
   Sarcomatoid carcinoma
   With trophoblastic differentiation
   With pseudosarcomatous stroma or with
       osseous/cartilaginous metaplasia
2. *Squamous cell carcinoma*
3. *Adenocarcinoma*
   Variants
   Typical intestinal type
   Mucinous (including colloid)
   Signet-ring cell
   Clear cell
   Not otherwise specified
4. *Undifferentiated carcinoma*
   Variants
   Small cell carcinoma
   Giant cell carcinoma
   Lymphoepithelioma

---

but, in our own personal experience, variants, whether common (with squamous or gland differentiation) (84–87) or uncommon, are most often seen in the urinary bladder.

Papillary Transitional Cell Carcinoma

Macroscopic Appearances

The appearance of these lesions varies greatly. Some are barely visible, small papillary excrescences whereas others are huge, confluent papillary masses that may have a "cauliflower-like" appearance (88) and may fill, or almost fill, the bladder lumen or renal pelvis, or may obstruct the uterer. In one study (89) 41% and in another (90) 31% of the tumors in the bladder were more than 3 cm in greatest dimension. They are typically soft, delicate, and friable and may be creamy-white, tan, or pink to red. The delicate papillae are appreciable on gross examination (Fig. 19.18). In one series (89) multiple bladder tumors were present in 40% of the cases and in another 49% were multiple with 21% of patients having four or more tumors (90). In noninvasive tumors a sharp interface with the underlying normal bladder is apparent on sectioning. Tumors of the upper tract may be present synchronously or asynchronously in patients with bladder neoplasm.

Histologic Appearances

These tumors are characterized by papillae that are usually tall and often branch (Fig. 19.19). The papillae may be separate from each other or may be adherent to each other, particularly near their bases. The papillae are usually covered by hyperplastic urothelium that is often more than seven layers. The cells covering the papillae vary from almost normal in appearance to highly atypical. They typically have moderate amounts of pale eosinophilic cytoplasm but sometimes the cytoplasm is more abundant and densely eosinophilic or clear. Papillary carcinomas are graded using conventional cytologic

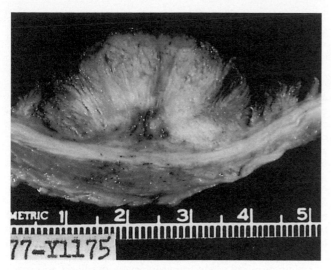

FIGURE 19.18. Papillary transitional cell carcinoma, noninvasive. Delicate tall papillae are appreciable, particularly at the lateral edges of the specimen. The well-circumscribed, noninvasive margin of the base of the neoplasm is apparent.

criteria, something with major prognostic significance (91). Grade I lesions show an increase in the number of layers of urothelial cells and slight cytologic atypia; mitotic figures are rare. Grade II lesions usually show areas of moderate cytologic atypia, and readily found mitotic figures (Fig. 19.20). Grade III lesions show at least focal high-grade nuclear atypia and mitotic figures are frequent. "Micropapillary transitional cell carcinomas" occur in which numerous small cellular papillae are present, producing an appearance similar to that of ovarian serous carcinoma (92). Glandular and squamous differentiation are uncommon in noninvasive papillary carcinoma. The cores of the papillae are usually slender and moderately vascular and composed of connective tissue with occasional inflammatory cells. They occasionally are edematous causing the lesion to appear polypoid rather than papillary. In some cases, the stroma or blood vessel walls within it are extensively hyalinized.

The features of the invasive tumor derived from papillary carcinoma are similar to those seen in nonpapillary carcinoma described below. Because invasion is very rare in case of grade I papillary carcinoma, it should not be diagnosed unless it is unequivocal. Assessment of invasion in cases of papillary carcinoma may be difficult. Tangential sectioning of the bases of papillae

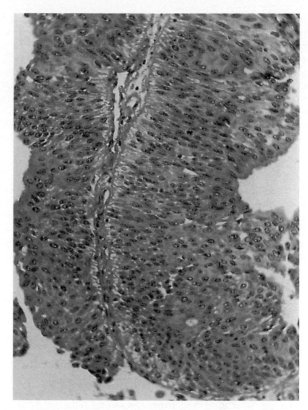

FIGURE 19.20. Papillary transitional cell carcinoma, grade II. A papilla is lined by hyperplastic urothelial cells. The cytologic features are relatively bland but mitotic figures were easily found in this specimen, which was considered a grade II neoplasm on that basis.

may simulate invasion by giving the appearance of detached nests of cells in the lamina propria. The presence of blood vessels within these foci may be a clue that they represent the edge of a papilla. Papillary carcinomas may be associated with noninvasive carcinoma in von Brunn's nests mimicking invasion. The well-circumscribed contour of these round to oval structures facilitates their distinction from true invasion (93). Occasionally, the bases of the papillae of papillary carcinoma are bulbous and protrude with a pushing border into the underlying stroma, occasionally causing attenuation of the lamina propria and approaching the muscularis propria (93). This is not to be considered invasion. When invasion occurs, it usually is seen at the bases of the papillae but, rarely, invasion of the cores of the papillae is seen.

Differential Diagnosis

Cases occur in which it is debatable whether the diagnosis of urothelial hyperplasia or early papillary carcinoma is most appropriate. These are usually seen in patients with a history of papillary carcinoma and this problem does not generally cause clinical difficulty in these patients who remain under observation. It is important to see unequivocal fibrovascular papillary cores before diagnosing papillary carcinoma. Sarma's elegant studies (94) showed that papillary carcinoma evolved on a background of urothelial hyperplasia with the development of small blood vessels gradually leading to the development of the stromal cores of papillary formations which, when not fully developed, are descriptively best considered papillary urothelial hyperplasia (95).

Papillary carcinoma must be distinguished from papillary or polypoid cystitis (96), or the equivalent lesion in the pelvis or ureters. This is a reactive lesion in which papillae are covered by normal urothelium and often have a prominent

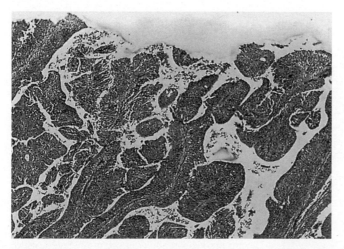

FIGURE 19.19. Papillary transitional cell carcinoma. Tall, finger-like papillae from which smaller papillae branch are conspicuous.

layer of umbrella cells, a feature which is uncommon in papillary carcinoma. The frequent branching of small papillae from large papillae seen in papillary carcinoma is not a feature of either papillary or polypoid cystitis. The broad fronds of polypoid cystitis are much thicker than the thin papillae of most papillary carcinomas and the stromal cores of papillary and polypoid cystitis generally are more intensely inflamed and vascular than those of carcinomas. The clinical setting, such as the presence of an in-dwelling catheter or a vesical fistula, both of which may be associated with the entity, may be helpful in the bladder.

A controversial area concerns the existence, or otherwise, of exophytic papillomas of the bladder, which can be reliably distinguished from low-grade papillary transitional cell carcinomas. We believe a distinction can be made because a small subset of papillary lesions have a different appearance from that of the typical papillary carcinoma (33). These lesions, which sometimes occur in patients younger than the typical patient who gets a papillary carcinoma, do not exhibit such prominent, tall, branching papillae as seen in papillary carcinoma, are covered by urothelium that is not hyperplastic, is not atypical, does not exhibit appreciable mitotic activity, and is generally covered by a relatively complete layer of umbrella cells. Most tumors reported as papillomas in the older literature have more recently been considered grade I papillary carcinomas.

Inverted papillomas are well-known benign lesions that most often occur in the bladder (34) but may also be seen in the renal pelvis and exceptionally in the ureter. They should be carefully distinguished from carcinoma with an inverting pattern (93).

The classification of transitional (urothelial) cell neoplasms of the urinary bladder proposed by the World Health Organization and the International Society of Urological Pathology (97) recommends that what have most often been referred to in the recent literature as papillary carcinoma, grade I, be referred to as papillary neoplasm of low-malignant potential. This is because of a desire to avoid having the word "carcinoma" in the report in cases which are noninvasive and grade I and are associated with such an excellent outcome. For reasons presented elsewhere arguing against the "papilloma" designation for low-grade malignant papillary lesion (77), we still prefer to use the grade I papillary transitional carcinoma terminology.

Transitional Cell Carcinoma (Nonpapillary)

Transitional Cell Carcinoma *In Situ*

A spectrum of atypical lesions occurs in nonpapillary urothelium, ranging from mild cytologic changes to cells with obviously malignant cytologic features characterizing transitional cell carcinoma *in situ*. Mild degrees of atypicality in which the cells have the cytologic features of grade I papillary transitional cell carcinoma are considered mild dysplasia but this diagnosis should be made sparingly because of problems with pathologists consistently recognizing low-grade cytologic abnormalities (97). Cells with the features of a grade II lesion are called moderate dysplasia, and lesions with the cytologic features of a grade III carcinoma are called severe dysplasia or transitional cell carcinoma *in situ* (97–100), the latter term being used when the abnormal cells are present throughout all layers and show a marked loss of polarity (Fig. 19.21) (99). Mitotic figures are easily found in severe dysplasia and carcinoma *in situ*. As is the case with premalignant epithelial lesions elsewhere in the body, considerable subjectivity exists in the interpretation of these lesions (97,101), although this is less so for high-grade lesions. From the viewpoint of patient care the most important concern in this area is making sure that high-grade lesions falling in the category of severe dysplasia or transitional cell carcinoma *in situ* are not overlooked. This diagnosis is, practically speaking, only made with appreciable frequency in specimens from the bladder.

On gross inspection, mucosa involved by transitional cell carcinoma *in situ* usually is erythematous and may be slightly granular, or edematous due to the frequent associated edema of the lamina propria. Microscopically, the abnormal urothelium may vary in thickness from a single layer of cells, to normal, to hyperplastic. Loss of intercellular cohesion and adherence to the basement membrane with resultant urothelial denudation frequently occur. This may result in only a single layer of cells being present, and in some cases considerable areas of the mucosa are denuded completely. When examining biopsies with denudation, one must be careful not to overlook even a small number of highly atypical cells. Even when only one layer of cells is present, the diagnosis of carcinoma *in situ* of the bladder may be made on the basis of severe cytologic atypia. In the past, patients with carcinoma *in situ* and marked

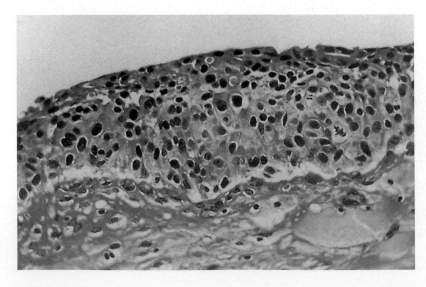

FIGURE 19.21. Transitional cell carcinoma *in situ*. There is marked variability in size of the nuclei, which are hyperchromatic and exhibit loss of polarity. Note mitotic figure (*lower right*).

urothelial denudation have sometimes been followed for long periods of time with the diagnosis of nonspecific or interstitial cystitis. Deeper sections are often indicated in these cases, as is close correlation with the findings of urine cytology as malignant cells are often present in cytologic specimens from cases of carcinoma *in situ*. In many cases, a low-power clue to the diagnosis of transitional cell carcinoma *in situ* is a very edematous, inflamed, hypervascular lamina propria.

Invasive Transitional Cell Carcinoma

Macroscopic Appearances

As invasive tumors arise from both papillary and sessile precursors, the gross appearance of invasive transitional cell carcinoma is variable. They may be strikingly papillary, nodular (Fig. 19.22) or polypoid (Fig. 19.23), sessile and ulcerated, or in some cases cause only subtle abnormalities in the form of a granular or velvety mucosa. The size of the lesions is also variable, ranging from a few millimeters in diameter to huge masses that may fill the renal pelvis, ureteral lumen, or bladder lumen. The tumors may be hemorrhagic and necrotic, although generally these features are not striking. The appearance of the underlying tissue depends upon the extent of invasion; in deeply invasive bladder neoplasms the bladder wall is typically replaced by firm, white tumor tissue and, in similarly extensive renal pelvic neoplasms, a sometimes scirrhous mass is often present that may replace most or all of medullary and cortical tissue in the involved region (Fig. 19.24) with extension to hilar fat or even, on rare occasions, pericortical fat. That such renal tumors are of renal pelvic origin, as opposed to renal cortical origin, is not always easy to discern from gross inspection.

Microscopic Appearances

Many invasive cancers are associated with overlying epithelial abnormalities from which they arise, specifically, papillary transitional cell carcinoma or transitional cell carcinoma *in situ*, as already described. However, not all invasive carcinomas are

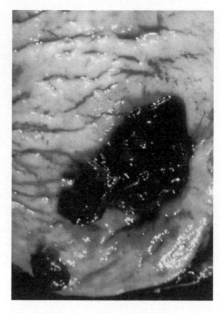

FIGURE 19.23. Invasive transitional cell carcinoma, sarcomatoid variant. Two hemorrhagic polypoid nodules project from the mucosa.

associated with an abnormality of the overlying epithelium, at least as assessed at the light microscopic level (102). In our experience, this is most often seen in the case of carcinomas with deceptive histologic features, as discussed below.

Several specific variants (103) will be described after the common forms of invasive transitional cell carcinoma are

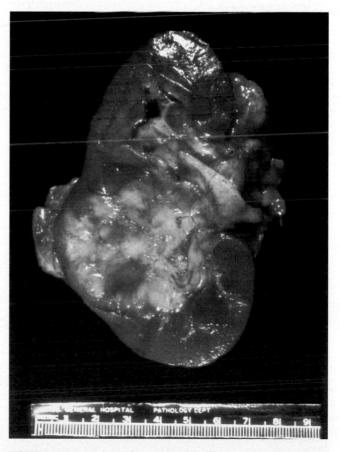

FIGURE 19.24. High-grade transitional cell carcinoma of renal pelvis with extensive effacement of renal parenchyma.

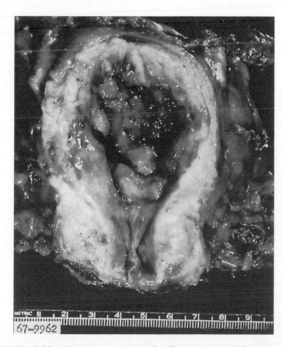

FIGURE 19.22. Invasive transitional cell carcinoma. The mucosa of the bladder shows many irregular nodular masses of tumor.

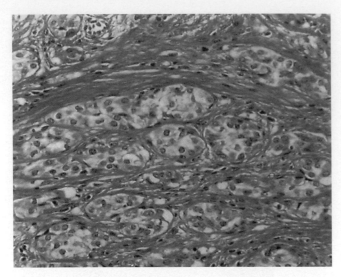

FIGURE 19.25. Invasive low-grade transitional cell carcinoma. Small nests of cells are closely apposed to one another. The cells in this case exhibit only mild atypia. Occasionally, invasive tumors with these low-grade features are misdiagnosed as benign.

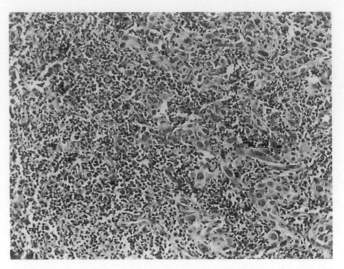

FIGURE 19.27. Invasive transitional cell carcinoma with marked lymphocytic infiltrate. The inflammatory cell infiltrate partially obscures the underlying neoplastic cells.

discussed. Most frequently there are nests (Fig. 19.25), small clusters (Fig. 19.26) and single neoplastic cells irregularly dispersed in the lamina propria, and muscularis propria, if invasion of the latter is present. The tumor sometimes grows in a diffuse pattern, but even in these cases focal nests and clusters are generally present. Rarely, the tumor is uniformly diffuse. Occasional carcinomas are associated with a pronounced chronic inflammatory cell infiltrate which sometimes partially obscures the underlying tumor cells (Fig. 19.27). Invasion usually occurs in the form of irregular infiltration but sometimes the nests of invasive tumors are well circumscribed.

The neoplastic cells are usually of medium size and have modest amounts of pale to slightly eosinophilic cytoplasm. In some tumors the cytoplasm is more abundant and may be clear or strikingly eosinophilic. The transitional (urothelial) character of the cells, including the presence of focal longitudinal nuclear grooves, is often appreciable, at least focally, in low-grade tumors and in some high-grade lesions. At least moderate, and frequently marked, cytologic atypia is present

but occasional tumors are composed of cells with only mild cytologic atypia. Bizarre, hyperchromatic nuclei may be seen, particularly in patients whose tumors have been treated with radiation therapy. The mitotic rate is variable and related to the grade of the tumor. Focal necrosis is common in high-grade tumors; hemorrhage is uncommon. Lymphatic or vascular invasion is seen to varying degrees, occasionally being striking. In some tumors, nests of cells lie in spaces that are artifactual. This should not be misdiagnosed as vascular invasion. These spaces, which have been described as a particular feature of "micropapillary" tumors (92), are not lined by endothelial cells.

The assessment of the presence or absence of invasion, and if present, its depth may be difficult for the pathologist. Many bladder specimens are fragmented as a result of the transurethral resection procedure, and cautery artifact often adds to the difficulties in interpretation. Furthermore, specimens from the ureter or renal pelvis often procure a small amount of tissue. In most cases in which there is invasion of the lamina propria the appearances are not subtle and invasion of the lamina propria is a straightforward interpretation.

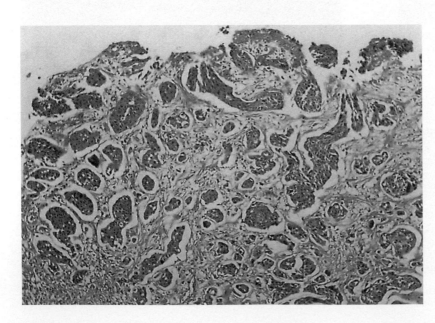

FIGURE 19.26. Invasive transitional cell carcinoma. The tumor cells are growing in irregular clusters of varying sizes and shapes and as single cells in a focally desmoplastic stroma.

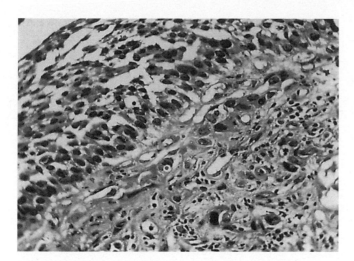

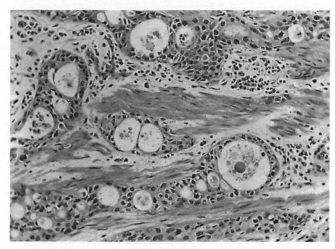

FIGURE 19.28. Microinvasive transitional cell carcinoma. The superficial lamina propria contains a few small clusters of invasive carcinoma. The invasion in this case was restricted to this small focus. Note the highly atypical overlying urothelium.

FIGURE 19.29. Transitional cell carcinoma with gland differentiation. The numerous cells of transitional cell type surrounding the gland lumens are features helpful to distinguish it from a pure adenocarcinoma.

Occasional transitional cell carcinomas have very small foci of early invasion which is possible to overlook (Fig. 19.28). These have been referred to as "microinvasive" transitional cell carcinomas (104,105). When invasion of the lamina propria is present, the pathologist then must assess whether there is invasion of the muscularis propria. If there is not, the pathologist then must assess whether the muscularis propria is present in submitted tissue and, if it is not, note this. Evaluation of muscularis propria invasion is difficult due to the artifact already referred to in some cases, and fibrosis and inflammatory changes may sometimes make the interpretation even more difficult. It is best for the pathologist to be conservative when assessing muscularis propria invasion and to require the presence of unequivocal involvement of well-organized muscle bundles. This is to prevent the misdiagnosis of invasion of the muscularis mucosae (106–109) as involvement of the muscularis propria. As the term "muscle invasion" is not in and of itself discriminatory between involvement of the muscularis mucosae and muscularis propria, it is better not just to say "muscle invasion" but rather "invasion of the muscularis propria" so that the clinician knows the pathologist is specifically referring to involvement of that muscle. The muscle of the latter tends to occur in smaller less well-organized bundles than that of the muscularis propria, enabling them to be distinguished. It is self-evident that the assessment of invasion of the muscularis propria is dependent on the urologist submitting a deep biopsy. In a transurethral resection specimen it is relatively infrequent for the pathologist to be able to make an accurate assessment as to the depth of invasion of the muscularis propria. In some well-oriented pieces of tissue one can discern that the involvement is only superficial whereas in other similarly well-oriented specimens one can see that the invasion is deep. However, the fragmentary nature of many specimens precludes a definitive interpretation of the depth of involvement of the muscularis propria in many instances.

Approximately 10% of transitional cell carcinomas of the bladder contain foci of glandular or squamous differentiation (Fig. 19.29). The glands are variable in appearance, occasionally being small and tubular. Glandular differentiation is usually found in moderate- to high-grade, often deeply invasive tumors, but it is occasionally seen in well-differentiated, superficially invasive tumors. Since glandular and squamous differentiation have no clear-cut prognostic significance, by convention the primary diagnosis remains transitional cell carcinoma but squamous and/or glandular differentiation should

be recorded. Rarely, transitional cell carcinomas contain microcysts (110).

Some high-grade transitional cell carcinomas contain areas composed of atypical spindle cells meriting the descriptive designation "sarcomatoid carcinoma" (Fig. 19.30) (111). This is seen most often in the bladder (111–114) but is rarely seen in the upper tract (115). The neoplastic cells in these cases may grow in a variety of patterns. Most commonly, fascicles impart a resemblance to leiomyosarcoma or there is a storiform pattern reminiscent of that seen in malignant fibrous histiocytoma. A resemblance to rhabdomyosarcoma results when pleomorphic, round, or elongated cells with abundant eosinophilic cytoplasm are present. Usually there is moderate to severe nuclear atypia and mitotic figures are typically frequent. Some tumors are myxoid or sclerotic, which rarely leads to their initial misinterpretation as a benign lesion, the inflammatory pseudotumor (111). The sarcomatoid areas usually merge with either invasive or *in situ* transitional cell carcinoma. While generous sampling usually reveals the urothelial nature of these tumors, occasionally immunohistochemistry is helpful since the spindle cells may stain for cytokeratin and epithelial membrane antigen but are negative for mesenchymal markers (114).

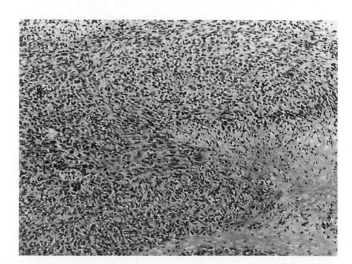

FIGURE 19.30. Sarcomatoid transitional cell carcinoma. The neoplastic cells are uniformly spindle shaped in this illustration. They merged elsewhere with recognizable foci of transitional cell carcinoma.

Rare transitional cell carcinomas that are high-grade have areas resembling choriocarcinoma (116,117). Immunohistochemical studies have shown human chorionic gonadotropin (hCG) and its beta subunit in the cells of morphologically typical transitional cell carcinomas, invasive or *in situ*, in approximately 30% of the cases (118). That hCG production is common in high-grade transitional cell carcinomas and well-documented cases in which choriocarcinoma has evolved from or coexisted with high-grade urothelial carcinoma suggest that most vesical tumors with trophoblastic elements are transitional cell carcinomas in which trophoblastic differentiation has occurred, rather than being of germ cell origin.

The stroma in transitional cell carcinomas may exhibit some degree of desmoplasia but an extremely desmoplastic reaction is unusual. The stroma occasionally contains significant numbers of atypical, but benign, mesenchymal cells, so-called transitional cell carcinomas with pseudosarcomatous stroma (119,120). The stroma of transitional cell carcinoma may also undergo osseous or cartilaginous metaplasia (121,122) and rarely contains osteoclast-type giant cells (120).

Differential Diagnosis

The usual invasive transitional cell carcinoma generally does not pose much diagnostic difficulty. There is a small subset of cases, less than 5% of the total, in which the tumors are grade I and these occasionally cause some difficulty in their distinction from von Brunn's nests (123–125). It is helpful that nests of well-differentiated carcinoma of this type usually grow in more closely packed aggregates and are more irregular in size and shape than von Brunn's nests, which are invariably round or oval and generally have an orderly distribution (126,127) which contrasts with the disorderly architecture of most carcinomas. In our experience, von Brunn's nests may be particularly exuberant in the renal pelvis when they may additionally be elongated more so than in the bladder.

Transitional cell carcinomas with squamous and/or glandular differentiation are usually grade II or III and their distinction from non-neoplastic lesions is rarely difficult. Rarely the glandular component takes the form of small, relatively regular, tubules, suggesting the tubules of a nephrogenic adenoma (128). However, the association of the tubules with foci of conventional transitional cell carcinoma usually facilitates the correct diagnosis, and there is often a peripheral layer of transitional cells, something absent in nephrogenic adenomas. A similar comment pertains in the occasionally difficult distinction between transitional cell carcinoma with larger gland-like structures and cystitis glandularis (128). In both these situations there are generally irregularities of architecture which are inconsistent with the benign lesions they are occasionally misdiagnosed as.

Grade III transitional cell carcinomas often have a relatively nondescript appearance which viewed in isolation cannot be distinguished from poorly differentiated carcinomas of other types. A poorly differentiated bladder, ureteral, or renal pelvis cancer is considered to be of transitional cell type unless there is good evidence to the contrary. The possibility of prostate carcinoma should be borne in mind with poorly differentiated bladder neck tumors in males. Immunohistochemistry may be very helpful in these cases as most prostate carcinomas will stain for prostate-specific antigen and prostatic acid phosphatase. Occasional poorly differentiated transitional cell carcinomas without an obvious epithelial pattern may superficially resemble malignant lymphoma (129), but small foci of epithelial differentiation and high power scrutiny of the neoplastic cells to recognize that their cytologic features are not typical of those of malignant lymphoma are usually helpful. Immunohistochemistry for epithelial and lymphoid markers may be of help in cases which are difficult to distinguish on the basis of routine stains.

The tumors that enter into the differential diagnosis in cases of sarcomatoid carcinomas are sarcomas, mainly leiomyosarcoma, malignant fibrous histiocytoma and pleomorphic rhabdomyosarcoma, carcinosarcomas, and transitional cell carcinomas with pseudosarcomatous stroma. Although it is occasionally difficult, a distinction between sarcomatoid carcinomas and sarcomas can usually be made by evaluating their features in routinely stained slides. The pathologic feature that is diagnostic of the former tumor is the presence of recognizable epithelial elements of various types that merge imperceptibly with the sarcomatoid areas. However, a small specimen may contain only the sarcomatoid component and immunohistochemistry may be helpful in disclosing the epithelial nature of the tumor cells in such cases. Carcinosarcomas often exhibit heterologous differentiation of the sarcomatous component, including skeletal muscle or chondro-osseous tissue, elements that exclude the diagnosis of sarcomatoid carcinoma.

Squamous Cell Carcinoma

Squamous cell carcinoma accounts for approximately 5% of bladder carcinomas in areas where schistosomiasis is not endemic (130), but for approximately 75% of bladder carcinomas where schistosomiasis is endemic. The male-to-female ratio is lower than it is in cases of transitional cell carcinoma but the age distribution is similar. These tumors account for approximately 20% of cases arising within diverticula, 50% of cancers occurring in patients with nonfunctioning bladders, and 15% of cancers in patients who have had renal transplants. These tumors are rarely primary in the renal pelvis and even more exceptionally in the ureter.

The gross appearance of squamous cell carcinomas varies from sessile and ulcerated to papillary, polypoid, or nodular (Fig. 19.31). They are usually large and deeply invasive even

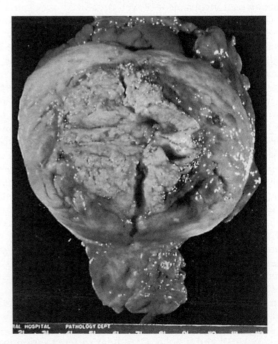

FIGURE 19.31. Squamous cell carcinoma. The mucosa is largely replaced by a predominantly sessile tumor that was white in the fresh state. [From Young, RH. Unusual variants of primary bladder carcinoma and secondary tumors of the bladder. Chapter 3 in: *Pathology of the Urinary Bladder* (Young RH, ed), Vol. 13 in *Contemporary Issues in Surgical Pathology* (Roth LM, ed). Churchill Livingstone, New York, 1989, with permission.]

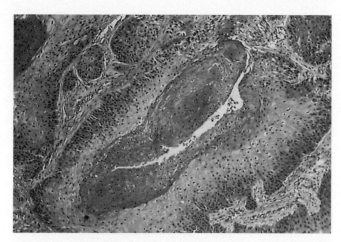

FIGURE 19.32. Squamous cell carcinoma of the bladder. Note the keratinization. [From Young, RH. Unusual variants of primary bladder carcinoma and secondary tumors of the bladder. Chapter 3 in: *Pathology of the Urinary Bladder* (Young RH, ed), Vol. 13 in *Contemporary Issues in Surgical Pathology* (Roth LM, ed). Churchill Livingstone, New York, 1989, with permission.]

when well differentiated. Their microscopic appearance is similar to that of squamous cell carcinomas arising elsewhere. Most are moderately or well differentiated and they often are abundantly keratinized (Fig. 19.32). These tumors often are associated with keratinizing squamous metaplasia (so-called leukoplakia) (131,132) of the adjacent mucosa and are distinguished from it by either their greater degree of atypia and/or the presence of invasion.

Adenocarcinoma

Adenocarcinoma accounts for from 0.5% to 2 percent of bladder carcinomas (133–140). They may be of urachal origin (Fig. 19.33) (141), associated with exstrophy (Fig. 19.34) (142), or endometriosis (143), or unassociated with either of the aforementioned. The last is the most common situation (Figs. 19.35, 19.36). In one large series one-third of the tumors were urachal and two-thirds, nonurachal (140). Adenocarcinomas account for approximately 90% of urachal cancers, the remaining tumors being divided, more or less equally, between those of transitional and squamous type. Renal pelvic tumors of this type are rare and ureteral tumors even more so.

The age distribution and male-to-female ratio of adenocarcinoma is similar to that of transitional cell carcinoma, the neoplasms usually arising in male patients over 50 years old. The clinical presentation usually mimics that of transitional cell carcinoma but occasionally patients present with mucinuria. Adenocarcinoma, like squamous cell carcinoma, accounts for a greater than normal percentage of bladder cancers in some clinical settings. They have accounted for approximately 15% of tumors arising in a patient with a nonfunctioning bladder and 85% of those associated with exstrophy. Adenocarcinoma of the bladder generally has a poor prognosis. The outlook for signet-ring cell carcinoma, which is typically high stage at presentation, is worse than for other types. Urachal tumors have a better prognosis than nonurachal tumors.

On gross examination these tumors vary considerably in appearance according, in part, to whether they are urachal (Fig. 19.33), complicate exstrophy (Fig. 19.34), or have neither association (Figs. 19.35, 19.36). Tumors of the last type may involve any part of the mucosa. They vary from papillary or polypoid, to nodular, to sessile and ulcerative. The neo-

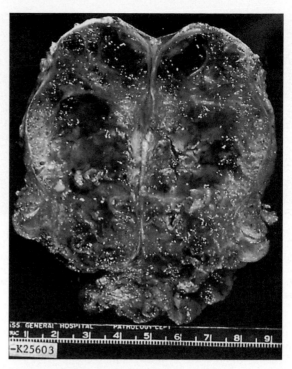

FIGURE 19.33. Adenocarcinoma of the urachus. The tumor has a prominent gelatinous cut surface. [From Eble JN. Abnormalities of the urachas. Chapter 6 in: *Pathology of the Urinary Bladder* (Young RH, ed), Vol. 13 in *Contemporary Issues in Surgical Pathology* (Roth LM, ed), Churchill Livingstone, New York, 1989, with permission.]

plastic tissue is usually soft and often mucoid (Fig. 19.33); foci of hemorrhage and necrosis are common. In cases of signet-ring cell adenocarcinoma, which account for from 3% to 5% of vesical adenocarcinomas (144,145), the mucosa often appears edematous and in most cases is ulcerated, but sometimes it is grossly normal. Some cases have the diffuse

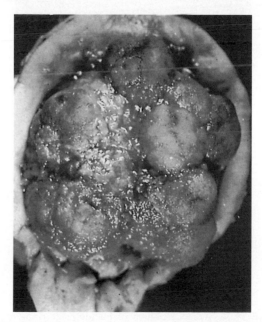

FIGURE 19.34. Adenocarcinoma complicating exstrophy. A large, multinodular-mass projects from the abdominal wall. (Courtesy of Dr. Fred Askin). [From Young, RH. Unusual variants of primary bladder carcinoma and secondary tumors of the bladder. Chapter 3 in: *Pathology of the Urinary Bladder* (Young RH, ed), Vol. 13 in *Contemporary Issues in Surgical Pathology* (Roth LM, ed). Churchill Livingstone, New York, 1989, with permission.]

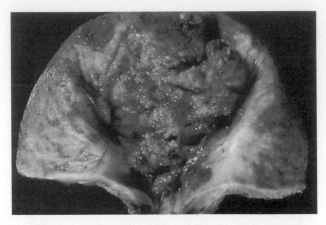

FIGURE 19.35. Adenocarcinoma, intestinal type. Papillary to polypoid tissue replaces much of the bladder mucosa. [From Young RH, Parkhurst EC. Mucinous adenocarcinoma of bladder. Case associated with extensive intestinal metaplasia of urothelium in patient with nonfunctioning bladder for 12 years. *Urology* 1984;23:192–195, with permission.]

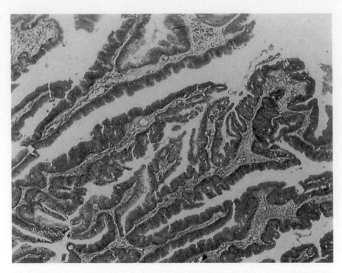

FIGURE 19.37. Adenocarcinoma of bladder, not otherwise specified. The neoplasm has a focally papillary pattern.

fibrosis and mural thickening typical of linitis plastica of the stomach (Fig. 19.36).

Urachal tumors are typically submucosal masses at the bladder dome and often extensively infiltrate the surrounding muscle of the bladder wall and extend superiorly in the space of Retzius towards the umbilicus (Fig. 19.33). There is usually some degree of overlying mucosal ulceration or abnormality of some type but this is variable. On sectioning, the tumors

often are cystic or if solid have a gelatinous surface (Fig. 19.33). Tumors that complicate exstrophy (rarely seen now) are remarkable primarily for their presence on the anterior abdominal wall (Fig. 19.34).

Vesical adenocarcinomas are subclassified into the following microscopic groups, with respective frequency in one large series included in parentheses (140): adenocarcinoma, not otherwise specified (27.8%); mucinous (23.6%); enteric (19.4%); signet-ring cell (16.7%); and mixed (12.5%). Microscopic examination generally shows a predominantly glandular pattern (Fig. 19.37), although in poorly differentiated tumors areas of solid growth may be encountered. The glands frequently resemble those of intestinal adenocarcinoma of typical or colloid type (Fig. 19.38). Their lining epithelium may have a prominent mucinous character. Urachal tumors tend to be more often mucinous than nonurachal tumors and have a greater tendency to be cystic. The differentiation of mucinous epithelium covers a spectrum from benign to atypical to carcinomatous, and invasive foci of the latter may be documented only after thorough sampling. Papillary tumors accounted for 8% of the tumors in one series (56).

Microscopic examination in signet-ring cell tumors usually shows the typical features of a signet-ring cell adenocarcinoma (Fig. 19.39) but the signet-ring cells may be embedded in lakes

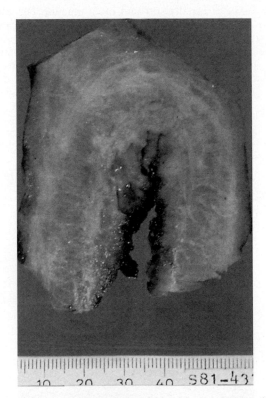

FIGURE 19.36. Adenocarcinoma of bladder, signet-ring cell type. There is marked thickening of the bladder wall which was rigid in the fresh state. (Courtesy of Professor Max N. I. Walters.) [From Young, RH. Unusual variants of primary bladder carcinoma and secondary tumors of the bladder. Chapter 3 in: *Pathology of the Urinary Bladder* (Young RH, ed), Vol. 13 in *Contemporary Issues in Surgical Pathology* (Roth LM, ed). Churchill Livingstone, New York, 1989, with permission.]

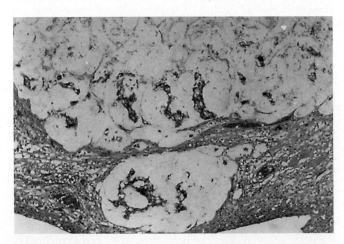

FIGURE 19.38. Colloid adenocarcinoma of bladder. Small aggregates of tumor cells are embedded in abundant mucus.

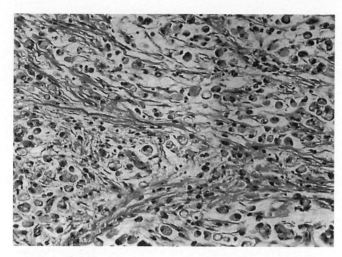

FIGURE 19.39. Signet-ring cell adenocarcinoma. Numerous cells have eccentric nuclei and vacuolated cytoplasm that stained positively with mucin stains.

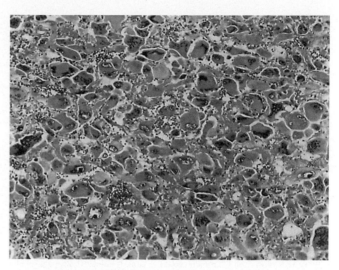

FIGURE 19.41. Undifferentiated carcinoma, giant-cell type. Large pleomorphic multinucleate giant cells with abundant cytoplasm are conspicuous. A few epulis-type giant cells representing a reactive stromal component are also present.

of extracellular mucus and the tumor is occasionally admixed with a component of adenocarcinoma of another type. Tumors consisting entirely of signet-ring cells have a worse prognosis than those admixed with another component.

Undifferentiated Carcinoma Including Small Cell Carcinoma

Undifferentiated carcinomas of the urinary tract are rare and have the nonspecific features of undifferentiated carcinomas of other sites. Small-cell undifferentiated carcinomas that are similar histologically to pulmonary tumors of this type occur occasionally (Fig. 19.40) (146–150). The tumors are typically large, often polypoid, and frequently ulcerated. Histologically they are composed of sheets of small, oat-shaped cells with hyperchromatic nuclei as well as slightly larger cells with more

variation in nuclear chromatin, comparable to the intermediate cell type of pulmonary small cell carcinoma, or mixtures of the two cell types. Other forms of carcinoma, usually either *in situ* or invasive transitional cell carcinoma, but occasionally squamous cell carcinoma or adenocarcinoma, are often present. Small-cell carcinomas may be confused with lymphoma, particularly in a small biopsy specimen. Immunohistochemical stains for lymphoid and epithelial markers may be helpful in these cases. Primary small-cell carcinomas of the urinary tract should be distinguished from a metastasis from the lung, or rarely elsewhere. Occasional undifferentiated carcinomas of the bladder are composed purely or predominantly of large pleomorphic cells with abundant eosinophilic or amphophilic cytoplasm and have a conspicuous component of malignant giant cells (Fig. 19.41) (151). Finally, rare carcinomas have the features of a lymphoepithelioma (152).

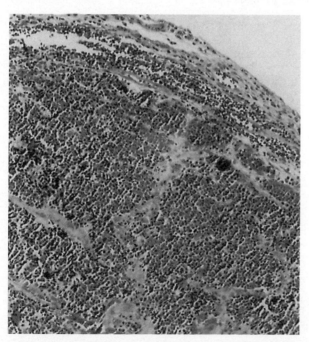

FIGURE 19.40. Small cell undifferentiated carcinoma of bladder. The lamina propria is occupied by large aggregates of small cells with scant cytoplasm and hyperchromatic nuclei.

References

1. Sanders WR. Cancer of the bladder. Fragments forming urethral plugs discharged in the urine, concentric colloid bodies. *Ed J Med* 1864;10:273.
2. Papanicoloau GN, Marshall VF. Urine sediment: a diagnostic procedure in cancers of the urinary tract. *Science* 1945;101:519–521.
3. Trott PA. Cytological screening for cancer of the bladder. *Proc R Soc Med* 1976;69:496.
4. Howell ADN, Smith SR, Butterly DQ, et al. Diagnosis and management of BK polyomavirus interstitial nephritis in renal transplant recipients. *Transplantation* 1999;68:1279–1288.
5. Corey HE, Alfonso F, Hamele-Bena D, et al. Urine cytology and the diagnosis of renal allograft rejection. II. Studies using immunostaining. *Acta Cytol* 1997;41:1742–1746.
6. Kitamoto Y, Tomita M, Akamine M, et al. Differentiation of haematuria using a uniquely-shaped red cell. *Nephron* 1993;64:32–36.
7. Goldwasser P, Antiguani A, Mittman N, et al. Urinary red cell size: diagnostic value and determinants. *Am J Nephrol* 1990;10:148–156.
8. Tsukahara H, Yoshimoto M, Morikawa K, et al. Mean cellular volume of urinary red blood cells in investigation of haematuria. *Acta Paediatr Jpn* 1989;31:476–479.
9. Harris MJ, Schwinn CP, Morrow JW, et al. Exfoliative cytology of the urinary bladder irrigation specimen. *Acta Cytol* 1971;15:385–399.
10. Bastacky S, Ibrahim S, Wilczynski SP, et al. The accuracy of urinary cytology in daily practice. *Cancer* 1999;87:118–128.
11. Paez A, Coba JM, Murillo N, et al. Reliability of the routine cytological diagnosis in bladder cancer. *Eur Urol* 1999;35(1):228–232.
12. Geisse LJ, Tweeddale DN. Pre-clinical cytological diagnosis of bladder cancer. *J Urol* 1978;120:51–56.
13. Pask CH, Britsch C, Uson AG, et al. Reliability of positive exfoliative cytology study of the urine in urinary tract malignancy. *J Urol* 1969;102:91.

14. Trott PA, Edwards L. Comparison of bladder washings and urine cytology in the diagnosis of bladder cancer. *J Urol* 1973;110:664–666.

15. Farrow GM. Urine cytology in the detection of bladder cancer: a critical approach. *J Occup Med* 1990;32:817–821.

16. Luthra UK, Dey P, George J, et al. Comparison of ThinPrep and conventional preparations: urine cytology evaluation. *Diagn Cytopathol* 1999; 21(5):364–465.

17. Matzkin H, Moinuddin S, Soloway M. Value of urine cytology vs. bladder washings in bladder cancer. *Urology* 1992;39:201–203.

18. Lebret T, Bohin D, Kassardijian Z, et al. Recurrence, progression and success in stage Ta grade 3 bladder tumours treated with low dose Bacillus Calmette-Guerin instillation. *J Urol* 2000;163(1):63–67.

19. Sharma N, Prescott S. BCG vaccine in superficial bladder cancer [Editorial]. *BMJ* 1994;308:801–802.

20. Betz SA, See WA, Cohen MB. Granulomatous inflammation in bladder wash specimens after intravesical Bacillus Calmette-Guerin therapy for transitional cell carcinoma of the bladder. *Am J Clin Pathol* 1993;99:244–249.

21. Cohen J-M, Szporn AJ, Unger P, et al. Noncaseating granulomata of the bladder following intravesical adjinistration of Bacille Calmette-Guerin. *Acta Cytol* 1991;35:600.

22. Dalbagni G, Rechtschaffen T, Herr HW. Is transurethral biopsy of the bladder necessary after 3 months to evaluate response to Bacillus Calmette-Guerin therapy? *J Urol* 1999;162(3 Pt 1):708–709.

23. Bhan R, Pisharodi LR, Gudlaugsson E, et al. Cytological, histological and clinical correlations in intravesical Bacillus Calmette-Guerin immunotherapy. *Ann Diagn Pathol* 1998;2(1):55–60.

24. Drachenberg CB, Beskow CO, Cangro CB, et al. Human polyomavirus in renal allograft biopsies: morphological findings and correlation with urine cytology. *Hum Pathol* 1999;30(8):970–977.

25. Kupper T, Stoffels U, Pawlita M, et al. Morphological changes in urothelial cells replicating human polyomavirus BK. *Cytopathol* 1993;4:361–368.

26. Thal SM, DeBellis CC, Iversm SA, et al. Comparison of dysmorphic erythrocytes with other urinary sediment parameters of renal bleeding. *Am J Clin Pathol* 1986;86:784–787.

27. Pellet H, Buenerd A, Mirairie E, et al. Clinical prevalence of glomerular haematuria: a nine year retrospective study. *Diagn Cytopathol* 1991;7: 27–31.

28. Fassett RG, Horgan BA, Mathew TH. Detection of glomerular bleeding by phase-contrast microscopy. *Lancet* 1982;1:1432–1434.

29. Janssens PMW, Kornaat N, Tieleman F, et al. Localizing the site of haematuria by immunochemical staining of erythrocytes in urine. *Clin Chem* 1992;38:216–222.

30. Pollock C, Pei-Ling L, Gijory AZ, et al. Dysmorphism of urinary red blood cells—value in diagnosis. *Kidney Int* 1989;36:1045–1049.

31. Kannan V, Gupta D. Calculus artefact. A challenge in urinary cytology. *Acta Cytol* 1999;43(5):794–800.

32. Murphy WM, Beckwith JB, Farrow GM. Tumors of the urinary bladder. In: Rosai J, Sobin LH, eds. *Tumors of the kidney, bladder, and related urinary structures, Atlas of Tumor Pathology,* Fascicle 11. Washington, DC: Armed Forces Institute of Pathology, 1994:282.

33. McKenney JK, Amin MB, Young RH. Urothelial (transitional cell) papilloma of the urinary bladder: a clinicopathologic study of 26 cases. *Mod Pathol* 2003;16:623–629.

34. Kunze E, Schauer A, Schmitt M. Histology and histogenesis of two different types of inverted urothelial papilloma. *Cancer* 1983;51:348–358.

35. Murphy WM. Current status of urinary cytology in the evaluation of bladder neoplasms. *Hum Pathol* 1990;21:886–895.

36. Farrow GM. Urine cytology in the detection of bladder cancer: a critical approach. *J Occup Med* 1990;32:817–821.

37. Koss G. Tumors of the urinary tract and prostate in urinary sediment. In: Koss LG, ed. *Diagnostic cytology and its histologic basis,* 4th ed. Philadelphia, PA: JB Lippincott, 1992.

38. Shenoy UA, Colby TV, Schumann GB. Reliability of urinary cytodiagnosis in urothelial neoplasms. *Cancer* 1985;56:2041–2045.

39. Heney NM, Szyfelbein WM, Daly JJ. Positive urinary cytology in patients without evident tumour. *J Urol* 1977;117:223–224.

40. Kannan V. Papillary transitional cell carcinoma of the upper urinary tract: a cytological review. *Diagn Cytopathol* 1990;6:204–209.

41. Highman WJ. Transitional carcinoma of the upper urinary tract: a histological and cytological review. *J Clin Pathol* 1986;39:297–305.

42. Stella F, Battistelli S, Marcheggianni F, et al. Urothelial cell changes due to busulphan and cyclophosphamide treatment in bone marrow transplantation. *Acta Cytol* 1990;34:885–890.

43. Stella F, Battistelli S, Marcheggianni F, et al. Urothelial toxicity following conditioning therapy in bone marrow transplantation and bladder cancer: morphologic and morphometric comparison using exfoliation urinary cytology. *Diagn Cytopathol* 1992;8:216–221.

44. Stillwell TJ, Benson RC. Cyclophosphamide-induced haemorrhagic cystitis. A review of 100 patients. *Cancer* 1988;61:451–457.

45. Fanning CV, Staerkl GA, Sneige N, et al. Spindling artefact of urothelial cells in post-laser treatment urinary cytology. *Diagn Cytopathol* 1993;9: 279–281.

46. Ali SZ, Reuter V, Zakowski MF. Small cell neuroendocrine carcinoma of the urinary bladder. A clinicopathologic study with emphasis on cytologic features. *Cancer* 1997;79:356–361.

47. Borghi L, Bianchini E, Atlavilla G. Undifferentiated small-cell carcinoma of the urinary bladder: report of two cases with a primary urinary cytodiagnosis. *Diagn Cytopathol* 1995;13(1):61–65.

48. McRae S, Garcia BM. Cytologic diagnosis of a primary pure oat cell carcinoma of the bladder in voided urine. A case report. *Acta Cytol* 1997; 41(Suppl. 4):1279–1283.

49. Edgerton ME, Hoda RS, Gupta PK. Cytologic diagnosis of metastatic ovarian adenocarcinoma in the urinary bladder: a case report and review of the literature. *Diagn Cytol* 1999;20(3):156–159.

50. Wolinska WH, Melamed MR. Urinary conduit cytology. *Cancer* 1973;32: 100–106.

51. Magnusson B, Carlen B, Bak-Jensen B, et al. Ileal conduit stenosis—an enigma. *Scan J Urol Nephrol* 1996;30(3):193–197.

52. Mitchell ME, Yoder IC, Pfister RC, et al. Ileal loop stenosis: a late complication of urinary diversion. *J Urol* 1977;118:957–961.

53. Malone MJ, Izes JK, Hurley LJ. Carcinogenesis: the fate of intestinal segments used in urinary reconstruction. *Urol Clin North Am* 1997;34(4): 723–725.

54. Shokeir AA, Smama M, el-Mekresh MM, et al. Late malignancy in bowel segments exposed to urine without fecal stream. *Urol* 1995;46(5):657–661.

55. Stewart M. Urinary diversion and bowel cancer. *Ann R Coll Surg Engl* 1986;68(2):98–102.

56. Buchumensky V, Klein A, Zemer R, et al. Cytokeratin 20: a new marker for early detection of bladder carcinoma? *J Urol* 1998;160(6 Pt 1):1971–1974.

57. McKenney JK, Desai S, Cohen C, et al. Discriminatory immunohistochemical staining of urothelial carcinoma in situ and non-neoplastic epithelium. *Am J Surg Pathol* 2001;25:1075–1078.

58. Mian C, Pycha A, Wiener H, et al. Immunocyt: a new tool for detecting transitional cell cancer of the urinary tract. *J Urol* 1999;161(5):1486–1489.

59. Swana HS, Grossman D, Anthony JN, et al. Tumor content of the anti-apoptosis molecule surviving and recurrence of bladder cancer. *N Engl J Med* 1999;341:453–453.

60. Smith SD, Wheeler MA, Plescia J, et al. Urine detection of surviving and diagnosis of bladder cancer. *JAMA* 2001;285:324–328.

61. Heino A, Aaltoman S, Ala-Opas M. BTA test is superior to voided urine cytology in detecting malignant bladder tumours. *Ann Chir Gynaecol* 1999;84(4):304–307.

62. Leigh H, Marberger M, Conort P, et al. Comparison of the BTA stat test with voided urine cytology and bladder wash cytology in the diagnosis and monitoring of bladder cancer. *Eur Urol* 1999;35(2):52–56.

63. Nasuti JF, Gomella LG, Ismail M, et al. Utility of the BTA stat test for bladder cancer screening. *Diagn Cytol* 1999;21(1):27–29.

64. Zippe C, Pandrangi L, Potto JM, et al. NMP22: a sensitive cost-effective test in patients at risk for bladder cancer. *Anticancer Res* 1999;19(4A): 2621–2623.

65. Grocela JA, McDougal WS. Utility of nuclear matrix protein in the detection of bladder cancer. *Urol Clin North Am* 2000;27:47–51.

66. Lokeshwar VB, Obek C, Pham HT, et al. Urinary hyaluronic acid and hyaluronidase markers for bladder cancer detection and evaluation of grade. *J Urol* 2000;1:348–356.

67. Dalbagri G, Han W, Zlang AF, et al. Evaluation of the telomeric repeat amplification protocol (TRAP) assay for telomerase as a diagnostic modality in recurrent bladder cancer. *Clin Cancer Res* 1997;3(9):1593–1598.

68. Melamed MR, Klein FA. Flow cytometry of urinary bladder irrigation specimens. *Hum Pathol* 1984;15:362–365.

69. Deitch AD, Andersen KA, de Vere White RW. Evaluation of DNA flow cytometry as a screening test for bladder cancer. *J Occup Med* 1990;32: 898–903.

70. Giella JG, Ring C, Olsson CA. The predictive value of flow cytometry and urinary cytology in the follow up of patients with transitional cell carcinoma of the bladder. *J Urol* 1992;148:293–296.

71. Mellon K, Shenton BK, Neal DE. Is voided urine suitable for flow cytometric DNA analysis? *Br J Urol* 1991;67:48–53.

72. Hermansen DC, Badalament RAM, Bretton RR, et al. Voided flow cytometric in screening high-risk patients for the presence of bladder cancer. *J Occup Med* 1990;32:894–897.

73. Koss LG, Wersto RP, Simmons DA, et al. Predictive value of DNA measurements in bladder washings. *Cancer* 1989;64:916–924.

74. Gerber WL, Lenahan PJ, Kendall AR, et al. Computer-assisted microfluorometric detection of individual malignant bladder cells. *Urology* 1991;38: 466–472.

75. Junker K, Werner W, Mueller C. Interphase cytogenetic diagnosis of bladder cancer on cells from urine and bladder washing. *Int J Oncol* 1999;14(2): 309–313.

76. Brown FM. Urine cytology. It is still the gold standard for screening. *Urol Clin North Am* 2000;27:25–37.

77. Eble JH, Young RH. Benign and low-grade papillary lesions of the urinary bladder: a review of the papilloma-papillary carcinoma controversy, and a report of five typical papillomas. *Semin Diagn Pathol* 1989;6:351–371.

78. Thomas GJ, Regnier EA. Tumors of the kidney pelvis and ureter. *J Urol* 1924;11:205–238.

79. MacLean JT. Pathology of tumors of the renal pelvis and ureter. *J Urol* 1956;75:384–415.

80. Auld CD, Grigor KM, Fowler JW. Histopathological review of transitional cell carcinoma of the upper urinary tract. *J Urol* 1984;56:485–489.

81. Highman WJ. Transitional carcinoma of the upper urinary tract: a histological and cytopathological study. *J Clin Pathol* 1986;39:297–305.

82. Lauritzen AF, Kvist E, Bredesen J, et al. Primary carcinoma of the upper urinary tract. *Acta Pathol Microbiol Immunol Scand Sect A* 1987;95:7–10.

83. Davis BW, Hough AJ, Gardner WA. Renal pelvic carcinoma: morphological correlates of metastatic behavor. *J Urol* 1987;137:857–861.

84. Utz DC, McDonald JR. Squamous cell carcinoma of the kidney. *J Urol* 1957;78:540–552.

85. Kandemir O, Tatlisen A, Kontas O, et al. Sarcomatoid squamous cell carcinoma of the right renal pelvis with liver metastasis: case report. *J Urol* 1995;153:1895–1896.

86. Aufderheide AC, Streitz JM. Mucinous adenocarcinoma of the renal pelvis. Report of two cases. *Cancer* 1974;33:167–173.

87. Ackerman LV. Mucinous adenocarcinoma of the pelvis of the kidney. *J Urol* 1946;55:36–45.

88. Royce RK, Ackerman LV. Carcinoma of the bladder: clinical therapeutic and pathologic aspects of 135 cases. *J Urol* 1951;65:66–86.

89. Lerman RI, Hutter RVP, Whitmore WF. Papilloma of the urinary bladder. *Cancer* 1970;25:333–342.

90. Prout GR, Bassil B, Griffin P. The treated histories of patients with Ta grade I transitional-cell carcinoma of the bladder. *Arch Surg* 1986;121:1463–1468.

91. Gilbert HA, Logan JL, Kagan AR, et al. The natural history of papillary transitional cell carcinoma of the bladder and its treatment in an unselected population on the basis of histologic grading. *J Urol* 1978;119:488–492.

92. Amin MB, Ro JY, Troncoso P, et al. Micropapillary (ovarian serous carcinoma-like) variant of transitional cell carcinoma of the urinary bladder. *Am J Surg Pathol* 1994;18:1224–1232.

93. Amin MB, Gomez JA, Young RH. Urothelial transitional cell carcinoma with endophytic growth patterns. A discussion of patterns of invasion and problems associated with assessment of invasion in 18 cases. *Am J Surg Pathol* 1997;21:1057–1068.

94. Sarma KP. Genesis of papillary tumors: histological and microangiographic study. *Br J Urol* 1981;53:228–236.

95. Taylor DC, Bhagavan BS, Larsen MP, et al. Papillary urothelial hyperplasia. A precursor to papillary neoplasms. *Am J Surg Pathol* 1996;20:1481–1488.

96. Young RH. Papillary and polypoid cystitis. A report of eight cases. *Am J Surg Pathol* 1988;12:542–546.

97. Epstein JI, Amin MB, Reuter VR, Bladder Concensus Conference Committee. The World Health Organization/International Society of Urological Pathology Consensus Classification of urothelial (transitional cell) neoplasms of the urinary bladder. *Am J Surg Pathol* 1998;22:1435–1448.

98. Koss LG, Nakanishi I, Freed SZ. Nonpapillary carcinoma in situ and atypical hyperplasia in cancerous bladders. Further studies of surgically removed bladders by mapping. *Urology* 1977;9:442–455.

99. Prout GR, Griffin PP, Daly JJ, et al. Carcinoma in situ of the urinary bladder with and without associated vesical neoplasms. *Cancer* 1983;52:524–532.

100. Murphy WM, Soloway MS. Developing carcinoma (dysplasia) of the urinary bladder. *Pathol Annu* 1982;17(Pt I):197–217.

101. Robertson AJ, Beck JS, Burnett RA, et al. Observer variability in histopathological reporting of transitional cell carcinoma and epithelial dysplasia in bladders. *J Clin Pathol* 1990;43:17–21.

102. Amin MB, Young RH. Intraepithelial lesions of the urinary bladder with a discussion of the histogenesis of urothelial neoplasia. *Semin Diagn Pathol* 1997;14:84–97.

103. Young RH, Eble JN. Unusual forms of carcinoma of the urinary bladder. *Hum Pathol* 1991;22:948–965.

104. Farrow GM, Utz DC. Observations on microinvasive transitional cell carcinoma of the urinary bladder. *Clin Oncol* 1982;1:609–615.

105. McKenney JK, Gomez JA, Desai S, et al. Morphologic expression of urothelial carcinoma in situ. A detailed evaluation of its historical patterns with emphasis on carcinoma in situ with microinvasion. *Am J Surg Pathol* 2001;25:356–362.

106. Ro JY, Ayala AG, El-Naggar A. Muscularis mucosa of urinary bladder. Importance for staging and treatment. *Am J Surg Pathol* 1987;11:668–673.

107. Keep JC, Piehl M, Miller A, et al. Invasive carcinomas of the urinary bladder. Evaluation of tunica muscularis mucosae involvement. *Am J Clin Pathol* 1989;91:575–579.

108. Weaver MG, Abdul-Karim FW. The prevalence and character of the muscularis mucosae of the human urinary bladder. *Histopathology* 1990;17:563–566.

109. Younes M, Sussman J, True LD. The usefulness of the level of the muscularis mucosae in the staging of invasive transitional cell carcinoma of the urinary bladder. *Cancer* 1990;66:543–548.

110. Young RH, Zukerberg L. Microcystic transitional cell carcinomas of the urinary bladder. A report of four cases. *Am J Clin Pathol* 1991;96:635–639.

111. Young RH, Wick MR, Mills SE. Sarcomatoid carcinoma of the urinary bladder. A clinicopathologic analysis of 12 cases and review of the literature. *Am J Clin Pathol* 1988;90:653–661.

112. Jones EC, Young RH. Myxoid and sclerosing sarcomatoid transitional cell carcinoma of the urinary bladder: a clinicopathologic and immunohistochemical study of 25 cases. *Mod Pathol* 1997;10:908–916.

113. Ro JY, Ayala AG, Wishnow KI, et al. Sarcomatoid bladder carcinoma: clinicopathologic and immunohistochemical study on 44 cases. *Surg Pathol* 1988;1:359–374.

114. Wick MR, Brown BA, Young RH, et al. Spindle-cell proliferations of the urinary tract. An immunohistochemical study. *Am J Surg Pathol* 1988;12:379–389.

115. Suster S, Robinson MJ. Spindle cell carcinoma of the renal pelvis. Immunohistochemical and ultrastructural study of a case demonstrating

116. Burry AF, Munn SR, Arnold EP, et al. Trophoblastic metaplasia in urothelial carcinoma of the bladder. *Br J Urol* 1986;58:143–146.

117. Morton KD, Burnett RA. Choriocarcinoma arising in transitional cell carcinoma of bladder: a case report. *Histopathol* 1988;12:325–328.

118. Martin JE, Jenkins BJ, Zuk RJ, et al. Human chorionic gonadotropin expression and histological findings as predictors of response to radiotherapy in carcinoma of the bladder. *Virchows Arch (A)* 1989;414:273–277.

119. Young RH, Wick MR. Transitional cell carcinoma of the urinary bladder with pseudosarcomatous stroma. *Am J Clin Pathol* 1988;89:216–219.

120. Mahadevia PS, Alexander JE, Rojas-Corona R, et al. Pseudosarcomatous stromal reaction in primary and metastatic urothelial carcinoma. A source of diagnostic difficulty. *Am J Surg Pathol* 1989;13:782–790.

121. Eble JN, Young RH. Stromal osseous metaplasia in carcinoma of the bladder. *J Urol* 1991;145:823–825.

122. Zukerberg LR, Armin A-R, Pisharodi L, et al. Transitional cell carcinoma of the urinary bladder with osteoclast-type giant cells: a report of two cases and review of the literature. *Histopathology* 1990;17:407–411.

123. Talbert ML, Young RH. Carcinomas of the urinary bladder with deceptively benign-appearing foci. A report of three cases. *Am J Surg Pathol* 1989;13:374–381.

124. Drew PA, Furman J, Civantos F, et al. The nested variant of transitional cell carcinoma: an aggressive neoplasm with innocuous histology. *Mod Pathol* 1996;9:989–994.

125. Lin O, Cardillo M, Dalbagni G, et al. Nested variant of urothelial carcinoma: a clinicopathologic and immunohistochemical study of 12 cases. *Mod Pathol* 2003;16:1289–1298.

126. Young RH. Non-neoplastic epithelial abnormalities and tumor-like lesions. In: Young RH, Roth LM, eds. *Pathology of the urinary bladder*, Vol. 13. Chapter 1 in *Contemporary Issues in Surgical Pathology*. New York: Churchill Livingstone, 1989.

127. Volmar KE, Chan TY, DeMarzo AM, et al. Florid von Brunn nests mimicking urothelial carcinoma. A morphologic and immunohistochemical comparison to the nested variant of urothelial carcinoma. *Am J Surg Pathol* 2003;27:1243–1252.

128. Young RH, Oliva E. Transitional cell carcinomas of the urinary bladder that may be underdiagnosed. A report of four invasive cases exemplifying the homology between neoplastic and non-neoplastic transitional cell lesions. *Am J Surg Pathol* 1996;20:1448–1454.

129. Zukerberg LR, Harris NL, Young RH. Carcinomas of the urinary bladder simulating malignant lymphoma: a report of five cases. *Am J Surg Pathol* 1991;15:569–576.

130. Friedell GH, Bell JR, Burney SW, et al. Histopathology and classification of urinary bladder carcinoma. *Urol Clin North Am* 1976;3:53–70.

131. Connery DB. Leukoplakia of the urinary bladder and its association with carcinoma. *J Urol* 1953;69:121–127.

132. Benson RC, Swanson SK, Farrow GM. Relationship of leukoplakia to urothelial malignancy. *J Urol* 1984;131:507–511.

133. Mostofi FK, Thomson RV, Dean AL Jr. Mucous adenocarcinoma of the urinary bladder. *Cancer* 1955;8:741–758.

134. Thomas DG, Ward AM, Williams JL. A study of 52 cases of adenocarcinoma of the bladder. *Br J Urol* 1971;43:4–15.

135. Jacobo E, Loening S, Schmidt JD, et al. Primary adenocarcinoma of the bladder: a retrospective study of 20 patients. *J Urol* 1977;117:54–56.

136. Anderstrom C, Johansson SL, von Schultz L. Primary adenocarcinoma of the urinary bladder. A clinicopathologic and prognostic study. *Cancer* 1983;52:1273–1280.

137. Bennett JK, Wheatley JK, Walton KN. 10-year experience with adenocarcinoma of the bladder. *J Urol* 1984;131:262–263.

138. Abenoza P, Manivel C, Fraley EE. Primary adenocarcinoma of urinary bladder. Clinicopathologic study of 16 cases. *Urology* 1987;29:9–14.

139. Young RH, Parkhurst EC. Mucinous adenocarcinoma of bladder. Case associated with extensive intestinal metaplasia of urothelium in patient with nonfunctioning bladder for twelve years. *Urology* 1984;24:192–195.

140. Grignon DG, Ro JY, Ayala AG, et al. Primary adenocarcinoma of the urinary bladder: a clinicopathologic analysis of 72 cases. *Cancer* 1991;67:2165–2172.

141. Sheldon CA, Clayman RV, Gonzalez R, et al. Malignant urachal lesions. *J Urol* 1984;131:1–8.

142. O'Kane HOJ, Megaw JMcI. Carcinoma in the exstrophic bladder. *Br J Surg* 1968;55:631–635.

143. Chor PJ, Gaum LD, Young RH. Clear cell adenocarcinoma of the urinary bladder: report of a case of probable Mullerian origin. *Mod Pathol* 1993;6:225–228.

144. Saphir O. Signet-ring cell carcinoma of the urinary bladder. *Am J Pathol* 1955;31:223–231.

145. Grignon DJ, Ro JY, Ayala AG, et al. Primary signet-ring carcinoma of the urinary bladder. *Am J Clin Pathol* 1991;95:13–20.

146. Ordonez NG, Khorsand J, Ayala AG, et al. Oat cell carcinoma of the urinary tract. An immunohistochemical and electron microscopic study. *Cancer* 1986;58:2519–1530.

147. Mills SE, Wolfe JT III, Weiss MA, et al. Small cell undifferentiated carcinoma of the urinary bladder. A light-microscopic, immunocytochemical, and ultrastructural study of 12 cases. *Am J Surg Pathol* 1987;11:606–617.

148. Grignon DJ, Ro JY, Ayala AG, et al. Small cell carcinoma of the urinary bladder. A clinicopathologic analysis of 22 cases. *Cancer* 1992;69:527–536.

149. Podesta AH, True LD. Small cell carcinoma of the bladder: report of five cases with immunohistochemistry and review of the literature with evaluation of prognosis according to stage. *Cancer* 1989;64:710–714.

150. Blomjous CEM, Vos W, De Voogt HJ, et al. Small cell carcinoma of the urinary bladder: a clinicopathologic, morphometric, immunohistochemical, and ultrastructural study of 18 cases. *Cancer* 1989;64:1347–1357.

151. Komatsu H, Kinoshita K, Mikata N, et al. Spindle and giant-cell carcinoma of the bladder. Report of 3 cases. *Eur Urol* 1985;11:141–144.

152. Amin MB, Ro JY, Lee KM, et al. Lymphoepitheloma-like carcinoma of the urinary bladder. *Am J Surg Pathol* 1994;18:466–473.

CHAPTER 20 ■ MOLECULAR BIOLOGY AND PROGNOSTIC MARKERS IN BLADDER CANCER

RICHARD J. COTE, SETH P. LERNER, AND RAM H. DATAR

INTRODUCTION

There have been significant advances in our understanding of molecular biology of bladder cancer progression and response to therapy. Thus, there is the exciting possibility that both existing and new therapies can be tailored to benefit patients based on the risk of progression and molecular alterations specific to a patient's tumor. Targeted therapy—a therapy that targets molecular mechanism and risk—can now be conceived for bladder cancer. We review here the potential for rational therapeutic intervention utilizing the available knowledge of the molecular biology of cell-cycle regulation, signal transduction, apoptosis, and angiogenesis in bladder cancer.

BLADDER CANCER: THE DISEASE

Bladder cancer comprises a broad spectrum of tumors that include urothelial carcinomas (UCs, also known as transitional cell carcinomas or TCCs), squamous cell carcinomas (SCCs), adenocarcinomas, and a few other tumor types that are less frequent. UCs are by far the more prevalent tumors and represent nearly 90% of all bladder cancers in the United States (1). In Western countries, only about 2% of bladder cancers are squamous cell carcinomas, and adenocarcinomas comprise about 1% to 2% of bladder cancers (2). A primary risk factor for bladder cancer in the West is smoking (3). However, the etiology and the prevalent type of bladder cancer can vary dramatically in different geographical regions; for example, in Egypt, where the dominant etiology is schistosomiasis, SCC is the most prevalent histologic subtype of bladder cancer. UCs are subdivided into noninvasive papillary and invasive carcinoma types that are believed to originate from different genetic alterations. Superficial papillary UCs correspond to 70% of all UCs and usually are of low grade and noninvasive at the time of presentation. These tumors begin as areas of hyperplasia that later undergo a process of dedifferentiation (2). Invasive tumors may arise from these lesions, and are more poorly differentiated neoplasms (i.e., those with higher histologic grade) having a higher tendency to invade and metastasize. Superficial papillary UCs are characterized by multiple recurrences, and 10% to 30% of these will progress to invasive disease. In general, multifocal recurrent superficial papillary tumors provide a unique model system to study the molecular mechanisms underlying the various steps involved in cancer development, and offer a valuable source of material to search for specific markers for early tumor detection and prognosis. Most invasive carcinomas are believed to develop from carcinoma *in situ* (CIS), a flat lesion that has a high propensity to progress to a high-grade invasive tumor. Added to the complexity of the UCs is the fact that high-grade lesions can undergo metaplasia (squamous and/or glandular) as well as epithelial-mesenchymal transitions. The variability in manifestation and the histology of the UCs underscores the need to study the molecular biology of the disease.

MOLECULAR BASIS FOR THE DEVELOPMENT AND PROGRESSION OF BLADDER CANCER: EVOLVING MODEL OF BLADDER CANCER PROGRESSION

Advances in molecular biology over the last decade have led to the identification of many genetic alterations in bladder cancer and a better understanding of its malignant evolution and progression. Alterations in chromosomes 9 and 17 appear to play important roles in the development and progression of bladder cancer (4). Approximately 60% to 65% of all transitional cell tumors are characterized by loss of heterozygosity (LOH) on chromosome 9. Chromosomal analysis of various stages of UC has revealed that allelic loss only on chromosome 9 is found exclusively in early-stage, well-differentiated tumors, while in more advanced lesions, other genetic changes are frequently observed. LOH on chromosome 9 is thus considered to be an early event in bladder tumorigenesis (5). Two main categories of genes are considered to be responsible for malignant transformation—oncogenes and tumor suppressor genes. Transformation of a proto-oncogene into an oncogene results in overexpression that may be caused by a mutation, gene amplification, promoter methylation, or insertion of viral genetic material into the human DNA. Activation of the proto-oncogene results in derangement of cell cycle control, thereby stimulating malignant transformation. Tumor suppressor genes have two alleles and since they are recessive in function, both must be inactivated in order to induce tumorigenesis. The proposed mechanisms for this event are via loss of or mutation in both alleles, or the LOH in one and mutation in the sequence of (or methylation-mediated silencing of) the remaining allele (6). Many studies have been conducted to identify the proto-oncogenes and tumor suppressor genes contributing to the development and progression of bladder cancer. The tumor suppressor genes on chromosome 9 (marked by allelic losses seen in both 9p and 9q, and deletions between the region 9p12-9q34.1 that spans the $p16^{INK4A}$ locus) have been implicated in the formation of UC. These tumors have a good prognosis, and a low propensity to invade and metastasize. In contrast, loss of genetic material on chromosome 17p (the location of *p53* gene) is associated with flat lesions, or CIS (7).

These tumors demonstrate a more aggressive behavior (2). These studies indicate the existence of at least two divergent pathways of bladder tumor progression that identify morphologically and biologically distinct subsets of UC that can be defined by unique patterns of molecular alterations. Based on the consistent and frequent genetic defects found in bladder tumors in studies from a number of groups and increasing understanding of the role of cell-cycle regulation in tumor behavior, a detailed and sophisticated model of important molecular events in bladder cancer has been established (Figure 20.1).

Many of the genetic defects described in bladder cancer actually represent alterations in cell cycle regulation. The normal cell cycle consists of a series of highly structured and sequential events, culminating in cell growth and eventual division into two daughter cells. The cell's chromatin (chromosomal DNA and associated proteins) is the most important structure that must double in size in preparation for cell division. The active cell cycle is divided into four phases: M (mitosis), G1 (gap phase 1), S (DNA synthetic phase), and G2 (gap phase 2); the time spent outside of M (i.e., G1, S, and G2) is referred to as "interphase." In order to protect from propagation of genetic lesions that may result from any replicative DNA damage, the normal cell has several intrinsic checkpoints for interrupting the cell cycle if such DNA damage occurs. The different checkpoints include DNA damage checkpoints, which occur before the cell enters S phase (a G_1 checkpoint), during S phase itself, and after DNA replication (a G_2 checkpoint); a check on completion of S phase when the cell is believed to monitor the presence of Okazaki fragments on the lagging strand during DNA replication (the cell is not permitted to proceed in the cell cycle until these have disappeared); and spindle checkpoints that act through a variety of mechanisms to detect any failure of spindle fibers to attach to kinetochores and arrest the cell in metaphase, detect improper alignment of the spindle itself and block cytokinesis, and trigger apoptosis if the damage is irreparable.

Alterations in the normal cell cycle can occur due to numerous reasons and they have been implicated in a variety of cancers. Disruption of the normal cell division cycle has been reported to be crucial in the development and progression of bladder cancer (8). These disruptions can occur singly or in combination, suggesting the importance of studying the entire pathway of cell cycle regulation in order to understand the molecular mechanisms leading to bladder tumorigenesis. Furthermore, the cell cycle is not an autonomous pathway; it is guided by extraneous signals from apoptotic and signal transduction pathways. Hence, understanding alterations in the cell cycle in the context of other cellular pathways is critical in elucidating mechanisms underlying the development of bladder cancer.

MOLECULAR STAGING OF BLADDER CANCER

Standard methods of bladder cancer assessment are based on histologic grade and stage of the tumor. Pathologic staging systems are based on depth of invasion and assessment of regional and systemic spread of tumor. For bladder cancer, stage is based on the depth of invasion of the tumor to involve specific anatomic areas of the bladder wall and is the basis for the tumor/nodes/metastasis (TNM) system (9–12). However, whereas these histopathologic criteria can provide us with reliable and reproducible information about populations of patients, they are unable to specify risk for progression or response to treatment for the individual patient with bladder cancer. Bladder tumors are grouped into various clinical stages based on the depth of tumor invasion, lymph node involvement, and presence/absence of distant metastasis. The type of treatment administered to patients with UC is currently based on this staging system, and the therapy can result in significant morbidity and financial burden to the patient. Thus, it is essential to develop a system of staging that can optimize the therapy administered to bladder cancer patients (2).

Over the past decade, there have been enormous advances in our understanding of the molecular basis for bladder cancer tumorigenesis and progression (Fig. 20.1). We now are beginning to translate this information to develop methods to assess cancer at the cellular and molecular level in ways that were inconceivable only a few years ago (4). The increased understanding of the molecular basis for bladder cancer is leading to

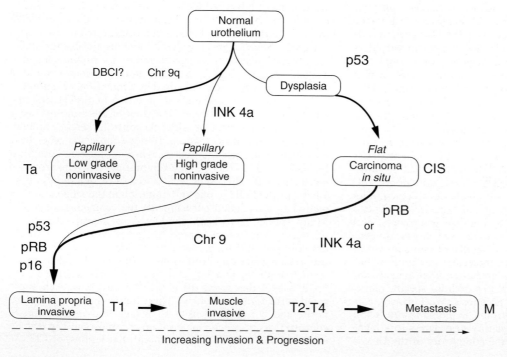

FIGURE 20.1. A model of molecular pathways of bladder cancer progression.

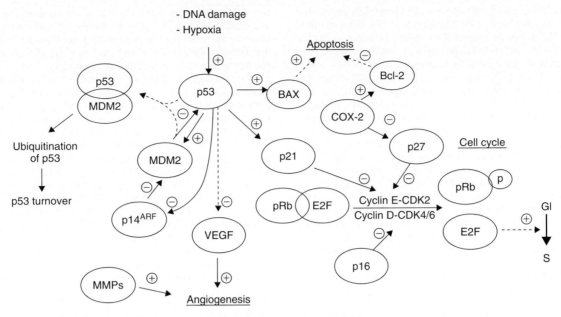

FIGURE 20.2. Molecular pathways prone to alteration during bladder cancer progression, which can be targeted therapeutically, are depicted.

the development of a new wave of therapeutic interventions targeted at specific cellular mechanisms. Many molecular pathways that are altered in bladder cancer and can be targeted therapeutically are depicted in Figure 20.2 (13). The studies described below show that understanding molecular alterations in UC can add greater specificity to the determination of outcome. Molecular profiling can facilitate a molecular staging of bladder tumors. Furthermore, this "ultrastaging" can lead to identification of specific molecular classes, which may respond better to specific chemotherapeutic agents. This will eventually lead to targeted therapy tailored toward specific molecular defects, thereby significantly lowering the morbidity associated with bladder cancer. The future goal therefore will be to approach each individual tumor as a specific entity and to identify the molecular characteristics that make each tumor unique. Specific management strategies and therapeutic modalities most efficacious for each individual patient may then be determined.

ALTERATIONS IN p53 PATHWAY

p53

The protein encoded by the *p53* tumor suppressor gene, located on chromosome 17p13.1, is a 393 amino acid, 53-kDa nuclear phosphoprotein. The *p53* gene (genotype) and protein (phenotype) play a critical role in regulation of the normal cell cycle and apoptotic response. The functional loss of *p53* tumor suppressor gene is implicated in a complex array of aberrations in growth regulatory functions involving cell cycle, apoptotic, senescence, and angiogenic pathways.

The p53 protein plays a key role in mediating growth arrest and repairing DNA damage at the G1/S transition. In response to DNA damage, p53 protein expression is up-regulated, which in turn up-regulates its downstream target, a cyclin-dependent kinase inhibitor (cdki) called p21/WAF1, thereby arresting cell cycle progression. Once the DNA damage is repaired, accumulated p53 protein levels are abrogated by MDM2, an upstream regulator of p53 expression. Alternatively, in cells where an effective cell cycle arrest cannot be mediated in response to

DNA damage, the p53 protein has been shown to initiate and execute an apoptotic response (14). The tumor suppressor function of the p53 protein occurs at the G1/S transition as well as the G2/M checkpoint, thereby making it as Levine describes in his 1997 review "a guardian or gatekeeper of the cell cycle" (15).

In accordance with the important role of *p53* in bladder carcinogenesis, the majority of UCs display a loss of one allele of 17p (LOH). Mutation in the remaining allele following LOH is an important mechanism of tumor suppressor gene inactivation. The wild type p53 protein (wt p53) has a short half-life of less than 30 minutes. However, the mutated protein has a prolonged half life due to decreased ubiquitination. This increased half life leads to nuclear accumulation, allowing for nuclear levels for p53 adequate for detection by immunohistochemistry. Hence, nuclear accumulation of p53 protein as detected by immunostaining has been hypothesized to correlate with p53 mutations and thus a loss of p53 function.

While mutations in the *p53* gene have been thought to be at least partially responsible for the nuclear accumulation of p53 (altered p53 phenotype), there are reports to suggest that this is not always the case (16). In addition, the absence of nuclear accumulation of p53 protein does not rule out *p53* gene alterations. In fact, nonsense mutations may produce unstable transcripts or truncated proteins that lack the nuclear localization signal, thereby giving negative results on immunostaining. These events have been reported to contribute to approximately 20% of the *p53* gene mutations detected in particular tumor types such as head-and-neck cancers (17).

Previous reports indicate that not all cases with a nuclear accumulation of p53 have a loss of function of p53. It has also been shown that not all cases with a wt phenotype have intact p53 function (18,19). Thus the p53 phenotype is not completely predictive of p53 function. One of the major reasons for this finding could be the discordance between the p53 phenotype and corresponding genotype. Previous studies have investigated the relationship between p53 phenotype and genotype in bladder UC (20,21). These studies, however, were limited by either small cohort size and/or lack of specificity of the technology used to investigate mutations in the *p53* gene.

Recently, we examined the p53 genotype in bladder cancer in archival paraffin embedded tissue sections by complete exonic sequencing using Affymetrix p53 GeneChip in collaboration with Roche Molecular Diagnostics. We demonstrated that tumor DNA can be analyzed for gene mutations using the valuable resource of archival paraffin-embedded tissues, and that such analysis can provide important information about the p53 genotype (22). Significant concordance exists between the p53 phenotype and the genotype, although a substantially minor fraction of cases demonstrates discordance. The possible explanations for the discordance seen in some cases (where no nuclear accumulation of p53 protein could be detected despite the p53 gene mutations identified by the GeneChip analysis) include the following: (a) not all p53 mutations result in nuclear accumulation because the resultant protein is still effectively degraded; (b) specific p53 gene polymorphisms do not interfere with the normal p53 phenotype; (c) nonsense mutations result in unstable transcripts or truncated protein that lacks the nuclear localization signal; and (d) mutations generate stop codons resulting in negative immunostaining. When p21 expression was examined to understand the relationship of gene mutations on downstream p53 function, the cases with a mutated p53 genotype and wt phenotype had an up-regulated p21 expression, suggesting the existence of a functional p53 protein in majority of these cases. Conversely, cases with no evidence of mutation by the GeneChip analysis which demonstrate a nuclear accumulation of p53 protein could possibly be a result of failure of normal turnover of p53 in spite of a wt genotype due to alterations in proteins involved in wt p53 protein degradation pathways (such as MDM2 or p14), or failure of mutation detection due to lack of sufficient tumor DNA in the extracts from the archival paraffin-embedded tissue sections. These findings may underscore the significance of determining both p53 genotype and p53 phenotype in assessing bladder cancer.

Several studies have addressed the impact of immunohistochemical p53 accumulation in predicting tumor recurrence in patients with superficial papillary bladder cancer. p53 expression has been shown to be associated with progression of Ta disease (23,24), T1 disease (25,26), and CIS (27). However, these studies are complicated by methodologic differences in the immunohistochemical and statistical analysis and critically in the definition of progressive disease. While some of the smaller studies have shown a correlation between p53 accumulation and tumor recurrence by univariate analysis, none of these studies reported p53 accumulation to provide additional information compared to clinical parameters, and the actual question still remains open (28).

We investigated whether the nuclear accumulation of p53 protein was an important factor in predicting the clinical behavior of bladder cancer, and demonstrated that detection of nuclear accumulation of p53 protein is significantly associated with an increased risk of recurrence of bladder cancer and a decreased overall survival (19). More specifically, we analyzed histologic specimens from 243 patients with bladder cancer who were treated by radical cystectomy. p53 nuclear reactivity was analyzed in relation to time to recurrence and overall survival. In patients with UC confined to the bladder following cystectomy and no evidence of perivesical invasion or lymph node metastases, detection of nuclear p53 protein was significantly associated with a decreased survival independent of grade and tumor stage (Table 20.1). Based on this data, patients with organ-confined bladder UC demonstrating a p53 alteration may not be cured with surgery alone and may benefit from adjuvant treatment strategies. The detection of nuclear p53 was significantly associated with an increased risk of recurrence ($P < .001$) and a decreased overall survival rate ($P < .001$) (Fig. 20.3). In patients with organ-confined bladder carcinoma, the rates of recurrence for stage pT1, pT2, and pT3a tumors that had no detectable nuclear reactivity were similar at 5 years and significantly lower than for pT1, pT2, and pT3a tumors that demonstrated p53 immunoreactivity. In a multivariable analysis stratified according to grade, pathologic stage, and lymph node status, nuclear p53 accumulation was an independent predictor (and in cancer confined to the bladder, the only independent predictor) of recurrence free and overall survival ($P < .001$). These results support the hypothesis that within organ-confined carcinoma, it is not the depth of bladder wall invasion that determines survival, but the presence or absence of nuclear accumulation of p53 protein (i.e., a p53 alteration/mutation).

Another study also demonstrated that bladder tumors with p53 alterations behaved more aggressively than those tumors with a wt p53 gene (25). In this study, superficial (T1) bladder

TABLE 20.1

ASSOCIATION OF p53 IMMUNOREACTIVITY WITH GRADE AND PATHOLOGIC STAGE OF BLADDER CANCER AND PRESENCE OR ABSENCE OF LYMPH-NODE METASTASES IN 190 PATIENTS NOT PREVIOUSLY TESTED FOR p53 ALTERATION

Variable	No. of patients	Nuclear p53 reactivity Negative Number (percent)	Positive	P Value
Grade				
2	9	7 (78)	2 (22)	
3	122	79 (65)	43 (35)	
4	59	33 (56)	26 (44)	0.20
Stage				
Metastases absent				
Pa or Pis	15	12 (80)	3 (20)	
P1	39	30 (77)	9 (23)	
P2	29	19 (66)	10 (34)	
P3a	20	11 (55)	9 (45)	
P3b	36	21 (58)	15 (42)	
P4	9	7 (78)	2 (22)	
Metastases present	42	19 (45)	23 (55)	0.003

Adapted from Esrig D, Elmajian D, Groshen S, et al. Accumulation of nuclear p53 and tumor progression in bladder cancer. N Engl J Med 1994;331:1259–1264.

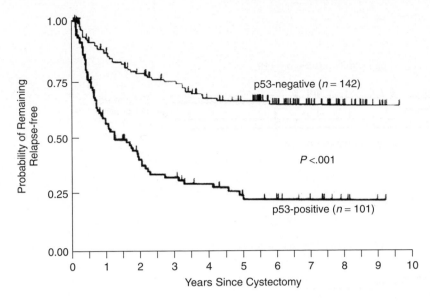

FIGURE 20.3. Probability of remaining relapse-free in 243 patients with bladder cancer and either p53-positive or p53-negative tumors. (Adapted from Esrig D, Elmajian D, Groshen S, et al. Accumulation of nuclear p53 and tumor progression in bladder cancer. *N Engl J Med* 1994;331:1259–1264.)

tumors with p53 mutations were found to progress more quickly and in higher percentages than similar tumors with no p53 alterations. The authors suggest that superficial tumors with p53 mutations may be considered candidates for early cystectomy. These two studies investigating the clinical behavior of bladder tumors based on the presence or absence of a p53 alteration suggest that organ-confined tumors demonstrating a p53 alteration progress more quickly than tumors with no p53 alteration, and that these patients are at high risk for recurrence and may be considered for adjuvant treatment strategies.

While many studies in bladder cancer have concluded that p53 immunohistochemistry (IHC) can provide independent prognostic information, others have failed to show this relationship as independent from known prognostic factors. The importance of p53 mutations in tumor biology, particularly bladder cancer progression, is irrefutable. Numerous retrospective studies have indicated association between p53 alterations with adverse clinical outcomes in superficial as well as muscle-invasive bladder cancer; these studies have been reviewed recently (29). Despite many such studies, however, there is some ambiguity about the clinical impact of p53 mutations. Schmitz-Drager et al. have performed a meta-analysis of 138 publications reporting on 43 studies comprising 3,764 bladder cancer patients (30). This comparison yielded considerable differences in the conclusions of clinical outcome, which the authors have ascribed to technical aspects of p53 immunohistochemistry (such as selection of antibodies and use of different cutoff values), study design, and patient selection. They contend that further retrospective investigations are unlikely to offer any solution, and that prospective multicenter clinical trials examining the utility of p53 alterations is needed.

p21

p21 WAF1 is a downstream effector of p53 and belongs to the Cip1/Kip1 family of cdkis (see below). Thus, it is a potential tumor suppressor gene and likely plays an important role in tumor development. Although Chen et al. have reported that polymorphism of p21 codon 31 is associated with development of bladder cancer (31), Lancombe et al. found WAF1 mutations in only 2 of the 27 primary bladder tumors and concluded that *p21/WAF1* gene aberrations are infrequent in bladder cancer (32).

Although loss of p21 expression has been consistently associated with a poor outcome in patients with muscle-invasive

bladder cancer (see below) (33), Shariat et al. suggested that its function in patients with bladder CIS was different (34). They found that in CIS without muscle-invasive disease, positive p21 expression was independently associated with bladder cancer recurrence and progression, which is counterintuitive to the general protective function of p21 against disease progression. One possible explanation provided is that in CIS, p21 expression may be modulated by molecular events different from those involved in muscle-invasive bladder cancer (i.e., p53-independent pathways).

Reduced expression of p21WAF1 has been reported to have prognostic value in several human malignancies. Loss of p21 expression and subsequent loss of cell cycle control is thought to be a mechanism by which p53 alterations may influence tumor progression. However, it has been demonstrated that p21 expression may be mediated through p53-independent pathways (35). This indicates that p21 expression can be maintained despite p53 alterations. p53-altered tumors that are p21-negative demonstrate a significantly increased probability of recurrence and significantly decreased probability of overall survival in patients compared to those who maintain expression of p21 (Fig. 20.4) (33). The association between p21 status and prognosis in p53-altered bladder tumors was independent of tumor grade, pathologic stage, and lymph node status. The strongest association between p21 status and tumor progression was demonstrated in patients with organ-confined (CIS, T1, T2, T3a) and extravesical (T3b, T4) disease with no evidence of lymph node metastases. Loss of p21 expression was strongly associated with an increased probability of recurrence and decreased probability of survival in patients with lymph node–negative organ-confined and lymph node–negative extravesical disease. In fact, p21 was the only independent predictor of disease progression in p53-altered bladder tumors in a multivariate analysis of p21 status, histologic grade, and pathologic stage. Maintenance of p21 expression appeared to abrogate the deleterious effects of p53 alterations on bladder cancer progression (33). The pivotal role of the p53/p21 pathway in bladder cancer progression has been further confirmed by recent studies by Chatterjee et al. and Shariat et al. (36,37).

MDM2

The MDM2 gene is located on chromosome 12q14.3-q15. It is involved in an autoregulatory feedback loop with p53 (38).

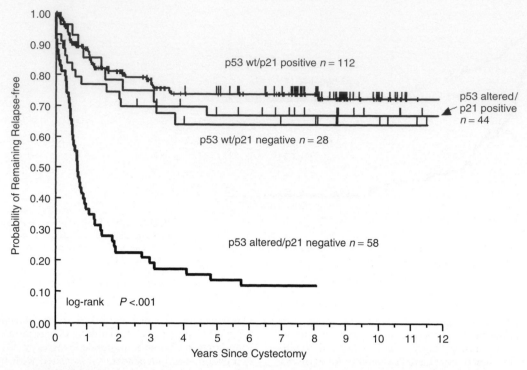

FIGURE 20.4. Probability of remaining recurrence-free in 242 patients with bladder tumors stratified by p53 and p21 status: p53 wt, no detectable p53 nuclear reactivity (p53 wt phenotype); p53-altered, nuclear p53 reactivity detected (p53-altered phenotype); p21-positive, p21 nuclear expression detected; p21-negative, no detectable p21 nuclear expression. The patients were stratified into four groups on the basis of p53 status and p21 status of their tumors. Patients with p53-altered/p21-negative tumors had a significantly higher rate of recurrence (two-sided P <.00001) in comparison with other patients. 95% confidence intervals and number of patients at risk are provided at 5 years. Each tick mark represents a patient who had no evidence of tumor recurrence or who was alive at the time of last follow-up. The log-rank test was used to compare the time to tumor recurrence and survival among the patient groups. (Adapted from Stein JP, Ginsberg DA, Grossfeld GD, et al. Effect of p21WAF1/CIP1 expression on tumor progression in bladder. *J Natl Cancer Inst* 1998;90:1072–1079.)

An increase in the level of p53 leads to transactivation of the MDM2 promoter, thereby upregulating the expression of MDM2. MDM2 in turn binds p53 and transports it to the proteasome for polyubiquitination and subsequent degradation; MDM2 levels are reduced when p53 levels are lowered (Figure 20.2) (39).

MDM2 gene amplification has been reported in bladder cancer. The frequency of this amplification increased with stage (Ta to T4) and grade (low grade to high grade) (40). Lianes et al. reported a >20% nuclear staining with MDM2 IHC in 30% of 87 bladder tumors (66/87 were T2-T4) and found an association with low grade and stage (41). MDM2 overexpression was also associated with positive p53 nuclear reactivity in 16 tumors in this study. In contrast, there was no correlation between p53 positivity and MDM2 expression in 25 tumors studied by Barbareschi et al. They proposed that a combined MDM2/p53 evaluation might be of prognostic relevance (42). Multivariate analysis in a set of 21 patients with T1 disease who had subsequently progressed and 17 patients with T1 disease who had remained progression-free showed that both p53 and MDM2 IHC were independent predictors of reduced progression-free intervals (43).

Novel forms of MDM2 with alternatively spliced transcripts have been reported in bladder cancer and these appear to be more common in muscle-invasive disease (44). The biologic importance of these alternate forms and their relationship to MDM2 IHC remains to be established. Evaluation of the expression of MDM2 in bladder cancer is likely to be important and its simultaneous use with p53 IHC for the prediction of prognosis in bladder cancer needs to be pursued further.

ALTERATIONS IN THE RETINOBLASTOMA GENE AND PROTEIN

The *RB* gene, the first tumor suppressor gene to be identified, is localized to band q14 on chromosome 13 (13q14), and its product is a nuclear phosphoprotein (pRb). Phosphorylation of pRb plays a central role in the regulation of the cell cycle. pRb interacts with multiple cell cycle regulatory proteins that are involved at the G1/S transition (45,46). The active nonphosphorylated form of pRb binds to and sequesters the transcription factor E2F. During late G1, pRb is phosphorylated and inactivated by cyclin D1-cdk4/6 complex, and releases E2F. Free E2F can transcribe genes such as thymidylate synthase (*TS*), which are required for DNA synthesis. Cyclin-dependent kinase (cdk) inhibitors such as p16, p21, and p27 inhibit cdk activity and regulate pRb phosphorylation.

The most commonly known inactivation of *RB* gene function in bladder tumors is deletion of chromosome 13q. The frequency of *RB* gene inactivation in invasive bladder cancers varies considerably between different investigations. Depending on the method used, frequencies between 14% and 80%

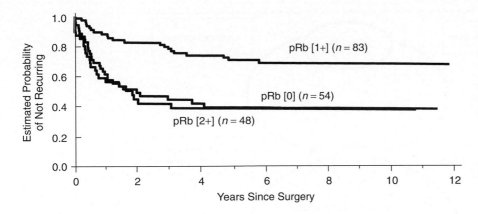

FIGURE 20.5. Probability of remaining relapse-free in 185 patients with invasive urothelial cancer according to pRb status. pRb 0 (no detectable nuclear reactivity); pRb 1+ (1-50% nuclear reactivity); and pRb2+ (>50% nuclear reactivity). (Adapted from Chatterjee SJ, Shi SR, Datar RH, et al. Hyperphosphorylation of pRb: a mechanism for RB tumor suppressor pathway inactivation in bladder cancer. *J Pathol* 2004;203:762–770.)

have been reported. Miyamoto et al. examined the entire coding region of the *RB* gene using polymerase chain reaction followed by single strand conformation polymorphism (PCR-SSCP) analysis. Of 30 samples obtained from patients with bladder cancer, 8 (27%) were found to have *RB* gene mutations (47). DNA sequencing of the PCR products revealed five cases with single-point mutations and three cases with small deletions. Mutations were detected in 21% (4 of 19) noninvasive (Ta and T1) tumors and 36% (4 of 11) invasive (pT2 or greater) tumors. These results suggest that *RB* gene mutations are involved in low-grade and noninvasive bladder cancers as well as in high-grade and invasive cancers. Acikbas et al. have suggested that detection of LOH of the *RB1* gene by polymerase chain reaction followed by restriction fragment length polymorphism (PCR-RFLP) can be a good adjunctive test for evaluation of the bladder cancer (48).

The role of pRb inactivation in noninvasive bladder tumors has rarely been addressed. Grossman et al. studied p53 accumulation along with Rb expression in 45 patients with T1 bladder cancer (49). Patients with abnormal expression of either or both proteins had a significant increase in tumor progression ($P < .04$ and $P = .005$ respectively), while no patients with normal expression of both the proteins progressed.

Loss of expression of Rb tumor suppressor protein has been regarded as the only indicator of loss of pRb function; such loss has been shown to be important in bladder cancer progression (50–52). Rb alterations have been thought to take place only at the gene level, resulting in loss of protein expression. However, we have shown that a significant proportion of tumors expressing Rb show clinical consequences of loss of pRb function. Patients with tumors expressing the highest levels of pRb have clinical outcomes virtually identical to those with no detectable pRb (Fig. 20.5). These patients have significantly lower recurrence-free survival and overall survival compared with patients with tumors expressing moderate levels of pRb (52).

We have recently demonstrated the biologic basis for this observation. We show that tumors with pRb overexpression demonstrate pRb hyperphosphorylation, and that hyperphosphorylation is associated with loss of p16 expression and/or cyclin D1 overexpression (53). Thus, we have shown the biologic basis for the reliability of immunohistochemical evaluation of pRb as an indicator of loss of RB function; not only loss of pRb expression, but aberrant overexpression of pRb also indicates a disrupted RB pathway. In order to examine whether or not pRb hyperphosphorylation is a mechanism of RB inactivation in bladder tumors overexpressing pRb, we chose to evaluate pRb hyperphosphorylation without regard to cdk-specific phosphorylation sites. Thus, we were able to evaluate pRb hyperphosphorylation which might occur due to cdks other than cdk-4. Cell line models have shown that pRb expression increases as cells enter the cell cycle. Although tumor cells are expected to be in different phases of the cell cycle, and as such are expected to express varying amounts of hyperphosphorylated pRb, we

observed that most tumors with moderate pRb expression expressed an underphosphorylated form.

Based on our findings, we propose a model for the relationship between the critical factors involved in the Rb tumor suppressor pathway: pRb, p16, and cyclin D1 (Fig. 20.6). Genetic alterations of Rb leading to loss of a functional protein result in increased p16 expression through feedback mechanisms within the cell, which attempt to "brake" the cell cycle. In this situation, cyclin D1 expression appears to be redundant. On the other hand, loss of p16 through genetic or epigenetic mechanisms in the presence of an intact *Rb* gene results in the inactivation of the Rb protein through constitutive hyperphosphorylation. This change in pRb function is reflected as cells having a high pRb phenotype. In this scenario, p16 induction, at least *in vitro*, results not only in decreased phosphorylation of pRb, but also in a change in the pRb phenotype from high to moderate; the moderate pRb phenotype indicates a functional Rb tumor suppressor pathway. Overexpression of cyclin D1 can result in similar inactivation of RB even when p16 expression is maintained. Other factors such as cyclins (cyclin D1 in particular), cdks, and cdk inhibitors must also play a role. This mechanism of posttranslational modification of pRb leading to its inactivation may also be important in other tumors.

These studies clearly demonstrate that the analysis of tumor suppressor function must take place at the gene as well as at the protein level, and through an understanding of the pathways in which these gene products are involved. Inferences regarding the prognostic implications of tumor suppressor expression must not be taken out of context, but rather need to be assessed in the context of the pathway in which that product plays a role. Thus, understanding the pathways involved in controlling tumor behavior will provide more information than simply assessing a single genetic event.

ALTERATIONS IN CYCLINS, CYCLIN DEPENDENT KINASES, AND CDK INHIBITORS

In a normal cell, transition through G1 to S phase is regulated by cdks, which, when bound to cyclin molecules, are activated by cdk-activating kinase (54). This active cdk/cyclin complex then acts to phosphorylate the tumor suppressor retinoblastoma protein (pRb), which releases bound transcription factors such as the E2F family proteins. The net result is transcription of gene-encoding proteins necessary for progression through S phase (55). The ability of cdk/cyclin to drive the cell cycle forward can be blocked by members of two families of inhibitory proteins: the CIP (p21, p27, p57) or KIP (p15, p16, p18, p19) families (56).

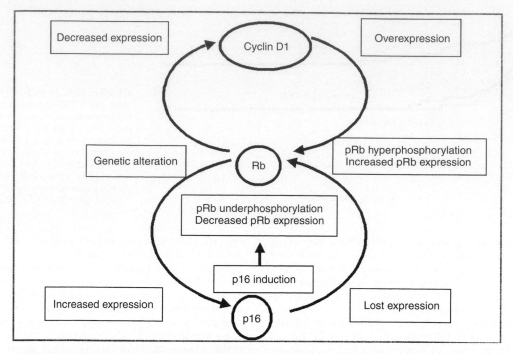

FIGURE 20.6. Proposed model showing the interrelationships between pRb, p16, and cyclin D1 in bladder cancer. Genetic alterations in RB result in increased p16 expression and decreased cyclin D1 expression. In cells with an intact RB gene, loss of p16 expression and/or increased cyclin D1 expression leads to hyperphosphorylation of pRb, resulting in high pRb expression. This phenotype is associated with increased cell proliferation and poor clinical outcome. Induction of p16 in cells with an intact RB gene leads to a decrease in the levels of hyperphosphorylated pRb, resulting in moderate pRb expression. This phenotype is associated with decreased cell proliferation and improved clinical outcome. (Adapted from Chatterjee SJ, Shi SR, Datar RH, et al. Hyperphosphorylation of pRb: a mechanism for RB tumor suppressor pathway inactivation in bladder cancer. *J Pathol* 2004;203:762–770.)

Cyclin D1, the major cyclin involved in transition from G1/S phase, is thought to act primarily via its association with cdk4 and cdk6 (57). The cyclin *D1* gene (CCND1) is located on chromosome 11q13, and both gene activation (due to amplification or chromosomal rearrangement such as translocation) and/or protein overexpression of cyclin D1 have been described in a variety of tumor types (58–60). In a recent fluorescent *in situ* hybridization (FISH) analysis of peripheral blood lymphocytes from 100 bladder cancer patients and matched 100 normal individuals, CCND1 translocation and amplification were observed only in bladder cancer patients (61). As discussed above, we have shown that cyclin D1 overexpression, possibly in conjunction with loss of p16, may result in pRb hyperphosphorylation and its functional inactivation (53). Takagi et al. have reported that immunohistochemical detection of cyclin D1 protein expression could be used as an inverse indicator for the level of invasiveness of bladder cancer, but not as an independent prognostic factor (62).

The cyclin *E* gene (CCNE), encoding a regulatory protein that binds cdk2, has been mapped to 19q13. Richter et al. investigated the role of cyclin E alterations in bladder cancer, using a high-throughput tissue microarray of 2,317 specimens from 1,842 bladder cancer patients (63). CCNE amplification was analyzed by fluorescence *in situ* hybridization and for cyclin-E protein overexpression by immunohistochemistry. The frequency of protein expression increased from stage pTa to pT1 but decreased for stage pT2-T4. Low cyclin E expression was associated with poor overall survival in all patients but had no prognostic impact independent of stage. Makiyama et al. have reported that cyclin E protein expression may be associated with aggressive tumor growth, and may have a relationship

with p27 (Kip1) for the regulation of cell cycle progression in transitional cell bladder carcinoma (64).

CDK4, CDK6, and cyclin D1 together predominantly phosphorylate the retinoblastoma protein at the G1/S transition. *CDK4* gene amplification has been reported in bladder cancer. The frequency of amplification has been observed to increase with stage (pTa to pT1-T4) and grade (low grade to high grade) (40).

The four major cdkis relevant to bladder cancer progression include p16, p14, p27, and p21. Of these, the role of p21 has been described above in context with p53. The chromosomal locus 9p21 harbors genes that encode cdkis such as CDKN2A and CDKN2B. LOH analysis by use of microsatellite markers established that CDKN2A microdeletion is the predominant mechanism of 9p21 inactivation in bladder cancer (65). Using an alternative reading frame, the CDKN2A locus encodes two proteins, p16[INK4a] and p14[ARF] (human homolog of the mouse p19[ARF]), both of which inhibit the cell cycle (66). The p16[INK4a] acts as a cdk inhibitor and prevents phosphorylation of pRb during cell cycle progression (67). The p14[ARF] protein does not directly bind and inhibit but appears to function upstream of p53 (68). This arrangement facilitates coordinated regulation of two key cell cycle regulatory pathways, namely the RB and p53 pathways from a single locus (66). Alterations in p16[INK4a] and p14[ARF] both at the gene level and protein level have elicited great interest due to their key cell cycle regulatory functions and have been extensively investigated in bladder cancer.

Deletions and methylation of the *INK4A* gene occur frequently in noninvasive bladder tumors. However, only those deletions that affect both p16[INK4a] and p14[ARF] have been shown to correlate with clinicopathologic parameters of worse prognosis (69). Inactivation of the *p16* gene through homozygous deletion appears to be a contributing factor for the development and progression of urothelial cancers, while point mutations appear to be an uncommon mechanism in inactivating this gene (70). Orlow et al. showed that homozygous deletion of the *INK4A* gene correlated with a lower recurrence-free survival ($P = .040$) (69). The inactivation of CDKN2A locus, including homozygous deletions, is probably an early event in TCC since no association is established between occurrence of genetic aberrations at 9p21 and tumor stage or grade (71). A report from Chang et al. indicates that p14^{ARF} is a primary target of homozygous deletion, whereas p16^{INK4a} is the hot spot of hypermethylation on the 9p21 region in bladder cancer (72). (See the section "DNA Methylation" later in this chapter.)

p27 Kip1 is a member of the Cip1/Kip1 family of cdkis and is a potential tumor suppressor gene. A significant correlation has been reported between low expression of p27 Kip1 and decreased disease-free survival and overall survival in bladder cancer (73). Low p27 expression is more common in poorly differentiated muscle-invasive UCs and is a major player in cell cycle control in these neoplasms (74). Loss of expression of p27 Kip1 protein has been reported to be associated with the subsequent development of invasive disease; this predictive value was enhanced significantly when combined with overexpression of caspase 3 protein (75).

ALTERATIONS IN ANGIOGENESIS PATHWAY IN BLADDER CANCER

The ability to induce new blood vessel growth is a tightly regulated process in normal tissues. Dysregulation of this process is a key feature of tumors. The prognostic significance of tumor angiogenesis, as determined by microvessel density (MVD), has been investigated in a variety of tumor systems, including bladder cancer, by us and many other investigators (76–78). The regulation of angiogenesis in normal tissue occurs through a complex, finely balanced interaction of stimulatory and inhibitory processes of neovascularization, which is imbalanced in malignant tissues. Thrombospondin-1 (TSP-1), a potent inhibitor of angiogenesis, is a 450 kD protein that is a normal constituent of extracellular matrix. Loss of TSP-1 expression has been shown to be a characteristic molecular event during bladder cancer progression, such that an inverse relationship exists between TSP-1 expression and MVD, a measure of tumor angiogenesis. On the other hand, vascular endothelial growth factor (VEGF) and basic fibroblast growth factor (bFGF) appear to be the most relevant pro-angiogenic factors for bladder cancer (79). Significantly higher amounts of VEGF are expressed in bladder tumors than in normal tissues, which may induce tumor angiogenesis and accelerate tumor growth.

The expression of factors regulating angiogenesis may be important prognostically as well as therapeutically. TSP-1 is transcriptionally activated by normal p53, while mutated or functionally inactive p53 (denoted by its nuclear accumulation) is unable to activate TSP-1. We found that the tumors that retain TSP-1 expression have better clinical outcome than those that have lost TSP-1 expression (80,81). Tumors with altered p53 were significantly more likely to express low levels of TSP. Conversely, tumors with wt p53 were significantly more likely to express moderate or high levels of TSP. Also, TSP-1 expression was found to inversely correlate with microvessel density. Tumors with low TSP expression were significantly more likely to demonstrate high microvessel density counts, whereas tumors with moderate or high TSP expression were significantly more likely to demonstrate low MVD counts. These observations link p53 with tumor angiogenesis, and hence with tumor metastasis (82,83). They also suggest a variety of therapeutic strategies targeted at negative regulation of angiogenesis. Thus VEGF, for example, provides a useful therapeutic target.

When various angiogenesis inhibitors become available for clinical use in cancer patients, these new therapeutic agents can be added to chemotherapy or to radiotherapy, or used in combination with immunotherapy or vaccine therapy (84).

ALTERATIONS IN GROWTH FACTOR RECEPTORS AND OTHER MARKERS IN BLADDER CANCER PROGRESSION

Receptor tyrosine kinases include growth factor receptors such as epidermal growth factor (EGF), and Her2/neu (ErbB-2), as well as VEGF. Many of these have been found overexpressed in UCs. Epidermal growth factor receptor (EGF-R), a transmembrane glycoprotein that mediates the mitogenic response of cells to epidermal growth factor, is highly expressed on malignant human bladder cancer cells (85). Since EGF signaling is well known to be involved in tumor survival, and overexpression of EGF-R is attributed to decreased responsiveness to many available therapies in cancer treatment, negative regulation of EGF-R assumes therapeutic implications. Many bladder cancer cell lines have been shown to demonstrate elevated EGF-R expression, and inhibitors of the EGF-R family of tyrosine kinase, such as 4,5-dianilinophthalimides, have been tested successfully for their antitumor potential in these cell lines. EGF-R thus may provide an important target for bladder cancer therapy (86,87).

Another possibly useful target could be the protein product of the c-ERB-B2 oncogene (Her2/neu), which is frequently found to be elevated in urinary bladder carcinoma (88). Clinical relevance of this Her2/neu overexpression, however, is controversial. Some studies found correlation between the protein overexpression and increasing tumor grade, cancer-specific survival, and incidence of metastatic disease (88,89), suggesting that Her2/neu was a significant and independent prognostic factor of tumor specific survival. Other studies conclude that determination of Her2/neu provided no additional prognostic information over tumor stage and grade for bladder cancer (90,91). If additional studies bear out the hypothesis that Her2/neu overexpression is indeed clinically relevant, then this protein may provide an additional rational therapeutic target. Attention is being drawn to assessing monoclonal antibody drugs and small molecule inhibitory drugs in patients with bladder cancer following the success seen with Herceptin, and EGF-receptor-targeted agents such as IMC-C225 Cetuximab, ZD1389 Iressa, OSI-774 Tarceva, and GW 57016 in other cancers.

TGF-ß is a 25-kDa pleiotropic growth factor that is expressed by many cell lines and tissue types. There are three ubiquitously expressed TGF-ß receptors—type I, II, and III (TßR-I, TßR-II, and TßR-III, respectively). TßR-III is a membrane proteoglycan that has a very short cytoplasmic tail and lacks any signaling motif, whereas TßR-I and TßR-II are serine/threonine kinases (92,93). Both TßR-I and TßR-II are required for TGF-ß signal transduction (94,95). TGF-ß usually acts as a potent growth inhibitor in most cells, especially those of the epithelial lineage. However, malignant cells are frequently resistant to the growth inhibitory effects of TGF-ß (96). An accumulating body of evidence suggests that alteration in the expression of TßRs may play a critical role in rendering malignant cells resistant to TGF-ß (97,98). We studied 59 bladder cancer specimens using immunohistochemistry and demonstrated loss of TßR-I in 31% and loss of TßR-II in 44% of cases (99). Loss of expression correlated with tumor grade, pathologic stage, and lymph node status. Only loss of TßR-I was associated with progression and decreased survival.

Cadherins, the primary mediators of cell–cell adhesion found universally in all tissues, are typically located at adherence junctions such that a cadherin molecule on one cell binds to a similar cadherin molecule on the neighboring cell to form a homodimer via members of the catenin family of molecules (100). E-cadherin is expressed by all normal epithelia and anchors to the actin cytoskeleton via its binding with α, β, and γ catenins (101). The loss of membranous expression of E-cadherin has been attributed to an aggressive phenotype of primary bladder cancer, with an independently predictive role for the marker (102–106).

Extracellular matrix degradation is mediated by several proteinases through proteolysis by serine proteases such as urokinase plasminogen activator (uPA) and its receptor (uPAR) (107–114), and the large family of matrix metalloproteases (MMPs) (115–118). Although an independent prognostic role for MMP-2 and MMP-9 levels by IHC in invasion and metastasis is not widely accepted, their correlation with traditional prognostic factors is well established (120–121). MMP-1 may be a promising marker of unfavorable prognosis (119). Similarly, high expression of uPA and uPAR has been shown to correlate with an unfavorable prognosis in invasive bladder cancer (113,122–127).

Tenascin-C (Tn-C) is an extracellular matrix glycoprotein that is up-regulated in malignant tumors. Tn-C promotes cell growth, cell migration, and angiogenesis. It has been suggested to be a prognostic factor in various cancers. In a recent study of 106 patients with Bladder cancer who were followed up for 126 months, Brunner et al. found that the patients with diffuse Tn-C staining in the tumor stroma had a significantly worse overall survival rate than those with negative staining or only moderate Tn-C expression ($P = .025$) (128). Patients with cytoplasmic expression of Tn-C had a significantly better overall survival than those without ($P = .001$). This study indicates that Tn-C may provide important prognostic information in bladder cancer.

Cyclooxygenase-2 is overexpressed in a majority of bladder cancers and is a therefore a highly relevant therapeutic target (129). A multicenter group is evaluating the selective COX-2 inhibitor Celecoxib as a chemopreventive agent following treatment with Bacillus Calmette-Guerin (BCG) in patients with non–muscle-invasive Bladder cancer. Another example is targeting overexpression of the EGF receptor. At University of California—Los Angeles, EGFR antagonists are currently being tested in combination with green tea plyphenols for chemoprevention of non–muscle-invasive cancers, while investigators at M.D. Anderson Cancer Center are examining such antagonists in combination with cytotoxic chemotherapy agents in metastatic disease.

BLADDER CANCER: A MULTISTEP GENETIC PROCESS

While alterations in single determinants have important predictive and prognostic value in bladder cancer, they have a limited role given the multifactorial nature of the disease. A number of studies have attempted to evaluate the utility of evaluating multiple determinants, particularly those relevant to specific pathways, in order to improve the predictive value of such markers in bladder cancer. Alterations in oncogenes and tumor suppressor genes can be grouped according to their functional role within independent cascades of the cell cycle control machinery, and such alterations at multiple points in a pathway may show cooperative or synergistic effects on clinical outcome.

We have demonstrated that alteration in both p53 and pRb may act in cooperative or synergistic ways to promote bladder

tumor progression (52). The combination of p53 and p21 status may provide additional clinical outcome information that is superior to that obtained from a single determinant (33). However in a series of 173 patients treated with cystectomy for advanced bladder cancer, Jahnson et al. have shown that altered expression for pRb and/or p53 was not correlated with cancer-specific death and hence could not be used as predictors of treatment outcome after cystectomy (130).

Loss of expression of p27 Kip1 protein has been reported to be associated with the subsequent development of invasive disease; this predictive value was enhanced significantly when combined with overexpression of caspase 3 protein (75). Low p27 expression is more common in poorly differentiated muscle-invasive UCs and is a major player in cell cycle control in these neoplasms. Further, in a multivariate analysis, when the tumor tissue sections were stained immunohistochemically for p27Kip1 and Ki-67 antigen (a marker of cell proliferation), Ki-67/p27 status had the strongest bearing on the overall survival of muscle-invasive UCs (74).

Altered expressions of p53, p21, or Rb are independent predictors of bladder cancer progression when examined as individual determinants (33,52,53). We and other researchers have reported that alterations in p53, p21, and Rb act in cooperative or synergistic ways to promote tumor progression in bladder cancer (36,37). By examining these determinants in combination, patients were categorized into four groups: group I (no alteration in any marker, 47 patients), group II (alteration in any one marker, 51 patients), group III (alteration in any two markers, 42 patients), and group IV (alteration in all three markers, 24 patients) (Fig. 20.7) (36). The 5-year recurrence rates in these groups were 23%, 31%, 60%, and 93%, respectively, and the 5-year survival rates were 68%, 56%, 28%, and 8%, respectively. Shariat et al. evaluated the expression of p53, p21, and pRb/p16 and found that the incremental number of altered markers was independently associated with an increased risk of bladder cancer progression and mortality (37). These reports suggest that examining markers in combination provides additional information above the use of a single determinant alone.

MOLECULAR DETERMINANTS OF RESPONSE TO CHEMOTHERAPY

Data from different laboratories, including ours, point toward a multifactorial basis for the chemosensitivity of urothelial cancers. Various cellular pathway components, most notably proteins from the p53 pathway, may influence the efficacy of chemotherapy. Retrospective studies have demonstrated the importance of cell cycle regulatory proteins in the development and progression of UC; some of these proteins also have a role in predicting response to therapy in bladder cancer. Numerous studies have been performed to identify molecular markers, which are reliable predictors of chemo-response in bladder cancer.

Kielb et al. have demonstrated *in vitro* that p53 mutations are required for paclitaxel to induce cell death in human bladder cell lines, while this agent did not affect cells with wt p53; however, the cytotoxic action of gemcitabine was not modulated by p53 status (131). This suggests a differential response to cytotoxic agents based on cellular genotype. The clinical significance of p53 mutations modulating chemo-response in the context of cytotoxic chemotherapy is a controversial issue. Studies from Memorial Sloan-Kettering Cancer Center (MSKCC) have suggested that p53 mutation is associated with resistance to neoadjuvant chemotherapy with the MVAC regimen (132). Conversely, Cote et al. have reported that in patients with tumors that did not demonstrate p53 alterations,

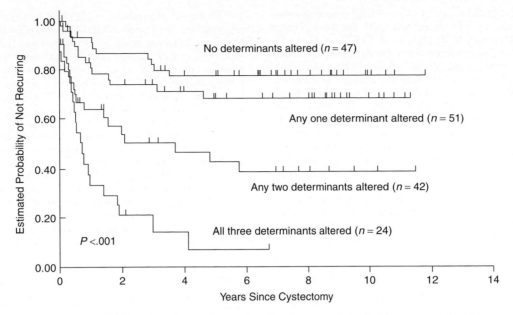

FIGURE 20.7. Probability of recurrence-free survival, based on cumulative incidence curves, for 164 patients with bladder cancer who underwent radical cystectomy, based on alterations in p53, p21, and/or pRb expression. (From Chatterjee SJ, Datar R, Youssefzadeh D, et al. Combined effects of p53, p21, and pRb expression in the progression of bladder transitional cell carcinoma. *J Clin Oncol* 2004;22: 1007–1013.)

adjuvant chemotherapy conferred no recurrence or survival benefit. However, in patients with p53-altered tumors, adjuvant chemotherapy resulted in a 3-fold decreased risk of recurrence and a 2.6-fold increased chance of survival (133) (Table 20.2). The molecular basis for this observation can be found in the studies by Waldman et al. (134). They showed that following DNA damage, the cells with mutated p53 and lacking p21 expression experience an uncoupling of S and M phases. Hence, they are able to traverse through S phase, showing aneuploidy without cell division, culminating into apoptosis. Siu et al., however, have demonstrated in a detailed study on invasive bladder cancer patients treated with MVAC regimen that the immunohistochemical expression of p53 did not predict survival (135). Thus, the question still remains unanswered and the ongoing p53 Targeted Therapy Trial (see below) may provide conclusive evidence in this matter.

As discussed previously, the treatment options for bladder cancer include surgery, often combined with chemotherapy,

radiation, and/or immunotherapy. While adjuvant therapy has been shown to be effective for patients with locally advanced bladder cancer, such treatment is not standard in patients with invasive organ-confined disease, as only a proportion of such patients are at risk for progression. Thus, there is substantial need to better define those patients that are most likely to progress and those who would benefit from systemic adjuvant chemotherapy. An international randomized p53 targeted therapy trial, led by investigators at the University of Southern California Keck School of Medicine, Baylor College of Medicine, and the University of Chicago, is currently underway to study the effects of three cycles of adjuvant MVAC (methotrexate, vinblastin, adriamycin, cisplatin) chemotherapy after radical cystectomy for pathological T1-T2 tumors with negative lymph nodes and expression of altered p53. Based on the data that p53 alterations identify tumors at increased risk for progression and identify bladder cancers that selectively respond to chemotherapy containing cisplatin, we

TABLE 20.2

RELATIVE RISK OF BLADDER CANCER RECURRENCE AND PATIENT DEATH WITH RESPECT TO p53 ALTERATIONS p53 AND TREATMENT OF BLADDER CANCER

Tumor p53 status	Pts observed	Pts treated[a]	Relative risk of recurrence (95% CI)[b]	Relative risk of death (95% CI)[c]
No alteration	32	18	1.1 $P = .88$ (0.8–1.5)	1.1 $P = .94$ (0.7–1.3)
Altered	24	14	3.0 $P = .006$ (1.4–6.5)	2.6 $P = .005$ (1.4–4.7)

[a]Treated with adjuvant chemotherapy using DNA-damaging agents.
[b]Relative risk of recurrence and death of untreated versus treated patients.
[c]P values for treated versus untreated.
Adapted from Cote RJ, Esrig D, Groshen S, et al. p53 and treatment of bladder cancer. *Nature* 1997;385:123–125.

designed the first bladder cancer clinical trial targeting a molecular lesion—that is, p53 alterations (p53-Targeted Therapy Trial in Bladder Cancer, NCI Grant #CA-71921).

Combining our own observation of increased chance of survival following adjuvant MVAC chemotherapy in patients with p53-altered tumors (133) with the data by Waldman et al. showing that genetic aberrations in p53 impart upon cells increased sensitivity to DNA-damaging chemotherapeutic agents (134), it was apparent that not only do p53 alterations predict prognosis by serving as a stratifier for risk of progression, but also may identify patients with bladder cancer who show selective response to chemotherapy containing cisplatin. In the p53-Targeted Therapy Trial in Bladder Cancer, patients with organ-confined invasive bladder cancers treated with radical cystectomy and bilateral pelvic lymphadenectomy whose tumors demonstrate p53 alterations by immunohistochemistry are randomized to either observation (the standard treatment) or three courses of adjuvant MVAC chemotherapy (Fig. 20.8). Patients with no evidence of p53 alterations are observed. This trial compares the progression-free survival of bladder cancer patients with p53 alteration randomized to three cycles of MVAC chemotherapy to similar patients who are observed. We hope that this trial will resolve the issues pertaining to the prognostic value of p53 in patients with organ-confined bladder cancer and the effect of systemic chemotherapy on the survival of high-risk patients with altered p53 immunoreactivity. The ability to determine the population of patients that require therapy based on the risk of progression and to predict the response of individual tumors to cytotoxic agents will profoundly alter the way therapy is determined for patients.

There are reports suggesting a role for additional cell cycle regulators in modulating chemo-response in bladder cancer. Koga et al. have reported that negative p53/positive p21 immunostaining is a predictor of favorable chemotherapeutic response in bladder cancer patients treated with intraarterial chemotherapy (IAC) comprising 100 mg/m^2 of cisplatin (CDDP)

and 40 mg/m^2 of pirarubicin (THP) (136). Qureshi et al. have reported that p53 and/or MDM2 immunopositivity were not predictive of tumor response or patient survival after systemic chemotherapy in bladder cancer; however, patients with p53-positive tumors were observed to derive survival benefit from salvage therapy, and those with concomitant p53 and MDM2 positivity received the most benefit (137). Jankevicius et al. have reported that positive p21 protein expression confers a survival advantage to patients receiving systemic adjuvant chemotherapy for locally advanced bladder cancer (138).

One of the suggested mechanisms for drug resistance in solid tumors is the phenomenon of multidrug resistance modulated by the *MDR* gene. The protein responsible for the action is a P-glycoprotein, but a broader family of MDR proteins has been identified, and the expression of proteins in this family are correlated with resistance to the taxanes, vinca alkaloids, and anthracycline antibiotics. Petrylak et al. have demonstrated an increased expression of P-glycoprotein in pretreatment and posttreatment biopsies of human tumors that were treated with the MVAC regimen (139). Interestingly, the highest proportion of tumor cells expressing P-glycoprotein was observed in metastases from patients who were treated with six or more cycles of chemotherapy.

There is now a growing body of information regarding the predictive versus lack of predictive value of cell cycle regulatory molecules in modulating chemo-response in bladder (and other) cancers. Detailed clinical trials (such as the p53-Targeted Therapy Trial in Bladder Cancer) are necessary to identify molecular targets, which can predict chemo-response in an efficacious manner. The future design of clinical trials needs to incorporate parameters that will take into account the significant differences in drug metabolism systems among individuals (such as those caused by age and sex) and also among population groups. These differences are likely to account for many of the unexplained inconsistencies in drug response, toxicity, and long-term outcomes of treatment with conventional and novel cytotoxic regimens. The increasing demographic heterogeneity of the

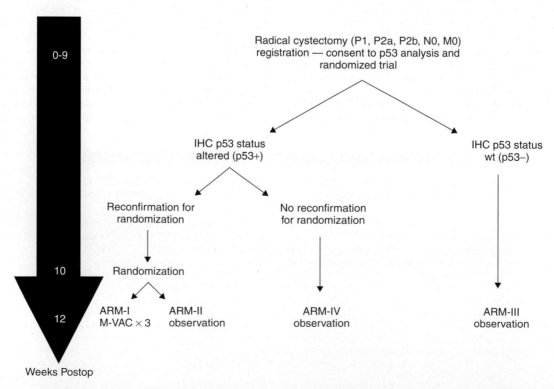

FIGURE 20.8. A schematic representation of the multi-institutional p53-Targeted Therapy Clinical Trial in Bladder Cancer.

population receiving these chemotherapeutic regimens warrants consideration of such variables while designing large-scale clinical trials.

DNA METHYLATION

Significant changes in the global levels and regional patterns of DNA methylation are among the earliest and most frequent events known to occur in human cancers (140). Alterations in DNA methylation have a direct impact on both the mutational and epigenetic components of neoplastic transformation. Important effects of DNA methylation on the genome include mutational burden of 5-methylcytosine, epigenetic effects of promoter methylation on gene transcription, and potential gene activation and induction of chromosomal instability by DNA hypomethylation (141,142). Hypermethylation of CpG islands is associated with transcriptional repression, while hypomethylation may lead to increased potential for gene activity or chromosomal instability. CpG islands located in tumor suppressor gene promoters are normally unmethylated. Abnormal methylation of these regions may lead to progressive reduction in gene expression, thus transcriptionally silencing suppressor genes by a variety of mechanisms, including remodeling of local chromatin structure or inhibition of transcription factor binding, ultimately altering normal cellular growth properties. Application of novel molecular biologic techniques has increased our appreciation of the widespread changes in methylation patterns that occur during urinary bladder carcinogenesis. Epigenetic events such as methylation occur throughout all stages of tumorigenesis, including the early phases, and are increasingly recognized as major mechanisms involved in silencing tumor suppressor genes.

A large number of genes have been reported to be hypermethylated in bladder cancer. The frequency of such events suggests that widespread alterations in the patterns of DNA methylation are common in bladder carcinogenesis. Some examples include the *p16* gene (at CDKN2A^{INK4a} locus on chromosome 9p21), *E-cadherin* gene (CDH1, encoding a transmembrane glycoprotein that modulates calcium-dependent intercellular adhesion), and *RASSF1A* gene (ras association domain family gene 1, isoform A) (72,143,144). Diminished CDH1 expression may lead to increase in beta-catenin activity and proliferation in UCs (145). Aside from deletion and mutation, the p16 gene has been shown to be inactivated by promoter methylation (146–149). Mutation or deletion of one p16 allele and hypermethylation of the remaining allele may be sufficient for loss of functional activity. Progressive inhibition of p16 expression by DNA methylation may result in loss of adequate growth regulatory function. Methylation of p16 has been observed in 27% to 60% of primary UCs (150,151). Both p16^{INKa} and p14^{ARF} hypermethylation may be involved in bladder carcinogenesis (152). p14^{ARF} promoter hypermethylation in plasma DNA may also be an indicator of disease recurrence in bladder cancer patients (153).

A variety of techniques are available for assessment of DNA methylation. Methylation-specific polymerase chain reaction (MS PCR) (154) and methylation-sensitive single nucleotide primer extension (Ms-SNuPE) (155) are among the most widely utilized techniques for identification and characterization of novel methylation changes associated with bladder carcinogenesis. This method has been used to detect methylation differences between the genomes of normal and tumor bladder cancer tissues and cell lines (156). The development of MethyLight technology has further improved the ability to assess the methylation patterns in a high-throughput manner (157). Gene expression microarray analysis has also been utilized to characterize methylation changes in bladder cancer cells following treatment with 5-Aza-CdR (158). Since DNA-based tumor markers can be characterized by unique specificity, they make an attractive target for molecular diagnosis of cancer in body fluids such as blood serum, plasma, and urine. Methylation changes in DNA isolated from bodily fluids such as urine or blood may serve as useful adjuncts to current techniques for disease detection or surveillance. Potential clinical value of DNA-based analysis of body fluids for the initial diagnosis and the follow-up of urologic cancer patients has been reviewed by Goessl et al. (159).

Catto et al. have recently analyzed hypermethylation at 11 CpG islands in a large cohort of upper urinary tract transitional cell carcinomas (UTT) and lower-tract (bladder) UCs, and have provided some interesting insights into differential epigenetic features of the two types of malignancies (160). Despite morphologic similarities between the two, more extensive promoter hypermethylation was found in UTT (96%) than in the UC (76%). Compared to tumors without methylation, the presence of methylation was significantly associated with advanced stage, higher tumor progression, and mortality rates. The authors have presented evidence to show that methylation occurs more extensively in UTT compared to bladder UC. Further, there is evidence to indicate an association between methylation and advanced tumor stage. The authors have also shown an association between methylation at the RASSF1A and DAPK loci and cumulative survival, suggesting their utility as potential predictive and prognostic markers and likely therapeutic targets. In combining the data regarding the genes studied here with that from numerous publications reporting the role of methylation in many other genes relevant in bladder cancer, it is becoming obvious that not only these "marker" genes, but also the process of aberrant methylation itself, may provide a therapeutic target in bladder cancer.

Because of its global role in cancer progression, there has been intense interest in the process of DNA methylation as a potential therapeutic target. Inhibitors of DNA methylation act through reactivation of the expression of genes that have undergone epigenetic silencing. Initially developed as cytotoxic agents, the methylation inhibitors like 5-azacytidine (5-aza-CR) and 5-aza-2′-deoxycytidine (5-aza-CdR) have been shown to induce gene expression and differentiation *in vitro* (161). When incorporated in place of cytosine into replicating DNA, such nucleoside analogues serve as powerful mechanism-based inhibitors of DNA methylation active only in S-phase cells, heritably demethylating DNA. Recent additions of other analogues include 5-fluorocytosine, pseudoisocytosine or zebularine (5-fluoro-2′-deoxycytidine), and azacytosine. Of these, zebularine might be orally active (162). Another approach to target the process of hypermethylation is to block the activity of DNA methyltransferases; clinical trials with antisense oligonucleotides that target these enzymes are also underway (163). Decitabine, 2′-deoxy-5-azacytidine, has been shown to inhibit DNA methyltransferases and reverse epigenetic silencing of aberrantly methylated genes (164). Because multiple genes become methylated in individual cancers (165), it may be possible to target multiple candidate genes with one drug.

An opposite scenario, however, may present itself when one considers genes such as MDR1, an encoding P-gp protein responsible for multidrug resistance in many cancers. Hypomethylation of the MDR1 promoter has been observed to be a clinically important event in patients with recurrent bladder cancers that are resistant to therapy (166). When expression of the *MDR1* gene in bladder cancer was examined, the tumors that recur after treatment with chemotherapy had 3.5- to 5.7-fold higher mRNA levels of the *MDR1* gene compared with untreated tumors. Furthermore, the *MDR1* gene was overexpressed in the majority of tumors (89%) that later recurred, whereas overexpression was observed in 25% of the tumors that did not recur (and thus responded to chemotherapy). Overexpression of the *MDR1* gene in cancers is shown to be inversely correlated with DNA methylation at CpG sites in the promoter, such that promoter hypomethylation results in increased expression. Thus, hypomethylation of the MDR1 promoter may result in development of a multidrug resistant phenotype in patients with bladder cancer. Recent use of siRNAs targeted to CpG islands within the promoter of a specific gene, which induce transcriptional gene silencing by means of DNA-methyltransferase-dependent methylation of DNA, may serve to help resolve such situations (167). In summary, targeting aberrant promoter hypermethylation may become a potential therapeutic modality in bladder cancer management (168).

EXPRESSION PROFILING IN BLADDER CANCER

The lack of ability of a single marker or even a limited number of markers in providing a comprehensive understanding of the biology of neoplasia has ushered in an era of high-throughput expression profiling. The need for expression profiling has resulted in the development of new expression-profiling techniques and advancement of currently available technologies. Detailed description of expression profiling techniques has been provided by Pagliarulo et al. (169). In 2003, Dyrskjot et al. reported the identification of clinically relevant subclasses of bladder carcinoma using expression microarray analysis of 40 well-characterized bladder tumors (170). Using hierarchical clustering, they identified three major stages, Ta, T1 and T2-4, with further classification of the Ta tumors into subgroups. The 32-gene molecular classifier that they built using a cross-validation approach was able to classify benign and muscle-invasive tumors with close correlation to pathologic staging in an independent test set of 68 tumors. They employed supervised learning classification to correctly discriminate between recurring and nonrecurring Ta tumors in 75% of the samples. Modlich et al. analyzed 20 invasive and 22 superficial bladder tumors from 34 patients with known outcome regarding disease recurrence and progression by filter-based cDNA arrays containing 1,185 genes (171). They found that a two-way clustering algorithm using different subsets of gene expression data classified tumor samples according to clinical outcome as superficial, invasive, or metastasizing. Several gene clusters that characterized invasive or superficial tumors were identified. While in superficial bladder tumors increased mRNA levels of genes encoding transcription factors, protein synthetic and metabolic machinery, and some proteins involved in cell cycle progression and differentiation were observed, the invasive tumors showed up-regulation of transcripts for immune, extracellular matrix, adhesion, peritumoral stroma and muscle tissue components, proliferation, and cell cycle regulators. The investigators therefore concluded that gene expression profiling of human bladder cancers provides insight into the biology of bladder cancer progression and identifies patients with distinct clinical phenotypes. Another recent study used microarray expression profiling to examine the gene expression patterns in superficial transitional cell carcinoma with surrounding CIS (13 patients), without surrounding CIS lesions (15 patients), and in muscle-invasive carcinomas (13 patients) (172). They used a supervised learning approach to build a 16-gene molecular CIS classifier, which was able to classify superficial TCC samples according to the presence or absence of surrounding CIS with a high accuracy. They contended that identification of such an expression signature could provide guidance for the selection of therapy and follow-up regimen in patients with early stage bladder cancer.

Expression profiling technologies such as microarrays for relatively smaller, defined subsets of genes may provide a modality to identify clinically important tumor subtypes and molecular targets not identified using standard methods (173,174). Willey et al. have developed a modified quantitative method for standardized competitive RT-PCR that allows simultaneous measurement of many genes using nanogram amounts of cDNA (175,176). The transcript levels are expressed as numerical values per million molecules of β-actin, thus allowing intrasample and intersample comparisons. We have used this analytical tool to obtain transcript profiles of 66 bladder tumors from various pathological stages for over 70 genes that are crucial in pathways such as cell cycle regulation, apoptosis, signal transduction, invasion, metastasis, angiogenesis, and so forth. Our preliminary analysis shows that a medium-throughput transcript-profiling approach can allow identification of informative subsets of genes that could be used in molecular class prediction and prediction of clinical outcome. Moreover, these analyses may also identify subgroups of patients at highest risk of cancer progression who will benefit from either adjuvant therapy or, based upon unique, patient-specific targets, individualized treatment regimens. Generation of a molecular profile in an individual tumor may provide a number of advantages: (a) it can provide an understanding of the deregulation occurring in multiple pathways; (b) it may help identification of gene expression patterns specific to given tumors; (c) it may help detection of novel targets for therapy; and (d) it can aid in rational drug design directed against these specific targets. The expression-profiling studies are thus expected to both add to our understanding of the mechanisms of carcinogenesis as well as improve our ability to diagnose and treat bladder cancer.

EVOLVING ANTICANCER STRATEGIES

Based upon patient-specific aberrations in pathways or known markers, both existing and new therapies can be tailored to benefit patients based on the risk of progression and molecular alterations specific to a patient's tumor. Targeted therapy, therefore, can be defined as therapy that targets both mechanism and risk. Potential therapeutic targets for rational drug development can be identified utilizing the available knowledge of the molecular biology of cell-cycle regulation, signal transduction, apoptosis, and angiogenesis in bladder cancer.

CONCLUDING REMARKS

It is clear that bladder cancer tumorigenesis and progression is a process involving multiple genetic defects and pathways. Thus, knowledge of the status of multiple pathways will be important in assessing the prognosis of patients with bladder cancer, and for evaluating the expression of potential therapeutic targets. The ultimate goal of studying molecular determinants of bladder cancer outcome is to better define risk and response for the individual patient. Bladder cancer is a model of modern cancer management, where advances in pathology, surgery, oncology, and basic science have converged to produce the possibility of a more rational, biologically based approach. Furthermore, our understanding of molecular pathways is leading to the development of an increasing array of untraditional treatment possibilities. All these factors are increasingly leading us to the point of patient-specific management of bladder cancer.

ACKNOWLEDGMENTS

The authors would like to gratefully acknowledge Peter Jones, Ph.D., Donald Skinner, MD, and Susan Groshen, Ph.D. (all from USC/Norris Comprehensive Cancer Center, Los Angeles) for their valuable input during the manuscript preparation.

They would also like to acknowledge the funding support of National Institutes of Health Grants CA-65726, CA-70903, CA-71921, and CA-86871, which supported the authors' research described in this chapter.

References

1. Skinner DG, Lieskovsky GL. Management of invasive and high-grade bladder cancer. In: Lieskovsky GL, ed. *Diagnosis and management of genitourinary cancer*. Philadelphia, PA: WB Saunders, 1988:295–312.
2. Cote RJ, Soni RA, Amin MB. Bladder and Urethra. In: Weidner N, Cote RJ, Suster S, et al., eds. *Modern surgical pathology*, Vol. 2. Philadelphia, PA: WB Saunders, 2003:1102–1147.
3. Landman J, Droller MJ. Risk factors in clonal development from superficial to invasive bladder cancer. *Cancer Surv* 1998;31:5–15.
4. Knowles MA. What we could do now: molecular pathology of bladder cancer. *J Clin Pathol: Mol Pathol* 2001;54:215–221.
5. Ruppert JM, Tokino K, Sidransky D. Evidence for two bladder cancer suppressor loci on human chromosome 9. *Cancer Res* 1993;53:5093–5095.
6. Sidransky D, Frost P, Von Eschenbach A, et al. Clonal origin bladder cancer. *N Engl J Med* 1992;326:737–740.
7. Presti JC Jr, Reuter VE, Galan T, et al. Molecular genetic alterations in superficial and locally advanced human bladder cancer. *Cancer Res* 1991;51: 5405–5409.
8. Nobori T, Miura K, Wu DJ, et al. Deletions of the cyclin-dependent kinase-4 inhibitor gene in multiple human cancers. *Nature* 1994;368:753–756.
9. Jewett HJ, Strong GH. Infiltrating carcinoma of the bladder. Relation of the depth of penetration of the bladder wall to incidence of local extension and metasis. *J Urol* 1946;55:336–372.
10. Jewett HJ. Carcinoma of the bladder. Influence of depth infiltration on the 5-year results following complete extirpation of the primary growth. *J Urol* 1952;67:672–676.
11. Marshall VF. The relation of the preoperative estimate to all the pathologic demonstration of the extent of vesical neoplasms. *J Urol* 1952;68:714–723.
12. Fleming ID, Cooper JS, Henson DE, et al. Urinary bladder. In: Fleming ID, ed. *AJCC cancer staging manual*. Philadelphia, PA: Lippincott-Raven, 1997:241–243.
13. Cote RJ, Datar RH. Therapeutic approaches to bladder cancer: identifying targets and mechanisms. *Crit Rev Oncol Hematol* 2003;46:S67–S83.
14. Vousden KH, Lu X. Live or let die: the cell's response to p53. *Nat Rev Cancer* 2002;2:594–604.
15. Levine AJ. p53, the cellular gatekeeper for growth and division. *Cell* 1997; 88:323–331.
16. Cordon-Cardo C, Sheinfeld J, Dalbagni G. Genetic studies and molecular markers of bladder cancer. *Semin Surg Oncol* 1997;13:319–327.
17. Taylor D, Koch WM, Zahurak M, et al. Immunohistochemical detection of p53 protein accumulation in head and neck cancer: correlation with p53 gene alterations. *Hum Pathol* 1999;10:1221–1225.
18. Dalbagni G, Cordon-Cardo C, Reuter V, et al. Tumor suppressor gene alterations in bladder carcinoma. Translational correlates to clinical practice. *Surg Oncol Clin N Am* 1995;4:231–240.
19. Esrig D, Elmajian D, Groshen S, et al. Accumulation of nuclear p53 and tumor progression in bladder cancer. *N Engl J Med* 1994;331:1259–1264.
20. Esrig D, Spruck CH, Nichols PW, et al. p53 nuclear protein accumulation correlates with mutations in the p53 gene, tumor grade, and stage in bladder cancer. *Am J Pathol* 1993;143:1389–1397.
21. Erill N, Colomer A, Verdu M, et al. Genetic and immunophenotype analyses of TP53 in bladder cancer: TP53 alterations are associated with tumor progression. *Diagn Mol Pathol* 2004;13:217–223.
22. George B, Datar RH, Wu L, et al. Complete p53 multi-exon sequencing by GeneChip complements use of p53 immunohistochemistry for prediction of clinical outcome in invasive bladder cancer. Orlando, FL: American Society for Clinical Oncology, March 27–31, 2004.
23. Sarkis AS, Zhang ZF, Cordon-Cardo C. p53 nuclear overexpression and disease progression in Ta bladder carcinoma. *Int J Oncol* 1993;3:355–360.
24. Casetta G, Gontero P, Russo R, et al. p53 expression compared with other prognostic factors in OMS grade-I stage-Ta transitional cell carcinoma of the bladder. *Eur Urol* 1997;32:229–236.
25. Sarkis AS, Dalbagni G, Cordon-Cardo C, et al. Nuclear overexpression of p53 protein in transitional cell bladder carcinoma: a marker for disease progression. *J Natl Cancer Inst* 1993;85:53–59.
26. Serth J, Kuczyk MA, Bokemeyer C, et al. p53 immunohistochemistry as an independent prognostic factor for superficial transitional cell carcinoma of the bladder. *Br J Cancer* 1995;71:201–205.
27. Sarkis AS, Dalbagni G, Cordon-Cardo C, et al. Association of p53 nuclear overexpression and tumor progression in carcinoma in situ of the bladder. *J Urol* 1994;152:388–392.
28. Masters JRW, Vani UD, Grigor KM, et al. Can p53 staining be used to identify patients with aggressive superficial bladder cancer? *J Pathol* 2003; 200:74–81.
29. Smith ND, Rubenstein JN, Eggener SE, et al. The p53 tumor suppressor gene and nuclear protein: basic science review and relevance in the management of bladder cancer. *J Urol* 2003;169:1219–1228.
30. Schmitz-Drager BJ, Goebell PJ, Ebert T, et al. p53 immunohistochemistry as a prognostic marker in bladder cancer. Playground for urology scientists? *Eur Urol* 2000;38:691–699.
31. Chen W-C, Wu H-C, Hsu C-D, et al. p21 gene codon 31 polymorphism is associated with bladder cancer. *Urol Oncol* 2002;7:63–66.
32. Lacombe L, Orlow I, Silver D, et al. Analysis of p21WAF1/CIP1 in primary bladder tumors. *Oncol Res* 1996;8:409–414.
33. Stein JP, Ginsberg DA, Grossfeld GD, et al. Effect of p21WAF1/CIP1 expression on tumor progression in bladder. *J Natl Cancer Inst* 1998;90: 1072–1079.
34. Shariat SF, Kim J, Raptidis G, et al. Association of p53 and p21 expression with clinical outcome in patients with carcinoma in situ of the urinary bladder. *Urology* 2003;61:1140–1145.
35. Li D, Tian Y, Ma Y, et al. p150(Sal2) is a p53-independent regulator of p21(WAF1/CIP). *Mol Cell Biol* 2004;24:3885–3893.
36. Chatterjee SJ, Datar R, Youssefzadeh D, et al. Combined effects of p53, p21, and pRb expression in the progression of bladder transitional cell carcinoma. *J Clin Oncol* 2004;22:1007–1013.
37. Shariat SF, Tokunaga H, Zhou J, et al. p53, p21, pRB, and p16 expression predict clinical outcome in cystectomy with bladder cancer. *J Clin Oncol* 2004;22:1014–1024.
38. Wu X, Bayle JH, Olson D, et al. The p53-mdm-2 autoregulatory feedback loop. *Genes Dev* 1993;7:1126–1132.
39. Yang Y, Li CC, Weissman AM. Regulating the p53 system through ubiquitination. *Oncogene* 2004;23:2096–2106.
40. Simon R, Struckmann K, Schraml P, et al. Amplification pattern of 12q13-q15 genes (MDM2, CDK4, GLI) in urinary bladder cancer. *Oncogene* 2002;21:2476–2483.
41. Lianes P, Orlow I, Zhang ZF, et al. Altered patterns of MDM2 and TP53 expression in human bladder cancer. *J Natl Cancer Inst* 1994;86:1325–1330.
42. Barbareschi M, Girlando S, Fellin G, et al. Expression of mdm-2 and p53 protein in transitional cell carcinoma. *Urol Res* 1995;22:349–352.
43. Keegan PE, Griffiths TRL, Marsh C, et al. MDM2 and p53 immunoreactivity: independent predictors of stage progression in pT1 bladder cancer (TCC). *Br J Urol* 1998;81(Suppl. 4):16.
44. Sigalas I, Calvert AH, Anderson JJ, et al. Alternatively spliced mdm2 transcripts with loss of p53 binding domain sequences: transforming ability and frequent detection in human cancer. *Nat Med* 1996;2:912–917.
45. Cordon-Cardo C. Mutations of cell cycle regulators. Biological and clinical implications for human neoplasia. *Am J Pathol* 1995;147:545–560.
46. Cote RJ, Chatterjee SJ. Molecular determinants of outcome in bladder cancer. *Cancer J Sci Am* 1999;5:2–15.
47. Miyamoto H, Shuin T, Torigoe S, et al. Retinoblastoma gene mutations in primary human bladder cancer. *Br J Cancer* 1995;71:831–835.
48. Acikbas I, Keser I, Kilic S, et al. Detection of LOH of the RB1 gene in bladder cancers by PCR-RFLP. *Urol Int* 2002;68:189–192.
49. Grossman HB, Liebert M, Antelo M, et al. p53 and RB expression predict progression in T1 bladder cancer. *Clin Cancer Res* 1998;4:829–834.
50. Cordon-Cardo C, Wartinger D, Petrylak D, et al. Altered expression of the retinoblastoma gene product: prognostic indicator in bladder cancer. *J Natl Cancer Inst* 1992;84:1251–1256.
51. Logothetis CJ, Xu HJ, Ro JY, et al. Altered expression of retinoblastoma protein and known prognostic variables in locally advanced bladder cancer. *J Natl Cancer Inst* 1992;84:1256–1261.
52. Cote RJ, Dunn MD, Chatterjee SJ, et al. Elevated and absent pRb expression is associated with bladder cancer progression and has cooperative effects with p53. *Cancer Res* 1998;58:1090–1094.
53. Chatterjee SJ, Shi SR, Datar RH, et al. Hyperphosphorylation of pRb: a mechanism for RB tumor suppressor pathway inactivation in bladder cancer. *J Pathol* 2004;203:762–770.
54. Morgan DO. Principles of CDK regulation. *Nature* 1995;374:131–134.
55. Sellers WR, Kaelin WG Jr. Role of the retinoblastoma protein in the pathogenesis of human cancer. *J Clin Oncol* 1997;15:3301–3312.
56. Grana X, Reddy EP. Cell cycle control in mammalian cells: role of cyclins, cyclin dependent kinases (CDKs), growth suppressor genes and cyclin-dependent kinase inhibitors (CKIs). *Oncogene* 1995;11:211–219.
57. Sherr CJ. Cancer cell cycles. *Science* 1996;274:1672–1677.
58. Bartkova J, Lukas J, Muller H, et al. Abnormal patterns of D-type cyclin expression and G1 regulation in human head and neck cancer. *Cancer Res* 1995;55:949–956.
59. Arber N, Hibshoosh H, Moss SF, et al. Increased expression of cyclin D1 is an early event in multistage colorectal carcinogenesis. *Gastroenterology* 1996;110:669–674.
60. Musgrove EA, Lee CS, Buckley MF, et al. Cyclin D1 induction in breast cancer cells shortens G1 and is sufficient for cells arrested in G1 to complete the cell cycle. *Proc Natl Acad Sci U S A* 1994;91:8022–8026.
61. Shao L, Lerner SL, Bondaruk J, et al. Specific chromosome aberrations in peripheral blood lymphocytes are associated with risk of bladder cancer. *Genes Chromosomes Cancer* 2004;41:379–389.
62. Takagi Y, Takashi M, Koshikawa T, et al. Immunohistochemical demonstration of cyclin D1 in bladder cancers as an inverse indicator of invasiveness but not an independent prognostic factor. *Int J Urol* 2000;7: 366–372.
63. Richter J, Wagner U, Kononen J, et al. High-throughput tissue microarray analysis of cyclin E gene amplification and overexpression in urinary bladder cancer. *Am J Pathol* 2000;157:787–794.

64. Makiyama K, Masuda M, Takano Y, et al. Cyclin E overexpression in transitional cell carcinoma of the bladder. *Cancer Lett* 2000;151:193–198.
65. Cairns P, Shaw ME, Knowles MA. Preliminary mapping of the deleted region of chromosome 9 in bladder cancer. *Cancer Res* 1993;53:1230.
66. Clurman BE, Groudine M. The CDKN2A tumor-suppressor locus—a tale of two proteins. *N Engl J Med* 1998;338:910–912.
67. Rocco JW, Sidransky D. p16(MTS-1/CDKN2/INK4a) in cancer progression. *Exp Cell Res* 2001;264:42–55.
68. Zhang Y, Xiong Y, Yarbrough WG. ARF promotes MDM2 degradation and stabilizes p53: ARF-INK4a locus deletion impairs both the Rb and p53 tumor suppression pathways. *Cell* 1998;92:725–734.
69. Orlow I, LaRue H, Osman I, et al. Deletions of the INK4A gene in superficial bladder tumors. Association with recurrence. *Am J Pathol* 1999;155:105–113.
70. Wu W-J, Huang C-H, Huang C-N, et al. Homozygous deletion of p16/cdkn2/mts1 gene in human urothelial carcinomas. *Br J Urol* 1997;80(Suppl. 2):67.
71. Berggren P, Kumar R, Sakano S, et al. Detecting homozygous deletions in the CDKN2A (p16(INK4a))/ARF(p14(ARF)) gene in urinary bladder cancer using real-time quantitative PCR. *Clin Cancer Res* 2003;9:235–242.
72. Chang L-L, Yeh W-T, Yang S-Y, et al. Genetic alterations of p16INK4a and p14ARF genes in human bladder cancer. *J Urol* 2003;170:595–600.
73. Sgambato A, Migaldi M, Faraglia B, et al. Cyclin D1 expression in papillary superficial bladder cancer: its association with other cell cycle-associated proteins, cell proliferation and clinical outcome. *Int J Cancer* 2002;97:671–678.
74. Korkolopoulou P, Christodoulou P, Konstantinidou AE, et al. Cell cycle regulators in bladder cancer: a multivariate survival study with emphasis on p27Kip1. *Hum Pathol* 2000;31:751–760.
75. Burton PB, Anderson CJ, Corbishly CM. Caspase 3 and p27 as predictors of invasive bladder cancer. *N Engl J Med* 2000;343:1418–1420.
76. Bochner BH, Cote RJ, Weidner N, et al. Angiogenesis in bladder cancer: relationship between microvessel density and tumor prognosis. *J Natl Cancer Inst* 1995;87:1603–1612.
77. Dickson AJ, Fox SB, Persad RA, et al. Quantification of angiogenesis as an independent predictor of prognosis in invasive bladder carcinomas. *Br J Urol* 1994;74:762–766.
78. Jaeger TM, Weidner N, Chew K, et al. Tumor angiogenesis correlates with lymph node metastases in invasive bladder cancer. *J Urol* 1995;154:69–71.
79. Shao ZM, Nguyen M. Angiogenic factors and bladder cancer. *Front Biosci* 2002;7:e33–e35.
80. Grossfeld GD, Ginsberg DA, Stein JP, et al. Thrombospondin-1 expression in bladder cancer: association with p53 alterations, tumor angiogenesis, and tumor progression. *J Natl Cancer Inst* 1997;89:219–227.
81. Reiher FK, Ivanovich M, Huang H, et al. The role of hypoxia and p53 in the regulation of angiogenesis in bladder cancer. *J Urol* 2001;165(Pt 1):2075–2081.
82. Rastinejad F, Polverini PJ, Bouck NP. Regulation of the activity of a new inhibitor of angiogenesis by a cancer suppressor gene. *Cell* 1989;56:345–355.
83. Dameron KM, Volpert OV, Tainsky MA, et al. Control of angiogenesis in fibroblasts by p53 regulation of thrombospondin-1. *Science* 1994;265:1582–1584.
84. Kerbel R, Folkman J. Clinical translation of angiogenesis inhibitors. *Nat Rev Cancer* 2002;2:727–739.
85. Ravery V, Grignon D, Angulo J, et al. Evaluation of epidermal growth factor receptor, transforming growth factor alpha, epidermal growth factor and c-erbB2 in the progression of invasive bladder cancer. *Urol Res* 1997;25:9–17.
86. Dinney CP, Parker C, Dong Z, et al. Therapy of human transitional cell carcinoma of the bladder by oral administration of the epidermal growth factor receptor protein tyrosine kinase inhibitor 4,5-dianilinophthalimide. *Clin Cancer Res* 1997;3:161–168.
87. van der Poel HG, Molenaar B, van Beusechem VW, et al. Epidermal growth factor receptor targeting of replication competent adenovirus enhances cytotoxicity in bladder cancer. *J Urol* 2002;168:266–272.
88. Sato K, Moriyama M, Mori S, et al. An immunohistologic evaluation of c-erb-B2 gene product in patients with urinary bladder carcinoma. *Cancer* 1992;70:2493–2498.
89. Moriyama M, Akiyama T, Yamamoto T, et al. Expression of c-erb-B2 gene product in urinary bladder cancer. *J Urol* 1991;145:423–427.
90. Underwood M, Bartlett J, Reeves J, et al. C-erb-B2 gene amplification: a molecular marker in recurrent bladder tumors? *Cancer Res* 1995;55:2422–2430.
91. Mellon JK, Lunec J, Wright C, et al. c-erb-B-2 in bladder cancer: molecular biology, correlation with epidermal growth factor receptors and prognostic value. *J Urol* 1996;155:321–326.
92. Lin HY, Wang XF, Ng-Eaton E, et al. Expression cloning of the TGF-beta type II receptor, a functional transmembrane serine/threonine kinase. *Cell* 1992;68:775–785.
93. Franzen P, ten Dijke P, Ichijo H, et al. Cloning of a TGF beta type I receptor that forms a heteromeric complex with the TGF beta type II receptor. *Cell* 1993;75:681–692.
94. Chen F, Weinberg RA. Biochemical evidence for the autophosphorylation and transphosphorylation of transforming growth factor ß receptor kinases. *Proc Natl Acad Sci U S A* 1995;92:1565–1569.
95. Wrana JL, Attisano L, Wieser R, et al. Mechanism of activation of the TGF-beta receptor. *Nature* 1994;370:341–347.
96. Kim IY, Ahn HJ, Zelner DJ, et al. Genetic change in transforming growth factor beta (TGF-beta) receptor type I gene correlates with insensitivity to TGF-beta 1 in human prostate cancer cells. *Cancer Res* 1996;56:44–48.
97. Wang J, Sun L, Myeroff L, et al. Demonstration that mutation of the type II transforming growth factor ßreceptor inactivates its tumor suppressor activity in replication error-positive colon carcinoma cells. *J Biol Chem* 1995;270:22044–22049.
98. Park K, Kim S-J, Bang Y-J, et al. Genetic changes in the transforming growth factor ß (TGF-ß) type II receptor gene in human gastric cancer cells: correlation with sensitivity to growth inhibition by TGF-ß. *Proc Natl Acad Sci U S A* 1994;91:8772–8776.
99. Tokunaga H, Lee D-H, Kim IY, et al. Decreased expression of transforming growth factor ß receptor type I is associated with poor prognosis in bladder transitional cell carcinoma patients. *Clin Cancer Res* 1999;5:2520–2525.
100. Takeichi M. Cadherin cell adhesion receptors as a morphogenetic regulator. *Science* 1991;22:1451–1455.
101. Smith MEF, Pignatelli M. The molecular histology of neoplasia: the role of the cadherin/catenin complex. *Histopathology* 1997;31:107–111.
102. Popov Z, Gil-Diez de Medina S, Lefrere-Belda MA, et al. Low E-cadherin expression in bladder cancer at the transcriptional and protein level provides prognostic information. *Br J Cancer* 2000;83:209–214.
103. Imao T, Koshida K, Endo Y, et al. Dominant role of E-cadherin in the progression of bladder cancer. *J Urol* 1999;161:692–698.
104. Shariat SF, Pahlavan S, Baseman AG, et al. E-cadherin expression predicts clinical outcome in carcinoma in situ of the urinary bladder. *Urology* 2001;57:60–65.
105. Byrne RR, Shariat SF, Brown R, et al. E-cadherin immunostaining of bladder transitional cell carcinoma, carcinoma in situ and lymph node metastases with long-term follow up. *J Urol* 2001;165:1473–1479.
106. Sun W, Herrera GA. E-cadherin expression in urothelial carcinoma in situ, superficial papillary transitional cell carcinoma and invasive transitional cell carcinoma. *Hum Pathol* 2002;33:996–1000.
107. Dvorak HF. Tumours: wounds that do not heal. Similarities between tumour stroma generation and wound healing. *N Engl J Med* 1986;315:1650–1659.
108. Dano K, Andreason PA, Grondahl-Hansen J, et al. Plasminogen activators, tissue degradation, and cancer. *Adv Cancer Res* 1985;44:139–166.
109. Ossowski L, Clunie G, Masucci MT, et al. In vivo paracrine interaction between urokinase and its receptor: effect on tumour cell invasion. *J Cell Biol* 1991;115:1107–1112.
110. Moller LB. Structure and function of the urokinase receptor. *Blood Coagul Fibrinolysis* 1993;4:293–303.
111. Hollas W, Blasi F, Boyd D. Role of the urokinase receptor in facilitating extracellular matrix invasion by cultured colon cancer. *Cancer Res* 1991;51:3690–3695.
112. Allgayer H, Heiss MM, Riesenberg R, et al. Urokinase plasminogen activator receptor (uPA-R)—one potential characteristic of metastatic phenotypes in minimal residual tumor disease. *Cancer Res* 1997;57:1394–1399.
113. Hasui Y, Marutsuka K, Nishi S, et al. The content of urokinase-type plasminogen activator and tumour recurrence in superficial bladder cancer. *J Urol* 1994;151:16.
114. Reuning U, Magdolen V, Wilhelm O, et al. Multifunctional potential of the plasminogen activation system in tumour invasion and metastasis. *Int J Oncol* 1998;13:893–906.
115. Stetler-Stevenson WG, Krutzsch HC, Liotta LA. Tissue inhibitor of metalloproteinase (TIMP-2). A new member of the metalloproteinase inhibitor family. *J Biol Chem* 1989;264:17374–17378.
116. Kleiner DE, Stetler-Stevenson WG. Matrix metalloproteinases and metastasis. *Cancer Chemother Pharmacol* 1999;43:S42–S51.
117. Kanayama H, Yokota K, Kurokawa Y, et al. Prognostic values of matrix metalloproteinase-2 and tissue inhibitor of metalloproteinase-2 expression in bladder cancer. *Cancer* 1998;82:1359–1366.
118. Grignon DJ, Sakr W, Toth M, et al. High levels of tissue inhibitor of metalloproteinase-2 (TIMP-2) expression are associated with poor outcome in invasive bladder cancer. *Cancer Res* 1996;56:1654–1659.
119. Papathoma AS, Petraki C, Grigorakis A, et al. Prognostic significance of matrix metalloproteinases 2 and 9 in bladder cancer. *Anticancer Res* 2000;20:2009–2013.
120. Hara I, Miyake H, Hara S, et al. Significance of matrix metalloproteinases and tissue inhibitors of metalloproteinase expression in the recurrence of superficial transitional cell carcinoma of the bladder. *J Urol* 2001;165:1769–1772.
121. Inuoe K, Kamada M, Slaton JW, et al. The prognostic value of angiogenesis and metastasis-related genes for progression of transitional cell carcinoma of the renal pelvis and ureter. *Clin Cancer Res* 2002;8:1863–1870.
122. Hasui Y, Suzumiya J, Marutsuka K, et al. Comparative study of plasminogen activators in cancers and normal mucosa of human urinary bladder. *Cancer Res* 1989;49:1067–1070.
123. Hasui Y, Marutsuka K, Asada Y, et al. Prognostic value of urokinase-type plasminogen activator in patients with superficial bladder cancer. *Urology* 1996;47:34–37.
124. Hasui Y, Marutsuka K, Suzumiya J, et al. The content of urokinase-type plasminogen activator antigen as a prognostic factor in urinary bladder cancer. *Int J Cancer* 1992;50:871–873.

125. McGarvey TW, Kariko K, Barnathan ES, et al. The expression of urokinase-related genes in superficial and invasive transitional cell carcinoma. *Int J Oncol* 1998;12:175–180.

126. Seddighzadeh M, Steineck G, Larsson P, et al. Expression of UPA and UPAR is associated with the clinical course of urinary bladder neoplasms. *Int J Cancer* 2002;99:721–726.

127. Casella R, Shariat SF, Monoski MA, et al. Urinary levels of urokinase-type plasminogen activator and its receptor in the detection of bladder carcinoma. *Cancer* 2002;95:2494–2499.

128. Brunner A, Mayerl C, Tzankov A, et al. Prognostic significance of tenascin-C expression in superficial and invasive bladder cancer. *J Clin Pathol* 2004;57:927–931.

129. Wulfing C, Eltze E, von Struensee D, et al. Cyclooxygenase-2 expression in bladder cancer: correlation with poor outcome after chemotherapy. *Eur Urol* 2004;45:46–52.

130. Jahnson S, Karlsson MG. Predictive value of p53 and pRB immunostaining in locally advanced bladder cancer treated with cystectomy. *J Urol* 1998;160:1291–1296.

131. Kielb SJ. Functional p53 mutation as a molecular determinant of paclitaxel and gemcitabine susceptibility in human bladder cancer. *J Urol* 2001;166:482–487.

132. Sarkis A, Bajorin D, Reuter V, et al. Prognostic value of p53 nuclear overexpression in patients with invasive bladder cancer treated with neoadjuvant MVAC. *J Clin Oncol* 1995;13:1384–1390.

133. Cote RJ, Esrig D, Groshen S, et al. p53 and treatment of bladder cancer. *Nature* 1997;385:123–125.

134. Waldman T, Lengauer C, Kinzler KW, et al. Uncoupling of S phase and mitosis induced by anticancer agents in cells lacking p21. *Nature* 1996;81:713–716.

135. Siu LL, Banerjee D, Khurana RJ, et al. The prognostic role of p53, metallothionein, P-glycoprotein, and MIB-1 in muscle-invasive urothelial transitional cell carcinoma. *Clin Cancer Res* 1998;4:559–565.

136. Koga F, Kitahara S, Arai K, et al. Negative p53/positive p21 immunostaining is a predictor of favorable response to chemotherapy in patients with locally advanced bladder cancer. *Jpn J Cancer Res* 2000;91:416–423.

137. Qureshi KN, Griffiths TRL, Robinson MC, et al. TP53 and MDM2 immunoreactivity as predictors of response in muscle-invasive bladder cancer treated by systemic chemotherapy. *BJU Int* 1999;84:140–141.

138. Jankevicius F, Goebell P, Kushima M, et al. p21 and p53 immunostaining and survival following systemic chemotherapy for urothelial cancer. *Urol Int* 2002;69:174–180.

139. Petrylak DP, Scher HI, Reuter V, et al. P-glycoprotein expression in primary and metastatic transitional cell carcinoma of the bladder. *Ann Oncol* 1994;5:835–840.

140. Jones PA, Baylin SB. The fundamental role of epigenetic events in cancer. *Nat Rev Genet* 2002;3:415–428.

141. Gonzalgo ML, Jones PA. Mutagenic and epigenetic effects of DNA methylation. *Mutat Res* 1997;386:107–118.

142. Jones PA, Gonzalgo ML. Altered DNA methylation and genome instability: a new pathway to cancer? *Proc Natl Acad Sci U S A* 1997;94:2103–2105.

143. Chan MW, Chan LW, Tang NL, et al. Frequent hypermethylation of promoter region of RASSF1A in tumor tissues and voided urine of urinary bladder cancer patients. *Int J Cancer* 2003;104:611–616.

144. Horikawa Y, Sugano K, Shigyo M, et al. Hypermethylation of an E-cadherin (CDH1) promoter region in high grade transitional cell carcinoma of the bladder comprising carcinoma in situ. *J Urol* 2003;169:1541–1545.

145. Thievessen I, Seifert HH, Swiatkowski S, et al. E-cadherin involved in inactivation of WNT/beta-catenin signalling in urothelial carcinoma and normal urothelial cells. *Br J Cancer* 2003;88:1932–1938.

146. Spruck CH, Gonzalez-Zulueta M, Shibata A, et al. p16 gene in uncultured tumors. *Nature* 1994;370:183–184.

147. Herman JG, Merlo A, Mao L, et al. Inactivation of the CDKN2/p16/MTS1 gene is frequently associated with aberrant DNA methylation in all common human cancers. *Cancer Res* 1995;55:4525–4530.

148. Gonzalez-Zulueta M, Bender CM, Yang AS, et al. Methylation of the 5′ CpG island of the p16/CDKN2 tumor suppressor gene in normal and transformed human tissues correlates with gene silencing. *Cancer Res* 1995;55:4531–4535.

149. Serrano M, Hannon GJ, Beach D. A new regulatory motif in cell-cycle control causing specific inhibition of cyclin D/CDK4. *Nature* 1993;366:704–707.

150. Chan MW, Chan LW, Tang NL, et al. Hypermethylation of multiple genes in tumor tissues and voided urine in urinary bladder cancer patients. *Clin Cancer Res* 2002;8:464–470.

151. Chang LL, Yeh WT, Yang SY, et al. Genetic alterations of p16INK4a and p14ARF genes in human bladder cancer. *J Urol* 2003;170:595.

152. Dominguez G, Silva J, Garcia JM, et al. Prevalence of aberrant methylation of p14ARF over p16INK4a in some human primary tumors. *Mutat Res* 2003;530:9–17.

153. Dominguez G, Carballido J, Silva J, et al. p14ARF promoter hypermethylation in plasma DNA as an indicator of disease recurrence in bladder cancer patients. *Clin Cancer Res* 2002;8:980–985.

154. Herman JG, Graff JR, Myohanen S, et al. Methylation-specific PCR: a novel PCR assay for methylation status of CpG islands. *Proc Natl Acad Sci U S A* 1996;93:9821–9826.

155. Gonzalgo ML, Jones PA. Rapid quantitation of methylation differences at specific sites using methylation-sensitive single nucleotide primer extension (Ms-SNuPE). *Nucleic Acids Res* 1997;25:2529–2531.

156. Liang G, Salem CE, Yu MC, et al. DNA methylation differences associated with tumor tissues identified by genome scanning analysis. *Genomics* 1998;53:260–268.

157. Eads CA, Danenberg KD, Kawakami K, et al. MethyLight: a high-throughput assay to measure DNA methylation. *Nucleic Acids Res* 2000;28:E32.

158. Liang G, Gonzales FA, Jones PA, et al. Analysis of gene induction in human fibroblasts and bladder cancer cells exposed to the methylation inhibitor 5-aza-2′-deoxycytidine. *Cancer Res* 2002;62:961–966.

159. Goessl C, Muller M, Straub B, et al. DNA alterations in body fluids as molecular tumor markers for urological malignancies. *Eur Urol* 2002;41:668–676.

160. Catto JW, Azzouzi AR, Rehman I, et al. Promoter hypermethylation is associated with tumor location, stage, and subsequent progression in transitional cell carcinoma. *J Clin Oncol* 2005;23(13):2903–2910.

161. Jones PA, Taylor SM. Cellular differentiation, cytidine analogs and DNA methylation. *Cell* 1980;20:85–93.

162. Cheng JC, Matsen CB, Gonzales FA, et al. Inhibition of DNA methylation and reactivation of silenced genes by zebularine. *J Natl Cancer Inst* 2003;95:399–409.

163. Yan L, Nass SJ, Smith D, et al. Specific inhibition of DNMT1 by antisense oligonucleotides induces re-expression of estrogen receptor-α (ER) in ER-negative human breast cancer cell lines. *Cancer Biol Ther* 2003;2:552–556.

164. Brown R, Plumb JA. Demethylation of DNA by decitabine in cancer chemotherapy. *Expert Rev Anticancer Ther* 2004;4:501–510.

165. Esteller M, Corn PG, Baylin SB, et al. A gene hypermethylation profile of human cancer. *Cancer Res* 2001;61:3225–3229.

166. Tada Y, Wada M, Kuroiwa K, et al. MDR1 gene overexpression and altered degree of methylation at the promoter region in bladder cancer during chemotherapeutic treatment. *Clin Cancer Res* 2000;6:4618–4627.

167. Kawasaki H, Taira K. Induction of DNA methylation and gene silencing by short interfering RNAs in human cells. *Nature* 2004;431:211–217.

168. Cote RJ, Laird PW, Datar RH. Promoter hypermethylation: a new therapeutic target emerges in urothelial cancer. *J Clin Oncol* 2005;23(13):2879–2881.

169. Pagliarulo V, Datar RH, Cote RJ. Role of genetic and expression profiling in pharmacogenomics: the changing face of patient management. *Curr Issues Mol Biol* 2002;4:101–110.

170. Dyrskjot L, Thykjaer T, Kruhoffer M, et al. Identifying distinct classes of bladder carcinoma using microarrays. *Nat Genet* 2003;33:90–96.

171. Modlich O, Prisack HB, Pitschke G, et al. Identifying superficial, muscle-invasive, and metastasizing transitional cell carcinoma of the bladder: use of cDNA array analysis of gene expression profiles. *Clin Cancer Res* 2004;10:3410–3421.

172. Dyrskjot L, Kruhoffer M, Thykjaer T, et al. Gene expression in the urinary bladder: a common carcinoma in situ gene expression signature exists disregarding histopathological classification. *Cancer Res* 2004;64:4040–4048.

173. Sanchez-Carbayo M, Cordon-Cardo C. Applications of array technology: identification of molecular targets in bladder cancer. *Br J Cancer* 2003;89:2172–2177.

174. Sanchez-Carbayo M, Socci ND, Lozano JJ, et al. Gene discovery in bladder cancer progression using cDNA microarrays. *Am J Pathol* 2003;163:505–516.

175. Apostolakos MJ, Schuermann WH, Frampton MW, et al. Measurement of gene expression by multiplex competitive polymerase chain reaction. *Anal Biochem* 1993;213:277–284.

176. Crawford EL, Warner KA, Khuder SA, et al. Multiplex standardized RT-PCR for expression analysis of many genes in small samples. *Biochem Biophys Res Commun* 2002;293:509–516.

CHAPTER 21 ■ SCREENING, EARLY DETECTION, AND PREVENTION OF BLADDER CANCER

JORDAN R. STEINBERG, COLIN P. N. DINNEY, AND H. BARTON GROSSMAN

SCREENING AND EARLY DETECTION

Bladder cancer is the fourth most-common cancer in men and the 10th most common cancer in women in the United States (1). An estimated 57,400 new cases of bladder cancer were diagnosed in 2003. The lifetime probability of developing bladder cancer, based on epidemiologic studies between 1997 and 1999, is 3.45% (1 in 29) for men and 1.14% (1 in 88) for women. The vast majority of patients with newly diagnosed bladder cancers have superficial, low-grade neoplasms with an excellent prognosis. However, these tumors have a 30% to 70% recurrence rate and may progress to invasive cancers in 10% to 30% of patients (2–4). For this reason, patients with bladder cancer are closely monitored with cystoscopy and urinary cytology to detect early recurrence and progression and enable early therapeutic intervention. The risk of tumor recurrence is related to several clinical and histological factors including tumor grade, tumor stage, and cystoscopic findings at the first 3-month follow-up cystoscopy. Patients at high risk for recurrence and progression are often treated with intravesical chemotherapy or immunotherapy to lower their risks.

Superficial noninvasive papillary disease (Ta) is usually more of a nuisance than a threat to the patient, as the risk of recurrence far outweighs the risk of progression. Invasive, high-grade tumors portend a much poorer outcome despite aggressive treatment. Most patients with muscle-invasive disease present as such at the time of their first bladder cancer episode (5). Death from bladder cancer rarely occurs in the absence of metastatic disease, and metastatic disease rarely occurs in the absence of muscle invasion (6). Therefore, early detection, while the tumor is confined to the superficial layers of the bladder, should decrease bladder cancer mortality.

Bladder cancer is a symptomatic disease with most patients presenting with hematuria (macroscopic or microscopic), urinary symptoms, or both. In contrast to other cancers, bladder tumors are rarely found at autopsy. Bladder cancer represents a serious health risk and cost concern to both the patient and society. These observations support the hypothesis that screening and early detection would improve the outcome for patients with bladder cancer.

Ideally, screening and early detection tools should be relatively inexpensive, easy to use, provide reproducible results, and have acceptable performance characteristics. "Sensitivity," defined as the percentage of patients with the disease for whom the test is positive, should approach 100%. "Specificity," defined as the percentage of patients without the disease for whom the test is negative, should also approach 100%.

Although it is currently not realistic to achieve complete accuracy in detecting bladder cancer, minimizing false-positive and false-negative rates is important. In addition to sensitivity and specificity, the positive and negative predictive values of the test must be considered. These parameters are influenced by the prevalence of the disease in the population. A test may perform relatively well in a selected population, for example, patients with a history of bladder cancer, but have low-positive predictive value for population-based screening. Tests with high-positive predictive value can be used to initiate an intervention to diagnose and treat bladder cancer. On the other hand, tests with high-negative predictive value can be used to indicate that aggressive surveillance is not necessary.

General screening for bladder cancer is associated with several practical problems. With a population-based incidence rate of less than 5% and a preponderance of superficial low-grade tumors, demonstrating a reduction in bladder cancer mortality would require massive screening efforts and high costs. As such, most screening and early detection studies have focused on high risk individuals, namely patients with a prior history of bladder cancer or occupational exposure to known or suspected bladder carcinogens.

The gold standard for diagnosing bladder cancer is cystoscopy. However, this standard is flawed. Whereas it has long been recognized that cystoscopy can fail to detect carcinoma *in situ*, recent experiments with fluorescence cystoscopy demonstrate that papillary tumors can also escape conventional cystoscopic detection. Current bladder cancer surveillance protocols are based on 3-month to 6-month cystoscopic evaluation. The examination is invasive, relatively expensive, and often a source of patient anxiety. These concerns have driven the search for noninvasive screening and detection tools.

The two most commonly used tests for bladder cancer screening are urinalysis for hematuria and urinary cytology. Both tests have inherent strengths and weaknesses and are often combined with other investigations to maximize bladder cancer detection. Neither test is an ideal screening tool, but rather a means of directing further diagnostic evaluation.

Hematuria is present in virtually all cases of cystoscopically detectable bladder cancer, and painless hematuria is the presenting symptom in 85% of patients (7). The current methods of detecting hematuria are sensitive, inexpensive, and reproducible. These methods include microscopic examination of the urinary sediment and dipstick analysis of the uncentrifuged specimen. Microscopic analysis, although technically more demanding and time consuming, avoids the potential false-positives caused by hemoglobinuria and myoglobinuria. Benign inflammatory, traumatic, and iatrogenic conditions often produce variable amounts of hematuria and contribute to the poor specificity of this test in bladder cancer detection. In fact, less than 5% of patients who present with hematuria have bladder cancer (8,9).

Urine cytology is performed by microscopic assessment of shed urothelial cells. High-grade malignant cells have a characteristic appearance and can be readily differentiated from normal urothelium; however, low-grade bladder cancers are more difficult to detect. Most contemporary series report sensitivities in the 70% to 85% range for high-grade tumors and in the 30% to 40% range for low-grade tumors (10). With an experienced observer, the specificity of cytology is excellent, with published values typically exceeding 90% (11–13). However, the use of urine cytology as a screening test for bladder cancer is hindered by its poor sensitivity. Its clinical use, for the most part, has been limited to the surveillance of patients with bladder cancer as an indicator of occult carcinoma *in situ*.

Few large studies have addressed the issue of bladder cancer screening in asymptomatic general populations. Britton et al. (9) evaluated the efficacy of urine dipsticks in the early detection of bladder cancer in a group of men from Leeds, England. A group of 2,356 asymptomatic men over 60 years of age were evaluated at baseline with dipstick urinalysis followed by weekly home dipstick testing for 10 weeks. Of this group, 474 (20.1%) were found to have hematuria. Of these 474 men, 295 (12.5%) had hematuria identified at the initial screening evaluation, and 179 (7.6%) had at least one positive test during the subsequent period of home testing. Only 265 of the 474 patients completed the urologic evaluation. Bladder tumors were diagnosed in 17 patients and were subsequently treated. Abnormal urine cytology was found in 10 of the 17 patients. The authors concluded that the urine dipsticks provided an inexpensive, simple, and acceptable test for bladder cancer and acknowledged that this screening method produced large numbers of patients with false-positive test results for whom additional evaluations were necessary. They proposed the addition of urine cytology to this screening strategy.

In a similar study, Messing et al. (8) screened 1,240 healthy men 50 years or older for bladder cancer with home dipstick testing. The participants tested their urine daily for 14 consecutive days. At least one episode of hematuria was documented in 283 men (21.1%). Of the 192 hematuria-positive participants who completed the urologic evaluation, 16 (8.3%) were found to harbor urologic cancers, 9 of which were transitional cell carcinoma of the bladder. Another 47 participants (24.5%) were found to have other hematuria-causing diseases that required treatment. These authors concluded that home screening for hematuria was a feasible and economical tool for the early detection of urinary tract cancers and other diseases and that the quantity and frequency of hematuria were not related to disease severity. In an earlier study by Messing et al. (14), home screening for 1 full year revealed hematuria in 44 (18.7%) of 235 asymptomatic men 50 years of age and older. Of these patients, 31 underwent full urologic evaluation, and 8 were found to have urinary cancers (5 transitional cell cancers and 3 renal cell cancers).

The rationale for screening is improvement in disease outcome. Importantly, there have been no prospective randomized studies evaluating bladder cancer screening in a population of asymptomatic adults. To address this, Messing et al. (15) compared bladder tumor characteristics and outcomes in patients with tumors detected by hematuria screening with those of a comparable population of unscreened patients from the Wisconsin Tumor Registry. The proportion of advanced-stage cancers (T2 or higher) was significantly lower in the screened group compared with the unscreened group. In addition, no patients in the screened group died of disease (3 to 9 years of follow-up) compared with a 16.4% mortality rate among patients in the unscreened group (within 2 years of diagnosis). Caution should be practiced when interpreting this nonrandomized study. However, it does suggest that bladder cancer screening could be beneficial.

Screening studies in high-risk groups have yielded promising results as well. Theriault et al. (16) evaluated a bladder screening protocol (using annual urinary cytology) among aluminum production workers in Quebec who were exposed to coal-tar-pitch volatiles, a known bladder carcinogen. Cases detected after the screening program was introduced (1980s) were compared to cases diagnosed earlier (1970s). The proportion of cases identified at earlier stages favored the screening group and a trend toward improved survival was noted as well. Although tumor grade did not appear to differ, the percentage of superficial lesions diagnosed in the screening group was 63% compared with 39% in the nonscreened group.

Mason et al. (17) evaluated a home self-test for microscopic hematuria in a group of subjects working at the DuPont Chambers Works in Deepwater, New Jersey. These workers were exposed to β-naphthylamine, benzidine, and other suspected bladder cancer carcinogens. Every 6 months, subjects tested their urine at home for 14 consecutive days for the presence of blood. In addition, urine cytologies were periodically performed. Through the first seven periods of screening, two new cases and one recurrence of transitional cell carcinoma of the bladder were detected.

Marsh et al. (18) recently reported the 15-year bladder cancer screening results from the Drake Health Registry Study (DHRS). This study was initiated in 1986 by the University of Pittsburgh to screen employees of the Drake Chemical Company in Lock Haven, Pennsylvania. Workers employed by the company had been exposed to β-naphthylamine. In a previous cohort analysis, Marsh et al. (19) found a 20- to 30-fold excess bladder cancer mortality risk in this patient population. DHRS participants were screened annually with urinalysis for hematuria, Papanicolaou cytology, and quantitative fluorescence image analysis. Newer biomarkers, including M344 and G-actin, were added in 1995. Over the course of 15 years, DHRS screened over 350 individuals and identified 51 people eligible for further diagnostic evaluation. Of 41 people who underwent cystoscopy, one was diagnosed with carcinoma *in situ*, two with transitional cell papilloma, 14 with dysplasia, and two with transitional cell carcinoma. Bladder abnormalities such as chronic cystitis, atypia, and hyperplasia were identified in 26 individuals. The authors concluded that the DHRS identified early stage bladder cancer and other abnormalities among workers exposed to β-naphthylamine. In addition, they emphasized the importance of ongoing screening in these patients, as the median latency period for this cohort (including cases detected prior to screening) was 25 years.

As with the screening studies conducted in the general population, assessment of benefit in the targeted studies is limited due to the lack of randomized controlled populations. The data suggest that the screening tests are detecting bladder cancers at lower stages. Nevertheless, in the absence of randomized prospective trials, screening and early detection policies for the general population cannot be recommended.

The recent emergence of sensitive markers for bladder cancer has provided new opportunities for early bladder cancer detection. There are currently more than 20 urine-based markers (UBMs) in various stages of development. A comprehensive review of all UBMs is beyond the scope of this chapter. Evaluation of these markers has been conducted almost exclusively in patients with bladder cancer or patients presenting with signs and symptoms of bladder cancer. Assays currently available in the United States include BTA *stat*, BTA TRAK, NMP22 and NMP22 BladderChek, DD23, ImmunoCyt, and UroVysion.

The BTA *stat* and TRAK tests are immunoassays that recognize human complement factor H related protein, a protein produced by several bladder cancer cell lines and found in the urine of patients with transitional cell bladder cancer (20). These assays differ from the original BTA test, which was

TABLE 21.1

CURRENTLY AVAILABLE URINE-BASED MARKERS FOR BLADDER CANCER

Test	Marker/Antigen	Testing situation	% Sensitivity	% Specificity	Reference
Hematuria	Hemoglobin	Point of care	70 to 90	Low	(8,9,14)
Cytology	Shed tumor cell	Laboratory	30 to 40	90 to 100	(10)
BTA *Stat*	Human complement factor H related protein	Point of care	60 to 70	50 to 75	(21–24)
BTA TRAK	Human complement factor H related protein	Laboratory	60 to 70	50 to 75	(21–24)
NMP22	Nuclear mitotic apparatus protein	Laboratory	60 to 75	70 to 85	(21,25–27)
DD23	Protein dimer	Laboratory	80	60	(29)
ImmunoCyt	High molecular weight CEA and mucins	Laboratory	70 to 95	70 to 85	(30–32)
UroVysion	Chromosomal probes	Laboratory	70 to 100	90	(33,34)

designed to detect a basement membrane-protein antigen released into the urine of patients with bladder cancer. BTA *stat* is a qualitative point-of-care test, whereas BTA TRAK is quantitative and requires laboratory analysis. Most published series report the sensitivity for both tests as 60% to 70% and the specificity as 50% to 75% (21–24). The NMP22 is based on a nuclear mitotic apparatus protein that is an abundant component of the nuclear matrix. This apparatus is released from cancer cells and detected by an enzyme-linked immunoassay that uses two monoclonal antibodies. NMP22 is a quantitative test with reported sensitivity and specificity of 60% to 75% and 70% to 85%, respectively (21,25–27). NMP22 BladderChek is a recently developed point-of-care assay. DD23 is an IgG1 monoclonal antibody that recognizes a protein dimer found in bladder cancer cells (28). Sensitivity and specificity of DD23 have been reported as 80.5% and 59.7%, respectively (29). Combining DD23 with cytology significantly enhances the performance of cytology alone, especially in low-grade cancers. The ImmunoCyt test combines an immunofluorescence assay with urinary cytology. Using three monoclonal antibodies, the test detects a high molecular weight form of carcinoma embryonic antigen and several mucins that are expressed preferentially on bladder cancer cells. The reported sensitivity and specificity is 70% to 95% and 70% to 85%, respectively (30–32). UroVysion is a fluorescence *in situ* hybridization (FISH) test composed of three chromosome enumeration probes (CEP17, CEP3, and CEP7) and a single locus-specific indicator probe (9p21). Bladder cancers are associated with a number of cytogenetic changes, including increased copy numbers of chromosomes. UroVysion has a reported sensitivity of 70% to 100% and a specificity

of approximately 90% (33,34). Markers in development, showing promising signs of clinical applicability, include BLCA-4, cytokeratins, hyaluronic acid/hyaluronidase, proteomics, and microsatellite assays. Microsatellite assays detect genomic instability by comparing DNA from tumor cells with normal cells, for example, shed urothelial carcinoma cells with peripheral blood lymphocytes. The loss of heterozygosity (LOH) indicates a specific locus where a tumor suppressor gene may be present. Using multiple microsatellite markers, the likelihood of detecting a malignancy can be improved. Sidransky and colleagues (35) tested 13 microsatellite markers in the urine of 25 patients presenting with signs and symptoms suggestive of bladder cancer. Genetic alterations were detected in 19 of 20 patients who were subsequently found to have histologically confirmed bladder cancer. Five patients without neoplasia (controls) did not show any microsatellite changes. Tables 21.1 and 21.2 present the test and performance characteristics outlined above as well as those of other select UBMs.

There has been no consensus regarding the clinical application of UBMs. A recent meta-analysis by Lotan and Roehrborn (10) compared 20 UBMs with cytology. The review included 54 publications with 338 distinct patient groups and over 10,000 patients. They concluded that all UBMs are more sensitive than cytology, especially for low-grade disease, but cannot match cytology regarding specificity. Glas et al. (46) recently evaluated 42 studies specifically addressing UBMs in the diagnosis of primary bladder cancer. Cytology was found to be the most specific marker at 94%, whereas telomerase had the best sensitivity at 75%. They caution against the routine use of UBMs as a screening tool in the diagnosis of primary bladder cancer because overall sensitivity is not high enough.

TABLE 21.2

OTHER UBMS IN DEVELOPMENT

Test	Marker/Antigen	Testing situation	% Sensitivity	% Specificity	Reference
Telomerase	Telomeres	Laboratory	70 to 85	80 to 95	(13,36,37)
FDPs	FDPs	Point of care	78 to 91	75 to 90	(27,38)
BLCA-4	Nuclear matrix protein	Point of care/Laboratory	96	100	(39)
Cytokeratins	Cytokeratins	Laboratory	85 to 95	75 to 90	(40–42)
Hyaluroric acid/ Hyaluronidase	HA-HAase	Laboratory	80 to 100	70 to 90	(43–45)

At the present time, UBMs cannot replace cystoscopy for patients who present with signs and symptoms of bladder cancer. The problems encountered when screening the general population have already been discussed. UBMs are indicated for the follow-up of patients with superficial bladder cancer. Their high sensitivity results in a high negative predictive value, suggesting that they could be used to increase the interval between cystoscopies. Using decision analysis models, Lotan and Roehrborn (47) demonstrated cost-effectiveness in a protocol in which tumor marker testing was alternated with cystoscopy compared with cystoscopy (and cytology) every 3 months. Their finding was found to be true for a wide range of marker sensitivies, and was based on a 20% to 80% yearly recurrence rate and a 2% to 40% yearly progression rate. Jewett and colleagues (48) also demonstrated a cost reduction when using urinary marker testing for follow-up of patients with superficial bladder cancer. They constructed a decision analysis model based on a cohort of 361 patients previously diagnosed with superficial bladder cancer. The cost benefit over standard care was apparent as early as 6 months and increased with longer follow-up. The clinical significance of delaying the time to the diagnosis of a superficial low-grade tumor recurrence is minimal. High-grade/high-stage lesions are less likely to produce false-negative tests, as the sensitivity for most UBMs in detecting these lesions exceeds 85% to 90%. However, safety cannot be effectively modeled. A randomized trial is needed to document the safety and cost efficiency of this strategy.

PREVENTION

Bladder cancer prevention can be broadly classified into two main categories: (a) avoidance strategies focus on the reduction or elimination of known risk factors, and (b) chemoprevention strategies entail the administration of chemical agents, either locally or systemically. Cancers can be prevented by reducing exposures to initiators or by suppressing promotional activity in initiated cells (49). Bladder cancer is characterized by a long latency period and provides a potentially long window for chemoprevention. As was the case for screening and early detection, targeting patients at high risk for developing bladder tumors facilitates the evaluation of such strategies.

Avoidance Strategies

Cigarette smoking has long been recognized as a leading risk factor for the development of bladder cancer. Smokers have up to a fourfold higher incidence of bladder cancer than do nonsmokers (50–52). The risk can further be correlated with frequency of cigarette smoking, degree of inhalation, duration of smoking, and type of cigarette (53,54). Smoking is believed to be responsible for approximately 50% of cases of bladder cancer in the United States (55) and possibly a higher percentage in less-developed countries where smoking is more prevalent. As opposed to other smoking related malignancies and illnesses, a reduction of this risk down to baseline takes nearly 20 years after cessation (56). Other published reports are unclear with respect to the risk reduction relative to the time since quitting, and question whether this risk is ever truly eliminated (57). Leistikow et al. (58) analyzed and correlated the United States National Cancer Institute's Surveillance Epidemiology and End Results (SEER) database with the California Cancer Registry (CCR) from 1988 to 1997 and found that the incidence of bladder cancer decreased 0.5% per year faster in the state of California as compared to other states in the United States. They attributed this reduction to the remarkable decrease in smoking during the same time period. Strategies for smoking cessation should be offered to all smokers with a history of bladder cancer.

Occupational exposure to aromatic amines is strongly associated with bladder cancer. 2-naphthylamine and benzidine are the most widely recognized compounds responsible for the excesses of bladder cancer observed in workers in dye, rubber, and textile industries. These chemicals likely affect both the early and late stages of bladder tumorigenesis (59,60). There is a long latency period, typically measured in decades, between exposure and clinical onset of bladder cancer. Although government regulation has improved the safety of the workplace, the long latency period suggests that some individuals remain at risk and need to be closely monitored.

The reduction in use or avoidance of various foods has been debated since the early 1970s. Cole (61) and Fraumeni et al. (62) first reported an association between bladder cancer and coffee consumption. Multiple studies, either supporting or disputing this claim, have emerged over the last 3 decades, adding further uncertainty to this contentious topic. Whereas some studies demonstrate a mildly increased relative risk of bladder cancer in coffee drinkers, they fail to consistently demonstrate a dose- or duration-related effect (63–65). Overall, the published data suggest that recommending coffee reduction or elimination as a means of preventing bladder cancer is unjustified. A recent Medline review concluded that there was no significant association between the two (66). Studies addressing the consumption of tea have been similarly conflicting. Artificial sweeteners, including saccharin and cyclamates, have been shown to promote bladder cancer in experimental rodent studies (67–69). This concern led to a ban on cyclamate in the United States in 1970 and restrictions on its use in other countries. These findings, however, have not been reproducible in animal models using physiologic doses and exposure patterns. More importantly, the association between artificial sweeteners and bladder cancer has not been substantiated in human case-control studies (70–72).

Phenacetin-containing analgesics have been strongly implicated in the development of bladder cancer. Consequently, other analgesics have been the focus of more recent studies. Castelao et al. (73) conducted a population-based case-control study in Los Angeles, involving 1,514 incident bladder cancer cases and an equal number of matched controls. Regular use of analgesics was not associated with an increased risk of bladder cancer in either men or women. In fact, regular analgesic users compared to nonusers or irregular users were at decreased risk for bladder cancer overall (odds ratio = 0.81). As expected, phenacetin intake was positively related to bladder cancer risk in a dose-dependent manner. Acetaminophen, the major metabolite of phenacetin, was not associated with an increased risk of bladder cancer, whereas the intake of all classes of nonsteroidal anti-inflammatory drugs (NSAIDs), except pyrazolon derivatives, was associated with a protective effect. These findings are in keeping with earlier studies that have consistently demonstrated an inhibitory and protective effect of NSAIDs in both *in vitro* and *in vivo* animal models (74–76).

Chemoprevention

The ideal chemopreventive agent must be well tolerated, inexpensive, readily available, and free of adverse side effects. Newer strategies focus on the chemopreventive effects of diet and nutrition. Because of the lack of drugs proven to be effective and the large resources required for primary chemoprevention studies, promising drugs are initially tested in a secondary chemoprevention strategy. Patients with superficial bladder cancer present an outstanding opportunity for evaluating secondary chemoprevention strategies. They are frequently evaluated with cytology and cystoscopy and have a high frequency of tumor recurrence in a relatively short period.

Fluid Intake

The bladder mucosa is in constant contact with urinary toxins and potential carcinogens. Diluting the urine and promoting increased urinary frequency would intuitively decrease the risk of carcinogen-related tumors. Michaud et al. (77) examined the relationship between total fluid intake and the risk of bladder cancer over a period of 10 years in 47,909 participants from the Health Professional Follow-up Study. During the follow-up period, 252 new cases of bladder cancer were diagnosed. Total daily fluid intake was inversely associated with the risk of bladder cancer. The multivariate relative risk (RR) was 0.51 for the highest quintile of daily fluid intake (>2531 mL/day) compared with the lowest quintile (<1290 mL/day). This risk decreased by 7% for each 240 mL increment of daily fluid consumption recorded. The consumption of water contributed to a lower risk (RR of 0.49 for >6 cups/day vs. <1 cup/day), as did the consumption of other fluids (RR of 0.63 for >9 cups/day vs. <3.7 cups/day). However, the Netherlands Cohort Study failed to demonstrate a significant association between total fluid consumption and bladder cancer risk (78). The RR for men and women was 0.87, comparing the highest to lowest quintiles of total fluid consumption. A multicenter case-control study from France detected a slightly increased risk of bladder cancer associated with total fluid intake in men (79). They attributed this finding to the high consumption of coffee and other nonalcoholic drinks. No relation between bladder cancer risk and fluid intake was identified in women. Donat et al. (80) recently examined the association between fluid intake and the risk of tumor recurrence in patients with superficial bladder cancer. They prospectively evaluated 267 patients undergoing routine bladder cancer surveillance and failed to demonstrate a relationship between fluid intake and tumor recurrence. Whereas the average daily intake was quite high (2,654 mL or 13.3 cups), multivariate analysis failed to show a protective effect against recurrence at any level of fluid intake. These findings suggest that reducing urinary contact time and diluting carcinogens are unlikely to decrease tumor recurrence rate in patients already diagnosed with bladder cancer.

Vitamins

Laboratory and epidemiologic studies suggest that vitamin supplements may be beneficial in the prevention of several malignancies. Although there are only a handful of clinical trials evaluating this potential, the largely unregulated marketing and sale of vitamin and herbal supplements have flooded the public with unproven claims.

Lamm et al. (81) evaluated the efficacy of megadose multivitamins in reducing tumor recurrence in bladder cancer patients. They conducted a phase III trial using a 2 × 2 design. Sixty-five patients with biopsy-confirmed transitional cell carcinoma of the bladder were initially randomized to intravesical bacillus calmette-geurin (BCG) with or without the administration of percutaneous BCG. Patients were subsequently randomized to therapy with multiple vitamins in the recommended daily allowance (RDA) versus RDA multivitamins plus 40,000 units of vitamin A, 100 mg of vitamin B6, 2,000 mg of vitamin C, 400 units of vitamin E, and 90 mg of zinc. The rates of tumor recurrence for the two groups were identical for the first 10 months but diverged significantly thereafter. Overall recurrence was detected in 24 (80%) of 30 patients in the RDA arm and 14 (40%) of 35 patients in the megadose arm. The 5-year estimates of tumor recurrence were 91% and 41% in the RDA and megadose arms, respectively (P = .0014). The addition of percutaneous BCG did not significantly reduce tumor occurrences.

The impact of individual vitamins has been studied as well. Vitamin B6 (pyridoxine) is thought to correct abnormalities of tryptophan metabolism in patients with bladder cancer. Byar et al. (82) prospectively randomized 121 patients with stage I bladder cancer to placebo, pyridoxine, or intravesical thiotepa. Pyridoxine was significantly better than placebo at reducing the recurrence rate once patients with fewer than 10 months of follow-up or tumor recurrences within the first 10 months were excluded (P = .03). The european organization for research and treatment of cancer (EORTC) GU Group conducted a double-blind, randomized, phase III trial evaluating the effect of pyridoxine administration on the recurrence of Ta and T1 tumors of the bladder (83). The trial accrued 291 patients and failed to demonstrate a significant difference between the pyridoxine and placebo groups with respect to time-to-first-recurrence or recurrence rate.

Vitamin C is a potent reducing agent and water-soluble antioxidant. It inhibits the *in vivo* production of N-nitroso compounds and acts as a free radical scavenger preventing DNA damage (84). Shibata et al. (85) followed a cohort of 11,580 cancer-free residents from a retirement community. With 8 years of follow-up, 1,335 incident cancer cases were diagnosed. An inverse relationship between vitamin C supplement use and bladder cancer risk was observed (0.59 relative risk). In a case-control study based on 261 cases, Nomura et al. (86) demonstrated a decrease in lower urinary tract cancers in women with increasing levels of vitamin C consumption. However, a recent analysis of 991,522 adults from the Cancer Prevention Study II failed to demonstrate an association between regular vitamin C supplement use and bladder cancer mortality (87). Studies in rats have addressed a possible dose and concentration threshold beyond which vitamin C could promote tumorigenesis (88,89). The relevance of these observations to man is unclear.

Vitamin E (α tocopherol) is another potent free radical scavenger that reduces the formation of nitroso compounds. As opposed to vitamin C, it is lipid soluble and capable of diffusing into the cell membrane where it can exert a local protective effect. In addition, vitamin E has been shown to stimulate immunologic function and enhance antibody production and resistance to infection (90). Clinical studies, however, have failed to consistently demonstrate a protective effect. The Alpha-Tocopherol Beta-Carotene (ATBC) Cancer Prevention Study assessed the effect of supplemental vitamin use on the incidence of lung cancer and other cancers among 29,133 male smokers 50 to 69 years of age (91). With a median of 6.1 years of follow-up, vitamin E supplementation was not associated with a protective role against bladder cancer (RR 1.27). A recent postintervention follow-up study of the same group of participants revealed similar findings (92). The ATBC study results, however, cannot be generalized to nonsmokers. Nonetheless, vitamin E chemoprevention for bladder cancer is unproven.

Retinoids are natural and synthetic analogues of vitamin A. They play a key role in cell differentiation and the maintenance of epithelial integrity. Animal studies have demonstrated the inhibitory effects of retinoids on multiple tumors, including transitional cell carcinoma of the bladder (93). Although the mechanisms of retinoid-induced inhibition are not completely understood, it appears that the therapeutic effects result from inducing differentiation, decreasing growth, and inducing apoptosis. Lower vitamin A intake and plasma levels have been linked with an increased risk of bladder cancer in several epidemiologic studies (94,95). Studer et al. (96) conducted a prospective randomized double-blind multicenter trial evaluating the adjuvant use of a vitamin A analogue (etretinate) after transurethral resection (TUR) of superficial bladder tumors. Seventy-nine patients in whom Ta or T1 tumors had recently been resected were randomized to receive either 25 mg of etretinate or a placebo daily for a minimum of 2 years.

The time to first recurrence was similar in the two groups; however, the mean interval to subsequent tumor recurrence was significantly longer in the etretinate group (12.7 months in the placebo group and 20.3 months in the etretinate group, $P = .006$). The number of TUR per patient-year was also significantly reduced in the etretinate group ($P <.001$). Decensi et al. (97) assessed the activity of fenretinide in superficial bladder cancer using DNA flow cytometry and conventional cytology as surrogate biomarkers in 99 patients with resected pTa or pT1 bladder cancers. The patients were randomized to either 200 mg/day of oral fenretidine for 24 months or no intervention. Recurrence-free survival was comparable between the two groups (27 events in the fenretidine arm and 21 events in the control arm, $P = .36$). In addition, fenretidine showed a lack of effect on DNA content distribution and the morphology of urothelial cells obtained in bladder washings. Adding to the uncertainty of vitamin A as a chemopreventive agent is the well-documented toxicity associated with the ingestion of excessive doses. Side effects include cheilosis, conjunctivitis, pruritis, arthralgia, ophthalmic pain, and visual disturbances. In general, the synthetic retinoids and retinamides are associated with fewer side effects. Carotenes, derived from vegetable sources, have also been studied as chemopreventive agents and found to be of little benefit in preventing bladder cancer. In fact, there is evidence that β-carotene supplementation in smokers increases the risk for lung cancer and cancer mortality (92).

Other Agents

Difluoromethylornithine (DFMO) is an irreversible inhibitor of ornithine decarboxylase, the key enzyme in mammalian polyamine biosynthesis. Ornithine decarboxylase is thought to regulate growth and apoptosis in multiple cell systems and has been implicated in the development of several cancers. DFMO has been shown to reduce the incidence of N-butyl-N-(4-hydroxybutyl)-nitrosamine-induced papillary tumors in rodents (98,99). In vitro studies of human transitional cell carcinoma cell lines have also showed an inhibitory effect (100). Clinical data supporting the use of DFMO is lacking. A multicenter trial evaluating its efficacy has been completed.

Soy foods, particularly isoflavones, have generated tremendous interest owing to their effect against breast, colon, and prostate cancers. Metabolites of isoflavones are excreted in the urine where they can inhibit bladder carcinogenesis. Using these compounds, Su et al. (101) induced apoptosis and inhibited the growth of J82 bladder cancer cells. Zhou et al. (102) evaluated the in vitro effects of pure soy isoflavones and soy phytochemical concentrate on growth curves, cell-cycle progression, and apoptosis in human and murine bladder cancer cell lines. Soy products reduced angiogenesis, increased apoptosis, and slightly reduced proliferation and showed no histopathologic effects on the normal bladder mucosa. These data suggest that soy isoflavones can inhibit bladder tumor growth through a combination of direct effects on tumor cells and indirect effects on the tumor neovasculature. Limited studies addressing the clinical impact of isoflavones on bladder cancer have been discouraging. Sun et al. (103) recently reported the results of the Singapore Chinese Health Study, a population-based cohort study with 329,848 person-years of follow-up. High intake of soy foods was significantly related to an elevated risk of bladder cancer. The highest quartile of total soy intake (≥ 92.5 g/1000 Kcal), relative to the lowest quartile of total soy intake (<36.9 g/1000 Kcal), was associated with a 2.3-fold increase in bladder cancer risk. Similar results were obtained for intakes of soy protein and soy isoflavones. In addition, the soy–cancer relationship became stronger when the analysis was restricted to subjects

with longer follow-up duration (≤ 3 years). Further clinical studies are needed to clarify the chemopreventive role of soy products.

Selective cyclooxygenase-2 (COX-2) inhibitors have received increasing attention for their role in the prevention and treatment of different cancers. COX-2 is an inducible enzyme that is upregulated in inflammation, angiogenesis, and neoplasia. NSAIDs inhibit both COX-1 and COX-2. The toxicity of NSAIDs has been attributed to the inhibition of COX-1. Therefore, selective COX-2 inhibitors were developed as potentially less toxic agents. The different COX-2 inhibitors, such as celecoxib and rofecoxib, exhibit various degrees of efficacy in inducing apoptosis, decreasing microvascular density, and decreasing the expression of vascular endothelial growth factor (VEGF). Celecoxib has been shown to inhibit bladder tumor formation in mice and rats treated with N-butyl-N-(4-hydroxybutyl)-nitrosamine (104). Nimesulide, another COX-2-specific inhibitor, has demonstrated chemopreventive effects in a rat bladder carcinogenesis model (105). To evaluate the possible involvement of COX-2 in human bladder cancer, Komhoff et al. (106) examined the expression of COX isoforms in benign and malignant tissue specimens. Paraffin-embedded tissues from 75 patients with urothelial carcinomas were immunostained with specific antibodies against COX-1 and COX-2. COX-2 immunoreactivity was absent in benign tissue and in specimens with low-grade urothelial carcinoma (0 of 23). In contrast, expression of COX-2 was detected in malignant epithelial cells in 36% (17 of 47) of specimens with high-grade urothelial carcinomas. Gee et al. (107) detected COX-2 in 11 of 16 TCC tumors examined from Egyptian patients. Shariat et al. (108) demonstrated COX-2 overexpression in 62 (78%) of 80 transitional cell carcinoma specimens and found that COX-2 overexpression was associated with pathologically staged muscle-invasive disease. Shirahama et al. (109) demonstrated by multivariate analysis that COX-2 expression correlated with invasion but was not an independent prognostic factor. Although clinical evidence has demonstrated that celecoxib reduces the incidence of colonic polyps in patients with familial adenomatous polyposis, the role of COX-2 inhibitors in bladder cancer chemoprevention remains to be determined. A multi-institutional randomized study of celecoxib for secondary chemoprevention of bladder cancer is nearing completion.

Despite encouraging preclinical data with a number of drugs, clinical documentation of efficacy is minimal or absent. At this time, it is prudent to recommend smoking cessation and a balanced diet to all patients with bladder cancer. These patients are highly motivated to reduce the morbidity associated with further recurrences and are eager to play a more active role in their disease management. Laboratory studies continue to identify specific pathways and targets for prevention and expand our understanding of bladder carcinogenesis. Ongoing and future chemoprevention trials will ultimately guide the clinical applicability of this approach.

References

1. Jemal A, Murray T, Samuels A, et al. Cancer statistics, 2003. CA Cancer J Clin 2003;53(1):5–26.
2. Rubben H, Lutzeyer W, Fischer N, et al. Natural history and treatment of low and high risk superficial bladder tumors. J Urol 1988;139(2):283–285.
3. Heney NM, Ahmed S, Flanagan MJ, et al. Superficial bladder cancer: progression and recurrence. J Urol 1983;130(6):1083–1086.
4. Millan-Rodriguez F, Chechile-Toniolo G, Salvador-Bayarri J, et al. Primary superficial bladder cancer risk groups according to progression, mortality and recurrence. J Urol 2000;164(3 Pt 1):680–684.
5. Kaye KW, Lange PH. Mode of presentation of invasive bladder cancer: reassessment of the problem. J Urol 1982;128(1):31–33.
6. Babaian RJ, Johnson DE, Llamas L, et al. Metastases from transitional cell carcinoma of urinary bladder. Urology 1980;16(2):142–144.

7. Varkarakis MJ, Gaeta J, Moore RH, et al. Superficial bladder tumor. Aspects of clinical progression. *Urology* 1974;4(4):414–420.
8. Messing EM, Young TB, Hunt VB, et al. Home screening for hematuria: results of a multiclinic study. *J Urol* 1992;148(2 Pt 1):289–292.
9. Britton JP, Dowell AC, Whelan P, et al. A community study of bladder cancer screening by the detection of occult urinary bleeding. *J Urol* 1992;148(3):788–790.
10. Lotan Y, Roehrborn CG. Sensitivity and specificity of commonly available bladder tumor markers versus cytology: results of a comprehensive literature review and meta-analyses. *Urology* 2003;61(1):109–118; discussion 118.
11. Planz B, Synek C, Deix T, et al. Diagnosis of bladder cancer with urinary cytology, immunocytology and DNA-image-cytometry. *Anal Cell Pathol* 2001;22(3):103–109.
12. Leyh H, Marberger M, Conort P, et al. Comparison of the BTA stat test with voided urine cytology and bladder wash cytology in the diagnosis and monitoring of bladder cancer. *Eur Urol* 1999;35(1):52–56.
13. Ito H, Kyo S, Kanaya T, et al. Detection of human telomerase reverse transcriptase messenger RNA in voided urine samples as a useful diagnostic tool for bladder cancer. *Clin Cancer Res* 1998;4(11):2807–2810.
14. Messing EM, Young TB, Hunt VB, et al. Urinary tract cancers found by home screening with hematuria dipsticks in healthy men over 50 years of age. *Cancer* 1989;64(11):2361–2367.
15. Messing EM, Young TB, Hunt VB, et al. Comparison of bladder cancer outcome in men undergoing hematuria home screening versus those with standard clinical presentations. *Urology* 1995;45(3):387–396; discussion 396–397.
16. Theriault GP, Tremblay CG, Armstrong BG. Bladder cancer screening among primary aluminum production workers in Quebec. *J Occup Med* 1990;32(9):869–872.
17. Mason TJ, Walsh WP, Lee K, et al. New opportunities for screening and early detection of bladder cancer. *J Cell Biochem Suppl* 1992;16I:13–22.
18. Marsh GM, Cassidy LD. The Drake Health Registry Study: findings from fifteen years of continuous bladder cancer screening. *Am J Ind Med* 2003;43(2):142–148.
19. Marsh GM, Leviton LC, Talbott EO, et al. Drake Chemical Workers' Health Registry Study: I. Notification and medical surveillance of a group of workers at high risk of developing bladder cancer. *Am J Ind Med* 1991;19(3):291–301.
20. Lokeshwar VB, Soloway MS. Current bladder tumor tests: does their projected utility fulfill clinical necessity? *J Urol* 2001;165(4):1067–1077.
21. Sozen S, Biri H, Sinik Z, et al. Comparison of the nuclear matrix protein 22 with voided urine cytology and BTA stat test in the diagnosis of transitional cell carcinoma of the bladder. *Eur Urol* 1999;36(3):225–229.
22. Priolo G, Gontero P, Martinasso G, et al. Bladder tumor antigen assay as compared to voided urine cytology in the diagnosis of bladder cancer. *Clin Chim Acta* 2001;305(1–2):47–53.
23. Mahnert B, Tauber S, Kriegmair M, et al. BTA-TRAK—a useful diagnostic tool in urinary bladder cancer? *Anticancer Res* 1999;19(4Λ):2615–2619.
24. Heicappell R, Muller M, Fimmers R, et al. Qualitative determination of urinary human complement factor H-related protein (hcfHrp) in patients with bladder cancer, healthy controls, and patients with benign urologic disease. *Urol Int* 2000;65(4):181–184.
25. Lee KH. Evaluation of the NMP22 test and comparison with voided urine cytology in the detection of bladder cancer. *Yonsei Med J* 2001;42(1):14–18.
26. Giannopoulos A, Manousakas T, Gounari A, et al. Comparative evaluation of the diagnostic performance of the BTA stat test, NMP22 and urinary bladder cancer antigen for primary and recurrent bladder tumors. *J Urol* 2001;166(2):470–475.
27. Ramakumar S, Bhuiyan J, Besse JA, et al. Comparison of screening methods in the detection of bladder cancer. *J Urol* 1999;161(2):388–394.
28. Grossman HB, Washington RW Jr, Carey TE, et al. Alterations in antigen expression in superficial bladder cancer. *J Cell Biochem Suppl* 1992;16I:63–68.
29. Sawczuk IS, Pickens CL, Vasa UR, et al. DD23 Biomarker: a prospective clinical assessment in routine urinary cytology specimens from patients being monitored for TCC. *Urol Oncol* 2002;7(5):185–190.
30. Feil G, Zumbragel A, Paulgen-Nelde HJ, et al. Accuracy of the Immuno-Cyt assay in the diagnosis of transitional cell carcinoma of the urinary bladder. *Anticancer Res* 2003;23(2A):963–967.
31. Fradet Y, Lockhard C. Performance characteristics of a new monoclonal antibody test for bladder cancer: ImmunoCyt trade mark. *Can J Urol* 1997;4(3):400–405.
32. Mian C, Pycha A, Wiener H, et al. Immunocyt: a new tool for detecting transitional cell cancer of the urinary tract. *J Urol* 1999;161(5):1486–1489.
33. Bubendorf L, Grilli B, Sauter G, et al. Multiprobe FISH for enhanced detection of bladder cancer in voided urine specimens and bladder washings. *Am J Clin Pathol* 2001;116(1):79–86.
34. Friedrich MG, Toma MI, Hellstern A, et al. Comparison of multitarget fluorescence in situ hybridization in urine with other noninvasive tests for detecting bladder cancer. *BJU Int* 2003;92(9):911–914.
35. Mao L, Schoenberg MP, Scicchitano M, et al. Molecular detection of primary bladder cancer by microsatellite analysis. *Science* 1996;271(5249):659–662.
36. Kavaler E, Landman J, Chang Y, et al. Detecting human bladder carcinoma cells in voided urine samples by assaying for the presence of telomerase activity. *Cancer* 1998;82(4):708–714.
37. Rahat MA, Lahat N, Gazawi H, et al. Telomerase activity in patients with transitional cell carcinoma: a preliminary study. *Cancer* 1999;85(4):919–924.
38. Johnston B, Morales A. Re: comparison of screening methods in the detection of bladder cancer. *J Urol* 1999;162(4):1388–1389.
39. Konety BR, Nguyen TS, Brenes G, et al. Clinical usefulness of the novel marker BLCA-4 for the detection of bladder cancer. *J Urol* 2000;164(3 Pt 1):634–639.
40. Sanchez-Carbayo M, Herrero E, Megias J, et al. Initial evaluation of the new urinary bladder cancer rapid test in the detection of transitional cell carcinoma of the bladder. *Urology* 1999;54(4):656–661.
41. Sanchez-Carbayo M, Herrero E, Megias J, et al. Initial evaluation of the diagnostic performance of the new urinary bladder cancer antigen test as a tumor marker for transitional cell carcinoma of the bladder. *J Urol* 1999;161(4):1110–1115.
42. Sanchez-Carbayo M, Herrero E, Megias J, et al. Comparative sensitivity of urinary CYFRA 21-1, urinary bladder cancer antigen, tissue polypeptide antigen, tissue polypeptide antigen and NMP22 to detect bladder cancer. *J Urol* 1999;162(6):1951–1956.
43. Pham HT, Block NL, Lokeshwar VB. Tumor-derived hyaluronidase: a diagnostic urine marker for high-grade bladder cancer. *Cancer Res* 1997;57(4):778–783.
44. Lokeshwar VB, Obek C, Pham HT, et al. Urinary hyaluronic acid and hyaluronidase: markers for bladder cancer detection and evaluation of grade. *J Urol* 2000;163(1):348–356.
45. Lokeshwar VB, Schroeder GL, Selzer MG, et al. Bladder tumor markers for monitoring recurrence and screening comparison of hyaluronic acid-hyaluronidase and BTA-Stat tests. *Cancer* 2002;95(1):61–72.
46. Glas AS, Roos D, Deutekom M, et al. Tumor markers in the diagnosis of primary bladder cancer. A systematic review. *J Urol* 2003;169(6):1975–1982.
47. Lotan Y, Roehrborn CG. Cost-effectiveness of a modified care protocol substituting bladder tumor markers for cystoscopy for the followup of patients with transitional cell carcinoma of the bladder: a decision analytical approach. *J Urol* 2002;167(1):75–79.
48. Nam RK, Redelmeier DA, Spiess PE, et al. Comparison of molecular and conventional strategies for followup of superficial bladder cancer using decision analysis. *J Urol* 2000;163(3):752–757.
49. Kamat AM, Lamm DL. Chemoprevention of bladder cancer. *Urol Clin North Am* 2002;29(1):157–168.
50. Augustine A, Hebert JR, Kabat GC, et al. Bladder cancer in relation to cigarette smoking. *Cancer Res* 1988;48(15):4405–4408.
51. Hartge P, Silverman DT, Schairer C, et al. Smoking and bladder cancer risk in blacks and whites in the United States. *Cancer Causes Control* 1993;4(4):391–394.
52. Morrison AS, Buring JE, Verhoek WG, et al. An international study of smoking and bladder cancer. *J Urol* 1984;131(4):650–654.
53. Burch JD, Rohan TE, Howe GR, et al. Risk of bladder cancer by source and type of tobacco exposure: a case-control study. *Int J Cancer* 1989;44(4):622–628.
54. Wynder EL, Augustine A, Kabat GC, et al. Effect of the type of cigarette smoked on bladder cancer risk. *Cancer* 1988;61(3):622–627.
55. Moyad MA. Potential lifestyle and dietary supplement options for the prevention and postdiagnosis of bladder cancer. *Urol Clin North Am* 2002;29(1):31–48, viii.
56. Messing EM. Urothelial tumors of the urinary tract. In: Walsh PC, Retik AB, Vaughan ED et al., eds. *Campbell's urology*, 8th ed., Vol. 4. Philadelphia, PA: Elsevier Science, 2003:2732–2784.
57. Negri E, La Vecchia C. Epidemiology and prevention of bladder cancer. *Eur J Cancer Prev* 2001;10(1):7–14.
58. Leistikow BN, Smith WE. California's reductions in smoking and bladder cancer incidence: a success story. *J Urol* 2001;165:28.
59. Day NE, Brown CC. Multistage models and primary prevention of cancer. *J Natl Cancer Inst* 1980;64(4):977–989.
60. Piolatto G, Negri E, La Vecchia C, et al. Bladder cancer mortality of workers exposed to aromatic amines: an updated analysis. *Br J Cancer* 1991;63(3):457–459.
61. Cole P. Coffee-drinking and cancer of the lower urinary tract. *Lancet* 1971;1(7713):1335–1337.
62. Fraumeni JF Jr, Scotto J, Dunham LJ. Coffee-drinking and bladder cancer. *Lancet* 1971;2(7735):1204.
63. Hartge P, Hoover R, West DW, et al. Coffee drinking and risk of bladder cancer. *J Natl Cancer Inst* 1983;70(6):1021–1026.
64. Morrison AS, Buring JE, Verhoek WG, et al. Coffee drinking and cancer of the lower urinary tract. *J Natl Cancer Inst* 1982;68(1):91–94.
65. Tavani A, La Vecchia C. Coffee and cancer: a review of epidemiological studies, 1990–1999. *Eur J Cancer Prev* 2000;9(4):241–256.
66. Zeegers MP, Kellen E, Buntinx F, et al. The association between smoking, beverage consumption, diet and bladder cancer: a systematic literature review. *World J Urol* 2003;17:17.
67. Bryan GT, Erturk E. Production of mouse urinary bladder carcinomas by sodium cyclamate. *Science* 1970;167(920):996–998.
68. Price JM, Biava CG, Oser BL, et al. Bladder tumors in rats fed cyclohexylamine or high doses of a mixture of cyclamate and saccharin. *Science* 1970;167(921):1131–1132.
69. Whysner J, Williams GM. Saccharin mechanistic data and risk assessment: urine composition, enhanced cell proliferation, and tumor promotion. *Pharmacol Ther* 1996;71(1–2):225–252.

70. Morrison AS, Buring JE. Artificial sweeteners and cancer of the lower urinary tract. *N Engl J Med* 1980;302(10):537–541.

71. Ohno Y, Aoki K, Obata K, et al. Case-control study of urinary bladder cancer in metropolitan Nagoya. *Natl Cancer Inst Monogr* 1985;69:229–234.

72. Ahmed FE, Thomas DB. Assessment of the carcinogenicity of the nonnutritive sweetener cyclamate. *Crit Rev Toxicol* 1992;22(2):81–118.

73. Castelao JE, Yuan JM, Gago-Dominguez M, et al. Non-steroidal anti-inflammatory drugs and bladder cancer prevention. *Br J Cancer* 2000;82(7):1364–1369.

74. Droller MJ, Gomolka D. Indomethacin and poly I:C in the inhibition of carcinogen-induced bladder cancer in an experimental animal model. *J Urol* 1984;131(6):1212–1217.

75. Klan R, Knispel HH, Meier T. Acetylsalicylic acid inhibition of n-butyl-(4-hydroxybutyl)nitrosamine-induced bladder carcinogenesis in rats. *J Cancer Res Clin Oncol* 1993;119(8):482–485.

76. Wang Z, Chen Y, Zheng R, et al. In vitro effects of prostaglandin E2 or indomethacin on the proliferation of lymphokine-activated killer cells and their cytotoxicity against bladder tumor cells in patients with bladder cancer. *Prostaglandins* 1997;54(5):769–779.

77. Michaud DS, Spiegelman D, Clinton SK, et al. Fluid intake and the risk of bladder cancer in men. *N Engl J Med* 1999;340(18):1390–1397.

78. Zeegers MP, Dorant E, Goldbohm RA, et al. Are coffee, tea, and total fluid consumption associated with bladder cancer risk? Results from the Netherlands Cohort Study. *Cancer Causes Control* 2001;12(3):231–238.

79. Geoffroy-Perez B, Cordier S. Fluid consumption and the risk of bladder cancer: results of a multicenter case-control study. *Int J Cancer* 2001;93(6):880–887.

80. Donat SM, Bayuga S, Herr HW, et al. Fluid intake and the risk of tumor recurrence in patients with superficial bladder cancer. *J Urol* 2003;170(5):1777–1780.

81. Lamm DL, Riggs DR, Shriver JS, et al. Megadose vitamins in bladder cancer: a double-blind clinical trial. *J Urol* 1994;151(1):21–26.

82. Byar D, Blackard C. Comparisons of placebo, pyridoxine, and topical thiotepa in preventing recurrence of stage I bladder cancer. *Urology* 1977;10(6):556–561.

83. Newling DW, Robinson MR, Smith PH, et al. EORTC Genito-Urinary Tract Cancer Cooperative Group. Tryptophan metabolites, pyridoxine (vitamin B6) and their influence on the recurrence rate of superficial bladder cancer. Results of a prospective, randomised phase III study performed by the EORTC GU Group. *Eur Urol* 1995;27(2):110–116.

84. Schlegel JU. Proposed uses of ascorbic acid in prevention of bladder carcinoma. *Ann N Y Acad Sci* 1975;258:432–437.

85. Shibata A, Paganini-Hill A, Ross RK, et al. Intake of vegetables, fruits, beta-carotene, vitamin C and vitamin supplements and cancer incidence among the elderly: a prospective study. *Br J Cancer* 1992;66(4):673–679.

86. Nomura AM, Kolonel LN, Hankin JH, et al. Dietary factors in cancer of the lower urinary tract. *Int J Cancer* 1991;48(2):199–205.

87. Jacobs EJ, Henion AK, Briggs PJ, et al. Vitamin C and vitamin E supplement use and bladder cancer mortality in a large cohort of US men and women. *Am J Epidemiol* 2002;156(11):1002–1010.

88. Fukushima S, Imaida K, Sakata T, et al. Promoting effects of sodium L-ascorbate on two-stage urinary bladder carcinogenesis in rats. *Cancer Res* 1983;43(9):4454–4457.

89. Chen TX, Wanibuchi H, Wei M, et al. Concentration dependent promoting effects of sodium L-ascorbate with the same total dose in a rat two-stage urinary bladder carcinogenesis. *Cancer Lett* 1999;146(1):67–71.

90. Beisel WR, Edelman R, Nauss K, et al. Single-nutrient effects on immunologic functions. Report of a workshop sponsored by the Department of Food and Nutrition and its Nutrition Advisory Group of the American Medical Association. *JAMA* 1981;245(1):53–58.

91. The Alpha-Tocopherol, Beta Carotene Cancer Prevention Study Group. The effect of vitamin E and beta carotene on the incidence of lung cancer and other cancers in male smokers. *N Engl J Med* 1994;330(15):1029–1035.

92. Virtamo J, Pietinen P, Huttunen JK, et al. Incidence of cancer and mortality following alpha-tocopherol and beta-carotene supplementation: a postintervention follow-up. *JAMA* 2003;290(4):476–485.

93. Sporn MB, Squire RA, Brown CC, et al. 13-cis-retinoic acid: inhibition of bladder carcinogenesis in the rat. *Science* 1977;195(4277):487–489.

94. Mettlin C, Graham S. Dietary risk factors in human bladder cancer. *Am J Epidemiol* 1979;110(3):255–263.

95. Hicks RM. The scientific basis for regarding vitamin A and its analogues as anti-carcinogenic agents. *Proc Nutr Soc* 1983;42(1):83–93.

96. Studer UE, Jenzer S, Biedermann C, et al. Adjuvant treatment with a vitamin A analogue (etretinate) after transurethral resection of superficial bladder tumors. Final analysis of a prospective, randomized multicenter trial in Switzerland. *Eur Urol* 1995;28(4):284–290.

97. Decensi A, Torrisi R, Bruno S, et al. Randomized trial of fenretinide in superficial bladder cancer using DNA flow cytometry as an intermediate end point. *Cancer Epidemiol Biomarkers Prev* 2000;9(10):1071–1078.

98. Boone CW, Kelloff GJ, Malone WE. Identification of candidate cancer chemopreventive agents and their evaluation in animal models and human clinical trials: a review. *Cancer Res* 1990;50(1):2–9.

99. Uchida K, Seidenfeld J, Rademaker A, et al. Inhibitory action of alpha-difluoromethylornithine on N-butyl-N-(4-hydroxybutyl)nitrosamine-induced rat urinary bladder carcinogenesis. *Cancer Res* 1989;49(19):5249–5253.

100. Messing EM, Hanson P, Reznikoff CA. Normal and malignant human urothelium: in vitro response to blockade of polyamine synthesis and interconversion. *Cancer Res* 1988;48(2):357–361.

101. Su SJ, Yeh TM, Lei HY, et al. The potential of soybean foods as a chemoprevention approach for human urinary tract cancer. *Clin Cancer Res* 2000;6(1):230–236.

102. Zhou JR, Mukherjee P, Gugger ET, et al. Inhibition of murine bladder tumorigenesis by soy isoflavones via alterations in the cell cycle, apoptosis, and angiogenesis. *Cancer Res* 1998;58(22):5231–5238.

103. Sun CL, Yuan JM, Arakawa K, et al. Dietary soy and increased risk of bladder cancer: the Singapore Chinese Health Study. *Cancer Epidemiol Biomarkers Prev* 2002;11(12):1674–1677.

104. Grubbs CJ, Lubet RA, Koki AT, et al. Celecoxib inhibits N-butyl-N-(4-hydroxybutyl)-nitrosamine-induced urinary bladder cancers in male B6D2F1 mice and female Fischer-344 rats. *Cancer Res* 2000;60(20):5599–5602.

105. Okajima E, Denda A, Ozono S, et al. Chemopreventive effects of nimesulide, a selective cyclooxygenase-2 inhibitor, on the development of rat urinary bladder carcinomas initiated by N-butyl-N-(4-hydroxybutyl)nitrosamine. *Cancer Res* 1998;58(14):3028–3031.

106. Komhoff M, Guan Y, Shappell HW, et al. Enhanced expression of cyclooxygenase-2 in high grade human transitional cell bladder carcinomas. *Am J Pathol* 2000;157(1):29–35.

107. Gee JR, Montoya RG, Khaled HM, et al. Cytokeratin 20, AN43, PGDH, and COX-2 expression in transitional and squamous cell carcinoma of the bladder. *Urol Oncol* 2003;21(4):266–270.

108. Shariat SF, Matsumoto K, Kim J, et al. Correlation of cyclooxygenase-2 expression with molecular markers, pathological features and clinical outcome of transitional cell carcinoma of the bladder. *J Urol* 2003;170(3):985–989.

109. Shirahama T, Arima J, Akiba S, et al. Relation between cyclooxygenase-2 expression and tumor invasiveness and patient survival in transitional cell carcinoma of the urinary bladder. *Cancer* 2001;92(1):188–193.

CHAPTER 22 ■ BLADDER CANCER STAGING

THERESA M. KOPPIE AND BERNARD H. BOCHNER

Cancer-staging systems provide a uniform means by which the extent of a tumor can be communicated to others and should highlight those characteristics which best define tumor specific behavior. Staging information should assist in therapeutic decision making and prognostication, and should facilitate the evaluation of clinical outcomes. It is now well established that bladder cancer constitutes at least two distinct clinical entities with unique clinical behavior, molecular phenotypes, and responses to therapy. Superficial disease is characterized by frequent recurrences of superficial lesions that possess a low overall risk of progression. In contrast, invasive bladder tumors are characterized by a propensity for local invasion, regional extension, and the development of metastatic disease. The vastly differing clinical behavior of these tumors and therapeutic options for their management underlies the importance of accurate clinical staging of disease prior to assignment of therapy.

The landmark observations of Jewett and Strong in 1946 relating the association of increasing risk of regional and distant metastases with increasing depth of invasion of the primary bladder tumor clearly documented the natural pathways of progression of invasive bladder cancer (1). These observations served as the basis for the present staging criteria for bladder tumors. Jewett subsequently reported the correlation between the depth of bladder wall invasion and 5-year survival, validating the utility of clinical staging in estimating the prognosis of bladder cancer (2). The Jewett-Strong-Marshall system was revised by Marshall in 1952 (3).

Currently, bladder tumors are staged according to the AJCC (American Joint Committee on Cancer) TNM (Tumor-Nodes-Metastasis) system. The AJCC TNM classification system recognizes that cancers of the same anatomic site and histology share similar growth patterns which dictate clinical outcomes (4). The bladder cancer TNM staging system allows for precise and simultaneous description of primary tumor extent (T), status of the lymph nodes (N), and extent of metastatic disease (M) (Table 22.1). The most recent revision of the TNM staging system for bladder cancer in 1997 combined all muscularis propria invasion into the T2 category (T2a for superficial muscle invasion, T2b for deep muscle invasion), and designated all perivesical fat invasion into the T3 category (T3a for microscopic fat invasion, T3b for gross fat invasion) (Fig. 22.1). The AJCC system was designed for flexibility, and has the potential for staging throughout the clinical course of a tumor (Table 22.2).

The goals of this chapter are to outline approaches to clinical (cTNM) and pathologic (pTNM) staging of bladder cancer. Clinical staging is based on data collected prior to definitive therapy and provides useful information to guide the selection of primary therapy. Pathologic staging is based on pathologic assessment of the specimen removed during surgery performed for definitive therapy. The pathologic stage can guide adjuvant therapy, prognostication, and outcome reporting.

CLINICAL STAGING OF BLADDER CANCER

Precise staging information for bladder cancer is obtained through a combination of endoscopic inspection, histologic evaluation of endoscopically obtained biopsy material, physical examination under anesthesia, and radiographic imaging for examination of local, regional, and distant progression. (Table 22.3)

Cystoscopy

While there are several techniques by which urothelial cancer can be identified, only cystoscopy provides reliable, direct visualization and localization of a bladder tumor. Cystoscopy, which remains the gold standard for the detection of bladder cancer, provides the opportunity for initial assessments of tumor grade and stage. Studies have demonstrated that an experienced urologist can distinguish high-grade from low-grade tumors as well as superficial from grossly invasive disease (5). In general, low-grade, noninvasive tumors appear papillary, contacting the surface of the bladder on a narrow stalk. Carcinoma *in situ*, a noninvasive, high-grade tumor, appears as a flat velvety lesion, arising in isolated areas or involving large regions of the urothelial lining. High-grade, invasive tumors lose their papillary configuration, frequently appearing as sessile, solid, or nodular lesions. Few studies address the utility of cystoscopy alone in the local staging of bladder cancer. Satoh et al. performed 275 cystoscopies on 165 patients in order to evaluate cystoscopic features which predict muscle invasion (6). They found that size, stalk (sessile vs. pedunculated), and configuration (nonpapillary vs. papillary) were independent predictors of muscle invasion. Cina et al. (7) evaluated the ability of the trained urologist to determine grade and stage of bladder cancer by cystoscopy alone, reporting a sensitivity and specificity of predicting low-grade tumor of 91% and 46%. In contrast, the sensitivity and specificity was poor for the detection of high-grade tumors, lamina propria invasion, or muscle invasion. Others have reported a similar sensitivity for the cystoscopic detection of low-grade noninvasive tumors in a select population of patients undergoing surveillance for superficial bladder cancer (5).

Examination Under Anesthesia

The bimanual examination of the bladder, prostate, rectum, and gynecologic organs is an important part of the overall

TABLE 22.1

TNM STAGING SYSTEMS

Primary tumor (T)	Tx	Primary cannot be assessed
	T0	No evidence of primary tumor
	Ta	Noninvasive papillary tumor
	Tis	Carcinoma *in situ*
	T1	Tumor invades subepithelial connective tissue
	T2	Tumor invades muscle
	PT2a	Tumor invades superficial muscle (inner half)
	PT2b	Tumor invades deep muscle (outer half)
	T3	Tumor invades perivesical tissue
	PT3a	Tumor invades perivesical tissue microscopically
	PT3b	Tumor invades perivesical tissue macroscopically (extravesical mass)
	T4	Tumor invades any of the following: prostate, uterus, vagina, pelvic wall, abdominal wall
	T4a	Tumor invades prostate, uterus, vagina
	T4b	Tumor invades pelvic wall, abdominal wall
Regional lymph nodes (N)	NX	Regional lymph nodes cannot be assessed
	N0	No regional lymph node metastases
	N1	Metastasis in a single lymph node, 2 cm or less in greatest dimension
	N2	Metastasis in a single lymph node, more than 2 cm but not more than 5 cm in greatest dimension; or multiple lymph nodes, none more than 5 cm in greatest dimension
	N3	Metastasis in a lymph node, more than 5 cm in greatest dimension
Distant metastasis (M)	MX	Distant metastasis cannot be assessed
	M0	No distant metastases
	M1	Distant metastasis

evaluation of the bladder cancer patient. The examination under anesthesia (EUA) can detect locally advanced disease, which may present as gross extravesical extension, invasion of adjacent organs, or pelvic sidewall extension. It is a useful adjunct to imaging in assessing tumor operability. However, the EUA is relatively insensitive for the staging of tumors confined to the bladder. The presence of grossly palpable disease or tumor fixation to adjacent structures or the pelvic side walls may predict a worse survival in patients with bladder cancer (8,9). False positives may result from changes related to previous surgery, pelvic radiation, or inflammatory disease.

Transurethral Resection

The role of transurethral resection (TUR) includes the provision of tissue for diagnosis and removal of tumor that may be therapeutic. The clinical stage and grade of a bladder tumor is strongly associated with its risk of both local and distant progression. Treatment varies dramatically based on the staging information provided prior to determination of definitive management. Distinguishing superficial bladder cancer (Ta, T1) from muscle-invasive bladder lesions (≥T2) is the most important task of clinical tumor staging. To date, no technique achieves this better than TUR of a bladder tumor.

Invasive tumors frequently extend into bladder wall as a collection of fingerlike projections rather than as a solid tumor front. To assure accurate clinical staging and the most complete resection possible, it is important that a TUR is carried deep to the tumor and into the muscularis propria, and extended widely on either side of the tumor base. Sampling the tumor base with a separate specimen by loop or cold cup can confirm complete resection. Finally, careful evaluation of the surrounding bladder for carcinoma *in situ* should be performed as well.

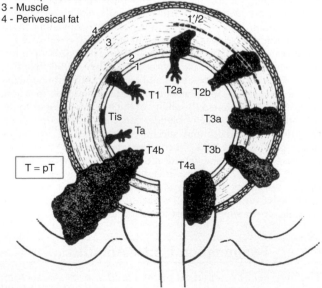

1 - Epithelium
2 - Subepithelial connective tissue
3 - Muscle
4 - Perivesical fat

FIGURE 22.1. Local tumor (T) staging of bladder cancer.

TABLE 22.2

FOUR PHASES OF TNM STAGING

Staging system	Time	Assessment	Goal
Clinical (cTNM)	Prior to primary definitive treatment	Physical examination Imaging Endoscopy Biopsy Surgical exploration	Selection of primary therapy Evaluation of primary therapy
Pathologic (pTNM)	Definitive surgery	Clinical staging data Pathologic examination of surgical specimen Primary tumor resection sufficient to evaluate the highest T category Node dissection sufficient to evaluate the highest N category	Estimating prognosis and evaluating outcomes
Retreatment (rTNM)	Prior to secondary treatment after a disease free interval	Biopsy Imaging	Outcomes assessment
Autopsy (aTNM)	After death	Autopsy	Assess outcomes and confirm cause of death

TABLE 22.3

CLINICAL STAGING RECOMMENDATIONS

Cystoscopy
TURBT
Examination under anesthesia
CT scan of the abdomen and pelvis
Chest x-ray or CT scan of the chest
Liver function studies including
    serum alkaline phosphatase level
Bone scan

TURBT, transurethral resection of a bladder tumor; CT, computed tomography.

The role of repeat transurethral resection following an initial diagnostic or therapeutic resection has been evaluated in several studies. Initial TUR understages T1 disease in up to 30% to 40% of lesions, particularly when no muscle is identified in the initial TUR specimen (10–12). Even in the absence of upstaging, repeat resection in this setting frequently reveals residual Ta or T1 disease which should be removed prior to intravesical therapy. Repeat resection plays an important role for patients with T1 disease for whom conservative management is considered. Dalbagni et al. showed that a second TUR performed at 6 to 8 weeks after initial TUR allows for a more complete resection and improved staging accuracy of clinical T1 tumors (13).

As a diagnostic procedure, the goals of a TUR are to provide evaluable material to the pathologist which allows for a histologic diagnosis of cell type, tumor grade, and depth of invasion, if present. Proper technique should aim to minimize cautery or crush artifact and, when appropriate, provide anatomical orientation. Cautery artifact may be minimized by performing tumor resection using a cutting current. Using a finer diameter loop cut with a more concentrated current can minimize cautery artifact as well, but provides less hemostasis than larger-diameter loops. Technologic advances in bipolar equipment may provide improved resection performance by allowing cutting at lower temperatures to enhance tissue preservation while still providing adequate hemostasis. Cold-cup biopsy can sample the urothelium without cautery artifact but provides a less controlled resection, limiting its therapeutic effectiveness.

As T1 bladder tumors comprise a heterogeneous group of cancers with widely variable clinical behaviors, some have advocated further stratification of clinical T1 tumors to improve bladder cancer staging. Subclassification of T1 tumors according to their depth of invasion within the lamina propria and their association with the muscularis mucosae (MM) has been recommended. Several studies suggest that invasion into or beyond the muscularis mucosae is associated with an increased likelihood of progression and overall mortality (14–19). However, subclassification of T1 according to MM invasion is not feasible in 6% to 42% of tumors due to the discontinuous nature of the MM, increasing the technical challenge of an accurate pathologic evaluation (16–20).

Rather than focus on tumor association with the muscularis mucosae, Bostwick has suggested T1 tumor subclassification according to the distance of bladder cancer microinvasion as described by Farrow and Utz (21). He found that in T1 tumors, microscopic invasion of ≤1.5 mm was associated with a significantly higher (93%) 5-year progression-free survival rate than those with invasion ≥1.5 mm (67%) (22).

Subclassification of T1 bladder tumors remains controversial and has not been incorporated into the World Health Organization (WHO) International Society of Urological Pathology (ISUP) consensus classification (23). It is instead recommended that pathologists provide an assessment of the extent of lamina propria invasion by characterizing the invasion as focal or extensive. When describing muscularis invasion, pathologists are urged to clearly state that the process represents muscularis mucosae or muscularis propria invasion.

Clinical T2 disease is identified on TUR when tumor is noted to infiltrate the thick smooth muscle bundles of the muscularis propria. Distinguishing muscularis propria invasion (T2) from invasion of the muscularis mucosa within the lamina propria (T1) is critical, as treatment recommendations may vary dramatically. The presence of characteristic blood vessels within the muscularis mucosae aid in distinguishing this layer from the muscularis propria. A pathologist may also employ Masson stains or actin immunohistochemistry to facilitate the diagnosis. While the staging system subdivides T2 tumors into those with superficial and deep muscle invasion, this subclassification may not be reliably obtained using transurethral biopsy material. The diagnosis of extravesical disease (T3) relies on the identification of tumor in the perivesical fatty tissues. This diagnosis may also be difficult to reliably obtain on TUR specimens. Lamina propria fat can be mistaken for perivesical fat, leading to inadvertent upstaging (24). Transurethral evaluation of the prostate should also be performed if prostatic urethral, ductal, or stromal invasion is suspected. For definitive staging purposes, transurethral biopsies are relatively insensitive for the detection of prostatic stromal invasion (T4a) (25).

Radiographic Imaging

The radiographic imaging of the patient with bladder cancer plays a central role in staging and should provide information on the extent of local invasion/extension, the presence of regional metastases, and the presence, extent, and location of distant disease. While not specifically relevant to bladder cancer staging, appropriate imaging can also be used to evaluate the upper urinary tracts, which is a necessary part of the workup of a newly diagnosed bladder tumor.

Evaluation of Local Disease Extent

When performed prior to TUR, computed tomography (CT) and magnetic resonance imaging (MRI) can be used to determine the extent of bladder wall invasion with an overall accuracy of 40% to 85% (26–28). Recent reports have suggested improved sensitivity and specificity of gadolinium-enhanced MRI in the detection of muscle invasion by tumor, with a sensitivity of 96% and a specificity of 83% (29). However, these results have not been routinely reproduced (30). Staging of a bladder tumor with MRI and CT relies on the disruption of normal tissue planes. Similar changes within the bladder wall and perivesical tissues can be observed whether related to a malignant or benign inflammatory process (such as the reaction to a prior transurethral biopsy). After TUR, bladder wall cross-sectional images are distorted by postprocedural artifact. Consequently, CT and MR imaging have limited ability to distinguish between superficial disease, muscle invasion, and perivesical infiltration in this setting.

CT and MRI are perhaps most useful in distinguishing gross extravesical extension from organ-confined disease. The sensitivity of CT in detecting extravesical disease ranges from 60% to 96%, while the specificity ranges from 66% to 93% (31). Unlike CT, MRI is able to obtain images in multiple planes and therefore can better demonstrate perivesical fat and tissue planes. Despite these advantages, the reported sensitivity and specificity of MRI for extravesical disease extension is similar to that of CT, ranging from 60% to 100% (32,33). Regardless of imaging modality, the greatest limitation in accurate staging relates to the inability to distinguish inflammatory changes in the bladder wall and surrounding perivesical tissues from actual tumor infiltration.

Upper tract imaging with CT, MRI, IVP, or US can detect the presence of hydronephrosis, a finding that suggests muscle-invasive bladder cancer. Furthermore, the presence of hydronephrosis in patients with invasive bladder cancer has been shown to correlate with poor outcome following definitive local therapy (34,35). Moreover, these modalities can detect upper tract transitional cell carcinomas which may occur in 2% to 4% of bladder cancer patients (36).

Determination of Nodal and Distant Metastatic Disease

The most common sites of metastasis for invasive bladder cancer include the regional lymph nodes, liver, lung, and bone (37). Both CT and MRI rely on size criteria to detect regional lymphadenopathy. Lymph nodes greater than 1 cm in size are considered clinically suspicious for metastatic disease. Since microscopic tumor involvement of regional nodes are not detected by cross-sectional imaging, the overall staging accuracy for lymph node involvement by CT or MRI ranges from 50% to 92% (26,38).

Alternative imaging strategies that rely on tumor specific characteristics are being investigated to improve lymph node staging accuracy. One area of investigation is that of positron emission tomography (PET) in the detection of metastatic bladder cancer. Local staging of bladder cancer with standard PET agents such as fluorine-2-D-deoxyglucose (FDG) is complicated by the excretion of tracer in the bladder, which confounds accurate local evaluation. For the detection of lymph node metastases, PET has a reported sensitivity of 67%, a specificity of 86%, and an accuracy of 80% (39). Currently, PET agents that rely on alternative metabolic pathways and undergo limited urinary excretion are being investigated as possible tools in the staging of bladder cancer.

Whole-body bone scans should be considered if the history and/or physical examination suggest the possibility of bone metastases or if the serum alkaline phosphatase level is elevated (40). The utility of bone scans in the evaluation of the asymptomatic patient with presumed organ-confined bladder cancer and an elevated serum alkaline phosphatase level remains controversial (39,41).

PATHOLOGIC STAGING OF BLADDER CANCER

The pathologic stage (pTNM) of a tumor represents a summary of clinical staging data collected preoperatively as well as additional data acquired from pathological evaluation of the surgical specimen (bladder, perivesical tissues, surrounding organs, and regional lymph nodes). Pathologic staging of bladder cancer provides the data necessary for the most accurate risk stratification, and, therefore, identifies those patients who may benefit from adjuvant therapies. To optimize staging accuracy, the surgical specimen should contain a full-thickness bladder resection that includes the adjacent perivesical tissues and regional lymph nodes.

Local Tumor (T) Staging

The AJCC classifies the local bladder cancer staging according to the level of bladder tumor invasion. Papillary tumors confined to the epithelium are classified as stage Ta. Flat *in situ* tumors are classified as Tis. Tumors which invade the lamina propria are classified as stage T1. Those which invade the muscularis propria are classified as T2a (superficial muscle invasion) or T2b (deep muscle invasion). Tumors which have extended into the perivesical fat are classified as stage T3a (microscopic) or T3b (gross). Tumors which invade pelvic organs are classified as T4a (prostate, uterus, and vagina) and T4b (pelvic and abdominal wall). The level of invasion of the primary tumor carries important implications with respect to both prognosis and treatment. The established correlation between the depth of primary tumor invasion and recurrence-free survival and disease-specific survival was an early observation that has been corroborated in contemporary experience (42–46). Moreover, the depth of tumor invasion is associated with the likelihood of lymph node metastases. Regional lymph node metastases have been noted in 20% to 30% of patients with organ-confined disease, and in as many as 30% to 66% of patients with disease which extends into the perivesical fat (47).

In the current AJCC staging system, all muscle-invasive bladder tumors are classified as T2, and bladder tumors which extend beyond the muscle wall into the perivesical fat are classified as T3. This represents a change from the previous AJCC system, in which T2 tumors invaded the superficial muscle and T3a tumors invaded the deep muscle. The decision to incorporate muscle-invasive tumors into a single stage was made based on the challenges of differentiating the level of muscle invasion, particularly in TUR specimens, and because no convincing evidence exists that the level of muscle invasion predicts outcome. The present clinical subclassification of T2 tumors into those with superficial (T2a) and deep (T2b) muscle is somewhat subjective, and rarely alters clinical decision making. Similarly, T3 disease, which is subcategorized into those tumors with either microscopic or gross perivesical fat extension, can be difficult to accurately identify prior to definitive resection. Studies to date suggest that outcomes for patients with perivesical fat invasion, with or without gross disease, do not significantly differ (46,48).

Extension of bladder cancer into the prostate in men or the vagina, cervix, or uterus in women is classified as pT4a. Though not specified in the current TNM staging system, differentiating the specific type of prostatic involvement may provide clinically useful information. Bladder cancer which directly invades the prostatic stroma appears to portend a worse prognosis when compared to tumor which lies within the prostatic urethra and intraprostatic ducts (49,50). The pathway of prostatic invasion also appears to have an influence on outcomes after cystectomy. Pagano et al. found that patients with prostatic invasion from a noncontiguous transitional cell carcinoma of the prostate had improved 5-year survival when compared to patients with contiguous invasion of the prostate from a bladder tumor which had invaded through the bladder wall into the prostate (46% vs. 7%, $P < .001$) (51).

Nodal (N) and Metastatic (M) Disease

Currently, the AJCC TNM staging system categorizes nodal stage based on the size and multiplicity of positive regional lymph nodes. Regional lymph nodes are defined as the nodes of the true pelvis, which lie below the bifurcation of the common iliac arteries. Stage N1 is defined as metastatic disease in a single regional lymph node, which is 2 cm or less in greatest dimension. Stage N2 is defined as metastasis(es) in either a single regional lymph node greater than 2 cm but less than 5 cm in size, or multiple regional lymph nodes, none more than 5 cm in greatest dimension. N3 staging is reserved for metastasis to a regional lymph node, which is greater than 5 cm in greatest dimension. Distant metastases are designated as M1.

For adequate staging of the regional node status, submitted material should include a sufficient number of lymph nodes to address the highest nodal stage. Presently the optimal number of lymph nodes that should be evaluated for adequate staging has yet to be defined. By current AJCC nodal staging criteria, lymph nodes that are outside of the true pelvis are staged as distant metastases, rather than as regional lymph nodes. Yet recent studies have demonstrated improved survival for bladder cancer patients who have had more lymph nodes removed at the time of radical cystectomy and lymphadenectomy (52–54) and for those who have undergone more extensive lymph

node dissections that include nodal regions outside of the true pelvis (55). The number of positive lymph nodes (55,56) within the specimen has been shown to affect bladder cancer survival with four to five positive lymph nodes suggested as the optimal cut point (54–57). Additional data support that the extent of the lymph node dissection, considered simultaneously with the number of positive lymph nodes, may also provide independent prognostic information (55,56). Moreover, a wide variation exists in the techniques and extent of nodal evaluation among urologists and pathologists, including extent of anatomic boundaries and the method of submission of nodal tissues (en bloc vs. separate packets) (54,58,59). Establishing standards for the lymph node dissection will better clarify the most appropriate dissection required for adequate pathologic staging as well as any potential therapeutic advantage. Widely accepted standards of bladder cancer staging will also be critical for the identification of appropriate candidates for combined modality treatment as well as entry into clinical trials. Modification of the AJCC nodal staging system to incorporate such data may improve its value as a clinical tool and aid in minimizing staging variation.

References

1. Jewett HJ. Infiltrating carcinoma of the bladder: relation of the depth of penetration of the bladder wall to incidence of local extension and metastasis. *J Urol* 1946;55:366.
2. Jewett HJ. Carcinoma of the bladder: influence of depth of infiltration on the 5-year results following complete extirpation of the primary growth. *J Urol* 1952;67:672.
3. Marshall V. The relation of the preoperative estimate to the pathologic demonstration of the extent of vesical neoplasms. *J Urol* 1952;68:714.
4. American Joint Committee on Cancer. Urinary bladder. In: Fleming I, ed. *AJCC cancer staging manual*. Philadelphia, PA: Lippincott Williams & Wilkins, 1997:241.
5. Herr HW, Donat SM, Dalbagni G. Correlation of cystoscopy with histology of recurrent papillary tumors of the bladder. *J Urol* 2002;168:978.
6. Satoh E, Miyao N, Tachiki H, et al. Prediction of muscle invasion of bladder cancer by cystoscopy. *Eur Urol* 2002;41:178.
7. Cina SJ, Epstein JI, Endrizzi JM, et al. Correlation of cystoscopic impression with histologic diagnosis of biopsy specimens of the bladder. *Hum Pathol* 2001;32:630.
8. Fossa SD, Ous S, Berner A. Clinical significance of the "palpable mass" in patients with muscle-infiltrating bladder cancer undergoing cystectomy after pre-operative radiotherapy. *Br J Urol* 1991;67:54.
9. Hendry WF, Rawson NS, Turney L, et al. Computerisation of urothelial carcinoma records: 16 years' experience with the TNM system. *Br J Urol* 1990;65:583.
10. Herr HW. The value of a second transurethral resection in evaluating patients with bladder tumors. *J Urol* 1999;162:74.
11. Vogeli TA, Grimm MO, Simon X, et al. [Prospective study of effectiveness. Reoperation (re-TUR) in superficial bladder carcinoma.] *Urologe A* 2002; 41:470.
12. Dutta SC, Smith JA Jr, Shappell SB, et al. Clinical under staging of high risk nonmuscle invasive urothelial carcinoma treated with radical cystectomy. *J Urol* 2001;166:490.
13. Dalbagni G, Herr HW, Reuter VE. Impact of a second transurethral resection on the staging of T1 bladder cancer. *Urology* 2002;60:822.
14. Younes M, Sussman J, True LD. The usefulness of the level of the muscularis mucosae in the staging of invasive transitional cell carcinoma of the urinary bladder. *Cancer* 1990;66:543.
15. Hasui Y, Osada Y, Kitada S, et al. Significance of invasion to the muscularis mucosae on the progression of superficial bladder cancer. *Urology* 1994;43:782.
16. Hermann GG, Horn T, Steven K. The influence of the level of lamina propria invasion and the prevalence of p53 nuclear accumulation on survival in stage T1 transitional cell bladder cancer. *J Urol* 1998;159:91.
17. Angulo JC, Lopez JI, Grignon DJ, et al. Muscularis mucosa differentiates two populations with different prognosis in stage T1 bladder cancer. *Urology* 1995;45:47.
18. Smits G, Schaafsma E, Kiemeney L, et al. Microstaging of pT1 transitional cell carcinoma of the bladder: identification of subgroups with distinct risks of progression. *Urology* 1998;52:1009.
19. Holmang S, Hedelin H, Anderstrom C, et al. The importance of the depth of invasion in stage T1 bladder carcinoma: a prospective cohort study. *J Urol* 1997;157:800.
20. Platz CE, Cohen MB, Jones MP, et al. Is microstaging of early invasive cancer of the urinary bladder possible or useful? *Mod Pathol* 1996;9: 1035.

21. Farrow G, Utz DC. Observation on microinvasive transitional cell carcinoma of the urinary bladder. *Clin Oncol* 1982;1:609.

22. Cheng L, Weaver AL, Neumann RM, et al. Substaging of T1 bladder carcinoma based on the depth of invasion as measured by micrometer: a new proposal. *Cancer* 1999;86:1035.

23. Epstein JI, Amen MB, Reuter VR et al, The World Health Organization. International Society of Urological Pathology (ISUP) consensus classification of urothelial (transitional cell) lesions. Neoplasms of the urinary bladder. *Am J Surg Pathol* 1998;22:1435.

24. Bochner BH, Nichols PW, Skinner DG. Overstaging of transitional cell carcinoma: clinical significance of lamina propria fat within the urinary bladder. *Urology* 1995;45:528.

25. Donat SM, Wei DC, McGuire MS, et al. The efficacy of transurethral biopsy for predicting the long-term clinical impact of prostatic invasive bladder cancer. *J Urol* 2001;165:1580.

26. Amendola MA, Glazer GM, Grossman HB, et al. Staging of bladder carcinoma: MRI-CT-surgical correlation. *AJR Am J Roentgenol* 1986;146:1179.

27. Husband JE, Olliff JF, Williams MP, et al. Bladder cancer: staging with CT and MR imaging. *Radiology* 1989;173:435.

28. Fisher MR, Hricak H, Tanagho EA. Urinary bladder MR imaging. Part II. Neoplasm. *Radiology* 1985;157:471.

29. Tanimoto A, Yuasa Y, Imai Y, et al. Bladder tumor staging: comparison of conventional and gadolinium-enhanced dynamic MR imaging and CT. *Radiology* 1992;185:741.

30. Kim B, Semelka RC, Ascher SM, et al. Bladder tumor staging: comparison of contrast-enhanced CT, T1- and T2-weighted MR imaging, dynamic gadolinium-enhanced imaging, and late gadolinium-enhanced imaging. *Radiology* 1994;193:239.

31. Bryan PJ, Butler HE, LiPuma JP, et al. CT and MR imaging in staging bladder neoplasms. *J Comput Assist Tomogr* 1987;11:96.

32. Nishimura K, Hida S, Nishio Y, et al. The validity of magnetic resonance imaging (MRI) in the staging of bladder cancer: comparison with computed tomography (CT) and transurethral ultrasonography (US). *Jpn J Clin Oncol* 1988;18:217.

33. See WA, Fuller JR. Staging of advanced bladder cancer. Current concepts and pitfalls. *Urol Clin North Am* 1992;19:663.

34. Haleblian GE, Skinner EC, Dickinson MG, et al. Hydronephrosis as a prognostic indicator in bladder cancer patients. *J Urol* 1998;160:2011.

35. Kachnic LA, Kaufman DS, Heney NM, et al. Bladder preservation by combined modality therapy for invasive bladder cancer. *J Clin Oncol* 1997;15:1022.

36. Malkowicz SB. Management of superficial bladder cancers. In: Campbell MF, Walsh PC, Retik AB, eds. *Campbell's urology*, 8th ed. Vol. 4 of 4. Philadelphia, PA: WB Saunders, 2002:4 v (xl, 3954, 3128).

37. Messing E. Urothelial tumors of the urinary tract. In: Campbell MF, Walsh PC, Retik AB, eds. *Campbell's urology*, 8th ed. Vol. 4 of 4. Philadelphia, PA: WB Saunders, 2002:4 v (xl, 3954, 3128).

38. Koss JC, Arger PH, Coleman BG, et al. CT staging of bladder carcinoma. *AJR Am J Roentgenol* 1981;137:359.

39. Bachor R, Kotzerke J, Reske SN, et al. Lymph node staging of bladder neck carcinoma with positron emission tomography. *Urologe A* 1999;38:46.

40. Berger GL, Sadlowski RW, Sharpe JR, et al. Lack of value of routine preoperative bone and liver scans in cystectomy candidates. *J Urol* 1981;125:637.

41. Braendengen M, Winderen M, Fossa SD. Clinical significance of routine pre-cystectomy bone scans in patients with muscle-invasive bladder cancer. *Br J Urol* 1996;77:36.

42. Ghoneim MA, el-Mekresh MM, el-Baz MA, et al. Radical cystectomy for carcinoma of the bladder: critical evaluation of the results in 1,026 cases. *J Urol* 1997;158:393.

43. Mathur VK, Krahn HP, Ramsey EW. Total cystectomy for bladder cancer. *J Urol* 1981;125:784.

44. Skinner DG, Lieskovsky G. Contemporary cystectomy with pelvic node dissection compared to preoperative radiation therapy plus cystectomy in management of invasive bladder cancer. *J Urol* 1984;131:1069.

45. Stein JP, Lieskovsky G, Cote R, et al. Radical cystectomy in the treatment of invasive bladder cancer: long-term results in 1,054 patients. *J Clin Oncol* 2001;19:666.

46. Dalbagni G, Genega E, Hashibe M, et al. Cystectomy for bladder cancer: a contemporary series. *J Urol* 2001;165:1111.

47. Pressler L, Petrylak D, Olsson C. *Invasive transitional cell carcinoma of the bladder: prognosis and management*. Philadelphia, PA: WB Saunders, 1997:xix,822.

48. Quek ML, Stein JP, Clark PE, et al. Natural history of surgically treated bladder carcinoma with extravesical tumor extension. *Cancer* 2003;98:955.

49. Herr HW, Donat SM. Prostatic tumor relapse in patients with superficial bladder tumors: 15-year outcome. *J Urol* 1999;161:1854.

50. Esrig D, Freeman JA, Elmajian DA, et al. Transitional cell carcinoma involving the prostate with a proposed staging classification for stromal invasion. *J Urol* 1996;156:1071.

51. Pagano F, Bassi P, Ferrante GL, et al. Is stage pT4a (D1) reliable in assessing transitional cell carcinoma involvement of the prostate in patients with a concurrent bladder cancer? A necessary distinction for contiguous or noncontiguous involvement. *J Urol* 1996;155:244.

52. Leissner J, Ghoneim MA, Abol-Enein H, et al. Extended radical lymphadenectomy in patients with urothelial bladder cancer: results of a prospective multicenter study. *J Urol* 2004;171:139.

53. Leissner J, Hohenfellner R, Thuroff JW, et al. Lymphadenectomy in patients with transitional cell carcinoma of the urinary bladder; significance for staging and prognosis. *BJU Int* 2000;85:817.

54. Herr HW. Extent of surgery and pathology evaluation has an impact on bladder cancer outcomes after radical cystectomy. *Urology* 2003;61:105.

55. Poulsen AL, Horn T, Steven K. Radical cystectomy: extending the limits of pelvic lymph node dissection improves survival for patients with bladder cancer confined to the bladder wall. *J Urol* 1998;160:2015.

56. Vieweg J, Gschwend JE, Herr HW, et al. Pelvic lymph node dissection can be curative in patients with node positive bladder cancer. *J Urol* 1999;161:449.

57. Stein JP, Cai J, Groshen S, et al. Risk factors for patients with pelvic lymph node metastases following radical cystectomy with en bloc pelvic lymphadenectomy: concept of lymph node density. *J Urol* 2003;170:35.

58. Lopez-Beltran A, Bassi PF, Pavone-Macaluso M, et al. Handling and pathology reporting of specimens with carcinoma of the urinary bladder, ureter, and renal pelvis. A joint proposal of the European Society of Uropathology and the Uropathology Working Group. *Virchows Arch* 2004;445:103.

59. Herr HW, Faulkner JR, Grossman HB, et al. Pathologic evaluation of radical cystectomy specimens: a cooperative group report. *Cancer* 2004;100:2470.

CHAPTER 23 ■ IMAGING OF TRANSITIONAL CELL CARCINOMA

ALEXANDER R. GUIMARAES AND MUKESH G. HARISINGHANI

Bladder carcinoma remains the second most-common malignancy of the urinary tract in men, accounting for approximately 2% of all malignancies (1,2). Approximately 90% to 95% of urinary bladder and upper urothelial malignancies are transitional cell carcinomas, the remaining being squamous cell and adenocarcinomas, with rare sarcomas and metastases from primary tumors (1). As transitional cell carcinomas usually present with painless hematuria, radiology has played an important role in the diagnosis of transitional cell carcinoma, but until recently remained low in sensitivity and specificity in grading and staging. Recent improvements in computed tomography (CT) and magnetic resonance imaging (MRI), however, have improved detection and staging accuracy.

This chapter will provide an overview of radiographic assessment and will provide detailed extant technological improvements in imaging transitional cell carcinomas with a focus on current cross sectional imaging modalities of CT and MRI.

PLAIN RADIOGRAPHY

Plain radiography as a modality has high spatial resolution, but extremely poor soft-tissue contrast. As a result, plain radiography remains a poor means of diagnosing transitional cell carcinomas. Plain radiography may detect the presence of mottled or irregularly shaped calcification, which is present in 2% of renal transitional cell carcinoma and 0.7% to 6% of bladder transitional cell carcinoma. Although the etiology of the calcification may be secondary to malignancy, it is often secondary to superimposed infection with dystrophic calcification, cystic degeneration, necrosis, or hemorrhage (3–6). Plain radiography has largely been replaced by CT, since CT provides increased sensitivity for detection and localization of calcification (Fig. 23.1).

ULTRASONOGRAPHY

Ultrasound examination of the kidneys and urinary bladder is a noninvasive imaging modality, whose precise role in the evaluation of transitional cell carcinomas remains undetermined. The benefits and advantages of ultrasound in the evaluation of hematuria, which is the most common presenting sign in patients with bladder and upper tract transitional cell carcinoma, include the following: (a) ultrasound is readily available, cost effective, and requires no patient preparation; and (b) ultrasound examination of the urinary bladder does not require any use of intravenous contrast and, therefore, minimizes the associated risk that accompanies intravenous, iodinated contrast. The disadvantages include poor spatial resolution, poor soft-tissue contrast, operator dependence, and lack of full volumetric coverage. As a screening modality, ultrasound is effective in detecting indirect signs of transitional cell carcinomas (TCCs) such as obstruction of the collecting system. In the setting of mild pelvicaliectasis, filling defects within the proximal collecting systems may be visualized against the background of anechoic urine (Fig. 23.2). In the absence of obstructive hydronephrosis and hydroureter, the ureters are not well visualized with ultrasound. Therefore, subtle infiltrating lesions may go unnoticed (Fig. 23.3). Within the bladder, however, ultrasound has demonstrated increased sensitivity secondary to the contrast in the background of an anechoic bladder (Fig. 23.4). In a study of 1,007 patients complaining of hematuria, Datta et. al. demonstrated that the sensitivity of ultrasound with respect to bladder cancer was 63% and specificity was 99%. The odds ratio of diagnosing cancer in patients with visible hematuria compared to microscopic or unspecified hematuria was 3.3 (7). Dibb et al. retrospectively analyzed the ultrasonographic features of bladder tumors during transabdominal ultrasonography. Of 109 patients reviewed, 104 had transitional cell carcinoma, 3 adenocarcinoma, 1 carcinosarcoma, and 1 prostatic carcinoma. The most common appearance was a polypoid

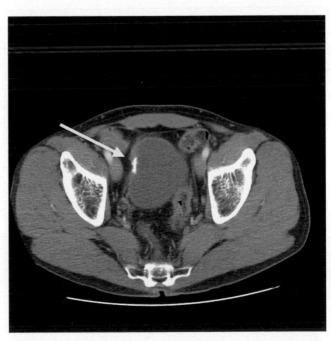

FIGURE 23.1. Axial contrast-enhanced CT image within the pelvis that demonstrates dystrophic calcification within the right aspect of the bladder wall. Biopsy confirmed the diagnosis of transitional cell carcinoma (TCC).

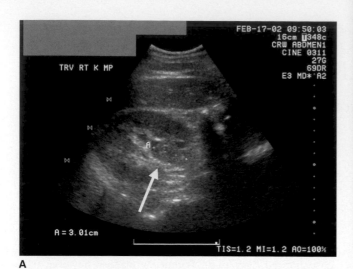

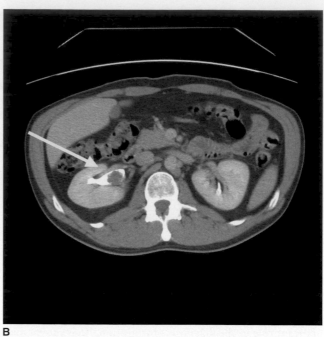

FIGURE 23.2. A: Transabdominal ultrasound examination, which is in a transverse orientation with respect to the midpole of the right kidney, and demonstrates a solid, echogenic filling defect within the right proximal collecting system. **B:** Contrast-enhanced computed tomography (CT) examination with delayed phase imaging demonstrates a hypodense, irregular mass within the proximal, contrast-filled collecting system of the right kidney.

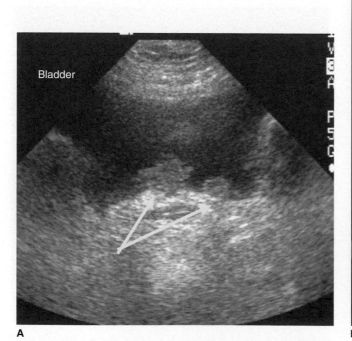

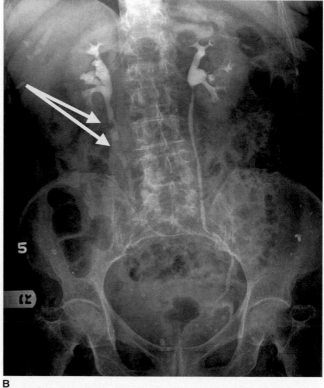

FIGURE 23.3. A: Transabdominal ultrasound imaging examination of the bladder, which demonstrates multiple solid, echogenic masses within the bladder with a background of anechoic urine within the bladder. **B:** Intravenous urogram (IVU) of the same patient, which demonstrates multiple filling defects within the right collecting system and ureter. These lesions were not identified on the ultrasound examination. Note that the right kidney does not demonstrate any evidence of hydronephrosis.

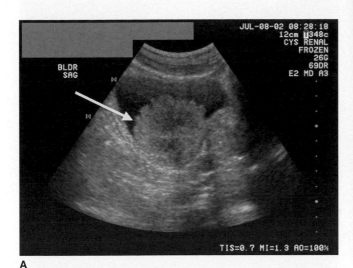

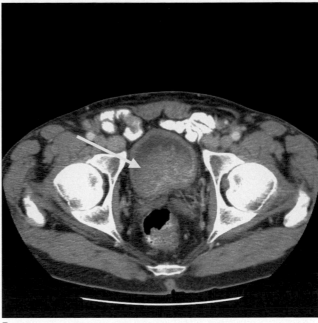

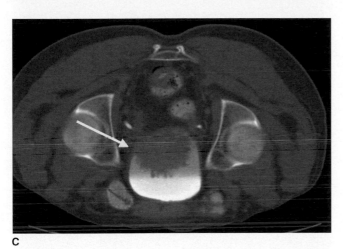

FIGURE 23.4. A: Transabdominal image in an axial orientation through a filled bladder. There is a solid, irregular lesion at the bladder base that causes a filling defect within the anechoic urine of the bladder. **B:** Supine contrast enhanced computed tomography (CT) examination in an early phase that demonstrates early enhancement of the mass relative to the hypodense urine within the bladder. Note that the bladder wall also enhances. **C:** Prone contrast-enhanced CT examination in a late phase that demonstrates partial filling of the bladder with contrast. The mass is represented by a hypodense filling defect within the relatively hyperdense urine of the contrast filled bladder.

lesion arising from the trigone, but there was much variation in the ultrasonographic features of bladder tumors (8).

Transabdominal ultrasound imaging is limited in diagnosing tumors of the bladder neck, dome, and anterior wall. Transrectal and transvaginal approaches, secondary to both the improved proximity to the urinary bladder, as well as the increased probe frequency used, have significantly improved the detection sensitivity in this regard. Furthermore, endoluminal (transurethral) ultrasound techniques have evolved and provide intravesicular imaging with high frequency (20 MHz) miniature probes. Although limited, these techniques have demonstrated excellent correlation with stage pTa or pT1 disease, but decreased sensitivity in stage II disease, likely secondary to lack of penetration with the high frequency probe. Furthermore, these techniques suffer from being invasive, and often require sedation for administration. In some studies endoluminal, transurethral ultrasound demonstrated lower sensitivity than cystoscopy, bimanual examination, and biopsy (9).

CONTRAST ENHANCED UROGRAPHY

Intravenous, Antegrade, and Retrograde Urography

Until very recently, intravenous urography or pyelography (IVP) was considered the most sensitive initial screening method for

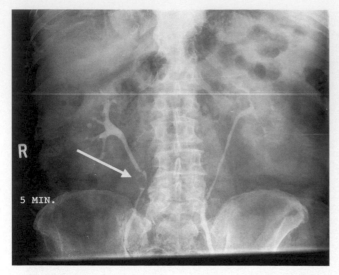

FIGURE 23.5. Intravenous urogram (IVU) which demonstrates contrast within the collecting systems, bilaterally. Within the proximal right ureter, there is an irregular filling defect that demonstrates the characteristic "goblet sign," which refers to accumulation of contrast in a prestenotic cup-shaped dilated ureter. There is no evidence of obstruction of the right kidney.

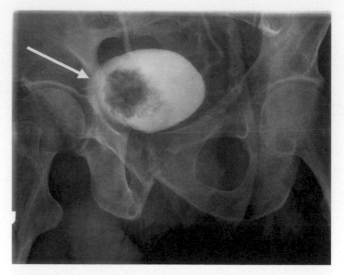

FIGURE 23.7. Right anterior oblique view of the pelvis from an intravenous urogram, which demonstrates an irregular, frondlike filling defect of the right aspect of the bladder. The ureters are seen in the background, bilaterally.

patients presenting with painless hematuria, or with cytology suspicious of malignancy. The intravenous pyelogram is performed by injecting iodinated contrast, followed by imaging with both plain radiography and tomography of the contrast-filled collecting system, ureters, and bladder. As 6% of transitional cell carcinoma appears within the upper urothelial tract, it is important to investigate not only the bladder, but the collecting system and ureters (Fig. 23.5) (10). Masses may appear as nodular, well-demarcated filling defects, or frondlike and irregular filling defects within the collecting system, ureter, or bladder (Figs. 23.6

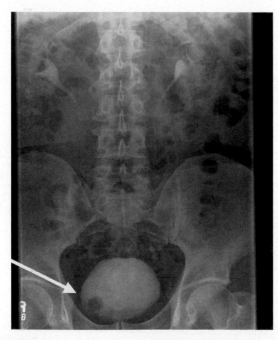

FIGURE 23.6. Anterior posterior view from an intravenous urogram, which demonstrates a filling defect within a right base of a contrast filled bladder. Cystoscopic evaluation and eventual biopsy confirmed the diagnosis of transitional cell carcinoma (TCC).

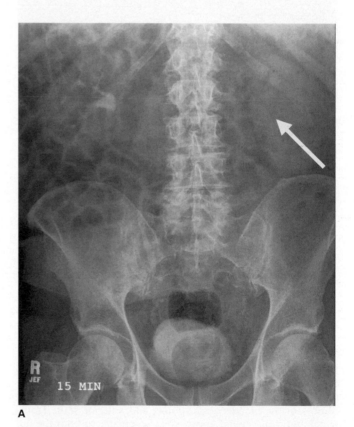

A

FIGURE 23.8. A: AP view from an intravenous urogram (IVU), which demonstrates contrast within the bladder, as well as the right collecting system and ureter. Note the absence of contrast within the left collecting system. B: Axial image from a contrast-enhanced computed tomography (CT) examination in the delayed phase confirms a lack of contrast within the collecting system of the left kidney. C: Axial image from the same CT examination, which demonstrates contrast within the bladder and thickening of the bladder extending into the left distal ureter. The findings were consistent with transitional cell carcinoma (TCC) of the bladder. The mass invades into the distal left ureter and causes obstruction of the left kidney.

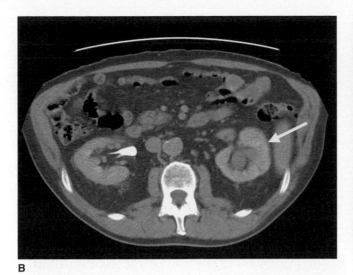

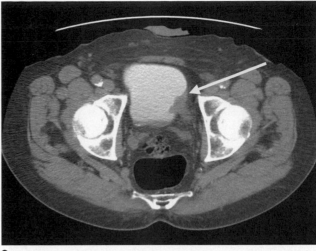

B

C

FIGURE 23.8. (Continued).

and 23.7). Asymmetric thickening of the bladder and ureters should also be viewed with some level of suspicion and should be further investigated cystoscopically. Masses within the infundibulum or proximal collecting system may also present with asymmetric enhancement of the entire renal parenchyma with obstructive hydronephrosis, or part of the kidney with infundibular stenosis during the nephrographic phase (Fig. 23.8).

Retrograde pyelography is an invasive means of examining the collecting system, ureter, and bladder in patients allergic to intravenous contrast. Being invasive, this technique requires catheterization and cystoscopic selection of the ureters. The morphologic findings associated with malignancy are similar

to those with IVP and include filling defects within the bladder, ureters, and collecting system (Fig. 23.9).

Although urography remains sensitive to large mass occupying lesions, it is insensitive to smaller lesions or carcinoma *in situ*. Furthermore, the depth of invasion, which is the most important prognostic indicator and requisite for accurate staging of TCC, is not accurately assessed. Only with associated sequelae, such as hydronephrosis and hydroureter, is muscular invasion inferred. This sign as well is anatomically dependent, and is only noted in 92% of cases (11,12).

The improvement in imaging technology, most notably within MRI and CT, has improved the detection sensitivity and the staging of TCC.

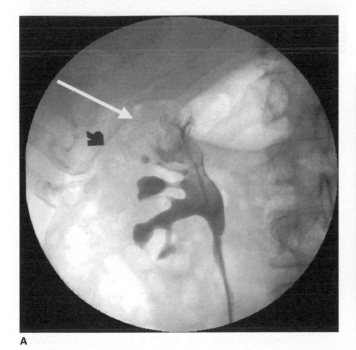

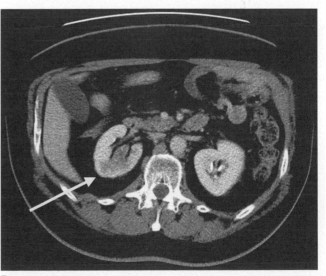

A

B

FIGURE 23.9. A: Spot view from a retrograde urogram which demonstrates a catheter within the partially filled right collecting system. There is an irregular, frondlike filling defect within the upper pole of the right kidney. B: Axial slice from contrast-enhanced computed tomography (CT) confirms an irregular lesion within the upper pole collecting system of the right kidney, extending to and invading the right renal parenchyma.

COMPUTED TOMOGRAPHY

In addition to urinalysis, the evaluation of painless hematuria usually includes a combination of imaging and cystoscopy (13). Until very recently, the radiologic evaluation of painless hematuria involved contrast urography or a combination of regrograde urography and cystoscopy in patients who are intolerant of intravenous contrast. However, many recent studies have both demonstrated the superiority of CT in the evaluation of both urinary tract calculi and renal masses (14–17). The spatial resolution in the axial dimension, concurrent with improvements in computing technology, has demonstrated similar improvements in the evaluation of the urothelium in delayed, urographic phase CT imaging. Recent studies demonstrate comparable sensitivity of excretory phase helical CT with intravenous urography in patients with painless hematuria (18).

The evaluation of painless hematuria has now shifted in many institutions to utilizing CT as the primary screening modality. A typical hematuria protocol is detailed in the Appendix. The advent of multislice CT allows for postprocessing collimation to a slice thickness of 1.25 mm. Coronal reformatted images are then rendered with maximum intensity projection (MIP), or volume rendered (VR) images of the collecting system, distal ureters, and bladder are performed which allow for interpretation in both the axial and coronal planes. The coronal plane allows better visualization of the bladder dome as well.

Criteria for mass lesions applied to intravenous urography are similar for excretory phase contrast-enhanced CT. Primary tumors may appear as filling defects within the ureters (Fig. 23.10),

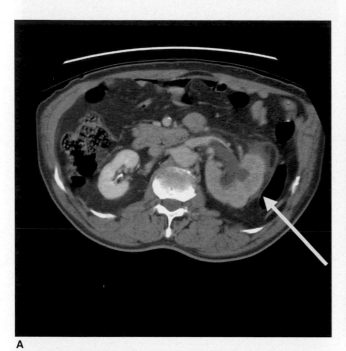

A

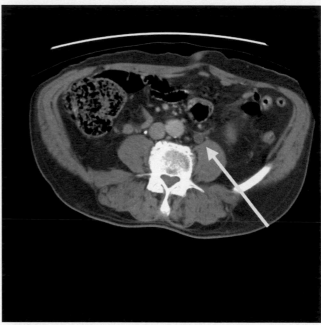

B

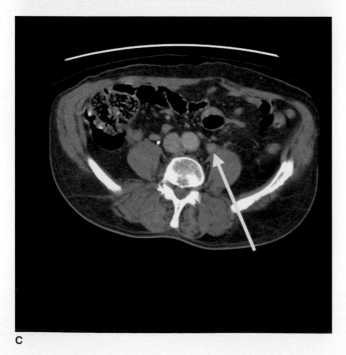

C

FIGURE 23.10. A: Axial slice from a delayed phase, contrast-enhanced computed tomography (CT) examination at the level of the renal midpole, which demonstrates asymmetric enhancement of the left kidney relative to the right kidney. The hydronephrosis is secondary to obstructive hydronephrosis of the left kidney, with stranding of the perinephric fat. **B:** Axial slices from the same CT examination demonstrate contrast within a nondilated right ureter, but no evidence of contrast within the dilate-tissue density within the ureter immediately distal to the obstructed, nonopacified right ureter, consistent with transitional cell carcinoma (TCC).

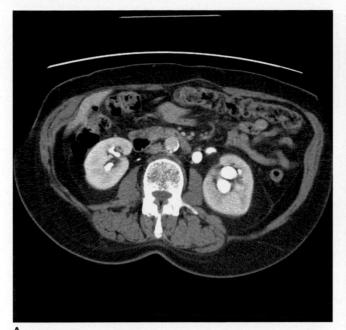

A

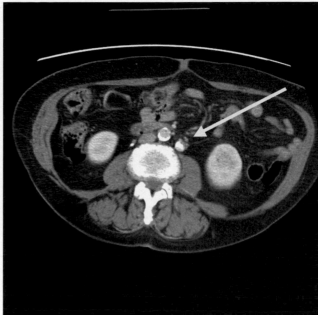

B

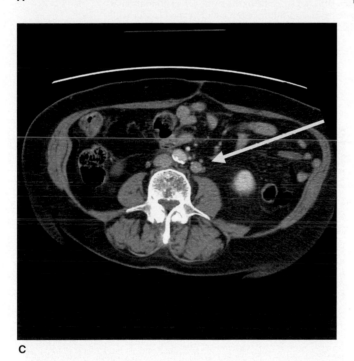

C

FIGURE 23.11. A: Axial slice from a delayed phase, contrast-enhanced computed tomography (CT) examination at the level of the midpole of the left kidney demonstrates mild dilatation of the left collecting system with mild asymmetry in enhancement of the left kidney relative to the right kidney. **B:** Axial slices from the same CT examination demonstrate contrast within a nondilated right ureter and asymmetric soft-tissue thickening along the left anterior aspect of the dilated left ureter. **C:** Axial slices demonstrate stricture of the left ureter from circumferential thickening of the left ureter secondary to transitional cell carcinoma (TCC).

asymmetric soft-tissue density within the collecting system and distal ureters (Fig. 23.11), or multicentric thickening of the ureters or bladder wall (Fig. 23.12). Furthermore, as a result of ~5% of transitional cell carcinomas containing calcification (19), nodular or arched surface calcifications may be visualized on noncontrast or within the early phase of a contrast- enhanced CT examination (Fig. 23.10).

The hematuria protocol images the collecting system, ureters, and bladder in two different phases of contrast administration. This varies the amount of contrast within the bladder. Masses are usually noted as filling defects and are most often seen in a later phase of imaging when the bladder is filled with contrast (Fig. 23.13). Masses can also show changes in relative contrast depending on the phase of imaging

utilized as well as the amount of urine extant within the bladder, which can dilute the contrast. This is well demonstrated in Figure 23.14 (case 1), where a mass at the right ureterovesical junction has penetrated and has extended into the distal right ureter. These changes in enhancement and the phase of imaging could mask a lesion if it is not imaged in the correct phase. For instance, some masses are more easily distinguished during the early phase of contrast administration and could easily be missed during a later phase of imaging when there is more contrast within the bladder. This is illustrated in Figures 23.15 and 23.16.

Unlike intravenous urography, however, CT demonstrates increased sensitivity in staging TCC. When a tumor has penetrated the serosa and has extended into the perivesicular fat,

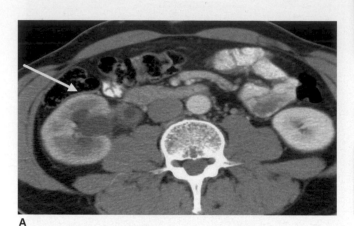

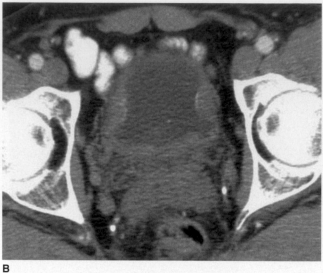

FIGURE 23.12. A: Axial slice from a delayed phase, contrast-enhanced computed tomography (CT) examination at the level of the midpole of the kidneys demonstrates asymmetric enhancement of the right kidney relative to the left secondary to obstructive hydronephrosis of the right kidney, with stranding of the perinephric fat. Note the thickened proximal ureter. **B:** Axial slices from the same CT examination at the level of the bladder demonstrating multiple enhancing masses/filling defects within the bladder wall consistent with TCC. The enhancing masses are evident within an unopacified bladder.

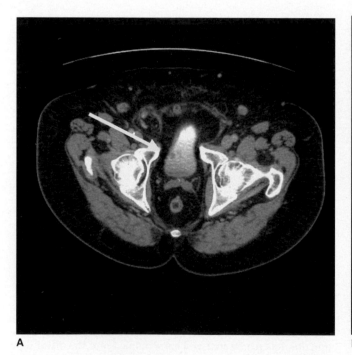

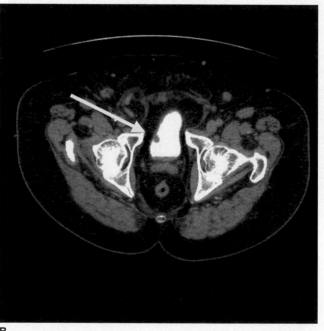

FIGURE 23.13. A: Axial slice at the level of the bladder in a delayed phase of contrast administration. There is a gradient of contrast, which is posterior to anterior within the bladder, secondary to the dilution from urine. Note the subtle filling defect within the right aspect of the bladder. **B:** At a later phase, an axial slice at the same level demonstrates decrease in the contrast gradient. The mass is easily distinguished as a filling defect surrounded by high-density contrast.

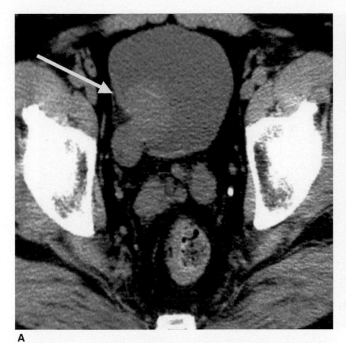

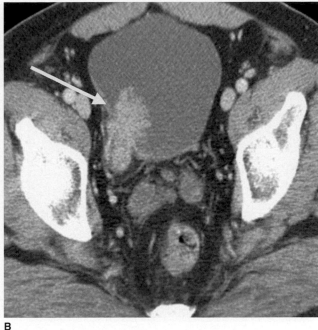

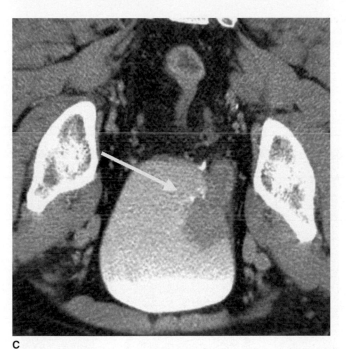

FIGURE 23.14. A: Axial slice from a noncontrast enhanced examination demonstrating a slightly hyperdense mass at the right uretero-vesical junction extending into the bladder as well as retrograde into the distal right ureter. Note that the mass demonstrates relatively low contrast relative to the hypodense urine. **B:** The mass demonstrates early contrast enhancement relative to the hypodense urine and is thus more easily discernible. **C:** Prone examination during the delayed phase of imaging, where the bladder is normally filled with contrast, demonstrates the mass as a relatively hypodense filling defect surrounded by hyperdense contrast that has filled the bladder.

the stage has increased to 3b. This is seen as stranding or "haziness" of the perivesicular fat. Figure 23.17 demonstrates a mass extending from the left uretero-vesical junction (UVJ) into the left ureter, with extension to the perivesicular fat with the presence of adenopathy confirming a diagnosis of stage T3bN1 disease. Asymmetric or diffuse thickening of the bladder, as well, is often viewed with suspicion and can represent malignancy. These findings, however, are not specific. Figure 23.18 demonstrates multiple axial slices from the early phase of enhancement of a contrast-enhanced CT examination at the level of the bladder. The images demonstrate abnormal thickening and dystrophic calcification within the bladder wall consistent with TCC. Thickening of the bladder can also be post-infectious, postradiation therapy as

well as postchemotherapy (20). Subtle, flat tumors of the bladder, however, remain a challenge with CT urography and should be investigated cystoscopically. As multiplanar and volume CT techniques advance, however, these subtle discriminations may be possible.

The presence of lymphadenopathy and metastases also has significant bearing on the staging, prognosis, and management of transitional cell carcinoma. The extant evaluation of lymph nodes includes short-axis measurement by CT criteria and the presence of a single lymph node of <2 cm in greatest dimension equivalent to a stage N1 tumor (Fig. 23.19). The combination of these advances has led to multiple studies to assess the wide variance in the staging of primary cancer of the bladder and upper urothelial tract ranging from 55% to 92% (21–27).

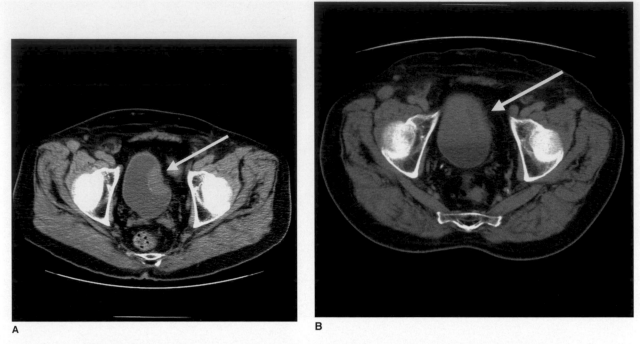

FIGURE 23.15. A: Axial slice from a contrast-enhanced computed tomography (CT) examination at the level of the bladder. There is an enhancing mass relative to the hypodense urine extending from the left bladder wall. **B:** During a later phase of imaging this mass is not easily discernible and could easily be missed.

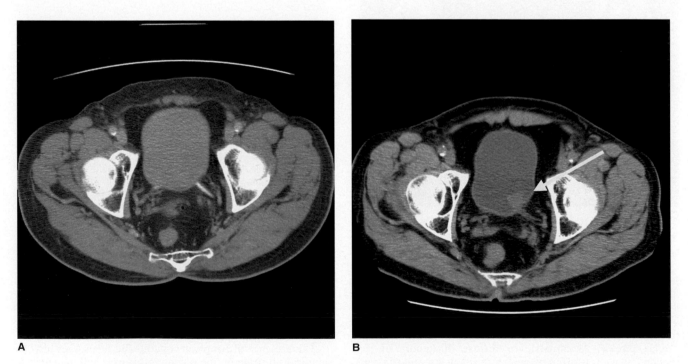

FIGURE 23.16. A: Axial slice from a contrast-enhanced CT examination at the level of the bladder. The distal ureters are easily identified and are filled with contrast. The contrast within the bladder is diluted by urine. **B:** Imaging done at an earlier phase when there was no contrast within the bladder demonstrates an early enhancing mass within the bladder extending from the left uretero-vesical junction (UVJ).

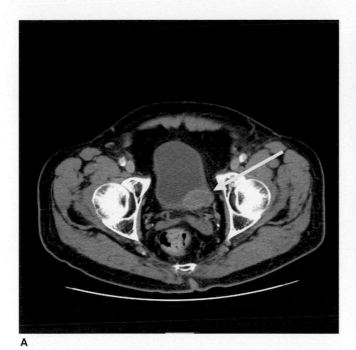

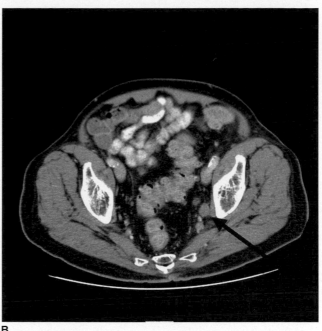

A   B

FIGURE 23.17. A: Axial slice from a contrast-enhanced examination during the early phase of contrast administration which demonstrates a mass at the left UVJ extending into and involving the distal left ureter. Note that there is haziness of the perivesicular fat, which may designate stage IIIb disease. **B:** A slice superior to the previous demonstrates an enlarged lymph node in the left obturator lymph node chain.

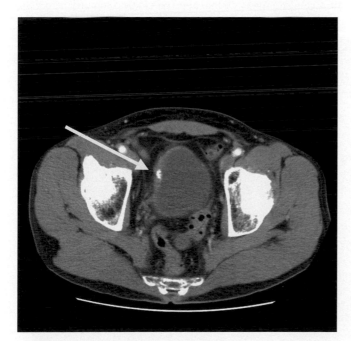

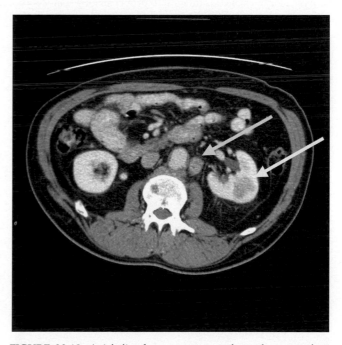

FIGURE 23.18. Axial slice from a contrast-enhanced computed tomography (CT) examination at the level of the bladder. There is mild right-sided, asymmetric thickening to the bladder where there is a region of dystrophic calcification. Cystoscopic biopsy from within this region confirmed the diagnosis of TCC.

FIGURE 23.19. Axial slice from a contrast-enhanced computed tomography (CT) examination at the level of the left midpole. There is a hypodense mass within the proximal left collecting system extending into the left renal parenchyma. Note the large lymph node adjacent to the aorta in the left pararenal/paraaortic space.

MAGNETIC RESONANCE IMAGING

MRI is a multiplanar, noninvasive imaging technique that produces high spatial resolution images based on the water content of the tissue being investigated. Soft-tissue contrast, which is superior to any other imaging technique, is based on the molecular properties of the tissues as well as the relaxation properties being exploited within the imaging technique. The standard imaging techniques that are utilized exploit differences in the T1 and T2 relaxivity of the tissues. In a T1-weighted image, fluid has low signal intensity, fat has high signal intensity, and organs and muscles have intermediate signal intensity. Conversely, in a T2-weighted image, fluid has high signal intensity and many soft tissues have intermediate to low signal intensity. Fat, however, can appear bright or dark depending on the choice of pulse sequence being utilized. For instance, fat appears bright on a fast-spin-echo T2-weighted pulse sequence, but is dark on a standard T2-weighted spin-echo pulse sequence. On T1-weighted imaging, tumor is nonspecific, being either isointense to slightly hyperintense to normal renal parenchyma. Likewise, on T2-weighted imaging, tumor is isointense to slightly hyperintense to normal renal parenchyma.

The multiplanar capabilities and exquisite soft-tissue contrast of MRI make it an excellent choice in imaging of the urinary bladder. The investigation of the urinary bladder includes axial, coronal, and sagittal T2-weighted imaging and T1-weighted imaging, without gadolinium and following the administration of gadolinium contrast administration. Postcontrast imaging is performed at an early phase (20-second and 70-second delay) to better differentiate the early enhancement of the tumor relative to normal bladder with a background of T1 hypointense urine within the bladder. Chemical fat saturation allows for adequate differentiation of enhancing tumor from the perivesicular fat, which is integral to proper staging (Fig. 23.20).

However, similar to CT, if imaging is done at a later phase, the contrast that is administered is excreted in the urine and shortens the T1 of the urine. The urine within the bladder will therefore appear bright on T1-weighted and T2-weighted imaging (Fig. 23.21). The enhancing tumor may also allow the differentiation of invasion within the muscular layers of the bladder as well as the perivesicular fat or surrounding structures, which would allow differentiation of stage T1 from T4 disease. Figure 23.22 illustrates a case of a TCC within a bladder diverticulum that extends into and invades the iliac vasculature. Invasive findings can be subtle, however. Figure 23.23 demonstrates a case of a tumor thrombus within the right external iliac vein from bladder TCC. The combination of multiplanar imaging and soft-tissue contrast has demonstrated MRI to be an excellent study for staging bladder carcinoma, with studies demonstrating an accuracy of between 73% and 96% (28). However, MRI has not supplanted CT as an initial screening modality for painless hematuria at many institutions secondary to cost and availability.

The evaluation of the upper urinary tract poses unique technical considerations with MRI. MR urography is composed of delayed T2-weighted sequences in the coronal phase by using fast T2-weighted imaging sequences (HASTE or RARE), or their equivalent on other platforms, to produce T2 contrast by static contrast from the renal pelvis and collecting system as compared to surrounding structures (29,30). Although static MR urography is excellent in differentiating filling defects and anomalies in dilated collecting systems, the relatively poorer spatial resolution of MRI as compared to CT in a nondilated system may obscure subtle filling defects in a nondilated pelvis. Excretory phase MR urography has been a welcome addition to the evaluation of the upper urinary tract and the addition of furosemide has minimized the T2* effect of concentrated contrast within the collecting system. Current technological approaches to excretory MR urography include the intravenous administration of low-dose furosemide (5 mg to 10 mg) approximately 5 minutes before the

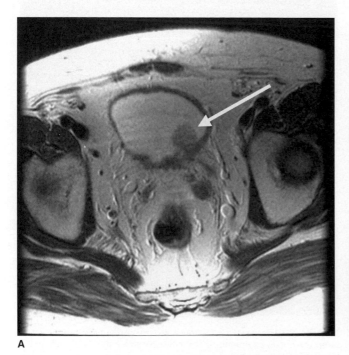 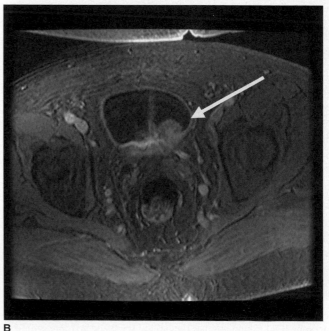

A   B

FIGURE 23.20. A: Axial T2-weighted image at the level of the urinary bladder. The bladder is filled with T2 hyperintense urine. At the left UVJ there is a relatively T2 hypointense mass extending into the bladder consistent with a transitional cell carcinoma (TCC). **B:** Chemical shift fat saturation easily distinguishes enhancing tumor from the urine, which is low in T1 signal intensity secondary to an early phase of imaging. Note that there is no evidence of abnormal enhancement in the perivesicular fat, which implies that there is no evidence of perivesicular extension.

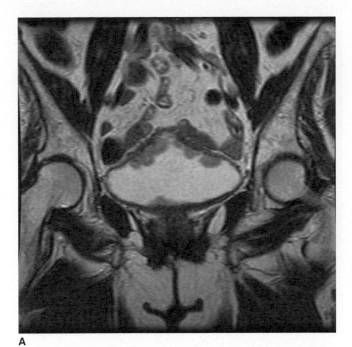

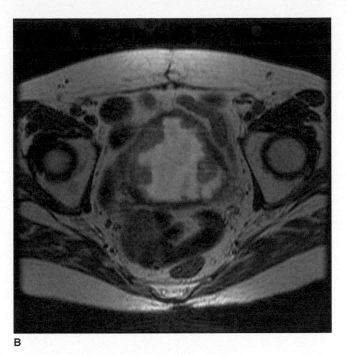

A   B

FIGURE 23.21. A: Coronal T1-weighted image following gadolinium contrast administration. The urine within the bladder is bright in signal intensity secondary to excretion of gadolinium within the urine and a delayed phase of imaging. Note the multiple filling defects within the urinary bladder consistent with multifocal transitional cell carcinoma (TCC). **B:** Axial T2-weighted image from the same patient demonstrates multiple T2 hypointense lesions within the T2 hyperintense urine within the bladder.

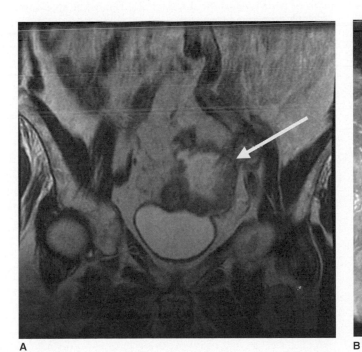

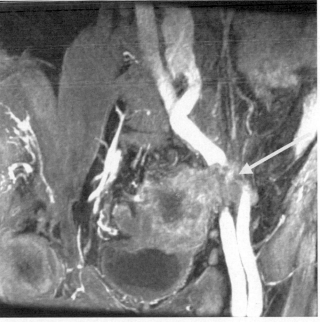

A   B

FIGURE 23.22. A: Coronal T1-weighed image postgadolinium contrast administration centered at the level of the pelvis. There is an enhancing mass within a left-sided bladder diverticulum extending to and possibly invading the iliac vessels. **B:** The addition of fat saturation into an angiographic study (coronal T1-weighted gradient echo examination) that opacifies the iliac vasculature confirms the invasive nature of the transitional cell carcinoma (TCC) within the left-sided bladder diverticulum.

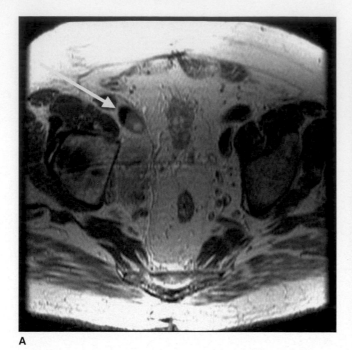

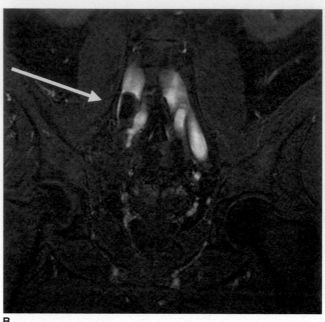

FIGURE 23.23. **A:** Axial T1-weighted image at the level of the acetabulum which demonstrates a T1 hyperintense filling defect, which is suspicious for tumor thrombus, within the right external iliac vein in a patient with known transitional cell carcinoma (TCC) of the urinary bladder. **B:** Coronal angiographic images confirm the diagnosis of thrombosis within the right external iliac vein.

administration of 0.1 mmol of Gd-DTPA (30,31). Approximately 5 minutes after the administration of gadolinium contrast, breathhold, coronal 3D gradient echo images are obtained to allow for reconstruction of the entire renal pelvis and distal collecting system (30). Similar morphologic findings noted on extretory-phase contrast urography are utilized for denoting pathology on MR excretory-phase contrast urograms. The vast majority of malignancies involving the upper urinary tract are transitional cell carcinomas and present as filling defects, which are hypointense relative to the hyperintense surrounding contrast-filled renal pelvis or dilated ureters. Characteristic findings include the following: ballooning of a tumor-filled calyx ("oncocalix"), obstruction of a caliceal infundibulum with preserved excretion of the affected calyx ("amputation") or ceased function "phantom calyx," or the "goblet sign" in the ureter, which refers to accumulation of contrast in a prestenotic cup-shaped dilated ureter (30,31). The combination of T2-weighted static and excretory MR urography has demonstrated itself capable of diagnosing advanced intrinsic tumor growth within the upper urothelial tract, but there remain no prospective studies of the sensitivity, specificity, or accuracy of these modalities with nonobstructive, early tumors.

LYMPHANGIOGRAPHY

In the past, evaluating lymph node metastases required the use of lymphangiography, which involved the injection of radio-opaque dye into the lymphatic system. Although this technique evaluated nodes based on their architecture, the procedure was invasive and was limited in its ability to visualize completely the primary lymph node groups. Hence it has been supplanted by cross-sectional modalities like CT and MRI, which use size criteria for differentiating lymph nodes. However, size criteria have been shown to be inadequate for evaluating involved lymph nodes. With respect to adenopathy, previous studies did not demonstrate a relative increase in the

sensitivity of MRI versus CT in assessing the presence of one or more lymph nodes that measured >2 cm, which is the hallmark of nodal metastatic disease (32). The recent application of lymphotrophic contrast agents, ultrasmall superparamagnetic iron oxide (USPIO—Combidex), to genitourinary cancers has demonstrated improved sensitivity of 90.5% as compared to conventional MRI sensitivity of 35.4% in distinguishing malignant from benign lymphadenopathy (33). USPIO has a long intravascular half-life and is taken up into the lymphatics. If a lymph node does not demonstrate the normal signal drop secondary to uptake of the USPIO, then it is metastatic. These findings are illustrated in Figure 23.24. This may have a significant impact on the noninvasive staging of transitional cell carcinoma.

DISTANT METASTASIS

The evaluation of distant metastases arising from transitional cell carcinoma also remains clinically relevant secondary to staging considerations. Hematogenous spread is less frequent than lymphatic spread of disease, secondary to extensive lymphatic supply. Therefore, lymph node involvement is paramount in staging evaluation, although metastases occur to the skeleton, lung, and liver with direct extension to the retroperitoneum occurring as well. Multiple imaging modalities are currently utilized for assessing the presence or absence of distant metastasis. Of particular interest within this aspect of staging is nuclear scintigraphy.

Positron Emission Tomography

Positron emission tomography (PET) exploits short half-life positrons that have extremely short path lengths before annihilation into two gamma rays of equal energy. The metabolite that has received the most recent attention is clearly ^{18}F-fluorodeoxyglucose (FDG), a positron-emitting analog of glucose. The increased metabolic rate associated with most

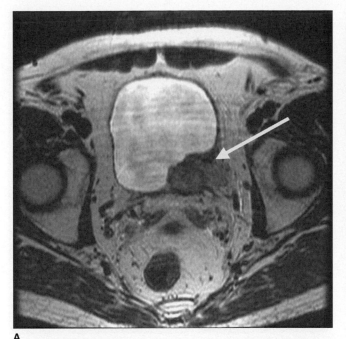

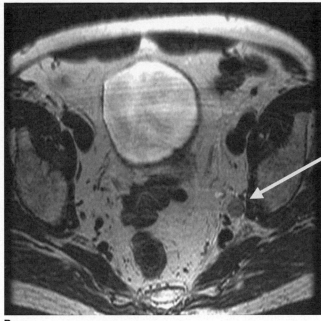

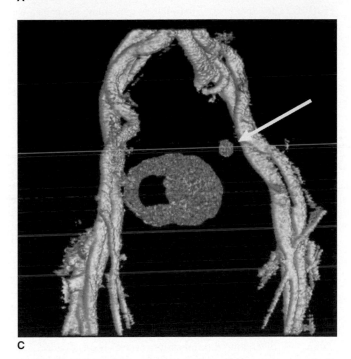

FIGURE 23.24. **A:** Axial T2*-weighted examination at the level of the acetabulum which demonstrates a T2* hyperintense, mildly enhancing, lobulated mass at the left base of the bladder. **B:** Axial T2*-weighted image from a level more superior demonstrates a rounded lymph node along the left internal iliac chain that does not enhance with USPIO contrast. The radiographic determination of malignant involvement was confirmed pathologically. **C:** 3D representation of the mass, colored in green, within the bladder, lymph node, which is colored in red, and superimposing vasculature, colored in white. The long-lived intravascular properties of USPIO allow for excellent angiographic mapping, which benefits surgical planning.

neoplasms is therefore detected and imaged. The technique is of limited spatial resolution, but has been utilized in the detection of transitional cell carcinoma. Furthermore, because a whole-body scan is routinely performed, the presence of distant metastasis is readily available. In a study Kosuda et al. studied 10 patients with histologically proven bladder carcinoma. Their study demonstrated that FDG-PET scanning was true-positive in eight patients (66.7%), but false-negative in four (33.3%). Furthermore, FDG-PET scanning detected all of 17 distant metastatic lesions and two of three proven regional lymph node metastases (34). Their results, although preliminary, suggested the feasibility of detecting bladder cancer. However, one of the strong limitations was the intense signal within the bladder from urinary accumulation. This intense signal, which could mask a hyperintense bladder tumor as well as the inherently poor spatial resolution of PET, make

this technique not as desirable as MRI or CT in tumor detection. However, the utility in nodal involvement and distant metastasis continues to be studied (35).

Nuclear Imaging

^{99m}Tc-labeled diphosphonates remain a very valuable and sensitive means of detecting metastasis to the axial skeleton in patients suffering from various malignancies. In bladder cancer, however, the incidence of axial metastasis in invasive carcinoma remains low, and in two studies there was only impact on 1% of patients (36,37). Further evidence has also demonstrated that MRI may be more sensitive and specific to the presence of bone marrow metastasis, which may prove valuable in a universal, noninvasive staging examination.

POSTOPERATIVE SURVEILLANCE

Depending on the stage of the malignancy, the primary treatment secondary to TCC varies from cystoscopic resection for local disease to a combination of chemotherapy, radiation therapy, and cystectomy with or without the creation of a diversionary loop for more advanced disease. The multifocal nature of transitional cell carcinoma in combination with the sequelae of chemotherapy and radiation therapy, which can mimic neoplasms, therefore results in a need for continued surveillance. There is, however, no widely agreed upon routine for surveillance imaging following radical cystectomy (38).

Patients undergoing radical cystectomy for advanced, invasive disease can either undergo the creation of an ileal loop diversion or the creation of an orthotopic neobladder. In the setting of many ileal loop diversions, there has been cutaneous diversion of the efferent urine flow into a stoma. However, there has been increased utility and interest in anastomosing to the primary urethra, without cutaneous diversion for preserving continence, and thus enhancing quality of life. Excretory urography and CT remain the mainstay in surveillance in patients that have orthotopic neobladder construction (39,40). Excretory urography allows for visualization of the orthotopic neobladder, which is often in the right lower quadrant and often preserves the mucosal folding pattern of the loop of ileum. The presence or absence of minimal to mild pelvicaliectasis is a normal finding and should not be viewed with suspicion. In comparison, severe hydronephrosis should be regarded with high suspicion, as it is usually associated with ureteral stricture or tumor recurrence (39,40). Yet, if the dilatation is a transient phenomenon, which can occur secondary to the normal, decreased peristaltic activity of the reservoir, then the level of suspicion can be lowered, but continued surveillance is recommended (39,40). MRI has also demonstrated increased utility in surveillance, postoperatively. Figure 23.25 demonstrates an axial T2-weighted image from a patient that is status post-creation of a neobladder. At the anastamosis there is a T2 hypointense region surrounded by T2 hyperintense urine consistent with TCC recurrence.

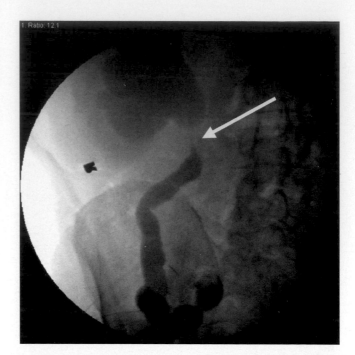

FIGURE 23.26. Spot image from an ileography study. The patient has a history of transitional cell carcinoma (TCC) of the bladder and renal cell carcinoma of the left kidney and is status post-left-nephroureterectomy and cystectomy with creation of an ileal loop diversion. The image demonstrates stricture at the ureteropelvic junction.

When a cutaneous diversion is performed a retrograde study should be performed (39). The stoma is accessed with a catheter and, similar to a cystogram, contrast material is then instilled retrograde into the reservoir under fluoroscopic guidance. Pressures are monitored, to avoid exceeding 30 cm H_2O. The exam is completed when reflux is noted bilaterally into the collecting systems of the kidneys. Proper interrogation of the anastamoses bilaterally must be performed to exclude a ureteral stricture, which may be a sign of tumor recurrence (Fig. 23.26). Lack of reflux into one ureter should be viewed with high suspicion, as this may represent a complete, distal ureteral stricture. The reservoir itself while distended should be studied for any abnormal filling defects that could represent tumor recurrence.

CT scans allow for interrogation of the reservoir as well as for obstructive uropathy, but because CT scans contain axial images they are superior to excretory urography or retrograde pyelography and ureterography in the evaluation of postoperative complications, both early and late, following orthotopic or cutaneous diversion. Complications have been divided into those that occur early, which include postoperative extravasation and fluid collections including urinomas, hematomas, abscesses, and lymphoceles. Late complications include obstructive hydronephrosis, fistulas, urethral strictures, and ureteral strictures as well as necrosis (39,40). Furthermore, given the increased incidence of tumor recurrence, which reaches approximately 20% in the literature, CT examination of the abdomen and pelvis is requisite to assess for either local or distant recurrence in the form of adenopathy or distant metastatic disease (39,40).

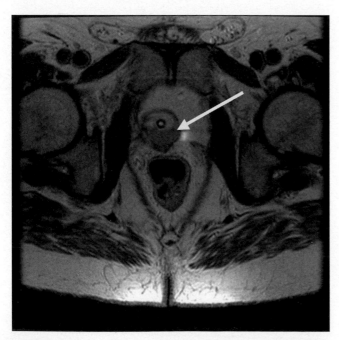

FIGURE 23.25. Axial T2-weighted image from a patient that is status post-bladder resection and creation of neobladder. At the anastamosis there is a T2 hypointense region surrounded by T2 hyperintense urine consistent with transitional cell carcinoma (TCC) recurrence.

SUMMARY

In summary, bladder cancer remains the second most common malignancy affecting the urinary tract in men, and 90% to 95% of these malignancies are transitional cell carcinoma. As the most common complaint of patients with transitional cell carcinoma remains painless hematuria, the initial radiologic evaluation remains a mainstay in early and proper diagnosis and staging. Recent advances have increased the role of CT in both characterizing renal masses and assessing the collecting system, distal ureters, and bladder in a complete urographic assessment of hematuria. These findings have allowed for CT to supplant IV urography in our institution for screening patients with painless hematuria. Furthermore, CT imaging allows for a complete evaluation of the abdomen and pelvis within the same setting. This may allow for evaluation of distant metastatic disease in the setting of bladder cancer to the liver and lung as well as assessing for possible lymph node involvement by using extant pathologic criteria (>2 cm in size). However, advances in MRI have demonstrated that in patients with known genitourinary cancers, lymphotrophic, susceptibility contrast-agents show increased sensitivity and specificity to pathologic lymph node involvement. These data may prove that MRI may be more efficacious in staging for both possible lymph node involvement and distant metastatic disease.

These combinations of advances in imaging technology will provide the urologist with an increased armamentarium in the diagnosis of possible early bladder carcinoma and increased accuracy in staging, which may alter treatment strategies.

APPENDIX

Hematuria
Patient orientation: Supine
Landmark: Xyphoid
Oral contrast: None
Scan type: I−   I−   I+   I+

Range	Liver to symphysis pubis	Through renal stones only	Pt. under 40 -> radiologist	
Pt. Position	Supine	Supine		Prone
Slice thickness	5 mm	1.25 mm		5 mm
Image spacing	5 mm	1.25 mm	If I+ (or over 40)	5 mm
Mode	High speed	High speed	1. 30 cc contrast	High speed
KvP	140	140	2. 100 cc saline	140
mA	Variable	Variable	Over 10 min	Variable
Time	0.8	0.8	3. wait 5 min	0.8
Scan fov	Large	Large		Large
Display fov	Variable	Target to kidney	total wait = 15 min	Variable
Contrast	None	None		3 cc/sec for 100 sec
				300 mg/mL, 100 sec delay

References

1. Borden L, Clark P, Hall M. Bladder cancer. *Curr Opin Oncol* 2003;15:227–233.
2. Greenlee R, Hill-Harmon M, Murray T, et al. Cancer statistics. *CA Cancer J Clin* 2001;51:15–36.
3. Phillips T, Chin F, Palubinskas A. Calcification in renal masses: an eleven year survey. *Radiology* 1963;80:786–794.
4. Cannon A, Zanon B, Karras B. Cystic calcifications in the kidney. Its occurance in malignant renal tumors. *Am J Roentgenol* 1962;84:837–848.
5. Daniel W, Harman G, Witten D, et al. Calcified renal masses: a review of ten years experience at the Mayo Clinic. *Radiology* 1972;103:503–508.
6. Ferris E, O'Connor S. Calcification in urinary bladder tumors. *Am J Roentgenol* 1965;95:447–449.
7. Datta S, Allen G, Evans R, et al. Urinary tract ultrasonography in the evaluation of hematuria—a report of over 1,000 cases. *Ann R Coll Surg Engl* 2002;84(3):203–205.
8. Dibb M, Noble D, Peh W, et al. Ultrasonographic analysis of bladder tumors. *J Clin Imaging* 2001;25:416–420.
9. Schulze S, Holm-Neilsen A, Morgensen P. Transurethral ultrasound scanning in the evaluation of invasive bladder cancer. *Scand J Urol Nephrol* 1991;25:215–217.
10. Barentsz J, Wickstrom M, Ruijs J. What is new in bladder cancer imaging. *Urol Clin North Am* 1997;24(3):583–602.
11. Hatch T, Barry J. The value of excretory urography in staging bladder cancer. *J Urol* 1986;135:49.
12. Badalmant R, Ryan P, Bahn D. Imaging for transitional cell carcinoma. In: Vogelzang NJ, Shipley WU, Scardino PT, et al., eds. *Comprehensive textbook of genitourinary oncology*. 2nd ed. Baltimore, MD: Lippincott Williams & Wilkins 2000:356–365.
13. Webb J. Imaging in haematuria. *Clin Imaging* 1997;52:167–171.
14. Street L, Warshauer D, McCarthy S, et al. Detection of renal masses: sensitivities and specifities of excretory urography/linear tomography, US and CT. *Radiology* 1988;169:363–365.
15. Choe K, Smith R, Rosenfield A, et al. Acute flank pain: comparison of noncontrast enhanced CT and intravenous urography. *Radiology* 1995;194:789–794.
16. Smith R, Verga M, McCarthy S, et al. Diagnosis of acute flank pain: value of unenhanced helical CT. *Am J Roentgenol* 1996;166:97–101.
17. Freed K, Shaefor D, Hertzberg B, et al. Nonenhanced helical CT and US in the emergency evaluation of patients with renal colic: prospective comparison. *Radiology* 2000;217:792–797.
18. O'Malley M, Hahn P, Yoder I, et al. Comparison of excretory phase, helical computed tomography with intravenous urography in patients with painless hematuria. *Clin Radiol* 2003;58(4):294–300.
19. Moon W, Kim S, Cho J, et al. Calcified bladder tumors. CT features. *Acta Radiol* 1992;33(5):440–443.
20. Ramchandani P, Pollack H. Radiology of drug-related genitourinary disease. *Semin Roentgenol* 1995;30:77–87.
21. Amendola M, Glazer G, Grossman H, et al. Staging of bladder carcinoma: MRI-CT-surgical correlation. *Am J Roentgenol* 1986;146(6):1179–1183.
22. Bryan P, Butler H, LiPuma J, et al. CT and MR imaging in staging bladder neoplasms. *J Comput Tomogr* 1987;11:96–101.
23. Husband J, Oliff J, Williams M, et al. Bladder cancer: staging with CT and MR imaging. *Radiology* 1989;173:435–440.
24. Tanimoto A, Yusa Y, Imai Y, et al. Bladder tumor staging: comparison of conventional and gadolinium-enhanced dynamic MR imaging and CT. *Radiology* 1992;185:741–747.
25. Vock P, Haertel M, Fuchs W, et al. Computed tomography in staging carcinoma of the urinary bladder. *Br J Urol* 1982;54:158–163.
26. Caterino M, Giunta S, Finocchi V, et al. Primary cancer of the urinary ladder: CT evaluation of the T parameter with different techniques. *Abdom Imaging* 2001;26:433–438.
27. Kundra V, Silverman P. Imaging in the diagnosis, staging, and follow-up of cancer of the urinary bladder. *Am J Roentgenol* 2003;180:1045–1054.
28. Tekes A, Kamel I, Imam K, et al. MR imaging features of transitional cell carcinoma of the urinary bladder. *Am J Roentgenol* 2003;180(3):771–777.
29. Roy C, Saussine C, Jacqmin D. Magnetic resonance urography. *BJU Int* 2000;86(Suppl. 1):42–47.
30. Nolte-Ernsting C, Adam G, Gunther R. MR urography: examination techniques and clinical applications. *Eur Radiol* 2001;11:355–372.
31. Nolte-Ernsting C, Bucker A, Adam G, et al. Gadolinium-enhanced excretory MR urography after low-dose diuretic injection: comparison with conventional excretory urography. *Radiology* 1998;209:147–157.
32. Sobin L, Wittekind C, eds. *TNM classification of malignant tumours*. Baltimore, MD: Wiley-Liss, 1997.
33. Harisinghani M, Barentsz J, Hahn P, et al. Noninvasive detection of clinically occult lymph-node metastases in prostate cancer. *N Engl J Med* 2003;348(25):2491–2499.
34. Kosuda S, Kison P, Greenough R, et al. Preliminary assessment of fluorine-18 fluorodeoxyglucose positron emission tomography in patients with bladder cancer. *Eur J Nucl Med Mol Imaging* 1997;24(6):615–620.
35. Hain S, Maisey M. Positron emission tomography for urological tumors. *BJU Int* 2003;92(2):159–164.

36. Lindner A, deKernion J. Cost effective analysis of pre-cystectomy radioisotope scans. *J Urol* 1982;128:1181–1182.

37. Berger G, Sandlowski R, Sharpe J, et al. Lack of value of routine preoperative bone and liver scans in cystectomy candidate. *J Urol* 1981;125:637–639.

38. Montie J. Follow-up after cystectomy for carcinoma of the bladder. *Urol Clin North Am* 1994;21:639–643.

39. Koegan M. Radiology of urinary diversions. *Curr Opin Urol* 2000;10(2):117–122.

40. Heaney M, Francis I, Cohan R, et al. Orthotopic neobladder reconstruction: findings on excretory urography and CT. *Am J Roentgenol* 1999;172:1213–1220.

CHAPTER 24 ■ UPPER TRACT TUMORS

CHAPTER 24A
Management of Upper Tract Tumors

R. Houston Thompson and Bradley C. Leibovich

Treatment of urothelial tumors of the upper tract has traditionally been radical nephroureterectomy with bladder cuff excision. However, management of upper-tract malignancies, most commonly transitional cell carcinoma (TCC), has undergone considerable changes in the last decade. Retrograde endoscopic and percutaneous treatment of upper-tract TCC was initially reserved for a subset of patients needing renal preservation. More recent evaluation has supported renal sparing treatment in a select group of patients with normal contralateral kidneys. Systemic chemotherapy, historically reserved for patients with metastatic lesions, is now often used for locally advanced disease in the absence of metastasis. Nephroureterectomy with bladder cuff resection remains the gold standard of treatment, but the lack of prospective randomized trials on a relatively rare cancer does not allow for absolute treatment conclusions. Currently, treatment is guided by perceived tumor risk, efficacy of treatment, and patient health status. This chapter will focus on the presentation and diagnosis of upper-tract TCC and discuss the various treatment modalities and complications thereof.

INCIDENCE

Tumors of the renal pelvis and ureter are relatively uncommon, accounting for approximately 5% of all urologic malignancies (1). The incidence of upper-tract tumors is increasing, but whether this is a true increase or is related to improved endoscopy, imaging, and surveillance is not well quantified. Similar to their counterparts in the bladder, upper-tract urothelial tumors occur most commonly in the sixth and seventh decade and appear in men more often than in women with a ratio of approximately 3:1 (2,3). Over a 15-year period at the authors' institution, there were 296 upper-tract tumors compared with over 5,000 bladder tumors, a ratio of 1:17 (4).

Urothelial tumors occur throughout the renal collecting system and are slightly more common in the pelvis compared with the ureter. However, among ureteral tumors, distal tumors are more frequent than proximal tumors, with a ratio of 70:20:10 for the distal, middle, and proximal ureter, respectively (5).

Like TCC of the bladder, upper-tract tumors represent a field change to the urothelium with the predilection for multiple recurrences. Upper tract tumors occur with equal frequency in each kidney; however, the field change is generally confined to the ipsilateral renal unit and bladder, as the incidence of TCC in the contralateral renal unit is only 3% (6,7).

An exception is found among patients with Balkan nephropathy, in whom 10% of cases are bilateral (8). These lesions tend to be of lower grade and renal sparing procedures are more frequently necessary (8).

Following radical cystectomy for bladder TCC, recurrence in the upper tracts occurs in about 3% to 4% of patients (9). More recently, Herr reported on 307 bladder tumor patients followed for a median of 12 years. The cumulative risk of upper-tract tumors in these patients were 10%, 26%, and 34% at 5 years, 5 to 10 years, and 15 years of follow-up, respectively (10).

ETIOLOGY

Evidence suggests that causes of upper-tract TCC are similar to those of bladder TCC. Environmental factors, including cigarette smoking and exposure to industrial chemicals such as those used in the rubber and textile industries, are particularly important (11). Prolonged high-dose exposure to the anti-inflammatory agent phenacetin produces a characteristic nephropathy along with upper-tract urothelial cancers (12).

Chronic infection, inflammation, obstruction, and stone disease are associated with adenocarcinoma and squamous cell carcinoma of the upper urinary tract (13,14). Cyclophosphamide use has been implicated in upper-tract and bladder TCC, as has consumption of caffeine (15). Hereditary factors also have been implicated through studies of familial cancer syndromes (15–17).

Multiple transurethral resections of bladder tumors have more recently been implicated as an etiologic factor. Elliot et al. reported that 70% of patients with pelvis TCC and 95% of patients with ureteral TCC treated ureteroscopically had previous resections of bladder tumors (18). It is not clear if these findings are due to the biology of the tumor and host or is secondary to iatrogenic causes from repeated instrumentation and resection.

PATHOLOGY

TCC, also known as urothelial carcinoma, represents greater than 90% of all upper-tract urothelial cancers (19,20). The morphology of these tumors is similar to that of lesions found in the bladder, and the histologic grading scale is demonstrated in Table 24A.1 (21). Squamous cell carcinomas account for less than 10% of renal pelvic and ureteral carcinomas. They tend to present at a higher stage and thus carry a poor prognosis (22,23). Adenocarcinoma represents less than 1% of upper-tract urothelial malignancies, and when it is identified, the possibility of metastatic disease from a gastrointestinal source should be ruled out (23). True primary adenocarcinomas are associated with chronic infection (15), occur equally in men and women, and are uniformly associated with a poor outcome. Nonurothelial cancers of the upper urinary tract, such as sarcomas and lymphoma, are quite rare and are not discussed.

HISTOLOGIC GRADE

Grades	Description
Grade 1	Well differentiated
Grade 2	Moderately differentiated
Grades 3–4	Poorly differentiated or undifferentiated

DIAGNOSIS AND STAGING

Presenting signs and symptoms are similar to those of other genitourinary malignancies and include gross hematuria (60% to 75%), flank pain (30% to 40%), and, rarely, a mass. Systemic symptoms such as weight loss, anorexia, and bone pain are usually associated with regional or distant metastasis. Ten percent to 15% of patients are asymptomatic.

TCC of the upper tracts is most often discovered as a radiolucent filling defect on excretory urography (EXU). Obstruction of varying degrees and nonvisualization may be seen in 10% to 30% of patients (24). The differential diagnosis of such filling defects includes radiolucent calculi, blood clots, external compression, fungal balls, pyelitis or ureteritis cystica, tuberculosis, endometriosis, and sloughed papillae (25). Therefore, additional diagnostic studies are needed to confirm the diagnosis of TCC.

Standard evaluation of a filling defect on EXU usually includes cystoscopy, retrograde ureteropyelography, voided urine cytology, and selective upper-tract cytology. Computerized tomography (CT) has a limited role in diagnosis of upper-tract TCC but is commonly used for delineating calculus causes of filling defects and staging advanced TCC. Cystoscopy during an episode of gross hematuria is useful to both localize the site of bleeding and evaluate the bladder for concomitant lesions. The presence of vermiform clots is indicative of upper tract origin. Retrograde ureteropyelography serves mainly to confirm the presence of a filling defect but is particularly informative in patients with high-grade obstruction resulting in a poorly visualized collecting system on excretory urography or in patients who are allergic to systemic contrast agents. A properly performed retrograde study should not be associated with absorption of contrast medium and can safely be done in patients with a contrast allergy. Characteristically on retrogrades, there is a local dilation distal to the intraluminal lesion, described as goblet or meniscus shaped.

Cytologic studies have variable benefit in the evaluation of upper tract disease. As is the case with bladder TCC, the sensitivity of cytology varies directly with tumor grade. Selective cytology for high-grade TCC and carcinoma *in situ* (CIS) of the upper tract has a reported accuracy rate as high as 80% (26,27). Conversely, in the presence of low-grade TCC, a washing from the renal pelvis often yields abnormal cells although their cytologic features are not sufficiently altered for a diagnosis of cancer (28). Voided urine cytology from low-grade lesions can have a false-negative rate as high as 96%, and even selective upper-tract cytology in the setting of well-differentiated tumors has an accuracy rate of only 10% to 40% (26,29–31). The use of saline barbotage to shed poorly cohesive superficial cells may improve diagnostic yield, but the pitfalls of cytology must be considered as a false-positive rate as high as 10% can be associated with inflammation and stone disease.

Retrograde brush biopsy has some utility for obtaining superficial tissue from the upper tract. This method has been associated with a high-positive predictive value (75% to 100%), sensitivity (91%), and specificity (88%) (32). Others have reported a 50% under-grading rate with brush biopsy (33)

and a false-negative rate of 16% (34,35). Fluoroscopically guided retrograde brush biopsy has now largely been replaced by ureteropyeloscopy and direct vision biopsy.

Ureteropyeloscopy has been assuming an ever-increasing role in the evaluation and management of upper-tract urothelial tumors. The standard diagnostic evaluation of upper-tract filling defects including EXU, cystoscopy, retrograde ureteropyelography, and voided and selective cytology, has shortcomings now demonstrated by many studies. Utilizing the standard evaluation including selective use of brush biopsies, ultrasonography, and CT scanning yields a correct diagnosis in only 58% of cases (36). Adding rigid ureteropyeloscopy to the evaluation increases the diagnostic accuracy to 83% with diagnostic failure usually due to inaccessibility of lesions with the rigid ureteroscope (36). With the advent of smaller, flexible ureteroscopes, the diagnostic accuracy can now be achieved in nearly every case in experienced hands (37,38).

Clearly, ureteropyeloscopy has become the standard of care in the diagnosis of upper-tract filling defects. It allows direct visualization within a closed system and offers the opportunity to biopsy encountered lesions, confirming the pathologic disease process. Keeley et al. reported on 51 patients who underwent ureteroscopic biopsy followed by nephroureterectomy. There were 90% and 92% agreement on grade with ureteroscopic biopsy and the final pathologic specimen for low-moderate and poorly differentiated tumors, respectively (39). Determining stage on ureteroscopic biopsy is limited by the thin wall of the upper-tract urothelium and the need to avoid violating the urinary tract integrity in the setting of TCC.

The 2002 American Joint Committee on Cancer (AJCC) staging system for upper-tract urothelial neoplasms is depicted in Tables 24A.2 and 24A.3 (21). Many authors have demonstrated a strong correlation between stage and grade of upper-tract TCC and survival, with stage being the single most important determinant (40). CT scanning has limited usefulness in determining TCC stage with a sensitivity and specificity for fat invasion of 67% and 44%, respectively (41). CT evidence of frank tumor extension beyond the wall of the pelvis or ureter is reported to be as high as 100% accurate (42). However, in the same study, CT false-negatives for pathologically confirmed invasive disease occurred in 59% of patients (42). As previously stated, ureteroscopic biopsy is also unreliable in determining stage (43). However, several studies have reported a strong correlation between grade and stage of upper-tract TCC (16,30). At the Mayo Clinic, 47 of 49 patients who had grade 1 upper-tract TCC also had stage I or superficial disease (30), and this correlation has subsequently been confirmed at different institutions (44,45). It is therefore reasonable to assume that patients with upper-tract TCC who have low-grade disease on biopsy and lack frank extension on CT scan have superficial disease.

Tumor multifocality and DNA ploidy has also been reported to be of prognostic significance. Among 198 patients with upper-tract TCC, 79% of multifocal tumors compared with 50% of solitary tumors were found to be invasive (46). Of 109 patients at the Mayo Clinic treated with nephroureterectomy for renal pelvis TCC, the 5-year and 10-year survival rates of DNA diploid patterns was significantly higher compared to aneuploid or tetraploid tumors (47).

MANAGEMENT

Radical Nephroureterectomy

In patients with a normal contralateral kidney, radical nephroureterectomy with resection of a bladder cuff remains the gold standard for organ-confined renal pelvis and proximal

TABLE 24A.2

2002 AMERICAN JOINT COMMITTEE ON CANCER (AJCC) TNM CLINICAL CLASSIFICATION FOR RENAL PELVIS AND URETER TUMORS

Primary Tumor (T)	Description
TX	Primary tumor cannot be assessed
T0	No evidence of primary tumor
Ta	Papillary noninvasive carcinoma
Tis	Carcinoma *in situ*
T1	Tumor invades subepithelial connective tissue
T2	Tumor invades muscularis
T3	Tumor invades beyond muscularis into periureteric fat (for ureter only) or peripelvic fat or the renal parenchyma (for renal pelvis only)
T4	Tumor invades adjacent organs, or through the kidney into the perinephric fat

Regional Lymph Nodes (N)	Description
NX	Regional lymph nodes cannot be assessed
N0	No regional lymph node metastasis
N1	Metastasis in a single lymph node, 2 cm or less in greatest dimension
N2	Metastasis in a single lymph node, more than 2 cm but not more than 5 cm in greatest dimension; or multiple lymph nodes, none more than 5 cm in greatest dimension
N3	Metastasis in a lymph node, more than 5 cm in greatest dimension

Distant Metastasis (M)	Description
MX	Distant metastasis cannot be assessed
M0	No distant metastasis
M1	Distant metastasis

TABLE 24A.3

AJCC TNM STAGE GROUPING

Stages	Description		
Stage 0a	Ta	N0	M0
Stage 0is	Tis	N0	M0
Stage I	T1	N0	M0
Stage II	T2	N0	M0
Stage III	T3	N0	M0
Stage IV	T4	N0	M0
	Any T	N1, N2, N3	M0
	Any T	Any N	M1

ureteral TCC that is either grade 3 or invasive (neoadjuvant chemotherapy for patients with locally advanced or metastatic disease at presentation is discussed below). Grade 2, noninvasive TCC of the pelvis or proximal ureter, also requires radical nephroureterectomy when they are large, multifocal, or rapidly recurring. The rationale for this management is based on the multifocal and recurrent nature of TCC, low incidence of contralateral disease (6,7), and a high rate of urothelial recurrence in the ureteral stump (20% to 84%) when nephrectomy alone is performed (6,48–50).

The technique of open radical nephroureterectomy entails removal of the entire kidney along with its perinephric fat, Gerota's fascia, and ureter with 1 cm of normal bladder mucosa surrounding the ureteral orifice. The procedure may be performed using a variety of incisions or combination of incisions and is largely one of surgeon preference. Generally, a flank or subcostal incision for the nephrectomy followed by a Gibson or midline incision for the distal ureteral resection provides excellent exposure. Alternatively, a single, long midline incision with intraperitoneal exposure can be used, although left-sided kidney exposure is limited with this approach.

The entire kidney is mobilized outside Gerota's fascia and the hilar vessels are divided. The adrenal gland is usually left intact unless there is concern for locally advanced disease. The ureter may be divided at a location that is free of tumor, or preferably removed intact with the kidney and cuff of bladder wall. The entire ureter, including the intramural portion, and a 1-cm circumferential cuff of bladder mucosa around the orifice is subsequently removed with the specimen. In cases of urinary diversion, a cuff of uretero-enteric anastomosis should accompany the distal ureteral resection.

A regional lymphadenectomy is then performed, especially for patients with high-grade tumors. Pelvis and upper ureteral TCC initially spreads to the para-aortic and paracaval nodes, while distal ureteral TCC spreads to pelvic nodes.

At the authors' institution, laparoscopic nephroureterectomy has largely replaced the open procedure. See Chapter 24B for a detailed discussion on laparoscopic management.

Partial Ureterectomy

Distal ureterectomy is recommended for grade 2-3 or invasive tumors of the distal ureter provided the proximal upper tract is free of disease. The rationale for this management stems from the knowledge that ipsilateral tumor recurrence occurs in a proximal to distal direction and that recurrence proximal to the original lesion is rare (40). Especially in patients with borderline renal function who might require adjuvant platinum-based chemotherapy, renal preservation is paramount. In Mazeman's classic review, the incidence of locoregional failure was similar for patients treated with nephroureterectomy (246 patients) versus distal ureterectomy (44 patients) (50).

A low midline incision provides adequate exposure. The distal ureter is removed in a similar fashion as described previously with care to avoid tumor contamination. If a direct ureteroneocystostomy is unable to be accomplished, then a psoas hitch should provide adequate length to bridge the gap. If a boari flap is anticipated, then incisions for the flap should be made before making the cystotomy for the psoas hitch.

A segmental ureterectomy and ureteroureterostomy are rarely indicated. An exception would be proximal or midureteral TCC that is either high-grade or invasive or too large for endoscopic ablation in a patient with a functional solitary kidney.

Outcome

The limited number of patients with upper tract TCC makes organization of randomized, prospective trials improbable. Consequently, outcome information must be obtained from retrospective observations. While few studies include >100 patients, most report that outcome following surgical extirpation is dependent on stage and grade, with stage being the single most important determinant. At the University of Texas, Southwestern, Hall et al. reported their 30-year experience with 252 patients treated surgically for upper tract TCC (51). In this large cohort, only stage and patient age correlated with disease-specific survival in a multivariate analysis. The 5-year actuarial survival rates by primary tumor classification are demonstrated in Table 24A.4. While grade is an important predictor of outcome, it is not uniformly reported to be an independent prognostic indicator (51). Perhaps the association of grade and survival is related to the strong correlation between grade and stage. Nevertheless, patients with grade 1 TCC generally have low stage TCC with >80% 5-year survival, while patients with grade 3–4 TCC generally have high stage TCC with <25% 5-year survival (Table 24A.5) (52). Outcome in patients with grade 2 TCC is highly variable (Table 24A.5).

ENDOUROLOGIC MANAGEMENT

Endoscopic treatment of upper-tract TCC initially emerged from the need to preserve renal function in patients with anatomic or functional solitary kidneys, bilateral upper-tract TCC, and patients with significant chronic renal insufficiency. With the advent of sophisticated endourologic techniques, including improved optics, small caliber actively deflecting telescopes, and applicable laser technology, enthusiasm for conservative management

TABLE 24A.4

5-YEAR SURVIVAL OF PATIENTS WITH UPPER-TRACT TRANSITIONAL CELL CARCINOMA TREATED WITH NEPHROURETERECTOMY ACCORDING TO PATHOLOGIC STAGE

Stage	5-year survival (%)
pTis/pTa	>90
pT1	90
pT2	70
pT3	40
pT4	<5

TABLE 24A.5

5-YEAR SURVIVAL OF PATIENTS WITH UPPER-TRACT TRANSITIONAL CELL CARCINOMA TREATED WITH NEPHROURETERECTOMY ACCORDING TO TUMOR GRADE

Tumor grade	5-Year survival (%)
G1	>80
G2	30 to 90
G3–4	<25

of upper-tract TCC has grown appreciably. The field of upper-tract TCC is now open to a variety of innovative approaches. Endoscopic resection of low-risk tumors in patients with categorical indications for renal sparing surgery have demonstrated low progression and mortality rates, and recurrences were amenable to endoscopic retreatment in a majority of cases (18). Subsequently, more recent reports have supported endoscopic treatment of low-risk superficial TCC in patients with normal contralateral kidneys (53).

The Mayo Clinic reported on 21 patients with upper-tract TCC and normal contralateral kidneys that were managed conservatively with either retrograde ureteroscopy or antegrade percutaneous tumor ablation (53). All tumors were solitary, small (<2 cm), low grade, and completely visible and no patient had a categorical indication for nephron-sparing surgery. Of the 21 patients followed for a mean of 6.1 years, 33% had a recurrence, although no recurrence was of higher grade. Nineteen percent of patients required nephroureterectomy due to recurrence, but 81% of renal units were preserved. Only one patient in the series died due to TCC, and that patient developed invasive bladder cancer after conservative treatment of his upper-tract TCC.

Currently, endourologic management of upper-tract TCC is reserved for patients with a solitary kidney, poor renal function, bilateral disease, or panurothelial predisposition to recurrent TCC, or in patients who are poor operative risks. Select patients with normal contralateral kidneys, who have small, low-risk tumors, can also be safely treated conservatively.

Retrograde Ureteropyeloscopy

The advantage of a retrograde ureteroscopic approach is lower morbidity and the ability to maintain urothelial integrity. It is best applied to patients with small tumors in accessible locations.

Both rigid and flexible ureteroscopes can be used for treatment of upper-tract TCC. The intramural tunnel and distal ureter are easier to inspect with a rigid scope while the evaluation of the proximal ureter and pelvis are more satisfactory with the deflectable, flexible endoscopes. The ureteral orifice will usually accept a small caliber rigid instrument (<7.5 Fr) without dilation. This allows inspection of the intramural and distal ureter prior to trauma from a wire or balloon dilator. It is often helpful to rotate the rigid ureteroscope 90 to 180 degrees as it enters the ureter, enabling the beveled tip of the instrument to lift the upper lip of the orifice and permit smooth insertion. A floppy-tip wire can then be inserted through the rigid instrument to the renal pelvis. If dilation of the intramural ureter is needed, this is usually accomplished by passing a balloon dilating catheter over the wire and across the ureteral orifice and intramural tunnel. Contrast instilled into the balloon can be watched fluoroscopically with the endpoint occurring when the balloon reaches its full cylindrical configuration. Dilation expands the safety margin as ureteroscopes are passed, and dilating to 15 Fr is both sufficient and has no detrimental effect on the structure or function of the orifice (54–56).

Prior to passing the flexible ureteroscope, it is recommended to place a second safety wire, which can be done through a dual access lumen. If multiple ureteroscopic passes are expected, we will also advance an access sheath over one of the wires. The flexible ureteroscope is then advanced over the guidewire and into the ureter using fluoroscopic monitoring to ensure proper positioning. Once the ureteroscope is in the ureter, the irrigation fluid is attached and direct visual advancement is performed over the guidewire. When the area of concern is encountered or the ureteroscope is in the pelvis, the wire is removed.

Biopsies within the ureter or pelvis are functionally different than bladder biopsies. In the bladder, the forceps can be applied perpendicularly to the area being biopsied, while the ureter requires the forceps to be applied parallel to the mucosa. A biopsy should be performed during the initial pass of the ureteroscope to prevent avulsing or traumatizing the lesion during instrument passage. A 3-Fr or 5-Fr cup forceps is carefully advanced with its jaws parallel to the ureteral wall. The intraluminal portion of the lesion is then grasped with the jaws and pulled free from the ureter. Only intraluminal tumor is resected and no attempt is made to take deep bites into the ureteral wall. Alternatively, a stone basket (1.9 or 2.4 Fr) may be used to snare exophytic tumors. It is recommended that the entire instrument be removed with the biopsy specimen as withdrawing the specimen through the instrument channel often leads to disappointment. The size of the biopsy is minute and should be placed at once into fixative (57). The base of the tumor is then fulgurated with a Bugbee or bipolar electrode while using an irrigant such as glycine or sorbitol.

The neodymium: yttrium-aluminum-garnet (Nd:YAG) and the holmium: yttrium-aluminum-garnet (Ho:YAG) lasers can also be utilized in place of electrocautery and fulguration. The Nd:YAG has a depth penetration of 5 mm to 6 mm and is used predominantly for deep tissue ablation with a recommended setting of 20 watts for one second (57,58). Higher settings, including 35 watts for two seconds, have caused transmural necrosis of the canine ureter (59). Optimal function requires that the laser fiber not be in actual contact with the tumor, or charring of the tip will occur. When applied parallel to the urothelial lumen, there is little risk for perforation. Complete mucosal healing has been demonstrated after 3 weeks (60). In contrast to the Nd:YAG, the Ho:YAG has a tissue penetration depth of 0.5 mm and should be kept in contact or very close to the tissue being ablated. The primary advantages of the Ho:YAG are for superficial ablation in the thin-walled ureter, aid in coagulation and hemostasis, and the ability to open the lumen of an occluding ureteral neoplasm (57). Most common settings for the Ho:YAG laser are 0.6 to 1.0 joules with a frequency of 8 to 10 hertz. Using the Nd:YAG laser for tumor debulking and the Ho:YAG laser for superficial ablation and coagulation, Keeley et al. reported eight recurrences in 41 renal units (19.5%) after a mean follow-up of 35.1 months (61). The ultimate role for lasers in endourologic management of upper-tract TCC remains to be determined, and at this time there is no clear difference between laser and electrocautery.

Complications of Retrograde Ureteropyeloscopy

Perforation of the ureter occurs at a reported rate of 0 to 10.2% (18,61,62). All reported cases were successfully managed conservatively with either a ureteral stent or nephrostomy tube. No long-term adverse sequelae have been reported following ureteral perforation, although there is a theoretical risk of extraluminal seeding or dissemination. This concern was first highlighted by Zincke's group, who reported on local recurrences in the renal fossa in two of 18 patients following nephroureterectomy for noninvasive TCC (63). Intraoperative pyeloscopy was performed in these patients during open exploration for indeterminate renal pelvis filling defects and the authors raised the concern about extraluminal seeding as a consequence of pyeloscopy. In addition, Lim et al. reported on submucosal lymphovascular invasion of TCC in a nephroureterectomy specimen immediately following ureteropyeloscopy (64). The authors suggested that the ureteroscopic procedure, utilizing pressurized saline irrigation at 200 mmHg, caused migration and seeding of the upper-tract TCC. In contrast to these studies, numerous others have reported no instances of extraluminal tumor implantation following ureteropyeloscopy, open pyeloscopy, or ureteral perforation during management of TCC (18,61,62,65,66). It is generally felt that risk for extraluminal seeding or TCC dissemination during retrograde management of upper-tract TCC is very small.

The reported stricture rate in large series following retrograde management of upper-tract TCC is 4.9% to 13.6% (18,61,62). Most of these are managed endoscopically with stent placement, Ho:YAG laser incision, or balloon dilation. Some authors have reported a decreased stricture rate with the use of lasers rather than electrocautery (57,59,61), although others have found no appreciable difference (62).

An unusual complication of endoscopic management is intrarenal pelvic explosion. Andrews and Segura reported on this case and suggested that minimizing the amount of continuous coagulation and subsequent intraluminal hydrogen formation can avoid this problem (67).

Percutaneous Management

If endourologic management is selected, it is our practice to approach all tumors using retrograde ureteropyeloscopy. If the tumor is not completely resectable, then an antegrade approach is performed. A percutaneous approach offers several practical advantages over retrograde ureteropyeloscopy, including better visibility, ability to use larger instrumentation, and improved access to virtually any renal unit including infundibulocalyceal tumors and in patients with prior urinary diversion. A number of centers have now used percutaneous management of upper-tract TCC with a success rate at least comparable to retrograde management.

At the authors' institution, percutaneous access is established in the radiology department under local anesthesia and intravenous sedation. We favor access under the 12th rib, as supracostal approaches have an increased risk of pleural injury. A 22-guage needle is passed through the posterior axillary line into the appropriate calyx with the patient in the prone position. A guidewire is then maneuvered down the ureter and an angiographic catheter is passed over the wire. A urinary catheter is left indwelling, and the patient is then brought to the endourology suite where general anesthesia is administered. This method has worked well in over 2,000 patients with stone disease and is easily adaptable (68).

In the prone position, a guidewire is placed down the angiographic catheter, which is then discarded. The tract is dilated to 30 Fr using flexible Amplatz dilators. Concentric steel dilators are preferred if there is dense scar tissue surrounding the kidney or if the tract is unstable due to long stretches of retroperitoneal fat. A second safety guidewire is then placed down the ureter and the rigid nephroscope is introduced into the collecting system.

If the tumor has not already been sampled, cold cup biopsies are obtained including the surrounding mucosa. The remaining intraluminal tumor is then removed with either the cold cup forceps or resectoscope. Because of the small renal pelvis capacity, the specimen must be removed and irrigation drained after each loop of resection. As with the retrograde approach, the loop excursion must avoid deep bites of the thin pelviocaliceal system and lack of supporting muscle. The tumor bed is then fulgurated with electrocautery. An angiographic catheter is advanced down the ureter and a 24 Fr nephrostomy tube is placed. The catheter is removed the following day after an antegrade pyelogram and the nephrostomy tube is pulled after tolerating a clamping trial. If there is concern for residual unresected disease or plans for topical therapy (see below), the percutaneous access is left in place.

Complications of Percutaneous Management

Violation of the urothelial lumen increases the potential risk of extraluminal seeding, particularly along the nephrostomy tube tract. At least two case reports have been published on nephrostomy tract seeding by high-grade TCC following percutaneous pyeloscopy and/or manipulation (69,70). However, in both of these cases, complete resection of the tumor was not performed and no adjuvant therapy was administered. Numerous other series have been reported where the primary tumor was resected at the time of percutaneous manipulation, all reporting no cases of nephrostomy tract seeding (18,62,71–82).

Single stage access, dilation, and tumor resection is recommended to reduce the risk of nephrostomy tract seeding (58). Furthermore, maintaining low intrarenal pressures by keeping the irrigation solution less than 40 cm above the patient is also beneficial (83). Access tract radiation with a commercial high-dose rate radiation delivery system or iridium wire is advocated by some investigators (75,79).

Other complications of percutaneous management are similar to those encountered in percutaneous management of stone disease. These include infection, bleeding, hemothorax, electrolyte abnormalities, injury to adjacent viscera, and perforation. No case of extraluminal seeding has been demonstrated. In contrast to retrograde management, the risk of stricture appears to be much less, with only one case of ureteropelvic junction stricture in 73 renal units (18,62,78,79).

Outcome Following Endourologic Management

The Mayo Clinic reported on 44 patients treated endourologically (37 ureteroscopy, 7 percutaneous) for upper-tract TCC (18). With a mean follow-up of 5 years, 38.6% patients had a local recurrence with six (14%) requiring nephroureterectomy. No tumor progressed in grade and only one recurrent tumor progressed in stage during follow-up. Of note, one patient had a local recurrence 64 months after initial treatment, emphasizing the need for long-term surveillance.

In 1997, Tawfiek and Bagley summarized 14 modern series of upper-tract TCC treated endourologically and found a recurrence rate of 33% for 61 renal pelvic tumors, 31.2% for 144 ureteral tumors, with recurrent bladder TCC occurring in 43.2% of patients (57). A more recent review of series published since 1996 on ureteroscopic treatment of upper-tract TCC found similar results: 22 of 60 (37%) tumors in the renal pelvis recurred, while 33 of 77 (43%) ureteral tumors recurred, and 19 of 137 (14%) patients ultimately required nephroureterectomy during surveillance (84). These recurrence rates are lower than rates from earlier studies of open nephron sparing surgery, where recurrences from renal pelvic tumors were as high as 62% (48). The most frequent site of recurrence following both endourologic management and nephroureterectomy is the bladder, and the risk for bladder recurrence does not appear to differ between the two treatments (27,30,48).

Recurrence is dependent on tumor grade. Average recurrences for grade 1 and 2 TCC are 16% (5% to 33%) and 22% (6% to 66%), respectively (78,79,82,85,86). Despite recurrence, death from low-grade TCC is rare (48). In contrast, grade 3 TCC carries a poor prognosis regardless of management. Lee et al. found no significant survival difference in patients with grade 3 disease treated with nephroureterectomy or initial percutaneous resection (85).

Because of frequent recurrence, patients need rigorous and lifelong follow-up after endourologic treatment. Although long-term recurrence (more than 5 years) can occur, most develop in the first 3 years after initial treatment (87). Provided no recurrence develops, we recommend cystoscopy and voided cytology every 3 months for 1 year, every 6 months for another year, then annually. Annual contralateral imaging with an EXU or retrograde is also recommended, although these lack sensitivity compared with ureteropyeloscopy (61,88). Thus, we recommend ureteropyeloscopy of the affected upper-tract unit be performed every 6 months for 3 years, then annually.

ADJUVANT TOPICAL THERAPY

Because at least one-third of patients managed endoscopically will develop a local recurrence, adjuvant topical chemotherapy and immunotherapy has been utilized. The most common method for adjuvant topical therapy delivery is via a nephrostomy tube. Other novel approaches include bladder instillation with an indwelling refluxing ureteral stent, a surgically manipulated refluxing system, or direct irrigation of a suprapubic externalized single J ureteral catheter.

Although the results of nonrandomized trials have varied, most authors have used intracavitary bacillus calmette–guerin (BCG) or mitomycin C. Orihuela and Smith found that patients treated with BCG via a nephrostomy tube had a recurrence rate of 16.6% compared to 80% recurrence for patients who did not receive BCG (74), although an update of their series did not demonstrate a survival advantage (78). Other studies have not shown a significant difference with adjuvant topical therapy compared with endoscopic treatment alone (18,61). The variability of these studies is likely due to selection bias and nonrandomized methods, and the true efficacy of adjuvant therapy awaits prospective randomized trials.

While the efficacy of adjuvant topical therapy is debated, most studies report that it is generally safe and well tolerated. The most common complication is bacterial sepsis. Maintaining low intrarenal pressures during administration and documenting a lack of obstruction or extravasation prior to instillation help prevent potential serious complications.

NEOADJUVANT SYSTEMIC CHEMOTHERAPY

Recently, enthusiasm for neoadjuvant platinum-based combination chemotherapy for invasive bladder cancer has emerged. For some time, neoadjuvant chemotherapy has been thought to offer some therapeutic advantages over surgical care alone. First, patients are better able to tolerate chemotherapy prior to debilitating surgical procedures. Second, giving chemotherapy before blood supply to the tumor has been altered offers the potential to deliver the drugs more effectively and at higher doses than in the adjuvant setting. Finally, many patients subsequently relapse in part due to undetectable metastases at the time of presentation, and earlier chemotherapy to smaller metastases offers improved susceptibility. Therefore, neoadjuvant chemotherapy offers the potential to deliver the drugs more effectively and at higher doses than the adjuvant setting.

Vale and colleagues from the Advanced Bladder Cancer Meta-analysis Collaboration recently reported on a systematic review of all relevant randomized trials of neoadjuvant chemotherapy for invasive bladder cancer (89). The results from this collaboration demonstrated a 5% 5-year improved survival in patients treated with neoadjuvant platinum-based chemotherapy. This validated the largest US trial of neoadjuvant chemotherapy prior to cystectomy, where among 317 patients with locally advanced bladder cancer, survival for patients receiving neoadjuvant chemotherapy was 77 months compared to 46 months for surgery alone (90).

Clinical regression rates of metastatic urothelial carcinoma from the upper urinary tract appear to be similar to those reported by investigators treating metastatic bladder cancer, although patients who have undergone nephroureterectomy appear to be at a distinct disadvantage (91). There is no data available to show that removal of the primary lesion in the presence of metastatic disease improves survival, and nephroureterectomy requires chemotherapy dose reductions potentially adversely affecting outcome (92).

CONCLUSION

Nephroureterectomy with bladder cuff resection remains the gold standard for treatment of upper-tract TCC. However, to say that all patients with upper-tract TCC need nephroureterectomy is analogous to saying that all patients with carcinoma of the bladder need cystectomy. Distal ureterectomy, or, more rarely, segmental ureterectomy, can provide regional control with renal preservation. The advent of sophisticated endourologic techniques has improved diagnostic accuracy, allowed pathologic confirmation of tumor grade, and can potentially stage upper-tract TCC. The results of endourologic management have been encouraging and can often be the first line of therapy in patients with a functional solitary kidney, bilateral disease, or those at risk for dialysis following organ removal. In patients with a normal contralateral kidney, endourological management can successfully be accomplished in a select group with low-grade, solitary, accessible lesions. Endourologic management has high recurrence rates, although usually not of increased grade or stage, and requires lifelong diligent surveillance. The role of adjuvant topical chemotherapy or immunotherapy appears well tolerated, but reports of efficacy are uncontrolled and anecdotal. Neoadjuvant chemotherapy should be considered in patients with localized high-grade invasive disease prior to surgical extirpation.

References

1. Munoz JJ, Ellison LM. Upper tract urothelial neoplasms: incidence and survival during the last 2 decades. *J Urol* 2000;164:1523–1525.
2. Gittes RF. Management of transitional cell carcinoma of the upper tract: case for conservative local excision. *Urol Clin North Am* 1980;7:559–568.
3. Bennington JL, Beckwith JB. Tumors of the kidney, renal pelvis, and ureter. *Atlas of tumor pathology, second series, fascicle 12.* Washington, DC: Armed Forces Institute of Pathology, 1975.
4. Blute ML. Endourology: management of upper tract genitourinary pathology. *Curr Probl Urol* 1991;1:4.
5. McDonald MW, Zincke H. Urothelial tumors of the upper urinary tract. In: deKernion JR, Paulson DF, eds. *Genitourinary cancer management.* Philadelphia, PA: Lea & Febiger, 1987:1–39.
6. Charbit L, Gendreau MC, Mee S, et al. Tumors of the upper urinary tract: 10 years experience. *J Urol* 1991;146:1243–1246.
7. Shinka T, Uekado Y, Aoshi H, et al. Occurrence of uroepithelial tumors of the upper urinary tract after the initial diagnosis of bladder cancer. *J Urol* 1988;140:745–748.
8. Petkovic SD. Conservation of the kidney in operations for tumors of the renal pelvis and calyces: report of 26 cases. *Br J Urol* 1972;44:1–8.
9. Zincke H, Garbeff PJ, Beahrs JR. Upper urinary tract transitional cell cancer after radical cystectomy for bladder cancer. *J Urol* 1984;131:50–52.
10. Herr HW. Long-term results of BCG therapy: concern about upper tract tumors. *Semin Urol Oncol* 1998;15:13–16.
11. Jensen OM, Knudsen JB, McLaughlin JL, et al. The Copenhagen case-control study of renal pelvis and ureter cancer: role of smoking and occupational exposures. *Int J Cancer* 1988;41:557–561.
12. Palvio DH, Anderson JC, Falk E. Transitional cell tumors of the renal pelvis and ureter associated with capillarosclerosis indicating analgesic abuse. *Cancer* 1987;59:972–976.

13. Babaian RJ, Johnson DE. Primary carcinoma of the ureter. *J Urol* 1980; 123:357–359.
14. Stein A, Sova Y, Lurie M, et al. Adenocarcinoma of the renal pelvis: report of two cases, one with simultaneous transitional cell carcinoma of the bladder. *Urol Int* 1988;43:299–301.
15. Ross RK, Paganini-Hill A, Landolph J, et al. Analgesics, cigarette smoking, and other risk factors for cancer of the renal pelvis and ureter. *Cancer Res* 1989;49:1045–1048.
16. Frischer Z, Waltzer WC, Fonder MJ. Bilateral transitional cell carcinoma of the renal pelvis in the cancer family syndrome. *J Urol* 1985;134:1197–1198.
17. Orphali SI, Shols GW, Hagewood T, et al. Familial transitional cell carcinoma of renal pelvis and upper ureter. *Urology* 1986;27:394–396.
18. Elliott DS, Blute ML, Patterson DE, et al. Long-term follow-up of endoscopically treated upper urinary tract transitional cell carcinoma. *Urology* 1996;47:819–825.
19. Melamed MR, Reuter VE. Pathology and staging of urothelial tumors of the kidney and ureter. *Urol Clin North Am* 1993;20:333–347.
20. Say CS, Jori JM. Transitional cell carcinoma of the renal pelvis: experience from 1940-1972 and literature review. *J Urol* 1974;112:438–442.
21. Greene FL, Page DL, Fleming ID, et al. *AJCC cancer staging manual,* 6th ed. New York: Springer-Verlag, 2002.
22. Li MK, Cheung WL. Squamous cell carcinoma of the renal pelvis. *J Urol* 1987;138:269–271.
23. Peterson RO. *Urologic pathology.* Philadelphia, PA: J.B. Lippincott, 1986:762.
24. Auld CD, Grigor KM, Fowler JW. Histopathological review of transitional cell carcinoma of the upper urinary tract. *Br J Urol* 1984;56:485–489.
25. Malek RS, Aquilo JJ, Hattery RR. Radiolucent filling defects of the renal pelvis: classification and report of unusual cases. *J Urol* 1975;114:508–513.
26. Zincke J, Aquilo JJ, Farrow GM, et al. Significance of urine cytology in the early detection of transitional cell cancer of the upper urinary tract. *J Urol* 1976;116:781–783.
27. Murphy DM, Zincke H, Furlow WL. Management of high-grade transitional cell cancer of the upper urinary tract. *J Urol* 1981;135:25–29.
28. Grace DA, Taylor WN, Taylor JN, et al. Carcinoma of the renal pelvis: a 15-year review. *J Urol* 1997;98:566–569.
29. Farrow GM, Utz DC, Rife CC. Morphological and clinical observations of patients with early bladder cancer treated with total cystectomy. *Cancer Res* 1976;36:2495–2501.
30. Murphy DM, Zincke H, Furlow WL. Primary grade 1 transitional cell carcinoma of the renal pelvis and ureter. *J Urol* 1980;123:629–631.
31. Sarnacki CT, McCormick LJ, Kiser WS, et al. Urinary cytology and the clinical diagnosis of urinary tract malignancy: a clinicopathologic study of 1400 patients. *J Urol* 1971;106:761–764.
32. Sheline M, Amendola MA, Pollack HM, et al. Fluoroscopically guided retrograde brush biopsy in the diagnosis of transitional cell carcinoma of the upper urinary tract: results in 45 patients. *AJR Am J Roentgenol* 1989; 153:313–316.
33. Huffman JL, Morse MJ, Herr HW, et al. Ureteropyeloscopy: the diagnosis and therapeutic approach to upper tract urothelial tumors. *World J Urol* 1985;3:58.
34. Gill WB, Lu CT, Thomsen S. Retrograde brushing: a new technique for obtaining histologic and cytologic material from ureteral, renal pelvic and renal caliceal lesions. *J Urol* 1973;109:573–578.
35. Blute RD Jr, Gittes RR, Gittes RF. Renal brush biopsy: survey of indications, techniques and results. *J Urol* 1981;126:146–149.
36. Streem SB, Pontes J, Novick AC, et al. Ureteropyeloscopy in the evaluation of upper tract filling defects. *J Urol* 1986;136:383–385.
37. Bagley DH, Rivas D. Upper urinary tract filling defects: flexible ureteroscopic diagnosis. *J Urol* 1990;143:1196–2000.
38. Bagley DH, Rivas D. Flexible ureteropyeloscopy: diagnosis and treatment in the upper urinary tract. *J Urol* 1987;138:280–285.
39. Keeley FX, Kulp DA, Bibbo M, et al. Diagnostic accuracy of ureteroscopic biopsy in upper tract transitional cell carcinoma. *J Urol* 1997;157:33–37.
40. Sagalowsky AI, Jarrett TW. Management of urothelial tumors of the renal pelvis and ureter. In: Walsh PC, Retik AD, Vaughan ED, et al., eds. *Campbell's urology,* 8th ed. Philadelphia, PA: WB Saunders, 2002:2845–2875.
41. McCoy M, Honda H, Resnick M, et al. Computed tomography for detection and staging of localized and pathologically defined upper tract urothelial tumors. *J Urol* 1991;146:1500–1503.
42. Badalament RA, Bennett WF, Bova JG, et al. Computed tomography of primary transitional cell carcinoma of upper urinary tracts. *Urology* 1992; 40:71–75.
43. Huffman JL, Bagley DH, Lyon ES, et al. Endoscopic diagnosis and treatment of upper-tract urothelial tumors. A preliminary report. *Cancer* 1985;55: 1422–1428.
44. Heney NM, Nocks BN, Daly JJ, et al. Prognostic factors in carcinoma of the ureter. *J Urol* 1981;125:632–636.
45. Chesko SB, Gray GF, McCarron JP. Urothelial neoplasia of the upper urinary tract. In: Sommers SC, Rosen PP, eds. *Pathology annual,* Part 2. New York: Appleton Century-Crofts, 1981:127–153.
46. Krogh J, Kvist E, Rye B. Transitional cell carcinoma of the upper urinary tract: prognostic variables and post-operative recurrences. *Br J Urol* 1991; 67:32–36.
47. Blute ML, Tsushima K, Farrow GM, et al. Transitional cell carcinoma of the renal pelvis: nuclear deoxyribonucleic acid ploidy studied by flow cytometry. *J Urol* 1988;140:944–949.

48. Zincke H, Neves RJ. Feasibility of conservative surgery for transitional cell cancer of the upper urinary tract. *Urol Clin North Am* 1984;11:717–724.

49. Abercrombie GF, Eardley I, Payne SR, et al. Modified nephro-ureterectomy: long-term follow-up with particular reference to subsequent bladder tumors. *Br J Urol* 1988;61:198–200.

50. Mazeman I. Tumors of the upper urinary tract, calyces, renal pelvis and ureter. *Eur Urol* 1976;2:120–126.

51. Hall MC, Womack S, Sagalowsky AI, et al. Prognostic factors, recurrence and survival in transitional cell carcinoma of the upper urinary tract: a 30-year experience in 252 patients. *Urology* 1998;52:594–601.

52. Guinan P, Vogelzang NJ, Randazzo R, et al. Renal pelvic cancer: a review of 611 patients treated in Illinois 1975–1985. *Urology* 1992;40:393–399.

53. Elliott DS, Segura JW, Lightner D, et al. Is nephroureterectomy necessary in all cases of upper tract transitional cell carcinoma? Long-term results of conservative endourologic management of upper tract transitional cell carcinoma in individuals with a normal contralateral kidney. *Urology* 2001;58:174–178.

54. Greene LF. The renal and ureteral changes induced by dilating the ureter. An experimental study. *J Urol* 1944;52:505–521.

55. Ford TF, Parkinson MC, Wickham JE. Clinical and experimental evaluation of ureteric dilatation. *Br J Urol* 1984;56:460–463.

56. Huffman JL, Bagley DH. Balloon dilation of the ureter for ureteroscopy. *J Urol* 1988;140:954–956.

57. Tawfiek ER, Bagley DH. Upper-tract transitional cell carcinoma. *Urology* 1997;50:321–329.

58. Clark PE, Streem SB. Endourologic management of upper tract transitional cell carcinoma. *AUA Update Series* 1999;16:122–127.

59. Smith JA Jr, Lse RG, Dixon JA. Tissue effects on neodymium:YAG laser photoradiation of canine ureters. *J Surg Oncol* 1984;27:168–171.

60. Schilling A, Bowering R, Keiditsch E. Use of the neodymium-YAG laser in the treatment of ureteral tumors and urethral condylomata accuminata. *Eur Urol* 1986;12(Suppl. 1):30–33.

61. Keeley FX Jr, Bibbo M, Bagley DH. Ureteroscopic treatment and surveillance of upper urinary tract transitional cell carcinoma. *J Urol* 1997;157:1560–1565.

62. Martinez-Pineiro JA, Matres MJG, Martinez-Pineiro L. Endourological treatment of upper tract urothelial carcinomas: analysis of a series of 59 tumors. *J Urol* 1996;156:377–385.

63. Tomera KM, Leary FJ, Zincke H. Pyeloscopy in urothelial tumors. *J Urol* 1982;127:1088–1089.

64. Lim DJ, Shattuck MC, Cook WA. Pyelovenous lymphatic migration of transitional cell carcinoma following flexible ureteroscopy. *J Urol* 1993;149:109–111.

65. McCarron JP, Mills C, Vaughan ED Jr. Tumors of the renal pelvis and ureter: current concepts and management. *Semin Urol* 1983;1:75–81.

66. Kulp DA, Bagley DH. Does flexible ureteropyeloscopy promote local recurrence of transitional cell carcinoma? *J Endourol* 1994;8:111–113.

67. Andrews PA, Segura JW. Renal pelvic explosion during conservative management of upper tract urothelial cancer. *J Urol* 1991;146:407–408.

68. Blute ML, Segura JW. Percutaneous nephrolithotomy. In: Marshall FF, ed. *Operative urology*, Chap. 80. Philadelphia, PA: WB Saunders, 1991.

69. Huang A, Low RK, White RD. Nephrostomy tract tumor seeding following percutaneous manipulation of a ureteral carcinoma. *J Urol* 1995;153:1041–1042.

70. Yamada Y, Kobayashi Y, Yao A, et al. Nephrostomy tract tumor seeding following percutaneous manipulation of a renal pelvic carcinoma. *Acta Urologica Japonica* 2002;48:415–418.

71. Gerber GS, Lyon ES. Endourologic management of upper tract urothelial tumors. *J Urol* 1993;150:2–7.

72. Streem SB, Pontes EJ. Percutaneous management of upper tract transitional cell carcinoma. *J Urol* 1986;135:773–775.

73. Woodhouse CRJ, Kellett MJ, Bloom HJ. Percutaneous renal surgery and local radiotherapy in the management of renal pelvic transitional cell carcinoma. *Br J Urol* 1986;58:245–249.

74. Orihuela E, Smith AD. Percutaneous treatment of transitional cell carcinoma of the upper urinary tract. *Urol Clin North Am* 1988;15:425–431.

75. Nolan RL, Nickel JC, Froud PI. Percutaneous endourologic approach for transitional cell carcinoma of the renal pelvis. *Urol Radiol* 1988;9:217–219.

76. Blute ML, Segura JW, Patterson DE, et al. Impact of endourology on the diagnosis and management of upper urinary tract urothelial cancer. *J Urol* 1989;141:1298–1301.

77. Tasca A, Zattoni F, Garbeglio A, et al. The case for a percutaneous approach to transitional cell carcinoma of the renal pelvis. *J Urol* 1990;143:902–904.

78. Jarrett TW, Sweester PM, Weiss GH, et al. Percutaneous management of transitional cell carcinoma of the renal collecting system: 9-year experience. *J Urol* 1995;154:1629–1635.

79. Patel A, Soonawalla P, Shepherd SF, et al. Long term outcome after percutaneous treatment of transitional cell carcinoma of the renal pelvis. *J Urol* 1996;155:868–874.

80. Tasca A, Zattoni F, Garbeglio A, et al. Endourologic treatment of transitional cell carcinoma of the upper urinary tract. *J Endourol* 1992;6:253–256.

81. Schoenberg MP, Van Arsdalen KN, Wein AJ. The management of transitional cell carcinoma in solitary renal units. *J Urol* 1991;146:700–703.

82. Clark PC, Streem SB, Geisinger MA. 13-year experience with percutaneous management of upper tract transitional cell carcinoma. *J Urol* 1999;161:772–775.

83. Streem SB. Percutaneous management of upper-tract transitional cell carcinoma. *Urol Clin North Am* 1995;22:221–229.

84. Chen GL, Bagley DH. Ureteroscopic surgery for upper tract transitional-cell carcinoma: complications and management. *J Endourol* 2001;15:399–404.

85. Lee BR, Jabbour ME, Marshall FF, et al. 13-year survival comparison of percutaneous and open nephroureterectomy approaches for management of transitional cell carcinoma of renal collecting system: equivalent outcomes. *J Endourol* 1999;13:289–294.

86. Jabbour ME, Desgrandchamps F, Cazin S, et al. Percutaneous management of grade II upper urinary tract transitional cell carcinoma: the long-term outcome. *J Urol* 2000;163:1105–1107.

87. Mills IW, Laniado ME, Patel A. The role of endoscopy in the management of patients with upper urinary tract transitional cell carcinoma. *BJU Int* 2001;87:150–162.

88. Chen GL, El-Gabry EA, Bagley DH. Surveillance of upper urinary tract transitional cell carcinoma: the role of ureteroscopy, retrograde pyelography, cytology, and urinalysis. *J Urol* 2000;164:1901–1964.

89. Advanced Bladder Cancer Meta-analysis Collaboration. Neoadjuvant chemotherapy in invasive bladder cancer: a systematic review and meta-analysis. *Lancet* 2003;361:1927–1934.

90. Grossman HB, Natale RB, Tangen CM, et al. Neoadjuvant chemotherapy plus cystectomy compared with cystectomy alone for locally advanced bladder cancer. *N Engl J Med* 2003;349:859–866.

91. Blute ML. Treatment of upper urinary tract transitional cell carcinoma. In: Smith AD, ed. *Smith's textbook of endourology*. St. Louis, MO: Quality Medical Publications, 1996:352–365.

92. Lerner SE, Blute ML, Richardson RL, et al. Platinum-based chemotherapy for advanced transitional cell carcinoma of the upper urinary tract. *Mayo Clin Proc* 1996;71:945–950.

CHAPTER 24B
Laparoscopic Management of Upper Tract Tumors

Erik S. Weise and Howard N. Winfield

INTRODUCTION

The standard treatment for upper-tract transitional cell carcinoma (TCC) has been open nephroureterectomy with ipsilateral bladder cuff excision. Laparoscopic nephroureterectomy was first described by Clayman et al. in 1991 (1), based on their pioneering work with laparoscopic nephrectomy (2,3). The procedure was replicated shortly thereafter by other centers around the world (4,5), and is now considered a new standard of care at many centers dedicated to minimally invasive surgery. However, accrual of large series has occurred slowly due to the relative rarity of upper-tract TCC.

PATIENT PRESENTATION AND EVALUATION

Gross or microscopic hematuria is the most common presentation of upper-tract TCC. Flank pain, caused by obstructing tumor or blood clot, may occur. Asymptomatic lesions may be found on upper tract imaging that is mandatory with diagnosis and follow-up of bladder cancer, or as an incidental finding on imaging for other reasons. We prefer intravenous urography in all patients to characterize the suspicious lesion and evaluate the contralateral upper tract. Computerized tomography with a urographic phase (Fig. 24B.1) is an alternative that is gaining in popularity with radiologists, and may add staging information. Evaluation of a patient with suspected upper-tract transitional cell cancer usually includes a diagnostic procedure, which begins with careful urethrocystoscopy. Upper-tract urinary cytology is obtained with the aid of a

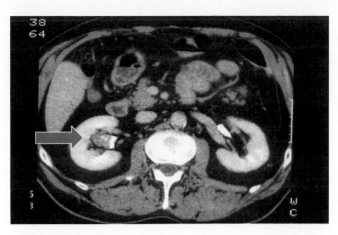

FIGURE 24B.1. Transitional cell carcinoma (TCC) of the right renal pelvis (*arrow*) on excretory phase of computed tomography.

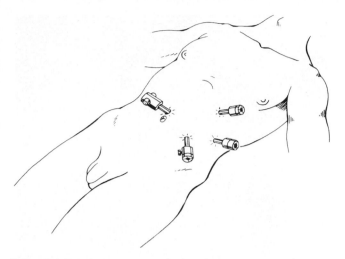

FIGURE 24B.2. Laparoscopic radical nephroureterectomy: placement of umbilical camera port, two working ports in the midclavicular line, and a port for assistance in the anterior axillary line.

ureteral catheter. Retrograde pyelography is then performed, followed by ureteropyeloscopy and biopsy of any lesions. For limited disease of low-grade appearance, endoscopic management is a consideration. Manipulation of the contralateral upper tract is avoided to prevent possible seeding with tumor cells. Metastatic evaluation is completed. Contraindications to laparoscopic nephroureterectomy are the same as for open surgery. The open surgical approach is recommended for select patients, in which segmental ureterectomy or distal ureterectomy and reimplantation is indicated.

PREOPERATIVE MANAGEMENT

Patients who are to undergo laparoscopic nephroureterectomy observe a clear liquid diet the day before their operation and administer a Fleet enema the evening prior to surgery. A first generation cephalosporin is administered preoperatively and continued for 24 hours. All patients wear venous compression stockings and lower extremity serial compression devices throughout their hospital stay. The procedure is performed under general endotracheal anesthetic without the use of nitrous agents. Foley catheter is placed. Orogastric tube is maintained on suction and removed with extubation.

TECHNIQUE

Laparoscopic nephroureterectomy consists of three distinct parts: (a) radical nephrectomy; (b) management of distal ureter and bladder cuff; and (c) specimen extraction. For the first, well-developed techniques exist for standard transperitoneal laparoscopy, hand-assisted laparoscopy, standard retroperitoneoscopy, and hand-assisted retroperitoneoscopy. For the second, many alternatives have been described and no universally accepted technique has emerged. Specimen extraction is also of critical importance to the oncologic safety of this operation.

Radical Nephrectomy

Standard Transperitoneal Technique

We normally perform the nephrectomy portion first, using a transperitoneal approach. The patient is initially placed in a 70-degree decubitus position. In most patients four to five trocars are used. The camera port is placed at the umbilicus, two working ports are placed in the midclavicular line above and

below the camera, and a port for assistance is placed in the anterior axillary line (Fig. 24B.2). An additional port is placed in the midaxillary line to allow for liver retraction in right-sided cases (Fig. 24B.3). The colon is reflected medially by incision along the white line of Toldt. Having entered into the retroperitoneal space, the renal hilum is dissected. Once the renal artery and vein are isolated, they are clipped and transected. Normally we doubly clip the renal artery with Hemolock clips (Weck, Baxter Healthcare Corp., Deerfield, IL) on the body side and singly on the kidney side (Fig. 24B.4). The renal vein is stapled and transected with an EndoGIA-30 vascular stapler (U.S. Surgical-Tyco Healthcare Group, Norwalk, CT). The kidney with investing perirenal fat and Gerota's fascia is then mobilized. When indicated, the adrenal gland is spared. The proximal ureter is quickly identified and clipped, but not transected. The ureter is then dissected distally using a pure laparoscopic technique. Normally we can dissect the ureter down in this fashion to the bladder. Crossing structures such as the gonadal vein, obliterated umbilical ligament, and vas deferens/round and broad ligaments are mobilized or transected as necessary. Lymph node dissection is carried out if preoperative evaluation or intraoperative findings are suspicious.

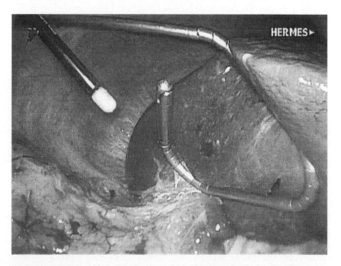

FIGURE 24B.3. Liver retraction with Diamond Flex snake retractor (Snowden Pencer, Tucker, GA) through 5-mm midaxillary port.

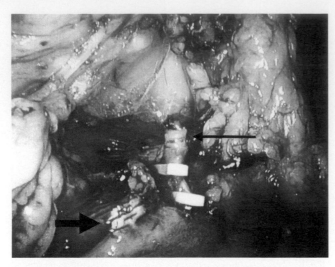

FIGURE 24B.4. The renal artery has been doubly clipped with He-molock clips on the body side, and transected (*thin arrow*). The renal vein has been transected with the endo GIA stapler; three rows of sta-ples are visible on the renal vein stump (*thick arrow*).

Hand-assisted Transperitoneal Technique

Hand-assisted nephrectomy was developed by Nakada et al. (6) and was later applied to nephroureterectomy by Keeley et al. (7). Various sites for the hand port have been described, including flank, supra- or infraumbilical midline, or iliac re-gions (8–10). Increasing numbers of hand port devices are now commercially available (11). The operative steps are analogous to standard laparoscopy and have recently been re-viewed in detail (12).

Retroperitoneal Technique

Modern retroperitoneoscopy began when Gaur developed a retroperitoneal dilation balloon (13) and reported the first retroperitoneal nephrectomy (14). Nephroureterectomy by this approach was first performed for benign indications (15) and subsequently for malignant disease in 1996 (16). With the pa-tient in full flank position, a finger is inserted through a small incision at the tip of the 12th rib, and a space is created be-tween the psoas muscle and Gerota's fascia (17). A trocar-mounted distention device that allows direct observation with the laparoscope (U.S. Surgical-Tyco Healthcare Group, Nor-walk, CT) is used to create a retroperitoneal working space, displacing the kidney anteriorly. Two or three working ports are placed and the hilum is dissected from the posterior as-pect, followed by mobilization of the kidney and ureter.

Hand-assisted retroperitoneal approach has been devel-oped (18) whereby the incision for the hand port is made ini-tially in a vertical pararectus position. Manual dissection of the retroperitoneal space is followed by the creation of the pneumoretroperitoneum.

Management of the Distal Ureter and Bladder Cuff

Authors' Technique

In our practice, dissection of the most distal portion of the ureter is performed by hand assistance. We use a small Pfan-nenstiel incision with a vertical fascial incision, creating a cru-ciate-type opening, which essentially becomes sealed by the surgeon's forearm, obviating the need for a hand port device. Under digital manipulation the remaining ureter is dissected to

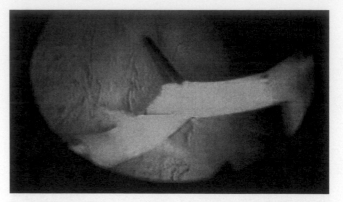

FIGURE 24B.5. The ureteral orifice and remnant ureter are unroofed with the Collins' knife.

the bladder and partially out of its intramural tunnel. With the ureterovesical junction almost fully dissected and with gentle traction on the ureter, an endoscopic GIA stapler is used to lig-ate and transect the ureter, taking also a small bladder cuff. The specimen (kidney, ureter, and bladder cuff) is then ex-tracted intact through the hand port.

After completion of the laparoscopic portion, the patient is placed in dorsal lithotomy position and the involved hemitrigone is inspected cystoscopically. If the endo-GIA sta-ple line is immediately visualized, the overlying mucosa is ex-tensively fulgurated for a circumference of 1 cm and the procedure is terminated. If a remnant of ureteral tunnel is ob-served, it is unroofed with a Collins' knife (Fig. 24B.5) until the staple line is visible and the mucosa of the intramural ureter and its surroundings are extensively fulgurated with a roller ball electrode.

Ureteral Unroofing

Our technique is based on the Washington University tech-nique, which itself has been modified (19) and now consists of standard laparoscopic dissection of the distal ureter and trans-section with the endoscopic GIA followed by transurethral unroofing and fulguration of the ureteral tunnel remnant (20). Another similar technique consists of antegrade dissec-tion of the ureterovesical junction and transection with the endo-GIA stapler, without hand assistance or adjunct cys-toscopy (21). The use of endo-GIA titanium staples in the bladder raises concern for encrustation, as observed with uri-nary diversion. Application in patients was preceded by the observation that no problems arose in the porcine model (22). We have not seen stone formation in our patients over the course of a decade, an experience shared by Shalhav et al. (20). Another author reported an exposed and nonencrusted staple line on 6-month surveillance and removed all staples without sequelae (23).

Transurethral Resection or Excision of the Ureteral Orifice ("Pluck" Technique)

Transurethral resection of the ureteral orifice with a loop elec-trode prior to nephroureterectomy—the so-called "pluck" technique—was described by McDonald et al. in 1952 (24). Chiu et al. combined it with laparoscopic nephroureterectomy (4). Rassweiler described transurethral excision of the orifice using a hot knife (5). Whether resection or excision is used, the goal of this technique is to completely detach the ureter from the bladder, so that it can be "plucked" during subse-quent antegrade dissection. Others have described transection of the ureter with distal intussusception and extraction aided by transurethral manipulation (25).

Open Technique

Standard open technique to mobilize and remove the distal ureter with a bladder cuff has been used following (16) or preceding (26) the laparoscopic portion. This technique is well described in urologic textbooks (27) and can usually be accomplished through the small Pfannenstiel midline incision that has been described previously.

Transvesical Technique

Gill et al. developed a transvesical approach, using two needle-scopic ports (2 mm) placed directly into the bladder and a transurethral resectoscope to excise the ureteral orifice with a Collins' knife (28). The distal ureter is occluded with a 2 mm endoloop. This is usually followed by a retroperitoneal nephroureterectomy. Three authors described modification of this approach to the distal ureter for use with hand assistance. Stifelman et al. used one transvesical trocar and a resectoscope (10). Gonzales et al. favored a transvesical nephroscope to circumscribe the ureteral orifice after the laparoscopic portion (29). Transurethral manipulation and ureteral occlusion are omitted. Wong et al. described transurethrally excising the ureteral orifice after the nephrectomy portion, coming full circle from the pluck technique, with the difference that it is performed after the nephrectomy portion and immediately precedes removal of the specimen (30).

Specimen Extraction

Initial reports of laparoscopic nephroureterectomy for TCC described specimen entrapment in an impermeable sac (Lap-Sac, Cook Urological, Spencer, IN) and subsequent morcellation and extraction with an electric tissue morcellator or a finger (1,5). Morcellation was rapidly abandoned (31), as there were important concerns for tumor spillage with this approach. Removing the specimen intact allows for improved assessment of pathologic stage, grade, and margin status, factors that have import in determining adjuvant treatment. Intact specimen removal with or without (32) a sac is now widely practiced. We strongly recommend using a sac, especially if the specimen size significantly exceeds the size of the extraction incision. Three port site recurrences have been reported (33–35). In one case, the specimen was not entrapped and in another the entrapment device ruptured. In the third case the ureteral stent was protruding from the renal pelvis during laparoscopy. It is our experience that the LapSac is the most robust on the market. We extract our specimens through the Pfannenstiel incision. Other sites for extraction may include midline, subcostal, Gibson, and flank (16,31,36,37).

POSTOPERATIVE MANAGEMENT

Routine pain management includes intravenous ketorolac, if appropriate for the individual patient, initiated at the conclusion of the procedure and continued for 5 doses. Supplemental narcotics are given as needed. Postoperatively, on the day of surgery, patients are encouraged to ambulate and receive clear liquid diet, which is advanced if tolerated.

OUTCOMES

Perioperative Outcomes

Several single institution series have compared laparoscopic to open nephroureterectomy. Estimated blood loss was lower in the laparoscopic patients in all but one study. Operative times were usually comparable between the groups. In a minority of studies the laparoscopic approach took longer. Laparoscopic time was shorter in one study using the retroperitoneal approach. Parameters of convalescence consistently demonstrated a benefit in the laparoscopic groups. Conversion to open surgery was an uncommon event. There was no consistent excess of complications in either group (18,26,36–43). Perioperative outcomes in series comparing standard and hand-assisted to open nephroureterectomy are summarized in Tables 24B.1 and 24B.2, respectively.

Two comparisons between standard and hand-assisted laparoscopy have been published. No statistically significant differences were identified in the small series. There was a trend toward longer operative time and shorter convalescence in the standard laparoscopy group in one study (44). The authors of the other study noticed increased wound complications in the hand-assisted group and abandoned the technique in favor of standard laparoscopy (45).

Two series evaluated the financial aspects of laparoscopic nephroureterectomy. While both showed higher operating room charges for laparoscopy, they calculated similar overall hospital cost (39,46), demonstrating that minimally invasive procedures can be performed in dedicated centers of excellence

---

TABLE 24B.1

COMPARATIVE SERIES OF LAPAROSCOPIC (L) VERSUS OPEN (O) NEPHROURETERECTOMY FOR UPPER-TRACT TRANSITIONAL CELL CARCINOMA

	No. of patients L/O	EBL (cc)	OR time (min)	Hospital stay (d)	Time to oral intake (d)	Analgesic use (mg)	Normal activity (wk)	Convalescence (wk)
Shalhav et al. (20) Transperitoneal	25/17	199/441[a]	462/234[a]	6.1/12	1/4.8[a]	37/144[a]	2.8/10	
Gill et al. (36) Retroperitoneal	42/35	242/696[a]	225/280[a]	2.3/6.6[a]	1.6/3.2[a]	26/228[a]	4.7/8.2[a]	8/14.4[a]
McNeill et al. (38) Transperitoneal	25/42		165/165	9.1/10.7				
Matsui et al. (43) Retroperitoneal	17/17	151/300[a]	287/240[a]	2.7/4.2[a]	2.2/2.5	75/178	2.3/2.8[a]	
Klinger et al. (42) 14 Trans./5 Retro.	19/15	282/532[a]	198/220	8.1/13.3[a]		190/590[a]		

EBL, estimated blood loss; OR, odd ratio.
[a]$P < .05$.

TABLE 24B.2

COMPARATIVE SERIES OF HAND-ASSISTED LAPAROSCOPIC (L) VERSUS OPEN (O) NEPHROURETERECTOMY
FOR UPPER-TRACT TRANSITIONAL CELL CARCINOMA

	No. of patients L/O	EBL (cc)	OR time (min)	Hospital stay (day)	Time to oral intake (day)	Analgesic use (mg)	Normal activity (wk)	Convalescence (wk)
Seifman et al. (39) Transperitoneal	16/11	557/345	320/199[a]	3.9/5.2[a]	1.4/1.6[a]	48/81	2.7/5.6[a]	
Stifelman et al. (40) Transperitoneal	11/11	147/311[a]	291/232	4.6/6.1[a]	1.3/2.3	45/44		
Chen et al. (26) Transperitoneal	7/15	140/455[a]	224/216	7.9/9.1[a]	1.4/2.6[a]	38/70[a]		3.7/5.6[a]
Li et al. (41) Transperitoneal	9/35	146/546[a]	267/273	7.6/10.8[a]	2.6/2.1	69/158[a]		
Kawauchi et al. (18) Retroperitoneal	34/34	236/427[a]	263/259	13.8/21.1[a]	1.8/2.1[a]	2.1/1.4[a,b]	3.4/4.4[a]	

EBL, estimated blood loss; OR, odd ratio.
[a]$P < .05$.
[b]analgesia frequency.

in a financially equivalent manner. This does not take into account the monetary value of earlier return to productivity and improved convalescence associated with laparoscopy.

Oncologic Outcomes

Long-term reports of cancer-specific outcomes are emerging. The only available 5-year data was published in abstract form (47). Cancer-specific survival in 65 patients who underwent laparoscopic nephroureterectomy was 94% at 1 year and 91% at 5 years, compared to 95% at 1 year and 83% at 5 years in 44 patients who underwent the open operation. Two comparative series (37,38) found similar survival with 2-year to 3-year follow-up in the laparoscopic group and longer follow-up in the open group. Two other studies comparing laparoscopic and open nephroureterectomy reported no difference in the cancer-specific survival, adjusted for shorter follow-up in the laparoscopic cohort (36,43); median follow-up in the laparoscopic patients was under 1 year in both studies. In a multicenter review of 116 patients with laparoscopic nephroureterectomy, the 1-year and 2-year cancer-specific survival was 92% and 83%, respectively, comparable to reports of open surgery (48).

While the available data indicates oncologic effectiveness comparable to the open standard nephroureterectomy, larger long-term studies are necessary before laparoscopic nephroureterectomy can be considered equivalent.

CONTROVERSY: MANAGEMENT OF THE DISTAL URETER

From an oncologic perspective, optimal management of the distal ureter should primarily: (a) provide an intact specimen consisting of kidney, ureter, and bladder cuff; (b) avoid leakage of urine from the affected kidney, which may be laden with tumor cells and (c) avoid leakage of urine from the bladder. Tumor cells from the ipsilateral upper tract may be present in the bladder. Also, there is potential for occult lesions in the bladder and the contralateral upper tract as TCC is a pan-urothelial disease. Finally, such a technique should be time-efficient and straightforward to perform.

The standard open technique yields an optimal specimen, good control of proximal leakage, and allows for careful handling of the cystotomy to minimize spillage of bladder urine.

Our technique, as described, of transection of the bladder cuff with the endo-GIA stapler after completion of the nephrectomy portion followed by cystoscopic assessment and unroofing and fulguration of any remnant ureter should completely avoid leakage of urine. However, in our experience the quality of the bladder cuff is not consistently optimal. Other authors have evaluated a similar technique and have reported the absence of any ureteral remnants on postoperative cystoscopy (21). Even so, the stapler is almost 10 mm wide, resulting in an approximately 5-mm cuff of opposing mucosa incorporated in the staple line. Any transitional cell neoplasm arising from this mucosa, even biologically superficial, would constitute extravesical disease and not be amenable to transurethral treatment.

Initial transurethral excision of the ureteral orifice would be expected to lead to extravasation of urine from the affected kidney, even if the ureter is clipped early in the nephrectomy portion. Indeed, several recurrences at the site of the resected ureteral orifice following the pluck technique have been reported (49–54). Another concern is the potential difficulty in confirming that the entire ureter has been plucked (28). Transurethral excision at the conclusion of the operation, as has been described in combination with hand-assisted laparoscopy, would seem equivalent to the open standard with regard to proximal leakage. However, leakage from the bladder is not controlled.

The transvesical technique provides an optimal bladder cuff and good occlusion of the ureter; however, integrity of the bladder is not maintained and concern of irrigant extravasation has been voiced.

These considerations are theoretical and deduced from oncologic principals, concerned with preventing contamination of the operative field with urothelial cancer cells. The only available report comparing techniques is a retrospective single-institution study published in abstract form that concluded the transvesical technique was associated with improved survival when compared to laparoscopic stapling (55). The role of local recurrences at the site of the ureteral orifice remained unclear.

SUMMARY

Laparoscopic nephroureterectomy is a maturing procedure that is performed routinely at many dedicated centers of minimally invasive surgery. Standard and hand-assisted laparoscopy as well as the transperitoneal and retroperitoneal approaches are becoming well established. No conclusions can be drawn regarding the superiority of one laparoscopic technique over another. Several techniques are practiced to manage the distal ureter and bladder cuff, none of which are optimal. Reports of long-term oncologic outcomes are emerging and appear comparable to open nephroureterectomy. Large long-term studies are necessary before laparoscopic nephroureterectomy is established as equivalent.

References

1. Clayman RV, Kavoussi LR, Figenshau RS, et al. Laparoscopic nephroureterectomy: initial clinical case report. *J Laparoendosc Surg* 1991;1: 343–349.
2. Clayman RV, Long SL, Kavoussi LR, et al. Laparoscopic nephrectomy in the pig: technique and results. *J Endourol* 1990;4:247–252.
3. Clayman RV, Kavoussi LR, Soper NJ, et al. Laparoscopic nephrectomy [Letter]. *N Engl J Med* 1991;324:1370.
4. Chiu AW, Chen M-T, Huang WJS, et al. Case report: laparoscopic nephroureterectomy and endoscopic excision of bladder cuff. *Minim Invasive Ther Allied Technol* 1992;1:299–303.
5. Rassweiler JJ, Henkel TO, Potempa DM, et al. The technique of transperitoneal laparoscopic nephrectomy, adrenalectomy and nephroureterectomy. *Eur Urol* 1993;23:425–430.
6. Nakada SY, Moon TD, Gist M, et al. Use of the pneumo sleeve as an adjunct in laparoscopic nephrectomy. *Urology* 1996;49:612–613.
7. Keeley FX, Tolley DA Jr. Laparoscopic nephroureterectomy: making management of upper-tract transitional-cell carcinoma entirely minimally invasive. *J Endourol* 1998;12:139–141.
8. Nakada SY. Hand-assisted laparoscopic nephrectomy. *J Endourol* 1999; 13:9–15.
9. Keeley FX, Sharma NK, Tolley DA. Hand-assisted laparoscopic nephroureterectomy. *BJU Int* 1999;83:504–505.
10. Stifelman MD, Sosa RE, Andrade A, et al. Hand-assisted laparoscopic nephroureterectomy for the treatment of transitional cell carcinoma of the upper urinary tract. *Urology* 2000;56:741–747.
11. Rane A, Dasgupta P. Prospective experience with a second-generation hand-assisted laparoscopic device and comparison with first-generation devices. *J Endourol* 2003;17:895–897.
12. Munver R, Del Pizzo JJ, Sosa RE. Hand-assisted laparoscopic nephroureterectomy for upper urinary-tract transitional-cell carcinoma. *J Endourol* 2004;18:351–358.
13. Gaur DD. Laparoscopic operative retroperitoneoscopy: use of new device. *J Urol* 1992;148:1137–1139.
14. Gaur DD, Agarwal DK, Purohit KC. Retroperitoneal laparoscopic nephrectomy: initial case report. *J Urol* 1993;149:103–105.
15. Henkel TO, Rassweiler J, Alken P. Ureteral laparoscopic surgery. *Ann Urol (Paris)* 1995;29:61–72.
16. Doublet JD, Barreto HS, Degremont AC, et al. Retroperitoneal nephrectomy: comparison of laparoscopy with open surgery. *World J Surg* 1996;20: 713–716.
17. Savage SJ, Gill IS. Laparoscopic radical nephroureterectomy. *J Endourol* 2000;14:859–864.
18. Kawauchi A, Fujito A, Ukimura O, et al. Hand assisted retroperitoneoscopic nephroureterectomy: comparison with the open procedure. *J Urol* 2003;169: 890–894.
19. Shalhav AL, Elbahnasy AM, McDougall EM, et al. Laparoscopic nephroureterectomy for upper tract transitional-cell cancer: technical aspects. *J Endourol* 1998;12:345–353.
20. Shalhav AL, Portis AJ, McDougall EM, et al. Laparoscopic nephroureterectomy. A new standard for the surgical management of upper tract transitional cell cancer. *Urol Clin North Am* 2000;27:761–773.
21. Yoshino Y, Ono Y, Hattori R, et al. Retroperitoneoscopic nephroureterectomy for transitional cell carcinoma of the renal pelvis and ureter: Nagoya experience. *Urology* 2003;61:533–538.
22. Kerbl K, Chandhoke P, McDougall E, et al. Laparoscopic stapled bladder closure: laboratory and clinical experience. *J Urol* 1993;149:1437–1440.
23. Baughman SM, Sexton W, Bishoff JT. Multiple intravesical linear staples identified during surveillance cystoscopy after laparoscopic nephroureterectomy. *Urology* 2003;62:351.
24. McDonald HP, Upchurch WE, Sturdevant CE, et al. Nephroureterectomy: a new technique. *J Urol* 1952;67:804–809.
25. McDonald DF. Intussusception ureterectomy: a method of removal of the ureteral stump at time of nephroureterectomy without an additional incision. *Surg Gynecol Obstet* 1953;97:565–568.
26. Chen J, Chueh SC, Hsu WT, et al. Modified approach of hand-assisted laparoscopic nephroureterectomy for transitional cell carcinoma of the upper urinary tract. *Urology* 2001;58:930–934.
27. Sagalowski AI, Jarrett TW. Management of urothelial tumors of the renal pelvis and ureter. In: Walsh PC, Retik AB, Vaughan ED Jr, et al., eds. *Campbell's urology*, 8th ed., Vol. 4. Philadelphia, PA: WB Saunders, 2002: 2845–2875.
28. Gill IS, Soble JJ, Miller SD, et al. A novel technique for management of the en bloc bladder cuff and distal ureter during laparoscopic nephroureterectomy. *J Urol* 1999;161:430–434.
29. Gonzalez CM, Batler RA, Schoor RA, et al. A novel endoscopic approach towards resection of the distal ureter with surrounding bladder cuff during hand assisted laparoscopic nephroureterectomy. *J Urol* 2001;165:483–485.
30. Wong C, Leveillee RJ. Hand-assisted laparoscopic nephroureterectomy with cystoscopic en bloc excision of the distal ureter and bladder cuff. *J Endourol* 2002;16:329–333.
31. Kerbl K, Clayman RV, McDougall EM, et al. Laparoscopic nephroureterectomy: evaluation of first clinical series. *Eur Urol* 1993;23:431–436.
32. Rassweiler J, Tsivian A, Kumar AV, et al. Oncological safety of laparoscopic surgery for urological malignancy: experience with more than 1,000 operations. *J Urol* 2003;169:2072–2075.
33. Ong AM, Bhayani SB, Pavlovich CP. Trocar site recurrence after laparoscopic nephroureterectomy. *J Urol* 2003;170:1301.
34. Ahmed I, Shaikh NA, Kapadia CR. Track recurrence of renal pelvic transitional cell carcinoma after laparoscopic nephrectomy. *Br J Urol* 1998;81: 319.
35. Otani M, Irie S, Tsuji Y. Port site metastasis after laparoscopic nephrectomy: unsuspected transitional cell carcinoma within a tuberculous atrophic kidney. *J Urol* 1999;162:486–487.
36. Gill IS, Sung GT, Hobart MG, et al. Laparoscopic radical nephroureterectomy for upper tract transitional cell carcinoma: the Cleveland Clinic experience. *J Urol* 2000;164:1513–1522.
37. Shalhav AL, Dunn MD, Portis AJ, et al. Laparoscopic nephroureterectomy for upper tract transitional cell cancer: the Washington University experience. *J Urol* 2000;163:1100–1104.
38. McNeill SA, Chrisofos M, Tolley DA. The long-term outcome after laparoscopic nephroureterectomy: a comparison with open nephroureterectomy. *BJU Int* 2000;86:619–623.
39. Seifman BD, Montie JE, Wolf JS Jr. Prospective comparison between hand-assisted laparoscopic and open surgical nephroureterectomy for urothelial cell carcinoma. *Urology* 2001;57:133–137.
40. Stifelman MD, Hyman MJ, Shichman S, et al. Hand-assisted laparoscopic nephroureterectomy versus open nephrectomy for the treatment of transitional-cell carcinoma of the upper urinary tract. *J Endourol* 2001; 15:391–397.
41. Li CC, Chou YH, Shen JT, et al. Comparison of hand-assisted laparoscopic nephroureterectomy with open surgery for upper urinary tract tumor. *Kaohsiung J Med Sci* 2001;17:615–619.
42. Klingler HC, Lodde M, Pycha A, et al. Modified laparoscopic nephroureterectomy for treatment of upper urinary tract transitional cell cancer is not associated with an increased risk of tumour recurrence. *Eur Urol* 2003;44:442–447.
43. Matsui Y, Ohara H, Ichioka K, et al. Retroperitoneoscopy-assisted total nephroureterectomy for upper tract transitional cell carcinoma. *Urology* 2002;60:1010–1015.
44. Landman J, Lev RY, Bhayani S, et al. Comparison of hand assisted and standard laparoscopic radical nephroureterectomy for the management of localized transitional cell carcinoma. *J Urol* 2002;167:2387–2391.
45. Okeke AA, Timoney AG, Keeley FX. Hand-assisted laparoscopic nephrectomy: complications related to the hand-port site. *BJU Int* 2002;90:364–367.
46. Meraney AM, Gill IS. Financial analysis of open versus laparoscopic radical nephrectomy and nephroureterectomy. *J Urol* 2002;167:1757–1762.
47. Hattori R, Ono Y, Gotoh M, et al. Retroperitoneoscopic nephroureterectomy for transitional cell carcinoma of the renal pelvis and ureter: Nagoya experience [Abstract]. *J Urol* 2003;169(Suppl. 4):77.
48. El Fettouh HA, Rassweiler JJ, Schulze M, et al. Laparoscopic radical nephroureterectomy: results of an international multicenter study. *Eur Urol* 2002;42:447–452.
49. Hetherington JW, Ewing R, Philp NH. Modified nephroureterectomy: a risk of tumor implantation. *Br J Urol* 1986;58:368–370.
50. Jones DR, Moisey CU. A cautionary tale of the modified "pluck" nephroureterectomy. *Br J Urol* 1993;71:486.
51. Abercrombie GF, Eardley I, Payne SR, et al. Modified nephro-ureterectomy. Long-term follow-up with particular reference to subsequent bladder tumors. *Br J Urol* 1988;61:198–200.
52. Carr T, Powell H, Ramsden PD, et al. Re: the risk of tumor implantation following "Abercrombie" modified nephroureterectomy [Letter]. *Br J Urol* 1987;59:99–100.
53. Fernandez Gomez JM, Barmadah SE, Perez Garcia J, et al. Risk of tumor reseeding after nephroureterectomy combined with endoscopic resection of the ureteral meatus. *Arch Esp Urol* 1998;51:829–831.
54. Arango O, Biesla O, Carles J, et al. Massive tumor implantation in the endoscopic resected area in modified nephroureterectomy. *J Urol* 1997;157:1839.
55. Matin S, Gill IS. Laparoscopic radical nephrectomy with various forms of bladder cuff control II. Patterns of survival [Abstract]. *J Endourol* 2003; 17(Suppl. 1):A74.

CHAPTER 25 ■ RISK ASSESSMENT AND TREATMENT OF SUPERFICIAL BLADDER CANCER

CHAPTER 25A
Natural History and Initial Management Based on Prognostic Factors

J.A. Witjes and Frans M.J. Debruyne

INTRODUCTION

Over 95% of bladder tumors are transitional cell carcinomas. As discussed in Chapter 18, bladder cancer is among the 10 most common cancers in men in most Western countries, and the situation in the Netherlands is no different. In 2000, for example, it was the fourth most-common invasive cancer in men after prostate, lung, and colon. However, if superficial tumors are included, bladder cancer is the third most common in men (3497) and seventh in women (961). Incidence of invasive tumors has become stable over the last 10 years; however, incidence of superficial tumors is still rising. Consequently, bladder cancer is an important topic of study for both sexes. Another often-overlooked point is that because of the high recurrence rates of superficial tumors, the number of patients under treatment or check-up for bladder cancer is even higher. Conservative estimates for the Dutch situation, based on the number of transurethral resections and data on the number of outpatient coagulations of superficial recurrences, reveals that the prevalence of superficial bladder cancer is approximately two to three times the incidence of these tumors. This means that in the Netherlands there are approximately 6,000 to 8,000 patients with superficial bladder cancer, which makes superficial bladder cancer one of the most common cancers in the country. This underlines the need for good understanding of the natural history of invasive and superficial bladder cancer. It is especially important in superficial disease to decide on potential additional treatment after transurethral resection (TUR), with consequently significant impact on the costs of health care.

The natural history can be determined by so-called prognostic factors. In Chapter 20, molecular biology with regard to prognostic factors is discussed, so the topic will only be mentioned briefly in this chapter. Here, predominantly clinical and histological factors will be discussed, as well as their potential implication in the formation of risk groups and general guidelines based on these risk groups. Initial surgical management is discussed briefly. An additional treatment called intravesical therapy is discussed in more detail in Chapter 25B.

NATURAL HISTORY OF SUPERFICIAL PAPILLARY (TA AND T1) BLADDER CANCER

Superficial bladder cancer is typically characterized by a high risk of recurrence (30% to 85%), with maximal incidence in the first years, and 10% to 20% risk of progression to muscle-invasive tumors. However, as is shown in Chapter 19, superficial bladder carcinoma includes a broad spectrum of tumors. On one end of the spectrum there are troublesome low-grade Ta tumors, which almost never have adverse consequences for survival. On the other end there are life-threatening T1 grade III tumors, invading into the submucosa or lamina propria, posing a major challenge to the urologist and the patient.

This risk-group classification, a subdivision of the natural history of the disease, is based on prognostic factors, and has consequences for the therapy, follow-up, and final outcome of patients. However, the real (i.e, untreated) natural history can only be derived from older series, since in the last decades additional therapy after TUR is standard of care, and that logically influences the natural history, for example, by lowering the recurrence rates.

From a large unselected group of Dutch bladder-cancer patients, Kiemeney et al. described patients' characteristics in 1993 (1). In all, 1,745 of the 2,805 patients registered had Ta and T1 bladder tumors. Carcinoma *in situ* (CIS) was excluded. Since in the registration period (1983–1990) adjuvant intravesical therapy was not standard of care, 64% were treated by TUR only. Interestingly, and important for the natural course of the disease, there was a clear shift toward a higher disease stage with increasing age. No differences with regard to sex were found, but Mungan et al. also found a worse stage of the disease in women at presentation, as well as a worse cancer-specific survival, even after correction for other prognostic factors (2,3). The large Dutch registry found an actuarial risk of recurrent disease after primary treatment in superficial bladder cancer of nearly 60% within 5 years. This risk was 33% after 1 year. In the second year of follow-up, this risk was 47% among patients with, as compared to 18% among patients without, recurrence in the first year of follow-up.

In a multivariate proportional hazards regression model, adjusted for the potential distorting effect of adjuvant intravesical therapy, tumor stage, grade, extent, and multiplicity had statistically significant independent prognostic value with regard to the risk of first recurrence. Intravesical therapy reduced the 3-year risk of recurrence from 55% to 49% ($P = .005$). Surprisingly, patients with the most favorable prognostic score still had a 3-year risk of recurrence of 37%, compared to 77% in the prognostically least favorable group. Progression, as defined by a shift to muscle-invasive disease or the development of metastases, was seen in 10.2% (95% CI: range 8.6% to 11.8%) after 3 years, and hardly increased thereafter. Again, tumor stage, grade, and multiplicity had prognostic significance for the risk of progression in a multivariate model. Additionally, age of >70 years was significant for progression (12.7% vs. 7.4%, $P = .001$), as was the presence or absence of CIS (21% vs. 7%, $P <.001$). Intravesical instillations did not lower the risk of progression. The excess risk of dying from superficial bladder cancer within 5 years was approximately 14%.

Two earlier series studied patients who did not have additional therapy after TUR at all. Heney et al. reported on 249 Ta and T1 patients (4). High tumor-grade, stage T1, biopsy atypia, positive urinary cytology, tumor multiplicity, and size were associated with early recurrences. Progression was significantly different in stages Ta and T1, and grades I, II, and III: 4%, 30%, 2%, 11%, and 45%, respectively. Fitzpatrick et al. followed 188 patients for >5 years, of which 54% experienced recurrences (5). This group consisted of relatively low-risk patients: all patients were pTa grade 1 or 2 and only 16% had multiple tumors. Patients free of tumor at 3 months had an 80% chance of having no further recurrences and this rate remained the same up to 2 years from the start of the disease. The importance of the 3-month recurrence was confirmed later by Parmar et al. (6).

The risk of recurrences for low-risk tumors were confirmed by a recent European Organization for the Research and Treatment of courier (EORTC) meta-analysis on the impact of one immediate instillation of chemotherapy after TUR on the risk of recurrence in patients with Ta and T1 bladder tumors (7). After a median follow-up of 3.4 years 36.7% of 728 patients receiving one postoperative instillation had a recurrence compared to 48.4% of 748 patients with TUR alone ($P <.0001$). This study not only indicates the value of one immediate post TUR instillation, but also shows that the untreated recurrence rate of these low-risk tumors is substantial. For all Ta and T1 tumors, similar figures were found in a combined analysis of EORTC and medical research council (MRC) superficial bladder cancer trial (8).

To study the impact of intravesical therapy on the recurrence and progression rates of Ta and T1 bladder cancer, a combined analysis of several older trials was performed, in which 2,535 were treated adjuvant after TUR, but 906 were not. In both groups almost all recurrences were seen in the first 4 years. At 4 years, approximately 52% of patients with additional therapy had recurrences, as compared to approximately 58% in the control (untreated) group. At 8 years, these figures were 55.1% and 63.3% ($P <.01$). The progression rates after 8 years were not significantly different: 11% for the untreated group versus 13% for the treated group. Unfortunately, no subanalysis for different risk groups was made.

In most of these series patients with CIS were not included. CIS is a distinct entity, which is defined as a flat (e.g., nonpapillary) high-grade non-invasive transitional cell carcinoma. The untreated natural history indicates a more-than-50% progression rate in 5 years and an even higher recurrence rate (9). In the case of concomitant high-grade pT1 papillary tumors, the chance of progression seems even worse. Furthermore, it seems that cellular changes that can be seen in CIS are one of the pathways through which patients are prone to invasive disease. Another aspect of CIS that is important for the natural history of patients with this disease is the finding that the urothelium outside the bladder, the upper urinary tract, and the urethra also seem more at risk in patients with bladder CIS (10,11).

In summary, the natural untreated history of superficial bladder cancer clearly shows a substantial risk of recurrent disease in 3 years, ranging from 35% to 40% in the lowest-risk tumors to 70% to 80% in the highest-risk tumors. The risk of tumor progression to muscle-invasive disease varies depending on the risk category of the patient, but is on average 10% in 3 years.

The 5-year cancer-specific survival is somewhat under 90%. This last observation suggests that many of the patients with superficial bladder tumors that have progression to muscle-invasive disease do die of their disease. This indeed was confirmed by Schier et al., indicating that risk-adapted therapy is very important (12).

For this risk-adapted therapy after TUR, some clinical and histological factors have been shown to be important. For recurrence, these are especially stage, grade, multiplicity, size, intravesical therapy, and a recurrence at 3 months after TUR. Additional factors are cytology and the result of biopsies. For progression stage, grade and the presence of CIS are important, as are to a lesser extent multiplicity, sex, and age.

The ideal situation would be if the prognoses of patients could be predicted based on these clinical and histological factors to tailor therapy and follow-up. Indeed, some authors have tried to do so, specifically in patients with superficial bladder cancer.

RISK GROUPS

In 1989, Parmar et al. looked at recurrences of primary Ta and T1 tumors from a combination of two large, randomized British Medical Research Council studies (6). In a multivariate analysis the 3-month cystoscopy results after the initial TUR was the most important prognostic factor, together with tumor multiplicity. With these two factors, three risk groups were constructed. According to this stratification, risk-adapted follow-up could reduce the number of cystoscopies and costs for the large proportion of patients who have a low risk of recurrence.

In 1995, Kurth et al. (13) grouped 576 Ta and T1 patients into three different risk categories. In the multivariate model, three factors remained significant: tumor size, grade, and prior recurrence rate/year. Based on these three factors and their association with invasion and death due to malignant disease, an index was computed reflecting the risk of both early invasion and death due to malignant disease. The observed rate of tumor progression and death due to malignant disease was 7.1% and 4.3%, respectively, in the low-risk group vs. 41.6% and 36.1%, respectively, in the high-risk group. According to the authors this system was easy to apply and had clear therapeutic consequences, such as early aggressive therapy in high-risk patients.

In 1998, Allard et al. studied 333 patients with primary Ta and T1 tumors and proposed a simple prognostic index (14). Multivariate analysis revealed multiplicity, size, stage, and grade to be significant prognostic factors for early recurrence. With these four so-called adverse tumor characteristics (ATCs) the clinical course within 3 years of the first TUR could be predicted. For example, in case of no ATCs, the recurrence-free probability at 1 and 2 years was 86% and 69%, respectively, and no progression was expected. In case of 3 or 4 ATCs these figures were 30% and 19%, respectively, and 7% had progression within 35 months of follow-up. Again, this index is easy to apply and the individual factors are available from routine urological practice. However, the authors themselves concluded that it is premature to use the index in routine urological practice and that further validation in future studies was needed.

Most recently Millan-Rodríguez et al. identified risk groups for recurrence, progression, and mortality based on data on a cohort of 1,529 patients with primary superficial bladder cancer (15). Recurrence was influenced by multiplicity, size, bacillus calmette-guerin (BCG) therapy, and the presence of CIS. The main predictor of progression and survival was grade. Three risk groups were constructed with these factors. The rates of recurrence, progression, and mortality were 37%, 0%, and 0% in the low-risk group; 45%, 1.8%, and 0.73% in the intermediate-risk group; and 54%, 15%, and 9.5% in the high-risk group, respectively. These authors also concluded that risk-group differentiation is possible, with potential impact on management and prognosis of these patients.

These four studies clearly show that risk-group formation is very feasible based on prognostic factors that are derived from daily urological practice. However, there are several drawbacks in these studies. Most of the studies are small and have different endpoints. Also, none of them included all patient categories. For example, CIS was excluded in the first three studies, and all studies only looked at primary patients. Also, not all studies come to a clear conclusion based on their own results and it is doubtful whether indexes as proposed are really used in daily practice. Last but not least, with these studies risk classification on group level may be possible, but prediction of individual patient outcome—the ultimate goal—remains questionable. This was clearly shown by Kiemeney et al. (16). They not only wanted to discriminate between risk groups, but also tried to optimize prediction of disease outcome in individual patients. After a multivariate analysis, several patient and tumor characteristics of 1,674 cases of primary pTa or pT1 bladder cancer were used to construct a prognostic index. Subsequently, they evaluated the reliability of the prognostic index by comparing the observed and predicted actuarial risks of tumor recurrence and progression. The reliability seemed useful on a group level, but on an individual level predictability was highly inaccurate—indeed, no better than the flip of a coin.

DISCUSSION AND CONCLUSION

In spite of some limitations, the conclusion of the results of the abovementioned studies appears to be that prediction of the natural history is feasible on a group level, although not yet on an individual level. Factors which can be used are stage, grade, and multiplicity in most models, whereas size, presence of CIS, and age are not studied or relevant in all models. A potential prognostic factor that is not mentioned in these studies is the level of invasion of T1 tumors in the submucosa (17). Still, these prognostic models or indices are hardly ever used in daily practice. Nevertheless, an important application has been implementation of these factors in guidelines, such as the American urological association (AUA) and European association of urology (EAU) guidelines, where advice is given with respect to therapy and follow-up based on risk stratification. In the EAU guideline, for example, patients are differentiated in low-risk (single Ta, G1, ≤3-cm diameter), high-risk (T1, G3, multifocal or highly recurrent, CIS), and intermediate-risk (all other tumors, Ta-1, G1-2, multifocal, >3-cm diameter) (18).

Initial treatment advice is given based on these risk groups. Basically, initial treatment is a complete TUR with biopsies, if there is an indication such as abnormal cytology. The additional value of random biopsies has been studied extensively and considered to be low (19,20). In case of an incomplete resection, or any doubts about the completeness, especially in case of T1 tumors when conservative treatment is planned, a second TUR within 2 to 4 weeks after the first one should be considered (21). According to the EAU guidelines, low-risk tumors need one additional intravesical instillation and no further treatment. Intermediate-risk tumors can be treated after TUR with a course of four to eight sessions of chemotherapy. Maintenance intravesical chemotherapy is not worthwhile. In high-risk tumors, intravesical BCG is advised; in CIS, even maintenance BCG. Intravesical therapy is discussed in detail in Chapter 25B.

A potential answer to the question of risk prediction on an individual level is the application of molecular markers from urine or tissue. Some urinary markers can be used for diagnosis, but their prognostic value still is unknown. Molecular factors were recently reviewed by Quek et al. (22); although in the future a panel of markers may be able to predict tumor recurrence or progression of superficial tumors and much research is ongoing, the authors conclude "accurate predictions of tumor behavior based on molecular markers is yet to be realized." Finally, the value of the most-studied molecular marker, p53, was recently reviewed by Schmitz-Dräger et al. (23). Based on the results of 43 trials including 3,764 patients, they found a correlation between p53 immunohistochemistry and tumor stage and grade, but could not clarify whether p53 had independent prognostic information. This topic is discovered further in Chapter 20.

In conclusion, even with the limitations of clinical and histological prognostic factors for prediction on an individual level, these are the only factors that can currently be applied in clinical practice to decide on adjuvant treatment after the initial TUR.

References

1. Kiemeney LALM, Witjes JA, Verbeek ALN, et al. The clinical epidemiology of superficial bladder cancer. *Br J Cancer* 1993;67:806–812.
2. Mungan NA, Kiemeney LALM, van Dijck JAAM, et al. Gender differences in stage distribution of bladder cancer. *Urology* 2000;55:368–371.
3. Mungan NA, Aben KKH, Schoenberg MP, et al. Gender differences in stage-adjusted bladder cancer survival. *Urology* 2000;55:876–880.
4. Heney NM, Ahmed S, Flanagan MJ, et al. Superficial bladder cancer: progression and recurrence. *J Urol* 1983;130:1083–1086.
5. Fitzpatrick JM, West AB, Butler MR, et al. Superficial bladder tumors (stage pTa, grades 1 and 2): the importance of recurrence pattern following initial resection. *J Urol* 1986;135:920.
6. Parmar MK, Freedman LS, Hargreave TB, et al. Prognostic factors for recurrence and followup policies in the treatment of superficial bladder cancer: report from the British Medical Research Council Subgroup on Superficial Bladder Cancer (Urological Cancer Working Party). *J Urol* 1989;142:284–288.
7. Sylvester RJ, Oosterlinck W, van der Meijden AP. A single immediate postoperative instillation of chemotherapy decreases the risk of recurrence in patients with stage Ta-T1 bladder cancer: a meta-analysis of published-results of randomized clinical trials. *J Urol* 2004;171:2186–2190.
8. Pawinski A, Sylvester R, Kurth KH, et al. A combined analysis of EORTC and MRC randomized clinical trials for the prophylactic treatment of stage Ta-T1 bladder cancer. *J Urol* 1996;156:1934–1941.
9. Witjes JA. Bladder CIS in 2003, state of the art. *Eur Urol* 2004;45:142–146.
10. Zincke H, Garbeff PJ, Beahrs JR. Upper urinary tract transitional cell cancer after radical cystectomy for bladder cancer. *J Urol* 1984;131:50–52.
11. Nixon RG, Chang SS, Lafleur BJ, et al. Carcinoma in situ and tumor multifocality predict the risk of prostatic urethral involvement at radical cystectomy in men with transitional cell carcinoma of the bladder. *J Urol* 2002;167:502–505.
12. Schrier BPH, Hollander MP, van Rhijn BWG, et al. Prognosis of muscle invasive bladder cancer: difference between primary and progressive tumors: possible implications for therapy. *Eur Urol* 2004;45:292–296.
13. Kurth KH, Denis L, Bouffioux C, et al. Factors affecting recurrence and progression in superficial bladder tumors. *Eur J Cancer* 1995;31A:1840–1846.
14. Allard P, Bernard P, Fradet Y, et al. The early clinical course of primary Ta and T1 bladder cancer: a proposed prognostic index. *Br J Urol* 1998;81:692–698.
15. Millan-Rodriguez F, Chechile-Toniolo G, Salvador-Bayarri J, et al. Primary superficial bladder cancer risk groups according to progression, mortality and recurrence. *J Urol* 2000;164:680–684.
16. Kiemeney LA, Witjes JA, Heijbroek RP, et al. Predictability of recurrent and progressive disease in individual patients with primary superficial bladder cancer. *J Urol* 1993;150:60–64.
17. Smits G, Schaafsma E, Kiemeney L, et al. Microstaging of pT1 transitional cell carcinoma of the bladder; identification of subgroups with distinct risks for progression. *Urology* 1998;52:1009–1014.
18. Oosterlinck W, Lobel B, Jakse G, et al. Guidelines on bladder cancer. *Eur Urol* 2002;41:105–112.
19. Kiemeney LA, Witjes JA, Heijbroek RP et al. Members of the Dutch South-East Co-Operative Urological Group. Should random urothelial biopsies be taken from patients with primary superficial bladder cancer? A decision analysis. *Br J Urol* 1994;73:164–171.
20. van der Meijden A, Oosterlinck W, Brausi M et al. EORTC-GU Group Superficial Bladder Committee. Significance of bladder biopsies in Ta,T1 bladder tumors: a report from the EORTC Genito-Urinary Tract Cancer Cooperative Group. *Eur Urol* 1999;35:267–271.
21. Jakse G, Algaba F, Malmstrom PU, et al. A second-look TUR in T1 transitional cell carcinoma: why? *Eur Urol* 2004;45:539–546.
22. Quek ML, Quinn DI, Daneshmand S, et al. Molecular prognostication in bladder cancer—a current perspective. *Eur J Cancer* 2003;39:1501–1510.
23. Schmitz-Drager BJ, Goebell PJ, Ebert T, et al. p53 immunohistochemistry as a prognostic marker in bladder cancer. Playground for urology scientists? *Eur Urol* 2000;38:691–699.

CHAPTER 25B
Intravesical Therapy
Guido Dalbagni and Michael O'Donnell

Seventy percent of bladder tumors are superficial at presentation, and 60% to 70% of superficial tumors recur (1), with 20% to 30% progressing to a higher stage or grade (2). The high recurrence rate and the unpredictability of the progression pattern have led to the widespread use of intravesical therapy as a supplement to transurethral resection (TUR). Superficial bladder cancer lends itself to intravesical therapy owing to direct contact of the chemotherapeutic agent with the bladder mucosa and tumor. Furthermore, some agents can be used at high doses with minimal systemic side effects due to lack of absorption (e.g., mitomycin C is given at a dose of 40 mg weekly for 8 weeks).

Intravesical agents are used:

1. *To eradicate existing disease that cannot be controlled endoscopically.* This is particularly relevant to carcinoma *in situ* (CIS), which is usually a diffuse process. It also applies to the rare situation of extensive papillary tumors that cannot be completely removed cystoscopically. The intravesical agent is used to ablate residual small volumes.
2. *To prevent recurrences in patients at risk.* Recurrence rates over several years range from 67% to 73% in different series, depending on the patient population. Factors predictive of recurrence, based on retrospective data, include the depth of invasion, tumor grade, multiplicity of tumors, size of tumor, presence of concomitant CIS, and the time interval between the first tumor and subsequent recurrence (3).
3. *To prevent progression in patients at risk.* Progression is defined as the development of muscle invasion or metastasis. It occurs in 20% to 30% of patients who present with superficial disease (3).

CHEMOTHERAPY

Chemotherapeutic Agents

Triethylenethiophosphoramide (thiotepa) is an alkylating agent known to cross-link DNA and prevent the cells from replicating. Thiotepa has a molecular weight of 189 kd, which makes it readily absorbed into systemic circulation. It is given at a concentration of 1 mg/mL for 4 to 8 weeks. Lamm reported the results of nine randomized trials comparing thiotepa to TUR alone. The average incidence of recurrence was 61% in the control population versus 49% among the patients treated with thiotepa, an advantage of a 12% decrease in tumor recurrence (4). The major systemic side effect is myelosuppression (5). Irritative voiding symptoms have been reported in a third of the patients (5).

Doxorubicin is an anthracycline produced by the *Streptomyces* species. Anthracyclines have several mechanisms of action, the most important of which is interaction with topoisomerase II. Doxorubicin is usually given at a concentration of 1 mg/mL. Seven controlled, randomized trials comparing doxorubicin to TUR alone have been performed. The average recurrence rate was 58% in the control group versus 38% in the doxorubicin arm, a 20% improvement in tumor recurrence (6). There is minimal absorption due to the large size of the drug (580 kd). Chemical cystitis has been reported in up to 56% of the patients, with a decreased bladder capacity in 16%

and hematuria in 40%. Systemic reactions, including fever and allergy, have been reported in 5% (7).

Epirubicin (4'-epi-doxorubicin) is a synthetic derivative of doxorubicin. The most common dose is 50 mg/50 mL for 4 to 8 weeks. Epirubicin is effective in the prophylaxis of superficial tumors (8–10). Its therapeutic efficacy is similar to that of doxorubicin, but it has a better toxicity profile (11). In four controlled trials using epirubicin, a decrease in recurrence rate from 55% for TUR to 27% for epirubicin was reported (6). Adverse events are mild, the most common being cystitis and hematuria.

Mitomycin C (MMC) is an alkylating agent derived from the *Streptomyces* species with a molecular weight of 334 kd. The most effective dose is 40 mg in 20 mL of distilled water given for 8 consecutive weeks (12). Nilsson et al. reported the results of 1,774 patients in nine randomized trials comparing MMC to TUR alone, only five of which showed statistical significance. The average recurrence rate was 54% in the control group versus 38% in the MMC arm, a 16% overall improvement in tumor recurrence (6). Dysuria and frequency occur in 41% of the patients (7).

Chemotherapy Delivery

The role of intravesical chemotherapy in decreasing recurrences is well established. However, there is no consensus on the best drug, schedule, dose, and timing of the instillation.

Comparison of Different Chemotherapeutic Agents

The majority of randomized trials comparing different chemotherapeutic agents have failed to show the superiority of one drug over others. Thiotepa and MMC were found to be equally effective for ablating any residual tumor (chemoresection) (5), achieving a complete response (CR) in 26% and 39%, respectively. Patients with Tis disease had equal responses (Table 25B.1). A 356-patient European Organization for Research and Treatment of Cancer (EORTC) study comparing thiotepa, doxorubicin, and cisplatin showed recurrence rates per year of 0.50, 0.54, and 0.58, respectively (13). There was no difference in the recurrence rate or in progression after a mean follow-up of 41 months; however, some patients receiving cisplatin developed a severe anaphylactic reaction (13). A Japanese multicenter trial found similar recurrence rates among patients randomized to epirubicin or doxorubicin (14). Shinohara reported no differences among doxorubicin, epirubicin, or pirarubicin (15). Conversely, an Egyptian randomized study comparing epirubicin to doxorubicin, although at different schedules and different doses, observed a better outcome in patients receiving epirubicin (11).

Current data suggest that all current intravesical chemotherapeutic agents are similar in efficacy but differ in toxicity.

Dose and Concentration

Most studies evaluating different chemotherapeutic agents have lacked standardization in the dose and concentration. Thiotepa has been shown to be an effective prophylactic agent, and yet a large Medical Research Council (MRC) trial did not show a decrease in recurrence rate (20). In this trial, the patients received 30 mg of thiotepa diluted in 50 mL, a dose comparable to other studies but at a much lower concentration, suggesting that, unlike systemic chemotherapy, response to intravesical chemotherapy is proportional to the concentration rather than to the total dose of the drug. In a pharmacokinetic study of thiotepa, Masters et al. suggested that systemic exposure depends on the total dose, but tumor exposure depends on the concentration (21). It is therefore possible to increase the efficacy of the drug without increasing its systemic toxicity by decreasing the volume of the diluent. Similarly, Gao et al. indicated that tumor uptake of MMC was proportional to the drug

TABLE 25B.1

RANDOMIZED TRIALS COMPARING DIFFERENT CHEMOTHERAPEUTIC AGENTS

	Arm A	N	Recurrence	Arm B	N	Recurrence	P
Zincke (16)	Thiotepa	30	30% at 3 mo	Doxorubicin	31	32% at 3 mo	NS
Zincke (17)	Thiotepa	41	78% at 12 mo	Mitomycin C	42	67% at 12 mo	NS
Flanigan (18)	Thiotepa	15	0.45/100 patient-mo	Mitomycin C	25	1.19/100 patient-mo	NS
Heney (5)[a]	Thiotepa	73	26%	Mitomycin C	76	39%	NS
Martinez-Pineiro (19)	Thiotepa	56	43% (median follow-up 3 yr)	Doxorubicin	53	36% (median follow-up 3 yr)	NS
Bouffioux (13)	Thiotepa	109	0.50 recurrence rate/yr	Doxorubicin	112	0.54 recurrence rate/yr	NS
Eto (14)	Epirubicin	60	11% at 2 yr	Doxorubicin	54	18% at 2 yr	NS
Shinohara (15)	Epirubicin	79	—	Doxorubicin	80	—	NS
Ali-el-Dein (11)	Epirubicin	64 low[b]	0.83	Doxorubicin	60	1.18/100 patient-mo	.02
		68 high[b]	0.60 (per 100 patient-mo)				

NS, not stated.
[a]Chemoresection application.
[b]low: low dose (50 mg in 50 mL); high: high dose (80 mg in 50 mL).

concentration (22). In an attempt to optimize MMC delivery, a multi-institutional phase III trial was carried out. Patients in the optimized arm received a 40-mg dose in 20 mL of sterile water, as well as manipulations to reduce urine production and alkalinize the urine. Patients in the optimized arm showed a decrease in recurrence from 75% to 49% at 5 years. Median time to recurrence was increased from 12 to 29 months (12).

Despite these results, more concentrated drug is not always better. The optimal concentration needs to be evaluated for each individual drug. In a randomized trial of 122 patients, Masters et al. concluded that 2 mg/mL epirubicin was no better than 1 mg/mL (23). In two Japanese studies, epirubicin at a concentration of 0.5 mg/mL did not decrease recurrences compared to TUR alone (24), and the efficacy of the drug at 40 mg/40 mL was better than at 20 mg/40 mL (25). These studies indicate that there is a threshold below which some drugs are not effective and, similarly, an upper limit beyond which more drug is superfluous.

Perioperative Single-dose Instillation

Several randomized studies of thiotepa as an adjuvant agent have shown a decrease in the recurrence rate. The greatest decrease in tumor recurrence was noted in the studies using a single, early postoperative instillation (16,26), suggesting that this schedule is a viable alternative to multiple instillations. Although a large multicenter trial including patients with primary superficial tumors failed to show a benefit for postoperative thiotepa over TUR alone (27), the negative outcome of this trial was attributed to the low concentration of thiotepa used. Several randomized studies comparing different chemotherapeutic agents have since confirmed the efficacy of a single prophylactic postoperative instillation (9,28–30). An EORTC study comparing epirubicin to water showed that patients with a primary and solitary Ta tumor had a 50% decrease in the recurrence rate in the epirubicin group (9). These results were confirmed by a randomized controlled trial using MMC for patients with a single, primary or recurrent, non–muscle-invasive tumor (29). The benefits were mainly noted during the first 12 months, suggesting a beneficial effect of a single instillation in preventing tumor cell implantation (29). In a randomized multicenter study comparing TUR alone versus interferon-alpha (IFN-α) versus epirubicin, Rajala et al. noted that interferon had no effect on

recurrence. Epirubicin showed a durable effect in preventing tumor recurrences in patients overall (31), but failed to produce a decrease in recurrences in a subset of patients with multiple tumors (32). In contrast, two prospective randomized studies showed a positive effect among patients with multiple as well as solitary papillary tumors (28,30).

Intravesical chemotherapy should be given within the first day after TUR, preferably within the first 6 hours. It is well tolerated (28), with 10% of patients reporting irritative lower tract symptoms (9). In a recent meta-analysis of seven randomized trials on 1,476 patients with 3.4 years median follow-up, Sylvester et al. demonstrated a 39% reduction in the odds of recurrence (36.7% recurrence vs. 48.4% recurrence) when a single dose of cytotoxic chemotherapy was delivered postoperatively after TUR (33). Patients either with single tumors or multiple tumors benefited; however, 65% of patients with multiple tumors eventually had a recurrence, compared to 36% with single tumors. These data strongly support the postoperative instillation of a chemotherapeutic agent in the immediate postoperative period in patients with a solitary low-grade papillary tumor. Although patients with multiple lesions also benefit from a single instillation, a more intensive adjuvant regimen is recommended.

Maintenance

While the rationale for a perioperative instillation is to prevent tumor cell implantation, the role of maintenance therapy is to prevent new occurrences by altering tumor diathesis. In a prospective multicenter study, Huland et al. did not find a significant difference in recurrence rate among patients treated with and without maintenance MMC or doxorubicin (34). Two EORTC prospective randomized trials comparing early (the day of resection) versus delayed (7 to 15 days after resection) and short-term (6 months) versus long-term (12 months) treatment with MMC and doxorubicin found no significant difference in the disease-free interval among all groups. However, the recurrence rate was worse among patients who started treatment late and received no maintenance (35), suggesting that maintenance is not beneficial when treatment is given within the first 24 hours. This was further confirmed by a randomized trial of early instillation of epirubicin with maintenance versus no maintenance, showing no difference in recurrence (36). In contrast, Koga et al. reported a higher efficacy for long-term instillation of epirubicin versus short-term instillation. In a prospective randomized trial, the patients received their first treatment within 24 hours, followed by epirubicin for 3 months or 12 months. The 3-year recurrence rate was 36% in the first group versus 15% in the second (37). Conrad et al. similarly found that 3 years of monthly MMC maintenance was superior to no maintenance (recurrence 14% vs. 31%) in Ta G2/3 and T1 G1-3 tumors at median follow-up of 2.9 years (38). In a meta-analysis of 11 randomized trials, Huncharek suggested that chemotherapy for 2 years had the greatest effect on decreasing the recurrence rates (39).

Given these mixed results, a role for maintenance chemotherapy is not yet clear. Further prospective randomized trials are needed.

Dwell Time and pH

Very few studies have evaluated the importance of the dwell time in efficacy of the chemotherapeutic agent. In a randomized trial comparing different dwell times of MMC, De Bruijn reported a recurrence rate of 36% for 30 minutes of dwell time versus 14% for 60 minutes of dwell time (40), without an increase in toxicity.

The effects of pH *in vitro* have been more extensively evaluated. Doxorubicin and epirubicin are more cytotoxic in alkaline media, while thiotepa and MMC are more cytotoxic in acidic media (41). MMC is, however, less stable in acidic media, requiring alkalinization of the urine to optimize its efficacy (12).

Technological Advances in Drug Delivery

Local microwave hyperthermia in conjunction with MMC (20 mg/50 cc) was compared in a multicenter randomized trial to intravesical MMC alone in 83 patients (42). Hyperthermia was delivered at a temperature of 42°C for at least 40 minutes. At a minimum follow-up of 24 months, the hyperthermia group had a statistically significant reduction in recurrences (17.1% for the thermochemotherapy group vs. 57.5% for chemotherapy alone). Thermochemotherapy has also been used in treating patients with high-grade superficial bladder cancer (Ta/T1 G3) as a prophylactic (40 mg MMC) or ablative (80 mg MMC) protocol by Gofrit et al. (43). Among 24 patients given the prophylactic protocol, 62.5% were recurrence-free after a mean follow-up of 35.3 months. The ablative protocol was administered to 28 patients, with complete ablation of the tumor in 75% and a recurrence-free rate of 80.9% at a mean follow-up of 20 months.

Electromotive intravesical mitomycin C (eMMC) has been proposed as a method to improve drug delivery across biological membranes and to increase accumulation in bladder tissue. Di Stasi et. al. randomized three groups of patients with CIS to 40 mg eMMC instillation with 20 mA electric current for 30 minutes, 40 mg passive MMC with a dwell time of 60 minutes, or 81 mg bacillus Calmette-Guerin (BCG) with a dwell time of 120 minutes (44). Patients were scheduled for an initial 6 weekly treatments; responders then received 10 monthly treatments, while nonresponders received a further 6 weekly treatments. The CR rate at 6 months for eMMC (58%) was statistically significantly superior to that of passive MMC (31%). The response rate of eMMC approached that of BCG (64%). Peak plasma MMC was significantly higher after eMMC than after passive MMC (43 vs. 8 ng/mL), supporting the hypothesis that electromotive MMC increases tissue levels.

Sequential Therapy

Alternative approaches have been investigated to improve the efficacy of intravesical therapy. Several investigators have explored the use of BCG combined with chemotherapy. The rationale for giving chemotherapy prior to BCG is to induce

sloughing of the urothelium, allowing BCG to better interact with fibronectin and initiating an immune response. However, BCG immediately after epirubicin is not well tolerated. Erol reported that over a third of patients discontinued treatment due to severe cystitis (45).

Rintala et al. reported a novel approach of alternating MMC and BCG for prophylaxis of superficial papillary bladder cancer (46). After an induction course of MMC, 188 patients with recurring Ta or T1 tumors were randomly assigned to maintenance MMC versus alternating MMC and BCG instillations (Pasteur Strain). The patients were treated for 2 years, and the mean follow-up was 34 months. Alternating MMC and BCG was equal in efficacy to MMC and was clearly superior to transurethral resection alone. For CIS, Rintala et al. reported that alternating BCG with MMC was superior to MMC (47). The superiority of BCG and MMC could, however, be attributed to the presence of BCG in one arm and not the other rather than the alternating mode of delivery. More importantly, no significant side effects developed in the alternating group. A different randomized prospective trial of sequential BCG and eMMC was reported by DiStasi et al. (48), who compared 6 weekly BCG instillations followed by 1 year of monthly maintenance to a program of 9 weekly instillations in the sequence BCG, BCG, eMMC, and nine monthly maintenance instillations in the sequence eMMC, eMMC, BCG. The sequential program resulted in a statistically significant decrease in recurrence at 5 to 6 years, from 47% to 28%. In contrast, Kaasinen reported that alternating BCG with IFN-α after an induction course of MMC was inferior to BCG after MMC (49).

A randomized phase III trial of intermediate-risk and high-risk superficial bladder cancer comparing sequential MMC for 4 weeks followed by weekly BCG versus weekly MMC showed no difference in recurrence or progression (50). BCG alternating with epirubicin was not superior to BCG alone, but had fewer side effects (51).

BCG monotherapy was superior to an induction course of MMC followed by alternating MMC and BCG instillations in patients with Tis disease (52). The recurrence-free survival and progression-free survival were also superior in the patients treated with BCG only.

The results from trials of combination therapy are summarized in Table 25B.2. As yet, it is not possible to determine whether mixed chemoimmunotherapy programs will dependably improve outcomes.

Impact on Recurrence and Progression

The long-term goals of intravesical chemotherapy are to decrease the recurrence rate and prevent progression. Several studies have addressed the performance of intravesical intervention in terms of these goals. Lamm reported an absolute decrease of tumor recurrence averaging 14%, yet no effect on tumor progression among 3,899 patients enrolled in 22 prospective randomized studies comparing intravesical chemotherapy versus surgery alone (53). Pawinsky et al. analyzed four previous EORTC and two MRC randomized clinical trials comparing prophylactic intravesical chemotherapy versus surgery alone for Ta and T1 transitional cell carcinoma (TCC). They observed a significant improvement in disease-free survival and no effect on progression among 2,535 patients receiving adjuvant therapy (54). Huncharek et al. performed a meta-analysis of 11 randomized trials of patients receiving intravesical chemotherapy for primary resection; patients with recurrent disease were excluded from the analysis (39). The analysis demonstrated a relative decrease in tumor recurrence risk of 44% at 1 year. Patients receiving chemotherapy for 2 years showed the greatest decrease in recurrence rates (39). In a follow-up meta-analysis of eight

TABLE 25B.2

RANDOMIZED TRIALS USING COMBINATION THERAPY

First Author	Pathology	N	Arm A	CR or RR	N	Arm B	CR or RR	Follow-up	P
Rintala (47)	Tis	40	MMC	47% at 24 mo	28	Weekly MMC followed by MMC alternating with BCG	74% at 24 mo	Mean = 33 mo	.043
Rintala (46)	Recurrent Ta/T1	93	MMC	22%	95	Weekly MMC followed by MMC alternating with BCG	19%	Mean = 34 mo	NS
Di Stasi (48)	T1 G2/3	92	BCG + monthly BCG	47%	93	Weekly BCG, BCG, eMMC X3 monthly eMMC, eMMC, BCG	28%	64 vs. 71 mo	.001
Kaasinen (49)	Recurrent Ta/T1	118	MMC followed by BCG	33%	118	Weekly MMC followed by BCG alternating with interferon-alpha	78%	Median = 31 mo	<.00001
Witjes (50)	High- and intermediate-risk pap TCC Ta/T1	92	MMC	46%	90	MMC followed by BCG	39%	Median = 32 mo	NS
Ali-El-Dein (51)		58	BCG	21%	56	BCG alternating with epirubicin	11%	Median = 30 mo	NS
Kaasinen (52)	Tis	145	BCG	54% at 5 yr	159	MMC followed by BCG alternating with MMC	41% at 5 y	Median = 56 mo	.03

CR, complete response; RR, recurrence rate; pap, papillary; TCC, transitional cell carcinoma; MMC, mitomycin C; BCG, bacillus Calmette-Guerin; NS, not stated.

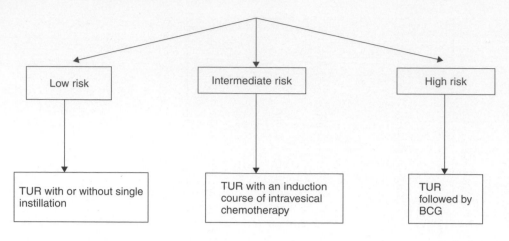

FIGURE 25B.1. Treatment of superficial bladder cancer.

chemotherapy studies enrolling patients with recurrent tumors, Huncharek et al. found a 38% reduction in relative 1-year tumor recurrence risk that was further improved at 2 and 3 years (55). Doxorubicin appeared to be less effective in the longer term.

Although earlier reports suggested that the beneficial effects of adjuvant intravesical chemotherapy are temporary (53), several studies have since demonstrated durable effects. An MRC trial comparing one and five instillations of MMC versus TUR alone demonstrated a decrease in the recurrence rate after a median follow-up of 7 years (28). Similarly, a phase III trial comparing a standard versus an optimized dose of MMC showed a decreased recurrence rate at 5 years for the optimized dose (12).

Figure 25B.1 shows treatment recommendations for superficial disease.

Conclusion

Intravesical chemotherapy decreases tumor recurrence. All current chemotherapeutic agents are similar in efficacy. A single postoperative instillation is effective in patients with low-grade papillary tumors, while postoperative instillation along with a more intensive regimen is recommended for patients with multiple or recurrent lesions. The role of maintenance chemotherapy and sequential chemoimmunotherapy remains unclear. New technologies such as microwave thermochemotherapy and electromotive thermochemotherapy are showing promise. Intravesical chemotherapy does not affect progression.

IMMUNOTHERAPY

Unlike chemotherapy, which relies on the direct cytotoxic effect of the drug, immunotherapy requires the induction of an inflammatory immune response in the bladder to achieve an anticancer effect. While multiple immunostimulating agents have been variably tried in the past, only BCG has reproducibly resulted in substantial improvements in all three categories of therapeutic use: eradication of existing disease, prevention of recurrence, and reduction in disease progression.

Brief History of Bacillus Calmette-Guerin Use

BCG was developed by Albert Calmette and Camille Guèrin in 1921 at the Pasteur Institute in France by attenuating the cow tuberculosis bacillus, *Mycobacterium bovis* (56). Used worldwide (except in the United States and Canada) as a live vaccine against tuberculosis, laboratory and clinical studies subsequently suggested BCG might be able to act against a wide range of malignancies (57–60). In 1976, Morales et al. reported the first successful treatment in 7 of 9 patients with recurrent superficial stage Ta/T1 TCC using intravesical BCG once a week for 6 weeks BCG (61). It is noteworthy that the choice of dose, interval, dwell time, and number of treatments was arbitrary, without the benefit of phase I or II studies. In the early 1980s both the Southwest Oncology Group (SWOG) and Memorial Sloan-Kettering Cancer Center verified the efficacy of the Morales regimen against TCC, which led to the clinical acceptance of this treatment scheme during the ensuing two decades (62,63). Currently there are multiple substrains of BCG in use for superficial bladder cancer throughout the world, including Pasteur, Armand-Frappier, TICE, RIVM, Glaxo, and Tokyo among others. There are no conclusive clinical studies showing superiority of one BCG substrain over another.

Mechanism of Action

BCG evokes a complex immune response in the bladder, beginning with its binding to fibronectin and integrin-mediated ingestion by urothelial cells with subsequent elaboration of various chemokines and pro-inflammatory cytokines (64). Within the first few hours of instillation, neutrophils are recruited into the urine, followed by monocytes, macrophages, T cells, and natural killer (NK) cells, some of which take up transient residence in the bladder submucosa as granuloma. With successive BCG instillations this process is greatly accentuated, leading to development of a local type 1 cellular immune response characterized by high levels of urinary cytokines, such as tumor necrosis factor, interleukin-2, and interferon-gamma. Irritative urinary symptoms peak at the same time as the inflammatory response and likewise usually resolve within 12 to 24 hours. In response to the inflammatory process, the urothelial and tumor cells upregulate the expression of important surface proteins, such as major histocompatibility antigens, adhesion molecules, and death receptors; this response endures for 3 to 6 months. The immune cell type responsible for actual TCC elimination is unknown, but research studies suggest multiple cells, including neutrophils, macrophages, T cells, and NK cells, may be responsible (65). Despite the involvement of T cells, there is no evidence that systemic immunity to bladder cancer cells occurs. Tumors outside the physical contact zone for BCG, such as in the upper tract and prostatic ducts, do not reliably respond to BCG instillation unless BCG is mechanically delivered to these sanctuary sites.

BCG for Residual Disease

One of the most demonstrable examples of intravesical BCG's anticancer activity is its ability to ablate existing bladder tumors either following incomplete TUR (residual tumor) or in place of TUR as primary therapy (immunoresection) (66–75). While the ablative effect of one course of BCG on residual papillary tumors varies between 15% and 70%, the total CR rate is consistently approximately 60% if at least one additional course of therapy is included. Those studies providing 1-year to 3-year follow-up show only a marginal drop-off over time, but this is difficult to interpret given the tendency to use various regimens of maintenance therapy. Results from these trials also suggest it is prudent to (a) perform debulking TUR whenever possible, especially if tumor burden exceeds 3 cm, (b) institute therapy within 3 weeks after TUR, and (c) use caution when treating residual T1 grade 2-3 disease since these tumors appear to be less responsive to BCG ablation alone and are often clinically understaged (76).

Numerous BCG therapy trials for CIS have reported aggregate CR rates between 70% and 75%, if up to two induction cycles are used (77). In one study the ultimate complete response of CIS to BCG followed a delayed time course, whereby the 6-month CR was increased another 11% above that of the 3-month CR (from 56.9% to 68.1%) even in the absence of additional therapy (78). These impressive results have made BCG the therapy of choice for primary CIS, secondary CIS, and concomitant CIS (79). Over half of complete responders remain disease-free over 5 years from the start of therapy, resulting in a substantial reduction in the need for alternative therapy, primarily cystectomy (80–82).

BCG for Prophylaxis

Multiple clinical trials directly comparing TUR alone to TUR plus BCG for tumor prophylaxis (i.e., no CIS or obvious residual disease) have demonstrated a statistically significant benefit in the reduction of bladder cancer recurrence rates, ranging between 20% and 57% at median follow-ups of 2 to 7 years (83–90). In aggregate, this amounts to an estimated net benefit of about 32% versus surgery alone, an amount over twice that reported for intravesical chemotherapy by Lamm using a similar comparison technique (4). Relative risk for recurrence was found to be reduced to 0.39 in the large Spanish Primary Bladder Tumor Registry (91) and 0.3 at 12 months in an even larger British meta-analysis (92). Interestingly, the greatest clinical benefits appear to be derived by those patients with more recurrent or aggressive disease, including prior chemotherapy failures (83,84,93). The median duration of disease freedom is 2 to 4 years, over twice that expected for surgery alone, along with a threefold to fourfold reduction in recurrence index (number of separate recurrence episodes divided by follow-up time).

Impact of BCG on Progression

Reduction in true disease progression has been difficult to demonstrate in any single clinical trial with BCG, partly owing to the low event rate and long follow-up time required. A nonrandomized Spanish registry study showed a reduction in relative risk of progression to 0.3 with BCG therapy (91). Likewise, Solsona et al. reported a progression rate of 12% for BCG versus 29% for chemotherapy, a statistically significant difference, in the composite analysis of two randomized trials of high-risk adjuvant intravesical therapy (94). The most persuasive evidence to date comes from an even larger meta-analysis involving 4,863 patients in 24 trials, in which a statistically significant 27% reduction in the odds of progression (9.8% vs. 13.8%) was found for patients receiving BCG at a mean follow-up of 2.5 years (95). The size of the treatment effect was similar in patients with either papillary disease or CIS. Death due to bladder cancer favored BCG by 19%, but the difference was not statistically significant.

The Role of BCG Maintenance Therapy

Many modern BCG treatment programs incorporate some form of time-limited continuous retreatment with BCG, even for patients with no demonstrable disease. This practice probably derives from the recognized benefit of additional courses of BCG reinduction therapy (68,72,73,84,96) and the steady relapse rate of initial complete responders over time. Only recently has there been sufficient evidence to support such a policy.

Two early randomized controlled studies using either one dose of BCG every 3 months or one dose monthly for 2 years failed to demonstrate a statistical advantage to maintenance therapy (97,98). Furthermore, patients in both trials had additional local toxicity attributable to BCG. Studies from other countries have been equally disappointing. Tachibana et al. did see favorable results in 12-month and 18-month maintenance groups, but statistical significance was not achieved (99). Palou et al. in a large randomized Spanish trial, reported an 11% overall benefit to routine 6-week courses every 6 months for 2 years in patients with no evidence of disease 6 months after TUR and induction BCG, but this difference did not reach statistical significance (100).

Results of the SWOG 8507 trial specifically designed to answer the maintenance question indicate an alternative schedule is useful (78). Using miniseries of three weekly treatments administered at 3 and 6 months, then every 6 months to 3 years, there was a statistically significant difference in favor of maintenance therapy over a 1 year follow-up. For 233 randomized patients with CIS, 84% ultimately achieved a CR with maintenance versus 68% without ($P = .004$). For 254 patients with papillary disease and complete resection at the time of randomization, 87% were disease-free at 2 years in the maintenance arm compared to 57% without maintenance. A differential of at least 20% persisted up to 5 years. For patients with CIS or papillary disease, median recurrence-free survival was roughly doubled from 36 to 77 months. Even disease worsening was improved in the maintenance group by a statistically significant 6%. However, one quarter of patients on maintenance experienced significant grade 3 toxicity, and less than half completed more than three cycles, with only 16% completing all seven planned cycles. Since the maintenance group as a whole benefited even without most patients completing a full 3 years of therapy, maximum benefit may have been achieved earlier. These results have been reproduced in a smaller nonrandomized study with only 19% completing the entire 3-year maintenance schedule (101).

Additional support for BCG maintenance has indirectly come from large meta-analyses of prior clinical trials. In the analysis of reduction of progression, Sylvester et al. found that only trials employing maintenance therapy contributed to the observed benefit of BCG (95). Similarly, Boehle et al. found that a statistically significant improvement favoring BCG versus mitomycin for tumor recurrence was apparent only in trials using at least 1 year of BCG maintenance (102). Collectively, the scales have tipped in the direction of routine BCG maintenance, especially for patients with high-risk disease.

BCG Toxicity

The toxic effects of BCG occur both locally and systemically. The vast majority of patients experience self-limited cystitis that escalates with later treatments (103,104). Symptoms usually begin 2 to 4 hours after instillation, peak between 6 to 10 hours, and resolve rapidly over the next 24 to 48 hours. Microscopic hematuria and pyuria are common, while occasional gross hematuria also occurs. Systemic manifestations of the inflammatory response follow a similar time course and include fevers, chills, a flu-like malaise, and occasional arthralgias. During re-induction or maintenance cycles, all of these symptoms tend to be more intense, occur sooner after the instillation, and reach the highest level by the second or third treatment. Most symptoms can be controlled with the appropriate use of acetaminophen, nonsteroidal anti-inflammatories, urinary analgesics, and antispasmodics. Routine administration of antibiotics with catheterization is not recommended. If clinically indicated for nonBCG infection, penicillins, cephalosporins, trimethoprim/sulfa, and nitrofurantoin are preferred, while fluoroquinolones, azithromycin, and doxycycline are to be avoided since they can kill BCG and could affect efficacy (105,106). Conversely, short courses of antiBCG antibiotics such as isoniazid (INH) and rifampin have not been shown to diminish either the associated symptomatology or the incidence of serious BCG infection (106).

Clinical signs of a more serious process, such as BCG intravasation into the bloodstream (BCGosis), include exaggerated manifestations of systemic effects, particularly if they occur early during the initial course of induction therapy, within 2 hours after BCG instillation, or in the setting of traumatic catheterization. A fever of over 102.5°F, while a cause for concern, is not in itself a definite sign of BCGosis, especially if it occurs at the expected peak time and resolves within 24 hours (107). Such patients need evaluation but, in the absence of other signs, may be treated initially with fluoroquinolone antibiotics and antipyretics. Conversely, fevers that begin after 24 hours, persist more than 48 hours, or relapse in a diurnal pattern (usually in the early evening) are more indicative of an established BCG infection (BCGitis). Organ-specific manifestations may be present, suggesting epididymal orchitis, pneumonitis, and hepatitis. These patients usually require hospitalization and the administration of triple-drug therapy such as INH, rifampin, and ethambutol. A fluoroquinolone may also be added, since it covers most gram-negative rods and has moderate activity against BCG. Failure to improve on such therapy, or significant clinical deterioration, should prompt institution of systemic steroids (e.g., prednisone 40 mg/day tapered over 2 to 6 weeks), which has been shown to be life-saving in such instances (108–110). BCG is resistant to both pyrazinamide and cycloserine. Antituberculosis drugs should be continued for 3 to 6 months depending on the severity of the presenting illness.

Prolonged symptomatic BCG cystitis and/or prostatitis can become a troubling problem during therapy and in the postBCG observation period. This situation is best avoided by withholding BCG treatment until all significant symptoms from the prior instillation have subsided. A delay of 1 to 2 weeks has not been shown to reduce BCG efficacy in such a setting. Reinstitution of BCG at a lower dose or premature termination of further treatment for this cycle may also be appropriate. If localized severe cystitis does occur and conservative measures fail, this condition can be treated with oral fluoroquinolones (3 to 12 weeks) or oral INH. A short 2-week to 3-week oral steroid taper sandwiched between antibiotic coverage has also been shown to be helpful in refractory cases (111). Rarely, a noninfectious hypersensitivity known as Reiter's syndrome (urethritis, arthritis, conjunctivitis) may occur during BCG treatment and should prompt cessation of further treatment (112).

New Prospectives for BCG Dosing

Dose Reduction

Efforts to decrease BCG toxicity while maintaining or enhancing efficacy are currently under study for all subgroups of patients treated with BCG. Several recent clinical trials have shown that decreasing the dose of BCG to one-half or one-third in the induction phase will lower the local toxicity by about 50%. However, controversy exists as to whether efficacy is sacrificed, especially in patients with multifocal or the more high-risk CIS or stage T1/grade 3 disease (84,113–118). Cancer results were worse in some studies, but in others they were actually better. The routine use of reinduction courses and extended maintenance regimens may have obscured weaker induction courses. Some of this discrepancy may also be due to differences in BCG sensitivity among various patient populations, either genetic or from prior BCG immunization. For example, populations in the US and Canada, unlike much of the world, are rarely vaccinated with BCG and have had little exposure to tuberculosis. This may explain why a Canadian study on BCG dose reduction for first-time treatment showed a substantial reduction in efficacy (116). Until this controversy is resolved, a more sensible approach may be to reduce the BCG dose during the maintenance phase to increase treatment tolerability, an option that has shown efficacy in combined BCG plus interferon trials (104).

Slow Dosing

There is at least one preliminary report that every-other-week BCG dosing for low-risk to intermediate-risk patients may be as effective as the conventional weekly dosing scheme, but with reduced side effects (119). This may be especially appropriate for patients with low-risk or intermediate-risk papillary tumors.

Regimen Modifications

The conventional BCG treatment regimen has come under increased scrutiny with the emerging knowledge about BCG's effect on the human immune system. Studies monitoring lymphoproliferative responses to BCG antigens, for instance, suggest preimmunized patients may peak after just four induction treatments, while nonimmunized patients may require more than six (120). During reinduction therapy for BCG failures, plateau urinary IL-2 is reached by treatment three, suggesting two cycles of 3 weekly retreatments may be better than one cycle of 6. Similarly, since immune parameters peak most commonly with the second weekly treatment during maintenance therapy, 2-week minicycles every 2 to 3 months may be better than either monthly maintenance or 3-week miniseries given every 3 to 6 months (121). Formal studies to prospectively investigate such strategies are in development.

BCG versus Intravesical Chemotherapy

BCG intravesical immunotherapy has been compared to several different chemotherapeutic agents in terms of efficacy and toxicities (Table 25B.3). In a SWOG study comparing BCG to doxorubicin, 262 patients with recurrent Ta/T1 disease or with CIS were randomly assigned to receive either Connaught strain BCG intravesically and percutaneously or doxorubicin. The median follow-up was 65 months. BCG produced more adverse side effects than doxorubicin, but the efficacy was superior with BCG. Of the patients with CIS assigned to BCG, 70% achieved a CR and 45% were estimated to be free of disease at 5 years. Of the patients assigned to doxorubicin, 34% achieved a CR and 18% were free of disease at 5 years. The

TABLE 25B.3

INTRAVESICAL CHEMOTHERAPY VERSUS BACILLUS CALMETTE-GUERIN

	Chemo agent	Pathology	Authors	No. Pts chemo	CR or RR chemo[a]	Median follow-up	No. Pts BCG	CR or RR BCG[a]	Median follow-up
Lamm et al. (122)	DOX	Ta/T1 CIS	No	68	17% 5 yr	65 mo	63	67% 5 yr	65 mo
SWOG		CIS		67	34%		64	70%	
Rintala et al. (123)	MMC	Ta/T1 CIS		46 12	70% 58%	N/A	45 10	88% 40%	N/A
Vegt et al. (124)	MMC	Ta/T1 CIS	No	136	57%	36 mo[b]	Tice 117 RIVM 134	36% 54%	36 mo[b] 36 mo[b]
Krege et al. (125)	MMC	Ta/T1		113	0.508[c]	20.2 mo	102	0.618[c]	20.2 mo
Lundholm et al. (126)	MMC	CIS Ta T1		42 51 32	33% 35%	39 mo	41 53 31	54% 48%	39 mo
Malmstrom et al. (127)	MMC	Ta/T1/ CIS		125	66%	64 mo	125	53%	64 mo
Melekos et al. (128)	EPI	Ta/T1		48	45.8%	35.2 mo[b]	46	34.8%	35.1 mo[b]

CR, complete response; RR, recurrence rate; DOX, doxorubicin; MMC, mitomycin C; EPI, epirubicin; CIS, carcinoma *in situ*; BCG, bacillus Calmette-Guerin; N/A, not applicable.
[a]Patients with papillary tumors were treated prophylactically and the primary endpoint was recurrence. Patients with CIS were treated therapeutically and the primary endpoint was CR as defined by lack of persistent CIS or positive cytology.
[b]Mean follow-up.
[c]Risk of recurrence relative to TUR alone.

recurrence rate for the patients with Ta or T1 disease without CIS was 63% for the BCG-treated patients and 82% for the doxorubicin-treated patients (122).

Melekos et al. (128) reported a randomized trial of epirubicin versus BCG for prophylaxis in patients with multiple superficial bladder tumors. This prospective study showed no difference in the recurrence rate after a mean follow-up of 35.1 months. However, in patients with T1 and high-grade tumors, BCG was superior to epirubicin.

Numerous studies have compared BCG to MMC, with mixed results. In a randomized trial, the Finnbladder Group showed that BCG Pasteur strain was superior to MMC in 91 patients with recurrent superficial bladder cancer. After a follow-up of 6 months, 70% of patients had a CR to MMC and 88% to BCG; at 12 months CR was observed in 79% and 97%, respectively (123). Among patients with CIS, the CR rate was 58% in the mitomycin group and 40% in the BCG group.

In a three-arm, prospective randomized trial, the Dutch Southeast Cooperative Urological Group compared the efficacy of MMC chemotherapy to BCG-RIVM strain and BCG-Tice strain in patients with Ta, T1, or CIS. MMC was given in a 30-mg dose once a week for 4 weeks, followed by a monthly dose for a total of 6 months. Both strains of BCG were given once a week for 6 consecutive weeks. Time to recurrence was the primary endpoint. The study enrolled 469 patients with a mean follow-up of 36 months (range, 2 to 81 months). For stages Ta/T1 without CIS, recurrence was observed in 58 of 136 (43%) evaluable patients treated with MMC, 62 of 134 (46%) treated with BCG-RIVM, and 75 of 117 (64%) treated with BCG-Tice. MMC and BCG-RIVM were equally effective, while MMC was more effective than BCG-Tice. For patients with CIS, the CR rate was 67% for MMC, 60% for BCG-RIVM, and 74% for BCG-Tice. Progression in tumor stage was noted in eight (6%) of the MMC group, eight (6%) of the BCG-RIVM group, and seven (5%) of the BCG-Tice group. Due to the small number of patients, this study does not address the efficacy of MMC versus the two strains of

BCG in CIS (124). MMC was discontinued in 8.6% of patients and BCG instillations in 19.6%, due to side effects.

More recently, Krege et al. (125) reported a randomized multicenter trial of adjuvant therapy of TUR only versus TUR plus MMC versus TUR plus BCG. The study included 337 patients with Ta or T1 disease. MMC was given every 2 weeks at a dose of 20 mg per instillation. At a median follow-up of 20.2 months, there was no significant difference in recurrence rates between the MMC and BCG instillations, and the progression rate was similar in all three therapy groups. The relative risk of recurrence, compared to TUR alone, was 0.508 after MMC and 0.618 after BCG.

Lundholm et al. (126) reported the results of the Swedish-Norwegian Bladder Cancer Study Group, which enrolled 261 patients with CIS, T1 grade 3, or multiple recurrent Ta/T1 grade 1 or 2 disease. Patients were randomized to MMC 40 mg or BCG Pasteur strain instilled weekly for 6 weeks, followed by monthly instillations for 1 year and every 3 months for another year. The median follow-up was 39 months and the disease-free rate was 49% for BCG and 33% for MMC. Among Ta/T1 patients the disease-free rates for BCG and mitomycin were 48% and 35%; among patients with CIS rates were 54% and 33%. Although BCG was superior to MMC in preventing recurrence, no significant difference in progression was observed. Patients receiving BCG had more frequent side effects.

Malmstrom et al. reported a randomized study comparing MMC to BCG (127). After a median follow-up of 5 years, 34% in the MMC group and 47% in the BCG group were free of disease ($P = 0.04$). There was no difference in progression or survival between the two arms.

The results from three large meta-analyses help to put the BCG versus MMC question in proper perspective. Using 11 clinical trials involving approximately 2,800 patients in aggregate, Bohle et al. reported an overall statistical superiority of BCG over mitomycin in reducing tumor recurrence rate by an odds ratio of 0.56 (38.6% for BCG vs. 46.4% for MMC)

(102). Importantly, only studies using BCG maintenance contributed to this advantage (odds ratio of 0.43). The trade-off, though, was a 1.8-fold increase in associated cystitis for BCG (53.8% vs. 39.2%). With regard to superficial TCC progression, the results are less clear. Sylvester et al. could not demonstrate a statistically significant advantage to BCG versus MMC for progression (overall 14% difference favoring BCG). However, Bohle et al. using a larger database including non-English studies, did find a statistically significant reduction in odds risk of progression for BCG compared to maintenance to MMC (OR Odd ratio = 0.66) (129). Because these studies with MMC did not routinely incorporate more recent modifications optimizing efficacy, this conclusion may no longer be applicable. At this time, MMC should still be considered a viable option for patients with papillary tumors at low-intermediate risk of progression. However, BCG with maintenance should be viewed as the agent of choice for the management of CIS and higher-risk bladder cancer.

Intravesical Chemotherapy After Failure of BCG

Although BCG is highly effective for bladder cancer, the problem of BCG failure is significant. For these patients, radical cystectomy is the gold standard. Patients are, however, sometimes reluctant to undergo major surgery for a condition that does not pose an immediate threat to their lives. Furthermore, radical cystectomy is not suitable for a subset of patients with severe comorbidities. A number of alternatives have been developed.

In evaluating salvage therapies for use after BCG failure, comparisons between therapies have been hampered by the lack of standard definitions for BCG failure and BCG-refractory transitional cell carcinoma (TCC). Some series have defined BCG failure after a single induction course of BCG (130,131),

others after two courses (132). In addition, the methods of reporting the results have been inconsistent. Most studies have included all patients who received one or more courses of BCG (133–136). Investigators have often combined patients with persistent disease (nonresponders) and patients with recurrent Tis after an initial response (130,132), and a few studies have combined patients who were nonresponders to BCG and patients who could not complete BCG therapy because of toxicity (BCG intolerant) (132,133). Furthermore, most studies have combined all patients with papillary tumors with and without Tis. Finally, most studies did not indicate the disease-free interval after the last BCG course. These inconsistencies have led to comparisons of outcome in a very heterogeneous population. As shown in Figure 25B.2, we recommend defining BCG failure as persistence of disease after two consecutive courses of BCG, or any other situation associated with a high risk of progression: recurrent Tis within less than 6 months of achieving a CR after one or two courses of BCG, recurrent Tis while on maintenance therapy, or relapse with T1 disease.

Intravesical Valrubicin

Valrubicin is an analogue of adriamycin [N-trifluoroacetyladriamycin-14-valerate (AD32)], an anthracycline with a mechanism of action different from the parent compound. Valrubicin inhibits nucleotide incorporation into DNA and RNA, leading to chromosomal damage (137). In a phase I study of 32 patients with superficial TCC, 13 patients (41%) achieved a CR to valrubicin treatment. The drug had only minor systemic side effects, and the serum levels of unmetabolized valrubicin and its two primary metabolites were very low. However, 29 patients (91%) had mild to severe irritative symptoms, which persisted for several days after each instillation (138).

The efficacy of valrubicin was demonstrated in a phase II study of 90 patients with Tis after failure of multiple courses

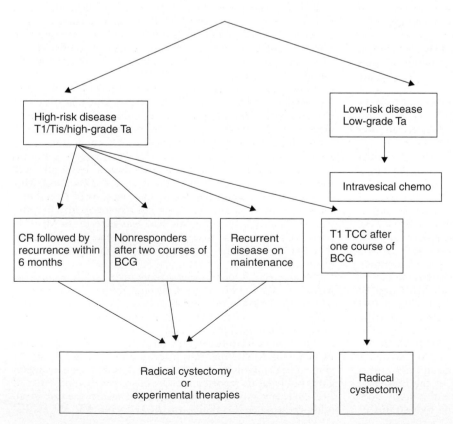

FIGURE 25B.2. Treatment of BCG-refractory bladder cancer.

of intravesical therapy, including at least one course of BCG. Patients received 800 mg of valrubicin weekly for 6 weeks. Nineteen patients (21%) had a CR, defined as no evidence of recurrence for at least 6 months from the initiation of therapy, and 7 of these 19 had a durable response, with a median follow-up of 30 months. Forty-four patients underwent radical cystectomy (six of whom had stage pT3 disease at cystectomy), and 4 patients died of bladder cancer during follow-up. Most patients (90%) had mild to moderate local bladder symptoms, with urinary frequency in 66%, urinary urgency in 63%, and dysuria in 60% (136).

In 1997, valrubicin was approved by the FDA for the treatment of BCG-refractory Tis in patients who refuse cystectomy. Unfortunately, its clinical availability has been severely curtailed.

Intravesical Gemcitabine

Gemcitabine (2',2'-difluoro-2'-deoxycytidine, Gemzar; Eli Lilly and Co, Indianapolis, IN) is a novel deoxycytidine analog with a broad spectrum of antitumor activity. Gemcitabine has a molecular weight of 299.66, and, after intracellular activation, the active metabolite is incorporated into DNA, resulting in inhibition of further DNA synthesis. Gemcitabine may also inhibit ribonucleotide reductase and cytidine deaminase as part of its cytotoxic activity (139). Gemcitabine is highly effective (overall response rates ranging from 22.5% to 28%) and well tolerated as both first-line and second-line, single-agent therapy for the treatment of metastatic TCC (140–142). Studies have reported a low incidence of systemic side effects. A randomized, multicenter, phase III study demonstrated that patients with unresectable or metastatic disease treated with gemcitabine plus cisplatin (GC) had a similar survival to patients treated with MVAC [methotrexate, vinblastine, doxorubicin (Adriamycin), and cisplatin], and GC had a better safety profile and tolerability (143). Based on its excellent clinical activity, patient tolerability, and chemical characteristics, gemcitabine represents a logical candidate for intravesical therapy.

Dalbagni et al. reported a phase I study of intravesical gemcitabine twice a week for 3 weeks, followed by a second cycle after a week of rest, in a heavily pretreated population with BCG-refractory TCC. This study demonstrated that intravesical gemcitabine was well tolerated with minimal bladder irritation and acceptable myelosuppression. Serum levels of gemcitabine were undetectable at concentrations of 5 mg/mL, 10 mg/mL, and 15 mg/mL. However, serum gemcitabine was detected at a concentration of 20 mg/mL. CR, as defined by a negative post-treatment cystoscopy including a biopsy of the urothelium and a negative cytology, was achieved in seven of 18 patients (39%) (133). This was followed by a phase II study of patients with BCG-refractory TCC to determine the efficacy of gemcitabine as an intravesical agent. Twenty-eight patients completed therapy, and 16 achieved a CR (144).

Laufer et al. reported a phase I study of weekly intravesical gemcitabine in 15 patients who received prior intravesical therapy. Serum gemcitabine levels were undetected at concentrations of 5 mg/mL, 10 mg/mL, 15 mg/mL, and 20 mg/mL, while low concentrations were present in all patients receiving 40 mg/mL. However, the metabolite dFdU (2'2'-difluorodeoxyuridine) was detectable in plasma of patients receiving gemcitabine at concentrations of 15 mg/mL or higher, implying minimal absorption of gemcitabine at lower doses. The authors concluded that intravesical gemcitabine is well tolerated, with minimal toxicity. Furthermore, no evidence of recurrence at 12 weeks was noted in nine of 13 evaluable patients (145).

In a recent phase I study, De Berardinis reported no systemic detection of gemcitabine at a concentration of 40 mg/mL. However, the inactive metabolite was detected in plasma. They were able to demonstrate activity of deoxycytidine kinase in tissue samples, a enzyme that produces 2',2'-difluoro-deoxycytidine triphosphate, the active metabolite of gemcitabine (146).

All reports published thus far confirm the low systemic absorption of gemcitabine, the good tolerability with minimal local and systemic toxicity, and, more importantly, its efficacy as an intravesical agent, even in heavily pretreated patients. This agent warrants further investigation in a large cohort of patients, especially to determine the long-term durability.

Intravesical BCG and Interferon-alpha

Interferons are glycoproteins that mediate immune responses such as stimulation of phagocytes, cytokine release, enhanced natural killer cell activity, and activation of T and B lymphocytes. Intravesical IFN-α has demonstrated activity in patients with superficial bladder cancer (147). Among 9 patients with Tis enrolled in a randomized trial after failure of prior intravesical therapy, 2 had a CR to IFN-α (131). Intravesical IFN-α has been shown to have moderate ($\geq$40%) dose-dependent (better for doses at or above 80 MU) clinical activity against papillary bladder cancer both in postTUR (prophylactic) and in marker lesion (ablative) settings (148,149).

A phase I study of low-dose BCG with different doses of IFN-α demonstrated that this combination is well tolerated (150). O'Donnell et al. reported the efficacy of the combination in a cohort of patients who had received one or more induction courses of BCG. Of 40 patients enrolled, 63% and 53% were disease-free at 12 and 24 months, respectively (134). The response for patients in whom a single course of BCG failed was similar to the response of those in whom multiple courses failed. There was a trend toward worse outcomes in patients with an early relapse after the induction course of BCG (134). Punnen et al. reported a durable response to low-dose BCG plus IFN-α in 6 of 12 patients with superficial TCC who received one or more courses of BCG (151). Lam et al. treated 32 patients with superficial bladder cancer, including patients whose disease recurred after BCG. After a follow-up of 22 months, 66% were disease free (152). O'Donnell et al. also recently reported the interim results of 490 intermediate-high risk patients treated with BCG plus IFN-α followed for a median of 24 months. For BCG-naïve patients receiving standard dose BCG plus IFN-α the 2-year disease-free estimate was 57%, while for prior BCG failures it was 42% on low-dose BCG + IFN-α. About a 50% decrease in BCG toxicity as seen in the low-dose BCG regimen. No increase in early progression or cystectomy rate was noted for BCG failures (153).

Photodynamic Therapy

Investigators have reported the efficacy of photodynamic therapy in managing superficial tumors. This approach has also been tested in patients with BCG-refractory tumors. Nseyo et al. reported the results of a multicenter trial for assessing the safety and efficacy of porfimer sodium photodynamic therapy in patients in whom prior intravesical therapy for Tis failed. Of the 36 patients enrolled, 34 had received more than one intravesical therapy, including thiotepa, mitomycin, and doxorubicin. At 3 months, 58% achieved a CR, but 10 of the 21 responders had a recurrence during follow-up, which averaged 12 months. Fourteen patients (39%) underwent a radical cystectomy for persistent or recurrent disease, and 22% had muscle-invasive disease. Significant urinary symptoms developed, and seven patients developed bladder contractures (154).

Photodynamic therapy after oral administration of 5-aminolevulinic acid was performed in 24 patients with recurrent superficial TCC after BCG. At a median follow-up of 36 months, three of five patients with Tis and four of 19 with papillary TCC were free of disease (155).

Other alternative therapies have been investigated, including oral bropirimine, an immunostimulant that has produced remission in patients with Tis after prior intravesical therapy (132). CR was detected in 30% of the evaluable patients who were BCG-resistant. Progression to muscle-invasive or metastatic disease was documented in 6% of the patients (132). This agent was abandoned for further clinical use.

Radical cystectomy still remains the standard of care for patients with BCG-refractory Tis. Salvage therapy for patients who refuse cystectomy is still under investigation. New promising strategies and agents warrant further investigation.

References

1. Reuter VE, Melamed MR. The lower urinary tract. In: Sternberg S, ed. *Diagnostic surgical pathology*, New York: Raven Press, 1994:1764–1805.
2. Soloway MS. Overview of treatment of superficial bladder cancer. *Urology* 1985;26:18–26.
3. Heney NM, Ahmed S, Flanagan MJ, et al. Superficial bladder cancer: progression and recurrence. *J Urol* 1983;130:1083–1086.
4. Lamm DL. Long-term results of intravesical therapy for superficial bladder cancer. *Urol Clin North Am* 1992;19:573–580.
5. Heney NM, Koontz WW, Barton B, et al. Intravesical thiotepa versus mitomycin C in patients with Ta, T1 and TIS transitional cell carcinoma of the bladder: a phase III prospective randomized study. *J Urol* 1988;140:1390–1393.
6. Nilsson S, Ragnhammar P, Glimelius B, et al. A systematic overview of chemotherapy effects in urothelial bladder cancer. *Acta Oncol* 2001;40:371–390.
7. Thrasher JB, Crawford ED. Complications of intravesical chemotherapy. *Urol Clin North Am* 1992;19:529–539.
8. Okamura K, Murase T, Obata K, et al. A randomized trial of early intravesical instillation of epirubicin in superficial bladder cancer. The Nagoya University Urological Oncology Group. *Cancer Chemother Pharmacol* 1994;35:S31–S35.
9. Oosterlinck W, Kurth KH, Schroder F, et al. A prospective European Organization for Research and Treatment of Cancer Genitourinary Group randomized trial comparing transurethral resection followed by a single intravesical instillation of epirubicin or water in single stage Ta, T1 papillary carcinoma of the bladder. *J Urol* 1993;149:749–752.
10. Melekos MD, Dauaher H, Fokaefs E, et al. Intravesical instillations of 4-epi-doxorubicin (epirubicin) in the prophylactic treatment of superficial bladder cancer: results of a controlled prospective study. *J Urol* 1992;147:371–375.
11. Ali-el-Dein B, el-Baz M, Aly AN, et al. Intravesical epirubicin versus doxorubicin for superficial bladder tumors (stages pTa and pT1): a randomized prospective study. *J Urol* 1997;158:68–73; discussion 73–74.
12. Au JL, Badalament RA, Wientjes MG, et al. Methods to improve efficacy of intravesical mitomycin C: results of a randomized phase III trial. *J Natl Cancer Inst* 2001;93:597–604.
13. Bouffioux C, Denis L, Oosterlinck W, et al. Adjuvant chemotherapy of recurrent superficial transitional cell carcinoma: results of a European Organization for Research on Treatment of Cancer randomized trial comparing intravesical instillation of thiotepa, doxorubicin and cisplatin. The European Organization for Research on Treatment of Cancer Genitourinary Group. *J Urol* 1992;148:297–301.
14. Eto H, Oka Y, Ueno K, et al. Comparison of the prophylactic usefulness of epirubicin and doxorubicin in the treatment of superficial bladder cancer by intravesical instillation: a multicenter randomized trial. Kobe University Urological Oncology Group. *Cancer Chemother Pharmacol* 1994;35:S46–S51.
15. Shinohara N, Nonomura K, Tanaka M, et al. Prophylactic chemotherapy with anthracyclines (adriamycin, epirubicin, and pirarubicin) for primary superficial bladder cancer. The Hokkaido University Bladder Cancer Collaborative Group. *Cancer Chemother Pharmacol* 1994;35:S41–S45.
16. Zincke H, Utz DC, Taylor WF, et al. Influence of thiotepa and doxorubicin instillation at time of transurethral surgical treatment of bladder cancer on tumor recurrence: a prospective, randomized, double-blind, controlled trial. *J Urol* 1983;129:505–509.
17. Zincke H, Benson RC Jr, Hilton JF, et al. Intravesical thiotepa and mitomycin C treatment immediately after transurethral resection and later for superficial (stages Ta and Tis) bladder cancer: a prospective, randomized, stratified study with crossover design. *J Urol* 1985;134:1110–1114.
18. Flanigan RC, Ellison MF, Butler KM, et al. A trial of prophylactic thiotepa or mitomycin C intravesical instillation in patients with recurrent or multiple superficial bladder cancers. *J Urol* 1986;136:35–37.
19. Martinez-Pineiro JA, Jimenez Leon J, Martinez-Pineiro L Jr, et al. Bacillus Calmette-Guerin versus doxorubicin versus thiotepa: a randomized prospective study in 202 patients with superficial bladder cancer. *J Urol* 1990;143:502–506.
20. Medical Research Council Working Party on Urological Cancer. The effect of intravesical thiotepa on the recurrence rate of newly diagnosed superficial bladder cancer: an MRC study. *Br J Urol* 1985;57:680.
21. Masters JR, McDermott BJ, Harland S, et al. ThioTEPA pharmacokinetics during intravesical chemotherapy: the influence of dose and volume of instillate on systemic uptake and dose rate to the tumour. *Cancer Chemother Pharmacol* 1996;38:59–64.
22. Gao X, Au JL, Badalament RA, et al. Bladder tissue uptake of mitomycin C during intravesical therapy is linear with drug concentration in urine. *Clin Cancer Res* 1998;4:139–143.
23. Masters JR, Popert RJ, Thompson PM, et al. Intravesical chemotherapy with epirubicin: a dose response study. *J Urol* 1999;161:1490–1493.
24. Igawa M, Urakami S, Shirakawa H, et al. Intravesical instillation of epirubicin: effect on tumour recurrence in patients with dysplastic epithelium after transurethral resection of superficial bladder tumour [see Comments]. *Br J Urol* 1996;77:358–362.
25. Kuroda M, Niijima T, Kotake T, et al. Effect of prophylactic treatment with intravesical epirubicin on recurrence of superficial bladder cancer—The 6th trial of the Japanese Urological Cancer Research Group (JUCRG): a randomized trial of intravesical epirubicin at dose of 20 mg/40 ml, 30 mg/40 ml, 40 mg/40 ml. *Eur Urol* 2004;45:600–605.
26. Burnand KG, Boyd PJ, Mayo ME, et al. Single dose intravesical thiotepa as an adjuvant to cystodiathermy in the treatment of transitional cell bladder carcinoma. *Br J Urol* 1976;48:55–59.
27. Medical Research Council Working Party on Urological Cancer, Subgroup on Superficial Bladder Cancer. The effect of intravesical thiotepa on tumour recurrence after endoscopic treatment of newly diagnosed superficial bladder cancer. A further report with long-term follow-up of a Medical Research Council randomized trial. *Br J Urol* 1994;73:632–638.
28. Tolley DA, Parmar MK, Grigor KM, et al. The effect of intravesical mitomycin C on recurrence of newly diagnosed superficial bladder cancer: a further report with 7 years of follow up. *J Urol* 1996;155:1233–1238.
29. Solsona E, Iborra I, Ricos JV, et al. Effectiveness of a single immediate mitomycin C instillation in patients with low risk superficial bladder cancer: short and long-term followup. *J Urol* 1999;161:1120–1123.
30. Ali-el-Dein B, Nabeeh A, el-Baz M, et al. Single-dose versus multiple instillations of epirubicin as prophylaxis for recurrence after transurethral resection of pTa and pT1 transitional-cell bladder tumours: a prospective, randomized controlled study [see Comment]. *Br J Urol* 1997;79:731–735.
31. Rajala P, Kaasinen E, Raitanen M, et al. Perioperative single dose instillation of epirubicin or interferon-alpha after transurethral resection for the prophylaxis of primary superficial bladder cancer recurrence: a prospective randomized multicenter study—FinnBladder III long-term results. *J Urol* 2002;168:981–985.
32. Rajala P, Liukkonen T, Raitanen M, et al. Transurethral resection with perioperative instillation on interferon-alpha or epirubicin for the prophylaxis of recurrent primary superficial bladder cancer: a prospective randomized multicenter study—Finnbladder III. *J Urol* 1999;161:1133–1135; discussion 1135–1136.
33. Sylvester RJ, Oosterlinck W, van der Meijden AP. A single immediate postoperative instillation of chemotherapy decreases the risk of recurrence in patients with stage Ta/T1 bladder cancer: a meta-analysis of published results of randomized clinical trials. *J Urol* 2004;171:2186–2190, quiz 2435.
34. Huland H, Kloppel G, Feddersen I, et al. Comparison of different schedules of cytostatic intravesical instillations in patients with superficial bladder carcinoma: final evaluation of a prospective multicenter study with 419 patients. *J Urol* 1990;144:68–71; discussion 71–72.
35. Bouffioux C, Kurth KH, Bono A, et al. Intravesical adjuvant chemotherapy for superficial transitional cell bladder carcinoma: results of 2 European Organization for Research and Treatment of Cancer randomized trials with mitomycin C and doxorubicin comparing early versus delayed instillations and short-term versus long-term treatment. European Organization for Research and Treatment of Cancer Genitourinary Group. *J Urol* 1995;153:934–941.
36. Okamura K, Kinukawa T, Tsumura Y, et al. A randomized study of short-versus long-term epirubicin instillation for superficial bladder cancer. Nagoya University Urological Oncology Group. *Eur Urol* 1998;33:285–288; discussion 289.
37. Koga H, Kuroiwa K, Yamaguchi A, et al. A randomized controlled trial of short-term versus long-term prophylactic intravesical instillation chemotherapy for recurrence after transurethral resection of Ta/T1 transitional cell carcinoma of the bladder. *J Urol* 2004;171:153–157.
38. Conrad S, Friedrich MG, Schwaibold H. Long term prophylaxis with mitomycin C (MMC) further reduces tumor recurrence compared to short term prophylaxis with MMC or bacillus Calmette-Guerin (BCG) [Abstract]. *J Urol* 2004;171:271.
39. Huncharek M, Geschwind JF, Witherspoon B, et al. Intravesical chemotherapy prophylaxis in primary superficial bladder cancer: a meta-analysis of 3703 patients from 11 randomized trials. *J Clin Epidemiol* 2000;53:676–680.
40. De Bruijn EA, Sleeboom HP, van Helsdingen PJ, et al. Pharmacodynamics and pharmacokinetics of intravesical mitomycin C upon different dwelling times. *Int J Cancer* 1992;51:359–364.
41. Groos E, Walker L, Masters JR. Intravesical chemotherapy. Studies on the relationship between pH and cytotoxicity. *Cancer* 1986;58:1199–1203.
42. Colombo R, Da Pozzo LF, Salonia A, et al. Multicentric study comparing intravesical chemotherapy alone and with local microwave hyperthermia for prophylaxis of recurrence of superficial transitional cell carcinoma. *J Clin Oncol* 2003;21:4270–4276.

43. Gofrit ON, Shapiro A, Pode D, et al. Combined local bladder hyperthermia and intravesical chemotherapy for the treatment of high-grade superficial bladder cancer. *Urology* 2004;63:466–471.

44. Di Stasi SM, Giannantoni A, Stephen RL, et al. Intravesical electromotive mitomycin C versus passive transport mitomycin C for high risk superficial bladder cancer: a prospective randomized study. *J Urol* 2003;170:777–782.

45. Erol A, Ozgur S, Basar M, et al. Trial with bacillus Calmette-Guerin and epirubicin combination in the prophylaxis of superficial bladder cancer. *Urol Int* 1994;52:69–72.

46. Rintala E, Jauhiainen K, Kaasinen E, et al. Alternating mitomycin C and bacillus Calmette-Guerin instillation prophylaxis for recurrent papillary (stages Ta to T1) superficial bladder cancer. Finnbladder Group [see Comments]. *J Urol* 1996;156:56–59; discussion 59–60.

47. Rintala E, Jauhiainen K, Rajala P, et al. Alternating mitomycin C and bacillus Calmette-Guerin instillation therapy for carcinoma in situ of the bladder. The Finnbladder Group. *J Urol* 1995;154:2050–2053.

48. Di Stasi SM, Giannantoni A, Stephen RL. Sequential intravesical bacillus Calmette-Guerin and electromotive mitomycin-C for high risk superficial bladder cancer: a prospective controlled study [Abstract]. *J Urol* 2004; 171:280.

49. Kaasinen E, Rintala E, Pere AK, et al. Weekly mitomycin C followed by monthly bacillus Calmette-Guerin or alternating monthly interferon-alpha2B and bacillus Calmette-Guerin for prophylaxis of recurrent papillary superficial bladder carcinoma. *J Urol* 2000;164:47–52.

50. Witjes JA, Caris CT, Mungan NA, et al. Results of a randomized phase III trial of sequential intravesical therapy with mitomycin C and bacillus Calmette-Guerin versus mitomycin C alone in patients with superficial bladder cancer [see Comment]. *J Urol* 1998;160:1668–1671; discussion 1671–1672.

51. Ali-El-Dein B, Nabeeh A, Ismail EH, et al. Sequential bacillus Calmette-Guerin and epirubicin versus bacillus Calmette-Guerin alone for superficial bladder tumors: a randomized prospective study. *J Urol* 1999;162:339–342.

52. Kaasinen E, Wijkstrom H, Malmstrom PU, et al. Alternating mitomycin C and BCG instillations versus BCG alone in treatment of carcinoma in situ of the urinary bladder: a Nordic study. *Eur Urol* 2003;43:637–645.

53. Lamm DL, Riggs DR, Traynelis CL, et al. Apparent failure of current intravesical chemotherapy prophylaxis to influence the long-term course of superficial transitional cell carcinoma of the bladder. *J Urol* 1995;153:1444–1450.

54. Pawinski A, Sylvester R, Bouffioux C, et al. A combined analysis of EORTC/MRC randomized clinical trials for the prophylactic treatment of TaT1 bladder cancer. EORTC Genito-Urinary Tract Cancer Cooperative Group and the Medical Research Council Working Party on Superficial Bladder Cancer. *Acta Urol Belg* 1996;64:27.

55. Huncharek M, McGarry R, Kupelnick B. Impact of intravesical chemotherapy on recurrence rate of recurrent superficial transitional cell carcinoma of the bladder: results of a meta-analysis. *Anticancer Res* 2001; 21:765–769.

56. Crispen R. History of BCG and its substrains. *Prog Clin Biol Res* 1989; 310:35–50.

57. Mathe G, Amiel JL, Schwarzenberg L, et al. Active immunotherapy for acute lymphoblastic leukaemia. *Lancet* 1969;1:697–699.

58. Morton D, Eilber FR, Malmgren RA, et al. Immunological factors which influence response to immunotherapy in malignant melanoma. *Surgery* 1970;68:158–163; discussion 163–164.

59. Coe JE, Feldman JD. Extracutaneous delayed hypersensitivity, particularly in the guinea-pig bladder. *Immunology* 1966;10:127–136.

60. Zbar B, Bernstein ID, Bartlett GL, et al. Immunotherapy of cancer: regression of intradermal tumors and prevention of growth of lymph node metastases after intralesional injection of living Mycobacterium bovis. *J Natl Cancer Inst* 1972;49:119–130.

61. Morales A, Eidinger D, Bruce AW. Intracavitary bacillus Calmette-Guerin in the treatment of superficial bladder tumors. *J Urol* 1976;116:180–183.

62. Lamm DL, Thor DE, Harris SC, et al. Bacillus Calmette-Guerin immunotherapy of superficial bladder cancer. *J Urol* 1980;124:38–40.

63. Pinsky CM, Camacho FJ, Kerr D, et al. Intravesical administration of bacillus Calmette-Guerin in patients with recurrent superficial carcinoma of the urinary bladder: report of a prospective, randomized trial. *Cancer Treat Rep* 1985;69:47–53.

64. Alexandroff AB, Jackson AM, O'Donnell MA, et al. BCG immunotherapy of bladder cancer: 20 years on. *Lancet* 1999;353:1689–1694.

65. Bohle A, Brandau S. Immune mechanisms in bacillus Calmette-Guerin immunotherapy for superficial bladder cancer. *J Urol* 2003;170:964–969.

66. Douville Y, Pelouze G, Roy R, et al. Recurrent bladder papillomata treated with bacillus Calmette-Guerin: a preliminary report (phase I trial). *Cancer Treat Rep* 1978;62:551–552.

67. Morales A, Ottenhof P, Emerson L. Treatment of residual, non-infiltrating bladder cancer with bacillus Calmette-Guerin. *J Urol* 1981;125:649–651.

68. Brosman SA. BCG in the management of superficial bladder cancer. *Urology* 1984;23:82–87.

69. deKernion JB, Huang MY, Lindner A, et al. The management of superficial bladder tumors and carcinoma in situ with intravesical bacillus Calmette-Guerin. *J Urol* 1985;133:598–601.

70. Heney NM, Koontz WW, Weinstein R. BCG in superficial bladder cancer. *J Urol* 1986;135(Suppl.):184A.

71. Schellhammer PF, Ladaga LE, Fillion MB. Bacillus Calmette-Guerin for superficial transitional cell carcinoma of the bladder. *J Urol* 1986;135:261–264.

72. Pansadoro V, De Paula F. Intravesical bacillus Calmette-Guerin in the treatment of superficial transitional cell carcinoma of the bladder. *J Urol* 1987;138:299–301.

73. Kavoussi LR, Torrence RJ, Gillen DP, et al. Results of 6 weekly intravesical bacillus Calmette-Guerin instillations on the treatment of superficial bladder tumors. *J Urol* 1988;139:935–940.

74. Khanna OP, Son DL, Mazer H, et al. Multicenter study of superficial bladder cancer treated with intravesical bacillus Calmette-Guerin or adriamycin. *Urology* 1990;35:101–108.

75. Akaza H. BCG treatment of existing Ta, T1 tumours or carcinoma in situ of the bladder. *Eur Urol* 1995;27(Suppl 1):9–12.

76. Ozen H, Ekici S, Uygur MC, et al. Repeated transurethral resection and intravesical BCG for extensive superficial bladder tumors. *J Endourol* 2001;15:863–867.

77. Hudson MA, Herr HW. Carcinoma in situ of the bladder. *J Urol* 1995; 153:564–572.

78. Lamm DL, Blumenstein BA, Crissman JD, et al. Maintenance bacillus Calmette-Guerin immunotherapy for recurrent TA, T1 and carcinoma in situ transitional cell carcinoma of the bladder: a randomized Southwest Oncology Group Study. *J Urol* 2000;163:1124–1129.

79. Jakse G. Intravesical instillation of BCG in carcinoma in situ of the urinary bladder. EORTC protocol 30861. EORTC-GU Group. *Prog Clin Biol Res* 1989;310:187–192.

80. Herr HW, Wartinger DD, Fair WR, et al. Bacillus Calmette-Guerin therapy for superficial bladder cancer: a 10-year followup. *J Urol* 1992;147: 1020–1023.

81. Nadler RB, Catalona WJ, Hudson MA, et al. Durability of the tumor-free response for intravesical bacillus Calmette-Guerin therapy. *J Urol* 1994; 152:367–373.

82. Lamm DL, Blumenstein BA, Crawford ED, et al. A randomized trial of intravesical doxorubicin and immunotherapy with bacille Calmette-Guerin for transitional-cell carcinoma of the bladder. *N Engl J Med* 1991;325: 1205–1209.

83. Lamm DL. Bacillus Calmette-Guerin immunotherapy for bladder cancer. *J Urol* 1985;134:40–47.

84. Pagano F, Bassi P, Milani C, et al. A low dose bacillus Calmette-Guerin regimen in superficial bladder cancer therapy: is it effective? *J Urol* 1991; 146:32–35.

85. Melekos MD, Chionis H, Pantazakos A, et al. Intravesical bacillus Calmette-Guerin immunoprophylaxis of superficial bladder cancer: results of a controlled prospective trial with modified treatment schedule. *J Urol* 1993;149:744–748.

86. Yang DA, Li SQ, Li XT. Prophylactic effects of zhuling and BCG on postoperative recurrence of bladder cancer. *Zhonghua Wai Ke Za Zhi* 1994; 32:433–434.

87. Zhang S, Li H, Cheng H. The preventive recurrent results of postoperative intravesical instillation therapy in bladder cancer. *Zhonghua Wai Ke Za Zhi* 1995;33:304–306.

88. Krege S, Giani G, Meyer R, et al. A randomized multicenter trial of adjuvant therapy in superficial bladder cancer: transurethral resection only versus transurethral resection plus mitomycin C versus transurethral resection plus bacillus Calmette-Guerin. Participating clinics. *J Urol* 1996;156: 962–966.

89. Tkachuk VN, al-Shukri A, al-Khani F. The use of BCG vaccine for preventing recurrences of superficial bladder cancer. *Urol Nefrol (Mosk)* 1996;(2):23–25.

90. Iantorno R, Nicolai M, Mastroprimiano G, et al. Randomized prospective study comparing long-term intravesical instillation of BCG after transurethral resection and transurethral resection alone in patients with superficial bladder cancer. *J Urol* 1999;161:[Abstract 1100]284.

91. Millan-Rodriguez F, Chechile-Toniolo G, Salvador-Bayarri J, et al. Multivariate analysis of the prognostic factors of primary superficial bladder cancer. *J Urol* 2000;163:73–78.

92. Shelley MD, Court JB, Kynaston H, et al. Intravesical bacillus Calmette-Guerin in Ta and T1 bladder cancer (Cochrane review). *The Cochrane Library*. Chichester: John Wiley and Sons, 2000.

93. Witjes JA, Fransen MP, van der Meijden AP, et al. Use of maintenance intravesical bacillus Calmette-Guerin (BCG), with or without intradermal BCG, in patients with recurrent superficial bladder cancer. Long-term followup of a randomized phase 2 study. *Urol Int* 1993;51:67–72.

94. Solsona E, Iborra I, Dumont R, et al. The 3-month clinical response to intravesical therapy as a predictive factor for progression in patients with high risk superficial bladder cancer. *J Urol* 2000;164:685–689.

95. Sylvester RJ, van der MA, Lamm DL. Intravesical bacillus Calmette-Guerin reduces the risk of progression in patients with superficial bladder cancer: a meta-analysis of the published results of randomized clinical trials. *J Urol* 2002;168:1964–1970.

96. Okamura T, Tozawa K, Yamada Y, et al. Clinicopathological evaluation of repeated courses of intravesical bacillus Calmette-Guerin instillation for preventing recurrence of initially resistant superficial bladder cancer. *J Urol* 1996;156:967–971.

97. Hudson MA, Ratliff TL, Gillen DP, et al. Single course versus maintenance bacillus Calmette-Guerin therapy for superficial bladder tumors: a prospective, randomized trial. *J Urol* 1987;138:295–298.

98. Badalament RA, Herr HW, Wong GY, et al. A prospective randomized trial of maintenance versus nonmaintenance intravesical bacillus Calmette-Guerin therapy of superficial bladder cancer. *J Clin Oncol* 1987;5:441–449.

99. Tachibana M, Jitsukawa S, Iigaya T, et al. Comparative study on prophylactic intravesical instillation of bacillus Calmette-Guerin (BCG) and

adriamycin for superficial bladder cancers. *Nippon Hinyokika Gakkai Zasshi* 1989;80:1459–1465.

100. Palou J, Laguna P, Millan-Rodriguez F, et al. Control group and maintenance treatment with bacillus Calmette-Guerin for carcinoma in situ and/or high grade bladder tumors. *J Urol* 2001;165:1488–1491.

101. Saint F, Irani J, Patard JJ, et al. Tolerability of bacille Calmette-Guerin maintenance therapy for superficial bladder cancer. *Urology* 2001;57:883–888.

102. Bohle A, Jocham D, Bock PR. Intravesical bacillus Calmette-Guerin versus mitomycin C for superficial bladder cancer: a formal meta-analysis of comparative studies on recurrence and toxicity. *J Urol* 2003;169: 90–95.

103. Orihuela E, Herr HW, Pinsky CM, et al. Toxicity of intravesical BCG and its management in patients with superficial bladder tumors. *Cancer* 1987; 60:326–333.

104. Berry DL, Blumenstein BA, Magyary DL, et al. Local toxicity patterns associated with intravesical bacillus Calmette-Guerin: a Southwest Oncology Group Study. *Int J Urol* 1996;3:98–100; discussion 101.

105. van der Meijden PM, van Klingeren B, Steerenberg PA, et al. The possible influence of antibiotics on results of bacillus Calmette-Guerin intravesical therapy for superficial bladder cancer. *J Urol* 1991;146:444–446.

106. Durek C, Rusch-Gerdes S, Jocham D, et al. Sensitivity of BCG to modern antibiotics. *Eur Urol* 2000;37(Suppl 1):21–25.

107. Lamm DL, Steg A, Boccon-Gibod L, et al. Complications of bacillus Calmette-Guerin immunotherapy: review of 2602 patients and comparison of chemotherapy complications. *Prog Clin Biol Res* 1989;310:335–355.

108. Steg A, Leleu C, Debre B, et al. Systemic bacillus Calmette-Guerin infection in patients treated by intravesical BCG therapy for superficial bladder cancer. *Prog Clin Biol Res* 1989;310:325–334.

109. Durek C, Jurczok A, Werner H, et al. Optimal treatment of systemic bacillus Calmette-Guerin infection: investigations in an animal model. *J Urol* 2002;168:826–831.

110. Case records of the Massachusetts General Hospital. Weekly clinicopathological exercises. Case 29-1998. A 57-year-old man with fever and jaundice after intravesical instillation of bacille Calmette-Guerin for bladder cancer. *N Engl J Med* 1998;339:831–837.

111. Wittes R, Klotz L, Kosecka U. Severe bacillus Calmette-Guerin cystitis responds to systemic steroids when antituberculous drugs and local steroids fail. *J Urol* 1999;161:1568–1569.

112. Shoenfeld Y, Aron-Maor A, Tanai A, et al. BCG and autoimmunity: another two-edged sword. *J Autoimmun* 2001;16:235–240.

113. Lebret T, Gaudez F, Herve JM, et al. Low-dose BCG instillations in the treatment of stage T1 grade 3 bladder tumours: recurrence, progression and success. *Eur Urol* 1998;34:67–72.

114. Mack D, Frick J. Five-year results of a phase II study with low-dose bacille Calmette-Guerin therapy in high-risk superficial bladder cancer. *Urology* 1995;45:958–961.

115. Hurle R, Losa A, Ranieri A, et al. Low dose Pasteur bacillus Calmette-Guerin regimen in stage T1, grade 3 bladder cancer therapy. *J Urol* 1996; 156:1602–1605.

116. Morales A, Nickel JC, Wilson JW. Dose-response of bacillus Calmette-Guerin in the treatment of superficial bladder cancer. *J Urol* 1992;147: 1256–1258.

117. Martinez-Pineiro JA, Solsona E, Flores N, et al. Improving the safety of BCG immunotherapy by dose reduction. Cooperative Group CUETO. *Eur Urol* 1995;27(Suppl 1):13–18.

118. Pagano F, Bassi P, Piazza N, et al. Improving the efficacy of BCG immunotherapy by dose reduction. *Eur Urol* 1995;27(Suppl 1):19–22.

119. Bassi P, Spinadin R, Carando R, et al. Modified induction course: a solution to side-effects? *Eur Urol* 2000;37(Suppl 1):31–32.

120. Zlotta AR, van Vooren JP, Huygen K, et al. What is the optimal regimen for BCG intravesical therapy? Are six weekly instillations necessary? *Eur Urol* 2000;37:470–477.

121. de Reijke TM, De Boer EC, Kurth KH, et al. Urinary interleukin-2 monitoring during prolonged bacillus Calmette-Guerin treatment: can it predict the optimal number of instillations? *J Urol* 1999;161:67–71.

122. Lamm DL, Blumenstein BA, Crawford ED, et al. A randomized trial of intravesical doxorubicin and immunotherapy with bacille Calmette-Guerin for transitional-cell carcinoma of the bladder. *N Engl J Med* 1991;325: 1205–1209.

123. Rintala E, Jauhiainen K, Alfthan O, et al. Intravesical chemotherapy (mitomycin C) versus immunotherapy (bacillus Calmette-Guerin) in superficial bladder cancer. *Eur Urol* 1991;20:19–25.

124. Vegt PD, Witjes JA, Witjes WP, et al. A randomized study of intravesical mitomycin C, bacillus Calmette-Guerin tice and bacillus Calmette-Guerin RIVM treatment in pTa-pT1 papillary carcinoma and carcinoma in situ of the bladder. *J Urol* 1995;153:929–933.

125. Krege S, Giani G, Meyer R, et al. A randomized multicenter trial of adjuvant therapy in superficial bladder cancer: transurethral resection only versus transurethral resection plus mitomycin C versus transurethral resection plus bacillus Calmette-Guerin. Participating clinics [see Comments]. *J Urol* 1996;156:962–966.

126. Lundholm C, Norlen BJ, Ekman P, et al. A randomized prospective study comparing long-term intravesical instillations of mitomycin C and bacillus Calmette-Guerin in patients with superficial bladder carcinoma [see Comments]. *J Urol* 1996;156:372–376.

127. Malmstrom PU, Wijkstrom H, Lundholm C, et al. 5-year followup of a randomized prospective study comparing mitomycin C and bacillus Calmette-Guerin in patients with superficial bladder carcinoma. Swedish-Norwegian Bladder Cancer Study Group. *J Urol* 1999;161: 1124–1127.

128. Melekos MD, Zarakovitis I, Dandinis K, et al. BCG versus epirubicin in the prophylaxis of multiple superficial bladder tumours: results of a prospective randomized study using modified treatment schemes. *Int Urol Nephrol* 1996;28:499–509.

129. Bohle A, Bock PR. Intravesical bacille Calmette-Guerin versus mitomycin C in superficial bladder cancer: formal meta-analysis of comparative studies on tumor progression. *Urology* 2004;63:682–686; discussion 686–687.

130. Klein EA, Rogatko A, Herr HW. Management of local bacillus Calmette-Guerin failures in superficial bladder cancer. *J Urol* 1992;147: 601–605.

131. Glashan RW. A randomized controlled study of intravesical alpha-2b-interferon in carcinoma in situ of the bladder. *J Urol* 1990;144:658–661.

132. Sarosdy MF, Manyak MJ, Sagalowsky AI, et al. Oral bropirimine immunotherapy of bladder carcinoma in situ after prior intravesical bacille Calmette-Guerin. *Urology* 1998;51:226–231.

133. Dalbagni G, Russo P, Sheinfeld J, et al. Phase I trial of intravesical gemcitabine in bacillus Calmette-Guerin-refractory transitional-cell carcinoma of the bladder [see Comment]. *J Clin Oncol* 2002;20:3193–3198.

134. O'Donnell MA, Krohn J, DeWolf WC. Salvage intravesical therapy with interferon-alpha 2b plus low dose bacillus Calmette-Guerin is effective in patients with superficial bladder cancer in whom bacillus Calmette-Guerin alone previously failed. *J Urol* 2001;166:1300–1304; discussion 1304–1305.

135. Luciani LG, Neulander E, Murphy WM, et al. Risk of continued intravesical therapy and delayed cystectomy in BCG-refractory superficial bladder cancer: an investigational approach. *Urology* 2001;58:376–379.

136. Steinberg G, Bahnson R, Brosman S, et al. Efficacy and safety of valrubicin for the treatment of Bacillus Calmette-Guerin refractory carcinoma in situ of the bladder. The Valrubicin Study Group. *J Urol* 2000;163: 761–767.

137. Kuznetsov DD, Alsikafi NF, O'Connor RC, et al. Intravesical valrubicin in the treatment of carcinoma in situ of the bladder. *Expert Opin Pharmacother* 2001;2:1009–1013.

138. Greenberg RE, Bahnson RR, Wood D, et al. Initial report on intravesical administration of N-trifluoroacetyladriamycin-14-valerate (AD 32) to patients with refractory superficial transitional cell carcinoma of the urinary bladder. *Urology* 1997;49:471–475.

139. Hurle R, Losa A, Manzetti A, et al. Upper urinary tract tumors developing after treatment of superficial bladder cancer: 7-year follow-up of 591 consecutive patients. *Urology* 1999;53:1144–1148.

140. Burris HA III, Moore MJ, Andersen J, et al. Improvements in survival and clinical benefit with gemcitabine as first-line therapy for patients with advanced pancreas cancer: a randomized trial [see Comments]. *J Clin Oncol* 1997;15:2403–2413.

141. Stadler WM, Kuzel T, Roth B, et al. Phase II study of single-agent gemcitabine in previously untreated patients with metastatic urothelial cancer. *J Clin Oncol* 1997;15:3394–3398.

142. Lorusso V, Pollera CF, Antimi M, et al. A phase II study of gemcitabine in patients with transitional cell carcinoma of the urinary tract previously treated with platinum. Italian Co-operative Group on Bladder Cancer. *Eur J Cancer* 1998;34:1208–1212.

143. von der Maase H, Hansen SW, Roberts JT, et al. Gemcitabine and cisplatin (GC) versus methotrexate, vinblastine, adriamycin, and cisplatin (MVAC) chemotherapy in advanced or metastatic transitional cell carcinoma (TCC) of the urothelium: a large randomized multicenter, multinational phase II study. *Proc ASCO* 2000;19:329a.

144. Dalbagni G, Mazumdar M, Russo P, et al. Phase II trial of intravesical gemcitabine in BCG-refractory transitional cell carcinoma of the bladder. *J Urol* 2004;171:72, Abstract 274.

145. Laufer M, Ramalingam S, Schoenberg MP, et al. Intravesical gemcitabine therapy for superficial transitional cell carcinoma of the bladder: a phase I and pharmacokinetic study. *J Clin Oncol* 2003;21:697–703.

146. De Berardinis E, Antonini G, Peters GJ, et al. Intravesical administration of gemcitabine in superficial bladder cancer: a phase I study with pharmacodynamic evaluation. *BJU Int* 2004;93:491–494.

147. Torti FM, Shortliffe LD, Williams RD, et al. Alpha-interferon in superficial bladder cancer: a Northern California Oncology Group Study. *J Clin Oncol* 1988;6:476–483.

148. Giannakopoulos S, Gekas A, Alivizatos G, et al. Efficacy of escalating doses of intravesical interferon alpha-2b in reducing recurrence rate and progression in superficial transitional cell carcinoma. *Br J Urol* 1998;82: 829–834.

149. Malmstrom PU. A randomized comparative dose-ranging study of interferon-alpha and mitomycin-C as an internal control in primary or recurrent superficial transitional cell carcinoma of the bladder. *BJU Int* 2002; 89: 681–686.

150. Stricker P, Pryor K, Nicholson T, et al. Bacillus Calmette-Guerin plus intravesical interferon alpha-2b in patients with superficial bladder cancer. *Urology* 1996;48:957–961; discussion 961–962.

151. Punnen SP, Chin JL, Jewett MA. Management of bacillus Calmette-Guerin (BCG) refractory superficial bladder cancer: results with intravesical BCG and interferon combination therapy. *Can J Urol* 2003;10: 1790–1795.

152. Lam JS, Benson MC, O'Donnell MA, et al. Bacillus Calmete-GuA(C)rin plus interferon-alpha2B intravesical therapy maintains an extended treatment plan for superficial bladder cancer with minimal toxicity. *Urol Oncol* 2003;21:354–360.

153. O'Donnell MA, Lilli K, Leopold C, National Bacillus Calmette-Guerin/Interferon Phase 2 Investigator Group. Interim results from a national multicentre phase II trial of combination bacillus Calmette-Guerin plus interferon alpha-2b for superficial bladder cancer. Alpha[Clinical Trial. Clinical Trail, Phase II, Journal Article, Multicenter Study]. *J Urol* 2004;172(3):888–893.Title at MSK,WMC.

154. Nseyo UO. Photodynamic therapy in the management of bladder cancer. *J Clin Laser Med Surg* 1996;14:271–280.

155. Waidelich R, Stepp H, Baumgartner R, et al. Clinical experience with 5-aminolevulinic acid and photodynamic therapy for refractory superficial bladder cancer. *J Urol* 2001;165:1904–1907.

CHAPTER 26 ■ INVASIVE BLADDER CANCER

CHAPTER 26A
Role of Radical Cystectomy in Patients with Advanced Bladder Cancer

Harry W. Herr and S. Machele Donat

INTRODUCTION

Radical cystectomy is the mainstay of treatment for invasive bladder cancer. The curative intent of radical cystectomy is to remove all cancer in the bladder, pelvis, and regional lymph nodes. Radical cystectomy with a pelvic lymphadenectomy cures the majority of patients with invasive tumors confined to the bladder (stage pT1-2), about half with microscopic tumor spread outside the bladder (stage pT3a), and a significant minority with low-volume positive (N1) pelvic lymph nodes (1–3). Radical cystectomy alone rarely cures locally advanced (stage pT3b-4), extensive node-positive (N2-3), or metastatic (M+) bladder cancer (4). The role of surgery as an adjunct to chemotherapy, even in patients with locally advanced bulky pelvic tumors, grossly positive lymph nodes, unresectable bladder tumors, or distant metastases, is currently evolving coincident with developments of newer, more effective chemotherapy regimens.

DEFINITION OF ADVANCED BLADDER CANCER

We define advanced bladder cancer as significant pelvic tumor invasion outside the bladder or metastasis to regional or distant sites. Such tumors include bulky extravesical pelvic tumor (stage pT3b-4), grossly positive pelvic and/or regional lymph nodes (N2-3), unresectable bladder cancer (fixed bladder mass), and distant nodal (retroperitoneal), soft tissue, or visceral metastases. Radical surgery plays a role in each of these clinical scenarios representing increasing tumor volume and burden. Radical cystectomy may provide local control for locally advanced pelvic and regional disease, and postchemotherapy surgery may salvage some patients with unresectable or metastatic bladder cancer.

RADICAL CYSTECTOMY FOR ADVANCED EXTRAVESICAL (PT3B-4) BLADDER CANCER

Locally advanced (stage pT3b-4) nonmetastatic bladder cancer is rare and rarely cured by surgery alone. Radical cystectomy cures less than half the patients with measurable extravesical tumor spread, owing to high-volume pelvic disease, positive lymph nodes in 40% or more, and pre-existing distant metastases, collectively accounting for tumor relapse and surgical failure. Table 26A.1 (1–9) shows the outcomes from contemporary cystectomy series in which the 5-year survival rates vary between 26% and 44% after radical cystectomy, with higher survival noted among patients with resectable pelvic masses but negative lymph nodes. Patients with pathologic stage pT3b-4 tumors associated with microscopic positive nodes have a 20% 5-year survival rate, but fewer than 5% with high-volume nodal metastasis survive (10).

RADICAL CYSTECTOMY FOR GROSSLY POSITIVE LYMPH NODES

The possibility of surgical cures among patients with high-volume nodal metastasis is low, ranging only between 13% and 29% in contemporary series (Table 26A.1). Due to the inaccuracies of clinical staging, the nodal status and pathologic stage of a bladder cancer is unknown at the time of laparotomy and thus provides little help to the surgeon faced with deciding whether or not to proceed with surgery when palpable, grossly positive lymph nodes are encountered. We addressed the surgeon's dilemma from this perspective by analyzing the long-term outcome of patients undergoing cystectomy and resection of extensive nodal disease (7). Of a total of 84 patients with gross positive nodes discovered at cystectomy, 20 (24%) survived 10 years after surgery alone (Fig. 26A.1). Of 53 patients with clinical stage T2 (organ-confined) primary tumors, 17 (32%) survived versus three of 31 (10%) with stage T3 (extravesical) tumors. The University of Southern California (USC) group has shown a similar 27% 10-year survival rate among 84 patients with five or more positive nodes (1), indicating that some patients with grossly positive but resectable lymph nodes can be cured with surgery. However, our earlier experience demonstrated that of the subset of patients with locally advanced (pT3b-4) node-positive bladder cancer, fewer than 20% survived 5 years (11). Collectively, the data suggest that few patients with bulky pelvic tumors and positive lymph nodes are cured with surgery alone, and argue for a multimodality therapy combining a systemic chemotherapeutic intervention with radical cystectomy and extended pelvic lymphadenectomy.

NEOADJUVANT CHEMOTHERAPY FOR LOCALLY ADVANCED BLADDER CANCER

Following radical cystectomy for locally advanced bladder cancer, there is a significant rate of tumor recurrence, most commonly as distant metastases but also pelvic recurrence.

TABLE 26A.1

SURVIVAL AFTER RADICAL CYSTECTOMY ALONE FOR LOCALLY ADVANCED (MACROSCOPIC EXTRAVESICAL TUMOR) AND REGIONALLY METASTATIC (GROSSLY NODE-POSITIVE) BLADDER CANCER

Series (ref., first author)	Yr	Stage pT3b-4 N0 (no. pts)	5-year survival, %	Stage N2-3 (no. pts)	5-year survival, %
Stein (1)	2001	254	44	86	24
Dalbagni (2)	2001	129	26	39	13
Zincke (6)	2002	0	—	24	15
Herr (7)	2002	0	—	84	24
Mills (8)	2002	0	—	60	29
Studer (3)	2003	111	38	44	26
Herr (9)	2003	353	42	108	28

Pts, patients.

Most patients who suffer tumor relapse die of bladder cancer. For this reason, systemic chemotherapy has been explored in both neoadjuvant (preoperative) and adjuvant (postoperative) settings. Recent studies show that neoadjuvant chemotherapy improves the survival of patients who are potentially curable by cystectomy. These encouraging results also suggest that therapeutic chemotherapy may improve survival after radical cystectomy, even for more advanced bladder cancer.

A cooperative, group, randomized study [Southwest Oncology Group (SWOG) 8710, Intergroup-0080] of 307 patients with muscle-invasive bladder cancer (stage cT2-T4a) found a significant and clinically meaningful improvement in survival among patients who received neoadjuvant chemotherapy over cystectomy alone (12). With more than 8 years follow-up, the median survival time was 46 months among patients in the cystectomy group versus 77 months of the combination group ($P = .04$). At 5 years, 57% of the patients in the chemotherapy plus cystectomy group were alive, as compared with 43% of those in the cystectomy group ($P = .06$). There were 77 deaths from bladder cancer in the cystectomy group and 54 deaths in the combination therapy group ($P = .002$), translating into a 14% reduction in absolute mortality and a 5% improvement in 5-year survival rate. In both groups, the survival benefit of neoadjuvant methotrexate, vinblastine, doxorubicin, and cisplatin (M-VAC) was strongly related to down-staging of the tumor to pT0. In the neoadjuvant M-VAC patients, 38% had no evidence of cancer at cystectomy (pT0), as compared with 15% of the patients in the cystectomy-alone group ($P <.001$). Overall, the patients who were pT0 at surgery demonstrated an 85% five-year survival rate.

Of particular relevance to treatment strategies for advanced bladder tumor, patients entered on the SWOG trial with extravesical disease (stage T3 or T4) derived significant benefit from neoadjuvant MVAC chemotherapy. Figure 26A.2 shows a median survival time of 65 months among 92 locally advanced disease patients after MVAC + cystectomy compared with 24 months in 93 patients after cystectomy alone ($P = .04$). Among advanced-disease patients, there was a 10% reduction in mortality in the combination therapy group compared with the cystectomy alone group. For patients with clinical T2 tumors, the 5-year survival was improved by only 5%, whereas patients with stage T3b-T4 tumors had a 20% improvement in 5-year survival.

The M.D. Anderson Cancer Center also addressed combined chemotherapy and surgery in patients suspected to have pathologic extravesical tumor extension and nodal involvement (13). A total of 140 patients (including 94 with T3b-4 tumors) were randomly assigned to receive either two courses of neoadjuvant M-VAC followed by cystectomy plus three additional cycles of chemotherapy, or, alternatively, to have initial cystectomy followed by five cycles of adjuvant chemotherapy. Although there was no difference in outcome between the two groups by intent-to-treat, 81 patients (58%) remained disease-free, with a median follow-up of 6.8 years. Of particular relevance was the finding of a nearly 40% cure rate among patients with pathologically proven lymph node metastasis, better than any reported outcome with surgery alone in a similar cohort. Of note, all patients in this study with pathologically confirmed extravesical extension also had nodal involvement. These findings support an improved cure fraction among patients with locally advanced bladder cancer by a combination of multiagent chemotherapy and surgery.

Meta-analyses of all randomized trials in more than 3,000 patients confirm that neoadjuvant chemotherapy improves survival of patients with muscle-invasive bladder cancer

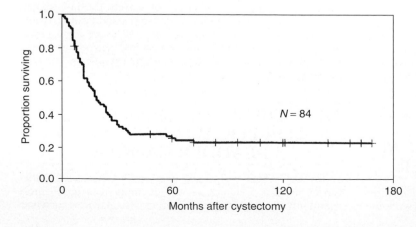

FIGURE 26A.1. Disease-specific survival of 84 patients with grossly node-positive bladder cancer after radical cystectomy and extended lymph node dissection (includes 20, or 24%, who survived more than 5 years).

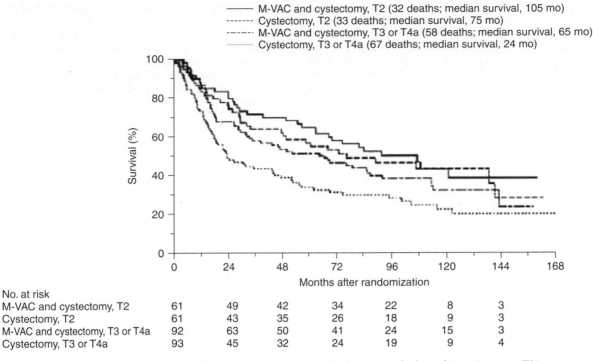

FIGURE 26A.2. Survival according to treatment group and whether patients had muscle invasion (stage T2) or more advanced disease (stage T3 or T4a).

treated by cystectomy (14,15). Platinum-based combination chemotherapy has a 5% absolute survival benefit at 5 years and a 13% reduction in risk of death from bladder cancer among patients undergoing cystectomy. These collective results, as well as the dismal outcome associated with cystectomy alone, argue strongly for integrating systemic chemotherapy and cystectomy, especially in patients with locally advanced and metastatic bladder cancer.

Although radical cystectomy is usually advised after combination chemotherapy for most invasive bladder cancers (16), selected patients may be treated by partial cystectomy if they achieve a major reduction in tumor size and a complete cystoscopic response to neoadjuvant chemotherapy. Of 26 patients who underwent a partial cystectomy after M-VAC, 17 (65%) survived beyond 5 years, including 14 (54%) with an intact functioning bladder (17). Patients with no tumor (pT0) in their surgical specimens had a 5-year survival rate of 87% (14 of 16) compared with 30% (3 of 10) among patients with residual invasive cancer. Twelve patients (46%) developed bladder recurrences, which were invasive in 5 (18%) and superficial in 7 (26%). Neoadjuvant chemotherapy may permit bladder sparing in highly selected patients who have significant downsizing of their tumors located in sites favorable to partial cystectomy. The bladder remains at risk for new tumors, but the majority of local recurrences can be treated successfully by local therapy or salvage cystectomy.

We believe that therapeutic platinum-based combined chemotherapy (at least four cycles) should be given before cystectomy in patients who have clinical evidence of extravesical pelvic tumor (palpable mass, hydronephrosis) and a high likelihood of nodal or silent distant metastases (Hydronephrosis is not so much an indicator of extravesical disease as one of muscle-invasive disease. Unlike palpable mass, hydronephrosis has not been used by most as an indicator for neoadjuvant chemotherapy.) Additional efforts at improving our ability to accurately identify locally advanced and regional/pelvic nodal disease are needed to allow for better selection of patients for preoperative chemotherapy.

RATIONALE FOR POSTCHEMOTHERAPY SURGERY

Platinum-based chemotherapy is the primary treatment of metastatic bladder cancer (18). Various combined regimens have yielded major response proportions ranging from 39% to 72%, including complete pathologic remission in 20% to 36% of cases (19). However, the median survival time from the identification of metastatic disease remains at about 1 year, with only 3% to 7% of patients surviving longer than 5 years (20). Lymph node metastases and pelvic soft-tissue tumors respond more favorably than tumors involving the lung, liver, or bone (19). Longer survival is seen in patients with lymph node and soft tissue disease, and a substantially worse prognosis is found in those with visceral involvement. Tumor relapse in the bladder, pelvis, and distant sites is common, even after a complete clinical response to chemotherapy (21). Based on these findings, the primary tumor and regional or retroperitoneal nodes would appear to be most amenable to surgical cure with extended lymph node dissection and radical cystectomy. Selected tumors in the lung, liver, and even bone may also be amenable for complete postchemotherapy surgical resection. Lastly, a complete response to chemotherapy alone or chemotherapy plus surgery is the best correlate of prolonged survival and is a prerequisite for cure in advanced bladder cancer (19). These observations provide a rationale for postchemotherapy surgery that may benefit selected patients with locally advanced, initially unresectable, or inoperable primary or metastatic bladder cancers.

POSTCHEMOTHERAPY SURGERY FOR UNRESECTABLE AND NODE-POSITIVE BLADDER CANCER

When the M-VAC regimen became established in 1983 as effective chemotherapy against metastatic bladder cancer (22), oncologic logic persuaded us to combine chemotherapy and surgery for patients with locally advanced but inoperable disease. We initially treated 41 consecutive patients with unresectable or extensive node-positive bladder cancer (stage pT4b, N2-3, M0) with M-VAC followed by an attempt at postchemotherapy radical cystectomy (23). Of the 41 patients, 29 underwent surgical exploration and cystectomy was accomplished in 24. Cystectomy was not performed in 17 patients due to lack of response to chemotherapy or patient refusal. After a minimum follow-up of 4 years (range, 4 to 7 years), 9 patients (22%) survived, including 7 with no cancer (pT0) left in the bladder (complete response to chemotherapy) and 2 after resection of residual viable bladder cancer (complete response to M-VAC plus surgery) (Fig. 26A.3A). Overall survival according to whether surgery was performed showed 8 of 24 patients alive after cystectomy versus only 1 of 17 without cystectomy (Fig. 26A.3B, $P = .009$). We concluded from this initial experience that patients with advanced unresectable bladder cancer who did not have a surgical option initially may benefit from combination chemotherapy (M-VAC) when down-staging allows potentially curative surgery to be performed as combined modality strategy.

An update of our experience with postchemotherapy surgery from 1984 to 1999 (24) showed that of the 207 patients with unresectable and regionally metastatic bladder cancer treated with cisplatin-based chemotherapy regimens, 80 (39%) underwent surgery, 12 (6%) refused surgery although clinically deemed resectable, and 115 (55%) did not undergo cystectomy secondary to either tumor progression or poor performance status (24). Postchemotherapy surgery was designed to resect all pelvic and metastatic nodal sites of disease documented before chemotherapy with a radical cystectomy and a bilateral pelvic and retroperitoneal lymph dissection. En bloc resection of extravesical soft tissue pelvic masses was included with the bladder and adjacent contiguous organs. Response to chemotherapy

was documented as shrinkage of measurable tumor in the bladder and nodes on follow-up computed tomography (CT) scans, and evaluation under anesthesia and transurethral resection biopsies of tumor sites showing down-staging of local tumor invasion or no evidence of residual tumor.

Of the 80 operated patients, 34 (42%) survived 9 months to 5 years, including 20 of 49 (41%) with resection of residual viable disease (Table 26A.2). Of these, 60 patients who had received M-VAC and had mature follow-up of 5 years or more, 19 (32%) survived 5 years, including 10 of 34 (29%) after resection of persistent tumor. Only one of 12 patients (8%) who refused surgery survived longer than 1 year, and died of disease at 3 years post chemotherapy. Of the patients who failed to achieve a major clinical response to chemotherapy, none achieved any survival benefit from postchemotherapy surgery. In addition, although technically challenging, there were no operative mortalities or surgical morbidity requiring reoperation, indicating that postchemotherapy surgery may be performed safely in experienced hands. Our experience demonstrates that postchemotherapy surgery may benefit a subset of patients with unresectable or regionally metastatic bladder cancer who achieve a major response to chemotherapy.

The M.D. Anderson Cancer Center recently reported the survival results in 11 patients who underwent postchemotherapy cystectomy plus retroperitoneal lymph node dissection for non-visceral metastasis restricted to the retroperitoneal nodes (25). Although all 11 patients showed major clinical responses to chemotherapy, 9 had residual viable tumor in the retroperitoneal nodes. Four-year disease-specific and recurrence-free survival rates were 36% and 27%, respectively. These two series from major tertiary cancer centers demonstrate that postchemotherapy surgical resection of metastatic bladder cancer can be curative in selected patients (24,25). Furthermore, the inaccuracy of clinical methods for assessing a complete response to chemotherapy

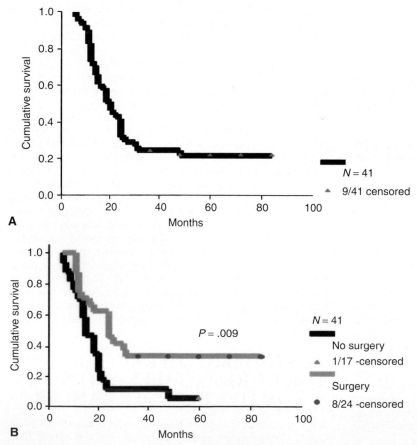

FIGURE 26A.3. A: Survival of complete responders (CR) to chemotherapy. **B:** Overall survival according to postchemotherapy surgery versus no surgery.

TABLE 26A.2

MEMORIAL SLOAN-KETTERING CANCER CENTER (MSKCC) EXPERIENCE: POSTCHEMOTHERAPY SURGERY
FOR UNRESECTABLE PRIMARY AND NODE-POSITIVE BLADDER CANCER 1983–1999

Pathologic findings at surgery	Number of patients (%)	Response to	Chemotherapy	Number of patients NED (%)[a]
Residual cancer	49 (61)	9 CR	35 PR, 5 NR	20 (41)
No residual cancer	24 (30)	15 CR	7 PR, 2 NR	14 (58)
Unresectable disease	7 (9)	0 CR	2 PR, 5 NR	0 (0)
Refused surgery	12 (6)	10 CR	2 PR	1 (8)
Overall	80	24 (30%)	56 (70%)	34 (42)

NED, no evidence of disease at last follow-up; CR, complete response; PR, partial response; NR, no response.
[a]Survival 9 months to 5 years (32% of patients with a minimum of 5 years of follow-up are alive at 5 years).
From Herr HW, Donat SM, Bajorin DF. Post-chemotherapy surgery in patients with unresectable or regionally metastatic bladder cancer. *J Urol* 2001;165:811–814.

alone is emphasized in the M.D. Anderson series where only 1 of 7 (14%) patients thought to be clinical complete responders were indeed without evidence of disease at surgery (25). This suggests that in select patients who respond to chemotherapy, a surgical resection of prechemotherapy sites of locoregional disease may improve relapse-free survival.

POSTCHEMOTHERAPY SURGERY FOR METASTATIC BLADDER CANCER

The role of postchemotherapy surgery for patients with metastatic bladder cancer is controversial. Although the use of postchemotherapy surgery to resect viable residual cancer to

achieve complete response is well defined in other genitourinary tumors, it is not established in urothelial cancer. In the original M-VAC series (26), 13 patients who underwent complete postchemotherapy resection of viable metastatic tumor achieved a median survival of 25 months and several survived 5 years. We have since treated and evaluated 203 patients with unresectable primary tumors and metastatic transitional cell carcinoma who received therapeutic M-VAC chemotherapy (27). Fifty responding patients underwent postchemotherapy surgery for suspected or known residual disease. In 17 patients, no viable tumor was found at surgery, pathologically confirming a complete response to chemotherapy. In 30 patients, residual, viable bladder cancer was completely resected, which resulted in a complete response to chemotherapy plus surgery. Figure 26A.4 shows that 10 of these 30 patients (33%) remained alive at 5 years, similar to results observed

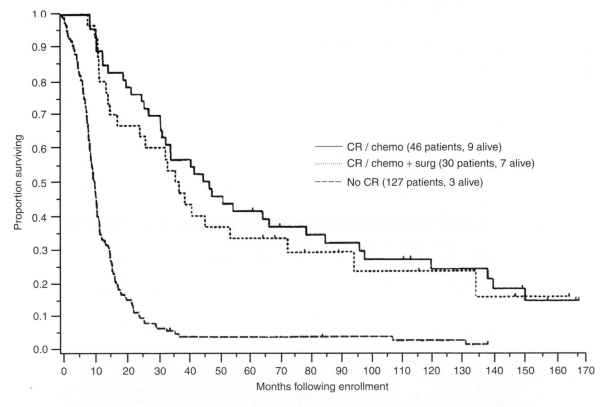

FIGURE 26A.4. Overall survival rate of patients with advanced bladder cancer after chemotherapy.

TABLE 26A.3

MSKCC POSTCHEMOTHERAPY SURGERY OUTCOMES FOR UNRESECTABLE OR METASTATIC BLADDER CANCER

Pathologic findings at surgery	Number of patients clinically resectable postchemotherapy	Response to chemotherapy (number of patients)	Disease at surgery (site)	Number patients alive (3–5 yr), (%)
Residual cancer	54	7 CR 42 PR 5 NR	30 bladder, 24 lymph nodes, 9 pelvic mass, 11 visceral met	18 (33)
No residual cancer	27	14 CR 11 PR 2 NR	No residual disease	12 (44)
Unresectable disease	8	2 PR 6 NR	Fixed bladder and lymph nodes	0 (0)
Refused surgery	14	10 CR 4 PR		1 (7)
Overall	103/276 (37%)	CR 30%, PR 57%, NR 13%		31/103 (30)

CR, complete response; PR, partial response; NR, no response; met, metastases.
From Herr HW, Donat SM, Bajorin DF. Bladder cancer, the limits of surgical excision: when/how much? *Urol Oncol* 2001;6:221–224.

for patients who attained a complete response to chemotherapy (41%) (27). Patients with unresectable primary tumors and metastases restricted to lymph node sites were most likely to survive 5 years. Of 7 patients who underwent postchemotherapy resection of visceral metastasis, 3 survived after thoracotomy to resect residual lung disease. Postchemotherapy surgical resection of residual cancer may result in 5-year disease-free survival in some patients who would otherwise succumb to disease. Optimal surgical candidates include patients whose prechemotherapy sites of disease are restricted to the pelvis or lymph node sites (and perhaps the lung) and who have a major response to chemotherapy.

Table 26A.3 shows our collective experience among patients who underwent postchemotherapy surgery after cisplatin-based chemotherapy to assess overall impact on survival (28). Of a total of 276 patients, 103 (37%) were deemed to be candidates for postchemotherapy surgery after they were downstaged from inoperable or unresectable to resectable primary tumors and achieved major responses in nodal or distant metastatic sites. Of these, 89 (32%) patients agreed to and subsequently underwent postchemotherapy surgery. Thirty of the 89 patients (34%) survived 5 years after postchemotherapy surgery. In 27 patients, no viable tumor was found in the resected specimen, confirming a complete response to chemotherapy. In 54 patients, residual, viable cancer was completely resected, resulting in a complete response to chemotherapy plus surgery. Eighteen of these 54 patients (33%) remain alive at 5 years, similar to the

results observed for patients who attained a complete response to chemotherapy alone (44%). Of the 14 responding patients who refused surgery, only one (7%) survived for 3 years. Conclusions were that postchemotherapy surgical resection of residual cancer may result in 5-year disease-free survival in a subset of patients who would otherwise succumb to disease. Optimal candidates include patients whose postchemotherapy sites of disease are restricted to the bladder or pelvis, lymph nodes, or solitary visceral metastases and who have a major response to chemotherapy.

Table 26A.4 (27,29,30) summarizes survival outcome reported by three reported series of patients after postchemotherapy resection of residual viable local or metastatic bladder cancer. About a third of resected patients survive up to 5 years, with many including resection of both pelvic and distant metastatic sites of disease. The M.D. Anderson experience is particularly significant since they focused on 31 patients with metastatic bladder cancer who underwent metastasectomy (22 after chemotherapy) with intent of rendering them free of disease (30). All gross disease was completely resected in 30 patients (97%). The most frequently resected location was lung in 24 cases (77%), followed by distant lymph nodes in 4 (13%), brain in 2 (7%) and a subcutaneous metastasis in 1 (3%). The results in this highly selected cohort, with 33% alive at 5 years after metastasectomy, suggest that resection of metastatic disease is feasible and may contribute to long-term disease control, especially when integrated with combination chemotherapy.

TABLE 26A.4

OUTCOME OF POSTCHEMOTHERAPY SURGERY AMONG PATIENTS WITH RESECTED VIABLE RESIDUAL BLADDER CANCER

Series	Number of patients	3- to 5-year survival (%)	Median survival time (mo)	Site of metastasis (number of patients)	
				Pelvis	Distant
MSKCC (27)	30	33	37	20	10
Stanford (29)	14	46	30	10	4
MDACC (30)	22	33	31	4	18[a]

[a]predominantly lung resections.

SELECTION OF PATIENTS FOR POSTCHEMOTHERAPY SURGERY

Selection of patients who should undergo and are most likely to benefit from postchemotherapy surgery is evolving. Experience suggests several generalizations can be made. First, patients should achieve a major clinical response (complete or partial) to chemotherapy. No patient who achieved less than a major response to chemotherapy survived 5 years in any of the series reported, despite postchemotherapy surgery (23–25,27–30). Second, visceral metastasis (especially liver and bone) portends a poor outcome, even with surgery, in contrast to patients with locally advanced primary, pelvic soft-tissue, and regional or distant nodal disease. Third, limited nodes (one or two positive nodes) or a solitary visceral/lung lesion (rather than multiple) is most likely to benefit from surgical resection. Fourth, long-term survival is greatest when disease is restricted to the bladder, pelvis, and regional nodes. Almost all of our patients with residual tumor after chemotherapy in both distant sites and the bladder experienced rapid recurrence and death. Lastly, patients who refuse definitive postchemotherapy surgery, even if they achieve a complete clinical response to chemotherapy, with shrinkage of tumor on CT scans and have no tumor found in the bladder on transurethral resection (TUR) biopsy, inevitably relapse and die of disease.

The latter observation is important in patient management, in that postchemotherapy clinical evaluation (biopsy and scans) are poor substitutes for surgical resection, unless such studies clearly show progression of metastatic tumor. Unlike neoadjuvant chemotherapy given to patients with operable tumors confined to the bladder, TUR biopsies and CT images to evaluate advanced bladder cancer generally confirm absence of tumor progression (but not pathologic tumor response) and are not always useful or accurate in selecting patients for postchemotherapy surgery (16). Residual disease in the bladder, pelvis, or nodes has been reported in up to 86% of patients despite complete clinical response in these sites to chemotherapy (16,23–25,27–30).

SURGICAL RESECTION OF METASTATIC BLADDER CANCER REFRACTORY TO CHEMOTHERAPY

Surgical resection of metastatic deposits failing to respond to chemotherapy is rarely reported nor practiced, except to achieve palliation in selected cases. German surgeons resected metastatic bladder cancer in 70 patients (76% multiple and 24% solitary sites) that failed to respond to M-VAC chemotherapy (31). Metastatic tumors were removed in lymph nodes, peritoneum, skin, bone, lung, and liver. The median survival time was 7 months, and 30% and 19% survived 1 and 2 years, respectively. Although it is unlikely that surgery prolonged survival in these patients, 42 of the 51 patients (83%) with symptomatic secondary cancer did benefit from surgery in terms of tumor-related symptoms and performance score. The World Health Organization (WHO) performance score changed from 3.3 to 2.1 (P = .005). The authors reported no major adverse effects of surgery in such patients, although asymptomatic patients felt worse after surgery.

CONCLUSION

Patients with unresectable primary bladder tumors and regionally metastatic bladder cancer are the best candidates for postchemotherapy surgery. Tumors restricted to these sites respond better than visceral metastases. Tumor relapse in the bladder, pelvic soft tissue, and lymph nodes is common even after a complete clinical response to chemotherapy. The primary tumor and regional or retroperitoneal lymph nodes are the most amenable to surgical cure with extended lymph node resection and radical cystectomy. Clinical complete or partial response to chemotherapy does not correlate well enough with disease in the final pathologic specimen to defer surgery since a large proportion of patients who achieve a complete response will be found to have residual invasive or metastatic disease (23–25,27–30). Selected patients with isolated solitary visceral metastasis may benefit from postchemotherapy surgical resection.

Current data show that many patients with advanced bladder cancer have residual viable cancer even after achieving a major response to chemotherapy. Known or suspected sites of residual disease can be completely resected with up to 33% of these patients who are rendered disease-free by chemotherapy plus surgery surviving up to 5 years of follow-up. They would likely have died of recurrent bladder cancer since, in our experience, 92% of patients who refuse surgery after a major response to chemotherapy died of metastatic bladder cancer. Patients who do not achieve a major response to chemotherapy or have disease progression while on chemotherapy do not appear to benefit from postchemotherapy surgery with few, if any, surviving 5 years even with surgery. In addition, of all complete responders in our collective postchemotherapy patient population, more than half (61%) were achieved by the combination of chemotherapy followed by surgery removing all sites of pretreatment disease, with 41% surviving free of tumor recurrence for up to 5 years (24).

Newer chemotherapy regimens portend greater response rates in patients with locally advanced and metastatic bladder cancer. However, many patients fail to respond completely to chemotherapy or relapse at prior sites of responding disease. The increasingly integrative role of surgery in the multimodality management of bladder cancer will demand of the surgeon higher levels of decision analysis and skill in the future. Surgeons are being asked more frequently to resect locally advanced and metastatic bladder cancer after chemotherapy. The risks may be high, but survival may be prolonged significantly in some patients by postchemotherapy surgery, and palliation may be achieved in many more.

References

1. Stein JP, Lieskovsky G, Skinner DG. Radical cystectomy in the treatment of invasive bladder cancer: long-term results in 1,054 patients. *J Clin Oncol* 2001;19:666–675.
2. Dalbagni G, Genega E, Herr HW, et al. Cystectomy for bladder cancer: a contemporary series. *J Urol* 2001;165:1111–1116.
3. Maderbacher S, Hochreiter W, Studer UE. Radical cystectomy for bladder cancer today: homogeneous series without neoadjuvant therapy. *J Clin Oncol* 2003;21:690–696.
4. Quek ML, Stein JP, Clark PE, et al. Natural history of surgically treated bladder carcinoma with extravesical tumor extension. *Cancer* 2003;98:955–961.
5. Hall MC, Dinney CPN. Radical cystectomy for stage T3b bladder cancer. *Semin Urol Oncol* 1996;14:73–80.
6. Frank I, Cheville JC, Zincke H. Transitional cell carcinoma of the urinary bladder with regional lymph node involvement treated by cystectomy. *Cancer* 2003;97:2425–2431.
7. Herr HW, Donat SM. Outcome of patients with grossly node positive bladder cancer after pelvic lymph node dissection and radical cystectomy. *J Urol* 2001;165:62–64.
8. Mills RD, Turner WH, Fleischmann A, et al. Pelvic node metastases from bladder cancer: outcome in 83 patients after radical cystectomy and pelvic lymphadenectomy. *J Urol* 2001;166:19–23.
9. Herr HW. Superiority of ratio based lymph node staging for bladder cancer. *J Urol* 2003;169:943–945.
10. Stein JP, Skinner DG. Results with radical cystectomy for treating bladder cancer: a 'reference standard' for high-grade, invasive bladder cancer. *BJU Int* 2003;92:12–17.

11. Vieweg J, Gschwend JE, Herr HW. Pelvic lymph node dissection can be curative in patients with node-positive bladder cancer. *J Urol* 1999;161:449–454.
12. Grossman HB, Natale RB, Tangen CM, et al. Neoadjuvant chemotherapy plus cystectomy compared with cystectomy alone for locally advanced bladder cancer. *N Engl J Med* 2003;349:859–866.
13. Millikan R, Dinney C, Swanson D, et al. Integrated therapy for locally advanced bladder cancer: final report of a randomized trial of cystectomy plus adjuvant M-VAC versus cystectomy with both preoperative and postoperative M-VAC. *J Clin Oncol* 2001;19:4005.
14. Advanced Bladder Cancer (ABC) Meta-analysis Collaboration. Neoadjuvant chemotherapy in invasive bladder cancer: a systematic review and meta-analysis. *Lancet* 2003;361:1927–1934.
15. Winquist E, Kirchner TS, Segal R, et al. Neoadjuvant chemotherapy for transitional cell carcinoma of the bladder: a systematic review and meta-analysis. *J Urol* 2004;171:561–569.
16. Schultz PK, Herr HW, Zhang Z-F, et al. Neoadjuvant chemotherapy for invasive bladder cancer: prognostic factors for survival of patients treated with M-VAC with 5-year follow-up. *J Clin Oncol* 1994;12:1394.
17. Herr HW, Scher HI. Neoadjuvant chemotherapy and partial cystectomy for invasive bladder cancer. *J Clin Oncol* 1994;12:975–980.
18. Raghavan D. Progress in the chemotherapy of metastatic cancer of the urinary tract. *Cancer* 2002;97:2050–2055.
19. Bajorin DF, Dodd PM, Mazumdar M, et al. Long-term survival in metastatic transitional cell carcinoma and prognostic factors predicting outcome of therapy. *J Clin Oncol* 1999;17:3173–3181.
20. Saxman SB, Propert KJ, Einhorn LH, et al. Long-term followup of a phase III intergroup study of cisplatin alone or in combination with VAC in patients with metastatic urothelial carcinoma. *J Clin Oncol* 1997;15:2564–2569.
21. Dimopoulos MA, Finn L, Logothetis CJ. Pattern of failure and survival of patients with metastatic urothelial tumors relapsing after cis-platinum chemotherapy. *J Urol* 1994;151:598.
22. Sternberg CN, Yagoda A, Scher HI, et al. Preliminary results of M-VAC for transitional cell carcinoma of the urothelium. *J Urol* 1985;133:403–407.
23. Donat SM, Herr HW, Bajorin DF. M-VAC chemotherapy and cystectomy for unresectable bladder cancer. *J Urol* 1996;156:368–371.
24. Herr HW, Donat SM, Bajorin DF. Post-chemotherapy surgery in patients with unresectable or regionally metastatic bladder cancer. *J Urol* 2001;165:811–814.
25. Sweeney P, Millikan R, Donat SM, et al. Is there a therapeutic role for post-chemotherapy retroperitoneal lymph node dissection in metastatic transitional cell carcinoma of the bladder? *J Urol* 2003;169:2113–2117.
26. Sternberg CN, Yagoda A, Scher HI, et al. M-VAC for advanced transitional cell carcinoma of the urothelium. *Cancer* 1989;64:2448.
27. Dodd PM, McCaffrey JA, Herr HW, et al. Outcome of post-chemotherapy surgery after treatment with M-VAC in patients with unresectable or metastatic transitional cell carcinoma. *J Clin Oncol* 1999;17:2546–2552.
28. Herr HW, Donat SM, Bajorin DF. Bladder cancer, the limits of surgical excision: when/how much? *Urol Oncol* 2001;6:221–224.
29. Miller RS, Freiha FS, Torti FM. Cisplatin, methotrexate and vinblastine plus surgical restaging for patients with advanced transitional cell carcinoma of the urothelium. *J Urol* 1993;150:65.
30. Siefker-Radtke AO, Walsh GL, Pisters LL, et al. Is there a role for surgery in the management of metastatic urothelial cancer? The M.D. Anderson experience. *J Urol* 2004;171:145–148.
31. Otto T, Krege S, Suhr J, et al. Impact of surgical resection of bladder cancer metastases refractory to systemic therapy on performance score: a phase II trial. *Urology* 2001;57:55–59.

CHAPTER 26B
Selective Bladder Preservation in the Treatment of Muscle-invasive Bladder Cancer

Donald S. Kaufman, Anthony L. Zietman, and William U. Shipley

The treatment options for muscularis propria-invasive bladder tumors can broadly be divided into those that involve removing the bladder and those that spare it. In the United States, radical cystectomy with pelvic lymph node dissection is the standard method used to treat patients with this tumor.

Radical cystectomy for stage T2 to T4a muscle-invading bladder cancer is an approach that results in 90% local control at 5 years, but only 40% to 60% 5-year overall survival. It is likely that the low cure rate is due to micrometastatic disease present at the time of cystectomy, and patients so afflicted are therefore destined to die of distant metastases. An analysis of cystectomy by investigators at Memorial Sloan-Kettering Cancer Center (MSKCC) demonstrated a disease-specific survival of 67% and a median overall survival of only 45% with a median follow-up of 65 months (1). Several studies have established that the clinical and pathologic stage of the disease is important in predicting long-term survival. At the University of Southern California (USC), the 5-year recurrence-free survival for muscle-invasive bladder cancer was 89% in P2 node-negative tumors, 50% in P4 node-negative tumors, and 35% in patients with node-positive tumors (2). The effects of cystoprostatectomy on quality of life in males have been carefully studied. Modern surgical techniques of nerve sparing that may preserve male potency and help increase the likelihood of continence with orthotopic urinary diversions have made cystectomy more tolerable, but even the most enthusiastic proponents of orthotopic bladder construction agree that a naturally functioning bladder is superior to any reconstructed bladder devised in the past decade and currently being offered to patients.

EXTERNAL BEAM RADIATION THERAPY ALONE

The advances in bladder preservation by trimodality therapy had their beginnings in various types of monotherapy.

Over the last three decades the most common method of bladder-sparing treatment has been external beam radiation therapy. In this country, radiation treatment has generally been reserved for patients judged unfit for cystectomy on the basis of age, comorbid conditions, or disease extent. These negative-selection criteria may have contributed somewhat to the poor results achieved with radiation therapy alone (3–9) (Table 26B.1). In addition, approximately 15% of the patients are excluded from treatment by radical surgery because at the time of operation previously unrecognized extravesical tumor is found. Thus in cystectomy series, but not in radiation series, some patients with advanced local spread of tumor are excluded. By 1985, of four randomized trials that compared cystectomy (and preoperative radiation therapy) with external beam treatment alone, only one reported a statistically significant survival advantage for immediate cystectomy (Table 26B.2). Dr. David Wallace led a prospective multicenter trial under the auspices of the Institute of Urology in London. Patients were randomized to undergo either 4,000 cGy of radiation followed by total cystectomy or 6,000 cGy of radiation followed by salvage cystectomy for persistent or recurrent tumor (9). This trial showed no difference in the 5-year and 10-year survival rates for the 98 patients randomized to immediate cystectomy (39% and 19%, respectively), compared to the 91 patients randomized to radiation with salvage surgery with the comparable figures 28% and 15%. In 1991, the Danish national bladder cancer group reported no statistical survival difference in overall survival in two arms of a similar study that involved 183 patients. The pelvic failure rate was, however, significantly lower in the group treated by immediate cystectomy compared to those treated by radiation therapy. The incidence of metastatic disease was similar in both groups, 32% and 34% at 5 years (7).

The National Bladder Cancer Group reported a randomized trial of 72 patients in which there was no difference in the 5-year survival rate or the rate of distant metastasis for patients randomized to immediate cystectomy (27% and 38%, respectively) compared with those undergoing primary radiation therapy

TABLE 26B.1

RESULTS OF RADICAL RADIATION THERAPY ALONE (MONOTHERAPY): MUSCLE-INVADING BLADDER CANCER

Study	Number	5-year survival rates		
		T2	T3(±T4a)	All Stages
M.D. Anderson Cancer Center (3)	32		22%	
National Bladder Cancer Group[a]	35			40%
Edinburgh (4)	889	40%	26%	36%
London Hospital (5)	182	46%	35%	40%
Princess Margaret Hospital (6)	121	59%	39%	45%
Danish National Study (7)	95		23%	
Norway (8)	308	38%	14%	24%
UK Cooperative Group (9)	91		28%	

[a]SD Cutler, National Cancer Institute, unpublished observations, 1983.
Modified from Zietman et al. Organ-conserving approaches to muscle-invasive bladder cancer: future alternatives to radical cystectomy. *Ann Med* 2000;32:42–47.

with cystectomy only for recurrence (40% and 31%, respectively). The median follow-up of that phase III study was 66 months (Table 26B.2). Thus, in the two trials that reported the incidence of the subsequent development of distant metastases, there was no increased rate among those patients receiving radiation with deferred cystectomy for salvage, and in only one of the four randomized trials comparing immediate cystectomy to radical radiation therapy with cystectomy deferred for salvage was there a statically significant survival advantage and that was in the smallest trial (67 patients) and those with advanced stage T3 tumors (3).

Twice-a-day (accelerated) radiation regimens may be more effective than once-a-day regimens in eradicating a primary bladder tumor (10). However, in a randomized phase III trial testing once-a-day versus twice-a-day radiation at the Royal Marsden Hospital with radiation as monotherapy there was no significant difference (11).

Radiation treatment schedules that use a relatively large dose per fraction (more than 2 Gy) have been shown to produce a late toxicity rate in the bladder and intestine of 20% to 25% (12). This is distinctly less satisfactory than the excellent bladder tolerance achieved with conventional radiation.

Interstitial Radiation Therapy

Interstitial radiation therapy (brachytherapy) allows for the delivery of a higher biologic dose of radiation to a limited area of the bladder within a short period, and remote after-loading techniques decrease the radiation hazard to hospital personnel. This approach has been reported by investigators in the Netherlands, Belgium, and France. The majority of the reported series of patients also underwent maximum tumor debulking either by partial cystectomy or transurethral resection. In addition, external beam radiation doses of 30 Gy or more were used in combination with implant doses of 40 Gy. This approach has generally been reserved for patients with solitary bladder tumors less than 4 cm in diameter. Five-year survival rates of 72% to 84% have been reported, with disease-specific survivals of approximately 80% (12,13). The data suggest

TABLE 26B.2

RANDOMIZED TRIALS OF IRRADIATION THAT DID OR DID NOT DEFER RADICAL CYSTECTOMY FOR SALVAGE OF RECURRENCE IN MUSCLE-INVASIVE BLADDER CANCER

Study (reference) Treatment	Patients n	Clinical stage	5-year survival (%)	10-year survival (%)	Distant metastases (%)
M.D. Anderson Cancer Center (3)					
50 Gy + cystectomy	35	T3	46	—	—
60 Gy + salvage cystectomy	32	T3	22	—	—
National Danish Trial (7)					
40 Gy + radical cystectomy	88	T3	29	—	34
60 Gy + salvage cystectomy	95	T3	23	—	32
UK Cooperative Group (9)					
40 Gy + radical cystectomy	98	T3	39	19	—
60 Gy + salvage cystectomy	91	T3	28	15	—
National Bladder Cancer Group[a]					
40 Gy + radical cystectomy	37	T2-T4a	27	—	38
60 Gy + salvage cystectomy	35	T2-T4a	40	—	31

[a]SD Cutler, National Cancer Institute, unpublished observations, 1983.

that in carefully selected patients, interstitial radiation produces high local control rates and results in excellent survival. However, without a randomized trial comparing the results and toxicity of brachytherapy with those of radical external beam radiation therapy, firm conclusions cannot be drawn.

COMBINED MODALITY TREATMENT WITH BLADDER SPARING

Conservative management with organ preservation is now the standard of care in numerous malignancies, including carcinomas of the breast, the anus, and the head and neck region, where radical surgery can be avoided in most patients without compromising survival. There are several reports from North America and Europe of long-term survival using multimodality treatment of muscularis propria-invading bladder cancer, with appropriate safeguards for early cystectomy should the bladder preservation treatment fail. For bladder conserving therapy to be more widely accepted, however, the treatment approach must have a high likelihood of eradicating the primary tumor, must preserve good organ function, and must not result in compromised patient survival.

Modern radiation treatment techniques are employed as one key element of treatment in bladder-sparing approaches which also include debulking transurethral surgery and chemotherapy. Radiation is delivered to the whole small pelvis, with the external and internal iliac lymph nodes in the target volume, for a total dose of 40 Gy to 45 Gy in 1.8 to 2.0 Gy fractions over 4 to 5 weeks. Subsequently, the target volume is reduced to deliver a final boost 20 Gy to 25 Gy in 10 to 15 fractions to the primary tumor. Some protocols call for partial bladder radiation at the boost volume, if the location of the tumor in the bladder can be satisfactorily determined by use of cystoscopic mapping, selective mucosal biopsies, and imaging information from CT or MRI. When twice-a-day radiation protocols are to be used, a dose per fraction of 1.5 Gy to 1.6 Gy has been shown to be quite well tolerated when combined with concurrent cisplatin-containing chemotherapy (14,15). With concurrent cisplatin-containing chemotherapy, total whole bladder doses from 50 Gy to 55 Gy and total doses to the bladder tumor volume of 65 Gy have been widely used. In the United Kingdom, daily doses of 2.5 Gy to 2.75 Gy per fraction over 4 weeks to a total dose of 50 Gy to 55 Gy have been the rule. However, available information suggests that the higher dose per fraction leads to a higher rate of serious late bladder complications.

Because the bladder is not a fixed organ, its location and volume can vary considerably from day to day. This results in a number of logistic problems which require the careful attention of the radiation oncologist to ensure adequate coverage of the bladder tumor. Recent studies have identified substantial movement of the bladder during the course of external beam radiation therapy, and as a result of these findings a minimum margin of 2 cm to 2.5 cm around the target volume to the edge of the light field is necessary (16,17). When 3D conformal external beam radiation therapy is to be used, treating the patient with an empty bladder minimizes bladder motion. The clinical target volume (CTV) expansion to the planning target volume (PTV) should be 1.5 cm to 2.0 cm and possibly even greater superiorly (17). Total bladder tumor doses of higher than 65 Gy seem appropriate, especially in light of the higher doses now used in CT-planned prostate cancer patients. However, because of the increased problems with bladder organ motion and with the fact that the majority of patients are now treated with concurrent cisplatin-containing chemotherapy, escalation in total dose above 65 Gy should be done only in the investigational setting.

Present-day combined-modality treatment and selective bladder preservation by early response evaluation differ from previous approaches utilizing monotherapy. These older approaches included: (a) transurethral resection alone done selectively for patients with small tumors, which represented less than 20% of all muscle-invading bladder tumors, (b) external beam radiation therapy as monotherapy, and (c) systemic multidrug chemotherapy as monotherapy. Local control rates with radiation alone for muscle-invading tumors have been disappointingly low, and radiation as monotherapy has largely been abandoned (see below) (5,6,18,19). It is now clear that monotherapies of various types are in general unsuccessful in curing patients of invasive bladder cancer. Barnes et al. reported a 27% 5-year survival in 85 patients with well-differentiated and moderately differentiated T2 transitional cell carcinomas treated with transurethral resection alone (20). Sweeney et al. found that only 19% of patients with muscle-invasive tumors were selected for treatment by partial cystectomy, and these had a local recurrence rate of 38% to 78% (21). Hall and Roberts reported a 19% 3-year freedom from recurrence with chemotherapy alone in 27 patients with localized disease, utilizing cisplatin, methotrexate, vinblastine, and epirubicin (22). The local control rates for the monotherapies noted above are inadequate when compared to radical cystectomy with its local control rate of 90%.

Attempts at bladder sparing must be selective, as not all patients are candidates for that approach. One must make certain that a complete response (CR) following initial chemoradiation induction is achieved, as measured by follow-up cytology and cystoscopic biopsies. Only if there is a CR to induction therapy is consolidation chemotherapy recommended and that is followed by adjuvant chemotherapy only in those patients who have negative bladder biopsies following consolidation radiochemotherapy. If residual disease is found, cystectomy is recommended as an immediate step in treatment, followed by adjuvant chemotherapy.

The combination of transurethral resection, radiation, and chemotherapy has yielded better results than any of the monotherapies, with an improved clinical CR rate (Tables 26B.3 and 26B.4). Moreover, substantial improvements in local control have been achieved with combined modality therapy (23–26). This generally consists of transurethral resection of the tumor for debulking, with the goal a visibly complete tumor removal, followed by radiation treatment with concurrent radiosensitizing chemotherapy. In the studies reported, the most commonly used radiosensitizing drugs were cisplatin, 5-fluorouracil, and paclitaxel, used either singly or in various combinations.

The results of trimodality therapy for muscle-invasive bladder cancer have led to further studies utilizing trimodality treatment with improved radiation techniques and the use of newer chemotherapeutic agents in innovative combinations in attempts to improve on the CR rate as well as the long-term control rate in the treatment of muscle-invasive bladder cancer.

Despite promising results, there is reluctance among urologic surgeons to accept trimodality therapy as an alternative to cystectomy even in selected patients. In part, this is due to improvements in urinary diversion in patients undergoing cystectomy, but, more importantly, concern persists among urologists that only cystectomy has the potential to rid the patient of the disease permanently. Urologists have expressed the following widely held views as arguments against bladder sparing:

a. Superficial relapse is common and very difficult to treat after radiochemotherapy.
b. Radiation burns the bladder, rendering it useless, with bleeding and scarring associated with frequency, urgency, nocturia, and perineal pain.
c. Innovative surgical techniques including neobladders, continent diversion, and other technical advances have

TABLE 26B.3

RECENT RESULTS OF MULTIMODALITY TREATMENT FOR MUSCLE-INVASIVE BLADDER CANCER

Multimodality therapy used	Number of patients	5-year overall survival (%)	5-year survival with intact bladder (%)	Study location	References
External beam radiation + cisplatin	42	52	42	RTOG 8512	Tester et al. 1993 (23)
TURBT, external beam radiation + cisplatin	79	52	41	University of Erlangen	Dunst et al. 1994 (24)
TURBT, MCV, external beam radiation + cisplatin	91	62 (4 yr)	44 (4 yr)	RTOG 8812	Tester et al. 1996 (25)
TURBT, 5-FU, external beam radiation + cisplatin	120	63	NA	University of Paris	Housset et al. 1997 (27)
TURBT, external beam radiation + cisplatin or carboplatin	162 (93—cisplatin; 69—carboplatin)	55	44	University of Erlangen	Sauer et al. 1998 (28)
TURBT, +/−MCV, external beam radiation + cisplatin	123	49	38	RTOG 8903	Shipley et al. 1998 (29)
TURBT, MCV, external beam radiation + cisplatin	190	54	45	MGH	Shipley et al. 2002 (26)
TURBT, MCV, external beam radiation + cisplatin	123	49	NA	RTOG 9706	Hagan et al. 2001 (14)

TURBT, transurethral resection of bladder tumor; 5-FU, 5-fluorouracil; MCV, methotrexate, cisplatin, vinblastine; RTOG, Radiation Therapy Oncology Group; MGH, Massachusetts General Hospital; NA, not available.

been successful and are subject to continuing improvement, making bladder-sparing efforts unnecessary.

d. Once the patient has been treated with chemotherapy and radiation to the bladder, radical cystectomy becomes more difficult to perform and is associated with considerable morbidity.

e. Chemotherapy, with its attendant nausea, anorexia, weight loss, and malaise, is permanently destructive of the quality of life.

f. Delay in cystectomy risks patients' lives.

It is important to note that each of the above statements has been negated by appropriate studies.

Investigators have become interested in clinical trials with the demonstration that some older as well as newer drugs have considerable activity against metastatic bladder cancer (Tables 26B.5 and 26B.6). The list includes cisplatin, methotrexate, vinblastine, ifosfamide, doxorubicin, gemcitabine, and paclitaxel as the principal agents. Not surprisingly, combinations of these drugs have been shown to be more effective than single agents in the percentage of CRs achieved. With the use of combination chemotherapy in advanced measurable disease, CR has become a common achievement as compared to a 15% to 20% rate of partial remission utilizing a variety of single drugs, and with complete remissions only rarely observed with single-agent treatments.

Successful bladder-sparing treatment is and should be very selective, with frequent examinations of patients' bladders for signs of persistence or recurrence of disease. All protocols explicitly direct discontinuation of the bladder-sparing effort in favor of radical cystectomy at the earliest sign of failure of local control. And further, all of our protocols have required for acceptance that patients be medically fit and willing to undergo cystectomy if deemed medically necessary.

Successful approaches have evolved over the last two decades following the initial reports of the effectiveness of cisplatin against transitional cell carcinoma and reports of added efficacy when it is given concurrently with radiation. From 1981

TABLE 26B.4

RTOG BLADDER PROTOCOLS (1985–2002): TRIMODALITY THERAPY WITH CYSTECTOMY ONLY FOR POORLY RESPONDING/RELAPSING PATIENTS

Protocol (ref.)	Induction treatment	Patients (out of 426)	5-year survival	Complete response
8512 (30)	TURBT, CP + XRT	42	52%	66%[a]
8802 (31)	TURBT, MCV, CP + XRT	91	51%	75%[a]
8903 (29)	TURBT, ±MCV then CP + XRT	123	49%	59%
9506 (32)	TURBT, 5-FU plus CP + XRT	34	NA	67%
9706 (33)	TURBT, CP + BID XRT adj. MCV	52	NA	74%
9906 (n.a.)	TURBT, TAX plus CP + XRT; adj. CP + GEM	84	NA	NA

TURBT, transurethral resection of bladder tumor; XRT, external beam radiation; CP, cisplatin; 5-FU, 5-fluorouracil; MCV, methotrexate, cisplatin, vinblastine; TAX, paclitaxel; GEM, gemcitabine; NA, not available.
[a]Urine cytology not evaluated as a response criterion.

SINGLE-AGENT ACTIVITY IN BLADDER CANCER—OLDER AGENTS

Drug	Response rate
Cisplatin	12%–28%
Methotrexate	29%–45%
Doxorubicin	17%
5-fluorouracil	15%–17%
Vinblastine	15%
Mitomycin C	13%–20%

SINGLE-AGENT ACTIVITY IN BLADDER CANCER—NEWER AGENTS

Drug	Response rate
Paclitaxel	42%–56%
Ifosfamide	20%–31%
Gemcitabine	23%–28%
Carboplatin	13%–15%
Docetaxel	13%

to 1986 the National Bladder Cancer Group first used cisplatin as a radiation sensitizer in 68 patients with muscularis propria-invading bladder cancer who were unsuitable for cystectomy. In a multicenter protocol this approach was shown to be feasible and safe (30). Furthermore, the long-term survival rate with stage T2 tumors (64%) and even for stage T3-T4 tumors (22%) was encouraging. This early result with concurrent cisplatin and pelvic irradiation was validated by the NCI-Canada randomized trial of radiation (either definitive or precystectomy) with or without concurrent cisplatin for patients with T3 bladder cancer. The Canadian study showed

a significant improvement in pelvic tumor control (67% vs. 47%) in the patients who were assigned cisplatin (34). Moreover, single-institution studies showed that the combination of a visibly complete transurethral resection of tumor (TURBT) followed by radiation therapy or radiation therapy concurrent with chemotherapy led to improved local control (24,35). These findings led the Radiation Therapy Oncology Group (RTOG) to develop the algorithm for bladder preservation of an initial TURBT of as much of the bladder tumor as is safely possible followed by a combination of radiation with concurrent radiosensitizing chemotherapy. One key to the success of

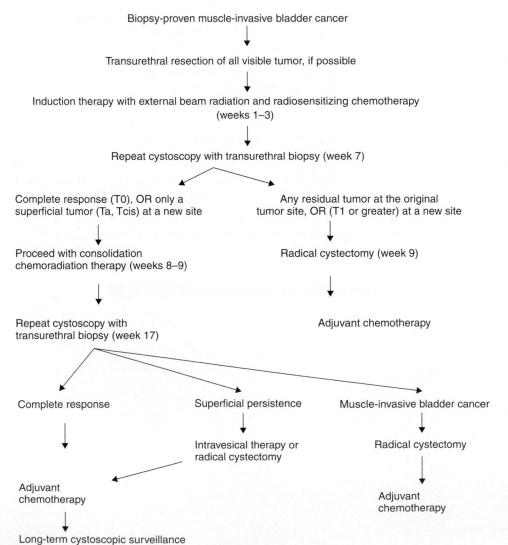

FIGURE 26B.1. Current schema for trimodality treatment of muscle-invasive bladder cancer with selective bladder preservation.

such a program is the selection of patients for bladder preservation on the basis of the initial response of each individual patient's tumor to therapy. Thus, bladder conservation was reserved for those patients who had a clinical CR to concurrent chemotherapy and radiation. Prompt cystectomy was recommended for those patients whose tumors responded only incompletely or who subsequently developed an invasive tumor (Fig. 26B.1). All of the protocols developed at the Massachusetts General Hospital (MGH) or within RTOG since 1986 call for radical cystectomy at the first sign of failure of local control. More than one-third of the patients entering a potential bladder-preserving protocol with trimodality therapy (initial TURBT followed by concurrent chemotherapy and radiation) will require radical cystectomy (26).

Eligibility criteria for bladder sparing include: (a) histologic proof of invasion of the muscularis propria, (b) normal upper tracts, (c) the absence of hydronephrosis, (d) adequate renal function, (e) a normal hemogram, (f) medical fitness for cystectomy, and (g) the absence of malignant lymphadenopathy on imaging studies utilizing computed tomography (CT) or magnetic resonance imaging (MRI), with biopsy as necessary.

Protocols carried out between 1986 and 2002 at the Massachusetts General Hospital Cancer Center included as complete a TURBT as possible, followed by radiation and concomitant chemotherapy (36). In an early protocol, we utilized neoadjuvant multidrug systemic chemotherapy in an effort to reduce the appearance of distant metastases. However, the 5-year and 10-year metastasis-free survival rates were not influenced by the addition of two cycles of neoadjuvant methotrexate, vinblastine, and cisplatin (MCV) chemotherapy. We have not used neoadjuvant chemotherapy in subsequent protocols, directing our attention instead to adjuvant chemotherapy.

Phase II and phase III protocols with concurrent radiochemotherapy are listed in Table 26B.4 and are described here. The first Radiation Therapy Oncology Group (RTOG) study, RTOG 8512, included 42 patients treated with once-daily radiation treatment and concurrent cisplatin, yielding a 5-year survival of 52% (23). This treatment was well tolerated and resulted in 42% of the patients achieving long-term survival with an intact bladder. RTOG studies 8802 and 8903 utilized MCV chemotherapy as neoadjuvant treatment. In the latter study, patients were treated on a phase III trial with or without two cycles of MCV prior to the combination of cisplatin and once-a-day radiation (25). There was no improvement in survival or in local tumor eradication as a result of neoadjuvant therapy (29). With a median follow-up of 5 years the overall survival was 48% in patients treated with MCV and 49% in patients who received no neoadjuvant treatment. The cystoscopic CR rate was 61% in the MCV arm and 55% in the control arm, not statistically significant. At 5 years, metastases were present in 35% of the patients who received MCV and 42% of the patients who received no neoadjuvant chemotherapy. This difference was not statistically significant. The toxicity of the MCV arm was considerable, with only 67% of patients able to complete the planned treatment. This phase III study was not sufficiently powered to settle the question of the place of neoadjuvant chemotherapy in patients undergoing bladder-preserving therapy, but neither RTOG nor MGH has revisited the question of the effectiveness of neo-adjuvant chemotherapy. (See adjuvant chemotherapy, below.)

Houssett et al. from the University of Paris reported on 120 patients with stage T2-T4a bladder cancer. The treatment consisted of TURBT followed by cisplatin and 5-fluorouracil (5-FU) given concurrently with twice-a-day hypofractionated radiation. They reported a 63% overall survival rate (27).

Investigators at the University of Erlangen recently updated the largest bladder-sparing study to date, 415 patients treated from 1982 to 2000 (37). This report included 126 patients who received radiation without any chemotherapy and 89 patients who were not clinical stage T2 to T4 but classified as

"high-risk T1." The CR rate of all 415 patients was 72% and local control of the bladder tumor after the CR without a muscle invasive relapse was maintained in 64% of the patients at 10 years. The 10-year disease-specific survival was 42% and more than 80% of these survivors preserved their bladder. This series, not randomized, included sequential use of radiation with no chemotherapy (126 patients) followed by concurrent cisplatin (145 patients), concurrent carboplatin (95 patients), and concurrent cisplatin plus 5-FU (49 patients). The CR rates in these four sequential treatment protocols were 51%, 81%, 64%, and 87%, respectively (38,39). The 5-year actuarial survival with an intact bladder in these four protocols were 38%, 47%, 41%, and 54%, respectively. These results suggest strongly that radiochemotherapy when given concurrently is superior to radiation therapy alone, that carboplatin is less radiosensitizing than cisplatin, and that cisplatin plus 5-FU may be superior to cisplatin alone. The authors recognized that their study was compromised by the absence of randomized trial data.

From 1994 to 1998, twice-daily radiation therapy was introduced into RTOG protocols with concurrent cisplatin or with cisplatin plus 5-FU as radiosensitizers (40). From 1999 to 2002, twice-a-day radiation concurrent with cisplatin and paclitaxel as radiosensitizers along with adjuvant cisplatin and gemcitabine was evaluated. The latest North American protocol for bladder-sparing treatment (RTOG 0233) recently opened. This is a randomized phase II study comparing two combinations of radiosensitizing chemotherapy (cisplatin plus paclitaxel vs. cisplatin plus 5-FU), each given concurrently with an induction course of twice-daily radiation treatment. This is followed in patients whose tumors initially responded completely by consolidation chemoradiation and in those with incompletely responding tumors by radical cystectomy. All patients are then to undergo a three-drug adjuvant treatment consisting of cisplatin, gemcitabine, and paclitaxel (40).

The MGH experience with 190 patients with invasive bladder cancers with clinical stages T2-T4a entered on successive prospective protocols has recently been updated (26). A common feature of all the protocols was early bladder tumor response evaluation and the selection of patients for bladder conservation on the basis of their initial response to TURBT combined with chemotherapy and radiation. Bladder conservation was reserved for those who had a complete clinical response at the midpoint in therapy (after a radiation dosage of 40 Gy). Approximately two-thirds of the total then received consolidation with additional chemotherapy and radiation to a total tumor dose of 64 Gy to 65 Gy. Incomplete responders were advised to undergo radical cystectomy, as were patients whose invasive tumors persisted or recurred after treatment.

In these phase II and phase III protocols, the scheduling of the chemoradiation varied. In the one phase III study, all patients underwent TURBT with patients then randomized to neoadjuvant or no neoadjuvant chemotherapy. All patients then were treated with concurrent cisplatin and radiation therapy.

The median follow-up for all surviving patients was 6.7 years with 81 patients having been followed for 5 or more years, and 28 patients for 10 or more years (26). The 5-year and 10-year actuarial overall survival rates were 54% and 36%, respectively (stage T2, 62% and 41%; stage T3-T4a, 47% and 31%). The 5-year and 10-year disease-specific survivals are 63% and 59% (T2, 74% and 66%; stage T3-T4a, 53% and 52%). The 5-year and 10-year disease-specific survivals with an intact bladder are 46% and 45% (T2, 57% and 50%; T3-T4a, 35% and 34%). The pelvic failure rate was 8.4%. No patient required cystectomy due to bladder morbidity.

The overall survival rate is provided in Figure 26B.2 and the disease-specific survival rate stratified by clinical stage in Figure 26B.3. The current schema for multimodality treatment

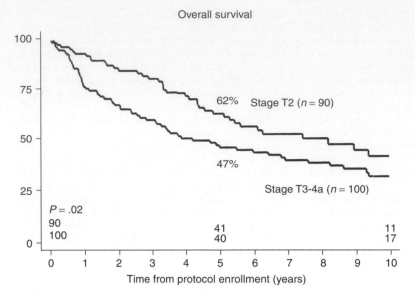

FIGURE 26B.2. Overall survival.

of muscle-invasive bladder cancer is provided in Figure 26B.1 and the risk of relapse with a superficial tumor following multimodality treatment in Figure 26B.2.

The actuarial 5-year and 10-year overall survival and disease-specific survival for all 190 patients and for some clinically important subgroups are shown in Table 26B.7. The clinical stage (Figs. 26B.2 and 26B.3) significantly influences overall survival ($P = .02$) and disease-specific survival ($P = .01$) as well as CR rate (stage T2, 71%; T3-T4a, 50%; $P = .04$) and the rate of subsequent distant metastases (T2, 22%; T3-T4a, 37%; $P = .03$). We also found a higher 5-year and 10-year disease-specific survival with an intact bladder for stage T2 patients, 57% and 50%, respectively, than for T3-T4a patients, 35% and 24%, respectively, with a p value of 0.008. Neither the tumor grade nor the use of neoadjuvant chemotherapy significantly improved the CR rate (64%), overall survival, disease-specific survival, or distant metastasis-free survival. The presence of hydronephrosis significantly reduces the CR rate, 37% versus 68%, $P = .002$. The 5-year and 10-year disease-specific survival for all 66 patients undergoing cystectomy are 48% and 41%, indicating the important contribution of this procedure in those patients treated with this

approach. The tumor stage did not influence the 5–year and 10-year disease-specific survival in the 66 patients undergoing either an immediate cystectomy or a salvage cystectomy, (stage T2, 57% and 39%; T3-T4a, 42% and 42%).

The current schema for trimodality treatment of muscle-invading bladder cancer is provided in Figure 26B.1. The 5-year and 10-year disease-specific survival rate for the 66 patients undergoing cystectomy is 48% and 41%, respectively. This indicates the very important contribution of prompt salvage cystectomy for disease control in the 66 patients who required salvage cystectomy.

Of the 121 patients who were complete responders after induction therapy, 73 developed no further bladder tumors, 32 (26%) subsequently developed a superficial occurrence and 16 developed an invasive tumor (41). Twenty-nine patients with superficial recurrence were treated conservatively by TURBT and intravesical chemotherapy and three underwent immediate cystectomy. However, 7 of the 29 patients required subsequent cystectomy for additional superficial (4 patients) or invasive (3 patients) recurrence. For these patients the overall survival was comparable to the 73 who had no failure. However, one third of these patients required a salvage cystectomy.

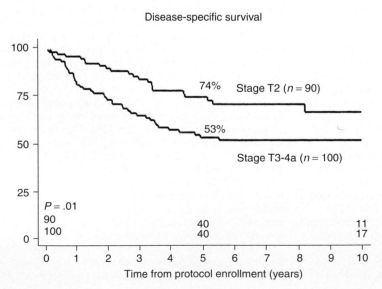

FIGURE 26B.3. Disease-specific survival.

TABLE 26B.7

SURVIVAL OUTCOMES BY PATIENT AND TUMOR CHARACTERISTICS

Patient group	n	Overall survival (%)			Disease-specific survival (%)		
		5 yr	10 yr	P value	5 yr	10 yr	P value
All patients	190	54 ± 7.5^a	36 ± 8.3^a		63 ± 7.5^a	59 ± 8.0^a	
Age at entry (yr)							
<75	155	55	40	0.04	65	60	NS
>75	35	51	22	56	56		
Sex							
Female	47	59	40	0.67	60	52	0.50
Male	143	52	34		64	62	
Clinical stage							
T2	90	62	41	0.02	74	66	0.01
T3-T4a	100	47	31		53	52	
Hydronephrosis							
No	163	55	37	0.15	64	61	0.09
Yes	27	48	29		53	49	

NS, not stated.
^{a}95% confidence interval.

The pelvic recurrence rate of all 190 patients was 8.4%. This includes 6 of the 41 patients who underwent immediate cystectomy and 6.7% of the remainder, with a median follow-up of 7.3 years.

Comparing our results to those of contemporary radical cystectomy series is confounded by the discordance between clinical TURBT staging and pathological (cystectomy) staging. A recent prospective evaluation from Stockholm (42) has documented that clinical staging is more likely to undercvaluate the extent of the disease with regard to penetration into muscularis propria or beyond than is pathological staging. Thus, if any favorable outcome bias exists, it is in favor of the pathologically reported radical cystectomy series. The University of Southern California recently reported on 633 patients undergoing radical cystectomy with pathologic stages T2 to T4a with an actuarial overall survival rate at 5 years of 48% and

TABLE 26B.8

INVASIVE BLADDER CANCER—SURVIVAL OUTCOMES IN CONTEMPORARY SERIES

Series	Stages	Number	Overall survival	
			5 yr	10 yr
Cystectomy				
USC (2)				
(2001)	P2-P4a	633	48%	32%
MSKCC (1)				
(2001)	P2-P4a	181	36%	27%
Selective bladder preservation				
Erlangen (37)				
(2002)	cT2-T4	326	45%	29%
MGH (26)				
(2001)	cT2-T4a	190	54%	36%
RTOG (29)				
(1998)	cT2-T4	123	49%	—

USC, University of Southern California; MSKCC, Memorial Sloan-Kettering Cancer Center; MGH, Massachusetts General Hospital; RTOG, Radiation Therapy Oncology Group.

10 years of 32% (2). The Memorial Sloan-Kettering Cancer Center (MSKCC) Contemporary Radical Cystectomy series showed that in 184 patients with tumors of pathologic stage P2-P4, the 5-year overall survival rate was 36%. The actuarial 5-year survival rate of all 269 patients undergoing radical cystectomy with pathologic stages ranging from P0 to P4 in this series was 45% (1). The results of these contemporary cystectomy series for muscle-invading bladder cancer are similar to the MGH series as well as those from the University of Erlangen (37) and the RTOG (29) (Table 26B.8). This similarity in survival is likely in part due to the prompt use of salvage cystectomy when necessary in the selective bladder-preservation series. The disease-specific survival rate of 40% at 10 years in the MGH series for patients having cystectomy underscores the need for close urologic follow-up with cystoscopic surveillance and prompt bladder removal when clinically indicated.

One of the concerns with bladder-sparing therapy is the risk of subsequent superficial relapses within the intact bladder, which could progress to life-threatening malignancy once again for those patients. Long-term follow-up from the MGH series has examined this issue in detail in the 121 patients with a CR (Fig. 26B.4). Sixty percent of patients did not have evidence of relapse after a median follow-up of 7.1 years. Of the 32 superficial recurrences, 10 required cystectomy and 18 were treated conservatively with tumor-free bladders. Thus, with a median follow-up of over 7 years, 91 (75%) of the 121 complete responding patients have tumor-free bladders. The overall survival of those patients with a superficial recurrence is the same as those CR patients without a bladder recurrence (41).

Lifelong surveillance with cystoscopy is therefore crucial in patients treated with bladder-sparing therapy, and prompt salvage therapy for either superficial or recurrent invasive disease results in no survival disadvantage.

EVOLVING STANDARDS FOR SYSTEMIC CHEMOTHERAPY

Neoadjuvant Chemotherapy

There is strong evidence that invasive transitional cell cancer of the bladder is associated with occult metastases, with the

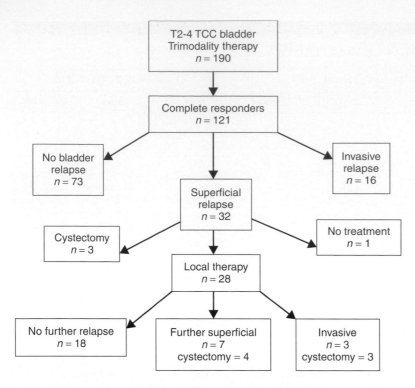

FIGURE 26B.4. Outcome of 121 patients with clinical T2-4 transitional cell carcinoma of the bladder who had a complete response (CR).

likelihood that micrometastases are present, in many cases, at the time of initial discovery of the bladder tumor. Randomized studies utilizing single-agent neoadjuvant chemotherapy have failed to demonstrate a survival benefit or a reduction in the development of distant metastases.

Despite more than two decades of clinical experience and investigation with neoadjuvant chemotherapy, followed either by radiochemotherapy as part of bladder-sparing or radical cystectomy, there is still uncertainty as to whether treatment, timed in this way, affects survival. There were, in fact, some hopeful results from early phase I-II trials of single-agent chemotherapy, but several phase II studies done subsequently using multiagent chemotherapy, several randomized studies, and a meta-analysis all failed to demonstrate a survival benefit. In advanced disease, combination chemotherapy is superior to single-agent chemotherapy. Data from studies in patients with measurable metastatic disease clearly showed the superiority of M-VAC over single-agent cisplatin on survival (43). Recently published randomized trials have given conflicting results, but there are now several studies which demonstrated a survival benefit from neoadjuvant combination chemotherapy. These results, however, as interesting and important as they are, do not effectively make the case for neoadjuvant chemotherapy as a new standard of treatment in muscularis propria-invasive bladder cancer, either as part of a bladder-sparing approach or precystectomy.

The Medical Research Council (MRC) and the European Organization for the Research and Treatment of Cancer (EORTC), with R. R. Hall as coordinator (44), began in 1989 a prospective randomized trial of neoadjuvant cisplatin, methotrexate, and vinblastine in patients undergoing cystectomy or full-dose external beam radiotherapy for muscularis propria bladder cancer. The authors of the study acknowledged that the equivalence of radiotherapy and cystectomy had not been proved by all the historical randomized trials. The type of local radical treatment, surgery or radiation treatment, was chosen by the individual doctors.

In order to detect an absolute improvement in survival of 10% (i.e., 50% increased to 60%), a total of 915 patients was planned. It is important, in assessing the results of this study,

to note that in 6 years 976 patients were recruited from more than 100 institutions in 20 countries. The median length of follow-up was 4 years. Further, out of 491 patients assigned chemotherapy, 99 did not receive all three cycles for a variety of reasons, and 26% of patients required dose decreases or delay. Out of 561 patients, 76 did not undergo a planned cystectomy; 32.4% of patients underwent (optional) cystoscopy and biopsy after chemotherapy, and the biopsy confirmed endoscopic CR in 44%. The median survival for the chemotherapy group was 44 months versus 37.5 months for the cystectomy-only group, and the difference was not considered statistically significant when this study was published.

This, then, represents the largest randomized trial of neoadjuvant cisplatin-based chemotherapy for muscularis propria-invasive bladder cancer. The study was powered to detect a 10% improvement in survival, but the study results showed only a possible 5% difference in 3-year survival, and to confirm this benefit statistically would require 3,500 patients. The authors concluded, therefore, that though they observed a possible improvement in 3-year survival, "this conclusion is not certain because this very large multicenter trial had sufficient power to detect only a larger survival benefit." We cannot conclude from this study—and the authors do not suggest—that neoadjuvant chemotherapy should be considered the new standard of care in the treatment of muscularis propria bladder cancer based on these data.

This MRC/EORTC study was updated in a presentation at the meeting of the American Society of Clinical Oncology in May 2002 (45). Based on their interpretation of the data as presented, Sharma et al. stated that a significantly improved survival was seen in all patients receiving chemotherapy (46). Overall survival was superior for patients who received chemotherapy at 3 years (55% vs. 50%), 5 years (50% vs. 44%), and 8 years (43% vs. 37%), with a median follow-up of 7 years. There was also an improved disease-free survival ($P = .012$) and locoregional progression-free survival ($P = .003$). Publication of these data will allow for critical review by oncologists to determine whether the additional years of follow-up of this large clinical trial will merit a change in the standard of care of invasive bladder cancer. This published update should clarify the extent of the benefit of neoadjuvant MCV by type of planned local therapy because this was cystectomy in only about one half of the 976 patients.

Raghavan et al. published a meta-analysis of all completed randomized trials (47) of neoadjuvant chemotherapy for invasive bladder cancer. Their analysis, comprising 2,688 patients, led the authors to the following conclusions: single-agent neoadjuvant chemotherapy is ineffective and should not be used; and current combination chemotherapy regimens improve the 5-year survival by 5%, which reduces the risk of death by 13% compared with the use of definitive local treatment alone (i.e., from 43% to 38%). Though each of the studies cited above was adequately designed and sufficiently powered to settle the question as to whether neoadjuvant chemotherapy should be considered the new standard of care in invasive bladder cancer, a careful review of all of the published material on this subject suggests the following conclusion:

While the published data on neoadjuvant chemotherapy do not meet the required standard to declare neoadjuvant chemotherapy the new standard of care in muscularis propria bladder cancer, the data in support of benefit are sufficiently compelling that patients should be informed of the potential benefits versus the risks of neoadjuvant chemotherapy as part of the discussion leading to a decision to proceed with cystectomy. The possible role of adjuvant chemotherapy should also be discussed with these patients (vida infra).

ADJUVANT CHEMOTHERAPY

The obvious advantage of adjuvant, as opposed to neoadjuvant, chemotherapy is that pathologic staging allows for a more accurate selection of patients. This approach facilitates the separation of patients in stage pT2 from those in stages pT3 or pT4 or node-positive disease, all at a high risk for progression (1,2). The major disadvantage is the delay in systemic therapy for occult metastases while the primary tumor is being treated. It is not possible to assess response to treatment, as there is no clinical endpoint except for clinically detectable disease progression. Pathologic staging has been used to advantage in breast cancer and colon cancer, two diseases in which adjuvant chemotherapy has been demonstrated to increase disease-free survival. The parallel continues in breast cancer, colon cancer, and bladder cancer, as drugs for use in the adjuvant setting have been selected on the basis of their demonstrated activity in advanced, measurable metastatic disease.

Adjuvant chemotherapy has been studied in two major clinical settings: (a) following bladder-sparing chemo-irradiation, and (b) postradical cystectomy. In the former case, it became clear in our early bladder-sparing studies that bladder cancer is a systemic disease, and simply rendering the bladder free of invasive cancer is not sufficient to prevent death from metastatic disease in the majority of patients whose bladders were cured of the primary tumor (48). Unlike our earlier studies, which utilized cisplatin alone as the radiosensitizing drug, MCV in a total of three 28-day cycles was used as the treatment of choice for the adjuvant phase of treatment. The adjuvant regimen of choice in our later studies consisted of four cycles of cisplatin plus gemcitabine (29). In our current study, the adjuvant regimen of choice consists of four cycles of cisplatin, gemcitabine, and paclitaxel, a potent and well-tolerated regimen in the treatment of metastatic disease (49).

The results thus far of the contribution of adjuvant chemotherapy in affecting survival in patients undergoing bladder-sparing treatment are uncertain. There is currently no study in progress prospectively comparing adjuvant chemotherapy versus no adjuvant chemotherapy in patients undergoing bladder-preserving treatment.

Another important adjuvant trial is underway, which is an example of the convergence of biologic predictors and chemotherapy in the search for improved treatment of bladder cancer. This is a multiinstitutional Southwest Oncology Group (SWOG) phase III trial, sponsored by the National Cancer Institute and led by the University of Southern California. The purpose of the study is to evaluate the therapeutic and prognostic significance of altered p53 expression by the tumor p53 following radical cystectomy in patients whose tumors are pT1 or pT2 and assessed for p53 status. For patients with p53 (−) tumors, the treatment is observation. For those with p53 (+) tumors, the patients are randomized to M-VAC or observation. The possible significance of other genes, including p21, pRB, c-erb B-2, and others may prove to be important as relates to prognosis and possible benefit for chemotherapy postcystectomy or as part of bladder-sparing treatment (50). Until the completion of a well-designed and well-executed clinical trial(s), sufficiently powered to settle the question, the place of adjuvant chemotherapy will necessarily remain uncertain. The place of newer drug combinations, already determined to be active in advanced bladder cancer, remains to be determined.

Please refer to Chapter 29 for further discussion of neoadjuvant chemotherapy, including neoadjuvant chemotherapy followed by TURBT or partial cystectomy, as well as patients subjected to radical cystectomy. The chapter also weighs the evidence for and against adjuvant chemotherapy following cystectomy.

QUALITY OF LIFE AFTER THERAPY FOR INVASIVE BLADDER CANCER

Evaluating the quality of life in long-term survivors of bladder cancer has been difficult and only recently have attempts been made to assess this in an objective and quantitative fashion (15,51–58). A number of problems arise in the interpretation of the published studies. Tools to assess quality of life variables were developed early for common prostate and gynecologic cancers but no such instruments exist for bladder cancer. The instruments now used in bladder cancer are thus adaptations of uncertain validity. The published studies are all cross-sectional and patients have follow-up of varying lengths. This may matter in a surgical series in which functional outcome improves with time and a radiation series in which it may deteriorate. All studies are hampered by incomplete accrual of all potential participants. It is never clear whether the nonparticipants are those who have had a worse outcome or are the most satisfied. Despite these limitations some conclusions can now be drawn.

Radical cystectomy causes changes in many areas of quality of life, including urinary, sexual, and social function, daily living activities, and satisfaction with body image (51–55). Sexual function has been particularly emphasized because of the high prevalence of erectile dysfunction. Researchers have, over the last decade, concentrated on the relative merits of continent and noncontinent diversions. Available data have been mixed with some groups, surprisingly, reporting few differences between the quality of life of those with an ileal conduit and those with continent diversions. Until recently little comparative data has been available on those who have neobladders. Hart et al. have compared outcome in cystectomy patients who have either ileal conduits, cutaneous Koch pouches, or urethral Koch pouches (55). Of 1,074 patients undergoing cystectomy for bladder cancer at the University of Southern California, 368 were eligible for study because they were alive, spoke English, and had no major health issues that might affect global quality of life. Sixty-one percent of these completed self-reporting questionnaires. Regardless of the type of urinary diversion the majority of patients reported good overall quality of life, little emotional distress, and few problems with social, physical, or functional activities. Problems with their diversions and with sexual function were the most commonly reported. After controlling for age, no significant differences were seen among urinary diversion subgroups in any quality of life area. It might be anticipated that those receiving the urethral Koch diversions would be the most satisfied and the explanation why this is not so is unclear. It may be that the subgroups were too small to detect differences but perhaps it is more likely that each group adapts in time to the specific difficulties presented by that type of diversion.

Zietman et al. have performed a study on patients receiving TURBT, chemotherapy, and radiation in the treatment of their bladder cancer at MGH (15). Of 221 patients with clinical T2-4a cancer of the bladder treated at MGH from 1986 to 2000, 71 were alive with their native bladders and disease free in 2001. These patients were asked to undergo an urodynamic study (UDS) and to complete a quality of life questionnaire. Sixty-nine percent participated in some component of this study, with a median time from trimodality therapy of 6.3 years. This long follow-up is sufficient to capture the majority of late radiation effects. Seventy-five percent of patients had normally functioning bladders by UDS. Reduced bladder compliance, a recognized complication of radiation, was seen in 22% but in only one-third of these was it reflected in distressing symptoms. Two of 12 women showed bladder hypersensitivity, involuntary detrusor contractions, and incontinence. The questionnaire showed that bladder symptoms were uncommon, especially among men, with the exception of control problems. These were reported by 19%, with 11% wearing pads (all women). Distress from urinary symptoms was half as common as their prevalence. Bowel symptoms occurred in 22%, with only 14% recording any level of distress. The majority of men retained sexual function. Global health-related quality of life was high. The great majority of patients treated by trimodality therapy therefore retain good bladder function. It was concluded that there is a small but detectable level of lasting bowel dysfunction and distress and that this might be judged the additional price that these patients have had to pay to retain their bladders. A prospective multicenter study from France has recently been presented. It tracks voiding symptoms and quality of life in 53 patients from before their trimodality treatment. Thirty-three retained their bladders and these were interviewed 6, 12, and 24 months later. Levels of urinary symptoms were very high, with only 5% reporting any EORTC grade 3 symptom. It was also notable that most patients experienced improvement of symptoms over the 2 years after treatment presumably because of the eradication of a symptomatic tumor.

Two recent cross-sectional questionnaire studies, one from Sweden and one from Italy, have compared the outcome following radiation with the outcome following cystectomy (57,58). The questionnaire results for urinary function following radiation were very similar to those recorded in the MGH study. Over 74% of patients reported good urinary function. Both studies compared bowel function in irradiated patients with that seen in patients undergoing cystectomy. In both, the bowel symptoms were greater for those receiving radiation than for those receiving cystectomy (10% vs. 3% and 32% vs. 24% respectively), but in neither was this statistically significant.

In the assessment of sexual function, most women in the MGH study preferred not to answer the questions and no data was therefore available for them. Almost all men, however, did. In contrast to patients who have been irradiated for prostate cancer, the majority of male bladder-sparing patients reported adequate erectile function (full or sufficient for intercourse), and only 8% reported dissatisfaction with their sex lives. These are in line with those obtained in the Swedish and Italian series in which 38% and 25% of men retained useful

erections as compared with 13% and 8% of cystectomized controls. The MGH series allowed the use of sildenafil, probably contributing to the better outcome.

NEWER CHEMOTHERAPEUTIC AGENTS

In an attempt to improve safety as well as to increase efficacy, newer studies of multimodality therapy, utilizing newer chemotherapeutic agents, have recently shown a high degree of activity in metastatic transitional cell tumors, and these newer drugs are appropriately utilized as adjuvant treatment following the initial phases of bladder-sparing with TURB, radiosensitizing chemotherapy, and radiation therapy. The major drugs in this category are gemcitabine and paclitaxel. Many recent studies have suggested that paclitaxel is an active agent in transitional cell carcinomas and a phase II study of the combination of cisplatin and paclitaxel demonstrated a 50% response rate in 52 patients with metastatic disease (59). Three phase II trials demonstrated that gemcitabine combined with cisplatin is a well-tolerated active regimen (60–62). The combination of cisplatin and gemcitabine has been compared to methotrexate, vinblastine, doxorubicin, and cisplatin (M-VAC) in a phase III study, and the two combinations were shown to have similar efficacy in metastatic disease. The gemcitabine/cisplatin combination, however, was better tolerated and led to fewer hospital days for the treatment of toxic side effects (61). It is, therefore, considered by many to represent the new standard of care for metastatic transitional cell carcinoma and is under investigation in the adjuvant setting as well.

The latest national protocol for bladder sparing treatment (RTOG 0233) was approved in January 2003. This is a randomized phase II study comparing two combinations of radiosensitizing chemotherapy, each given concurrently with a short course of twice-daily radiation treatment. Patients received either the combination of fluorouracil and cisplatin or paclitaxel and cisplatin. This is followed, in patients whose tumors are successfully controlled with chemotherapy and radiation, by a three-drug adjuvant treatment program utilizing cisplatin, gemcitabine, and paclitaxel. This regimen has shown the highest response rate yet observed in published reports in advanced measurable bladder cancer (49).

CONCLUSION

The 10-year overall survival and disease-specific survival rates in our bladder-sparing protocols are comparable to the results reported with contemporary radical cystectomy. For patients of similar clinical and pathologic stage, one-third of patients treated on protocol with the goal of bladder sparing ultimately required a cystectomy. A trimodality approach with bladder preservation based on the initial tumor response is therefore safe and appropriate treatment with the majority of long-term survivors retaining functional bladders. It is clear, however, that life-long bladder surveillance is essential because only prompt salvage therapy can prevent a focus of new or recurrent bladder cancer from disseminating.

We would conclude that selective bladder sparing should be one of the approaches considered in the treatment of invasive bladder cancer. While it is not suggested that it will replace radical cystectomy, sufficient data now exist from many international prospective studies to demonstrate that it represents a valid alternative. This approach contributes significantly to the quality of life of patients so treated and represents a unique opportunity for urologic surgeons, radiation oncologists, and medical oncologists to work hand in hand in a joint effort to provide patients with the best treatment for this disease.

References

1. Dalbagni G, Genega E, Hashibe M, et al. Cystectomy for bladder cancer: a contemporary series. *J Urol* 2001;165:1111–1116.

2. Stein JP, Lieskovsky G, Cote R, et al. Radical cystectomy in the treatment of invasive bladder cancer: long-term results in 1,054 patients. *J Clin Oncol* 2001;9:666–675.

3. Miller LS. Bladder cancer: superiority of preoperative radiation in cystectomy in clinical stage T3. *Cancer* 1977;39:973–980.

4. Duncan W, Quilty PM. The result of a series of 963 patients with transitional cell carcinoma of the urinary bladder primarily treated by radical megavoltage x-ray therapy. *Radiother Oncol* 1986;7:299–310.

5. Jenkins BJ, Caulfield MJ, Fowler CG, et al. Reappraisal of the role of radical radiotherapy and salvage cystectomy in the treatment of invasive (T2-T3) bladder cancer. *Br J Urol* 1988;62:343–346.

6. Gospodarowicz MK, Hawkins NV, Rawlings GA, et al. Radical radiotherapy for muscle invasive transitional cell carcinoma of the bladder: failure analysis. *J Urol* 1989;142:1448–1453.

7. Sell A, Jakobsen A, Nerstrom B, et al. Danish Vesical Cancer Group. Treatment of advanced bladder cancer category T2,T3,T4a. A randomized multicenter study of preoperative indication and cystectomy versus salvage cystectomy for residual tumor. DAVECA protocol 8201. *Scand J Urol Nephrol Suppl* 1991;39:937–943.

8. Fossa SD, Waehre H, Aass N, et al. Bladder cancer: definitive radiation therapy of muscle invasive bladder cancer. A retrospective analysis of 317 patients. *Cancer* 1993;72:3036–3043.

9. Horwich A, Pendleburg S, Dearnaley DP. Organ conservation in bladder cancer. *Eur J Cancer* 1995;31(Suppl. 6):208.

10. Cole DJ, Durrant KR, Roberts JT, et al. A pilot study of accelerated fractionation in the radiotherapy of invasive carcinoma of the bladder. *Br J Radiol* 1992;65:792–798.

11. Horwich A, Dearnaley DP, Huddart R, et al. A trial of accelerated fractionation in fractionation in T2-T3 bladder cancer. *Int J Radiat Oncol Biol Phys* 1998;42(Suppl. 1):204. Abstract 160.

12. Gosparodarowicz MK, Blandy JP. Radiation therapy alone for organ conservation for invasive bladder cancer. In: Vogelzang NJ, Scardino PT, Shipley WU et al., eds. *Comprehensive textbook of genitourinary oncology*, 3rd ed. Philadelphia, PA: Lippincott Williams & Wilkins, 2000:487–496.

13. Moonen LM, Hornblas S, Van der Voet JC, et al. Bladder conservation in selective T1G3 and muscle invasive T2-T3z bladder carcinoma using combination therapy of surgery and iridium-192 implantations. *Br J Urol* 1994;74:322–327.

14. Hagan MP, Winter KA, Kaufman DS, et al. RTOG 97-06; initial report of a phase I-II trial of selective bladder conservation using TURBT, twice-daily accelerated irradiation sensitized with cisplatin, and adjuvant MCV combination chemotherapy. *Int J Radiat Oncol Biol Phys* 2003;57:665–672.

15. Zietman AL, Sacco D, Skowronski U, et al. Organ-conservation in bladder cancer treated by transurethral resection, chemotherapy, and radiation: results of urodynamic and quality of life study on long-term survivors. *J Urol* 2003;170:1772–1776.

16. Turner S, Swindell R, Bowl N, et al. Bladder movement during radiation therapy for bladder cancer: implications for treatment planning. *Int J Radiat Oncol Biol Phys* 1994;30:191–204.

17. Muren LP, Smaalan R, Dahl O. Organ motion set-up variation and treatment margins in radical radiotherapy of urinary bladder cancer. *Radiother Oncol* 2003;69:291–304.

18. Mameghan H, Fisher R, Mameghan J, et al. Analysis of failure following definitive radiotherapy for invasive transitional cell carcinoma of the bladder. *Int J Radiat Oncol Biol Phys* 1995;31:247–254.

19. DeNeve W, Lybeert ML, Goor C, et al. Radiotherapy for T2 and T3 carcinoma of the bladder: the influence of overall treatment time. *Radiol Oncol* 1995;36:183–188.

20. Barnes RW, Dick AL, Hadley HL, et al. Survival following transurethral resection of bladder carcinoma. *Cancer Res* 1977;37:2895–2898.

21. Sweeney P, Kursh ED, Resnick MI. Partial cystectomy. *Urol Clin North Am* 1992;2(Suppl. 2):75–87.

22. Hall RR, Robert JT, Marsh MM. Radical transurethral surgery in chemotherapy aiming at bladder preservation. In: Splinter WE, Scher HI, eds., *Neoadjuvant Chemotherapy in Invasive Bladder Cancer*. New York: Wiley Liss, 1990:169–174.

23. Tester W, Porter A, Asbell S, et al. Combined modality program with possible organ preservation for invasive bladder carcinoma: results of RTOG protocol 85-12. *Int J Radiat Oncol Biol Phys* 1993;25:783–790.

24. Dunst J, Sauer R, Schrott KM, et al. Organ-sparing treatment of advanced bladder cancer. A 10-year experience. *Int J Radiat Oncol Biol Phys* 1994;30:261–266.

25. Tester W, Porter A, Heaney J, et al. Neoadjuvant combined modality therapy with possible organ preservation for invasive bladder cancer. *J Clin Oncol* 1996;14:119–126.

26. Shipley WU, Kaufman DS, Zehr E, et al. Selective bladder preservation by combined modality protocol treatment: long-term outcomes of 190 patients with invasive bladder cancer. *Urology* 2002;60:62–68.

27. Housset M, Dufour B, Maulard C. Concomitant 5-fluorouracil-cisplatin and bifractionated split course radiation therapy for invasive bladder cancer. *Proc Am Soc Clin Oncol* 1997;16:319a.

28. Sauer R, Birkenhake S, Kuhn R, et al. Efficacy of radiochemotherapy with platin derivatives compared to radiotherapy alone in organ-sparing treatment of bladder cancer. *Int J Radiat Oncol Biol Phys* 1998;40:121–127.

29. Shipley WU, Winter KA, Kaufman DS, et al. A phase III trial of neoadjuvant chemotherapy in patients with invasive bladder cancer treated with selective bladder preservation by combined radiation therapy and chemotherapy: initial results of RTOG 89-03. *J Clin Oncol* 1998;16:3576–3583.

30. Shipley WU, Prout GR Jr, Einstein AB Jr, et al. Treatment of invasive bladder cancer by cisplatin and irradiation in patients unsuited for surgery: a high success rate in clinical stage T2 tumors in a National Bladder Cancer Group trial. *JAMA* 1987;258:931–935.

31. Tester W, Caplan R, Heaney J, et al. Neoadjuvant combined modality program with selective organ preservation for invasive bladder cancer: results of RTOG phase III trial 8802. *J Clin Oncol* 1996;14:119–126.

32. Kaufman DS, Winter KA, Shipley WU, et al. The initial results in muscle-invading bladder cancer of RTOG 95-06: phase I/II trial of transurethral surgery plus radiation therapy with concurrent cisplatin and 5-fluorouracil followed by selective bladder preservation or cystectomy depending on the initial response. *Oncologist* 2000;5:471–476.

33. Hagan MP, Winter KA, Kaufman DS, et al. RTOG 9706: initial report of a phase I/II trial of bladder conservation employing TURBT, accelerated irradiation sensitized with cisplatin followed by adjuvant MCV chemotherapy [Abstract]. *Int J Radiat Oncol Biol Phys* 2001;51:20.

34. Coppin CM, Gospodarowicz MK, James K, et al. Improved local control of invasive bladder cancer by concurrent cisplatin and preoperative or definitive radiation. *J Clin Oncol* 1996;14(11):2901–2907.

35. Shipley WU, Prout GR Jr, Kaufman SD, et al. Invasive bladder carcinoma. The importance of initial transurethral surgery and other significant prognostic factors for improved survival with full-dose irradiation. *Cancer* 1987; 60:514–520.

36. Prout GR Jr, Shipley WU, Kaufman DS, et al. Preliminary results in invasive bladder cancer with transurethral resection, neoadjuvant chemotherapy and combined pelvic irradiation plus cisplatin chemotherapy. *J Urol* 1990;144:1128–1136.

37. Rodel C, Grabenbaer GG, Kuhn R, et al. Combined modality treatment and selective organ preservation in invasive bladder cancer: long-term results. *J Clin Oncol* 2002;20:3061–3071.

38. Rodel C, Grabenbaer GG, Kuhn R, et al. Organ preservation in patients with invasive bladder cancer: initial results of an intensified protocol of transurethral surgery and radiation therapy plus concurrent cisplatin and 5-fluorouracil. *Int J Radiat Oncol Biol Phys* 2002;52(5):1303–1309.

39. Rodel C, Grabenbauer CB, Kuhn R, et al. Invasive bladder cancer: organ preservation by radiochemotherapy. *Front Radiat Ther Oncol* 2002;36: 118–130.

40. Shipley WU, Kaufman DS, Tester WJ, et al. An overview of bladder cancer trials in the Radiation Therapy Oncology Group (RTOG). *Cancer* 2003; 97(Suppl. 8):2115–2119.

41. Zietman AL, Grocela J, Zehr E, et al. Selective bladder conservation using transurethral resection, chemotherapy and radiation: the management and consequences of Ta, T1, Tis recurrence within the retained bladder. *Urol* 2001;58:380–385.

42. Wijkstrom H, Norning U, Lagerkvist M, et al. Evaluation of clinical staging before cystectomy for transitional cell bladder carcinoma, a long-term follow-up of 276 consecutive patients. *Br J Urol* 1998;81:686–691.

43. Vogelzang NJ. Editorial: neoadjuvant M-VAC: the long and winding road is getting shorter and straighter. *J Clin Oncol* 2001;19:4003.

44. Hall RR. Neoadjuvant cisplatin, methotrexate, and vinblastine chemotherapy for muscle-invasive bladder cancer: a randomized controlled trial. *Lancet* 1999;354:533–540.

45. Hall R. On behalf of the International Collaboration of Trialists of the MRC Advanced Bladder Cancer Group. Updated results of a randomised controlled trial of neoadjuvant cisplatin (C), methotrexate (M) and vinblastine (V) chemotherapy for muscle-invasive bladder cancer. *Proc Am Soc Clin Oncol* 2002; 21: (Abstr 178).

46. Sharma P, Bajorin D. Controversies in neoadjuvant and adjuvant chemotherapy for muscle-invasive urothelial cancer and clinical research initiatives in locally advanced disease. *Am Soc Clin Oncol* 2003; *Educational Book for 39th Annual Meeting* 478–487.

47. Raghavan D, Quinn D, Skinner DG, et al. Surgery and adjunctive chemotherapy for invasive bladder cancer. *Surg Oncol* 2002;11:55–59.

48. Prout GR Jr, Griffin PP, Shipley WU. Bladder carcinoma as a systemic disease. *Cancer* 1979;43:2532–2539.

49. Bellmunt J, Guillem V, Paz-Ares L, et al. Phase I-II study of paclitaxel, cisplatin and gemcitabine in advanced transitional-cell carcinoma of the urothelium. *J Clin Oncol* 2000;18(8):3247–3255.

50. Al-Sukhun S, Hussain M. Current understanding of the biology of advanced bladder cancer. *Cancer* 2003;97(Suppl):2064–2075.

51. Boyd SD, Feinberg SM, Skinner DG, et al. Quality of life survey of urinary diversion patients: comparison of ileal conduits versus continent Koch urinary reservoirs. *J Urol* 1987;138:1386–1389.

52. Mansson A, Johnson G, Mansson W. Quality of life after cystectomy: comparison between patients with conduit and those with caecal reservoir urinary diversion. *Brit J Urol* 1988;62:240–245.

53. Raleigh ED, Berry M, Monite JE. A comparison of adjustments to urinary diversions: a pilot study. *J Wound Ostomy Continence Nurs* 1995;22:58–63.

54. Bjerre BD, Johansen C, Steven K. Health related quality of life after cystectomy: bladder substitution compared with ileal conduit diversion. A questionnaire survey. *Brit J Urol* 1995;75:200–205.

55. Hart S, Skinner EC, Meyerowitz BE, et al. Quality of life after radical cystectomy for bladder cancer in patients with an ileal conduit, or cutaneous or urethral Koch pouch. *J Urol* 1999;162:77–81.

56. Chauvet JL, Lagrange L, Geoffrois, V, et al. GETUG. Quality of life assessment after concurrent chemoradiation for invasive bladder cancer: preliminary results of a French multicentric prospective study. *Int J Radiat Oncol Biol Phys* 2003;57(Suppl. 2):177; Abstract 88.

57. Caffo O, Fellin G, Graffer U, et al. Assessment of quality of life after cystectomy or conservative therapy for patients with infiltrating bladder carcinoma. *Cancer* 1996;78:1089–1097.

58. Henningsohn L, Wijkstrom H, Dickman PW, et al. Distressful symptoms after radical radiotherapy for urinary bladder cancer. *Radiother Oncol* 2002;60:215–225.

59. Dreicer R, Manola J, Roth B, et al. Phase II study of cisplatin and paclitaxel in advanced carcinoma of the urothelium: an Eastern Cooperative Oncology Group (ECOG) study. *J Clin Oncol* 2000;18:1056–1061.

60. Kaufman DS, Raghavan D, Carducci M, et al. Phase II trial of gemcitabine plus cisplatin in patients with metastatic urothelial cancer. *J Clin Oncol* 2000;18:1921–1927.

61. Von der Maase H, Hansen SW, Roberts JT, et al. Gemcitabine and cisplatin versus methotrexate, vinblastine, doxorubicin, and cisplatin in advanced or metastatic bladder cancer: results of a large, randomized, multicenter, phase III study. *J Clin Oncol* 2000;18(17):3068–3077.

62. Moore MJ, Winquist EW, Murray N, et al. Gemcitabine plus cisplatin, an active regimen in advanced urothelial cancer: a phase II trial of the National Cancer Institute of Canada Clinical Trials Group. *J Clin Oncol* 1999; 287(17):876–881.

CHAPTER 26C
Radical Cystectomy

John Peter Stein and Donald G. Skinner

INTRODUCTION

In the United States, bladder cancer is the fourth most common cancer in men and the eighth most common cancer in women, with transitional cell carcinoma (TCC) comprising nearly 90% of all primary bladder tumors. In 2002, it was estimated that 56,500 new patients were diagnosed with bladder cancer, with 12,500 projected deaths from the disease (1). Although the majority of patients present with superficial bladder tumors, 20% to 40% of patients will either present with or develop muscle-invasive disease. Invasive bladder cancer is a lethal malignancy. If left untreated, over 85% of patients die of the disease within 2 years of the diagnosis (2). Furthermore, a certain percentage of patients with high-grade bladder tumors involving the lamina propria (T1) will recur/progress and/or fail intravesical management and may be best treated with an earlier cystectomy when survival outcomes are optimal (3).

The rationale for an aggressive treatment approach employing radical cystectomy for high-grade, invasive bladder cancer is based on several important observations. First, the best long-term survival rates coupled with the lowest local recurrences are seen following radical cystectomy (4,5). Second, the morbidity and mortality of radical cystectomy has significantly improved over the past several decades. Third, TCC tends to be resistant to radiation therapy even at high doses. Fourth, chemotherapy alone or in combination with bladder sparing protocols has yet to demonstrate equivalent long-term survival rates comparable to cystectomy (6). Fifth, radical cystectomy provides accurate pathologic staging of the primary bladder tumor (p-stage) and regional lymph nodes, thus selectively determining the need for adjuvant

therapy based on precise pathologic evaluation. Last, improvements in lower urinary tract reconstruction (particularly orthotopic diversion) have improved the quality of life of patients requiring bladder removal, eliminating the need for urostomy appliances, cutaneous stomas, and the need for catheterization in most instances (7). For the aforementioned reasons, radical cystectomy has become a standard therapy for high-grade, invasive bladder cancer.

Improvements in urinary diversion have now provided appropriately selected men and women the opportunity to safely undergo orthotopic lower urinary tract reconstruction to the native intact urethra following cystectomy (7). Orthotopic reconstruction most closely resembles the original bladder in both location and function, provides a continent means to store urine, and allows volitional voiding per urethra. The orthotopic neobladder eliminates the need for a cutaneous stoma, urostomy appliance, and the need for intermittent catheterization, in most cases. These efforts have improved the quality of life of patients requiring removal of their bladder and have also stimulated patients and physicians to consider radical cystectomy at an earlier, more curable stage for high-grade, invasive bladder cancer (8).

At the University of Southern California (USC), a dedicated effort has been made to improve the technique of radical cystectomy and to provide an acceptable form of urinary diversion without compromising a sound cancer operation (9–11). Certain technical issues regarding radical cystectomy and an appropriate extended bilateral pelvic iliac lymphadenectomy are critical in order to minimize local recurrence and positive surgical margins and to maximize cancer-specific survival. Attention to surgical detail is important in optimizing the successful clinical outcomes of orthotopic diversion, maintaining the rhabdosphincter mechanism and urinary continence in these patients (11). Here we describe the detailed surgical approach and technical aspects of radical cystectomy. Although it is emphasized that the importance of a properly performed lymphadenectomy is critical to the outcomes of patients, the technique of a pelvic iliac lymphadenectomy will be described elsewhere. There appears to be a growing body of evidence to suggest that a more extended lymphadenectomy is beneficial in both lymph node positive and lymph node negative patients (12–16). We strongly recommend that the limits of the lymphadenectomy include initiation at the level of the inferior mesenteric artery (superior limits of dissection), extending laterally over the inferior vena cava to the genitofemoral nerve (lateral limits of dissection), and distally to the lymph node of Cloquet medially (on Cooper's ligament) and the circumflex iliac vein laterally. This dissection should also include bilaterally all obturator, hypogastric, and presciatic lymph nodes, as well as the presacral lymph nodes.

DEFINITION

Radical cystectomy implies the removal of the pelvic-iliac lymph nodes with the pelvic organs anterior to the rectum: the bladder, urachus, prostate, seminal vesicles, and visceral peritoneum in men, and the bladder, urachus ovaries, fallopian tubes, uterus, cervix, vaginal cuff, and the anterior pelvic peritoneum in women. The perivesical fat and pelvic and iliac lymph nodes are also removed with the specimen. The absolute extent of the lymphadenectomy is currently a matter of debate and will be covered elsewhere.

PREOPERATIVE EVALUATION

Complete clinical staging for bladder cancer should evaluate the retroperitoneum and pelvis along with the most common metastatic sites including the lungs, liver, and bone. A chest x-ray, liver function tests, and serum alkaline phosphatase should be obtained routinely. Patients with an elevated serum alkaline phosphatase or with/without complaints of bone pain should undergo a bone scan. Computed tomography (CT) scanning of the chest is obtained when pulmonary metastases are suspected by history or because of an abnormal chest x-ray. A CT scan of the abdomen and pelvis is routinely performed to evaluate the pelvis and retroperitoneum for any significant lymphadenopathy or local contiguous spread. This radiographic study should also be performed in patients with suspected metastases, elevated liver function tests, a bladder tumor associated with hydronephrosis, or in patients with an extensive primary bladder tumor that is either nonmobile or fixed, the results of which may affect the decision for neoadjuvant therapy. However, a CT scan of the primary bladder is neither sensitive nor specific enough to evaluate the degree of bladder wall tumor invasion or to accurately determine pelvic lymph node involvement with tumor (17,18).

SURGICAL TECHNIQUE OF RADICAL CYSTECTOMY

Preoperative Preparation

Patients undergoing radical cystectomy are admitted the morning prior to surgery. Patients undergo a mechanical and antibacterial bowel preparation the day prior to surgery. Intravenous hydration should be considered in these patients to prevent dehydration upon arrival to the operating room. In addition, all patients should be evaluated and counseled by the enterostomal therapy nurse prior to surgery. A clear-liquid diet may be consumed until midnight, at which time the patient takes nothing by mouth. We have employed a standard modified Nichols bowel prep (19) which is initiated the morning of admission: 120 mL of Neoloid po at 9:00 a.m., 1 gram of neomycin po at 10:00 a.m., 11:00 a.m., 12:00 p.m., 1:00 p.m., 4:00 p.m., 8:00 p.m., and 12:00 a.m., and 1 gram of erythromycin base po at 12:00 p.m., 4:00 p.m., 8:00 p.m., and 12:00 a.m. This regimen is well tolerated, obviates the need for enemas, and maintains nutritional and hydration support. Intravenous crystalloid fluid hydration is initiated in the evening prior to surgery in those patients admitted to the hospital the day prior to surgery, and maintained to ensure an adequate circulating volume as the patient enters the operating room. This may be particularly important in the elderly, frail patient with associated comorbidities.

Patients over 50 years of age should be considered for prophylactic digitalization prior to cystectomy unless a specific contraindication exists. Patients younger than 50 years of age are not routinely digitalized. Digoxin is given orally: 0.5 mg at 12:00 p.m., 0.25 mg at 4:00 p.m., and 0.125 mg at 8:00 p.m. Our experience with preoperative digitalization in patients undergoing cystectomy has been positive. There is some evidence suggesting that preoperative digitalization may decrease the risk of perioperative dysrhythmias and congestive heart failure in the elderly patient undergoing an extensive operative procedure (20,21). Attention to fluid management is important in these elderly patients, particularly on postoperative day 3 and day 4 when mobilization of third-space fluid is highest, subsequently necessitating liberal use of diuretics. In addition, intravenous broad-spectrum antibiotics are administered en route to the operating room, providing adequate tissue and circulating levels at the time of incision.

Preoperative evaluation and counseling by the enterostomal therapy nurse is a critical component to the successful care of all patients undergoing cystectomy and urinary diversion. Patients determined to be appropriate candidates for orthotopic reconstruction are instructed how to catheterize per urethra should it be necessary postoperatively. All patients are site marked for a cutaneous stoma, instructed in the care of a cutaneous diversion (continent or incontinent form), and instructed in proper catheterization techniques should medical, technical, or oncologic factors preclude orthotopic reconstruction. The ideal cutaneous stoma site is determined only after the patient is examined in the supine, sitting, and standing position. Proper stoma site selection is important to patient acceptance, and to the technical success of lower urinary tract reconstruction should a cutaneous form of diversion be necessary. Incontinent stoma sites are best located higher on the abdominal wall, while stoma sites for continent diversions can be positioned lower on the abdomen (hidden below the belt line) since they do not require an external collecting device. The use of the umbilicus as the site for catheterization may be employed with excellent functional and cosmetic results.

Patient Positioning

The patient is placed in the hyperextended supine position with the superior iliac crest located at the fulcrum of the operating table (Fig. 26C.1). The legs are slightly abducted so that the heels are positioned near the corners of the foot of the table. In the female patient considering orthotopic diversion, the modified frogleg or lithotomy position is employed allowing access to the vagina. Care should be taken to ensure that

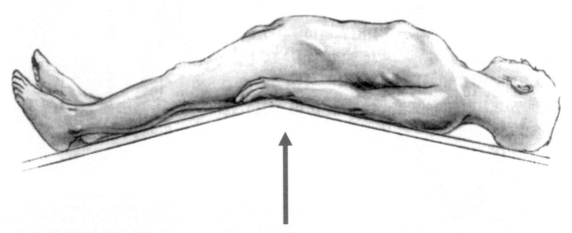

FIGURE 26C.1. Proper patient positioning for cystectomy in the male patient. Note the iliac crest is located at the break of the table.

all pressure points are well padded. Reverse Trendelenburg position levels the abdomen parallel with the floor and helps to keep the small bowel contents in the epigastrium. A nasogastric tube is placed, and the patient is prepped from nipples to midthigh. In the female patient the vagina is fully prepped. After the patient is draped, a 20 F Foley catheter is placed in the bladder and drainage is left to gravity. A right-handed surgeon stands on the patient's left-hand side of the operating table.

Incision

A vertical midline incision is made extending from the pubic symphysis to the cephalad aspect of the epigastrium. This incision allows for proper exposure when performing the extended lymphadenectomy. The incision should be carried lateral to the umbilicus on the contralateral side of the marked cutaneous stoma site. When considering the umbilicus as the site for a catheterizable stoma, the incision should be directed 2 to 3 cm lateral to the umbilicus at this location. The anterior rectus fascia is incised, the rectus muscles retracted laterally, and the posterior rectus sheath and peritoneum entered in the superior aspect of the incision. As the peritoneum and posterior fascia are incised inferiorly to the level of the umbilicus, the urachal remnant (median umbilical ligament) is identified, circumscribed, and removed en bloc with the cystectomy specimen (Fig. 26C.2). This maneuver prevents early entry into a high-riding bladder, and ensures complete removal of all bladder remnant tissue. Care is taken to remain medial and avoid injury to the inferior epigastric vessels (lateral umbilical ligaments) which course posterior to the rectus muscles. If the patient has had a previous cystotomy or segmental cystectomy, the cystotomy tract and cutaneous incision should be circumscribed full-thickness and excised en bloc with the bladder

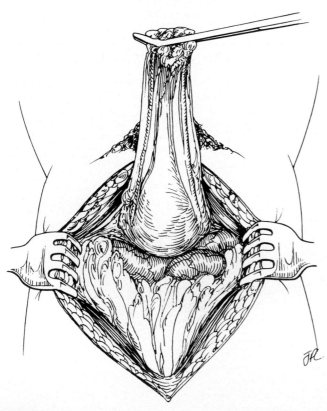

FIGURE 26C.2. Wide excision of the urachal remnant and medial umbilical ligaments en bloc with the cystectomy specimen.

specimen. The medial insertion of the rectus muscles attached to the pubic symphysis can be slightly incised if necessary for maximizing pelvic exposure throughout the operation.

Abdominal Exploration

A careful, systematic intra-abdominal exploration is performed to determine the extent of disease and to evaluate for any hepatic metastases or gross retroperitoneal lymphadenopathy. The abdominal viscera are palpated to detect any concomitant unrelated disease. If no contraindication exists at this time, all adhesions should be incised and freed.

Bowel Mobilization

The bowel is mobilized beginning with the ascending colon. A large right-angle Richardson retractor elevates the right abdominal wall. The cecum and ascending colon are reflected medially to allow incision of the lateral peritoneal reflection along the avascular/white line of Toldt. The mesentery to the small bowel is then mobilized off its retroperitoneal attachments cephalad (toward the ligament of Treitz) until the retroperitoneal portion of the duodenum is exposed. This mobilization facilitates a tension-free urethroenteric anastomosis if orthotopic diversion is performed. Combined sharp and blunt dissection facilitates mobilization of this mesentery along a characteristic avascular fibroareolar plane. Conceptually, the mobilized mesentery forms an inverted right triangle: the base formed by the third and fourth portions of the duodenum, the right edge represented by the white line of Toldt along the ascending colon, the left edge represented by the medial portion of the sigmoid and descending colonic mesentery, and the apex represented by the ileocecal region (Fig. 26C.3). This mobilization is critical in setting up the operative field and facilitates proper packing of the intra-abdominal contents into the epigastrium.

The left colon and sigmoid mesentery are then mobilized to the region of the lower pole of the left kidney by incising the peritoneum lateral to the colon along the avascular/white line of Toldt. The sigmoid mesentery is then elevated off the sacrum, iliac vessels, and distal aorta in a cephalad direction up to the origin of the inferior mesenteric artery (Fig. 26C.4).

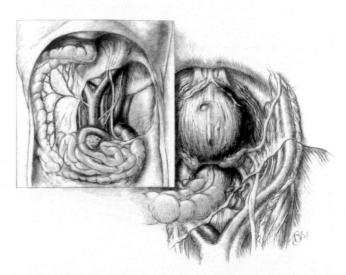

FIGURE 26C.3. View of the pelvis from overhead, after the ascending colon and peritoneal attachments of the small bowel mesentery have been mobilized up to the level of the duodenum. This mobilization allows the bowel to be properly packed in the epigastrium and exposes the area of the aortic bifurcation which is the starting point of the lymph node dissection.

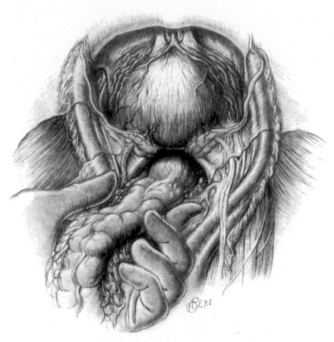

FIGURE 26C.4. View of the pelvis from overhead, after the ascending colon and small bowel have been packed in the epigastrium. Note that the sigmoid mesentery is mobilized off the sacral promontory and distal aorta up to the origin of the inferior mesenteric artery.

This maneuver provides a wide mesenteric window through which the left ureter will pass (without angulation or tension) for the ureteroenteric anastomosis at the terminal portions of the operation. This sigmoid mobilization also facilitates retraction of the sigmoid mesentery while performing the extended lymph node dissection. Care should be taken to dissect along the base of the mesentery and avoid injury to the inferior mesenteric artery and blood supply to the sigmoid colon.

Following mobilization of the bowel, a self-retaining retractor is placed. The right colon and small intestine are carefully packed into the epigastrium with three moist lap pads, followed by a moistened towel rolled to the width of the abdomen. The descending and sigmoid colon are not packed and remain as free as possible, providing the necessary mobility required for the ureteral and pelvic lymph node dissection.

Successful packing of the intestinal contents is an art and prevents their annoying spillage into the operative field. Packing begins by sweeping the right colon and small bowel under the surgeon's left hand along the right sidewall gutter. A moist open lap pad is then swept with the right hand along the palm of the left hand, under the viscera along the retroperitoneum and sidewall gutter. In similar fashion, the left sidewall gutter is packed ensuring not to incorporate the descending or sigmoid colon. The central portion of the small bowel is packed with a third lap pad. A moist rolled towel is then positioned horizontally below the lap pads, but cephalad to the bifurcation of the aorta. Occasionally, prior to placement of the first moist lap pad, a mobile greater omental apron can be used to facilitate packing of the intestinal viscera in a similar fashion to the lap pad. After the bowel has been packed, a wide Deaver retractor is placed with gentle traction on the previous packing to provide cephalad exposure.

Ureteral Dissection

The ureters are most easily identified in the retroperitoneum just cephalad to the common iliac vessels. They are carefully dissected into the deep pelvis (several centimeters beyond the iliac vessels) and divided between two large hemoclips. A section of the proximal cut ureteral segment (distal to the proximal hemoclip) is sent for frozen section analysis to ensure the absence of carcinoma *in situ* or overt tumor. The ureter is then slightly mobilized in a cephalad direction and tucked under the rolled towel to prevent inadvertent injury. Frequently, an arterial branch from the common iliac artery or the aorta needs to be divided to provide adequate ureteral mobilization. In addition, the rich vascular supply emanating laterally from the gonadal vessels should remain intact and undisturbed. These attachments are an important blood supply to the ureter and they ensure an adequate vascular supply for the ureteroenteric anastomosis at the time of diversion. This is particularly important in irradiated patients. Leaving the proximal hemoclip on the divided ureter during the exenteration allows for hydrostatic ureteral dilation, and facilitates the ureteroenteric anastomosis. In women, the infundibulopelvic ligaments are ligated and divided at the level of the common iliac vessels.

Extended Lymphadenectomy

We advocate a meticulous, extended lymph node dissection when performing a radical cystectomy. The extent of the lymphadenectomy may vary depending on the patient and surgeon preference. When performing a salvage procedure following definitive radiation treatment (greater then 5000 rads), care should be taken as the lymphadenectomy may be difficult and associated with a significant risk of iliac vessel and obturator nerve injury (22).

Ligation of the Lateral Vascular Pedicle to the Bladder

After completion of the lymphadenectomy, specifically following dissection of the obturator fossa and dividing the obturator vessels, the lateral vascular pedicle to the bladder is isolated and divided. Developing this plane isolates the lateral vascular pedicle to the bladder, a critical maneuver in performing a safe cystectomy with proper vascular control. Isolation of the lateral vascular pedicle is performed with the left hand. The bladder is retracted toward the pelvis, placing traction and isolating the anterior branches of the hypogastric artery. The left index finger is passed medial to the hypogastric artery, posterior to the anterior visceral branches, and lateral to the previously transected ureter. The index finger is directed caudally toward the endopelvic fascia, parallel to the sweep of the sacrum. This maneuver defines the two major vascular pedicles to the anterior pelvic organs: the lateral pedicle, anterior to the index finger, composed of the visceral branches of the anterior hypogastric vessel, and the posterior pedicle, posterior to the index finger, composed of the visceral branches between the bladder and rectum.

With the lateral pedicle entrapped between the left index and middle fingers, firm traction is applied vertically and caudally. This facilitates identification and allows individual branches off the anterior portion of the hypogastric artery to be isolated (Fig. 26C.5). The posterior division of the hypogastric artery including the superior gluteal, ilio-lumbar, and lateral sacral arteries is preserved to avoid gluteal claudication. Distal to this posterior division, the hypogastric artery may be ligated for vascular control, but should not be divided since the lateral pedicle is easier to dissect if left in continuity. The largest and most consistent anterior branch to the bladder, the superior vesical artery, is usually isolated and individually ligated and divided easily. The remaining anterior

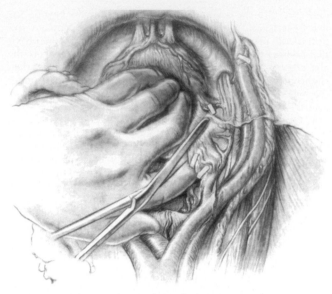

FIGURE 26C.5. Isolation of the lateral vascular pedicle. The left hand is used to define the right lateral pedicle, extending from the bladder to the hypogastric artery. This plane is developed by the index finger (medial) and the middle finger (lateral), exposing the anterior branches of the hypogastric artery. This vascular pedicle is clipped and divided down to the endopelvic fascia. Traction with the left hand defines the pedicle, allows direct visualization, and protects the rectum from injury.

branches of the lateral pedicle are then isolated and divided between hemoclips down to the endopelvic fascia, or as far as is technically possible. With blunt dissection the index finger of the left hand helps identify this lateral pedicle, and protects the rectum as it is pushed medially. Right angle hemoclip appliers are ideally suited for proper placement of the clips. Each pair of hemoclips are positioned as far apart as possible to ensure that 0.5 to 1 cm of tissue projects beyond each clip when the pedicle is divided. This prevents the hemoclips from being dislodged resulting in unnecessary bleeding. Occasionally, in patients with an abundance of pelvic fat, the lateral pedicle may be thick and require division into two manageable pedicles. The inferior vesicle vein serves as an excellent landmark as the endopelvic fascia is just distal to this structure. The endopelvic fascia just lateral to the prostate may then be incised which helps identify the distal limit of the lateral pedicle.

Ligation of the Posterior Pedicle to the Bladder

Following division of the lateral pedicles, the bladder specimen is retracted anteriorly exposing the cul-de-sac (pouch of Douglas). The surgeon elevates the bladder with a small gauze sponge under the left hand, while the assistant retracts on the peritoneum of the rectosigmoid colon in a cephalad direction. This provides excellent exposure to the recess of the cul-de-sac, and places the peritoneal reflection on traction facilitating the proper division. The peritoneum lateral to the rectum is incised and extended anteriorly and medially across the cul-de-sac to join the incision on the contralateral side (Fig. 26C.6).

An understanding of the fascial layers is critical for the appropriate dissection of this plane. The anterior and posterior peritoneal reflections converge in the cul-de-sac to form Denonvilliers' fascia, which extends caudally to the urogenital diaphragm (Fig. 26C.7, large arrow). This important anatomic boundary in the male separates the prostate and seminal vesicles anterior to the rectum posterior. The plane between the

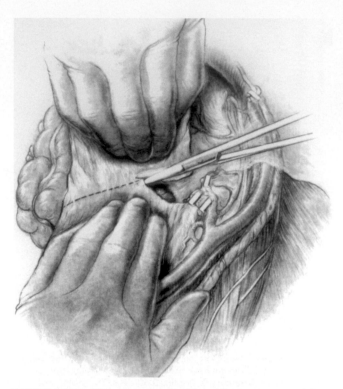

FIGURE 26C.6. The peritoneum lateral to the rectum is incised down into the cul-de-sac, and carried anteriorly over the rectum to join the opposite side. Note that the incision should be made precisely so the proper plane behind Denonvilliers' fascia can be developed safely.

prostate and seminal vesicles and the anterior sheath of Denonvilliers' will not develop easily. However, the plane between the rectum and the posterior sheath of Denonvilliers' (Denonvilliers' space) should develop easily with blunt and sharp dissection. Therefore, the peritoneal incision in the

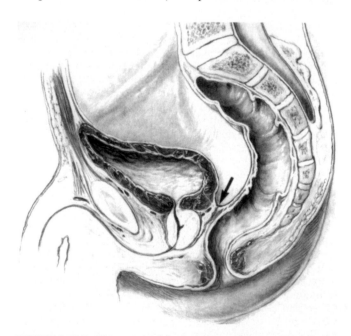

FIGURE 26C.7. Illustration of the formation of Denonvilliers' fascia. Note that it is derived from a fusion of the anterior and posterior peritoneal reflections. Denonvilliers' space lies behind the fascia. To successfully enter this space and facilitate mobilization of the anterior rectal wall off Denonvilliers' fascia, the incision in the cul-de-sac is made close to the peritoneal fusion on the anterior rectal wall side, and not on the bladder side.

performed under direct vision. To prevent a rectal injury is to avoid blunt dissection with the finger in areas where normal tissue planes have been obliterated by previous surgery or radiation. Sharp dissection under direct vision will dramatically reduce the potential for rectal injury. If a rectotomy occurs, a two-layer or three-layer closure is recommended. A diverting proximal colostomy is not routinely required unless gross contamination occurs or if the patient has received previous pelvic radiation therapy. If orthotopic diversion or vaginal reconstruction is planned, an omental interposition is recommended to prevent fistulization between suture lines.

Once the posterior pedicles have been defined, they are clipped and divided to the endopelvic fascia in the male patient. The endopelvic fascia is then incised adjacent to the prostate, medial to the levator ani muscles (if not done previously), to facilitate the apical dissection. In the female patient, the posterior pedicles including the cardinal ligaments are divided 4 to 5 cm beyond the cervix. With cephalad pressure on a previously placed vaginal sponge stick, the apex of the vagina can be identified, and incised posteriorly just distal to the cervix. The vagina is then circumscribed anteriorly with the cervix attached to the cystectomy specimen. If there is concern about an adequate surgical margin at the posterior or base of the bladder, then the anterior vaginal wall should be removed en bloc with the bladder specimen, subsequently requiring vaginal reconstruction if sexual function is desired. It is our preference to spare the anterior vaginal wall if orthotopic diversion is planned. This eliminates the need for vaginal reconstruction, which helps maintain the complex musculofascial support system and helps prevent injury to the pudendal innervation to the rhabdosphincter proximal urethra, both important components to the continence mechanism in women. The anterior vaginal wall is then sharply dissected off the posterior bladder down to the region of the bladder neck (vesicourethral junction) which is identified by palpating the Foley catheter balloon. At this point, the specimen remains attached only at the apex in men and vesicourethral junction in women.

Anterior Apical Dissection in the Male Patient

Only after the cystectomy specimen is completely free and mobile posteriorly is attention directed anteriorly to the pelvic floor and urethra. All fibroareolar connections between the anterior bladder wall, prostate, and undersurface of the pubic symphysis are divided. The endopelvic fascia is incised adjacent to the prostate and the levator muscles are carefully swept off the lateral and apical portions of the prostate. The superficial dorsal vein is identified, ligated, and divided. With tension placed posteriorly on the prostate, the puboprostatic ligaments are identified and only slightly divided just beneath the pubis, lateral to the dorsal venous complex which courses between these ligaments. Care should be made in avoiding any extensive dissection in this region along the pelvic floor. The puboprostatic ligaments need only to be incised enough to allow for a proper apical dissection of the prostate. The apex of the prostate and membranous urethra now becomes palpable.

Several methods can be performed to properly control the dorsal venous plexus. One may carefully pass an angled clamp beneath the dorsal venous complex, anterior to the urethra (Fig. 26C.9). The venous complex can then be ligated, with a 2-0 absorbable suture, and divided close to the apex of the prostate. If bleeding occurs from the transected venous complex, it can be oversewn with an absorbable (2-0 polyglycolic acid) suture. In slightly different fashion, the dorsal venous complex may be gathered at the apex of the prostate with a long Allis clamp (Fig. 26C.10). This may help to better define the plane between the dorsal venous complex and anterior urethra. A figure-of-eight 2-0 absorbable suture can then be

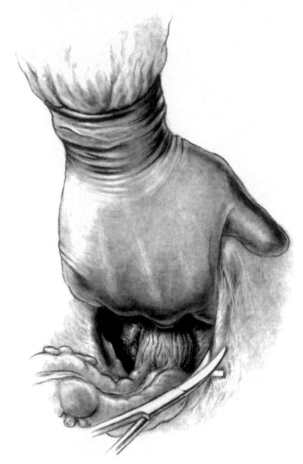

FIGURE 26C.8. After the peritoneum of the cul-de-sac has been incised, the anterior rectal wall can be swept off the posterior surface of the Denonvilliers' fascia. This effectively defines the posterior pedicle that extends from the bladder to the lateral aspect of the rectum on either side.

cul-de-sac must be made slightly on the rectal side rather than the bladder side (Fig. 26C.7, small arrow). This allows proper and safe entry and development of Denonvilliers' space between the anterior rectal wall and the posterior sheath of Denonvilliers' fascia (Fig. 26C.8). Employing a posterior sweeping motion of the fingers, the rectum can be carefully swept off the seminal vesicles, prostate, and bladder in men, and off the posterior vaginal wall in women. This sweeping motion, when extended laterally, helps to thin and develop the posterior pedicle which appears like a collar emanating from the lateral aspect of the rectum. Care should be taken as one develops this posterior plane more caudally as the anterior rectal fibers often are adherent to the specimen and can be difficult to bluntly dissect. In this region, just cephalad (proximal) to the urogenital diaphragm, sharp dissection may be required to dissect the anterior rectal fibers off the apex of the prostate in order to prevent rectal injury at this location.

Particular mention should be made concerning several situations which may impede the proper development of this posterior plane. Most commonly, when the incision in the cul-de-sac is made too far anteriorly, proper entry into Denonvilliers' space is prevented. Improper entry can occur between the two layers of Denonvilliers' fascia, or even anterior to this, making the posterior dissection difficult, increasing the risk of rectal injury. Furthermore, posterior tumor infiltration or previous high-dose pelvic irradiation can obliterate this plane making the posterior dissection difficult. To prevent injury to the rectum in these situations, only sharp dissection should be

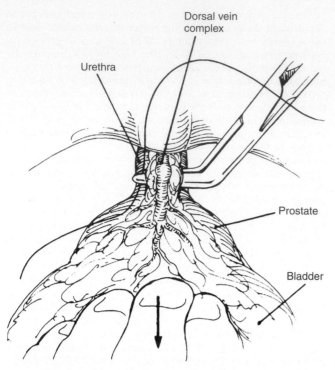

FIGURE 26C.9. Control of the dorsal venous complex. A right-angled clamp can be passed posterior to the venous complex and anterior to the urethra. An absorbable suture can be passed to ligate the complex distal to the apex of the prostate.

placed under direct vision anterior to the urethra (distal to the apex of the prostate) around the gathered venous complex (Fig. 26C.11). This suture is best placed with the surgeon facing the head of the table and holding the needle driver perpendicular to the patient. The suture is then tagged with a hemostat. This maneuver also avoids the unnecessary passage of any instruments between the dorsal venous complex and rhabdosphincter, which could potentially injure these structures

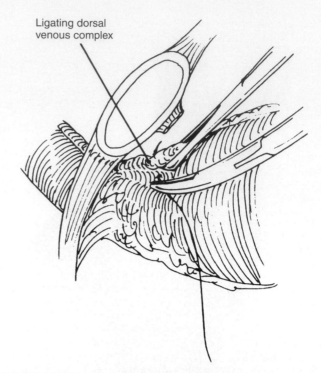

FIGURE 26C.11. An absorbable suture is carefully passed in a figure-of-eight fashion anterior to the urethra around the gathered dorsal venous complex to control the vascular structure.

and compromise the continence mechanism. After the complex has been ligated, it can be sharply divided with excellent exposure to the anterior surface of the urethra. Once the venous complex has been severed, the suture can be used to further secure the complex. The suture is then used to suspend the venous complex anteriorly to the periosteum to help reestablish anterior fixation of the dorsal venous complex and puboprostatic ligaments (Fig. 26C.12). This may enhance continence recovery. The anterior urethra is now exposed.

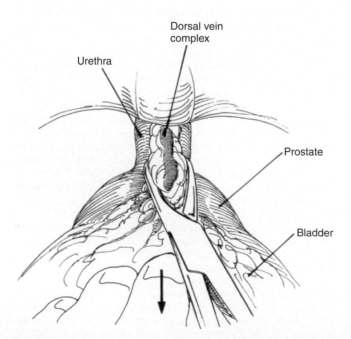

FIGURE 26C.10. The dorsal venous complex is gathered with an Allis clamp distal to the apex of the prostate. This maneuver will define the plane between the dorsal venous complex and urethra.

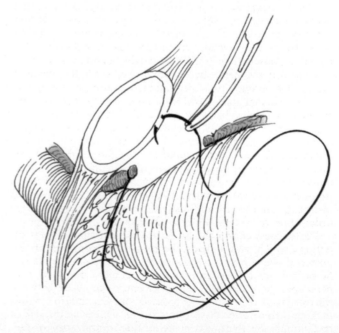

FIGURE 26C.12. The dorsal venous complex is completely divided. The previously placed suture is then used to further secure the venous complex. The complex is then fixed anteriorly to the periosteum.

Regardless of the aforementioned technique to control the dorsal venous complex, the urethra is then incised 270 degrees just beyond the apex of the prostate. A series of 2-0 polyglycolic acid sutures are placed in the anterior urethra, carefully incorporating only the mucosa and submucosa of the striated urethral sphincter muscle anteriorly, the urethra incorporating the rectourethralis muscle or the caudal extent of Denonvilliers' fascia posteriorly. Following this, the posterior urethra is divided and the specimen removed.

Alternatively, the dorsal venous complex can be sharply transected without securing vascular control of the dorsal venous complex. Cephalad traction on the prostate elongates the proximal and membranous urethra, and allows the urethra to be skeletonized laterally by dividing the so-called "lateral pillars," extensions of the rhabdosphincter. The anterior two-thirds of the urethra is divided, exposing the urethral catheter. The urethral sutures are then placed. Six 2-0 polyglycolic acid sutures are placed equally spaced into the urethral mucosa and lumen anteriorly. The rhabdosphincter, the edge of which acts as a hood overlying the dorsal venous complex, is included in these sutures if the dorsal venous complex was sharply incised. This maneuver compresses the dorsal vein complex against the urethra for hemostatic purposes. The urethral catheter is then drawn through the urethrotomy, clamped on the bladder side, and divided. Cephalad traction on the bladder side with the clamped catheter occludes the bladder neck, prevents tumor spill from the bladder, and provides exposure to the posterior urethra. Two additional sutures are placed in the posterior urethra, again incorporating the rectourethralis muscle or distal Denonvilliers' fascia. The posterior urethra is then divided and the specimen removed. Bleeding from the dorsal vein is usually minimal at this point. If additional hemostasis is required, one or two anterior urethral sutures can be tied to stop the bleeding. Regardless of the technique, frozen section analysis of the distal urethral margin of the cystectomy specimen is then performed to exclude tumor involvement.

If a cutaneous form of urinary diversion is planned, urethral preparation is slightly modified. Once the dorsal venous complex is secured and divided, the anterior urethra is identified. The urethra is mobilized from above as far distally as possible into the pelvic diaphragm. With cephalad traction, the urethra is stretched above the urogenital diaphragm, and a curved clamp is placed as distal on the urethra as feasible and divided distal to the clamp. Care must be taken to avoid rectal injury with this clamp. This is prevented by placing gentle posterior traction with the left hand or index finger on the rectum and ensuring the clamp is passed anteriorly. The specimen is then removed. Mobilization of the urethra as distally as possible facilitates a late urethrectomy should it be necessary. The levator musculature can then be reapproximated along the pelvic floor to facilitate hemostasis.

Anterior Dissection in the Female

The wide female pelvis allows for better anterior exposure in a woman, particularly at the vesicourethral junction. However, urologists may be less familiar with pelvic surgery in women than in men. In addition, paravaginal vascular control may be troublesome in women, and the venous plexus anterior to the urethra is less well defined in women. When considering orthotopic diversion in female patients undergoing cystectomy, several technical issues are critical to the procedure in order to maintain the continence mechanism in these women.

When developing the posterior pedicles in women, the posterior vagina is incised at the apex just distal to the cervix (Fig. 26C.13). This incision is carried anteriorly along the lateral and anterior vaginal wall forming a circumferential incision. The anterior-lateral vaginal wall is then grasped with

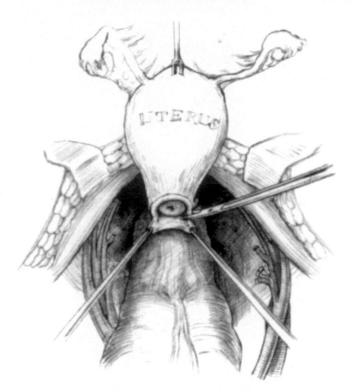

FIGURE 26C.13. In women, the vagina is incised distal to the cervix. Note that cephalad traction on the posterior aspect of the vagina facilitates the incision of the anterior vaginal wall. Slight dissection of the posterior vaginal wall off the rectum provides mobility to the vaginal cuff.

curved Kocher clamps. This provides counter-traction and facilitates dissection between the anterior vaginal wall and the bladder specimen. Careful dissection of the proper plane will prevent entry into the posterior bladder and also reduce the amount of bleeding in this vascular area (Fig. 26C.14). Development of this posterior plane and vascular pedicle is best

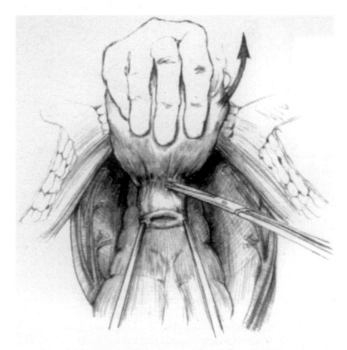

FIGURE 26C.14. Dissection of the anterior vaginal wall off of the bladder. Note caudal traction of the cystectomy specimen with counter-traction applied to the vagina in a cephalad direction.

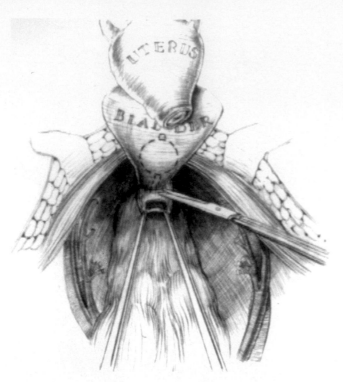

FIGURE 26C.15. Dissection continues only slightly distal to the vesicourethral junction. This can be identified by palpation of the Foley balloon in the bladder.

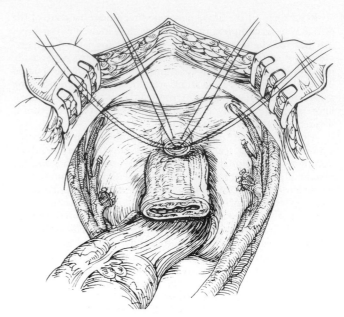

FIGURE 26C.16. View of the female pelvis from above with open vaginal cuff and urethral suture placement.

performed sharply and carried just distal to the vesicourethral junction (Fig. 26C.15). Palpation of the Foley catheter balloon assists in identifying this region. This dissection effectively maintains a functional vagina.

In the case of a deeply invasive posterior bladder tumor in a woman, with concern of an adequate surgical margin, the anterior vaginal wall should be removed en bloc with the cystectomy specimen. After dividing the posterior vaginal apex, the lateral vaginal wall subsequently serves as the posterior pedicle and is divided distally. This leaves the anterior vaginal wall attached to the posterior bladder specimen. The Foley catheter balloon again facilitates identification of the vesicourethral junction. The surgical plane between the vesicourethral junction and the anterior vaginal wall is then developed distally at this location. A 1-cm length of proximal urethra is mobilized while the remaining distal urethra is left intact with the anterior vaginal wall. Vaginal reconstruction by a clam shell (horizontal) or side-to-side (vertical) technique is required. Other means of vaginal reconstruction may include a rectus myocutaneous flap, detubularized cylinder of ileum, a peritoneal flap, or an omental flap.

It is emphasized that no dissection be performed anterior to the urethra along the pelvic floor. The endopelvic fascia should remain undisturbed and not opened in women considering orthotopic diversion. This prevents injury to the rhabdosphincter region and corresponding innervation which is critical in maintaining the continence mechanism. Anatomic studies have demonstrated that the innervation to this rhabdosphincter region in women arises from branches off the pudendal nerve that course along the pelvic floor posterior to the levator muscles (23,24). Any dissection performed anteriorly may injure these nerves and compromise the continence status.

When the posterior dissection is completed (being certain to dissect just distal to the vesicourethral junction), a Statinski vascular clamp is placed across the bladder neck. The Statinski vascular clamp placed across the catheter at the bladder neck prevents any tumor spill from the bladder. With gentle

traction the proximal urethra is completely divided anteriorly, distal to the bladder neck and clamp. The female urethra is situated more anteriorly then in men, and the urethral sutures can be placed easily after the specimen is completely removed (Fig. 26C.16). A total of 10 to 12 sutures are placed. Frozen section analysis is performed on the distal urethral margin of the cystectomy specimen to exclude tumor. Once hemostasis is obtained the vaginal cuff may be closed in two layers with absorbable sutures. The vaginal cuff is then anchored via a colposacralpexy using a strut of Marlex mesh to the sacral promontory. This fixates the vagina without angulation or undue tension. Note that, at the terminal portions of the operation, a well-vascularized omental pedicle graft is placed between the reconstructed vagina and neobladder and secured to the levator ani muscles to separate the suture lines and prevent fistulization (Fig. 26C.17).

If a cutaneous diversion is planned in the female patient, the posterior pedicles are developed as previously mentioned. Attention is then directed anteriorly and the pubourethral ligaments are divided. A curved clamp is placed across the urethra and the anterior vaginal wall is opened distally and incised circumferentially around the urethral meatus. The vaginal cuff is closed as previously described and suspended. Alternatively, a perineal approach may be used for this dissection with complete removal of the entire urethra.

Following removal of the cystectomy specimen, the pelvis is irrigated with warm sterile water. The presacral nodal tissue previously swept off the common iliac vessels and sacral promontory into the deep pelvis is collected and sent separately for pathologic evaluation. Nodal tissue in the presciatic notch, anterior to the sciatic nerve, is also sent for histologic analysis. Hemostasis is obtained and the pelvis is packed with a lap pad while attention is directed to the urinary diversion.

The use of various tubes and drains postoperatively are important. The pelvis is drained for urine or lymph leak with a 1-inch Penrose drain for 3 weeks and a large suction Hemovac drain for the evacuation of blood for 24 hours. A gastrostomy tube with an 18 French Foley catheter is routinely placed utilizing a modified Stamm technique which incorporates a small portion of omentum (near the greater curvature of the stomach) interposed between the stomach and the abdominal wall (25). This provides a simple means to drain the stomach, and

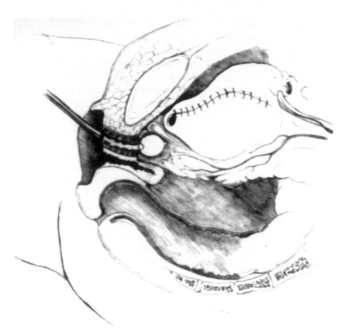

FIGURE 26C.17. Sagittal section of the female pelvis. Note that a vascularized omental pedicle graft is situated between the reconstructed vagina/vaginal cuff and the neobladder. The graft is secured to the pelvic floor to prevent fistulization.

prevents the need for an uncomfortable nasogastric tube while the postoperative ileus resolves.

POSTOPERATIVE CARE

A detailed, team-oriented approach to the care of these generally elderly patients undergoing radical cystectomy helps reduce perioperative morbidity and mortality. Patients are best monitored in the surgical intensive care unit (ICU) for at least 24 hours or until stable. Careful attention to fluid management is imperative as third-space fluid loss in these patients can be tremendous and deceiving. Patients with compromised cardiac or pulmonary function may require invasive cardiac monitoring with a pulmonary artery catheter placed prior to surgery to precisely ascertain the cardiac response to fluid shifts. A combination of crystalloid and colloid fluid replacement is given on the night of surgery and converted to crystalloid on postoperative

day 1. Prophylaxis against stress ulcer is initiated with an H_2 blocker. Intravenous broad-spectrum antibiotics are continued in all patients and subsequently converted to oral antibiotics as the diet progresses. Pulmonary toilet is encouraged with incentive spirometry, deep breathing, and coughing.

Prophylaxis against deep vein thrombosis is important in these patients undergoing extensive pelvic operations for malignancies. The anticoagulation is initiated in the recovery room with 10 mg of sodium warfarin via a nasogastric or the gastrostomy tube. The daily dose is adjusted to maintain a prothrombin time in the range of 18 to 22 seconds. If the prothrombin time exceeds 22 seconds, 2.5 mg of vitamin K is administered intramuscularly to prevent bleeding. No systemic anticoagulation is used. Pain control by a patient-controlled analgesic system provides comfort and enhances deep breathing and early ambulation. If digoxin was given preoperatively, it is continued until discharge. The gastrostomy tube is generally removed on postoperative day 7, or later if bowel function is delayed. Some patients may develop a prolonged ileus or develop some other complication which delays the return bowel function and oral intake, in which case the tube gastrostomy remains and avoids the need for nasogastric tube decompression. The catheter and drain management is specific to the form of urinary diversion.

DISCUSSION

Understanding that invasive bladder cancer is a lethal disease, we have adopted an early and aggressive surgical approach for these patients (3,4). This includes a meticulous, radical cystectomy with an extended bilateral pelvic iliac lymph node dissection. We believe radical cystectomy provides the best local pelvic control of the disease. In addition, radical cystectomy provides accurate evaluation of the primary bladder tumor (p-stage), along with the regional lymph nodes. This pathologic evaluation allows the application of adjuvant treatment strategies based on clear histopathologic determination and not clinical staging, which has been associated with significant errors in 30% to 50% of patients (3,17,18,26,27). This, coupled with the evolution of orthotopic lower urinary tract reconstruction, has provided patients a more acceptable means to store and eliminate urine (7).

Generally, most invasive TCCs are high-grade tumors. Bladder tumors originate in the bladder mucosa and progressively invade the lamina propria and sequentially into the muscularis propria, perivesical fat, and contiguous pelvic structures, with an increasing incidence of lymph node involvement with disease progression (Table 26C.1) (4,16,28,29). Radical cystectomy

TABLE 26C.1

INCIDENCE OF LYMPH NODE METASTASIS FOLLOWING RADICAL CYSTECTOMY IN CONTEMPORARY SERIES: CORRELATION TO PRIMARY BLADDER TUMOR

Series (ref., first author)	Period	Total no. of patients	No (%) LN metastasis	Bladder tumor stage[a] no. (%)				
				P0, Pis, Pa, P1	P2a	P2b	P3	P4
Poulsen (16)	1990–1997	191	50 (26%)	2 (3%)	4 (18%)	7 (25%)	33 (51%)	4 (44%)
Vieweg[b] (28)	1980–1990	686	193 (28%)	10 (10%)	12 (9%)	22 (23%)	97 (43%)	52 (41%)
Leissner[c] (29)	1999–2002	290	81 (28%)	1 (2%)	5 (13%)	12 (22%)	53 (44%)	10 (50%)
Stein (4)	1971–1997	1054	246 (24%)	19 (5%)	21 (18%)	35 (27%)	113 (45z%)	58 (43%)
Totals		2221	570 (25%)					

[a]TNM Staging System 1997 AJCC.
[b]Six patients with Cis of prostatic ducts with LN positive disease classified as Pis.
[c]Multicenter trial.

with an appropriate lymphadenectomy effectively removes the primary bladder tumor and the regional lymph nodes that may contain metastases in up to 25% of patients undergoing the procedure. In the USC series of 1,054 patients undergoing radical cystectomy for TCC, the incidence of lymph node metastases correlated with the primary bladder tumor stage (Table 26C.1) (4). Patients with nonmuscle-invasive tumors demonstrated a 5% incidence of node-positive disease, compared to 18% with superficial muscle-invasive bladder tumors (P2), 27% with deep muscle-invasive bladder tumors (P3a), and approximately 45% of patients with extravesical tumor extension of the primary bladder tumor (P3b and P4).

The early results and outcomes of radical cystectomy were disappointing. Lack of universal acceptance of this procedure was attributed to the considerable morbidity and the need for improvements in urinary diversion. Prior to 1970, the perioperative complication rate of radical cystectomy was approximately 35%, with a mortality rate of nearly 20%. With contemporary medical, surgical, and anesthetic techniques, the mortality and morbidity from radical cystectomy have dramatically decreased. A 3% mortality rate in the USC series (Table 26C.2) (4) is comparable to other contemporary series of radical cystectomy (5,16,26–29). We have found that the administration of preoperative therapy (radiation and/or chemotherapy), and the form of urinary diversion performed (continent or incontinent), does not significantly alter the mortality rate of radical cystectomy (4). Neoadjuvant radiation therapy has not routinely been employed and may be considered only in those patients who had a previous partial cystectomy or extravesical tumor spill at the time of endoscopic treatment of the primary bladder tumor (30).

The early complication rate following radical cystectomy should not be underestimated in this elderly group of patients often with associated comorbidities. In the USC series, 28% of patients developed an early complication within the first 3 months of surgery (Table 26C.2). These early complications included all those related to the cystectomy, perioperative care, and urinary diversion. The administration of preoperative therapy (radiation and/or chemotherapy), and the form of urinary diversion performed, did not apparently alter the early complication rate in these patients. It is emphasized that most early complications following cystectomy can be appropriately managed nonoperatively, without further sequelae. Strict attention to perioperative details, along with a dedicated and meticulous surgical approach, is critical to minimize the morbidity and mortality and to ensure the best clinical outcomes following radical cystectomy.

The pathologic stage of the primary bladder tumor and the presence of lymph node metastases are perhaps the most important survival determinant in patients undergoing cystectomy for bladder cancer (Table 26C.3) (4). These pathologic determinants can be categorized into certain pathologic subgroups that provide risk stratification. Pathologic evaluation and subgroup stratification may also direct the need for adjuvant therapy. In the USC series, 56% of patients demonstrated pathologically organ-confined, lymph node negative bladder tumors (4). The survival results in this subgroup of patients were excellent (Table 26C.3, Fig. 26C.18). The recurrence-free survival in this pathologic subgroup of organ-confined, lymph node negative bladder tumors was 85% at 5 years and 82% at 10 years. Importantly, we found that no significant survival difference was observed when comparing superficially noninvasive (Pis, Pa), lamina propria invasive (P1), and muscle invasive (P2, P3a) tumors, as long as the tumor was confined to the bladder and there was no evidence of lymph node tumor involvement. Similar outcomes for patients with pathologic superficial bladder tumors following cystectomy have been previously reported (5,27). These data support the notion that the ideal outcome for patients with high-grade, invasive bladder cancer is when the primary bladder tumor is confined to the bladder, without evidence of extravesical extension or lymph node metastases. Therefore, significant delays in patients with muscle-invasive bladder cancer should be avoided. There is evidence to suggest prolonged delays may lead to more advanced stages and decreased survival in patients with muscle-invasive bladder cancer (31). Furthermore, care should be taken in delaying a more definitive therapy in patients with superficial tumors that do not appropriately respond to conservative forms of therapy (3).

Non-organ-confined (extravesical), lymph node negative tumors were found in approximately 20% of our patients undergoing cystectomy in series (Table 26C.3, Fig. 26C.18) (4). In this pathologic subgroup, no obvious survival differences between extravesical P3b and P4 tumors were observed. The recurrence-free survival in the pathologic subgroup of extravesical, non-organ-confined, lymph node negative tumors was 58% at 5 years and 55% at 10 years. It is clear that patients with locally advanced disease have higher recurrence rates and

TABLE 26C.2

PERIOPERATIVE MORTALITY AND EARLY COMPLICATION RATE FOLLOWING CYSTECTOMY AT USC

Form of urinary diversion		Number of patients	Perioperative mortality[a]	Early complication[b]
	Conduit[c]	278 (26%)	8 (3%)	83 (30%)
	Continent[d]	776 (74%)	19 (2%)	209 (27%)
Preoperative Adjuvant Therapy	None	884 (84%)	26 (3%)	247 (28%)
	Radiation Only	108 (10%)	1 (1%)	30 (30%)
	Chemotherapy Only	49 (5%)	0	12 (25%)
	Radiation and Chemotherapy	13 (1%)	0	3 (23%)
Totals		1,054	27 (3%)	292 (28%)

[a]Any death within 30 days of surgery or prior to discharge.
[b]Any complications within the first 3 months postoperative.
[c]Including ileal and colon conduits.
[d]Including continent cutaneous, orthotopic, and rectal reservoirs.
From Stein JP, Lieskovsky G, Cote R, et al. Radical cystectomy in the treatment of invasive bladder cancer: long-term results in 1054 patients. *J Clin Oncol* 2001;19:666–675, with permission.

TABLE 26C.3

THE PATHOLOGICAL STAGE AND SURVIVAL OF 1,054 PATIENTS UNDERGOING RADICAL CYSTECTOMY FOR BLADDER CANCER

Variable		No. of patients	Recurrence-free 5 yr	Survival (%) 10 yr	Overall survival (%) 5 yr	10 yr
Pathologic stage	P0	66 (6%)	92	86	84	67
	Pls	100 (9%)	91	89	89	72
	Pa	42 (4%)	79	74	80	56
	P1	194 (19%)	83	78	76	52
	P2	94 (9%)	89	87	77	57
	P3a	98 (9%)	78	76	64	44
	P3b	135 (13%)	62	61	49	29
	P4	79 (7%)	50	45	44	23
Lymph node−	all patients	308 (76%)	78	75	69	49
Lymph node+	all patients	246 (24%)	35	34	31	23
	1-4 nodes	160	41	40	39	32
	≥5 nodes	86	24	24	17	8
	organ confined (p-stage)	75	46	44	47	37
	estravesical (p-stage)	171	30	30	24	19
Pathologic subgroups	organ confined[a]	594 (56%)	85	82	78	56
	extravesical[b]	214 (20%)	58	55	47	27
Entire group		1054	68	66	60	43

[a]Including P0, Pls, Pa, P1, P2, P3a (lymph node negative).
[b]Including P3b, P4 (lymph node negative).
From Stein JP, Lieskovsky G, Cote R, et al. Radical cystectomy in the treatment of invasive bladder cancer: long-term results in 1054 patients. *J Clin Oncol* 2001;19:666–675, with permission.

decreased survival compared to the subgroup of patients with organ-confined, lymph node negative tumors (32). In view of this, one should consider adjuvant treatment strategies for this pathologic subgroup of patients.

Despite an aggressive treatment philosophy and approach to bladder cancer, 24% of our patients demonstrated lymph node positive disease at the time of cystectomy (Table 26C.3, Fig. 26C.18) (4). This underscores the virulent and metastatic capabilities of high-grade, invasive bladder cancer. Although

patients with lymph node tumor involvement are a high-risk group of patients, nearly one-third of these patients were alive at 5 years and 23% alive at 10 years. It is possible that the surgical approach (which includes an extended pelvic iliac lymph node dissection) may provide some advantage with long-term survival in selected individuals with node positive disease. The impact of adjuvant therapy in this group of patients, although difficult to assess and subject to selection bias, may also play a role in the outcomes of patients with lymph

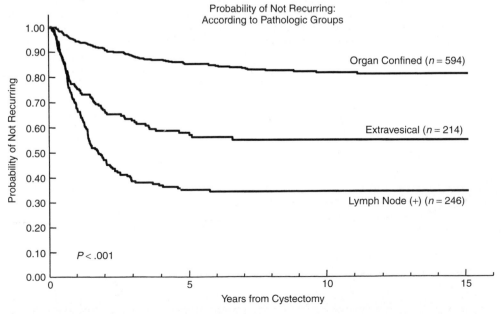

FIGURE 26C.18. Recurrence-free survival in 1,054 patients following radical cystectomy stratified by pathologic subgroups (organ-confined, extravesical, and lymph node positive).

node positive disease (4). In fact, in a separate analysis of lymph node positive patients, we found that the administration of adjuvant chemotherapy was a significant and independent predictor for recurrence and overall survival in these patients with lymph node positive disease (13).

The prognosis in patients with lymph node positive disease can be stratified by the number of lymph nodes involved (tumor burden), and by the p-stage of the primary bladder tumor (Table 26C.3) (4). In our cystectomy series, patients with less than five positive lymph nodes had improved survival rates compared to patients with five or more lymph nodes involved. A significant difference was also observed when stratifying patients by their primary bladder stage. Patients with lymph node positive disease and organ-confined bladder tumors had a significant, improved recurrence-free survival compared to those with non-organ-confined, lymph node positive tumors. Similar results with lymph node positive disease following cystectomy have been previously reported (5,32).

It is clear that the number of lymph nodes involved with tumor, as well as the extent of the lymph node dissection, are both important variables for patients undergoing cystectomy for bladder cancer. We have recently reexamined our 246 patients with lymph node tumor involvement following radical cystectomy (13) to evaluate other prognostic factors in this high-risk group of patients. This reevaluation has led to the concept of *lymph node density,* an important prognostic factor which may better stratify lymph node positive patients following radical cystectomy. Lymph node density (defined as the total number of positive lymph nodes divided by the total number of lymph nodes removed) accounts for the extent of the lymph node dissection (number of lymph nodes removed) and the tumor burden (number of positive lymph nodes) following radical cystectomy for patients with lymph node positive disease. Therefore, lymph node density incorporates these concepts simultaneously.

If lymph node tumor burden and the extent of the lymphadenectomy are important variables in patients with lymph node positive disease, it would only be logical that lymph node density should also be important. In fact, we found that lymph node density was a significant and independent prognostic variable in patients with lymph node metastases and that it may best stratify this high-risk group of patients (Fig. 26C.19) (13). It is possible that future staging systems and the application of adjuvant therapies in clinical trials should consider applying these concepts to help better stratify these high-risk groups of patients following radical cystectomy. Regardless, patients with any lymph node involvement remain at high risk for disease recurrence and should be considered for adjuvant treatment strategies.

Radical cystectomy provides the best local (pelvic) control of the disease. An overall local pelvic recurrence rate of 7% was observed in the USC cystectomy series (4). Patients with organ-confined, lymph node negative tumors demonstrated only a 6% local recurrence rate, compared to a 13% local recurrence rate in those with non-organ-confined, lymph node negative tumors. Even those at highest risk of a local recurrence (lymph node positive disease) had only a 13% local recurrence rate following cystectomy. The use of high-dose, short-course preoperative radiation therapy does not reduce the risk of pelvic recurrence (30). Nearly all patients suffering a pelvic recurrence following cystectomy will die of their disease despite additional therapeutic efforts.

Clinical staging errors in patients with invasive bladder cancer have been reported to occur in 30% to 50% of patients (3,17,18,26,27). Unlike other therapies, radical cystectomy pathologically stages the primary bladder tumor and regional lymph nodes. This histologic evaluation provides important prognostic information and may help identify high-risk patients who may benefit from adjuvant therapy. Our data suggest that patients with extravesical tumor extension or with lymph node positive disease appear to be at increased risk for recurrence and may be considered for adjuvant treatment strategies. Additionally, the recent application of molecular markers based on pathologic staging and analysis may also serve to identify patients at risk for tumor recurrence who may benefit from adjuvant forms of therapy (33).

The clinical results and outcomes following radical cystectomy demonstrate good survival, with excellent local recurrence rates for high-grade, invasive bladder cancer. These results provide sound data, and a standard to which other forms of therapy for invasive bladder cancer can be compared. Furthermore, improvements in orthotopic urinary diversion have improved the quality of life in patients following cystectomy. Continence rates following orthotopic diversion are good and provide patients a more natural voiding pattern per urethra. Contraindications to orthotopic urinary diversion include the presence of tumor within the urethra or extending to the urethral margin as determined by frozen section analysis of the distal surgical margin at the time of cystectomy, compromised renal function (creatinine greater than 2.5 ng/mL), or the presence of inflammatory bowel disease. Even in patients with locally advanced disease, orthotopic diversion can be employed without concern over subsequent tumor related reservoir complications.

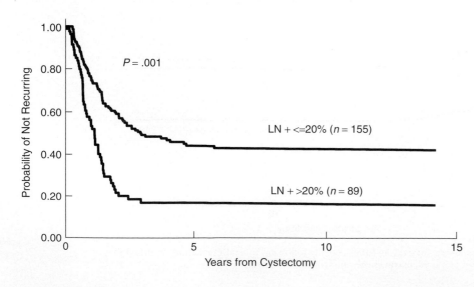

FIGURE 26C.19. Recurrence-free survival in 244 patients with lymph node positive disease following radical cystectomy stratified by lymph node density (20% or less versus greater than 20%).

The question whether patients have a better quality of life following cystectomy or following bladder-sparing protocols, which require significant and prolonged treatment to the bladder with the potential for tumor recurrence, has not been elucidated. Currently, orthotopic diversion should be considered the diversion of choice in all cystectomy patients, and the urologist should have a specific reason why an orthotopic diversion is *not* performed. Patient factors such as frail general health, motivation, or comorbidity and the cancer factor of a positive urethral margin may disqualify some patients. Nevertheless, the option of lower urinary tract reconstruction to the intact urethra has been shown to decrease physician reluctance and increase patient acceptance to undergo earlier cystectomy when the disease may be at a more curable stage (8).

In conclusion, a properly performed radical cystectomy with an appropriate lymphadenectomy provides the best survival rates with the lowest reported local recurrence rates for high-grade invasive bladder cancer. The surgical technique is critical to optimize the best clinical and technical outcomes in patients with this procedure. Advances in lower urinary tract reconstruction provide a reasonable alternative for patients undergoing cystectomy and have improved the quality of life of these patients requiring removal of their bladder.

References

1. Jemal A, Thomas A, Murray T, et al. Cancer statistics 2002. *CA Cancer J Clin* 2002;52:23–47.
2. Prout G, Marshall VF. The prognosis with untreated bladder tumors. *Cancer* 1956;9:551–558.
3. Stein JP. Indications for early cystectomy. *Urology* 2003;62:591–595.
4. Stein JP, Lieskovsky G, Cote R, et al. Radical cystectomy in the treatment of invasive bladder cancer: long-term results in 1054 patients. *J Clin Oncol* 2001;19:666–675.
5. Ghoneim MA, El-Mekresh MM, El-Baz MA, et al. Radical cystectomy for carcinoma of the bladder: critical evaluation of the results in 1,026 cases. *J Urol* 1997;158:393–399.
6. Montie JE. Against bladder sparing surgery. *J Urol* 1999;162:452–455.
7. Stein JP, Skinner DG. Orthotopic bladder replacement. In: Walsh PC, Retik AB, Vaughan ED et al., eds. *Campbell's urology*, 8th ed. Philadelphia, PA: WB Saunders, 2002:3835–3864.
8. Hautmann RE, Paiss T. Does the option of the ileal neobladder stimulate patient and physician decision toward earlier cystectomy? *J Urol* 1998;159:1845–1850.
9. Stein JP, Skinner DG. Radical cystectomy in the female. In: *Atlas of the urologic clinics of North America*: Philadelphia, PA: WB Saunders, 1997:5(2)37–64.
10. Stein JP, Skinner DG, Montie JE. Radical cystectomy and pelvic lymphadenectomy in the treatment of infiltrative bladder cancer. Droller MJ, ed. *Bladder cancer: current diagnosis and treatment*. Towanta, NJ: Humana Press, 2001:267–307.
11. Stein JP, Quek MD, Skinner DG. Contemporary surgical techniques for continent urinary diversion: continence and potency preservation. In: *Atlas of the urologic clinics of North America*: Philadelphia, PA: WB Saunders, 2001:147–173.
12. Stein JP. The role of lymphadenectomy in bladder cancer. *Am J Urol Rev* 2003;1:146–148.
13. Stein JP, Cai J, Groshen S, et al. Risk factors for patients with pelvic lymph node metastases following radical cystectomy with en bloc cystectomy: the concept of lymph node density. *J Urol* 2003;170:35–41.
14. Herr HW, Bochner BH, Dalbagni G, et al. Impact of the number of lymph nodes retrieved on outcome in patients with muscle invasive bladder cancer. *J Urol* 2002;167:1295–1298.
15. Leissner J, Hohenfellner R, Thuroff JW, et al. Lymphadenectomy in patients with transitional cell carcinoma of the urinary bladder; significance for staging and prognosis. *Brit J Urol Int* 2000;85:817–823.
16. Poulsen AL, Horn T, Steven K. Radical cystectomy: extending limits of pelvic lymph node dissection improves survival for patients with bladder cancer confined to the bladder wall. *J Urol* 1998;160:2015–2019.
17. Voges GE, Tauschke E, Stockle M, et al. Computerized tomography: an unreliable method for accurate staging of bladder tumors in patients who are candidates for radical cystectomy. *J Urol* 1989;142:972–974.
18. Pagano F, Bassi P, Galetti TP, et al. Results of contemporary radical cystectomy for invasive bladder cancer: a clinicopathological study with an emphasis on the inadequacy of the tumor, nodes and metastases classification. *J Urol* 1991;145:45–50.
19. Nichols RL, Broido P, Condon RE, et al. Effect of preoperative neomycin-erythromycin intestinal preparation on the incidence of infectious complications after colon surgery. *Ann Surg* 1973;178:453–462.
20. Pinaud MLJ, Blanloeil YAG, Souron RJ. Preoperative prophylactic digitalization of patients with coronary artery disease—a randomized echocardiographic and hemodynamic study. *Anesth Analg* 1983;62:685–689.
21. Burman SO. The prophylactic use of digitalis before thorocotomy. *Ann Thorac Surg* 1972;14:359–368.
22. Crawford ED, Skinner DG. Salvage cystectomy after radiation failure. *J Urol* 1980;123:32–34.
23. Colleselli K, Stenzl A, Eder R, et al. The female urethral sphincter: a morphological and topographical study. *J Urol* 1998;160:49–50.
24. Grossfeld GD, Stein JP, Bennett CJ, et al. Lower urinary tract reconstruction in the female using the Koch ileal reservoir with bilateral ureteroileal urethrostomy: update of continence results and flurourodynamic findings. *Urology* 1996;48:383–388.
25. Buscarini M, Stein JP, Lawrence MA, et al. Tube gastrostomy following radical cystectomy and urinary diversion: surgical technique and experience in 709 patients. *Urology* 2000;56:150–152.
26. Frazier HA, Robertson JE, Dodge RK, et al. The value of pathologic factors in predicting cancer-specific survival among patients treated with radical cystectomy for transitional cell carcinoma of the bladder and prostate. *Cancer* 1993;71:3993–4001.
27. Amling CL, Thrasher JB, Frazier HA, et al. Radical cystectomy for stages Ta, Tis and T1 transitional cell carcinoma of the bladder. *J Urol* 1994;151:31–35.
28. Viewig J, Gschwend JE, Herr HW, et al. The impact of primary stage on survival in patients with lymph node positive bladder cancer. *J Urol* 1999;161:72–76.
29. Leissner J, Ghoneim MA, Abol-Enein H, et al. Extended radical lymphadenectomy in patients with urothelial bladder cancer: results of a prospective multicenter study. *J Urol* 2004;171:139–144.
30. Skinner DG, Lieskovsky G. Contemporary cystectomy with pelvic node dissection compared to preoperative radiation therapy plus cystectomy in management of invasive bladder cancer. *J Urol* 1984;131:1069–1072.
31. Sanchez-Ortiz RF, Huang WC, Mick R, et al. An interval longer than 12 weeks between the diagnosis of muscle invasion and cystectomy is associated with worse outcome in bladder carcinoma. *J Urol* 2003;169:110–115.
32. Quek ML, Stein JP, Clark PE, et al. Microscopic and gross extravesical extension in pathologic staging of bladder cancer. *J Urol* 2004;171:640–645.
33. Stein JP, Grossfeld GD, Ginsberg DA, et al. Prognostic markers in bladder cancer: a contemporary review of the literature. *J Urol* 1999;160:645–659.

CHAPTER 27 ■ ROLE OF THE LYMPHADENECTOMY IN BLADDER CANCER

BERNARD H. BOCHNER

INTRODUCTION

The surgical management of invasive bladder cancer has undergone a significant evolution since its initial introduction into clinical practice. Changes to the technique have been implemented as a direct result of an improved understanding of the natural history of invasive bladder cancer. Clinical observations of the biology of high-grade bladder cancer have characterized its propensity for local invasion and regional pelvic lymph node involvement with the subsequent formation of distant metastases. The relatively frequent observation of involved regional lymphatics in the absence of distant dissemination and the high rate of pelvic recurrences with surgical approaches that ignored the regional nodes suggested a potential role for surgical removal of the regional lymph nodes as a means to improve outcome. The potential benefits that can be obtained if a thorough regional lymphadenectomy is performed include establishing a more accurate pathologic stage, enhanced local disease control, and possibly improved disease-specific survival. While no clearly established standard for the pelvic lymphadenectomy performed at the time of cystectomy for bladder cancer exists, this chapter will highlight the available information on its role in treatment and prognosis.

EARLY EXPERIENCE WITH CYSTECTOMY FOR BLADDER CANCER

The initial surgical approach to removal of the bladder for cancer consisted of a two-stage procedure that included initial urinary diversion (uretero-enterostomies) followed by what would be considered today as a simple cystectomy. This approach was associated with significant perioperative mortality, reported as high as 30% to 40%. As improvements in perioperative management and increased surgical experience emerged, surgical mortality for cystectomy decreased to a range that was comparable to that of other major contemporary surgical procedures. As the percentage of patients surviving the perioperative period increased, the efficacy of the procedure was better delineated. In 1950 Leadbetter and Cooper published a focused review of the literature on the initial disease control experience with cystectomy (1). Of the 429 patients reported from surgical series between 1939 and 1948, 342 survived the procedure and were evaluable for both local and distant disease control. Overall 33% (range 22.8% to 53.3%) of surviving patients died of recurrent disease, typically within the first 1 to 2 years after surgery. Although the patterns of failure were not particularly well documented in these

early series, local recurrences were frequently reported. Local extension of disease into the perivesical tissues that were incompletely excised was likely responsible for many locally recurrent lesions; however, regionally metastatic deposits that were present in the pelvic lymphatics and not controlled at cystectomy also represented a source of subsequent local failure. Orr, Carson, and Novak collected data on 26,811 cases of bladder cancer and noted that the operative surgeons in this series identified evidence of regional lymphatic involvement at the time of surgery in 47% of patients (2). It must be highlighted that most initial surgical approaches to cystectomy made no attempt at controlling the regional lymphatics.

PATHOLOGIC CONFIRMATION OF PATTERNS OF BLADDER CANCER PROGRESSION

As the early experience with cystectomy progressed, several autopsy studies provided additional supportive evidence to document the natural pathways of progression of invasive bladder cancer. Several large reports demonstrated that involvement of the regional lymphatics was a frequent finding in patients with advanced bladder cancer and occasionally represented the only site of metastatic disease. Cunningham reported on the autopsy findings of 411 patients with advanced bladder cancer and noted that 24% of patients had evidence of regional lymph node involvement (3). This number most certainly underestimated the true rate of nodal involvement given that these data were collected without detailed microscopic evaluations of the nodes and more accurately represented the percentage of patients with obvious or grossly involved nodes. Distant metastases were present in approximately one-third of patients in this series with nodal involvement observed in the majority. Spooner reported on 163 autopsy cases performed in patients with carcinoma of the bladder from the Mayo Clinic between 1914 and 1931 (4). Twenty-nine percent of patients had evidence of metastatic disease at the time of autopsy with the regional lymph nodes noted as the most frequent site of metastases. In 24% of cases the regional lymph nodes represented the only site of metastatic disease. Colston and Leadbetter reported their observations of 98 autopsy cases, over 50% of whom had recognized metastatic disease (5). Of those with metastases, 25% had involvement of the pelvic or retroperitoneal lymph nodes as their only site of metastatic disease. Similar to the above-noted series, limitations in the extent of microscopic review of the regional lymph nodes likely underestimated the complete extent of regionally metastatic disease within these populations.

The relationship between the relative risk of regional nodal involvement and the extent of disease within the bladder was a landmark association provided by autopsy data from Jewett and Strong in 1946 (6). These investigators reported the autopsy findings of 107 patients with infiltrating bladder tumors in which patients were grouped by the extent of invasion by the primary tumor: Group A consisted of three cases and represented lesions involving the submucosal layer only; Group B included 15 patients with invasion into the detrusor muscle but confined to the bladder; and Group C included 89 patients with disease extension into the perivesical tissues. No patient in Group A had evidence of metastatic disease; however, 11% of Group B and 52 of the 89 (58%) patients in Group C were found to have evidence of either regional or distant spread. Of the 52 Group C patients with metastatic disease, 33 (63%) had regional lymph node involvement. Six of the 52 (12%) had regional pelvic lymph node involvement as their only site of metastatic disease. The relationship between depth of invasion of the primary tumor and risk of regional lymph node involvement has been corroborated in contemporary radical cystectomy series. The risk of regional lymph node involvement ranges from 6% to 10% for organ-confined, invasive tumors to 42% to 75% for lesions that involve the perivesical fat or adjacent organs (7–9).

Based on the disappointing rates of local disease control of the early surgical series and autopsy data that clearly documented that the pathways of progression for invasive disease included involvement of the regional pelvic lymphatics, it became apparent that alterations in the surgical approach toward invasive bladder cancer was needed to improve outcome. Indeed, in 1950 Marshall and Whitmore concluded after reporting a 38% local failure rate in 100 consecutive patients undergoing cystectomy for bladder cancer that "the implication seems unavoidable that a more radical procedure might be worthy of trial" (10). The basis of this more radical approach would incorporate a formal attempt at controlling the regional lymphatics via a pelvic lymphadenectomy at the time of cystectomy, thus defining the contemporary radical cystectomy procedure.

ANATOMY OF LYMPHATIC DRAINAGE OF THE BLADDER

Anatomic studies performed around the turn of the 19th century, both in Europe and the United States, provided detailed descriptions of the lymphatic drainage of the urinary bladder. The classic descriptions of the lymphatic pathways within the bladder include a rich subepithelial lymphatic plexus which provides drainage through the detrusor musculature to the exterior of the bladder. Efferent lymphatic channels drain into perivesical lymph nodes that lie on the anterior, posterior, and lateral aspects of the bladder and perivesical tissues. Larger lymphatic channels then pass to nodal basins located along the external iliac vessels, hypogastric vessels, and lateral sacral/sacral promontory. These basins form a ring of pelvic nodes and constitute the primary drainage sites. All primary landing sites subsequently drain into the more proximal common iliac node chain.

EXPERIENCE WITH RADICAL CYSTECTOMY AND LYMPHADENECTOMY

Following the identification of the primary and secondary lymphatic drainage basins of the bladder within the pelvis, it remained to be determined whether a therapeutic advantage could be gained through their excision at the time of cystectomy. Experience with a similar radical surgical approach for cervical cancer, in which a therapeutic pelvic lymphadenectomy

was combined with a total exenterative procedure, not only demonstrated that it could safely be executed but that it also potentially improved outcome (11). Early experience with radical cystectomy and regional lymphadenectomy for patients with nodal metastases suggested that despite a more aggressive surgical approach, most node-positive patients experienced an exceedingly poor long-term outcome. In 1956, Whitmore and Marshall published their experience of 100 consecutive bladder cancer patients undergoing radical cystectomy and a regional pelvic lymphadenectomy (12). In 32 patients with node-positive disease, only 22% were reported alive at 1 year. Three patients (9%), the majority of whom developed metastatic disease, survived 2 years and only one (3%) was alive at 3 years. While these data represented an overall improvement in outcome in node-positive patients, the poor rate of survival among patients with regionally advanced disease led many to question whether radical cystectomy was indicated in the presence of positive regional nodes.

Supported by reports of success with the Wertheim technique for cervical cancer, Leadbetter proposed inclusion of a thorough pelvic lymph node dissection that included the hypogastric, external iliac, presacral, and common iliac lymphatics at cystectomy (1). Subsequently Skinner championed the benefits of a thorough lymph node dissection at the time of cystectomy and presented evidence supporting its therapeutic benefits (13). Contemporary experience with patients whose bladder cancer has involved the regional pelvic lymph nodes establishes a significantly more favorable outcome following radical cystectomy and pelvic lymphadenectomy compared with early published experiences. Current reports note that approximately 25% to 33% of all patients with invasive bladder cancer involving the regional lymph nodes will be rendered disease free following radical cystectomy and a thorough pelvic lymph node dissection (7,9,14,15). Updated data from Stein and colleagues reported in their series of 1,054 bladder cancer patients, 246 with pathologic evidence of regional lymph node involvement revealed that at 5 and 10 years, 35% and 34% of all lymph node positive bladder cancer patients were found to be free of disease following radical cystectomy and an extended pelvic lymphadenectomy that included all nodes from the aortic bifurcation distally to the inguinal ligament (9). The Memorial Sloan-Kettering experience with 193 contemporary node-positive bladder cancer patients that received radical cystectomy and a more limited PLND (proximal limit at the bifurcation of the common iliac vessels) reported a 31% disease-specific survival and 25% overall survival at 5 years (14). Ghoneim et al. found 188 node-positive patients out of 1,026 (18%) patients with bladder cancer. A 23.4% 5-year survival was reported in the 188 node-positive patients who received a lymphadenectomy at cystectomy that included the nodes at the distal common iliac vessels (7). Mills et al. reported a 29% overall survival in 83 node-positive patients that underwent cystectomy and a pelvic lymphadenectomy that included nodes from the bifurcation of the common iliac distally (15). Other groups have similarly documented that overall approximately one-quarter to one-third of all patients with regionally metastatic bladder cancer can be expected to survive 5 years following radical cystectomy and PLND.

Subgroups of patients with regionally metastatic disease may actually demonstrate a significantly better prognosis and can be identified by having a lower volume of disease both at the level of the primary tumor and the regional lymph nodes. The survival for node-positive patients whose primary tumors are confined to the bladder is significantly better than that observed in node-positive patients with more invasive primary tumors. Vieweg et al. reported a 51% 5-year overall survival in 44 P0-P3a, LN+ patients compared to a 17% 5-year survival in 149 patients with P3b-P4, N+ disease (16). The USC group reported a 46% versus 30% 5-year recurrence-free survival in node-positive patients with organ-confined versus non-organ-confined primary tumors, respectively (17). A similar stratification of outcome can be observed when considering the volume of disease at the level of the regional lymph nodes. If the number of positive nodes or size of the involved node(s) is considered as a measure of the extent of tumor involvement of the regional nodes, patients with fewer involved nodes or smaller tumor-bearing nodes have been found to have an improved outcome. Vieweg et al. reported the 5-year disease-specific survival of 193 node-positive patients that underwent cystectomy based on TNM node staging (1987 system) as 44%, 27%, and 0% for N1, N2, and N3 patients, respectively. The median survival for these three groups was 3.1, 1.9, and 0.9 years, respectively ($P = .0006$). The number of involved lymph nodes has been reported as an independent prognostic indicator following radical cystectomy (14). Lerner et al. noted that patients with fewer than six involved lymph nodes exhibited a significantly improved 5-year survival compared to patients with greater than six positive nodes (18). An update of this series found that eight or fewer nodes involved was an optimized cutoff in that patients with eight or fewer involved nodes ($n = 193$) demonstrated a 41% 5-year recurrence-free survival and 37% overall 5-year survival compared with 10% and 4%, respectively, in patients with greater than eight involved nodes ($n = 51$, $P < .001$) (17). Other series have confirmed similar differences in outcome, as noted by Mills et al. in which patients with fewer than five involved lymph nodes did significantly better compared with those with more involved nodes (5-year survival of approximately 50% vs. 10%) (15).

Additional measurements of the burden of disease, such as the size of the involved nodes or the presence of extracapsular lymph node extension by tumor within the regional lymph nodes, may also prove to be prognostically important. Mills et al. reported that patients with involved nodes greater than 0.5 cm or the presence of extracapsular extension within the involved nodes demonstrated a lower survival. Multivariate analysis of the relative importance of the number of positive nodes, size of involved nodes, or the presence of extracapsular lymph node perforation demonstrated that only the presence of extracapsular perforation remained independently predictive of outcome, with a hazard ratio of 2.6 (15).

While the number of lymph nodes involved with disease contains important prognostic information, simultaneous consideration of the extent of the lymphadenectomy performed appears to enhance the prognostic significance of such data. For example, consider two patients, both with four positive lymph nodes identified after cystectomy. Patient one had a total of 10 lymph nodes evaluated pathologically while patient two had 40 lymph nodes analyzed. Should both patients be considered similarly staged? Would both patients have a similar anticipated outcome? Data from both University of Southern California and Memorial Sloan-Kettering Cancer Center (MSKCC) would suggest that evaluation of the number of involved nodes in the context of the total number of lymph nodes removed provides a more accurate means to identify higher-risk node-positive patients (17,19). Using information obtained from the ratio of positive lymph nodes to the total number of lymph nodes evaluated (density of positive lymph nodes), both institutions have independently demonstrated an improved stratification of node-positive patients into differing risk groups. Using 20% as a cutoff for the percentage of involved lymph nodes, a 44% versus 17% 5-year recurrence-free survival was observed for patients with less than compared with greater than 20% of their total nodes involved with disease, respectively. An even greater difference in outcome was reported using a ratio-based analysis in a series of 162 node-positive patients who had undergone cystectomy and lymphadenectomy. The 5-year disease-specific survival of patients with <20% of total nodes involved was approximately 65% compared with 5% for patients with >20% of evaluated

lymph nodes involved with tumor. Positive-node ratio provided improved prognostic information compared to 1997 TNM nodal staging criteria or total number of involved lymph nodes.

IMPORTANCE OF EXTENT OF LYMPHADENECTOMY

Given the importance in staging information provided by the lymphadenectomy, the question of the extent of the dissection required for adequate staging or therapeutic value remained to be clarified. An established set of necessary anatomic boundaries and extent (number of lymph nodes) of the lymph node dissection that would provide optimal staging and therapeutic efficacy for bladder cancer is presently not available. A lack of prospectively validated studies has led to ongoing controversy regarding the necessary extent of dissection.

Wishnow et al. attempted to determine the rate of involvement of the pelvic lymph nodes within the common iliac chain or more distally in the obturator, hypogastric, and external iliac nodes in bladder cancer patients undergoing radical cystectomy (20). In a series of 130 patients with grossly negative lymph nodes at the time of cystectomy, 88% of whom had common iliac nodes resected, 14% of patients were identified with microscopically involved nodes. Seventeen of the 18 patients with microscopically involved lymph nodes had one or two positive nodes. None of the 17 patients with one or two microscopically involved nodes had common iliac or lateral external iliac lymph nodes involved. Based on these findings, the authors recommended limiting the proximal limit of the lymph node dissection to the bifurcation of the common iliac vessels for patients with no evidence of grossly positive lymph nodes. More recently at MSKCC, a series of 144 bladder cancer patients undergoing radical cystectomy were prospectively evaluated to determine the site of regional lymph node involvement. Eighteen patients (14%) were found to have microscopically involved regional lymph nodes including four with disease involving the common iliac nodes. In this series all but one patient with common iliac nodes had simultaneous involvement of a more distal lymph node region (hypogastric, obturator, or external iliac) suggesting that excision of the common iliac nodes would benefit a subset of microscopically LN positive patients. Additional information on the distribution of positive pelvic nodes is provided by a multicenter, prospective trial in which all patients underwent an extended pelvic lymph node dissection (proximal limits of dissection at or above the bifurcation of the aorta) (21). Of the 290 patients evaluated in this series, 81 (27.9%) demonstrated evidence of tumor involvement in 599 pelvic nodes. Involved nodes above the bifurcation of the common iliac vessels comprised 35% of all positive nodes. A total of 20 patients (6.9%) demonstrated involvement of the common iliac nodes without evidence of disease within the more distal nodal regions (obturator, hypogastric, or external iliac). While exact information on the nature of the nodes (gross or microscopically enlarged) was not available, in the 29 patients with only a single lymph node metastasis, 10% were located above the bifurcation of the common iliac vessels providing further strong support for the need to extend the dissection to minimally include the common iliac chain.

TECHNIQUE FOR PELVIC LYMPHADENECTOMY AT THE TIME OF RADICAL CYSTECTOMY

The technique for the extended pelvic lymphadenectomy can be performed either before or after the cystectomy has been completed. The author prefers completing the lymph node dissection as the initial part of the procedure as it facilitates the cystectomy by improving access to the vascular pedicles.

The procedure is started by exposing the lower retroperitoneum and pelvic sidewalls. The ascending colon is mobilized by incising the white line of Toldt. This is carried around the base of the cecum in a cephalad direction, up the root of the small bowel mesentery to the crossing of the third portion of the duodenum. The sigmoid colon is then mobilized off the sacral promontory. An opening in the base of the sigmoid mesentery below the inferior mesenteric vessels is made and carried cephalad to the region of the take-off of the inferior mesenteric artery from the aorta. This provides optimal exposure of the lower aorta and its bifurcation. The small bowel is packed in the upper abdomen and the sigmoid colon and its mesentery are retracted laterally. The extended lymphadenectomy is initiated 2 cm above the bifurcation of the aorta. All lymphatic tissues are clipped proximally at this level out to the genitofemoral nerves, which represent the lateral limits of dissection. All lymphatic tissues are split and rolled off the lower aorta and vena cava. The common iliac vessels are then skeletonized, sweeping all tissues distally toward its bifurcation. At this point the distal limits of the dissection are delineated. The medial aspect of the distal external iliac vein is identified. The lymphatics medial to the vein are traced to Cooper's ligament where the node of Cloquet is identified, clipped, and divided. A row of clips is placed medial to lateral along the external iliac vein and artery at the level of the crossing of the circumflex iliac vein. Care is taken to avoid injury to the genitofemoral nerve fibers lateral to the artery. The lymphatics overlying the external iliac artery and vein are split and rolled to completely free both vessels circumferentially. Psoas branches from both vessels can be found on their lateral aspects near their midpoint, where they should be secured and divided. A small sponge is then passed lateral to the external artery and vein between the psoas muscle and gently pushed distally into the obturator fossa. This allows for complete clearance of all tissues in the groove between the external iliac artery and psoas. The vein is then retracted anteriorly and the obturator nerve freed from all lymphatics. This allows for isolation of the obturator vessels that typically are secured and divided as they exit the obturator foramen. The remaining lymphatics overlying the hypogastric vessels are then swept medially to completely free the hypogastric branches leading to the anterior pelvic organs. The remaining nodal region that requires clearance is the presacral chain, which can be freed from below the bifurcation of the common iliac vessels and swept off the entirety of the sacral promontory. Separate submissions for each nodal region are recommended to optimize the number of nodes reported (22).

OUTCOMES BASED ON EXTENT OF DISSECTION

Data describing the relationship between the extent of the node dissection and outcome are provided by single-institution, retrospective reviews. Poulsen et al. reported a comparative analysis of two consecutive series of bladder cancer patients undergoing either a limited (proximal limit at the bifurcation of the common iliac vessels) or extended (included the nodes up to the level of the bifurcation of the aorta) lymphadenectomy performed at the time of radical cystectomy (23). Previously untreated bladder cancer patients were included in the study in which 126 underwent an extended (between 1993 and 1997) and 68 received a limited (between 1990 and 1993) LN dissection. The two groups were well matched demographically, with a slightly higher percentage of extravesical tumors in the extended lymphadenectomy group. As anticipated, the extended node dissection yielded a greater number of lymph nodes compared to the more limited excision (25 vs. 14, $P < .001$). Both groups had a similar proportion of node-positive patients, 27% in the extended and 24% in the limited LN groups. Despite the increased number of more advanced tumors in the extended dissection group, a similar 5-year recurrence-free survival, risk of local recurrence, and risk of distant metastasis was observed. In the subgroup of patients with organ-confined primary tumors, however, patients that underwent an extended dissection benefited with an improved 5-year recurrence (85% vs. 64%, $P < .02$).

Leissner and colleagues presented their analysis of 302 patients who received an extended lymph node dissection at the time of radical cystectomy for bladder cancer. They noted that patients with a greater number of lymph nodes reported in their pathology report had an improved disease-free and overall survival as well as improved local tumor control. At 5 years, 51% of patients with ≤15 lymph nodes removed were alive and disease-free compared to 65% for those with ≥16 lymph nodes evaluated. The improvement in local control was also significant, with pelvic recurrences identified in 27% compared to 17% of patients with ≤15 and ≥16 lymph nodes evaluated, respectively ($P < .01$) (8). Herr et al. confirmed a similar improved outcome in 322 patients, in which those that underwent a more extensive node dissection, as represented by a greater number of lymph nodes identified in the pathology report, exhibited an improved overall survival. All patients underwent cystectomy without preoperative radiation or neoadjuvant or adjuvant chemotherapy. Of the 258 patients with negative nodes, the median number of nodes evaluated was eight and for the 64 node-positive patients the median number of nodes was 11. The 5-year overall survival for node-positive patients was 84% versus 40% for those with greater or less than eight lymph nodes evaluated, respectively. For patients with node-positive disease, approximately 50% versus 20% of patients with greater or less than 11 lymph nodes removed were alive at 5 years, respectively (24). Additional supportive data obtained from a national cohort of patients is provided by a multivariate analysis of Surveillance, Epidemiology, and End Results (SEER) registry data on 1,923 radical cystectomy patients. This retrospective study found that the number of lymph nodes examined was positively associated with an improved survival, particularly in patients with higher-stage disease. Patients with at least four lymph nodes evaluated demonstrated an improved outcome. However, patients with 10 to 14 nodes reported exhibited the greatest improvement in overall survival (25).

The ability to limit the dissection to the ipsilateral side of the pelvis in patients with tumors located on one side of the bladder has also been proposed. It is apparent, however, that despite a clear laterality location of the primary bladder tumor, contralateral nodal involvement will frequently be identified. Data from Leissner et al. found that of 32 node-positive patients with primary tumors located specifically to one side of the bladder, the risk of contralateral lymph node involvement was only slightly less than that found for the ipsilateral nodes (21). Sentinal node studies have also confirmed that the initial node region involved with disease may be located in the contralateral side of the primary tumor (26).

SURGICAL STANDARD FOR BLADDER CANCER AND CURRENT PRACTICE

The establishment of the minimum number of lymph nodes needed for adequate staging, prognosis, or improved outcome would provide a surgical standard that could be widely applied. Much work to establish such standards for the surgical management of colorectal, breast, and gastric cancers has been completed (27–29). To date no such standard has been established for the lymphadenectomy for bladder cancer. Major difficulties in establishing such a standard include the wide variation in reported node yields following either limited or extended dissections and the lack of prospective studies validating any such "standard." The variable extent of surgical dissection and differing techniques used for pathologic review contribute to the differences in reported median node number as well as individual anatomic variation in the number of nodes present (30), surgeon, patient age, and pretreatment. While increasing data support that surgeon experience is related to outcome following major surgical procedures (31), Leissner et al. demonstrated that node yield following radical cystectomy was not related to surgical experience (8). In this series, some surgeons with the highest surgical volume reported the lowest node yields. Recent data from MSKCC evaluating the factors associated with node yield variability in a series of 144 consecutive radical cystectomies demonstrated that only the extent of the dissection was associated with overall node yield within a group of four experienced surgeons. Patient age, neoadjuvant systemic chemotherapy, the time from transurethral resection (TUR), or prior use of Bacillus Calmette-Guerin (BCG) use did not exhibit a statistically significant association with node count (32). In contrast, others have found that increasing patient age is associated with lower node yields after an extended dissection (21). The way in which the nodes are submitted to pathology also affects the number of nodes reported. By sending separate nodal packets from the different anatomic node regions as opposed to an en bloc submission with the main specimen, Bochner et al. reported a 3.5-fold increase in the number of reported nodes for a standard dissection and a 1.6-fold increase in node yield for an extended dissection (22).

Despite evidence supporting the importance of the lymphadenectomy for both improved prognosis and possible therapeutic benefit, national data on surgical practice suggest that many surgeons limit or avoid the node dissection at cystectomy. SEER registry data that included 1,923 patients who underwent cystectomy in the United States between 1988 and 1996 indicated that 53% of reported cystectomies had three or fewer lymph nodes reviewed in the final pathologic report (25).

CONCLUSION

Anatomic and clinical experience with invasive bladder cancer has established the natural pathways of disease progression. Decades of experience with radical surgery for the management of muscle invasive bladder cancer clearly emphasizes the role that surgical quality may play in patient outcome. Future advances in establishing surgical standards for the treatment of bladder cancer will require well-controlled prospective trials that directly compare varying extents of surgery with their ability to provide local and distant disease control as well as disease-specific survival. This will set the stage for clear benchmarks that can then be broadly applied to clinical practice.

References

1. Leadbetter WF, Cooper J. Regional gland dissection for carcinoma of the bladder: a technique for one-stage cystectomy, gland dissection, and bilateral uretero-enterostomy. *J Urol* 1950;63:242–260.
2. Orr L, Carson R, Novak W. *J Urol* 1939;42:778.
3. Cunningham J. Tumors of the bladder. *J Urol* 1931;25:559.
4. Spooner A. *Trans Am Assoc G-U Surg* 1934;27:86.
5. Colston J, Leadbetter WF. Infiltrating carcinoma of the bladder. *J Urol* 1936;36:669.
6. Jewett H, Strong G. Infiltrating carcinoma of the bladder: relation of depth of penetration of the bladder wall to incidence of local extension and metastases. *J Urol* 1946;55:366–372.
7. Ghoneim MA, el-Mekresh MM, el-Baz MA, et al. Radical cystectomy for carcinoma of the bladder: critical evaluation of the results in 1,026 cases. *J Urol* 1997;158:393–399.
8. Leissner J, Hohenfellner R, Thuroff JW, et al. Lymphadenectomy in patients with transitional cell carcinoma of the urinary bladder; significance for staging and prognosis. *BJU Int* 2000;85:817–823.
9. Stein JP, Lieskovsky G, Cote R, et al. Radical cystectomy in the treatment of invasive bladder cancer: long-term results in 1,054 patients. *J Clin Oncol* 2001;19:666–675.
10. Marshall VF, Whitmore WF. Simple cystectomy for cancer of the urinary bladder: one hundred consecutive cases: two years later. *J Urol* 1950;63:232–241.
11. Brunschwig A. Complete excision of pelvic viscera for advanced carcinoma. *Cancer* 1948;1:177–183.
12. Whitmore WF, Marshall VF. Radical surgery for carcinoma of the urinary bladder: one hundred consecutive cases four years later. *Cancer* 1956;3:596–608.
13. Skinner DG. Management of invasive bladder cancer: a meticulous pelvic node dissection can make a difference. *J Urol* 1982;128:34–36.
14. Vieweg J, Gschwend JE, Herr HW, et al. Pelvic lymph node dissection can be curative in patients with node positive bladder cancer. *J Urol* 1999;161:449–454.
15. Mills RD, Turner WH, Fleischmann A, et al. Pelvic lymph node metastases from bladder cancer: outcome in 83 patients after radical cystectomy and pelvic lymphadenectomy. *J Urol* 2001;166:19–23.
16. Vieweg J, Gschwend JE, Herr HW, et al. The impact of primary stage on survival in patients with lymph node positive bladder cancer. *J Urol* 1999;161:72–76.
17. Stein JP, Cai J, Groshen S, et al. Risk factors for patients with pelvic lymph node metastases following radical cystectomy with en bloc pelvic lymphadenectomy: the concept of lymph node density. *J Urol* 2003;170:35–41.
18. Lerner SP, Skinner DG, Lieskovsky G, et al. The rationale for en bloc pelvic lymph node dissection for bladder cancer patients with nodal metastases: long-term results. *J Urol* 1993;149:758–764; discussion 764–765.
19. Herr HW. Superiority of ratio based lymph node staging for bladder cancer. *J Urol* 2003;169:943–945.
20. Wishnow KI, Johnson DE, Ro JY, et al. Incidence, extent and location of unsuspected pelvic lymph node metastasis in patients undergoing radical cystectomy for bladder cancer. *J Urol* 1987;137:408–410.
21. Leissner J, Ghoneim MA, Abol-Enein H, et al. Extended radical lymphadenectomy in patients with urothelial bladder cancer: results of a prospective multicenter study. *J Urol* 2004;171:139–144.
22. Bochner BH, Herr HW, Reuter VE. Impact of separate versus en bloc pelvic lymph node dissection on the number of lymph nodes retrieved in cystectomy specimens. *J Urol* 2001;166:2295–2296.
23. Poulsen J, Krarup T. Pelvic lymphadenectomy (staging) in patients with bladder cancer: laparoscopic versus open approach. *Scand J Urol Nephrol Suppl* 1995;172:19–21.
24. Herr HW, Bochner BH, Dalbagni G, et al. Impact of the number of lymph nodes retrieved on outcome in patients with muscle invasive bladder cancer. *J Urol* 2002;167:1295–1298.
25. Konety BR, Joslyn SA, O'Donnell MA. Extent of pelvic lymphadenectomy and its impact on outcome in patients diagnosed with bladder cancer: analysis of data from the Surveillance, Epidemiology and End Results Program data base. *J Urol* 2003;169:946–950.
26. Sherif A, De La Torre M, Malmstrom PU, et al. Lymphatic mapping and detection of sentinel nodes in patients with bladder cancer. *J Urol* 2001;166:812–815.
27. Mathiesen O, Carl J, Bonderup O, et al. Axillary sampling and the risk of erroneous staging of breast cancer. An analysis of 960 consecutive patients. *Acta Oncol* 1990;29:721–725.
28. Caplin S, Cerottini JP, Bosman FT, et al. For patients with Dukes' B (TNM Stage II) colorectal carcinoma, examination of six or fewer lymph nodes is related to poor prognosis. *Cancer* 1998;83:666–672.
29. Siewert JR, Bottcher K, Stein HJ, et al. Relevant prognostic factors in gastric cancer: ten-year results of the German Gastric Cancer Study. *Ann Surg* 1998;228:449–461.
30. Weingartner K, Ramaswamy A, Bittinger A, et al. Anatomical basis for pelvic lymphadenectomy in prostate cancer: results of an autopsy study and implications for the clinic. *J Urol* 1996;156:1969–1971.
31. Birkmeyer JD, Stukel TA, Siewers AE, et al. Surgeon volume and operative mortality in the United States. *N Engl J Med* 2003;349:2117–2127.
32. Bochner B. *J Urol* 2004 *(in press)*.

CHAPTER 28 ■ URINARY DIVERSIONS AND RECONSTRUCTIONS AND ORTHOTOPIC BLADDER SUBSTITUTION

CHAPTER 28A
Urinary Diversions and Reconstructions

Edward M. Gong and Gary D. Steinberg

INTRODUCTION

Over the years, the problem of how to divert the urinary stream after radical cystectomy has been solved with many methods. From simply establishing a direct tract from the ureters to the skin surface to performing complex bladder reconstructions, almost every method imaginable has been attempted. Despite the attempt by urologic oncologists, no perfect bladder replacement currently exists. However, several goals for urinary diversion have been established. Ideally, a urinary diversion will closely match the function of the native bladder (1,2). The native bladder is a structure that should provide low-pressure filling, high compliance, storage with perfect continence, and complete voluntary emptying (3). Inherent to the native bladder are other criteria, such as nonrefluxing ureteral orifices, no absorption of urine electrolytes, and sterility of urine (Table 28A.1). Currently, three basic categories of urinary reconstruction exist which adequately, if not perfectly, meet these goals: the urinary conduit, the cutaneous continent diversion, and the orthotopic urinary diversion.

TYPES OF URINARY DIVERSION

Before discussion of specifics associated with the use of various intestinal segments, benefits of each diversion, quality of life (QOL), etc., this section will first familiarize the reader with the various forms of urinary diversions and the most common types of diversion within each form. Though over the years, many creative methods have been developed to best divert the urinary stream, these methods essentially boil down to three major categories: the noncontinent cutaneous diversion, the continent cutaneous diversion, and the continent orthotopic diversion.

As the name for the first category of urinary diversion implies, this method is noncontinent, requiring an external collection appliance similar to that for bowel diversions such as the ileostomy or colostomy. The second category is a continent diversion that consists of a larger internal reservoir made of various bowel segments and a continent stoma at the skin level that requires catheterization to drain urine. Finally, the orthotopic diversion also has a larger internal reservoir; however, the continence method is derived from the orthotopic position that allows the use of the native urethral sphincter.

Noncontinent Cutaneous Diversions

The noncontinent cutaneous diversion consists of two portions. The first is a short segment of intestine, known as the "conduit," which bridges urine from the ureters through the abdominal wall to the skin level. The second is a cutaneous stoma that allows free drainage of urine from this conduit to an external collection appliance attached to the skin via an adhesive that prevents leakage of urine. Two major forms of the conduit exist, one made of ileum and one made of colon. To date, these diversions are the most common and should be part of every urologic surgeon's armamentarium. In our institution, ileal conduits are performed on patients with diminished renal function, bulky extravesical or nodal disease, the inability to care for a continent reservoir, or significant comorbidities to shorten surgical time.

The advantage to noncontinent cutaneous diversions lies in their simplicity in construction, shorter operative time, and decreased perioperative and postoperative complications. Stoma positioning is extremely crucial to success because poor stoma placement can lead to urinary leakage, skin breakdown, and poor QOL. Preoperative and postoperative support from an enterostomal therapist help patients more readily adapt to their new body image. Complications associated with conduits include parastomal hernias, stomal stenosis, stomal retraction, pyelonephritis, and long-term deterioration of the upper tracts. Approximately one third of patients will undergo some degree of upper tract deterioration after conduit diversion, with 6% requiring dialysis. Factors that are responsible for this include ureteral-ileal conduit strictures, chronic bacteriuria and reflux nephropathy, stomal stenosis, serious metabolic acidosis, and preexisting renal damage due to obstruction from bladder cancer. Though the urinary drainage appliance does require care and maintenance, this device can be changed once every several days, versus a catheter every 4 hours for the patient with a catheterizable continent diversion, greatly reducing the burden to family or caregivers.

Ileal Conduit

Since its introduction by Bricker in 1950, the ileal conduit has been the gold standard of urinary diversions (4). It is created using a 15 to 20 cm segment of ileum at least 15 cm from the ileo-cecal valve to prevent complications such as bile salt and vitamin B_{12} malabsorption. The segment is taken out of bowel continuity and the remaining ileum is anastomosed to preserve bowel continuity. The proximal end of the ileal segment to be used as the conduit is sutured closed (in a watertight fashion) and the ureters anastomosed in an end-to-side fashion to that end using a refluxing technique. The open end of the ileal segment is brought to the skin level through the rectus fascia of the anterior abdominal

TABLE 28A.1

CRITERIA FOR AN IDEAL URINARY DIVERSION

Metabolic stability
Easy to construct/minimal morbidity
Preservation of upper tract
Nonrefluxing
Continent at all times
Natural cycling
No malignant changes
Sterile urine
Easy endoscopic access
Applicable to both genders
Catheterless
Stomaless
Valveless
Psychologically acceptable

wall and anastomosed, usually as end "rosebud" stoma (5,6) (Fig. 28A.1A,B). However, in the markedly obese patient, the end stoma is difficult to create due to the thick abdominal wall and tethered mesentery preventing a protruding stoma. In this situation a loop end urostomy or modified Turnball stoma may be easier to perform, albeit with a higher parastomal hernia rate (Fig. 28A.1C,D).

Colon Conduit

The colon conduit is an excellent alternative for patients in whom the ileum is not a viable option for use in diversion. Patients who have undergone extensive pelvic radiation may have radiation damage to the ileum, elevating their risk of postoperative complications. In this population, the transverse colon is usually a radiation-spared segment of bowel. Electrolyte abnormalities differ little between ileum and colon and a nonrefluxing ureteral implantation using the taenia is easier in colonic segments. In general, ileum and colon conduits are fairly comparable segments of bowel for use in conduits, and

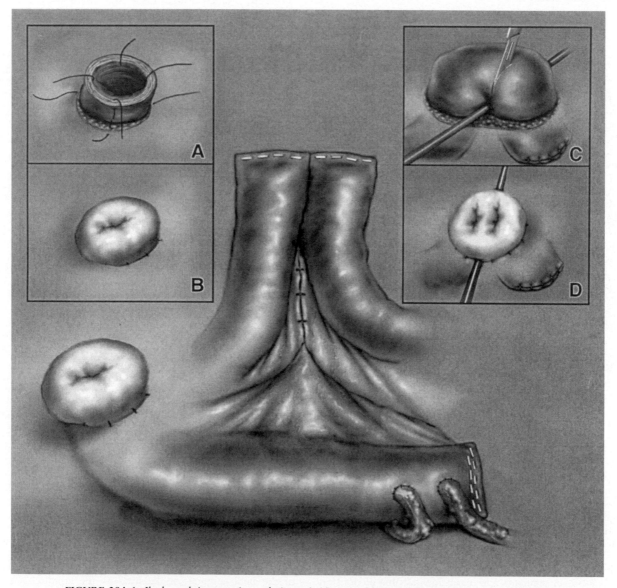

FIGURE 28A.1. Ileal conduit operative technique. A 15 cm to 20 cm segment of ileum is isolated and closed at the antiperistaltic end. The remainder of the bowel is closed in a stapled side-to-side fashion. The stoma is brought out through the anterior abdominal wall. **A and B:** "Rosebud" stoma. **C and D:** Turnbull loop stoma. (Reprinted from Droller MJ, ed. *Current clinical urology: bladder cancer: current diagnosis and treatment.* Totowas, NJ: Humana Press, 2001:347, with permission.)

both provide a safe and reliable means of urinary diversion for patients who require bladder removal (7).

Continent Cutaneous Urinary Diversions

Despite the effectiveness of the ileal conduit urinary diversion, the need for an external collection device remains an inconvenience to patients and may alter body image, especially in young patients. Though a continent catheterizable diversion was first introduced by Gilchrist in the 1950s, it was not until the early 1980s that a push toward continent diversion of the urinary stream led to various techniques of fashioning bowel reservoirs for urinary storage (8). The basic concept of the continent cutaneous diversion consists of a detubularized bowel reservoir and a leakproof stoma that requires catheterization to release urine. The bowel is detubularized to destroy peristaltic integrity and maximize volume per surface area of intestine (5). Many techniques for the creation of the continent catheterizable stoma exist. However, these are typically based on three major categories of stoma. The first utilizes the small caliber appendix or a tapered length of bowel (Mitrofanoff or Monti technique); the second is the terminal ileum to take advantage of the nonrefluxing ileocecal valve; and the third is a nipple or flap valve (Kock or Mainz pouch) (9). Despite the advent of orthotopic urinary diversion, continent cutaneous diversions are still an excellent alternative for patients with contraindications to use the native urethra such as previous surgery or radiation to the pelvis, or cancer at the bladder neck/prostatic urethra. Today, though many forms of continent cutaneous urinary diversion exist, the Indiana Pouch is the easiest to perform and the most popular.

Indiana Pouch

First introduced by Drs. Rowland and Mitchell in 1985 (10), the Indiana pouch has undergone multiple modifications since its original description. Currently the Indiana Pouch consists of a plicated terminal ileum to the level of the ileocecal valve that acts as a continent catheterizable stoma and a detubularized right colon fashioned into a low-pressure reservoir with absorbable sutures (11). The authors use the entire right colon and approximately 8–10 cm of the terminal ileum (Fig. 28A.2).

The clinical results for the Indiana pouch in combination with its technical simplicity make it the mainstay for continent cutaneous urinary diversions. Long-term follow-up data in 150 patients by Bihrle showed 98% continence with low reoperation and complication rates (12). This data compares favorably with other catheterizable reservoirs. Blute, in a study of 194 women who underwent Indiana pouch creation, demonstrated a 15% reoperation rate and late complications in 17% of patients, including pouch calculi, stomal stenosis, incontinence, stomal hernia, small bowel obstruction, and renal insufficiency (13). In our institution, 2 of 60 patients required an augmentation of their Indiana pouch with a 20-cm "ileal patch" because of uninhibited contractions and urge incontinence of the pouch. Incontinence was resolved in both patients after augmentation. In patients with a thick abdominal wall, the authors will bring the catheterizable stoma through the umbilicus.

Koch Pouch

The Koch pouch was introduced in 1982, and its creation stimulated interest in creating a continent urinary diversion (9). Due to high complication and reoperation rates, combined with the technical difficulty of creating the pouch, its use has diminished in popularity. However, we mention the Koch pouch due to its historical significance and its preservation of the ileocecal valve in creating a continent catheterizable stoma.

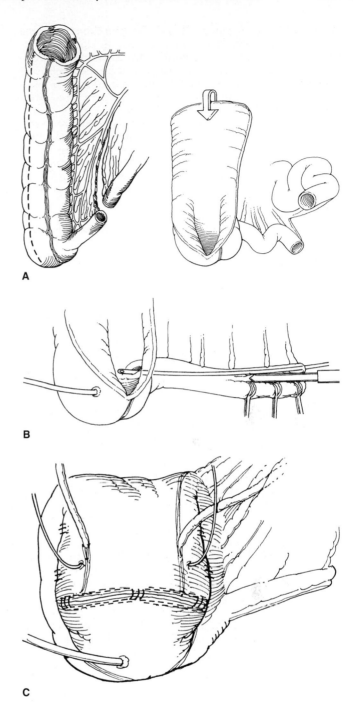

FIGURE 28A.2. Indiana Pouch operative technique. **A:** The entire right colon and 8 to 10 cm of terminal ileum are isolated. The colonic segment is detubularized along the antimesenteric surface and folded upon itself. **B:** A continent catheterizable limb is created by tapering the efferent limb with a stapling device. **C:** The ureters are implanted into the pouch.

An intussuscepted nipple valve is utilized for urine continence and antireflux technique.

Orthotopic Continent Diversions

After the creation of continent cutaneous urinary diversion, it was only a matter of time before the development of orthotopic urinary reconstruction. Although the catheterizable stoma provides a significant improvement over the external urinary drainage appliance, the patient is still subjected to the psychological stigma associated with frequent clean intermittent catheterizations. The orthotopic diversion preserves relatively normal volitional voiding and may provide improved body image, sexuality, sociability, and a global sense of well-being (14). The orthotopic neobladder most closely resembles the original bladder in form and function.

Over the past 15 years, numerous reconstructive procedures to create an orthotopic neobladder have been introduced (Table 28A.2). However, as yet there is no consensus to the best form of orthotopic diversion, much less to the segment of bowel used or the need for a nonrefluxing or refluxing ureteral implantation. Described here are several of the more popularly used orthotopic reconstructions.

Hautmann Neobladder and Chimney Modification

First described by Hautmann at the University of Ulm in Germany, this neobladder consists of 60 cm to 80 cm of detubularized ileum that has been oriented into the shape of a "W" and then refashioned into a spherical pouch (15). The ureters are implanted directly into this spherical pouch, or into an isoperistaltic "chimney" of tubularized ileum (16,17). Presently, the author is using 4 limbs of 12 cm and a chimney limb of 8 cm to 12 cm in length (for a total of 50 cm to 60 cm) depending on the length of the ureters. The necessity to prevent neobladder-ureteral reflux is controversial. Long-term studies have demonstrated the potential deleterious effects of ureteral reflux over a 30-year period in patients who underwent ileal conduits as children; however, the renal nephron loss is less significant in the adult cancer population. In our practice, renal functional loss is more commonly related to ureteral-neobladder stricture.

Many techniques have been described to prevent ureteral strictures. One is the chimney modification, which simplifies the ureteral-neobladder anastomosis. By extending the chimney toward the kidneys, a tension-free ureteral anastomosis that minimizes ureteral ischemia with less mobilization and more proximal resection of the ureters can be performed. The chimney will also prevent competition with the bowel mesentery for access to the posterior wall of the neobladder, decrease the risk of ureteral angulation and obstruction with distention of the neobladder, and allow for easier repair and revision. Additionally, the short iso-peristaltic segment will assist in preventing ureteral reflux. Finally, the pouch is anastomosed to the urethra, utilizing the properties of a low pressure, high compliance reservoir and the native urethral sphincter as the continence mechanism (Fig. 28A.3). Because no detrusor activity is present, voiding occurs passively via relaxation of the urinary sphincter, with a coordinated valsalva maneuver.

Results from the first 290 patients yielded continence rates exceeding 95%, with 3.9% requiring clean intermittent

catheterization. However, the number of patients requiring clean intermittent catheterization increases with long-term follow-up. Early and late neobladder-related complications occurred in 15.4% and 23.4% of patients, respectively. Reoperation rates, however, were fairly low, with 0.3% and 4.4% requiring further surgery in the early and late phases of postoperative care (15). Complication rates have been comparable with all forms of urinary diversion (18).

Studer Neobladder

The Studer neobladder was developed and popularized at the University of Bern. It consists of a 60-cm segment of ileum in which the distal 40 cm is detubularized and folded over onto itself to form a U-shaped pouch. The proximal 20 cm remains as an isoperistaltic limb into which the ureters are implanted in a refluxing method (Fig. 28A.4). Studer reported daytime continence rates of 92% at 1 year and nighttime continence of 80% after 2 years. Complication rates are comparable with other urinary diversions, with 15% of patients experiencing major complications (19). The long isoperistaltic limb serves as an antireflux mechanism and also allows for the creation of a tension-free ureteral anastomosis in the case of distal ureteral involvement of urothelial tumor.

Sigmoid Pouch (Reddy)

The Sigmoid pouch, first described by Reddy and Lange at the University of Minnesota, utilizes a detubularized U-shaped 30-cm sigmoid segment for bladder replacement (20). The use of sigmoid allows for a simpler urethral anastomosis (because the pouch is already in close approximation with the membranous urethra), and nonrefluxing ureteral implantation. Contraindications to the use of sigmoid colon for a reservoir include diverticulosis, colon polyps, or inflammatory large bowel disease. Therefore, the colon must be thoroughly examined by barium enema or colonoscopy (17) (Fig. 28A.5). In addition, it is our impression that the rate of nocturnal enuresis and uninhibited contractions is higher when using sigmoid rather than ileum.

DIVERSION CONSIDERATIONS

Selection of Bowel Segment

Though any bowel segment can be used to fashion a urinary reservoir, each type of intestine has associated electrolyte abnormalities. These differences can be significant and may affect the type of bowel segment used in a particular patient. Factors such as renal function, previous abdominal surgery, and type of diversion will affect the intestinal segment utilized.

Stomach

The use of the stomach has advantages and disadvantages compared to other bowel segments for urinary diversion. Of all bowel segments, the stomach has the lowest permeability to urinary solutes. In addition, the stomach has been reported to have lower rates of bacteriuria due to acidified urine (21). Due to proton and chloride secretion, the stomach will acidify the urine, producing a hypochoremic metabolic alkalosis. Typically, with normal renal function, this does not pose a significant problem. However, if impairment of bicarbonate excretion exists, such as in patients with renal insufficiency, the stomach should be avoided. In addition, patients may develop hematuria-dysuria syndrome due to excess acid production by the stomach portion utilized.

TABLE 28A.2

RECONSTRUCTIVE PROCEDURES TO CREATE AN ORTHOTOPIC BLADDER

Types of orthotopic neobladder procedure	Segment of bowel
Camey	Ileum
Hautmann with chimney	Ileum
Studer	Ileum
Hemi-Koch	Ileum
T-Pouch	Ileum
Mainz	Ileocolic
LeBag	Right colon
Reddy	Sigmoid colon

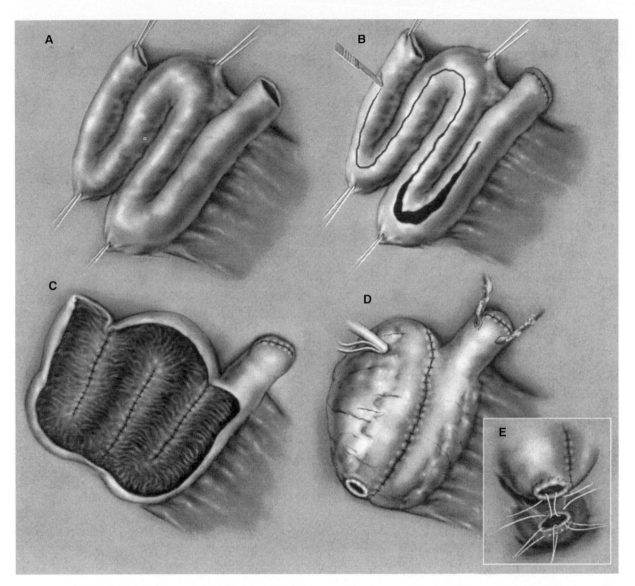

FIGURE 28A.3. Hautmann neobladder with chimney modification operative technique. **A:** A 60-cm segment of ileum is isolated and positioned in to a "W" configuration, leaving an extra 8 cm as a "chimney." **B:** The bowel is detubularized along the antimesenteric border. **C:** The posterior plate is sewn together using absorbable running sutures. **D:** The neobladder is fully closed, the ureters are implanted, and the mucosa at the urethral opening everted. **E:** The neobladder to urethra anastomosis is created. (Reprinted from Droller MJ, ed. *Current clinical urology: bladder cancer: current diagnosis and treatment.* Totowa, NJ: Humana Press, 2001:357, with permission.)

Jejunum

The use of the jejunum for urinary diversion is typically avoided due to the significant side effects. Use of the jejunum results in severe electrolyte imbalance secondary to increased sodium and chloride secretion combined with potassium and hydrogen ion reabsorption. This leads to hyponatremia, hypochoremia, hyperkalemia, and acidosis. Sodium and chloride loss is associated with water and volume loss, resulting in severe dehydration. These problems are more prominent when the proximal jejunum is used.

Ileum/Colon

The ileum and colon are often used for urinary diversion. Both segments are easily mobilized, have good mesenteric blood supply, and cause minimal electrolyte problems. The electrolyte abnormalities that occur with the use of the ileum and the colon are similar. Most patients will develop a hyperchloremic metabolic acidosis secondary to ammonium chloride reabsorption (22). This usually does not pose a problem for patients with normal renal function (serum creatinine <2.0 mg/dL), but in severe cases may cause lethargy, loss of appetite, and weight loss. Treatment involves alkalinizing medications or chloride transport blockers or maintaining adequate hydration and minimizing urinary stasis. Specific complications from the use of ileum include vitamin B_{12} malabsorption, fat malabsorption, and diarrhea. The use of colon typically will not encounter nutritional problems unless the ileocecal valve is removed from bowel continuity. In those cases, diarrhea and bacterial colonization of the ileum with associated fluid and bicarbonate loss may occur.

Selection of Diversion Type

The decision process involved in the selection of a urinary diversion involves many factors and cannot be reduced to a simple

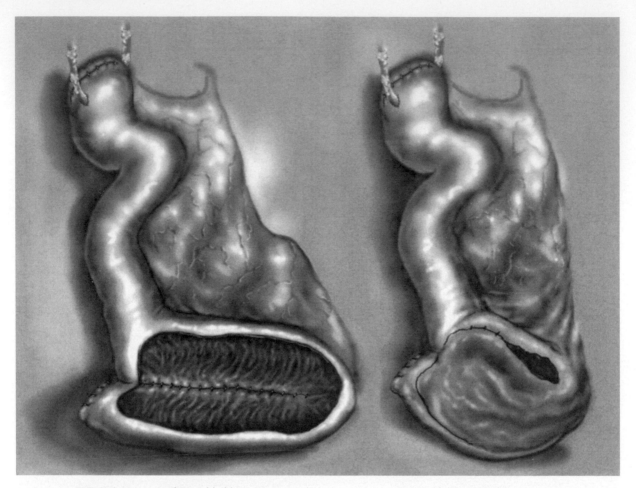

FIGURE 28A.4. Studer neobladder operative technique. A 60-cm segment of ileum is isolated and the distal 40 cm are detubularized and fashioned into a "U" configuration. B: The "U" is closed with running absorbable sutures and the ureters implanted into the isoperistaltic limb. (Reprinted from Droller MJ, ed. *Current clinical urology: bladder cancer: current diagnosis and treatment.* Totowa, NJ: Humana Press, 2001:349, with permission.)

algorithm. Patient, family, and physician discussion is encouraged. Important factors in the decision tree include the goal of surgery, patient physical and mental status, previous treatment history, surgical margins, and the method of diversion itself. With proper planning, all forms of urinary diversion can be well accepted (23).

If palliation is the primary goal of surgery, then the simplest surgical procedure is probably the best option (24). However, if cure is the goal, then any diversion is acceptable as long as cancer cure is not compromised (1). The stage and location of the patient's tumor can play a major role in the choices available. In women, urethral and anterior vaginal wall involvement with cancer is a contraindication to orthotopic neobladder reconstruction. Stein et al., in an extensive histological review, found that involvement of the bladder neck with cancer is a significant risk factor for urethral and anterior vaginal wall involvement (25). Frozen-section analysis of the distal surgical margin is sufficient for determining risk of concomitant urethral urothelial cancer and possibly of recurrence (26); however, long-term follow-up is necessary to assess the risk of recurrence. In men, a positive urethral margin or prostatic stromal involvement with urothelial carcinoma are contraindications for neobladder reconstruction secondary to the increased risk of urethral disease bladder recurrence (27).

Though the idea of a continent urinary diversion is attractive to most patients, several limitations exist as to who may receive these forms of reconstruction. These can be separated into absolute and relative contraindications and are listed in Table 28A.3. Patients must have both the physical and mental agility to perform self-catheterization before consideration of any continent diversion. This is obvious for patients with catheterizable stomas. Patients with orthotopic neobladders may have an increased risk of requiring long-term intermittent catheterization (especially women) and must be determined preoperatively to be able to do so (28).

In any form of reconstruction in which the bowel serves as a reservoir, absorption of urinary solutes occurs. Therefore, renal reserve must be able to compensate for this degree of absorption. In addition, free water loss will occur in bowel reservoirs and any patient with compromised urine-concentrating ability may have problems with dehydration. The minimum accepted creatinine clearance for continent diversion is 40–50 mL/min and any patient with a serum creatinine level greater than 2.0 mg/dL should be further evaluated (9). In patients whose serum creatinine exceeds 2.0 mg/dL, a detailed assessment of renal function is necessary. Such patients may still be candidates for orthotopic diversion if they can produce a urinary pH of <5.8 following an ammonium chloride load, can concentrate their urine to greather than 600 mOsm/kg in response to water restriction, have minimal proteinuria, and have a glomerular filtration rate of greater than 35 mL/min. Renal deterioration

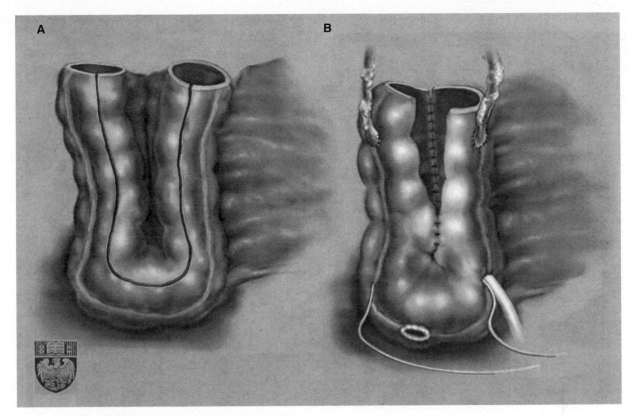

FIGURE 28A.5. Reddy sigmoid neobladder operative technique. **A:** A 30-cm segment of sigmoid colon is isolated, detubularized along the antimesenteric border, and fashioned into a "U" configuration. **B:** The pouch is sewn closed with absorbable running sutures, the ureters implanted, and the urethral anastomosis created. (Reprinted from Droller MJ, ed. *Current clinical urology: bladder cancer: current diagnosis and treatment*. Totowa, NJ, Humana Press, 2001:361, with permission.)

after intestinal diversion has been shown to vary between 10% and 60%.

Several relative contraindications to continent diversion have since been dispelled. Advanced patient age (greater than 70) is not necessarily a factor when considering continent diversion. A differentiation must be made between physiologic

TABLE 28A.3

INDICATIONS FOR EXTERNAL COLLECTING DEVICE DIVERSION

Absolute Indications
Impaired renal function
Impaired hepatic function
Impaired physical ability to perform self-catheterization
  (quadriplegia, severe multiple sclerosis)
Inability to understand the significance of and possible
  complications associated with a continent diversion
Inability or unwillingness to comply with patient demands
  associated with continent diversion

Relative Indications
Advanced age
Postoperative chemotherapy
Radiation to pelvis
Bowel disease (colitis, regional enteritis, cancer)
Body habitus
Abnormal urethra
Impaired functional status

age and chronological age in the decision-making process. Recent studies have shown that age is not significant in determining continence after undergoing orthotopic diversion (29). However, inability to void to completion and risk of nocturnal enuresis may be increased in patients over the age of 70.

Until recently, orthotopic neobladder was solely performed in men. It was thought that women were at greater risk for urinary incontinence and local tumor recurrence. As previously discussed, urethral involvement of tumor is rare in the absence of bladder neck involvement. The early fear of urinary incontinence is also unfounded as more recent studies have shown that in reality hypercontinence is a greater risk, with as many as 20% to 40% of women requiring clean intermittent catheterization (30). The etiology of hypercontinence is presently unknown, but may be due to angulation of the urethral neobladder neck angle due to increased pelvic floor descent with filling of the neobladder with urine. However, with the appropriate selection criteria, orthotopic neobladder substitution in women provides excellent long-term functional results.

Little difference exists in the selection criteria for orthotopic and continent cutaneous urinary diversions. Patients who qualify for continent cutaneous diversion usually also qualify for orthotopic diversion unless preoperative urethral involvement is noted or a urethral margin is discovered at the time of cystectomy.

Comparison

Currently, the morbidity and mortality rates of continent and noncontinent urinary diversions have been shown to be similar

(23,31–33). Therefore, assessing the QOL after urinary tract reconstruction has become increasingly important. Despite the effort to create a urinary diversion that most closely mimics the form and function of the original bladder, very little data exists to prove the benefits of one type of urinary diversion over another. One study reported diversion related problems in 62% of all patients after radical cystectomy, with urinary leakage and odor the most prevalent complaint (34).

Continence

Although many facets must be met in restoring normal urinary function after urinary reconstruction, perhaps the most important is the prevention of urinary leakage. In our institution, patients with severe incontinence from other causes will often opt for a conduit diversion rather than tolerate the odor and difficulty of urinary leakage. In part, continent urinary diversions were developed to minimize the detrimental effects associated with stomal leakage.

Conduit diversions can be associated with leakage from loose-fitting appliances, poorly positioned stomas, and nocturnal leakage. This risk can be minimized with proper enterostomal care including preoperative and perioperative visits from an enterostomal therapist. Also, continuous improvements are being made in the external appliances and surgical techniques used.

Continent urinary diversions can also be associated with episodes of incontinence. The Indiana Pouch is associated with a low risk of urinary leakage from the stoma; however, it is also associated with a risk of catheterization problems and a 15% to 20% reoperation rate for all complications. In general, the efferent limb ("catheterizable" portion) of the Indiana pouch should be no more than 8 cm to 10 cm in length and be a "straight shot" from the skin to the pouch to avoid kinking and redundancy of the efferent limb. The orthotopic neobladder has been found to have daytime continence rates of up to 95%. However, approximately 4% to 10% of male patients and up to 40% of female patients develop "hypercontinence" and require clean intermittent catheterization (15). Nocturnal enuresis is more problematic in patients with orthotopic diversion and is present in up to 25% of patients. The etiology is multifactorial and includes increased urine output at night with aging, increased urine output due to reabsorption of hypertonic acidic urine, decreased urethral closing pressure, pelvic floor relaxation, injury to the rhabdosphincter, loss of spinal reflexes governing sphincteric contraction during sleep, medications taken at nighttime, or uninhibited contractions. In general, most patients need to void 2 to 3 times during the night to maintain nocturnal continence. In an unpublished comparison study between female patients undergoing radical cystectomy with either orthotopic neobladder or Indiana pouch, Katz et al. found that continence rates were similar. Mild stress incontinence can be seen in orthotopic neobladders and can be simply managed with light urinary pads. Hypercontinence in the case of neobladders can be managed by clean intermittent catheterization, but this leads to significantly higher reports of anxiety and depression compared with patients who volitionally void by valsalva alone. However, overall well-being and subjective QOL scores are similar in the two groups (35).

Mucus production from the intestinal segment used to create the urinary diversion can occasionally cause urethral obstruction or impair conduit/pouch emptying. It is thought that the mucus production decreases with time, especially with small bowel segments. In a study by N'Dow, the majority of patients with neobladder formation had some degree of mucus obstruction, while patients with ileal conduits rarely developed mucus obstruction. In fact, approximately 13% of patients with neobladders underwent surgery for mucus-related problems, while no patients with ileal conduit did (36). However, with time, mucus production decreases and urethral obstruction with mucus plugs becomes rare. In our experience, most patients with orthotopic diversion can void mucus plugs per urethra satisfactorily.

Quality of Life

Cystectomy has been shown to adversely affect most aspects of a patient's life. Therefore the surgeon must carefully consider an individual's desires and needs when planning the proper urinary diversion (37). Each patient must receive individualized treatment and receive the maximum information on outcomes for various treatment modalities. These outcomes must include not only cancer cure and survival, but also the patient's QOL after cystectomy.

Few measurements of QOL based on the type of urinary diversion the patient received after cystectomy exist. Many factors go toward measuring a patient's post-treatment satisfaction, and no general consensus has been reached on the best method to measure QOL. Studies that have attempted to determine health-related QOL following cystectomy run into similar design flaws. Most older studies utilize nonvalidated questionnaires, while newer studies only use portions of validated questionnaires in combination with nonvalidated forms in order to make the inventory more specific to urinary diversion.

Currently, there is no validated questionnaire to specifically measure QOL in patients with urinary diversion. However, several generic validated questionnaires have been utilized to measure QOL after radical cystectomy and urinary diversion. These include the general health SF-36 Quality of Life Survey and Sickness Impact Profile (SIP) surveys, as well as the cancer-specific QLQ-C30 and Functional Assessment of Cancer Therapy general score (FACT-G) surveys (38–41). Recently, Mansson and Mansson introduced a bladder cancer–specific questionnaire; however, it is not yet shown whether this will yield different results than in previous studies with generic questionnaires (42).

Since urinary leakage is a significant complaint after cystectomy, one would assume that a continent diversion would have less impact on a patient's lifestyle and health-related satisfaction (43). Despite this notion that patients with a continent diversion have improved QOL compared to patients with ileal or colon conduits, published reports have not substantiated this belief (Table 28A.4). Several studies comparing ileal conduit with orthotopic neobladder urinary diversion have shown no significant difference in health related QOL (44,45).

Conversely, other studies have shown a significant benefit with an orthotopic neobladder compared with ileal conduit. Dutta et al. reported a trend toward improved QOL scores for patients with orthotopic neobladders. Both groups appear satisfied with their type of diversion; however, emotional and functional well-being was improved with a neobladder (46). One study of 102 patients after cystectomy and either orthotopic neobladder ($n = 69$) or ileal conduit ($n = 33$) demonstrated significantly higher QOL for neobladder patients than for ileal conduit patients using the QLQ-C30 and an additional supplement. They further reported that 97% of neobladder patients would recommend the same urinary diversion to other patients needing a cystectomy, while only 36% of conduit patients would do so (31).

Sexual Function

One of the primary complaints following cystectomy with any form of urinary diversion is sexual dysfunction (34). Patients experience an overall decrease in sexual desire, interaction with their partners, and sexual activities. Previously, this had been shown to be more profound in patients with ileal conduits compared with continent cutaneous diversions (52). Embarrassment about wearing an appliance during sexual intercourse can inhibit patients. This reaction can be limited by proper preoperative and postoperative counseling.

TABLE 28A.4

COMPARISON OF DIVERSIONS

Authors	Number of points	Number of points per diversion	Questionnaire type	QOL results	Significance
Hara et al. (2002) (44)	85	IC–37 NB–48	SF-36	NB = IC	
Dutta et al. (2002) (46)	72	IC–23 NB–49	SF-36 FACT-G	NB > IC	NS
Hobisch et al. (2000) (31)	102	IC–33 NB–69	EORTC QLQ-C30 and supplement	NB > IC	Signif
Fujisawa et al. (2000) (45)	56	IC–20 NB–36	SF-36	NB = IC	
McGuire et al. (2000) (47)	92	IC–38 CR–16 NB–38	SF-36	NB = CR > IC	Signif
Hart et al. (1999) (34)	221	IC–25 CR–93 NB–103	4 adapted, validated questionnaires	NB > CR > IC	Signif
Kitamura et al. (1999) (48)	79	IC–36 CR–22 NB–21	Nonvalidated questionnaire	NB = CR = IC	
Weijerman et al. (1998) (14)	56	CR–23 NB–33	Sickness impact profile + supplement	NB > CR	NS
Sullivan et al. (1998) (43)	55	CR–10 NB–45	Nonvalidated questionnaire	NB = CR	
Gerharz et al. (1997) (49)	192	IC–131 CR–61	Nonvalidated questionnaire	CR > IC	NS
Bjerre et al. (1994) (50)	76	IC–50 CR–26	Nonvalidated questionnaire	CR > IC	Signif
Mansson et al. (1988) (51)	60	IC or CC–40 CR–20	Nonvalidated questionnaire	CR > IC	Signif
Boyd et al. (1987) (52)	172	IC–87 NB or CR–85	4 adapted, validated questionnaires	NB > IC	NS

IC, ileal conduit; CC, colon conduit; CR, continent reservoir; NB, neobladder; NS, not significant.

Inherent to cystectomy in men is the risk of erectile dysfunction caused by damage to the autonomic nerves from the sacral parasympathetic plexus to the corpora cavernosa. This has been improved after the discovery of nerve-sparing cystectomy by Schlegel, as first reported in 1987 (53). Nerve-sparing techniques have not been associated with greater risk of cancer recurrence (54). Restoration of sexual function can be seen in up to 70% of patients and is dependent on patient age, size and location of the tumor, and surgical technique. In patients who fail sexual function preservation, Hart has shown a significant improvement in sexual function and satisfaction in patients who received penile implants (34).

Anterior pelvic exenteration in women can cause vaginal scarring, decreased vault size, and reduced vaginal lubrication, resulting in painful intercourse and loss of sexual function. This can be managed with the creation of a "neovagina" using myocutaneous muscle flaps or intestine. Women of childbearing age with an ileal conduit must be informed that there is a decrease in the absorption of oral birth control pills, and therefore other forms of contraception are recommended. Furthermore, the displacement of the stoma by the enlarging uterus can occur, causing difficulty in managing the stoma.

CONCLUSION

Though no form of diversion currently exists that can precisely mimic the function of the native bladder, many viable options exist for the diversion and reconstruction of the urinary tract. Each of these forms of urinary diversion offered in this chapter has met the test of durability and patient tolerance. Selection of the proper urinary reconstruction is based upon patient and physician discussion, with important patient-specific and cancer-specific criteria that must be met. However, with the proper counseling and preparation of patient expectations, any of these urinary diversions can provide patients with an excellent QOL after cystectomy.

References

1. Hautmann RE, Bachor R. Bladder substitutes for continent urinary diversion. *Monogr Urol* 1994;15:47–59.
2. Benson MC, Olsson CA. Urinary diversion. *Urol Clin North Am* 1992;19: 779–795.

3. Wein AJ. Pathophysiology and categorization of voiding dysfunction. In: Walsh PC, Retik AB, Vaughan ED et al., eds. *Campbell's urology*, 8th ed. Philadelphia, PA: WB Saunders, 2002:887–899.

4. Bricker E. Bladder substitution after pelvic evisceration. *Surg Clin North Am* 1950;30:1511.

5. Hinman F. Selection of intestinal segments for bladder substitution: physical and physiological characteristics. *J Urol* 1988;139:519.

6. Persky L. Large and small bowel urinary conduits. In: Glenn JF, ed. *Urologic surgery*, 4th ed. Philadelphia, PA: JB Lippincott Co, 1991:1 004–1012.

7. Bachor R, Hautmann R. Options in urinary diversion: a review and critical assessment. *Semin Urol* 1993;11:235–250.

8. Gilchrist RK, Merricks JW, Hamlin HH, et al. Construction of a substitute bladder and urethra. *Surg Gynecol Obstet* 1950;90:752–760.

9. Benson MC, Olsson CA. Cutaneous continent urinary diversion. In: Walsh PC, Retik AB, Vaughan ED et al., eds. *Campbell's urology*, 8th ed. Philadelphia, PA: WB Saunders, 2002:3789–3834.

10. Rowland RG, Mitchell ME, Bihrle R, et al. The cecoileal continent urinary reservoir. *World J Urol* 1985;3:185.

11. Rowland RG, Kropp BP. Evolution of the Indiana continent urinary reservoir. *J Urol* 1994;152:2247–2251.

12. Bihrle R. The Indiana pouch continent urinary reservoir. *Urol Clin North Am* 1997;24:773–779.

13. Steinberg GD, Rinker-Schaeffer CW, Sokoloff MH, et al. Highlights of the Urologic Oncology Meeting June 2, 2001. *J Urol* 2002;168: 653–659.

14. Weijerman PC, Schurmans JR, Hop WC, et al. Morbidity and quality of life in patients with orthotopic and heterotopic continent urinary diversion. *Urol* 1998;51(1):51–56.

15. Hautmann RE, Depetriconi R, Gottfried H, et al. The ileal neobladder: complications and functional results in 363 patients after 11 years of follow-up. *J Urol* 1999;161:422–428.

16. Lippert CM, Theodorescu D. The Hautmann neobladder with chimney: a versatile modification. *J Urol* 1997;158:1510–1512.

17. Hollowell CM, Steinberg GD, Rowland RG. Current concepts of urinary diversion in men. In: Droller MJ, ed. *Current clinical urology: bladder cancer: current diagnosis and treatment*, Totowa, NJ: Humana Press, 2001: 343–366.

18. Stein JP, Skinner DG. Orthotopic urinary diversion. In: Walsh PC, Retik AB, Vaughan ED, eds. *Campbell's urology*, 8th ed. Philadelphia, PA: WB Saunders, 2002:3835–3867.

19. Studer UR, Danuser H, Merz VW, et al. Experience in 100 patients with an ileal low pressure bladder substitute combined with an efferent tubular isoperistaltic segment. *J Urol* 1995;154:49–56.

20. Reddy PK. Detubularized sigmoid reservoir for bladder replacement after cystoprostatectomy. *Urol* 1987;29(6):625–628.

21. Kurzrock EA, Baskin LS, Kogan BA. Gastrocystoplasty: is there a consensus? *World J Urol* 1998;16(4):242–250.

22. McDougal WS, Stampfer DS, Kirley S, et al. Intestinal ammonium transport by ammonium and hydrogen exchange. *J Am Coll Surg* 1995;181(3): 241–248.

23. Carlin BI, Rutchik SD, Resnick MI. Comparison of the ileal conduit to the continent cutaneous diversion and orthotopic neobladder in patients undergoing cystectomy: a critical analysis and review of the literature. *Semin Urol Oncol* 1997;15(3):189–192.

24. Montie JE, Pontes JE, Smyth EM. Selection of the type of urinary diversion in conjunction with radical cystectomy. *J Urol* 1987;137: 1154–1155.

25. Stein JP, Cote RJ, Freeman JA, et al. Indications for lower urinary tract reconstruction in women after cystectomy for bladder cancer: a pathological review of female cystectomy specimens. *J Urol* 1995;154(4): 1329–1333.

26. Stein JP, Esrig D, Freeman JA, et al. Prospective pathologic analysis of female cystectomy specimens: risk factors for orthotopic diversion in women. *Urol* 1998;51(6):951–955.

27. Iselin CE, Robertson CN, Webster GD, et al. Does prostate transitional cell carcinoma preclude orthotopic bladder reconstruction after radical cystoprostatectomy for bladder cancer? *J Urol* 1997;158(6): 2123–2126.

28. Steven K, Poulsen AL. The orthotopic Kock ileal neobladder: functional results, urodynamic features, complications and survival in 166 men. *J Urol* 2000;164:288.

29. Elmajian DA, Stein JP, Esrig D, et al. The Kock ileal neobladder: updated experience in 295 male patients. *J Urol* 1996;156(3):920–925.

30. Stein JP, Stenzl A, Grossfeld GD, et al. The use of orthotopic neobladders in women undergoing cystectomy for pelvic malignancy. *World J Urol* 1996; 14(1):9–14.

31. Hobisch A, Tosun K, Kinzl J, et al. Quality of life after cystectomy and orthotopic neobladder versus ileal conduit urinary diversion. *World J Urol* 2000;18:338–344.

32. Laven BA, O'Connor RC, Steinberg GS, et al. Long-term results of antegrade endoureterotomy using the holmium laser in patients with ureterointestinal strictures. *Urology* 2001;58(6):924–929.

33. Gburek B, Lieber M, Blute M. Comparison of Studer ileal neobladder and ileal conduit urinary diversion with respect to perioperative outcome and late complications. *J Urol* 1998;160(3-1):721–723.

34. Hart S, Skinner E, Meyerowitz B, et al. Quality of life after radical cystectomy for bladder cancer in patients with an ileal conduit, or cutaneous or urethral Koch pouch. *J Urol* 1999;162(1):77–81.

35. Henningsohn L, Steven K, Kallestrup EL, et al. Distressful symptoms and well-being after radical cystectomy and orthotopic bladder substitution compared with a matched control population. *J Urol* 2002;168: 168–175.

36. N'Dow J, Robson CN, Matthews JN, et al. Reducing mucus production after urinary reconstruction: a prospective randomized trial. *J Urol* 2001; 165(5):1433–1440.

37. Mansson A, Caruso A, Capovilla S, et al. Quality of life after radical cystectomy and orthotopic bladder substitution: a comparison between Italian and Swedish men. *BJU Int* 2000;85:26–31.

38. Ware JE. *S7-36: Health Status Questionnaire*. Boston: Quality Quest Inc., 1989.

39. Aaronson NK, Ahmedzai S, Bergman B, et al. The European Organization for Research and Treatment of Cancer QLQ-C30: a quality-of-life instrument for use in international clinical trials in oncology. *J Natl Cancer Inst* 1993;85(5):365.

40. Da Silva FC, Fossa SD, Aaronson NK, et al. The quality of life of patients with newly diagnosed prostate cancer: experience with EORTC clinical trial 30853. *Eur J Cancer* 1996;32A:72.

41. Bergner M, Bobbitt RA, Carter WB, et al. The Sickness Impact Profile: development and final revision of a health status measure. *Med Care* 1981;19(8):787–805.

42. Mansson A, Mansson W. When the bladder is gone: quality of life following different types of urinary diversion. *World J Urol* 1999;17: 211–218.

43. Sullivan LD, Chow VDW, Ko DSC, et al. An evaluation of quality of life in patients with continent urinary diversions after cystectomy. *Br J Urol* 1998; 81:699–704.

44. Hara I, Miyake H, Hara S, et al. Health-related quality of life after radical cystectomy for bladder cancer: a comparison of ileal conduit and orthotopic bladder replacement. *BJU Int* 2002;89:10–13.

45. Fugisawa M, Isotani S, Gotoh A, et al. Health-related quality of life with orthotopic neobladder versus ileal conduit according to the SF-36 survey. *Urol* 2000;55(6):862–865.

46. Dutta SA, Chang SS, Coffey CS, et al. Health related quality of life assessment after radical cystectomy: comparison of ileal conduit with continent orthotopic neobladder. *J Urol* 2002;168:164–167.

47. McGuire MS, Grimaldi G, Grotas J, et al. The type of urinary diversion after radical cystectomy significantly impacts on the patient's quality of life. *Ann Surg Oncol* 2000;7(1):4–8.

48. Kitamura H, Miyao N, Yanase M, et al. Quality of life in patients having an ileal conduit, continent reservoir or orthotopic neobladder after cystectomy for bladder carcinoma. *Int J Urol* 1999;6:393–399.

49. Gerharz E, Weingartner K, Dopatka K, et al. Quality of life after cystectomy and urinary diversion: results of a retrospective interdisciplinary study. *J Urol* 1997;158(3):778–785.

50. Bjerre BD, Johansen C, Steven K. Health-related quality of life after urinary diversion: continent diversion with Koch pouch compared with ileal conduit. A questionnaire study. *Scand J Urol Nephrol Suppl* 1994;157: 113–118.

51. Mansson A, Johnson G, Mansson W. Quality of life after cystectomy. Comparison between patients with conduit and those with continent caecal reservoir urinary diversions. *Br J Urol* 1988;62(3):240–245.

52. Boyd SD, Feinberg SM, Skinner DG, et al. Quality of life survey of urinary diversion patients: comparison of ileal conduits versus continent Kock ileal reservoirs. *J Urol* 1987;138(6):1386–1389.

53. Schlegal PN, Walsh PC. New anatomical approach to radical cystoprostatectomy with preservation of sexual function. *J Urol* 1987;138: 1402.

54. Brendler CB, Steinberg GD, Marshall FF, et al. Local recurrence and survival following nerve sparing radical cystoprostatectomy. *J Urol* 1990;144: 1137.

CHAPTER 28B
Orthotopic Bladder Substitution

Richard E. Hautmann

INTRODUCTION

Choosing the best type of orthotopic diversion and enteric segment should include the consideration of multiple factors including volume capacity, pressure characteristics and urodynamic behavior of the reservoir, vesicoureteral reflux (VUR), renal function, upper tract safety, metabolic safety, previous surgical and/or radiation history, and potential for complications (1).

The primary goal of orthotopic reconstruction is to improve the quality of life. Consequently continence is the single most important factor. Continence is determined by sphincteric competence as well as reservoir behavior.

VOLUME CAPACITY

Perioperatively, reservoirs constructed from ileum have a volume of approximately 100 cc, while reservoirs made from large bowel have a capacity of 200 to 300 cc, given that the taenia has been divided in several places. At 1 month postoperatively both types of reservoirs have an almost identical maximal volume capacity of about 300 cc. During the first year following its construction, an ileal reservoir increases to 600 to 700 cc, while reservoirs from large bowel reach 400 cc. Usually the expansion of all types of reservoirs ends after 4 to 12 months, unless obstruction occurs or the patient tries to expand the reservoir capacity intentionally.

In summary: In reservoirs constructed from large bowel, the final volume is significantly smaller than in ileal reservoirs (2).

PRESSURE CHARACTERISTICS

Contraction pressure waves appear in all types of reservoirs. They are seen when an ileal reservoir has been distended to 50% ± 20% of the maximal volume capacity and the highest pressure waves 1 year postoperatively are about 40 cm water.

In reservoirs made from large bowel, contraction pressure waves appear at all filling volumes. The amplitude and frequency of the pressure waves increase with greater volumes in the reservoir but do not change with an increasing time interval after the operation. The amplitude of the highest pressure wave recorded at one year postoperatively is about 90 cm water. Berglund and Kock (2) calculated the motor activity as the area under the pressure curves expressed in cm². The motor activity increased with larger filling volumes in all types of reservoirs. The motor activity decreased significantly during the first postoperative year in reservoirs made from ileum but not in reservoirs from large bowel. Ileal as well as cecal reservoirs had a low basal pressure during filling, even though the pressure in the large bowel reservoir was significantly higher when volumes were in excess of 400 cc. There was, however ten times more motor activity in large bowel reservoirs than in ileal reservoirs.

Long-lasting obstruction to urinary flow leads to renal deterioration. Pyelorenal backflow occurs as a result of obstruction even, to some extent, at a pelvic pressure of approximately 20 cm of water. With increasing pressure there is a substantial increase of the backflow. Glomerular net filtration pressure is calculated to be 25 to 30 cm of water, and the amplitude of the peristaltic waves in the ureters is normally less than 10 cm of

water. In view of these figures, long-lasting periods with pressure exceeding about 25 cm of water in the urinary receptacle will in the long run probably impair renal function by impeding the urine flow. Patients with a continent ileal reservoir for urinary diversion utilize approximately 60% of the maximal volume capacity during the daytime, that is, about 300 to 500 cc. At this reservoir volume, the pressure exceeds zero by more than 25 cm water during only about 2 minutes per hour (2).

At volumes of 300 to 500 cc in the cecal reservoir, the percentage of recorded time when pressure exceeded zero by more than 25 cm water was about 20 munutes per hour. In order to avoid exceeding 2 minutes per hour, which was the case for the ileal reservoir at the corresponding degree of filling, the volume in the cecal reservoir should not exceed 100 cc. It is obvious that these differences in pressure characteristics between the ileal and cecal reservoirs are of great importance and should be considered when a receptacle for urine is requested (2). An interesting comparison of the properties of different gut smooth muscles was made by Hohenfellner et al. (3), who examined the ileal and cecal segments incorporated into a canine model of the Mainz bladder substitution. Sonomicrometry transducers were implanted in the circular and longitudinal muscular layers to allow measurements of their properties. It was found that the circular ileal layer was most distensible, followed by the colonic circular and longitudinal ileal layers. The longitudinal layer of the colonic segment was relatively indistensible.

In summary: The detubularized ileal reservoir for either continent stomal diversion or bladder replacement would seem to constitute the ideal low pressure reservoir (4,5) (Table 28B.1).

URODYNAMICS/CONTINENCE

Most investigators have reported on a single type of orthotopic diversion. Santucci et al. (6) performed six different continent

---

TABLE 28B.1

CAPACITY AND PRESSURE CHARACTERISTICS OF RESERVOIRS

	Ileum	Colon
Volume increase		
Initially		Advantage
Late	Advantage	
Capacity		
First contraction	Advantage	
Maximum contraction	Advantage	
Involuntary contractions		
Maximum amplitude	Advantage	
Motor activity (calculated)		10–20 × higher
Distensibility		
ICL > CCL > ILL > CLL	Advantage	
Compliance	Advantage	

ICL, ileal circular layer; CCL, colonic circular layer; ILL, ileal longitudinal layer; CLL, colonic longitudinal layer.
Data from Berglund B, Kock NG. Volume capacity and pressure characteristics of various types of intestinal reservoirs. *World J Surg* 1987; 11:798; Hohenfellner M, Buerger R, Schad H, et al. Reservoir characteristics of Mainz pouch studied in animal model osmolality of filling solution an effect of oxybutinin. *Urology* 1993;42:741; Colding-Jørgensen M, Poulsen AL, Steven K. Mechanical characteristics of tubular and detubularised bowel for bladder substitution: theory, urodynamics and clinical results. *Br J Uro* 1993;72:586; Goldwasser B, Madgar I, Hanani Y. Urodynamic aspects of continent urinary diversion. Review. *Scand J Urol Nephrol* 1987;21:245.

urinary reconstructions and reported their continence and uro-dynamic parameters: stomal urinary reservoirs had the best continence rates: Indiana pouch, 100%; Mainz pouch 91%. Neobladder continence rates were as follows: Hautmann, 80%; Mainz, 75%; sigmoid, 50%; and gastric, 33%. Day and night incontinence rates were nearly identical. Compared with the other pouches, gastric and sigmoid reconstructions had the smallest capacity, were the least compliant, and were the most contractile (8).

Santucci et al. (6) concluded that stomal urinary reservoirs using ileocecal valve and right colon, with or without an over-lying patch of ileum, provide similar excellent results. Continence approached 100% in compliant patients without the need for revision. Patients with neobladders were less continent, although those with ileal or ileocecal configurations still had very good continence rates. Neobladders of sigmoid or stomach can be used when necessary, but with greater incontinence rates. This poorer continence can be explained by the decreased capacity, decreased compliance, and a tendency toward high pressure spikes despite detubularization.

Metabolic Considerations

Potential metabolic consequences in the early postoperative period, as well as long term, remain a serious problem. Because the absorptive and secretory capacities of each portion of intestine are different, each portion results in a different clinical syndrome. Furthermore, the severity of metabolic complications after urinary reconstruction with any of the segments is directly related to mucosal physiology, duration of contact between urine and intestinal mucosa, surface area of mucosa in contact with urine, urine solute concentration, and underlying physiologic state of the host (7). Complications related to disruption of the normal gastrointestinal tract also occur (Table 28B.2).

Stomach

Hypochloremic metabolic alkalosis can occur when portions of stomach are utilized in urinary reconstruction. HCl secretion by the gastric segment is coupled with systemic bicarbonate release. Renal bicarbonate excretion (compensation) is impaired in persons with compromised renal function, and this condition exacerbates alkalosis. For this reason, the isolated use of stomach for urinary reconstruction is discouraged in persons with renal function impairment. When stomach is utilized in orthotopic bladder reconstruction, acid production may cause dysuria which, when fulminant, can manifest as the dysuria-hematuria syndrome. Both hyperaciduria and symptomatic metabolic alkalosis are effectively treated with histamine (H_2) receptor antagonists or by blocking the potassium/hydrogen exchanger itself with omeprazole (8).

Jejunum

The jejunal segment, exposed to a hyperosmotic, potassium-rich urine, loses more sodium and water while reabsorbing potassium, perpetuating the cycle. Jejunum is the least desirable bowel segment for urinary reconstruction because metabolic derangements are often more severe than with ileum or colon. Approximately 25% to 40% of patients with jejunum interposed in the urinary tract manifest metabolic abnormalities, more commonly with the proximal than with the distal segments. In its most severe form (the jejunal conduit syndrome, which results from the aforementioned imbalances), the patient presents with nausea, emesis, anorexia, lethargy, muscle weakness, and fever. Treatment of this condition involves correction of acidosis with bicarbonate and salt repletion, as well as continued maintenance with sodium chloride supplementation (8).

Ileum and Colon

The rather theoretical differences between small and large bowel are validated by clinical experience. Hyperchloremic acidosis is most prevalent following ureterosigmoidostomy, as urine may come in contact with the whole colonic mucosa. The frequency and severity of metabolic complications after ureterosigmoidostomy were major stimuli for the development of alternative procedures. Comparative studies of ileal and colonic pouches are limited because the absorptive surface areas are difficult to calculate. However, in the colon, chloride absorption and bicarbonate excretion are more pronounced, and evidence suggests that inherent chloride absorption is maintained when the colon is in contact with urine. Therefore, it may be preferable to use ileum rather than colon for bladder reconstruction to reduce the risk of hyperchloremic acidosis, particularly in the presence of renal impairment. Whichever segment of bowel is used, regular voiding or drainage to completion is important (9).

TABLE 28B.2

SUMMARY OF COMPLICATIONS AND TREATMENTS FOR RESERVOIRS MADE FROM STOMACH, JEJUNUM, AND ILEUM/COLON

Segment	Complications	Treatment
Stomach	Hypochloremic metabolic alkalosis Hypokalemia Hypochloremia Ulcers Dysuria hematuria syndrome (orthotopic)	H_2 blocker Omeprazole Do not use in renal impairment
Jejunum	Hypochloremic metabolic acidosis Hyperkalemia Dehydration, azotemia	NaCl Volume substitution
Ileum/colon	Hyperchloremic metabolic acidosis Hypokalemia (colon > ileum)	Alkalinizing agents Na and K citrate Block chloride transport Chlorpromazine Nicotinic acid

Adapted from Stampfer DS, McDougal WS, McGovern FJ. The use of bowel in urology. Metabolic and nutritional complications. *Urol Clin North Am* 1997;24(4):715.

Summary: Metabolic and nutritional complications of urinary diversion through bowel or stomach segments are common, but fortunately not often severe. When metabolic abnormalities are problematic, deterioration or baseline insufficiency in renal function is the most likely cause. Deterioration is most commonly associated with obstruction or infection. The urologist should be acutely aware of the potential for metabolic derangements when the prediversion creatinine level is greater than 2.0 mg/dL (8).

There are clear differences between ileum and colon in regard to metabolic consequences, but this is only one consideration when planning continent diversion. No clear advantage has yet been demonstrated for one bowel segment over another. Some doubt remains about the long-term consequences, particularly in regard to bone metabolism and secondary neoplasm. Many metabolic effects may be subtle, and only with continued follow-up, particularly of patients most at risk, will the consequences become known. As far as we can tell, and provided these caveats are rigorously respected, continent urinary diversion is an inherently safe procedure after cystectomy (9).

LENGTH OF ILEUM SEGMENT

The optimum length of the ileum segment to be used is a subject of considerable controversy.

Making the reservoir from 60 cm of ileum, what we recommend, instead of the 40 cm that Studer, Skinner, and Ghoneim (39,52,12) recommend, has the advantage that, with a 50% increase in bowel surface, almost double the capacity can be obtained. This results in prolonged micturition intervals, particularly at night, and less postoperative urinary incontinence because of more favorable pressure characteristics with a larger reservoir (law of Laplace). Our results show that improved urinary continence parallels the increase in functional capacity. The functional capacity of a reservoir made of 60 cm of ileum increases within days and, in elderly patients (who require more time to regain urinary continence), within weeks from approximately 150 cc to 650 cc.

The advocates of 40 cm ileum for the reservoir itself actually also use a 60 cm ileal segment (and an additional 20 cm for valves or afferent loops!), thus having the same surface and the same potential for metabolic complications. They claim to avoid the increased risk of a chronically infected reservoir, residual urine, or even the need for lifelong intermittent self-catheterization [Clean Intermittent Catherization (CIC)]. Moreover, if larger reservoirs were filled to the leaking point (with a pressure of 40 cm of water, for example, corresponding to the outlet resistance of the membranous urethra), then the tension on the reservoir's wall would be significantly higher than in smaller reservoirs with the same intraluminal pressure. Inevitably, therefore, larger reservoirs have an increased risk of urinary retention and of so-called "spontaneous" rupture, which did not occur in our patients (10).

Clinically, however, the opposite seems to be true. The largest reservoir (ileal neobladder 60 cm) has the lowest reported CIC rate, 3.9 % (11), as compared to the 8.8 % CIC rate of reservoirs made from 40 cm ileum (12). To understand this phenomenon one must remember that the pressure in a given reservoir begins to rise once the reservoir is "unfolded," that is to say, the geometric capacity has been reached. This occurs significantly later in the larger reservoir. On the other hand it is apparent that overdistension, which occurs significantly earlier in the smaller reservoir, reduces the pressure rise produced by partial contractions, and this pressure reduction may lead to better urinary retention (4).

A reservoir made from only 30 cm of ileum, 25% less than 40 cm, theoretically has a significantly decreased volume, from 500 cc down to 300 cc. This is confirmed by clinical experience showing that such patients have less satisfactory results with

regard to functional capacity, voiding intervals, and time to achieve urinary continence.

Summary: We use 60 cm of bowel for construction of the reservoir, and we do not recommend using less.

DETUBULARIZATION

Although it would be ideal if the bowel segment could contribute to voluntary voiding, in reality this does not seem to happen, and a highly compliant neobladder is the desired outcome (13). Detubularized bowel segments provide greater capacity at lower pressure, and require a shorter length of intestine than do intact segments. Four factors account for their superiority: (i) their configuration takes advantage of the geometric fact that volume increases by the square of the radius, so that a pouch has a larger diameter than a tube, (ii) they accommodate to filling more readily because, as Laplace law states, the container with the greater radius and, thus, the greater mural tension will hold larger volumes at lower pressure, (iii) compliance is superior to that of the tubular bowel, and (iv) contractile ability is blunted by the failure of contractions to encompass the entire circumference (14). These theoretical considerations are consistent with clinical observations showing that detubularization increases reservoir capacity substantially and delays the onset and reduces the amplitude of the pressure rise produced by contractions. These findings account for the markedly improved nocturnal continence (80% versus 17% at 2 years), the longer voiding intervals (4 versus 2.5 hours at 1 year), and the predisposition to urinary retention (25% versus 0% at 1 year) with detubularized bladder substitution. Altering the shape of a reservoir from spherical to ellipsoid is calculated to have only a slight effect on its mechanical characteristics. Consequently the essence of detubularization is to create a reservoir with high capacity, while shape is of secondary importance (15).

COMPARISON OF ILEAL, ILEOCOLIC, RIGHT COLIC, AND SIGMOID RESERVOIRS

There are clear differences between ileum and colon in regard to metabolic consequences. Due to the reduced absorption of electrolytes in ileal urinary reservoirs, it seems that ileum is preferable to large bowel for storing urine, at least in patients with decreased kidney function and increased risk for metabolic disorders. However, this is only one consideration when planning orthotopic reconstruction.(9,16).

An obvious advantage of the sigmoid reservoir is its ease of accessibility. However there is the substantial disadvantage of high reservoir pressures, as compared to those in cecum or ileum reservoirs, that is confirmed by most urodynamic studies (6,17). We, like others, use a sigmoid reservoir only in cases in which ileum or right colon are not available (18). An advantage of the ileocolonic reservoir is its greatest initial volume of a reservoir. However, it requires mobilization of the entire right colon and is potentially the most tedious procedure to perform (18). The greatest disadvantage of the procedure is the loss of the ileocecal valve, leading to the chronic loss of bile acids with the potential risks of hyperoxaluria and gall bladder stone formations, as well as diarrhea (9). There is also a greater risk of vitamin B_{12} deficiency secondary to resection of terminal ileum. Most investigators have reported on one single type of diversion, but Santucci et al. performed six different continent urinary reservoir operations which revealed remarkably different continence rates and urodynamic data. Their experience suggests that neobladders composed of stomach or sigmoid should be used only under unusual circumstances because of high rates of incontinence (6).

Ileal reservoirs are the most common form of neobladders used worldwide. There are three major categories:

The hemi Kock, originally developed by Kock, was popularized by Skinner and associates (19). The most recent modification (T pouch) is technically complex, unnecessarily time consuming, and has yet to be widely adopted.

The second type of ileal reservoir, initially described by Studer et al., has the advantage of an afferent limb that facilitates placement of the ileoureterostomies but without any valve formation (20).

The third type of ileal reservoir is the ileal neobladder, a W-shaped reservoir as described by Hautmann et al. (21–23). Its obvious advantage is that it has the best continence rate of all reservoirs as a consequence of having the greatest volume. This technique makes feasible both incorporation of an afferent or efferent limb for ureteral anastomosis and orthotopic anastomosis of the ureters directly into the reservoir, with or without antireflux technique (18,23–25). In our experience, difficulty reaching the urethral remnant occurs less often with this type of reservoir.

Of course, other patient and surgeon issues might supersede these guidelines. Surgeon's preference, length of surgery, ease of construction, potential need for revision, the patient's body image, and other characteristics of the patient are among the many factors that must be considered when choosing which type of orthotopic reconstruction to provide each individual.

REFLUX PREVENTION

Controversy exists about the importance of an antireflux mechanism (1,26–31). The benefits are not easy to define. It is clear that the need for reflux prevention is not the same as in a ureterosigmoidostomy conduit or continent diversion. Reflux prevention in neobladders is even less important than in a normal bladder (see list below). Many reports have revealed a high incidence (13% to 41%) of renal deterioration associated with a refluxing ileal conduit, as evaluated using serum creatinine and urography (32). However, after a long-term follow-up (mean, 13 years) of patients with colonic conduits, significantly more renal units not showing reflux on the cystogram of neobladder remained normal on urography than did units with reflux (33).

In deciding whether reflux prevention in neobladders is as important as it is in a normal bladder, one should consider (2,28) that in neobladders:

- There are no coordinated contractions during micturition
- Pressure increases simultaneously in neobladder, abdomen, kidney and pelvis during the Valsaalva maneuver
- An ileourethrostomy acts as a safety valve (leak point) in case of high pressure

Because obstruction may occur at the level of the fascia immediately superfical to the external oblique muscle, conduits are not always low-pressure systems. This situation, coupled with the presence of infected urine, means that high-pressure reflux may occur. It has become recognized over the past two decades that this reflux, or alternatively, ureteroileal obstruction, may contribute to the gradual deterioration in renal function in these patients.

The rationale for implanting the ureters in an antireflux fashion into orthotopic bladder substitutes or continent reservoirs is to prevent the upper urinary tract from retrograde hydrodynamically transmitted pressure peaks and from ascending bacteriuria. However, the routine of antireflux ureter implantation into intestinal urinary reservoirs was born in the era before creation of designated low-pressure reservoirs.

Glomerular filtration pressure is calculated to be 25 to 30 cm of water, and the amplitude of the peristaltic waves in the ureters is normally less than 10 cm of water. In view of these figures, long-lasting periods with pressure exceeding about 25 cm of water in the urinary receptacle will, in the long run, probably impair renal function by impeding the urine flow. Patients with a continent ileal reservoir for urinary diversion utilize approximately 60% of the maximal volume capacity during the daytime, that is, about 300 to 500 cc. At this reservoir volume, the pressure exceeds zero by more than 25 cm of water only during about 2 minutes per hour (2).

Use of nonrefluxing techniques raises the risk of obstruction to at least twice that following a direct anastomosis, irrespective of type or bowel segment used. Half of these strictures require secondary procedures (34).

In a recent study the reported obstruction rate following direct anastomoses was 1.7%, which is significantly lower than the 13% rate of nonrefluxing techniques (30). Among the latter, the LeDuc technique resulted in the highest incidence of postoperative strictures. Studer and Zingg reported a 3% obstruction rate using ureteral direct anastomosis, compared to 13% postoperative strictures in patients for whom Coffey flap valves were used (35). Likewise, Roth et al. reported 3.6% and 20.4% obstruction rate, respectively, comparing ureteral direct anastomoses to an afferent loop with the LeDuc antireflux anastomoses (36). Moreover, the reported obstruction rate was 3.8% for the nipple valve of the Koch pouch (12), but 9.3% for the LeDuc antireflux anastomoses of the Hautmann neobladder (34). For the latter antireflux technique, an obstruction rate up to 29% has been reported (37).

We conclude that obstruction from anastomotic strictures has greater potential as a source of short- and long-term morbidity than does reflux. Direct techniques are easier to perform, and they preserve renal function as well as non-refluxing methods. We see no justification for any antireflux mechanism in neobladders.

Since 1996 we have been using a freely refluxing, open-end-to-side ureteroileal anastomosis, a "chimney modification," which is the simplest surgery employing small bowel (23). Our 9.5% stenosis rate with the LeDuc procedure (the first 363 out of a total of 558 neobladders) went down to 1.0% among the next 195 patients with our current procedure. Table 28B.3 presents advantages of this chimney modification.

TABLE 28B.3
ADVANTAGES OF NEOBLADDER SURGERY WITH CHIMNEY MODIFICATION
Extra length to reach ureteral stump
Ease of surgery (antirefluxing techniques)
Tension-free anastomosis (no ureteral ischemia)
No risk of angulation with neobladder filling
Simplified revisional surgery (flank access)
Lowest possible stenosis rate
Resection of ureter far above the bladder (addressing concern about distal ureteral carcinoma *in situ*)

Data from Hautmann RE. The ileal neobladder. *Atlas Urol Clin North Am* 2001;9:85; Hollowell CMP, Christiano AP, Steinberg GD. Technique of Hautmann ileal neobladder with chimney modification: interim results in 50 patients. *J Urol* 2000;163:47; Lippert MC, Theodorescu D. The Hautmann neobladder with a chimney: a versatile modification. *J Urol* 1997;158:1510.

UPPER URINARY TRACT PRESERVATION

In a prospective, randomized study of patients undergoing conduit or continent reservoir diversion, renal function was evaluated after a mean follow-up of 10 years (29). Renal units subjected to obstruction were excluded. Patients scheduled for conduit diversion were randomized as to the type of intestinal segment and technique for ureterointestinal anastomosis. There was a moderate decrease in the preoperative total glomerular filtration rate (GFR) in the ileal and colonic conduit groups (17 and 19 mL per minute, respectively). Part of the change in GFR is probably a normal age-related decrease, which has been estimated to be about 1 mL/min/yr at ages >50 and 0.5 mL/min/yr in younger people (38). If a fall in GFR of 25% or more is defined as renal deterioration, then it occurred in 34% of patients after a conduit diversion (40% colonic, 28% ileal) and in 28% of those with a continent cecal reservoir. Similar results were reported in patients with a Koch pouch observed for 5–11 years and in patients with an ileal bladder substitute (28,35,39,40).

In a study on upper tract preservation published in 2000, Jonsson et al. presented 25 years of follow-up on kidney function in 126 patients with a Kock reservoir (31). They reached two significant conclusions:

First: Kidney function is not impaired by the diversion per se, provided stenosis is recognized and managed.

Second: The patient's health status is more influenced by the underlying disease than by the diversion.

VOIDING DYSFUNCTION

Improved quality of life following orthotopic bladder substitution as compared to alternative forms of diversion fails to be realized when voiding dysfunction arises. Functional results should be reported in accordance with the International Continence Society standards established for intestinal urinary reservoirs (40).

A comparison of the severity and prevalence of voiding dysfunction in many surgical series is confounded by variability in endpoints, definitions, length of follow-up, patient age, patient sex, and surgical technique. Moreover, lower urinary tract symptoms, incontinence, or retention have rarely been assessed with validated outcome instruments and/or voiding diaries. Despite these obvious limitations, some general observations can be made and are reviewed in this report.

Failure to Store: Daytime Incontinence

In a review of 2,238 patients with a follow-up of 26 ± 18 months, daytime incontinence occured in 13.3% ± 13.6% of patients (41). Functional urethral length correlates with daytime urinary incontinence. This has also been shown to be true after radical prostatectomy (42). Because the cause of urinary incontinence is multifactorial (reservoir shape, reservoir volume, functional urethral length, age, nerve supply, mental status), care must be taken not to overinterpret results which do not show a difference, particularly if data from different centers are pooled (41). Patients with a short functional urethra typically experience dribbling when walking with full neobladder, but not when coughing or sneezing. Because the neobladder enlarges over time, these patients may become continent 6 months to a year following surgery. Evaluation should be postponed until after this period. Risk factors for the development of daytime urinary incontinence include advanced patient age, the use of colonic segments and, in some series, a lack of nerve sparing techniques (43,44).

Daytime continence rates decrease gradually during the 4 to 5 years following bladder substitution (45). One factor is declining external urethral sphincter function with age (46). Age is an important factor; in one series the mean age of the patients 5 and 10 years after surgery was 68 years and 73 years, respectively. It is noteworthy that in this age group 10% to 15% of healthy men normally report urinary incontinence (47). Urethral sensitivity, which generally decreases after radical cystectomy, might be an additional factor. Hugonett has demonstrated that the sensory threshold in the membranous urethra was lower in incontinent patients (48).

Failure to Store: Nocturnal Leakage

Some degree of nocturnal leakage is a constant finding in most reports, even despite a technically sound operation. Nocturnal incontinence following replacement cystoplasty, which is more common and lasts longer than daytime incontinence, is a feature shared by all forms of neobladders. Nocturnal enuresis plagues nearly 28% of patients (range, 0 to 67%)(40). Unlike patients after radical prostatectomy, and also unlike a person with a normal bladder, several unexpected mechanisms are involved (Table 28B.4) (49). Similar to daytime incontinence, nighttime incontinence resolves as the functional capacity

---

TABLE 28B.4

VOIDING DYSFUNCTION: NOCTURNAL LEAKAGE IN NEOBLADDERS

Lack of detrusor spincteric reflex (increases urethral closure pressure as bladder pressure increases)
Lack of sensory vesical feedback to the brain to alert the patient when the reservoir is full, particularly at night (overflow incontinence)
New sensation of (new) bladder fullness
Loss of the afferent limb (sensory innervation of the urethra from intrapelvic branches of pudendal nerve/branches of pelvic plexus) may result in loss of an external sphincter guarding reflex stimulated by urinary leakage into proximal urethra
Gradual decline of continence with age
Decreased muscle tone during night
Increased nighttime diuresis
  – secretion of hyperosmotic urine at night (ADH secretion during nighttime)
  – shift of free water from the neobladder into the concentrated urine to obtain iso-osmolality
Interdependence among urine osmolality, neobladder distensibility, peristaltic contractions, and generation of pressure waves

ADH, antidiuretic hormone.
Data from Hohenfellner M, Buerger R, Schad H, et al. Reservoir characteristics of Mainz pouch studied in animal model osmolality of filling solution an effect of oxybutinin. *Urology* 1993;42:741; Studer UE, Zingg EJ. Ileal orthotopic bladder substitutes: what have we learned from 12 years' experience with 200 patients. *Urol Clin North Am* 1997;24:781; Jagenburg R, Kock NG, Norlen L. Clinical significance of changes in composition of urine during collection and storage in continent ileum reservoir urinary diversion. *Scand J Urol Nephrol* 1978;49:43.

increases over time. As long as the functional capacity is lower than the (increased) nocturnal urinary output, the use of an alarm clock at night is recommended until the patient has learned to be awakened by the new sensation of bladder fullness (35).

Failure to Empty

Between 4% and 25% of male patients must perform intermittent self-catheterization for incomplete emptying of the neobladder (41). The reported functional outcome in female patients differs among series, particularly in regard to voiding ability. Some reported a 53% (50) and some a 41% (51) rate of intermittent catheterization, whereas others noted a much lower rate of 0 (52) and 3% (53). The precise pathogenesis of urinary retention or elevated residual urine requiring CIC remains uncertain (Table 28B.5). In the postoperative period voiding reduction is of paramount importance. Patients must clearly understand the principle that lowering outlet resistance is the key to success. Increasing intraabdominal pressure does not by itself allow voiding. Instruction on pelvic floor relaxation, regular voiding to prevent overdistention of the reservoir, and regular follow-up are essential (54–59).

COMPLICATIONS

The complications of both continent catheterizable reservoirs and orthotopic bladder substitutes in the hands of the most experienced surgeons have been considered in detail (60). Reoperation for early complications overall reportedly occurred in 3% of continent, catheterizable reservoirs and in 7% of orthotopic bladder substitutions. Reoperation for late complications overall occurred in about 30% of continent, catheterizable reservoirs and in 13% of orthotopic bladder substitutions. We

TABLE 28B.5

VOIDING DYSFUNCTION IN THE NEOBLADDER: FAILURE TO EMPTY

Angulation of urethra (pouchocele)
Elongation/lengthening of bladder neck
Neobladder outlet not at most caudal portion of reservoir
No funneling on abdominal straining
Preserved but dysfunctional bladder neck
Denervated (floppy) proximal urethra
Inadequate pelvic floor relaxation
Inability to sustain abdominal straining
Collapse of reservoir wall toward outlet
Reservoir too big (floppy bag)
  – the greater the radius of the reservoir, the lower the pressure (law of Laplace)
  – intraluminal pressure too low to allow evacuation by gravity alone

Data from Mills RD, Studer UE. Female orthotopic bladder substitution: a good operation in the right circumstances. *J Urol* 2000;163:1501; Ali-El-Dein B, El-Sobky E, Hohenfeller M, et al. Orthotopic bladder substitution in women: functional evaluation. *J Urol* 1999;161:1875; Smith E, Yoon J, Theodorescu D. Evaluation of urinary continence and voiding function: early results in men with neourethral modification of the Hautmann orthotopic neobladder. *J Urol* 2001;166:1346; Mikuma M, Hirose T, Yokoo A, et al. Voiding dysfunction in ileal neobladder. *J Urol* 1997;158:1365; Aboseif SR, Borirakchanyavat S, Lue TF, et al. Continence mechanism of the ileal neobladder in women: a urodynamic study. *World J Urol* 1998;16:400; Arai Y, Okubo K, Konami T. Voiding function of orthotopic ileal neobladder in women. *Urology* 1999;54:44.

TABLE 28B.6

MUCUS FORMATION IN ILEAL RESERVOIRS

Dramatic increase in mucus secretion in response to chronic urinary irritation
Mucus formation constant ≤8 years
Relative increase in goblet cells
Shift in secretive pattern towards sialomucins
Less viscous mucus
Increase due to UTI
First clinical sign of bacterial colonization of reservoir

UTI, urinary tract infection.
Data from Leibovitch IJ, Ramon J, Chaim JB, et al. Increased urinary mucus production: a sequela of cystography following enterocystoplasty. *J Urol* 1991;145:736; Gatti R, Ferretti S, Bucci G, et al. Histological adaptation of orthotopic ileal neobladder mucosa: 4-year follow-up of 30 patients. *Eur Urol* 1999;36:588.

believe that the morbidity of orthotopic bladder substitutes is actually similar to, or lower than, the true rates of morbidity after conduit formation, contrary to the popular view that conduits are simple and safe (10,61–63).

There are several new complications that were unknown when there were no alternatives to conduit surgery: incisional hernias as a consequence to the Valsalva maneuver, neobladder-intestinal and neobladder-cutaneous fistulas, neobladder rupture, and mucus formation in ileal reservoirs (64,65) (Table 28B.6).

Spontaneous late rupture of neobladders is a rare but potentially life-threatening complication (66,67) (Table 28B.7). Physicians must be aware of the risk of rupture.

METABOLIC SAFETY

Metabolic and nutritional complications of urinary diversions through bowel segments are common, but fortunately, not often severe. When metabolic abnormalities are problematic, deterioration or baseline insufficiency in renal function is the most likely cause. Deterioration is most commonly associated with obstruction or infection (7–9,68–71). The urologist should be acutely aware of the potential for metabolic derangements when the prediversion creatinine is greater than 2.0 mg/dL. The longer the segment of ileum used for reservoir construction is, the higher the incidence of postoperative metabolic acidosis is. The absence of this problem is the greatest advantage a conduit has over a neobladder.

When patients switch from intravenous supplementation to oral feeding, one may see a hypovolemic salt-losing state with subsequent acidosis, hypochloremia, and hyperkalemia. Clinically, these metabolic disturbances may result in lethargy, nausea, abdominal pain, vomiting, dehydration, and muscular weakness, and these symptoms may develop soon after catheter removal. The appropriate means for prevention are monitoring of body weight and generous sodium bicarbonate supplementation (9).

CHANGE IN PARADIGM FOR URINARY DIVERSION

The goal of patient counseling about urinary diversion should be to find the method that would be the safest for cancer control, has the fewest complications in both the short and long term, and provides the easiest adjustment for the patient's lifestyle, that is, for supporting the best quality of life. The paradigm for choosing a urinary diversion has changed substantially. In 2005

TABLE 28B.7

SPONTANEOUS LATE RUPTURE OF NEOBLADDER

Etiology
Acute/chronic stretch
Secondary to distension
Micro tearing/minor blunt trauma

Pathophysiology
Risk of rupture is highest where the radius of the
   reservoir is smallest
Compromised blood supply ileocolic artery
Fall in blood flow
Arteriovenous (a-v) oxygen difference

Patient characteristics
Obstruction (mucus)
Bacterial infection
Excellent continence
No voiding on regular time intervals
Anesthesia (character drainage)

Typical location of rupture site
Upper right corner
Most distensible/mobile part
Dome shaped top (law of pressure chamber)

Diagnosis
Cystogram (misleading in 2/3 of patients)

Treatment
High index of suspicion
Early aggressive surgery

Prevention
Compliance and patient education
Regular voiding, especially at bedtime
Clean Intermittent Cathcterizations (CIC) for residual urine

Data from Desgrandchamps F, Cariou G, Barthelemy Y, et al. Spontaneous rupture of orthotopic detubularized ileal bladder replacement: report of 5 cases. *J Urol* 1997;158:798; Nippgen JB, Hakenberg OW, Manseck A, et al. Spontaneous late rupture of orthotopic detubularized ileal neobladders: report of five cases. *Urology* 2001;58:43.

all cystectomy patients are candidates for a neobladder, and we should identify patients in whom orthotopic reconstruction may be less than ideal (1). The proportion of cystectomy patients receiving a neobladder has increased at medical centers to 50% to 90% (18,26,34,35).

Patient Selection Criteria

Absolute and Relative Contraindications

Compromised renal function as a result of long-standing obstruction or chronic renal failure, with serum creatinine >150 to 200 μmol/L, is an absolute contraindication to continent diversion of any type. Severe hepatic dysfunction is also a contraindication to continent diversion. Patients with compromised intestinal function, particularly inflammatory bowel disease, may be better served by a bowel conduit.

Orthotopic reconstruction is absolutely contraindicated in all patients who are candidates for simultaneous urethrectomy, based on their primary tumor (27,72).

The number of relative contraindications and comorbidity is steadily decreasing. However, some of them, like mental impairment, external sphincter dysfunction, or recurrent urethral strictures, deserve serious consideration.

Patient Factors for the Neobladder

The primary factor is the patient's desire for a neobladder. The patient needs a certain motivation to tolerate the initial and sometimes lasting inconveniences of nocturnal incontinence associated with a neobladder. Most patients readily accept some degree of nocturnal incontinence for the benefit of avoiding an external stoma and pouch, but not all patients do, and realistic expectations of the functional outcome are essential for both the surgeon and the patient (73). The psychological damage and stigma experienced by a patient who enters surgery expecting a neobladder, but awakens with a stoma, is increasingly recognized. It should always be remembered that in many parts of the world, a bag may be either socially unacceptable or economically unrealistic as a long-term solution. These realities lead the urologist toward some from of continent urinary diversion, and although rectal pouches have been utilized widely as an alternative to conduits, continent catheterizable reservoirs, or orthotopic bladder substitutes in particular, represent attractive options.

Patient Factors against the Neobladder

There are still patients who are better served with a conduit. The following factors would argue against a neobladder:

- The patient's main motivation is to "get out of the hospital as soon as possible" and resume normal, rather sedentary activities. Many frail patients undergoing cystectomy will have less disruption of normal activities with a well-functioning conduit than an orthotopic reservoir associated with less than ideal continence.
- The patient is old and living in social isolation.
- The possibility of regular follow-up or patient compliance is low, or the patient is of an advanced age.
- The patient is unconcerned about body image. Most older patients do not have the same concerns that a younger patient might have, and their main goal is returning to their previous lifestyle, which is often quite sedentary (74).

Patient Selection Criteria: Oncologic Factors

Following cystectomy, the rhabdosphincter must remain intact. Nevertheless the cancer operation must not be compromised. This concern applies to two aspects of selection: urethral tumor recurrence in men and the use of orthotopic replacement in women.

One of the first deterrents to orthotopic diversion that the surgeon encounters is the risk for urethral recurrence of cancer. Historically, this risk following cystectomy has been 10% (75). The best predictor of the risk for urethral disease is the presence and extent of carcinoma *in situ* (CIS) in the prostatic urethra, ducts, or stroma. In cases with diffuse CIS in the ducts and invasion of the stroma, the risk for urethral disease has historically been 25% to 35 % (76), thus discouraging the use of the urethra. Lesser amounts of CIS confer a lesser degree of risk. Our aggressive approach for neobladder diversion relies only on a frozen section of the urethral margin at the time of surgery. A conservative approach would disqualify patients with any prostatic involvement. In our view, neither multifocal bladder tumors nor CIS of the bladder are indications for urethrectomy. The frequency of urethral recurrence after orthotopic diversions is much lower than might be anticipated. Freeman et al. (75) and others (34,35) provide data that show a 2% to 4% frequency of urethral recurrence after orthotopic diversion.

Orthotopic bladder substitution in women with invasive bladder cancer has been popularized recently (50,77,78). Analysis of pathologic specimens has supported its use in women who have no evidence of tumor at the bladder neck (79,80). Indeed, the majority of the invasive cancers are located in the area of the trigone, making a wide excision together with the anterosuperior part of the vagina and the dorsomedial bladder pedicle in the paravaginal region necessary.

Increasing experience with orthotopic reconstruction supports *less restriction of patient selection based on tumor stage.* Should extensive pelvic disease, a palpable mass, or positive but resectable lymph nodes preclude a neobladder because of the high propensity for a pelvic recurrence or eventual relapse? We have studied local recurrence and complications related to diversion in a series of 435 patients. The local recurrence rate was the expected 10%. There is no convincing evidence that a patient with an orthotopic diversion tolerates adjuvant chemotherapy less well, or that a pelvic recurrence is any more difficult to manage in a patient with a neobladder than in one with an ileal conduit. Patients can anticipate normal neobladder function for the rest of their lives (81).

Our approach respects the patient's desire for a neobladder; if the patient is strongly motivated, he or she gets a neobladder. Even when the patient has a poor prognosis and relapse is likely to occur, we still try to construct the diversion he or she wants. Previous radiation therapy, especially with an advanced cancer, usually militates against an orthotopic diversion, but does not absolutely preclude it. However, all patients should be informed that diversion to the skin, either by a continent reservoir or ileal conduit, may be necessary due to unexpected tumor extent, and an appropriate stoma site should be marked on the abdominal wall beforehand.

Current Practice

Despite the fact that orthotopic bladder replacement provides the ideal method of urinary diversion after cystectomy, many patients treated outside centers that are dedicated to neobladder reconstruction receive an ileal conduit. Why? The answer is that the selection criteria for patients to receive a conduit are very broad: more advanced age, more comorbidity, and more previous cancer therapy or a desperation cystectomy for cancer that was previously deemed unresectable or that had failed to respond to combined radiation and chemotherapy regimes (74).

Thus despite a strong desire to offer orthotopic diversion whenever possible, some patients do not qualify on the basis of current clinical judgment. An ileal conduit remains an expedient, safe, and appropriate method of diversion in these patients. Many factors go into the decision to perform a urinary diversion and they all must be kept in mind while discussing the pros and cons of each method with the patient and his or her family.

CONCLUSION

Our experience suggests that neobladders composed of stomach or sigmoid should be used only under unusual circumstances because of the high rates of incontinence. The major benefit of the neobladder is the ability to void without a catheter, but at a small risk of being incontinent. Of course, other factors affecting the patient and surgeon may supersede these guidelines. The surgeon's preference, length of surgery, ease of construction, potential need for stomal revision, the patient's body image, and other characteristics of the patient are among the many factors that must be considered when choosing which continent urinary diversion to provide to each individual patient (1).

References

1. Hautmann RE. Urinary diversion: ileal conduit to neobladder. *J Urol* 2003; 169:834–842.
2. Berglund B, Kock NG. Volume capacity and pressure characteristics of various types of intestinal reservoirs. *World J Surg* 1987;11:798.
3. Hohenfellner M, Buerger R, Schad H, et al. Reservoir characteristics of Mainz pouch studied in animal model: osmolality of filling solution an effect of oxybutinin. *Urology* 1993;42:741.
4. Colding-Jørgensen M, Poulsen AL, Steven K. Mechanical characteristics of tubular and detubularised bowel for bladder substitution: theory, urodynamics and clinical results. *Br J Urol* 1993;72:586.
5. Goldwasser B, Madgar I, Hanani Y. Urodynamic aspects of continent urinary diversion. [Review]. *Scand J Urol Nephrol* 1987;21:245.
6. Santucci RA, Park CH, Mayo ME, et al. Continence and urodynamic parameters of continent urinary reservoirs: comparison of gastric, ileal, ileocolic, right colon, and sigmoid segments. *Urology* 1999;54:252.
7. Chang SS, Koch MO. The metabolic complications of urinary diversion. *Urol Oncol* 2000;5:60.
8. Stampfer DS, McDougal WS, McGovern FJ. The use of bowel in urology. Metabolic and nutritional complications. *Urol Clin North Am* 1997; 24(4):715.
9. Mills RD, Studer UE. Metabolic consequences of continent urinary diversion. *J Urol* 1999;161:1056.
10. Turner WH, Bitton A, Studer UE. Reconstruction of the urinary tract after radical cystectomy: the case for continent urinary diversion. *Urology* 1997; 49:663.
11. Hautmann RE, de Petriconi R, Gottfried HW, et al. The ileal neobladder: complications and functional results in 363 patients after 11 years of followup. *J Urol* 1999;161:422–428.
12. Elmajian DA, Stein JP, Esrig D, et al. The Kock ileal neobladder: updated experience in 295 male patients. *J Urol* 1996;156:920.
13. Moore JA, Brading AF. Gastrointestinal tissue as a substitute for the detrusor. *World J Urol* 2000;18:305.
14. Sandberg Tschopp AB, Lippuner K, Jaeger P, et al. No evidence of osteopenia 5 to 8 years after ileal orthotopic bladder substitution. *J Urol* 1996; 155:71–75.
15. Deane AM, Woodhouse CRJ, Constance Parkinson M. Histological changes in ileal conduits. *J Urol* 1984;132:1108.
16. Åkerlund S, Forssell-Aronsson E, Jonsson O, et al. Decreased absorption of ^{22}Na and ^{36}Cl in ileal reservoirs after exposure to urine. An experimental study in patients with continent ileal reservoirs for urinary or fecal diversion. *Urol Res* 1991;19:249.
17. Lytton B, Green DF. Urodynamic studies in patients undergoing bladder replacement surgery. *J Urol* 1989;141:1394.
18. Montie JE, Wie JT. Formation of an orthotopic neobladder following radical cystectomy: historical perspective, patient selection and contemporary outcomes. *J Pelvic Surg* 2002;8(3):141–147.
19. Stein JP, Lieskovsky G, Ginsberg DA, et al. The T pouch: an orthotopic ileal neobladder incorporating a serosal lined ileal antireflux technique. *J Urol* 1998;159:1836.
20. Studer UE, Danuser H, Merz VW, et al. Experience in 100 patients with an ileal low pressure bladder substitute combined with an afferent tubular isoperistaltic segment. *J Urol* 1995;154:49.
21. Hautmann RE, Egghart G, Froheberg D, et al. The ileal neobladder. *J Urol* 1988;139:39.
22. Hautmann RE. The ileal neobladder to the female urethra. *Urol Clin North Am* 1997;24:827.
23. Hautmann RE. The ileal neobladder. *Atlas Urol Clin North Am* 2001;9:85.
24. Hollowell CMP, Christiano AP, Steinberg GD. Technique of Hautmann ileal neobladder with chimney modification: interim results in 50 patients. *J Urol* 2000;163:47.
25. Lippert MC, Theodorescu D. The Hautmann neobladder with a chimney: a versatile modification. *J Urol* 1997;158:1510.
26. Stein JP, Skinner DG. Application of the T-mechanism to an orthotopic (T-pouch) neobladder: a new era of urinary diversion. *World J Urol* 2000; 18:315.
27. Studer UE, Hautmann RE, Hohenfellner M, et al. Indications for continent diversion after cystectomy and factors affecting long-term results. *Urol Oncol* 1998;4:172.
28. Studer UE, Danuser H, Thalmann GN, et al. Antireflux nipples or afferent tubular segments in 70 patients with ileal low pressure bladder substitutes: long-term results of a prospective randomized trail. *J Urol* 1996;156:1913.
29. Kristjánsson A, Månsson W. Refluxing or nonrefluxing ureteric anastomosis. *BJU Int* 1999;84:905.
30. Pantuck AJ, Han KR, Perrotti M, et al. Ureteroenteric anastomosis in continent urinary diversion: long-term results and complications of direct versus nonrefluxing techniques. *J Urol* 2000;163:450.
31. Jonsson O, Olofsson G, Lindholm E, et al. Long-time experience with the Kock ileal reservoir for continent urinary diversion. *Eur Urol* 2001;40:632.
32. Pernet FP, Jonas U. Ileal conduit urinary diversion: early and late results of 132 cases in a 25-year period. *World J Urol* 1985;3:40.
33. Elder DD, Moisey CU, Rees RWM. A long-term followup of the colonic conduit operation in children. *Br J Urol* 1979;51:462.
34. Hautmann RE, de Petriconi R, Gottfried HW, et al. The ileal neobladder: complications and functional results in 636 patients after 11 years of followup. *J Urol* 1999;161:422.
35. Studer UE, Zingg EJ. Ileal orthotopic bladder substitutes: what have we learned from 12 years' experience with 200 patients. *Urol Clin North Am* 1997;24:781.
36. Roth S, van Ahlen H, Semjonow A, et al. Does the success of ureterointestinal implantation in orthotopic bladder substitution depend more on surgeon level of experience or choice of technique? *J Urol* 1997;157:56.

37. Shaaban AA, Gaballah MA, El-Diasty TA, et al. Urethral controlled bladder substitute: a comparison between the intussuscepted nipple valve and the technique of Le Duc as antireflux procedures. *J Urol* 1992;148:1156.

38. Granerus G, Aurell M. Reference values for ^{51}Cr EDTA clearance as a measure of glomerular filtration rate. *Scand J Clin Lab Invest* 1981;41:611.

39. Studer UE, Danuser H, Moehrle K, et al. Results in the upper urinary tract in 220 patients with an ileal low pressure bladder substitute combined with an afferent tubular segment. *J Urol* 1999;161(4 Suppl. 91):A350.

40. Thüroff JW, Mattiasson A, Andersen JT, et al. The standardization of terminology and assessment of functional characteristics of intestinal urinary reservoirs. *Br J Urol* 1996;78:516.

41. Steers WD. Voiding dysfunction in the orthotopic neobladder. *World J Urol* 2000;18:330.

42. Hammerer P, Huland H. Urodynamic evaluation of changes in urinary control after radical retropubic prostatectomy. *J Urol* 1997;157:233–236.

43. Park JM, Montie JE. Mechanisms of incontinence and retention after orthotopic neobladder diversion. *Urology* 1998;51:601.

44. Porru D, Madeddu G, Campus G, et al. Urodynamic analysis of voiding dysfunction in orthotopic ileal neobladder. *World J Urol* 1999;17:285.

45. Madersbacher S, Moehrle K, Burkhard F, et al. Long-term voiding pattern of patients with ileal orthotopic bladder substitutes. *J Urol* 2002;167:2052.

46. Hammerer P, Michl U, Meyer-Moldenhauser WH, et al. Urethral closure pressure changes with age in men. *J Urol* 1996;156:1741.

47. Temml C, Haidinger G, Schmidbauer J. Urinary incontinence in both sexes: prevalence rates and impact on quality of life and sexual life. *Neurourol Urodyn* 2000;19:259.

48. Hugonnet CL, Danuser H, Springer JP, et al. Decreased sensitivity in the membranous urethra after orthotopic ileal bladder substitute. *J Urol* 1999;161:418.

49. Jagenburg R, Kock NG, Norlen L. Clinical significance of changes in composition of urine during collection and storage in continent ileum reservoir urinary diversion. *Scand J Urol Nephrol* 1978;49:43.

50. Hautmann RE, Paiss T, de Petriconi R. The ileal neobladder in women: 9 years of experience with 18 patients. *J Urol* 1996;155:76.

51. Linn JF, Hohenfellner M, Roth S, et al. Treatment of intestinal cystitis: comparison of subtrigonal and supratrigonal cystectomy combined with orthotopic bladder substitution. *J Urol* 1998;159:774.

52. Ghoneim MA. Orthotopic bladder substitution in women following cystectomy for bladder cancer. *Urol Clin North Am* 1997;24:225.

53. Stenzl A, Colleselli K, Bartsch G. Update for urethra-sparing approaches in cystectomy in women. *World J Urol* 1997;15:134.

54. Mills RD, Studer UE. Female orthotopic bladder substitution: a good operation in the right circumstances. *J Urol* 2000;163:1501.

55. Ali-El-Dein B, El-Sobky E, Hohenfeller M, et al. Orthotopic bladder substitution in women: functional evaluation. *J Urol* 1999;161:1875.

56. Smith E, Yoon J, Theodorescu D. Evaluation of urinary continence and voiding function: early results in men with neo-urethral modification of the Hautmann orthotopic neobladder. *J Urol* 2001;166:1346.

57. Mikuma M, Hirose T, Yokoo A, et al. Voiding dysfunction in ileal neobladder. *J Urol* 1997;158:1365.

58. Aboseif SR, Borirakchanyavat S, Lue TF, et al. Continence mechanism of the ileal neobladder in women: a urodynamic study. *World J Urol* 1998;16:400.

59. Arai Y, Okubo K, Konami T. Voiding function of orthotopic ileal neobladder in women. *Urology* 1999;54:44.

60. Rowland RG. Complications of continent cutaneous reservoirs and neobladders—series using contemporary techniques. *AUA Update Ser* 1995;14 (lesson 25):201.

61. Benson MC, Slawin KM, Wechsler MH. Analysis of continent versus standard urinary diversion. *Br J Urol* 1992;69:156.

62. Gburek B, Lieber MM, Blute ML. Comparison of studer ileal conduit diversion with respect to perioperative outcome and late complications. *J Urol* 1998;160:271.

63. Jahnson S, Pedersen J. Cystectomy and urinary diversion during twenty years—complications and metabolic implications. *Eur Urol* 1993;24:343.

64. Leibovitch IJ, Ramon J, Chaim JB, et al. Increased urinary mucus production: a sequela of cystography following enterocystoplasty. *J Urol* 1991;145:736.

65. Gatti R, Ferretti S, Bucci G, et al. Histological adaptation of orthotopic ileal neobladder mucosa: 4-year follow-up of 30 patients. *Eur Urol* 1999;36:588.

66. Desgrandchamps F, Cariou G, Barthelemy Y, et al. Spontaneous rupture of orthotopic detubularized ileal bladder replacement: report of 5 cases. *J Urol* 1997;158:798.

67. Nippgen JB, Hakenberg OW, Manseck A, et al. Spontaneous late rupture of orthotopic detubularized ileal neobladders: report of five cases. *Urology* 2001;58:43.

68. McDougal WS. Metabolic complications of urinary intestinal diversion. *J Urol* 1992;147:1199.

69. Matsui U, Topoll B, Miller K, et al. Metabolic long-term followup of the ileal neobladder. *Eur Urol* 1993;24:197.

70. Lockhart JL, Davies R, Persky L, et al. Acid-base changes following urinary tract reconstruction for continent diversion and orthotopic bladder replacement. *J Urol* 1994;152:338.

71. Kristjánsson A, Davidson T, Månsson W. Metabolic alterations at different levels of renal function following continent urinary diversion through colonic segments. *J Urol* 1997;157:2099.

72. Skinner DG, Studer UE, Okada K, et al. Which patients are suitable for continent diversion or bladder substitution following cystectomy or other definitive local treatment? *Int J Urol* 1995;2(Suppl. 2):105.

73. Hautmann RE. Editorial: 15 Jahre Erfahrung mit der Ileumneoblase. Was haben wir gelernt? *Urologe A* 2001;40:360.

74. Montie JE. Ileal conduit diversion after radical cystectomy: pro. *Urology* 1997;49:659.

75. Freeman JA, Tarter TA, Esrig D, et al. Urethral recurrence in patients with orthotopic ileal neobladders. *J Urol* 1996;156:1615.

76. Hardeman SW, Soloway MS. Urethral recurrence following radical cystectomy. *J Urol* 1990;144:666.

77. Stein JP, Stenzl A, Esrig D, et al. Lower urinary tract reconstruction following cystectomy in women using the Kock ileal reservoir with bilateral ureteroileal urethrostomy: initial clinical experience. *J Urol* 1994;152:1404.

78. Stenzl A, Draxl H, Posch K, et al. The risk of urethral tumors in female bladder cancer: can the urethra be used for orthotopic reconstruction of the lower urinary tract? *J Urol* 1995;153:950.

79. Stein JP, Cote RJ, Freeman JA, et al. Indications for lower urinary tract reconstruction in women after cystectomy for bladder cancer: a pathological review of female cystectomy specimens. *J Urol* 1995;154:1329.

80. Coloby PJ, Kakizoe T, Tobisu K, et al. Urethral involvement in female bladder cancer patients: mapping of 47 consecutive cystourethrectomy specimens. *J Urol* 1994;152:1438.

81. Hautmann RE, Simon J. Ileal neobladder and local recurrence of bladder cancer: patterns of failure and impact on function in men. *J Urol* 1999;162:1963.

CHAPTER 29 ■ NEOADJUVANT AND ADJUVANT CHEMOTHERAPY IN MUSCLE-INVASIVE BLADDER CANCER

CORA N. STERNBERG

Muscle-invasive bladder cancer is one of the most aggressive epithelial tumors, with a high rate of early systemic dissemination. Five-year survival rates depend principally upon pathologic stage and nodal status. With increasing T stage, and especially when cancer extends outside the bladder wall, the prognosis worsens. Failure is usually due to occult metastatic disease present at the time of the initial diagnosis.

SURVIVAL IN CYSTECTOMY SERIES

Cystectomy series from major academic centers report 5-year survivals after cystectomy of 36% to 54% (1–4). In addition, for high-risk patients with pathologic stage pT3 to pT4 and/or pN+ M0 bladder cancer, 5-year survival is only 25% to 35%. With the advent of orthotopic bladder substitutions and better postoperative medical care, radical cystectomy is the ideal treatment for muscle-invasive bladder cancer.

RATIONALE, ADVANTAGES, AND DISADVANTAGES OF NEOADJUVANT CHEMOTHERAPY

Neoadjuvant chemotherapy was designed for patients with operable clinical stage cT2 to cT4a muscle-invasive disease. The rationale for giving upfront chemotherapy prior to cystectomy or definitive radiation therapy (RT) is based on the intent to improve survival by treating micrometastatic disease that is present but not detected at initial staging. Neoadjuvant chemotherapy has also been proposed in some programs with the intention of saving the bladder (5,6). Systemic therapy is delivered early when the burden of metastatic disease is minimal, and it is usually well tolerated prior to surgery or radiation. The toxicity of neoadjuvant therapy is less for patients without metastatic disease than it is for patients with metastatic disease since patients without metastatic disease generally have a better performance status and localized disease. It is not known whether three or four cycles are needed as no study has ever systematically evaluated this question.

The principal disadvantage of neoadjuvant chemotherapy relates to the difficulty in assessing response in the primary tumor, due to the differences between clinical and pathologic staging of approximately 30% (6,7). Another disadvantage is that cystectomy or RT is delayed during the time that chemotherapy is administered. This presents a particular problem for nonresponding patients.

Toxicity in the neoadjuvant setting can be determined from two large randomized trials. In the European Organization for Research and Treatment of Cancer/Medical Research Council (EORTC/MRC) international trial of neoadjuvant CMV (cisplatin, methotrexate, and vinblastine) chemotherapy, a 1% mortality was due to CMV chemotherapy (8). In the American Southwest Oncology Group (SWOG) trial, no deaths were attributable to M-VAC (methotrexate, vinblastine, adriamycin, and cisplatin) (9).

RANDOMIZED NEOADJUVANT CHEMOTHERAPY TRIALS

Randomized trials have tried to definitively establish whether or not neoadjuvant chemotherapy prior to cystectomy or RT improves survival. Initial trials used single-agent cisplatin, but more modern studies have employed cisplatin-containing combination chemotherapy. The benefit from neoadjuvant chemotherapy should theoretically occur irrespective of the method of local definitive treatment (RT or cystectomy). In the United States and in most of Europe, radical cystectomy is the preferred option for "fit" patients.

Many neoadjuvant chemotherapy trials show either a trend toward a small benefit or no benefit in survival. However, the majority of trials may not have enrolled sufficient numbers of patients to detect statistically significant differences in survival. Results from randomized trials in the literature can be found in Table 29.1.

The EORTC/MRC trial randomized patients to three cycles of CMV neoadjuvant chemotherapy prior to cystectomy or RT versus cystectomy or RT alone. Since this is the largest trial in the literature, it should be examined more carefully. In this trial 976 patients were accrued over a 5.5-year period from 106 institutions in 20 countries. When first published in 1999, this trial did not reveal a statistically significant improvement in survival, although a small difference in survival in favor of the CMV chemotherapy group was observed (8). In an update of this trial presented at the American Society of Clinical Oncology (ASCO) in 2002, with a longer follow-up of 7.4 years, the data have just reached statistical significance ($P = .048$), with a 5.5% benefit in favor of patients treated with neoadjuvant CMV (20). A better 5-year survival of 50% versus 44% was observed in the patients treated with neoadjuvant CMV. In addition, survival at 8 years was 43% in the CMV arm as opposed to 37%. The investigators concluded that the results showed no change in absolute benefit, although patients treated with CMV chemotherapy had a consistent survival benefit that was maintained over time.

TABLE 29.1

RANDOMIZED PHASE III TRIALS OF NEOADJUVANT CHEMOTHERAPY

Study group	Neoadjuvant arm	Standard arm	Patients	Survival
Cisplatin Chemotherapy Trials				
Australia/UK (10)	DDP/RT	RT	255	No difference
Canada/NCI (11)	DDP/RT or preop RT + Cyst	RT or preop RT + Cyst	99	No difference
Spain (CUETO) (12)	DDP/Cyst	Cyst	121	No difference
Combination Chemotherapy Trials				
EORTC/MRC (8)	CMV/RT or Cyst	RT or Cyst	976	5.5% difference in favor of CMV ($P = .048$)
SWOG Intergroup (13)	M-VAC/Cyst	Cyst	298	Trend toward benefit M-VAC (HR = 1.33; $P = .06$)
Italy (GUONE) (14)	M-VAC/Cyst	Cyst	206	No difference
Italy (GISTV) (15)	M-VEC/Cyst	Cyst	171	No difference
Genoa (16)	DDP/5FU/RT/Cyst	Cyst	104	No difference
Nordic 1 (17)	ADM/DDP/RT/Cyst	RT/Cyst	311	15% benefit for T3–T4a ($P = .03$)
Nordic 2 (18)	MTX/DDP/Cyst	Cyst	317	No difference
Abol-Enein et al. (19)	CarboMV/Cyst	Cyst	194	Benefit with CarboMV

5-FU, 5-fluorouracil; DDP or C, cisplatin; MTX, methotrexate; ADM, doxorubicin; E, epirubicin; V, vinblastine; Carbo, carboplatin; Cyst, cystectomy; RT, radiation therapy; NCI, National Cancer Institute; M-VAC, methotrexate, vinblastine, adriamycin, and cisplatin; M-VEC, methotrexate, vinblastine, epirubicin, and cisplatin; HR, hazard ratio; GUONE, Gruppo Uro Oncologico del Nord Est; GISTV, Gruppo Italiano per lo Studio dei Tumori della Vescica; CUETO, Spanish Oncology Group.

The American Southwest Oncology Group (SWOG) Intergroup trial similarly randomized patients between three cycles of neoadjuvant M-VAC chemotherapy prior to cystectomy versus cystectomy alone (9). Patients that were clinical cT2 to cT4a from 126 institutions were enrolled over an 11-year period. Patients were stratified according to age (<65 years or ≥65 years) and stage (cT2 versus cT3 or cT4a). Of the 317 patients enrolled, 307 were considered eligible. Median survival among those randomized to surgery alone was 46 months, compared to 77 months for patients who received neoadjuvant M-VAC chemotherapy ($P = .06$; 2-sided stratified log rank test). In part due to the very long accrual period and follow-up, these results have also achieved borderline statistical significance. The estimated risk of death was reduced by 25% (HR 1.33) in patients treated with neoadjuvant M-VAC (21).

Similar to the EORTC/MRC trial, improved survival in the SWOG trial was found in patients who had no cancer remaining in the cystectomy specimen (pT0). More patients in the M-VAC arm had no residual disease (38%) than did patients treated with cystectomy alone (15%) ($P < .001$). Not all patients underwent the cystectomy as planned. In the M-VAC group 82% and in the surgery group 81% actually underwent cystectomy.

The SWOG trial is an important trial in favor of neoadjuvant M-VAC chemotherapy, but it represents only a portion of the patients randomized in neoadjuvant chemotherapy trials. An almost identical Northern Italian trial by the GUONE Group trial randomized 206 patients over a 6.5-year period to four cycles of M-VAC prior to cystectomy versus cystectomy alone (14). Survival at 3 years was 62% for the M-VAC arm and 68% for the cystectomy-alone arm. In this smaller trial, no clear difference in survival was demonstrated.

The Nordic cystectomy 1 trial gave neoadjuvant adriamycin, cisplatin, and preoperative RT prior to cystectomy versus preoperative RT and cystectomy alone. At 5 years the overall survival was 59% in the chemotherapy group and 51% in the control group ($P = .1$). The corresponding cancer-specific survival rates were 64% and 54%, respectively (17). No difference was observed for stages T1 to T2 disease, while a 15% difference was observed in overall survival for patients with stages T3 to T4a disease ($P = .03$).

The same cooperative group was unable to confirm these results in a subsequent Nordic cystectomy 2 trial (18). In 317 patients with muscle-invasive disease who were treated with methotrexate and cisplatin and no RT, no survival advantage occurred with neoadjuvant chemotherapy. However, by combining these two trials in an ad hoc meta-analysis, the same investigators were able to demonstrate positive results in favor of neoadjuvant chemotherapy (22).

The actual situation is that more than 3,000 patients have been entered into randomized clinical trials in an attempt to determine whether or not neoadjuvant chemotherapy improves survival in patients with locally advanced muscle-invasive bladder cancer, and no definitive answer as to the true value of this chemotherapy has yet been determined (23). A meta-analysis of 10 neoadjuvant chemotherapy trials was performed. This meta-analysis included 88% of patients from all known randomized trials (24). Unfortunately, data from the SWOG trial was not included, and the majority of patients in the meta-analysis are from the EORTC/MRC trial. Overall survival for the whole group was not affected by neoadjuvant chemotherapy, and patients treated with single-agent cisplatin did not benefit by neoadjuvant chemotherapy. Only in a subgroup analysis of patients treated with cisplatin-containing combination chemotherapy, in the context of an overall result that was insignificant, was a 5% (95% confidence interval 1%–7%) hint of activity in favor of neoadjuvant chemotherapy shown. This difference was not very large, and reflected a change in survival from 45% to 50% ($P = .16$, HR = .87; .78 to .98), which is also consistent with only a 1% difference in survival. Since the majority of patients in this analysis were from the EORTC/MRC trial, it is not very surprising that the results were similar.

Another meta-analysis of randomized neoadjuvant chemotherapy trials has produced similar results (25). Of 16 eligible trials in 3,315 patients identified in the literature, 11 (2,605 patients) provided data for a meta-analysis of overall survival. The pooled HR was 0.90 (95%, CI 0.82 to 0.99, $P = .02$). Eight trials used cisplatin-based combination chemotherapy, and the pooled HR was 0.87 (95%, CI 0.78 to 0.96, $P = .006$), consistent with an absolute overall survival benefit of 6.5% (95% CI, 2% to 11%) from 50% to 56.5%.

Neoadjuvant cisplatin-based chemotherapy improves overall survival in muscle-invasive transitional cell carcinoma (TCC). The size of the effect is modest, and combination chemotherapy can be administered safely without adverse outcomes resulting in delayed local therapy. An optimal chemotherapy regimen has not been identified, and newer regimens have not been tested in randomized clinical trials.

NEOADJUVANT CHEMOTHERAPY AND BLADDER PRESERVATION

Since the advent of orthotopic bladder substitutions, many urologists prefer early cystectomy with a continent urinary diversion. Organ conservation has been used in the management of several solid tumors, and bladder preservation has been the subject of several phase II studies. Bladder preservation influences quality of life as it means less surgery, no need for a urinary diversion, and a normal sexual life. Following neoadjuvant chemotherapy, bladder preservation may be possible in highly selected cases who respond to chemotherapy. This concept has been championed at Memorial Sloan-Kettering in New York, by investigators in Rome, Italy, and by radiation oncologists for patients who attain complete remission (6,26,27).

In the SWOG trial, the pT0 rate in M-VAC patients was 38%. The pT0 rate in the EORTC/MRC trial was 33% after CMV. Likewise, after two cycles of neoadjuvant M-VAC chemotherapy, the pT0 rate was 40% in the M.D. Anderson trial of neoadjuvant and adjuvant versus adjuvant M-VAC (28). It appears that response to chemotherapy is an important prognostic factor (5,6,9,20). However, this may represent patient selection factors, as it is possible that patients who do well have characteristics that would make them survive longer whether or not they were treated with chemotherapy. In fact, these may also be exactly the same patients who would benefit from a bladder preservation strategy.

In Rome, 104 patients with cT2 to cT4 N0M0 of the bladder were treated with three cycles of neoadjuvant M-VAC (6). After clinical restaging, 52 patients underwent transurethral resection of the bladder (TURB) alone, 13 patients had a partial cystectomy, and 39 patients had a radical cystectomy. Median survival for the entire group was 7.49 years (95%, CI 4.86 to 10.0 years). At the TURB following M-VAC, 49 patients (49%) were T0. Responding patients underwent TURB or partial cystectomy alone following chemotherapy. Of the patients who had M-VAC and TURB alone, 60% were alive at a median follow-up of 56+ months (10 to 160+). Of the patients in the TURB group, 44% maintained an intact bladder. Of the responding patients with monofocal lesions who underwent partial cystectomy, only one required salvage cystectomy and 5-year survival was 69%.

In 77 patients who had downstaging to T0 or superficial disease, 5-year survival was 69%. This is in contrast to 5-year survival of only 26% in 27 patients who failed to respond and were T2 or greater after chemotherapy. Median survival for 27 elderly patients who are more than 70 years old (median 73 years; 70 to 82 years) was surprisingly long: 90 months (7.5 years). For elderly patients who underwent TURB and partial cystectomy, 5-year survival was 67% with a median survival of 9 years; 47% kept their bladders intact.

Bladder sparing in selected patients on the basis of response to neoadjuvant chemotherapy is a feasible approach that should be confirmed in prospective randomized trials. Selected elderly patients are candidates for this approach.

Herr reviewed the 10-year outcomes in 111 surgical candidates who received neoadjuvant M-VAC chemotherapy followed by a bladder-sparing surgery at Memorial Sloan-Kettering (26). Sixty (54%) achieved a complete clinical response (T0) at TURB, and 28 had TURB alone, 15 had a partial cystectomy, and 17 underwent elective radical cystectomy. Patients were followed for a median of 10 years (range, 8 to 13 years). Of 43 patients who had bladder-sparing surgery, 32 (74%) were alive at the 10-year point, including 25 (58%) with an intact functioning bladder. Twenty-four patients (56%) developed bladder tumor recurrences that were invasive in 30% and superficial in 26%. The authors concluded that the majority of patients with invasive bladder tumors who achieved T0 status after neoadjuvant M-VAC chemotherapy preserved their bladders for up to 10 years after bladder-sparing surgery. The bladder remained at risk for new invasive tumors. Cystectomy salvaged the majority, but not all, relapsing patients.

The use of such new chemotherapeutic agents as gemcitabine and the taxanes in the neoadjuvant setting is experimental but is being incorporated into treatment protocols. The SWOG is evaluating neoadjuvant gemcitabine, paclitaxel, and carboplatin followed by observation or immediate cystectomy in a phase II study in 95 patients with T2 to T4a, N0 bladder cancer. Molecular markers, recurrence rates, and cystectomy-free survival are studied. This study will determine feasibility, tolerability, and toxicity of this triplet combination in an intergroup setting.

Patients who undergo a bladder-preservation approach must be extremely well informed and accept frequent follow-up, multiple invasive procedures, the possibility that cystectomy may eventually become necessary, and the uncertainty of tumor relapse.

NEOADJUVANT CHEMOTHERAPY AND RADIATION THERAPY

Combining systemic chemotherapy with RT is an alternative approach to bladder preservation. Chemotherapy can sensitize the tumor to RT and may be able to irradiate occult metastases as well. Trials of combined neoadjuvant chemotherapy and RT are detailed in Table 29.2.

Selection criteria for chemoradiation are similar to those that predict a good prognosis at cystectomy. Patients with small T2 to T3 lesions without evidence of hydronephrosis who undergo a thorough TURB tend to do the best. Most series are characterized by TURB, followed by chemoradiation, with re-staging TURB followed by consolidative RT for responding patients or cystectomy for nonresponding patients. Five-year survival rates of 42% to 63%, with organ preservation in approximately 40% of patients, have been reported.

Many studies have been piloted by the Radiation Therapy Oncology Group (RTOG) and by investigators at the Massachusetts General Hospital (MGH) (27). The RTOG has recently reported on twice-daily accelerated irradiation (RT) and methotrexate, cisplatin, and vinblastine (MCV) chemotherapy after aggressive TURB in an attempt to preserve the bladder (37). Fifty-two patients with stage T2 to T4a N0M0 disease from 17 institutions were entered into the trial. The protocol required TURB within 6 weeks of the initiation of induction therapy. Induction treatment involved concomitant boost RT, 1.8 Gy to the pelvis in the morning followed by 1.6 Gy to the tumor 4 to 6 hours later. For sensitization, low-dose cisplatin was given on the first 3 days of each treatment week. Three to 4 weeks after induction, patients were evaluated by cystoscopy for residual disease.

TABLE 29.2

TRIALS OF COMBINED NEOADJUVANT CHEMOTHERAPY AND RADIOTHERAPY

Series	Year	n	Chemo	5-year survival	5-year survival with intact bladder
RTOG—study 85-12 (29)	1993	42	DDP	52%	42%
RTOG—study 85-72 (30)	1996	91	MCV and RT and DDP	62%[a]	44%
RTOG—study 89-03 (31)	1998	123	MCV and RT and DDP	48%	36%
University of Erlangen (32,33)	2001	199	DDP or Carbo	52%	41%
University of Paris (34,35)	2001	120	DDP/5-FU	63%	
MGH (36)	2002	190	MCV or DDP/5-FU	54%	46%
RTOG—study 97-06 (37)	2003	47	MCV and BID accelerated RT and DDP	48%[b]	

RTOG, Radiation Therapy Oncology Group; MGH, Massachusetts General Hospital; DDP or C, cisplatin; RT, radiation therapy; Carbo, carboplatin; MCV, methotrexate, cisplatin, and vinblastine; 5-FU, 5-fluorouracil; BID, twice daily.
[a]4-year survival data.
[b]Projected 3-year survival data.

Therapy was well tolerated and resulted in a complete remission (CR) rate of 74%, similar to that in previous bladder-sparing trials. Projected 2-year values for locoregional control, bladder-intact survival, and overall survival were consistent with previously reported trials of bladder-sparing treatment. However, only 45% of patients completed three cycles of MCV as it was poorly tolerated by most patients in this multi-institutional cooperative group study.

Although survival is similar to that in contemporary cystectomy series, the combined morbidity of chemotherapy and RT can be significant and should be considered in planning treatment.

RATIONALE, ADVANTAGES, AND DISADVANTAGES OF ADJUVANT CHEMOTHERAPY

Radical cystectomy remains the standard treatment for patients with muscle-invasive bladder cancer. Adjuvant chemotherapy is given after cystectomy to patients at high risk for relapse. Adjuvant chemotherapy is widely used in patients with pT3 to pT4a and/or pN+ M0 disease in an effort to delay recurrence and prolong survival. This approach of giving chemotherapy after local treatment has led to increases in survival in patients with several solid tumors (5,38,39).

The rationale for giving adjuvant, as opposed to neoadjuvant, chemotherapy is that the local definitive treatment is performed immediately (40). There is no delay in surgery and no time is wasted, especially for those patients who do not respond to chemotherapy. Treatment decisions are based on pathologic criteria, after careful examination of the cystectomy specimen. Micrometastases are treated when at a really low volume. Orthotopic bladder substitutions and the decreased morbidity of cystectomy have been cited as reasons to perform cystectomy and adjuvant chemotherapy.

The major disadvantage of adjuvant chemotherapy is that preservation of the bladder is not possible. A delay is necessary in giving systemic therapy for occult metastases while treating the primary tumor. Response cannot be easily evaluated, and the only clinical endpoint that can be assessed is time to recurrence. An additional disadvantage may be that it is more difficult to administer chemotherapy following cystectomy.

In one of the first adjuvant trials, Logothetis et al. divided patients into three groups: low-risk controls, high-risk controls who had one high-risk pathological finding (refused, not offered, or had medical contraindications to adjuvant chemotherapy), and high-risk patients treated with adjuvant chemotherapy

(41,42). Clearly, patients at high risk who received adjuvant cisplatin, cychlophosphamide, and adnamycin (CISCA) chemotherapy benefited. Although this study was provocative, it was not a randomized trial. Patients were selected for treatment based upon their compliance and general medical conditions. The study was, however, the first that suggested a benefit for adjuvant chemotherapy in highly selected patients. Unfortunately, relatively few randomized trials have systematically evaluated adjuvant chemotherapy. These can be found in Table 29.3.

Two studies in the literature have received an inordinate amount of attention. The study from Skinner et al. in California was the first phase III prospective trial that showed a significant increase in time to progression and survival in patients who were randomized to receive chemotherapy following cystectomy (44). This study has often been criticized for its retrospective use of subgroup analyses and its methodology. The statistical analysis may have provided artificial results in the context of the survival curves that crossed over with follow-up. While chemotherapy appeared to prolong the median time to recurrence by 14 months, no residual advantage was observed at 2 years.

Stockle published another adjuvant study that has been highly publicized and quoted (45,49). Patients were randomized to either cystectomy or cystectomy followed by M-VAC or M-VEC. The population had poor risk factors: 60% had positive nodes and most were stage T4. Since this study was performed in two small towns, the results became readily known to the participants and the study was subsequently closed prematurely. Only a small number of patients were entered after an interim analysis revealed a benefit for those randomized to chemotherapy. There was a 27% progression rate in the treated patients compared to an 82% progression rate in the control patients. Survival was markedly different between the two groups, as patients who relapsed in the observation arm were not offered chemotherapy at the time of relapse. In an intent-to-treat analysis, 5-year progression-free survival was 59% after the recommendation to receive chemotherapy versus 13% after being recommended cystectomy alone (49). It is of interest that in a more recent German series comparing M-VEC to observation after cystectomy, no difference in survival was confirmed (50).

Due to the difficulty of interpreting these adjuvant chemotherapy trials, a systematic review of published randomized trials of adjuvant cisplatin-containing combination chemotherapy in locally advanced bladder cancer was undertaken. Although trials appeared to show a difference in favor of adjuvant chemotherapy, serious methodologic flaws were found. Major deficiencies were found in sample size, early stopping of patient entry, statistical analyses, reporting of results, and drawing conclusions (51).

TABLE 29.3

TRIALS OF ADJUVANT CHEMOTHERAPY FOLLOWING CYSTECTOMY

Investigator	Year	Chemo	n, Chemo	n, No Chemo	Randomized	Results
Einstein et al. (43)	1984	DDP	41	39	Yes	Preop RT; no benefit; single-agent DDP, few patients finished therapy
Logothetis et al. (41,42)	1988	CISCA	62	71	No	Benefit, but not randomized
Skinner et al. (44)	1991	CAP	47	44	Yes	Benefit, but too few patients received therapy
Stockle et al. (45)	1992	M-VAC/ M-VEC	23	26	Yes	Benefit, small patient numbers, premature closure, no treatment at relapse
Studer et al. (46)	1994	DDP	40	37	Yes	No benefit, single-agent therapy probably inadequate
Bono et al. (47)	1995	CM	48	35	Yes	No benefit for N0M0
Freiha et al. (48)	1996	CMV	25	25	Yes	Benefit in relapse-free survival
Otto et al. (49)	2001	M-VEC	55	53	Yes	No benefit

DDP, cisplatin; CMV, cisplatin, methotrexate, and vinblastine; RT, radiation therapy; CISCA, cisplatin, cychlophosphamide, and adriamycin; CAP, cychlophosphamide, adriamycin, and cisplastin; M-VAC, methotrexate, vinblastine, adriamycin, and cisplatin; M-VEC, methotrexate, vinblastine, epirubicin, and cisplatin.

For this reason, these trials provide insufficient evidence to support the routine use of adjuvant chemotherapy in clinical practice due to small sample sizes, confusing analyses and terminology, and the reporting of questionable conclusions. Analyses of the duration of survival were either not done or were inconclusive, and quality of life was not considered.

Based on the desire to treat only patients who are at high risk, the EORTC/MRC and many other international groups throughout the world have begun collaborating on a large adjuvant trial that plans to enlist patients worldwide. This study evaluates four cycles of immediate chemotherapy versus therapy at the time of relapse in high-risk patients with pT3 to pT4 or node-positive disease. Three different chemotherapy regimens are permitted: M-VAC, high-dose M-VAC (HD-M-VAC), and gemcitabine/cisplatin (GC) (52–54).

Another multicenter US and international adjuvant trial seeks to evaluate patients with low-stage T1 to T2 tumors who are randomized after surgery to M-VAC versus observation based upon p53 status. Following radical cystectomy, eligible patients are those with pT1 to pT2 disease, or those who have had pT1 to pT2 on the TURB and are pT0 at the cystectomy. These patients are then evaluated for p53 status. Patients with wild-type p53 are entered on the study and observed, and patients with mutant p53 are randomized between three cycles of M-VAC and observation.

This study is based upon the University of Southern California (USC) experience that tumors expressing alterations in pRb and p53 had significantly increased rates of recurrence (P <.0001) and decreased survival (P <.0001), compared to patients without alterations in pRb and p53 (55,56). They have also found that patients with altered p53 are more likely to benefit from chemotherapy. Although the USC results concerning who may benefit from chemotherapy may be questioned (57,58), this is an important study in that it seeks to use molecular markers to determine outcome of patients with locally advanced bladder cancer.

CONCLUSION

Muscle-invasive bladder cancer is a chemoresponsive disease. Response to neoadjuvant chemotherapy is an important prognostic factor, but this may represent patient selection factors.

Efforts to identify those patients most likely to benefit from neoadjuvant therapy are necessary to optimize its use.

Despite the fact that neoadjuvant chemotherapy may provide a small survival advantage based upon the EORTC/MRC, SWOG trials, and meta-analyses, this approach has not been universally accepted. In part, this is due to the increased use of orthotopic bladder substitutions and the desire to not overtreat patients based only on clinical staging. Neoadjuvant chemotherapy may also be useful in programs of bladder preservation, which remains a controversial topic, as radical cystectomy is still regarded as the gold standard.

Whether it is best to give chemotherapy in the neoadjuvant or adjuvant setting has not been clearly determined. Adjuvant studies in the literature have been less definitive than neoadjuvant studies; however, pathologic staging and the ability to evaluate molecular prognostic markers such as p53 have led to new adjuvant chemotherapy trials.

The international adjuvant chemotherapy trial coordinated by the EORTC (Protocol #30994) will hopefully clarify some of the unanswered questions concerning whether or not adjuvant chemotherapy immediately following cystectomy improves survival.

An optimal chemotherapy regimen has not been identified, and chemotherapy regimens incorporating newer agents have not been sufficiently investigated or tested in randomized clinical trials.

References

1. Stein JP, Lieskovsky G, Cote R, et al. Radical cystectomy in the treatment of invasive bladder cancer: long-term results in 1,054 patients. *J Clin Oncol* 2001;19(3):666–675.
2. Dalbagni G, Genega E, Hashibe M, et al. Cystectomy for bladder cancer: a contemporary series. *J Urol* 2001;165(4):1111–1116.
3. Bassi P, Ferrante GD, Piazza N, et al. Prognostic factors of outcome after radical cystectomy for bladder cancer: a retrospective study of a homogeneous patient cohort. *J Urol* 1999;161(5):1494–1497.
4. Ghoneim MA, el-Mekresh MM, el-Baz MA, et al. Radical cystectomy for carcinoma of the bladder: critical evaluation of the results in 1,026 cases. *J Urol* 1997;158(2):393–399.
5. Sternberg CN. Current perspectives in muscle invasive bladder cancer. *Eur J Cancer* 2002;38(4):460–467.
6. Sternberg CN, Pansadoro V, Calabro F, et al. Can patient selection for bladder preservation be based on response to chemotherapy? *Cancer* 2003; 97(7):1644–1652.
7. Herr HW, Scher HI. Surgery of invasive bladder cancer: is pathologic staging necessary? *Semin Oncol* 1990;17:590–597.

8. International Collaboration of Trialists. Neoadjuvant cisplatin, methotrexate, and vinblastine chemotherapy for muscle-invasive bladder cancer: a randomised controlled trial. *Lancet* 1999;354 (9178):533–540.

9. Grossman HB, Natale RB, Tangen CM, et al. Neoadjuvant chemotherapy plus cystectomy compared with cystectomy alone for locally advanced bladder cancer. *N Engl J Med* 2003;349(9):859–866.

10. Wallace DM, Raghavan D, Kelly KA, et al. Neo-adjuvant (pre-emptive) cisplatin therapy in invasive transitional cell carcinoma of the bladder. *Br J Urol* 1991;67:608–615.

11. Coppin CM, Gospodarowicz MK, James K et al. The National Cancer Institute of Canada Clinical Trials Group. Improved local control of invasive bladder cancer by concurrent cisplatin and preoperative or definitive radiation. *J Clin Oncol* 1996;14(11):2901–2907.

12. Martinez Pineiro JA, Gonzalez Martin M, Arocena F. Neoadjuvant cisplatin chemotherapy before radical cystectomy in invasive transitional cell carcinoma of the bladder: prospective randomized phase III study. *J Urol* 1995;153:964–973.

13. Natale RB, Grossman HB, Blumenstein B, et al. SWOG 8710 (INT-0080): randomized phase III trial of neoadjuvant M-VAC and cystectomy versus cystectomy alone in patients with locally advanced bladder cancer. *Proc Am Soc Clin Oncol* 2001;20(1):2a Ref Type: Abstract.

14. Bassi P, Pagano F, Pappagallo G, et al. Neo-adjuvant M-VAC of invasive bladder cancer: the G.U.O.N.E. multicenter phase III trial. *Eur Urol* 1998;33(Suppl. 1):142 Ref Type: Abstract.

15. GISTV (Italian Bladder Cancer Study Group). Neoadjuvant treatment for locally advanced bladder cancer: a randomized prospective clinical trial. *J Chemother* 1996;8:345–346.

16. Orsatti M, Curotto A, Canobbio L. Alternating chemo-radiotherapy in bladder cancer: a conservative approach. *Int J Radiat Oncol Biol Phys* 1995;33:173–178.

17. Malmstrom PU, Rintala E, Wahlqvist R, et al. Five year follow-up of a prospective trial of radical cystectomy and neoadjuvant chemotherapy. *J Urol* 1996;155:1903–1906.

18. Sherif A, Rintala E, Mestad O, et al. Neoadjuvant cisplatin-methotrexate chemotherapy of invasive bladder cancer—Nordic cystectomy trial 2. *Scand J Urol Nephrol* 2002;36(6):419–425.

19. Abol-Enein H, El Makresh M, El Baz M, et al. Neo-adjuvant chemotherapy in treatment of invasive transitional bladder cancer: a controlled, prospective randomised study. *Br J Urol* 1997;80(Suppl. 2):49.

20. Hall RR. Updated results of a randomised controlled trial of neoadjuvant cisplatin (C), methotrexate (M) and vinblastine (V) chemotherapy for muscle-invasive bladder cancer. *Proc Annu Meet Am Soc Clin Oncol* 2002; 21(1):178a Ref by: Abstract.

21. Grossman HB, Natale RB, Tangen CM, et al. Errata corrige for: "Neoadjuvant chemotherapy plus cystectomy compared with cystectomy alone for locally advanced bladder cancer," published in *N Engl J Med* 2003 Aug 28;349(9):859–866. Erratum in: *N Engl J Med* 2003;349(19):1880.

22. Sherif A, Rintala E, Mestad O, et al. Neoadjuvant platinum based combination chemotherapy improves overall survival in patients with locally advanced bladder cancer: a meta-analysis of two Nordic collaborative studies of 620 patients. *J Urol* 2003;169:307 Ref Type: Abstract.

23. Sternberg CN, Parmar MKB. Neo-adjuvant chemotherapy is not (yet) standard treatment for muscle invasive bladder cancer. *J Clin Oncol* 2001; 19(Suppl. 1):21S–26S.

24. Advanced Bladder Cancer Meta-Analysis Collaboration. Neoadjuvant chemotherapy in invasive bladder cancer: a systematic review and meta-analysis. *Lancet* 2003;361(9373):1927–1934.

25. Winquist E, Kirchner TS, Segal R, et al. On behalf of the Genitourinary Cancer Disease Site Group of the Cancer Care Ontario Program in Evidence-based Care Practice Guidelines Initiative. Neoadjuvant chemotherapy for transitional cell carcinoma of the bladder: A systematic review and meta-analysis. *J Urol* 2004;171(2):561–569.

26. Herr HW, Bajorin DF, Scher HI. Neoadjuvant chemotherapy and bladder sparing surgery for invasive bladder cancer: ten-year outcome. *J Clin Oncol* 1998;16(4):1298–1301.

27. Shipley WU, Kaufman DS, Tester WJ et al. Radiation Therapy Oncology Group. Overview of bladder cancer trials in the Radiation Therapy Oncology Group. *Cancer* 2003;97(Suppl. 8):2115–2119.

28. Millikan R, Dinney C, Swanson D, et al. Integrated therapy for locally advanced bladder cancer: final report of a randomized trial of cystectomy plus adjuvant M-VAC versus cystectomy with both preoperative and postoperative M-VAC. *J Clin Oncol* 2001;19:4005–4013.

29. Tester W, Porter A, Asbell S. Combined modality program with possible organ preservation for invasive bladder carcinoma: Results of RTOG protocol 85-12. *Int J Radiat Oncol Biol Phys* 1993;25:783–790.

30. Tester W, Caplan R, Heaney J. Neoadjuvant combined modality program with selective organ preservation for invasive bladder cancer: Results of Radiation Therapy Oncology Group phase II trial 8802. *J Clin Oncol* 1996;14(1):119–126.

31. Shipley WU, Winter KA, Kaufman DS, et al. Phase III trial of neoadjuvant chemotherapy in patients with invasive bladder cancer treated with selective bladder preservation by combined radiation therapy and chemotherapy: initial results of Radiation Therapy Oncology Group 89-03. *J Clin Oncol* 1998;16(11):3576–3583.

32. Sauer R, Birkenhake S, Kühn R, et al. Muscle-invasive bladder cancer: Transurethral resection and radiochemotherapy as an organ-sparing treatment option. In: Petrovich Z, Baert L, Brady LW, eds. *Carcinoma of the Bladder*: Berlin, Heidelberg: Springer, 1998:205–214.

33. Sauer R, Rodel C. Biological selection for organ conservation. *Eur J Cancer* 2001;37(Suppl. 6):S286.

34. Housset M, Dufour B, Maulard-Durdux C, et al. Concomitant fluorouracil (5-FU)-cisplatin (CDDP) and bifractionated split course radiation therapy (BSCRT) for invasive bladder cancer. *Proc Am Soc Clin Oncol* 1997;16:319A.

35. Durdux C, Housset M, Dufour B. Altered fractionation in chemo-radiation for bladder cancer. *Eur J Cancer* 2001;37(Suppl. 6):S286.

36. Shipley WU, Kaufman DS, Zehr E, et al. Selective bladder preservation by combined modality protocol treatment: Long-term outcomes of 190 patients with invasive bladder cancer. *Urol* 2002;60(1):62–67.

37. Hagan MP, Winter KA, Kaufman DS, et al. RTOG 97-06: initial report of a phase I–II trial of selective bladder conservation using TURBT, twice-daily accelerated irradiation sensitized with cisplatin, and adjuvant MCV combination chemotherapy. *Int J Radiat Oncol Biol Phys* 2003;57(3):665–672.

38. Sternberg CN. Neo-adjuvant and adjuvant chemotherapy of bladder cancer: is there a role? *Ann Oncol* 2002;13(Suppl. 4):273–279.

39. De Braud F, Maffezzini M, Vitale V, et al. Bladder cancer. *Crit Rev Oncol Hematol* 2002;41(1):89–106.

40. Sternberg CN. Current treatment strategies in transitional cell carcinoma of the bladder. *Crit Rev Oncol Hematol* 2003;47(2):81–82.

41. Logothetis CJ, Johnson DE, Chong C, et al. Adjuvant chemotherapy of bladder cancer: a preliminary report. *J Urol* 1988;139:1207–1211.

42. Logothetis CJ, Johnson DE, Chong C, et al. Adjuvant cyclophosphamide, doxorubicin, and cisplatin chemotherapy for bladder cancer: an update. *J Clin Oncol* 1988;6:1590–1596.

43. Einstein AB, Shipley W, Coombs J, et al. Cisplatin as adjunctive treatment for invasive bladder carcinoma: tolerance and toxicities. *Urol* 1984; 23(Suppl. 4):110–117.

44. Skinner DG, Daniels JR, Russell CA, et al. The role of adjuvant chemotherapy following cystectomy for invasive bladder cancer: a prospective comparative trial. *J Urol* 1991;145:459–467.

45. Stockle M, Meyenburg W, Wellek S, et al. Advanced bladder cancer (stages pT3b, pT4a, pN1 and pN2): improved survival after radical cystectomy and 3 adjuvant cycles of chemotherapy: results of a controlled prospective study. *J Urol* 1992;148:302–307.

46. Studer UE, Bacchi M, Biedermann C. Adjuvant cisplatin chemotherapy following cystectomy for bladder cancer: results of a prospective randomized trial. *J Urol* 1994;152:81–84.

47. Bono AV, Benvenuti C, Reali L et al. Italian Uro-Oncologic Cooperative Group. Adjuvant chemotherapy in advanced bladder cancer. *Prog Clin Biol Res* 1989;303:533–540.

48. Freiha F, Reese J, Torti FM. A randomized trial of radical cystectomy versus radical cystectomy plus cisplatin, vinblastine and methotrexate chemotherapy for muscle invasive bladder cancer. *J Urol* 1996;155(2):495–499.

49. Stockle M, Meyenburg W, Wellek S. Adjuvant polychemotherapy of nonorgan-confined bladder cancer after radical cystectomy revisited: long term results of a controlled prospective study and further clinical experience. *J Urol* 1995;153:47–52.

50. Otto T, Börgemann C, Krege S, et al. Adjuvant chemotherapy in locally advanced bladder cancer (PT3/PN1-2,M0): a phase iII study. *Eur Urol* 2001;39(Suppl 5):147.

51. Sylvester R, Sternberg C. The role of adjuvant combination chemotherapy after cystectomy in locally advanced bladder cancer: what we do not know and why. *Ann Oncol* 2000;11(7):851–856.

52. Sternberg CN, Yagoda A, Scher HI, et al. M-VAC for advanced transitional cell carcinoma of the urothelium: efficacy, and patterns of response and relapse. *Cancer* 1989;64:2448–2458.

53. Sternberg CN, de Mulder PHM, Schornagel JH, et al. Randomized phase III trial of high dose intensity methotrexate, vinblastine, doxorubicin, and cisplatin (MVAC) chemotherapy and recombinant human granulocyte colony-stimulating factor versus classic MVAC in advanced urothelial tract tumors: European Organization for Research and Treatment of Cancer protocol no. 30924. *J Clin Oncol* 2001;19(10):2638–2646.

54. Von der Maase H, Hansen SW, Roberts JT, et al. Gemcitabine and cisplatin versus methotrexate, vinblastine, doxorubicin, and cisplatin in advanced or metastatic bladder cancer: results of a large, randomized, multinational, multicenter, phase III study. *J Clin Oncol* 2000;18(17):3068–3077.

55. Cote RJ, Esrig D, Groshen S, et al. p53 and treatment of bladder cancer. *Nature* 1997;385(6612):123–125.

56. Cote RJ, Dunn MD, Chatterjee SJ, et al. Elevated and absent pRb expression is associated with bladder cancer progression and has cooperative effects with p53. *Cancer Res* 1998;58(6):1090–1094.

57. Williams SG, Gandour-Edwards R, Deitch AD, et al. Differences in gene expression in muscle-invasive bladder cancer: a comparison of Italian and American patients. *Eur Urol* 2001;39(4):430–437.

58. McShane LM, Aamodt R, Cordon-Cardo C, et al. National Cancer Institute, Bladder Tumor Marker Network. Reproducibility of p53 immunohistochemistry in bladder tumors. *Clin Cancer Res* 2000;6(5): 1854–1864.

CHAPTER 30 ■ CHEMOTHERAPY FOR METASTATIC BLADDER, ALONE OR IN COMBINATION WITH OTHER TREATMENT

MATTHEW D. GALSKY AND DEAN F. BAJORIN

Transitional cell carcinoma (TCC) of the urinary bladder is the second most common genitourinary malignancy in the United States. Each year in the United States, more than 56,000 patients will develop TCC, and more than 12,000 will die of the disease. As a result, intense efforts over the past two decades have focused on the development of active chemotherapeutic regimens for this disease.

INITIAL EXPERIENCE WITH CISPLATIN AND OTHER SINGLE AGENTS

Cisplatin is the most active single-agent in urothelial TCC. During the late 1970s, several trials of single-agent cisplatin in patients with advanced TCC reported overall response (OR) rates ranging from 26% to 65% (1–8). Although uncommon, complete responses (CRs) were also observed (5% to 16%). These early trials served as the basis for the inclusion of cisplatin in the multiagent regimens that have subsequently become standards of care in TCC. Of note, in later randomized trials that included single-agent cisplatin as a treatment arm, results were somewhat less impressive, with OR rates and CR rates of 9% to 31% and 3% to 9%, respectively. The median survival of patients treated with single-agent cisplatin in these trials was 8 to 9 months (9–11).

During the late 1970s and early 1980s, additional single agents were found to have activity in urothelial TCC. The most active of these agents included methotrexate (OR 30%), doxorubicin (OR 17%), and vinblastine (OR 22%) (12–24). Despite the modest activity of these agents, CRs were extremely rare and response durations were typically 3 to 6 months.

COMBINATION CHEMOTHERAPY AND THE DEVELOPMENT OF M-VAC

Multiagent chemotherapeutic regimens were developed during the 1980s in an attempt to improve the results of single-agent therapy. In 1985, investigators at Memorial Sloan-Kettering Cancer Center (MSKCC) reported a landmark trial using the combination of methotrexate, vinblastine, doxorubicin, and cisplatin (M-VAC). In the initial report, 24 patients with advanced or unresectable urothelial TCC were treated with methotrexate (30 mg/m^2) on days 1, 15, and 22; vinblastine (3 mg/m^2) on days 2, 15, and 22; doxorubicin (30 mg/m^2) on day 2; and cisplatin (70 mg/m^2) on day 2 (25). Remarkably, responses were observed in 71% [95% confidence interval (CI),

53% to 89%] of those treated with complete clinical responses in 50% (95% CI, 30% to 70%). At the time of the report, the median duration of response had not been reached at a median follow-up of 9.5 months. A second study from the same investigators confirmed the preliminary results with M-VAC in a larger patient population (26).

Subsequently, several other groups published their experiences with the M-VAC regimen. In these small phase II studies, response rates were somewhat lower, with OR rates ranging from 40% to 57% and CRs in 13% to 19% (27–29).

EARLY RANDOMIZED TRIALS WITH M-VAC

In addition to M-VAC, several other cisplatin-based regimens were extensively studied during the 1980s, including CISCA (cyclophosphamide, cisplatin, and doxorubicin) and CMV (cisplatin, methotrexate, and vinblastine). In phase II trials, these regimens were all associated with similar CR and OR rates. Given the significant activity of these regimens, and the superior median survivals when compared with historical single-agent trials, randomized trials were performed to further define a standard of care (Table 30.1).

M-VAC versus Cisplatin

In an intergroup trial reported by Loehrer et al., M-VAC was compared with single-agent cisplatin (11). Of the 246 assessable patients, 126 were randomized to cisplatin alone and 120 were randomized to M-VAC. At a median follow-up duration of 19.7 months, the M-VAC regimen resulted in a significantly greater response rate (39% vs. 12%; $P < .0001$) and overall survival (12.5 months vs. 8.2 months; $P = .0002$). As expected, treatment with M-VAC was more toxic, causing more drug-related deaths (4% vs. 0%), febrile neutropenia (10% vs. 0%), grade 3 or 4 nausea/vomiting (12% vs. 1%), and mucositis (17% vs. 0%).

M-VAC versus CISCA

A prospective randomized trial compared M-VAC with CISCA (30). Of the 110 patients enrolled, 55 were randomized to CISCA and 55 were randomized to M-VAC. Treatment with M-VAC was associated with a superior OR rate (65% vs. 46%; $P < .05$) and median survival duration (48.3 weeks vs. 36.1 weeks; $P = .0003$). The toxicity associated with these two regimens was comparable.

TABLE 30.1

RANDOMIZED TRIALS OF CISPLATIN-BASED CHEMOTHERAPY IN ADVANCED
TRANSITIONAL CELL CARCINOMA

Regimens	Reference	OR	CR	Survival (mo)	P
M-VAC	(11)	36%	13%	12.5	<.0002
Cisplatin		11%	3%	8.2	
M-VAC	(30)	65%	35%	12.6	<.05
CISCA		46%	25%	10.0	
M-VAC	(31)	59%	24%	12.5	.17
FAP		42%	10%	12.5	
M-VAC	(32)	58%	9%	14.1	.122
HD-M-VAC		72%	21%	15.5	
M-VAC	(33)	46%	12%	14.8	.746
Gemcitabine + cisplatin		50%	12%	13.8	
M-VAC	(34)	54%	23%	14.2	.025
Docetaxel + cisplatin		37%	13%	9.3	
[a]M-VAC	(35)	40%	13%	14.2	.41
Paclitaxel + carboplatin		28%	3%	13.8	

M-VAC, methotrexate, vinblastine, doxorubicin, cisplatin; CISCA, cyclophosphamide, cisplatin, doxorubicin; FAP, 5-fluorouracil, interferon-alpha-2b, cisplatin; HD-M-VAC, high-dose M-VAC; OR, overall response.
[a]Trial terminated early with only 85 patients.

CMV versus MV

Despite the popularity of CMV, this regimen was never directly compared with M-VAC. A randomized trial was conducted comparing CMV with MV (methotrexate and vinblastine) (36). Of the 214 patients enrolled, 108 were randomized to CMV and 106 to MV. The hazard ratio was 0.68 (95% CI, .51–.90; $P = .0065$) in favor of the CMV arm. While the CMV regimen proved superior, underscoring the importance of cisplatin in combination chemotherapy for TCC, the median survival with this regimen was only 7 months.

LIMITATIONS OF M-VAC

It was concluded from these initial randomized trials that cisplatin-based combination chemotherapy should be considered for patients with metastatic/unresectable urothelial TCC requiring chemotherapy and that M-VAC should be considered the treatment of choice. However, despite the superiority of M-VAC in phase III trials, the limitations of this regimen were readily apparent. Although many patients responded to treatment, median survival rates were consistently less than 13 months. Furthermore, the long-term durability of CRs was poor, with only 3.7% of patients remaining continuously free of disease in a reported intergroup trial comparing M-VAC with cisplatin (37).

Perhaps the most limiting factor associated with M-VAC was the associated toxicity. In the reported trials, febrile neutropenia occurred in up to 25% of patients and grade 2 to grade 3 mucositis developed in up to 50%. Other prominent toxicities included decreased renal function, hearing loss, and peripheral neuropathy. Treatment-related deaths occurred in 2% to 4% of patients. Given the elderly patient population with metastatic TCC, and their comorbid conditions, this side-effect profile is particularly relevant. However, the regimen also proved toxic in patients with a good renal function and preserved performance status.

ATTEMPTS TO IMPROVE M-VAC

In an effort to decrease the toxicity and improve the efficacy of M-VAC, several investigators evaluated the use of altered doses/schedules with colony-stimulating factor support. In a study utilizing standard dose M-VAC, treatment with granulocyte colony-stimulating factor (GCSF) after chemotherapy was associated with a reduction in both hematopoietic toxicity and mucositis (38). Given the feasibility of this approach, and the dose response relationship suggested by studies with cisplatin and doxorubicin, several phase II trials of dose-escalated M-VAC with colony-stimulating factor support were initiated. While it was shown that the dose of M-VAC could be increased as much as 60%, there was no increase in response rate compared with historical controls and some investigators reported increased toxicity (39–42). As a result, this approach was largely abandoned in the United States.

Based on promising phase II data with standard dose M-VAC given every 2 weeks with GCSF support (43), the European Organization for Research and Treatment of Cancer (EORTC) conducted a prospective randomized trial comparing this regimen to M-VAC administered every 4 weeks (32). A total of 263 chemotherapy-naïve patients with metastatic/advanced TCC were enrolled. With the biweekly schedule, it was possible to deliver twice the doses of cisplatin and doxorubicin in half the time and with less toxicity. While there was a significant difference in the CR rates (21% vs. 9%, $P = .009$) and progression-free survival ($P = .037$; hazard ratio 0.75; 95% CI, 0.58 to 0.98) favoring the biweekly schedule, there was no significant difference in median overall survival. Of note, this trial was powered to detect a 50% difference in median survival, and thus a lesser benefit with this dose-dense regimen may have been missed.

TABLE 30.2

RESULTS WITH NEWER SINGLE AGENTS IN PATIENTS WITH ADVANCED
BLADDER CANCER

Agent (refs.)	First-line		Previously treated	
	OR	95% CI	OR	95% CI
Paclitaxel (47–49)	42%	23% to 63%	9%	0% to 17%
Docetaxel (50,51)	31%	14% to 48%	13%	4% to 30%
Ifosfamide (52–54)	33%	20% to 46%	20%	10% to 32%
Gemcitabine (55,56)	26%	16% to 36%	23%	8% to 38%

OR, overall response; CI, confidence interval.

THE IMPACT OF PROGNOSTIC FACTORS

The importance of pretreatment prognostic factors in predicting outcomes has been underscored by several analyses of patients with metastatic TCC treated with M-VAC (11,37,44,45). In one such study, a database of 203 patients with unresectable/metastatic TCC was retrospectively subjected to multivariate analysis to determine which patient characteristics predicted survival (44). Two factors, KPS ≤80% and visceral (lung, liver, or bone) metastases, had independent prognostic significance. The median survival times for patients with zero, one, or two risk factors were 33, 13.4, and 9.3 months, respectively ($P = .0001$). This report highlighted that the median survival of patient cohorts could vary from 9 to 26 months simply by altering the proportion of patients from different risk categories.

Clearly, attention to these baseline prognostic factors is critical when comparing median survivals among different phase II studies, and stratification of phase III trials should be based on these variables. Notably, the same two prognostic factors have proven to be independent predictors of survival in patients treated with more modern chemotherapeutic regimens (46).

NEW SINGLE-AGENTS IN METASTATIC TCC

With the M-VAC experience, it became apparent that improvements in efficacy and/or reduction of toxicity would require the development of new agents. Over the past decade, several new agents with activity in TCC have been identified, including gemcitabine, the taxanes, and ifosfamide (Table 30.2). These new agents differ from the older drugs in several ways: (a) They have moderate activity both as first-line and second-line therapy, (b) they are associated with more favorable toxicity profiles, and (c) many of these agents can be administered in patients with poor renal function.

NEW DOUBLETS IN METASTATIC TCC: RANDOMIZED TRIALS

In an attempt to further improve the efficacy and tolerability of chemotherapeutic regimens for advanced TCC, various combinations of old and new active drugs have been explored (Table 30.3). The combinations of gemcitabine plus cisplatin, docetaxel plus cisplatin, and paclitaxel plus carboplatin have been compared with M-VAC in randomized phase III trials.

Gemcitabine and Cisplatin: A New Standard of Care

Based on encouraging initial results with the gemcitabine plus cisplatin (GC) combination (62–64), a multicenter randomized phase III trial was performed to compare GC with M-VAC in patients with advanced/metastatic TCC (33). Of the 405 chemotherapy-naïve patients enrolled, 203 were randomized to GC (gemcitabine 1,000 mg/m² on days 1, 8, and 15; cisplatin 70 mg/m² on day 2) and 202 were randomized to standard M-VAC. Treatment on both arms was administered

TABLE 30.3

PHASE II TRIALS OF NEWER DOUBLETS AS FIRST-LINE TREATMENT IN METASTATIC TRANSITIONAL CELL CARCINOMA (CUMULATIVE RESULTS, DATA COMPLIED IRRESPECTIVE OF DOSE AND SCHEDULE)

Regimen (refs.)	N	OR (95% CI)	CR (95% CI)
Paclitaxel + cisplatin (57,58)	86	45% (34% to 55%)	16% (2% to 24%)
Docetaxel + cisplatin (59–61)	129	43% (34% to 52%)	23% (16% to 30%)
Gemcitabine + cisplatin (62–64)	112	46% (37% to 55%)	21% (13% to 29%)
Paclitaxel + carboplatin (65–69)	153	45% (37% to 53%)	18% (12% to 24%)
Gemcitabine + carboplatin (70–72)	90	56% (46% to 66%)	8% (2% to 13%)
Paclitaxel + ifosfamide (73)	13	31% (6% to 56%)	23% (0% to 46%)
Paclitaxel + gemcitabine (74)	39	56% (40% to 72%)	8% (0% to 17%)

OR, overall response; CR, complete response.

every 28 days for a maximum of six cycles. The response rates on both arms were similar with 12% CRs and 37% partial responses (PRs) on the GC arm and 12% CRs and 34% PRs on the M-VAC arm ($P = .51$). Similarly, median overall survival was similar: 13.8 months with GC and 14.8 months with M-VAC (HR 1.04; 95% CI, .82 to 1.32; $P = .75$). Importantly, GC was associated with a better safety profile and tolerability. While GC was associated with more grade ≥ 3 anemia and thrombocytopenia, M-VAC was associated with more neutropenic fever (14% vs. 2%), neutropenic sepsis (12% vs. 1%), grade ≥ 3 mucositis (22% vs. 1%), and treatment-related deaths (3% vs. 1%).

This randomized trial was not adequately powered to determine the therapeutic equivalence of these two regimens. However, these data can be interpreted as showing that, in terms of survival, GC is comparable to M-VAC. In addition, GC appears to be associated with a more favorable risk-benefit ratio. Given the results of this trial, and the ease of administration of this regimen, GC has become a widely used standard treatment regimen for patients with metastatic urothelial TCC.

Docetaxel and Cisplatin

A phase III randomized trial comparing docetaxel plus cisplatin (DC) with M-VAC has been reported by the Hellenic Cooperative Oncology Group (34). Patients randomized to DC received docetaxel 75 mg/m^2 and cisplatin 75 mg/m^2 repeated every 3 weeks. Both treatment arms received GCSF support. Of the 224 patients enrolled, 109 were randomized to M-VAC and 111 were randomized to DC. Although DC was associated with less hematologic toxicity and febrile neutropenia, OR rate (54.2 vs. 37.4; $P = .017$), median time to progression (9.4 vs. 6.1 months; $P = .003$), and median survival (14.2 vs. 9.3 months; $P = .026$) favored the M-VAC arm.

Paclitaxel and Carboplatin

The results of Eastern Cooperative Oncology Group (ECOG) 4897, a phase III trial comparing M-VAC with paclitaxel plus carboplatin, have recently been reported (35). This trial randomized patients with previously untreated advanced/metastatic TCC to either standard M-VAC or paclitaxel (225 mg/m^2) plus carboplatin area under the curve (AUC 6) administered every 21 days. Notably, after 2.5 years, the study was terminated due to slow accrual. Of the planned 330 patients, only 85 were enrolled at the time of the analysis. Compared with carboplatin/paclitaxel (CP), patients treated with M-VAC had more severe myelosuppression, mucositis, and renal toxicity.

Interestingly, a quality-of-life instrument revealed no significant differences between the two arms. At a median follow-up of 32.5 months, there was no significant difference in response rate (35.9% M-VAC versus 28.2% CP, $P = .34$) or median survival (15.4 months M-VAC versus 13.8 months CP, $P = .41$) between the two arms. However, given that the trial was severely underpowered, definitive conclusions are not possible.

CARBOPLATIN VERSUS CISPLATIN

Given the renal, neurologic, and auditory toxicity associated with cisplatin, and the elderly patient population with advanced TCC, it was hoped that carboplatin would be equivalent to cisplatin in this disease. Carboplatin may be administered to patients with impaired renal function, is more feasible in patients with multiple comorbidities, and is more easily administered in the outpatient setting. While carboplatin has a greater risk of myelosuppression, this toxicity can be managed easily by adjusting the dose according to the patient's creatinine clearance. In a review of 327 patients with advanced/metastatic TCC treated during 13 trials with single-agent carboplatin, 14% of patients achieved objective responses (3% CRs and 11% PRs) (75). These reports suggested efficacy similar to single-agent cisplatin but with a more favorable toxicity profile.

Despite the similar response proportions of single-agent carboplatin compared with historical controls treated with single-agent cisplatin, controversy still exists regarding the relative efficacy of carboplatin in TCC, particularly in combination regimens. Several randomized phase II trials have been performed in an attempt to address this issue (70,76,77) (Table 30.4). While these trials have limitations, they do consistently report higher overall and CR rates for the cisplatin-containing regimens. As a result, in patients with advanced TCC with favorable prognostic factors and adequate renal function, cisplatin-based therapy should be considered the treatment of choice.

NEW TRIPLETS IN METASTATIC TCC

Cisplatin, Paclitaxel, and Ifosfamide

The three-drug regimen of ifosfamide, paclitaxel, and cisplatin (ITP) has been explored in a phase II trial (78,79). Of 44 assessable patients treated with this regimen (68%; 95%

TABLE 30.4

RANDOMIZED PHASE II TRIALS COMPARING CISPLATIN- AND CARBOPLATIN-BASED COMBINATIONS

Treatment arms	Reference	OR	P	CR
M-VAC	(77)	52%	.3	13%
M-CAVI		39%		0%
MVE-cisplatin	(76)	71%	.04	25%
MVE-carboplatin		41%		11%
[a]Gemcitabine + cisplatin	(70)	66%	NP	23%
Gemcitabine + carboplatin		59%		9%

M-VAC, methotrexate, vinblastine, doxorubicin, cisplatin; M-CAVI, methotrexate, carboplatin, vinblastine; MVE, methotrexate, vinblastine, epirubicin; NP, not provided; OR, overall response; CR, complete response.
[a]Preliminary results.

CI, 52% to 81%), 30 demonstrated a major response, with 10 (23%) demonstrating CRs. Overall, myelosuppression was the predominant toxicity (45% grade 3 to 4 neutropenia), although the risk of febrile neutropenia was low (3.3% of all cycles). Grade 3 neuropathy and renal insufficiency occurred in 9% and 11%, respectively. The median survival of patients treated with ITP was 20 months. This survival is among the best reported results for patients with metastatic/advanced TCC, and it is greater than the previously observed results with M-VAC (12 to 13 months). However, the impact of baseline prognostic factors and aggressive post-treatment surgery cannot be discounted and may have contributed to the favorable results. The majority (>90%) of patients had either no poor risk factors (i.e., KPS ≥80 and no visceral metastases) or 1 poor prognosis feature (either KPS <80 or visceral metastases).

Cisplatin, Gemcitabine, and Ifosfamide

In a pilot trial at M. D. Anderson Cancer Center (MDACC), the combination of cisplatin, gemcitabine, and ifosfamide was explored (80). Fifty-one previously treated patients received cisplatin (30 mg/m^2), gemcitabine (800 mg/m^2), and ifosfamide (1 g/m^2) given on day 1 and then repeated on days 8 and 15 unless there was dose-limiting toxicity. Treatment cycles were repeated every 28 days. Of the 51 patients enrolled, 48 (94%) had dose-limiting hematologic toxicity on day 8 or 15. Despite the difficulty delivering this regimen, there were two CRs (4%) and 18 PRs (37%).

Cisplatin, Gemcitabine, and Paclitaxel

The combination of paclitaxel, gemcitabine, and cisplatin has been investigated in a phase I/II study (81). Among the 58 patients evaluated for response, there were 16 CRs (28%) and 29 PRs (50%) for an OR rate of 77.6% (95% CI, 60% to 98%). Toxicities consisted mainly of asthenia, thrombocytopenia, and neutropenia, with 11 cases (22%) of febrile neutropenia and 1 toxic death. The median survival time for the phase I portion was 24 months, and the median survival time of the whole group had not been reached at the time of the report. This regimen is currently being compared with gemcitabine plus cisplatin in an international randomized phase III trial conducted by the EORTC.

NOVEL APPROACHES TO THE TREATMENT OF TCC

Sequential "Dose-Dense" Therapy

Despite the promising activity and improved tolerability of the newer combination regimens in TCC, the majority of patients still succumb to their disease, necessitating new approaches to treatment. Simply adding additional agents may not prove beneficial given the expected degree of overlapping myelosuppression. A novel approach to combination chemotherapy is based on the Norton-Simon hypothesis, a mathematical prediction model of chemotherapy sensitivity based on Gompertzian growth rates displayed by malignant tumors (82). This hypothesis suggests that cytotoxic agents should be administered at the shortest possible interval to minimize tumor regrowth between cycles. This "dose density" is most feasible with a sequential schedule of administration. For example, if using therapies A and B, in which each letter depicts a single drug or combination, maintaining the dose intensity and dose density of both A and B is best achieved with sequenced therapy (A-A-A-B-B-B) rather than with an alternating (A-B-A-B-A-B) or a standard combination (AB-AB-AB-AB) schedule. This model has been extremely well studied in breast cancer and has been found to affect survival in the adjuvant chemotherapy setting (83).

Given the promising results with the ITP regimen, a study of sequenced therapy with doxorubicin and gemcitabine (AG) followed by ITP was initiated (84). In a pilot trial, 15 patients were treated with six cycles of AG (at five dose levels) repeated every 2 weeks with GSCF support. Two weeks after completing AG, ITP was given for four cycles every 21 days (paclitaxel 200 mg/m^2, cisplatin 70 mg/m^2, ifosfamide 1500 mg/m^2 on day 1; ifosfamide repeated on days 2 and 3) with GCSF support. This trial determined that a regimen of doxorubicin 50 mg/m^2 and gemcitabine 2000 mg/m^2 given every 2 weeks, followed by ITP, was feasible. Notably, there was no grade 3 or 4 myelosuppression with this dose and schedule of AG. Toxicity experienced with ITP included ≥ grade 3 neutropenia in 4 patients and grade 3 nausea/vomiting in 3 patients. After completion of the AG–ITP sequence, 9 of 14 evaluable patients (64%) had a major response (3 CRs and 6 PRs).

This regimen has been studied subsequently in a phase II trial that has recently completed accrual. A preliminary analysis of 21 patients has been reported with a major response seen in 18 patients (87%; 95% CI, 71% to 100%) and 43% of patients achieving a CR (95% CI, 22% to 64%) (85). Notably, the sequential use of ITP increased the rates of CR and PR seen after the initial AG doublet. More patients and longer follow-up are needed to determine this regimen's suitability for further study.

Targeting the Epidermal Growth Factor Receptor

The ErbB, or human epidermal growth factor receptor (EGFR), family of tyrosine kinases is an important mediator of cell growth, survival, and differentiation. Ligand binding to EGFR (or c-ErbB1) leads to homodimerization or heterodimerization with other members of the receptor subfamily (including c-ErbB2 or Her-2). These interactions result in autophosphorylation of the intracellular domain of EGFR leading to signaling through the mitogen-activated protein kinase pathway. Expression of EGFR and Her-2 has been variably demonstrated in bladder cancer specimens, depending on the methodology used and the criteria utilized to define expression. EGFR has also been implicated as a prognostic factor in bladder cancer. As a result, this receptor family has been a prime target for novel treatment strategies in TCC (86).

Trastuzumab is a humanized murine monoclonal antibody directed against the extracellular domain of Her-2. A Cancer and Leukemia Group B (CALGB) trial is currently exploring weekly single-agent trastuzumab in patients with previously treated TCC whose tumors overexpress Her-2 (87). A phase II evaluation of trastuzumab given in combination with paclitaxel, carboplatin, and gemcitabine has been reported in preliminary form (88). Patients with advanced/metastatic TCC and overexpression of Her-2 were eligible for enrollment. Treatment was administered as follows: trastuzumab (4 mg/kg on cycle 1 followed by 2 mg/kg with each subsequent cycle; days 1, 8, and 15), paclitaxel (200 mg/m^2 on day 1), carboplatin AUC 5 (on day 1), and gemcitabine (800 mg/m^2 on days 1 and 8). Fifty-three patients were evaluated for Her-2 status with overexpression by immunohistochemistry detected in 47%. Of 18 patients treated, there was 1 complete response (CR) and 14 PRs. This regimen is being further evaluated in a Southwest Oncology Group trial. The selective EGFR tyrosine kinase inhibitor ZD1839, in combination with either gemcitabine/cisplatin or gemcitabine/carboplatin, is being explored as first-line therapy in two CALGB phase II trials.

SPECIAL CONSIDERATIONS IN METASTATIC TCC

Post-chemotherapy Surgery

Several studies have highlighted the importance of post-chemotherapy surgery in the setting of minimal residual disease after achieving a "near" CR to chemotherapy (89–91). In a retrospective study of 203 patients treated on five trials with M-VAC, 50 patients underwent post-chemotherapy surgery for suspected or known residual disease (89). In 17 patients, no viable tumor was found at post-chemotherapy surgery, and 3 patients had unresectable disease. In the remaining 30 patients, residual TCC was completely resected, resulting in a CR to chemotherapy plus surgery. Of these 30 patients, 10 (33%) remained alive at 5 years, similar to results attained for patients achieving a CR to chemotherapy alone (41%). Optimal candidates were those patients with pre-chemotherapy disease limited to the primary site or lymph nodes.

Second-line Therapy

For patients with progressive TCC after first-line chemotherapy, prognosis is generally poor. However, several trials have indicated activity of both single-agents and combinations in patients with refractory or recurrent disease (47,50,52,92–95). In patients with a preserved functional status, treatment with one of these agents/combinations may be considered.

Treatment of Patients with Impaired Renal Function

Despite the high frequency of comorbidities and renal dysfunction in patients with advanced/metastatic TCC, few studies have specifically addressed the efficacy and tolerability of chemotherapy in this patient population. Bellmunt et al. reported a trial of the combination of gemcitabine and carboplatin in patients "unfit" for cisplatin due to a World Health Organization (WHO) performance status of 2 and/or a creatinine clearance of below 60 ml/min (71). For the 16 evaluable patients, the OR rate was 44%, with 1 CR and 6 PRs. A randomized trial of this regimen versus M-CAVI (methotrexate, vinblastine, and carboplatin) in patients with impaired renal function is being organized by the EORTC.

The ECOG performed a phase II trial of paclitaxel and carboplatin in patients with advanced TCC and renal dysfunction as defined by a serum creatinine of 1.6 to 4.0 mg/dL (65). Forty-two patients were accrued, and 37 were treated. Paclitaxel (225 mg/m^2) and carboplatin (AUC 6) were administered every 3 weeks for up to six cycles. Granulocytopenia (60%) and neurotoxicity (35%) were the most common ≥ grade 3 toxicities. The regimen resulted in an objective response rate of 24.3% (95% CI, 11.9% to 41.7%).

Given the promising initial results with "dose-dense" sequenced therapy, a pilot trial was performed at Memorial Sloan-Kettering Cancer Center evaluating a regimen of doxorubicin plus gemcitabine followed by paclitaxel plus carboplatin in patients with advanced/metastatic TCC and creatinine clearance of ≤60 mL/min (96). Preliminary results of this trial have been reported. Twenty-one patients were treated: 16 patients with metastatic or unresectable disease and 5 patients in the adjuvant setting. Grade 3 or grade 4 toxicity was primarily hematologic, with 73% neutropenia (1 patient with fever), 33% anemia, and 17% thrombocytopenia. Of the 7 evaluable patients at the time of the preliminary analysis, there was 1 CR and 4 PRs.

The Role of Radiation Therapy in Metastatic or Recurrent Disease

Although the initial treatment for most patients with metastatic disease is systemic multidrug chemotherapy, which has become very effective over the last two decades, many patients present with localized symptoms due to their metastatic TCC and may be helped by additional aggressive local therapy, such as external beam radiation therapy or surgery. Most of the local symptoms, such as pain or neurologic deficits, are the result of the bulk of the metastatic deposit, which can often be reduced by palliative radiation therapy. The underlying therapeutic goal is to improve or maintain quality of life while minimizing treatment-related toxicities. In these instances, treatment should be directed not toward long-term control of all sites of disease but rather to the alleviation of troubling symptoms and prevention of impending difficulties. Radiation therapy plays an important role in this regard in metastatic transitional cell carcinoma in a variety of sites (97). The precise radiation dose and technique need to be individualized. Radiation should be, whenever possible, delivered in a modest or short period of time, from 1 to 3 weeks, with acceptable acute morbidity and a good response rate (98).

The Treatment of Brain Metastases

Brain metastases from transitional cell carcinomas are uncommon but not rare. With whole-brain external beam radiation therapy alone, neurologic dysfunction from brain metastases is improved for between 50% and 70% of patients, and the median survival is increased by 3 to 6 months, compared with supportive care alone. The Radiation Therapy Oncology Group (RTOG) has conducted several studies evaluating the efficacy of various radiation fractionation schedules. No innovative schedule has been shown to be superior to the standard radiation treatment schedules used in most centers, which give a total dose of 30 Gy administered in 10 fractions. The solitary brain metastatic deposits can be treated with either surgery or focused radiation. However, subsequent failure in other regions of the brain will occur in 40% to 80% of patients (99,100). The addition of whole-brain radiation treatment to surgical resection or to stereotactic radiation treatment of the solitary lesion reduces the risk of cerebral recurrence to approximately 20% (101,102). Stereotactic radiation is a single-day procedure that produces a focal distribution of radiation to obliterate or control relatively small metastatic tumors in the brain. Metastases are often an ideal target for stereotactic radiosurgery because they are radiographically discrete and usually not invasive into the surrounding brain tissue. In the absence of any randomized data involving specifically metastatic TCC to the brain, it is most reasonable to treat patients with controlled systemic metastases and a single metastatic brain lesion with surgery or stereotactic radiosurgery plus whole brain radiotherapy, whereas whole-brain radiotherapy alone seems most reasonable for patients with multiple brain metastases or those with solitary brain metastases and other uncontrolled metastatic sites.

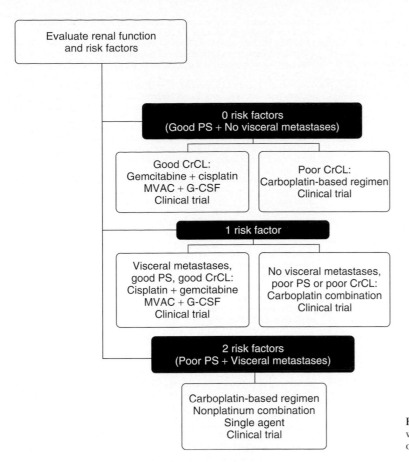

FIGURE 30.1. Algorithm for the management of patients with advanced/metastatic transitional cell carcinoma based on baseline prognostic factors and renal function.

Treatment of Metastatic Disease to Bone

External beam radiation therapy to painful bony metastases is an excellent form of palliative treatment resulting in pain relief in more than 70% of patients, but often the pain relief is not complete and its durability is less than 6 months (103,104). Before irradiating bony metastases that present with the threat of an impending pathologic fracture, orthopedic stabilization should precede radiation therapy (105). Combined concurrent chemotherapy and radiation for patients with metastatic or recurrent disease should now be considered because the dose of radiation that can be safely administered in many clinical settings is limited by constraints of adjacent normal tissues. Radiosensitizing doses of concurrent chemotherapy with cisplatin or 5-fluorouracil (5-FU) may be appropriate when trying to palliate bony pain or palliate symptoms from pelvic recurrent disease following radical cystectomy. However, certain chemotherapeutic agents given concurrently with radiation, such as gemcitabine or methotrexate, may cause excessive normal tissue reaction and should be avoided.

CONCLUSIONS

The last 20 years have brought significant advances in the management of metastatic TCC. This disease has proven to be chemotherapy-sensitive, and long-term survival has been achieved in a select subgroup of patients. Recently, regimens with preserved efficacy and improved tolerability have been introduced. In addition, the importance of baseline prognostic factors, comorbidities, and post-chemotherapy surgery has been recognized. Integrating this information has allowed the development of rational approaches to the treatment of individual patients (Figure 30.1). Novel approaches to the administration of combination chemotherapy and the addition of agents targeting critical signal transduction pathways may further improve the outlook for patients with this disease.

References

1. Herr HW. Cis-diamminedichloride platinum II in the treatment of advanced bladder cancer. *J Urol* 1980;123:853–855.
2. Yagoda A. Phase II trials with cis-dichlorodiammineplatinum (II) in the treatment of urothelial cancer [Review]. *Cancer Treat Rep* 1979;63:1565–1572.
3. Peters PC, O'Neill MR. Cis-diamminedichloroplatinum as a therapeutic agent in metastatic transitional cell carcinoma. *J Urol* 1991;121:375–377.
4. Merrin C. Treatment of advanced bladder cancer with cis-diamminedichloroplatinum (II) (NSC 119875): a pilot study. *J Urol* 1978;119: 493–495.
5. Soloway MS, Ikard M, Ford K. Cis-diamminedichloroplatinum (II) in locally advanced and metastatic urothelial cancer. *Cancer* 1981;47:476–480.
6. De Lena M, Lorusso V, Iacobellis U, et al. Cis-diamminedichloroplatinum activity in bidimensionally measurable metastatic lesions of the bladder. *Tumori* 1984;70:85–88.
7. Oliver RTD, Newlands ES, Wiltshaw E, et al. The London and Oxford Co-operative Urological Cancer Group. A phase 2 study of cis-platinum in patients with recurrent bladder carcinoma. *Br J Urol* 1981;55:444–457.
8. Rossof AH, Talley RW, Stephens R, et al. Phase II evaluation of cis-dichlorodiammineplatinum (II) in advanced malignancies of the genitourinary and gynecologic organs: a Southwest Oncology Group Study. *Cancer Treat Rep* 1979;63:1557–1564.
9. Soloway MS, Einstein A, Corder MP, et al. A National Bladder Cancer Collaborative Group Study. A comparison of cisplatin and the combination of cisplatin and cyclophosphamide in advanced urothelial cancer. *Cancer* 1983;51:767–772.
10. Hillcoat BL, Raghavan D, Matthews J, et al. A randomized trial of cisplatin versus cisplatin plus methotrexate in advanced cancer of the urothelial tract. *J Clin Oncol* 1989;7:706–709.

11. Loehrer PJ Sr, Einhorn LH, Elson PJ, et al. A randomized comparison of cisplatin alone or in combination with methotrexate, vinblastine, and doxorubicin in patients with metastatic urothelial carcinoma: a cooperative group study. *J Clin Oncol* 1992;10:1066–1073.

12. Oliver RT. Methotrexate as salvage or adjunctive therapy for primary invasive carcinoma of the bladder. *Cancer Treat Rep* 1981;65(Suppl. 1):179–181.

13. Oliver RT, England HR, Risdon RA, et al. Methotrexate in the treatment of metastatic and recurrent primary transitional cell carcinoma. *J Urol* 1984;131:483–485.

14. Turner AG, Hendry WF, Williams GB, et al. The treatment of advanced bladder cancer with methotrexate. *Br J Urol* 1977;49:673–678.

15. Turner AG. Methotrexate in advanced bladder cancer. *Cancer Treat Rep* 1981;65(Suppl. 1):183–186.

16. Natale RB, Yagoda A, Watson RC, et al. Methotrexate: an active drug in bladder cancer. *Cancer* 1981;47:1246–1250.

17. Gad-el-Mawla N, Hamsa R, Cairns J, et al. Phase II trial of methotrexate in carcinoma of the bilharzial bladder. *Cancer Treat Rep* 1978;62:1075–1076.

18. Hall RR. Methotrexate treatment for advanced bladder cancer. A review after 6 years. *Br J Urol* 1980;52:403.

19. Pavone-Macaluso M. Single-drug chemotherapy of bladder cancer with adriamycin, VM-26 or bleomycin. *Eur Urol* 1976;2:138–141.

20. O'Bryan RM, Baker LH, Gottlieb JE. Dose response evaluation of adriamycin in human neoplasia. *Cancer* 1977;39:1940.

21. Yagoda A, Watson RC, Whitmore WF, et al. Adriamycin in advanced urinary tract cancer. Experience in 42 patients and review of the literature. *Cancer* 1977;39:279–285.

22. Knight EW, Pagand M, Hahn RG, et al. Comparison of 5-FU and doxorubicin in the treatment of carcinoma of the bladder. *Cancer Treat Rep* 1983;67:514–515.

23. Gagliano R, Levin H, El-Bolkainy MN, et al. A Southwest Oncology Group Study. Adriamycin versus adriamycin plus cis-diamminedichloroplatinum (DDP) in advanced transitional cell bladder carcinoma. *Am J Clin Oncol (CCT)* 1983;6:215–218.

24. Blumenreich MS, Yagoda A, Natale RB, et al. Phase II trial of vinblastine sulfate for metastatic urothelial tract tumors. *Cancer* 1982;50:435–438.

25. Sternberg CN, Yagoda A, Scher HI, et al. Preliminary results of M-VAC (methotrexate, vinblastine, doxorubicin and cisplatin) for transitional cell carcinoma of the urothelium. *J Urol* 1985;133:403–407.

26. Sternberg CN, Yagoda A, Scher HI, et al. Methotrexate, vinblastine, doxorubicin, and cisplatin for advanced transitional cell carcinoma of the urothelium. Efficacy and patterns of response and relapse. *Cancer* 1989;64:2448–2458.

27. Tannock I, Gospodarowicz M, Connolly J, et al. M-VAC (methotrexate, vinblastine, doxorubicin and cisplatin) chemotherapy for transitional cell carcinoma: the Princess Margaret Hospital experience. *J Urol* 1989;142:289–292.

28. Igawa M, Ohkuchi T, Ueki T, et al. Usefulness and limitations of methotrexate, vinblastine, doxorubicin and cisplatin for the treatment of advanced urothelial cancer. *J Urol* 1990;144:662–665.

29. Boutan-Laroze A, Mahjoubi M, Droz JP, et al. M-VAC (methotrexate, vinblastine, doxorubicin and cisplatin) for advanced carcinoma of the bladder. The French Federation of Cancer Centers experience. *Eur J Cancer* 1991;27:1690–1694.

30. Logothetis CJ, Dexeus F, Sella A, et al. A prospective randomized trial comparing CISCA to MVAC chemotherapy in advanced metastatic urothelial tumors. *J Clin Oncol* 1990;8:1050–1055.

31. Siefker-Radtke AO, Millikan RE, Tu SM, et al. Phase III trial of fluorouracil, interferon alpha-2b, and cisplatin versus methotrexate, vinblastine, doxorubicin, and cisplatin in metastatic or unresectable urothelial cancer. *J Clin Oncol* 2002;20:1361–1367.

32. Sternberg CN, de Mulder PH, Schornagel JH, et al. Randomized phase III trial of high-dose-intensity methotrexate, vinblastine, doxorubicin, and cisplatin MVAC chemotherapy and recombinant human granulocyte colony-stimulating factor versus classic MVAC in advanced urothelial tract tumors: European Organization for Research and Treatment of Cancer Protocol no. 30924. *J Clin Oncol* 2001;19:2638–2646.

33. Von der Maase H, Hansen SW, Roberts JT, et al. Gemcitabine and cisplatin versus methotrexate, vinblastine, doxorubicin, and cisplatin in advanced or metastatic bladder cancer: results of a large, randomized, multinational, multicenter, phase III study. *J Clin Oncol* 2000;18:3068–3077.

34. Bamias A, Aravantinos G, Deliveliotis C, et al. Docetaxel and cisplatin with granulocyte colony-stimulating factor (G-CSF) versus MVAC with G-CSF in advanced urothelial carcinoma: a multicenter, randomized, phase III study from the Hellenic Cooperative Oncology Group. *J Clin Oncol* 2004;22:220–228.

35. Dreicer R, Manola J, Roth BJ, et al. Phase III trial of methotrexate, vinblastine, doxorubicin, and cisplatin versus carboplatin and paclitaxel in patients with advanced carcinoma of the urothelium. *Cancer* 2004;100:1639–1645.

36. Mead GM, Russell M, Clark P, et al. A randomized trial comparing methotrexate and vinblastine (MV) with cisplatin, methotrexate and vinblastine (CMV) in advanced transitional cell carcinoma: results and a report on prognostic factors in a Medical Research Council study. MRC Advanced Bladder Cancer Working Party. *Br J Cancer* 1998;78:1067–1075.

37. Saxman SB, Propert KJ, Einhorn LH, et al. Long-term follow-up of a phase III intergroup study of cisplatin alone or in combination with methotrexate,

vinblastine, and doxorubicin in patients with metastatic urothelial carcinoma: a cooperative group study. *J Clin Oncol* 1997;15:2564–2569.

38. Gabrilove JL, Jakubowski A, Scher H, et al. Effect of granulocyte colony-stimulating factor on neutropenia and associated morbidity due to chemotherapy for transitional-cell carcinoma of the urothelium. *N Engl J Med* 1988;318:1414–1422.

39. Logothetis CJ, Finn LD, Smith T, et al. Escalated MVAC with or without recombinant human granulocyte-macrophage colony-stimulating factor for the initial treatment of advanced malignant urothelial tumors: results of a randomized trial. *J Clin Oncol* 1995;13:2272–2277.

40. Logothetis CJ, Dexeus FH, Sella A, et al. Escalated therapy for refractory urothelial tumors: methotrexate-vinblastine-doxorubicin-cisplatin plus unglycosylated recombinant human granulocyte-macrophage colony-stimulating factor. *J Natl Cancer Inst* 1990;82:667–672.

41. Seidman AD, Scher HI, Gabrilove JL, et al. Dose-intensification of methotrexate, vinblastine, doxorubicin, and cisplatin with recombinant granulocyte-colony stimulating factor as initial therapy in advanced urothelial cancer. *J Clin Oncol* 1992;11:414–420.

42. Loehrer PJ Sr, Elson P, Dreicer R, et al. Escalated dosages of methotrexate, vinblastine, doxorubicin, and cisplatin plus recombinant human granulocyte colony-stimulating factor in advanced urothelial carcinoma: an Eastern Cooperative Oncology Group trial. *J Clin Oncol* 1994;12:483–488.

43. Sternberg CN, de Mulder PH, van Oosterom AT, et al. Escalated M-VAC chemotherapy and recombinant human granulocyte-macrophage colony stimulating factor (rhGM-CSF) in patients with advanced urothelial tract tumors. *Ann Oncol* 1993;4:403–407.

44. Bajorin DF, Dodd PM, Mazumdar M, et al. Long-term survival in metastatic transitional-cell carcinoma and prognostic factors predicting outcome of therapy. *J Clin Oncol* 1999;17:3173–3181.

45. Geller NL, Sternberg CN, Penenberg D, et al. Prognostic factors for survival of patients with advanced urothelial tumors treated with methotrexate, vinblastine, doxorubicin, and cisplatin chemotherapy. *Cancer* 1991;67:1525–1531.

46. Bellmunt J, Albanell J, Paz-Ares L, et al. Pretreatment prognostic factors for survival in patients with advanced urothelial tumors treated in a phase I/II trial with paclitaxel, cisplatin, and gemcitabine. *Cancer* 2002;95:751–757.

47. Vaughn DJ, Broome CM, Hussain M, et al. Phase II trial of weekly paclitaxel in patients with previously treated advanced urothelial cancer. *J Clin Oncol* 2002;20:937–940.

48. Roth BJ, Dreicer R, Einhorn LH, et al. Significant activity of paclitaxel in advanced transitional-cell carcinoma of the urothelium: a phase II trial of the Eastern Cooperative Oncology Group. *J Clin Oncol* 1994;12:2264–2270.

49. Papamichael D, Gallagher CJ, Oliver RT, et al. Phase II study of paclitaxel in pretreated patients with locally advanced/metastatic cancer of the bladder and ureter. *Br J Cancer* 1997;75:606–607.

50. McCaffrey JA, Hilton S, Mazumdar M, et al. Phase II trial of docetaxel in patients with advanced or metastatic transitional-cell carcinoma. *J Clin Oncol* 1997;15:1853–1857.

51. De Wit R, Kruit WH, Stoter G, et al. Docetaxel (Taxotere): an active agent in metastatic urothelial cancer; results of a phase II study in non-chemotherapy-pretreated patients. *Br J Cancer* 1998;78:1342–1345.

52. Witte RS, Elson P, Bono B, et al. Eastern Cooperative Oncology Group phase II trial of ifosfamide in the treatment of previously treated advanced urothelial carcinoma. *J Clin Oncol* 1997;15:589–593.

53. Gad el Mawla N, Hamza MR, Zikri ZK, et al. Chemotherapy in invasive carcinoma of the bladder: a review of phase II trials in Egypt. *Acta Oncol* 1989;28:73–76.

54. Otaguro K, Ueda K, Niijima T, et al. Clinical evaluation of Z4942 (ifosfamide) for malignant urological tumors. *Acta Urol Jpn* 1981;27:459–469.

55. Stadler WM, Kuzel T, Roth B, et al. Phase II study of single-agent gemcitabine in previously untreated patients with metastatic urothelial cancer. *J Clin Oncol* 1997;15:3394–3398.

56. Moore MJ, Tannock IF, Ernst DS, et al. Gemcitabine: a promising new agent in the treatment of advanced urothelial cancer. *J Clin Oncol* 1997;15:3441–3445.

57. Dreicer R, Manola J, Roth BJ, et al. Phase II study of cisplatin and paclitaxel in advanced carcinoma of the urothelium: an Eastern Cooperative Oncology Group study. *J Clin Oncol* 2000;18:1058–1061.

58. Burch PA, Richardson RL, Cha SS, et al. Phase II study of paclitaxel and cisplatin for advanced urothelial cancer. *J Urol* 2000;164:1538–1542.

59. Garcia del Muro X, Marcuello E, Guma J, et al. Phase II multicentre study of docetaxel plus cisplatin in patients with advanced urothelial cancer. *Br J Cancer* 2002;86:326–330.

60. Sengelov L, Kamby C, Lund B, et al. Docetaxel and cisplatin in metastatic urothelial cancer: a phase II study. *J Clin Oncol* 1998;16:3392–3397.

61. Dimopoulos MA, Bakoyannis C, Georgoulias V, et al. Docetaxel and cisplatin combination chemotherapy in advanced carcinoma of the urothelium: a multicenter phase II study of the Hellenic Cooperative Oncology Group. *Ann Oncol* 1999;10:1385–1388.

62. Von der Maase H, Andersen L, Crino L, et al. Weekly gemcitabine and cisplatin combination therapy in patients with transitional cell carcinoma of the urothelium: a phase II clinical trial. *Ann Oncol* 1999;10:1461–1465.

63. Kaufman D, Raghavan D, Carducci M, et al. Phase II trial of gemcitabine plus cisplatin in patients with metastatic urothelial cancer. *J Clin Oncol* 2000;18:1921–1927.

64. Moore MJ, Winquist EW, Murray N, et al. Gemcitabine plus cisplatin, an active regimen in advanced urothelial cancer: a phase II trial of the National Cancer Institute of Canada Clinical Trials Group. *J Clin Oncol* 1999;17:2876–2881.

65. Vaughn DJ, Manola J, Dreicer R, et al. Phase II study of paclitaxel plus carboplatin in patients with advanced carcinoma of the urothelium and renal dysfunction (E2896): a trial of the Eastern Cooperative Oncology Group. *Cancer* 2002;95:1022–1027.

66. Redman BG, Smith DC, Flaherty L, et al. Phase II trial of paclitaxel and carboplatin in the treatment of advanced urothelial carcinoma. *J Clin Oncol* 1998;16:1844–1848.

67. Zielinski CC, Schnack B, Grbovic M, et al. Paclitaxel and carboplatin in patients with metastatic urothelial cancer: results of a phase II trial. *Br J Cancer* 1998;78:370–374.

68. Pycha A, Grbovic M, Posch B, et al. Paclitaxel and carboplatin in patients with metastatic transitional cell cancer of the urinary tract. *Urology* 1999; 53:510–515.

69. Small EJ, Lew D, Redman BG, et al. Southwest Oncology Group study of paclitaxel and carboplatin for advanced transitional-cell carcinoma: the importance of survival as a clinical trial end point. *J Clin Oncol* 2000; 18:2537–2544.

70. Carteni G, Dogliotti L, Crucitta A, et al. Phase II randomized trial of gemcitabine plus cisplatin and gemcitabine plus carboplatin in patients with advanced or metastatic transitional cell carcinoma of the urothelium. *Proc Am Soc Clin Oncol* 2003;22:384 (Abstract 1543).

71. Bellmunt J, de Wit R, Albanell J, et al. A feasibility study of carboplatin with fixed dose of gemcitabine in "unfit" patients with advanced bladder cancer. *Eur J Cancer* 2001;37:2212–2215.

72. Carles J, Nogue M. Gemcitabine/carboplatin in advanced urothelial cancer. *Semin Oncol* 2001;28:19–24.

73. Sweeney CJ, Williams SD, Finch DE, et al. A phase II study of paclitaxel and ifosfamide for patients with advanced refractory carcinoma of the urothelium. *Cancer* 1999;86:514–518.

74. Meluch AA, Greco FA, Burris HA III, et al. Paclitaxel and gemcitabine chemotherapy for advanced transitional-cell carcinoma of the urothelial tract: a phase II trial of the Minnie Pearl Cancer Research Network. *J Clin Oncol* 2001;19:3018–3024.

75. Mottet-Auselo N, Bons-Rosset F, Costa P, et al. Carboplatin and urothelial tumors. *Oncology* 1993;50(Suppl. 2):28–36.

76. Petrioli R, Frediani B, Manganelli A, et al. Comparison between a cisplatin-containing regimen and a carboplatin-containing regimen for recurrent or metastatic bladder cancer patients: a randomized phase II study. *Cancer* 1996;77:344–351.

77. Bellmunt J, Ribas A, Eres N, et al. Carboplatin-based versus cisplatin-based chemotherapy in the treatment of surgically incurable advanced bladder carcinoma. *Cancer* 1997;80:1966–1972.

78. Bajorin DF, McCaffrey JA, Hilton S, et al. Treatment of patients with transitional-cell carcinoma of the urothelial tract with ifosfamide, paclitaxel, and cisplatin: a phase II trial. *J Clin Oncol* 1998;16:2722–2727.

79. Bajorin DF, McCaffrey JA, Dodd PM, et al. Ifosfamide, paclitaxel, and cisplatin for patients with advanced transitional cell carcinoma of the urothelial tract: final report of a phase II trial evaluating two dosing schedules. *Cancer* 2000;88:1671–1678.

80. Pagliaro LC, Millikan RE, Tu SM, et al. Cisplatin, gemcitabine, and ifosfamide as weekly therapy: a feasibility and phase II study of salvage treatment for advanced transitional-cell carcinoma. *J Clin Oncol* 2002;20:2965–2970.

81. Bellmunt J, Guillem V, Paz-Ares L, et al. Spanish Oncology Genitourinary Group. Phase I-II study of paclitaxel, cisplatin, and gemcitabine in advanced transitional-cell carcinoma of the urothelium. *J Clin Oncol* 2000; 18:3247–3255.

82. Norton L, Simon R. The Norton-Simon hypothesis revisited. *Cancer Treat Rep* 1986;70:163–169.

83. Citron ML, Berry DA, Cirrincione C, et al. Randomized trial of dose-dense versus conventionally scheduled and sequential versus concurrent combination chemotherapy as postoperative adjuvant treatment of node-positive primary breast cancer: first report of Intergroup Trial C9741/Cancer and Leukemia Group B Trial 9741. *J Clin Oncol* 2003;21:1431–1439.

84. Dodd PM, McCaffrey JA, Hilton S, et al. Phase I evaluation of sequential doxorubicin gemcitabine then ifosfamide paclitaxel cisplatin for patients with unresectable or metastatic transitional-cell carcinoma of the urothelial tract. *J Clin Oncol* 2000;18:840–846.

85. Maluf F, Hilton S, Nanus D, et al. Sequential doxorubicin/gemcitabine and ifosfamide, paclitaxel, and cisplatin chemotherapy in patients with metastatic or locally advanced transitional cell carcinoma of the urothelium. *Proc Am Soc Clin Oncol* 2000;19:342(Abstract 1344).

86. Bellmunt J, Hussain M, Dinney CP. Novel approaches with targeted therapies in bladder cancer. Therapy of bladder cancer by blockade of the epidermal growth factor receptor family. *Crit Rev Oncol Hematol* 2003; 46(Suppl.1):85–104.

87. Small EJ, Halabi S, Dalbagni G, et al. Overview of bladder cancer trials in the Cancer and Leukemia Group B. *Cancer* 2003;97:2090–2098.

88. Hussain M, Smith DC, Vaishampayan U, et al. Trastuzumab, paclitaxel, carboplatin and gemcitabine in patients with advanced urothelial cancer and overexpression of HER-2. *Proc Am Soc Clin Oncol* 2003;22:391 (Abstract 1569).

89. Dodd PM, McCaffrey JA, Herr H, et al. Outcome of postchemotherapy surgery after treatment with methotrexate, vinblastine, doxorubicin, and cisplatin in patients with unresectable or metastatic transitional cell carcinoma. *J Clin Oncol* 1999;17:2546–2552.

90. Donat SM, Herr HW, Bajorin DF, et al. Methotrexate, vinblastine, doxorubicin and cisplatin chemotherapy and cystectomy for unresectable bladder cancer. *J Urol* 1996;156:368–371.

91. Miller RS, Freiha FS, Reese JH, et al. Cisplatin, methotrexate and vinblastine plus surgical restaging for patients with advanced transitional cell carcinoma of the urothelium. *J Urol* 1993;150:65–69.

92. Lorusso V, Pollera CF, Antimi M, et al. A phase II study of gemcitabine in patients with transitional cell carcinoma of the urinary tract previously treated with platinum. Italian Co-operative Group on Bladder Cancer. *Eur J Cancer* 1998;34:1208–1212.

93. Dreicer R, Manola J, Schneider DJ, et al. Phase II trial of gemcitabine and docetaxel in patients with advanced carcinoma of the urothelium: a trial of the Eastern Cooperative Oncology Group. *Cancer* 2003;97:2743–2747.

94. Sternberg CN, Calabro F, Pizzocaro G, et al. Chemotherapy with an every-2-week regimen of gemcitabine and paclitaxel in patients with transitional cell carcinoma who have received prior cisplatin-based therapy. *Cancer* 2001;92:2993–2998.

95. Bellmunt J, Cos J, Cleries R, et al. Feasibility trial of methotrexate-paclitaxel as a second line therapy in advanced urothelial cancer. *Cancer Invest* 2002; 20:673–685.

96. Novick S, Higgins G, Hilton S, et al. Phase I/II sequential doxorubicin plus gemcitabine followed by paclitaxel plus carboplatin in patients with transitional cell carcinoma and impaired renal function. *Proc Am Soc Clin Oncol* 2000;19:342 (Abstract 1423).

97. Petrovich Z, Jozsef G, Brady LW. Radiotherapy for carcinoma of the bladder: a review. *Am J Clin Oncol* 2001;24:1–9.

98. Duchesne GM, Bolger JJ, Griffiths GO, et al. A randomized trial of hypofractionated schedules of palliative radiotherapy in the management of bladder carcinoma: results of Medical Research Council trial BA09. *Int J Radiat Oncol Biol Phys* 2000;47:379–388.

99. Rosenstein M, Wallner K, Scher H, et al. Brain metastases from transitional cell carcinoma of the bladder. *J Urol* 1993;149:480–483.

100. Anderson RS, El-Mahdi AM, Kuban DA, et al. Brain metastases from transitional carcinoma of urinary bladder. *Urology* 1992;39:17–20.

101. DeAngelis LM, Mandell LR, Thaler HT, et al. The role of postoperative radiotherapy after resection of single brain metastasis. *Neurosurgery* 1989;24:798–805.

102. Andrews DW, Scott CB, Sperduto PW, et al. Whole brain radiation therapy with or without stereotactic radiosurgery boost for patients with one to three brain metastases: phase III results of RTOG 9508 randomized trial. *Lancet* 2004;363:1665–1672.

103. Kabalin JN, Freiha FS, Torti FM. Brain metastases from transitional cell carcinoma of urinary bladder. *J Urol* 1988;140:820–824.

104. Bates T, Yarnold JF, Blitzer P, et al. Bone metastasis consensus statement. *Int J Radiat Oncol Biol Phys* 1992;23:215–216.

105. Townsend PW, Smalley SR, Cozad SC, et al. Is radiation therapy beneficial after orthopedic stabilization of impending or pathologic fracture due to metastatic disease? *Int J Radiat Oncol Biol Phys* 1993;27:159.

CHAPTER 31 ■ TESTIS CANCER: CLINICAL SIGNS AND SYMPTOMS

STEPHEN D. W. BECK AND JOHN P. DONOHUE

Testicular cancer, although relatively rare, is the most common malignancy among men aged 15 years to 35 years. Prior to the introduction of cisplatin-based chemotherapy in the mid-1970s, testicular cancer accounted for 11.4% of all cancer deaths in the 25-year to 34-year age group (1). With platinum-based regimens, it is now expected that 95% of patients with early stage testicular cancer, and up to 70% to 80% of patients with advanced disease, will survive. The American Cancer Society estimates that in the year 2005, about 8,010 new cases of testicular cancer will be diagnosed in the United States. An estimated 390 men will die of testicular cancer in the year 2005.

The diagnosis of testicular cancer is typically not difficult. Over 95% of solid testicular masses are neoplastic, and combined serum tumor markers alpha-fetoprotein (AFP) and human chorionic gonadotripin (HCG) are elevated in 90% of patients (2,3). For the vast majority of patients, the diagnosis of testicular cancer can be included or excluded with scrotal examination and serum tumor markers. What can be difficult is remembering that germ-cell cancer is a potential diagnosis and including it in the differential diagnosis for a wide spectrum of clinical signs and symptoms that may seem unrelated to a testicular primary neoplasm.

SIGNS AND SYMPTOMS

Scrotum

The most common presentation of testicular cancer relates to the site of origin and typically presents as a nodule or painless swelling in one gonad (Table 31.1). A painful testis is the next most common symptom, and in 10% this pain is acute on onset (4). Testicular pain at presentation is possibly secondary to hemorrhage or mass effect and has been linked to rapid tumor growth observed in nonseminomatous germ cell tumors (NSGCT). Seminomas have a slower growth rate and more often present with a painless mass. Sandeman reported testicular pain as the initial presenting symptom in 47% and 38% of nonseminoma and seminoma patients, respectively (5).

Trauma is observed in only 10% of patients with testicular cancer (7,9). Trauma was once regarded as a risk factor, because the enlarged gonad secondary to malignancy is more prone to injury and injury itself leads to recognition of the pre-existing tumor. Other red herrings, including epididymo-orchitis, torsion, hydrocele, and hernias, all lead to misdiagnosis and delay in diagnosis. Although nearly two-thirds of patients with testicular cancer have an abnormal semen analysis at presentation, infertility as an initial complaint is uncommon (<5%) (10–12).

Retroperitoneum

The primary landing zone for metastatic spread in testicular cancer is the retroperitoneum, which is the most common location of lymphatic disease. Though frequently involved with tumor, retroperitoneal disease is typically asymptomatic and most commonly identified at the time of metastatic workup, after the diagnosis of testicular cancer is reached. However, approximately 10% to 20% of patients do present with symptoms of distant metastases, with the retroperitoneum the most common site of disease (7,8). At Indiana University, back pain was the presenting symptom in over 10% of patients, and half of such patients presented with retroperitoneal malignancy greater than 10 cm. Other signs and symptoms of abdominal malignancy include gastrointestinal disturbance or hemorrhage, weight loss, or palpable mass. Flank pain from ureteral obstruction is not uncommon.

Supradiaphragmatic Disease

Metastatic disease above the diaphragm can present on examination with pulmonary symptoms including shortness of breath or hemoptysis, or radiographically with pleural effusions. Enlargement or tenderness of the breast was noted in 33 of 1044 patients at Indiana University. Daniels and Layer reported on 175 men who presented to a breast clinic with gynecomastia, of whom 4 had testicular cancer (13). Secretion of beta-HCG by germ-cell tumors stimulates estrogen secretion from Leydig cells with resultant gynecomastia. Leydig cell tumors have a higher incidence of gynecomastia (10% to 20%) than do other metastatic tumors, secondary to direct production and secretion of estrogens from the tumor. Other locations of metastatic spread include the neck (about 10%) and other supraclavicular locations and, less commonly, the cerebrum. In the report of the International Germ Cell Cancer Collaborative Group (IGCCCG), initial brain metastases were observed in only 70 of 5,862 patients with metastatic germ cell cancer (1.2%) (14).

Biologic Significance

Clinical signs and symptoms of metastases at initial diagnosis may reflect biologic aggressiveness and predict outcome. Size of the primary tumor, although an integral part in most oncologic staging systems, is not included in the TNM staging of testis tumors (15). However, Warde et al. reported the effect of tumor size on relapse in patients with clinical stage 1 seminoma. The 5-year relapse-free rate for 317 patients with primary tumor size of 4 cm or smaller and for 281 patients with tumor size larger than 4 cm was 86.6% and 75.9%, respectively

TABLE 31.1

SIGNS AND SYMPTOMS OF PATIENTS PRESENTING WITH TESTICULAR CANCER (%)

Registry (Ref.)	Painless mass	Painful mass	Associated with trauma	Symptoms and signs of metastases	Back pain	Breast complaints
Toronto, Canada (6) ($n = 360$)	56.9	26.4	13.0	5.2	NS	NS
Peter MacCallum Hospital, Melbourne, Australia (5) ($n = 502$)	54.0	42.0	NS	NS	NS	NS
Irish Testicular Tumour Registry (7) ($n = 217$)	32.0	31.0	10.0	19.0	2.0	2.0
University of Minnesota (8) ($n = 335$)	NS	45.0	11.2	10.7	NS	5.0
Indiana University[a] ($n = 1044$)	42.5	17.2	3.0	22.3	13.9	3.2

NS, not specified.
[a]Unpublished data.

($P = .003$) (16). At Indiana University, reviewing 779 patients with clinical stage 1 NSGCT, we were unable to demonstrate this same predictive value of primary tumor size for the non-seminoma group (17).

Initial risk stratification models incorporated clinical signs and symptoms as predictive of outcome; they included palpable abdominal disease [Indiana University and National Cancer Institute (NCI) models], pleural effusion, and obstructive uropathy (NCI model). Additional risk assessment for Indiana University, NCI, and the European Organisation for the Research and Treatment of Cancer (EORTC) included liver, osseous, and CNS metastases. To standardize risk stratification, the IGCCCG evaluated data on 5,202 patients with NSGCT and 660 patients with pure seminoma. For NSGCT the following independent adverse factors were identified: mediastinal primary, degree of serum tumor marker elevation, and presence of nonpulmonary visceral metastases. For seminoma, the predominant adverse feature was the presence of nonpulmonary visceral metastases (14). No signs or symptoms were evaluated for prognostic significance in this multinational collaboration. Quantifying such factors would be difficult and open to wide interpretational variability. Despite these limitations, clinical symptoms and signs remain an important tool for the astute clinician for diagnosis, evaluating response to therapy, and identifying relapse.

Delay in Diagnosis

Despite the external location of the male gonad, allowing accessibility for both self-exam and physician-performed exam, delay of diagnoses for testicular cancer continues to occur. Delay in diagnosis is not uncommon, with a reported mean delay time of over 5 weeks (18,19). Some investigators have reported a significant relation between survival and delay in diagnosis (7,20). However, others have shown no impact on survival (21). With germ-cell tumors showing rapid growth rate, a delay in diagnosis would theoretically allow for tumor spread and presentation at advanced stage of disease; conversely, early diagnosis offers a chance to identify disease at a lower stage. Moul et al. reported a decrease in survival rate for nonseminoma patients with a delay of diagnosis greater than 16 weeks (22). When controlling for chemotherapy, however, delay in diagnosis did not impact survival. Because of the chemosensitivity of germ-cell tumors, despite advanced disease curability remains high, though advanced disease may require more cycles or more intensive chemotherapy, adding to patient morbidity.

Delay in diagnosis may be related to patient reluctance to seek health care or misdiagnosis by the physician. Many young men delay medical care with explanations including embarrassment, fear, guilt, and ignorance. Delay on the part of the physician in initiating diagnosis may also be considerable. Common initial diagnoses include trauma, hydrocele, and infection. With the presumed diagnoses of orchitis/epididymitis, re-evaluation in the clinic is necessary to monitor response to antibiotics.

Retroperitoneal mass identified in the young adult male is typically not a diagnostic dilemma, and metastatic germ-cell tumor or primary retroperitoneal germ-cell tumor is first on a rather short differential including lymphoma and sarcoma. Multiple case reports have described exploratory laparotomy for unsuspected germ-cell tumor (23–26). Memorial Sloan-Kettering Cancer Center (MSKCC) recently reported the impact of surgery on therapeutic delay and cancer therapy in 40 patients managed with initial exploratory laparotomy for unsuspected metastatic germ-cell tumor (27). The median interval from laparotomy to chemotherapy was 29 days, and in 48% of the patients the delay was 30 days or more. Of patients with a delay longer than 30 days, 60% required chemotherapy dose intensification, compared with 26% with a delay of 30 days or fewer ($P = .01$). Germ-cell tumor should be considered as a potential etiology for a retroperitoneal mass in all male patients regardless of age.

CONCLUSION

Prompt diagnosis and treatment of germ-cell cancer requires the awareness of both patient and physician. Young men require education on the importance of testicular self-examination. They should be familiar with performing this examination and encouraged to seek medical attention upon a suspicious finding, most often a solid, painless, testicular mass. Testicular cancer can present with a wide array of symptoms and signs seemingly unrelated to a primary gonadal neoplasm. Physicians, often confronted with this spectrum of patient complaints and physical findings, must recognize germ-cell cancer as at least a candidate in the differential diagnoses, to be excluded with testicular examination and serum tumor marker evaluation to prevent delay in diagnosis.

Despite remarkable advances in the management of germ-cell cancer over the past 30 years, with this being the most common neoplasm in the young adult male, public awareness has remained limited. Annual visits to the physician should instill into young men both the importance and proper technique of testicular self-examination to limit delay in diagnosis of this very curable neoplasm.

References

1. Twito DI, Kennedy BJ. Treatment of testicular cancer. *Ann Rev Med* 1975;26:235–243.
2. Kressel K, Schnell D, Dettmann R, et al. Diagnosis and therapy of non-germ cell testicular tumors. Organ preservation or orchiectomy? *Urologe A* 1993;32:237–241.
3. Fowler JJ, Taylor G, Blom J, et al. Experience with serum alpha-fetoprotein and human chorionic gonadotropin in non-seminomatous testicular tumors. *J Urol* 1980;124:365–368.
4. Richie JP. Advances in the diagnosis and treatment of testicular cancer. *Cancer Invest* 1993;11:670–675.
5. Sandeman TF. Symptoms and early management of germinal tumours of the testis. *Med J Aust* 1979;2:281–284.
6. Robson CJ, Bruce AW, Charbonneau J. Testicular tumors: a collective review from the Canadian Academy of Urological Surgeons. *J Urol* 1965;94:440–444.
7. Thornhill JA, Fennelly JJ, Kelly DG, et al. Patients' delay in the presentation of testis cancer in Ireland. *Br J Urol* 1987;59:447–451.
8. Bosl GJ, Vogelzang NJ, Goldman A, et al. Impact of delay in diagnosis on clinical stage of testicular cancer. *Lancet* 1981;2:970–973.
9. Patton JF, Hewitt CB, Mallis N. Diagnosis and treatment of tumors of the testis. *JAMA* 1959;171:2194–2198.
10. Petersen P, Skakkebaek N, Vistisen K, et al. Semen quality and reproductive hormones before orchiectomy in men with testicular cancer. *J Clin Oncol* 1999;17:941–947.
11. Jacobsen R, Bostofte E, Engholm G, et al. Risk of testicular cancer in men with abnormal semen characteristics: cohort study. *BMJ* 2000;321:789–792.
12. Honig S, Lipshultz L, Jarrow J. Significant medical pathology uncovered by a comprehensive male infertility evaluation. *Fertil Steril* 1994;62:1028–1034.
13. Daniels IR, Layer GT. Testicular tumours presenting as gynaecomastia. *Eur J Surg Oncol* 2003;29:437–439.
14. International Germ Cell Cancer Collaborative Group. International Germ Cell Consensus Classification: a prognostic factor-based staging system for metastatic germ cell cancers. *J Clin Oncol* 1997;15:594–603.
15. Fleming I, Cooper J, Henson D. *AJCC cancer staging manual*, 5th ed. Philadelphia, PA: Lippincott–Raven, 1997.
16. Warde P, Specht L, Horwich A, et al. Prognostic factors for relapse in stage I seminoma managed by surveillance: a pooled analysis. *J Clin Oncol* 2002;20:4448–4452.
17. Beck S, Foster R, Bihrle R, et al. Significance of primary tumor size and pre-orchiectomy serum tumor marker level in predicting retroperitoneal pathology at primary retroperitoneal lymph node dissection. In: *North Central Section 78th Annual Conference*, American Urologic Association. October 4-9, 2004. Palm Beach, FL.
18. Chilvers CE, Saunders M, Bliss JM, et al. Influence of delay in diagnosis on prognosis in testicular teratoma. *Br J Cancer* 1989;59:126–128.
19. Nikzas D, Champion AE, Fox M. Germ cell tumours of testis: prognostic factors and results. *Eur Urol* 1990;18:242–247.
20. Oliver RT. Factors contributing to delay in diagnosis of testicular tumours. *Br Med J (Clin Res Ed)* 1985;290:356.
21. Fossa SDKO, Elgjo RF, Eliassen G, et al. The effect of patient delay and doctor delay in patients with malignant germ cell tumours. *Int J Androl* 1981;4:134–145.
22. Moul JW, Paulson DF, Dodge RK, et al. Delay in diagnosis and survival in testicular cancer: impact of effective therapy and changes during 18 years. *J Urol* 1990;143:520–523.
23. Prout GR Jr, Griffin PP. Testicular tumors: delay in diagnosis and influence on survival. *Am Fam Physician* 1984;29:205–209.
24. Post GJ, Belis JA. Delayed presentation of testicular tumors. *South Med J* 1980;73:33–35.
25. Moul JW, Moellman JR. Unnecessary mastectomy for gynecomastia in testicular cancer patient. *Mil Med* 1992;157:433–434.
26. Lassmann J, Wille A, Wiechen K, et al. Diagnostic difficulties before definitive treatment of an extragonadal retroperitoneal germ cell tumor. *Urology* 2001;58:281.
27. Stephenson AJ, Russo P, Kaplinsky R, et al. Impact of unnecessary exploratory laparotomy on the treatment of patients with metastatic germ cell tumor. *J Urol* 2004;171:1474–1477.

CHAPTER 32 ■ EPIDEMIOLOGY OF TESTIS CANCER

CHAPTER 32A
Epidemiology of Testis Cancer: A Clinical Perspective

R. T. D. Oliver

This chapter reviews current understanding of the development of germ cell cancer arising in the testis from a clinical perspective. For completeness when appropriate, mention is also made of extragonadal germ cell cancers as a proportion of these arise after rejection of a primary tumor of the testis (1,2). The remainder (apart from the ovary) are thought to arise from germ cells that are lost in midline structures such as the brain, mediastinum, retroperitoneum, or sacrum during their passage during embryogenesis from the yolk sac into the gonad (3).

With the incidence of germ cell cancer of the testis increasing throughout the Western world (4) coincident with declining sperm counts (5,6), the hypothesis that testis atrophy is the final common pathway by which several well-established etiologic factors are involved in testis tumor development is increasingly accepted (7,8). Testis atrophy, whether induced by intra-uterine exposures such as excessive estrogens or smoking or postpubertal events such as trauma, infection, chemical damage, or heat, reduces feedback inhibition of the hypothalamus due to lack of inhibin production. This increases gonadotropin release, particularly the release of follicle-stimulating hormone (FSH), which accelerates cellular proliferation of the remaining spermatogonia. A similar mechanism has been thought to explain the development of thyroid tumors that develop in patients with raised thyroid stimulating harmone (TSH) (9). Reduced time for repair of incidental DNA damage provides the driving force for clonal evolution, with transformation from the precancerous carcinoma *in situ* (CIS) cells into invasive germ cell cancer (10) and also possibly the progression from seminoma to nonseminoma (11). The results of cytogenetic studies on bowel cancer (12) and bladder cancer (13) have led to increasing acceptance of the premise that cancers develop due to an accumulation of deletions of tumor-suppresser genes and mutations in cellular oncogenes. The observation that CIS cells have a median ploidy value of near tetraploid and that seminomas have a median ploidy value intermediate between that of CIS cells and nonseminomas (14–16) provides evidence that clonal development is relevant to the development of germ cell cancer of the testis and explains why tumors with both seminoma and nonseminoma elements behave in a manner intermediate between seminoma and nonseminoma (11). Recent evidence from immunochemistry marker studies of CIS in normal tubules surrounding an established tumor suggest that the step from seminoma to embryonal cancer can occur within the tubule. Berney et al. (17) found that 3% of seminomas, 25% of combined seminomas/nonseminomas, and 65% of nonseminomas

showed the nonseminoma marker CD30 expressed by scattered *in situ* cells. These data would suggest that though clonal evolution from CIS to seminoma to nonseminoma occurs for a minority of nonseminomas, for the majority there can be early genetic change of sufficient magnitude (such as a loss of a supressive gene on chromosome 15) (18) to allow nonseminoma to emerge without the development of a macroscopic seminoma, possibly by escape of immune surveillance machanisms (19).

Little dispute now remains about the increasing evidence that a prenatal factor influences the early development of these tumors (20,21). One group of factors involved are the estrogens and xeno-estrogens, though there is also evidence for involvement of maternal but not paternal smoking habits (22). There remains more controversy about the relative importance of prenatal verses postpubertal factors in their development (23).

This chapter reviews the evidence and relative importance of these two extreme mechanisms and their potential contribution to an understanding of how to prevent these tumors and the associated male infertility.

DEMOGRAPHIC FACTORS ASSOCIATED WITH GERM CELL CANCERS OF THE TESTIS

Dieckmann and Pichlmeier's (24) comprehensive overview has recently summarized the evidence for clinical factors involved in the development of these tumors. Germ cell cancers of the testis are the most frequent malignancy in white men between the ages of 20 and 34, when the lifetime risk is 1 in 500 (25). Three observations can be made from the geographic epidemiology of germ cell cancer that, although far from totally explained, do expand our horizons in trying to understand the development of these cancers. The first is that testicular germ cell cancers are rare in Asian and African populations (26). The New Zealand Maori are the one exception to this observation (27), and this population has one of the highest frequencies in the world. This observation remains unexplained, although this population also has a high incidence of diabetes and obesity.

The second geographic association relates to the relative frequency of testicular and ovarian germ cell cancers in Africans, Asians, and Europeans living in the same country (28). In Kenya, which has minority European and Asian populations and an African majority, the ratio of ovarian to testis germ cell cancers in Africans is approximately 1:1, whereas in Europeans and Asians the ratio is 1:2 or greater, similar to that in Western populations (Table 32A.1). The frequency of ovarian germ cell cancer in Europe is 0.2 per 100,000 (29) and is the same as that of testis and ovarian germ cell cancer in Africa today (26). The figure of 0.2 per 100,000 is also the frequency of testis cancer in the United Kingdom at the beginning of the 20th century (25). This observation has led Kamdar et al. (28) to speculate that physical factors, such as

TABLE 32A.1

INCIDENCE OF OVARIAN CANCER AND TESTICULAR GERM CELL CANCER BY GEOGRAPHICAL ANCESTRY

	Total	European	Asian	African
Ovarian GCC (Nairobi)	19	—	—	19
Testicular GCC (Nairobi)	24	2	3	19
Ratio O:T	1:126	>1.2	1:3	1:1
Ovarian GCC (London)	22	15	4	3
Testicular GCC (London)	610	585	22	3
Ratio O:T	1:28	1:42	1:5.5	1:1

GCC, germ cell cancer; O:T, ovarian to testicular.
Data are from three hospitals in Nairobi, Kenya, during the period 1989 to 1995, and from the Royal London Hospital and St. Bartholomew's Hospital, London, 1978 to 1995.

an increasingly sedentary lifestyle which affects the external location of the testes, may be an additional factor to estrogens and xeno-estrogens contributing to the rise in incidence of testis cancer in the West since 1900. If the cause were totally a rising incidence of chemical pollution that influences intrauterine development, then the incidence of germ cell cancer might be expected to be increased in both males and females equally.

The final clue from geographic epidemiology comes from study of central nervous system germ cell cancers. Although the central nervous system is the rarest of the main sites, the highest frequency of occurrence is in the Far East in Japan (30), Korea (31), and China (32), where testis germ cell cancer is particularly rare. Because no statistics are available for the era before the atomic explosions in Nagasaki or Hiroshima, greater insight may come from more careful epidemiology studies on the regional occurrence of this tumor in the Far East.

MOLECULAR MARKERS AND CYTOGENETICS OF GERM CELL CANCER DEVELOPMENT

Expression of p53 (33) and Bcl-2 (34) are known to be two critical factors in regulating cell proliferation and suppressing programmed cell death (apoptosis). Under normal conditions, very little or no p53 is detectable in normal cells (35); however, because its function is primarily to act as the guardian of the genome, p53 is rapidly induced when cells are exposed to DNA damage or mutation. Under such circumstances, p53 causes mitotic arrest until the DNA damage is repaired or, if the damage is too great to repair, switches on programmed cell death (apoptosis) via the p21/Ras pathway. This is blocked in some malignancies by inappropriate expression of Bcl-2 (blocking apoptosis) or overexpression of mdm 2 (stabilising p53 and blocking its action).

Mutation of the p53 gene has been shown to be a frequent event in various malignancies. In most instances, this mutation correlates with poor prognosis and poor response to chemotherapy and radiotherapy (36–38). In most of these cases, mutation leads to overexpression of nonfunctional p53 protein, which, because normal breakdown processes do not eliminate it, can be detected using immunohistochemical assay.

Study has now shown that not all p53 detectable by immunohistochemical assay in tumor cells is mutated (39). This phenomenon has been most noticeable in testicular germ cell cancers, both seminomas and nonseminomas (40,41). Sequencing of the p53 gene in these tumors has shown no mutation (42), and studies of apoptosis has proven that the gene is fully functional (43). Schwartz et al. (44), by demonstrating that p53 is switched on during normal spermatogenesis, have demonstrated a possible reason why unmutated p53 expression is universal in spermatogenesis. This group demonstrated that p53 is detectable only during the brief period that the tetraploid pachytene spermatocyte is in existence. Presumably at this stage it is responsible for a final check of the genome after meiotic recombination before the reduction division that leads to development of the sperm. The observation that the tetraploid pachytene cell may be the primary stem cell for all germ cell cancers (23,45) provides an explanation for why unmutated p53 is overexpressed in all germ cell cancers. Some authors studying other tumor types that have unmutated p53 constitutively expressed have noted that these tumors retain sensitivity to chemotherapy and radiotherapy (36–38). The fact that p53 is functionally expressed in a tetraploid dose in germ cell cancer cells and that those cells require little triggering to undergo apoptosis because they are also deficient in DNA repair capacity (46) could go a long way toward explaining why germ cell cancers are so exquisitely sensitive to radiation and chemotherapy and also why germ cells are so sensitive to environmental toxins. The demonstration that seminomas have less frequent MDM2 expression than nonseminomas has been speculated as a possible cause of the differential chemo and radiation sensitivity between seminoma and nonseminoma (47) though none of the mdm2 studies have distinguished embryonal cell from teratocarcinoma cell mdm2 expression.

These observations support the view that germ cell cancers are derived from the tetraploid pachytene spermatocyte (23,46) and help to explain the observation that CIS cells have a near tetraploid DNA ploidy value, whereas seminoma ploidy value is intermediate between that of CIS and nonseminoma (16,44). The report that fewer copies of chromosome 15 are found in nonseminoma than in seminoma (18) raises the question of whether this chromosome contains suppressor genes whose loss is associated with the clonal evolution from seminoma to nonseminoma (Table 32A.2). The observation that chromosome 11 contains a suppressor gene which influences expression of teratocarcinoma phenotype (48) provides

TABLE 32A.2

LOSS OF TOTAL DNA AND SPECIFIC CHROMOSOMES IN GERM CELL CANCER CLONAL EVOLUTION

	Number of cases	Median DNA ploidy value	Centromeric analysis[a] #1	#12	#15
CIS areas next to seminoma	6	1.59	2.7	3.2	2.0
Seminoma tumor	6	1.55	2.7	3.5	3.0
CIS areas next to nonseminoma	5	1.57	2.4	2.5	1.9
Nonseminoma tumor	5	1.47	3.0	3.58	1.8

CIS, carcinoma in situ
#1, #12, #15 = chromosome 1, chromosome 2, chromosome 15.
[a]In situ hybridization of interphase nuclei; values indicate mean number of centromeres identified.
Modified from Oosterhuis JW, Gillis AJM, van Putten WJL, et al. Interphase cytogenetics of carcinoma in situ of the testis. Eur J Urol 1993;23:16–22.

an additional demonstration of the mechanisms for a genetic clone to influence clonal evolution of the multiple phenotypic variants seen in these patients. The expression of the c-kit receptor predominantly on seminomas (49) and the production of the ligand by nonseminomas (50) provides a possible molecular mechanism, namely, the loss of suppressor genes to mediate the clonal evolution. A further example of such a mechanism is the overexpression of cyclin D2 which has been suggested as an early step in the transformation of the p53-arrested tetraploid pachytene spermatocyte to malignancy (23,46,51). Though there is confirmation of its expression in early stages of germ cell cancer (52), study of the "RB pathway" demonstrates that the *in utero* changes occur earlier (53). The demonstration in gene knock out mice that cyclin D2 is regulated by FSH (54) links the genetic changes induced during tumor development to the endocrine changes associated with atrophy.

ENDOCRINE FACTORS AND GERM CELL CANCER

Apart from the small peak that occurs in the first year of life (presumably reflecting the influence of the intrauterine hormone milieu), the peak of the age-incidence curve for germ cell cancers coincides precisely with the period of maximum sexual activity in the male. Despite this, apart from one intriguing paper from 1973 (55), there has been little focus on the dependence of germ cell cancer on hormones. Considerably more attention has been paid to the role of hormones in the causation of germ cell cancer. This attention has been most extensive with respect to the role of intrauterine estrogens and xenestrogens in infertility and germ cell cancer. There is also increasing attention being paid to the links between postpubertal testicular atrophy induced gonadotropin drive and germ cell cancer development following the demonstration that FSH levels at the time of orchidectomy predict the risk of subsequent development of a tumor in the contralateral testis. The next sections address these two issues in detail.

Intrauterine Endocrine Environment

The first evidence to suggest that intrauterine estrogen might be a factor in the development of testis cancer was the observation of an increased incidence of cryptorchidism and testis cancer in the sons of mothers who used the estrogen-supplement pregnancy testing kit or took estrogen supplements to protect fetuses that threatened to miscarry (56). Subsequently, research using animal models demonstrated that such supplements induced infertility and cryptorchidism (57). In addition, evidence has continued to accumulate that shows a link between declining sperm count and rising testis cancer rates as well as increased cryptorchidism, hypospadias, and a reversal of the sex ratio of infants born over the last 40 years (58). Speculation that this might be a product of transplacental xenestrogenic effects of organochlorine pesticides (59) was supported by animal studies and observations of humans accidentally exposed to spillage. Three other indirect observations were made that favored the intrauterine rather than postpubertal influence of these agents. The first was the observation that the rising testis cancer rate fit a birth cohort effect and that the temporary dip in germ cell cancer incidence in Europe in those conceived during World War II was possibly explained by a decrease in levels of circulating maternal estrogens due to inadequate nutrition during the war (21). The second observation was that dizygotic twins had a higher risk of germ cell cancer than monozygotic twins, presumably because

of the higher level of circulating estrogens associated with the larger placenta (60,61). The third indirect observation supporting primacy of intrauterine endocrine effect in development of testis cancer is the observation that Finnish immigrants to Sweden, whatever their age, have a lower incidence than native Swedes and closer to that of low-incidence native Finnish population (62).

Recently some exciting new insights into how estrogens may be acting have been published. The first is a report that c-kit mutations were found in 93% of 57 bilateral tumors but only 1.3% of unilateral tumors (63). A second smaller series confirmed these findings, though it a lower frequency (29% vs. 2.6%) (64). In this second series no germ-line mutations of c-kit were found in the patients with a c-kit mutation in their tumor or their relatives (63). This suggests that the mutation is occuring *in utero*. Moreover as the same mutation was found in both tumors (63), it must have occurred while the germ cells were migrating in a midline location before migrating to one or other testis (i.e., before 16 weeks). Even more interesting is a special study in two patients with bilateral tumors who did not have a c-kit mutation in either of their bilateral tumors (even after microdissection of tumor tissue). Both had a c-kit mutation found in the normal tubules surrounding these tumors when they were microdissected (63), suggesting that the prenatal genetic damage is being lost after subsequent genetic change (possibly postpuberty) has established immortilization. The conclusion from this is that tumor development is possible without the primary initiating c-kit mutation [in a manner similar to the hit-and-run association of some tumor viruses with tumor initiation (65)].

Some uncertainty remains as to whether the mutations produced by excess intrauterine estrogens are capable of primary transformation sufficient to generate *in situ* carcinoma cells. They certainly eliminate germ cells and contribute to infertility. More controversial, however, is Skakkebaek's view that they might actually induce carcinoma *in situ*. This hypothesis is based on reports that CIS-like cells have been observed before puberty, although the only study of p53 expression in infantile germ cell cancer shows a different pattern from that seen in the adult variety (66). With new observations on ejaculates demonstrating a variable level of aneuploidy in infertile males (67), the possibility is raised that prenatal estrogen could increase the "stickiness" of germ cells, thereby increasing their risk of developing tetraploid arrest during spermatogenesis. Alternatively, it could increase their susceptibility to viruses that can induce cell fusion, as is well known to occur with the Sendai virus and has also been observed with mumps virus. However, how a cell normally committed to meiosis after tetraploidy switches to mitosis and perpetuates the near-tetraploid phenotype is becoming clearer. The work of Chaganti's group on the role of cyclin D_2 (23,46,51) in regulating the cell cycle is possibly providing an explanation. They suggest that a chance aberrant recombinant event occurring during meiotic arrest at the time of the tetraploid pachytene spermatocyte leads to an amplification of the il2p segment of the 12 chromosome. Overexpression of cyclin D_2 then occurs as this gene is on p12, functioning as an oncogene, switching tetraploid meiotically arrested cells into mitosis. Evidence from cyclin D2 gene knock out animals shows that cyclin D2 is regulated by FSH (54) thus providing an important link beween the endocrine changes in the patient and the genetic changes occuring during the clonal evolution of the malignant process.

Postpubertal Endocrine Effects

The peak of the age-incidence curve of testicular germ cell cancer in adults corresponds with the period of maximum sexual activity in men. Coincident with earlier onset of puberty

TABLE 32A.3

IMPACT OF YEAR OF BIRTH ON AGE OF FIRST SEXUAL INTERCOURSE AND PEAK INCIDENCE OF TESTICULAR CANCER

Year of birth	First sexual intercourse before age 18[a] (%)	Peak age of incidence of testicular cancer[b] (yr)
1968 or later	58	NA
1958–1967	46	29
1948–1957	44	29
1938–1947	41	31
Before 1938	NA	35

NA, not available.
[a]Data from Forman D, Chilvers C. A survey of sexual characteristics of young and middle aged males in England and Wales. *BMJ* 1989;298:1137.
[b]Data from office population census studies.

(68) and earlier onset of regular sexual activity (69), the incidence has begun to peak earlier (Table 32A.3). That the primary stem cell of all germ cell cancers of the testis—the spermatogonium—is endocrine-dependent is beyond dispute. The most convincing evidence that endocrine drive is important in the development of testicular germ cell tumors is the detection of elevated levels of gonadotropins, particularly FSH, in a substantial proportion of patients with germ cell cancers of the testis (46% in one series of stage I patients who were followed for more than 2 years after orchidectomy without any other treatment) (70). Further support for the idea that FSH-driven overstimulation of spermatogonia is a risk factor for development of germ cell cancers came from a study of Hoff Wanderas et al. (71), who showed that elevated FSH levels after orchidectomy were predictive of risk of developing a tumor in the remaining testis (Table 32A.4). This data has been confirmed in two subsequent studies (72,73) and by a study showing a fivefold increased risk of testis cancer on follow-up of men operated on for gynecomastia that is also associated with raised FSH (74).

Additional support for involvement of postpubertal endocrine factors has emerged from an epidemiologic study in the United Kingdom (75,76). This study demonstrated that the early onset of puberty, trauma, and increased sexual activity is associated with an increased risk (Table 32A.5), whereas regular exercise appeared to reduce the risk of germ cell cancer of the testis and a sedentary lifestyle was associated with an increased risk (Table 32A.6). Similar reports have been published of the benefits of exercise for both breast cancer (77) and bowel cancer (78). One study of women showed that

TABLE 32A.4

FSH LEVEL AND RISK OF CONTRALATERAL TUMOR AFTER UNILATERAL ORCHIDECTOMY

	Number of cases	Elevated FSH level
Patients with second tumor	13	77%
Control patients	26	15%

FSH, follicle-stimulating hormone.
Modified from Hoff Wanderas E, Fossa SD, Heilo A, et al. Serum follicle-stimulating hormone—predictor of cancer in the remaining testis in patients with unilateral testicular cancer. *Br J Urol* 1990;66:315–317.

TABLE 32A.5

RELATION OF PUBERTAL CHARACTERISTICS AND SEXUAL BEHAVIOR TO TESTIS TUMOR INCIDENCE

	Number in group		χ^2 for trend
Age voice broke		Age ≤13	
Testis tumor group	552	18%	6.7
Neighborhood control group	550	15%	
Age started shaving		Age ≤16	
Testis tumor group	749	49%	7.2
Neighborhood control group	757	43%	
Age at first nocturnal emission		Age ≤14	
Testis tumor group	652	57%	4.6
Neighborhood control group	628	51%	
Frequency of sexual activity at age 20		Every 2–3 weeks	
Testis tumor group	689	72%	4.9
Neighborhood control group	692	67%	

Adapted from Forman D, Chilvers C, Oliver R, et al. The aetiology of testicular cancer: association with congenital abnormalities, age at puberty, infertility and exercise. *BMJ* 1994;308:1393–1399.

regular exercise suppressed gonadotrophin secretion and this could explain how it can delay puberty and reduce ovulation (79); this provides a possible mechanism that would be relevant in testis cancer.

Study of the effect of heat on survival of germ cells has provided a possible explanation of the association of a sedentary lifestyle with an increased risk of testis cancer. The speculation has long been made that, because testicular temperature is lower than core body temperature in most mammals (80), this difference is critical to fertility. Several studies have shown that sitting, particularly sitting with legs together, produces a higher intratesticular temperature than standing and reduces the difference between the testis temperature and core body temperature by approximately 30% (81). Evidence that testicular heating damages sperm count comes from both animal and

TABLE 32A.6

RELATION OF WEEKLY EXERCISE AND TIME SEATED PER DAY TO TESTIS CANCER INCIDENCE

	Number of patients		χ^2 for trends
Exercise at time of diagnosis		4 hr/wk	
Testis cancer group	794	73%	3.4
Neighborhood control group	793	69%	
Hours seated per day at time of diagnosis		>10 hr/d	
Testis cancer group	793	29%	7.9
Neighborhood control group	794	23%	

Modified from Forman D, Chilvers C, Oliver R, et al. The aetiology of testicular cancer: association with congenital abnormalities, age at puberty, infertility and exercise. *BMJ* 1994;308:1393–1399.

human studies. In experimental animals, studies have demonstrated that the most sensitive cell is the pachytene spermatocyte (82), which is known to express p53 (45). Studies in mice demonstrate that the *p53* gene lowers germ cell numbers in response to heat by inducing apoptosis (83).

In humans, the most critical experiment demonstrating the link between raised scrotal temperature and reduced sperm count comes from an experiment in which a group of nine men wore specially designed underwear that lifted the testes up out of the scrotum and localized them close to the external inguinal ring for 16 hours a day (84). After 11 months using a less reliable scrotal support and 3.5 months using a more effective technique, the sperm count had fallen to subfertile levels, and the couples stopped taking contraceptive precautions (Table 32A.7). After a period of 8 to 49 months (median, 24 months), the heating was stopped and sperm counts recovered, albeit slightly more slowly in those individuals who had used the more effective technique.

The degree to which such heating is a real contributing factor in the declining sperm count and rising testis cancer rate is uncertain. The clues suggest, however, that it could be more important than previously appreciated. Thonneau et al. examined time from first attempt to conception in a group of French women. This study showed significantly slower time to conception among women whose husbands were seated for more than 3 hours per day in a vehicle (85). A second study by same group showed that after 160 minutes driving in a car, scrotal temperature rose by 1.7 to 2.2°C (86). Possible confirmatory data (87) comes from comparing average sperm counts in highly automobile-commuting Californians (73×10^6/mL) and more pedestrian New Yorkers (132×10^6/mL). Reports from this group are important for another reason, because they are one of the most significant series not supporting the view that sperm count has been declining over the last 25 years (88). The actual data are more interesting, however, and show an initial decline until 1970 to 1975, followed by a reversal coincident with the institution of antipollution measures and the development of jogging as a major activity (Fig. 32A.1).

TABLE 32A.7

EFFECT OF TESTICULAR HEATING ON SPERM COUNT

	Scrotal support technique 1 (n = 3)	Scrotal support technique 2 (n = 6)
Pretreatment sperm count	50.2	40.2
Time to sperm count nadir	11 mo	3 mo
Sperm count at nadir (8 to 36 mo)	1.86	0.12
Cycles of contraceptive use (pregnancies)	42(1)	117 (0)
Posttreatment sperm count, 0 to 6 mo	51	26.5
Posttreatment sperm count, 7 to 18 mo	98.7	36.3

For sperm counts, mean sperm count = value shown $\times 10^6$.
Data from Mieusset R, Bujan L. The potential of mild testicular heating as a safe, effective and reversible contraceptive method for men. *Int J Androl* 1994;17:186–191.

The very gentle decline that began after 1984 and still continues coincides with relaxed antipollution measures and declining rates of jogging.

ATROPHIC EVENTS AND DEVELOPMENT OF TESTICULAR GERM CELL TUMORS

The previous section has demonstrated that intrauterine estrogen can induce mutations in immature germ cells prior to puberty. In addition, postpubertal gonadotropins clearly

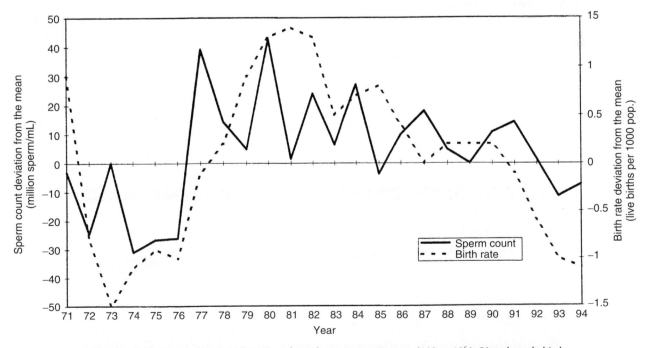

FIGURE 32A.1. Yearly absolute deviations from the mean sperm count (102×10^6/mL) and yearly birth rate in Minnesota (mean 15.4 live births per 1,000 population). (Reprinted with permission from Fisch H, Andrews H, Hendricks J, et al. Olson C. The relationship of sperm counts to birth rates: a population-based study. *J Urol* 1997;157(3):840–843.)

contribute to accelerating additional genetic changes necessary for the development of fully developed testicular germ cell tumors. They also suggest that, though the first step is happening *in utero*, the critical event of tetraploidization might be a postpubertal event. The next sections assess the conditions involved in magnifying testicular atrophy postpuberty and their contribution to the development of germ cell tumors.

Cryptorchidism has been the most consistently associated risk factor for the development of testis cancer (89). It is also well recognized to be associated with a low sperm count, which may explain why a significant but not marked increased risk of testis germ cell cancer is noted in the contralateral testis in men with unilateral cryptorchidism (89).

Until recently, considerable uncertainty existed about whether surgical correction of cryptorchidism had any effect on the occurrence of testis tumor or the incidence of low sperm count. The most convincing data come from the case-control study of Forman et al. (75), which suggested that if cryptorchidism is corrected before puberty, the risk of testis cancer is little different from that of men without cryptorchidism. Another interesting observation is that, if the defect is corrected surgically (90–92), any tumor that develops is less likely to be a seminoma (Table 32A.8). These observations could be interpreted as indicating that surgically induced traumatic atrophy may have an accelerating effect on transition from normal cell to malignant tumor and that, after surgery, the increased atrophy accelerates the transition from seminoma to nonseminoma.

Chemicals as Postpubertal Atrophy-inducing Agents (Atrophogens)

The previous section reviewed some of the studies that have demonstrated an association between the development of germ cell cancer and levels of maternal estrogen, usually due to the use of exogenous estrogen as part of a now discredited approach to preventing repeated miscarriage (56). These observations have been confirmed in animal studies that have demonstrated actual germ cell loss. These studies also have suggested that estrogen could be a factor in the development of cryptorchidism, because they have demonstrated that prenatal exposure to estrogen induces abnormalities of testicular descent (93).

These observations led Carlsen et al. (5) to speculate that the increasing use of estrogens both to fatten poultry and to prevent conception in women could be a factor in declining sperm counts and the rising incidence in germ cell cancer of the testis. These authors also speculated that increased agricultural use of pesticides and herbicides, some of which have estrogenic effects, could also be involved. Direct evidence that this might be true comes from studies undertaken to investigate why military working dogs in Vietnam had an excess of seminomas and impaired spermatogenesis. An epidemiologic

case-control study of patients being treated for testicular germ cell cancer in the Washington area found evidence for impaired spermatogenesis in men exposed to the defoliant Agent Orange while in Vietnam (94); the incidence of impaired spermatogenesis was twice as high among men who had served in Vietnam than among matched controls. The relative risk of testis cancer was 3.0 in those younger than 35 years at the time of diagnosis and 1.1 in those older than 35 at time of diagnosis.

As many of these xenostrogens are fat soluble, they could also explain some confounding associations such as increased milk-drinking in puberty increasing the risk and the association of a high-fat diet. This latter effect has been less apparent in recent studies as the 60-year legacy of organochlorine is phased out by newer chemicals (59), and the presumed protective effect of dietary vitamin A and D leads to improved immune surveillance. It may also explain evidence for associations of height and testis cancer (24).

TRAUMA AS POSTPUBERTAL ATORPHOGENS

Whether trauma is an etiologic risk factor for testis cancer has long been debated as it has with regard to several other tumors, such as breast tumors and osteosarcoma. It is now 90 years since Joynes and Rous first observed that traumatic injury accelerated cancer growth (95).

Support for the view that the intensity of trauma and, therefore, presumably the degree of cytokine or growth factor release determines the relation of scrotal traumatic events to induction of testis cancer comes from the United Kingdom epidemiologic study, which demonstrated an association between germ cell cancer and traumatic events, and that there was a stronger association with the more intense degree of trauma (Table 32A.9). Even more interesting, in light of the finding that surgical correction increases the incidence of nonseminoma in cryptorchid patients (91,92) and in adults who had a hernia correction as a child, is the observation that the association of trauma with testicular germ cell cancer is more marked in patients with nonseminoma (76,91, 92). Trauma as a factor in testis cancer epidemiology is controversial because it could draw attention of the patient to a preexisting tumor and encourage recall bias, though there is only one study to investigate this thoroughly. That study reported an odds ratio of 3.49 for an association of trauma and development of testis cancer. However, by examining medical records of the patients, the authors found that only three of 21 patients with history of trauma had sought medical attention at the time compared to 11 of 20 controls (96). As this was the reverse of the observations of Chilvers et al. (76), who reported a stronger association the more severe the trauma was in terms of days off work, further studies need to be done.

TABLE 32A.8

EFFECT OF SURGICAL CORRECTION OF UNDESCENDED TESTIS ON HISTOLOGY OF SUBSEQUENT TUMOR

	Number of cases	Incidence of seminoma (%)	Number of cases	Incidence of seminoma (%)
Normal descent	729	50	319	37
Undescended testis, operated	34	44	12	17
Undescended testis, nonoperated	12	67	16	75

Forman D, Chilvers C, Oliver R, et al. The aetiology of testicular cancer: association with congenital abnormalities, age at puberty, infertility and exercise. *Br Med J* 1994;308:1393–1399.
Raja MA, Oliver RT, Badenoch D, et al. Orchidopexy and transformation of seminoma to non-seminoma [Letter]. *Lancet* 1992;339(8798):930.

TABLE 32A.9

EPIDEMIOLOGIC RISK FACTORS AND GERM CELL CANCER SUBTYPE

	Number of cases	Seminoma (%)	Significance test[a]
All cases	794	50	—
Unilateral cryptorchidism, uncorrected	12	67	—
Unilateral cryptorchidism, corrected	34	44	0.16
No injury	759	51	—
Testis/groin injury	35	34	0.023
No STD	715	51	—
History of STD	76	41	0.018

STD, sexually transmitted disease.
[a]Significance test calculated using likelihood ratio test in comparison to two groups of cases.
From Coupland CA, Chilvers CE, et al. Risk factors for testicular germ cell tumors by histological tumor type. *Br J Cancer* 1999;80:1859–1863.

Idiopathic or Unexplained Atrophy

Many series have commented that, in some patients with testis cancer, a period of testicular shrinkage occurs before onset of swelling. In my own series, there were three cases of testicular atrophy so gross that the patient noted it. Although one man had been investigated for fertility and found to be azoospermia, the other two men had fathered a total of five children without any conception problems. Evidence supporting the finding that the occurrence of secondary atrophic events may be more frequent than previously believed comes from the epidemiologic study of Forman et al. (75) who observed that more patients than controls were aware of a difference in the size of their two testicles for several years before interview. Paradoxically, in 15% of patients the side that developed the tumor was not the smaller side.

Viruses As Testicular Atrophogens

The mumps virus is the only virus known to induce testicular atrophy and to have an association with development of testis tumor (97). The study finding this association, however, reported only a small number of testis tumors, four in a series of 132 patients with mumps virus–induced atrophy. Although the follow-up was limited, this number was 15 times higher than the currently accepted lifetime risk of 1 in 500. Mumps virus is not known to cause malignant transformation and is not known to cause proliferation of germ cells. A plausible hypothesis is that tumor induction is due to an indirect mechanism, with atrophy leading to diminished pituitary suppression of gonadotropin release, followed by increased FSH drive that acts as an augmented proliferative signal. Although the series of Beard et al. (97) established that atrophy induced by postpubertal mumps virus infection is associated with an increased risk of testis cancer, mumps is not a common cause, for no testis tumor series has reported more than 10% of patients with such a history. Furthermore, not all epidemiologic studies that have reported on this factor found the incidence of mumps to be significantly higher in cancer patients than in controls. Finally, the incidence of clinical mumps orchitis has declined rapidly with widespread vaccination, though there are no cohort studies of testis tumors in vaccinated populations as yet.

The excess of patients with orchitis not related to the mumps virus in the United Kingdom Testicular Cancer Study Group (76) possibly could be explained by an excess of unrecognized mumps virus infections, because only 37% of patients with laboratory-proven mumps infection had classic parotitis (98). Alternatively, patients could have been infected with other viruses, such as Coxsackie, or even with bacteria.

Other possible testis-tropic infectious agents are the retroviruses. Two separate observations raise interest in these viruses. The first relates to the increasing evidence that individuals infected with human immunodeficiency virus 1 (HIV-1) have an increased incidence of seminomas (99). Although HIV is not thought to be directly oncogenic, the excess of seminoma is thought to reflect the fact that spontaneously arising seminomas have a high level of lymphocyte infiltration, which influences the prognosis. Reduced T cell function in HIV-infected individuals would reduce the lymphocyte infiltration and hence the hypothetical "need" of the cells to mutate to nonseminoma to escape immune surveillance.

The second observation related to retroviruses is the discovery that endogenous (i.e., transmitted via the germ line) retroviral sequences are expressed in germ cell but not in the somatic elements in these tumors (100). As these sequences are also reported in normal placentas, whether this is just an epiphenomenon or a critical factor in tumor development is not clear. Further work is required on the role of endogenous viral infections in testis cancer, particularly teratocarcinoma and the immune response.

Other Infectious Agents as Atrophogens

Although several other authors have investigated the association between the occurrence of testis cancer and a past history of sexually transmitted disease, only the report of the United Kingdom Testicular Cancer Study Group (see Table 32A.9) found a significant association, particularly with nonspecific sexually transmitted diseases (76). These results could be due to a recall bias, but the association of stomach cancer with persistent infection with *Helicobacter pylori* (101) provides a possible model for how a low-grade pathogenic bacterium could be involved in the development of malignant disease. The observation that patients with testis cancer have a high incidence of persistent relapsing tender testicles on follow-up after orchidectomy (Table 32A.10) could reflect either a low-grade persistent infection or autoimmune orchitis in these patients. Because no one has done sperm culture systematically on testis tumor patients, such a study possibly is worth initiating.

GENETIC FACTORS AND TESTICULAR GERM CELL DEVELOPMENT

Human Lymphocyte Antigen–Linked Immune Hyporesponsiveness To Atrophogenic Viruses As A Factor In Testicular Atrophy

Clear evidence exists that susceptibility and resistance linked to human lymphocyte antigen (HLA) influences the behavior

TABLE 32A.10

ASSOCIATION BETWEEN FLUCTUATING PAIN AND SIZE OF CONTRALATERAL TESTIS IN PATIENTS PREVIOUSLY TREATED FOR GERM CELL CANCER

Testis size	Number of cases	Adult mumps (%) ($n = 2$)	Fluctuating testis pain (%) ($n = 12$)[a]	Elevated FSH, >7 IU/L (%) ($n = 21$)	Elevated FSH + Testis Pain (%) ($n = 7$)
Small (<10 cm^3)	13	100	58	52	86
Intermediate (10–15 cm^3)	13	—	33	33	14
Large (>15 cm^3)	13	—	8	14	—

FSH, follicle-stimulating hormone.
[a]Percentage of this number.

of oncogenic viruses involved in the development of at least four tumor types: hepatoma induced by hepatitis B virus (102), Hodgkin disease (103) and nasopharyngeal cancer (104) induced by Epstein-Barr virus, and cervical cancer induced by human papillomavirus (105).

In testis cancer, although some evidence exists for an HLA association in unrelated individuals (106,107), the association has not been confirmed in studies of families (108). This raises doubt about the hypothesis of a testicular atrophy–inducing virus susceptibility gene linked to the HLA complex. However, continued investigation of the hypothesis is justified because, despite the fact that at least three causes of testicular atrophy exist other than viruses—namely, trauma, heat, and chemical exposure—evidence from the study of human papillomavirus–induced cervix cancer demonstrates that the HLA antigen association is strongest in the CIS stage. This may be the same with testis cancer as it is the earlier pathological stages of germ cell cancer that show the strongest evidence for an immune response (19). As shown by the studies of atrophy induced by mumps, many more patients develop atrophy than develop testis cancer (97). A clearer insight into the role of HLA may come from studying HLA type in patients with testicular atrophy and CIS. Support for this approach comes from a study published some time ago demonstrating that, after reversal of vasectomy, the subgroup with infertility from autoallergic reaction to the testis demonstrated an association with HLA (109).

One observation, which may indicate that atrophy is linked to immune response and autoimmunity, is the fact that more than 80% of patients with retroperitoneal germ cell cancer have evidence of atrophic change in the testes, with or without CIS. The concept of spontaneous regression of primary germ cell cancer after development of metastases was first suggested by Azzopardi and Hoffbrand (110) to have an immunologic basis. Study of these cases is now relatively easy because of improved biopsy techniques (111), and using modern T lymphocyte receptor technology to investigate the link with endogenous retrovirus expressions (100) could give a clearer insight into the mechanism involved.

Family Studies

Little doubt exists that a genetic influence in families affects the risk of developing germ cell cancer (Table 32A.11). However, the observation that the risk for siblings is double the risk for father to son (75,112–114) provides further support for the idea that postfertilization genetic mutation via maternal estrogens may be augmenting the actual inherited risk. The observation that the risk is higher in dizygotic twins, who have a larger placenta and higher level of maternal estrogens than monozygotic twins, provides further evidence for this concept (60,61). These

findings may explain why genome screening has been disappointing in terms of achieving progress toward identification of the specific locus involved in the inherited risk. However, a 2000 report found evidence for an X-linked genetic linkage with familial testis tumor, particularly those with undescended testis (115).

The preceding description of risk factors shows that genetic factors could be involved thorough at least three mechanisms of atrophy: via an immune response gene influencing response to an atrophogenic virus, via a gene influencing detoxification of a gonadotoxic agent, and via a gene influencing expression of an endogenous retrovirus. Clearly, further studies linking functional assays to genotype are requested to fully explain the subtleties of familial testes cancer is inherited. As evidence now exists that infertility has a genetic component (116), studies to clarify which subgroups of infertile males are at risk of testis cancer are needed. However, it is unlikely that all X-linked genes associated with infertility cause testis cancer.

RISK FACTORS FOR PROGRESSION FROM CARCINOMA *IN SITU* TO DIFFERENT HISTOLOGIC SUBTYPES

There have now been three reports showing that the rising incidence of germ cell cancer over the last 30 years mainly effects one histological subtype more than the other (117–119). As two of these reported more seminomas than nonseminomas and the third reported the reverse, further studies in these and other populations might reveal clues to factors leading to the different tumor type.

TABLE 32A.11

RELATIVE RISK OF GERM CELL CANCER OF THE TESTIS IN FAMILY MEMBERS

Study	Number of patients	Father and son	Brother and brother
Forman et al. (59)	794	4.0	8.0
Heimdahl et al. (93)	922	4.3	10.2
Westergaard et al. (94)	2,113/702	1.96	12.3
Hemminki and Li (114)	4082	4	8.0

Little is known about the effects of genes on the clinical development of germ cell cancer subtypes, although a review of the case reports of familial testis cancer (120) showed some evidence that identical twin pairs were more likely than dizygotic twin, sibling, and father-son pairs to show a similar histologic subtype (80% vs. 64% vs. 65%, respectively). This finding suggests that activation and transcription of some genes may influence germ cell cancer morphology. Surgical correction of cryptorchidism and trauma may increase the risk of nonseminoma. Biopsy at the time of orchidopexy, a type of trauma, is also associated with an increased risk of testis cancer as an adult (121).

The other epidemiological evidence to support this interpretation of the clonal evolution from seminoma to nonseminoma comes from the study of tumors arising in immunosuppressed individuals (Table 32A.12). In HIV-infected individuals, immunosuppression is associated with an increased risk of seminoma but not of nonseminoma, whereas among kidney transplant patients treated with alkylating agents who have testis tumors, an excess of nonseminomas is seen (122) compared to that seen in spontaneous tumors (123). Seminoma is the tumor with one of the highest levels of lymphocytic infiltration (19). Loss of T lymphocyte surveillance would facilitate tumor expansion (124,125) at the seminoma stage, and the need for immune selection to drive evolution to nonseminoma would decrease. In contrast, agents used to suppress the immune response in transplant recipients are often mutagens and hypothetically could accelerate the transition from seminoma to nonseminoma.

The differences identified in these studies are undoubtedly small and only hypothesis-generating. Little is known about the driving force of clonal evolution in germ cell cancer or most other cancers. Placental alkaline phosphatase and c-kit are tissue markers for seminoma (126), and CD30 is a marker for embryonal carcinoma (127). Both markers identify these cellular changes in a larger proportion of patients than does conventional morphology. A pathologic review of the cases from a large epidemiological study using immunohistochemical assay for placental alkaline phosphatase and CD30 would be of value. The aim would be better definition of the intermediate

(combined seminoma and nonseminoma) group (11). If this proved possible, an analysis could then be attempted to investigate whether this group was indeed intermediate with respect to the risk factors that have been identified as possibly involved in clonal evolution, such as trauma, mutagenic chemical exposure, immunosurveillance, smoking, and family history.

CONCLUSION

Review of testicular germ cell tumor epidemiological studies identifies three groups of epidemiological factors: prenatal, postpubertal and genetic (Fig. 32A.2). The first group includes those factors acting *in utero* during fetal gonadal development. These are predominantly excess estrogens or estrogen-mimicking chemicals. However, that other chemicals may act in the same way is suggested by the data that show that maternal but not paternal smoking is associated with testis cancer development (22). Although these factors are demonstrated in experimental models to eliminate germ cells and interfere with testicular descent, a critical area of uncertainty remains as to whether these prenatal events actually induce transformation, that is, tetraploidization of the primitive germ cell precursor en route to the gonad. It is now clear that from the recent studies that intrauterine estrogen does produce a mutation in the intrauterine germ cells but it is still unclear whether tetraploidization occurs *in utero* or after puberty. Overexpression of nonmutant p53 is a marker of postpubertal germ cells at the pachytene spermatocyte. Tetraploidization is demonstrable in the CIS cell after puberty that is now known to precede all subtypes of germ cell cancer (128). A possible interpretation is that spermatogonia exposed to excess estrogen *in utero* are more prone to the postpubertal events that initiate mitosis in the meiotically arrested tetraploid pachytene spermatocyte. Such an event is overexpression of the FSH-regulated gene, cyclin D2. This gene is present on chromosome 12, also involved in producing the i12p post pubertal marker of germ cell tumors.

The second group of risk factors in testicular germ cell tumor epidemiology are those postpubertal factors such as viral orchitis, testicular trauma, heat, or postnatal chemical

---

TABLE 32A.12

IMMUNOSUPPRESSION AND GERM CELL CANCER

Histologic subtype	Number of cases	Seminoma (%)
AIDS-linked[a]	92	54
Posttransplantation[b]	20	40
Spontaneous[b]	342	45

Clinical stage	Number of cases	Stage 1 (%)
AIDS-linked	60	28
Posttransplantation	18	28
Spontaneous	153	50

Disease-free survival	Number of cases	Disease free[c] (%)
AIDS-linked	66	85
Posttransplantation	20	72
Spontaneous	453	92

AIDS, acquired immunodeficiency syndrome.
[a]Modified from Leibovitch I, Baniel J, Rowland RG, et al. Malignant testicular neoplasms in immunosuppressed patients. *J Urol* 1996;155:1938–1942.
[b]Modified from Oliver RTD, Ong J, Blandy JP, Altman DG. Testis conservation in germ cell cancer justified by improved primary chemotherapy response and reduced delay 1978–1994. *Br J Urol* 1996;78:119–124.
[c]Noncancer deaths excluded.

Prenatal Factors

Estrogens / xenoestrogens

Maternal smoking (? and diet)

X linked gene (Xq27) and cryptorchidisn (? estrogen induced)

C-Kit gene mutation (Induced by excessive *inutero estrogen*)

Postpubertal Factors

Increasing FSH / cyclin D2 switch on

CIS → seminoma → non seminoma (non s.)

4.0N ↑ 3.6N ↑ 2.7N

↓ p53 ↑ bcl2 ↑ mdm2 ↑ DNA repair activity

Trauma / surgery cryptorchidism non S. > seminoma

HIV immunosuppression seminoma > non S.

Azothiopine immunosuppress non S > seminoma

Orchitis / atrophy secondary to viruses e.g. mumps,

Diet

High-fatdiets increase xenoestrogenic chemical exposure.

Low-fatdiets decrease vitamin A and D producing immunosuppression.

FIGURE 32A.2. Summary of prenatal and postpubertal environmental and genetic factors in germ cell cancer epidemiology.

exposure that induce testicular atrophy leading to loss of hypothalamic suppression. This increases FSH gonadotropin drive and accelerates the DNA loss from the genetically unstable near-tetraploid CIS cell. This leads to the clonal development of the multiplicity of phenotypes that are seen in germ cell cancers.

The third group of epidemiological factors are the genetic factors. Increasing evidence is found that constitutive expression of p53 and suppression of mdm2 during spermatogenesis at the immediately premeiotic tetraploid pachytene spermatocyte stage plays a critical role. This is presumed to ensure that recombination during that stage does not lead to a major genetic defect in the fetus. It also seems to play a critical role in making spermatogenesis sensitive to the atrophogenic effects of both external toxins and testicular heat. The latter, an important byproduct of our sedentary lifestyle, is gaining increasing recognition as an important risk factor for germ cell tumor development. Evidence is also increasing that p53 may also play a critical role in determining the exquisite sensitivity of these tumors to both chemotherapy and radiation. The final dimension of genetic influence in germ cell cancers relates to the clear evidence for increased risk in families, but as yet no definite chromosomal linkage is found in genome screening studies. The demonstration that the risk is twice as high in sibling–sibling pairs than in father–son pairs provides an indication that the interaction between environment and genetic factors must be evaluated for a full understanding of the etiology of these tumors.

References

1. Oliver RTD. Clues from natural history and results of treatment supporting the monoclonal origin of germ cell tumours. *Cancer Surv* 9:1990;332–368.
2. Daugaard G, Rortu M, Vandernaase H, et al. Management of extragonadal germ cell tumours and the signficiance of bilateral testicular biopsies. *Ann Oncol* 1992;3:288–289.
3. Wylie C. The biology of primordial germ cells. In: Skakkebaek N, Grigor K, Giwercman A et al., eds. *Management and biology of carcinoma in situ and cancer of the testis.* Copenhagen: Karger, 1993:62–67.
4. Moller H. Clues to the aetiology of testicular germ cell tumours from descriptive epidemiology. *Eur Urol* 1993;23:8–13.
5. Carlsen E, Giwercman A, Keiding N, et al. Evidence for decreasing quality of semen during the past 50 years. *Br Med J* 1992;305:609–612.
6. Richthoff J, Rylander L, Hagmar L, et al. Higher sperm counts in Southern Sweden compared with Denmark. *Hum Reprod* 2002;17(9):2468–2473.
7. Oliver RTD. Atrophy, hormones, genes and viruses in aetiology of germ cell tumours. *Cancer Surv* 1990;9(2):263–268.
8. Oliver RT, Oliver JC. Endocrine hypothesis for declining sperm count and rising incidence of cancer [Letter]. *Lancet* 1996;347:339–340.
9. Pacini S, de Groot LJ, et al. *Thyroid neoplasia in endocrinology.* Philadelphia, 2004.
10. Skakkebaek NE, Berthelsen JG, Giwercman A, et al. Carcinoma-in-situ of the testis: possible origin from gonocytes and precursor of all types of germ cell tumours except spermatocytoma. *Int J Androl* 1987;10:19–28.
11. Oliver RTD, Leahy M, Ong J. Combined seminoma/non-seminoma should be considered as intermediate grade germ cell cancer (GCC). *Eur J Cancer* 1995;31A:1392–1394.
12. Vogelstein B, Fearon ER, Hamilton SR, et al. Genetic alterations during colorectal-tumor development. *N Engl J Med* 1988;319:527–532.
13. Dalbagni G, Presti G, Reuter J, et al. Genetic alterations in bladder cancer. *Lancet* 1993;342:469–471.
14. Muller J, Skakkebaek NE. Microspectrophotometric DNA measurements of carcinoma-in-situ germ cells in the testis. *Int J Androl* 1981;4:211–221.
15. Atkin NK, Kay R. Prognostic significance of modal DNA value and other factors in malignant tumours, based on 1465 cases. *Br J Cancer* 1979; 40: 210–214.
16. Oosterhuis JW, Sergio MMJ, Castedo S. Ploidy of subtypes of primary germ cell tumours of the testis. Pathogenetic and clinical relevance. *Lab Invest* 1989;4:14–21.
17. Berney D, Lee A, Randle SJ, et al. The frequency of intratubular embryonal carcinoma: implications for the pathogenesis of germ cell tumours. *Histopathology* 2004;45:155–161.
18. van-Echten J, Oosterhuis J, Looijenga L. Cytogenetics of seminomas and non seminomas. *Genes Chromosomes Cancer* 1995;14:133–144.
19. Oosterhuis JW, Kersemaekers AM, Jacobsen GK, et al. Morphology of testicular parenchyma adjacent to germ cell tumours. An interim report. *APMIS* 2003;111(1):32–40.
20. Sharpe RM. The 'oestrogen hypothesis'—where do we stand now? *Int J Androl* 2003;26(1):2–15.
21. Moller H. Decreased testicular cancer risk in men born in wartime. *J Natl Cancer Inst* 1989;81(21):1668–1669.
22. Pettersson A, Kaijser M, Richiardi L, et al. Women smoking and testicular cancer: one epidemic causing another? *Int J Cancer* 2004;109(6):941–944.
23. Chaganti RSK, Houldsworth J. The cytogenetic theory of the pathogenesis of human adult male germ cell tumours. *APMIS* 1998;106:80–84.
24. Dieckmann KP, Pichlmeier U. Clinical epidemiology of testicular germ cell tumours. *World J Urol* 2004;22(1):2–14.
25. Davies JM. Testicular cancer in England and Wales; some epidemiological aspects. *Lancet* 1981;2:928.
26. Parkin DM, Pisani P, Ferlay J. Global cancer statistics. *CA Cancer J Clin* 1999;49:33–64.
27. Wilkinson TJ, Colls BM, Schluter PJ. Increased incidence of germ cell testicular cancer in New Zealand Maoris. *Br J Cancer* 1992;65:769–771.
28. Kamdar R, Oliver R, Otheino-Abinya N. Geographic epidemiology of ovarian and testicular germ cell cancers. *Br J Cancer* 1998;78(11):1401–1402.
29. Westhoff C, Pike M, Vessey M. Benign ovarian teratomas: a population-based case-control study. *Br J Cancer* 1988;58:93–98.
30. Koide O, Watanabe Y, Sato K. Pathological survey of intracranial germinoma and pinealoma in Japan. *Cancer* 1980;45:2119–2130.
31. Choi J, Kim D, Chung S, et al. Treatment of germ cell tumours in the pineal region. *Childs Nerv Syst* 1998;14(1–2):41–48.
32. Ho D, Liu H. Primary intracranial germ cell tumour. *Cancer* 1992;70: 1577–1584.
33. Lane DP. p53, guardian of the genome. *Nature* 1992;358(6381):15–16.
34. Bishop JM. Molecular themes in oncogenesis. *Cell* 1991;64(2):235–248.
35. Alberts B, Bray D, Lewis J, et al. *Molecular biology of the cell.* New York: Garland, 1994:1281–1289.
36. Esrig D, Elmajian D, Groshen S, et al. Accumulation of nuclear p53 and tumor progression in bladder cancer [see Comments]. *N Engl J Med* 1994; 331(19):1259–1264.
37. Dowell SP, Wilson PO, Derias NW, et al. Clinical utility of the immunocytochemical detection of p53 protein in cytological specimens. *Cancer Res* 1994;54(11):2914–2918.
38. Dee S, Haskogan D, Israel M. Inactivation of p53 is associated with decreased levels of radiation induced apoptosis in medulloblastoma cell lines. *Cell Death Differ* 1995;2:267–275.
39. Elledge RM, Clark GM, Fuqua SA, et al. p53 protein accumulation detected by five different antibodies: relationship to prognosis and heat shock protein 70 in breast cancer. *Cancer Res* 1994;54(14):3752–3757.
40. Bartkova J, Bartek J, Lukas J, et al. p53 protein alterations in human testicular cancer including pre-invasive intratubular germ-cell neoplasia. *Int J Cancer* 1991;49(2):196–202.
41. Nouri A, Oliver R. Tetraploid arrest with over expressed non-mutated p53 in germ cell cancers. Relevance to their chemosensitivity and possible application in non germ cell cancers. *Int J Oncol* 1997;11:1167–1371.
42. Schenkman NS, Sesterhenn IA, Washington L, et al. Increased p53 protein does not correlate to p53 gene mutations in microdissected human testicular germ cell tumors. *J Urol* 1995;154(2 Pt 1):617–621.
43. Huddart RA, Titley J, Robertson D, et al. Programmed cell death in response to chemotherapeutic agents in human germ cell tumour lines. *Eur J Cancer* 1995;31A(5):739–746.
44. Schwartz D, Goldfinger N, Rotter V. Expression of p53 protein in spermatogenesis is confined to the tetraploid pachytene primary spermatocytes. *Oncogene* 1993;8(6):1487–1494.
45. Chaganti R, Rodriguez E, Mathew S. Origin of adult male mediastinal germ-cell tumours. *Lancet* 1994;343:1130–1132.
46. Koberle B, Grimaldi KA, Sunters A, et al. DNA repair capacity and cisplatin sensitivity of human testis tumour cells. *Int J Cancer* 1997;70(5):551–555.
47. Oliver RT, Shamash J, Berney DM. p53 and MDM2 in germ cell cancer treatment response. *J Clin Oncol* 2002;20(18):3928–3929.
48. Prost S, Droz J, Gabillot M, et al. The human foetal H19 gene in germ cell tumours of the testis. *Eur J Cancer (Proc ECCO)* 1993;7:29A Abstract 1345.
49. Bokemeyer C, Kuczyk M, Dunn T, et al. Expression of stem-cell factor and its receptor c-kit protein in normal testicular tissue and malignant germ cell tumours. *J Cancer Res Clin Oncol* 1996;122:301–306.
50. Murty VVVS, Houldsworth J, Baldwin S, et al. Allelic deletions in the long arm of chromosome 12 identify sites of candidate tumour suppressor genes in male germ cell tumours. *Proc Natl Acad Sci U S A* 1992;89:11006–11010.
51. Houldsworth J, Reuter V, Bosl GJ, et al. Aberrant expression of cyclin D2 is an early event in human male germ cell tumorigenesis. *Cell Growth Differ* 1997;8(3):293–299.
52. Bartkova J, Rajpert-de Meyts E, Skakkebaek NE, et al. D-type cyclins in adult human testis and testicular cancer: relation to cell type, proliferation, differentiation, and malignancy. *J Pathol* 1999;187(5):573–581.
53. Bartkova J, Thullberg M, Meyts ER-D, et al. Lack of p19INK4d in human testicular germ cell tumours contrasts with high expression during normal spermatogenesis. *Oncogene* 2000;19(36):4146–4150.
54. Sicinski P, Donaher JL, Geng Y, et al. Cyclin D2 is an FSH-responsive gene involved in gonadal cell proliferation and oncogenesis. *Nature* 1996; 384(6608):470–474.
55. Bloom H, Hendry W. Possible roles of hormones in treatment of metastatic testicular teratomas; tumour regression with medroxyprogesterone acetate. *Br Med J* 1973;3(880):563–567.

56. Depue RH, Pike MC, Henderson BE. Estrogen exposure during gestation and risk of cancer of the testis. *J Natl Cancer Inst* 1983;71:1151–1155.

57. Newbold R, Bullock B, McLachlan B. Testicular tumours in mice exposed in utero to diethylstilboestrol. *J Urol* 1987;138:1446–1450.

58. Moller H. Trends in sex-ratio, testicular cancer and male reproductive hazards: are they connected? *APMIS* 1998;106:232–239.

59. Sharpe R. Reproductive biology — another DDT connection. *Nature* 1995;375: 538–539.

60. Braun M, Ahlbom A, Floderus B, et al. Effect of twinship on incidence of cancer of the testis, breast and other sites (Sweden). *Cancer Causes Control* 1995;6:519–524.

61. Swerdlow A, Stavola B, Swanwick M, et al. Risks of breast and testicular cancers in young adult twins in England and Wales: evidence on prenatal and genetic aetiology. *Lancet North Am Ed* 1997;350:1723–1728.

62. Ekbom A, Richiardi L, Akre O, et al. Age at immigration and duration of stay in relation to risk for testicular cancer among Finnish immigrants in Sweden. *J Natl Cancer Inst* 2003;95(16):1238–1240.

63. Looijenga LH, de Leeuw H, van Oorschot M, et al. Stem cell factor receptor (c-KIT) codon 816 mutations predict development of bilateral testicular germ-cell tumors. *Cancer Res* 2003;63(22):7674–7678.

64. Rapley EA, Hockley S, Warren W, et al. Somatic mutations of KIT in familial testicular germ cell tumours. *Br J Cancer* 2004;90(12):2397–2401.

65. McDougall JK. "Hit and run" transformation leading to carcinogenesis. *Dev Biol* 2001;106:77–82.

66. Hawkins E, Heifetz SA, Giller R, et al. The prepubertal testis (prenatal and postnatal): its relationship to intratubular germ cell neoplasia: a combined Pediatric Oncology Group and Children's Cancer Study Group. *Hum Pathol* 1997;28(4):404–410.

67. Lahdetie J, Saari N. Incidence of aneuploid spermatoza among infertile men studied by multicolour fluoresecence in situ hybridization. *Am J Med Genet* 1997;71(1):115–121.

68. Tanner J. Secular trends for puberty between 1860–1970. In: Tanner JM, ed. *Foetus into man.* London: Castlemead Publications, 1989:156–162.

69. Forman D, Chilvers C. A survey of sexual characteristics of young and middle aged males in England and Wales. *Br Med J* 1989;298:1137.

70. Hansen PV, Hansen SW. Gonadal function in men with testicular germ cell cancer: the influence of cisplatin-based chemotherapy. *Eur Urol* 1993;23(1):153–156.

71. Hoff Wanderas E, Fossa SD, Heilo A, et al. Serum follicle stimulating hormone—predictor of cancer in the remaining testis in patients with unilateral testicular cancer. *Br J Urol* 1990;66:315–317.

72. Oliver R, Mason M, Von der Masse H, et al. A randomised comparison of single agent carboplatin with radiotherapy in the adjuvant treatment of stage I seminoma of the testis, following orchidectomy: MRC TE19/EORTC 30982. *J Clin Oncol* 2004;23(Suppl):385, (Abstract 4517).

73. Jacobsen KD, Fossa SD, Bjoro TP, et al. Gonadal function and fertility in patients with bilateral testicular germ cell malignancy. *Eur Urol* 2002;42:229–238.

74. Olsson H, Bladstrom A, Alm P. Male gynecomastia and risk for malignant tumours—a cohort study. *BMC Cancer* 2002;2(1);16.

75. Forman D, Chilvers C, Oliver R, et al. The aetiology of testicular cancer: association with congenital abnormalities, age at puberty, infertility and exercise. *Br Med J* 1994;308:1393–1399.

76. Chilvers CEO, Forman D, Oliver RTD, et al. Social, behavioural and medical factors in the aetiology of testicular cancer—results from the UK study. *Br J Cancer* 1994;70(3):513–520.

77. Friosh RE, Wyshak G, Albright NL. Lower prevalence of breast cancer and cancers of the reproductive system amongst former college atheletes compared to non-atheletes. *Br J Cancer* 1985;52:885–891.

78. Gerhardsson M, Floderus B, Norell S. Physical activity and colon cancer risk. *Int J Epidemiol* 1988;17:743–746.

79. Bernstein L, Ross RK, Lobo RA, et al. The effects of moderate physical activity on menstrual cycle patterns in adolescence: implications for breast cancer prevention. *Br J Cancer* 1987;55(6):681–685.

80. Dahl E, Herrick J. A vascular mechanism for maintaining testicular temperature by counter-current exchange. *Surg Gynecol Obstet* 1959;108:697–705.

81. Mieusset R, Bujan L. Testicular heating and its possible contributions to male infertility: a review. *Int J Androl* 1995;18:169–184.

82. Setchell B. Naturally occurring and induced dysfunctions of the testis. In: Setchell B, ed. *The mammalian testis.* London: Elck Books, 1978:359–378.

83. Socher S, Yin Y, Dewolf W, et al. Temperature-mediated germ cell loss in the testis is associated with altered expression of the cell-cycle regulator p53. *J Urol* 1997;157(5):1986–1989.

84. Mieusset R, Bujan L. The potential of mild testicular heating as a safe, effective and reversible contraceptive method for men. *Int J Androl* 1994;17:186–191.

85. Thonneau P, Ducot B, Bujan L, et al. Heat exposure as a hazard to male fertility. *Lancet* 1996;347:204–205.

86. Bujan L, Daudin M, Charlet JP, et al. Increase in scrotal temperature in car drivers. *Hum Reprod* 2000;15(6):1355–1357.

87. Fisch H, Goluboff ET, Olson JH, et al. Semen analyses in 1,283 men from the United States over a 25-year period: no decline in quality [see Comments]. *Fertil Steril* 1996;65(5):1009–1014.

88. Fisch H, Andrews H, Hendricks J, et al. The relationship of sperm counts to birth rates: a population based study. *J Urol* 1997;157(3):840–843.

89. Chilvers C, Dudley NE, Gough MH. Undescended testis: the effect of treatment of subsequent risk of subfertility and malignancy. *J Pediatr Surg* 1986;21:691.

90. Jones B, Thornhill J, O'Donnell B, et al. Influence of prior orchiopexy on stage and prognosis of testicular cancer. *Eur Urol* 1991;19(3):201–203.

91. Coupland C, Chilvers C, Forman D, et al. Risk factors for testicular cancer by histological tumour type. *Br J Cancer* 1999;80(11):1859–1863.

92. Raja MA, Oliver RT, Badenoch D, et al. Orchidopexy and transformation of seminoma to non-seminoma [Letter]. *Lancet* 1992;339(8798):930.

93. Grocork LA, Charlton HM, Pyke MC. Role of foetal pituitary in cryptorchidism induced by exogenous oestrogen during pregnancy in mice. *J Reprod Fertil* 1988;83:295–300.

94. Destefano F, Annest JL, Kresnow M. Semen characteristics of Vietnam veterans. *Reprod Toxicol* 1989;3:165–173.

95. Joynes F, Rous P. On the cause of localisation of secondary tumour at points of injury. *J Exp Med* 1914;20:404–412.

96. Merzenich H, Ahrens W, Stang A, et al. Sorting the hype from the facts in testicular cancer: is testicular cancer related to trauma? *J Urol* 2000;164(6):2143–2144.

97. Beard CM, Benson RC, Kelalis PP. The incidence and outcome of mumps orchitis in Rochester, Minnesota 1935-1974. *Mayo Clin Proc* 1977;52:3–7.

98. Johnstone JA, Ross CAC, Dunn M. Meningitis and encephalitis associated with mumps infection: a 10 year survey. *Arch Dis Child* 1972;47:647–651.

99. Powles T, Bower M, Daugaard KG, et al. Multicenter study of human immunodeficiency virus-related germ cell tumours. *J Clin Oncol* 2003;21(10):1922–1927.

100. Herbst H, Sauter M, Mueller-Lantzsch N. Expression of human endogenous retrovirus K elements in germ cell and trophoblastic tumors. *Am J Pathol* 1996;149(5):1727–1735.

101. Isaacson PG. Gastric lymphoma and Helicobacter Pylori. *N Engl J Med* 1994;330:1310–1311.

102. Pol S, Legendre C, Mattlinger B. Genetic basis of non-response to hepatitis B vaccine in hemodialyzed patients. *J Hepatol* 1990;11:385.

103. Hors J, Dausset J. HLA and susceptibility to Hodgkin's disease. *Immunol Rev* 1983;70:167.

104. Lu SJ, Day NE, Degos L. Linkage of a nasopharyngeal carcinoma susceptibility locus to the HLA region. *Nature* 1990;346:470.

105. Davies DH, Stauss H. The significance of human leukocyte antigen associations with cervical cancer. *Papillomavirus Report* 1997;8(2):43–50.

106. Oliver RTD. HLA phenotype and clinicopathological behaviour of germ cell tumours—possible evidence for clonal evolution from seminomas to nonseminomas. *Int J Androl* 1987;10:85–93.

107. Dieckmann KP, Klan R, Bunte S. HLA antigens, Lewis antigens, and blood groups in patients with testicular germ cell tumors. *Oncology* 1993;50:252–258.

108. Forman D, Oliver RTD, Brett AR, et al. Familial testicular cancer: a report of the UK Family register, estimation of risk and an HLA class I sib-pair analysis. *Br J Cancer* 1992;65:255–262.

109. Law HY, Bodmer WF, Matthews JD, et al. The immune response to vasectomy and its relation to the HLA system. *Tissue Antigens* 1979;14:115–139.

110. Azzopardi JG, Hoffbrand AV. Retrogression in testicular seminoma with viable metastases. *J Clin Pathol* 1965;18:135.

111. Fossa SD, Aass N, Heilo A, et al. Testicular carcinoma in situ in patients with extragonadal germ-cell tumours: the clinical role of pretreatment biopsy. *Ann Oncol* 1412;14(9):1412–1418.

112. Heimdal K, Olsson H, Tretli S, et al. Familial testicular cancer in Norway and southern Sweden. *Br J Cancer* 1996;73:964–969.

113. Westergaard T, Olsen J, Frisch M, et al. Cancer risk in fathers and brothers of testicular cancer patients in Denmark—a population-based study. *Int J Cancer* 1996;66:627–631.

114. Hemminki K, Li X. Familial risks of cancer as a guide to gene identification and mode of inheritance. *Int J Cancer* 2004;110(2):291–294.

115. Rapley E, Crockford G, Teare D, et al. Localisation of a susceptibility gene for testicular germ cell tumours. *Nat Genet* 2000;24:197–200.

116. Lilford R, Jones A, Bishop D, et al. Case-control study of whether subfertility in men is familial. *BMJ* 1994;309:570–573.

117. McGlynn KA, Devesa SS, Sigurdson AJ, et al. Trends in the incidence of testicular germ cell tumors in the United States. *Cancer* 2003;97(1):63–70.

118. Powles T, Shamash J, Ong J, et al. The rising incidence of stage 1 seminoma; a reflection of earlier diagnosis of germ cell cancer of the testis in last 20 years. *J Clin Oncol* 2004;23(Suppl):388 (Abstract 452).

119. Post PN, Casparie MK, ten Kate FJ, et al. [The epidemiology of tumors of the testes in the Netherlands: accurate rendering by the Registry of Histopathology and Cytopathology (PALGA)]. *Ned Tijdschr Geneeskd* 1150;148(23):1150–1154.

120. Dieckmann KP, Becker T, Jonas D. Inheritance and testicular cancer. *Oncology* 1987;4:367.

121. Swerdlow AJ, Huttly SRA, Smith PG. Is the incidence of testis cancer related to trauma or temperature? *Br J Urol* 1988;61:518–521.

122. Leibovitch I, Baniel J, Rowland RG, et al. Malignant testicular neoplasms in immunosuppressed patients. *J Urol* 1996;155(6):1938–1942.

123. Oliver RT, Ong J, Blandy JP, et al. Testis conservation studies in germ cell cancer justified by improved primary chemotherapy response and reduced delay, 1978-1994. *Br J Urol* 1996;78(1):119–124.

124. Oliver RTD, Nouri AME. T cell immune response to cancer in humans and its relevance for immunodiagnosis and therapy. *Cancer Surv* 1992;13:173–204.

125. Thackray AC, Crane WAJ. Seminoma. In: Pugh RCB, ed. Pathology of testes tumours. Oxford: Blackwell Scientific Publications, 1976:164–168.
126. Epenetos AA, Travers P, Gatter KC, et al. An immunohistological study of testicular germ cell tumours using two different monoclonal antibodies against placental alkaline phosphatase. Br J Cancer 1984;49:11–15.
127. Leroy X, Augusto D, Leteurtre E, et al. CD30 and CD117 (c-kit) used in combination are useful for distinguishing embryonal carcinoma from seminoma. J Histochem Cytochem 2002;50(2):283–285.
128. Oosterhuis JW, Gillis AJM, van Putten WJL, et al. Interphase cytogenetics of carcinoma in situ of the testis. Eur Urol 1993;23:16–22.

CHAPTER 32B
Hereditary Testicular Cancer

Joan L. Kramer and Mark H. Greene

INTRODUCTION

Although testicular cancer is rare, accounting for only 1% of all cancers in men, its importance exceeds its frequency. It is the most common cancer in men aged between 20 and 35, putting young men at risk of morbidity and mortality during their most productive years. While treatment for testicular germ cell tumors (TGCT) has evolved rationally, with current cure rates of 85%, the survivors are still at risk of the delayed toxicities from therapy. Individuals with a history of testicular cancer have a 40% increase in their risk of (subsequent nongerm cell) malignancy (1). In addition, the risk of developing cardiovascular disease is more than twice as high in testicular cancer treatment survivors (2). Other toxicities from therapy include nephrotoxicity, neuropathy, and ototoxicity related to cisplatin, as well as pulmonary toxicity from bleomycin (3). Sexual dysfunction posttreatment is not uncommon (4). In addition, 5% of patients develop cancer of the contralateral testicle (5), while 15% of patients fail treatment and ultimately die of their disease.

In the United States, 8,980 new cases of TGCT are predicted to occur in 2004, with 360 deaths attributable to this disease (6). Epidemiologic studies have documented an increasing incidence of TGCT since the mid-20th century (7–9). Between 1973 and 1995, the incidence of testicular cancer increased by 50% in the United States. This increase in incidence correlates with the year in which patients were born, and thus is said to be related to birth cohort (10). The incidence peaks in white men between 30 and 35 years old, then declines rapidly until it exhibits a secondary increase again at age 65. The lifetime risk of TGCT in Caucasian men is estimated to be one in 500. It is the most common cancer in young men aged 20 to 35, but is significantly less common in African Americans (11,12).

RISK FACTORS

Genitourinary Anomalies

Cryptorchidism

A history of cryptorchidism (*Maldescendens Testis*) is found in 8% to 12% of testicular cancer patients (13–16), and is well-recognized as a risk factor for TGCT. Affected men experience from an 8-fold to a 16-fold increase in risk, compared with men who have normally-descended testes (13,17–19). In men with unilateral cryptorchidism, there is an increased risk of TGCT in *both* testes, with the risk in the undescended testis higher than that in the normally descended testis (13,16,19,20).

The effect of orchiopexy on this risk is still somewhat controversial. Early case reports of testicular cancer developing after successful orchiopexy are remarkable for the paucity of cases in which surgery was performed in childhood. For example, in a 1967 case report and literature review that cited 37 cases of testicular cancer occurring in men after orchiopexy, in only two cases was the surgery performed before the age of 10 years, with no case undergoing orchiopexy before the age of 2 years (21). Attempts to study this issue systematically have brought conflicting results. For example, in a case-control study by the United Kingdom Testicular Cancer Study Group (UKTCSG), the risk of TGCT was no different in those who had surgical correction of unilateral testicular maldescent prior to the age of 10 than in those without a history of cryptorchidism. Although this finding reached statistical significance, the analysis was based upon only six cases and 10 controls who had surgery prior to age 10 (16). In contrast, a larger study that examined a cohort of individuals diagnosed with cryptorchidism found that the age at orchiopexy had no significant effect on reducing the risk of testicular cancer ($P = .43$). In fact, for those with testicular descent between 5 and 9 years of age, the risk of testicular cancer was still 18 times that of the general population ($P < .001$) (18).

At present, management of cryptorchidism is largely guided by issues other than cancer risk, such as fertility and psychosocial factors (22,23). Histologic changes are visible in biopsies of testes which remain undescended after 1 year, including markedly decreased counts of adult dark spermatogonia (24,25). In addition, the risk of infertility becomes measurably greater as the age at correction increases (26), as do problems with body image (23). At present, orchiopexy prior to 2 years of age is the current standard in the United States (22).

Inguinal Hernia and Hydrocele

Other urogenital developmental anomalies resulting from anomalous closure of the processus vaginalis, such as inguinal hernia and hydrocele, have also been variably linked to an increased risk of testicular cancer. Evidence from case-control studies is inconsistent regarding a link between the risk of testicular cancer and a history of inguinal hernia repair. Some studies estimated a 1.5-fold to 3-fold increase in risk of testicular cancer in those with a history of inguinal hernia (16,27–29), but in other similarly designed studies, the increase did not reach statistical significance (15,20). In some of these analyses, the effect of inguinal hernia on risk lost statistical significance when individuals with cryptorchidism were excluded from the analysis, indicating that the effect of inguinal hernia may not be independent of the risk associated with cryptorchidism. This is not surprising given that inguinal hernia and cryptorchidism often coexist, and may share common etiologic factors (29,30).

Few studies have examined hydrocele as a risk factor for testicular tumors. In an early study, the excess of cases with a history of hydrocele was not statistically significant (17). In a later study, the excess reached statistical significance only in the subgroup of men older than 20 years of age (29).

Syndromes Associated with Increased Risk

Persistent Mullerian duct syndrome is a disorder in which males with normal external genitalia and a normal 46,XY karyotype also have internal Mullerian duct structures. Not uncommonly, an affected male will have fallopian tubes, a uterus, and an upper vagina, as well as cryptorchidism (31). Multiple case reports linking TGCT and persistent Mullerian duct syndrome have been published (32–39), but no systematic, quantitative studies have been published to date.

The association of polythelia (accessory breast nipples) and TGCT was described by one group (40). In addition, Klein has previously described a syndrome of renal dysgenesis, hypospadias, and testicular cancer, which is not associated with germline mutations in the Wilms tumor gene (WT1), and which appears to be a distinct clinical and genetic entity (41).

Hormonal Risk Factors

Many researchers have postulated a link between testicular cancer and hormone exposure *in utero*. Administration of diethylstilbestrol (DES) during pregnancy has been associated with genitourinary (GU) anomalies such as cryptorchidism and hypospadias which are, in turn, associated with TGCT. A study examining testicular cancer risk in those exposed to DES *in utero* suggested an increased relative risk (RR) of TGCT, but the finding did not reach statistical significance (42). Another study that grouped DES with other exogenous hormone exposures during pregnancy demonstrated a significantly increased risk, with an OR of 4.9 (43). Other factors that potentially relate to intrauterine estrogen exposure such as cigarette smoking (43) and birth order (43,44) [estrogen levels are highest during first pregnancies (45)] also increase TGCT risk.

Infertility

Over the last 4 to 5 decades, there has been a decrease in semen quality in the general population, coincident with the increase in testicular cancer incidence (46). Further, significantly lower sperm concentration and total sperm count have been documented prior to treatment in patients with testicular cancer compared with patients having nontesticular malignancies (47). In addition, a higher incidence of testicular cancer has been demonstrated in men with a history of infertility (48,49). Testicular atrophy is associated with a greater than threefold increase in the risk of testicular cancer: (OR 3.2 95% CI 2.3–4.5) (29). An increased risk associated with testicular atrophy persists after eliminating individuals with a history of cryptorchidism and/or inguinal hernia (OR = 2.8; 95% CI 1.8–4.2). In individuals with a history of testicular cancer, testicular atrophy is associated with a 4.3-fold increased risk of having contralateral testicular intraepithelial neoplasia (TIN) (50). These observations, combined with the association of testicular cancer with cryptorchidism and testicular dysgenesis, suggest that a common etiologic factor may link these genital abnormalities.

TESTICULAR INTRAEPITHELIAL NEOPLASIA

TIN (sometimes inaccurately referred to as "carcinoma *in situ*") is hypothesized by European investigators to be the precursor of the vast majority of testicular germ cell neoplasms. Atypical germ cells were first described in 1965, in a patient who developed a seminoma 3 years after his initial biopsy (51). TIN cells are felt to represent malignant gonadocytes arising during early fetal life *in utero*, and they are present in nearly all individuals destined to develop invasive TGCT in later life (52). TIN has been studied extensively by Danish investigators, who documented that the prevalence of TIN in the contralateral testis of men treated for unilateral testis cancer was 5% to 6%, a rate which corresponds to their lifetime risk of developing a contralateral TGCT (53).

TIN is reported much more frequently in the European literature (54,55) than in corresponding American reports (56). One possible explanation for this discrepancy is that while TIN is often a diffuse lesion within the testis, it may

not appear in all microscopy fields (56). If the pathologist does not routinely, systematically examine all sections made of a new testicular tumor, the TIN may be missed. In addition, the Europeans advocate large testicular biopsies (>3 mm^3), and employ special handling of the tissue to preserve the architecture and cytologic details of the testis (57).

TIN cells are shed into semen, and there have been a number of attempts to devise noninvasive diagnostic procedures to detect these cells based on immunohistochemistry, cytology, and cytogenetic examination of seminal fluid (58–61). Currently, however, testicular biopsy remains the gold standard for TIN diagnosis (58,59).

The risk of TIN progressing to an invasive TGCT has been estimated to be approximately 50% at 5 years (52,62). However, because spontaneous regression of TIN has never been documented, many European investigators believe that virtually all cases of untreated TIN will ultimately progress to invasive TGCT (63). Consequently, patients in Europe in whom this diagnosis is made are typically treated with either surgery or radiation. In selected cases, the affected gonad may be left *in situ,* while the patient is monitored with particular care. Both TIN and TGCT are associated with genital malformations, for example, cryptorchidism (64), ambiguous genitalia (65), and persistent Mullerian duct syndrome (34), suggesting a common etiology for these three entities.

Beginning in 1960, the pathological finding of testicular calcifications in conjunction with testicular malignancy in biopsy specimens led to speculation that such calcifications could serve as a marker for the presence of malignancy. Reports of testicular calcifications became more common as the use of scrotal/testicular sonography gained in popularity. Testicular microlithiasis (TM), defined as multiple, punctate, echogenic, intratesticular foci on ultrasound examination (66), was seen in 0.6% to 9% (67) of individuals undergoing scrotal sonography in various retrospective series (67–69). Testicular tumors were found in up to 50% of those with TM in those same series (68,69). TM is also associated with TIN in selected populations. For example, in subfertile men, TIN was diagnosed in 20% of those with bilateral TM, while only 0.5% of those without TM had TIN (70). More than 20% of men with a history of TGCT and the presence of TM in the contralateral testicle were found to have contralateral testicular neoplasia, giving an OR = 12.0 ($P = .002$), compared with those individuals lacking TM. Although these data provide evidence that TM frequently coexists with testicular neoplasia in high-risk populations, only one study has attempted to assess the risk associated with TM in low-risk, asymptomatic men. In a screening study of 1,504 young men (aged 18 to 35), 5.6% were found to have TM by ultrasound. None of the individuals with TM had a coexisting testicular mass (71).

FAMILIAL AGGREGATION

Familial clusters of testicular cancer have long been reported in the scientific literature; a family history of TGCT is associated with an increased risk of the disease in numerous epidemiologic studies. Sons of fathers with TGCT have a fourfold to sixfold increased risk of developing a testicular tumor compared with the general population. Brothers of affected siblings have a relative risk (RR) of eight to ten compared with the normal population (72). A twin study (without stratification by zygosity) reported a RR risk of 38 in twin brothers of affected men (73).

FAMILIAL TESTICULAR CANCER

Familial testicular cancer is defined as two or more cases of TGCT in blood relatives, and has a prevalence of 1% to 5%

(72,74–76). Over 90% of the affected families have only two cases of testicular cancer (72,75,76), with rare case reports of as many as five cases within a family (77,78). The most common presentation is that of affected brothers, which is seen at twice the rate of father-son pairs (72,75,76,79,80). There are also numerous reports of more distant relationships of affected pairs, such as cousins, uncle–nephew, or grandfather–grandson (72,76).

Age at Presentation

Familial testicular cancer cases presented at a younger age than sporadic cases in one study, with the mean age at diagnosis 29.0 years for familial cases and 32.5 for sporadic cases ($P <.01$) (72). Other studies noted a trend toward an earlier age at diagnosis, but the difference did not reach statistical significance (74,76,80). In families which show father–son inheritance, the average age at diagnosis for sons of testicular cancer cases is 16 years younger than the age at which their fathers presented, giving some evidence of genetic anticipation (74,81).

Laterality and Histology (FTC)

Bilateral tumors were seen significantly more frequently in multiple-case families in one study, 9.8% versus 2.8% ($P = .02$) (74). In other studies of familial testicular cancer, the proportion of bilateral cases varied from a low of zero (80) to a high of 17% (72,75,76,82). These data suggest, but do not definitively prove, that a bilateral presentation is one of the characteristics of familial testicular cancer.

To date, there is no evidence of concordance within each family in terms of which side (i.e., left or right) is affected (80), nor is there a significant difference in the proportion of left-sided and right-sided tumors overall (72). In addition, the overall histologic distribution seen in familial testicular cancer cases does not seem to differ significantly from that of sporadic cases (76), and the specific histologies within families are often discordant. However, the pathology of testicular germ cell tumors is very complex, and there has never been a systematic study of a series of familial versus sporadic cases conducted by expert pathologists. It is possible that significant differences in histology between familial and sporadic cases might be observed, were such a study to be done.

Associated Genitourinary Abnormalities

A history of cryptorchidism is found in 10% of familial testicular cancer cases (72,74,75) which, although elevated in comparison with the general population, is similar to the proportion seen in sporadic testicular cancer. In addition, there is no significant difference in the incidence of inguinal hernia between familial testicular cancer cases and unselected testicular cancer patients (72,75).

Other Cancers Seen in Familial Testicular Cancer Families

Although many different cancers have been reported in members of testicular cancer families (72,83), there has been little attempt to quantify these risks. One Swedish study did find a markedly increased incidence of colorectal cancer in mothers of multiple case families (79).

Genetics

Until recently, the mechanism of inheritance in these families was poorly defined, and no candidate-susceptibility gene had been identified. Unraveling the genetic basis of familial testicular cancer through traditional linkage studies has been difficult because: (a) multiple case families are very uncommon (unlike familial breast or colon cancer); and (b) families with many affected individuals (the type of family required for genetic linkage and gene mapping studies) are exceedingly rare. In fact, the vast majority of families with testicular cancer contain only two affected family members, as noted above.

Recently, a subset of testicular cancer families was recognized as having a pattern of inheritance consistent with X-linkage, and a testis cancer susceptibility gene (designated "TGCT1") was provisionally mapped to the X chromosome (X band q27) within these families (84). Although a number of candidate genes from this region have been evaluated, the gene itself has not yet been identified. TGCT1 was estimated to account for nearly all families featuring the occurrence of bilateral testicular cancer, but it accounted for only a third of all familial TGCT, suggesting that there are other susceptibility genes that remain to be discovered. Furthermore, a significant number of families in this analysis displayed "father-to-son transmission" of the disease trait, and thus had a pattern of inheritance that was clearly *not* compatible with X linkage.

Efforts are continuing to identify and clone the Xq27 gene, as well as to identify one or more additional autosomal susceptibility genes. The most recent analysis of the International Testicular Cancer Linkage Consortium (ITCLC) family set shows preliminary evidence for autosomal susceptibility loci on chromosomes 3, 14, 16, and 18 (85). These results have not reached statistical significance; current work is focused upon the ascertainment and analysis of additional new multiple-case families. It is estimated that at least 500 families will be required to achieve the statistical power required to identify these genes. The most recent ITCLC genome-wide linkage analysis was based upon 179 families (85).

BILATERAL TESTICULAR CANCER

Because the phenomenon of bilateral primary neoplasms in paired organs is considered a hallmark of hereditary cancer syndromes, patients with bilateral testicular cancer are often grouped with familial cases. A prior diagnosis of testicular cancer represents the single most significant risk factor in the subsequent development of testicular malignancy, with a RR of up to 45 (5,86–89). Although the median time between the diagnosis of the first and second GCTs is 5 years, second TGCTs have been documented after a lag of over 15 years (5,89,90). The overall incidence of bilateral TGCT is estimated at 1% to 5% (5,88,89,91–94). Bilateral TGCT patients tend to be younger at initial presentation (i.e., with their first tumor) than are unilateral cases, with those diagnosed at age <30 years at particularly elevated risk (5). In one study, the mean age at diagnosis (for the first cancer) was 29.1 for those who went on to develop bilateral disease, versus 34.2 for those individuals with only unilateral disease ($P = .02$) (95). In another study, the difference in age at presentation for bilateral testicular cancer as compared with unilateral was 6 years (79).

SECOND CANCERS

A large international study demonstrated a 40% increased risk of subsequent nongerm cell malignancy in testicular cancer survivors, with a standardized incidence ratio (SIR) of 1.43 (95% CI 1.36–1.51). A number of malignancies displayed at least a twofold excess among survivors of testicular cancer, including acute leukemias (both acute lymphocytic and acute myelogenous leukemias) as well as cancers of connective tissue, pancreas, and thyroid. In addition, more modest increases were seen for non-Hodgkin lymphoma and cancers of the stomach, colon, rectum, and kidney. Many of these malignancies were postulated to be related to cancer treatments, such as radiation and chemotherapy. The actuarial risk of developing a second non-GCT cancer was estimated at 22.6% after 30 years of follow-up, a 10% excess when compared with the general population (1). In the absence of chemotherapy, treatment of testicular cancer with radiotherapy carries with it an increased risk of both leukemia and solid tumors (88,96). Treatment with chemotherapy is also associated with an elevated risk of leukemia, with a cumulative 5-year incidence of up to 2% (97).

SUMMARY

The development of highly effective treatment for testicular cancer has led to a dramatic change in prognosis for this disease—from a cancer that is almost always fatal to a cancer that is almost always curable. Still, much remains unknown about the etiology of testicular cancer. That cryptorchidism, a well-established risk factor for testicular cancer, is present at birth suggests that the intrauterine environment may play a significant role in determining risk. The presence of TIN in the undescended testes of very young boys provides additional support for this hypothesis, as do some studies of intrauterine exposure to exogenous hormones.

One important unanswered question concerns the optimum management of testicular intraepithelial neoplasia. Is TIN truly a precancerous condition that will inevitably lead to cancer, or is it simply a marker of an increased risk of testicular cancer? Although European clinicians routinely biopsy the clinically uninvolved testis of newly diagnosed testicular cancer patients in a search for TIN, U.S. urologists do not. In Europe, a diagnosis of TIN often leads to treatment with radiotherapy, while there is no standard treatment for this condition in the U.S. Furthermore, the significance of testicular microlithiasis (and its relationship to TGCT) also remains to be elucidated.

Finally, the profound effect of family history on risk points to genetic factors in testicular cancer etiology. Ongoing studies of familial testicular cancer are actively searching for genetic clues to testicular cancer etiology, with the goal of finding the genes responsible for this disease. Studies currently underway at the Clinical Genetics Branch (CGB) of the National Cancer Institute are also attempting to clarify the full phenotype (both neoplastic and non-neoplastic) of the familial testicular cancer syndrome, seeking evidence of dysmorphic features in affected family members, searching for constitutional cytogenetic abnormalities, considering whether there exists a carrier phenotype for female family members of X-linked kindreds, and analyzing the behavioral and psychosocial consequences of being a member of a multiple-case TGCT family (see http://familial-testicular-cancer.cancer.gov/). In collaboration with the ITCLC, CGB investigators are quantifying the risk of cancers other than TGCT in these families, and conducting a formal pathology review of both familial and nonfamilial cases. Perhaps the next 5 to 10 years will witness an extension of the kind of dramatic progress previously observed in the treatment of TGCT to our understanding of the genetic component of TGCT etiology.

References

1. Travis LB, Curtis RE, Storm H, et al. Risk of second malignant neoplasms among long-term survivors of testicular cancer. *J Natl Cancer Inst* 1997; 89(19):1429–1439.
2. Huddart RA, Norman A, Shahidi M, et al. Cardiovascular disease as a long-term complication of treatment for testicular cancer. *J Clin Oncol* 2003;21(8):1513–1523.
3. Kollmannsberger C, Kuczyk M, Mayer F, et al. Late toxicity following curative treatment of testicular cancer. *Semin Surg Oncol* 1999;17:275–281.
4. van Basten JP, Jonker-pool G, van Driel M, et al. Sexual functioning after multimodality treatment for disseminated nonseminomatous germ cell tumor. *J Urol* 1997;158:1411–1416.
5. Wanderas EH, Fossa SD, Tretli S. Risk of a second germ cell cancer after treatment of a primary germ cell cancer in 2201 Norwegian male patients. *Eur J Cancer* 1997;33(2):244–252.
6. Jemal A, Tiwari RC, Murray T, et al. Cancer statistics, 2004. *Cancer J Clin* 2004;54(1):8–29.
7. Brown LM, Pottern LM, Hoover RN, et al. Testicular cancer in the United States: trends in incidence and mortality. *Int J Epidemiol* 1986;15(2): 164–170.
8. Bergstrom R, Adami HO, Mohner M, et al. Increase in testicular cancer incidence in six European countries: a birth cohort phenomenon. *J Natl Cancer Inst* 1996;88(11):727–733.
9. Zheng T, Holford TR, Ma Z, et al. Continuing increase in incidence of germ-cell testis cancer in young adults: experience from Connecticut, USA, 1935–1992. *Int J Cancer* 1996;65(6):723–729.
10. McKiernan JM, Goluboff ET, Liberson GL, et al. Rising risk of testicular cancer by birth cohort in the United States from 1973 to 1995. *J Urol* 1999;162(2):361–363.
11. Miller BA, Ries LAG, Hankey BF, et al. *SEER cancer statistics review: 1973-1990*, No. 93-2789. Bethesda, MD: National Cancer Institute, National Institutes of Health, 1993.
12. Swerdlow AJ. The epidemiology of testicular cancer. *Eur Urol* 1993; 23(Suppl. 2):35–38.
13. Strader CH, Weiss NS, Daling JR, et al. Cryptorchism, orchiopexy, and the risk of testicular cancer. *Am J Epidemiol* 1988;127(5):1013–1018.
14. Thornhill JA, Conroy RM, Kelly DG, et al. An evaluation of predisposing factors for testis cancer in Ireland. *Eur Urol* 1988;14(6):429–433.
15. Pottern LM, Brown LM, Hoover RN, et al. Testicular cancer risk among young men: role of cryptorchidism and inguinal hernia. *J Natl Cancer Inst* 1985;74(2):377–381.
16. United Kingdom Testicular Cancer Study Group. Aetiology of testicular cancer: association with congenital abnormalities, age at puberty, infertility, and exercise. *BMJ* 1994;308(6941):1393–1399.
17. Swerdlow AJ, Huttly SR, Smith PG. Testicular cancer and antecedent diseases. *Br J Cancer* 1987;55(1):97–103.
18. Swerdlow AJ, Higgins CD, Pike MC. Risk of testicular cancer in cohort of boys with cryptorchidism [see Comments] [published erratum appears in BMJ 1997 Nov 1;315(7116):1129]. *BMJ* 1997;314(7093):1507–1511.
19. Stone JM, Cruickshank DG, Sandeman TF, et al. Laterality, maldescent, trauma and other clinical factors in the epidemiology of testis cancer in Victoria, Australia. *Br J Cancer* 1991;64(1):132–138.
20. Prener A, Engholm G, Jensen OM. Genital anomalies and risk for testicular cancer in Danish men. *Epidemiology* 1996;7(1):14–19.
21. Altman BL, Malament M. Carcinoma of the testis following orchiopexy. *J Urol* 1967;97(3).498–504.
22. American Academy of Pediatrics. Timing of elective surgery on the genitalia of male children with particular reference to the risks, benefits, and psychological effects of surgery and anesthesia. *Pediatrics* 1996;97(4): 590–594.
23. Manley CB. Elective genital surgery at one year of age: psychological and surgical considerations. *Surg Clin North Am* 1982;62(6):941–953.
24. Huff DS, Fenig DM, Canning DA, et al. Abnormal germ cell development in cryptorchidism. *Horm Res* 2001;55(1):11–17.
25. Hadziselimovic F, Hecker E, Herzog B. The value of testicular biopsy in cryptorchidism. *Urol Res* 1984;12(3):171–174.
26. Hadziselimovic F, Herzog B, Buser M. Development of cryptorchid testes. *Eur J Pediatr* 1987;146(Suppl. 2):S8–S12.
27. Morrison AS. Cryptorchidism, hernia, and cancer of the testis. *J Natl Cancer Inst* 1976;56(4):731–733.
28. Gallagher RP, Huchcroft S, Phillips N, et al. Physical activity, medical history, and risk of testicular cancer (Alberta and British Columbia, Canada). *Cancer Causes Control* 1995;6(5):398–406.
29. Moller H, Prener A, Skakkebaek NE. Testicular cancer, cryptorchidism, inguinal hernia, testicular atrophy, and genital malformations: case-control studies in Denmark. *Cancer Causes Control* 1996;7(2):264–274.
30. Benson RC Jr, Beard CM, Kelalis PP, et al. Malignant potential of the cryptorchid testis. *Mayo Clin Proc* 1991;66(4):372–378.
31. Walsh PC, Retik AB, Vaughn ED et al., eds. *Campbell's urology*, 8th ed. Philadelphia, PA: WB Saunders, 2002.
32. Wu HC, Chen JH, Lu HF, et al. Persistent mullerian duct syndrome with seminoma: CT findings. *AJR Am J Roentgenol* 2000;174(1):102–104.
33. Berkmen F. Persistent mullerian duct syndrome with or without transverse testicular ectopia and testis tumours. *Br J Urol* 1997;79(1):122–126.
34. Williams JC, Merguerian PA, Schned AR, et al. Bilateral testicular carcinoma in situ in persistent mullerian duct syndrome: a case report and literature review. *Urology* 1994;44(4):595–598.
35. Eastham JA, McEvoy K, Sullivan R, et al. A case of simultaneous bilateral nonseminomatous testicular tumors in persistent mullerian duct syndrome. *J Urol* 1992;148(2 Pt 1):407–408.
36. Kulkarni JN, Bhansali MS, Tongaonkar HB, et al. Carcinoma in the third testis in a case of polyorchidism and persistent mullerian structure syndrome. *Eur Urol* 1992;22(2):174–176.

37. van Laarhoven CJ, Juttmann JR, Pijpers PM, et al. A testicular tumour in the left adnexa. The persistent mullerian duct syndrome with testicular malignancy. *Eur J Surg Oncol* 1991;17(1):97–98.

38. Melman A, Leiter E, Perez JM, et al. The influence of neonatal orchiopexy upon the testis in persistent Mullerian duct syndrome. *J Urol* 1981;125(6):856–858.

39. Duenas A, Saldivar C, Castillero C, et al. A case of bilateral seminoma in the setting of persistent mullerian duct syndrome. *Rev Invest Clin* 2001;53(2):193–196.

40. Goedert JJ, McKeen EA, Javadpour N, et al. Polythelia and testicular cancer. *Ann Intern Med* 1984;101:646–647.

41. Klein EA, Chen RN, Levin HS, et al. Testicular cancer in association with developmental renal anomalies and hypospadias. *Urology* 1996;47(1):82–87.

42. Strohsnitter WC, Noller KL, Hoover RN, et al. Cancer risk in men exposed in utero to diethylstilbestrol. *J Natl Cancer Inst* 2001;93(7):545–551.

43. Weir HK, Marrett LD, Kreiger N, et al. Pre-natal and peri-natal exposures and risk of testicular germ-cell cancer. *Int J Cancer* 2000;87(3):438–443.

44. Moller H, Skakkebaek NE. Testicular cancer and cryptorchidism in relation to prenatal factors: case-control studies in Denmark. *Cancer Causes Control* 1997;8(6):904–912.

45. Panagiotopoulou K, Katsouyanni K, Petridou E, et al. Maternal age, parity, and pregnancy estrogens. *Cancer Causes Control* 1990;1(2):119–124.

46. Carlsen E, Giwercman A, Keiding N, et al. Evidence for decreasing quality of semen during past 50 years [see Comments]. *BMJ* 1992;305(6854):609–613.

47. Petersen PM, Skakkebaek NE, Vistisen K, et al. Semen quality and reproductive hormones before orchiectomy in men with testicular cancer. *J Clin Oncol* 1999;17(3):941–947.

48. Moller H. Trends in sex-ratio, testicular cancer and male reproductive hazards: are they connected? *APMIS* 1998;106(1):232–238.

49. Jacobsen R, Bostofte E, Engholm G, et al. Risk of testicular cancer in men with abnormal semen characteristics: cohort study. *BMJ* 2000;321(7264):789–792.

50. Dieckmann KP, Loy V. Prevalence of contralateral testicular intraepithelial neoplasia in patients with testicular germ cell neoplasms. *J Clin Oncol* 1996;14(12):3126–3132.

51. Bunge RG, Bradbury JT. An early human seminoma. *J Am Med Assoc* 1965;193:960.

52. Skakkebaek NE, Berthelsen JG, Muller J. Carcinoma-in-situ of the undescended testis. *Urol Clin North Am* 1982;9(3):377–385.

53. Berthelsen JG, Skakkebaek NE, von der MH, et al. Screening for carcinoma in situ of the contralateral testis in patients with germinal testicular cancer. *Br Med J (Clin Res Ed)* 1982;285(6356):1683–1686.

54. Pryor JP, Cameron KM, Chilton CP, et al. Carcinoma in situ in testicular biopsies from men presenting with infertility. *Br J Urol* 1983;55(6):780–784.

55. Skakkebaek NE. Carcinoma in situ of the testis: frequency and relationship to invasive germ cell tumours in infertile men. *Histopathology* 1978;2(3):157–170.

56. Burke AP, Mostofi FK. Placental alkaline phosphatase immunohistochemistry of intratubular malignant germ cells and associated testicular germ cell tumors. *Hum Pathol* 1988;19(6):663–670.

57. Giwercman A, Berthelsen JG, Muller J, et al. Screening for carcinoma-in-situ of the testis. *Int J Androl* 1987;10(1):173–180.

58. Moore BE, Banner BF, Gokden M, et al. p53: a good diagnostic marker for intratubular germ cell neoplasia, unclassified. *Appl Immunohistochem Mol Morphol* 2001;9(3):203–206.

59. Salanova M, Gandini L, Lenzi A, et al. Is hyperdiploidy of immature ejaculated germ cells predictive of testis malignancy? A comparative study in healthy normozoospermic, infertile, and testis tumor suffering subjects. *Lab Invest* 1999;79(9):1127–1135.

60. Meng FJ, Zhou Y, Giwercman A, et al. Fluorescence in situ hybridization analysis of chromosome 12 anomalies in semen cells from patients with carcinoma in situ of the testis. *J Pathol* 1998;186(3):235–239.

61. Meng FJ, Zhou Y, Skakkebaek NE, et al. Detection and enrichment of carcinoma-in-situ cells in semen by an immunomagnetic method using monoclonal antibody M2A. *Int J Androl* 1996;19(6):365–370.

62. von der MH, Rorth M, Walbom-Jorgensen S, et al. Carcinoma in situ of contralateral testis in patients with testicular germ cell cancer: study of 27 cases in 500 patients. *Br Med J (Clin Res Ed)* 1986;293(6559):1398–1401.

63. Daugaard G, Giwercman A, Skakkebaek NE. Should the other testis be biopsied? *Semin Urol Oncol* 1996;14(1):8–12.

64. Giwercman A, Bruun E, Frimodt-Moller C, et al. Prevalence of carcinoma in situ and other histopathological abnormalities in testes of men with a history of cryptorchidism. *J Urol* 1989;142(4):998–1001.

65. Muller J, Skakkebaek NE. Testicular carcinoma in situ in children with the androgen insensitivity (testicular feminisation) syndrome. *Br Med J (Clin Res Ed)* 1984;288(6428):1419–1420.

66. Doherty FJ, Mullins TL, Sant GR, et al. Testicular microlithiasis. A unique sonographic appearance. *J Ultrasound Med* 1987;6(7):389–392.

67. Bach AM, Hann LE, Hadar O, et al. Testicular microlithiasis: what is its association with testicular cancer?. *Radiology* 2001;220(1):70–75.

68. Backus ML, Mack LA, Middleton WD, et al. Testicular microlithiasis: imaging appearances and pathologic correlation. *Radiology* 1994;192(3):781–785.

69. Hobarth K, Susani M, Szabo N, et al. Incidence of testicular microlithiasis. *Urology* 1992;40(5):464–467.

70. Gouveia Brazao CA, Pierik FH, Oosterhuis JW, et al. Bilateral testicular microlithiasis predicts the presence of the precursor of testicular germ cell tumors in subfertile men. *J Urol* 2004;171(1):158–160.

71. Peterson AC, Bauman JM, Light DE, et al. The prevalence of testicular microlithiasis in an asymptomatic population of men 18 to 35 years old. *J Urol* 2001;166(6):2061–2064.

72. Forman D, Oliver RT, Brett AR, et al. Familial testicular cancer: a report of the UK Family Register, estimation of risk and an HLA class 1 sib-pair analysis. *Br J Cancer* 1992;65(2):255–262.

73. Swerdlow AJ, De Stavola BL, Swanwick MA, et al. Risks of breast and testicular cancers in young adult twins in England and Wales: evidence on prenatal and genetic aetiology. *Lancet* 1997;350(9093):1723–1728.

74. Heimdal K, Olsson H, Tretli S, et al. Familial testicular cancer in Norway and Southern Sweden. *Br J Cancer* 1996;73(7):964–969.

75. Sonneveld DJ, Sleijfer DT, Schrafford KH, et al. Familial testicular cancer in a single-centre population. *Eur J Cancer* 1999;35(9):1368–1373.

76. Dieckmann KP, Pichlmeier U. The prevalence of familial testicular cancer: an analysis of two patient populations and a review of the literature. *Cancer* 1997;80(10):1954–1960.

77. Goss PE, Bulbul MA. Familial testicular cancer in five members of a cancer-prone kindred. *Cancer* 1990;66(9):2044–2046.

78. Cooper MA, Fellows J, Einhorn LH. Familial occurrence of testicular cancer. *J Urol* 1994;151(4):1022–1023.

79. Dong C, Lonnstedt I, Hemminki K. Familial testicular cancer and second primary cancers in testicular cancer patients by histological type. *Eur J Cancer* 2001;37(15):1878–1885.

80. Polednak AP. Familial testicular cancer in a population-based cancer registry. *Urol Int* 1996;56(4):238–240.

81. Han S, Peschel RE. Father-son testicular tumors: evidence for genetic anticipation? A case report and review of the literature. *Cancer* 2000;88(10):2319–2325.

82. Ondrus D, Kuba D, Chrenova S, et al. Familial testicular cancer and developmental anomalies. *Neoplasma* 1997;44(1):59–61.

83. Tollerud DJ, Blattner WA, Fraser MC, et al. Familial testicular cancer and urogenital developmental anomalies. *Cancer* 1985;55(8):1849–1854.

84. Rapley EA, Crockford GP, Teare D, et al. Localization to Xq27 of a susceptibility gene for testicular germ-cell tumours. *Nat Genet* 2000;24(2):197–200.

85. Rapley EA, Crockford GP, Easton DF, et al. Localisation of susceptibility genes for familial testicular germ cell tumour. *APMIS* 2003;111(1):128–133.

86. Colls BM, Harvey VJ, Skelton L, et al. Bilateral germ cell testicular tumors in New Zealand: experience in Auckland and Christchurch 1978–1994. *J Clin Oncol* 1996;14(7):2061–2065.

87. Ruther U, Dieckmann K, Bussar-Maatz R, et al. Second malignancies following pure seminoma. *Oncology* 2000;58(1):75–82.

88. van Leeuwen FE, Stiggelbout AM, Belt-Dusebout AW, et al. Second cancer risk following testicular cancer: a follow-up study of 1,909 patients. *J Clin Oncol* 1993;11(3):415–424.

89. Osterlind A, Berthelsen JG, Abildgaard N, et al. Risk of bilateral testicular germ cell cancer in Denmark: 1960–1984. *J Natl Cancer Inst* 1991;83(19):1391–1395.

90. Che M, Tamboli P, Ro JY, et al. Bilateral testicular germ cell tumors: twenty-year experience at M. D. Anderson Cancer Center. *Cancer* 2002;95(6):1228–1233.

91. Bokemeyer C, Schmoll HJ, Schoffski P, et al. Bilateral testicular tumours: prevalence and clinical implications. *Eur J Cancer* 1993;29A(6):874–876.

92. Scheiber K, Ackermann D, Studer UE. Bilateral testicular germ cell tumors: a report of 20 cases. *J Urol* 1987;138(1):73–76.

93. Thompson J, Williams CJ, Whitehouse JM, et al. Bilateral testicular germ cell tumours: an increasing incidence and prevention by chemotherapy. *Br J Urol* 1988;62(4):374–376.

94. van Basten JP, Hoekstra HJ, van Driel MF, et al. Cisplatin-based chemotherapy changes the incidence of bilateral testicular cancer. *Ann Surg Oncol* 1997;4(4):342–348.

95. Dieckmann KP, Loy V, Buttner P. Prevalence of bilateral testicular germ cell tumours and early detection based on contralateral testicular intraepithelial neoplasia. *Br J Urol* 1993;71(3):340–345.

96. Travis LB, Andersson M, Gospodarowicz M, et al. Treatment-associated leukemia following testicular cancer. *J Natl Cancer Inst* 2000;92(14):1165–1171.

97. Kollmannsberger C, Hartmann JT, Kanz L, et al. Therapy-related malignancies following the treatment of germ cell cancer. *Int J Cancer* 1999;83:860–863.

CHAPTER 33 ■ BIOLOGY AND GENETICS OF ADULT MALE GERM CELL TUMORS

JANE HOULDSWORTH, GEORGE J. BOSL, AND R. S. K. CHAGANTI

Germ cell tumors (GCTs) arise by transformation of a germ cell that during its normal lifespan undergoes a series of proliferation and differentiation events that culminate in the formation of gametes (1). They are the most common malignancy in young adult males of ages 15 to 40 presenting predominantly in the testis (2). Uniquely, transformed germ cells exhibit the potential to initiate molecular pathways resembling in part those occurring during normal human development, as evidenced by the array of histologies observed within tumor specimens (3). These histologies range from seminomas that resemble undifferentiated germ cells, to nonseminomas that resemble early zygotic differentiation (embryonal carcinoma), embryonic somatic differentiation (teratoma), and extraembryonic differentiation (yolk sac tumor, choriocarcinoma). Occasionally within differentiated components of teratoma, further malignant transformation can occur leading to the appearance of a non–germ cell malignancy (3). Clinically, more than 90% of newly diagnosed patients are cured, with 70% to 80% of advanced cases being cured with cisplatin based chemotherapy (2). Thus, GCTs represent an ideal system in which the molecular mechanisms underlying this exquisite sensitivity can be studied. In this chapter, a review is undertaken of the current state of knowledge of the biology and genetics of germ cell transformation, differentiation, and response to cisplatin.

LIFESPAN OF THE NORMAL HUMAN MALE GERM CELL

During gastrulation of the developing embryo, primordial germ cells (PGC)—as the embryonic precursors of gametes—are first recognized in the mouse as a cluster of alkaline phosphatase-positive cells that arise from the embryonic ectoderm (4). Upon proliferation, the PGCs migrate to the mesoderm of the primitive streak, to the endoderm via the base of the allantois, through the hindgut endoderm, and finally to the genital ridges. PGCs isolated at this stage are the source of embryonic germ cells that display pluripotentiality *in vitro* (5). In the genital ridges, the PGCs, along with Sertoli cells, are incorporated into the seminiferous cords and, along with other somatic cells such as Leydig cells, form the developing gonad by the seventh or eighth week of human fetal life (6). Once enclosed within the seminiferous tubules, the PGCs cease to proliferate and undergo differentiation into gonocytes. In the neonatal testis, gonocytes are easily recognized as large round cells centrally located within tubules (6). After birth, the gonocytes reinitiate proliferation, migrate to the tubular wall, and mature into undifferentiated Type A spermatogonia usually within 2 to 3 months of age. In the prepubertal testis and culminating at the onset of puberty induced by gonadotrophins, spermatogonial proliferation and maturation into Type B spermatogonia are evident with the onset of meiosis

leading to the appearance of fully differentiated spermatozoa in the tubules (7,8). In the pubertal and young adult testis, Type A dark type (d) and Type A pale type (p) spermatogonia usually exist as single, pairs, and chains of cells; by analogy with nonprimates, the single spermatogonia represent stem cells. Type Ad spermatogonia rarely divide and are thought to represent a reserve of stem cells in the case of germ cell loss. Type Ap spermatogonia actively divide, possibly representing renewing stem cells, though the true self-renewing stem cell in humans is still the subject of debate (7,8). Type B spermatogonia undergo only one mitotic division in humans that leads to primary spermatocytes. Premeiotic replication follows with entrance into meiosis comprising a protracted prophase (leptotene, zygotene, pachytene, diplotene, diakinesis) and mitoses I and II, resulting in four haploid gametes. These round spermatids then undergo spermiogenesis into spermatozoa. In humans, the entire cycle of spermatogenesis takes approximately 74 days, with waves of meiosis taking 26 days (6,7). Spontaneous apoptosis is normal in the adult male testis, occurring mostly in primary spermatocytes, spermatids, and few spermatogonia (7). In addition, apoptosis is thought to be involved in the control of the stem cell pool size, with some evidence for a mechanistic role of BCL2 family members (8).

Understanding of the genetic control of germ cell development and differentiation is limited in humans, based primarily on genetic disorders that lead to infertility (9). Microdeletions or translocations of the Y chromosome, in particular involving the SRY and AZF loci, imbalance of X and Y chromosome number, mutations of genes associated with gonadotrophin production, follicle-stimulating hormone (FSH) and luteinizing hormone (LH) function, and androgen synthesis and function can lead to oligospermia or azoospermia (7,9). It has been reported that multiple genes are expressed in specific stages of the germ cell lifespan and that their roles have often been indicated or confirmed in mutant or transgenic mice. With the advent of microarray-based expression analyses, the expression profiles of isolated populations of germ cells at different times during their lifespans have been performed, though the role of these genes in human germ cell development remains to be confirmed.

During their lifespans, germ cells undergo genetic and epigenetic modifications. Recombination between paired chromosomes during prophase of meiosis I is a specialized process for which the underlying enzymatic and structural machinery and regulatory checkpoints are being defined predominantly in lower eukaryotes, though often with homologs in mammals (10). Germ cells are also responsible for the inheritance of the paternal-specific epigenetic imprint of specific subsets of genes. Analysis of the methylation of CpG dinucleotides during human spermatogenesis has revealed that the methylation pattern inherited from the parents is initially erased in fetal spermatogonia prior to entry of meiosis (11). The parent-specific imprint is reestablished in adult spermatogonia and then maintained in spermatocytes and spermatozoa. Errors can occur in both forms of genomic modification, leading to miscarriage and birth defects.

PATHOBIOLOGY OF MALE GERM CELL TUMORS

Transformation of male germ cells gives rise to tumors that display an array of histopathologies in the adult. GCTs are broadly classified into two groups: seminomas and nonseminomas (3). The first recognizable lesion in the testis is intratubular germ cell neoplasia (ITGCN), where transformed germ cells are evident within the seminiferous tubules. ITGCN is generally accepted as the precursor of all invasive GCTs, although morphologically it more closely resembles seminomas than nonseminomas (3). Seminomatous GCTs retain the morphology of undifferentiated spermatogonial germ cells that frequently express protein markers of germ cells early in development, such as placental alkaline phosphatase, KIT, RET (GDNF receptor), and POU5F1 (OCT3/OCT4) (12–14). They exhibit low mitotic and apoptotic indices, as well as low metastatic potential, and are generally cured by a combination of orchiectomy and radiation therapy (RT) (2,3). Nonseminomas display a variety of histologies that resemble different stages and patterns of embryonic and extraembryonic differentiation that normally occur during human development. Embryonal carcinoma resembles zygotic cells early in embryonic development, consistent with the pluripotentiality displayed by embryonal carcinoma-derived cell lines in vitro (15). This histology displays the highest mitotic and apoptotic indices of all GCT components (3,16). Teratomas display multiple patterns of somatic differentiation normally seen in the three developing germ layers of the embryo. Components resembling incomplete differentiation (immature teratoma) or well-differentiated tissues (mature teratoma) are observed that tend to have both low mitotic and apoptotic indices (3,16). Mature teratomas on occasion will undergo malignant transformation of one of the histologic components, requiring subsequent tailoring of treatment to the malignant tissue counterpart (17). Yolk-sac tumors and choriocarcinomas express alpha-fetoprotein (AFP) and human chorionic gonadotrophin (HCG), respectively, and exhibit morphologies resembling extraembryonically differentiated tissues (3). Nonseminomas are cured in the majority of cases that combine surgery and cisplatin-based chemotherapy, although the relative resistance of teratomatous components to chemotherapy is well documented (2). With the exception of seminomas, GCTs of pure histology are rare, with the majority being a mixture of nonseminomatous histologic components. A combination of seminomatous and nonseminomatous components is also frequent.

GENETIC BASIS OF ADULT MALE GERM CELL TRANSFORMATION

In 1982, Atkin and Baker first reported the detection of an isochromosome of the short arm of chromosome 12 [i(12p)] in GCTs using conventional karyotypic analysis of metaphase chromosomes (18). This chromosomal abnormality has subsequently been recognized in 85% of GCTs (19). Using a 12p painting probe, fluorescence in situ hybridization (FISH) of GCTs that do not exhibit this marker chromosome revealed the presence of tandem duplications of 12p either in situ or in other chromosomes (20). Thus, the presence of extra copies of the short arm of chromosome 12 is diagnostic of GCTs, and FISH

analysis for this marker in interphase and metaphase tumor cells is used routinely for diagnostic purposes. This assay has been useful in the identification of some mediastinal tumors of uncertain histogenesis as GCTs, permitting appropriate treatment choices (21). Several studies have indicated that i(12p) is evident as early as in ITGCN, yet others have indicated that the appearance of this marker is associated with tumor invasion out of the tubules (22–25). An initial candidate gene approach identified CCND2 as a possible 12p target proto-oncogene in GCTs (26). This D-type cyclin, along with the cyclin-dependent kinases 4 and 6, regulates transition of the G1-S phase of the cell cycle (27). Perturbations in cell cycling due to overexpression of these cyclins have been noted in multiple tumor systems and the oncogenic capacity confirmed in transgenic murine models. For GCTs, cyclin D2 is aberrantly expressed in the transformed germ cells of ITGCN, with elevated expression also detected in seminoma and embryonal carcinoma (26). With somatic differentiation, the levels of cyclin D2 paralleled those detected in the normal tissue counterpart. Cyclin D2 expression was only rarely noted in spermatogonial cells of the normal adult testis, but examination of murine neonate testis showed that mitotically dividing spermatogonial cells express cyclin D2 (1). Thus, by analogy with cyclin D1 in breast cancer, increased 12p copy number may lead to aberrant expression of cyclin D2 in a germ cell that has previously expressed this D-type cyclin during its development but now with oncogenic potential. More recent studies have employed microarray-based expression analyses, where a number of genes along 12p exhibit overexpression in both seminomas and nonseminomas compared with normal testis including CCND2 (Fig. 33.1) (28). The role of these genes in germ cell tumorigenesis remains to be evaluated in murine transgenic models.

Chromosomal comparative genomic hybridization (CGH) analyses of GCTs have indicated that some GCTs (predominantly seminomas) exhibit a high-level amplification of the 12p11–12.2 region, in addition to gain of the entire short arm (30,31). Recently, molecular cytogenetic and global genomic screening methods have been employed to delineate the amplicon and identify potential candidates for the target gene(s) (28,29,32). As indicated by cDNA/EST and BAC array–CGH studies, the amplicon encompasses the region from approximately 20 Mbp on 12p to 30 Mbp (29,32). However, it would appear from higher resolution BAC arrays that structure of the amplicon between tumors within this region varies. Zafarana et al. (32) report that in 17 seminomas, 7 show high-level amplification of the entire region, with 3 showing a lower level of amplification in the center of the amplicon. In addition, 3 exhibited amplification predominantly at the centromeric border, 1 exhibited amplification at the telomeric border, and the remaining 6 showed two balanced peaks of amplification at the telomeric and centromeric regions. These results suggest two independently amplified subregions, each with a specific target gene. Microarray expression analysis of genes mapped within the entire 10 Mbp region have revealed several candidates, only some of which correlated with amplification (28,29). Thus, the target gene(s) of this amplified region in GCTs remain(s) to be identified and confirmed in in vitro and in vivo studies. It is also still unclear whether this region contains the responsible protooncogene that drives the gain of 12p observed in all GCTs or represents a subregional amplification involved predominantly in the progression of seminomas.

Extensive cytogenetic and molecular genetic studies have described other frequent chromosomal abnormalities in adult GCTs (24,25,31,33,34). Chromosomal CGH performed on microdissected ITGCN revealed gain of genetic material derived from chromosomes 1, 5, 7, 8, 12q, and X and loss of chromosome 18 material in these preinvasive lesions (24,25). Adjacent invasive tumors exhibited additional sites of gain including chromosomes 2, 3, 4, 6, 13q, 14q, 17q, 18q, 20, and

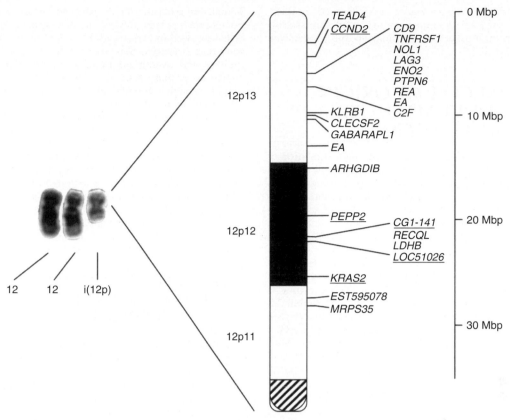

FIGURE 33.1. Candidate overexpressed cDNAs/ESTs mapped to 12p. All adult male GCTs exhibit extra copies of the entire p arm of chromosome 12 (approximately 35 Mbp), presenting as an isochromosome [i(12p)] in about 85% of cases. An i(12p) is shown on the left, along with two normal chromosome 12. From both published and unpublished microarray data using cDNA/EST arrays (28,29) and oligonucleotide arrays (JH, GJB, RSKC, unpublished data), the expression of 247 cDNAs/ESTs mapped to 12p have been evaluated in GCT specimens relative to that of normal testis. Of these, 24 show overexpression in >70% of tumors evaluated within the specific study and are listed relative to physical position on 12p. The sequences underlined are those for which the relative overexpression was confirmed in an independent assay.

21 and additional losses including chromosomes 1p, 4, 6q, 9, 11, 13q, and 19. For 17q, microarray-based expression studies have provided evidence for *GRB7* and *JUP* as the target genes of the regional gain (35). Conventional karyotype analysis revealed that, overall, GCTs are hypertriploid in chromosomal content and display recurrent chromosomal abnormalities, some of which are associated with histological subtype (33, 34). The most frequently observed nonrandom chromosomal aberrations were deletion/rearrangement of 12q, 1p32–36, and 7q, along with deletion at 6q13–25. Breakpoints involving 1p32–36 and 7q11.2 were associated significantly with a teratomatous histology, and 1p22 with yolk sac tumors. Comprehensive loss of heterozygosity (LOH) analyses of the chromosomal complement of GCTs has indicated a number of sites that may harbor tumor suppressor genes (36). These include regions containing known tumor suppressor genes (*RB1, DCC*, and *NME*), regions previously identified as containing putative tumor suppressor genes (1p, 3p, 5q, 9p, 10q, 11p, 11q, and 17p), and several novel sites (1q, 2q, 3q, 5p, 9q, 12q, 18p, and 20p). Molecular genetic analysis of the long arm of chromosome 12 has provided evidence for two putative tumor suppressor genes mapped at 12q13 and 12q22, and it narrowed the minimally deleted regions down to less than 1Mbp (37,38). For 5q, three common sites of loss have now been indicated (5q14, 5q21, and 5q34-qter), although the corresponding putative tumor suppressor genes remain to be identified (39). Silencing of expression of tumor suppressor genes can also be achieved by hypermethylation of the promoter of the respective gene. Examination of the methylation status and expression of candidate tumor suppressor genes in GCTs has been carried out by several investigators. Overall, seminomas displayed a much lower level of promoter methylation than nonseminomas, reflecting an epigenetic modification associated with differentiation rather than tumorigenesis (40–43). In addition, methylation of a gene did not always correlate with expression. However, it was apparent in two independent studies that expression of *MGMT* at 10q was regulated by methylation, implicating it as the candidate tumor suppressor gene at this locus (41,42). For the candidate on 3p, *RASSF1A*, the methylation status and associated expression were inconsistent between studies (42,43).

Mutations of *KRAS2* (44), *KIT* (45,46), and *SMAD4* (47) have been found in GCTs that may be involved in germ cell transformation. For *KIT*, activating somatic mutations have been found, which has recently been suggested to be predictive of bilateral GCT (46). In this study, activating mutations at codon 816 in *KIT* were identified in only 3 of 224 unilateral tumors (1.3%) but in 57 of 61 bilateral tumors (93%). Thus, screening of tumor DNAs for this mutation may be useful in identifying patients at risk for developing GCT in the contralateral testis, which occurs in approximately 2.5% to 5% of GCT patients. Interestingly, for 10 of the bilateral tumors, microdissected adjacent ITGCN was also available for analysis, and of these, 2 exhibited mutations in *KIT* additional to those detected for the invasive lesion, and 2 showed complete loss of mutation of *KIT* upon invasion. Thus, the precise role of this mutation in germ cell transformation and progression remains to be clarified.

GERM CELL OF ORIGIN OF ADULT MALE GERM CELL TUMORS

Expression and genetic studies have lead to the formulation of two models for the stage in the lifespan of a germ cell at which transformation occurs. For pediatric GCTs presenting prior to puberty, there is common acceptance that these tumors arise by transformation of a germ cell *in utero*. The genetics and biology of these prepubertal GCTs are distinct from those found in adult GCTs and have recently been reviewed (48). One model for the genesis of adult GCTs proposes that gonocytes in the developing embryo escape normal development into spermatogonia and undergo abnormal cell proliferation mediated through a paracrine loop involving KIT and its ligand (SCF), leading to ITGCN (49,50). Such gonocytes derailed in their normal development are then suggested to be susceptible to invasive growth mediated by postnatal and pubertal gonadotrophin stimulation. Data in support of this model include the shared expression of many genes between ITGCN aberrant germ cells and PGCs or gonocytes, the types of abnormal germ cells seen in developmental disorders that predispose to GCTs, and the epidemiology of GCT incidence (49,50). The second model takes into account various genetic and expression properties of GCTs (1,51). A zygotene/pachytene spermatocyte with a duplicated chromosomal complement and undergoing homologous recombination is postulated to be the germ cell of origin. During this phase of meiosis initiated at puberty, an aberrant recombinational event could lead to a chromosome abnormality with several exclusive outcomes: (1) act to trigger apoptosis leading to demise of the germ cell, (2) be transmitted to the zygote with or without obvious consequences to the embryo, or (3) in the specific case of increased 12p, lead to aberrant expression of cyclin D2, reinitiation of mitosis, and genomic instability portending tumor formation. Similarities between GCTs and zygotene/pachytene spermatocytes support this model, including the triploid–tetraploid chromosome complement of GCTs, and the abundant expression of wild-type p53 (33,34,52). With the current capacity to examine the global expression patterns of GCTs in relation to PGCs, gonocytes, and isolated populations of spermatogonia and spermatocytes in the adult testis, further insights may be gained into the germ cell of origin of adult GCTs.

GENETIC AND BIOLOGIC BASIS OF EXTRAGONADAL MALE GERM CELL TUMORS

While the majority of adult GCTs present in the testis, less than 10% present at extragonadal sites, including the retroperitoneum, mediastinum, sacrococcygeal region, and pineal region, predominantly exhibiting a nonseminomatous component (2). Retroperitoneal lesions are generally thought to represent metastatic lesions from primary testicular lesions. Extragonadal tumors presenting at the other sites have been proposed to arise by transformation of a PGC misplaced during the normal migration of germ cells through the developing embryo to the genital ridges (49). However, this hypothesis does not take into account several embryological and cytogenetic observations. Firstly, misplaced PGCs have not been detected in developing human embryos, and those identified in murine embryos undergo apoptosis presumably due to lack of surrounding supportive cells [reviewed in (1)]. In addition, karyotypic analysis of these tumors has revealed that they exhibit an increase in 12p copy number and overall nonrandom chromosomal abnormalities similar to primary testicular GCTs (53). Such genetic studies would argue that gonadal and extragonadal GCTs have a common germ cell of origin. As an alternative model for the origin of extragonadal GCTs, it has been suggested that a germ cell transformed in the testis can undergo reverse migration to regions, such as the thymus and pineal regions, where during development supportive environments would have existed (53). Such regions, while not supportive of normal germ cell development and differentiation, may support transformed germ cell growth. This argument has been based on germ cell migration and biology during development, as well as upon patterns of metastasis seen in patients with gonadal GCTs. Thus, at the present time, the true cell of origin of extragonadal GCTs is unclear.

GENETIC AND BIOLOGIC BASIS OF MALE GERM CELL TUMOR DIFFERENTIATION

Male GCTs display patterns of differentiation that recapitulate stages normally evident in the developing zygote (3). Such a totipotential capacity is suppressed in normal germ cells until fertilization with the acquisition of genetic and epigenetic contributions of a maternal complement. Thus, during the process of transformation germ cells undergo reprogramming from a germ cell normally destined to become a gamete to a pluripotent germ cell with the capacity to elicit extraembryonic and embryonic patterns of differentiation, albeit in a temporally and spatially aberrant manner. This reprogramming can also be achieved *in vitro*, in populations of normal PGCs isolated from the mouse and human where conversion into pluripotential cells (embryonic germ cells) occurs upon exposure to SCF (stem cell factor, the ligand for KIT), leukemia inhibitory factor (LIF), and basic fibroblast factor (bFGF) (5). Transformed germ cells, however, lose the inhibitory block to zygote-like differentiation and undergo conversion *in vivo*, although to varying extents. Seminomas, given their morphological resemblance to undifferentiated spermatogonial cells, would appear to have retained the ability to suppress the initiation of post-fertilization developmental programs. While studies examining the expression of select genes have confirmed the undifferentiated germ cell–like appearance of these cells, global comparison of the expression profiles of seminomas with those of normal germ cells at various stages of their lifespans should provide a clearer understanding of how closely this tumor type represents the presumptive normal counterpart. Nonseminomas, on the other hand, have lost a germ cell–like phenotype and have undergone conversion into a pluripotent cell capable of differentiation along embryonic and extraembryonic lineages. As these lineages appear, however, pluripotentiality of the transformed germ cell is lost, as would be expected during normal embryonic development. This is evidenced by the loss of expression of genes such as *KIT* and *POU5F1* (12,14) and by studies of derived embryonal carcinoma cell lines that retain pluripotentiality *in vitro* (15). Few molecular studies have been directed at understanding the genetic or epigenetic basis for the key developmental differences between seminomas and nonseminomas. This may result from loss or gain of function of receptor(s) or downstream effector(s), either by nondisjunctional loss of chromosomes or by subregional losses or mutations concurrent with tumor evolution. Alternatively, it may involve a disruption of the normally carefully monitored levels of key regulator proteins (factors and receptors) due to the aberrant reinitiation of cell cycling of the transformed germ cell.

Within nonseminomas, multiple patterns of differentiation are observed *in vivo*, reflecting the potential of these cells for somatic differentiation into all three germ layers (teratoma), as well as extraembryonic lineages (yolk sac and choriocarcinoma). Thus, GCTs provide a unique opportunity to study the molecular mechanisms that regulate cell fate and lineage decision events in the developing embryo. Again, it is unknown whether initiation of these developmental decisions in GCTs has an underlying genetic basis, arises due to a lack of the orchestrated signaling cues that would normally occur in the zygote and developing embryo, or is a combination of both. Evidence for a genetic basis comes from analysis of genomewide allelic loss in GCTs that showed an overall higher loss in the highly differentiated teratomas compared with the less differentiated embryonal carcinomas (36). These data suggested that genes mapped to the chromosomal sites of loss may be involved in induction of differentiation or lineage decision, though few genes have been followed up for a functional role. Notable among the genes deleted in teratomas were *NME1* and *NME2,* which have been reported to negatively regulate differentiation. Comparison of the levels of the NM23 proteins between teratomas and embryonal carcinomas revealed a four- to five-fold lower level in the former (54). In the second scenario, the transformed germ cells are "confused" as to which developmental decision to make and at which time, leading to disorganized patterns of multiple differentiation pathways, as is frequently exhibited within one tumor specimen. Understanding the mechanisms involved in making the correct cellular proliferation and cell fate and lineage decisions may lead then to elucidation of how these events are poorly regulated in GCTs. Much research effort has been focused on these goals by developmental biologists, and in recent years for humans this has mainly involved the use of isolated stem cells of varying differentiation potential (55). Embryonal carcinoma cell lines derived from GCTs also provide a resource of cells in which such studies can be performed. These cell lines are easily maintained *in vitro* in an undifferentiated state, display varying potential for spontaneous or morphogen-induced differentiation along multiple lineages, and exhibit an expression signature with many similarities to stem cell lines (15,56). Some embryonal carcinoma cell lines have the ability to differentiate along somatic and extraembryonic endodermal lineages, placing them as equivalents of cells derived from the inner cell mass in the developing embryo. Others exhibit the additional ability to differentiate into trophoblastic cells, placing them at an earlier stage in embryogenesis prior to trophoectodermal fate decision. In contrast, other embryonal carcinoma cell lines lack the ability to undergo spontaneous or morphogen-induced differentiation. Comparison of the cell lines both at the genetic and expression levels may lead to the identification of molecular regulators of cell fate/lineage decision, as well as identification of master regulators of differentiation induction in the developing zygote. Such studies have been enhanced with the use of microarray-based studies to identify transcriptional programs associated with specific differentiation pathways. The transcriptional response of the multipotential embryonal carcinoma cell line NTera2/Clone D1 (NT2/D1) upon all-*trans*-retinoic acid (RA)–induced neuronal differentiation has recently been reported (57,58). These studies identified distinct stages in the transition from an embryonal carcinoma cell to neuroprogenitor cells expressing patterning markers compatible with posterior hindbrain fates and to immature postmitotic neurons with an evolving synaptic apparatus (57). Comparison of the transcriptional program induced in the same cell line but along an epidermal/epithelial pathway by bone morphogenetic proteins-2 and -4 with that obtained for RA should yield clues as to how these agents in the same cell line similarly effect a decrease in proliferation associated with differentiation but differentially lead to the selection of distinct somatic cell fates. The functional role of candidate genes for specific lineage decision based on these studies can be assayed using exogenous overexpression of a specific gene(s) or down-regulation by RNA interference technology. The embryonal carcinoma cell line NCCIT is particularly well suited for such studies due to its demonstrated potential for differentiation along extraembryonic lineages, as well as along all three germ layers (59). Thus, embryonal carcinoma cell lines represent an *in vitro* system wherein the functional involvement of candidate genes in human cell fate/lineage decisions can be determined.

GENETIC AND BIOLOGIC BASIS OF CHEMORESISTANCE

Adult male GCTs are excellent models for a curable malignancy. Clinically, patients are risk-stratified according to criteria established by the International Germ Cell Cancer Consensus Group (IGCCCG), based on primary site, serum tumor marker levels, histology, and sites of metastasis (2). Treatment usually comprises surgical resection in combination with a cisplatin-based chemotherapeutic regime. Over 90% of newly diagnosed cases are cured. In patients with advanced disease requiring initial chemotherapy, 70% to 80% are cured. A complete understanding of the molecular basis for the exquisite sensitivity of these tumors to cisplatin-based treatment and identification of the genetic and biologic lesions that underlie resistance is lacking at the present time and is highly desirable. As is probably the case for most tumor systems, multiple pathways within cells will be affected in transformed cells that contribute to a resistant phenotype. Such pathways may comprise regulation of cell growth, cell death, differentiation, and cellular response to DNA damage. As expected, immunohistochemical analyses of GCTs for the expression of markers of cell proliferation (for example, Ki67, CDKN1A, and RB1) and of markers of susceptibility to apoptosis and resistance (for example, TP53, BCL2, BAX, BCLXL, ABCC1, ABCC2, and GSTP1), and terminal deoxynucleotidyl transferase (TdT)-mediated deoxyuridine triphosphate nick end-labeling TUNEL analyses for evaluation of spontaneous apoptotic cell death, have indicated a clear difference in the balance of cell growth and death between histological subtypes of GCTs (16,60,61). These studies have, in general, not led to the identification of specific markers or combination of markers that predict response to treatment. However, recent careful examination within a histological subtype—embryonal carcinoma—has identified a subgroup with a better survival that exhibits a comparatively higher level of cell proliferation and low spontaneous apoptosis (62).

As evidenced both *in vivo* and *in vitro*, the process of cellular differentiation in GCTs is associated with the acquisition of a resistant phenotype. Teratomas exhibiting differentiation along somatic lineages are relatively unresponsive to chemotherapy, and surgical resection is often required to remove this component (2). If left *in situ*, such lesions are susceptible to malignant transformation. *In vitro*, induction of differentiation of pluripotent embryonal carcinoma cell lines is also accompanied by loss of a chemosensitive phenotype. This is exemplified by NT2/D1, wherein undifferentiated cells exhibit a marked loss of viability and a large increase in cells undergoing apoptosis following treatment with cisplatin (63), (Fig. 33.2). On the other hand, RA-differentiated NT2/D1 neural cells showed a much attenuated response to cisplatin with little or no induction of apoptotic cell death (63), (Fig. 33.2). Among differentiated nonseminomas, differences in response to treatment are clinically known and may reflect the inherent sensitivity of the normal tissue counterpart. The molecular determinants of these differences are unknown and must be taken into consideration when using

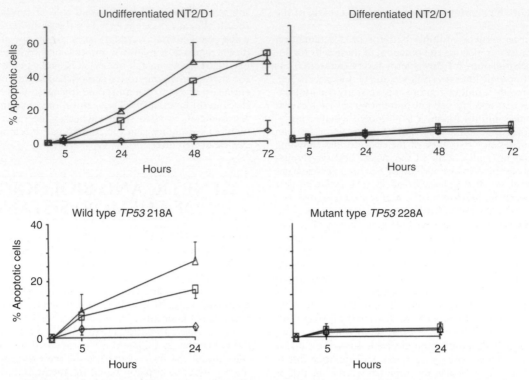

FIGURE 33.2. Effect of differentiation and *TP53* mutation on the apoptotic response of germ cell tumor (GCT) cell lines to cisplatin. GCT-derived cell lines were mock-treated (◇) or treated with 4 μg/mL (□) or 8 μg/mL (△) of cisplatin for 2 hours. Cultures were collected at the indicated times after treatment, and the cells were fixed and stained with Hoescht 33528 (64). Cells were considered apoptotic if two or more apoptotic bodies (representative of chromatin condensation) per cell were observed. At least 500 cells were counted per culture. Error bars represent the standard deviations of at least three independent experiments. The results obtained for NT2/D1 in an undifferentiated and retinoic acid (RA)–induced differentiated state and two cell lines 218A and 228A, with wild type and mutant *TP53* respectively, are shown. Undifferentiated NT2/D1 and 218A cells show a marked induction of apoptosis, while differentiated NT2/D1 and 228A cells exhibit little or no induction. Thus, differentiation and mutation of *TP53* represent two pathways by which the responses of normally highly sensitive GCTs can be subverted.

global screening expression methods to look for molecular markers of resistance within nonseminomas.

Examination of the response of GCT-derived cell lines to DNA-damaging agents has yielded a number of molecular clues involved in the sensitive/resistant phenotype of these tumors. Few reports have attributed the sensitivity of GCTs to reduced ability to repair DNA lesions induced by cisplatin resulting from either shielding lesions in DNA by high-mobility group domain proteins unique to germ cells (65) or by decreased levels of XPA involved in DNA damage recognition and facilitation of the DNA repair complex assembly (66). The tumor suppressor gene *TP53* is intimately involved in the activation of the cellular response to DNA damage, and it is perhaps one of the most well-studied genes for its role in GCT biology. This gene is rarely mutated in GCTs, unlike other tumor systems in which approximately 50% exhibit inactivating mutations or deletions (67,68). Mutations and deletions were, however, found in a subset of clinically resistant GCTs (64). A cell line that contained the same *TP53* mutation as the original tumor specimen from which it was derived exhibited a resistant response after exposure to cisplatin, compared to a cell line derived from a responsive tumor with no evidence of a mutation (64) (Fig. 33.2). Thus, inactivating mutations within *TP53* may comprise one molecular means by which GCTs can circumvent the usually rapid apoptotic response to DNA-damaging agents exhibited by most transformed germ cells and normal germ cells. One study has reported that one GCT cell line with mutant *TP53* displayed sensitivity to cisplatin in

culture, indicating that perhaps, in a minority of GCTs, *TP53* mutation may not confer resistance (69). Resistance to cisplatin-induced cell death has been attributed in another GCT cell line to failure to activate caspase-9 (activated downstream of cytochrome C release from mitochondria), independent of *TP53* expression (70). The genetic basis for this lack of activation is unknown. Other studies have suggested that GCTs may also employ the FAS-mediated cell death pathway following cisplatin exposure. An induction in the expression of FAS and recruitment of FADD and caspase-8 to FAS was noted in sensitive but not in resistant GCT cell lines after cisplatin treatment (71). Again, no underlying genetic defect has been identified as yet to explain the lack of response by the resistant cell lines. The common theme in these observations is the inherent capacity of these cells to rapidly activate, perhaps, multiple cell death pathways when exposed to DNA-damaging agents in both *TP53*-dependent and/or *TP53*-independent manners [reviewed in (72)]. In other cell types, such agents lead, rather, to cell cycle delays to permit assessment and repair of DNA lesions, followed by the decision of whether to undergo cell death or not. Identification of the biologic factors that predispose germ cells and consequently GCTs to apoptosis may have relevance in understanding the poorer responses of other tumor types to the same agents.

Of clinical relevance is the identification and development of genetic markers within GCTs for prognostic purposes. Few genetic markers portending resistance have been reported. As already discussed previously, one is *TP53* mutation/deletion. Another reported by us is high-level gene amplification, a genetic feature often associated in other tumor types with a poorer prognosis (31). CGH analysis revealed amplification of genetic material at multiple sites in 5 of 17 GCTs not cured by cisplatin-based therapy. No high-level amplification was detected by CGH in 17 cured GCTs other than at 12p. Follow-up studies to identify candidate target genes of the amplification events are being performed using a combination of array-CGH and expression array analyses. An example of such a follow-up study is described in the following section. Our previous chromosomal CGH analysis detected regional high-level amplification of 2p23–24 in GCT 231B, resected from a patient who succumbed to disease (31). This region represents approximately 20 Mbp of DNA, placed at 12.2 Mbp to 32.0 Mbp from the telomere on the short arm of chromosome 2. Array CGH was performed on DNA from GCT 231B in order to more accurately define the region of amplification. It was also performed on an additional 12 DNAs isolated from resistant GCTs and 6 from cured GCTs to determine if this region is amplified in other tumors that went previously undetected by chromosomal CGH, which has a resolution of approximately 20 Mbp for detecting amplified regions. Array-CGH analysis using cDNA/EST arrays with over 8,000 clones mapped over the entire chromosomal complement revealed that three resistant but no cured GCTs exhibited gain of this region. Furthermore, the size of

the amplicon could be narrowed to 10 Mbp at position 16 Mbp to 26 Mbp on 2p. Of the entire panel of 19 GCTs, RNA suitable for expression studies could be extracted from 12 specimens, comprising nine resistant and three cured. The RNAs were submitted to expression profiling using oligonucleotide arrays, in which 88 probe sets mapped to this 10 Mbp region on 2p. Comparison of the relative expression of these probe sets in the three GCTs exhibiting gain in this region versus six resistant without gain and three cured without gain revealed that *NMYC* is the most likely candidate target gene for this amplicon (Fig. 33.3). Expression of *NMYC* was detected in all but 2 of the 12 tumors assayed, consistent with prior reports of the expression of this gene in GCT (35). However in the three cases exhibiting gain of this region, *NMYC* was expressed at markedly higher levels. Thus, overexpression of *NMYC* in GCTs may represent one marker of resistance. Similar studies may suggest several possible expression markers of resistance that could be validated in independent tumor panels. Additional studies aimed at identifying expression markers of resistance not restricted to regions identified by molecular genetic studies are currently underway in several laboratories. Based on studies in other tumor types, adding a group of expression identifiers to the risk stratification of patients currently relying on clinical features alone presents exciting prospects.

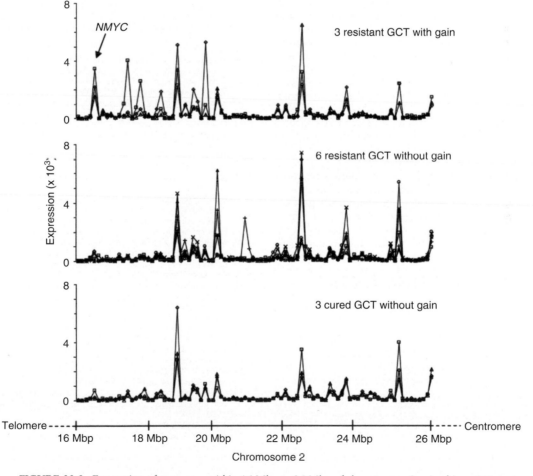

FIGURE 33.3. Expression of sequences within 16 Mbp to 26 Mbp of chromosome 2 gained in resistant germ cell tumors (GCTs). Expression profiling was performed on resistant and cured GCT specimens using oligonucleotide arrays (JH, GJB, RSKC, unpublished data), and those mapped and ordered within 16 Mbp to 26 Mbp on chromosome 2 are plotted. Three resistant GCTs with gain of the region individually exhibited higher expression of transcripts within the region than observed in other resistant or cured tumors, but *NMYC* was more highly expressed in all three resistant GCTs with 2p gain (including GCT 231B). Thus, *NMYC* may be the target gene of the 2p amplicon detected in resistant GCT specimens. Each symbol in each plot represents the relative expression of a transcript in a specimen.

GENETIC BASIS OF MALIGNANT TRANSFORMATION

Somatically differentiated teratomas can occasionally exhibit histologically non–germ cell malignancies whose GCT clonal origin has been confirmed by the presence of i(12p). Such "malignant transformation" of teratomas leads to aggressive malignancies displaying histologic differentiation along mesenchymal lineages such as sarcoma (in particular, rhabdomyosarcoma), hematopoietic lineages such as myeloid leukemia, epithelial lineages such as carcinoma, and neurogenic lineages such as primitive neuroectodermal tumor (PNET) (2). The transformed malignancy contains additional cytogenetic/genetic abnormalities not present in the original GCT, which may be characteristic of the differentiated malignant phenotype (73,74). This is exemplified by one case described by us in which resection of a post-chemotherapy anterior mediastinal mass revealed a cystic region that was composed mainly of teratoma and a solid region of embryonal rhabdomyosarcoma. The clonal karyotypes for the teratomatous lesion (203A) and the malignantly transformed lesion (203B) both exhibited i(12p), with the embryonal rhabdomyosarcoma component exhibiting additional chromosomal abnormalities including a translocation involving 2q37 and a deleted 6q (74). The latter abnormality has been observed in different tumor types, but the breakpoints in 2q have frequently been reported for de novo embryonal rhabdomyosarcomas. Mutation analysis revealed that both the teratomatous and the rhabdomyosarcoma specimens exhibited a common *TP53* deletion, implying acquisition of this genetic lesion prior to malignant transformation. It is not known if the mutation is de novo or treatment-induced since the specimen studied was post-chemotherapy (64). CGH analysis of the two components revealed high-level amplification only in the rhabdomyosarcoma component, indicating acquisition of this genetic lesion during or after malignant transformation (31). In 203B, three chromosomal sites were found to harbor amplified genes, including 7q21, 7q31, and 15q23 and 15q24. Both array CGH and southern hybridization have confirmed *MET* as a candidate-amplified target gene mapped to 7q31. There is clear evidence for a role of *MET* in rhabdomyosarcoma biology with respect to metastasis, as well as overexpression leading to enhancement of resistance to radiochemotherapy (75). Thus, studies of these malignantly transformed GCTs may aid in the understanding of the biology of the transformed counterpart.

ACKNOWLEDGMENTS

The reported studies were supported by the Byrne Fund and the Lance Armstrong Foundation.

References

1. Chaganti RSK, Houldsworth J. Genetics and biology of adult human male germ cell tumors. *Cancer Res* 2000;60:1475–1482.
2. Bosl GJ, Motzer RJ. Testicular germ-cell cancer. *N Engl J Med* 1997; 337:242–253.
3. Mostofi FK, Sesterhenn IA, Davis CJ Jr. Anatomy and pathology of testis cancer. In: Vogelzang NJ, Scardino PT, Shipley WU et al., eds. *Comprehensive textbook of genitourinary urology*, 2nd ed. Philadelphia: Lippincott Williams & Wilkins, 2000:909–926.
4. Ginsburg M, Snow MH, McLaren A. Primordial germ cells in the mouse embryo during gastrulation. *Development* 1990;110:521–528.
5. Donovan PJ, de Miguel MP. Turning germ cells into stem cells. *Curr Opin Genet Dev* 2003;13:463–471.
6. Setchell BP. *The mammalian testis*. Ithaca, NY: Cornell University, 1978.
7. Plant TM, Marshall GR. The functional significance of FSH in spermatogenesis and the control of its secretion in male primates. *Endocr Rev* 2001; 22:764–786.
8. De Rooij DG. Stem cells in the testis. *Int J Exp Pathol* 1998;79:67–80.
9. Brugh VM III, Maduro MR, Lamb DJ. Genetic disorders and infertility. *Urol Clin North Am* 2003;30:143–152.
10. Page SL, Hawley RS. Chromosome choreography: the meiotic ballet. *Science* 2003;301:785–789.
11. Kerjean A, Dupont JM, Vasseur C, et al. Establishment of the paternal methylation imprint of the human H19 and MEST/PEG1 genes during spermatogenesis. *Hum Mol Genet* 2000;9:2183–2187.
12. Rajpert-de Meyts E, Skakkebaek NE. Expression of the c-kit protein product in carcinoma-in-situ and invasive testicular germ cell tumours. *Int J Androl* 1994;17:85–92.
13. Tezel G, Nagasaka T, Shimono Y, et al. Differential expression of RET finger protein in testicular germ cell tumors. *Pathol Int* 2002;52:623–627.
14. Looijenga LH, Stoop H, de Leeuw HP, et al. POU5F1 (OCT3/4) identifies cells with pluripotent potential in human germ cell tumors. *Cancer Res* 2003;63:2244–2250.
15. Andrews PW. Teratocarcinomas and human embryology: pluripotent human EC cell lines: a review. *APMIS* 1998;106:158–168.
16. Soini Y, Paakko P. Extent of apoptosis in relation to p53 and bcl-2 expression in germ cell tumors. *Hum Pathol* 1996;27:1221–1226.
17. Motzer RJ, Amsterdam A, Prieto V, et al. Teratoma with malignant transformation: diverse malignant histologies arising in men with germ cell tumors. *J Urol* 1988;159:133–138.
18. Atkin NB, Baker MC. Specific chromosome change, i(12p), in testicular tumours? *Lancet* 1982;2:1349.
19. Chaganti RSK, Rodriguez E, Bosl GJ. Cytogenetics of male germ-cell tumors. *Urol Clin North Am* 1993;20:55–66.
20. Rodriguez E, Houldsworth J, Reuter VE, et al. Molecular cytogenetic analysis of i(12p)-negative human male germ cell tumors. *Genes Chromosomes Cancer* 1993;8:230–236.
21. Motzer RJ, Rodriguez E, Reuter VE, et al. Molecular and cytogenetic studies in the diagnosis of patients with poorly differentiated carcinomas of unknown primary site. *J Clin Oncol* 1995;13:274–282.
22. Vos A, Oosterhuis JW, de Jong B, et al. Cytogenetics of carcinoma in situ of the testis. *Cancer Genet Cytogenet* 1990;46:75–81.
23. Chaganti RSK, Murty VVVS, Bosl GJ. Molecular genetics of male germ cell tumors. In: Vogelzang NJ, Shipley WU, Scardino PT et al., eds. *Comprehensive textbook of genitourinary urology*. Baltimore: Williams & Wilkins, 1996:932–940.
24. Rosenberg C, Van Gurp RJ, Geelen E, et al. Overrepresentation of the short arm of chromosome 12 is related to invasive growth of human testicular seminomas and nonseminomas. *Oncogene* 2000;19:5858–5862.
25. Summersgill B, Osin P, Lu YJ, et al. Chromosomal imbalances associated with carcinoma in situ and associated testicular germ cell tumours of adolescents and adults. *Br J Cancer* 2001;85:213–220.
26. Houldsworth J, Reuter V, Bosl GJ, et al. Aberrant expression of cyclin D2 is an early event in human male germ cell tumorigenesis. *Cell Growth Differ* 1997;8:293–299.
27. Weinberg RA. The retinoblastoma protein and cell cycle control. *Cell* 1995; 81:323–330.
28. Rodriguez S, Jafer O, Goker H, et al. Expression profile of genes from 12p in testicular germ cell tumors of adolescents and adults associated with i(12p) and amplification at 12p11.2–p12.1. *Oncogene* 2003;22:1880–1891.
29. Bourdon V, Naef F, Rao PH, et al. Genomic expression analysis of the 12p11–p12 amplicon using EST arrays identifies two novel amplified and overexpressed genes. *Cancer Res* 2002;62:6218–6223.
30. Mostert MM, Van De Pol M, Olde Weghius D, et al. Comparative genomic hybridization of germ cell tumors of the adult testis: confirmation of karyotypic findings and identification of a 12p-amplicon. *Cancer Genet Cytogenet* 1996;89:146–152.
31. Rao PH, Houldsworth J, Palanisamy N, et al. Chromosomal amplification is associated with cisplatin resistance of human male germ cell tumors. *Cancer Res* 1998;58:4260–4263.
32. Zafarana G, Grygalewicz B, Gillis AJM, et al. 12p-Amplicon structure analysis in testicular germ cell tumors of adolescents and adults by array CGH. *Oncogene* 2003;22:7695–7701.
33. Rodriguez E, Mathew S, Reuter V, et al. Cytogenetic analysis of 124 prospectively ascertained male germ cell tumors. *Cancer Res* 1992;52:2285–2291.
34. Murty VVVS, Chaganti RSK. A genetic perspective of male germ cell tumors. *Semin Oncol* 1998;25:133–144.
35. Skotheim RI, Monni O, Mousses S, et al. New insights into testicular germ cell tumorigenesis from gene expression profiling. *Cancer Res* 2002;62: 2359–2364.
36. Murty VVVS, Bosl G, Houldsworth J, et al. Allelic loss and somatic differentiation in human male germ cell tumors. *Oncogene* 1994;9:2245–2251.
37. Murty VVVS, Houldsworth J, Baldwin S, et al. Allelic deletions in the long arm of chromosome 12 identify sites of candidate tumor suppressor genes in male germ cell tumors. *Proc Natl Acad Sci U S A* 1992;89: 11006–11011.
38. Murty VVVS, Montgomery K, Dutta S, et al. A 3-Mb high-resolution BAC, PAC contig of 12q22 encompassing the 830 kb consensus minimal deletion in male germ cell tumors. *Genome Res* 1998;9:662–671.
39. Peng HQ, Liu L, Goss PE, et al. Chromosomal deletions occur in restricted regions of 5q in testicular germ cell cancer. *Oncogene* 1999;18:3277–3283.
40. Smiraglia DJ, Szymanska J, Kraggerud SM, et al. Distinct epigenetic phenotypes in seminomatous and nonseminomatous testicular germ cell tumors. *Oncogene* 2002;21:3909–3916.

41. Smith-Sorensen B, Lind GE, Skotheim RI, et al. Frequent promoter hypermethylation of the O6-methylguanine-DNA methyltransferase (MGMT) gene in testicular cancer. *Oncogene* 2002;21:8878–8884.

42. Koul S, Houldsworth J, Mansukhani MM, et al. Characteristic promoter hypermethylation signatures in male germ cell tumors. *Mol Cancer* 2002;1:8.

43. Honorio S, Agathanggleou A, Wernert N, et al. Frequent epigenetic inactivation of the RASSF1A tumour suppressor gene in testicular tumours and distinct methylation profiles of seminoma and nonseminoma testicular germ cell tumours. *Oncogene* 2003;22:461–466.

44. Roelofs H, Mostert MC, Pompe K, et al. Restricted 12p amplification and RAS mutation in human germ cell tumors of the adult testis. *Am J Pathol* 2000;157:1155–1166.

45. Tian Q, Frierson HF Jr, Krystal GW, et al. Activating c-kit mutations in human germ cell tumors. *Am J Pathol* 1999;154:1643–1647.

46. Looijenga LHJ, de Leeuw H, van Oorschot M, et al. Stem cell factor receptor (c-KIT) codon 816 mutations predict development of bilateral testicular germ-cell tumors. *Cancer Res* 2003;63:7674–7678.

47. Bouras M, Tabone E, Bertholon J, et al. A novel *SMAD4* mutation in seminoma germ cell tumors. *Cancer Res* 2000;60:922–928.

48. Houldsworth J. Genetics and biology of male germ cell tumors. *Chest Surg Clin N Am* 2002;12:629–643.

49. Skakkebaek NE, Berthelsen JG, Giwercman A, et al. Carcinoma-in-situ of the testis: possible origin from gonocytes and precursors of all types of germ cell tumors except spermatocytoma. *Int J Androl* 1987;10:19–28.

50. Skakkebaek NE, Rajpert-de Meyts E, Jorgensen N, et al. Germ cell cancer and disorders of spermatogenesis: an environmental connection? *APMIS* 1998;106:3–12.

51. Chaganti RSK, Houldsworth J. The cytogenetic theory of pathogenesis of human adult male germ cell tumors. *APMIS* 1998;106:80–84.

52. Bartkova J, Bartek J, Lukas J, et al. P53 protein alterations in human testicular cancer including pre-invasive intratubular germ-cell neoplasia. *Int J Cancer* 1991;49:196–202.

53. Chaganti RSK, Rodriguez E, Mathew S. Origin of adult male mediastinal germ-cell tumours. *Lancet* 1994;343:1130–1132.

54. Backer JM, Mendola CE, Kovesdi I, et al. Chromosomal localization and nucleoside diphosphate kinase activity of human metastasis-suppressor genes NM23-1 and NM23-2. *Oncogene* 1993;8:497–502.

55. Trounson AO. The derivation and potential use of human embryonic stem cells. *Reprod Fertil Dev* 2001;13:523–532.

56. Sperger JM, Chen X, Draper JS, et al. Gene expression patterns in human embryonic stem cells and human pluripotent germ cell tumors. *Proc Natl Acad Sci USA* 2003;100:13350–13355.

57. Houldsworth J, Heath SC, Studer L, et al. Expression profiling of lineage differentiation in pluripotential human embryonal carcinoma cells. *Cell Growth Differ* 2002;13:257–264.

58. Freemantle SJ, Kerley JS, Olsen SL, et al. Developmentally-related candidate retinoic acid target genes regulated early during neuronal differentiation of human embryonal carcinoma. *Oncogene* 2002;21:2880–2889.

59. Damjanov I, Horvat B, Gibas Z. Retinoic acid-induced differentiation of the developmentally pluripotent human germ cell tumor-derived cell line, NCCIT. *Lab Invest* 1993;68:220–232.

60. Grobholz R, Zentgraf H, Kohrmann KU, et al. Bax, Bcl-2, fas and Fas-L antigen expression in human seminoma: correlation with the apoptotic index. *APMIS* 2002;110:724–732.

61. Mayer F, Stoop H, Scheffer GL, et al. Molecular determinants of treatment response in human germ cell tumors. *Clin Cancer Res* 2003;9:767–773.

62. Mazumdar M, Bacik J, Tickoo SK, et al. Cluster analysis of p53 and Ki67 expression, apoptosis, alpha-fetoprotein, and human chorionic gonadotrophin indicates a favorable prognostic subgroup within the embryonal carcinoma germ cell tumor. *J Clin Oncol* 2003;21:2679–2688.

63. Timmer-Bosscha H, de Vries EG, Meijer C, et al. Differential effects of all-trans-retinoic acid, docosahexaenoic acid, and hexadecylphosphocholine on cisplatin-induced cytotoxicity and apoptosis in a cisplatin sensitive and resistant human embryonal carcinoma cell line. *Cancer Chemother Pharmacol* 1998;41:469–476.

64. Houldsworth J, Xiao H, Murty VVVS, et al. Human male germ cell tumor resistance to cisplatin is linked to TP53 gene mutation. *Oncogene* 1998; 16:2345–2349.

65. Zamble DB, Mikata Y, Eng CH, et al. Testis-specific HMG-domain protein alters the responses of cells to cisplatin. *J Inorg Biochem* 2002;91: 451–462.

66. Koberle B, Masters JRW, Hartley JA, et al. Defective repair of cisplatin-induced DNA damage caused by reduced XPA protein in testicular germ cell tumours. *Curr Biol* 1999;9:273–276.

67. Heimdal K, Lothe RA, Lystad S, et al. No germline TP53 mutations detected in familial and bilateral testicular cancer. *Genes Chromosomes Cancer* 1993;6:92–97.

68. Peng H-Q, Hogg D, Malkin D, et al. Mutations of the p53 gene do not occur in testis cancer. *Cancer Res* 1993;53:3574–3578.

69. Burger H, Nooter K, Boersma AW, et al. Lack of correlation between cisplatin-induced apoptosis, p53 status and expression of Bcl-2 family proteins in testicular germ cell tumour cell lines. *Int J Cancer* 1997;73: 592–599.

70. Mueller T, Voigt W, Simon H, et al. Failure of activation of caspase-9 induces a higher threshold for apoptosis and cisplatin resistance in testicular cancer. *Cancer Res* 2003;63:513–521.

71. Spierings DC, de Vries EG, Vellenga E, et al. Loss of drug-induced activation of the CD95 apoptotic pathway in a cisplatin-resistant testicular germ cell tumor cell line. *Cell Death Differ* 2003;10:808–822.

72. Spierings DCJ, de Vries EGE, Vellenga E, et al. The attractive Achilles heel of germ cell tumours: an inherent sensitivity to apoptosis-inducing stimuli. *J Pathol* 2003;200:137–148.

73. Ladanyi M, Samaniego F, Reuter VE, et al. Cytogenetic and immunohistochemical evidence for the germ cell origin of acute leukemias associated with mediastinal germ cell tumors. *J Natl Cancer Inst* 1990;82:221–227.

74. Rodriguez E, Reuter VE, Mies C, et al. Abnormalities of 2q: a common genetic link between rhabdomyosarcoma and hepatoblastoma? *Genes Chromosomes Cancer* 1991;3:122–127.

75. Jankowski K, Kucia M, Wysoczynshki M, et al. Both hepatocyte growth factor (HGF) and stromal-derived factor-1 regulate the metastatic behavior of human rhabdomyosarcoma cells, but only HGF enhances their resistance to radiochemotherapy. *Cancer Res* 2003;63:7926–7935.

CHAPTER 34 ■ ANATOMY AND PATHOLOGY OF TESTIS CANCER

VICTOR E. REUTER

MORPHOLOGIC ANATOMY OF THE TESTIS

The adult testes are suspended by the spermatic cord and located within the scrotum. Each testis proper is surrounded by a thick connective tissue layer, the tunica albuginea, which itself is lined by the visceral tunica vaginalis (Fig. 34.1). In the posterior aspect of the gonad is the mediastinum testis, which contains blood vessels, lymphatics, nerves, and portions of the rete testis. The testis contains multiple fibrous septa that radiate from the mediastinum testis to the tunica albuginea, and these divide the organ into approximately 250 compartments that contain the seminiferous tubules (1,2). Surrounding the seminiferous tubules is the interstitium, which contains Leydig cells, blood vessels, lymphatics, and nerves. Each compartment of the testis contains a maximum of four seminiferous tubules that are very convoluted and usually empty into the straight portion of the rete (tubuli recti). Each seminiferous tubule is lined by a basement membrane and a thin lamina propria. Within the seminiferous tubule are Sertoli cells, as well as germ cells at different stages of differentiation.

Sertoli cells comprise 10% to 15% of cells within the tubule. They are columnar to pyramidal in shape with their long axis perpendicular to the basement membrane (Fig. 34.2). The cytoplasm is granular–eosinophilic and may contain fine vacuoles. The nuclei are round to oval with finely granular chromatin and are commonly located within a cell or two of the basement membrane. They contain a prominent nucleolus, the only normal cell within the tubule to do so. Intracytoplasmic Charcot-Bottcher crystalloids are characteristic but are seen preferentially by electron microscopy.

Sertoli cells have phagocytic capacity but also play an important role in regulating spermatogenesis. By immunohistochemistry they have been shown to express vimentin, cytokeratins 8, 18, and 19, and inhibin (3,4). Cytokeratin positivity is routinely observed in immature Sertoli cells, but expression of this intermediate filament is likely in adults in various conditions, including testicular atrophy, Sertoli cell tumors, and in Sertoli cells adjacent to germ cell tumors, orchitis, and infarct.

Germ cells originate in the yolk sac and migrate to the genital ridge during the first 7 weeks of gestation (5,6). They comprise 85% to 90% of cells within the seminiferous tubule and have the capacity to differentiate (mature). Spermatogonia are undifferentiated cells located adjacent to the basement membrane (Fig. 34.2). They have clear or basophilic cytoplasm, distinct cytoplasmic membranes, small round nuclei with dark chromatin, and no nucleoli. They have the capacity to proliferate and to give rise to primary spermatocytes. The latter cells are subclassified into preleptotene, leptotene, zygotene, pachytene, and diplotene spermatocytes based on their nuclear chromatin pattern. These subtle differences are difficult, if not impossible, to discern on routine histologic preparations and irrelevant when evaluating tumor-bearing gonads. In general, spermatocytes are larger than spermatogonia, have basophilic cytoplasm, indistinct nuclear borders, round nuclei with distinct chromatin patterns, and absent nucleoli (Fig. 34.2). Completion of the first meiotic division gives rise to secondary spermatocytes that have a short half-life and undergo a second meiotic division to form spermatids. Secondary spermatocytes are smaller than their progenitor cells and have denser chromatin. Spermatids are located toward the lumen of the tubule and have small nuclei with dense chromatin (Fig. 34.2). They transform into spermatozoa through metamorphosis.

Leydig cells are present in the interstitium as single cells or in clusters (Fig. 34.2). Interestingly, they also may be observed in the tunica albuginea, mediastinum testis, epididymis, and even along the spermatic cord, usually intimately associated with nerve bundles (5,7). Leydig cells have abundant eosinophilic cytoplasm and round, regular nuclei with prominent nucleoli. Intracytoplasmic lipofuscin pigment may be seen more commonly in older males. Intracytoplasmic Reinke crystalloids are characteristic of Leydig cells, rarely seen in normal cells, and more commonly observed by electron microscopy, where they appear as hexagonal prisms (8,9).

Leydig cells have the capacity to produce testosterone and share an important paracrine function with Sertoli cells (10). They express inhibin but not cytokeratins or vimentin by immunohistochemistry (11).

The rete testis collects the effluent from the seminiferous tubules. It is located within the hilus of the testis and includes the tubuli recti, the mediastinal rete, and the extratesticular rete (Fig. 34.1). The tubuli recti are short segments within the septa that connect the seminiferous tubules to the mediastinal rete. The mediastinal rete forms a series of epithelial-lined, interconnecting channels that lead to several dilated vesicular channels comprising the extratesticular rete, which anastomose to give rise to the efferent ducts or tubuli efferentia. The epithelium of the rete is low columnar and exhibits luminal microvilli. Every cell contains a flagellum that is not visible by routine light microscopy. The cells are immunoreactive for cytokeratins as well as vimentin (12).

The efferent tubules have an irregular (undulating) luminal contour. They receive the luminal content from the rete testis and are responsible for resorbing fluid. The epithelial lining is a mixture of ciliated and nonciliated columnar pseudostratified cells that express cytokeratin and variably vimentin by immunohistochemistry. The epithelial cells are surrounded by a thick basement membrane, which in turn is surrounded by a layer of smooth muscle. These tubules lead into the epididymis, a convoluted tubular structure that plays a role in the transport, maturation, and storage of sperm (7) (Fig. 34.1). Transport is aided by a thick smooth muscle layer that surrounds the epididymis. The epididymis is lined by a thick basement

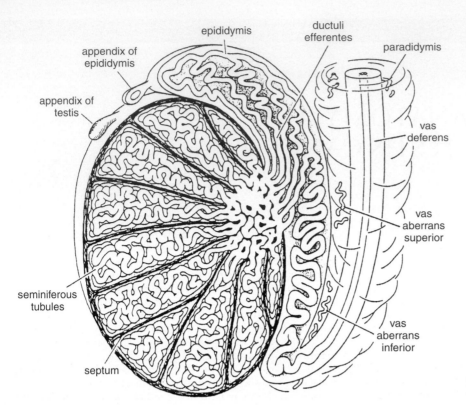

FIGURE 34.1. Schematic representation of the testis and its adnexa.

membrane and can be divided anatomically into three sections: head, body, and tail, with sperm storage and maturation occurring in the latter. The epithelial lining of the epididymis consists predominantly of tall columnar cells (principal cells), many of which exhibit esterocilia, but basal cells, clear cells, and luminal cells are also present. The luminal contour of the epididymis is rigid rather than undulating.

The vas deferens arises from the caudal portion of the epididymis, which joins proximally the excretory duct of the seminal vesicles to form the ejaculatory duct. The vas deferens is lined by pseudostratified, columnar epithelium and basal cells, the former containing long esterocilia. The luminal contour of the vas deferens is variably folded, and the epithelium is surrounded by loose connective tissue and a very thick smooth muscle layer.

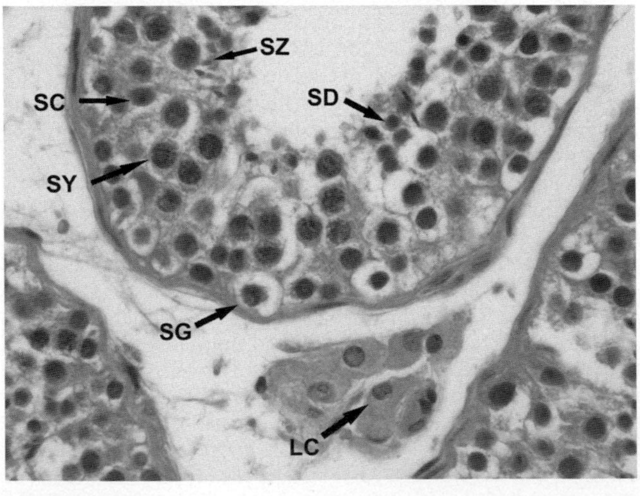

Several appendages may be encountered on the testis, testicular adnexa, or spermatic cord, the most common being the appendix testis and appendix epididymis (13,14) (Fig. 34.1). The appendix testis is a vestige of the Mullerian duct attached to the tunica vaginalis along the anterosuperior surface of the testis adjacent to the head of the epididymis. It is a small pedunculated structure lined by columnar nonciliated epithelium. The epithelium is undermined by richly vascular connective tissue. The appendix epididymis is a vestige of the mesonephric duct. It is a cystic, pedunculated structure attached to the head of the epididymis. The cyst is lined by low columnar epithelial cells and the external surface is lined by mesothelium. Two other types of appendages are present as incidental findings and represent remnants of mesonephric tubules. They appear as epithelial-lined tubular or cystic structures that are seen along the testicular adnexa or spermatic cord. Depending on their location, they are called vas aberrans or paradidymis (7,14).

TUMORS OF THE TESTIS

Germ Cell Tumors

Testicular germ cell tumors (GCT) comprise approximately 98% of all testicular neoplasms and are the most common malignancy in males between the ages of 15 and 35 years (15) (Table 34.1). They are relatively uncommon; approximately 5,500 to 6,000 new cases will be diagnosed in the United States during this calendar year. Because of their relative rarity, they present a diagnostic challenge to most practicing pathologists. It is remarkable that tumors of such diverse morphology and clinical behavior should be considered as variants of one entity. Nevertheless, circumstantial and laboratory evidence support this practice. First, these tumors tend to arise along the axial skeleton, be it the pineal gland, anterior

FIGURE 34.2. Normal seminiferous tubules in an adult containing spermatogonia (SG), spermatocytes (SY), spermatids (SD), spermatozoa (SZ), and Sertoli cells (SC). A cluster of Leydig cells (LC) is present in the interstitium (H&E stain, 100X).

TABLE 34.1

WHO HISTOLOGICAL CLASSIFICATION OF TESTIS TUMORS[a]

Germ Cell Tumors
Intratubular germ cell neoplasia, unclassified
Other types

Tumors of One Histological Type (Pure Forms)
Seminoma
    Seminoma with syncytiotrophoblastic cells
Spermatocytic seminoma
    Spermatocytic seminoma with sarcoma
Embryonal carcinoma
Yolk sac tumor
Trophoblastic tumors
    Choriocarcinoma
    Trophoblastic neoplasms other than choriocarcinoma
        Monophasic choriocarcinoma
        Placental site trophoblastic tumor
Teratoma
    Dermoid cyst
    Monodermal teratoma
    Teratoma with somatic type malignancies

Sex-cord/Gonadal Stromal Tumors (Pure Forms)
Leydig cell tumor
Sertoli cell tumor
    Sertoli cell tumor lipid-rich variant
    Sclerosing Sertoli cell tumor
    Large cell calcifying Sertolic cell tumor
Granulosa cell tumor
    Adult-type granulosa cell tumor
    Juvenile-type granulosa cell tumor
Tumors of the thecoma/fibroma group
Sex cord/gonadal stomal tumor
Incompletely differentiated tumor
Sex cord/gonadal stromal tumors, mixed forms
Malignant sex cord/gonadal stromal tumors
Tumors containing both germ cell and sex cord/gonadal
    stromal elements
        Gonadoblastoma
        Germ cell—sex cord/gonadal stromal tumor, unclassified

[a]Modified from Elbe JN, Sauter G, Epstien JI, Epstein et al., eds. WHO histological classification of testis tumours. *World Health Organization Classification of Tumours, Pathology & Genetics: Tumours of the Urinary System and Male Genital Organs.* Lyon, France: IARC Press, 2004:218.

mediastinum, retroperitoneum, or gonads. Second, mixed histologic patterns predominate over tumors with one histologic type. A third compelling piece of evidence relates to the so-called "precursor lesion." When these tumors arise in the gonad, irrespective of the morphology, one is likely to identify intratubular germ cell neoplasia (IGCN), also known in some circles as carcinoma *in situ*, in the adjacent seminiferous tubules. A fourth important piece of evidence linking these tumors comes to us from genetics, since approximately 80% of tumors, regardless of the primary site and histology, will have at least one isochromosome of the short arm of chromosome 12, which is known as i(12p). This genetic abnormality is not pathognomonic of germ cell neoplasia, yet it is a very useful diagnostic tool in selected circumstances due to its rare occurrence in other solid tumors (16–18).

Testicular germ cell tumors can be divided into three groups (infantile/prepubertal, adolescent/young adult, and spermatocytic

seminoma), each with its own constellation of clinical histology and molecular and clinical features (19,20). They originate from germ cells at different stages of development. The most common testicular cancers arise in postpubertal men, are characterized genetically by having one or more copies of i(12p), and exhibit other forms of 12p amplification and aneuploidy (21). The consistent gain of genetic material from chromosome 12 seen in these tumors suggests that it has a crucial role in their development. IGCN is the precursor to these invasive tumors. Their incidence is approximately 6.0 per 100,000 per year, with the majority being discovered in males between 15 and 40 years of age. Several factors have been associated with their pathogenesis, including cryptorchidism, elevated estrogens in utero, and gonadal dysgenesis. Tumors arising in prepubertal gonads are either teratomas or yolk sac tumors (YST), tend to be diploid, and are not associated with i(12p) or with IGCNU. The annual incidence is approximately 0.12 per 100,000. Spermatocytic seminoma (SS) arises in older patients. These benign tumors may be either diploid or aneuploid and have losses of chromosome 9 rather than i(12p). Intratubular SS is commonly encountered, but IGCN is not. Their annual incidence is approximately 0.2 per 100,000. The pathogenesis of prepubertal GCT and SS is poorly understood.

Intratubular Germ Cell Neoplasia

This term refers to the lesion initially described by Skakkebaek as "carcinoma *in situ*" (CIS), as well as to other "differentiated" forms of intratubular germ cell neoplasia (22–25). Strictly speaking, the lesion originally described by Skakkebaek is now called "intratubular germ cell neoplasia, unclassified" by most, at least in the Western Hemisphere.

The story of testicular CIS/intratubular germ cell neoplasia is fascinating and serves as a paradigm for the concept of progression from incipient or preinvasive neoplasia to invasive disease (24,26,27). In 1972 Skakkebaek reported atypical spermatogonia in two men undergoing testicular biopsies during a workup for infertility who subsequently developed invasive testicular germ cell tumor (TGCT). He hypothesized that these cells constituted CIS. Two subsequent seminal studies by his group proved that this was indeed the case. In 1978 he reported a series of 555 men who underwent testicular biopsies for infertility (26,27). The group identified 6 patients with evidence of CIS. With a median follow-up period of approximately 3 years, 3 of these patients developed evidence of an invasive germ cell tumor, one of them with bilateral disease. The remaining 449 patients were tumor free during the same follow-up period.

In 1986 Skakkebaek et al. reported their experience with contralateral biopsies in 500 patients with unilateral GCT (28). Twenty-seven patients (5.4%) were found to have CIS. Eight patients received systemic chemotherapy for advanced disease. Of the remaining 19 patients, 7 (37%) developed invasive GCT at this site within the follow-up period. Mathematical modeling suggested that 50% of biopsy-positive cases would develop disease within 5 years. Remarkably, not a single case of contralateral GCT developed in the remaining 463 biopsy-negative patients during the same follow-up period. In a subsequent report the authors revealed that at least 2 of the biopsy-positive cases that received systemic therapy subsequently developed contralateral tumors, suggesting that systemic therapy is not always effective against preinvasive disease (29).

It is clear that the original lesion described by Skakkebaek is the precursor to all types of germ cell tumors, at least for those that originate in postpubertal gonads, other than spermatocytic seminoma. In early 1980, a group of distinguished pathologists, including Drs. Robert Scully, Juan Rosai, F. K. K. Mostofi, and Robert Kurman, met in Minnesota to discuss nomenclature of incipient germ cell neoplasia. They agreed

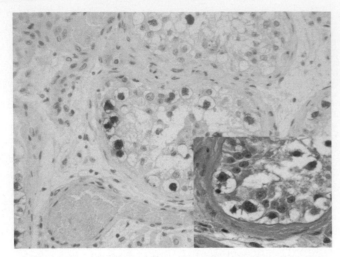

FIGURE 34.3. Intratubular germ cell neoplasia (IGCN). Insert shows atypical cells with irregular nuclei, coarse chromatin, prominent nucleoli, and perinuclear cytoplasmic clearing near the basement membrane (H&E stain, 200X). Background shows IGCN staining for POUSF1 (Oct 3/4) by immunohistochemistry (100X).

that CIS was a poor choice to describe this lesion since it had no features of epithelial differentiation. They suggested the term "intratubular germ cell neoplasia, unclassified" (IGCNU) because it was associated with all morphologic types of GCT with the exception of spermatocytic seminoma. It also underscores the fact that differentiated forms of intratubular germ cell neoplasia may occur, including intratubular embryonal carcinoma.

IGCN can be seen adjacent to invasive germ cell tumors in virtually all cases in which residual testicular parenchyma is present (22,30). As mentioned previously, it is present in up to 4% of cryptorchid patients, in up to 5% of contralateral gonads in patients with unilateral GCT, and in up to 1% of patients biopsied for oligospermic infertility. Its association with TGCT arising in prepubertal patients is still a source of controversy (19,31,32). While some authors suggest that it does not occur, others state that it does. In either case, we can state with reasonable certainty that, if IGCN does occur in childhood tumors, it is certainly less apparent.

IGCNU is characterized morphologically by the presence of enlarged, atypical germ cells located immediately above a usually irregularly thickened basement membrane (Fig. 34.3). The atypical cells either are isolated or form a single row along the basement membrane. They are typically larger than spermatogonia, the other cell that usually resides near the

basement membrane. IGCN cells have clear cytoplasm, irregular nuclear contours, coarse chromatin, and enlarged nucleoli that may be single or multiple. In comparison, spermatogonia may also have clear cytoplasm but the cells are small and have round and regular nuclear contours, densely packed chromatin, and absent nucleoli (Fig. 34.2). In most cases, tumor-bearing tubules do not have active spermatogenesis and contain mostly Sertoli cells. Sertoli cells may be displaced toward the tubular lumen. Characteristically, they contain a single nucleolus that is small and regular. The nuclei are oval or round with regular borders, and the chromatin is fine. The cytoplasm is amphophilic/eosinophilic and not vacuolated.

In essence, the cytologic features of classic IGCN are those of seminoma. The relationship is supported by the coexpression of a host of histochemical and immunohistochemical markers among both cell types. Further evidence comes from electron microscopy, which has shown that both share common ultrastructural features, including the absence of well-developed cytoplasmic intermediate filaments, inconspicuous organelles, glycogen particles, lack of mature desmosomes and cell junctions, and nucleoli with ropy nucleolonema. Tubules whose lumens are filled with these cells may be regarded as "intratubular seminomas."

IGCN may extend into the rete testis, usually undermining the epithelium in a pagetoid pattern. At times the epithelium may become hyperplastic, and in this setting it is important not to confuse this finding with the presence of nonseminomatous germ cell tumor.

IGCN cells contain glycogen and thus are p-aminosalicylic acid (PAS)-positive and diastase-sensitive. Rarely will other intratubular cells, either spermatogonia or Sertoli cells, show similar positivity. Placental-like alkaline phosphatase (PLAP) is one of the isoforms of alkaline phosphatase (Table 34.2). PLAP antibodies will stain IGCNU, as well as the majority of seminomas and embryonal carcinomas and a smaller percentage of yolk sac tumors. Immunoreactivity is seen in virtually all cases of IGCN, and the staining pattern is usually membranous or cytoplasmic. No other nonneoplastic intratubular cells are immunoreactive for PLAP, but immunoreactivity may be seen in other types of non–germ cell malignancies (33–36). c-kit (CD-117) is expressed in a large percentage of IGCN and seminomas but not in other germ cell tumors (37). Once again, the staining pattern is cytoplasmic/membranous. Despite the overexpression of this antigen, c-kit is rarely mutated in these tumors. Other antibodies that immunoreact with IGCNU but are rarely used in clinical practice include M2A and 43-F (36,38,39). POU5F1 (Oct3/4) is a very interesting marker that was recently described (40). The gene serves as a transcription factor, and its product is expressed in pluripotent mouse and human embryonic stem cells and is down-regulated during differentiation. Since the gene is also required for self-renewal of embryonic

TABLE 34.2

IMMUNOHISTOCHEMICAL PROFILE OF TESTICULAR TUMORS

Marker	IGCN	Seminoma	Spermatocytic seminoma	Embryonal carcinoma	Yolk Sac tumor	Trophoblastic tumors +++	Sex-cord gonadal stromal tumors ++
PLAP	+	+	−	+	+/−	−	−
CD-117 (c-kit)	+	+	+/−	−	−	−	−
Oct 3/4	+	+	−	+	−	−	−
AFP	−	−	−	−	+	−	−
Cytokeratin +	−	−	−	+	+	+	+/−
Inhibin	−	−	−	−	−	+/−	+
HCG	−	−	−	−	−	+	−

HCG, human chorionic gonadotropin; PLAP, placental-like alkaline phosphatase; AFP, alphafetoprotein; IGCN, intratubular germ cell neoplasia.

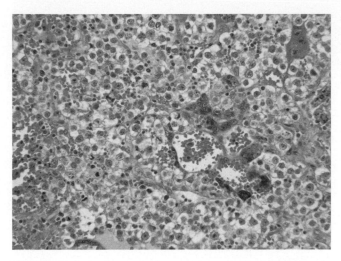

FIGURE 34.4. Seminoma with syncytiotrophoblasts (H&E stain, 100X).

stem cells, knocking out the gene is lethal. Early reports suggest that this antigen is expressed solely in IGCNU, seminoma, and embryonal carcinoma, suggesting that these are the types of GCT cells with pluripotency—that is, with capacity to differentiate. In any event, it provides us with yet another marker for IGCNU (Fig. 34.3).

It is important to keep in mind both that the presence of neoplastic cells within tubules does not always constitute IGCNU and that one must adhere strictly to the established diagnostic criteria. Besides intratubular seminoma, one can encounter intratubular embryonal carcinoma, intratubular spermatocytic seminoma, and even metastatic disease such as melanoma and prostatic carcinoma. Intratubular lymphoma and even mesothelioma may also be confused with IGCNU.

Seminoma

Seminomas are the most common germ cell tumors arising in the male gonad, whether they arise in a pure state or mixed with other morphologic types (41–47). "Pure" seminomas account for 27% to 30% of testicular GCT, and another 15% to 18% contain syncytiotrophoblasts. Approximately 1% to 2% are bilateral, and bilaterality can occur synchronously or asynchronously. Seminomas reach a peak incidence between the fourth and fifth decade of life, which is approximately one decade later than nonseminomatous germ cell tumors.

Macroscopic and Microscopic Features. Seminomas appear as fleshy, well-circumscribed, yellow-tan masses that, depending on size, may occupy a variable amount of testicular parenchyma or replace it entirely. Areas of necrosis may be observed grossly in 20% to 25% of cases. Some seminomas are associated with a granulomatous reaction, in which the tumor takes on a fibrous and nodular gross appearance. Microscopically, tumor cells are uniform and have round to vesicular nuclei with clear cytoplasm, prominent cytoplasmic membranes, and a centrally located, round nucleus with a prominent nucleolus (Fig. 34.4). These cells are arranged in sheets or nests separated by thin fibrovascular bands that contain mature lymphoid cells. Mitotic activity is variable. Some cases exhibit extensive fibrosis, particularly those associated with a granulomatous reaction or tumors that have undergone partial regression. Rarely, seminomas may exhibit unusual patterns such as cribriform, pseudoglandular, and tubular growth (48). These do not represent separate entities but rather histologic variants of classic seminoma. Less than 20% of cases contain syncytiotrophoblasts, but their presence may be associated with focal areas of hemorrhage and necrosis (Fig. 34.4). Seminomas with

syncytiotrophoblasts will be accompanied by serum elevation of human chorionic gonadotropin (HCG), but levels will rarely reach above 500 IU/mL (47).

Tumor cells contain glycogen (PAS-positive) and express PLAP and c-kit (CD-117) by immunohistochemistry (33,34, 49–55) but not cytokeratins, CD-30 or inhibin. A minority of seminoma cells may express focal and weak, dotlike or linear immunoreactivity for cytokeratin; however, they never express diffuse and strong staining throughout the cytoplasm. Like IGCN, seminoma cells express POU5F1 (Oct 3/4) in a nuclear distribution (33,37,56,57) (Table 34.2).

Some seminomas exhibit a significant degree of cytologic atypia (58–66), and this fact has led to the now-abandoned concept of "anaplastic seminoma" as a discrete entity with a worse prognosis (67,68). As described, this tumor was characterized by overall morphologic features of a seminoma, but one containing more pleomorphic cells with nonclear cytoplasm and abundant mitotic figures. Fibrovascular septa and lymphocytes were absent, and focal necrosis was commonly seen. This concept did not withstand the test of time since many series later showed that, stage for stage, there was no difference in clinical outcome between classic and anaplastic seminomas (43,58,69). In addition, it has become quite evident that mitotic activity in seminomas is quite variable and, in fact, may be quite high even in classical cases (60). Presently, tumors thought to be seminoma but exhibiting atypical histology should trigger consideration of a differential diagnosis of seminoma that includes (a) seminoma with "early carcinomatous differentiation," (b) solid variants of embryonal carcinoma or yolk sac tumor, (c) lymphoma, (d) sex-cord gonadal stromal tumor, and (e) metastatic disease, including poorly differentiated carcinoma and melanoma. Other causes of atypical histology in seminoma include poor fixation and faulty processing in the pathology laboratory. "Early carcinomatous differentiation" refers to areas of transition from seminoma to embryonal carcinoma. This concept suggests that seminoma cells are not terminally differentiated but rather, under certain poorly understood circumstances, may differentiate into other germ cell tumor types (47,63,70).

Spermatocytic Seminoma

Spermatocytic seminomas are rare, comprising less than 2% of testicular neoplasms (47,71,72). In fact, they account in our institution for significantly less than 1% of primary testicular tumors resected. Although classified as a variant of seminoma, in reality they represent an entirely separate and distinct clinicopathologic entity. The peak incidence is in the sixth decade of life; however, occurrence in younger patients as early as the third decade of life is reported. This tumor occurs only in the male gonad, may be unilateral or bilateral, and is not associated with cryptorchidism. It is a benign tumor with only one documented case having metastasized. An exception to this rule is the rare case of "spermatocytic seminoma with sarcoma" (73,74). These very rare tumors exhibit an undifferentiated or differentiated sarcoma component and are commonly associated with metastatic disease at the time of initial diagnosis. Prognosis is poor. Median survival is less than 1 year, with patients dying of widely metastatic disease.

Gross and Microscopic Features. Spermatocytic seminoma may be large, may be nodular, and may have a myxoid, mucoid, or fleshy appearance. Areas of hemorrhage, cystic degeneration, and necrosis are common. Microscopically, tumor cells are arranged in solid sheets or nests of round cells (Fig. 34.5). Occasionally the tumor cells may be arranged in nests or pseudoglandular arrangements within an edematous or mucoid stroma. Cytologically, it is possible to identify three distinct cell types (small, medium, and large), although cells of

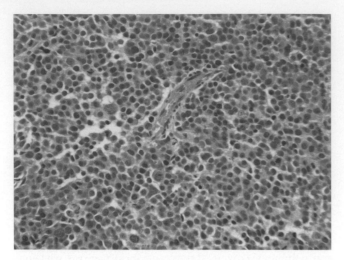

FIGURE 34.5. Spermatocytic seminoma. Notice the presence of small, intermediate, and large tumor cells, the latter with "spireme" chromatin (H&E stain, 100X).

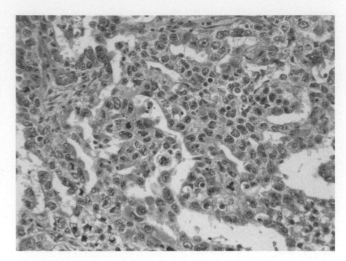

FIGURE 34.6. Embryonal carcinoma (H&E stain, 100X).

intermediate size predominate. The intermediate cells have a small amount of eosinophilic or amphophilic cytoplasm. The nuclei are round and contain coarse chromatin, at times exhibiting a "spireme" (filamentous or stringlike) pattern. The small cells have dark-staining nuclei and scant eosinophilic cytoplasm. The large cells have giant round or oval nuclei with a classic spireme chromatic distribution. All three cell types may be present within seminiferous tubules (intratubular spermatocytic seminomas). Mitoses are frequent, including atypical forms. These tumors rarely contain a lymphocytic infiltrate and are not associated with a granulomatous reaction.

Tumor cells do not contain glycogen (negative PAS stain). Immunohistochemical stains for PLAP are negative, although occasional cells may be weakly immunoreactive. Cytokeratins are negative, although occasional cells may exhibit dotlike cytoplasmic staining. CD-30 is negative, while some investigators have reported immunoreactivity for CD-117 (c-kit) (37,47,75,76) (Table 34.2).

Embryonal Carcinoma

Embryonal carcinomas comprise up to 3% of pure GCT, although they are common components of mixed germ cell tumors. They rarely present as pathologic stage I disease and are not associated with elevation of HCG or alphafetoprotein (AFP) (43,47).

Gross and Microscopic Features. Embryonal carcinomas (EC) may vary in size, color, and texture, are commonly hemorrhagic, and exhibit areas of cystic degeneration and necrosis (Fig. 34.6). Microscopically, tumor cells are large, irregular, and epithelioid. They exhibit scanty cytoplasm, large pleomorphic nuclei with coarse chromatin, and multiple irregular nucleoli. Common findings include nuclear overlap, individual cell necrosis, and apoptotic bodies. The pattern of growth is quite variable: glandlike, papillary, syncytial, and solid areas are commonly encountered. The solid variant of EC may be confused with "atypical" forms of seminoma, although the latter do not exhibit the same degree of cytologic anaplasia as embryonal carcinoma. Immunohistochemistry is useful in resolving this differential diagnosis. Embryonal carcinoma may have overlapping morphologic features with YST but, once again, close attention to subtle cytomorphologic differences and immunohistochemistry will resolve the majority of cases. Most ECs are immunoreactive for PLAP, low-molecular-weight cytokeratins, CD-30, and POU5F (Oct 3/4). They do not express CD-117, AFP, or HCG (37,76) (Table 34.2).

Large cell lymphoma and metastatic poorly differentiated carcinoma may also enter in the differential diagnosis. ECs are said to be negative with immunohistochemical stains for epithelial membrane antigen (EMA), carcinoembryogenic antigen (CEA), and B72.3 (77). All may be expressed in a subset of poorly differentiated non–germ cell carcinomas. Depending on the cell of origin, large cell lymphomas will be immunoreactive for B or T cell markers (33,34,49–51,53–55).

Yolk Sac (Endodermal Sinus) Tumor

YSTs are characterized by multiple patterns of growth that recapitulate the yolk sac, allantois, and extra embryonic mesenchyme. It has a bimodal age distribution: infants and young children and postpubertal males. In the latter group, it rarely presents in a pure form but is present in almost half of mixed germ cell tumors (47). In children it commonly presents in its pure form, usually within the first 2 years of life. These tumors are associated with serum elevation of AFP in the overwhelming majority of cases.

Gross and Microscopic Features. The gross appearance of YSTs is quite variable because YST components are usually closely admixed with other elements. If pure, they commonly appear grey-white with a myxoid or even mucoid appearance. Areas of hemorrhage and geographic necrosis are common. Microscopically these tumors are quite variable due to the multiple subtypes, which are usually intermixed (44,78):

- *Endodermal Sinus (Schiller-Duval):* This pattern exhibits Schiller-Duval bodies that are perivascular arrangements of cuboidal or low columnar epithelial cells with an intervening labyrinthlike network of extracellular spaces. This pattern is quite distinctive and recognized by most pathologists. Unfortunately, it is seen in only a minority of tumors.
- *Reticular or Microcystic* (Fig. 34.7): This is the most commonly encountered pattern and is characterized by round to oval tumor cells with variable amounts of cytoplasm surrounded by cysts. These cysts vary in size and may contain an amorphous eosinophilic or basophilic fluid.
- *Papillary*
- *Glandular–alveolar*
- *Myxomatous:* This pattern is quite common and is characterized by cords or nests of neoplastic cells embedded in a stoma rich in hyaluronic acid. This pattern is most commonly seen adjacent to microcystic and solid areas.
- *Enteric*

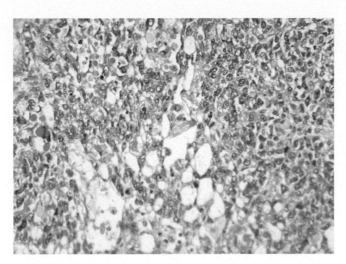

FIGURE 34.7. Yolk sac (endodermal sinus) tumor with microcystic and solid areas (H&E stain, 100X).

- *Macrocystic*
- *Polyvesicular vitelline*
- *Hepatoid*
- *Solid* (Fig. 34.7): This pattern may be confused with other germ cell tumors, particularly seminoma.

Tumor cells of YST are not as primitive or pleomorphic as those seen in EC. They have more abundant clear or weakly granular cytoplasm that is often vacuolated. Individual cell necrosis and apoptotic bodies are not as conspicuous as in EC. The cytoplasm may contain small, spherical, and densely eosinophilic intracytoplasmic droplets that are PAS positive and diastase resistant. These represent either AFP or, more commonly, alpha-1-antytrypsin deposition. Cells may be spindled or stellate, making them easily confused with mesenchyme. The extracellular matrix adjacent to YST is myxomatous, a feature that is rarely seen in EC.

Tumor cells of YST are usually immunoreactive for AFP and low-molecular-weight cytokeratins. PLAP staining is variable and may be absent. CD117 (c-kit) and CD-30 are usually negative, as is Oct 3/4 (33,34,37,49–51,53–55) (Table 34.2).

Choriocarcinoma

Choriocarcinoma is composed of syncytiotrophoblastic, cytotrophoblastic, and other trophoblastic cells. It comprises less than 1% of testicular GCT in its pure form; however, it may be encountered as a component of a mixed GCT in up to 10% of cases (43,47,79). In its pure form, these tumors occur in the second and third decades of life, are commonly associated with very high levels of serum HCG, and exhibit metastatic disease at the time of initial presentation. Small foci of choriocarcinoma within a mixed germ cell tumor do not alter the prognosis.

Gross and Microscopic Features. These tumors usually present as a hemorrhagic, necrotic mass with, in some instances, evidence of fibrosis and regression. Microscopically, these tumors exhibit an admixture of trophoblastic cells in varying proportions. Most cases will have syncytiotrophoblasts and cytotrophoblasts with occasional intermediate trophoblastic cells present (Fig. 34.8). The tumor cells are usually associated with such abundant hemorrhage and necrosis that many surgical sections are needed to see any viable disease. Very rare cases exhibit few syncytiotrophoblasts, containing predominantly cytotrophoblasts and intermediate trophoblastic cells. These tumors have been descriptively called "monophasic" variants of choriocarcinoma, have no association to a distinct clinical meaning, and are more likely

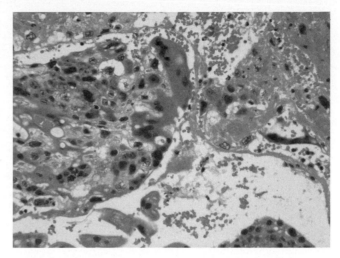

FIGURE 34.8. Choriocarcinoma. Syncytiotrophoblasts appear as multinucleated giant cells with abundant basophilic cytoplasm overlying cytotrophoblast (stain 100X).

encountered in the postchemotherapy setting (80,81). Another recently described and even rarer variant of trophoblastic disease is placental-site trophoblastic tumor (82). It is composed exclusively of intermediate trophoblastic cells. These cells are mononuclear and pleomorphic, and they exhibit eosinophilic cytoplasm. They are immunoreactive for human placental lactogen (HPL) and cytokeratins.

Syncytiotrophoblasts are immunoreactive with HCG as well as inhibin, epithelial membrane antigen, and low-molecular-weight cytokeratins. PLAP may be positive, but staining is variable (47) (Table 34.2).

Teratoma

The term "teratoma" refers to neoplasms composed of tissues that have differentiated along any of the three somatic pathways: ectoderm, mesoderm, or endoderm (43,44,47). Tumors composed of only one of these components are regarded as monodermal teratomas. Teratomas may be composed of mature tissues, embryonal-type tissues, or a mixture of both. Historically, they were subclassified as immature and mature forms based on their degree of differentiation. The World Health Organization now recommends that these morphologies be considered as a single entity based on their overlapping genetic features.

Teratomas have a bimodal incidence peak. They represent approximately one third of tumors in children and are benign. In adults, the incidence of pure teratoma is less than 7%. They are commonly found as a component of mixed GCT in adults. Teratomatous components may be the only remaining recognizable tumor after spontaneous regression or after systemic therapy.

Gross and Microscopic Features. Tumors are usually heterogeneous, firm, nodular, and well circumscribed. They may be solid or cystic, depending on their histologic components. Histologically, they may contain mature elements such as neural, glandular, and squamous tissues. Attempts at organ formation are common, particularly in children. Mesenchymal components such as smooth muscle cartilage are also common. Fetal-type tissues can emerge from any histologic type. Characteristically, all components—whether mature or fetal—are intermixed (Fig. 34.9). When one of the teratomatous components—whether mesenchymal (skeletal muscle), neural (primitive neuroepithelium), or epithelial (glandular or squamous)—predominate and form an expansile mass, the term "teratoma with somatic type malignancy" is used (47,83–87). These tumors were originally termed "teratoma with malignant

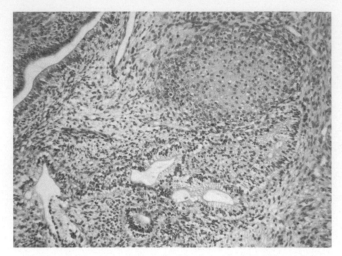

FIGURE 34.9. Teratoma. Notice that immature mesenchymal, glandular, and cartilaginous elements are intermingled (H&E stain, 100X).

transformation," a term no longer in use. The definition of what constitutes somatic-type malignancy is controversial, but most authors suggest that the expansile nodule should be equal or greater than a 4X microscopic field. The incidence of secondary somatic malignancy is approximately 3%. This phenomenon may be seen *de novo* in testicular GCT, more commonly in mediastinal primaries, and in retroperitoneal disease resected after chemotherapy (84,85). If limited to the gonad, it is not associated with a worse prognosis; the reverse is true when encountered in other sites.

Tumors of More than One Histologic Type

Mixed germ cell tumors comprise between 35% and 54% of GCT, exclusive of seminomas with trophoblastic cells and spermatocytic seminoma with sarcoma (43,47). They are rarely seen in prepubertal gonads. Cases containing a component of seminoma tend to occur later in life than those that do not. All the morphologic variants previously described, with the exception of spermatocytic seminoma, may be encountered. As expected, the gross and microscopic features are quite variable and will depend on the histologic components encountered. The term "teratocarcinoma" should be avoided since it lacks diagnostic specificity.

Epidermoid Cyst

Epidermoid cysts constitute 1% or less of all testicular neoplasms (47,88,89). Their histogenesis is unclear, although most investigators suggest that they represent monodermally differentiated mature teratoma, supported by the fact that a recent case with adjacent IGCNU was identified (90). Some have suggested that they arise from inclusion cysts, while others propose squamous metaplasia of seminiferous tubules or the rete testis (tumorlike condition). They are commonly discovered between the second and fourth decades of life and are often asymptomatic. These tumors may be as large as 10 cm, although most measure less than 2 cm.

Grossly, they appear as well-circumscribed cystic masses filled with keratinized debris similar to an epidermal inclusion cyst. The cyst wall is composed of fibrous tissue surrounding flattened squamous epithelium. No dermal adnexal elements or other teratomatous elements are present in the cyst wall or surrounding testicular parenchyma. These tumors are not associated with a testicular scar; furthermore, IGCN is not present except in the above-mentioned case.

These unusual neoplasms are invariably benign and should be managed conservatively. Nevertheless, the lesion should be thoroughly sampled and examined by the pathologist to rule out other elements of IGCNU.

Dermoid cysts have been described in the testis and are characterized by the presence of squamous epithelium overlying skin appendages (47,91). Occasionally other teratomatous components may be present. They are considered to be benign variants of cystic teratoma analogous to what is seen in the ovary. They are extremely rare and by definition are not associated with IGCNU.

Completely or Partially "Burned-out" Germ Cell Tumor

A possible explanation for most—if not all—presumed "primary" retroperitoneal GCT lies in the concept of partially or completely "burned-out" germ cell tumors. For many decades, pathologists have observed areas of regression within germ cell tumors. These usually take the form of a well-defined stellate fibrous scar at the periphery where sclerosed seminiferous tubules are evident (92–94). The scar may be accompanied by a sparse plasma cell infiltrate and aggregates of hemosiderin, and macrophages may be present. The scar is usually located well within the substance of the testis. It may abut the mediastinum testis but is rarely located toward the poles or directly below the tunica albuginea. The latter location suggests the possibility of a posttraumatic scar. Another occasional feature seen in burned-out lesions is the presence of peculiar hematoxyphilic deposits having an amorphous or granular structure. These deposits appear to be located within hyalinized seminiferous tubules. Infrequently, these hematoxylin staining bodies may be associated with scattered malignant germ cells. A burned-out lesion without any viable GCT may be the only evidence of a regressed testicular primary lesion. If viable germ cell components are present, they are usually in the form of teratoma, seminoma, or IGCN. Burned-out lesions may be very small, rendering them nonpalpable; nevertheless, they are usually discernible by testicular ultrasound.

Pathologic Prognostic Factors in Stage I Nonseminomatous Germ Cell Tumors

Until recently, the treatment of choice for stage I nonseminomatous germ cell tumors (NSGCT) was radical orchiectomy followed by retroperitoneal lymph node dissection (RPLND). Given the advent of highly effective chemotherapy, the availability of sensitive serum tumor markers, as well as more precise staging techniques, orchiectomy alone followed by close surveillance is a viable option for some patients. Overall, 20% to 25% of patients treated in this manner will recur, usually in the retroperitoneum and within a year of the orchiectomy. Many studies have shown that the presence of vascular invasion (VI) in the primary tumor is the best predictor of recurrence. In fact, the importance of vascular invasion in the primary tumor is reflected in the tumor, nodes, metastases (TNM) classification (Table 34.3). The impact of tumor histology on future relapse remains controversial, but most authors have suggested that a pure or predominant EC component also is more likely to metastasize (95–97).

Sex-cord Stromal (Gonadal Stromal) Tumors of the Testis

Sex-cord Sstromal (gonadal stromal) tumors are rare, comprising approximately 4.0% of testicular neoplasms (Table 34.1). Similar tumors may arise in the female gonads. The term refers to neoplasms containing Leydig (interstitial) cells, Sertoli cells, granulosa cells, or theca cells. Tumors may be made up of one or a combination of these cell types in varying

TABLE 34.3

TNM CLASSIFICATION OF GERM CELL TUMORS OF THE TESTIS

pTNM pathological classification

pT	Primary tumor
pTX	Primary tumor cannot be assessed
pT0	No evidence of primary tumor (e.g., histologic scar in testis)
pTis	Intratubular germ cell neoplasia (CIS)
pT1	Tumor limited to testis and epididymis without vascular/lymphatic invasion; tumor may invade tunica albuginea but not tunica vaginalis
pT2	Tumor limited to testis and epididymis with vascular/lymphatic invasion; or tumor extending through tunica albuginea with involvement of tunica vaginalis
pT3	Tumor invades spermatic cord with or without vascular/lymphatic invasion
pT4	Tumor invades scrotum with or without vascular/lymphatic invasion
pN	Regional lymph nodes
pNX	Regional lymph nodes cannot be assessed
pN0	No regional lymph node metastasis
pN1	Metastasis with a lymph node mass 2 cm or less in greatest dimension and 5 or fewer positive nodes, none more than 2 cm in greatest dimension
pN2	Metastasis with a lymph node mass more than 2 cm but not more than 5 cm in greatest dimension; or more than 5 nodes positive, none more than 5 cm; or evidence of extranodal extension to tumor
pN3	Metastasis with a lymph node mass more than 5 cm in greatest dimension

CIS, carcinoma *in situ*; TNM, tumor, nodes, metastasis.
Modified from Elbe JN, Sauter G, Epstein JI, eds. WHO histological classification of testis tumours. *World Health Organization Classification of Tumours, Pathology & Genetics: Tumours of the Urinary System and Male Genital Organs.* Lyon, France: IARC Press, 2004:219.

degrees of differentiation. The terminology used to describe these tumors is confusing and controversial, but it is best to adhere to the classification set forth by the World Health Organization (Table 34.1).

Leydig (Interstitial) Cell Tumor

Leydig cell tumors (LCT) are the most common pure testicular sex-cord stromal neoplasms and account for 1% to 3% of testicular neoplasms. They may occur at any age, although they are most common between the third and sixth decades of life (43,47,98–100). Between 15% and 20% of cases will present in prepubertal children. Approximately 10% will metastasize with metastasis occurring at an older age. LCTs usually arise in normally descended testes, although they have been described in cryptorchid gonads as well as in testes that have undergone orchiopexy. Only three cases have been reported in patients with Klinefelter syndrome.

Most, if not all, children with LCT present with isosexual precocity, which is characterized by deepening of the voice, appearance of body hair, penile enlargement, and advanced bone age. Often these physical changes are accompanied by excessive aggression or shyness. LCT must be considered in the differential diagnosis in all prepubertal patients with a testicular mass and precocious puberty. Painless testicular swelling is the most common manifestation in adults, followed by bilateral gynecomastia. It is not unusual for gynecomastia to precede the appearance of a testicular mass, and in 15% of cases the former is the only complaint at initial presentation. Approximately 25% of patients with gynecomastia experience a decrease in potency or libido. Given the low incidence of these tumors, endocrinological studies are limited and incomplete. Prepubertal patients will usually have elevated serum testosterone, as well as elevated urinary 17-ketosteroids. In adults, elevated estrogen levels have been documented in patients with, as well as without, gynecomastia. Testosterone levels may be low or normal in patients with gynecomastia and high levels of serum estradiol.

Gross and Microscopic Features. Grossly, LCT is a well-circumscribed, yellow-tan or brown-gray lobulated mass occasionally containing fibrous septa. Macroscopic evidence of hemorrhage or necrosis is rare. Microscopically, the tumor is made up of large polyclonal cells with abundant eosinophilic and granular cytoplasm (Fig. 34.10). Less frequently, the cytoplasm may be clear or vacuolated or microcystic (101,102). Nuclei are round or vesicular with delicate chromatin and a single prominent nucleolus. The cells usually exhibit a solid pattern of infiltration, although fibrous septa may give them a pseudotubular or trabecular appearance. Crystalloids of Reinke are present in 25% to 40% of cases but may require electron microscopic examination for their identification. With light microscopy, they appear as densely eosinophilic needlelike or rhomboid structures within the cytoplasm. LCTs are likely to be immunoreactive with inhibin and vimentin but not cytokeratins, CD-30, Oct 3/4, or PLAP (Fig. 34.10) (47,103–106) (Table 34.2).

It is difficult to determine histologically those tumors that will metastasize. Kim et al. reported their experiences with 40

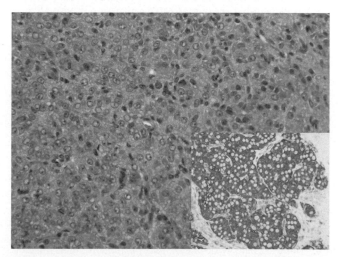

FIGURE 34.10. Leydig cell tumor (H&E stain). Insert shows strong cytoplasmic immunoreactivity for inhibin (100X).

cases, and they also reviewed the literature and confirmed that tumors larger than 5 cm, as well as those with infiltrative margins, vascular invasion, nuclear atypia, or increased mitotic rate, were associated with aggressive behavior (98). Interestingly, none of the malignant cases presented with endocrine manifestations or occurred in prepubertal children. Cheville et al. found that malignant Leydig cell tumors were more likely to have a high proliferation rate and to be nondiploid (107). The most common metastatic sites are retroperitoneal and inguinal lymph nodes, followed by the lungs and liver.

LCT must be distinguished from Leydig cell hyperplasia or nodular aggregates of Leydig cells that occur in atrophic testes (including patients with Klinefelter syndrome) and in testicular parenchyma adjacent to germ cell neoplasia. Here Leydig cells infiltrate between seminiferous tubules without displacing or obliterating them. LCT must also be distinguished from other sex-cord stromal tumors, especially when the former exhibits a cordlike or tubular pattern that may mimic a Sertoli cell tumor. Secondary lesions such as lymphoma, malignant melanoma, and poorly differentiated carcinoma may also enter into the differential diagnosis. LCT with microcystic features may be confused with yolk sac tumors (101). Similarly, one must not confuse LCT with malakoplakia or with the bilateral testicular masses seen in patients with untreated adrenogenital syndrome.

A lesion that must not be confused with LCT occurs in association with congenital adrenal hyperplasia (CAH, tumor of the adrenogenital syndrome) (43,47,108). CAH is due to a defect of any one of five enzymatic steps involved in steroid synthesis. This disorder is an inborn error of metabolism, has an autosomal recessive mode of inheritance, and is the most common cause of ambiguous genitalia in infants. Between 90% and 95% of cases are due to 21-hydroxylase deficiency. A small percentage may be due to 11-B-hydroxylase, 3-B-hydroxysteroid, 17-a-hydroxylase, or cholesterol desmolase deficiency.

Persistent stimulation of adrenal cortical tissue by adreno cortico tropic hormonc (ACTH) may give rise not only to hyperplasia but also, rarely, to adrenal cortical neoplasia (both adenomas and carcinomas). Heterotopic or accessory adrenal cortical tissue can also become hyperplastic and enlarged. A testicular "tumor" of adrenal cortical type is defined as a tumefactive lesion of uncertain histogenesis in the setting of CAH, which histologically resembles hyperplastic adrenal cortical cells stimulated by ACTH and in which endocrinological evaluation may reveal ACTH dependency. These tumors are thought to arise from primordial rests within the testicular hilum. These rests are a collection of cells morphologically resembling Leydig cells and are found in a large proportion of cases of well-studied CAH. Nodules of these cells may be clinically undetectable or demonstrated only through testicular ultrasound. Larger "tumors" are usually associated undiagnosed cases of CAH or patients who have demonstrated poor compliance with their treatments.

Testicular "tumors" in CAH usually occur in early adult life (average age of 22.5 years). Smaller tumors are seen in younger patients, typically located in the hilum of the testis. In adults, the lesions may measure up to 10 cm, and 83 percent of tumors are bilateral. In contrast, LCTs are bilateral in 3% or less of cases. The lesions are unencapsulated and are light tan-brown in color due to the absence of lipids and the presence of cytoplasmic lipochrome pigment. They are usually lobulated as a result of the presence of prominent bands of fibrous connective tissue. Occasionally, multiple extratesticular nodules measuring up to 1.5 cm in diameter have been described along the spermatic cord or adjacent to the epididymis. Microscopically, there are sheets and nests of cells with abundant granular cytoplasm and relatively distinct cell borders. Nuclei are uniform and round to oval with one or two prominent small nucleoli. Many of the tumor cells contain lipochrome pigment (lipofuscin). Mitoses are very uncommon.

As you might imagine from the microscopic description, there is great resemblance to Leydig cells. Indeed, Leydig cell tumor is the most common diagnosis made in these cases. Crystalloids of Reinke have not been described in tumors of CAH; however, they are seen in up to 40% of LCT. Ultrastructurally, the cells have features of steroid-producing cells with abundant smooth endoplasmic reticulum, numerous mitochondria, and accumulation of lipofuscin. The mitochondrial cristae may be lamellar or have a vesicular profile.

Sertoli Cell Tumor

Sertoli cell tumors (SCT) are rare, comprising less than 1% of testicular neoplasms (43,47,99,109,110). They were first described in the testis by Teilum who recognized their histologic similarity to Sertoli cell tumors of the canine testis. They may occur at any age, and approximately 15% develop in children. Patients characteristically present with a painless mass in a normally descended testis. Gynecomastia is evident in one third of patients. Hormonal alterations in patients with SCT have been poorly documented. Nevertheless, SCT should be in the differential diagnosis of all prepubertal patients presenting with a testicular mass and gynecomastia. Three cases have been reported in boys with Peutz-Jeghers syndrome (111).

Gross and Microscopic Features. Grossly, SCTs are well circumscribed, solid, and yellow-white or tan. The lesions may be lobulated and may contain small areas of hemorrhage. Microscopic examination reveals mostly tubules but also cords, nests, and masses of tumor cells in a fibrous stroma (Fig. 34.11). The neoplastic cells may contain abundant intracytoplasmic lipid that gives them a clear or vacuolated appearance. Electron microscopy may reveal Charcot-Boettcher filaments within the cytoplasm, which are characteristic of Sertoli cells. The classification of SCT should be reserved for tumors composed entirely of Sertoli cells. Those neoplasms composed only partially of these cells should be classified as mixed or incompletely differentiated sex-cord stromal tumors. SCT are immunoreactive for inhibin, vimentin, and cytokeratins (110) (Table 34.2). Markers typically seen in GCT are negative (47).

Metastases will occur in approximately 10% of SCT (110,112). Metastases are usually to inguinal or retroperitoneal lymph nodes, although skin and pulmonary involvement have been reported. Due to the rarity of this tumor, histologic criteria associated with malignant behavior are unreliable. The presence of metastasis remains as the best indicator of malignancy.

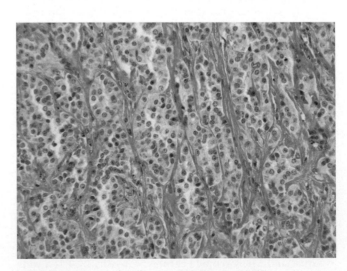

FIGURE 34.11. Sertoli cell tumor (H&E stain, 100X).

SCT must be distinguished from nonneoplastic, hyperplastic nodules of seminiferous tubules lined by Sertoli cells. These Sertoli cell nodules were previously mistakenly referred to as "adenomas." They may contain central hyaline material resembling Call-Exner bodies or laminated calcifications. The nodules are usually small and are most frequently encountered in cryptorchid testes, in atrophic scrotal testes, or adjacent to germ cell tumors. SCT are distinguished from other sex-cord stromal tumors by the predominantly tubular pattern in the former.

Radical orchiectomy is the treatment of choice and will be curative in the majority of cases. Since only 10% of cases will develop metastasis and no reliable criteria exist to predict an increased risk of metastasis, the role of primary retroperitoneal lymph node dissection is controversial. The role of radiation therapy and chemotherapy in patients with metastatic SCT is uncertain.

In 1980, Proppe and Scully described a subtype of SCT that they called "large cell calcifying Sertoli cell tumor" (LCCSCT) (113,114). It usually presents during the first three decades of life, although cases in older males have been described. While patients may present exclusively with a testicular mass, their initial symptomatology could be related to such other associated conditions as pituitary adenomas, bilateral adrenocortical hyperplasia, cardiac myxomas, or other sex-cord stromal tumors. Approximately one-third of LCCSCTs are bilateral and some will metastasize (115). These tumors are usually less than 5 cm in size and microscopically are characterized by large polygonal cells with abundant eosinophilic cytoplasm in a fibrous or myxoid stroma. Tumor cells within seminiferous tubules are present in 50% of cases. Microcalcifications are usually abundant. LCCSCTs are often mistaken for LCT, but the abundant calcifications, frequent intratubular growth, absence of crystalloids of Reinke, and unusual clinical associations should direct us toward the correct diagnosis.

Granulosa Cell Tumor

The adult variant of granulosa cell tumor very rarely develops in the testis (99,100,116,117). Variants have been described in males between the ages of 21 and 73 years who presented with testicular mass and gynecomastia. Urinary estrogen levels may be elevated. The tumors measure up to 13 cm in greatest diameter and microscopically are composed of neoplastic cells in a microfollicular and diffuse infiltrative pattern. The cells have scanty cytoplasm and angular, pale nuclei with longitudinal grooves. Call-Exner bodies may be evident in the microfollicular areas. Metastases are rare.

Granulosa cell tumors analogous to juvenile granulosa cell tumors of the ovary are the most common sex-cord stromal tumor of the infantile testis (43,118,119). They are usually present in the first 6 months of life, the oldest reported case being in a 21-month-old. Two cases have developed in undescended testes. Juvenile granulosa cell tumors may arise in patients with an abnormal karyotype and ambiguous genitalia. Tumors may be solid, cystic, or both, and the cysts frequently contain a gelatinous material. Microscopically, such tumors exhibit either a follicular or solid pattern and the cells are characterized by a moderate to large amount of eosinophilic cytoplasm and hyperchromatic nuclei. Stromal hyalinization is often extensive. Although mitoses may be plentiful, no testicular tumor of this type has metastasized (47,120).

Sex-cord Stromal and Gonadal Stromal Tumors, Mixed or Incompletely Differentiated Forms

As you might expect, these two categories include tumors with more than one identifiable sex-cord stromal element, as well as tumors in which the exact gonadal stromal cell of origin cannot be established with certainty (43,47,121). These neoplasms may occur at any age, although more than half of the patients are children or infants. Painless testicular enlargement is the most common presenting symptom that is infrequently associated with gynecomastia. Grossly, these tumors are similar to other sex-cord stromal neoplasms and their microscopic appearance is quite variable, ranging from predominantly epithelioid to predominantly stromal growth patterns. Frequently the cells are undifferentiated, making precise classification impossible. Approximately 30% of tumors presenting in patients older than 10 years of age are malignant, while tumors presenting in younger patients follow a benign course. Histologic predictors of aggressive clinical behavior have not been established. Radical orchiectomy is the treatment of choice, while retroperitoneal lymph node dissection should be given serious consideration in patients older than 10 years of age.

Tumors Containing Both Sex-cord Stromal and Germ Cell Elements

Gonadoblastoma. Gonadoblastomas are rare neoplasms composed of sex cord elements intimately admixed with germ cells (47,121). These tumors generally arise in chromosomally abnormal individuals with dysgenetic gonads; 20% of cases occur in phenotypic males. Patients usually present with cryptorchidism, hypospadia, and internal female genitalia, although two cases have been reported arising in a scrotal testis. One-third of cases are bilateral, and 60% are associated with malignant germ cell elements that are usually seminoma but may be yolk sac tumor or embryonal carcinoma. While gonadoblastomas do not metastasize, metastasis from the associated germ cell tumor may occur.

The microscopic appearance is distinctive and consists of tumor nests surrounded by connective-tissue stroma. The nests contain germ cells with clear cytoplasm and sex-cord elements resembling Sertoli cells, granulosa cells, or both. The nests may contain hyalinized eosinophilic structures resembling Call-Exner bodies.

Since gonadoblastomas are frequently bilateral, excision of the contralateral gonad is mandatory. With an associated germ cell tumor, the patient should be carefully worked up for metastatic disease.

Germ Cell/Sex-Cell Stromal–Gonadal Stromal Tumors, Unclassified

This is a controversial entity that is also composed of an admixture of germ cells and sex-cord stromal elements but that occurs in phenotypically and genotypically normal males (47,109,122,123). To date, no endocrine abnormalities have been described with this lesion. The tumor may be large, measuring up to 12 cm in diameter. It is usually solid, gray-white, and well-circumscribed. Microscopic examination reveals an admixture of germ cells and sex-cord stromal elements not arranged in nests, but instead having a trabecular, tubular, or haphazard infiltrative pattern. However, recent data question whether the germ cell component is neoplastic, in part due to the fact that the germ cells lack immunoreactivity for PLAP and CD-117 (124).

Miscellaneous Tumors

Tumors may arise within the rete testis, epididymis, and mesothelial lining of the tunica vaginalis, as well as the soft tissues surrounding the testicular hilum and spermatic cord. Hematopoietic tumors, as well as metastatic lesions, may also be encountered. These entities are beyond the scope of this chapter and the readers are directed to recent authoritative reviews on these subjects (43,47).

References

1. Trainer TD. Histology of the normal testis. *Am J Surg Pathol* 1987;11: 797–809.
2. Vilar O. Histology of the human testis from the neonatal period to adolescence. *Adv Exp Med Biol* 1970;10:95–111.
3. Aumuller G, Schulze C, Viebahn C. Intermediate filaments in Sertoli cells. *Microsc Res Tech* 1992;20:50–72.
4. Stosiek P, Kasper M, Karsten U. Expression of cytokeratins 8 and 18 in human Sertoli cells of immature and atrophic seminiferous tubules. *Differentiation* 1990;43:66–70.
5. Moore K, Persaud TVN. *The developing human.* Philadelphia, PA: WB Saunders, 1993.
6. Moore KL, Persaud TVN. *The developing human: clinically oriented embryology.* Philadelphia, PA: WB Saunders, 1998.
7. Trainer T. Testis and excretory duct system. In: Sternberg SS, ed. *Histology for pathologists.* Philadelphia, PA: Lippincott–Raven, 1997.
8. Schulze C. Sertoli cells and Leydig cells in man. *Adv Anat Embryol Cell Biol* 1984;88:1–104.
9. Nagano T, Otsuki I. Reinvestigation of the fine structure of Reinke's crystal in the human testicular interstitial cell. *J Cell Biol* 1971;51:148–161.
10. Davidoff MS, Schulze W, Middendorff R, et al. The Leydig cell of the human testis: a new member of the diffuse neuroendocrine system. *Cell Tissue Res* 1993;271:429–439.
11. Regadera J, Codesal J, Paniagua R, et al. Immunohistochemical and quantitative study of interstitial and intratubular Leydig cells in normal men, cryptorchidism, and Klinefelter's syndrome. *J Pathol* 1991;164:299–306.
12. Dinges HP, Zatloukal K, Schmid C, et al An immunohistochemical study: co-expression of cytokeratin and vimentin filaments in rete testis and epididymis. *Virchows Arch A Pathol Anat Histopathol* 1991;418:119–127.
13. Rolnick D, Kawanoue S, Szanto P, et al. Anatomical incidence of testicular appendages. *J Urol* 1968;100:755–756.
14. Srigley JR. The paratesticular region: histoanatomic and general considerations. *Semin Diagn Pathol* 2000;17:258–269.
15. Bosl GJ, Motzer RJ. Testicular germ-cell cancer. *N Engl J Med* 1997;337: 242–253.
16. Bosl GJ, Dmitrovsky E, Reuter VE, et al. Isochromosome of the short arm of chromosome 12: clinically useful markers for male germ cell tumors. *J Natl Cancer Inst* 1989;81:1874–1878.
17. Motzer RJ, Rodriguez E, Reuter VE, et al. Genetic analysis as an aid in diagnosis for patients with midline carcinomas of uncertain histologies. *J Natl Cancer Inst* 1991;83:341–346.
18. Mukherjee AB, Murty VV, Rodriguez E, et al. Detection and analysis of origin of i(12p), a diagnostic marker of human male germ cell tumors, by fluorescence in situ hybridization. *Genes Chromosomes Cancer* 1991;3:300–307.
19. Looijenga LH, Oosterhuis JW. Pathogenesis of testicular germ cell tumours. *Rev Reprod* 1999;4:90–100.
20. Oosterhuis JW, Looijenga LH. Current views on the pathogenesis of testicular germ cell tumours and perspectives for future research: highlights of the 5th Copenhagen Workshop on Carcinoma in situ and Cancer of the Testis. *Apmis* 2003;111:280–289.
21. Chaganti RS, Houldsworth J. Genetics and biology of adult human male germ cell tumors. *Cancer Res* 2000;60:1475–1482.
22. Dieckmann KP, Skakkebaek NE. Carcinoma in situ of the testis: review of biological and clinical features. *Int J Cancer* 1999;83:815–822.
23. Montironi R. Intratubular germ cell neoplasia of the testis: testicular intraepithelial neoplasia. *Eur Urol* 2002;41:651–654.
24. Gondos B, Berthelsen JG, Skakkebaek NE. Intratubular germ cell neoplasia (carcinoma in situ): a preinvasive lesion of the testis. *Ann Clin Lab Sci* 1983;13:185–192.
25. Skakkebaek NE. Atypical germ cells in the adjacent "normal" tissue of testicular tumours. *Acta Pathol Microbiol Scand [A]* 1975;83:127–130.
26. Skakkebaek NE. Carcinoma in situ of the testis: frequency and relationship to invasive germ cell tumours in infertile men. *Histopathology* 1978; 2:157–170; *Histopathology* 2002;41:2.
27. Skakkebaek NE. Carcinoma in situ of the testis: frequency and relationship to invasive germ cell tumours in infertile men. *Histopathology* 1978; 2:157–170.
28. Von der Maase H, Rorth M, Walbom-Jorgensen S, et al. Carcinoma in situ of contralateral testis in patients with testicular germ cell cancer: study of 27 cases in 500 patients. *Br Med J (Clin Res Ed)* 1986;293:1398–1401.
29. Von der Maase H, Meinecke B, Skakkebaek NE. Residual carcinoma-in-situ of contralateral testis after chemotherapy. *Lancet* 1988;1:477–478.
30. Jacobsen GK, Henriksen OB, von der Maase H. Carcinoma in situ of testicular tissue adjacent to malignant germ-cell tumors: a study of 105 cases. *Cancer* 1981;47:2660–2662.
31. Manivel JC, Simonton S, Wold LE, et al. A histochemical and immunohistochemical study: absence of intratubular germ cell neoplasia in testicular yolk sac tumors in children. *Arch Pathol Lab Med* 1988;112:641–645.
32. Hu LM, Phillipson J, Barsky SH. Intratubular germ cell neoplasia in infantile yolk sac tumor. Verification by tandem repeat sequence in situ hybridization. *Diagn Mol Pathol* 1992;1:118–128.
33. Manivel JC, Jessurun J, Wick MR, et al. Placental alkaline phosphatase immunoreactivity in testicular germ-cell neoplasms. *Am J Surg Pathol* 1987;11:21–29.

34. Wick MR, Swanson PE, Manivel JC. Placental-like alkaline phosphatase reactivity in human tumors: an immunohistochemical study of 520 cases. *Hum Pathol* 1987;18:946–954.
35. Burke AP, Mostofi FK. Intratubular malignant germ cells in testicular biopsies: clinical course and identification by staining for placental alkaline phosphatase. *Mod Pathol* 1988;1:475–479.
36. Giwercman A, Cantell L, Marks A. Placental-like alkaline phosphatase as a marker of carcinoma-in-situ of the testis: comparison with monoclonal antibodies M2A and 43-9F. *Apmis* 1991;99:586–594.
37. Leroy X, Augusto D, Leteurtre E, et al. CD30 and CD117 (c-kit) used in combination are useful for distinguishing embryonal carcinoma from seminoma. *J Histochem Cytochem* 2002;50:283–285.
38. Giwercman A, Lindenberg S, Kimber SJ, et al. Monoclonal antibody 43-9F as a sensitive immunohistochemical marker of carcinoma in situ of human testis. *Cancer* 1990;65:1135–1142.
39. Marks A, Sutherland DR, Bailey D, et al. Characterization and distribution of an oncofetal antigen (M2A antigen) expressed on testicular germ cell tumours. *Br J Cancer* 1999;80:569–578.
40. Looijenga LH, Stoop H, de Leeuw HP, et al. POU5F1 (OCT3/4) identifies cells with pluripotent potential in human germ cell tumors. *Cancer Res* 2003;63:2244–2250.
41. Mostofi FK, Sesterhenn I, Sobin LH. *Histological typing of testis tumours.* Berlin: Springer-Verlag, 1998.
42. Ulbright TM. Germ cell neoplasms of the testis. *Am J Surg Pathol* 1993; 17:1075–1091.
43. Ulbright TM, Amin MB, Young RH. Tumours of the testis, adnexa, spermatic cord, and scrotum. In: Rosai J, ed. *Atlas of tumor pathology.* Washington, DC: Armed Forces Institute of Pathology, 1999.
44. Ulbright TM. Testicular and paratesticular tumors. In: Sternberg SS, ed. *Diagnostic surgical pathology.* Philadelphia, PA: Lippincott Williams & Wilkins, 1999.
45. Jacobsen GK, von der Maase H, Specht L, et al. Histopathological features in stage I seminoma treated with orchiectomy only. *J Urol Pathol* 1995;3: 85–94.
46. Babaian RJ, Zagars GK. Testicular seminoma: the M. D. Anderson experience. An analysis of pathological and patient characteristics, and treatment recommendations. *J Urol* 1988;139:311–314.
47. Eble J, Sauter G, Epstein J, et al. *Pathology and genetics of tumours of the urinary system and male genital organs.* Lyon, France: IARC Press, 2004.
48. Ulbright TM. Morphologic variation in seminoma. *Am J Clin Pathol* 1994;102:395–396.
49. Jacobsen GK, Jacobsen M, Clausen PP. Distribution of tumor-associated antigens in the various histologic components of germ cell tumors of the testis. *Am J Surg Pathol* 1981;5:257–266.
50. Battifora H, Sheibani K, Tubbs RR, et al. Antikeratin antibodies in tumor diagnosis. Distinction between seminoma and embryonal carcinoma. *Cancer* 1984;54:843–848.
51. Jacobsen GK, Norgaard-Pedersen B, An immunohistochemical study: placental alkaline phosphatase in testicular germ cell tumours and in carcinoma-in-situ of the testis. *Acta Pathol Microbiol Immunol Scand [A]* 1984; 92:323–329.
52. Jacobsen GK, Jacobsen M. A prospective immunohistochemical study: alpha-fetoprotein (AFP) and human chorionic gonadotropin (HCG) in testicular germ cell tumours. *Acta Pathol Microbiol Immunol Scand [A]* 1983;91:165–176.
53. Mostofi FK, Sesterhenn IA, Davis CJ Jr. Immunopathology of germ tumors of the testis. *Semin Diagn Pathol* 1987;4:320–341.
54. Jacobsen GK. Histogenetic considerations concerning germ cell tumours: morphological and immunohistochemical comparative investigation of the human embryo and testicular germ cell tumours. *Virchows Arch A Pathol Anat Histopathol* 1986;408:509–525.
55. Eglen DE, Ulbright TM. The differential diagnosis of yolk sac tumor and seminoma: usefulness of cytokeratin, alpha-fetoprotein, and alpha-1-antitrypsin immunoperoxidase reactions. *Am J Clin Pathol* 1987;88: 328–332.
56. Jones TD, Ulbright TM, Eble JN, et al. OCT4 Staining in testicular tumors: a sensitive and specific marker for seminoma and embryonal carcinoma. *Am J Surg Pathol* 2004;28:935–940.
57. Niehans GA, Manivel JC, Copland GT, et al. Immunohistochemistry of germ cell and trophoblastic neoplasms. *Cancer* 1988;62:1113–1123.
58. Cockburn AG, Vugrin D, Batata M, et al. Poorly differentiated (anaplastic) seminoma of the testis. *Cancer* 1984;53:1991–1994.
59. Johnson DE, Gomez JJ, Ayala AG. Anaplastic seminoma. *J Urol* 1975; 114:80–82.
60. Von Hochstetter AR. Mitotic count in seminomas: an unreliable criterion for distinguishing between classical and anaplastic types. *Virchows Arch A Pathol Anat Histol* 1981;390:63–69.
61. Zuckman MH, Williams G, Levin HS. Mitosis counting in seminoma: an exercise of questionable significance. *Hum Pathol* 1988;19:329–335.
62. Denk H, Moll R, Weybora W, et al. Intermediate filaments and desmosomal plaque proteins in testicular seminomas and non-seminomatous germ cell tumours as revealed by immunohistochemistry. *Virchows Arch A Pathol Anat Histopathol* 1987;410:295–307.
63. Motzer RJ, Reuter VE, Cordon-Cardo C, et al. Blood group-related antigens in human germ cell tumors. *Cancer Res* 1988;48:5342–5347.

64. Srigley JR, Mackay B, Toth P, et al. The ultrastructure and histogenesis of male germ neoplasia with emphasis on seminoma with early carcinomatous features. *Ultrastruct Pathol* 1988;12:67–86.

65. Raghavan D, Heyderman E, Monaghan P, et al. Hypothesis: when is a seminoma not a seminoma? *J Clin Pathol* 1981;34:123–128.

66. Walt H, Arrenbrecht S, DeLozier-Blanchet CD, et al. A human testicular germ cell tumor with borderline histology between seminoma and embryonal carcinoma secreted beta-human chorionic gonadotropin and alpha-fetoprotein only as a xenograft. *Cancer* 1986;58:139–146.

67. Mostofi FK, Price EB. *Tumors of the male genital system*. Washington, DC: Armed Forces Institute of Pathology, 1973.

68. Mostofi FK. Pathology of germ cell tumors of testis: a progress report. *Cancer* 1980;45:1735–1754.

69. Tickoo SK, Hutchinson B, Bacik J, et al. Testicular seminoma: a clinicopathologic and immunohistochemical study of 105 cases with special reference to seminomas with atypical features. *Int J Surg Pathol* 2002;10:23–32.

70. Czaja JT, Ulbright TM. Evidence for the transformation of seminoma to yolk sac tumor, with histogenetic considerations. *Am J Clin Pathol* 1992;97:468–477.

71. Talerman A. Spermatocytic seminoma: clinicopathological study of 22 cases. *Cancer* 1980;45:2169–2176.

72. Eble JN. Spermatocytic seminoma. *Hum Pathol* 1994;25:1035–1042.

73. Floyd C, Ayala AG, Logothetis CJ, et al. Spermatocytic seminoma with associated sarcoma of the testis. *Cancer* 1988;61:409–414.

74. True LD, Otis CN, Rosai J, et al. Spermatocytic seminoma of testis with sarcomatous transformation. *Am J Surg Pathol* 1988;12:806.

75. Kraggerud SM, Berner A, Bryne M, et al. Spermatocytic seminoma as compared to classical seminoma: an immunohistochemical and DNA flow cytometric study. *Apmis* 1999;107:297–302.

76. Latza U, Foss HD, Durkop H, et al. CD30 antigen in embryonal carcinoma and embryogenesis and release of the soluble molecule. *Am J Pathol* 1995;146:463–471.

77. Ulbright TM, Goheen MP, Roth LM, et al. A light and electron microscopic study: the differentiation of carcinomas of teratomatous origin from embryonal carcinoma. *Cancer* 1986;57:257–263.

78. Ulbright TM, Roth LM, Brodhecker CA. Yolk sac differentiation in germ cell tumors: a morphologic study of 50 cases with emphasis on hepatic, enteric, and parietal yolk sac features. *Am J Surg Pathol* 1986;10:151–164.

79. Krag Jacobsen G, Barlebo H, Olsen J, et al. Testicular germ cell tumours in Denmark 1976–1980: pathology of 1058 consecutive cases. *Acta Radiol Oncol* 1984;23:239–247.

80. Ulbright TM, Loehrer PJ. Choriocarcinoma-like lesions in patients with testicular germ cell tumors: two histologic variants. *American Journal of Surgical Pathology* 1988;12:531–541.

81. Ulbright TM, Roth LM. A pathologic analysis of lesions following modern chemotherapy for metastatic germ-cell tumors. *Pathol Annu* 1990;25(Pt 1):313–340.

82. Ulbright TM, Young RH, Scully RE. Trophoblastic tumors of the testis other than classic choriocarcinoma: "monophasic" choriocarcinoma and placental site trophoblastic tumor: a report of two cases. *American Journal of Surgical Pathology* 1997;21:282–288.

83. Ulbright TM, Loehrer PJ, Roth LM, et al. The development of non-germ cell malignancies within germ cell tumors. A clinicopathologic study of 11 cases. *Cancer* 1984;54:1824–1833.

84. Motzer RJ, Amsterdam A, Prieto V, et al. Teratoma with malignant transformation: diverse malignant histologies arising in men with germ cell tumors. *J Urol* 1998;159:133–138.

85. Ahlgren AD, Simrell CR, Triche TJ, et al. Sarcoma arising in a residual testicular teratoma after cytoreductive chemotherapy. *Cancer* 1984;54:2015–2018.

86. Ahmed T, Bosl GJ, Hajdu SI. Teratoma with malignant transformation in germ cell tumors in men. *Cancer* 1985;56:860–863.

87. Michael H, Ulbright TM, Brodhecker CA. The pluripotential nature of the mesenchyme-like component of yolk sac tumor. *Arch Pathol Lab Med* 1989;113:1115–1119.

88. Malek RS, Rosen JS, Farrow GM. Epidermoid cyst of the testis: a critical analysis. *Br J Urol* 1986;58:55–59.

89. Price EB Jr. Epidermoid cysts of the testis: a clinical and pathologic analysis of 69 cases from the testicular tumor registry. *J Urol* 1969;102:708–713.

90. Younger C, Ulbright TM, Zhang S, et al. Molecular evidence supporting the neoplastic nature of some epidermoid cysts of the testis. *Arch Pathol Lab Med* 2003;127:858–860.

91. Ulbright TM, Srigley JR. Dermoid cyst of the testis: a study of five postpubertal cases, including a pilomatrixoma-like variant, with evidence supporting its separate classification from mature testicular teratoma. *Am J Surg Pathol* 2001;25:788–793.

92. Azzopardi JG, Mostofi FK, Theiss EA. Lesions of testes observed in certain patients with widespread choriocarcinoma and related tumors: the significance and genesis of hematoxylin-staining bodies in the human testis. *Am J Pathol* 1961;38:207–225.

93. Azzopardi JG, Hoffbrand AV. Retrogression in testicular seminoma with viable metastases. *J Clin Pathol* 1965;18:135–141.

94. Meares EM Jr, Briggs EM. Occult seminoma of the testis masquerading as primary extragonadal germinal neoplasms. *Cancer* 1972;30:300–306.

95. Sesterhenn IA, Weiss RB, Mostofi FK, et al. Prognosis and other clinical correlates of pathologic review in stage I and II testicular carcinoma: a report from the Testicular Cancer Intergroup Study. *J Clin Oncol* 1992;10:69–78.

96. Sogani PC, Perrotti M, Herr HW, et al. Clinical stage I testis cancer: long-term outcome of patients on surveillance. *J Urol* 1998;159:855–858.

97. Albers P, Siener R, Kliesch S, et al. Risk factors for relapse in clinical stage I nonseminomatous testicular germ cell tumors: results of the German Testicular Cancer Study Group Trial. *J Clin Oncol* 2003;21:1505–1512.

98. Kim I, Young RH, Scully RE. Leydig cell tumors of the testis: a clinicopathological analysis of 40 cases and review of the literature. *Am J Surg Pathol* 1985;9:177–192.

99. Lawrence WD, Young RH, Scully RE. Sex cord-stromal tumors. In: Talerman A, Roth LM, eds. *Pathology of the testis and its adnexa*. New York: Churchill Livingstone, 1986.

100. Cheville JC. Classification and pathology of testicular germ cell and sex cord-stromal tumors. *Urol Clin North Am* 1999;26:595–609.

101. Billings SD, Roth LM, Ulbright TM. Microcystic Leydig cell tumors mimicking yolk sac tumor: a report of four cases. *Am J Surg Pathol* 1999;23:546–551.

102. Ulbright TM, Srigley JR, Hatzianastassiou DK, et al. Leydig cell tumors of the testis with unusual features: adipose differentiation, calcification with ossification, and spindle-shaped tumor cells. *Am J Surg Pathol* 2002;26:1424–1433.

103. Augusto D, Leteurtre E, De La Taille A, et al. Calretinin: a valuable marker of normal and neoplastic Leydig cells of the testis. *Appl Immunohistochem Mol Morphol* 2002;10:159–162.

104. Zheng W, Senturk BZ, Parkash V. Inhibin immunohistochemical staining: a practical approach for the surgical pathologist in the diagnoses of ovarian sex cord-stromal tumors. *Adv Anat Pathol* 2003;10:27–38.

105. Cobellis L, Cataldi P, Reis FM, et al. Gonadal malignant germ cell tumors express immunoreactive inhibin/activin subunits. *Eur J Endocrinol* 2001;145:779–784.

106. Iczkowski KA, Bostwick DG, Roche PC, et al. Inhibin A is a sensitive and specific marker for testicular sex cord-stromal tumors. *Mod Pathol* 1998;11:774–779.

107. Cheville JC, Sebo TJ, Lager DJ, et al. Leydig cell tumor of the testis: a clinicopathologic, DNA content, and MIB-1 comparison of nonmetastasizing and metastasizing tumors. *Am J Surg Pathol* 1998;22:1361–1367.

108. Rutgers JL, Young RH, Scully RE. The testicular "tumor" of the adrenogenital syndrome: a report of six cases and review of the literature on testicular masses in patients with adrenocortical disorders. *Am J Surg Pathol* 1988;12:503–513.

109. Young RH, Talerman A. Testicular tumors other than germ cell tumors. *Semin Diagn Pathol* 1987;4:342–360.

110. Young RH, Koelliker DD, Scully RE. Sertoli cell tumors of the testis, not otherwise specified: a clinicopathologic analysis of 60 cases. *Am J Surg Pathol* 1998;22:709–721.

111. Cantu JM, Rivera H, Ocampo-Campos R, et al. Peutz-Jeghers syndrome with feminizing Sertoli cell tumor. *Cancer* 1980;46:223–228.

112. Krag Jacobsen G. Malignant Sertoli cell tumors of the testis. *J Urol Pathol* 1993;1:233–255.

113. Proppe KH, Scully RE. Large-cell calcifying Sertoli cell tumor of the testis. *Am J Clin Pathol* 1980;74:607–619.

114. Proppe KH, Dickersin GR. Large-cell calcifying Sertoli cell tumor of the testis: light microscopic and ultrastructural study. *Hum Pathol* 1982;13:1109–1114.

115. Kratzer SS, Ulbright TM, Talerman A, et al. Large cell calcifying Sertoli cell tumor of the testis: contrasting features of six malignant and six benign tumors and a review of the literature. *Am J Surg Pathol* 1997;21:1271–1280.

116. Wang BY, Rabinowitz DS, Granato RC Sr, et al. Gonadal tumor with granulosa cell tumor features in an adult testis. *Ann Diagn Pathol* 2002;6:56–60.

117. Mostofi FK, Theiss EA, Ashley DJ. Tumors of specialized gonadal stroma in human male patients: androblastoma, Sertoli cell tumor, granulosa-theca cell tumor of the testis, and gonadal stromal tumor. *Cancer* 1959;12:944–957.

118. Lawrence WD, Young RH, Scully RE. Juvenile granulosa cell tumor of the infantile testis. A report of 14 cases. *Am J Surg Pathol* 1985;9:87–94.

119. Young RH, Lawrence WD, Scully RE. Juvenile granulosa cell tumor—another neoplasm associated with abnormal chromosomes and ambiguous genitalia: a report of three cases. *Am J Surg Pathol* 1985;9:737–743.

120. Fagin R, Berbescu E, Landis S, et al. Juvenile granulosa cell tumor of the testis. *Urology* 2003;62:351.

121. Scully RE. Gonadoblastoma: a review of 74 cases. *Cancer* 1970;25:1340–1356.

122. Talerman A. A distinctive gonadal neoplasm related to gonadoblastoma. *Cancer* 1972;30:1219–1224.

123. Bolen JW. Mixed germ cell-sex cord stromal tumor: a gonadal tumor distinct from gonadoblastoma. *Am J Clin Pathol* 1981;75:565–573.

124. Ulbright TM, Srigley JR, Reuter VE, et al. Sex cord-stromal tumors of the testis with entrapped germ cells: a lesion mimicking unclassified mixed germ cell sex cord-stromal tumors. *Am J Surg Pathol* 2000;24:535–542.

CHAPTER 35 ■ STAGING AND IMAGING OF TESTIS CANCER

GRAEME S. STEELE, PHILIP KANTOFF, AND JEROME P. RICHIE

Testis cancer is a relatively rare tumor, accounting for 1% to 2% of all neoplasms in males, with an incidence of approximately 3 cases per 100,000. It is the most common malignancy in men in the 15- to 35-year age group and the second most common tumor in the 35- to 39-year group (1). Approximately 7,400 new cases of testis cancer were diagnosed in the United States in 1999 (2). In the United States, the incidence of testis cancer has gradually increased since the 1930s, due mainly to an increased incidence among white men (3). Moreover, a clear trend toward an increase in the incidence of testis tumors in the last 30 years in the majority of industrialized countries has been observed (4). Despite this, surprising differences in the incidence between neighboring countries have been reported: Finland 2.5/100,000 cases versus Denmark 9.2/100,000 cases.

Testis cancer is also one of the most curable solid neoplasms, and thus it can serve as a model for multimodal treatment of malignancies. Long-term survival rates of approximately 90% can be expected across all stages, and survival rates approaching 100% should be seen for low-stage disease. With such effective treatment available, the trend is to reduce the morbidity of therapy by a variety of techniques, including placing patients on surveillance protocols or reducing the amount and toxicity of chemotherapy. Accurate radiologic imaging plays an important role in clinical staging, in decisions to manage patients conservatively, and in patient surveillance. In this regard, the practitioner must be aware of the limitations of currently used imaging techniques.

EVALUATION OF THE TESTICULAR MASS

History

As with any illness, the staging and workup of a patient with a testicular mass begins with a thorough history. Although the usual presentation of a testis tumor is a palpable nodule, painless swelling, or testicular hardness, some patients complain of vague scrotal discomfort or a heaviness in the scrotum. Acute scrotal pain is the presenting complaint in approximately 10% of patients. Although up to one third of patients have metastases at presentation (5), symptoms attributable to metastatic disease are present in only 10%. Metastatic disease may be manifested as a palpable neck mass (supraclavicular adenopathy), gastrointestinal pain (bulky intraabdominal disease), lumbar back pain (retroperitoneal disease involving psoas muscle or nerve roots or both), bone pain (skeletal metastases), or central nervous system manifestations (central nervous system metastases). Approximately 5% of men have gynecomastia, resulting from either secretion of beta-human chorionic gonadotropin (beta-hCG), decreased androgen production, or increased estrogen production.

Crucial in the history is duration of symptoms. Delay in diagnosis is the rule rather than the exception in testis cancer, whether it be from patient fear or denial, or from misdiagnosis by the physician. Delay in diagnosis has been reported to correlate with stage at presentation (5) and with mortality (6). The need clearly exists for patient education through public health programs to emphasize the importance of testicular self-examination. Physician-related delays in diagnosis could also be reduced through continuing physician education; the greatest difficulty in making the diagnosis of a testis tumor seems to be in bringing the possibility of the diagnosis into one's mind (7).

Physical Examination

Physical examination of the testis begins with examination of the normal contralateral gonad. Careful palpation using the thumb and first two fingers of the examining hand gives a baseline of relative size and consistency. In the suspected testis, any firm or fixed area within the tunica albuginea should be considered suspicious for cancer until proved otherwise. Potential involvement of the epididymis, spermatic cord, or scrotal skin should also be assessed. A hydrocele may be present, which can make examination of the testis difficult or impossible. Scrotal masses should always be transilluminated.

The examination should also include abdominal palpation for bulky nodal disease, as well as inspection and auscultation of the chest for gynecomastia or intrathoracic disease. Palpation of the supraclavicular fossae may reveal adenopathy if the disease is advanced.

Differential Diagnosis

Included in the differential diagnosis of a testicular mass are epididymitis, epididymo-orchitis, and testicular torsion. Other less common entities include hernia or hydrocele, spermatocele, hematoma, and paratesticular masses. However, a firm, intratesticular mass should always be considered cancer until proved otherwise.

TESTICULAR IMAGING

Ultrasonography

Scrotal ultrasonography can sometimes be considered an extension of the physical examination. It is relatively easy to obtain in most centers, is noninvasive, and is inexpensive. The many indications for scrotal ultrasonography include evaluation of testicular masses, hydroceles, and varicoceles, as well as evaluation of extratesticular masses. Color Doppler ultrasonography has made possible the assessment of scrotal blood flow, which enables the sonographer to make specific diagnoses in cases of acute scrotal pain (8). When high-frequency transducers (5 to 10 MHz) are used, intratesticular lesions as small as 1 mm to 2 mm can confidently be identified. Intratesticular lesions can also be distinguished from extratesticular lesions with a high degree of accuracy; the sensitivity for tumor detection is likewise near 100% (9). Scrotal ultrasonography should always be performed whenever malignancy is suspected and whenever the presence of a hydrocele prohibits adequate testicular examination. A definite clinical impression of a testicular mass, however, can sometimes make the use of scrotal ultrasonography unnecessary.

The use of scrotal ultrasonography to determine the histology of a testis tumor has been investigated by a number of authors. Generally, seminomas have the most characteristic echo pattern, but the ultrasonographic scan is certainly not pathognomonic. Seminomas are characterized as well-defined, intratesticular, hypoechoic lesions without cystic areas (Fig. 35.1); 65% to 85% of seminomas demonstrate this pattern (10–13). In Benson's study, no cystic areas were identified, and only one of the 11 seminomas had a bright focus with shadowing, which suggested calcification (9). Likewise, Schwerk et al. found no echogenic foci and only rare, small cystic areas in 20 seminomas (11).

Nonseminomatous tumors, however, are characterized by the inhomogeneity of their echo patterns. These tumors may be hypoechoic, hyperechoic, or isoechoic. Calcification and cysts are common, and the border may be irregular and difficult to define (9–12). Reliably distinguishing among the different histologic types of nonseminomatous tumors using ultrasonography is nearly impossible. Marth et al. however, were able to correctly distinguish seminomatous from nonseminomatous tumors in 35 of 51 tumors studied (12).

Attempts have also been made to stage locally the primary tumor by ultrasonography. The tunica albuginea of the testis is not visualized by ultrasonography, and thus local invasion of this structure by the tumor may be difficult to appreciate. Seminomas, because of their well-defined border, are somewhat easier to stage, but results are still poor, with the correct stage being assigned in only 45% of cases (12,13). Nonseminomatous tumors are virtually impossible to stage by ultrasonography. In the study by Marth et al. the correct stage was

assigned to these tumors only 8% of the time (12). Although scrotal ultrasonography is often indispensable in the workup of a testicular mass, it cannot replace surgical intervention and pathologic scrutiny for histologic diagnosis and primary tumor staging.

Magnetic Resonance Imaging

As medical technology has rapidly advanced, magnetic resonance imaging (MRI) has become increasingly available. It should not be considered routine in the workup of a testicular mass, and its precise role has yet to be defined. With the use of a surface coil and scanning in the coronal plane, excellent images of the intrascrotal contents can be obtained. The coronal plane is preferred because both testes, as well as the epididymides and spermatic cords, are seen. Also, the coil is parallel to the imaging plane, so no signal dropout occurs (13,14). Other scanning planes can be used as needed.

In MRI, the normal testis is homogeneous in signal by both T1-weighted and T2-weighted imaging. Unlike in ultrasonography, the tunica albuginea can be easily identified with MRI. Relative to the normal testicular parenchyma, tumors are usually hypointense on T2-weighted images and show brisk and early enhancement after intravenous administration of gadolinium (15) (Fig. 35.2). On T1-weighted images, distinguishing intratesticular pathology can be very difficult. As with ultrasonography, seminomas are found to be mostly homogeneous but may have hyperintense foci. A pseudocapsule is sometimes visible around the tumor. Nonseminomatous tumors, in contrast, are markedly heterogeneous (Fig. 35.3). They may be isointense or hyperintense with hypointense foci. Differentiation of tumor types with MRI is difficult at best, and assessment of the primary tumor stage is problematic (13,14). In a study by Thurnher et al. the correct stage was assigned only 63% of the time (13). In terms of knowledge to be gained and cost, ultrasonography is the preferred imaging modality for suspected testis tumors at this time. If the ultrasonographic study is inconclusive or if the ultrasonographic

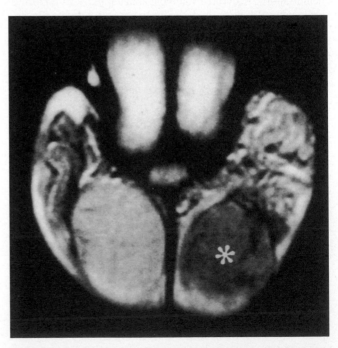

FIGURE 35.2. T2-weighted magnetic resonance image. Asterisk demonstrates tumor (seminoma). Note the decreased signal intensity of tumor. (Reprinted with permission from Hricak H, Carrington BM, eds. *MRI of the pelvis: A text atlas.* London: Martin Dunitz, 1994.)

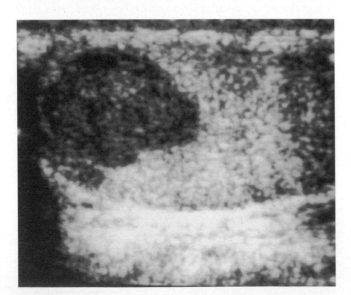

FIGURE 35.1. Ultrasonographic appearance of testis seminoma.

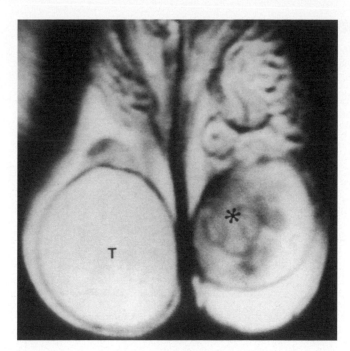

FIGURE 35.3. T2-weighted magnetic resonance image. Asterisk demonstrates tumor (nonseminoma). Note the heterogeneous signal intensity of tumor. (T, normal contralateral testis.) (Reprinted with permission from Hricak H, Carrington BM, eds. *MRI of the pelvis: A text atlas.* London: Martin Dunitz, 1994.)

results and the physical findings are discrepant, MRI can be used.

TUMOR MARKERS

A more detailed discussion of tumor markers in testis cancer can be found in Chapter 52. A brief discussion is necessary here, however, because measurement of marker levels is an integral part of the staging of testis tumors. The two most important markers are beta-hCG and alpha-fetoprotein (AFP). Others, such as lactate dehydrogenase (LDH) and placental-like alkaline phosphatase (PLAP), have more limited use at this time.

The marker beta-hCG is elevated in 40% to 60% of patients with testis cancer. All patients with choriocarcinoma have an elevated beta-hCG, as do 50% of patients with embryonal cell carcinoma and 10% to 25% of patients with pure seminoma. The serum half-life is 24 to 36 hours. If levels fail to decline as predicted by this half-life after orchiectomy, residual disease is practically a certainty. Also, a normal level does not necessarily imply absence of disease (16).

AFP level is elevated in 50% to 70% of patients with testis tumors. Embryonal cell carcinomas and yolk sac tumors both cause elevated AFP levels (12). Pure seminoma and choriocarcinoma do not. The half-life of AFP is 5 to 7 days. Again, post-orchiectomy levels should be monitored to determine if the AFP level is declining with the appropriate kinetics. As with beta-HCG, a normal level of AFP does not guarantee the absence of disease (16).

Other tumor markers used for testis cancer include LDH and PLAP. LDH (especially isoenzyme 1) is not specific for histologic type, and its degree of elevation correlates with the bulk of disease. In addition, rising levels of LDH are an accurate indicator of disease relapse. Serum levels of LDH-1 have correlated with the number of copies of chromosome arm 12p, which is often amplified in testis tumors (17). The LDH

gene is located on chromosome 12 (17). The sensitivity and specificity are limited, and therefore the clinical usefulness is also limited. Similarly, PLAP, expressed in fetal germ cells and in children younger than 1 year of age, is elevated in only 30% to 50% of low-stage seminomas. A greater percentage of patients with advanced seminoma have an elevated PLAP level. False-positive elevations of PLAP have occurred in smokers and in patients with other malignancies, such as breast, lung, or ovarian cancer (18).

Tumor marker levels should be measured during the initial evaluation of a patient with a testis mass and then remeasured at appropriate intervals after orchiectomy. This information, together with the pathologic and radiographic information, determines the course of therapy.

HISTOPATHOLOGY AND PROGNOSTIC SIGNIFICANCE

After a testicular mass has been identified by physical examination or ultrasonographic study and tumor markers have been tested, the patient must undergo a radical inguinal orchiectomy with early clamping of the spermatic cord. The orchiectomy specimen must be analyzed carefully by the pathologist because the local tumor stage and histologic findings have prognostic significance. The extent of the primary tumor can be staged according to the tumor, node, metastasis (TNM) system, as described by the American Joint Committee on Cancer (Table 35.1) (19). Histologic type can be divided initially into seminoma or nonseminoma. Nonseminomatous tumors can be further divided into embryonal carcinoma, teratoma, yolk sac tumor, choriocarcinoma, or a combination of types. Note that the mixture of embryonal carcinoma and teratoma is sometimes designated as teratocarcinoma.

In nonseminomatous tumors, the presence of certain elements within the primary tumor specimen have been found to place the patient at higher risk for having positive retroperitoneal lymph nodes or for relapsing in the retroperitoneum if placed on surveillance protocols. Rodriguez et al. retrospectively reviewed 120 patients (stages A through B3), all of whom underwent retroperitoneal lymph node dissection (RPLND) after radical orchiectomy. They demonstrated that increased primary stage (pT2 or greater) and the presence of vascular invasion in the orchiectomy specimen were highly predictive of disseminated disease (20). In a similar study, Fung et al. reviewed 60 patients who underwent RPLND for clinical stage I disease. Vascular invasion was again correlated with a higher likelihood of nodal disease, as was pathologic stage pT2 or greater. They also demonstrated that a high percentage (more than 50%) of teratoma in the primary specimen was protective against disseminated disease (21). A large study from the Swedish-Norwegian Testicular Cancer Group confirmed the importance of vascular invasion as a predictor for retroperitoneal disease. They noted the apparent protective benefit of teratoma or yolk sac elements in the primary tumor (22). More recently, the presence and percentage volume (greater than 30%) of embryonal carcinoma in the specimen have been added to the list of adverse prognostic features (22–26). Patients with these characteristics are therefore at greater risk for retroperitoneal disease.

Further assessment of the primary tumor with newer methods of molecular biology and cytogenetics may become prognostically significant in the near future. Cytogenetically, more than 80% of testicular tumors demonstrate an isochromosome of 12p [i(12p)]. In a report in 1989, Bosl et al. found that the copy number of i(12p) correlated with survival in patients with testis germ cell tumors (GCTs) (27). More recently, however, deGraaff et al. were unable to confirm the prognostic significance of such gross chromosomal changes (28). More subtle

TABLE 35.1

TESTICULAR CANCER STAGING SYSTEM OF THE AMERICAN JOINT COMMITTEE ON CANCER AND THE INTERNATIONAL UNION AGAINST CANCER: DEFINITION OF TUMOR, NODE, METASTASIS (TNM) SYSTEM

Primary tumor (T)	Description
pTX	Primary tumor cannot be assessed (if no radical orchiectomy has been performed, TX is used)
pT0	No evidence of primary tumor (e.g., histologic scar in testis)
pTis	Intratubular germ cell neoplasia (carcinoma *in situ*)
pT1	Tumor limited to the testis and epididymis and no vascular/lymphatic invasion. Tumor may invade the tunica albuginea but not the tunica vaginalis
pT2	Tumor limited to the testis and epididymis with vascular/lymphatic invasion or tumor extending through the tunica albuginea with involvement of tunica vaginalis
pT3	Tumor invades the spermatic cord with or without vascular/lymphatic invasion
pT4	Tumor invades the scrotum with or without vascular/lymphatic invasion

Regional lymph nodes (N)

Clinical

NX	Regional lymph nodes cannot be assessed
N0	No regional lymph node metastasis
N1	Lymph node mass 2 cm or less in greatest dimension; or multiple lymph node masses, none more than 2 cm in greatest dimension.
N2	Lymph node mass, more than 2 cm but not more than 5 cm in greatest dimension; or multiple lymph node masses, any one mass greater than 2 cm but not more than 5 cm in greatest dimension
N3	Lymph node mass more than 5 cm in greatest dimension

Pathologic

pN0	No evidence of tumor in lymph nodes
pN1	Lymph node mass, 2 cm or less in greatest dimension and ≤5 nodes positive, none >2 cm in greatest dimension
pN2	Lymph node mass, more than 2 cm but not more than 5 cm in greatest dimension; more than 5 nodes positive, none >5 cm; evidence of extranodal extension of tumor
pN3	Lymph node mass more than 5 cm in greatest dimension; more than 5 nodes positive, none >5 cm; evidence of extranodal extension of tumor

Distant metastases (M)

M0	No evidence of distant metastases
M1	Nonregional nodal or pulmonary metastases
M2	Nonpulmonary visceral metastases

Serum tumor markers (S)	LDH	hCG (mIU/mL)	AFP (ng/mL)
S0	≤N	≤N	≤N
S1	<1.5 N	<5,000	<1,000
S2	1.5–10 N	5,000–50,000	1,000–10,000
S3	>10 N	>50,000	>10,000

	Testis cancer			
Stage grouping	T	N	M	S
Stage 0	pTis	N0	M0	S0
Stage I	T1–T4	N0	M0	SX
IA	T1	N0	M0	S0
IB	T2	N0	M0	S0
	T3	N0	M0	S0
	T4	N0	M0	S0
IS	Any T	N0	M0	S1–3
Stage II	Any T	Any N	M0	SX
IIA	Any T	N1	M0	S0
	Any T	N1	M0	S1
IIB	Any T	N2	M0	S1
IIC	Any T	N3	M0	S0
	Any T	N3	M0	S1
Stage III	Any T	Any N	M1	SX
IIIA	Any T	Any N	M1	S0
	Any T	Any N	M1	S1
IIIB	Any T	Any N	M0	S2
	Any T	Any N	M1	S2
IIC	Any T	Any N	M0	S3
	Any T	Any N	M1a	S3
	Any T	Any N	M1b	Any S

AFP, alpha-fetoprotein; hCG, human chorionic gonadotropin; LDH, lactate dehydrogenase; N, upper limit of normal for the LDH assay.

changes, however, such as homogeneously staining regions, aberrantly banded regions, and double minutes, have been found more frequently in metastatic tumors (29).

Vergouwe et al. performed a meta-analysis of 23 publications involving 2,587 patients with a clinical stage I nonseminomatous germ cell tumor (NSGCT). Overall the 29.3% of patients had occult metastatic disease. The strongest predictor of metastatic disease was vascular invasion. In addition, immunohistochemical staining of primary tumor cells with MIB-1 monoclonal antibody showing proliferative activity was reported to be a promising predictor (30).

Loss-of-heterozygosity studies, which have been instrumental in identifying tumor suppressor genes in other tumors, have been performed on testis tumors. Two regions on the long arm of chromosome 12 (12q13 and 12q22) have demonstrated frequent loss of heterozygosity in testis cancers (31), but this finding has not been correlated with the stage of disease.

Flow cytometry studies have been used in an attempt at further prognostication. Because a high percentage of testis tumors have aneuploid stem lines, this finding in general has added little prognostic information (25,32), although at least one report has suggested that tumors with highly aneuploid stem lines or multiple aneuploid stem lines do have a worse prognosis (32). Mean percentage of S phase of the aneuploid cell lines and proliferative index have also been demonstrated to be significant for prediction of stage by univariate analysis. The association was lost by multivariate analysis (33). In those rare cases of stage I tumors with no aneuploid stem lines, the risk of relapse or recurrence is probably low (34).

Currently, the most reliable prognostic factors that can be assessed from the primary tumor are the local stage, the presence of vascular or lymphatic invasion, and the presence and percentage of embryonal carcinoma. Newer methods and markers show promise but are still in need of further investigation.

RETROPERITONEAL STAGING

After orchiectomy and evaluation of the primary tumor, the staging workup for metastatic disease commences. Testis GCTs metastasize predominantly through the lymphatic system, although vascular dissemination may occur, especially with choriocarcinoma. Donohue et al. elegantly defined the primary landing sites for right-sided and left-sided tumors after analysis of 275 specimens from RPLND. For right-sided tumors, the primary landing zones are the interaortocaval region, the precaval zone, and the paraaortic zone, in that order. More cross-metastases are seen in patients with right-sided tumors because of the drainage from right to left. In patients with left-sided tumors, the primary landing zones are the paraaortic and preaortic regions, with the interaortocaval zone involved in higher-stage disease (35) (Figs. 35.4 and 35.5). Iliac nodal involvement may be seen if the primary tumor has invaded the epididymis or spermatic cord, and inguinal metastases may be seen if the tunica albuginea has been invaded or the normal lymphatic flow has been disrupted from previous surgery. Suprahilar or retrocrural nodal involvement is seen primarily in advanced disease. Pulmonary, liver, central nervous system, and bone metastases may be seen late in the course of the disease.

Lymphangiography

Before the development of computed tomography (CT), the retroperitoneum was assessed primarily by physical examination, bipedal lymphangiography, and intravenous pyelography. Lymphangiography can identify abnormal architecture in normal-size lymph nodes but is rarely used today, with the

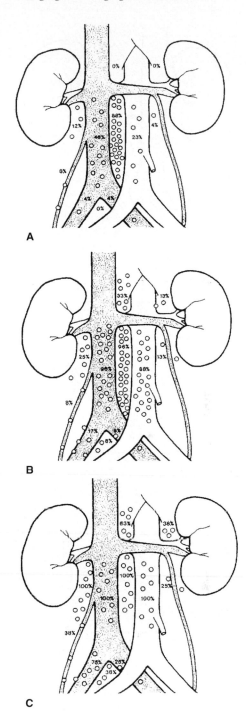

FIGURE 35.4. Mapping of metastatic landing zones for right-sided tumors. **A:** Stage B1. **B:** Stage B2. **C:** Stage B3. (Reprinted with permission from Donohue JP, Zachary JM, Maynard BR. Distribution of nodal metastases in nonseminomatous testis cancer. *J Urol* 1982;128: 315–320.)

exception of some centers where lymphangiography is used to define the limits of the radiation field in seminoma patients.

Ultrasonography

Ultrasonography has also been used to stage the retroperitoneum in testis cancer patients. Certainly less invasive and with less attendant morbidity than lymphangiography, ultrasonography is similarly accurate. One limitation of ultrasonographic staging of

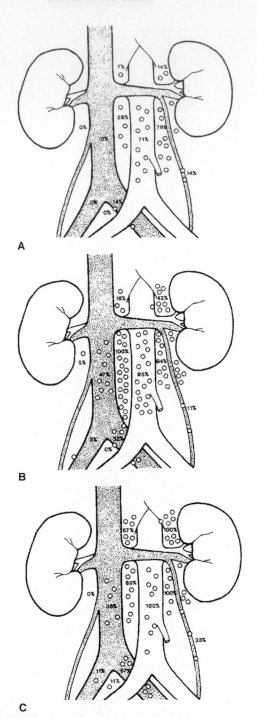

FIGURE 35.5. Mapping of metastatic landing zones for left-sided tumors. **A:** Stage B1. **B:** Stage B2. **C:** Stage B3. (Reprinted with permission from Donohue JP, Zachary JM, Maynard BR. Distribution of nodal metastases in nonseminomatous testis cancer. *J Urol* 1982;128: 315–320.)

the retroperitoneum is that 2% to 10% of the examinations are inadequate because of overlying bowel gas or patient obesity. Ultrasonography is also substantially operator dependent (9). In general, ultrasonography is highly accurate for bulky disease, with an accuracy of approximately 90%, but it is significantly less reliable for lower-stage disease, with an accuracy of 60% for nodes in the 2.0-cm to 2.5-cm range (36). Schwerk et al. noted an overall accuracy of 96%, but most patients in their series had bulky disease (11). Probably a more reasonable overall accuracy to be expected from this modality is 70% to

80% (36–38). As expected, the examination tends to understage patients, and ultrasonography is thus not recommended for retroperitoneal staging.

Computed Tomography

CT scanning is currently the imaging modality of choice for the retroperitoneum, although it is not perfect. Like other radiologic examinations, CT cannot detect micrometastases in the lymph nodes. As a result, a significant false-negative rate is always seen in staging with CT. Richie et al. reported a false-negative rate of 44% (39), and McLeod et al. reported a 59% false-negative rate (24). The arbitrary assignment of a nodal size that is to be considered abnormal can have significant implications. Socinski and Stomper, in a study of 51 patients, noted that when a cutoff of 5 mm was used to designate an abnormal node, the negative predictive value increased to 79%. However, this lowered the specificity of the test to 44%. When a cutoff of 15 mm was used, the negative predictive value was only 63%, but the specificity increased to 76% (40). If the lower criterion were used, more patients would thus be considered to have higher-stage disease and would perhaps undergo unnecessary therapy. If the higher cutoff were used, the false-negative rate would be higher, and patients with retroperitoneal disease would not receive therapy until their disease was more obvious and possibly at a higher, less curable stage. This problem has far-reaching implications, especially at a time when surveillance protocols are becoming more popular.

A number of reports have been published on the accuracy of CT determined by pathologic correlation after RPLND. The best results give an accuracy of 85% to 90%, with a sensitivity of approximately 90% and a specificity of 80% to 85% (41,42). Most reports, however, give slightly lower accuracies (70% to 80%) and sensitivities (50% to 70%), but similar specificities (24,36,39,43,44). The differences are probably due to different prevalence of higher-stage patients in each study population, as well as the cutoff size used for an abnormal node. Newer generations of scanners and techniques, such as spiral CT, should make this modality more accurate, but until micrometastases can be detected, a significant false-negative rate should be expected. Also, CT scanning cannot distinguish residual tumor from teratoma or fibrosis in patients with residual masses after chemotherapy (45) (Fig. 35.6).

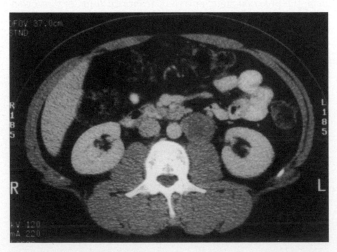

FIGURE 35.6. Computed tomography (CT) scan demonstrating large left paraaortic mass in patient with left-sided nonseminomatous tumor after chemotherapy. Pathologic study after retroperitoneal lymph node dissection revealed fibrosis.

Magnetic Resonance Imaging

With current techniques, MRI offers no advantage over CT for imaging and staging of the retroperitoneum in patients with testis cancer. Its reported accuracy is similar to that of CT (80%), and, like CT, it cannot detect micrometastases within normal-size lymph nodes. Another disadvantage is the longer scanning times and lack of oral contrast agents, which can lead to bowel motion artifact. Although tumor signal intensity and homogeneity vary significantly, no correlation is seen with histologic findings, nor can the change in signal intensity during chemotherapy predict the histology of residual masses (46,47).

Positron Emission Tomography

The use of positron emission tomography (PET) in the evaluation of radiographic abnormalities after chemotherapy has been reported (48–52). The proton-rich isotope 18F can be substituted into deoxyglucose, and radioactive decay of 18F leads to positron release. Fluoro-deoxyglucose (FDG) positron emission tomography has been shown to have significant advantages over anatomic imaging. FDG is taken up into cells in a way similar to glucose but accumulates within the cell because it is not metabolized. FDG-PET therefore uses differences in glucose metabolism between tumor and normal cells, such as differences in glucose uptake and glucose concentration by cells. Experimental data indicate that FDG is preferentially taken up by both seminomas and NSGCT. In most studies PET has a higher sensitivity and specificity than CT. However, FDG-PET scans are limited by low level of uptake in mature teratoma and by the potential for false-positives in scans performed immediately after chemotherapy.

PET scans have recently been combined with CT scans (PET/CT) to provide both functional and anatomic imaging studies and may prove to be another useful tool to determine the presence, location, and extent of occult disease in clinical stage I GCTs, as well in residual disease after chemotherapy. Further prospective studies are necessary to determine the role of this promising technology and its value to patients with GCTs (48–55).

Retroperitoneal Lymph Node Dissection (RPLND)

RPLND, which is discussed in separate chapters, plays an important role in identifying those patients with micrometastatic disease. The true gold standard for staging the retroperitoneum is an RPLND. Even with currently available staging techniques, including tumor marker measurement and radiographic imaging, a 15% to 20% error rate still exists in staging. RPLND thus identifies those patients with micrometastatic disease who are destined to fail if placed on surveillance. The small percentage of patients (5% to 10%) who relapse after RPLND have a high salvage rate with the available chemotherapy. Although controversy exists regarding the use of surveillance versus RPLND for clinical stage I patients, for the most accurate staging, RPLND should be performed. Modifications, such as template or prospective nerve sparing techniques, have markedly reduced or eliminated the problem of failure of ejaculation.

CHEST STAGING

Accurate staging of the chest is essential in testis cancer patients because the chest is the most common site of involvement after the retroperitoneal lymph nodes. If a patient relapses after an RPLND, the disease most commonly occurs in the chest. A variety of imaging methods exist to stage the chest, including chest radiography, whole-lung tomography, and chest CT. Jochelson et al. performed a prospective study on 120 patients with nonseminomatous testis tumors who underwent both plain radiography of the chest and whole-lung tomography. They found only one patient with a normal chest radiograph and an abnormal tomogram. They correctly concluded that tomography is not cost efficient for the initial staging or in subsequent follow-up of these patients (56).

See and Hoxie retrospectively reviewed patients with NS-GCTs regarding the incidence of disease in the chest. They found that only 4% of patients had intrathoracic involvement with normal abdominal CTs. If disease was present in the retroperitoneum, however, the chance of chest metastases was 40%. Because the pretest probability for chest involvement in the group with negative abdominal CT scan is low and the potential morbidity (i.e., chemotherapy) associated with a false-positive test is high, the ideal test would have high specificity. For these patients, then, plain radiography of the chest is recommended. On the other hand, if the pretest probability is high, sensitivity is of paramount importance. Thus, patients with positive abdominal CTs should undergo chest CT scanning (57). Similarly, in patients with seminoma, the risk of chest involvement in patients with little or no infradiaphragmatic disease is so low that chest CT scanning is not recommended (58).

Routine supraclavicular lymph node biopsy for patients with testis GCTs has been advocated (59). Because of low yield and potential morbidity, however, this practice has been abandoned. The incidence of supraclavicular nodal involvement in an impalpable node is approximately 5%, but if the node is palpable and its involvement would alter therapy, biopsy may be indicated (60).

STAGING SYSTEMS

Because of the differences in therapy, separate staging systems exist for seminomatous and NSGCTs of the testis. For nonseminomatous tumors, both clinical and pathologic staging systems exist to add to the confusion. Although there is no uniformly accepted clinical staging system, all systems are based on the system proposed by Boden and Gibb in 1951 (61). These investigators simply classified the disease as stage I for involvement of the testis alone, stage II for involvement of the retroperitoneum, and stage III for spread beyond the retroperitoneal nodes. Subsequent staging systems have modified this division somewhat, most frequently by subcategorizing stage II patients according to the amount of disease present by radiologic imaging. The differences in staging systems arose in response to the different treatment regimens at the various medical centers and the different methods used to assess disease. Some of the more common clinical staging systems for nonseminomatous testicular tumors are given in Table 35.1.

Patients with nonseminomatous tumors can also be staged pathologically when they undergo RPLND. As noted previously, a 15% to 20% staging error is seen with current methods of clinical staging. With RPLND, the error is removed. Some of the more common pathologic staging systems are given in Table 35.1. Note the pathologic distinction between stages B1 and B2. This distinction is important because most authors would agree that small-volume retroperitoneal disease identified by node dissection does not require adjuvant chemotherapy, as the relapse rate is low and the salvage rate is high. Patients with pathologic stage B2 disease or greater should be given adjuvant chemotherapy; the number of cycles depends on the institution.

Separate risk-stratification systems exist for patients with metastatic nonseminomatous tumors, based on the likelihood of the patient's being cured with conventional chemotherapy. Poor-risk patients as identified by these systems have a complete response rate of only approximately 50% and a high failure rate.

As noted, staging in seminoma patients is purely clinical. A comparison of the more commonly used systems is given in Table 35.1. As can be seen, most workers subdivide stage II according to the amount of retroperitoneal nodal involvement. Also, the Royal Marsden Hospital system differentiates supradiaphragmatic involvement (stage III) from visceral involvement (stage IV). Seminoma is exquisitely radiosensitive, and excellent results can be expected after radiotherapy for low-stage disease. Patients with bulky disease (5 to 10 cm) probably should receive initial cisplatin-based chemotherapy. Controversy surrounds the optimal treatment of patients with masses of 2 to 10 cm. While the standard therapy is generally considered to be radiotherapy, concerns regarding the long-term effects of even low-dose radiotherapy in young patients have led to the use of chemotherapy using three cycles of standard-dose cisplatin, etoposide, and bleomycin (BEP) (62). Testis GCTs represent one of the greatest success stories of modern oncology. Accurate imaging and staging have allowed patients with this disease to be appropriately stratified and their therapies to be refined so that morbidity and toxicity can be minimized. Although staging error still exists, its impact has been lessened by the efficacy of chemotherapy.

CONCLUSION

A complete staging workup for a patient with a testis GCT includes measurement of serum tumor marker levels, histologic assessment of the radical orchiectomy specimen, posteroanterior and lateral radiography of the chest, and abdominal CT. If the abdominal scan is positive, a chest CT scan should be obtained. With this information, tumor risk factors can be obtained and the disease can be staged according to one of a number of clinical staging systems. Thereafter, appropriate therapy can be initiated (63,64).

References

1. Richie JP. Detection and treatment of testicular cancer. *CA Cancer J Clin* 1993;43:161–175.
2. Landis SH, Murray T, Bolden S, et al. Cancer statistics, 1999. *CA Cancer J Clin* 1999;49:8–31.
3. Peterson GR, Lee JA. Secular trends of malignant tumors of the testes in white males. *CA Cancer J Clin* 1993;43:7–11.
4. Huyghe E, Matsuda T, Thonneau P. Increasing incidence of testicular cancer worldwide: A review. *Urology* 2003;170:5–11.
5. Bosl GJ, Vogelzang NJ, Goldman A. et al. Impact of delay in diagnosis on clinical stage of testicular cancer. *Lancet* 1981;2:970–973.
6. Nizkas D, Champion AE, Fox M. Germ cell tumors of testis: Prognostic factors and results. *Eur Urol* 1990;18:242–247.
7. Rowland RG, Donohue JP. Testicular cancer: Innovations in diagnosis and treatment. *Semin Urol* 1988;6:223–232.
8. Horstman WG. Scrotal imaging. *Urol Clin North Am* 1997;24(3):653–668.
9. Benson CB. The role of ultrasound in diagnosis and staging of testicular cancer. *Semin Urol* 1988;6:189–202.
10. Richie JP, Birnholz J, Garnick MB. Ultrasonography as a diagnostic adjunct for the evaluation of masses in the scrotum. *Surg Gynecol Obstet* 1982;154:695–698.
11. Schwerk WB, Schwerk WN, Rodeck G. Testicular tumors: Prospective analysis of real-time US patterns and abdominal staging. *Radiology* 1987;164:369–374.
12. Marth D, Scheidegger J, Studer UE. Ultrasonography of testicular tumors. *Urol Int* 1990;45:237–240.
13. Thurnher S, Hricak H, Carroll PR, et al. Imaging the testis: Comparison between MR staging and US. *Radiology* 1988;167:633–636.
14. Oyen R, Verellen S, Drochmans A, et al. Value of MRI in the diagnosis and staging of testicular tumors. *J Belge Radiol* 1993;76:84–89.
15. Hricak H, Hamm B, Kim B. *Imaging of the scrotum: Textbook and atlas.* New York: Raven Press, 1995:49–93.
16. Klein EA. Tumor markers in testis cancer. *Urol Clin North Am* 1993;20:67–73.
17. Von Eyben FE, de Graaff WE, Marrink J. Serum lactate dehydrogenase 1 activity in patients with testicular germ cell tumors correlates with the total number of copies of the short arm of chromosome 12 in the tumor. *Mol Gen Genet* 1992;235:140–144.
18. Dean CD, Moul JW. New tumor markers of testis cancer. *Urol Clin North Am* 1998;25(3):365–373.
19. Fleming ID, Cooper JS, Henson DE et al., eds. *AJCC cancer staging manual,* 5th ed. New York: Lippincott–Raven, 1997.
20. Rodriguez PN, Hafez GR, Messing EM. Nonseminomatous germ cell tumor of testicle: Does extensive staging of the primary tumor predict the likelihood of metastatic disease? *J Urol* 1986;136:604–608.
21. Fung CY, Kalish LA, Brodsky GL, et al. Stage I nonseminomatous germ cell testicular tumor: Prediction of metastatic potential by primary histopathology. *J Clin Oncol* 1988;6:1467–1473.
22. Klepp O, Olsson AM, Henrikson H, et al. Prognostic factors in clinical stage I nonseminomatous germ cell tumors of the testis: Multivariate analysis of a protective multicenter study. *J Clin Oncol* 1990;8:509–518.
23. Wishnow KI, Johnson DE, Swanson DA, et al. Identifying patients with low-risk clinical stage I nonseminomatous testicular tumors who should be treated by surveillance. *Urology* 1989;34:339–343.
24. McLeod DG, Weiss RB, Stablein DM, et al. Staging relationships and outcome in early stage testicular cancer: A report from the Testicular Cancer Intergroup Study. *J Urol* 1991;145:1178–1183.
25. Moul JW, Foley JP, Hitchcock CL, et al. Flow cytometric and quantitative histological parameters to predict occult disease in clinical stage I nonseminomatous testicular germ cell tumors. *J Urol* 1993;150:879–883.
26. Moul JW, McCarthy WF, Fernandez EB, et al. Percentage of embryonal carcinoma and vascular invasion predicts pathological stage in clinical stage I nonseminomatous testicular cancer. *Cancer Res* 1994;54:362–364.
27. Bosl GJ, Dmitrovsky E, Reuter VE, et al. Isochromosome of chromosome 12: Clinically useful marker for male germ cell tumors. *J Natl Cancer Inst* 1989;81:874–878.
28. De Graaff WE, van Echten-Arends J, Oosterhuis JW, et al. Cytogenetic abnormalities and clinical stage in testicular nonseminomatous germ cell tumors. *Cancer Genet Cytogenet* 1993;70:12–16.
29. Rodriguez E, Mathew S, Mukherjee AB, et al. Cytogenetic analysis of 124 prospectively ascertained male germ cell tumors. *Cancer Res* 1992;52:2285–2291.
30. Vergouwe Y, Steyerberg EW, Eijkemans MJ, et al. Predictors of occult metastasis in clinical stage I nonseminoma: A systematic review. *J Clin Oncol* 2003;21(22):4092–4099; Epub 2003 Oct 14. Comment in: Predictors of occult metastasis in clinical stage I nonseminoma: A systematic review. *J Clin Oncol* 2003;21(22):4075–4076.
31. Murty VV, Houldsworth J, Baldwin S, et al. Allelic deletions in the long arm of chromosome 12 identify sites of candidate tumor suppressor genes in male germ cell tumors. *Proc Natl Acad Sci U S A* 1992;89:11006–11010.
32. Austenfield MS, Bilhartz DL, Nativ O, et al. Flow cytometric DNA ploidy pattern for predicting metastasis of clinical stage I nonseminomatous germ cell testicular tumors. *Urology* 1993;41:379–383.
33. Fossa SD, Nesland JM, Waehre H, et al. DNA ploidy in the primary tumor from patients with nonseminomatous testicular germ cell tumors, clinical stage I. *Cancer* 1991;67:1874–1877.
34. De Graaff WE, Sleijfer DT, deJong B, et al. Significance of aneuploid stemlines in testicular nonseminomatous germ cell tumors. *Cancer* 1993;72:1300–1304.
35. Donohue JP, Zachary JM, Maynard BR. Distribution of nodal metastases in nonseminomatous testis cancer. *J Urol* 1982;128:315–320.
36. Poskitt KJ, Cooperberg CL, Sullivan LD. Sonography and CT in staging nonseminomatous testicular tumors. *Am J Roentgenol* 1985;144:939–944.
37. Williams RD, Feinberg SB, Knight LC, et al. Abdominal staging of testicular tumors using ultrasonography and computed tomography. *J Urol* 1980;123:872–875.
38. Chagnon S, Cochand-Priollet B, Gzall M, et al. Pelvic cancers: Staging of 139 cases with lymphangiography and fine-needle aspiration biopsy. *Radiology* 1989;173:103–106.
39. Richie JP, Garnick MB, Finberg H. Computerized tomography: How accurate for abdominal staging of testis tumors? *J Urol* 1982;127:715–717.
40. Socinski MA, Stomper PC. Radiologic evaluating of nonseminomatous germ cell tumor of the testis. *Semin Urol* 1988;6:203–215.
41. Vugrin D, Whitmore WF Jr, Nisselbaum J, et al. Correlation of serum tumor markers and lymphangiogram with degrees of nodal involvement in surgical stage II testis cancer. *J Urol* 1982;127:683–684.
42. Thomas JL, Bernardino ME, Bracken RB. Staging of testicular carcinoma: Comparison of CT and lymphangiography. *Am J Roentgenol* 1981;137:991–996.
43. Wilbert DM, Klose KJ, Alken P, et al. Tumor volume, CT scan, lymphangiography, sonography, intravenous pyelography and tumor markers in testis tumors. *Urol Int* 1989;44:15–19.
44. Samuelssom L, Fosberg L, Olsson AM. Accuracy of radiological staging procedures in nonseminomatous testis cancer compared with findings from surgical exploration and histopathological studies of extirpated tissue. *Br J Radiol* 1986;59:131–134.

45. Stomper PC, Jochelson MS, Garnick MB, et al. Residual abdominal masses after chemotherapy for nonseminomatous testicular cancer: Correlation of CT and histology. *Am J Roentgenol* 1985;145:743–746.

46. Ellis JH, Bies JP, Kopecky KK, et al. Comparison of MNR and CT imaging in the evaluation of metastatic retroperitoneal lymphadenopathy from testicular carcinoma. *J Comput Assist Tomogr* 1984;8:709–719.

47. Hogeboom WR, Hoekstra HJ, Mooyart EL, et al. Magnetic resonance imaging of retroperitoneal lymph node metastases of nonseminomatous germ cell tumours of the testis. *Eur J Surg Oncol* 1993;19:429–437.

48. Huddart RA. Use of FDG-PET in testicular tumours. *Clin Oncol (R Coll Radiol)* 2003;15(3):123–127.

49. Shvarts O, Han KR, Seltzer M, et al. Positron emission tomography in urologic oncology. *Cancer Control* 2002;9(4):335–342.

50. Sanchez D, Zudaire JJ, Fernandez JM, et al. 18F-fluoro-2-deoxyglucose-positron emission tomography in the evaluation of nonseminomatous germ cell tumours at relapse. *BJU Int* 2002;89(9):912–916.

51. Spermon JR, De Geus-Oei LF, Kiemeney LA, et al. The role of (18)fluoro-2-deoxyglucose positron emission tomography in initial staging and re-staging after chemotherapy for testicular germ cell tumours. *BJU Int* 2002;89(6):549–556.

52. Tsatalpas P, Beuthien-Baumann B, Kropp J, et al. Diagnostic value of 18F-FDG positron emission tomography for detection and treatment control of malignant germ cell tumors. *Urol Int* 2002;68(3):157–163.

53. Harns W, Bares R, Kamps H, et al. Therapy control of metastatic testicular carcinoma with F18-DOG PET. *J Nucl Med* 1995;36:198–202.

54. Stephens AW, Gonin R, Hutchins GD, et al. Positron emission tomography evaluation of residual radiographic abnormalities in postchemotherapy germ cell tumor patients. *J Clin Oncol* 1996;14:1637–1642.

55. Hoh CK, Seltzer MA, Franklin J, et al. Positron emission tomography in urological oncology. *J Urol* 1998;159:347–356.

56. Jochelson MS, Garnick MB, Balikian JP, et al. The efficacy of routine whole lung tomography in germ cell tumors. *Cancer* 1984;54:1007–1009.

57. See WA, Hoxie L. Chest staging in testis cancer patients: Imaging modality selection based upon risk assessment as determined by abdominal computerized tomography scan results. *J Urol* 1993;150:874–878.

58. Steinfeld AD, Macher MS. Radiologic staging of chest in testicular seminoma. *Urology* 1990;36:428–436.

59. Donohue RE, Pfister RR, Weigle JW, et al. Supraclavicular node biopsy in testicular tumors. *Urology* 1977;9:546.

60. Lynch DF, Richie JP. Supraclavicular node biopsy in staging testis tumors. *J Urol* 1980;123:39–40.

61. Boden G, Gibb R. Radiotherapy and testicular neoplasms. *Lancet* 1951;2:1195.

62. Schmoll HJ, Souchon R, Krege S, et al. European consensus on diagnosis and treatment of germ cell cancer: A report of the European Germ Cell Cancer Consensus Group—EGCCCG. *Ann Oncol* 2004;15:1377–1399.

63. Steele GS, Richie JR. Current role of retroperitoneal lymph node dissection in testicular cancer. *Oncology* 1997;11(5):717–737.

64. Einhorn LH, Donohue JP. Advanced testicular cancer. *J Urol* 1998;160:1964–1969.

CHAPTER 36 ■ SURVEILLANCE FOR LOW-STAGE TESTICULAR GERM CELL CANCERS

ALAN HORWICH

INTRODUCTION

Stage I germ cell tumors (GCTs) of the testis have an excellent prognosis. The current staging investigations post orchiectomy usually comprise a computed tomography (CT) scan of the thorax, abdomen, and pelvis and assays of the serum markers alpha-fetoprotein, human chorionic gonadotrophin, and lactate dehydrogenase. Due to the period of time required for physiologic clearing of markers that had been produced prior to the orchiectomy, it is conventional to monitor a sequence of marker assays if any are abnormal, to determine that they fall in concentration at an appropriate rate. The challenge of managing patients classified as having stage I testicular cancer derives from the insensitivity of this staging such that some 20% of patients with stage I seminoma and 30% with stage I nonseminoma will eventually relapse because of the presence following orchiectomy of microscopic subclinical metastases. Historically, the approach to managing this risk was based on early locoregional interventions with surgery or with radiotherapy. However, this approach has been revolutionized by the recognition of the high efficacy of systemic chemotherapy for these tumors. Not only does this introduce the possibility of adjuvant chemotherapy but also the possibility of reserving treatment for those who demonstrably need it for their recurrence, an approach that allows the majority of patients with stage I testicular cancer to avoid further anticancer treatment following an orchiectomy.

This chapter will review the evidence underpinning a surveillance approach and should be considered in conjunction with Chapter 39 by Smalley and Warde discussing adjuvant radiotherapy for stage I seminoma, Chapter 37 by Foster discussing the role of node dissection in stage I nonseminoma, and Chapter 38 by Culine discussing adjuvant chemotherapy. The issues are somewhat different for seminomas compared to nonseminomatous tumors. In particular, seminomas are considerably more sensitive to radiotherapy and have a lower potential for metastasis, especially metastasis beyond locoregional nodes. Seminomas have a slower pattern of disease proliferation and hence recurrence rate than nonseminomas, but seminomas are less likely to express serum markers as a sensitive indicator of recurrence. Thus pure seminomas and the group of nonseminomatous testicular germ cell tumors will be considered separately.

SEMINOMA OF THE TESTIS

Rationale for Surveillance

The traditional approach to managing the risk of recurrence in patients who have had an orchiectomy for stage I seminoma has been to irradiate the para-aortic and ipsilateral pelvic lymph nodes to a fairly modest radiation dose of 25 Gy to 30 Gy fractionated over 3 to 4 weeks. As described in Chapter 39, this clearly reduces the risk of relapse from about 20% (1) to approximately 3%. Even this 3% represents a group who can be successfully treated for relapse and thus cause-specific survival is very high and unlikely to be improved by any alternative management policy. The rationale for considering an alternative management policy is that the treated population is young and radiotherapy has potential long-term toxicities, such as carcinogenesis or cardiovascular events.

Second Cancer Risks

Extensive literature confirms carcinogenic risks of ionizing radiation deriving from children irradiated in utero (2), atomic bomb survivors (3), and radiotherapy for ankylosing spondylitis (4). The risk that therapeutic radiation for cancer might itself be carcinogenic may be obscured if treatment is for a malignancy with poor prognosis or if long-term follow-up information is not available. However, the risk has now become apparent for Hodgkin disease (5), and elevated risk has also been suggested in patients treated for seminoma.

The level of risk is not clear. Most reports either rely on epidemiologic records in which clinical details may be incomplete or inaccurate or have included patients with nonseminomas who often also had a variety of anticancer drugs and/or higher radiotherapy doses than are conventional for seminoma. The major epidemiologic study included 28,843 patients treated for testicular cancer between 1935 and 1993 who had been registered within population-based cancer registries in the United States, Canada, and Europe (6). A total of 7,476 men with seminoma were treated with radiotherapy initially and had an elevated risk of second cancers on long-term follow-up of 1.45. In 1,909 patients treated in the Netherlands between 1971 and 1985, 78 developed second cancers, but only 47.6 would have been expected in an age- and sex-matched general population. There appeared to be elevated risks particularly for stomach cancer and leukemia. An excess of contralateral testicular cancer was noted, but this was thought to be unrelated to radiation treatments.

Further difficulty in applying this data to current patients with stage I seminoma is that the adjuvant radiotherapy treatments upon which these figures are based was generally more extensive and at a higher dose than techniques employed today. For example, Fossa et al. (7) analyzed 876 patients treated at the Norwegian Radium Hospital between 1956 and 1977 and did identify a raised risk of second cancer (relative risk 1.58). However, patients with seminoma were treated to between 36 Gy and 40 Gy, and those with nonseminomas were treated to 50 Gy. Patients with metastases had additional mediastinal radiotherapy. For those 579 patients treated only with infradiaphragmatic radiotherapy, the relative risk of 1.32 was not statistically significant. Furthermore, a United

Kingdom study of 859 patients treated with infradiaphragmatic radiotherapy between 1961 and 1985 did not identify overall an excess of death from other causes (8). There were 20 deaths from second cancers, with 22.6 expected from an age- and sex-matched population.

Recently, a report from the M.D. Anderson Cancer Center presented an analysis of excess mortality in a cohort of 453 men previously cured of early seminoma by orchiectomy and radiotherapy (9). There was no significant excess mortality during the first 15 years of follow-up. However, beyond 15 years, the standardized mortality ratio was 1.85. The overall cancer specific standardized mortality ratio was 1.91, and this also was only significantly raised more than 15 years after treatment. The overall survival rates in this cohort are illustrated in Figure 36.1, and the analysis revealed that the use of prophylactic mediastinal irradiation significantly reduced survival.

Cardiovascular Events After Radiation

Cardiac radiotherapy has been linked to late-risk ischemic heart disease, cardiac events in Hodgkin disease (10,11), and left-sided breast cancer (12). Radiation doses used for Hodgkin disease are generally higher than those used for seminoma. However, some data suggest that even modest radiation doses may be hazardous in seminoma, such that prophylactic mediastinal irradiation is no longer employed (13,14). The analysis from the M.D. Anderson Cancer Center of mortality in patients cured of early Hodgkin disease by radiotherapy found a significantly increased cardiac-specific standardized mortality ratio of 1.61. It is a concern that the increase in cardiac deaths appeared also in those patients who had not had prophylactic mediastinal irradiation, especially in the time period more than 15 years after treatment. Though the pathologic mechanism whereby abdominal radiotherapy might lead to late cardiac events remains obscure, some support for its truth comes from the analysis of survivors following testicular cancer treatment at the Royal Marsden Hospital, which compared those treated with radiotherapy following orchiectomy with those managed by surveillance. Late cardiac events occurred in 9 of the 242 patients managed by surveillance, compared to 22 of the 230 patients managed by radiotherapy, an increased relative risk of 2.74. Even after adjusting for age differences in the two cohorts, the increased risk remains statistically significant (15).

Surveillance Technique

Monitoring must allow for the uncertain sensitivity of serum tumor markers, for the predominant pattern of relapse in the para-aortic region, and for the relatively indolent nature of seminoma. Thus programs of seminoma surveillance that were initiated in the mid-1980s usually incorporated regular outpatient visits for symptom review and tumor marker assay but also routine chest x-rays and abdominal CT scans. The Royal Marsden Hospital scheme is illustrated in Figure 36.2. This incorporates abdominal CT scan on an annual basis with additional 6-month scans in the first 2 years. Surveillance continues beyond 5 years but is based on investigation of symptoms rather than routine radiology. The program carried out in Denmark was similar with blood samples and chest x-rays every 2 months for the first year, every 4 months for the second year, then every 6 months for up to 5 years after orchiectomy. Follow-up radiographs after lymphangiography and/or CT scans were performed every 4 months for the first 2 years and then every 6 months for the next 3 years (16). Other major centers investigating seminoma surveillance were the Princess Margaret Hospital in Toronto (17) and the Royal London Hospital.

Results of Surveillance

Early reports from the Royal Marsden Hospital, the Princess Margaret Hospital, and the Danish National study are summarized in Table 36.1. In a total of 512 patients followed for a median of 48 to 62 months, the overall 4- to 5-year relapse-free survival (RFS) rates were 80% to 82%. Of the 89 recurrences, the pooled results indicated that 79 (88%) affected para-aortic nodes, 11 (12%) affected pelvic or inguinal nodes, 1 affected supradiaphragmatic nodes, and 2 involved the lungs. In 76 (85%) only the para-aortic nodes were involved.

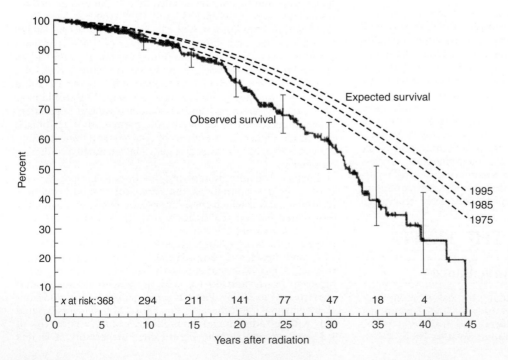

FIGURE 36.1. Survival of 453 nonrelapsing patients (with 95% confidence intervals) treated at the M.D. Anderson Cancer Center with radiotherapy for seminoma, compared to matched expected US male survivals in 1975, 1985, and 1995 (9).

Month	0	1	2	3	4	5	6	7	8	9	10	11	12	
OPD														
Markers (AFP, HCG, LDH)	√			√			√			√			√	Then as below
CXR	√			√			√			√			√	
CT Scan abdo+p	√						√						√	

Year 2	OPD q3/12	Markers q3/12	CXR q3/12	CT @ 18 &24/12
Year 3	OPD q4/12	Markers q4/12	CXR annually	CT @ 36/12
Year 4	OPD q6/12	Markers q6/12	CXR annually	CT @ 48/12
Year 5	OPD q6/12	Markers q6/12	CXR annually	CT @ 60/2

FIGURE 36.2. Seminoma surveillance schedule at the Royal Marsden Hospital.

In 68 of the recurrences, the initial treatment for recurrence was with radiotherapy alone. Of these patients, further relapse was seen in 11. Overall survival was high with 100% cause-specific survival in the Royal Marsden and Princess Margaret series. The Danish National study included 3 seminoma-related deaths, 1 due to progressive disease and 2 due to neutropenia following chemotherapy. Surveillance in stage I seminoma is now gaining in popularity (19–21).

To undertake a robust analysis of prognostic factors for relapse on surveillance, individual patient data were obtained from the Princess Margaret Hospital, the Danish Testicular Cancer Study Group, the Royal Marsden Hospital, and the Royal London Hospital for 638 patients (22). With a median follow-up of 7 years, 121 relapses had been observed (Fig. 36.3). The 5-year actuarial relapse-free rate was 82.3%, with most recurrences occurring within 2 years of orchiectomy. However, 8 (6.6%) of the recurrences occurred more than 6 years after diagnosis. Six patients died of disease or complications of treatment for relapse, giving a 5-year cause-specific survival rate of 99.3%. Analysis of candidate prognostic factors included tumor size, age, vascular invasion, classical versus anaplastic histology, and rete testis invasion. The univariate analysis of the impact of these variables on relapse is shown in Table 36.2, and showed that tumor size and rete testis invasion were important. Tumor size was also highly predictive when analyzed as a continuous variable, but at a cutoff of 4 cm in tumor diameter, patients with larger tumors were twice as likely to recur as those with smaller tumors. As shown in Figure 36.3, patients with both rete testis invasion and tumor size greater than 4 cm in diameter had a particularly high risk of recurrence: 31.5% by 5 years compared to 15.9% with one adverse factor and 12.2% with neither adverse factor.

Stratified Risk Management

The data suggest that either surveillance or adjuvant radiotherapy, usually to the para-aortic nodes alone, can be offered to patients following orchiectomy for stage I seminoma. There is a relatively high risk of recurrence in patients presenting with large primary tumors more than 4 cm in diameter that are invading the rete testis. Thus, to avoid both the stress of surveillance and the toxicity of salvage therapies, it seems logical to offer these patients adjuvant treatment. For those with one or no risk factors, the issue is less clear-cut since a significant risk remains of recurrence that some patients will prefer to manage by immediate adjuvant treatment, while others will prefer to avoid adjuvant treatment if possible. Clearly this decision would be helped if an adjuvant treatment were available that was both highly effective and did not carry long-term toxicity risks. With this in mind, adjuvant single-agent carboplatin has been investigated in patients with stage I seminoma (23–28) (Table 38.1 of Chapter 38). The recurrence rate overall after adjuvant carboplatin is 3.6% in 1,192 patients; 2.7% in 297 patients treated with two cycles, and 5.0% in 691 patients treated with one cycle. Tolerance of adjuvant carboplatin appears to be excellent. Steiner et al. (26) reported only three grade 3 myelosuppression toxicities in 108 patients, and

TABLE 36.1

SEMINOMA SURVEILLANCE

Series	Period of study	N	4- to 5-yr RFS	R	PA	RT
Horwich et al. 1992 (18)	1983–1988	103	82%	17	15	12
Warde et al. 1993 (17)	1984–1991	148	81%	23	20	19
Von der Maase et al. 1993 (16)	1985–1988	216	80%	49	41	37
Totals		512	815	89	76	68 (89.5%)

N, number of patients; RFS, relapse-free survival; R, number relapsing on surveillance; PA, relapse only in para-aortic nodes; RT, radiotherapy.

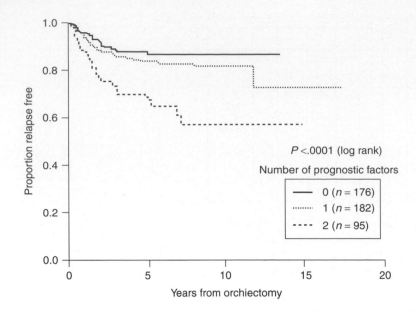

FIGURE 36.3. Relapse-free survival on surveillance for stage 1 seminoma comparing patients with 0, 1, or 2 risk factors (tumor diameter >4 cm, rete testis invasion); from a pooled analysis (22). (From Warde P, Specht L, Horwich A, et al. Prognostic factors for relapse in stage I seminoma managed by surveillance: A pooled analysis. *J Clin Oncol* 2002;20(22):4448–4452, with perimission.)

Reiter et al. (25) had no episodes of grade 3 myelosuppression in 107 patients.

A prospective randomized trial has been carried out comparing carboplatin and radiotherapy in the treatment of stage I seminoma under the auspices of the UK Medical Research Council and the European Organisation for Research and Treatment of Cancer (the EORTC). A total of 1,477 patients were randomized to either carboplatin or radiotherapy, and the results have so far been reported in abstract only (28). Carboplatin was administered in a single cycle to a dose to reach an area under the serum concentration × time curve (AUC) of 7 mg × min/mL. Radiotherapy was given to a para-aortic field in 87% of patients and a para-aortic + ipsilateral pelvic field in 13%; the median follow-up at the time of analysis was 3 years, and the relapse-free survival rates at 3 years were 96.6% for radiotherapy versus 95.4% for carboplatin.

A risk-adapted strategy in stage I seminoma has been evaluated by the Spanish Germ Cell Cancer Group and reported in abstract (27). Between January 1999 and December 2003, 300 patients with stage I seminoma were registered; 96 with no risk factors were managed by surveillance, and the remainder with one or two risk factors had two cycles of single-agent carboplatin at an AUC of 7. Grade 3 to grade 4 myelotoxicity was seen in 7% of patients, and grade 1 asthenia was seen in 19%. At a median follow-up of 20 months, 5 patients treated with adjuvant carboplatin relapsed and 4 of the 96 patients on surveillance relapsed. Overall 3-year survival was 100%.

Clinical Research Questions

It is reasonable at present to consider surveillance, adjuvant radiotherapy, or adjuvant chemotherapy in patients with stage I seminoma. The balance of this judgment could be affected by a number of areas of research. These include the role of positron emission tomography (PET) in initial staging, the development of more sensitive serum markers for seminoma, the evaluation of the long-term toxicities of modern radiotherapy techniques based on relatively low radiation doses and small radiation fields, development of less-intensive surveillance protocols, further evaluation of two cycles of adjuvant carboplatin, and long-term outcome and toxicity data on the use of carboplatin. Meanwhile, patients should understand the levels of efficacy and potential toxicities of adjuvant treatments before choosing this approach rather than surveillance. At the same time, salvage treatment for surveillance relapse carries the risk that more treatment may be needed than would have been required in the adjuvant setting. The need for long-term outcome data should encourage management of these patients within prospective studies.

NONSEMINOMA OF THE TESTIS

Rationale for Surveillance

Alternative management policies for patients with testicular nonseminoma who are found on CT scanning and analysis of serum markers to have stage I disease include surveillance, risk-adapted adjuvant chemotherapy, or retroperitoneal lymph node dissection (RPLND). As discussed in Chapters 37A and 37B, RPLND may be followed by observation or by a selection for adjuvant chemotherapy in those found to have involved retroperitoneal lymph nodes.

The rationale for surveillance derives in part from the efficacy of chemotherapy such that the subset of patients who progress and relapse can be salvaged successfully. Studies appear to show equivalently high cause-specific survivals of approximately 98% with any of these management approaches.

TABLE 36.2

SEMINOMA SURVEILLANCE: RELAPSE

Factor	Level	N	5-yr RFS	*P* Value
Tumor	≤4 cm	317	86.6	.003
Diameter	>4 cm	281	75.9	.003
Rete testis invasion	Yes	176	76.6	.003
	No	299	86.3	.003
Vascular invasion	Yes	191	77.3	.038
	No	384	85.6	.038
Histology	Classical	548	83.2	.056
	Anaplastic	50	71.4	.056

N, number of patients; RFS, relapse-free survival.
From Warde P, Specht L, Horwich A, et al. Prognostic factors for relapse in stage I seminoma managed by surveillance: A pooled analysis. *J Clin Oncol* 2002;20(22):4448–4452, with perimission.

TABLE 36.3

THEORETICAL TREATMENT BURDEN FOR ALTERNATIVE MANAGEMENT POLICIES FOR 100 PATIENTS WITH STAGE I TESTICULAR NONSEMINOMA

Policy	N	Relapse	BEPs by group	Total BEPs	Total RPLNDs
Surveillance	100	29	87	87	6
Path–RA	H(Ad) 50	1	104	122	2
	L(Ob) 50	6	18		
PET–RA	+ve 18Ad	0	36	60	2
	−ve 82Ob	8	24		
RPLND	100 Ob	15	45	45	100
RPLND	+Ad 15	0	30	54	100
	−Ob 85	8	24		

Ad, adjuvant chemotherapy; BEP, bleomycin, etoposide, and cisplatin; H, high pathological risk; L, low pathological risk; N, number of patients in group; Ob, observation; PET, positron emission tomography; RA, risk adapted; RPLND, retroperitoneal lymph node dissection.

However, the toxicity hazards are distinct, and therefore it is appropriate to consider the total burden of treatment to a population of patients with stage I nonseminoma as illustrated in Table 36.3. This table considers the early treatment consequences of different management approaches for 100 patients with stage I nonseminoma and is based on the following assumptions: (1) relapse will occur in 29% of patients managed by surveillance, but relapse on surveillance is likely to be of good prognosis and thus treated by three cycles of bleomycin, etoposide, and cisplatin (BEP) chemotherapy, (2) 20% of patients treated for metastatic disease by BEP chemotherapy will subsequently require a postchemotherapy RPLND, (3) relapse after adjuvant chemotherapy would require four cycles of chemotherapy and an RPLND, (4) adjuvant chemotherapy for high-risk patients will comprise two cycles of BEP chemotherapy, and (5) the sensitivity of PET scanning to detect involved nodes is 70% (29).

It can be seen from the analysis that a policy of routine RPLND tends to reduce chemotherapy usage and, in contrast, approaches based on surveillance or risk-adapted adjuvant chemotherapy all reduce dramatically the number of patients requiring RPLND. Though a policy of surveillance reduces surgery with only moderate increase in the use of chemotherapy, it is associated with the resource burden of the surveillance policy and a higher initial relapse rate than other policies. More recent studies have centred around risk-adapted therapy based either on pathologic risk factors such as vascular invasion in the primary tumor or on further staging with PET. Table 36.3 illustrates that PET imaging has considerable potential to reduce the overall burden of treatment and thus to reduce the risk of long-term toxicity in this young and highly curable patient population.

Method of Surveillance

When surveillance was first introduced (30), monitoring was intensive because of concern about relapse at an advanced stage. It then became apparent that the majority of recurrences were detected either by abnormalities of a serum marker or by symptoms prompting investigations (31). A recent medical research council (MRC) trial (TE08) has completed recruitment to a surveillance study in which patients are randomized to have either two scans or five scans as surveillance in stage I disease. The two scans were at 3 months and 12 months, and the five scans were at 3, 6, 9, 12, and 24 months. The trial has not yet been reported but indicates the range of current practice. Surveillance policies still involve frequent assessments in tumor marker assays, but the desire to avoid ionizing radiation has led to the questioning of the need for frequent chest x-ray (32), as well as investigation of reducing CT scans (19). Studies have shown that more than 90% of recurrences occur within 24 months of orchiectomy and 99% within 3 years. The majority of relapses are detected with small-volume metastatic disease. However, 1% to 2% of patients develop drug-resistant recurrences or suffer fatal treatment complications (32–37).

Results

Table 36.4 illustrates a selection of recent series describing the patterns of relapse in unselected patients managed by surveillance for stage I nonseminoma. In a range of series reported since 1986 and reviewed by Vergouwe et al. (38) comprising more than 2,000 patients, the risk of recurrence was approximately 29%. The early UK MRC studies identified that significant risk factors for recurrence included lymphatic vessel invasion, blood vessel invasion, the absence of yolk sac elements in the primary tumor, and the presence of undifferentiated embryonal tissue in the primary tumor. These factors appeared following univariate analysis of a large range of pathologic variables, and it was found that the presence of three or four of these factors indicated a >50% risk of relapse. However, this has not been used as the basis of identifying a high-risk group since only about one-fifth of patients with stage I seminoma have three or four of these risk factors.

TABLE 36.4

SURVEILLANCE FOR STAGE I NONSEMINOMA

Series	Study Period	N	Relapse
Read et al. 1992 (34)	1984–1987	373	100 (27%)
Gels et al. 1995 (37)	1982–1991	154	42 (27%)
Sogani et al. 1998 (35)	1979–1987	105	27 (26%)
Sharir et al. 1999 (32)	1980–1996	170	48 (28%)
Francis et al. 2000 (19)	1979–1996	183	52 (28%)
Roeleveld et al. 2001 (36)	1982–1994	90	23 (26%)
Daugaard et al. 2003 (21)	1984–2002	301	86 (29%)

N, number of patients in group.

Additionally, some difficulty was experienced in distinguishing lymphatic and blood vessel invasion on routine histology, and a more common result of subsequent surveillance analyses has been to identify the high-risk group as those with any vascular invasion. The presence of yolk sac elements has not consistently identified a reduced risk of metastasis, and such elements may be confounded by the associated presence of alpha-fetoprotein in the serum leading to delayed registration of patients with stage I disease as a consequence of the slow fall of this marker after orchiectomy. The proportion of primary tumor involved by embryonal carcinoma does appear to be a risk factor (36,39) as does the proliferation rate of cells in the primary tumor as judged by Mib-1 staining (36).

A detailed review of predictors of metastasis in clinical stage I nonseminoma identified 23 publications between 1979 and 2001 reporting on 2,587 patients, of whom 759 (29%) had occult metastases (38). These were either diagnosed by RPLND or by follow-up. The strongest indicator of occult metastasis was the presence of vascular invasion in the primary tumor (odds ratio 5.2). Mib-1 antibody positivity showed an odds ratio of 4.7, the presence of embryonal carcinoma in the primary tumor had an odds ratio of 2.9, and a T stage of 3 or 4 had an odds ratio of 2.6 (38).

Risk-adapted Management Strategies

Identification of the predictors of occult metastasis from surveillance studies has led to the development of risk-adapted policies for clinical stage I nonseminoma in which patients with a low predicted risk have been managed by surveillance and those with a high predicted risk have been treated with adjuvant chemotherapy (31,40–46). Some studies included RPLND for patients with intermediate risk (40,42). Adjuvant chemotherapy is reviewed in Chapter 38. The UK MRC multicenter trial required that patients have at least three of the four risk factors: blood vessel invasion, lymphatic invasion, embryonal carcinoma, and absence of yolk sac elements. Two cycles of adjuvant BEP were administered to 114 patients. There were two recurrences; however, one of these was found to have a carcinoma originally of the rete testis rather than a germ cell tumor. A subsequent MRC study based on the risk factor of any vascular invasion in 115 patients demonstrated similar efficacy of the combination of bleomycin, vincristine, and platinum (BOP) with the desire to avoid the leukemogenic risk of etoposide and with the hope that this would cause less alopecia. Again, the recurrence rate was 2%. However, moderate alopecia and also neuropathy (41) were observed. A number of different risk identifiers have been used to characterize intermediate and high-risk patients. Most studies have employed two cycles of adjuvant chemotherapy. Following this, 1% to 2% of patients will suffer recurrence. One study (45) used carboplatin rather than cisplatin and, in the setting of adjuvant treatment, this appears to be equivalent in efficacy. Of 68 patients treated with two cycles of carboplatin, etoposide, and bleomycin, no recurrences of undifferentiated germ cell cancer were seen, though one patient did develop teratoma differentiated that was resected at RPLND.

Research Approaches

Surveillance is an attractive option for managing patients with stage I NSGCT since it reserves treatment post orchiectomy for those who have demonstrated the need. However, concern exists about allowing progression of tumor, and this is especially a problem in patients who choose not to attend regularly the follow-up assessment. Furthermore, some patients find the threat of recurrence stressful; thus a more sensitive initial staging test would improve selection of patients for surveillance. It is possible that PET may fulfill this role (29); however, more extensive studies are required of this technology. The technique of surveillance appears safe, though radiation doses from multiple CT scans may themselves be carcinogenic. The MRC TE08 trial will demonstrate whether only two follow-up CT scans are sufficient within a surveillance program. Also, alternative surveillance technologies require evaluation, including abdominal MRI. Potential exists for evaluating new biomarkers to improve identification of risk or to provide even more sensitive serum assays for monitoring purposes. Finally, though the use of two cycles of adjuvant chemotherapy dramatically reduces risk of recurrence, little data have been collected as yet on whether this practice might be associated with long-term toxicities.

References

1. Duchesne GM, Horwich A, Dearnaley DP, et al. Orchidectomy alone for stage I seminoma of the testis. *Cancer* 1990;65(5):1115–1118.
2. Bithell JF, Stewart AM. Pre-natal irradiation and childhood malignancy: A review of British data from the Oxford Survey. *Br J Cancer* 1975;31(3):271–287.
3. Bizzozero OJ, Johnson KG, Ciocco A Jr. Radiation-related leukemia in Hiroshima and Nagasaki, 1946–1964. I. Distribution, incidence and appearance time. *N Engl J Med* 1996;274(20):1095–1101.
4. Smith PG, Doll R. Mortality among patients with ankylosing spondylitis after a single treatment course with x rays. *Br Med J (Clin Res Ed)* 1992;284(6314):449–460.
5. Van Leeuwen FE, Klokman WJ, Hagenbeek A, et al. Second cancer risk following Hodgkin's disease: A 20-year follow-up study. *J Clin Oncol* 1994;12(2):312–325.
6. Travis LB, Curtis RE, Storm H, et al. Risk of second malignant neoplasms among long-term survivors of testicular cancer. *J Natl Cancer Inst* 1997;89(19):1429–1439.
7. Fossa SD, Langmark F, Aass N, et al. Second non-germ cell malignancies after radiotherapy of testicular cancer with or without chemotherapy. *Br J Cancer* 1990;61(4):639–643.
8. Horwich A, Bell J. Mortality and cancer incidence following radiotherapy for seminoma of the testis. *Radiother Oncol* 1994;30(3):193–198.
9. Zagars GK, Ballo MT, Lee AK, et al. Mortality after cure of testicular seminoma. *J Clin Oncol* 2004;22(4):640–647.
10. Reinders JG, Heijmen BJ, Olofsen-van Acht MJ, et al. Ischemic heart disease after mantle field irradiation for Hodgkin's disease in long-term follow-up. *Radiother Oncol* 1999;51(1):35–42.
11. Corn BW, Trock BJ, Goodman RL. Irradiation-related ischemic heart disease. *J Clin Oncol* 1990;8(4):741–750.
12. Cuzick J, Mossman J, Stewart H. Cooperative breast cancer trials organized by the United Kingdom Co-ordinating Committee on Cancer Research. *Cancer* 1994;74(Suppl. 3):1160–1163.
13. Hanks GE, Peters T, Owen J. Seminoma of the testis: Long-term beneficial and deleterious results of radiation. *Int J Radiat Oncol Biol Phys* 1992;24(5):913–919.
14. Lederman GS, Sheldon TA, Chaffey JT, et al. Cardiac disease after mediastinal irradiation for seminoma. *Cancer* 1987;60(4):772–776.
15. Huddart RA. Improving treatment outcomes in testicular cancer: Strategies to reduce treatment related morbidity. *BJU Int* 2003;92(6):524–526.
16. Von der Maase H, Specht L, Jacobsen GK, et al. Surveillance following orchidectomy for stage I seminoma of the testis. *Eur J Cancer* 1993;29A(14):1931–1934.
17. Warde PR, Gospodarowicz MK, Goodman PJ, et al. Results of a policy of surveillance in stage I testicular seminoma. *Int J Radiat Oncol Biol Phys* 1993;27(1):11–15.
18. Horwich A, Alsanjari N, A'Hern R, et al. Surveillance following orchidectomy for stage I testicular seminoma. *Br J Cancer* 1992;65(5):775–778.
19. Francis R, Bower M, Brunstrom G, et al. Surveillance for stage I testicular germ cell tumors: Results and cost benefit analysis of management options. *Eur J Cancer* 2000;36(15):1925–1932.
20. Kakehi Y, Kamoto T, Kawakita M, et al. Follow-up of clinical stage I testicular cancer patients: Cost and risk benefit considerations. *Int J Urol* 2002;9(3):154–160.
21. Daugaard G, Petersen PM, Rorth M. Surveillance in stage I testicular cancer. *APMIS* 2003;111(1):76–83.
22. Warde P, Specht L, Horwich A, et al. Prognostic factors for relapse in stage I seminoma managed by surveillance: A pooled analysis. *J Clin Oncol* 2002;20(22):4448–4452.
23. Oliver RT, Edmonds PM, Ong JY, et al. Pilot studies of 2 and 1 course carboplatin as adjuvant for stage I seminoma: Should it be tested in a randomized trial against radiotherapy? *Int J Radiat Oncol Biol Phys* 1994;29(1):3–8.

24. Dieckmann KP, Bruggeboes B, Pichlmeier U, et al. Adjuvant treatment of clinical stage I seminoma: Is a single course of carboplatin sufficient? *Urology* 2000;55(1):102–106.
25. Reiter WJ, Brodowicz T, Alavi S, et al. Twelve-year experience with two courses of adjuvant single-agent carboplatin therapy for clinical stage I seminoma. *J Clin Oncol* 2001;19(1):101–104.
26. Steiner H, Holtl L, Wirtenberger W, et al. Long-term experience with carboplatin monotherapy for clinical stage I seminoma: A retrospective single-center study. *Urology* 2002;60(2):324–328.
27. Aparicio J, Germa JR, Garcia Del Muro X, et al. [Spanish Germ Cell Cancer Group (GG)]. Risk-adapted management of stage I seminoma: The second Spanish Germ Cell Cancer Group (GG) study. *Proc Am Soc Clin Oncol* 2004;22:385, Abstract 4518.
28. Oliver RT, Mason M, Von der Maase H, et al., on behalf of the MRC Testis Tumour Group & the EORTC GU Group. A randomised comparison of single agent carboplatin with radiotherapy in the adjuvant treatment of stage I seminoma of the testis, following orchidectomy: MRC TE19/EORTC 30982. *Proc Am Soc Clin Oncol* 2004:385, Abstract 4517.
29. Lassen U, Daugaard G, Eigtved A, et al. Whole-body FDG-PET in patients with stage I non-seminomatous germ cell tumour. *Eur J Nucl Med Mol Imaging* 2003;30(3):396–402.
30. Peckham MJ, Barrett A, Husband JE, et al. Orchidectomy alone in testicular stage I non-seminomatous germ-cell tumour. *Lancet* 1982;2(8300):678–680.
31. Cullen MH, Droz JP. Management of stage I non-seminoma: Surveillance. In: Alan Horwich, ed. *Testicular cancer–investigation and management*, 2nd ed. London, UK: Chapman & Hall Medical, 1996:165–178.
32. Sharir S, Jewett MA, Sturgeon JF, et al. Progression detection of stage I nonseminomatous testis cancer on surveillance: Implications for the followup protocol. *J Urol* 1999;161(2):472–475.
33. Freedman LS, Parkinson MC, Jones WG, et al. Histopathology in the prediction of relapse of patients with stage I testicular teratoma treated by orchidectomy alone. *Lancet* 1987;2(8554):294–298.
34. Read G, Stenning SP, Cullen MH, et al. Medical Research Council Testicular Tumors Working Party. Medical Research Council prospective study of surveillance for stage I testicular teratoma. *J Clin Oncol* 1992;10(11):1762–1768.
35. Sogani PC, Perrotti M, Herr HW, et al. Clinical stage I testis cancer: Long-term outcome of patients on surveillance. *J Urol* 1998;159(3):855–858.
36. Roeleveld TA, Horenblas S, Meinhardt W, et al. Surveillance can be the standard of care for stage I nonseminomatous testicular tumors and even high risk patients. *J Urol* 2001;166(6):2166–2170.
37. Gels E, Hoekstra HJ, Sleijfer DT, et al. Detection of recurrence in patients with clinical stage I nonseminomatous testicular germ cell tumors and consequences for further follow-up: A single-center 10-year experience. *J Clin Oncol* 1995;13:1188–1194.
38. Vergouwe Y, Steyerberg EW, Eijkemans MJ, et al. Predictors of occult metastasis in clinical stage I nonseminoma: A systematic review. *J Clin Oncol* 2003;21(22):4092–4099.
39. Fung CY, Kalish LA, Brodsky GL, et al. Stage I nonseminomatous germ cell testicular tumor: Prediction of metastatic potential by primary histopathology. *J Clin Oncol* 1988;6(9):1467–1473.
40. Klepp O, Dahl O, Flodgren P, et al. Risk-adapted treatment of clinical stage 1 non-seminoma testis cancer. *Eur J Cancer* 1997;33(7):1038–1044.
41. Dearnaley DP, Fossa SD, Kaye SB, et al. (MRC Testicular Tumour Working Party). Adjuvant bleomycin, vincristine and cisplatin (OP) for high risk clinical stage I (HRCS1) non-seminomatous germ cell tumours (NSCGCT): A Medical Research Council (MRC) Pilot Study. *Proc Am Soc Clin Oncol* 1998:309a, Abstract 1189.
42. Ondrus D, Matoska J, Belan V, et al. Prognostic factors in clinical stage I nonseminomatous germ cell testicular tumors: Rationale for different risk-adapted treatment. *Eur Urol* 1998;33(6):562–566.
43. Bohlen D, Borner M, Sonntag RW, et al. Long-term results following adjuvant chemotherapy in patients with clinical stage I testicular nonseminomatous malignant germ cell tumors with high risk factors. *J Urol* 1999;161(4):1148–1152.
44. Chevreau C, Mazerolles C, Soulie M, et al. Long-term efficacy of two cycles of BEP regimen in high-risk stage I nonseminomatous testicular germ cell tumors with embryonal carcinoma and/or vascular invasion. *Eur Urol* 2004;46(2):209–214.
45. Amato RJ, Ro JY, Ayala AG, et al. Risk-adapted treatment for patients with clinical stage I nonseminomatous germ cell tumor of the testis. *Urology* 2004;63(1):144–148.
46. Matoto-Rey P, Garcia Del Muro X, Paz-Ares L, et al. Risk adapted surveillance for stage I nonseminoma testicular tumour (NSCGT): Results of a prospective multicenter study. *Proc Am Soc Clin Oncol* 2004;72:386, Abstract 4524.

CHAPTER 37 ■ SURGICAL MANAGEMENT

CHAPTER 37A
Radical Orchiectomy and Retroperitoneal Lymph Node Dissection

Richard Foster, Richard Bihrle, and John P. Donohue

RADICAL ORCHIECTOMY

Patients who present with a definite intratesticular mass, which is usually hypoechoic on ultrasound, have a high probability of having germ cell testicular cancer. Approximately 95% of these patients will be found to have a germ cell tumor, with the remainder having either Sertoli or Leydig cell tumors or, alternatively, epidermoid cysts. Because of the probability of the diagnosis of germ cell cancer, the suggested treatment is radical inguinal orchiectomy. Historically, the reasoning behind this removal of the testis was a high ligation of the spermatic cord at the internal ring, which was believed to have a higher chance of containing lymphatic spread of the primary tumor. Though this was the initial rationale for the procedure, the so-called high ligation of the cord is probably not very important in the treatment of the disease.

The true rationale for performing radical inguinal orchiectomy is to limit the likelihood of spillage of the tumor at the time of the procedure. Because the incision is made away from the site of the primary disease, the probability of a surgical mistake leading to spillage of tumor is low. Additionally, early vascular control is obtained in an area that is not usually inflamed due to the tumor.

A review of the consequences of deviations in technique in orchiectomy for germ cell testicular cancer has been published (1). In this study from Indiana University, it was noted that the consequences of deviation in technique were minimal as long as there was no tumor spillage. Importantly, tumor spillage usually required subsequent chemotherapy. Therefore, though radical inguinal orchiectomy is advocated and is appropriate, an improper scrotal incision is not necessarily deleterious to the patient as long as there is no tumor spillage.

Technique

The patient is positioned supine and the lower abdomen and genitalia are antiseptically prepared and sterilely draped. An incision is made in Langer's lines and is carried down through Scarpa's fascia until the aponeurosis of the external oblique is identified. Similar to herniorrhaphy, the aponeurosis of the external oblique is opened from the external ring to the internal ring, exposing the cord and cremasteric fibers. Cremasteric fibers are sharply divided and the ileoinguinal nerve is dissected from the cord. If the decision has been made to commit to radical orchiectomy, the cord is encircled at the pubis and is dissected proximally to the internal ring. Many techniques exist for division of the cord. Our preference is to divide the cord into two separate sections with a right-angle clamp and then tie proximally and distally with permanent ligatures. In addition, suture ligatures are used proximally to control the vascular structures as they retract into the retroperitoneum. The divided end of the cord is then wrapped in a laparotomy pad and dissection is carried distally to mobilize the cord and testis up through the base of the scrotum. Digital pressure on the scrotum is used to delineate the gubernacular fibers, and they are divided sharply. The specimen is then delivered.

Special note should be given to those patients who have a very large primary tumor that cannot be mobilized easily through the base of the scrotum into the surgical incision. These patients should have the inguinal incision extended onto the scrotum so the tumor can be dissected from the scrotum without spillage of tumor contents. We are aware of several cases where the surgeon was unwilling to extend the incision and attempted to mobilize a very large tumor through a too-small base of the scrotum, resulting in spillage of the tumor in the wound. Germ cell testicular cancer characteristically implants and, as a result, usually requires systemic chemotherapy. Similarly, spillage of tumor contents in the inguinal area potentially contaminates another area of lymphatic drainage (the inguinal nodes); therefore, tumor rupture should be avoided. Though the morbidity of a retroperitoneal lymph node dissection is relatively low, the morbidity of a required postchemotherapy inguinal lymph node dissection is not minimal, so tumor spillage should be avoided.

After removal of the cord and testis, the wound is irrigated. Subsequently the aponeurosis of the external oblique is closed using interrupted permanent sutures. Scarpa's fascia is closed using a running absorbable suture. It is our preference to inject Marcaine as a field block prior to closure of the skin. Closure of the skin is done in a subcuticular fashion. Scrotal support is employed postoperatively to avoid venous bleeding into the scrotum and the patient is discharged from the hospital as a day-surgery case the same day.

If the pathologic diagnosis is germ cell cancer, the patient is scheduled for computed tomography (CT) scans of the chest, abdomen, and pelvis in order to properly stage the tumor. If serum alpha fetoprotein and beta human chorionic gonadotropin (HCG) were elevated prior to orchiectomy, these studies are again obtained after orchiectomy to determine whether these tumor markers are falling based upon appropriate half-lives. The half-life of beta HCG is approximately 1.5 days; the half-life of alpha fetoprotein is approximately 5 days.

RETROPERITONEAL LYMPH NODE DISSECTION

Rationale in Low-stage Disease

Germ cell testicular cancer is unique in many aspects. Perhaps the most unique behavioral component of this disease is its surgical curability, even after lymphatic metastasis has occurred (2). Though on rare occasions patients are cured with breast, colon, and other malignancies when lymphatic metastasis has occurred, only a few cancers are reliably cured surgically by the removal of the primary and the lymphatic metastases. Germ cell testicular cancer is certainly one of the most curable in this regard. Approximately 50% to 75% of patients who have retroperitoneal low- to moderate-volume metastases can be cured merely by the removal of the primary and the lymphatic metastases. Retroperitoneal lymph node dissection has been called a morbid and debilitating procedure. In low-stage disease, it has essentially the morbidity of a laparotomy (3).

Formerly, retroperitoneal lymph node dissection (RPLND) in low-stage disease also conferred a significant staging benefit. Because around 30% of patients with clinical stage I germ cell cancer have metastatic disease, RPLND served to clarify which patients had been clinically understaged. However, with the decreasing morbidity of systemic chemotherapy and with the realization that the deferred treatment of microscopic metastatic disease with chemotherapy has essentially the same cure rate, the staging benefit of RPLND has become less important over time.

Other developments in urologic oncology have solidified the usefulness of this operation as a therapeutic procedure. Recent studies have shown that although cisplatin-based chemotherapy is life-saving for many of these patients, some patients can have significant and clinically relevant long-term morbidity as a result of the chemotherapy (4). Studies from Europe have disclosed that patients who were treated with cisplatin-based chemotherapy have a higher chance of cardiovascular disease compared with controls (5). Other long-term side effects of chemotherapy include diminished fertility in the contralateral testis, high-frequency hearing loss, and some clinical evidence of renal deterioration over time (6). Though these side effects are certainly acceptable in a patient who requires chemotherapy for cure, some patients would like to avoid these potential side effects if there is an alternative to chemotherapy for cure. In low-stage disease, this alternative is retroperitoneal lymph node dissection.

Historically, one of the reasons to argue against retroperitoneal lymph node dissection was the attendant loss of emission and ejaculation due to interruption of retroperitoneal sympathetics. With the development of nerve-sparing techniques, virtually 100% of patients who undergo RPLND for low-stage disease should maintain emission and ejaculation and, therefore, potential fertility (7). Therefore, the argument against RPLND because of emission and ejaculation loss is not relevant at the beginning of the 21st century.

Finally, the acute morbidity of the procedure has fallen as a result of intrathecal narcotics, the recognition that not all of these patients develop an ileus, and the decrease in operative time because of increased experience with the procedure. Formerly, at Indiana University, patients were in the hospital 7 to 8 days as a result of a primary RPLND; currently, hospitalization for these patients averages 3 days.

Rationale for Postchemotherapy RPLND

Patients who are found to have high-volume disease to the retroperitoneum or distant metastatic disease at the time of initial staging are treated with systemic cisplatin-based chemotherapy. Though the nuances of selection of the chemotherapeutic regimen and the details of administration of the regimen are beyond the scope of this chapter, it is fair to say that studies have shown that carboplatin cannot substitute for cisplatin and that in so-called poor-risk disease (mediastinal primaries, very high alpha fetoprotein or beta HCG, or non-pulmonary visceral metastasis) high-dose chemotherapy with

stem cell rescue has become a mainstay of therapy (8). Currently a multinational trial is ongoing that randomizes so-called poor-risk patients between the standard four courses of bleomycin, etoposide, cisplatin, and high-dose chemotherapy with stem cell rescue. This is a very important trial that hopefully will enable us to determine appropriate therapy in these so-called poor-risk patients.

After the administration of systemic chemotherapy, if alpha fetoprotein and beta HCG have normalized and all radiographic disease has disappeared, patients are characteristically observed. Some groups from around the world will perform RPLND on patients who have complete clinical remissions because some studies have shown that up to 20% of these patients with no visible tumor radiographically will have microscopic teratoma or cancer pathologically (9) if RPLND is performed. At Indiana University, if these patients are followed, only a very small number will relapse. Therefore, the natural history of low-volume unresected teratoma is unknown, and this is why controversy continues to exist in the management of these patients.

What is generally agreed is that patients who normalize serum alpha fetoprotein and beta HCG and have residual retroperitoneal radiographic tumor should undergo retroperitoneal lymph node dissection. The reasoning behind this is that postchemotherapy resection of retroperitoneal tumor effectively restages the patient and is therapeutic if teratoma or viable carcinoma is removed. Approximately 40% of the time, what is found in these residual masses is only necrosis and fibrosis. It would be preferable to avoid surgery in these patients, but many studies looking at statistical methods of predicting necrosis, PET scanning, and CT scanning have shown that it is impossible to reliably select patients with necrosis and fibrosis who can be observed and not be subjected to RPLND (10). Therefore, all patients with normalization of markers and postchemotherapy tumor should undergo postchemotherapy RPLND.

Other groups of patients who are subjected to postchemotherapy RPLND are so-called desperation patients and patients with late relapse. Some patients will have only retroperitoneal localized disease after chemotherapy but will have clinical evidence of persistent carcinoma in the mass. Usually this means that patients have exhausted all chemotherapeutic alternatives and have elevated alpha fetoprotein, beta HCG, or both. These highly chemorefractory patients can be cured surgically merely by the removal of the nodes and the retroperitoneal mass. In the Indiana University experience, approximately 30% of such patients can be cured surgically who have resistant cancer in the retroperitoneum (11). Therefore, postchemotherapy RPLND is sometimes performed in patients who have elevated markers if all chemotherapeutic alternatives have been exhausted.

Technique

Low-stage Considerations

Nonseminoma patients in clinical stage I are those patients who have normal CT scans of the chest, abdomen, and pelvis and whose serum alpha fetoprotein and beta HCG have normalized or are normalizing according to appropriate half-lives. The approximate half-life of alpha fetoprotein is 4.5 to 5 days; for beta HCG, it is 1 to 1.5 days. Clinical stage I nonseminoma patients have various options for therapy. These include nerve-sparing RPLND, surveillance, or, as is practiced in some parts of the world, primary chemotherapy. Each of these methods of management is associated with a long-term cure rate of 98% to 99%, and, therefore, patient involvement in the appropriate choice of therapy is imperative. Characteristically, patients choose one or the other method of management based upon consideration of side effects, psychological issues, and access-to-care issues.

Formerly, full bilateral RPLND was performed for patients with clinical stage I disease. This involved the resection of all lymphatics from the crus of the diaphragm to the bifurcation of the common iliacs, from ureter to ureter. Subsequently, mapping studies were performed and illustrated the fact that if low-volume metastasis has occurred, it is characteristically unilateral (12). Therefore, so-called modified templates were developed based upon the clinical stage and the side of the primary. Hence, modified nerve sparing RPLND for a right-sided primary is a different operation compared with the procedure performed for a left-sided primary.

Right-modified Nerve-sparing RPLND. A midline incision is made, and the peritoneal cavity is entered. A self-retaining retractor is used, and general palpation and inspection are carried out. If there is retroperitoneal disease >2 cm in diameter or multiple obvious areas of metastasis, a full bilateral RPLND is performed. It is very unusual to encounter these findings in the modern era because of the quality of CT scanning. An incision is made in the posterior peritoneum from the cecum up to the area of the ligament of Treitz, which corresponds to roughly the area of the inferior mesenteric vein entering the splenic vein. The root of the small bowel and right colon are mobilized to the patient's right side. This nicely exposes the right pericaval, precaval, and interaortocaval zonal areas. The so-called split-and-roll maneuver is employed, whereby lymphatic tissue is split over the great vessels and rolled away from the great vessels. This split is carried out over the left renal vein, and tissue is rolled inferiorly. The 12 o'clock position on the aorta is identified, and lymphatic tissue is split from the crossing of the left renal vein distally to approximately the origin of the inferior mesenteric artery. This lymphatic tissue is then rolled into the interaortocaval area, which should expose any right-sided lower pole renal arteries. Next, the same split maneuver is performed over the vena cava from the origin of the renal veins distally to the crossing of the right common iliac artery. The origin of the right gonadal vein is identified, dissected, and divided between ties, and then it is dissected distally to the internal ring. The vas deferens is identified and divided, and the cord stump is mobilized from the internal ring. Thus, the first specimen of the right gonadal vein is taken. Attention is then turned back to the vena cava. Tissue is rolled medially and laterally off the vena cava, and the lumbar veins passing posteriorly are dissected and divided. This enables mobilization of the vena cava. The right-sided efferent sympathetic fibers are easily seen passing into the interaortocaval area from the sympathetic chain (Fig. 37A.1). They are dissected away from lymphatic tissue using fine scissors and placed in vessel loops. Attention is then returned to the aorta. The split maneuver over the distal aorta and the right common iliac artery is continued carefully avoiding efferent sympathetic fibers as they pass into the interiliac area. Tissue is rolled medially into the interaortocaval zone away from the aorta, and the right-sided lumbar arteries are identified, dissected, and divided between silk ties.

Superiorly, the right renal artery is dissected away from lymphatic tissue as it passes over the crus of the diaphragm. The right ureter is mobilized laterally setting up the right-sided border of the dissection. Next, the right pericaval and interaortocaval lymphatic zones are harvested from the posterior body wall. Lumbar arteries and veins are controlled with clips, cautery, or ties as they penetrate the posterior body wall medial to the right sympathetic chain or as in the case of the veins as they pass posterior to the aorta. At the crus of the diaphragm, clips are used to secure the lymphatics as they pass behind the crus to the cisterna chyli. Thus, a right-sided modified nerve sparing RPLND harvests three specimens: the right gonadal vein, the right pericaval nodes, and the interaortocaval nodes

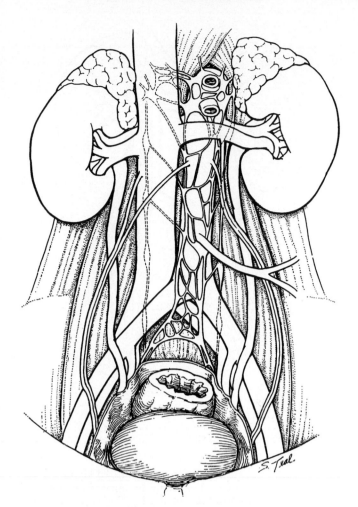

FIGURE 37A.1. The right-sided efferent sympathetic fibers.

(Fig. 37A.2). After completion of the dissection, the posterior peritoneum is closed using a running absorbable suture; subsequently, the midline incision is closed.

Left-modified Nerve-sparing RPLND. A midline incision is made, and the peritoneal cavity and retroperitoneum are inspected. As in the case for right-sided disease, if high-volume disease is not present in the retroperitoneum, a left-modified dissection is performed. The posterior peritoneum is entered laterally to the left colon, and the left colon is mobilized medially. The left renal vein is identified, and the split maneuver is performed over it; tissue is rolled inferiorly. The origin of the right gonadal vein is dissected and divided between silk ties. Around 40% of the time there will be a lumbar vein passing posteriorly from the left renal vein. This, too, is dissected and divided between silk ties. Next, the efferent sympathetic fibers are seen as they pass anterior to the left common iliac artery. They are dissected, placed in vessel loops, and then dissected proximally away from lymphatic tissue. The split maneuver is then performed on the aorta from the crossing of the left renal vein distally to the bifurcation of the left common iliac. Tissue is rolled into the left periaortic zone carefully avoiding efferent sympathetic fibers. The left-sided lumbar arteries are identified, dissected, and divided between silk ties. Superiorly, the left renal vein is identified as it passes to the left kidney. Lymphatic tissue is dissected away from it carefully, thus exposing the crus of the diaphragm on the left. The left gonadal vein is then dissected distally to the internal ring. The vas deferens is identified and divided, and the cord stump is mobilized from the internal ring. This specimen is harvested as the left

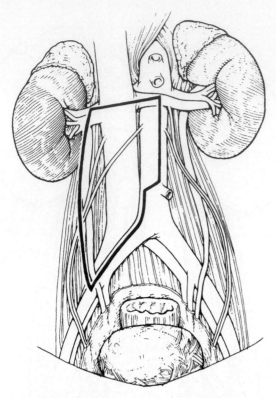

FIGURE 37A.2. Template of dissection for right-modified nerve-sparing retroperitoneal lymph node dissection is shown.

gonadal vein. Next, the left ureter is mobilized laterally away from the lymphatic tissue. Finally, the lymphatics are dissected away from the posterior body wall using clips, cautery, or ties to control lumbar arteries and veins as they penetrate the posterior body wall medial to the left sympathetic chain, or as the veins pass posterior to the aorta. At the crus of the diaphragm, clips are used in order to secure lymphatics. Hence, a left-modified nerve sparing RPLND entails the removal of two specimens; the left gonadal vein and the left periaortic lymphatics (Fig. 37A.3). The colon is then placed back in the anatomic position, and the midline incision is closed using a running looped absorbable suture.

Postchemotherapy Considerations

Patients who complete systemic chemotherapy for metastatic disease and have a residual radiographic mass on CT scanning are recommended to undergo postchemotherapy RPLND (Fig. 37A.4). Pathologically, one finds either fibrosis and necrosis, teratoma, or active carcinoma. Accurate clinical prediction of fibrosis and necrosis is not possible, and, therefore, all patients with a residual mass undergo RPLND.

Postchemotherapy RPLND is a vascular procedure. Conceptually, the idea is to dissect the great vessels away from the tumor and lymphatics and mobilize them away from the posterior body wall. The ureters, renal arteries, and renal veins are similarly dissected away from the lymphatics and tumor, then the tumor and lymphatics are removed from the posterior body wall. The cornerstone of such a procedure is the split-and-roll maneuver, whereby the initial steps in the procedure are to mobilize the great vessels and divide the lumbar veins passing posteriorly.

Various techniques of exposure of the retroperitoneum can be used. In low-volume residual disease, the same techniques of exposure of the posterior peritoneum used in low-stage disease can be used in postchemotherapy disease. Higher volume

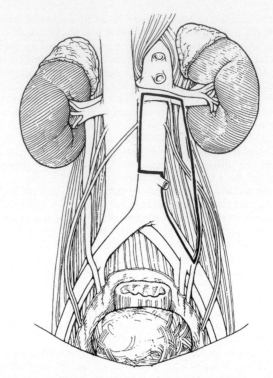

FIGURE 37A.3. Template of dissection for left-modified nerve-sparing retroperitoneal lymph node dissection is shown.

postchemotherapy disease, however, requires a complete mobilization of the right colon and root of the small bowel from the posterior body wall (Fig. 37A.5). This is performed by incising from the foramen of Winslow distally around the cecum and up to the area of the inferior mesenteric vein. The inferior mesenteric vein is then divided, which enables the right colon and root of the small bowel to be mobilized onto the patient's chest. Characteristically, a bowel bag is used to hold the bowel contents during the course of the procedure. Because the inferior mesenteric vein is divided, the pancreas can be mobilized superiorly and anteriorly.

Postchemotherapy RPLND involves the removal of all lymphatic tissue and tumor from the crus of the diaphragm distally to the bifurcation of the common iliacs from ureter to ureter. Modifications in this resection template certainly are used in

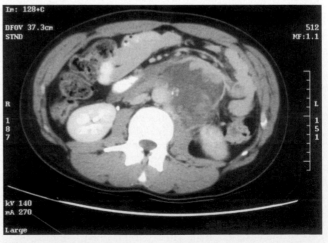

FIGURE 37A.4. Computed tomography (CT) scan showing a residual radiographic mass.

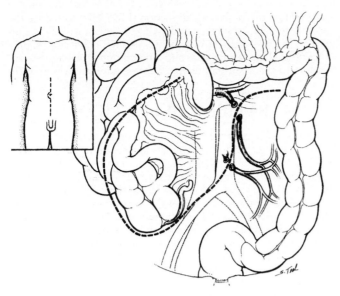

FIGURE 37A.5. Posterior peritoneal incision for a full bilateral retroperitoneal lymph node dissection is depicted.

patients with extremely high-volume disease. Some patients may require pelvic dissection, resection of retrocrural tumor, and sometimes resection of bowel (including duodenum) or en bloc resection of the kidney (Fig. 37A.6). Intraoperative judgments must be made in these patients with high-volume disease, and the experience of the surgeon in these complicated patients is very important. Similarly, surgeons attempting postchemotherapy RPLND should be thoroughly versed in techniques of vascular control and repair as sometimes there is a very dense reaction in the retroperitoneum that obliterates tissue planes.

Selected patients with postchemotherapy tumor are candidates for nerve sparing (13). Again, intraoperative judgment is extremely important in making the decision to save the nerves, as the primary consideration must be complete surgical removal of all retroperitoneal tumor and lymphatics. Similarly, because some of these patients have associated chest disease, combined procedures are performed, wherein an RPLND is done along with a thoracotomy under the same anesthetic. Again, experience and surgical judgment are very important in order to limit the perioperative morbidity.

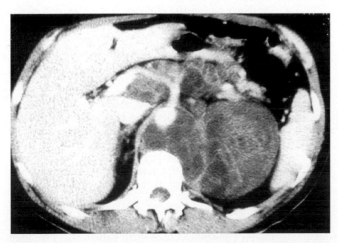

FIGURE 37A.6. High-volume teratoma in the retrocrural area is sometimes encountered.

Morbidity

In low-stage disease, the morbidity of the procedure is essentially that of a laparotomy. The most common complications include wound infection or postoperative incisional hernia, each of which occur <5% of the time. Currently, the average hospitalization for modified nerve sparing RPLND in low-stage disease is 3 days, and the return to full physical activity varies between 2 and 4 weeks, depending upon the age of the patient, his body habitus, etc.

Postchemotherapy retroperitoneal lymph node dissection is associated with a higher acute morbidity (14). Approximately 20% of patients will experience evidence of morbidity, but this, too, is dependent upon the general physical condition of the patient and the volume of tumor removed. Postchemotherapy patients with low-volume tumor have essentially similar morbidity to patients who undergo RPLND for low-stage disease. However, patients who have received multiple courses of chemotherapy or who have high-volume tumor have increased morbidity and a more lengthy hospitalization. Mortality after postchemotherapy RPLND is very rare but certainly occurs. The most common cause of postoperative mortality is adult respiratory distress syndrome, which has been linked to the use of bleomycin. Though rare, other devastating complications can occur, such as aorta duodenal fistula, chylous ascites, and paraplegia secondary to division of the vascular supply of the spinal cord during aortic mobilization.

LATE RELAPSE

Late relapse of testis cancer is defined as recurrence of disease later than 2 years after initial successful treatment. This entity is very important because it behaves differently compared with *de novo* testis cancer. Though it occurs in only 2% to 4% of all patients treated for testis cancer, it is important, biologically and clinically, because of its behavior (15).

Late relapse is represented histologically as either yolk sac tumor, teratoma, or degeneration into non–germ cell cancerous elements such as chondrosarcoma. Though yolk sac tumor at late relapse histologically appears very similar to *de novo* yolk sac tumor, it is not chemosensitive, and, therefore, late relapse is treated surgically. Most late relapses occur in the retroperitoneum, but late relapse can present in the chest, supraclavicular lymph nodes, pelvis, etc. Because yolk sac elements are common at late relapse, an elevated alpha fetoprotein is sometimes the initiating event that provokes a radiologic evaluation. Around 40% to 50% of patients with late relapse are cured, and the vast majority are cured surgically because of the lack of chemosensitive late relapse. Because of this entity, patients who are treated for testis cancer should be followed for the rest of their lives in order to identify patients at late relapse who are still curable surgically.

CONCLUSION

Testis cancer is not only chemosensitive, it is "surgery sensitive." Evolution of retroperitoneal lymph node dissection has resulted in a procedure that retains its clinical utility but is associated with much lower morbidity compared with previous decades. Both in low- and high-stage disease, this is a vascular procedure involving the mobilization of the great vessels away from retroperitoneal lymphatics, neural structures, and/or tumor. Surgeons who perform RPLND should be fully versed in techniques of vascular mobilization, repair, and control. Finally, intraoperative judgment is extremely important, especially in patients with high-volume postchemotherapy residual tumor.

References

1. Leibovitch I, Baniel J, Foster RS, et al. The clinical implications of procedural deviations during orchiectomy for nonseminomatous testis cancer. *J Urol* 1995;154:935.
2. Sweeney CS, Hermans BP, Heilman DK, et al. Results and outcome of retroperitoneal lymph node dissection for clinical stage I embryonal carcinoma-predominant testis cancer. *J Clin Oncol* 2000;18:358.
3. Baniel J, Foster RS, Rowland RG, et al. Complications of primary retroperitoneal lymph node dissection. *J Urol* 1994;152:424.
4. Bokemeyer C, Berger CC, Kuczyk MA, et al. Evaluation of long term toxicity after chemotherapy for testicular cancer. *J Clin Oncol* 1996;14:2923.
5. Huddart RA, Norman A, Shahidi M, et al. Cardiovascular disease as a long-term complication of treatment for testicular cancer. *J Clin Oncol* 2003;21:1513.
6. Lampe H, Horwich A, Norman A, et al. Fertility after chemotherapy for testicular germ cell cancers. *J Clin Oncol* 1997;15:239.
7. Foster RS, Donohue JP. Nerve sparing retroperitoneal lymphadenectomy. *Urol Clin North Am* 1993;20:117.
8. Krege S, Souchon R, Schmoll HJ. Interdisciplinary consensus on diagnosis and treatment of testicular germ cell tumors: result of an update conference on Evidence-Based Medicine (EBM). *Eur Urol* 2001;40:372.
9. Oldenburg J, Alfsen GC, Lien HH, et al. Post chemotherapy retroperitoneal surgery remains necessary in patients with nonseminomatous testicular cancer and minimal residual tumor masses. *J Clin Oncol* 2003;21:3310.
10. Steyerberg EW, Gerl A, Fossa SD, et al. Validity of predictions of residual retroperitoneal mass histology in nonseminomatous testicular cancer. *J Clin Oncol* 1998;16:269.
11. Beck SD, Foster RS, Bihrle R, et al. Post chemotherapy desperation retroperitoneal lymph node dissection for patients with elevated tumor markers. *J Urol* 2001;165:632A.
12. Donohue J, Zachary J, Maynard B. Distribution of nodal metastases in nonseminomatous testis cancer. *J Urol* 1982;128:315.
13. Wahle GR, Foster RS, Bihrle R, et al. Nerve sparing retroperitoneal lymphadenectomy after primary chemotherapy for metastatic testicular carcinoma. *J Urol* 1994;152:428.
14. Baniel J, Foster RS, Rowland RG, et al. Complications of post chemotherapy retroperitoneal lymph node dissection. *J Urol* 1995;153:976.
15. Baniel J, Foster RS, Gonin R, et al. Late relapse of testicular cancer. *J Clin Oncol* 1995;13:1170.

CHAPTER 37B
Laparoscopic Retroperitoneal Lymph Node Dissection

Nasser M. Albqami and Günter Janetschek

INTRODUCTION

Testicular cancer, although relatively rare, is the most common malignancy in men 15 to 35 years old and evokes widespread interest for several reasons. The combination of effective diagnostic techniques, improved tumor markers, effective chemotherapeutic regimens, and the modifications of surgical techniques led to a dramatic improvement in patient management and a decrease in patient mortality rates from >50% before 1970 to <5% in 1997 (1).

After radical orchiectomy, clinical staging is considered the first step in the management of all patients diagnosed with testicular cancer. About 25% to 30% of these patients will be clinically understaged, while some of them will be overstaged (2). Retroperitoneal lymphadenectomy is the most sensitive and specific method for testicular cancer staging with its therapeutic values.

Open surgical retroperitoneal lymph node dissection (RPLND) carries substantial morbidities with overall relapse rates up to 55% if it is used as a single therapeutic measure (3,4). We have replaced the open surgical technique by laparoscopic retroperitoneal lymph node dissection (LRPLND) to reduce the morbidities of open surgery. To have a convenient staging system to plan the management of patients with testicular cancer, they were divided into seminomas and nonseminomatous tumors, according to the main pathology of their orchiectomy specimen.

PATIENT SELECTION

In the management of nonseminomatous germ cell tumors (NSGCT) of the testis, RPLND has always been favored in our practice because it has a high diagnostic accuracy. Relapse rates after open RPLND alone are as high as 8% to 29% for stage IIA tumors (3,5) and 34% to 55% for stage IIB tumors (3,4). This rate falls to as low as 0% to 1% if two cycles of adjuvant chemotherapy are given (4,6); therefore, all our clinical stage I patients diagnosed as pathological stage II following open RPLND received chemotherapy as the definitive treatment.

In this concept, and because open RPLND has substantial morbidities, we replaced open surgery by laparoscopy.

LRPLND has been proved to be safe, with fewer postoperative morbidities, quicker convalescence, improved cosmetic results, and a diagnostic accuracy equal that of the open technique (7–10).

For patients diagnosed as NSGCT clinical stage I, surveillance, risk-adapted primary chemotherapy, and retroperitoneal lymphadenectomy are considered by urologists to manage this stage with overall disagreement on the optimal management (11,12).

We prefer RPLND by means of laparoscopy over the other options for the following reasons:

1. 15% to 20% of the patients under surveillance protocol will relapse (13,14), while up to 10% of these relapsing patients will die from the disease (15).
2. The main purpose of surveillance is to avoid the morbidities of open surgery, which were minimized by the introduction of LRPLND.
3. If risk-adapted primary chemotherapy was chosen for patients considered at high risk to develop retroperitoneal metastases (embryonic carcinoma as the primary tumor or tumors with vascular or lymphatic invasions), a relapse rate up to 2.7% was reported for patients who received chemotherapy because of chemoresistant cancer relapses and slow-growing retroperitoneal teratomas (13,16).

On the other hand, 50% of this group will be overtreated.

Our approach in the management of NSGCT is summarized in an algorithm (Fig. 37B.1) (7,17).

In our experience so far, 103 clinical stage I disease patients underwent LRPLND between August 1992 and June 2004 with a mean follow-up of 62 (6–113) months. Of the 103 patients, 26 had active tumor in the resected retroperitoneal lymph nodes and were, therefore, treated with adjuvant chemotherapy. During their follow-up, there was not a single recurrence observed.

Of the 103 patients, 77 had no tumor in the resected retroperitoneal lymph nodes, and 5 relapses were observed. One retroperitoneal recurrence occurred on the contralateral side outside the surgical field. Further investigations revealed that the tumor in the resected retroperitoneal lymph nodes was missed on histological examination. This patient was cured with two cycles of chemotherapy and contralateral laparoscopic RPLND.

Three other patients developed tumor recurrence in the lungs. Another patient had elevation of his tumor markers without an identifiable recurrence site. A sixth patient was treated in another center by primary chemotherapy and developed retroperitoneal relapse after one year of follow-up with negative

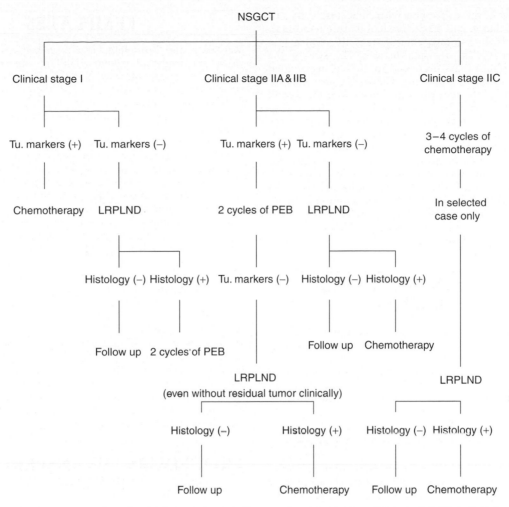

FIGURE 37B.1. Algorithm for the management of nonseminomatous germ cell tumors (NSGCT) clinical stage I and II.

tumor markers. Laparoscopic RPLND was performed, and the pathology revealed mature teratoma with immature ectodermal elements. Therefore, this patient was treated with two cycles of adjuvant chemotherapy, and he was free of recurrence during 16 months of follow-up. No further relapses occurred.

The most important statistic to prove the diagnostic accuracy of RPLND is the rate of retroperitoneal recurrence in pathological stage I.

Out of 239 NSGCT clinical stage I patients, 172 were identified as pathological stage I in a recent series of open RPLND (18). A retroperitoneal relapse rate of 1.2% was observed in this group. Our relapse rate of 1.15% compares favorably with that of open surgery and clearly demonstrates the oncologic efficacy of the procedure.

Patients with NSGCT clinical stage II are treated classically by either primary chemotherapy (3 to 4 cycles) followed by RPLND if residual retroperitoneal masses are observed or by open RPLND with or without adjuvant chemotherapy.

We adhered to the concept of primary chemotherapy for this stage, but we attempted to reduce its morbidity while maintaining its oncologic efficiency. It would be ideal to give the minimum dose required for complete tumor response and to avoid any overdose, which would only add morbidities without any therapeutic effect.

To achieve this goal, we reduced the dose of chemotherapy to two cycles of BEP in stage IIB patients (2–5 cm retroperitoneal tumors). However, to control the complete response,

RPLND becomes mandatory even if there is no residual tumor. Again, to reduce morbidity, open RPLND was replaced by laparoscopy. In our experience, morbidity of postchemotherapy LRPLND is clearly inferior to a third cycle of chemotherapy, and even more so for a fourth.

It has to be realized that the morbidities of chemotherapy are not increasing proportionally with the administrated dose, but these morbidities are increasing exponentially after each cycle of chemotherapy. Therefore, each patient will profit from this concept.

In our experience so far, 43 consecutive patients with clinical stage IIB disease treated with two cycles of primary chemotherapy underwent LRPLND between February 1995 and June 2004. Mean follow-up is 53 months. Over the same period, in 17 selected patients with clinical stage IIC disease, laparoscopic retroperitoneal residual mass excision was performed following 3 to 4 cycles of primary chemotherapy.

Out of the 43 patients with clinical stage IIB, 16 patients had mature teratomas, and 26 patients had no tumor in the resected lymph nodes. One patient had active tumor, which was a borderline case between stage IIB and IIC.

One patient with stage IIB disease had recurrence after 24 months of follow-up that was outside the surgical field at the external iliac lymph nodes close to the internal inguinal ring. This recurrence was again resected laparoscopically. The pathology of this node was mature teratoma, which was followed, and no further relapse was observed with a follow-up of 8 months. Out of the 16 patients with clinical stage IIC, 10 patients had no tumor, and 5 patients had mature teratomas.

One patient had seminoma clinical stage IIC, which was treated by three cycles of chemotherapy. The size of the retroperitoneal tumor mass decreased to 20% of its original size (from 30 cm down to 6 cm). Clinically there was no change in the size of the retroperitoneal mass after the second cycle of chemotherapy. A PET scan was done, and it was negative. LRPLND was then performed, and the pathology of the resected mass showed foci of viable tumor, and the patient was treated with two more cycles of chemotherapy.

There is a general consensus that there is no place for RPLND in the management of seminoma clinical stage I because the morbidities of alternative therapies are low and their efficacy is very high (19). RPLND for seminoma is considered only in exceptional cases for the removal of residual retroperitoneal masses after chemotherapy, which was proven to be feasible by laparoscopic means.

CONTRAINDICATIONS FOR LRPLND

The absolute contraindications are elevated tumor markers, severe pulmonary fibrosis that prevents pneumoperitoneum, and uncontrolled bleeding diathesis.

Patients with a higher body mass index benefit more from laparoscopy than slim patients in respect to postoperative pain and morbidity but do not experience more complications (20).

PREOPERATIVE PREPARATIONS

Low-fat diet with medium-chain triglycerides for 1 week preoperatively is continued 2 weeks postoperatively to prevent chylous ascites, which was observed after laparoscopic RPLND in some patients postchemotherapy. We have not seen this complication since this protocol was established.

As a mechanical bowel preparation, oral laxatives and clear liquid diet is started 1 day prior to surgery.

Two units of blood should be typed and cross-matched prior to surgery and be ready for transfusion, if needed.

Low-dose systemic antibiotic is given to the patient on call to surgery as prophylaxis against wound infection.

TECHNIQUE

RPLND is feasible endoscopically through a transperitoneal or extraperitoneal approach. In our practice, we use the transperitoneal approach exclusively. The extraperitoneal approach advocated by Le Blanc (21) is not going to be described in this chapter because we do not have experience with it.

Standard laparoscopic equipment is used, including a 3-chip video camera and a 30-degree laparoscope. The laparoscope is held and maneuvered by a robotic arm (manufactured by Computer Motion, Santa Barbara, CA). This has the advantage of providing stable video images even in lengthy procedures. Insufflation with a high flow rate has proved helpful because it prevents the pneumoperitoneum from collapsing during suction. All dissection is performed using bipolar grasping forceps and monopolar scissors. A small surgical sponge held with an atraumatic grasper is used for retraction, dissection, and haemostasis. A right-angled dissector (Aesculap, Tuttlingen, Germany) is applied for dissection of the vessels. We do not use metallic clips anymore and have replaced them with Hem-o-lok clips (Weck Closure System, Research Triangle, NC).

TEMPLATES

Weissbach and Boedefeld have described templates that include practically all primary landing sites of lymph node metastases for patients with NSGCT clinical stage I (22). The right template will hold 97% of all the primary landing sites of lymph node metastases, while the left template will hold 95% of all the primary landing sites of lymph node metastases in this stage.

The right template includes the interaortocaval lymph nodes, preaortic tissue between the left renal vein and the inferior mesenteric artery, precaval tissue, and all the tissues lateral to the vena cava and the right common iliac artery, while the lateral border of dissection is the ureter.

The left template includes preaortic tissue between the left renal vein and the inferior mesenteric artery, all the tissue lateral to the aorta and the left common iliac artery, and the interaortocaval lymph nodes, while the lymphatic tissue ventral to the aorta below the inferior mesenteric artery is preserved. The lateral border of dissection is the ureter (Fig. 37B.2).

We investigated the primary lymphatic metastatic spread in testicular cancer in 139 patients. All solitary metastases were detected ventral to the lumber vessels, whereas metastases dorsal to the lumber vessels were only detected in 3 out of 25 patients with multiple metastases who had ventral metastases as well. Therefore, it was concluded that the primary landing sites are invariably located ventral to the lumbar vessels, whereas dorsal metastases resulted from further tumor spread (23). Consequently, following the first 30 patients, we no longer routinely transect lumbar vessels for removal of dorsally located lymphatic tissue.

PROCEDURE (TRANSPERITONEAL APPROACH)

Positioning of the patient, trocar placement, and pneumoperitoneum are the first steps after general anaesthesia is established. A nasogastric tube and a urinary bladder catheter are inserted. The patient is placed with the ipsilateral side elevated 45 degrees off the operating table, so that he can be brought into supine or lateral decubitus positions simply by rotating the table rather than repositioning him. The operating table is flexed at the umbilicus, and the Trendlenburg or anti-Trendlenburg positions are used if necessary. A veress needle is used for the initial stab incision at the umbilicus to create the pneumoperitoneum, whereas Hasson cannula is used if indicated. The first trocar is placed at the umbilicus for the laparoscope, whereas two secondary trocars are placed at the lateral edge of the rectus muscle 8 cm above and below the umbilicus for the surgeon's instruments. A fourth trocar is placed at the anterior axillary line in the best point for retraction decided by the surgeon; 5 mm and 10 mm trocars are used.

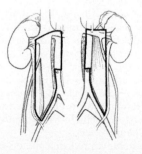

FIGURE 37B.2. Retroperitoneal template for laparoscopic lymph node dissection.

Right Side

The peritoneum is incised at the internal inguinal ring, then along the line of Toldt from the cecum to the right colic flexure. Cephalic dissection is carried out parallel to the transverse colon and lateral to the duodenum along the vena cava up to the hepato-duodenal ligament, while the caudal dissection is continued along the spermatic vessels down to the internal inguinal ring. In the next step the colon, duodenum, and the head of pancreas are reflected medially until the anterior surface of the vena cava, aorta, and left renal vein are completely exposed (Fig. 37B.3). A wide access to the retroperitoneal space is a prerequisite for LRPLND. The spermatic vein is dissected free along its entire course, clipped, and transected with much care so as not to be ruptured from the vena cava. Then the spermatic artery is clipped and transected at the point where it crosses over the vena cava; spermatic artery origin will be approached later. Those steps will make the right template fully accessible for dissection.

Cranial to caudal, the lymphatic tissue overlying the vena cava is split open, then the lateral and anterior surfaces of the vena cava are dissected free. Both renal veins are then dissected free (Fig. 37B.4). The lower border of the left renal vein must be completely freed at this point, as it might be easily injured during the dissection of the interaortocaval lymph node package from caudal in cephalic direction. Lymphatic tissue overlying the right common iliac artery is incised, and the dissection is continued from caudal in cephalic direction up to the origin of the inferior mesenteric artery. Lymphatic tissues in this area are dense and care must be taken not to injure the inferior mesenteric artery because it is a landmark to preserve the left sympathetic nerves. Cephalic to the inferior mesenteric artery dissection is continued upward along the left margin to the aorta. Thereby the ventral surface of the aorta is completely freed. Then the spermatic artery is clipped at its origin.

Cranial to caudal, the interaortocaval space is dissected, starting from the lower edge of the right renal artery down to the lumbar vessels, and the lymphatic tissue is removed step by step (Fig. 37B.5). The right renal vein and artery lateral to the vena cava delineate the cranial border of the dissection, while the caudal border of the dissection is the point where the ureter crosses the iliac vessels (Figs. 37B.6 and 37B.7). The lymphatic tissue is clipped distally, then the dissection is continued cephalic until the lymphatic package is freed, while the lumbar veins are exposed, but they are only transected in exceptional cases. Lymph nodes lateral to the vena cava and medial to the ureter are dissected free, and then the nodal package can be removed within a specimen retrieval bag. The colon and duodenum are returned to their anatomic position.

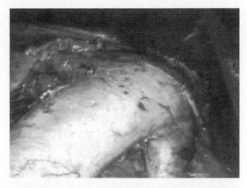

FIGURE 37B.4. Posterior peritoneum is dissected until the vena cava and both renal veins are dissected free.

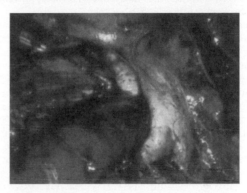

FIGURE 37B.5. The space is completely free of lymphatic tissue. The left renal vein and the right renal artery are the upper limit of dissection. The spine is seen in the interaortocaval space.

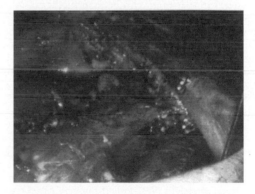

FIGURE 37B.6. The vena cava is retracted medially, and the aorta is seen underneath. The right renal vein and artery define the upper limit of dissection. The entire interaortocaval area and the tissue lateral to the vena cava are removed. A clipped lumbar vein is seen on the lateral side of the vena cava.

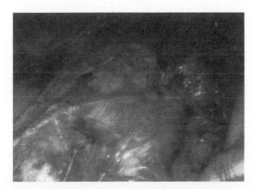

FIGURE 37B.3. Wide exposure of the right retroperitoneum. From right to left: the duodenum is reflected; left renal vein, aorta, and vena cava covered with posterior peritoneum. In the middle of the picture, the gonadal artery crosses the vena cava anteriorly.

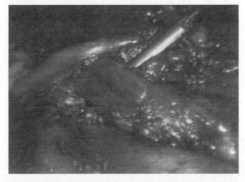

FIGURE 37B.7. Lower limit of dissection for the right template. The ureter is seen in the upper left corner of the picture crossing the common iliac vessels.

Then the colon is fixed in position with one stitch to the abdominal wall laterally which is tied extracorporeally. Drains are not required.

Left Side

The peritoneum is incised along the line of Toldt, starting from the left colonic flexure down to the pelvic brim and distally along the spermatic vein to the internal inguinal ring. The splenocolic ligament is transected, and the colon is dissected until the anterior surface of the aorta is exposed. In the next step, the spermatic vein is dissected along its entire course and excised, and then the ureter is identified laterally and separated from the lymphatic tissue carefully to preserve its blood supply. That step will facilitate left renal vein dissection until it is freed completely (Fig. 37B.8).

Dissection of the lymphatic template is started caudally at the crossing of the ureter with the common iliac vessels by splitting the lymphatic tissue over the anterior surface of the left common iliac artery in a cephalic direction along the lateral border of the aorta, circumventing the inferior mesenteric artery on the left side and preserving it. Cephalic to the inferior mesenteric artery dissection is continued along the anterior and medial surfaces of the aorta up to the left renal vein, and during this dissection the origin of the spermatic artery is clipped and transected. Next to that the lateral surface of the aorta is dissected down to the origin of the lumbar arteries. To gain access to the left renal artery, the lumbar vein draining into the left renal vein must be transected (Fig. 37B.9). Other lumbar vessels are dissected free from the lymphatic tissue to the point at which they disappear in the layer between the spine and psoas muscle (Fig. 37B.10), and then the sympathetic chain lateral to that point can be identified.

Although the left postganglionic fibers are readily identified, they are not preserved in template dissection because the right sympathetic chain remains intact, providing undisturbed antegrade ejaculations.

When the nodal package is completely freed, it can be retrieved within a laparoscopic retrieval bag. Then the colon is secured in its anatomic position with an extracorporeally tied suture. Drains are not required.

Preservation of Antegrade Ejaculation

Loss of antegrade ejaculation is the major long-term morbidity encountered after RPLND. This drawback can be overcome either by performing a template dissection as described by Weissbach (22) or by nerve-sparing RPLND (24). In clinical

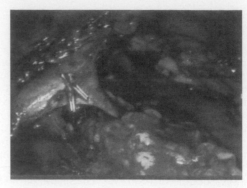

FIGURE 37B.9. Lumbar vein draining into left renal vein and a clipped gonadal vein.

stage I, the template dissection downscales the operative field, yet maintains acceptable sensitivity and, more important, doesn't increase relapse. We have followed this strategy in our work and, in 100 of our stage I patients, antegrade ejaculation rate was 100% (3 patients were lost during follow-up). In stage II patients, antegrade ejaculation was preserved in 57 out of 59 patients.

With the introduction of nerve-sparing RPLND, Donohue was able to improve the ejaculation rate from 70% to almost 100%. However, Donohue did not only introduce nerve-sparing dissection but also simultaneously limited the dissection to the unilateral template described by Weissbach (3,24).Using this template, the contralateral sympathetic nerves remain intact, and it has been known since 1951 that destruction of the sympathetic chain on one side doesn't result in aspermia (25). Therefore, nerve-sparing in addition to a unilateral template dissection is not necessary, as it cannot improve the favorable results for antegrade ejaculation preservation that already have been achieved through unilateral template dissection alone. Obviously, template dissection can be performed more precisely with laparoscopy than open surgery because anatomy is not disturbed by retractors.

Recently, Peschel et al. have shown that nerve-sparing RPLND is feasible by means of laparoscopy. They published an average operative time of 3.2 hours, a blood loss of 66 mL, and a hospital stay of 3.7 days for 5 patients. This required meticulous dissection and identification of the sympathetic chain and the post-ganglionic fibers in the retrocaval, the interaortocaval, and the para-aortic regions. Although, as we mentioned, antegrade ejaculation is routinely preserved when a nerve-sparing dissection is limited to a unilateral template, the development of a unilateral laparoscopic nerve-sparing technique is a step toward bilateral laparoscopic dissection (26).

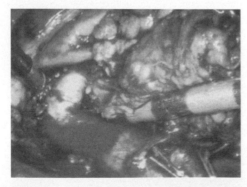

FIGURE 37B.8. Left template dissection: the anterior wall of the aorta is exposed with clipped gonadal artery. In the upper left corner of the picture, the renal artery and vein delineate the upper limit of dissection. Lymphatic package is seen lateral to the aorta.

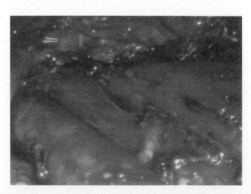

FIGURE 37B.10. Surgical template after left laparoscopic retroperitoneal lymph node dissection (LRPLND). Left upper corner: left renal vein; right lower corner: aorta. Middle of picture: a lumbar artery disappears between the spine and the psoas muscle.

Technical Tips

Adequate hemostasis is of crucial importance. Even minimal bleedings must be controlled and stopped instantly to provide a bloodless surgical field. Grasping forceps for bipolar coagulation and dissection is ideal for the dissection of delicate vessels such as the vena cava and renal veins. Broader bipolar forceps allow precise hemostasis without damaging the surrounding structures. The harmonic scalpel may also be used for a bloodless transection of the lymphatic tissue. A protruding segment of bowel can cause insufficient exposure and may render the operation difficult, dangerous, or even impossible. To gain exposure, a fan retractor can be used to retract the liver and the duodenum as well. Retraction of the bowel can be achieved by a surgical sponge held with a traumatic grasper. An additional trocar can be inserted in the mid-line just caudal to the costal margin for the introduction of a second fan retractor if required in exceptional cases. Exposure could be achieved in all instances, and we have never converted to open surgery because of insufficient exposure. Acute bleeding is the most frequent complication. A small surgical sponge that is held with a traumatic grasper can be a substitute for the surgeon's finger to be used for dissection, retraction, or pressure to control bleeding vessels so that subsequent measures can be taken without the pressure of time. Small defects in veins or even the vena cava can be sealed by direct application of fibrin glue. For larger defects, the edges should be approximated using a traumatic grasper without or with the use of endoscopic clips. Then the area of the defect is sealed by fibrin glue. Care must be taken when using endoscopic clips as they tend to fall off. The strength of the repair should be enhanced by the additional use of Surgicel (oxidized regenerated cellulose) or similar hemostatic substances such as Tachocomb to cover the area of the defect. In exceptional conditions, laparoscopic vascular suture repairs are feasible if needed (7,17,27). Instruments for general and vascular surgery must be available in the operating room in the event of bleeding that may not be controlled by endoscopic means.

RPLND PAST, PRESENT, AND FUTURE

To lower the morbidities of retroperitoneal lymphadenectomy, RPLND was modified over the past 35 years from extended suprahilar to bilateral infrahilar. Subsequently, a modified laparoscopic unilateral approach was introduced, followed by a nerve-sparing technique. There was no increase in relapse rates associated with the introduction of these operative refinements; significant factors for relapse were pathological stage (P <.001) and adjuvant chemotherapy in stage II disease (P <.001) (3).

In this respect, the future challenge is to develop a technique that could exactly locate the sentinel lymph node for testicular cancer. Thus the RPLND could be limited while maintaining its diagnostic accuracy and its therapeutic value (29).

In Europe, risk-adaptive primary chemotherapy is going to replace open RPLND in the management of NSGCT clinical stage I because of its high morbidity. We think that our concept of LRPLND and adjuvant chemotherapy for pathological stage II has many advantages over primary chemotherapy and may swing the pendulum back toward surgery.

SUMMARY

In our hands, LRPLND has demonstrated its surgical and oncologic efficacy. The morbidity and the complication rates are low. Adherence to the templates previously described allows for preservation of antegrade ejaculation in virtually all patients (3,24,25). It is a difficult procedure, but once the long and steep learning curve has been overcome, operative times are equal to or even shorter than those of open surgery. Thereafter, the costs will be in the range of open surgery. Survival and tumor recurrence rates after LRPLND are at least as low and equal to that of open surgery and chemotherapy. Patient satisfaction, however, is clearly higher with LRPLND, which we demonstrated in a recent extensive quality-of-life study (28).

References

1. Bost GJ, Motzer RJ. Testicular germ-cell cancer. *N Engl J Med* 1997;337: 242–253.
2. Bussar-Matz R, Weissbach L. Retroperitoneal lymph node staging of testicular tumours. TNM Study Group. *Br J Urol* 1993;72:234–240.
3. Donohue JP, Thornhill JA, Foster RS, et al. Retroperitoneal lymphadenectomy for clinical stage A testis cancer (1965–1989): modification of technique and impact on ejaculation. *J Urol* 1993;149:243–237.
4. Williams SD, Stablein DM, Einhorn LH, et al. Immediate adjuvant chemotherapy versus observation with treatment at relapse in pathological stage II testicular cancer. *N Engl J Med* 1987;317:1433–1438.
5. Richie JP, Kantoff PW. Is adjuvant chemotherapy necessary for patients with stage B1 testicular cancer? *J Clin Oncol* 1991;9:1393–1396.
6. Javadpour N. Predictors of recurrence in stage II nonseminomatous testicular cancer after lymphadenectomy: implications for adjuvant chemotherapy. *J Urol* 1984;135:629.
7. Steiner H, Peschel R, Janetschek G, et al. Long-term result of laparoscopic retroperitoneal lymph node dissection: a single-center 10 years experience. *Urology* 2004;63:550–555.
8. Corvin S, Kuczyk M, Anastasiadis A, et al. Laparoscopic retroperitoneal lymph node dissection for nonseminomatous testicular carcinoma. *World J Urol* 2004;22:33–36.
9. Rassweiler JJ, Frede T, Lenz E, et al. Long-term experience with laparoscopic retroperitoneal lymph node dissection in the management of low-stage testis cancer. *Eur Urol* 2000;37:251–260.
10. Bhayani SB, Allaf ME, Kavoussi LR. Laparoscopic retroperitoneal lymph node dissection for clinical stage I nonseminomatous germ cell testicular cancer: current status. *Urology Oncology* 2004;22:145–148.
11. Rassweiler JJ, Seemann O, Henkel TO, et al. Laparoscopic retroperitoneal lymph node dissection for non seminomatous germ cell tumour: indication and limitation. *J Urol* 1996;156:1108–1113.
12. Janetschek G. Laparoscopic RPLND. *Urol Clin North Am* 2001;28: 107–114.
13. Laguna MP, Klepp O, Horwich A, et al. Guidelines on testicular cancer. *Eur Assoc Urol* 2004.
14. Sogani PC, Perrotti M, Herr HW, et al. Clinical stage I testis cancer: long-term outcome of patients on surveillance. *J Urol* 1998;159:855–858.
15. Nicolai R, Pizzocaro G. A surveillance study of clinical stage I non-seminomatous germ cell tumours of the testis: 1-year follow up. *J Urol* 1995;154:1045–1049.
16. Gullen MH, Stenning SP, Parkinson MC, et al. High-risk stage I non-seminomatous germ cell tumours of the testis. A Medical Research Council Report. *J Clin Oncol* 1996;14:1106–1113.
17. Janetschek G, Hobisch A, Hittmair A, et al. Laparoscopic lymphadenectomy after chemotherapy for stage IIB nonseminomatous testicular carcinoma. *J Urol* 1999;161:477–481.
18. Heidenreich A, Albers P, Hartmann M, et al. Complications of nerve sparing retroperitoneal lymph node dissection for clinical stage I nonseminomatous germ cell tumours of the testis (experience of the German Testicular Cancer Study Group). *J Urol* 2003;169:1710–1714.
19. Steiner H, Holtl L, Wirtenberger W, et al. Long-term experience with carboplatin monotherapy for clinical stage I seminoma: a retrospective single-center study. *Urology* 2002;60:324–328.
20. Klingler HC, Remzi M, Janetschek G, et al. Benefits of laparoscopic renal surgery are more pronounced in patients with a high body mass index. *Eur Urol* 2003;43:522–527.
21. Le Blanc E, Caty A, Dargent D, et al. Extraperitoneal laparoscopic para-aortic lymph node dissection for early stage non seminomatous germ cell tumour of the testis with introduction of a nerve sparing technique: description and results. *J Urol* 2001;165:89–92.
22. Weissbach L, Boedefeld EA. Testicular Tumour Study Group: localization of solitary and multiple metastases in stage II non seminomatous testis tumour as basis for modified staging lymph node dissection in stage I. *J Urol* 1987;138:77–82.
23. Holtl L, Peschel R, Knapp R, et al. Primary lymphatic metastatic spread in testicular cancer occurs ventral to the lumbar vessels. *Urology* 2002;59: 114–118.
24. Donohue JP, Foster RS, Rowland RG, et al. Nerve-sparing retroperitoneal lymphadenectomy with preservation of ejaculation. *J Urol* 1990;144: 287–291.

25. Whitelaw GP, Smithwick RH. Some secondary effects of sympathectomy with particular reference to disturbance of sexual function. *N Engl J Med* 1951;245:212.
26. Peschel R, Gettman MT, Neururer R, et al. Laparoscopic retroperitoneal lymph node dissection: description of the nerve sparing technique. *Urology* 2002;60:339–343.
27. Janetschek G, Hobisch A, Peschel R, et al. Laparoscopic retroperitoneal lymph node dissection. *Urology* 2000;55:136–140.
28. Hobisch A, Tönnemann J, Janetschek G, et al. Morbidity and quality of life after open versus laparoscopic retroperitoneal lymphadenectomy for testicular tumour—the patient's view. In: Jones WG, Appleyard I, Harnden P et al., eds. *Germ cell tumours VI.* London: John Libbey, 1998:277.
29. Ohyama C, Chiba Y, Yamazaki T, et al. Lymphatic mapping and gamma probe guided laparoscopic biopsy of sentinel lymph node in patients with clinical stage I testicular tumour. *J Urol* 2002;168:1390–1395.

CHAPTER 37C
Postchemotherapy Retroperitoneal Lymph Node Dissection and Resection of Residual Masses for Germ Cell Tumors of the Testis

Joel Sheinfeld

The role, timing, and extent of postchemotherapy surgery in the management of patients with advanced germ cell tumors (GCT) has evolved significantly over the past two decades (1–3). Before the development of effective cisplatin-based chemotherapy regimens, surgical "debulking" was followed by ineffective chemotherapy. Not surprisingly, this resulted in high relapse rates, significant morbidity, and poor overall survival rates (4,5).

Improvements in radiographic staging modalities such as computed tomography (CT) and magnetic resonance imaging (MRI), a better appreciation of the role of serum tumor markers α-fetaprotein (AFP) and human chorionic gonadotropin (HCG) in clinical decision making, and the introduction of effective cisplatin and etoposide-based chemotherapy regimens have resulted in adjunctive postchemotherapy surgery comprising a critical role in the comprehensive management of patients with advanced GCT (1,6–9).

This multidisciplinary approach has resulted in cure rates of approximately 80% in patients with metastatic GCT (1,3,10). As the cure rates of patients with GCT have increased, emphasis has been placed on reducing treatment related toxicities (1). In advanced GCT, examples of this include prospective clinical trials that have resulted in the deletion of lengthy and toxic maintenance therapy, and reduction in the length of treatments and number of chemotherapeutic drugs required for effective systemic therapy (1,11–13). Similarly, investigators have attempted to identify patients whose residual masses in the retroperitoneum and/or other sites contain only necrosis following chemotherapy, thus identifying a group of patients for whom adjunctive surgery could be safely avoided, since surgery in this setting is generally felt to be of minimal therapeutic benefit (1).

With rare exceptions, the presence of persistently elevated serum tumor markers after chemotherapy is usually associated with unresectable viable GCT, and salvage chemotherapy is usually recommended. Conversely, the recommendations for postchemotherapy surgery for patients with appropriate normalization of serum tumor markers are variable (1–3). These recommendations range from observing all patients regardless of residual radiographic findings to surgical exploration of all patients following chemotherapy (14–16).

While most clinicians favor surgery for patients with normal tumor markers and residual radiographic abnormalities, at the present time there are no standard guidelines for observation rather than adjunctive surgery (1–3,17). Published variables for patients who can be safely managed by observation rather than adjunctive surgery include normal postchemotherapy CT scan, residual retroperitoneal masses less than 1.5 cm or 2.0 cm, greater than 90% volume reduction of the original prechemotherapy mass and the absence of teratoma in the orchiectomy specimen, and a normal postchemotherapy CT scan in patients without teratomatous elements in the primary specimen (18–21). Consequently, the proportion of patients undergoing surgery following chemotherapy varies significantly and has ranged from 28% to 73% (13,22–25).

POSTCHEMOTHERAPY RETROPERITONEAL LYMPH NODE DISSECTION FOLLOWING INDUCTION CHEMOTHERAPY FOR ADVANCED NONSEMINOMATOUS GERM CELL TUMORS

The early reports of the pathologic findings at retroperitoneal lymph node dissection (RPLND) following induction cisplatin-based chemotherapy and the normalization of serum tumor markers demonstrated that necrosis, teratoma, and persistent viable carcinoma were each found in approximately one third of cases (7,26). In the past 10 to 15 years, investigators have reported an increase in the proportion of patients with necrosis and a decrease in the number of patients with nonteratomatous GCT (1,16,27–31). This trend is felt to be the result of stage migration and improved chemotherapeutic regimens (1,32). Currently, the reported distribution of pathologic findings in the retroperitoneum following induction chemotherapy is necrosis, teratoma, and viable GCT in approximately 50%, 40% and 10%, respectively (Table 37C.1). However, it is important to note that the distribution of histologic findings following "salvage" chemotherapy is significantly different with viable GCT comprising approximately 50% of resected specimens, teratoma in 40% of cases, and necrosis in only 10% (33).

PREDICTING NECROSIS

Since approximately 50% of resected residual retroperitoneal specimens contain only necrotic debris, investigators have attempted to predict its presence and thus identify patients who could safely avoid postchemotherapy surgery (1,20,27,29,31).

COMPUTED TOMOGRAPHY CRITERIA

Observation has been recommended in patients whose tumor markers have normalized and the postchemotherapy CT scan is normal. Unfortunately, the definition of a normal CT scan is variable and includes no visible mass or lymph node diameters of ≤ 10 mm, 15 mm, or 20 mm (28,40–42). Furthermore, multiple investigators have shown that a significant proportion of resected specimens will contain teratoma and/or viable GCT despite strict CT criteria (6,15,16,39). Toner et al. reported

TABLE 37C.1

RETROPERITONEAL PATHOLOGIC FINDINGS IN PATIENTS FOLLOWING
INDUCTION CHEMOTHERAPY

Author, Yr	Number of patients	Necrosis (%)	Teratoma (%)	Carcinoma (%)
Donohue et al. (1982) (17)	51	16 (31%)	16 (31%)	19 (38%)
Tait et al. (1984) (34)	73	25 (34%)	32 (44%)	16 (22%)
Freiha et al. (1984) (35)	40	21 (55%)	18 (45%)	1 (2%)
Pizzocaro et al. (1985) (26)	36	16 (44%)	10 (28%)	10 (28%)
Donohue et al. (1987) (20)	80	35 (44%)	33 (41%)	12 (15%)
Gelderman et al. (1988) (21)	24	17 (71%)	7 (29%)	–
Harding et al. (1989) (36)	42	19 (45%)	14 (33%)	9 (22%)
Toner et al. (1990) (27)	122	57 (47%)	48 (39%)	17 (14%)
Mulder et al. (1990) (37)	55	31 (56%)	12 (22%)	12 (22%)
Aaas et al. (1991) (38)	173	85 (49%)	50 (29%)	38 (22%)
Fossa et al. (1992) (28)	78	51 (65%)	22 (28%)	5 (7%)
Steyerberg et al. (1995) (29)	556	250 (45%)	236 (42%)	70 (13%)
Stenning et al. (1998) (30)	153	45 (29%)	85 (56%)	23 (15%)
Steyerberg et al. (1998) (31)	172	77 (45%)	72 (42%)	23 (13%)
Oldenberg et al. (2003) (16)	87	58 (67%)	23 (26%)	6 (7%)
Patel et al. (2003) (39)	205	121 (56%)	79 (38%)	15 (6%)

that 8 of 39 (21%) patients with residual masses of <15 mm had viable GCT or teratoma resected. In 1992, Fossa et al. reported that 12 of 37 patients with normal serum markers and residual nodes >10 mm had teratoma and one patient had viable GCT in the resected specimen (15). In 2003, in an updated report from the same institution, Oldenberg noted that in spite of improved chemotherapy regimens and refinements in CT imaging, of 38 patients with residual masses ≤10 mm, 11 had teratoma and 5 had viable GCT. Therefore, they recommended postchemotherapy surgery regardless of CT findings (16).

Attenuation values of residual masses have been inconsistent in predicting necrosis (20,41,43). At the present time, there are no CT criteria reliable enough to distinguish necrosis from teratoma or viable GCT following chemotherapy.

Positron emission tomography (PET) has been evaluated as a technique to predict residual postchemotherapy histology; however, it cannot reliably distinguish teratoma from necrosis (44,45).

ADDITIONAL CLINICAL CRITERIA

In 1987, Donohue et al. (20) reported that none of the 15 patients without teratomatous elements in the orchiectomy specimen and a decrease greater than or equal to 90% in retroperitoneal tumor volume had viable GCT or teratoma in the resected RPLND specimen. Conversely, 7 of 9 patients with teratoma in the primary specimen had teratoma or viable GCT in the resected retroperitoneal specimen despite a 90% or greater volume reduction of the original mass (1). Consequently, the recommendation was to observe patients in whom there was a 90% decrease in volume of the retroperitoneal adenopathy following chemotherapy and the orchiectomy specimen did not contain teratoma (20). However, in a follow-up study from Indiana University, of 295 consecutive patients with advanced nonseminomatous germ cell tumor (NSGCT) treated with induction chemotherapy, Debono et al. (48) reported that 74% of 27 patients with teratoma-negative orchiectomy specimens who normalized their tumor markers and had a 90% or greater radiographic response were continuously free of disease without postchemotherapy surgery (1).

Furthermore, 4 of 6 patients with disease progression relapsed in the retroperitoneum (1,46). These investigators conclude that the management of these patients remains "complicated and controversial" and includes either postchemotherapy surgery or observation with sequential imaging and marker studies.

Although teratoma in the primary tumor predicts for the presence of teratoma or viable GCT in resected specimens following chemotherapy, regardless of the clinical response of the original masses, its absence in the orchiectomy specimen does not preclude its presence following chemotherapy (1). In a study of 105 patients treated at Memorial Sloan-Kettering Cancer Center (MSKCC), Toner et al. (27) found that 25 (33%) of 75 patients without teratoma in the primary tumor had teratomatous elements resected from metastatic sites. In a study of 51 patients with teratoma in postchemotherapy resections, Loehrer et al. (47) noted that 28% of the orchiectomy specimens were teratoma-negative. In an updated study from the same institution Beck et al. (48) reported that 48% of patients without teratoma in the primary had teratoma in the retroperitoneum.

Over the past 15 years a number of models have been developed in an effort to reliably predict necrosis in resected specimens (1–3). In a multivariate regression analysis, Toner et al. (27) identified the size, shrinkage of the prechemotherapy mass, and the prechemotherapy lactate dehydrogenase (LDH) and AFP levels as the best predictors of necrosis. There is a correlation between the histology and the degree of shrinkage of the tumors after chemotherapy, the size of the residual mass, or both (27). Thirty-one (79%) of 39 patients with a residual mass less than 1.5 cm had necrosis, five (13%) patients had teratoma, and three (8%) patients had viable GCT. Eighteen of 23 (78%) patients with 90% or greater volume reduction of metastatic disease had necrosis; however, 4 (17%) had teratoma and 3 (13%) had viable GCT. Of 17 patients with a residual mass less than 1.5 cm, 90% or greater tumor volume reduction, and no teratoma in the orchiectomy specimen, 3 (18%) had teratoma and 2 (12%) had viable GCT in the resected retroperitoneal specimens (1,27). The logistic regression model developed by using the four independent significant variables was able to predict necrosis in 83% of patients; however, the false-negative rate was 20%.

In 1995, Steyerberg et al. (29) developed a model to predict postchemotherapy histology by using an international data set collecting 556 patients. By using logistic regression analysis, the six variables predictive of necrosis were the absence of teratoma in the orchiectomy specimen, normal prechemotherapy AFP and HCG levels, elevated prechemotherapy LDH levels, a small prechemotherapy or postchemotherapy mass, and significant shrinkage following chemotherapy (28). However, the false-negative prediction was approximately 20% and, in a prospective follow-up study of 172 patients, the model's performance was poor in patients treated with chemotherapy regimens that included bleomycin, etoposide, and cisplatin (31).

Patient selection for observation following induction chemotherapy remains controversial. Although there are a number of models predictive of necrosis, the risk of a false-negative prediction remains approximately 20% (1,27,29,31). No single criterion or combination of criteria is sufficiently predictive of a negative histology to avoid the risk of unresected teratoma or viable GCT by obviating postchemotherapy surgery (1–3,17). Consequently, the decision to recommend postchemotherapy surgery depends on the frequency of viable GCT, the unpredictable biology of teratoma, and the morbidity of the RPLND (17).

POSTCHEMOTHERAPY RPLND

It is important to thoroughly reassess the postchemotherapy patient prior to surgery. Repeat serum tumor markers, complete blood count, and chemistries are drawn. Surgery is usually scheduled 3 to 4 weeks after the final cycle of chemotherapy to allow time for recovery of white blood cell (>3.5) and platelet ($>100,000$) counts into normal range (17). Patients who have undergone multiple chemotherapy regimens, salvage, and/or high-dose therapy may require an additional time interval prior to surgery.

Patients treated with bleomycin-containing regimens should undergo pulmonary function testing since restrictive pulmonary fibrosis may occur (49). This pulmonary fibrosis predisposes patients to alveolar edema if they are exposed to high oxygen concentrations and/or fluid overload (50,51). In a study of 77 patients, Donat and Levy (52) noted that the most predictive factors for pulmonary complications were blood transfusions and overall fluid requirements.

In general, the morbidity of RPLND after chemotherapy is higher than that of a primary RPLND (1,6). Baniel et al. (53) reported no deaths and 38 (8%) major complications in 478 patients who underwent primary RPLND compared to five deaths and 106 (18%) major complications in 603 patients after postchemotherapy RPLND (54). Although larger-volume residual disease, postchemotherapy desmoplastic reaction, prior exposure to bleomycin, and more extensive retroperitoneal resection increase the technical and perioperative demands of the procedure, a recent study from the same institution showed a significant decline in perioperative morbidity and hospital stay (55). Mosharafa et al. compared 150 patients who underwent postchemotherapy RPLND between July 2000 and July 2002 to 79 patients with similar clinical characteristics who underwent the same procedure between 1990 and 1992. They noted fewer intraoperative complications/additional procedures (44 of 150; 29%) compared to 41 (52%) of 79 ($P = .0008$), a trend toward lower postoperative complication rate (10/150; 7%) compared to 11 of 79 (14%) ($P = .07$), and shorter hospital stay (average 5.6 vs. 8.4 days; $P < .001$) (55). Chang et al. have also reported a significant decrease in the complication rate and hospital stay of postchemotherapy RPLND patients before and after 1997, and attribute this in part to the institution of clinical care pathways (56). In a study of 205 good-risk International Germ Cell Cancer Collaborative Group (IGCCCG) patients undergoing

postchemotherapy RPLND at MSKCC, the major complication rate was 4% (39). Careful monitoring of perioperative oxygen concentrations, meticulous fluid management with strict replacement criteria, and an emphasis on colloid rather than crystalloid have reduced pulmonary toxicity and the rare postoperative deaths from Adult Respiratory Distress Syndrome (ARDS). In tertiary referral centers with dedicated experts, most of the major complications occur in high-risk patients with either very large volume disease or in those patients after salvage chemotherapy or desperation RPLNDs (1).

The surgical principles of postchemotherapy RPLND include an in-depth knowledge of retroperitoneal anatomy, adequate exposure, and a thorough lymphadenectomy using "split-and-roll" technique (17).

The choice of incision is dictated by the tumor location and size. In general, either a transabdominal or thoracoabdominal approach will provide adequate exposure to the retroperitoneum. To prevent hepatic capsular tears, the falciform ligament is either divided between ligatures or excised en bloc with the properitoneal fat. The wound edges are spread with self retaining retractors and the abdomen, retroperitoneum, and pelvis are carefully explored. After the greater omentum and transverse colon are displaced onto the patient's chest between warm, moist pads, access to the retroperitoneum is achieved by incising the posterior parietal peritoneum from the ligament of Trietz, around the cecum, and up the right paracolic gutter to Winslow's foramen. The proper plane is along the medial aspect of the small bowel mesentery lateral to the right gonadal vein and its branches. The duodenum is kocherized, allowing cephalad mobilization and exteriorization of the small bowel, cecum, and right colon onto the chest where they can be placed in a Lahey bay or protected by moist laparotomy pads. Attachments between the undersurface of the duodenum and pancreas and the anterior surface of the left renal vein and inferior vena cava are divided to minimize traction and facilitate mobilization prior to placement of self-retaining retractors (Omni, Gallagher). Great care is taken to identify and protect the superior mesenteric artery (SMA). Mobilization of the distal pancreas can be achieved by extending the incision of the posterior parietal peritoneum cephalad to the ligament of Trietz to the duodenojejunal flexure and along the avascular plane between the inferior mesenteric vein (IMV) and the left gonadal vein. Alternatively, to gain additional mobility of the distal pancreas and access to the left renal hilum, the IMV can be doubly ligated and divided (17).

Additional exposure of the distal left para-aortic and left parailiac regions can be accomplished by further extending the incision in the left leaf of the parietal peritoneum inferiorly, and if needed, sacrificing the inferior mesenteric artery (IMA) between ligatures. The left colon can be reflected medially by incising the left white line of Toldt and developing the plane between the colonic mesentery and the anterior surface of Gerota's fascia (17).

Large left suprahilar masses may require a "visceral roll" to provide adequate exposure. The aorta can be exposed to the level of the diaphragmatic hiatus by incising the splenophrenic ligament and the parietal peritoneal attachments of the stomach and reflecting the descending colon, spleen, stomach, and tail of pancreas medially (17).

Injury to important structures can be minimized by identifying the ureters, renal vessels, SMA, IMA, and pancreas. Approximately 20% to 25% of patients have accessory renal arteries (17).

Split-and-roll technique is then used to perform lymphadenectomy and resection of residual mass(es). In properly selected candidates, nerve-sparing techniques may be feasible and prospective identification, dissection, and preservation of both sympathetic chains, postganglionic sympathetic fibers (L2, 3, 4), and the hypogastric plexus is necessary. To achieve this, the initial split should be along the anterior surface of the inferior vena cava (IVC), since dissection along the aorta before isolating and preserving these nerves results in their disruption (17,57). The oncologic aspects of the operation should not be compromised to preserve ejaculation. While performing split-and-roll technique, great care must be taken to prevent subadventitial dissection along the aorta as the mass and lymph nodes are separated from the great vessels. Direct invasion of the aorta or IVC may require graft interposition (58,59). Adjunctive procedures such as nephrectomy are sometimes necessary to achieve a complete resection. This is more common with left-sided primary tumors, and adequate function and preservation of the contralateral kidney must be assured prior to nephrectomy (60,61). Enterotomies or extensive serosal injury predispose patients to life-threatening fistulas, and omental interposition between the site of bowel resection or repair is advisable (17,61). Tumor encasement of the SMA, celiac axis, or porta hepatis usually precludes resection (17).

The recommended limits of postchemotherapy retroperitoneal surgery have ranged from resection or a residual mass only (62,63) to full bilateral RPLND (17). In a study of 113 patients who underwent a postchemotherapy RPLND at MSKCC, 9 patients would have had residual teratoma or viable GCT in the retroperitoneum without a bilateral dissection (64). Furthermore, excision of mass alone results in an inadequately controlled retroperitoneum with an increased risk of local recurrence, late relapse, malignant transformation of teratoma, and compromised clinical outcome (63,65). Similarly, modified templates, initially developed for patients with low-stage NSGCT in an effort to preserve ejaculation, are not recommended for patients with advanced disease who are at significantly higher risk for teratoma and/or viable GCT in contralateral nodal regions (1,6,17). Therefore, a standard bilateral RPLND should be performed. Extension into the retrocrural and posterior mediastinal areas is occasionally necessary to achieve a complete resection (61).

Following postchemotherapy surgery, the patients' prognosis and subsequent treatment are influenced by: (a) the biology of the original tumor as reflected by prior chemotherapeutic burden, pathology of the resected specimen(s), serum tumor marker level at the time of surgery; and (b) the adequacy of surgery (1,6,17).

Donohue et al. (66) analyzed 801 patients who underwent postchemotherapy RPLND at Indiana University and identified four, often interrelated, unfavorable prognostic variables: (a) salvage chemotherapy; (b) desperation surgery in patients with persistently elevated AFP and/or HCG levels; (c) unresectable patients; and (d) patients requiring reoperative surgery. The relapse and NED (no evidence of disease) rates of patients with one or more of these risk factors was 45% and 63% respectively, compared to 12% and 94% in patients without any risk factors (66).

Patients who required salvage chemotherapy prior to RPLND either relapsed or failed to achieve a complete response to induction cisplatin-based regimen. The chemorefractory nature of their disease is further reflected by a higher proportion (at least 50%) of residual viable nonteratomatous GCT in resected specimens. Unfortunately, these patients are also characterized by a lower rate of complete resection (1,17,67).

The second group of high-risk patients includes those undergoing RPLND with elevated serum tumor markers despite multiple chemotherapy regimens. In the past, surgery was avoided in this group of patients since they were felt to be unresectable and/or incurable (1–3). Several investigators have shown that carefully selected patients with elevated markers can achieve a cure with complete resection (68–71). Favorable variables included an elevated AFP rather than HCG, and a single nonvisceral site of disease (1,6,68,70). Wood et al. (68) reported that 7 of 15 (47%) patients with an elevated marker were cured with a

complete resection, while Eastham et al. (70) noted that 6 of 16 (37%) patients achieved cure following complete resection. Furthermore, patients with an elevated serum AFP level, teratomatous elements in the primary tumor, and a postchemotherapy cystic mass in the retroperitoneum following cisplatin-based induction therapy may benefit from RPLND rather than salvage chemotherapy. Investigators at MSKCC recently demonstrated that fluid from 11 consecutive retroperitoneum cystic teratoma specimens contained variably elevated levels of HCG and/or AFP in all patients and appeared to be independent of serum marker levels or marker decay. Complete resection resulted in normalization of serum AFP levels (71).

The outcome of patients deemed unresectable at the time of surgery is extremely poor (67). Several investigators have clearly demonstrated the adverse impact of an incomplete resection (30,66,67). Stenning et al. (27) reported that the risk for disease progression for patients without complete resection was approximately four times the risk for those undergoing complete resection (1). Furthermore, two-year progression-free survival rates were 88% and 60% for patients with and without complete resection, respectively (27).

The fourth high-risk group includes patients who require reoperative surgery. Investigators from Indiana University and MSKCC have clearly shown that patients undergoing redo-RPLND are significantly compromised regardless of other risk factors (66,72). Donohue et al. (66) reported that the relapse rates for primary versus redo postchemotherapy RPLND were 20.6% and 51.6%, respectively. Furthermore, the survival rates decrease from 84.1% in the primary postchemotherapy RPLND group to 55.3% in the redo group (1,66). Similarly, McKiernan (72) et al. reported a significant decrease in survival rates from 90% to 56% in patients requiring reoperative retroperitoneal surgery.

The data clearly demonstrate that complete initial postchemotherapy surgery is critically important in patient outcome (1,66,72). To assure complete resection it is sometimes necessary to perform adjunctive procedures including en bloc nephrectomy, bowel resection, and/or en bloc resection of a great vessel with graft interposition. These patients benefit from surgery in tertiary referral centers with dedicated surgeons with significant experience in postchemotherapy surgery (1–3).

The risk for relapse in patients with necrosis or teratoma in the retroperitoneal specimen is approximately 5% to 10%, and therefore no additional chemotherapy is needed (1,6,17). Conversely, the presence of viable nonteratomatous GCT is associated with a higher risk for relapse and decreased survival rates (1,6,17). Einhorn reported only two (9%) survivors of 22 patients with viable GCT following RPLND after cisplatin, bleomycin, vinblastine (PrB) (73). Fox et al. (67) reported that 18 of 27 (70%) patients who underwent complete postchemotherapy resection of viable GCT were disease-free if two additional cycles of postoperative chemotherapy were administered, compared to 0 of 7 without additional chemotherapy. Similarly Geller et al. (74) and Logothetis et al. (75) reported 12 of 18 (66%) and 9 of 17 (53%) survivors in patients undergoing complete resection of viable GCT and additional postoperative chemotherapy. More recently, Fizzazi et al. (76) challenged the therapeutic benefit of additional chemotherapy in completely resected GCT following induction cisplatin-based chemotherapy. In a multicenter, retrospective study using a multivariate analysis of 146 patients, they identified three independent prognostic variables for survival: (a) complete resection; (b) good risk IGCCCG classification; and (c) <10% viable malignant cells. Additional postoperative chemotherapy appeared to benefit only those patients with one risk factor, but not those without risk factors, or those with two or more risk factors. Fox et al. (67) reported that two additional cycles of chemotherapy did not have any therapeutic benefit in completely resected patients following salvage chemotherapy.

Teratoma

The finding of teratoma is unique to GCT (1). Despite the benign histologic appearance of teratoma, the biologic potential is unpredictable; therefore, there is significant benefit from complete resection (1,6,17).

Teratoma may grow, obstruct, or invade local structures (1,6,77,78). Since disease-free survival depends on completeness of resection, there are surgical advantages to performing the procedure in a lower-volume setting (1).

Second, there is a 6% to 8% risk of malignant transformation, i.e., the development of nongerm cell elements such as sarcoma or adenocarcinoma. These tumors are often chemorefractory, can recur in 58% to 86% of cases, and complete resection offers patients their best opportunity for cure (80–83). In addition to chromosomal abnormalities associated with the transformed histology, Motzer et al. (79) identified the isochrome 12p [i(12p)] in 11 patients confirming GCT clonality.

Third, teratoma may result in late relapse (46,84–87). Loehrer et al. reported that 19% (10 of 51) of patients with teratoma developed late relapse with no significant difference between mature or immature teratoma (46). Roth et al. reported that all 7 patients who developed late relapse had teratoma in the primary or retroperitoneal tumor (88). Investigators at MSKCC reported that almost 50% of retroperitoneal late relapses with teratoma had previously resected teratoma (87). Local late recurrence suggests incomplete resection and foci of residual disease with unpredictable biologic potential (1). It is important to emphasize that the most common site for late relapse of GCT is the retroperitoneum. These tumors are usually chemoresistant and survival rates are very poor (87,89,90).

Seminoma

The management of patients with pure seminoma and a residual mass following chemotherapy remains controversial. There are two important distinguishing features in this setting between seminoma and NSGCT. First, teratoma in the residual mass is extremely rare (6,17). Second, the perioperative morbidity is higher than that for NSGCT, and complete RPLND is frequently not technically feasible (17). This is secondary to the more severe desmoplastic reaction characteristic of seminoma patients treated with chemotherapy.

Whether the size of the residual mass is predictive of persistent malignancy remains controversial. In a study of 104 postchemotherapy seminoma patients, investigators at MSKCC reported that eight of 30 (27%) patients with a residual mass 3 cm or greater either relapsed or had residual seminoma, while only two of 74 (3%) of patients with masses less than 3 cm in diameter suffered a local recurrence when placed on an observation protocol (91,92). Conversely, other investigators have not found the size of the residual mass to be predictive of pathologic findings (93,94).

More recently, a FDG-PET study of 52 postchemotherapy seminoma patients was highly predictive of residual histology; all eight positive scans and 42 of 44 negative scans correlated with clinical outcome (95).

In summary, residual masses less than 3 cm should be observed (6,17). Management of masses ≥3 cm remains controversial. Observation is an option, and the role of FDG-PET scanning appears promising since identifying teratoma in this setting is not a significant concern. Although radiation to the area is feasible, 75% of patients are unnecessarily exposed to possible toxicity and local recurrence rates appear unaffected (96). Currently, surgery in experienced centers is associated with low morbidity and can direct immediate therapy if residual malignancy is identified (6). Factors such as patient age, comorbidity, size, location, and radiographic appearance of residual mass(es) affect the decisionmaking process.

Postchemotherapy Resection of the Lung and Mediastinum

Discordant pathologic findings between the retroperitoneum and the chest have ranged between 29% and 46% (97,99).

Tiffany et al. (98) reported on 23 patients who underwent postchemotherapy RPLND and thoracotomies and/or neck dissections, and found different histologies among different sites in 35% of cases. Hartmann et al. (99) noted a 30% discordance in four of eight patients having a less favorable pathology at the time of second resection.

Size of the pretreatment and the postchemotherapy pulmonary nodule do not correlate with the final histology, and different histologies may exist in each lung. Toner et al. (27) reported that six of 14 patients with nodules 1 cm or smaller had either teratoma or viable GCT, and three of eight patients who underwent bilateral thoracotomies had different histologies in each lung.

By using logistic regression, Steyerberg et al. (100) found necrosis in the retroperitoneum to be the most predictive variable of necrosis at the time of thoracotomy. However, Tognini et al. (101) reported that although retroperitoneal histology was predictive of thoracic histology, nine of 40 (22%) patients with necrosis in the retroperitoneum had teratoma or viable GCT in the chest. Excluding patients categorized as complicated (ie., those following salvage chemotherapy, elevated markers at the time of surgery, patients with late relapse, and/or patients who had undergone a prior unsuccessful attempt at resection) the predictive accuracy increased to 86%.

More recently, McGuire et al. (102) reported 93 patients who underwent RPLND and thoracotomy and noted pathologic discordance in 27 (29%) patients; 7 of 59 (14%) patients with fibrosis in the retroperitoneum had teratoma or viable GCT in the thoracic specimen.

OTHER PROCEDURES

Residual Neck Masses

Mohseni et al. (103) reported on 16 patients with a residual neck mass who underwent resection of 61 residual masses in multiple sites. Pathologic discordance in different sites was noted in seven of 16 (44%) patients, and 13 of 16 patients had teratoma (10) or viable GCT (3) in the neck. All 10 patients with teratoma in the residual neck mass and 1 of 3 with viable GCT have no evidence of disease after complete resection. No patient suffered relapse in the neck and there were no perioperative deaths.

Delayed Orchiectomy

Occasionally, patients with advanced GCT undergo systemic therapy prior to orchiectomy. Delayed orchiectomy at the time of postchemotherapy RPLND is indicated since a review of 160 patients reported that 40 (25%) patients had viable GCT and 50 (31%) had teratoma in the resected testicle (104). This can be accomplished either by manually dilating the inguinal ring and delivering the involved testicle into the operative field of the RPLND, or by standard inguinal incision.

Postchemotherapy Laparoscopic RPLND

In the postchemotherapy setting, with the exception of the Austrian group (105,106) who report minimal morbidity in carefully selected patients with low volume residual masses, the conversion rate to open surgery is high and very significant complications have been reported (106,107). Rassweiler et al. (107) converted 7 of 9 postchemotherapy stage II patients from laparoscopic to open RPLND, and Palese et al. (108) reported that 2 (28.5%) of 7 patients required open conversion. Furthermore, in the Johns Hopkins experience of 7 postchemotherapy laparoscopic RPLND (LRPLND) for residual masses with a mean size of 1.9 cm, the overall complication rate was 57% (108). Major complications included transection of the external iliac artery requiring bypass graft in a patient with a 1.5-cm residual mass, renal artery hematoma in a patient with mild adenopathy requiring aortorenal bypass, and a third patient with a 4.5-cm residual mass who suffered renal artery thrombosis requiring nephrectomy, subsequent duodenal perforation, necrotizing fasciitis, and a cerebral vascular event with neurologic sequelae (108). Consequently, in the postchemotherapy setting, laparoscopic RPLND cannot be endorsed as safe or standard, but rather as an operation to be evaluated in a formal prospective study by very experienced minimally invasive surgeons (6,17).

COMPLICATIONS

Perioperative morbidity is usually related to the complexity of the surgery and prior exposure to chemotherapeutic agents, particularly bleomycin. Large volume tumors and severe desmoplastic reactions make postchemotherapy RPLND one of the most challenging operations undertaken by urologists and therefore should be performed by experienced surgeons in tertiary centers who are comfortable with vascular techniques (17).

Lymphatic Complications

The incidence of chylous ascites is approximately 2% to 3%. Predisposing factors include suprahilar dissection, resection of the IVC, and/or hepatic resections. Patients should be initially managed with diuretics and dietary manipulation including low-fat diet with medium chain triglycerides. Total parenteral nutrition is occasionally required. Peritoneovenous shunting is indicated for persistent drainage of chyle that is refractory to conservative management. Reoperation to attempt to ligate leaking lymphatic is discouraged since it is associated with a high failure rate (17).

Most lymphoceles are asymptomatic and require no treatment; however, in the presence of infection, hydronephrosis, or bowel obstruction percutaneous drainage is highly effective. Persistent drainage may require a sclerosing agent. Knowledge of the lymphatic anatomy and meticulous lymphostasis minimize these complications (17).

Pulmonary Complications

The most common pulmonary complication is atelectasis, which is managed by respiratory therapy. Preoperative instruction, particularly in the use of incentive spirometry, is helpful in minimizing this problem. Pneumonia requires appropriate antibiotic therapy. Adult respiratory distress syndrome (ARDS) in bleomycin-treated patients may be lethal and requires mechanical ventilation and steroid therapy. It is critical to replace perioperative fluids very carefully and avoid exposure to high concentrations of oxygen (17,52).

Infectious Complications

Most infectious complications are superficial wound infections, which are usually managed with aggressive local care. Urinary tract infections are treated by the appropriate antibiotic(s) depending on culture results. Routine appendectomy at the time of RPLND was associated with a higher rate of infectious complications and is no longer performed (109).

Neurologic Complications

Careful positioning has minimized neural compression injuries. Spinal cord ischemia is, fortunately, very rare and usually associated with older age and simultaneous mediastinal and retroperitoneal dissections. The anterior spinal artery is usually at the T8 level and should be carefully identified if dissection in this area is necessary (110).

Vascular Complications

Severe injury to a great vessel may require graft interposition while minor injuries can be easily repaired with 4-0 or 5-0 vascular sutures. Injury to a renal artery may result in partial or total loss of a renal unit and possibly hypertension. To minimize the risk of transection of an accessory renal artery it is important to remember that approximately 20% of patients have multiple renal vessels. Renal vein thrombosis may require systemic anticoagulation.

Gastrointestinal Complications

Small-bowel obstruction is noted in approximately 2% of cases and usually responds to conservative management with nasogastric tube decompression (17). Prolonged ileus is usually self limiting but an underlying cause such as retroperitoneal hematoma, urinary extravasation, or bowel ischemia should be considered (17). Re-exploration is indicated if there are signs of toxicity or failure to respond to conservative measures in a timely fashion (17). Pancreatitis usually presents with hyperamylasemia and prolonged ileus and can usually be managed conservatively.

CONCLUSION

There is consensus that postchemotherapy surgical resection is indicated when serum tumor markers have normalized and residual radiographic abnormalities are present (6). The need for postchemotherapy RPLND in the face of a normal CT scan remains controversial. Several multivariate analyses show that, of patients predicted to have necrosis, approximately 20% will have teratoma or viable GCT (6). No single variable or combination of variables predicts a negative pathology with sufficient accuracy after induction chemotherapy to eliminate the risk for unresected teratoma or viable GCT. Residual teratoma has unpredictable biological potential that may result in rapid growth, malignant transformation, and/or late recurrence. By definition, unresected viable GCT is at least partially chemorefractory and will progress if left unresected.

Completeness of resection is an independent and consistent predictive variable of clinical outcome. Patients who are resected incompletely and require reoperative surgery are severely compromised. Given the high rate of histologic discordance between different sites, all residual disease generally should be resected regardless of the pathologic findings at the initial procedure. Surgical margins should not be compromised in an attempt to preserve ejaculation, although nerve-sparing dissections are possible with small residual masses. The size and location of residual masses, coupled with the postchemotherapy desmoplastic reaction often encountered, make RPLND a technically demanding procedure that should be performed by experienced surgeons in dedicated referral centers.

ACKNOWLEDGMENT

The author is grateful for the expert and invaluable assistance of Samantha M. Ford in the preparation of the manuscript.

References

1. Sheinfeld J. The role of adjunctive postchemotherapy surgery for nonseminomatous germ-cell tumors: current concepts and controversies. *Semin Urol Oncol* 2002;20:262–271.

2. Bajorin DF, Herr H, Motzer RJ, et al. Current perspectives on the role of adjunctive surgery in combined modality treatment for patients with germ cell tumors. *Semin Oncol* 1992;19:148–158.

3. Sheinfeld J, Bajorin D, Solomon M. Managment of postchemotherapy residual masses in advanced germ cell tumors. *AUA Update Series* 1997; 17:18–24.

4. Merrin C, Takita H, Becklye S, et al. Treatment of recurrent and widespread testicular tumor by radical reductive surgery and multiple sequential chemotherapy. *J Urol* 1976;117:291–295.

5. Donohue JP, Einhorn LH, Williams SD. Cytoreductive surgery for metastatic testis cancers. *J Urol* 1980;123:876–880.

6. Bosl G, Bajorin D, Sheinfeld J. Cancer of the testis. In: De Vita V, Hellman S, Rosenberg S et al., eds. *Cancer: principles and practice of oncology.* Philadelphia, PA: Lippincott, Williams & Wilkins, 2000:1491–1518.

7. Donohue JP, Roth LM, Zachary JM, et al. Cytoreductive surgery for metastatic testis cancer: tissue analysis of retroperitoneal masses after chemotherapy. *J Urol* 1982;127:1111–1114.

8. Donohue JP, Rowland RG. The role of surgery in advanced testis cancer. *Cancer* 1984;54:2716–2721.

9. Einhorn LH. Testicular cancer as a model for curable neoplasm. The Richard and Hinda Rosental Foundation Award Lecture. *Cancer Res* 1984;41: 3275–3280.

10. Bosl GJ, Gluckman R, Geller NL, et al. VAB-6: an effective chemotherapy regimen for patients with germ cell tumors. *J Clin Oncol* 1986;4:1493–1499.

11. Einhorn LH, Williams SD, Loehrer PJ, et al. Evaluation of optimal duration of chemotherapy in favorable-prognosis disseminated germ cell tumors: a Southeastern Cancer Study Group protocol. *J Clin Oncol* 1989;7:387–391.

12. Einhorn LH, Williams SD, Troner M, et al. The role of maintenance therapy in disseminated testicular cancer. *N Engl J Med* 1981;305:727–731.

13. Bosl GJ, Geller NL, Bajorin D, et al. A randomized trial of etoposide + cisplatin versus vinblastine + bleomycin + cisplatin + cyclophosphamide + dactinomycin in patients with good-prognosis germ cell tumors. *J Clin Oncol* 1988;6:1231.

14. Levitt MD, Reynolds PM, Sheiner HG, et al. Nonseminomatous germ cell testicular tumours: residual masses after chemotherapy. *Br J Surg* 1985; 72:19–22.

15. Fossa SD, Ous S, Lien HH, et al. Postchemotherapy lymph node histology in radiologically normal patients with metastatic nonseminomatous testicular cancer. *J Urol* 1989;141:557–559.

16. Oldenberg J, Alfsen GC, Lien HH, et al. Postchemotherapy retroperitoneal surgery remains necessary in patients with nonseminomatous testicular cancer and minimal residual tumor masses. *J Clin Urol* 2003;21:3310–3317.

17. Sheinfeld J, McKiernan J, Bosl GJ. Surgery of testicular tumors. In: Walsh PC, Retik AB, Vaughan ED et al., eds. *Campbell's urology*, 8th ed. Philadelphia, PA: WB Saunders, 2002:2920–2944.

18. Carter GE, Lieskovsky G, Skinner DG, et al. Reassessment of the role of adjunctives surgical therapy in the treatment of advanced germ cell tumors. *J Urol* 1987;138:1397–1401.

19. Stomper PC, Jochelson MS, Garnick M, et al. Residual abdominal masses after chemotherapy for nonseminomatous testicular cancer: correlation of CT and histology. *Am J Roentgenol* 1985;145:743–746.

20. Donohue JP, Rowland RG, Kopecky K, et al. Correlation of computerized tomographic changes and histological findings in 80 patients having radical retroperitoneal lymph node dissection after chemotherapy for testis tumor. *J Urol* 1987;137:1176–1179.

21. Gelderman WA, Schraffordt Koops H, Sleifer DT, et al. Results of adjuvant surgery in patients with stage III and IV nonseminomatous testicular tumors after cisplatin-vinblastine-bleomycin chemotherapy. *J Surg Oncol* 1988;38:227–232.

22. Levi JA, Thomson D, Dandeman T, et al. A prospective study of cisplatin-based combination chemotherapy in advanced germ cell malignancy: role of maintenance and long-term follow-up. *J Clin Oncol* 1988; 6:1154–1160.

23. Wozniak AJ, Samson MK, Shah NT, et al. A randomized trial of cisplatin, vinblastine, and bleomycin versus vinblastine, cisplatin, and etoposide in the treatment of advanced germ cell tumors of the testis: a southwest Oncology Group study. *J Clin Oncol* 1991;9:70–76.

24. Ozols RF, Ihde DC, Linehan WM, et al. A randomized trial of standard chemotherapy versus a high-dose chemotherapy regimen in the treatment of poor prognosis germ cell tumors. *J Clin Oncol* 1988;6:1031–1040.

25. Williams SD, Birch B, Einhorn D, et al. Treatment of disseminated germ cell tumors with cisplatin, bleomycin and either vinblastine or etoposide. *N Engl J Med* 1987;316:1435–1440.

26. Pizzocaro G, Salvioni R, Pasi M, et al. Early resection of residual tumor during cisplatin, vinblastine, bleomycin combination chemotherapy in stage II and bulky stage II nonseminomatous testicular cancer. *Cancer* 1985;56:249–255.

27. Toner GC, Panicek DM, Heelan RT, et al. Adjunctive surgery after chemotherapy for nonseminomatous germ cell tumors: recommendations for patient selection. *J Clin Oncol* 1990;8:1683–1694.

28. Fossa SD, Qvist H, Stenwig AK, et al. Is postchemotherapy retroperitoneal surgery necessary in patients with nonseminomatous testicular cancer and minimal residual tumor masses? *J Clin Oncol* 1992;10:569–573.

29. Steyerberg EW, Keizer HG, Fossa SD, et al. Prediction of residual retroperitoneal mass histology after chemotherapy for metastatic seminomatous germ cell tumor: multivariate analysis of individual patient data from six study groups. *J Clin Oncol* 1995;13:1177–1187.

30. Stenning SP, Parkinson MC, Fisher C, et al. Postchemotherapy residual masses in germ cell tumor patients: content, clinical features, and prognosis. *Cancer* 1998;83:1409–1419.

31. Steyerberg EW, Gerl A, Fossa SD, et al. Validity of predictions of residual retroperitoneal mass histology in nonseminomatous testicular cancer. *J Clin Oncol* 1998;16:269–274.

32. Bosl GJ, Geller NL, Chan EY. Stage migration and the increasing proportion of complete responders in patients with advanced germ cell tumors. *Cancer Res* 1988;48:3524–3527.

33. Fox EP, Weathers TD, Williams SD, et al. Outcome analysis for patients with persistent nonteratomatous germ cell tumor in postchemotherapy retroperitoneal lymph node dissections. *J Clin Oncol* 1993;11:1294–1299.

34. Tait D, Peckham MJ, Hendry WF, et al. Postchemotherapy surgery in advanced non-seminomatous germ-cell testicular tumors: the significance of histology with particular reference to differentiated (mature) teratoma. *Br J Cancer* 1984;50:601–609.

35. Freiha FS, Shortliffe LD, Rouse RV, et al. The extent of surgery after chemotherapy for advanced germ cell tumors. *J Urol* 1984;132:915–917.

36. Harding MJ, Brown IL, MacPherson SG, et al. Excision of residual masses after platinum based chemotherapy for non-seminomatous germ cell tumors. *Eur J Cancer Clin Oncol* 1989;25:1689–1694.

37. Mulder PFA, Oosterhof GON, Boetes C, et al. The importance of prognostic factors in the individual treatment of patients with disseminated germ cell tumors. *Br J Urol* 1990;66:425–429.

38. Aass N, Klepp O, Cavallin-Stahl E, et al. Prognostic factors in unselected patients with nonseminomatous metastatic testicular cancer: a multicenter experience. *J Clin Oncol* 1991;9:818–826.

39. Patel MI, Beck S, Bosl GJ, et al. Histology of good risk Non-seminomatous Germ Cell Tumor (NSGCT) patients following Retroperitoneal Lymph Node Dissection (PC-RPLND) after four cycles of Etoposide and Cisplatin (EP x 4). *J Urol* 2003;169:681A.

40. Richie JP, Garnick MB, Finberg H. Computerized tomography: how accurate for abdominal staging of testis tumors? *J Urol* 1982;127:715–717.

41. Stomper PC, Jochelson MS, Garnick M, et al. Residual abdominal masses after chemotherapy for nonseminomatous testicular cancer: correlation of CT and histology. *AM J Roentgenol* 1985;145:743–746.

42. Mead GM, Stenning SP, Parkinson MC, et al. The Second Medical Research Council Study of prognostic factors in nonseminomatous germ cell tumors. *J Clin Oncol* 1991;10:85–94.

43. Husband JE, Hawkes DJ, Peckham MJ, CT estimations of mean attention values and volume in testicular carcinoma. *Radiology* 1982;144:553–558.

44. Stephens AW, Gonin R, Hutchins GD, et al. Positron emission tomography evaluation of residual radiographic abnormalities in postchemotherapy germ cell tumor patients. *J Clin Oncol* 1996;14:1637–1641.

45. Cremerius U, Effert PJ, Adam G, et al. FDG PET for detection and therapy control of metastatic germ cell tumor. *J Nucl Med* 1998;39: 815–822.

46. Debono DJ, Heilman DK, Einhorn LH, et al. Decision analysis for avoiding postchemotherapy surgery in patients with disseminated nonseminomatous germ cell tumors. *J Clin Oncol* 1997;15:1455–1464.

47. Loehrer PJ Sr, Hui S, Clark S, et al. Teratoma following cisplatin-based combination chemotherapy for nonseminomatous germ cell tumors: a clinicopathological correlation. *J Urol* 1983;135:1183–1189.

48. Beck SD, Foster RS, Bihrle R, et al. Teratoma in the orchiectomy specimen and volume of metastasis are predictors of retroperitoneal teratoma in postchemotherapy nonseminomatous testis cancer. *J Urol* 2002;168: 1402.

49. Hay J, Shahzeidi S, Laurent G. Mechanisms of bleomycin-induced lung damage. *Arch Toxicol* 1991;65:81–94.

50. Goldiner PL, Carlon GC, Cvitkovic E, et al. Factors influencing postoperative morbidity and mortality in patients treated with bleomycin. *Br Med J* 1978;1:1664–1667.

51. Zwikler MP, Iancu D, Michel RP. Effects of pulmonary fibrosis on the distribution of edema. Morphometric analysis. *Am J Respir Crit Care Med* 1994;149:1276–1285.

52. Donat SM, Levy DA. Bleomycin associated pulmonary toxicity: is perioperative oxygen restriction necessary? *J Urol* 1998;160:1347–1352.

53. Baniel J, Foster RS, Rowland RG, et al. Complications of primary retroperitoneal lymph node dissection. *J Urol* 1994;152:424–427.

54. Baniel J, Foster RS, Rowland RG, et al. Complications of postchemotherapy retroperitoneal lymph node dissection. *J Urol* 1995;153:976–980.

55. Mosherafa AA, Foster RS, Bihrle R, et al. Does retroperitoneal lymph node dissection have a curative role for patients with sex cord-stromal testicular tumors? *Cancer* 2003;98:753–757.

56. Chang SS, Mohseni HF, Leon A, et al. Paracolic recurrence: the importance of wide excision of the spermatic cord at retroperitoneal lymph node dissection. *J Urol* 2002;167:94–96.

57. Klein EA. Nerve-sparing retroperitoneal lymphadenectomy. *Atlas Urol Clin* 1995;3:63–79.

58. Beck S, Foster R, Bihrle R, et al. Long term morbidity and survival in patients undergoing vena cava resection for metastatic germ cell tumors. *J Urol* 1999;161:607A.

59. Kelly R, Skinner D, Yellin AE, et al. En bloc aortic resection for bulky metastatic germ cell tumors. *J Urol* 1995;153:1849–1851.

60. Nash PA, Leibovitch I, Foster RS, et al. En bloc nephrectomy in patients undergoing postchemotherapy retroperitoneal lymph node dissection for nonseminomatous testis cancer: indications, implications and outcomes. *J Urol* 1998;159:707–710.

61. Chaganti RSK, Houldsworth J, Bosl GJ. Molecular genetics of adult male germ cell tumors. In: Vogelzang NJ, Scardino PT, Shipley WU et al., eds. *Comprehensive textbook of genitourinary oncology*, 2nd ed. Baltimore, MD: Lippincott Williams & Wilkins, 2000:891–896.

62. Hendry WF, A'hern RP, Hetherington JW, et al. Para-aortic lymphadenectomy after chemotherapy for metastatic non-seminomatous testicular tumours: prognostic value and therapeutic benefit. *Br J Urol* 1993;71:208–213.

63. Holzik MFL. A non-germ cell malignancy in a recurrent retroperitoneal tumor mass after combined treatment for a nonseminomatous testicular germ cell tumor. *Am J Urol Rev* 2003;6:263–266.

64. Wood DP Jr, Herr HW, Heller G, et al. Distribution of retroperitoneal metastases after chemotherapy in patients with nonseminomatous germ cell tumors. *J Urol* 1992;148:1812–1815.

65. Sheinfeld J. Risks of the uncontrolled retroperitoneum. *Ann Surg Oncol* 2003;10:100–101.

66. Donohue JP, Leviovitch I, Foster RS, et al. Integration of surgery and systemic therapy: results and principles of integration. *Semin Urol Oncol* 1998;16:65–71.

67. Fox EP, Weathers TD, Williams SD, et al. Outcome analysis for patients with persistent nonteratomatous germ cell tumor in postchemotherapy retroperitoneal lymph node dissections. *J Clin Oncol* 1993;11:1294–1299.

68. Wood DP Jr, Herr HW, Motzer RJ, et al. Surgical resection of solitary metastases after chemotherapy in patients with nonseminomatous germ cell tumors and elevated serum tumor markers. *Cancer* 1992;70:2354–2357.

69. Murphy BR, Breeden ES, Donohue JP, et al. Surgical salvage of chemorefractory germ cell tumors. *J Clin Oncol* 1993;11:324–329.

70. Eastham JA, Wilson TG, Russell C, et al. Surgical resection in patients with nonseminomatous germ cell tumor who fail to normalize serum tumor markers after chemotherapy. *Urology* 1994;43:74–80.

71. Beck SD, Patel MI, Sheinfeld J. Tumor marker levels in postchemotherapy cystic masses: clinical implications for patients with germ cell tumors. *J Urol* 2004;171:168–171.

72. McKiernan JM, Sheinfeld J, Bacik J, et al. Reoperative RPLND for germ cell tumor; clinical presentation, patterns of recurrence, and outcome. *Urology* 2003;62:732–736.

73. Einhorn LH, Williams SD, Mandelbaum I, et al. Surgical resection in disseminated testicular cancer following chemotherapeutic cytoreduction. *Cancer* 1981;48:904–908.

74. Geller N, Bosl G, Chan E. Prognostic factors for relapse after complete response in patients with metastatic germ cell tumors. *Cancer* 1989;63:440–445.

75. Logothetis C, Samuels M. Surgery in the management of stage III germinal cell tumors. Observations on the M. D. Anderson hospital experience, 1971–1979. *Cancer Treat Rep* 1984;11:27–37.

76. Fizazi K, Tjulandin S, Salvioni R, et al. Viable malignant cells after primary cell chemotherapy for disseminated nonseminomatous germ cell tumors: prognostic factors and role of postsurgery chemotherapy—results from an international study group. *J Clin Oncol* 2001;19:2647–2657.

77. Logothetis CJ, Samuels ML, Trindade A, et al. The growing teratoma syndrome. *Cancer* 1982;50:1629–1635.

78. Morgentaler A, Garnick MB, Richie JP. Metastatic testicular teratoma invading the inferior vena cava. *J Urol* 1988;140:149–150.

79. Motzer RJ, Amsterdam A, Prieto V, et al. Teratoma with malignant transformation: diverse malignant histologies arising in men with germ cell tumors. *J Urol* 1998;159:133–138.

80. Little JS Jr, Foster RS, Ulbright TM, et al. Unusual neoplasms detected in testis cancer patients undergoing post-chemotherapy retroperitoneal lymphadenectomy. *J Urol* 1994;152:1144–1149.

81. Ahmed T, Bosl GJ, Hajdu SI. Teratoma with malignant transformation in germ cell tumors in men. *Cancer* 1985;56:860–863.

82. Ahlgren AD, Simrell CR, Triche TJ, et al. Sarcoma arising in a residual teratoma after cytoreductive chemotherapy. *Cancer* 1984;54:2015–2018.

83. Ulbright TM, Loehrer PJ, Roth LM, et al. The development on non-germ cell malignancies with germ cell tumors. *Cancer* 1984;54:1824–1833.

84. Gelderman WA, Schraffordt Koops H, Sleijfer DT, et al. Results of adjuvant surgery in patients with stage III and IV nonseminomatous testicular tumors after cisplatin-vinblastine-bleomycin chemotherapy. *J Surg Oncol* 1988;38:227–232.

85. Borge N, Fossa SD, Ous S, et al. Late recurrence of testicular cancer. *J Clin Oncol* 1988;6:1248–1253.

86. Gerl A, Clemm C, Schmeller N, et al. Late relapse of germ cell tumors after cisplatin-based chemotherapy. *Ann Oncol* 1997;8:41–47.

87. Sheinfeld J. Late recurrence of testicular cancer. *AUA News* 2001;6:12–14.

88. Roth BJ, Greist A, Kubilis PS, et al. Cisplatin-based combination chemotherapy for disseminated germ cell tumors: long-term follow-up. *J Clin Oncol* 1988;6:1239–1247.

89. Baniel J, Roth B, Foster R, et al. Cost and risk benefit in the management of clinical stage II nonseminomatous testicular tumors. *Cancer* 1995;75:2897–2903.

90. George DW, Foster RS, Hromas RA, et al. Update on late relapse of germ cell tumor: a clinical and molecular analysis. *J Clin Oncol* 2003;21:113–122.

91. Puc HS, Heelan R, Mazumdar M, et al. Management of residual mass in advanced seminoma: results and recommendations from the memorial sloan-kettering cancer center. *J Clin Oncol* 1996;14:454–460.

92. Herr HW, Sheinfeld J, Puc HS, et al. Surgery for a post-chemotherapy residual mass in seminoma. *J Urol* 1997;157:860–862.

93. Loehrer PJ, Birch R, Williams SD, et al. Chemotherapy of metastatic seminoma: the Southeastern Cancer Study Group experience. *J Clin Oncol* 1987;5:1212–1220.

94. Fossa SD, Borge L, Gass N, et al. The treatment of advanced metastatic seminoma:experience in 55 cases. *J Clin Oncol* 1987;5:1071–1077.

95. Desantis PET, De Santis M, Bokemeyer C, et al. Predictive impact of 2-18fluoro-2-deoxy D-glucose positron emission tomography for residual postchemotherapy masses in patients with bulky seminoma. *Intern Med* 1997;242:421–423.

96. Horwich A, Paluchowska B, Norman A, et al. Residual mass following chemotherapy of seminoma. *Ann Oncol* 1997;8:37–40.

97. Mandelbaum I, Yaw PB, Einhorn LH, et al. The importance of one-stage median sternotomy and retroperitoneal node dissection in disseminated testicular cancer. *Ann Thorac Surg* 1983;36:524–528.

98. Tiffany P, Morse MJ, Bosl G, et al. Sequential excision of residual thoracic and retroperitoneal masses after chemotherapy for stage III germ cell tumors. *Cancer* 1986;57:978–983.

99. Hartmann JT, Candelaria M, Kuczyk MA, et al. Comparison of histological results from the resection of residual masses at different sites after chemotherapy for metastatic non-seminomatous germ cell tumors. *Eur J Cancer* 1997;33:843–847.

100. Steyerberg EW, Keizer HJ, Messemer JE et al. ReHiT Study Group. Residual pulmonary masses after chemotherapy for metastatic nonseminomatous germ cell tumor. Prediction of histology. *Cancer* 1997;79:345–355.

101. Tognini PG, Foster RS, McGraw P. et al. Combined postchemotherapy retroperitoneal lymph node dissection and resection of chest tumor under the same anesthetic is appropriate based on morbidity and tumor pathology [published erratum appears in *J Urol* 1998 Oct;160(4):1444]. *J Urol* 1998;159:1833–1835.

102. McGuire M, Rabbani F, Mohseni H, et al. The role of thoracotomy in the management of postchemotherapy residual thoracic masses. *J Urol* 1999;161:703A.

103. Mohseni HF, Rabbani F, Leon A, et al. Management and clinical outcome of patients with germ cell tumor and a postchemotherapy residual neck mass. *J Urol* 2002;167:693A.

104. Simmonds PD, Mead GM, Lee AH, et al. Orchiectomy after chemotherapy in patients with metastatic testicular cancer. Is it indicated? *Cancer* 1995;75:1018–1024.

105. Sheinfeld J. The case against laparoscopic RPLND. *AUA News* 2004;9:31–32.

106. Steiner H, Peschel R, Hotl L, et al. Ten years of laparoscopic retroperitoneal lymph node dissection. *J Urol* 2003;169:931A.

107. Rassweiler JJ, Seemann O, Henkel TO, et al. Laparoscopic retroperitoneal lymph node dissection for nonseminomatous germ cell tumors: indications and limitations. *J Urol* 1996;156:1108–1113.

108. Palese MA, Su L, Kavoussi LR. Laparoscopic retroperitoneal lymph node dissection after chemotherapy. *Urology* 2002;60:130–134.

109. Leibovitch I, Rowland RG, Goldwasser B, et al. Incidental appendectomy during urologic surgery. *J Urol* 1995;154:1110–1112.

110. Leibovitch I, Nash PA, Little JS Jr, et al. Spinal cord ischemia after postchemotherapy retroperitoneal lymph node dissection for nonseminomatous germ cell cancer. *J Urol* 1996;155:947–951.

CHAPTER 38 ■ ROLE OF CHEMOTHERAPY FOR LOW-STAGE TESTIS CANCER

STÉPHANE CULINE

Low-stage testis cancer usually includes stage I disease (tumor confined to the testis) and low-volume stage II disease (metastatic disease confined to the retroperitoneal lymph nodes with a maximum transverse diameter of 5 cm). In this chapter, the role of chemotherapy will be precisely reviewed in four different clinical situations: adjuvant chemotherapy for clinical stage I disease, adjuvant chemotherapy for patients with pathologic stage II disease (tumor evidenced by retroperitoneal lymph node dissection staging), primary chemotherapy for clinical stage II disease (retroperitoneal spread shown by radiologic assessment), and primary chemotherapy for biologic stage II disease (elevated tumor markers as only proof of metastatic disease after orchiectomy).

STAGE I DISEASE

Clinical stage I disease is defined as a tumor limited to the testis. Stage I patients are defined as patients with normal computed tomography scan of the thorax, abdomen, and pelvis and normalized serum tumor marker levels after inguinal orchiectomy. In patients with nonseminomatous germ cell tumors (NSGCT), the current management options following orchiectomy are retroperitoneal lymphadenectomy, surveillance, or adjuvant chemotherapy. In patients with pure seminomas, prophylactic retroperitoneal radiotherapy is the postorchiectomy standard of care in most countries. In recent years, the rationale for developing adjuvant chemotherapy was to define a less toxic modality than retroperitoneal dissection or radiotherapy and to eliminate the uncertainty of surveillance. The major disadvantage is to deliver a potentially toxic therapy without knowing the true extent of the disease and, therefore, to overtreat a significant number of patients.

Nonseminomatous Germ Cell Tumors

The trials of adjuvant chemotherapy for clinical stage I NSGCT patients are shown in Table 38.1. All of them have included patients with adverse prognostic factors (mainly vascular invasion in the primary tumor) and, therefore, a high risk (at least 50%) of disseminated disease. Less than 2% of patients relapsed. The overall survival rate, >98%, appears similar to that observed with retroperitoneal lymphadenectomy or surveillance. However, several points should be stressed. For one, the total number of patients reported so far in the literature is low. Also, the criteria used to define high-risk disease were not homogeneous, and the positive predictive value of around 50% associated with these criteria (1,2) means that more than one third of these patients have been overtreated. The long-term side effects of chemotherapy are not precisely known, although preliminary reports regarding fertility and sexual activity are rather reassuring (3). And finally, the risk of leaving behind

mature teratoma should be kept in mind. In daily practice, the treatment decision should take risk-group assessment, treatment options, and respective side effects as well as patient's choice and sociofamilial context into account. Chemotherapy clearly should be used only in patients with a high risk of disseminated disease defined by the presence of vascular invasion and a high percentage (>80%) of embryonal carcinoma in the primary tumor.

Pure Seminomas

Experiences with adjuvant chemotherapy for clinical stage I seminoma tumors that have been reported in the literature are listed in Table 38.2. All of them used carboplatin as chemotherapy, and the great majority of patients received one to two cycles. In these series, pathologic criteria for selecting patients were heterogeneous. The relapse rate was around 4%. The results of a randomized study comparing chemotherapy (one cycle of carboplatin) with radiotherapy (20 or 30 Gy) were recently reported. The relapse-free survival rates at 3 years (94.8% vs. 95.9%, respectively) suggest that an absolute increase in relapse rate in patients treated with chemotherapy can be excluded reliably (13). However, these results are not mature enough to consider adjuvant chemotherapy as a standard treatment, compared with prophylactic radiotherapy or surveillance.

STAGE II DISEASE

This section will consider NSGCT only, as low stage II pure seminomatous tumors are usually managed with radiotherapy.

Pathologic Stage II Disease

Adjuvant chemotherapy is a treatment option when retroperitoneal lymph nodes are confirmed by metastatic deposits to be involved after primary lymph node dissection. The results of series reported in the cisplatin area have shown that chemotherapy is almost universally effective in preventing relapses (Table 38.3). However, when considering the curative impact of retroperitoneal lymph node dissection alone (20), a surveillance approach is an alternative to the use of adjuvant chemotherapy. In a randomized trial comparing adjuvant chemotherapy to close observation with chemotherapy reserved for those patients who suffered a relapse, there was no difference in the survival rates (95%) at a median follow-up of 4 years. Only 1 of the 97 patients assigned to the adjuvant chemotherapy had a relapse. Of the 98 patients who were observed, 48 (49%) had a relapse (21). Therefore, two options exist in the management of patients with pathologic stage II

TABLE 38.1

CHEMOTHERAPY TRIALS IN CLINICAL STAGE I NONSEMINOMATOUS TUMORS OF THE TESTIS

Author	Number of patients	Prognostic factors	Chemotherapy	Number of relapses	Median follow-up (mo)
Madej and Pawinski (4)	30	VI or pT >1	3 PVB	0	36
Oliver et al. (5)	22	At least 2 of: VI, EC, no YS	2 BE$_{360}$P	1	43
Cullen et al. (6)	114	At least 2 of : VI, EC, no YS	2 BE$_{360}$P	1	48
Pont et al. (7)	29	VI	2 BE$_{500}$P	2 (including 1 MT)	79
Chevreau et al. (8)	38	VI or EC	2 PVB or 2 BE$_{360}$P	0	36
Klepp et al. (9)	32	VI and normal AFP level	3 BE$_{360}$P	1 MT	40
Dearnaley et al. (10)	115	At least 2 of : VI, EC, no YS	2 BOP	2	14
Ondrus et al. (11)	18	VI and EC	2 BE$_{360}$P	0	36
Böhlen et al. (12)	58	At least 2 of : VI, EC, pT >1	2 PVB or 2 BE$_{360}$P	1 MT	93
Total	456			8 (2%) (including 3 MT)	

VI, vascular invasion; pT, pathologic tumor stage; EC, embryonal carcinoma; AFP, alphafetoprotein; B, bleomycin; E, etoposide (360 or 500 refers to the total dose in mg delivered by cycle); P, cisplatin; V, vinblastine; O, vincristine; MT, mature teratoma; YS, yolk sac tumor.

disease. In daily practice, treatment decision should take into account prognostic factors that help to define the likelihood of relapse after retroperitoneal lymph node dissection. In patients with minimal nodal disease (fewer than six nodes involved, no node larger than 2 cm, no extranodal extension), observation alone can be considered, provided adherence to a rigorous follow-up schedule is assured because the probability of relapse is <10% (22). In other situations, chemotherapy

(two cycles combining etoposide and cisplatin with or without bleomycin) certainly is the optimal therapy.

Clinical Stage II Disease

From the largest experience reported by investigators at Indiana University with primary retroperitoneal lymph node dissection

TABLE 38.2

CHEMOTHERAPY TRIALS IN CLINICAL STAGE I PURE SEMINOMATOUS TUMORS OF THE TESTIS

Author	Number of patients	Carboplatin chemotherapy		Number of relapses	Median follow-up (mo)
		Doses/Cycle	Number of cycles		
Oliver et al. (13)	573	AUC = 7	1	29	48
Oliver et al. (14)	25	400 mg/m^2	1	0	29
	53	400 mg/m^2	2	1	51
Dieckmann et al. (15)	93	400 mg/m^2	1	8	48
	32	400 mg/m^2	2	0	
Reiter et al. (16)	107	400 mg/m^2	2	0	74
Steiner et al. (17)	108	400 mg/m^2	2	0	60
Aparicio et al. (18)	60	400 mg/m^2	2	2	52
Aparicio et al. (19)	204	AUC = 7	2	5	36
Total	1,255			45 (4%)	

AUC, area under curve.

TABLE 38.3

ADJUVANT CHEMOTHERAPY AFTER PRIMARY RETROPERITONEAL LYMPH NODE DISSECTION IN PATHOLOGICAL STAGE II NONSEMINOMATOUS TUMORS OF THE TESTIS

Author	Number of patients	Chemotherapy (number of cycles)	Number of relapses	Median follow-up (mo)
Vugrin et al. (23)	42	VAB-6 (at least 2 cycles)	1	24
Weissbach and Hartlapp (24)	112 109	PVB (2) PVB (4)	6 1	43
Gerl et al. (25)	85	PVB or BEP (2-4)	1	72
Kennedy, Torkelson, and Fraley (26)	37	PVB (4)	0	125
Culine et al. (27)	44	VAB-6 or EP (4)	0	72
Behnia et al. (28)	82	BEP (2)	1	85
Kondagunta et al. (29)	87	EP (2)	1	96
Total	598		11 (2%)	

VAB-6, vinblastine, actinomycin-D, bleomycin, cyclophosphamide, cisplatin; PVB, vinblastine, bleomycin, cisplatin; BEP, bleomycin, etoposide, cisplatin; EP, etoposide, cisplatin.

in patients with clinical stage II disease, three major points are important to highlight: (a) 65% of patients are expected to be cured with this surgical procedure alone; (b) about 20% of patients have histologically proven stage I disease; and (c) an incompressible rate of ejaculation is expected despite the development of modified templates of dissection (20). The other option in the management of patients is primary chemotherapy, the benefit of which would be to avoid lymph node dissection. The main drawbacks are the overtreatment of patients, considering the false-positive rates of radiological assessment, and the acute and long-term toxicities of chemotherapy. Five studies focused on the results of primary cisplatin-based chemotherapy in patients with low-volume clinical stage II disease (Table 38.4). High cure rates were observed, but postchemotherapy lymph node dissection was indicated in about 30% of patients.

In daily practice, there is no doubt that primary lymph node dissection or primary chemotherapy both yield excellent cure rates. However, neither surgery nor chemotherapy is entirely sufficient as monotherapy because approximately one-third of cases for each approach will need the other for achieving optimal results (35). In patients with normal serum tumor markers after orchiectomy, primary surgery certainly is the most appropriate way of staging and, therefore, the treatment to recommend. In patients with elevated tumor markers, treatment decisions could be based on cost/benefit and risk/benefit considerations, including relative toxicities and patient preference. These patients usually are considered to have metastatic disease and are treated with primary chemotherapy, according to the prognostic features of the International Germ Cell Consensus Classification for metastatic disease (36).

Biologic Stage II Disease

Patients with elevated serum tumor markers as the only evidence of disease following orchiectomy were historically managed

TABLE 38.4

EXPERIENCES WITH PRIMARY CHEMOTHERAPY IN PATIENTS WITH CLINICAL STAGE II NONSEMINOMATOUS TUMORS OF THE TESTIS

Author	Number of patients	Postchemotherapy retroperitoneal lymph node dissection (%)	Number of relapses	Median follow-up (mo)
Logothetis et al. (30)	30	5 (17)	2	33
Socinski et al. (31)	19	6 (32)	2 (including 1 MT)	22
Horwich et al. (32)	122	35 (29)	10 (including 5 MT)	66
Lerner et al. (33)	22	6 (27)	1	72
Culine et al. (34)	45	22 (49)	4 (including 2 MT)	72
Total	238		19 (8%) (including 8 MT)	

MT, mature teratoma.

with primary retroperitoneal lymph node dissection. Results clearly suggested that elevated markers usually reflect systemic metastases rather than retroperitoneal disease since a majority of these patients subsequently required chemotherapy (37,38). Reports of primary chemotherapy confirmed the efficacy of this approach. At Institut Gustave Roussy, 19 out of 20 patients who received various platinum-based chemotherapy remained free of disease 18 to 116 months after the end of treatment (39).

CONCLUSION

From the literature review concerning the role of chemotherapy in low-stage testicular cancer, the following conclusions can be drawn. Chemotherapy is a standard only for nonseminomatous tumors. Chemotherapy is a standard primary treatment following orchiectomy in patients with biologic stage II disease and in patients with clinical stage II disease and elevated serum tumor markers. Chemotherapy is a treatment option in patients with metastatic deposits at primary lymph node dissection. And finally, chemotherapy is a treatment option in patients with clinical stage I disease. Long-term results are excellent because >90% of patients are expected to be cured. However, it should be kept in mind that the use of chemotherapy should be restricted to patients with a high risk of disseminated disease when chemotherapy is only a treatment option in order to limit overtreatment.

References

1. Albers P, Siener R, Kliesch S, et al. Risk factors for relapse in clinical stage I nonseminomatous testicular germ cell tumors: results of the German Testicular Cancer Study Group trial. *J Clin Oncol* 2003;21:1505–1512.
2. Vergrouwe Y, Steyerberg EW, Eijkemans MJC, et al. Predictors of occult metastasis in clinical stage I nonseminoma: a systematic review. *J Clin Oncol* 2003;21:4092–4099.
3. Böhlen D, Burkhard FC, Mills R, et al. Fertility and sexual function following orchiectomy and 2 cycles of chemotherapy for stage I high risk nonseminomatous germ cell cancer. *J Urol* 2001;165:441–444.
4. Madej G, Pawinski A. Risk-related adjuvant chemotherapy for stage I non seminoma of the testis. *Clin Oncol* 1991;3:270–272.
5. Oliver RTD, Raja MA, Ong J, et al. Pilot study to evaluate impact of a policy of adjuvant chemotherapy for high risk stage 1 malignant teratoma on overall relapse rate of stage 1 cancer patients. *J Urol* 1992;148:1453–1456.
6. Cullen MH, Stenning SP, Parkinson MC, et al. Short-course adjuvant chemotherapy in high-risk stage I nonseminomatous germ cell tumors of the testis: a Medical Research Council report. *J Clin Oncol* 1996;14:1106–1113.
7. Pont J, Albrecht W, Postner G, et al. Adjuvant chemotherapy for high-risk clinical stage I nonseminomatous testicular germ cell cancer: long-term results of a prospective trial. *J Clin Oncol* 1996;14:441–448.
8. Chevreau C, Soulié M, Rischmann P, et al. Adjuvant chemotherapy in high risk stage I non-seminomatous germ cell tumors [Abstract]. *Proc Am Soc Clin Oncol* 1997;16:320a.
9. Klepp O, Dahl O, Flodgren P, et al. Risk-adapted treatment of clinical stage 1 non-seminoma testis cancer. *Eur J Cancer* 1997;33:1038–1044.
10. Dearnaley DP, Fossa SD, Kaye SB, et al. Adjuvant bleomycin, vincristine and cisplatin for high risk clinical stage I non-seminomatous germ cell tumours. A Medical Research Council pilot study [Abstract]. *Proc Am Soc Clin Oncol* 1998;17:309a.
11. Ondrus D, Matoska J, Belan V, et al. Prognostic factors in clinical stage I nonseminomatous germ cell testicular tumors: rationale for different risk-adapted treatment. *Eur Urol* 1998;33:562–566.
12. Böhlen D, Borner M, Sonntag RW, et al. Long-term results following adjuvant chemotherapy in patients with clinical stage I testicular nonseminomatous malignant germ cell tumors with high risk factors. *J Urol* 1999;161:1148–1152.
13. Oliver RT, Mason M, von der Maase H, et al. A randomised comparison of single agent carboplatin with radiotherapy in the adjuvant treatment of stage I seminoma of the testis, following orchiectomy: MRC TE19/EORTC 30982 [Abstract]. *Proc Am Soc Clin Oncol* 2004;23:385.
14. Oliver RT, Edmonds PM, Ong JY, et al. Pilot studies of 2 and 1 course carboplatin as adjuvant for stage I seminoma: should it be tested in a randomized trial against radiotherapy? *Int J Radiat Oncol Biol Phys* 1994;29:3–8.
15. Dieckmann KP, Bruggeboes B, Pichlmeier U, et al. Adjuvant treatment of clinical stage I seminoma: is a single course of carboplatin sufficient? *Urology* 2000;55:102–106.
16. Reiter J, Brodowicz T, Alavi S, et al. Twelve-year experience with two courses of adjuvant single-agent carboplatin therapy for clinical stage I seminoma. *J Clin Oncol* 2001;19:101–104.
17. Steiner H, Holtl L, Wirtenberger W, et al. Long-term experience with carboplatin monotherapy for clinical stage I seminoma: a retrospective single-center study. *Urology* 2002;60:324–328.
18. Aparicio J, Garcia del Muro X, Maroto P, et al. Multicenter study evaluating a dual policy of postorchiectomy surveillance and selective adjuvant single-agent carboplatin for patients with clinical stage I seminoma. *Ann Oncol* 2003;14:867–872.
19. Aparicio J, Germa GR, Garcia del Muro X, et al. Risk-adapted management of stage I seminoma: the second Spanish Germ Cell Cancer Group study [Abstract]. *Proc Am Soc Clin Oncol* 2004;23:385.
20. Donohue JP, Thornhill JA, Foster RS, et al. Clinical stage B non-seminomatous germ cell testis cancer: the Indiana University experience (1965–1989) using routine primary retroperitoneal lymph node dissection. *Eur J Cancer* 1995;31A:1599–1604.
21. Williams SD, Stablein DM, Einhorn LH, et al. Immediate adjuvant chemotherapy versus observation with treatment at relapse in pathological stage II testicular cancer. *N Engl J Med* 1987;317:1433–1438.
22. Richie JP, Kantoff PW. Is adjuvant chemotherapy necessary for patients with stage B1 testicular cancer? *J Clin Oncol* 1991;9:1393–1396.
23. Vugrin D, Whitmore WF, Herr H, et al. Adjuvant vinblastine, actinomycin D, bleomycin, cyclophosphamide and cis-platinum chemotherapy regimen with or without maintenance in patients with resected stage IIB testis cancer. *Cancer* 1982;128:715–717.
24. Weissbach L, Hartlapp JH. Adjuvant chemotherapy of metastatic stage II nonseminomatous testis tumor. *J Urol* 1991;146:1295–1298.
25. Gerl A, Clemm C, Kohl P, et al. Adjuvant chemotherapy of stage II non-seminomatous testicular cancer. *Oncol Rep* 1994;1:209–212.
26. Kennedy BJ, Torkelson JL, Fraley EE. Adjuvant chemotherapy for stage II nonseminomatous germ cell cancer of the testis. *Cancer* 1994;73: 1485–1489.
27. Culine S, Théodore C, Farhat F, et al. Cisplatin-based chemotherapy after retroperitoneal lymph node dissection in patients with pathological stage II nonseminomatous germ cell tumors. *J Surg Oncol* 1996;61: 195–198.
28. Behnia M, Foster R, Einhorn LH, et al. Adjuvant bleomycin, etoposide and cisplatin in pathological stage II non-seminomatous testicular cancer: The Indiana University experience. *Eur J Cancer* 2000;36:472–475.
29. Kondagunta GV, Sheinfeld J, Mazumdar M, et al. Relapse-free and overall survival in patients with pathologic stage II nonseminomatous germ cell cancer treated with etoposide and cisplatin adjuvant chemotherapy. *J Clin Oncol* 2004;22:464–467.
30. Logothetis CJ, Swanson DA, Dexeus F, et al. Primary chemotherapy for clinical stage II nonseminomatous germ cell tumors of the testis: a follow-up of 50 patients. *J Clin Oncol* 1987;5:906–911.
31. Socinski MA, Garnick MB, Stomper PC, et al. Stage II nonseminomatous germ cell tumors of the testis: an analysis of treatment options in patients with low volume retroperitoneal disease. *J Urol* 1988;140:1437–1441.
32. Horwich A, Norman A, Fisher C, et al. Primary chemotherapy for stage II nonseminomatous germ cell tumors of the testis. *J Urol* 1994;151:72–78.
33. Lerner SE, Mann BS, Blute ML, et al. Primary chemotherapy for clinical stage II nonseminomatous germ cell testicular tumors: selection criteria and long-term results. *Mayo Clin Proc* 1995;70:821–828.
34. Culine S, Théodore C, Court BH, et al. Evaluation of primary standard cisplatin-based chemotherapy for clinical stage II non-seminomatous germ cell tumours of the testis. *Br J Urol* 1997;79:258–262.
35. Culine S, Droz JP. Primary treatment in stage II non-seminomatous germ cell tumours of the testis: a matter of scalpel or drug infusion? *Eur J Cancer* 1996;32A:1641–1644.
36. International Germ Cell Cancer Collaborative Group. International Germ Cell Consensus Classification: a prognostic factor-based staging system for metastatic germ cell cancers. *J Clin Oncol* 1997;15:594–603.
37. Davis BE, Herr HW, Fair WR, et al. The management of patients with nonseminomatous germ cell tumors of the testis with serologic disease only after orchiectomy. *J Urol* 1994;152:111–114.
38. Saxman SB, Nichols CR, Foster RS, et al. The management of patients with clinical stage I nonseminomatous testicular tumors and persistently elevated serologic markers. *J Urol* 1996;155:587–589.
39. Culine S, Théodore C, Terrier-Lacombe MJ, et al. Primary chemotherapy in patients with nonseminomatous germ cell tumors of the testis and biological disease only after orchiectomy. *J Urol* 1996;155:1296–1298.

CHAPTER 39 ■ RADIATION THERAPY FOR TESTICULAR SEMINOMA

PADRAIG R. WARDE AND STEPHEN R. SMALLEY

INTRODUCTION

Testicular cancers are uncommon and the vast majority are primary germ cell tumors (GCTs). Approximately 45% of GCTs are pure seminomas and most patients (70% to 80%) present with no radiologic evidence of disease (stage I disease), 15% to 20% of patients have infradiaphragmatic lymph node involvement on radiologic investigation (stage II disease), and less than 5% of patients present with distant metastatic disease (stage III disease). Initial management is radical inguinal orchidectomy and surgery is both diagnostic and therapeutic by providing tissue to determine the diagnosis and assuring cure in a high proportion of patients with stage I disease.

Postorchidectomy treatment options in patients with stage I seminoma include surveillance (reserving treatment for those who relapse), adjuvant retroperitoneal radiation therapy (RT), and adjuvant chemotherapy. Adjuvant RT remains the treatment strategy of choice in most centers (1). However, largely because of concerns regarding the possible induction of second malignancies by RT, there is increasing interest in surveillance. Adjuvant chemotherapy using one to two cycles of carboplatin has recently been investigated as an alternative strategy. Current data indicate that two courses of carboplatin are necessary and the attractiveness of this approach is diminished with the use of more than one cycle of treatment (2). In addition, the long-term toxicity of this strategy is unknown and, except in high select cases, for example, patients with coincidental inflammatory bowel disease, it should only be used in a study setting.

Whichever treatment strategy is adopted, the cure rate in stage I disease is virtually 100%. The challenge in defining the optimal approach in these patients is how best to minimize toxicity while maintaining the excellent results seen with standard management.

Postorchidectomy treatment options in patients with stage II seminoma include RT, chemotherapy, and, in rare cases, retroperitoneal node dissection. RT is the treatment of choice in patients with low-bulk disease (most patients with stage IIA/B disease) and cisplatin-based chemotherapy regimens are used in patients with more advanced disease. Cure rates in modern series are in excess of 95% and again, as in stage I disease, minimizing toxicity of treatment while not compromising cure is the main challenge for physicians dealing with these patients.

RT has a small role in patients with more advanced disease, mostly in palliative management of metastatic disease. In patients with brain metastases, either seminoma or nonseminoma, RT can be curative in a small proportion of cases.

STAGING

The American Joint Committee on Cancer (AJCC) and International Union against Cancer (IUC) staging classification for testicular tumors is shown in Chapter 35 (3,4). Stage I disease includes patients with T1-T4 tumors with no evidence of nodal or distant spread following work-up. Stage II patients (retroperitoneal lymph node involvement) are subdivided into three substages based on the maximum transverse diameter of the largest lymph node mass: stage IIA ≤2 cm, stage IIB >2 cm to 5 cm, stage IIC >5 cm. Routine staging investigations following orchidectomy include abdominopelvic computed tomography (CT) scan, chest x-ray, and serum tumor markers [α-fetoprotein, (AFP), beta human chorionic gonadotrophin (B-HCG)]. In the absence of lymph node involvement, CT scanning of the chest is not necessary as pulmonary or mediastinal metastases are extremely rare. There is no proven role for the use of positron emission tomography (PET) in the initial assessment of patients with seminoma, but it may be useful in staging patients with stage II disease after treatment with chemotherapy (5–8).

Stage I Disease

The standard postorchidectomy management approach for patients with stage I seminoma remains adjuvant RT to the para-aortic and ipsilateral pelvic lymph nodes. In large (>100 cases) single or multi-institutional series in the modern era (all patients treated after 1970) the relapse rate has varied from 0.5% to 5%. Table 39.1 (9–14). In-field relapse is rare (<0.05% in above series) and when suspected, biopsy should be performed to rule out nonseminomatous tumor. The most common sites of relapse following adjuvant RT are the mediastinum, lungs, and supraclavicular fossa. A small proportion of patients, usually with predisposing factors, relapse in the inguinal nodes. Uncommon sites of isolated metastases, such as brain and tonsil, have been noted in case reports (15,16). For supradiaphragmatic relapse, chemotherapy is the treatment of choice and gives close to 100% cure. Inguinal relapse can often be treated successfully with RT to the involved area (17).

Most relapses occur within 2 years of RT (unlike on surveillance where late relapse frequently occurs) (18). In the Princess Margaret Hospital (PMH) series of 282 patients treated between 1981 and 1999, the median time to relapse was 18 months with the latest relapse occurring at 6 years. Follow-up efforts should therefore concentrate on the 2 years after RT and the current PMH follow-up policy is shown in Figure 39.1. This is similar to the policy used for patients on surveillance except that a CT abdomen and pelvis is done in addition at all visits.

The overall survival rate in most series ranges between 92% and 99% at 5 to 10 years with cause-specific survival approaching 100%. Most deaths are due to intercurrent illness but concern exists that premature death may be occurring from radiation-induced cancers or cardiac disease (19). With such excellent results the prognostic factors for relapse are difficult

TABLE 39.1

SUMMARY OF POSTORCHIDECTOMY RELAPSE RATES IN LARGE (>100 CASES)
SINGLE OR MULTI-INSTITUTIONAL SERIES IN THE MODERN ERA (ALL
PATIENTS TREATED AFTER 1970)

Author	Yr of study	Number of patients	% relapse	Cause-specific survival (%)
Bayens	(1975–1985)	132	4.5	99
Coleman	(1980–1995)	144	4.2	100
Fossa	(1989–1993)	242	3.7	100
Hultenschmidt	(1978–1992)	188	1	100
Santoni	(1970–1999)	487	4.3	99.4
Warde	(1981–1989)	282	5	100

to establish. One of the potential factors predicting relapse is the occurrence of anaplastic seminoma. In the Princess Margaret Hospital experience, eight of 55 patients with anaplastic seminoma relapsed compared to two of 116 patients with classical seminoma (14.5% vs. 1.7%) (17). The WHO criteria for the diagnosis of anaplastic seminoma (three or more mitosis per high-power field) are not uniformly used, and other series indicate that the prognosis for patients with anaplastic seminoma is similar to that for patients with classical seminoma (20). Other factors reported to be associated with a higher risk of relapse include tumor invasion of the tunica albuginea, epididymis and spermatic cord, advanced pT stage, as well as a raised preoperative human chorionic gonadotrophin level (21). The risk of recurrence in seminoma patients on surveillance can be stratified according to clinical and surgicopathologic factors. An analysis of 201 patients on surveillance at the Princess Margaret Hospital showed older age at diagnosis and large tumor size to have independent adverse prognostic significance, and the presence of small vessel invasion to be of marginal significance (22). Tumor size was the only factor independently associated with relapse in a series of 261 patients from the Danish Testicular Carcinoma Study Group, and small-vessel invasion was the only important factor among 103 patients at the Royal Marsden Hospital (23,24). Individual patient data from these three centers and from the Anglian Germ Cell Cancer Group was recently pooled to yield a cohort of 638 patients with a median follow-up on surveillance of 7 years. Age at diagnosis, tumor size, histologic subtype, and tumor invasion of small vessels, the rete testis, epididymis, tunica albuginea, and spermatic cord were examined as potential predictors of relapse. Tumor size and invasion of the rete testis were the only important factors by multivariate analysis (25).

RT Technique/Volume

For the past half century, the traditional management of stage I seminoma patients after orchiectomy has consisted of RT to the para-aortic and pelvic (retroperitoneal) lymph nodes. The lymphatic drainage of the testis is directly to the para-aortic lymph nodes, predominantly to those at the L1-L3 vertebral level. The left testicular vein drains to the left renal vein and the lymphatic drainage of the left testicle is primarily to the lymph nodes located around the left renal hilum. On the right side the testicular vein drains into the inferior vena cava below the level of renal vein and in right-sided tumors, paracaval and interaortocaval lymph nodes are the first to be involved. Crossover drainage from right to left occurs routinely but left to right nodal drainage occurs in only 15% to 25% of cases. Pelvic lymph node involvement is present in 1% to 3% of cases. Inguinal lymph node involvement is rare and usually limited to patients with factors leading to altered lymphatic drainage of the testis. The usual radiation technique involves treatment with parallel-opposed anteroposterior fields treated with 10 to 18 MeV linear accelerator photons. The clinical target volume includes the para-aortic lymph nodes and ipsilateral pelvic lymph nodes and is defined with the help of the information obtained from CT scan of the abdomen and pelvis to avoid irradiation of renal parenchyma. With left-sided tumors, the left renal hilum is included in the field by shaping the left lateral border of the RT portal. This classical

	Month 1	Month 2	Month 3	Month 4	Month 5	Month 6	Month 7	Month 8	Month 9	Month 10	Month 11	Month 12
Year 1				Markers CXR				Markers CXR				Markers CXR
Year 2				Markers CXR				Markers CXR				Markers CXR
Year 3						CXR						CXR
Year 4						CXR						CXR
Year 5						CXR						CXR
Year 6												CXR
Year 7												CXR
Year 8												CXR
Year 9												CXR
Year 10												CXR

FIGURE 39.1. Follow-up protocol at Princess Margaret Hospital for stage I seminoma treated with RT.

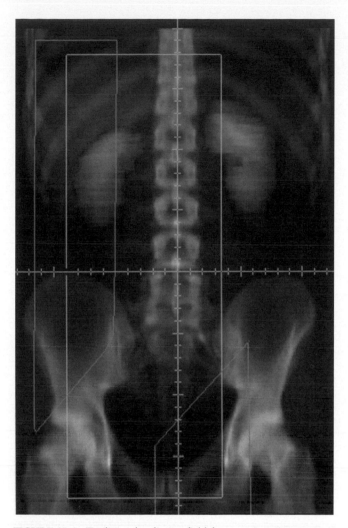

FIGURE 39.2. Traditional radiation field for stage I seminoma.

plan was called "hockey stick" in North America and "dog-leg" in the United Kingdom and Europe (Fig. 39.2). Classically, the radiation fields extended from the T10-11 vertebral body to the inguinal ligament and were typically 8 to 10 cm wide. The amount of cardiac tissue in the field should be minimized as there is increasing evidence that long-term survivors of seminoma treated with adjuvant retroperitoneal RT are at a significant excess risk of death from cardiac disease (19). No attempt was made to treat the hypogastric and contralateral pelvic lymph nodes. With this technique it is important to ensure that the penis is moved out of the field and, in addition, to place the contralateral testis in a scrotal shield to protect fertility and hormonal function. Verification, simulation, and port fields are routine. It is important to realize that in this field arrangement inguinal lymph nodes are not routinely treated. The inguinal lymph nodes may be treated in patients with risk factors for inguinal lymph node involvement, either by extending the radiation field inferiorly or by adding direct anterior field to cover the inguinal lymph nodes. In general, scrotal radiation is avoided even in patients with scrotal violation. The only instance where scrotal radiation may be recommended is in patients with very extensive local disease, incomplete surgery, and gross scrotal contamination prior to surgery.

One of the most important factors determining the radiation dosage to the remaining contralateral testis, and therefore the risk of infertility, is the distance from the inferior edge of the radiation field to the scrotum (26,27). This knowledge,

and the low incidence of pelvic lymph node involvement in stage I seminoma, has led to the investigation of adjuvant RT directed to the para-aortic lymph nodes alone. Reports from phase II trials and retrospective single-institutional experiences have shown excellent results with few pelvic failures (20,28). The Medical Research Council Testicular Study Group in the United Kingdom has conducted a prospective randomized trial of the traditional para-aortic and pelvic radiation versus para-aortic irradiation alone (29). The results of this study of 478 patients showed a 96% relapse-free survival for patients treated with para-aortic RT alone versus 96.6% relapse-free survival for those treated with the para-aortic and pelvic lymph nodes. Sperm counts after treatment were significantly higher in the para-aortic-alone group and there was some decrease in incidence of diarrhea in the patients treated to the para-aortic and pelvic lymph node RT. However, the 33% incidence of diarrhea in these patients likely reflects the use of a high dose per fraction (200 cGy per day) in this study as compared to the 125 cGy/d used in many other studies. All patients who received para-aortic and pelvic RT relapsed in supradiaphragmatic sites, but four patients (~2%) in the para-aortic-alone group failed with disease in the pelvis. This trial showed that reduced RT volume gives excellent results, but when used, a small risk of pelvic failure remains. Therefore, if this treatment approach is adopted, regular surveillance with CT of the pelvic lymph nodes should be performed to ensure that when pelvic relapse occurs it is detected early. Data from the Christie Hospital in Manchester where no routine CTs are performed after para-aortic radiation has shown that the median size of the pelvic lymph nodes at time of detection of relapse was 5 cm (range 2.5 to 9 cm) (20). The advantage of para-aortic RT alone is therefore diminished, particularly in comparison to surveillance.

Classically, the inferior border of the pelvic treatment field extended to the lower border of the obturator foramen. A compromise may be to irradiate the para-aortic and ipsilateral common iliac lymph nodes by positioning the inferior border of the radiation fields at midpelvis as is currently done at PMH (Fig. 39.3) (30). This encompasses the lymph nodes that are typically removed at lymphadenectomy in patients with nonseminomatous tumors (31). This approach may reduce the risk of second malignancy by reducing the integral dose of RT and has the potential to reduce the scatter dose to the remaining testis and preserve fertility without the requirement for ongoing pelvic surveillance (32). The upper border is placed at the superior aspect of T11.

Dose

The minimum dose of radiation required to control occult retroperitoneal disease has not been defined. Published reports include radiation doses ranging from 20 Gy to 40 Gy. At Princess Margaret Hospital in Toronto, a dose of 25 Gy prescribed at midline and delivered in 20 daily fractions of 1.25 Gy has been used for over 25 years with no in-field recurrences observed. While it is apparent from our experience that a dose greater than 25 Gy is unnecessary, the issue of whether a lesser dose would be sufficient has not been determined. Preliminary results from the Medical Research Council (MRC) TE18 trial comparing 20 Gy in 10 fractions to 30 Gy in 15 fractions to the para-aortic lymph nodes alone shows equivalent relapse rates in both arms with a median follow-up of 37 months (33). Further follow-up is necessary before this schedule can be adopted. Radiation doses of less than 20 Gy have been associated with in-field failures reported in the literature (34–36). A hypofractionated approach using 20 Gy in 8 fractions over 1.5 weeks has been advocated by Logue et al. from the Christie Hospital in Manchester. In 431 patients treated with this approach (para-aortic RT only)

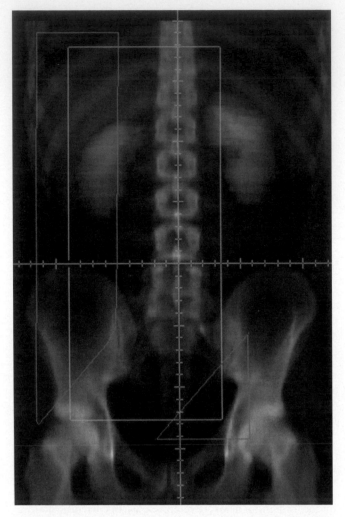

FIGURE 39.3. Recommended field for stage I seminoma, upper border T11, lower border mid-pelvis.

no infield recurrences were observed and the overall recurrence rate was 3.5% with a median follow-up of 62 months (20). The acute and late toxicity of treatment in this retrospective review was not well documented though it should be noted that 46% of patients developed nausea during treatment with 12% of patients reporting episodes of vomiting. With 1.25 Gy/d, as given at PMH, little acute toxicity is observed (17). However, patients may be willing to trade a higher acute toxicity for the convenience of a shorter treatment regimen.

Stage II Disease

At work-up after orchidectomy, about 15% to 20% of patients have radiologically involved para-aortic lymph nodes and are classified as having stage II disease. Patients are staged using the UICC/AJCC TNM classification, which divides patients into three groups depending on the transverse diameter of the largest retroperitoneal lymph node mass: <2 cm (stage IIA), 2.1 to 5 cm (stage IIB), and >5 cm (stage IIC) (3,4). Approximately 70% of stage II patients have small-bulk retroperitoneal disease at presentation with lymph nodes that are <5 cm. The definition of the substages of stage II seminoma has varied over time and the literature has to be interpreted cautiously. The number of patients with stage II disease is too small to mount phase III studies of management, and treatment decisions must be based on reports from single institutions where patients have been treated in a uniform fashion.

The most important prognostic factor in stage II seminoma is the bulk of retroperitoneal tumor, measured as the transverse diameter of the largest lymph node or lymph node mass visible on CT scan.

Lymph node size was the only factor that predicted recurrence in 95 patients with stage II seminoma treated with RT at PMH between 1981 and 1999 (37). The 5-year relapse-free rate in 79 patients with nodal disease of <5 cm (IIA/B) was 91% (7 of 79 patients), compared to 44% (9 of 16 patients) in patients with bulkier disease (IIC). Recurrence occurred most commonly in mediastinal or supraclavicular lymph nodes, lung, or bone. Thirteen patients were treated with chemotherapy at relapse, and nine were free of disease at last follow-up. Two patients had salvage RT in the early 1980s (they would now be treated with salvage chemotherapy) and one was free of disease on follow-up. These five patients plus one additional patient who refused salvage died of progressive seminoma. Thirty-one patients (23 Stage II C) received initial chemotherapy for Stage II disease with two relapses, one of whom was salvaged by second line chemotherapy. These results are similar to other series in the literature (Table 39.2) and support the continued use of primary RT in stage II patients with small-bulk lymphadenopathy (12,38–40). However, the high failure rate following RT in patients with bulky retroperitoneal disease, the fact that not all patients with recurrence were salvaged, and the apparently better outcome of similar patients who were treated with chemotherapy at diagnosis mandates primary chemotherapy instead of radiation in this population.

Staging should not be the only parameter used to decide on treatment of retroperitoneal disease in patients with stage II seminoma. Tumor bulk must also be considered, for example, a patient with nodal disease extending 8 to 9 cm from L1-L5 in the retroperitoneum with a maximum transverse diameter of 3.5 cm would be classified as having IIB disease. Patients with

TABLE 39.2

RESULTS OF RETROPERITONEAL RT IN STAGE II A/B SEMINOMA

Author (Yr of publication)	No. of patients	Yr of study	No. of relapse (%)	Cause-specific survival (%)
Bayens (1992)	29	1975–1985	7 (24%)	93
Chung (2004)	79	1981–1999	7 (8.8%)	97.5
Classen (2003)	87	1991–1994	4 (4.6%)	100
Vallis (1995)	48	1974–1989	3 (6%)	98
Zagars (2001)	37	1984–1999	5 (13.5%)	100
Bayens (1992)	29	1975–1985	7 (24%)	93

bulky disease such as this should be treated with chemotherapy rather than with RT. Other patient and tumor-related factors should also be taken into account. Lymph node masses that are situated laterally may necessitate irradiating a large volume of one or both kidneys or the liver in order to adequately encompass the tumor. The same situation may arise in cases of abnormal anatomy, such as with horseshoe or pelvic kidney. These patients are better treated with chemotherapy because of an unacceptably high risk of radiation toxicity. Patients in whom RT and chemotherapy are contraindicated or the diagnosis is uncertain should be considered for retroperitoneal lymph node dissection.

The technique of radiation in stage II seminoma is similar to that used in stage I disease. The treatment volume includes the gross tumor as well as the para-aortic and ipsilateral common and external iliac lymph nodes. The radiation dose is typically 25 Gy in 20 daily fractions plus a boost of a further 10 Gy in 5 to 8 fractions to the gross lymphadenopathy. At PMH, this boost is given concurrently with the large-field treatment. A CT scan with the patient in treatment position is used to ensure that the gross tumor is adequately encompassed by the radiation fields and that the minimal possible volume of kidney and liver are irradiated. The contralateral iliac lymph nodes may also be treated in cases where lymphadenopathy in the low para-aortic area is deemed to increase the risk of these nodes being involved by tumor. However, this is probably of most concern in patients with bulky retroperitoneal lymphadenopathy who are better treated with primary chemotherapy as discussed previously. Adjuvant radiation of supraclavicular lymph nodes in patients with stage II disease has been recommended by some, although it is not justified on a routine basis in view of the low risk of isolated supraclavicular recurrence (2 of 79 patients with IIA/B disease in the PMH series) (38,41). The ease with which supraclavicular lymph nodes can be followed clinically, the availability of effective salvage chemotherapy for these cases, the possibility of compromising bone marrow reserve for subsequent chemotherapy should it be necessary, and the potential for radiation-induced cardiac toxicity must be considered.

The use of combination carboplatin and RT in stage IIA/B seminoma has been suggested by Patterson et al. (42). She and her colleagues described a series of 30 patients treated with 1 course of carboplatin 4 to 6 weeks prior to RT. They reported a 5-year relapse survival rate of 96.9% as compared to 80.7% in a historical cohort (largely treated in the 1980s) treated with radiation alone. The major problems with this report include the possibility of stage migration improving the results in the combined therapy group as well as a low, by modern standards, control rate with RT alone. This approach cannot be accepted as routine practice without further data.

The most common sites of recurrence following (RT) in stage II patients with small-bulk lymph node metastases are mediastinal or supraclavicular nodes, lung, and bone. Most relapsing patients are cured with chemotherapy, which underscores the importance of regular follow-up with clinical examination and chest x-ray after radiation. CT imaging of the abdomen and pelvis is not necessary after complete resolution of abdominal disease. In the PMH series, two of the seven patients who recurred after RT had bone metastases, and both presented with spinal cord compression as the first sign of recurrence. Therefore, all patients with unexplained back pain require a bone scan to exclude metastases, and those with new onset neurologic deficits require urgent imaging of the spine with magnetic resonance imaging.

Residual Mass Following Radiation Therapy or Chemotherapy

Following treatment, patients with stage II disease require follow-up imaging of the abdomen after treatment until complete regression of disease has occurred. Residual retroperitoneal masses that may either regress slowly over time or remain stable are frequently seen. A stable, persistent mass often represents fibrosis or necrosis and only the minority contain active tumor. However, the possibility of a nonseminomatous component to explain the residual mass needs to be kept in mind even in patients whose primary tumors show pure seminoma. In addition, surgical extirpation of retroperitoneal nodes in the setting of seminoma is technically challenging and associated with a higher acute morbidity (43).

Therapeutic options for patients with residual masses after treatment include observation, surgical removal or, very rarely after chemotherapy, RT can be considered. PET scanning has been reported to be of little value in this setting by some authors, but others have reported it is a clinically useful predictor of tumor, especially in residual masses after chemotherapy, especially if the mass is greater than 3 cm in diameter (7,8). A small number of centers have reviewed their experience with surgery for residual masses in the setting of seminoma. The Memorial Sloan-Kettering Cancer Center (MSKCC) group published their data in 55 of 104 patients who demonstrated residual masses postchemotherapy (44). Of these 55 patients, 32 (58%) had a formal Retroperitoneal Lymph Node Dissection (RPLND) and 23 (42%) had multiple intraoperative biopsies performed, as the residual mass was deemed unresectable. Among patients with a mass >3 cm ($n = 27$), 8 (30%) had residual viable tumor. Interestingly, 2 of the 8 recurrences were teratoma and 6 were seminoma. No patients with tumors <3 cm had viable tumor at final pathology. Among the 8 patients with preoperative tumor masses >3 cm and positive pathologic findings, 6 remained with no evidence of disease at 47 months follow-up. Two patients, both with poorly defined masses on CT, died of disease. Given this high proportion of persistent malignancy, MSKCC investigators have recommended resection or biopsy of masses of 3 cm or larger. In contrast, Culine et al. have suggested that as long as the retroperitoneal mass continues to decrease in size after treatment, then continued observation is a reasonable strategy (45).

The use of RT in patients with postchemotherapy masses is often mentioned as a therapeutic option. Horwich et al. published their experience with both observation and radiotherapy for these masses and found that the recurrence rate was similar whether RT or observation was performed (46). The MRC Testicular Tumor Working Party published a retrospective pooled analysis assessing the role of RT for postchemotherapy residual mass among men with seminoma (47). Among the 123 patients with a residual abdominal residual mass 56% received consolidative RT. There was no significant difference in outcome among patients who did or did not receive RT. Given these data, it was concluded that routine RT is not indicated for a postchemotherapy residual mass.

It is clear that patients with a residual mass of 3 cm or less can safely be observed. For patients with bulkier disease, upfront surgery or observation can be instituted with therapy reserved for masses that increase in size. Using this approach at PMH, only six patients have required surgery over the past 15 years.

SPECIAL TREATMENT SITUATIONS

Seminoma in Patients with a Horseshoe Kidney

Horseshoe kidney occurs in approximately 1 in 400 of the general population. Patients with horseshoe kidneys are at an increased risk of testicular tumors because there is association between renal fusion abnormalities and cryptorchidism, a major risk factor for testicular neoplasms (48).

There are two main problems in the management of seminomas in patients with horseshoe or pelvic kidney. In many of these cases, a large part of the renal parenchyma directly overlies the regional lymph nodes and lies within the standard radiation volume. The delivery of a standard radiation dose would be associated with an unacceptable risk of radiation nephritis. The second problem is related to the possible abnormalities in lymphatic drainage of the testis and, therefore, the possibility of relapse when standard radiation fields are used. Unusual patterns of relapse have been observed in patients managed by surveillance, confirming concerns regarding abnormal lymphatic pathways. For these reasons, in patients with stage I seminoma, postorchidectomy surveillance is recommended. However, a retroperiteonal lymph node dissection (RPLD) is another option for patients unwilling to follow a surveillance program. In more advanced disease, chemotherapy should be used rather than RT.

Testicular Tumors Developing in Immunosuppressed Patients

Immunosuppressed patients, from HIV infection or posttransplant, have an increased risk of developing malignant germ cell neoplasms (49,50). Seminoma is the most common histologic type with a similar age on onset to that found in the general population (49). The majority of patients described in the literature have received standard treatment consisting of orchiectomy followed by surveillance, RT, or chemotherapy, as determined by stage. RT and chemotherapy appear to be well tolerated except in patients with very advanced immunosuppression (50). Most patients are cured of disease and overall survival is usually determined by the severity of immunosuppression and the complications of the acquired immunodeficiency syndrome (AIDS) rather than by seminoma (49,50).

Caution must be exercised as benign retroperitoneal adenopathy related to AIDS may be mistaken for metastasis from a testicular primary tumor. For those receiving chemotherapy, consideration should be given to concomitant prophylaxis for opportunistic infection. In transplant patients requiring retroperitoneal RT, the kidney or pancreatic allograft should be shielded wherever possible. If this cannot be safely achieved, then RPLD or chemotherapy should be used instead. Posttransplant patients appear to tolerate platinum-based chemotherapy without any problems. Overall, the clinical course of immunosuppressed patients with testicular tumors is similar to that of nonimmunosuppressed patients, and these patients should be offered standard oncologic therapy (49–51).

Central Nervous System Metastases

Approximately 2% to 3% of patients with metastatic GCT will present clinically with brain metastases and up to 40% of patients who die of progressive disease will have brain metastases at autopsy. Patients who present at time of diagnosis with brain metastases can achieve approximately 50% 5-year cause-specific survival with aggressive treatment (52). The optimal local therapy—RT or surgery—in patients with resectable tumors is unclear, but in those with unresectable disease RT to a dose of 40 to 45 Gy should be given to gross disease, preferably using a stereotactic approach. The role of total brain irradiation is unclear but, if given, the dose should not exceed 40 Gy. Patients who develop brain metastases during systemic chemotherapy have a very poor prognosis and should likely receive palliative RT only (53). Patients presenting with late relapse with CNS metastases should be treated aggressively, as long-term disease-free survival is possible (53).

Spermatocytic Seminoma

Spermatocytic seminoma is a rare testicular malignancy accounting for 1% to 2% of all seminomas, and is rarely associated with sarcomas of the testis (54,55). The usual age of diagnosis is 50 to 60 years, though it does occur in younger patients (56). It is distinct in its histologic characteristics with usually three different cell sizes, spherical nuclei, lack of cytoplasmic glycogen, and sparse or absent lymphocytic infiltrate when compared to classical seminoma (57,58). Unlike classic seminoma, it does not appear to arise from carcinoma in situ (CIS) and it occurs solely in the testis and has no ovarian equivalent. All patients presented as stage I and there is only one case in the literature that has been confirmed as developing subsequent metastatic disease (59). In the past it has been treated in a similar fashion to seminoma with adjuvant RT to the para-aortic and pelvic nodes, but the likelihood of benefit from this approach is low and all patients should be placed on surveillance (60).

Testicular Intraepithelial Neoplasia

Testicular intraepithelial neoplasia (TIN) is the precursor to all testicular GCTs except spermatocytic seminoma (61). Furthermore, virtually all cases of TIN in postpubertal men will progress to invasive cancer if given sufficient time (62). The incidence of TIN in the contralateral testis of men with a unilateral GCT is approximately 5%, in good agreement with the incidence of second testicular tumors (63–65). Therefore, it has been suggested that men with a unilateral tumor should undergo biopsy of the contralateral testis, preferably at the time of ipsilateral orchiectomy, with the aim of identifying and treating TIN before progression to invasive disease (66). Men with a normal testicular biopsy can be reassured that their risk of a contralateral tumor is <1% while those with a positive biopsy should be considered for testicular RT. A fractionated dose of 20 Gy has been reported to eradicate TIN and prevent the development of invasive cancer (67). Leydig cell function and androgen production appears to be preserved in most patients (62,68). Because of the risk of radiation-induced endocrinologic damage, attempts have been made to define the lowest effective dose in this setting. It would appear that 18 Gy to 20 Gy in 9 to 10 fractions gives reasonable control of TIN but that lower doses are likely ineffective (69). However, this approach remains controversial given that most second GCTs arising in the opposite testis are curable, and the fact that there are reports of second tumors arising in the contralateral testis after RT (69,70). In addition, the long-term effects of low-dose testicular radiation on androgen production are poorly documented.

Testicular biopsy should also be considered in other patients who are at high risk of having TIN, including those with a history of cryptorchidism, presumed primary extragonadal GCT, androgen insensitivity syndrome, or gonadal dysgenesis (60).

Second Testicular Germ Cell Tumors

Approximately 5% of patients will have bilateral testicular GCTs, either synchronously or metachronously (65,71). Frequent examination of the remaining testis after treatment of a unilateral tumor, including self-examination by patients, is important to assure that second GCTs are diagnosed when small and confined to the testis. Bilateral inguinal orchiectomy has been the standard management in this situation. However, patients then require life-long androgen replacement therapy, which may be associated with sexual dysfunction, mood swings, and a general impairment of quality of life. Tumor enucleation with preservation of normal testicular tissue and androgen production has been proposed as an alternative to orchiectomy (68). In 73 patients who underwent tumor enucleation, TIN was found in association with the invasive tumor in 56 cases and 46 of these patients received local irradiation of 18 to 20 Gy. Invasive tumor developed in the residual testicular tissue in only three patients, all of who had TIN and did not receive radiation. Eighty-five percent of patients had normal serum testosterone levels at last follow-up and did not require androgen replacement therapy.

Nonseminoma

With the exception of patients with brain metastases, there is little role for RT in patients with nonseminomatous tumors. However, RT is effective in eradicating microscopic disease in nonseminoma and should be considered in cases where microscopic residual disease is present following resection of tumor and chemotherapy is contraindicated (72). RT can also be effective as palliation in many circumstances, including bone metastases.

RADIATION TOXICITY

With the low-dose RT used in seminoma, acute complications are minor in most patients. Mild nausea and vomiting are common, and a small proportion of patients require regular antiemetics and are unable to complete daily tasks while receiving RT. Diarrhea develops in only a minority of patients, especially if low-dose per fraction radiation is used. Severe late radiation complications are rare and usually no severe complications are expected unless the patient has an underlying medical problem or a technical error occurs. Chronic fatigue has been reported in 16% of survivors of testicular cancer and some patients do experience severe psychological symptoms in the areas of sexual activity, infertility, distress, and social upheaval (73). Chronic gastrointestinal symptoms may develop and an increased incidence of peptic ulceration particularly after abdominal radiation doses in the range of 30 to 45 Gy has been reported (74,75).

Recent data from M.D. Anderson has suggested that long-term survivors of seminoma treated with postorchiectomy RT are at significant excess risk of death as a result of cardiac disease or second cancer (19). However, the relevance of this data to the modern practice of RT has been questioned (76).

LATE GONADAL TOXICITY

Oligospermia or azoospermia is reported in 20% or more of patients with testicular seminomas at diagnosis and if posttreatment fertility is a concern, then semen analysis should be performed prior to treatment (77). The testicular germinal epithelium is exquisitely sensitive to ionizing radiation. Although the contralateral testis is not located directly in the radiation field, scatter dose can be significant and may cause profound depression of spermatogenesis and compromise future fertility. A radiation dose between 20 and 50 cGy may produce temporary aspermia, and doses greater than 50 cGy may preclude recovery of spermatogenesis. The use of scrotal shielding reduces the scattered radiation dose to the testis, but cannot assure protection of spermatogenesis in all patients. In men who recover spermatogenesis after RT for seminoma, there is no evidence of an increased incidence of genetic abnormalities among offspring (78). Limiting RT target volume to the para-aortic and common iliac area does not eliminate concerns regarding RT-induced fertility. In the MRC randomized trial of para-aortic radiation alone versus para-aortics and pelvis, the median time to a normal posttreatment sperm count was 13 months in those patients treated to the para-aortics alone. This was significantly better than the patients treated to the para-aortic and pelvic lymph nodes (20 months). However, at 3 years of follow-up there was no significant difference in sperm counts between the two groups. Testicular shielding should be used in all patients who wish to retain fertility after treatment.

SECOND MALIGNANCY

A distinction must be made between second GCTs of the testis, which reflect a common risk factor for this disease, and unrelated malignancies, which may be treatment induced. An increased risk of second cancers has been documented in a number of studies, and since this increased risk is expressed more than 10 to 15 years following RT, it may not be apparent in series with shorter follow-up. The largest study of second cancers in long-term survivors of testicular cancer was conducted by Travis et al. at the National Cancer Institute Cancer Epidemiology Division (79). Over 28,000 patients with testis cancer, including over 15,000 with seminoma from 16 population-based registries worldwide, were evaluated. Overall, 1,406 second cancers, excluding contralateral testis tumors, occurred against 981 expected [observed/expected (O/E) = 1.43]. The actuarial risk of developing a second nontesticular malignancy increased over time from diagnosis of testicular cancer and was 18.2% at 25 years. Secondary leukemia was linked with RT and chemotherapy, while an excess of the stomach, bladder, and possibly pancreas tumors was associated with prior RT (79,80). Limitation of the RT field to the infradiaphragmatic region appears to result in a lower risk of second malignancy than more extensive fields and it is likely that limiting the treatment volume to the para-aortic area alone would decrease the risk further (81).

SUMMARY

Adjuvant radiation and surveillance are acceptable treatment options in stage I seminoma. Adjuvant chemotherapy should only be performed on a research protocol. If RT is chosen as the management strategy, then a dose of 25 Gy in 20 daily fractions over 4 weeks is appropriate and gives little acute toxicity. Patients should be advised that there is a potential carcinogenic risk with this approach. As regards treatment volume, it is reasonable to treat the para-aortic lymph nodes alone or para-aortics + pelvic lymph nodes. However, if the para-aortics alone are treated, then ongoing postradiation surveillance of the pelvis should be performed. In stage II seminoma, RT is the treatment of choice for low-tumor volume stage IIa/B cases with chemotherapy being preferred for more advanced disease. There is no role for adjuvant carboplatin off protocol. Combination RT and chemotherapy can be curative in patients with brain metastases from GCTs.

References

1. Choo R, Sandler H, Warde P, et al. Survey of radiation oncologists: practice patterns of the management of stage I seminoma of testis in Canada and a selected group in the United States. *Can J Urol* 2002;9:1479–1485.
2. Dieckmann KP, Bruggeboes B, Pichlmeier U, et al. Adjuvant treatment of clinical stage I seminoma: is a single course of carboplatin sufficient? *Urology* 2000;55:102–106.
3. Greene FL, Page DL, Fleming ID et al., eds. *AJCC cancer staging manual*, 6th ed. New York: Springer-Verlag, 2002.

4. Sobin LH, Wittekind CL, eds. *International union against cancer (UICC): TNM classification of malignant tumors*, 6th ed. New York: John Wiley and Sons, 2002.

5. Spermon JR, De Geus-Oei LF, Kiemeney LA, et al. The role of (18)fluoro-2-deoxyglucose positron emission tomography in initial staging and restaging after chemotherapy for testicular germ cell tumors. *BJU Int* 2002; 89:549–556.

6. Cremerius U, Effert PJ, Adam G, et al. FDG PET for detection and therapy control of metastatic germ cell tumor. *J Nucl Med* 1998;39:815–822.

7. De Santis M, Bokemeyer C, Becherer A, et al. Predictive impact of 2-18fluoro-2-deoxy-D-glucose positron emission tomography for residual postchemotherapy masses in patients with bulky seminoma. *J Clin Oncol* 2001;19:3740–3744.

8. Ganjoo KN, Chan RJ, Sharma M, et al. Positron emission tomography scans in the evaluation of postchemotherapy residual masses in patients with seminoma. *J Clin Oncol* 1999;17:3457–3460.

9. Hultenschmidt B, Budach V, Genters K, et al. Results of radiotherapy for 230 patients with stage I-II seminomas. *Strahlenther Onkol* 1996;172: 186–192.

10. Coleman JM, Coleman RE, Turner AR, et al. The management and clinical course of testicular seminoma: 15 years' experience at a single institution. *Clin Oncol (R Coll Radiol)* 1998;10:237–241.

11. Fossa SD, Horwich A, Russell JM, et al. Optimal planning target volume for stage I testicular seminoma: a Medical Research Council randomized trial. *J Clin Oncol* 1999;17:1146–1154.

12. Bayens YC, Helle PA, Van PW, et al. Orchidectomy followed by radiotherapy in 176 stage I and II testicular seminoma patients: benefits of a 10-year follow-up study. *Radiother Oncol* 1992;25:97–102.

13. Santoni R, Barbera F, Bertoni F, et al. Stage I seminoma of the testis: a bi-institutional retrospective analysis of patients treated with radiation therapy only. *BJU Int.* 2003;92(1):47–52.

14. Warde P, Gospodarowicz M, Panzarella T, et al. Surveillance is an appropriate management strategy for in-patients with stage I seminoma. *Int J Radiat Oncol Biol Phys* 2002;54 (2):61.

15. Rathmell AJ, Mapstone NP, Jones WG. Testicular seminoma metastasizing to palatine tonsil. *Clin Oncol* 1993;5:185–186.

16. Raina V, Singh SP, Kamble N, et al. Brain metastasis as the site of relapse in germ cell tumor of testis. *Cancer* 1993;72:2182–2185.

17. Warde P, Gospodarowicz MK, Panzarella T, et al. Stage I testicular seminoma: results of adjuvant irradiation and surveillance. *J Clin Oncol* 1995; 13:2255–2262.

18. Chung P, Parker C, Panzarella T, et al. Surveillance in stage I testicular seminoma – risk of late relapse. *Can J Urol* 2002;9:1637–1640.

19. Zagars GK, Ballo MT, Lee AK, et al. Mortality after cure of testicular seminoma. *J Clin Oncol* 2004;22:640–647.

20. Logue JP, Harris MA, Livsey JE, et al. Short course para-aortic radiation for stage I seminoma of the testis. *Int J Radiat Oncol Biol Phys* 2003;57: 1304–1309.

21. Allhoff EP, Liedke S, de Riese W, et al. Stage I seminoma of the testis. Adjuvant radiotherapy or surveillance? *Br J Urol* 1991;68:190–194.

22. Warde P, Gospodarowicz M, Banerjee D, et al. Prognostic factors for relapse in stage I testicular seminoma treated with surveillance. *J Urol* 1997; 157:1705–1709.

23. von der Maase H, Specht L, Jacobsen GK, et al. Surveillance following orchidectomy for stage I seminoma of the testis. *Eur J Cancer* 1993;14: 1931–1934.

24. Horwich A, Alsanjari N, A'Hern R, et al. Surveillance following orchidectomy for stage I testicular seminoma. *Br J Cancer* 1992;65:775–778.

25. Warde P, Specht L, Horwich A, et al. Prognostic factors for relapse in stage I seminoma managed by surveillance: a pooled analysis. *J Clin Oncol* 2002; 20:4448–4452.

26. Jacobsen KD, Olsen DR, Fossa K, et al. External beam abdominal radiotherapy in patients with seminoma stage I: field type, testicular dose, and spermatogenesis. *Int J Radiat Oncol Biol Phys* 1997;38:95–102.

27. Fraass BA, Kinsella TJ, Harrington FS, et al. Peripheral dose to the testes: the design and clinical use of a practical and effective gonadal shield. *Int J Radiat Oncol Biol Phys* 1985;11:609–615.

28. Melchior D, Hammer P, Fimmers R, et al. Long term results and morbidity of paraaortic compared with paraaortic and iliac adjuvant radiation in clinical stage I seminoma. *Anticancer Res* 2001;21:2989–2993.

29. Fossa S, Horwich A, Russell J, et al. Radiotherapy of testicular seminoma stage I; optimal field size. A Medical Research Council (UK) study. In: Joffe J, ed. *Germ cell tumors IV the proceedings of the fourth germ cell tumor conference leeds, November 1997*. London: John Libbey & Company, 1998: 121–129.

30. Thomas GM. Is "optimal" radiation for stage I seminoma yet defined? *J Clin Oncol* 1999;17:3004–3005.

31. Donohue J, Thornhill J, Foster R, et al. Retroperitoneal lymphadenectomy for clinical stage A testis cancer (1965-1989): modifications of technique and impact on ejaculation. *J Urol* 1993;149:237–243.

32. Schmidberger H, Bamberg M, Meisner C, et al. Radiotherapy in stage IIA and IIB testicular seminoma with reduced portals: a prospective multicenter study. *Int J Radiat Oncol Biol Phys* 1997;39:321–326.

33. Jones W, Fossa S, Meas G, et al. A randomised trial of two radiotherapy schedules in the adjuvant of stage I seminoma (MRC TE18): preliminary report. *Germ cell tumors*. London: V. Springer, 2002:235–236.

34. Gurkaynak M, Akyol F, Zorlu F, et al. Stage I testicular seminoma: para-aortic and iliac irradiation with reduced dose after orchiectomy. *Urol Int* 2003;71:385–388.

35. Dosoretz DE, Shipley WU, Blitzer PH, et al. Megavoltage irradiation for pure testicular seminoma: results and patterns of failure. *Cancer* 1981;48: 2184–2190.

36. Lester SG, Morphis J, Hornback NB. Testicular seminoma: analysis of treatment results and failures. *Int J Radiat Oncol Biol Phys* 1986;12: 353–358.

37. Chung PW, Gospodarowicz MK, Panzarella T, et al. Stage II testicular seminoma: patterns of recurrence and outcomes of treatment. *Eur Urol* 2004;45 (6):754–760.

38. Zagars GK, Pollack A. Radiotherapy for stage II testicular seminoma. *Int J Radiat Oncol Biol Phys* 2001;51:643–649.

39. Vallis KA, Howard GC, Duncan W, et al. Radiotherapy for stages I and II testicular seminoma: results and morbidity in 238 patients. *Br J Radiol* 1995;68:400–405.

40. Classen J, Schmidberger H, Meisner C, et al. Radiotherapy for stages IIA/B testicular seminoma: final report of a prospective multicenter clinical trial. *J Clin Oncol* 2003;21:1101–1106.

41. Chung PW, Warde PR, Panzarella T, et al. Appropriate radiation volume for stage IIA/B testicular seminoma. *Int J Radiat Oncol Biol Phys* 2003; 56:746–748.

42. Patterson H, Norman AR, Mitra SS, et al. Combination carboplatin and radiotherapy in the management of stage II testicular seminoma: comparison with radiotherapy treatment alone. *Radiother Oncol* 2001;59:5–11.

43. Mosharafa AA, Foster RS, Leibovich BC, et al. Is post-chemotherapy resection of seminomatous elements associated with higher acute morbidity? *J Urol* 2003;169:2126–2128.

44. Herr HW, Sheinfeld J, Puc HS, et al. Surgery for a post-chemotherapy residual mass in seminoma. *J Urol* 1997;157:860–862.

45. Culine S, Droz JP. Optimal management of residual mass after chemotherapy in advanced seminoma: there is time for everything. *J Clin Oncol* 1996; 14:2884–2885.

46. Horwich A, Paluchowska B, Norman A, et al. Residual mass following chemotherapy of seminoma. *Ann Oncol* 1997;8:37–40.

47. Duchesne GM, Stenning SP, Aass N, et al. Radiotherapy after chemotherapy for metastatic seminoma-a diminishing role. *Eur J Cancer* 1997;33:829–835.

48. Bauer SB, Perlmutter AD, Retik AB. Anomalies of the upper urinary tract. In: Vaughan ED Jr, ed. *Campell's urology*, 6th ed. Philadelphia, PA: WB Saunders, 1992:1357–1442.

49. Powles T, Bower M, Daugaard G, et al. Multicenter study of human immunodeficiency virus-related germ cell tumors. *J Clin Oncol* 2003;21: 1922–1927.

50. Leibovitch I, Baniel J, Rowland RG, et al. Malignant testicular neoplasms in immunosuppressed patients. *J Urol* 1996;155:1938–1942.

51. Fizazi K, Amato RJ, Beuzeboc P, et al. Germ cell tumors in patients infected by the human immunodeficiency virus. *Cancer* 2001;92:1460–1467.

52. Fossa SD, Bokemeyer C, Gerl A, et al. Treatment outcome of patients with brain metastases from malignant germ cell tumors. *Cancer* 1999;85: 988–997.

53. Bokemeyer C, Nowak P, Haupt A, et al. Treatment of brain metastases in patients with testicular cancer. *J Clin Oncol* 1997;15:1449–1454.

54. Floyd C, Ayala AG, Logothetis CJ, et al. Spermatocytic seminoma with associated sarcoma of the testis. *Cancer* 1988;61:409–414.

55. True LD, Otis CN, Delprado W, et al. Spermatocytic seminoma of testis with sarcomatous transformation. A report of five cases. *Am J Surg Pathol* 1988;12:75–82.

56. Pendlebury S, Horwich A, Dearnaley DP, et al. Spermatocytic seminoma: a clinicopathological review of ten patients. *Clin Oncol* 1996;8:316–318.

57. Masson P. Etude sur le seminome. *Rev Can Biol* 1946;5:361–387.

58. Damjanov I. Pathology of testicular tumors. In: Raghavan D, Scher HI, Leibel SA et al., eds. *Principles and practice of genitourinary oncology*. Philadelphia, PA: Lippincott–Raven Publishers, 1997:653–662.

59. Matoska J, Ondrus D, Hornak M. Metastatic spermatocytic seminoma. A case report with light microscopic, ultrastructural, and immunohistochemical findings. *Cancer* 1988;62:1197–1201.

60. Chung PW, Bayley AJ, Sweet J , et al. Spermatocytic seminoma: a review. *Eur Urol* 2004;45 (4):495–498.

61. Skakkebaek NE, Berthelsen JG, Giwercman A, et al. Carcinoma-in-situ of the testis: possible origin from gonocytes and precursor of all types of germ cell tumors except spermatocytoma. *Int J Androl* 1987;10:19–27.

62. Giwercman A, von der Maase H, Skakkebaek NE. Epidemiological and clinical aspects of carcinoma in situ of the testis. *Eur Urol* 1993;23: 104–110.

63. Dieckmann KP, Loy V. Prevalence of bilateral testicular germ cell tumors and early detection by testicular intraepithelial neoplasia. *Eur Urol* 1993; 2:22–23.

64. Osterlind A, Berthelsen JG, Abildgaard N, et al. Risk of bilateral testicular germ cell cancer in Denmark: 1960-1984. *J Natl Cancer Inst* 1991;83: 1391–1395.

65. Wanderas EH, Fossa SD, Tretli S. Risk of a second germ cell cancer after treatment of a primary germ cell cancer in 2201 Norwegian male patients. *Eur J Cancer* 1997;33:244–252.

66. Grigor KM, Rorth M. Should the contralateral testis be biopsied? Round table discussion. *Eur Urol* 1993;23:129–135.

67. Giwercman A, Skakkebaek NE. Carcinoma in situ of the testis: biology, screening and management. [Review]. *Eur Urol* 1993;2:19–21.
68. van der Schyff S, Heidenreich A. Tumor enucleation resection in testicular germ cell tumors: longterm follow-up (Abstract). *J Urol* 1999;161:182.
69. Classen J, Dieckmann KP. Radiotherapy of carcinoma-in-situ of the testis. *J Clin Oncol* 2002;20:3559–3560.
70. Dieckmann KP, Lauke H, Michl U, et al. Testicular germ cell cancer despite previous local radiotherapy to the testis. *Eur Urol* 2002;41:643–649; discussion 649–650.
71. Osterlind A, Berthelsen JG, Abildgaard N, et al. Incidence of bilateral testicular germ cell cancer in Denmark, 1960-84: preliminary findings. *Int J Androl* 1987;10:203–208.
72. Rorth M, Jacobsen GK, von der Maase H et al, Danish Testicular Cancer Study Group. Surveillance alone versus radiotherapy after orchiectomy for clinical stage I nonseminomatous testicular cancer. *J Clin Oncol* 1991;9: 1543–1548.
73. Fossa SD, Dahl AA, Loge JH. Fatigue, anxiety, and depression in long-term survivors of testicular cancer. *J Clin Oncol* 2003;21:1249–1254.
74. Hamilton CR, Horwich A, Bliss JM, et al. Gastrointestinal morbidity of adjuvant radiotherapy in stage I malignant teratoma of the testis. *Radiother Oncol* 1987;10:85–90.
75. Yeoh E, Horowitz M, Russo A, et al. The effects of abdominal irradiation for seminoma of the testis on gastrointestinal function. *J Gastroenterol Hepatol* 1995;10:125–130.
76. Horwich A. Radiotherapy in stage I seminoma of the testis. *J Clin Oncol* 2004;22:585–588.
77. Bussen S, Sutterlin M, Steck T, et al. Semen parameters in patients with unilateral testicular cancer compared to patients with other malignancies. *Arch Gynecol Obstet* 2003 2004;269(3):196–198.
78. Schover LR, Gonzales M, von Eschenbach A. Sexual and marital relationships after radiotherapy for seminoma. *Urology* 1986;27:117–123.
79. Travis L, Curtis R, Storm H, et al. Risk of second malignant neoplasms among long-term survivors of testicular cancer. *J Natl Cancer Inst* 1997; 89:1429–1439.
80. Travis L, Andersson M, Holowaty E, et al. Risk of leukemia following radiotherapy and chemotherapy for testicular cancer (Abstract). *J Clin Oncol* 1999;18:308a.
81. Fossa SD, Langmark F, Aass N, et al. Second non-germ cell malignancies after radiotherapy of testicular cancer with or without chemotherapy. *Br J Cancer* 1990;61:639–643.

CHAPTER 40 ■ RISK-ADAPTED THERAPY OF METASTATIC TESTIS CANCER

CHAPTER 40A
Risk-Adapted Therapy of Metastatic Testis Cancer: Good-Risk Patients

Stefan Sleijfer and Ronald de Wit

INTRODUCTION

Before the introduction of cisplatin-based multidrug chemotherapy, the outcome of most patients with disseminated germ cell tumor was very poor. In the 1970s, Einhorn and Donohue developed a regimen consisting of cisplatin, vinblastine, and bleomycin (PVB), yielding impressive results (1). The durable disease-free survival (DFS) rate obtained with this regimen was a major breakthrough in the treatment of this tumor entity, and since then, germ cell tumor has become a model for curable diseases (2). In 1987, a randomized phase III trial comparing two cisplatin-based therapies was reported by Williams et al. (3). This study revealed that four cycles of the combination of bleomycin, etoposide, and cisplatin (BEP) had a favorable toxicity profile and improved activity compared with four cycles of PVB (3). Following the report of this study, four cycles of BEP has become the standard first-line chemotherapeutic regimen for patients with disseminated germ cell tumor.

Shortly after the introduction of cisplatin-based chemotherapy, it was recognized that patients could be categorized into groups with different prognoses. Various prognostic factors were identified, including the primary site (gonadal vs. extragonadal), seminoma or nonseminoma, extent of disease, localization of metastatic disease, and the level of the tumor markers α-fetoprotein (AFP), β-human chorionic gonadotropin (β-HCG), and lactate dehydrogenase (LDH). Combination of two or more of these factors resulted in a wide number of classifications. By using these differential prognostic categories, studies were initiated in separate groups. For patients with good prognostic features, studies were designed to find new regimens with reduced toxicity but with the same treatment efficacy, whereas for patients with poor risk, studies aimed at enhancing antitumor activity by intensifying treatment. However, because large institutions and groups, such as Memorial Sloan-Kettering Cancer Center (MSKCC) (4), Indiana University (5), Australian Germ Cell Trial Group (6), the European Organization for Research and Treatment of Cancer (EORTC) (7), and the Medical Research Council (MRC) (8), used their own criteria of disease extent and serum markers cut-off values for determining risk status, including or excluding patients affected the response rates obtained in the various regimens. For example, the EORTC criteria for good prognosis nonseminomatous testicular cancer required that 90% of patients achieve a complete response rate with cisplatin-based therapy (7), whereas according to the early MSKCC criteria (4), good-risk patients only required a complete response rate probability of 50% or greater.

Because the diverse classification systems severely hampered intergroup study result comparisons, the International Germ Cell Cancer Collaborative Group (IGCCCG) was established in 1991 in order to develop a consensus classification. The IGCCCG system was formulated on the basis of the outcomes of almost 6,000 patients with disseminated germ cell tumor who were treated with cisplatin-based chemotherapy, and the system consisted of three groups with a good, an intermediate, and a poor prognosis (Table 40A.1). Because seminoma is more susceptible to chemotherapy than nonseminoma is and because seminoma consequently possesses a more favorable prognosis, none of the patients with seminoma fulfills the criteria for poor risk. For patients with nonseminomatous cancer, the 5-year survival rates of the good-, intermediate-, and poor-risk groups are 92%, 80%, and 48%, respectively, whereas these rates for patients with seminoma are 86% for the good-prognosis and 72% for the intermediate-prognosis groups (9).

This chapter addresses the treatment of patients with germ cell tumor who belong to the good-risk metastatic disease group. In particular, it focuses on those trials that form the basis of the current standard treatment. However, it should be noted that all studies except one (10) in this particular subgroup were done before the introduction of the IGCCCG classification; therefore, the translation of the results of the individual chemotherapeutic regimens in the studies is hampered. This chapter also provides guidelines on how treatment may be adapted in situations where the scheduled treatment plan has to be changed because of encountered toxicity.

RESULTS OF FOUR CYCLES BLEOMYCIN, ETOPOSIDE, AND CISPLATIN IN GOOD-PROGNOSIS DISEASE

Following initial trial results showing the efficacy of cisplatin-based chemotherapy and the subsequent recognition of the efficacy of etoposide (3), four cycles of BEP became standard treatment for all patients regardless the prognostic group. BEP consists of bleomycin (30 units) given weekly, etoposide (100 mg per m^2) given daily for 5 days, and cisplatin (20 mg per m^2) administered daily over a period of 5 days. Patients received these cycles at 3-week intervals. In Europe, initially, a lower dose of etoposide was given for a total dosage of 360 mg/m^2/cycle.

Irrespective of the prognostic classification used, the long-term DFS rates by BEP chemotherapy are impressive in patients who had a good prognosis. The rate of patients achieving a no-evidence-of-disease (NED) state either by BEP alone or after adjunctive resection of postchemotherapeutic

TABLE 40A.1

THE INTERNATIONAL GERM CELL CONSENSUS CLASSIFICATION (IGCCCG)

Prognosis	Nonseminoma	Seminoma
Good (5-yr 90%)	testis/retroperitoneal primary no nonpulmonary visceral metastases AFP <1,000 μg/L and β-HCG <5,000 U/L and LDH <1.5 × ULN	any primary site no nonpulmonary visceral metastases any β-HCG/LDH
Intermediate (5-yr 75%)	testis/retroperitoneal primary no nonpulmonary visceral metastases 1,000 <AFP <10,000 μg/L or 5,000 <β-HCG <50,000 U/L or 1.5 × N <LDH <10 × ULN	any primary site nonpulmonary visceral metastases any β-HCG/LDH
Poor (5-yr 50%)	mediastinal primary or nonpulmonary visceral metastases or AFP >10,000 μg/L or β-HCG >50,000 U/L or LDH >10 × ULN	

AFP, α-fetoprotein; β-HCG, β-human chorionic gonadotropin; LDH, lactate dehydrogenase; N, normal range; ULN, upper limit of normal range.

residual masses ranges from 90% to 95%. Relapses after obtaining the NED state occur in approximately 5% of patients, of which most relapses are encountered in the first 2 years after treatment (11). In addition, >50% of relapsing patients can be successfully treated by subsequent salvage chemotherapy. These favorable figures obtained by BEP are reflected in excellent long-term overall survival rates ranging from 90% to 95% (10,12–15).

SIDE EFFECTS OBTAINED WITH BLEOMYCIN, ETOPOSIDE, AND CISPLATIN

The impressive outcome of chemotherapeutic treatment with BEP, however, is at the expense of sometimes severe toxicity, both in the short term and in the long term. One of the most severe acute side effects of the use of bleomycin is the occurrence of bleomycin-induced pneumonitis (BIP). Clinically significant BIP occurs in approximately 10% of patients and has a fatal outcome in approximately 3% of all patients treated with bleomycin (16), thereby accounting for a substantial proportion of the total mortality in patients with good-prognosis disease. Several risk factors for the development of BIP have been identified, including the total bleomycin dose, renal dysfunction, age, extent of disease (17), smoking, and, probably, existing pulmonary comorbidity (16) (Table 40A.2). There are

TABLE 40A.2

RISK FACTORS FOR DEVELOPMENT OF BLEOMYCIN-INDUCED PULMONARY TOXICITY

Risk factors
Age above 40 years
Renal dysfunction
Stage IV according to the Royal Marsden classification
Cumulative bleomycin dose
Smoking
Pulmonary comorbidity

several indications that BIP develops through bleomycin-induced damage of the endothelium of the pulmonary vasculature. Another vascular side effect of bleomycin is the occurrence of Raynaud-like phenomenon, manifesting as painful digits and paresthesias, particularly following exposure to cold temperature (18). The reported incidence of this side effect, which may last for many years after completion of treatment, varies widely from 6% to up to 40% of the patients treated for testicular cancer, depending on the method of investigation (3,10,19). Other well-known side effects of bleomycin are fever, occurring several hours after infusion, and skin toxicity.

The characteristic side effect of the second compound of the BEP regimen, etoposide, is bone marrow depression. Severe myelosuppression, defined as neutropenia grade 4, neutropenic fever, and thrombopenia grade 4, occurs in about 20% of the patients at any point of time during treatment with four cycles of BEP (10). Late-term etoposide-related toxicity consists of an increased risk of acute leukemia (20). This risk is clearly dose related and is predominantly apparent at a total dose of >2 gm per m². In patients receiving a cumulative dose of <2 gm per m² of etoposide, this risk is still estimated to be increased 20-fold compared with the general population. However, because the risk of developing acute leukemia in the general population is rather small, the cumulative risk for patients treated with etoposide-based regimens is approximately .6% (21).

Cisplatin is regarded as the most active component of the BEP regimen. However, it is also one of the most emetogenic agents known. Nowadays, this disturbing side effect can be alleviated considerably by the introduction of the 5HT-antagonists and by the recent availability of the neurokinin-1-antagonist, aprepitant (22,23). Another serious side effect of cisplatin is nephrotoxicity. During cisplatin-based therapy, a median decrease of 20% in glomerular filtration rate (GFR) is observed. On long-term follow-up, a persistent impaired renal dysfunction defined as a GFR <70% of the lower normal range is found in 20% to 30% of the patients after receiving cisplatin-based treatment for germ cell tumor (25). Neurotoxicity manifesting as various forms, including peripheral sensory neuropathy, autonomic neuropathy, Lhermitte sign, and, sporadically, encephalopathy, is another side effect of cisplatin (26). The most predominant neuropathic symptom is paresthesia and is reported by approximately one-half of the patients (27). The exact underlying mechanism is uncertain, but accumulation of cisplatin in neurons is the probable mechanism. Cisplatin-induced vasospasms account probably for additional neurotoxic symptoms such as focal seizures or transient blindness. Ototoxicity, another form of cisplatin-mediated neurotoxicity, is caused by destruction of auditory neurons and outer hair cells in the organ of Corti. By pure-tone audiometry, disturbances at the higher frequencies are found in approximately 70% of patients treated with cisplatin-based chemotherapy for germ cell tumor (27). Fortunately, clinical neuropathy is to a great extent reversible and rarely impacts daily-life activities of the majority of patients.

In view of these severe treatment-related side effects and the excellent prognosis of patients with good-risk metastatic germ cell tumor, the trials carried out in this group aimed to reduce treatment toxicity without compromising efficacy. These studies focused particularly on elimination of bleomycin, substituting cisplatin by the less toxic component carboplatin, and reduction of the total drug dose by decreasing the number of cycles.

TRIALS STUDYING THE DELETION OF BLEOMYCIN FROM TREATMENT

Because of the severe side effects of bleomycin and doubts in the 1980s whether bleomycin provided a major contribution in cisplatin-based chemotherapy in germ cell tumor, several efforts have been made to find out if this component could be deleted from treatment. Three studies investigating this topic have been published.

In an Australian study, which was initiated before the superiority of etoposide over vinblastine was demonstrated by Williams et al. (3), 222 patients were randomized to receive treatment with cisplatin and vinblastine, 6 mg per m^2 on day 1 and day 2 every 3 weeks (PV), with or without bleomycin 30 units weekly for a maximum of 12 weeks (PVB) (28). Patients were classified as having good prognosis according to criteria of the Australian Germ Cell Trial Group. In the 218 evaluable patients, tumor-related mortality was significantly increased in the PV arm compared with those assigned to receive PVB (16 patients vs. 6 patients). Because of this increase, it was concluded that bleomycin could not be deleted from this regimen. Patients allocated to PVB experienced considerably more toxicity, resulting in six toxic deaths compared with one in the PV arm. Overall survival was similar for both arms after a minimum follow-up of 4 years (28).

Loehrer et al. (15) reported an Eastern Cooperative Oncology Group (ECOG) study comparing three cycles of BEP with three cycles of EP in 171 patients deemed to have a favorable prognosis according to the Indiana staging system. In both groups, the rate of patients achieving NED status after chemotherapy with or without subsequent resection of residual mass was similar. However, the number of relapses after obtaining NED was greater in the EP arm, which was translated into a significantly decreased overall survival (95% vs. 86%). These results clearly show that three cycles of BEP is superior to three cycles of EP and that bleomycin cannot be eliminated from treatment when three cycles of BEP are given.

The largest study investigating whether bleomycin could be eliminated from therapy was an EORTC study randomly assigning 419 patients to four cycles of BEP or four cycles of EP (14). Patients enrolled in this study were categorized as good prognosis according to the EORTC criteria that were in use at that time (7). Etoposide was given at a slightly reduced dose of 360 mg/m^2/cycle. The number of complete responses obtained by chemotherapy alone plus those achieving NED after additional surgery (95% vs. 87%) was clearly in favor of the BEP arm. The numbers of patients relapsing was identical in both

arms. As expected, the toxicity in this study was more pronounced in the BEP arm, particularly for pulmonary toxicity; neurotoxicity and Raynaud-like phenomenon were also encountered more frequently. Because of the relative low number of events, overall survival did not differ significantly. To place this study in full perspective, it must be noted that good-risk patients according to the EORTC classification (7) represents a group with an extremely good prognosis compared with other classification systems. Nevertheless, even in this group, the deletion of bleomycin resulted in a decrease in efficacy, underlining the importance of bleomycin in four cycles of BEP with etoposide at a dose of 360 mg/m^2/cycle.

In view of the congruent results of these three studies, it can be firmly concluded that bleomycin cannot be omitted without attenuating treatment efficacy from the following regimens: three cycles of BEP, four cycles of PVB, or four cycles of BEP (with etoposide at a dose of 360 mg/m^2/cycle). However, whether bleomycin can be deleted from four cycles of BEP, with etoposide dosed at 500 mg per m^2 per cycle, remains to be elucidated. By retrospectively analyzing two studies containing a treatment arm with four cycles of EP, Xiao et al. from MSKCC reported on the long-term efficacy of four cycles of EP in patients reclassified as having good prognosis according to IGCCCG classification (29). This update showing a 91% DFS indicated that four cycles of EP is a valid alternative.

Another strategy to circumvent bleomycin-mediated detrimental effects is by omitting this drug and by integrating another compound known to be active in germ cell malignancies. An example of such a drug is ifosfamide. Hinton et al. (30) reanalyzed an intergroup study in which patients with "advanced" metastatic disease, defined according to the Indiana staging system, were randomized to receive treatment with either four cycles of BEP or four cycles of ifosfamide, etoposide, and cisplatin (VIP). Applying the IGCCCG classification, 13.1% of the 286 evaluable patients enrolled belonged to the good prognosis group. In this group, as in the other risk groups, VIP yielded equivalent antitumor efficacy compared with BEP, but at the cost of increased myelosuppression. These findings are consistent with the results from a study comparing VIP versus BEP in patients with intermediate-risk disease (31). Therefore, although ifosfamide yields comparable efficacy as bleomycin in combination with etoposide and cisplatin, on the basis of the observed significant increase in myelosuppression, VIP should not be recommended as initial treatment of patients presenting with good-risk disease.

TRIALS ESTABLISHING WHETHER CISPLATIN CAN BE SUBSTITUTED BY CARBOPLATIN

As previously mentioned, cisplatin accounts for a substantial part of the encountered toxicity during treatment with BEP. Carboplatin is another platinum analog with proven activity against germ cell tumor. Its toxicity profile is predominantly featured by the occurrence of myelosuppression, but carboplatin is less emetogenic and lacks cisplatin-mediated toxicities such as ototoxicity, neurotoxicity, and renal deterioration.

At MSKCC, a trial was conducted that randomized 270 patients to receive four cycles of etoposide with either cisplatin (EP) or carboplatin (EC) (32). The dose of etoposide was 500 mg per m^2 per cycle in both regimens, and carboplatin was administered as a fixed dose of 500 mg per m^2. EP was given at 3-week interval, whereas EC was administered at 4-week interval because of the anticipation of more severe myelosuppression. The rate of complete responses obtained did not differ, but more patients assigned to EC experienced a relapse (12% vs. 3%). An unfavorable outcome defined as an incomplete response or relapse occurred in 24% in patients receiving EC, compared with 13% in those allocated to EP. In addition, the patients treated with EC were more frequently admitted because of neutropenic fever and encountered more thrombocytopenia (33). Because of successful salvage therapy in patients relapsing after EC, there was no difference in overall survival (32).

The largest study investigating whether cisplatin could be substituted by carboplatin is a collaborative study of the MRC and EORTC (34). In this study, 598 patients with nonseminoma were randomly allocated between either BEP or bleomycin, etoposide, and carboplatin (BEC). In both regimens, etoposide was administered at 360 mg per m^2. Bleomycin was given at 3-week interval. Carboplatin was dosed at an area under the curve (AUC) dosage of 5 mg/mL/min. A status of NED was achieved in more patients in the BEP group (94.4%) than in the BEC group (87.3%). In addition, there were more relapses on BEC, resulting in a significant difference in DFS in favor of the patients allocated to BEP. As expected, deterioration in renal function and audiometry was more pronounced in the BEP group. Myelosuppression, on the other hand, particularly thrombocytopenia, was more frequent in the patients receiving carboplatin. Most importantly, overall survival was significantly greater for the BEP group, with 3-year overall survival rates of 97% and 90% for patients receiving BEP and BEC, respectively.

Taken together, the data obtained by these two studies conclusively indicate that carboplatin cannot replace cisplatin with the used drugs and schedules for the treatment of patients with good prognosis nonseminoma. Obviously, the application of carboplatin results in an inferior outcome in this patient group compared with cisplatin-based regimens.

TRIALS INVESTIGATING THE FEASIBILITY OF REDUCING THE NUMBER OF CYCLES

Because many of the side effects associated with BEP are dose related, reduction in total drug dose is an important objective. The most straightforward manner to achieve this purpose is by reducing the number of cycles from four to three.

The first to do so were Einhorn et al. (12) for the Southeastern Cancer Study Group, which compared the efficacy of three versus four cycles of BEP in 184 patients with minimal and moderate disease according to the Indiana staging system. At a median follow-up of 19 months, it appeared that the antitumor efficacy of both schedules was similar in terms of achieved complete response rate, relapse rate, and DFS. Toxicity clearly favored the three cycles of BEP group. At a longer follow-up, a median of 10.1 years, both strategies exhibited comparable efficacy in terms of overall survival and DFS (13).

However, because this study was designed to detect a response rate difference >10%, a difference of anything <10% could not be excluded. Of note, in the clinical practice, a difference between 5% and 10% would be considered unacceptable because it may considerably increase the risk of failure to first-line chemotherapy and thereby the ultimate outcome. Therefore, a subsequent trial performed by the EORTC and MRC was designed to exclude a difference of 5% or more in 2-year progression-free survival (PFS) between three and four cycles of BEP (10). For patients allocated to four cycles, the final cycle was without bleomycin. This study, which began in 1995, is the only trial in which patients were entered with good-prognosis disease, according to the IGCCCG system. In this large trial, 812 patients were randomized to receive three or four cycles of BEP. The primary endpoint, 2-year PFS was equivalent at 90.7% (95% CI, 87.8% to 93.6%) and 89.1% (95% CI, 85.9% to 92.3%) for three and four

cycles, respectively. The achieved response rate and overall survival at 2 years, 97.0% versus 97.1% for three and four cycles, respectively, were identical as well, indicating that in terms of efficacy, these two regimens are equivalent. The large size of the trial allowed another question to be answered—whether a "condensed" 3-day regimen was equivalent to a 5-day regimen. By using a 2 × 2 factorial study design and a second randomization, therapeutic similarity between a condensed 3-day regimen and the conventional schedule was also assessed. Of the 812 patients entered on the study, 681 patients were also randomized for this purpose. The condensed 3-day BEP consisted of bleomycin, 30 units weekly for 9 weeks; etoposide, 165 mg per m^2 on days 1 through 3; and cisplatin, 50 mg per m^2 on days 1 and 2. The 5-day regimen comprised bleomycin, 30 units weekly for 9 weeks; etoposide, 100 mg per m^2 on days 1 through 5; and cisplatin, 20 mg per m^2 on days 1 through 5. Hence, the total doses administered per cycle were similar for both schedules. The two study arms yielded identical 2-year PFS, 89.5% (95% CI, 86.1% to 92.9%) for the 3-day schedule and 89% (95% CI, 85.5% to 92.5%) for the 5-day schedule, demonstrating equivalent efficacy for this comparison as well. In the patients assigned to the 5-day schedule, postponement of the next cycle and dose reduction of etoposide due to hematologic adverse events was more common, whereas nausea and late ototoxicity occurred more frequently in the 3-day arm. A second report on this study (35) described the quality of life in 666 participating patients. On the basis of questionnaire-based assessments, it was concluded that three cycles of either the 3- or the 5-day schedule of BEP were associated with acceptable toxicities. However, when four cycles were given, the 5-day schedule should be preferred over a 3-day schedule because of gastrointestinal toxicity and long-term risk for tinnitus with the 3-day schedule.

A third study aiming to establish the feasibility of dose reduction was conducted by Toner et al. (36) for the Australian and New Zealand Germ Cell Trial Group. In this study, three cycles of BEP (30 units bleomycin on days 1, 8, and 15; 100 mg per m^2 etoposide on days 1 to 5; 20 mg per m^2 cisplatin on days 1 to 5, given at 3-week interval) were compared with four cycles of BEP (30 units bleomycin on day 1; 120 mg per m^2 etoposide on days 1 to 3; 100 mg per m^2 cisplatin on day 1, at 3-week interval). Hence, the cumulative doses and dose intensities of the applied agents differ considerably between these two regimens. In total, 166 patients were enrolled. The study was terminated prematurely when an interim analysis revealed an inferior overall survival rate for those allocated to four cycles of BEP at a median follow-up of 33 months. These findings suggest that increasing the total dose of cisplatin does not compensate for lowering the total doses and dose intensities of bleomycin and etoposide. Drawing firm conclusions from this study, however, is hampered because of the multiple differences between the two regimens.

On the basis of the studies described in the preceding text, three cycles of BEP, with bleomycin given weekly and etoposide at a dose of 500 mg per m^2 per cycle, is equivalent to four cycles of BEP for good-risk patients and is accompanied by a more acceptable toxicity profile, more convenience for the patients, and reduced costs. Therefore, three cycles of BEP is recommended as standard therapy for patients with good-prognosis disease.

EFFICACY OF FOUR CYCLES OF ETOPOSIDE WITH CISPLATIN

The recommended standard regimen of three cycles of BEP is relatively contraindicated for patients at increased risk to develop bleomycin-related toxicities. For these patients, a regimen lacking bleomycin is warranted. In a retrospective

TABLE 40A.3

REPORTED DURABLE DISEASE-FREE SURVIVAL OR PROGRESSION-FREE SURVIVAL RATES OBTAINED IN PATIENTS WITH GOOD PROGNOSIS DISEASE

	Reference	Number of patients	Classification system	DFS/PFS
4 × BEP	12	96	Indiana	92%
3 × BEP–1 × EP	10	406	IGCCCG	89%
3 × BEP	12	88	Indiana	92%
	15	86	Indiana	86%
	10	406	IGCCCG	91%
	36	83	MSKCC	91%
4 × EP	29	148	IGCCCG (reclassified)	91%

DFS, disease-free survival; PFS, progression-free survival; BEP, bleomycin, etoposide, and cisplatin; IGCCCG, international germ cell cancer collaborative group; MSKCC, memorial sloan-kettering cancer center; EP, etoposide and cisplatin.

analysis, Xiao et al. (29) reported the outcomes of four cycles of EP with etoposide at 500 mg/m^2/cycle in good-risk patients, according to the MSKCC classification, on two randomized trials. One of these trials compared four cycles of EP with a regimen that was predominantly used as standard treatment at MSKCC, comprising cisplatin, vinblastine, bleomycin, dactinomycin, and cyclophosphamide (VAB-6) (37). This study revealed that EP was therapeutically equivalent but less toxic (37). The second study was a randomized comparison between etoposide with either cisplatin (EP) or carboplatin (EC) (32). In the long-term follow-up report of the 214 patients who had received EP in these two trials, a status of NED was achieved in 91%, whereas 86% were alive at a median follow-up of 7.6 years. Reclassification using the IGCCCG criteria showed that 148 (69%) of the patients belong to the good prognosis group. Outcome in this particular group was excellent, with 96% reaching complete response and 5% experiencing a relapse (29). In the light of these data, four cycles EP with etoposide given at 500 mg/m^2/cycle is a valid alternative in patients for whom there is concern for the risk to develop bleomycin-mediated side effects (Table 40A.2).

TREATMENT OF SEMINOMA VERSUS NONSEMINOMA

Because most studies conducted in disseminated germ cell tumor accrued patients with both nonseminomatous and seminomatous cancer, treatment of patients with pure seminoma does not differ from that of patients with nonseminoma from the same prognosis group. However, regarding the toxicity of BEP and the fact that patients with seminoma are generally 10 to 20 years older than patients with nonseminoma having more comorbidity, reduction of treatment-induced toxicity is especially important for these patients. The slightly greater chemosensitivity of seminoma over nonseminoma enables the assessment of potentially less toxic schedules. As a consequence, studies have been done focusing on patients with seminoma. However, most trials performed in patients with seminomatous cancer have been phase II because of the rarity of this disease; randomized data are therefore scarce. More than 90% of patients presenting with "advanced" seminoma are still categorized into the good-risk group according to the IGCCCG classification. The only randomized trial in this patient group published as a full paper is a study by Horwich et al. comparing four cycles EP with etoposide at a dose of

360 mg m^2 per cycle to four cycles single-agent carboplatin, 400 mg m^2 per cycle, adjusted to renal function (38). This study was intended to show equivalence for both schedules, but following publications that revealed inferiority of carboplatin-based schedules in patients with nonseminoma (32,34), enrollment declined considerably, so the study was terminated early, when 130 patients were entered in total. After a median follow-up of 4.5 years, the disease-free and overall survival at 3 years were in favor for those assigned EP, although these differences were not statistically significant. In view of the low power of this study because of the relatively small number of patients accrued, this outcome should not be regarded as an indication for similar efficacy between both regimens.

A number of phase II trials examining regimens yielding outcomes comparable to BEP have been published. Several of these were carboplatin-based multidrug regimens such as ifosfamide and carboplatin (39) and cyclophosphamide, vincristine, and carboplatin (40), the latter regimen with the advantage that it enables administration in an outpatient setting. Other regimens showing good efficacy in disseminated seminoma are four cycles of EP (41), cyclophosphamide and cisplatin (42), and cisplatin, vincristine, and ifosfamide that was, however, accompanied with severe toxicity, primarily hematologic (43). It should be emphasized, though, that none of these regimens have been compared with three cycles of BEP. Therefore, to date either 3 × BEP or 4 × EP should be regarded standard treatment for these patients.

ADJUSTING SCHEDULED TREATMENT PLAN BECAUSE OF TOXICITY

Treatment with BEP can be complicated by the occurrence of severe toxicity precluding further treatment according to the standard treatment plan. In such cases, it is warranted to adjust the chemotherapeutic treatment without seriously attenuating the ultimate outcome.

If bleomycin-related toxicities including severe skin reactions or pulmonary toxicity occur, further bleomycin administration is contraindicated. Also, the development of renal dysfunction, for example by the coadministration of cisplatin, can be a reason to stop further bleomycin therapy, as renal deterioration renders patients at greater risk for bleomycin-mediated side effects. This is underscored by the observation that patients with a compromised creatinine clearance <80 mL per min at the first bleomycin administration have a four times increased risk to develop bleomycin-induced pulmonary toxicity compared with patients with a normal renal function (17). Because bleomycin, as reported earlier in this chapter, is an essential component of the curative chemotherapy, withholding bleomycin treatment may compromise efficacy. However, the minimum dose of bleomycin remains to be established. Because, as discussed previously, three cycles of EP is inferior compared with three cycles of BEP with a cumulative dose of 270 units bleomycin (15), the critical minimum dose of bleomycin is unknown but lies somewhere between 30 and 270 units bleomycin. Should further bleomycin administration be contraindicated in the individual patient, there are several options. The first is simply to accept the omittance of the remaining bleomycin doses when most of the intended cumulative dose of bleomycin has been given, for example more than 180 units. In such a case, it is mandatory that both etoposide and cisplatin be administered full dose and on time for the full three cycles. This approach, however, adds some risk for attenuation of antitumor activity. On the basis of the outcomes obtained with four cycles of EP (29), probably the safest option is to continue with EP and to add an extra (fourth) cycle. An alternative strategy is to replace BEP with VIP during the remaining cycles. BEP and VIP are therapeutically equivalent, as has been shown in patients with disseminated disease, including a small group of patients with good prognosis features (30,31). This approach, however, is accompanied by more toxicity, in particular hematologic toxicity.

Another commonly occurring event during BEP is myelosuppression, predominantly because of the use of etoposide. Severe neutropenia with neutrophils $<.5 \times 10^9$ per L or platelets $<100 \times 10^9$ per L may necessitate postponement of a subsequent cycle. Treatment delay should preferably not exceed 3 to 7 days, and treatment should be continued at full dose following recovery above these values. To avoid further treatment delays in subsequent cycles, patients should be treated with granulocyte colony-stimulating factor (G-CSF) following any previous dose delays for reasons of prolonged neutropenia. The occurrence of neutropenic complications, such as neutropenic fever or sepsis, should also warrant the use of G-CSF rather than attenuation of etoposide dose and schedule adherence.

The most worrisome cisplatin-induced side effect hindering administration of chemotherapy according to appropriate guidelines is the development of renal dysfunction, which considerably decreases the clearance of both cisplatin and bleomycin. In fact, cisplatin is advised not to be given in the face of a creatinine clearance of <40 to 50 per mL. If the creatinine clearance begins to decrease, vigorous hydration measures should be used to avoid further deterioration of renal function. Only if forced by persistent severe renal dysfunction, the substitution of cisplatin for carboplatin may be considered. In view of the slightly higher chemosensitivity of seminoma, the use of carboplatin in elderly patients with seminoma who have worsening renal function during cisplatin-containing treatment may be of slightly lesser concern, whereas for patients with nonseminoma, the use of carboplatin-based regimens should be postponed whenever possible.

EMERGENCE OF A PREVIOUSLY UNDERESTIMATED LONG-TERM SIDE EFFECT

In addition to the long-term and well-known side effects associated with BEP, such as acute myeloid leukemia, ototoxicity, neurotoxicity, decline of renal function, and infertility, evidence is recently mounting that patients are also at a significant risk to experience cardiovascular events. This risk, which was reported in anecdotal fashion in the 1980s (44), is now estimated to be 2.5- to 7-fold greater than in the general population several years after treatment (45,46). In view of the considerable incidence of cardiovascular events in the general population, the risk for cardiovascular sequelae in the long term exceeds the risk for relapse or leukemia. The underlying responsible mechanisms have not been elucidated yet, but effects on the endothelium (possibly by bleomycin) exerted by chemotherapy may be involved. Additionally, in patients chemotherapeutically treated for germ cell tumor, the rate of cardiovascular risk factors such as hypertension, hypercholesterolemia, insulin resistance, overweight, and hypogonadism is increased compared with patients with stage I disease (45). Therefore, physicians involved in the follow-up of these patients should regularly screen for cardiovascular risk factors and treat accordingly.

Because it is currently unclear as to which exact treatment component is the main cause for this detrimental effect, further investigation is warranted in order to elucidate the responsible treatment compounds and to find means to circumvent this side effect. Until then, it remains uncertain which of the two recommended treatment options, three cycles of BEP or four cycles of EP, should be preferred over the other in view of the late-term cardiovascular risk.

CONCLUSION

The successful treatment of disseminated germ cell tumor has been a major challenge since the implementation of cisplatin-based multidrug chemotherapy. The subsequent recognition that patients can be classified into groups with different prognosis status has prompted investigators to develop regimens according to risk status. For patients with good risk features, the aim of such trials is to design regimens with an improved toxicity profile while maintaining efficacy. As a consequence of this goal, standard chemotherapy has been narrowed from four cycles of BEP to three cycles of BEP. A valid alternative option is treatment with four cycles of EP, in particular for those patients at increased risk to develop bleomycin-related side effects (Table 40A.2). In case of side effects necessitating adjustment of treatment, several strategies are available without comprising treatment efficacy.

Because it became clear that the risk for cardiovascular events presents the greatest long-term threat for patients cured from disseminated germ cell tumor, it is important to gain more insight into the underlying pathogenesis and exact cause of this particular adverse effect. This may enable further attenuation of treatment toxicity in the future. Therefore, efforts to minimize treatment-related toxicity without sacrificing the chance for cure should continue for patients with good-risk disease.

References

1. Einhorn LH, Donohue JP. Cis-diamminedichloroplatinum, vinblastine and bleomycin combination chemotherapy in disseminated testicular cancer. *Ann Intern Med* 1977;87:293–298.
2. Einhorn LH. Testicular cancer as a model for a curable neoplasm: the Richard and Hinda Rosenthal Foundation Award Lecture. *Cancer Res* 1981;41:3275–3280.
3. Williams SD, Birch R, Einhorn LH, et al. Treatment of disseminated germ-cell tumors with cisplatin, bleomycin, and either vinblastine or etoposide. *N Engl J Med* 1987;316:1435–1440.
4. Bosl GJ, Geller NL, Cirrincione C, et al. Multivariate analysis of prognostic variables in patients with metastatic testicular cancer. *Cancer Res* 1983; 43:3403–3407.
5. Birch R, Williams S, Cone A, et al. Prognostic factors for favorable outcome in disseminated germ cell tumors. *J Clin Oncol* 1986;4:400–407.

6. Levi JA, Thomson D, Sandeman T, et al. A prospective study of cisplatin-based combination chemotherapy in advanced germ cell malignancy: role of maintenance and long-term follow-up. *J Clin Oncol* 1988;6:1154–1160.

7. Stoter G, Sylvester R, Sleijfer DT, et al. Multivariate analysis of prognostic variables in patients with disseminated non-seminomatous testicular cancer: results from an EORTC Multi-institutional Study. *Cancer Res* 1987;47:2714–2718.

8. Medical Research Council Working Party On Testicular Tumours. Prognostic factors in advanced germ-cell tumours: results of a multicentre study. *Lancet* 1985;1:8–11.

9. International Germ Cell Cancer Collaborative Group. International germ cell consensus classification: a prognostic factor-based staging system for metastatic germ cell cancers. *J Clin Oncol* 1997;15:594–603.

10. De Wit R, Roberts JT, Wilkinson PM, et al. Equivalence of three or four cycles of bleomycin, etoposide, and cisplatin chemotherapy and of 3- or 5-day schedule in good-prognosis germ cell cancer: a randomized study of the European Organization for Research and Treatment of Cancer Genitourinary Tract Cancer Cooperative Group and the Medical Research Council. *J Clin Oncol* 2001;19:1629–1640.

11. Baniel J, Foster RS, Gonin R, et al. Late relapse of testicular cancer. *J Clin Oncol* 1995;13:1170–1176.

12. Einhorn LH, Williams SD, Loehrer PJ, et al. Evaluation of optimal duration of chemotherapy in favorable-prognosis disseminated germ cell tumors: a Southeastern Cancer Study Group Protocol. *J Clin Oncol* 1989;7:387–391.

13. Saxman SB, Finch D, Gonin R, et al. Long-term follow-up of a phase III study of three versus four cycles of bleomycin, etoposide, and cisplatin in favorable-prognosis germ-cell tumors: the Indiana University Experience. *J Clin Oncol* 1998;16:702–706.

14. De Wit R, Stoter G, Kaye SB, et al. Importance of bleomycin in combination chemotherapy for good-prognosis testicular non-seminoma: a randomized study of the European Organization for Research and Treatment of Cancer Genitourinary Tract Cancer Cooperative Group. *J Clin Oncol* 1997;15:1837–1843.

15. Loehrer PJ Sr, Johnson D, Elson P, et al. Importance of bleomycin in favorable-prognosis disseminated germ cell tumors: an Eastern Cooperative Oncology Group Trial. *J Clin Oncol* 1995;13:470–476.

16. Sleijfer S. Bleomycin-induced pneumonitis. *Chest* 2001;120:617–624.

17. O'Sullivan JM, Huddart RA, Norman AR, et al. Predicting the risk of bleomycin lung toxicity in patients with germ-cell tumours. *Ann Oncol* 2003;14:91–96.

18. Vogelzang N, Bosl GJ, Johnson K, et al. Raynaud's phenomenon-a common toxicity after combination chemotherapy for testicular cancer. *Ann Intern Med* 1981;95:288–292.

19. Berger CC, Bokemeyer C, Schneider M, et al. Secondary Raynaud's phenomenon and other late vascular complications following chemotherapy for testicular cancer. *Eur J Cancer* 1995;31A:2229–2238.

20. Nichols CR, Breeden ES, Loehrer PJ, et al. Secondary leukemia associated with a conventional dose of etoposide: review of serial germ cell tumor protocols. *J Natl Cancer Inst* 1993;85:36–40.

21. Bokemeyer C, Schmoll HJ. Treatment of testicular cancer and the development of secondary malignancies. *J Clin Oncol* 1995;13:283–292.

22. Hesketh PJ, Grunberg SM, Gralla RJ, et al. The oral neurokinin-1 antagonist aprepitant for the prevention of chemotherapy-induced nausea and vomiting: a multinational, randomized, double-blind, placebo-controlled trial in patients receiving high-dose cisplatin – the Aprepitant Protocol 052 Study Group. *J Clin Oncol* 2003;21:4112–4119.

23. De Wit R, Herrstedt J, Rapoport B, et al. Addition of the oral NK1 antagonist aprepitant to standard antiemetics provides protection against nausea and vomiting during multiple cycles of cisplatin-based chemotherapy. *J Clin Oncol* 2003;21:4105–4111.

24. Meijer S, Mulder NH, Sleijfer DT, et al. Nephrotoxicity of cis-diamminedichloride platinum (CDDP) during remission-induction and maintenance chemotherapy of testicular carcinoma. *Cancer Chemother Pharmacol* 1982;8:27–30.

25. Fosså SD, Aass N, Winderen M, et al. Long-term renal function after treatment for malignant germ-cell tumours. *Ann Oncol* 2002;13:222–228.

26. Cersosimo RJ. Cisplatin neurotoxicity. *Cancer Treat Rev* 1989;16:195–211.

27. Strumberg D, Brügge S, Korn MW, et al. Evaluation of long-term toxicity in patients after cisplatin-based chemotherapy for non-seminomatous testicular cancer. *Ann Oncol* 2002;13:229–236.

28. Levi JA, Raghavan D, Harvey V et al, Australian Germ Cell Trial Group. The importance of bleomycin in combination chemotherapy for good-prognosis germ cell carcinoma. *J Clin Oncol* 1993;11:1300–1305.

29. Xiao H, Mazumbar M, Bajorin DF, et al. Long-term follow-up of patients with good risk germ-cell tumors treated with etoposide and cisplatin. *J Clin Oncol* 1997;15:2553–2558.

30. Hinton S, Catalano PJ, Einhorn LH, et al. Cisplatin, etoposide and either bleomycin or ifosfamide in the treatment of disseminated germ cell tumors. *Cancer* 2003;97:1869–1875.

31. De Wit R, Stoter G, Sleijfer DT, et al. Four cycles of BEP vs four cycles of VIP in patients with intermediate prognosis metastatic testicular nonseminoma: a randomized study of the EORTC Genitourinary Tract Cancer Cooperative Group. *Br J Cancer* 1998;78:828–832.

32. Bajorin DF, Sarosdy MF, Pfister DG, et al. Randomized trial of etoposide and cisplatin versus etoposide and carboplatin in patients with good-risk germ cell tumors: a multiinstitutional study. *J Clin Oncol* 1993;11:598–606.

33. Bosl GJ, Bajorin DF. Etoposide plus carboplatin or cisplatin in good-risk patients with germ cell tumors: a randomized comparison. *Semin Oncol* 1994;21(5 suppl. 12):61–64.

34. Horwich A, Sleijfer DT, Fosså SD, et al. Randomized trial of bleomycin, etoposide, cisplatin compared with bleomycin, etoposide, carboplatin in good-prognosis metastatic nonseminomatous germ cell cancer: a Multiinstitutional Medical Research Council/European Organization for Research and Treatment of Cancer Trial. *J Clin Oncol* 1997;15:1844–1852.

35. Fosså SD, De Wit R, Roberts JT, et al. Quality of life in good prognosis patients with metastatic germ cell cancer: a prospective study of the European Organization for Research and Treatment of Cancer Genitourinary Group/Medical Research Council Testicular Cancer Study Group (30941/TE20). *J Clin Oncol* 2003;21:1107–1118.

36. Toner G, Stockler M. Comparison of two standard chemotherapy regimens for good prognosis germ cell tumours: a randomised trial. *Lancet* 2001;357:739–745.

37. Bosl GJ, Geller NL, Bajorin D, et al. A randomized trial of etoposide + cisplatin versus vinblastine + bleomycin + cisplatin + cyclophosphamide + dactinomycin in patients with good-prognosis germ cell tumors. *J Clin Oncol* 1988;6:1231–1238.

38. Horwich A, Oliver RTD, Wilkinson PM, et al. A medical research council randomised trial of single agent carboplatin versus etoposide and cisplatin for advanced metastatic seminoma. *Br J Cancer* 2000;83:1623–1629.

39. Amato RJ, Ellerhorst J, Banks M, et al. Carboplatin and ifosfamide and selective consolidation in advanced seminoma. *Eur J Cancer* 1995;31A:2223–2228.

40. Sleijfer S, Willemse PH, De Vries EG, et al. Treatment of advanced seminoma with cyclophosphamide, vincristine and carboplatin on an outpatient basis. *Br J Cancer* 1996;74:947–950.

41. Mencel PJ, Motzer RJ, Mazumdar M, et al. Advanced seminoma: treatment results, survival, and prognostic factors in 142 patients. *J Clin Oncol* 1994;12:120–126.

42. Logothetis CJ, Samuels ML, Ogden SL, et al. Cyclophosphamide and sequential cisplatin for advanced seminoma: long-term follow-up in 52 patients. *J Urol* 1987;138:789–794.

43. Fosså SD, Droz JP, Stoter G, et al. Cisplatin, vincristine and ifosphamide combination chemotherapy of metastatic seminoma: results of EORTC trial 30874. *Br J Cancer* 1995;71:619–624.

44. Samuels BL, Vogelzang NJ, Kennedy BJ. Severe vascular toxicity associated with vinblastine, bleomycin and cisplatin chemotherapy. *Cancer Chemother Pharmacol* 1987;19:253–256.

45. Meinardi MT, Gietema J, Van der Graaf WT, et al. Cardiovascular morbidity in long-term survivors of metastatic testicular cancer. *J Clin Oncol* 2000;18:1725–1732.

46. Huddart RA, Norman A, Shahidi M, et al. Cardiovascular disease as a long-term complication of treatment for testicular cancer. *J Clin Oncol* 2003;21:1513–1523.

CHAPTER 40B
Management and Treatment of Poor Prognosis and Relapsed Germ Cell Tumors

Gnanamba Varuni Kondagunta, George J. Bosl, and Robert J. Motzer

Seventy percent to 80% of patients with advanced germ cell tumors (GCTs) achieve a complete response to first-line cisplatin-based combination chemotherapy and adjunctive surgery. The remaining 20% to 30% of patients have disease that relapses or is resistant to initial treatment. Pretreatment identification and primary chemotherapy directed according to risk (i.e., "poor-risk") have determined treatment in this group of patients with advanced GCT. Because a relatively high proportion of patients with intermediate-risk GCT relapse (refer Table 40B.2), and most patients with poor-risk GCT die of disease, the goal of research in poor-risk and intermediate-risk patients (hereafter collectively referred to as poor prognosis) has been to improve treatment efficacy.

Conversely, for patients with a high likelihood of cure ("good risk"), the efforts focus on maintaining a high cure rate and on reducing chemotherapy-related toxicity.

Identification of more effective first-line therapy remains a challenge in patients with poor prognosis. Current standard therapy consisting of four cycles of bleomycin, etoposide, and cisplatin (BEP) chemotherapy achieves a durable complete response of 75% in intermediate-risk patients and of 40% in poor-risk patients. New chemotherapy combinations and dose-intensive programs have been studied in these patients in the hope of improving efficacy. Often, regimens found to show promise in second- or third-line therapy are moved into first-line therapy studies. The current therapeutic approach for previously untreated intermediate- and poor-risk patients and for second- and third-line treatment is outlined here.

PREDICTIVE CRITERIA FOR INTERMEDIATE- AND POOR-RISK (POOR PROGNOSIS) GERM CELL TUMOR

Before the development of the International Germ Cell Cancer Collaborative Group (IGCCCG) classification system, several prognostic classification systems were developed (Table 40B.1) (1). These models were used prospectively to drive Phase III clinical trials that defined the standard treatments used today. Each of the models listed in Table 40B.1 included specific clinical features that later were incorporated into the IGCCCG classification system (2–4). For example, the use of serum tumor markers as part of risk stratification was originally described in the mathematical model developed at Memorial Sloan-Kettering Cancer Center (MSKCC) (2).

The prognostic classification developed by the IGCCCG is the classification algorithm used exclusively in practice today. Data from collaborative groups in 10 countries were analyzed for more than 6,000 patients with metastatic GCT treated with platinum-based chemotherapy. A multivariate analysis of prognostic factors predicting survival was undertaken and then validated in an independent data set. For nonseminomatous GCT (NSGCT), the independent adverse factors were mediastinal primary site; high levels of α-fetoprotein (AFP), human chorionic gonadotropin (HCG), and lactate dehydrogenase (LDH); and presence of nonpulmonary visceral metastases. For seminoma, the only adverse prognostic factor was the presence of nonpulmonary visceral metastases (Table 40B.2) (1). The IGCCCG classification system has provided a widely accepted prognostic model, thereby making study populations more uniform and study results more amenable to comparison.

STANDARD MANAGEMENT

Treatment on a clinical trial is preferred for patients with intermediate- and poor-risk GCT because the percentage of patients who achieve a durable complete response (CR) to BEP chemotherapy is low. For patients who are not treated on a clinical trial, standard therapy is four cycles of BEP chemotherapy. Each cycle of chemotherapy is administered every 21 days with as few treatment delays as possible. Patients have serum tumor markers drawn the first week of each cycle, if not more frequently. If an inadequate decline in marker level is seen, patients are carefully monitored for evidence of tumor progression, possibly necessitating a change of therapy. In the setting of unsatisfactory marker decline or new symptoms of pain, reimaging is done.

Once serum marker values normalize after chemotherapy, the patient should undergo new imaging studies. Postchemotherapy resection of all residual disease is undertaken after recovery from chemotherapy, and the pathology from the surgical resection determines subsequent management. If necrosis/fibrosis or teratoma is found, the patient is closely observed. However, if viable GCT is found and serum tumor markers remain normal, the patient should receive two more cycles of cisplatin-based chemotherapy (usually cisplatin and etoposide). If surgical margins are positive, unresectable disease is present, or serum tumor markers are elevated, then salvage chemotherapy is required.

Clinical Trials in Poor risk Germ Cell Tumor

The studies in poor-risk patients have evaluated conventional dose regimens that have substituted new agents for an existing one or have intensified the dose of existing agents or both.

A randomized study compared BEP with cisplatin, vinblastine, and bleomycin (PVB), formerly the standard regimen for patients with advanced GCT. In this study, subcategorized by the Indiana University classification system, 72 poor-risk patients were randomized; 37 received PVB and 35 received BEP. There was a significant difference in the disease-free survival of the BEP subset of poor-risk (Indiana classification) patients (63% in the BEP arm vs. 38% in the PVB arm) (5). Although the arms showed similar myelosuppressive and pulmonary toxicity, the etoposide arm had less neurologic toxicity than the vinblastine arm. On the basis of this trial, BEP has remained the standard comparative arm for assessing new regimens in Phase III trials. Phase III trials conducted in poor-risk patients with BEP of high importance are summarized in Table 40B.3 (4–8).

TABLE 40B.1

COMPARISON OF FOUR POOR-RISK CLASSIFICATION ALGORITHMS

	Memorial Sloan-Kettering[2]	Indiana University[3]	EORTC[4]	International[1]
Histology	Yes	No	No	Yes
Primary site	Yes	Yes	No	Mediastinum
AFP	No	No	>1,000 IU/μL	>10,000 ng/mL
HCG	Continuous	No	>10,000 IU/μL	>50,000 ng/mL
LDH	Continuous	No	No	>10 × normal[a]
Metastatic sites	No	Bone, liver, brain	Bone, liver	Bone, liver, brain

AFP, α-fetoprotein; HCG, human chorionic gonadotropin; LDH, lactate dehydrogenase.
[a]Normal defined as the upper limit of normal for the specific assay.

TABLE 40B.2

GERM CELL TUMOR RISK CLASSIFICATION: INTERNATIONAL CONSENSUS[1]

	Seminoma	Nonseminoma
Good risk	Any HCG Any LDH Nonpulmonary visceral metastases absent Any primary site	AFP <1,000 ng/mL HCG <5,000 mIU/mL LDH <1.5 × upper limit of normal Nonpulmonary visceral metastases absent Gonadal or retroperitoneal primary tumor
Intermediate risk	Nonpulmonary visceral metastases present Any HCG Any LDH Any primary site	AFP 1,000–10,000 ng/mL HCG 5,000–50,000 mIU/mL LDH 1.5–10.0 × upper limit of normal Nonpulmonary visceral metastases absent Gonadal or retroperitoneal primary site
Poor risk	—	Mediastinal primary site Nonpulmonary visceral metastases present (e.g., bone, liver, brain) AFP ≥10,000 ng/mL HCG ≥50,000 mIU/mL LDH >10 × upper limit of normal

AFP, α-fetoprotein; HCG, human chorionic gonadotropin; LDH, lactate dehydrogenase.
From International Germ Cell Tumor Collaborative Group. International Germ Cell Consensus Classification: a prognostic factor-based staging system for metastatic germ cell tumors. *J Clin Oncol* 1997;15(2):594–603.

A small, randomized trial of standard chemotherapy with four cycles of PVB and treatment with twice the standard dose of cisplatin, vinblastine, bleomycin, etoposide (PVeBV) in poor-risk (NCI Classification) GCT showed a better 5-year survival in the high-dose arm (9) (48% vs. 78%) and disease-free survival (68% vs. 33%). However, myelosuppression and severe hearing loss were more prevalent. The increased efficacy of the PVeBV arm was thought to be because of the high-dose cisplatin, the addition of etoposide, or both, and it led to a multicenter Phase III trial.

The Southwest Oncology Group (SWOG) and Southeastern Oncology Group studied etoposide and bleomycin compared with either standard-dose cisplatin (100 mg per m²) or high-dose cisplatin (200 mg per m²) (6). There was no difference in response and overall survival between the two arms, and the authors concluded that dose escalation of cisplatin resulted only in increased toxicity (6). In retrospect, the higher efficacy of the PVeBV arm compared with PBV (9) was attributed to the addition of etoposide, not the dose escalation of cisplatin.

Additional studies have explored the efficacy of alternating and sequential regimens, the rationale being that administering non–cross resistant chemotherapies may decrease development of resistant disease. Alternating and sequential regimens such as POMB-ACE (cisplatin, vincristine, methotrexate, actinomycin D, cyclophosphamide, and etoposide) (10), CBOP-BEP (carboplatin, cisplatin, infusional bleomycin, and vincristine followed by three cycles of bleomycin, etoposide, and cisplatin) (11), and VIP/VB (etoposide, ifosfamide, cisplatin, vinblastine, and bleomycin) (12) were more toxic than standard therapy and did not confer a survival advantage. Although these regimens

TABLE 40B.3

RESULTS OF RANDOMIZED TRIALS IN PATIENTS WITH POOR-RISK GERM CELL TUMORS

Reference	Criteria	Treatment	Number of patients	Complete response (%)	Durable (%)	Benefit over standard arm
(4)	EORTC	PEB	102	74%	NS	
		PEB/PVB	102	75%	NS	No
(5)	Indiana	PVB	37	38%	NS	
		PEB	35	63%	NS	Yes[a]
(6)	Indiana	PEB	77	73%	61%	
		P(200)EB	76	68%	63%	No
(7)	Indiana	PEB	141	60%	57%	
		VIP	145	63%	56%	No
(8)	EORTC/MRC	BEP/EP	185	57	55%	No
		BOP/VIP-B	186	54	53%	

P, cisplatin 100 mg m⁻² P(200), cisplatin 200 mg m⁻²; V, vinblastine; B, bleomycin; E, etoposide; O, vincristine; I, ifosfamide; NS, not stated; EORTC, European Organization for the Research and Treatment of Cancer; NCI, National Cancer Institute; MRC, Medical Research Council; SWOG, Southwest Oncology Group.
[a]Subset analysis only. No difference in the clinical trial as a whole.

demonstrated better response rates than standard treatment with BEP in single-arm Phase II studies, efficacy has not been validated in prospective randomized trials.

As ifosfamide combination chemotherapy became more extensively studied in the second-line setting, efforts were made to incorporate ifosfamide into first-line therapy of patients with poor-risk GCT. In a randomized trial comparing four cycles of BEP with etoposide, ifosfamide, and cisplatin (VIP), response rates and survival were comparable, but the ifosfamide-containing arm had more hematologic toxicity (7). A recent update of this trial confirmed equivalent survival at a median follow-up of 7.3 years (13). VIP is an acceptable alternative for patients with poor-risk GCT with compromised pulmonary function or other pre-existing conditions that preclude treatment with the standard bleomycin-containing regimen.

Paclitaxel was shown to have efficacy in the second-line setting (see in subsequent text) in relapsed GCT. A small Phase I/II study of escalating doses of paclitaxel plus BEP (T-BEP) noted durable responses in intermediate- and poor-risk patients (14). This led to the current randomized Phase III trial, which is ongoing in Europe, comparing T-BEP to BEP in patients with IGCCCG intermediate-risk GCT.

Further studies are ongoing with new single agents and with dose intensification accompanied by stem cell support. However, until adequately powered randomized Phase III trials demonstrate a superior outcome, the standard therapy for poor-risk GCT remains four cycles of BEP chemotherapy.

First-Line High-Dose Therapy

Complete responses achieved with high-dose, carboplatin-containing regimens in the refractory setting (see subsequent text) led to the study of high-dose therapy (HDT) in the first-line setting. Single-arm Phase II trials were performed using HDT as first-line therapy in patients with poor-risk GCT (summarized in Table 40B.4) (15,16). When these results were compared to historical controls with conventional-dose therapy, a higher complete response proportion and improved survival was observed. Also, less cumulative toxicity was seen in this setting when compared with HDT given to heavily pre-treated patients (17–19). These findings led to Phase III trials evaluating the role of HDT in first-line treatment of poor-risk GCT.

In one randomized trial, previously untreated patients with poor-risk nonseminomatous GCT were given either three or four cycles of vinblastine, etoposide, bleomycin, and double-dose cisplatin (P2VeBV); or two cycles of P2VeBV followed by a single HDT treatment with cyclophosphamide, etoposide, and double-dose cisplatin followed by autologous stem cell transplantation (ASCT) (20). There was no benefit with HDT

in this trial. However, the high-dose arm used double-dose cisplatin, which has been shown to have no greater efficacy than single-dose cisplatin (9); the standard arm did not include BEP chemotherapy; and a significant proportion of patients in the high-dose arm did not complete HDT. Therefore, this trial did not adequately address the issue of first-line HDT in poor-risk GCT.

The German Testicular Cancer Study Group developed a sequential HDT regimen composed of VIP for four cycles with peripheral blood stem cell support. After a 4-year median follow-up, progression-free survival and disease-specific survival were 68% and 73%, respectively, at 5 years, with limited, severe toxicity (21). The Phase I/II trial demonstrated that this high-dose regimen was tolerable, achieved more responses than historical controls with conventional-dose therapy, and could be administered at multiple centers (21). In Europe, a randomized Phase III trial for patients with poor-risk GCT is studying four cycles of standard BEP versus high-dose VIP with autologous stem cell rescue on the basis of data from the German Testicular Cancer Study Group trial.

A randomized Phase III trial completed accrual in the United States to address the benefit of early dose intensification and autologous stem cell support versus standard BEP chemotherapy in previously untreated patients with poor- or intermediate-risk GCT. This was a multi-institutional study (MSKCC, Southwestern Oncology Group, Eastern Cooperative Oncology Group, and Cancer and Leukemia Group B). Patients in the high-dose arm received two cycles of BEP, after which they were treated with high-dose carboplatin, etoposide, and cyclophosphamide (CEC), followed by autologous stem cell support.

Rate of Tumor Marker Decline

The serum concentrations of AFP and/or HCG are elevated in 80% of patients with advanced GCT and in nearly all of those with poor-risk disease (22). The half-lives of decline for abnormally elevated AFP and HCG after complete surgical resection are approximately 5 days and 1 to 2 days, respectively. A significant deviation from these expected declines has been investigated as an early predictor of treatment failure. The significance of the decline in serum tumor markers AFP and HCG during the first two cycles of chemotherapy as a predictor of treatment outcome has been examined in retrospective studies.

In one study, patients with GCT with elevated AFP and/or HCG serum marker levels were retrospectively classified by IGCCCG criteria, and rate of marker decline was categorized as satisfactory or unsatisfactory. The marker half-life was calculated by a logarithmic transformation of all elevated marker values between days 7 and 56, and regressed over time. Unsatisfactory

TABLE 40B.4

SINGLE-ARM HIGH-DOSE CHEMOTHERAPY STUDIES IN THE FIRST-LINE SETTING

Reference	Regimen	Number of patients	Response rate	Conclusions
(16)	VAB-6 + 2 cycles HD Carboplatin and VP-16	22	54%	Better than historical control with conventional-dose therapy
(18)	VIP + CEC	14	57%	CEC tolerated and effective; further study necessary
(17)	BEP + 1 cycle of CEC	20	60%	Well tolerated and warrants further study
(20)	VIP + 3–4 cycles high dose VIP	221	73%	Up-front high-dose feasible; toxicity acceptable; randomized study ongoing

CEC, carboplatin, etoposide, cyclophosphamide; VAB-6, cisplatin, vinblastine, bleomycin, actinomycin, and cyclophosphamide; VIP, etoposide, ifosfamide, and cisplatin.

decline was defined as a half-life of more than 7 days for the AFP or more than 3.5 days for HCG. Analysis showed that satisfactory marker decline predicted improved complete response proportion (92% vs. 62%), 2-year event-free survival (91% vs. 69%), and 2-year overall survival (95% vs. 72%) (23). Outcome differences in the poor-risk category were the most pronounced in this analysis. However, other studies have not shown marker decline to be a useful predictor of treatment outcome (24–26). The role of marker decline as a posttreatment predictor of outcome is currently being studied as part of the large multi-institutional trial of poor-risk patients randomized to standard therapy or high-dose chemotherapy (HDT) with autologous stem cell transplantation described previously.

Salvage Therapy

Approximately 10% to 20% of patients have an incomplete response to first-line cisplatin-combination chemotherapy, and approximately 10% of patients will relapse after first attaining a complete response (22). For these patients, effective salvage therapy is required. Clinical trials using dose-intensive programs, new agents, and combinations of cisplatin and ifosfamide have been the focus of salvage therapies for GCT. Potentially, curative treatment options are available using both conventional-dose and HDT.

Cisplatin, Ifosfamide, and Vinblastine or Etoposide

One trial showed efficacy of single-agent ifosfamide in heavily pretreated refractory patients, with an objective response rate of 23% (27). Thereafter, ifosfamide was combined with cisplatin and etoposide (VIP) or cisplatin and vinblastine (VeIP) (Table 40B.5) (28–33). Complete response was achieved in 25% to 35% of patients who were heavily pretreated (28,29, 34). Nephrotoxicity and myelosuppression were the main toxicities seen with these regimens. After promising activity was seen in the third-line setting, VeIP was investigated as first-line salvage treatment (30,31). In this setting, between one-third and one-half of patients achieved a complete response, and approximately one-fourth of patients achieved durable complete responses. These studies established VeIP as standard second-line therapy in relapsed GCT.

High-Dose Chemotherapy for Refractory Tumors

The chemosensitivity of GCT, the dose-response phenomena of individual drugs and their synergistic action, the rare occurrence of bone marrow metastasis, and a young patient population prompted the study of HDT in GCT. The first trials of high-dose carboplatin and etoposide conducted in heavily pretreated patients with GCT yielded a small number of durable complete responses. In the initial studies, as growth factors were not available, toxicity and treatment-related deaths remained a significant issue. Later efforts focused on confirming activity, increasing the number of patients who achieved durable responses, and reducing toxicity. Selected studies of carboplatin-containing high-dose regimens in the salvage setting are summarized in Table 40B.6 (16,35–37). In an effort to improve efficacy, an oxazaphosphorine (cyclophosphamide or ifosfamide) was added to high-dose carboplatin and etoposide. One comprehensive review suggested that the complete response proportion improved (17), although these regimens were not studied in randomized trials, and a modified regimen of higher doses of carboplatin plus etoposide appears equally effective.

Efforts to improve efficacy include increasing the dose intensity/dose density of carboplatin and etoposide, and incorporating paclitaxel. In one trial, efforts were made to identify previously treated patients with GCT who were unlikely to achieve success with conventional-dose salvage chemotherapy. The patients enrolled in this trial all had cisplatin-refractory disease (failure to achieve a durable response to a cisplatin-based regimen) and had one or more of the following unfavorable prognostic factors for achieving a complete response: (a) extragonadal primary site, (b) progressive disease after an incomplete response to first-line therapy, or (c) poor or lack of response to prior treatment with cisplatin plus ifosfamide-containing conventional-dose therapy. These patients were treated with a dose-intensive program of rapidly recycling paclitaxel and ifosfamide followed by three cycles of carboplatin plus etoposide with stem cell support and dose escalation of carboplatin among patient cohorts (37). In this study, 61% of patients achieved a favorable response, showing that dose-intensive therapy with sequential, accelerated chemotherapy of paclitaxel/ifosfamide and carboplatin/etoposide administered with peripheral blood–derived stem cell (PBSC) support was relatively well tolerated. The durable complete response (CR) proportion was 41% in patients with unfavorable prognostic features for achieving durable complete response to conventional-dose salvage programs (37).

A randomized trial in Europe explored the efficacy of four cycles of conventional dose salvage therapy (VIP/VeIP) versus the use of three cycles of conventional dose therapy with one cycle of high-dose chemotherapy (carboplatin, etoposide, cyclophosphamide) and autologous stem cell transplantation. This trial reported no survival benefit in the high-dose arm (38). There is no randomized trial of one versus two cycles of high-dose therapy (HDT), but the data indicate that at least two cycles of HDT are necessary to cure refractory GCT.

TABLE 40B.5

VEIP/VIP SALVAGE REGIMENS FOR RELAPSED/REFRACTORY GERM CELL TUMORS

Reference	Regimen	Number of prior regimens	Evaluable	Complete response (%)	Durable complete response (%)
(28)	VIP	1	30	10 (33)	1 (3)
(30)	VeIP	1	124	56 (45)	29 (23)
(31)	VIP or VeIP	1 and ≥2	56	20 (36)	13 (23)
(29)	VIP or VeIP	≥2	56	20 (36)	15 (27)
(32)	VIP	1 and ≥2	19	9 (47)	NS
(33)	VIP	1	32	22 (69)	16 (50)

VIP, etoposide, ifosfamide, and cisplatin; VeIP, vinblastine, ifosfamide, and cisplatin; NS, not stated.

TABLE 40B.6

SELECTED SERIES OF HIGH-DOSE CARBOPLATIN-CONTAINING CHEMOTHERAPY IN PATIENTS WITH REFRACTORY, PROGRESSIVE GERM CELL TUMOR

Reference	(16)	(35)	(36)	(37)
Patients	40	58	68	37
Agents	Carboplatin, etoposide +/− ifosfamide	Carboplatin, etoposide, cyclophosphamide	Carboplatin, etoposide, ifosfamide	Carboplatin, etoposide, ifosfamide, paclitaxel
Complete Response (%)	30	40	51	57
Alive, Disease-Free (%)	15	21	37	41
Median Follow-up of Survivors (mo)	>24	28	NS	30

NS, not stated.

In an effort to intensify both the preparative regimen and the high-dose portion of therapy, patients were treated with paclitaxel, ifosfamide, and cisplatin followed by a single high-dose cycle of carboplatin, etoposide, and thiotepa with stem cell support (39). This regimen achieved a 25% response rate in a heavily pretreated population of patients with refractory and relapsed GCT. Another approach has been to incorporate two different high-dose cycles: sequential, dose-intensive etoposide and ifosfamide followed by one cycle of high-dose carboplatin and etoposide; and two cycles of carboplatin, cyclophosphamide, and thiotepa with autologous stem cell support (40). These studies established the feasibility and efficacy of HDT in the salvage setting. Finding the optimal dose-intensive regimen is the goal of continued study. The routine use of HDT and autologous bone marrow transplantation has also been studied in the setting of initial relapse. In a retrospective study of 65 patients with GCT treated with cisplatin-combination chemotherapy followed by two cycles of high-dose carboplatin and etoposide with autologous stem cell transplantation, 57% achieved a complete response to HDT with or without surgery at a median follow-up of more than 3 years (41). On the basis of the favorable results of this report compared with historical controls, first-line HDT is considered a standard approach by some investigators for routine treatment of first relapse. This approach seems to be most reasonable for patients with unresponsive mediastinal NSGCT after initial treatment and for patients with gonadal/retroperitoneal primary tumors who fail to achieve an initial CR, groups in which CR to standard-dose chemotherapy is very unlikely (<10%) (42).

Reducing Toxicity of High-Dose Regimens

Efforts to reduce toxicity with high-dose regimens have included the use of peripheral blood stem cells instead of autologous stem cell transplantation. A comparison study of autologous stem cell transplantation (ASCT) and peripheral blood-derived stem cells (PBSC) as rescue showed that patients who received PBSC had a significantly shorter neutrophil and platelet recovery time and fewer days to independence from red-cell transfusions. Overall and event-free survival were no different in the two groups (43,44). Toxicity of high-dose regimens has also been reduced by using growth factor support with granulocyte-colony stimulating factor (G-CSF) and by improvements in supportive care and antibiotics.

Toxicity has also been reduced with the introduction of HDT as first-line salvage therapy and as initial chemotherapy for poor-risk patients. These less heavily treated patients experience less cumulative toxicities, and their treatment mortality has been reduced. Prognostic factors help predict which patients will respond to HDT.

Paclitaxel Combination Chemotherapy

Paclitaxel has single-agent activity in patients with refractory GCT (45–48). Its activity as a single agent and preclinical data showing synergy with cisplatin led to a trial of paclitaxel and cisplatin plus ifosfamide as first-line salvage therapy. A Phase I/II trial explored the safety and feasibility of paclitaxel, ifosfamide, and cisplatin (TIP) in patients with previously treated GCT and favorable prognostic features. These favorable prognostic features were prior treatment limited to one program or six or fewer prior cycles of cisplatin, gonadal primary site, and either a complete or partial response for more than 6 months following chemotherapy and associated normal tumor markers (Table 40B.7) (49). The treatment program consisted of four cycles of paclitaxel (250 mg per m^2 by 24-hour continuous infusion), ifosfamide 5 gm per m^2, and cisplatin 100 mg per m^2 given 21 days apart, with G-CSF support. Out of 46 patients treated, 32 (70%) achieved a complete response to chemotherapy alone. Myelosuppression, the major toxicity, was managed with growth factor support. Notably, complete responses were observed in patients with "late relapse," a group generally thought to be resistant to salvage chemotherapy (50). On the

TABLE 40B.7

PACLITAXEL, IFOSFAMIDE, AND CISPLATIN SALVAGE CHEMOTHERAPY (50)

Treatment Program
4 cycles given 21 d apart
Paclitaxel 250 mg/m^2 24-h infusion d 1
Ifosfamide 1500 mg/m^2 daily infusion d 2–5
Cisplatin 25 mg/m^2 daily infusion d 2–5
Mesna 500 mg/m^2 before Ifosfamide and at 4 and 8 h after ifosfamide daily

Summary of Results

Criteria	Number of patients	Percent (%)
Evaluable	46	100
CR	32	70
To chemo alone	29	
To chemo + surgery	3	
PR (negative markers)	2	4
Relapse from CR	3	7
Alive	35	76

CR, complete response; PR, partial response.

basis of these findings, a randomized Phase III trial has been initiated to compare VeIP and TIP in the second-line setting.

Prognostic Factors: Salvage Chemotherapy

Prognostic factors have been studied in patients receiving conventional-dose salvage therapy (VeIP) and HDT. These criteria have been used to identify patients most likely to benefit from conventional-dose salvage chemotherapy, as well as to exclude some patients from HDT when the degree of potential treatment-related toxicity outweighs potential benefit. Patients who fail to achieve a complete response to first-line therapy and patients with an extragonadal primary (nonseminoma histology arising from the mediastinum) are unlikely to achieve a long-term survival with second-line VeIP therapy. These patients may be more appropriately managed with dose-intensive chemotherapy, clinical trials of new agents, or chemotherapy combinations.

In contrast, conventional-dose second-line treatment is curative for selected patients. Studies at MSKCC showed survival and response to salvage therapy were significantly enhanced in patients with a prior CR to first-line chemotherapy, testis primary site, normal LDH, normal HCG, and one site of metastasis (42). In patients selected by these favorable prognostic features, four cycles of TIP chemotherapy yielded a CR rate of 80% (48).

Also patients with an incomplete response to initial cisplatin-based chemotherapy have a <10% likelihood of a durable response to standard-dose second-line therapy with ifosfamide-based treatments (42). These patients may respond better to HDT regimens.

Several studies investigating prognostic factors with HDT found specific variables that predicted a poor outcome. In one high-dose study for refractory GCT, pretreatment levels of HCG (>100 × ULN) were found to predict short survival after treatment with HDT (35). In another analysis, patients with primary mediastinal nonseminomatous GCT who failed primary therapy were found to have a 5% survival rate or less despite salvage HDT (51). A third study found that patients with absolute refractory disease (defined as no marker response to initial treatment) have an especially poor response to high-dose chemotherapy in the salvage setting (52).

A multivariate analysis was performed on patients who received one cycle of HDT, and a nomogram was created to predict outcome to HDT (44). Progressive disease before HDT, mediastinal nonseminomatous GCT primary site, refractory or absolute refractory disease to conventional-dose cisplatin, and HCG levels >1,000 U per L were independent adverse prognostic indicators of survival after HDT. A scoring system based on risk factors was established to categorize individual patients as good (0 points), intermediate (up to 2 points), or poor prognosis (>2 points) Absolute refractory disease, a high HCG level prior to HDT, progressive disease prior to HDT, mediastinal primary tumor, and refractory disease received a score of one point each (44).

The authors of this analysis recommended that patients with high scores, usually characterized by progression within 1 month of cisplatin, high HCG levels, or nonseminomatous histology arising from a mediastinal primary site, generally do not achieve long-term benefit from HDT and should be considered for Phase II studies (44). In a later retrospective review of patients who received salvage HDT at Indiana University, favorable outcomes were reported in patients with the worst Beyer prognostic score (53). One possible explanation is the use of peripheral blood stem cell transplantation and growth factors, which allowed more patients to receive tandem transplants as first salvage treatment. Because this updated review includes a high percentage of patients who received multiple courses of HDT as well as less heavily pretreated patients, outcomes were improved.

Another analysis of prognostic factors in the setting of progression after conventional-dose cisplatin-based chemotherapy for nonseminoma yielded three independent variables of prognostic significance. These include progression-free interval, response to induction treatment, and serum marker levels (HCG and AFP) at relapse (54). This analysis differs from Beyer et al. where patients were in their first relapse after initial therapy, and not all were treated with HDT.

Surgery in the Salvage Setting

Surgical resection of residual disease after chemotherapy plays an integral role in the management of nonseminomatous GCT (NSGCT) patients following a response to cisplatin-based therapy. Standard management calls for surgical resection of residual disease when serum tumor marker levels have normalized. Necrotic tissue, fibrosis, teratoma, or viable GCT are possible findings at the time of surgery. The pathologic presence of necrotic tissue, fibrosis, or mature teratoma requires no further therapy, because only approximately 5% to 10% of patients will relapse.

In the salvage setting, histologic findings of resected masses following second-line chemotherapy show that viable tumor occurs in approximately 50% of specimens, teratoma in 40%, and necrosis in only 10% (55). Patients who have resection of viable tumor in the salvage setting have a worse prognosis compared with patients who have only mature teratoma or necrosis resected (56), and the risk of relapse despite resection of residual masses is approximately 50%. Additional standard-dose chemotherapy adds no benefit to patients who have viable NSGCT in the resected specimen after salvage chemotherapy. This contrasts with the benefit of two additional cycles following complete resection of NSGCT after first-line chemotherapy.

Surgical resection of metastasis in the setting of elevated serum tumor markers is performed in highly selected instances. Often referred to as "desperation surgery," surgery in this setting has curative potential in rare patients who are refractory to cisplatin. Patients with a solitary retroperitoneal mass or increased AFP alone seem to be the best candidates for this type of surgery. Resection of all disease seen on imaging studies and normalization of serum tumor markers predicted long-term survival (57). Patients with primary mediastinal nonseminomatous GCT rarely respond to conventional salvage chemotherapy, and, in some patients, surgical resection in the setting of elevated serum tumor markers can lead to long-term survival (58).

New Regimens

Several new agents have been recently studied in patients with refractory GCT (59–64). Agents that may be useful for palliation include oral etoposide, gemcitabine, paclitaxel, and oxaliplatin (45,65–67). Partial responses have been achieved in 10% to 15% of patients (Table 40B.8). Oral VP-16 was initially studied in a Phase II trial that showed activity in patients refractory to cisplatin-based therapies (65). Combination studies incorporating oral etoposide have not shown additional efficacy. However, oral VP-16 has remained a palliative option for patients who are refractory to all other available treatments. Gemcitabine is associated with response rates of 15% to 19% when used as a single agent in heavily pretreated patients with refractory GCT (66,68), and paclitaxel has shown a single-agent activity of approximately 26% (45,69). After preclinical data showed incomplete cross-resistance in

TABLE 40B.8

NOVEL AGENTS IN REFRACTORY GERM CELL TUMOR

Agent	Reference	Number of patients	Response rate
Oral etoposide (VP-16) 50 mg/m^2/d	(64)	22	14%
Gemcitabine 1,000 mg/m^2 weekly for 3 wk followed by 1 wk rest	(65)	35	19%
Oxaliplatin 60 mg/m^2 days 1,8,15 OR 130 mg/m^2 on d 1, 15	(66)	32	13%
Paclitaxel 250 mg/m^2 24-hr infusional	(44)	31	26%
Gemcitabine 1,000 mg m^{-2} on d 1, 8 and oxaliplatin 130 mg/m^2 on d 1	(72)	37	47%
Paclitaxel 110 mg m^{-2} and gemcitabine 1,000 mg/m^2 on d 1,8, 15	(73)	30	21%

cell lines between oxaliplatin and cisplatin, single-agent studies were performed that showed oxaliplatin activity in the same refractory GCT population.

Drug combinations have been studied in this refractory setting in the hope of improving outcome and response rates. In preclinical studies, synergy between gemcitabine and oxaliplatin was demonstrated, specifically for sequential treatment with gemcitabine followed by oxaliplatin (72). On the basis of this and safety data from an initial Phase I trial (70), a recent study of gemcitabine in combination with oxaliplatin was done and yielded a response rate of 44% in patients with cisplatin-refractory GCT (73). Also, in a Phase I study, a combination of gemcitabine and paclitaxel established safety (71). A Phase II trial then showed a 21% response rate, including three patients who had a complete response (74).

PRIMARY MEDIASTINAL GERM CELL TUMOR

The most common primary site of extragonadal GCT is the primary mediastinal germ cell tumor (PMGCT), which represents <5% of adult patients with GCT. PMGCT, which often presents with a bulky tumor and chemotherapy resistance, is classified by IGCCCG as poor risk. The 5-year overall survival rate for patients with primary mediastinal nonseminoma is 40%. This poor prognosis is limited to nonseminoma, as seminoma patients have a high chance of cure regardless of primary site.

In one retrospective analysis of patients with poor-risk GCT, primary mediastinal NSGCT patients were found to have the lowest CR rate (38%), more frequent relapses, and worse survival compared with patients with primary testicular tumors (75). Primary mediastinal NSGCT is highly resistant to high-dose carboplatin plus etoposide given in standard doses and schedules.

Surgical resection is an integral part of therapy for patients with primary mediastinal NSGCT because these patients nearly always have a bulky residual mass following chemotherapy. One feature that differs in the treatment of primary mediastinal NSGCT is highlighted by an analysis showing that postchemotherapy resection of residual tissue revealed viable tumor in 66%, teratoma in 22%, and necrosis in 12% of patients (58). Clinical characteristics associated with a shorter survival after surgery included the presence of viable tumor in a resected specimen and more than one site of disease resected at surgery. There was no statistically significant difference in survival for patients who underwent a surgical resection with normal markers compared with patients with elevated serum tumor markers. Patients with primary mediastinal NSGCT who fail first-line cisplatin-based therapy have a poor prognosis for

salvage chemotherapy. Because retrospective studies have shown that 0% to 7% of patients have a durable complete response to ifosfamide-based or high-dose salvage therapies (51,76), postchemotherapy surgery remains an integral part of treatment, even in the setting of elevated markers (58).

MALIGNANT TRANSFORMATION

GCTs have the potential to display totipotential differentiation, including pluripotential embryonal carcinoma, extraembryonic cell types (yolk sac tumor or choriocarcinoma), and somatic cell types (teratoma, mature or immature). Approximately 3% to 6% of teratomas are estimated to undergo malignant transformation (77,78). This represents the development of a tumor histology that is indistinguishable from a somatic malignancy. The types of tumors that can arise from teratomas include rhabdomyosarcoma, primitive neuroectodermal tumor, enteric adenocarcinoma, and leukemia. Acute leukemia occurs only in patients with primary mediastinal GCT, whereas carcinoma and sarcoma can arise in patients with teratoma arising from the primary site. Malignant transformation may be found incidentally on histopathologic analysis of a surgical specimen. However, malignant transformation should be suspected if the disease is not responsive to cisplatin-based chemotherapy or if serum tumor markers are normal and imaging studies reveal growth of disease despite cisplatin-based chemotherapy.

Chromosome analysis can identify the origin of malignant transformation in GCT. An isochromosome of chromosome 12, i(12p), is a specific marker of GCT (22). Identification of i(12p) or excess 12p copy number has established the clonal origin of malignant transformation. Although data are limited, the mainstay of treatment for transformed disease has been surgical resection; these tumors are resistant to cisplatin-based therapies. In a retrospective review of patients with malignant transformation of GCT, complete resection of disease was a favorable prognostic factor for survival (79). Patients who had distant metastases, malignant transformation arising from a mediastinal primary tumor or an incomplete resection of tumor, did poorly. However, chemotherapy for malignant transformation limited to a single cell type may result in a major response and long-term survival when treatment is directed toward the specific transformed histology cell type (80).

TUMOR BIOLOGY

Adult male GCT represents a unique system of pluripotent tumor cells that can manifest into various phenotypes. Recent studies of the molecular basis of GCT resistance and sensitivity, differentiation, and transformation revealed that overexpression of cyclin D2 is an early, possibly oncogenic event in GCT (81). Differentiation may be governed by various interacting pathways, such as loss of germ cell totipotentiality regulators and of embryonic development and genomic imprinting. Chemotherapy sensitivity and resistance are likely regulated by a p53-dependent apoptotic pathway.

Genetic analysis has revealed that virtually all GCT show an increased copy number of 12p, as one or more copies of i(12p), as tandem duplications of 12p, or transposed elsewhere in the genome. The gene *CCND2*, which encodes cyclin D2, mapped to 12p13, may be the abnormal driver responsible for GCT development. Abnormality in the *TP53* gene is present in the subset of cisplatin-resistant GCT, in contrast to the extreme platinum sensitivity of GCT with the wild-type *TP53* gene (82,83). It is possible that due to an abnormality in *TP53*, GCT cells are unable to properly follow apoptotic pathways after exposure to cisplatin. Studies applying comparative genomic hybridization to a set of cisplatin-sensitive tumors and a set of cisplatin-resistant tumors, and identifying specific genes involved in resistance, are ongoing. Identifying the function of these genes may help to further understand the mechanisms of cisplatin resistance in GCT.

References

1. International Germ Cell Cancer Collaborative Group. International Germ Cell Consensus Classification: a prognostic factor-based staging system for metastatic germ cell cancers. *J Clin Oncol* 1997;15(2):594–603.
2. Bosl GJ, Geller NL, Cirrincione C, et al. Multivariate analysis of prognostic variables in patients with metastatic testicular cancer. *Cancer Res* 1983; 43(7):3403–3407.
3. Birch R, Williams S, Cone A, et al. Prognostic factors for favorable outcome in disseminated germ cell tumors. *J Clin Oncol* 1986;4(3):400–407.
4. de Wit R, Stoter G, Sleijfer DT, et al. Four cycles of BEP versus an alternating regime of PVB and BEP in patients with poor-prognosis metastatic testicular non-seminoma; a randomised study of the EORTC Genitourinary Tract Cancer Cooperative Group. *Br J Cancer* 1995;71(6):1311–1314.
5. Williams SD, Birch R, Einhorn LH, et al. Treatment of disseminated germ-cell tumors with cisplatin, bleomycin, and either vinblastine or etoposide. *N Engl J Med* 1987;316(23):1435–1440.
6. Nichols CR, Williams SD, Loehrer PJ, et al. Randomized study of cisplatin dose intensity in poor-risk germ cell tumors: a Southeastern Cancer Study Group and Southwest Oncology Group protocol. *J Clin Oncol* 1991;9(7): 1163–1172.
7. Nichols CR, Catalano PJ, Loehrer PJ, et al. Randomized comparison of cisplatin and etoposide and either bleomycin or ifosfamide in treatment of advanced disseminated germ cell tumors: an Eastern Cooperative Oncology Group, Southwest Oncology Group, and Cancer and Leukemia Group B Study. *J Clin Oncol* 1998;16(4):1287–1293.
8. Kaye SB, Mead GM, Fossa S, et al. Intensive induction-sequential chemotherapy with BOP/VIP-B compared with treatment with BEP/EP for poor-prognosis metastatic nonseminomatous germ cell tumor: a Randomized Medical Research Council/European Organization for Research and Treatment of Cancer study. *J Clin Oncol* 1998;16(2):692–701.
9. Ozols RF, Ihde DC, Linehan WM, et al. A randomized trial of standard chemotherapy v a high-dose chemotherapy regimen in the treatment of poor prognosis nonseminomatous germ-cell tumors. *J Clin Oncol* 1988; 6(6):1031–1040.
10. Husband DJ, Green JA. POMB/ACE chemotherapy in non-seminomatous germ cell tumours: outcome and importance of dose intensity. *Eur J Cancer* 1992;28(1):86–91.
11. Christian JA, Huddart RA, Norman A, et al. Intensive induction chemotherapy with CBOP/BEP in patients with poor prognosis germ cell tumors. *J Clin Oncol* 2003;21(5):871–877.
12. Blanke C, Loehrer PJ, Nichols CR, et al. A phase II trial of VP-16, ifosfamide, cisplatin, vinblastine, and bleomycin in advanced germ-cell tumors. *Am J Clin Oncol* 1996;19(5):487–491.
13. Hinton S, Catalano PJ, Einhorn LH, et al. Cisplatin, etoposide and either bleomycin or ifosfamide in the treatment of disseminated germ cell tumors: final analysis of an intergroup trial. *Cancer* 2003;97(8):1869–1875.
14. de Wit R, Louwerens M, de Mulder PH, et al. Management of intermediate-prognosis germ-cell cancer: results of a phase I/II study of Taxol-BEP. *Int J Cancer* 1999;83(6):831–833.
15. Motzer RJ, Gulati SC, Crown J, et al. High-dose chemotherapy and autologous bone marrow rescue for patients with refractory germ cell tumors. Early intervention is better tolerated. *Cancer* 1992;69(2):550–556.
16. Broun ER, Nichols CR, Kneebone P, et al. Long-term outcome of patients with relapsed and refractory germ cell tumors treated with high-dose chemotherapy and autologous bone marrow rescue. *Ann Intern Med* 1992; 117(2):124–128.
17. Motzer RJ, Bosl GJ. High-dose chemotherapy for resistant germ cell tumors: recent advances and future directions. *J Natl Cancer Inst* 1992; 84(22):1703–1709.
18. Decatris MP, Wilkinson PM, Welch RS, et al. High-dose chemotherapy and autologous haematopoietic support in poor risk non-seminomatous germ-cell tumours: an effective first-line therapy with minimal toxicity. *Ann Oncol* 2000;11(4):427–434.
19. Motzer RJ, Mazumdar M, Bajorin DF, et al. High-dose carboplatin, etoposide, and cyclophosphamide with autologous bone marrow transplantation in first-line therapy for patients with poor-risk germ cell tumors. *J Clin Oncol* 1997;15(7):2546–2552.
20. Chevreau C, Droz JP, Pico JL, et al. Early intensified chemotherapy with autologous bone marrow transplantation in first line treatment of poor risk non-seminomatous germ cell tumours. Preliminary results of a French randomized trial. *Eur Urol* 1993;23(1):213–217; discussion 218.
21. Schmoll HJ, Kollmannsberger C, Metzner B, et al. Long-term results of first-line sequential high-dose etoposide, ifosfamide, and cisplatin chemotherapy plus autologous stem cell support for patients with advanced metastatic germ cell cancer: an extended phase I/II study of the German Testicular Cancer Study Group. *J Clin Oncol* 2003;21(22):4083–4091.
22. Bosl GJ, Motzer RJ. Testicular germ-cell cancer. *N Engl J Med* 1997; 337(4):242–253.
23. Mazumdar M, Bajorin DF, Bacik J, et al. Predicting outcome to chemotherapy in patients with germ cell tumors: the value of the rate of decline of human chorionic gonadotrophin and alpha-fetoprotein during therapy. *J Clin Oncol* 2001;19(9):2534–2541.
24. Stevens MJ, Norman AR, Dearnaley DP, et al. Prognostic significance of early serum tumor marker half-life in metastatic testicular teratoma. *J Clin Oncol* 1995;13(1):87–92.
25. de Wit R, Sylvester R, Tsitsa C, et al. Tumour marker concentration at the start of chemotherapy is a stronger predictor of treatment failure than marker half-life: a study in patients with disseminated non-seminomatous testicular cancer. *Br J Cancer* 1997;75(3):432–435.
26. Inanc SE, Meral R, Darendeliler E, et al. Prognostic significance of marker half-life during chemotherapy in non-seminomatous germ cell testicular tumors. *Acta Oncol* 1999;38(4):505–509.
27. Wheeler BM, Loehrer PJ, Williams SD, et al. Ifosfamide in refractory male germ cell tumors. *J Clin Oncol* 1986;4(1):28–34.
28. Harstrick A, Schmoll HJ, Wilke H, et al. Cisplatin, etoposide, and ifosfamide salvage therapy for refractory or relapsing germ cell carcinoma. *J Clin Oncol* 1991;9(9):1549–1555.
29. Loehrer PJ Sr, Lauer R, Roth BJ, et al. Salvage therapy in recurrent germ cell cancer: ifosfamide and cisplatin plus either vinblastine or etoposide. *Ann Intern Med* 1988;109(7):540–546.
30. Loehrer PJ Sr, Gonin R, Nichols CR, et al. Vinblastine plus ifosfamide plus cisplatin as initial salvage therapy in recurrent germ cell tumor. *J Clin Oncol* 1998;16(7):2500–2504.
31. McCaffrey JA, Mazumdar M, Bajorin DF, et al. Ifosfamide- and cisplatin-containing chemotherapy as first-line salvage therapy in germ cell tumors: response and survival. *J Clin Oncol* 1997;15(7):2559–2563.
32. Ghosn M, Droz JP, Theodore C, et al. Salvage chemotherapy in refractory germ cell tumors with etoposide (VP-16) plus ifosfamide plus high-dose cisplatin. A VIhP regimen. *Cancer* 1988;62(1):24–27.
33. Pizzocaro G, Salvioni R, Piva L, et al. Modified cisplatin, etoposide (or vinblastine) and ifosfamide salvage therapy for male germ-cell tumors. Long-term results. *Ann Oncol* 1992;3(3):211–216.
34. Motzer RJ, Bajorin DF, Vlamis V, et al. Ifosfamide-based chemotherapy for patients with resistant germ cell tumors: the Memorial Sloan-Kettering Cancer Center experience. *Semin Oncol* 1992;19(6 Suppl. 12):8–11.
35. Motzer RJ, Mazumdhar M, Bosl GJ, et al. High-dose carboplatin, etoposide, and cyclophosphamide for patients with refractory germ cell tumors: treatment results and prognostic factors for survival and toxicity. *J Clin Oncol* 1996;14(4):1098–1105.
36. Siegert W, Beyer J, Strohscheer I et al, The German Testicular Cancer Cooperative Study Group. High-dose treatment with carboplatin, etoposide, and ifosfamide followed by autologous stem-cell transplantation in relapsed or refractory germ cell cancer: a phase I/II study. *J Clin Oncol* 1994; 12(6):1223–1231.
37. Motzer RJ, Mazumdar M, Sheinfeld J, et al. Sequential dose-intensive paclitaxel, ifosfamide, carboplatin, and etoposide salvage therapy for germ cell tumor patients. *J Clin Oncol* 2000;18(6):1173–1180.
38. Rosti G, Pico JL, Wandt H, et al. High-dose chemotherapy (HDC) in the salvage treatment of patients failing first-line platinum chemotherapy for advanced germ cell tumors (GCT); first results of a prospective randomised trial of the European Group for Blood and Marrow Transplantation (EBMT): IT-94 study. *Am Soc Clin Oncol* 2002;21:716.
39. Rick O, Bokemeyer C, Beyer J, et al. Salvage treatment with paclitaxel, ifosfamide, and cisplatin plus high-dose carboplatin, etoposide, and thiotepa followed by autologous stem-cell rescue in patients with relapsed or refractory germ cell cancer. *J Clin Oncol* 2001;19(1):81–88.
40. Rodenhuis S, de Wit R, de Mulder PH, et al. A multi-center prospective phase II study of high-dose chemotherapy in germ-cell cancer patients

relapsing from complete remission. *Ann Oncol* 1999;10(12): 1467–1473.

41. Bhatia S, Abonour R, Porcu P, et al. High-dose chemotherapy as initial salvage chemotherapy in patients with relapsed testicular cancer. *J Clin Oncol* 2000;18(19):3346–3351.

42. Motzer RJ, Geller NL, Tan CC, et al. Salvage chemotherapy for patients with germ cell tumors. The Memorial Sloan-Kettering Cancer Center experience (1979–1989). *Cancer* 1991;67(5):1305–1310.

43. Beyer J, Schwella N, Zingsem J, et al. Hematopoietic rescue after high-dose chemotherapy using autologous peripheral-blood progenitor cells or bone marrow: a randomized comparison. *J Clin Oncol* 1995;13:1328–1335.

44. Beyer J, Kramar A, Mandanas R, et al. High-dose chemotherapy as salvage treatment in germ cell tumors: a multivariate analysis of prognostic variables. *J Clin Oncol* 1996;14(10):2638–2645.

45. Motzer RJ, Bajorin DF, Schwartz LH, et al. Phase II trial of paclitaxel shows antitumor activity in patients with previously treated germ cell tumors. *J Clin Oncol* 1994;12(11):2277–2283.

46. Bokemeyer C, Schmoll HJ, Natt F, et al. Preliminary results of a phase I/II trial of paclitaxel in patients with relapsed or cisplatin-refractory testicular cancer. *J Cancer Res Clin Oncol* 1994;120(12):754–757.

47. Bokemeyer C, Bokemeyer C, Beyer J, et al. Phase II study of paclitaxel in patients with relapsed or cisplatin-refractory testicular cancer. *Ann Oncol* 1996;7(1):31–34.

48. Sandler AB, Cristou A, Fox S, et al. A phase II trial of paclitaxel in refractory germ cell tumors. *Cancer* 1998;82(7):1381–1386.

49. Motzer RJ, Sheinfeld J, Mazumdar M, et al. Paclitaxel, ifosfamide, and cisplatin second-line therapy for patients with relapsed testicular germ cell cancer. *J Clin Oncol* 2000;18(12):2413–2418.

50. Donadio A, Sheinfeld SJ, Bacik J, et al. Paclitaxel, Ifosfamide, and Cisplatin (TIP): An effective second-line therapy for patients with relapsed testicular germ cell tumors (GCT). In: *American society of clinical oncology.* Chicago, IL: 2003;383.

51. Saxman SB, Nichols CR, Einhorn LH. Salvage chemotherapy in patients with extragonadal nonseminomatous germ cell tumors: the Indiana University experience. *J Clin Oncol* 1994;12(7):1390–1393.

52. Linkesch W, Greinix HT, Hocker P, et al. Longterm follow up of phase I/II trial of ultra-high carboplatin, VP-16, cyclophosphamide with ABMT in refractory or relapsed NSGCT. *Am Soc Clin Oncol* 1993;12:232.

53. Vaena DA, Abonour R, Einhorn LH. Long-term survival after high-dose salvage chemotherapy for germ cell malignancies with adverse prognostic variables. *J Clin Oncol* 2003;21(22):4100–4104.

54. Fossa SD, Stenning SP, Gerl A, et al. Prognostic factors in patients progressing after cisplatin-based chemotherapy for malignant non-seminomatous germ cell tumours. *Br J Cancer* 1999;80(9):1392–1399.

55. Fox EP, Weathers TD, Williams SD, et al. Outcome analysis for patients with persistent nonteratomatous germ cell tumor in postchemotherapy retroperitoneal lymph node dissections. *J Clin Oncol* 1993;11(7):1294–1299.

56. Rick O, Bokemeyer C, Christian J, et al. Residual tumor resection after high-dose chemotherapy in patients with relapsed or refractory germ cell tumors. *American society of clinical oncology.* Chicago, IL: 2003;389.

57. Habuchi T, Kamoto T, Hara I, et al. Factors that influence the results of salvage surgery in patients with chemorefractory germ cell carcinomas with elevated tumor markers. *Cancer* 2003;98(8):1635–1642.

58. Vuky J, Bains M, Bacik J, et al. Role of postchemotherapy adjunctive surgery in the management of patients with nonseminoma arising from the mediastinum. *J Clin Oncol* 2001;19(3):682–688.

59. Motzer RJ, Dmitrovsky E, Miller WH Jr, et al. Suramin for germ cell tumors. In vitro growth inhibition and results of a phase II trial. *Cancer* 1993;72(11):3313–3317.

60. Varuni Kondagunta G, Bacik J, Schwartz L, et al. Phase II trial of temozolomide in patients with cisplatin-refractory germ cell tumors. *Invest New Drugs* 2004;22(2):177–179.

61. Murphy BA, Motzer RJ, Bosl GJ. Phase II study of iproplatin (CHIP) in patients with cisplatin-refractory germ cell tumors; the need for alternative strategies in the investigation of new agents in GCT. *Invest New Drugs* 1992;10(4):327–330.

62. Puc HS, Bajorin DF, Bosl GJ, et al. Phase II trial of topotecan in patients with cisplatin-refractory germ cell tumors. *Invest New Drugs* 1995;13(2): 163–165.

63. Vuky J, McCaffrey J, Ginsberg M, et al. Phase II trial of pyrazoloacridine in patients with cisplatin-refractory germ cell tumors. *Invest New Drugs* 2000;18(3):265–267.

64. Kollmannsberger C, Rick O, Klaproth H, et al. Irinotecan in patients with relapsed or cisplatin-refractory germ cell cancer: a phase II study of the German Testicular Cancer Study Group. *Br J Cancer* 2002;87(7): 729–732.

65. Miller JC, Einhorn LH. Phase II study of daily oral etoposide in refractory germ cell tumors. *Semin Oncol* 1990;17(1 Suppl. 2):36–39.

66. Bokemeyer C, Gerl A, Schoffski P, et al. Gemcitabine in patients with relapsed or cisplatin-refractory testicular cancer. *J Clin Oncol* 1999;17(2): 512–516.

67. Kollmannsberger C, Rick O, Derigs HG, et al. Activity of oxaliplatin in patients with relapsed or cisplatin-refractory germ cell cancer: a study of the German Testicular Cancer Study Group. *J Clin Oncol* 2002;20(8): 2031–2037.

68. Einhorn LH, Stender MJ, Williams SD. Phase II trial of gemcitabine in refractory germ cell tumors. *J Clin Oncol* 1999;17(2):509–511.

69. Motzer RJ, Chou TC, Schwartz L, et al. Paclitaxel in germ cell cancer. *Semin Oncol* 1995;22(3 Suppl. 6):12–15.

70. Mavroudis D, Kourousis C, Kakolyris S, et al. Phase I study of the gemcitabine/oxaliplatin combination in patients with advanced solid tumors: a preliminary report. *Semin Oncol* 2000;27(1 Suppl. 2):25–30.

71. Rothenberg ML, Sharma A, Weiss GR, et al. Phase I trial of paclitaxel and gemcitabine administered every two weeks in patients with refractory solid tumors. *Ann Oncol* 1998;9(7):733–738.

72. Faivre S, Raymond E, Woynarowski JM, et al. Supraadditive effect of 2′,2′-difluorodeoxycytidine (gemcitabine) in combination with oxaliplatin in human cancer cell lines. *Cancer Chemother Pharmacol* 1999;44(2): 117–123.

73. Kollmannsberger C, Beyer J, Liersch R, et al. Combination chemotherapy with gemcitabine plus oxaliplatin in patients with intensively pretreated or refractory germ cell cancer: a study of the German Testicular Cancer Study Group. *J Clin Oncol* 2004;22(1):108–114.

74. Hinton S, Catalano P, Einhorn LH, et al. Phase II study of paclitaxel plus gemcitabine in refractory germ cell tumors (E9897): a trial of the Eastern Cooperative Oncology Group. *J Clin Oncol* 2002;20(7): 1859–1863.

75. Toner GC, Geller NL, Lin SY, et al. Extragonadal and poor risk nonseminomatous germ cell tumors. Survival and prognostic features. *Cancer* 1991;67(8):2049–2057.

76. Broun ER, Nichols CR, Einhorn LH, et al. Salvage therapy with high-dose chemotherapy and autologous bone marrow support in the treatment of primary nonseminomatous mediastinal germ cell tumors. *Cancer* 1991; 68(7):1513–1515.

77. Comiter CV, Kibel AS, Richie JP, et al. Prognostic features of teratomas with malignant transformation: a clinicopathological study of 21 cases. *J Urol* 1998;159(3):859–863.

78. Korfel A, Fischer L, Foss HD, et al. Testicular germ cell tumor with rhabdomyosarcoma successfully treated by disease-adapted chemotherapy including high-dose chemotherapy: case report and review of the literature. *Bone Marrow Transplant* 2001;28(8):787–789.

79. Motzer RJ, Amsterdam A, Prieto V, et al. Teratoma with malignant transformation: diverse malignant histologies arising in men with germ cell tumors. *J Urol* 1998;159(1):133–138.

80. Donadio AC, Motzer RJ, Bajorin DF, et al. Chemotherapy for teratoma with malignant transformation. *J Clin Oncol* 2003;21(23):4285–4291.

81. Houldsworth J, Reuter V, Bosl GJ, et al. Aberrant expression of cyclin D2 is an early event in human male germ cell tumorigenesis. *Cell Growth Differ* 1997;8(3):293–299.

82. Houldsworth J, Xiao H, Murty VV, et al. Human male germ cell tumor resistance to cisplatin is linked to TP53 gene mutation. *Oncogene* 1998; 16(18):2345–2349.

83. Houldsworth J, Reuter V, Bosl G, et al. ID gene expression varies with lineage during differentiation of pluripotential male germ cell tumor cell lines. *Cell Tissue Res* 2001;303(3):371–379.

CHAPTER 41 ■ CHRONIC TOXICITY FROM CHEMOTHERAPY FOR DISSEMINATED TESTICULAR CANCER

TIMOTHY DAVID GILLIGAN

INTRODUCTION

The high cure rate for testicular cancer and the young age of most patients has made late toxicities a major concern. The major potential long-term side effects of chemotherapy are infertility, pulmonary fibrosis, nerve damage, vascular toxicity, nephrotoxicity, and secondary malignancies.

INFERTILITY

Assessing the effect of treatment on fertility is complicated by the fact that most men with testicular cancer have abnormal semen analysis results at the time of diagnosis (1). Epidemiologic studies have documented that in the years before the diagnosis, patients with testicular cancer have lower fertility rates than the general population (2,3). Before orchiectomy, sperm counts in men with testicular cancer are about 20% of the counts in healthy controls, whereas follicle-stimulating hormone (FSH) levels are higher and inhibin levels are lower (4,5). Following orchiectomy, sperm counts fall further, but there is generally some subsequent improvement. To assess the impact of treatment on fertility, a study in Toulouse surveyed 446 patients and reported that 91% of patients who tried to father children before the treatment had been successful, compared with only 67% who tried after treatment (6). Fertility was substantially higher in men receiving cisplatin-based chemotherapy than in men undergoing radiation therapy (RT). Although cisplatin-based chemotherapy is associated with azoospermia at the completion of therapy, most patients recover their fertility subsequently. Among patients receiving chemotherapy, the risk factors for failure to recover sperm counts greater than 1 million per mL included low pretreatment sperm count, more than four cycles of chemotherapy, the use of cisplatin rather than carboplatin, and the use of a vinca alkaloids (7). A recent study reported that about 80% of patients treated with platinum-based chemotherapy achieve oligospermia or normospermia within 5 years of treatment (7). Patients receiving only two cycles of bleomycin, etoposide, cisplatin (BEP) have fertility rates no different from patients with testis cancer who are treated with orchiectomy alone (8). A study of patients with clinical stage I pure seminomas receiving adjuvant carboplatin reported that the percentage with normospermia increased from 35% before treatment to 68% 4 years after treatment, whereas azoospermia fell from 12% to 0% (9).

PULMONARY TOXICITY

Bleomycin-associated pulmonary toxicity represents one of the most feared acute complications of germ cell tumor chemotherapy. Although fatal bleomycin-induced pulmonary fibrosis represents the most well-known syndrome, milder toxicities also have been reported. Estimating the rate of bleomycin lung injury is difficult because of highly varying methods that trials have used to measure this toxicity. One 812-patient study conducted serial pulmonary function tests and reported a median acute decline in carbon monoxide diffusion capacity (DLCO) of 19% in men who received a cumulative dose of 270 units (10), but no long-term follow-up data was reported. Those studies that have only documented symptomatic or clinically obvious toxicity have often reported no pulmonary toxicity in such patients (11–13). Chronic declines in DLCO have not been shown. The toxic death rate for men receiving a cumulative dose of 270 units of bleomycin is <0.2% (13–19), and long-term follow-up has not shown evidence of clinically relevant impaired pulmonary function in this population (20). Among patients receiving 360 units of beomycin, the toxic death rate rises to between 1% and 2% (21,22). Unfortunately, we lack information on the early signs and symptoms of bleomycin pulmonary toxicity that are sensitive enough to eliminate the risk of severe complications. The development of an inspiratory lag, basilar rales, dyspnea on exertion, a dry cough, a 50% decline in DLCO, or a drop in vital capacity can all signal developing pulmonary fibrosis, but none has been shown to have high sensitivity or specificity (23,24). The practice of monitoring for pulmonary toxicity by performing serial pulmonary function tests is common but is not well supported by data. Because excellent alternative agents exist, bleomycin should be discontinued if signs of pulmonary toxicity are present and if a low threshold for such discontinuation is appropriate. For good-risk patients, the common practice is to exclude bleomycin from the regimen and to continue with etoposide and cisplatin alone but to give a total of four cycles of treatment rather than three. For intermediate- and poor-risk patients, ifosfamide can be substituted for bleomycin, as in the etoposide, ifosfamide, cisplatin (VIP) regimen. In addition to cumulative dose over 300 units, other risk factors identified in multivariate analysis include impaired renal function [glomerular filtration rate (GFR) <80 mL per minute], age over 40 years, and the presence of visceral metastases (19). Administration of bleomycin to patients with renal insufficiency should therefore be avoided when alternative agents are available (25). Cigarette smoking increases the risk of bleomycin pulmonary toxicity in animal models, but it has not been clearly demonstrated in humans (26–29).

Prior bleomycin exposure is associated with an increased risk of perioperative pulmonary complications, including potentially fatal acute respiratory distress syndrome. Patients undergoing postbleomycin surgery should have precautions taken, including judicious management of intravenous fluids and avoidance of high partial pressure of inspired oxygen (30–32). It is widely recommended that patients who have received bleomycin should never scuba dive because it entails exposure to oxygen at an elevated partial pressure.

NEUROTOXICITY

Cisplatin, ifosfamide, vinblastine, and paclitaxel are all associated with neurotoxicity. The most common manifestation is peripheral neuropathy, which affects about 25% to 50% of patients and can be chronic in 20% to 40% of patients (10,33, 34). Symptoms may include paresthesias, dysesthesias, pain, and reductions in strength and coordination. Activities of daily living may be impaired in severe cases, but such impairment is uncommon. Cisplatin is also associated with ototoxicity, which manifests as diminished high-pitch (4 to 8 kHz) hearing and tinnitus (35). Up to 25% of patients may have chronic symptoms, with transient symptoms in an additional 10% (34,36,37). The incidence of both peripheral neuropathy and ototoxicity correlate with cumulative cisplatin dose. In one study, every patient who received more than 650 mg per m^2 complained of persistent tinnitus or hearing loss (33). Effective treatment of neurotoxicity is lacking, but many patients experience improvement over time.

VASCULAR DISEASE

Cisplatin and bleomycin have both been associated with vascular toxicity, which takes the form of Raynaud phenomenon and cardiovascular disease. In carefully conducted studies with adequate follow-up, roughly 40% of patients are found to have symptoms of Raynaud phenomenon (33,38). Symptoms may not appear for many months after chemotherapy but are persistent for half or more of affected patients (37,39). Arteriograms have documented diffuse vascular narrowing in the hands of these patients (38). Although smoking may increase the risk of Raynaud following chemotherapy, this has not been conclusively demonstrated.

Hypertension and cardiovascular disease may also be the long-term side effects of platinum-based chemotherapy. Hannover University reported that in 90 patients followed up for a median of 58 months, the mean diastolic arterial blood pressure rose from 79 to 87 mm Hg (33). Out of the 55 men with reliable pre- and posttreatment data, 15% developed arterial hypertension after chemotherapy. A study from the Netherlands, with 10 years median follow-up, found that 24 of 62 (39%) patients treated with chemotherapy developed hypertension compared with 3 of 40 (8%) patients treated with orchiectomy alone (39). Hypercholesterolemia is a second risk factor for cardiovascular disease that has been associated with chemotherapy for germ cell tumors, with mean cholesterol levels increasing from 3.96 mmol per L to 6.12 mmol per L in one study (40). Compared with healthy controls and to men with stage I testicular cancer treated with surveillance, patients who have received chemotherapy have higher cholesterol and triglyceride levels and lower high-density lipoprotein levels (39,40). Several recent studies with a median follow-up of at least 10 years have documented an increased incidence of cardiovascular events in patients treated with RT and/or chemotherapy. A study of 87 men who had been treated with cisplatin-based chemotherapy reported that 5 men (6%) had either myocardial infarction or angina with proven myocardial ischemia (39). Compared with the general population, this represented a 7.1-fold increase over the expected number of events [95% confidence interval (CI) 1.9% to 18.3%]. The events occurred at 9 to 16 years after chemotherapy and at ages ranging from 30 to 42 years. A British study using a less

exacting definition of cardiovascular events similarly reported that among 992 men followed up for a median of 10.2 years, 9.6% of those receiving RT and 6.7% of those receiving chemotherapy experienced a cardiac event, compared with only 3.7% of those treated by orchiectomy alone (41). After adjusting for age, the relative risk (RR) was 2.59 for chemotherapy, 2.40 for radiotherapy, and 2.78 among those who received both therapies. No difference in risk was seen when comparing cisplatin with carboplatin chemotherapy. Increased cardiac mortality per se has not been demonstrated in patients treated with chemotherapy, but a report from the M.D. Anderson Cancer Center on 447 men treated between 1951 and 1999 found that RT for seminoma was associated with a 61% increase in cardiac-specific mortality compared with the general population (42). Whether modern RT, which uses lower doses and small fields, is associated with a similar risk remains unclear.

KIDNEY DAMAGE

Long-term decline in renal function following cisplatin chemotherapy and/or RT has been well documented (35,43). Vigorous intravenous hydration and forced diuresis reduces cisplatin nephrotoxicity, but even with these precautions, 20% to 30% of patients can be demonstrated to have long-term reduction in GFR. Evaluating more than 700 patients with a median follow-up of 10 years, the Royal Marsden National Health Service Trust reported that elevated creatinine levels were documented in 14% of those treated with chemotherapy, 13% of those treated with radiation, and 27% of those who received both modalities, compared with 7.5% of those treated only with orchiectomy.

SECONDARY MALIGNANCIES

Treatment of testicular cancer is associated with an increased risk of secondary non–germ cell cancers. This risk is distinct from the risk of a second primary (contralateral) testicular cancer seen in patients with testis cancer independent of treatment. Treatment-related cancers are primarily radiation-induced, with the exception that etoposide chemotherapy is associated with an increased risk of acute leukemias that are highly resistant to treatment.

Adequately powered studies with a sufficient follow-up have consistently reported an association between RT for germ cell tumors and an increased incidence of solid malignancies, with reported RR ranging from 1.45 to 7.5 (34,42, 44,45). M.D. Anderson Cancer Center reported that men with seminomas treated with radiation had an RR of death from secondary malignancies of 1.91 (95% CI, 1.30 to 2.71). The largest study was an international pooled analysis of population-based cancer registries including 28,843 men, with more than 3,300 men having survived the cancer for more than 20 years (44). Among men receiving radiation for seminoma, the RR of second tumors was 1.45 overall and was 1.65 among those with 20-year follow-ups. Twenty-five years following treatment, 18% of patients with seminoma had developed a secondary non–germ cell cancer compared with an expected incidence of 9.3%. The implication is that for every 100 men treated with radiation for seminoma, there will be 9 excess non–germ cell cancers. No increased risk of cancer was seen in men with seminomas who were treated with chemotherapy (RR = 0.90), although the number of such patients was too small to exclude an association. An analysis of 2,006 testicular cancer survivors in Norway, with a mean follow-up of 12 years, also reported that radiation (RR = 1.58; 95% CI 1.3 to 1.9) but not chemotherapy [odds ratio (OR) = 1/32, 95% CI 0.4 to 3.4] was associated with an increased risk of secondary malignancies

(46). However, the highest risk was seen among patients who had received both chemotherapy and radiation (RR = 3.54; 95% CI 2.0–5.8), an interaction that has been confirmed by other studies (47,48). A Dutch report of 1,909 testicular cancer survivors similarly reported that RT was associated with secondary cancers (RR = 1.8; 95% CI 1.4 to 2.2) but not with chemotherapy (RR = 0.83; 95% CI 0.10 to 3.0) (48). Malignancies associated with RT include leukemia, sarcomas, and cancers of the stomach, bladder, colon, and pancreas.

In contrast to other secondary malignancies, leukemia is more strongly associated with chemotherapy. Travis et al. (44) reported that among 2,664 patients receiving chemotherapy for nonseminomatous germ cell tumors (NSGCTs), six cases of leukemia were seen, representing an RR of 11 (95% CI = 4.18–25). The risk of leukemia in patients with germ cell tumor treated with modern chemotherapeutic regimens appears to be related primarily to etoposide, but cisplatin may contribute, as well (49,50). Carboplatin has not been associated with leukemia or other secondary malignancies. Etoposide-related leukemias are typically acute myeloid leukemias that occur

within 2 to 3 years following chemotherapy and are generally fatal. A review of published studies of secondary leukemias in this population reported that among patients receiving a cumulative dose of etoposide of up to 2 g per m² had an incidence of leukemia of .5%; those receiving more than 2 g per m² had an incidence of 2.6% (34). Standard first-line chemotherapy therefore carries a low risk of inducing secondary leukemia.

QUALITY OF LIFE

Studies of testicular cancer survivors have consistently documented considerable rates of anxiety, depression, sexual dysfunction, dissatisfaction with friends and family, chronic fatigue, and various psychosocial symptoms (51–54). However, studies have reached varying conclusions about whether rates of depression and fatigue are higher among testis cancer survivors, among healthy controls, or among the general population (51,52). Although most patients regain a good quality of life, roughly 10% suffer long-term psychological problems (53).

TABLE 41.1

CHRONIC TOXICITY FROM CHEMOTHERAPY FOR TESTICULAR GERM-CELL TUMORS

Organ system	Manifestation of toxicity
Cardiovascular	Increased risk of cardiovascular events (MI, angina, revascularization) • relative risk with long-term follow-up = 2.6–7.1 (39,41) • incidence with 10-year follow-up = 6%–6.7% (39,41) Raynaud phenomenon • incidence of chronic symptoms = 20%–30% (33,37,39) • associated most strongly with bleomycin dose and use of the PVB regimen Cardiac risk factors • inconclusive evidence of increased incidence of hypertension and dyslipidemia following chemotherapy (33,39–41)
Renal	Decreased renal function • increased serum creatinine in 7% to 16% (33,41) • decreased creatinine clearance and GFR in to 30% (39,43)
Neurologic	Peripheral neuropathy • acute in 25%–50% (10,33) • chronic in 13% to 17% (10,33,37) Ototoxicity • chronic tinnitus or subjective high-pitch hearing loss in 20% to 25% (33,37)
Endocrine	Elevated gonadotropin levels (LH and FSH) in 63% to 86% (40,55) Elevated dihydroepiandrosterone (55) Decreased serum testosterone levels in 5% to 10% (40,55)
Pulmonary	Dyspnea • No chronic dyspnea with cumulative dose of 270 units (37) Decreased DLCO and vital capacity • Immediately following chemotherapy, a 19% mean decline in DLCO has been documented (10) • Decline in vital capacity has been documented (23) • Chronic decline in DLCO has not been documented (56) Pulmonary fibrosis • With a cumulative bleomycin dose of 270 units or less, risk of pulmonary toxicity is about 2.5% and risk of fatal pulmonary toxicity is less than 0.2% (13–19) • With a cumulative bleomycin dose of 360 units, a fatal toxicity rate of 1% to 2% has been reported (21,22).
Gonadal	Infertility • Men with a history of testicular cancer have lower fertility rates than the general population as well as lower sperm counts and motility but these abnormalities precede treatment with chemotherapy • Sperm concentration and rate of azospermia are no different in patients undergoing surveillance or surgical treatment than in men receiving up to four cycles of standard-dose chemotherapy (57) • Men who receive more than four cycles of standard-dose chemotherapy have significantly decreased sperm counts (7,58)

MI, myocardial infarction; PVB, cisplatin, vinblastine, and bleomycin; GFR, glomerular filtration rate; LH, luteinizing hormone; FSH, follicle-stimulating hormone; DLCO, carbon monoxide diffusion capacity.

CONCLUSION

The major chronic side effects following chemotherapy for disseminated testicular cancer are peripheral neuropathy, ototoxicity, Raynaud phenomenon, and impaired fertility (Table 41.1). Most patients report no long-term side effects, and most are able to father children. Pulmonary toxicity for good-risk patients has been reduced by limiting chemotherapy to three cycles of bleomycin, etoposide, and cisplatin, but patients who have received bleomycin need to take lifelong precautions with regard to avoiding exposure to elevated partial pressures of oxygen (in medical, surgical, or recreational settings). Secondary malignancies are rare following chemotherapy.

Toxicity can best be minimized by avoiding overtreatment of patients and by carefully monitoring them during therapy. However, most side effects result from cisplatin, which is a crucial element of curative chemotherapy for disseminated germ cell tumors. Except in extreme cases, cisplatin is administered at full dose on schedule because of concerns that dose delays or reductions may compromise survival.

References

1. Hendry WF, Stedronska J, Jones CR, et al. Semen analysis in testicular cancer and Hodgkin's disease: pre- and post-treatment findings and implications for cryopreservation. *Br J Urol* 1983;55(6):769–773.
2. Jacobsen R, Bostofte E, Engholm G, et al. Fertility and offspring sex ratio of men who develop testicular cancer: a record linkage study. *Hum Reprod* 2000;15(9):1958–1961.
3. Richiardi L, Akre O, Montgomery SM, et al. Fecundity and twinning rates as measures of fertility before diagnosis of germ-cell testicular cancer. *J Natl Cancer Inst* 2004;96(2):145–147.
4. Petersen PM, Skakkebaek NE, Rorth M, et al. Semen quality and reproductive hormones before and after orchiectomy in men with testicular cancer. *J Urol* 1999;161(3):822–826.
5. Petersen PM, Skakkebaek NE, Vistisen K, et al. Semen quality and reproductive hormones before orchiectomy in men with testicular cancer. *J Clin Oncol* 1999;17(3):941–947.
6. Huyghe E, Matsuda T, Daudin M, et al. Fertility after testicular cancer treatments: results of a large multicenter study. *Cancer* 2004;100(4):732–737.
7. Lampe H, Horwich A, Norman A, et al. Fertility after chemotherapy for testicular germ cell cancers. *J Clin Oncol* 1997;15(1):239–245.
8. Pont J, Albrecht W, Postner G, et al. Adjuvant chemotherapy for high-risk clinical stage I nonseminomatous testicular germ cell cancer: long-term results of a prospective trial. *J Clin Oncol* 1996;14(2):441–448.
9. Reiter WJ, Kratzik C, Brodowicz T, et al. Sperm analysis and serum follicle-stimulating hormone levels before and after adjuvant single-agent carboplatin therapy for clinical stage I seminoma. *Urology* 1998;52(1):117–119.
10. de Wit R, Roberts JT, Wilkinson PM, et al. Equivalence of three or four cycles of bleomycin, etoposide, and cisplatin chemotherapy and of a 3- or 5-day schedule in good-prognosis germ cell cancer: a randomized study of the European Organization for Research and Treatment of Cancer Genitourinary Tract Cancer Cooperative Group and the Medical Research Council. *J Clin Oncol* 2001;19(6):1629–1640.
11. Loehrer PJ Sr, Johnson D, Elson P, et al. Importance of bleomycin in favorable-prognosis disseminated germ cell tumors: an Eastern Cooperative Oncology Group trial. *J Clin Oncol* 1995;13(2):470–476.
12. Bokemeyer C, Kohrmann O, Tischler J, et al. A randomized trial of cisplatin, etoposide and bleomycin (PEB) versus carboplatin, etoposide and bleomycin (CEB) for patients with 'good-risk' metastatic non-seminomatous germ cell tumors. *Ann Oncol* 1996;7(10):1015–1021.
13. Culine S, Theodore C, Terrier-Lacombe MJ, et al. Are 3 cycles of bleomycin, etoposide and cisplatin or 4 cycles of etoposide and cisplatin equivalent optimal regimens for patients with good risk metastatic germ cell tumors of the testis? The need for a randomized trial. *J Urol* 1997;157(3):855–858; discussion 858–859.
14. de Wit R, Roberts JT, Wilkinson PM, et al. Equivalence of three or four cycles of bleomycin, etoposide, and cisplatin chemotherapy and of a 3- or 5-day schedule in good-prognosis germ cell cancer: a randomized study of the European Organization for Research and Treatment of Cancer Genitourinary Tract Cancer Cooperative Group and the Medical Research Council. *J Clin Oncol* 2001;19:1629–1640.
15. Loehrer PJ Sr, Johnson D, Elson P, et al. Importance of bleomycin in favorable-prognosis disseminated germ cell tumors: an Eastern Cooperative Oncology Group trial, *J Clin Oncol.* 1995;13:470–476.
16. Bokemeyer C, Kohrmann O, Tischler J, et al. A randomized trial of cisplatin, etoposide and bleomycin (PEB) versus carboplatin, etoposide and bleomycin (CEB) for patients with 'good-risk' metastatic non-seminomatous germ cell tumors. *Ann Oncol* 1996;7:1015–1021.
17. Einhorn LH, Williams SD, Loehrer PJ, et al. Evaluation of optimal duration of chemotherapy in favorable-prognosis disseminated germ cell tumors: a Southeastern Cancer Study Group protocol. *J Clin Oncol* 1989;7(3):387–391.
18. Toner GC, Stockler MR, Boyer MJ, et al. Comparison of two standard chemotherapy regimens for good-prognosis germ-cell tumours: a randomised trial. Australian and New Zealand Germ Cell Trial Group. *Lancet* 2001;357:739–745.
19. O'Sullivan JM, Huddart RA, Norman AR, et al. Predicting the risk of bleomycin lung toxicity in patients with germ-cell tumours. *Ann Oncol* 2003;14(1):91–96.
20. Lehne G, Johansen B, Fossa SD. Long-term follow-up of pulmonary function in patients cured from testicular cancer with combination chemotherapy including bleomycin. *Br J Cancer* 1993;68(3):555–558.
21. Williams S, Birch R, Einhorn L, et al. Treatment of disseminated germ-cell tumors with cisplatin, bleomycin, and either vinblastine or etoposide. *N Engl J Med* 1987;316(23):1435–1440.
22. Nichols CR, Catalano PJ, Crawford ED, et al. Randomized comparison of cisplatin and etoposide and either bleomycin or ifosfamide in treatment of advanced disseminated germ cell tumors: an Eastern Cooperative Oncology Group, Southwest Oncology Group, and Cancer and Leukemia Group B Study [see comment]. *J Clin Oncol* 1998;16(4):1287–1293.
23. Sleijfer S, van der Mark TW, Schrafford Koops H, et al. Decrease in pulmonary function during bleomycin-containing combination chemotherapy for testicular cancer: not only a bleomycin effect. *Br J Cancer* 1995;71(1):120–123.
24. McKeage MJ, Evans BD, Atkinson C, et al. Carbon monoxide diffusing capacity is a poor predictor of clinically significant bleomycin lung. New Zealand Clinical Oncology Group. *J Clin Oncol* 1990;8(5):779–783.
25. Sleijfer S, van der Mark TW, Schrafford Koops H, et al. Enhanced effects of bleomycin on pulmonary function disturbances in patients with decreased renal function due to cisplatin. *Eur J Cancer* 1996;32A(3):550–552.
26. Cisneros-Lira J, Gaxiola M, Ramos C, et al. Cigarette smoke exposure potentiates bleomycin-induced lung fibrosis in guinea pigs. *Am J Physiol Lung Cell Mol Physiol* 2003;285(4):L949–L956.
27. Takada K, Takahashi K, Sato S, et al. Cigarette smoke modifies bleomycin-induced lung injury to produce lung emphysema. *Tohoku J Exp Med* 1987;153(2):137–144.
28. Osanai K, Takahashi K, Suwabe A, et al. The effect of cigarette smoke on bleomycin-induced pulmonary fibrosis in hamsters. *Am Rev Respir Dis* 1988;138(5):1276–1281.
29. Hansen SW, Groth S, Sorensen PG, et al. Enhanced pulmonary toxicity in smokers with germ-cell cancer treated with cis-platinum, vinblastine and bleomycin: a long-term follow-up. *Eur J Cancer Clin Oncol* 1989;25(4):733–736.
30. Donat SM, Levy DA. Bleomycin associated pulmonary toxicity: is perioperative oxygen restriction necessary? *J Urol* 1998;160(4):1347–1352.
31. Luis M, Ayuso A, Martinez G, et al. Intraoperative respiratory failure in a patient after treatment with bleomycin: previous and current intraoperative exposure to 50% oxygen. *Eur J Anaesthesiol* 1999;16(1):66–68.
32. Goldiner PL, Carlon GC, Cvitkovic E, et al. Factors influencing postoperative morbidity and mortality in patients treated with bleomycin. *Br Med J* 1978;1(6128):1664–1667.
33. Bokemeyer C, Berger CC, Kuczyk MA, et al. Evaluation of long-term toxicity after chemotherapy for testicular cancer. *J Clin Oncol* 1996;14(11):2923–2932.
34. Kollmannsberger C, Kuzyck M, Mayer F, et al. Late toxicity following curative treatment of testicular cancer. *Semin Surg Oncol* 1999;17(4):275–281.
35. Hartmann JT, Kollmannsberger C, Kanz L, et al. Platinum organ toxicity and possible prevention in patients with testicular cancer. *Int J Cancer* 1999;83(4):866–869.
36. Bokemeyer C, Berger CC, Hartmann JT, et al. Analysis of risk factors for cisplatin-induced ototoxicity in patients with testicular cancer. *Br J Cancer* 1998;77(8):1355–1362.
37. Fossa SD, de Wit R, Roberts JT, et al. Quality of life in good prognosis patients with metastatic germ cell cancer: a prospective study of the European Organization for Research and Treatment of Cancer Genitourinary Group/Medical Research Council Testicular Cancer Study Group (30941/TE20). *J Clin Oncol* 2003;21(6):1107–1118.
38. Vogelzang NJ, Bosl GJ, Johnson K, et al. Raynaud's phenomenon: a common toxicity after combination chemotherapy for testicular cancer. *Ann Intern Med* 1981;95(3):288–292.
39. Meinardi MT, Gietema JA, van der Graaf WT, et al. Cardiovascular morbidity in long-term survivors of metastatic testicular cancer. *J Clin Oncol* 2000;18(8):1725–1732.
40. Gietema JA, Sleijfer DT, Willemse PH, et al. Long-term follow-up of cardiovascular risk factors in patients given chemotherapy for disseminated nonseminomatous testicular cancer. *Ann Intern Med* 1992;116(9):709–715.
41. Huddart RA, Norman A, Shahidi M, et al. Cardiovascular disease as a long-term complication of treatment for testicular cancer. *J Clin Oncol* 2003;21(8):1513–1523.
42. Zagars GK, Ballo MT, Lee AK, et al. Mortality after cure of testicular seminoma. *J Clin Oncol* 2004;22(4):640–647.
43. Fossa SD, Aass N, Winderen M, et al. Long-term renal function after treatment for malignant germ-cell tumours. *Ann Oncol* 2002;13(2):222–228.

44. Travis LB, Curtis RE, Storm H, et al. Risk of second malignant neoplasms among long-term survivors of testicular cancer. *J Natl Cancer Inst* 1997; 89(19):1429–1439.

45. Bokemeyer C, Schmoll HJ. Secondary neoplasms following treatment of malignant germ cell tumors. *J Clin Oncol* 1993;11(9):1703–1709.

46. Wanderas EH, Fossa SD, Tretli S. Risk of subsequent non-germ cell cancer after treatment of germ cell cancer in 2006 Norwegian male patients. *Eur J Cancer* 1997;33(2):253–262.

47. Bachaud JM, Berthier F, Soulie M, et al. Second non-germ cell malignancies in patients treated for stage I-II testicular seminoma. *Radiother Oncol* 1999;50(2):191–197.

48. van Leeuwen FE, Stiggelbout AM, van den Belt-Dusebout AW, et al. Second cancer risk following testicular cancer: a follow-up study of 1,909 patients. *J Clin Oncol* 1993;11(3):415–424.

49. Bokemeyer C, Berger CC, Hartmann JT, et al. Analysis of risk factors for cisplatin-induced ototoxicity in patients with testicular cancer. *Br J Cancer* 1998;77:1355–1362.

50. Travis LB, Andersson M, Gospodarowicz M, et al. Treatment-associated leukemia following testicular cancer. *J Natl Cancer Inst* 2000;92(14): 1165–1171.

51. Kaasa S, Aass N, Mastekaasa A, et al. Psychosocial well-being in testicular cancer patients. *Eur J Cancer* 1991;27(9):1091–1095.

52. Fossa SD, Dahl AA, Loge JH. Fatigue, anxiety, and depression in long-term survivors of testicular cancer. *J Clin Oncol* 2003;21(7):1249–1254.

53. Heidenreich A, Hofmann R. Quality-of-life issues in the treatment of testicular cancer. *World J Urol* 1999;17(4):230–238.

54. Fegg MJ, Gerl A, Vollmer TC, et al. Subjective quality of life and sexual functioning after germ-cell tumour therapy. *Br J Cancer* 2003;89(12): 2202–2206.

55. Berger CC, Bokemeyer C, Schuppert F, et al. Endocrinological late effects after chemotherapy for testicular cancer. *Br J Cancer* 1996;73(9): 1108–1114.

56. Strumberg D, Brugge S, Korn MW, et al. Evaluation of long-term toxicity in patients after cisplatin-based chemotherapy for non-seminomatous testicular cancer. *Ann Oncol* 2002;13(2):229–236.

57. DeSantis M, Albrecht W, Holtl W, et al. Impact of cytotoxic treatment on long-term fertility in patients with germ-cell cancer. *Int J Cancer* 1999; 83(6):864–865.

58. Hansen SW, Berthelsen JG, von der Maase H. Long-term fertility and leydig cell function in patients treated for germ cell cancer with cisplatin, vinblastine, and bleomycin versus surveillance. *J Clin Oncol* 1990;8(10): 1695–1698.

CHAPTER 42 ■ SIGNS, SYMPTOMS, AND PARANEOPLASTIC SYNDROMES OF RENAL CELL CARCINOMA

HYUNG L. KIM, JOHN S. LAM, AND ARIE S. BELLDEGRUN

Renal cell carcinoma (RCC) is the fourth most common genitourinary malignancy (1). It was estimated that in 2004, more than 35,000 new cases would be diagnosed and more than 12,000 deaths would result from RCC. At the time of diagnosis, approximately one third of patients would have metastatic disease, and 25% to 50% of patients would eventually have recurrence of RCC following treatment of localized RCC (2–5). Historically, the frequency of presentation of the classic triad of hematuria, palpable mass, and pain has been quoted as 10% (6). However, in a modern RCC series, a palpable mass was noted in <5% of patients diagnosed with RCC (7), and with widespread use of ultrasonography and computerized tomography (CT) scan, approximately 15% to 48% of RCC is incidentally diagnosed during an evaluation of an unrelated disorder (8,9).

BIOLOGY AND CLINICAL BEHAVIOR OF RENAL CELL CARCINOMA

Although localized RCC may produce paraneoplastic signs and symptoms, most of these patients have asymptomatic presentations. Well-established predictors of prognosis include stage, grade, and performance status (10). RCC is most commonly staged according to the tumor node metastasis (TNM) staging criteria proposed by the American Joint Committee on Cancer. Tumor grade is determined using the Fuhrman grading system, which categorizes nuclear grade. Performance status is determined by the patient's ability to provide self-care and perform normal, day-to-day activities. Table 42.1 shows the relation between stage and grade in patients who have undergone nephrectomy at UCLA (University of California-Los Angeles).

TABLE 42.1

STAGE DISTRIBUTION AT PRESENTATION AND GRADE DISTRIBUTION FOR EACH STAGE

TNM stage		Fuhrman grade			
Stage	%	1 (%)	2 (%)	3 (%)	4 (%)
I	30	31	56	13	0
II	8	10	67	22	1
III	18	7	50	38	5
IV	44	3	36	51	10

TNM, tumor node metastasis.

RCC has the propensity to invade the venous system and is associated with venous tumor thrombus in 4% to 25% of cases (11–13). RCC associated with tumor thrombus often present with symptoms. In a study of 1,087 patients at UCLA, most patients with inferior vena cava (IVC) and renal vein (RV) extension were symptomatic at diagnosis, and the rate of incidental RCC was significantly lower in patients with tumor thrombus than in patients without tumor thrombus (14). Of the 130 patients with an IVC thrombus, 11 (8.5%) had an ipsilateral acute varicocele, and 31 (24%) had lower extremity edema. The mean number of symptoms increased in direct relation to the extent of the tumor thrombus—IVC extension was associated with significantly more symptoms than was RV extension (Table 42.2). Hypercalcemia and anemia also increased in direct relation to thrombus extent. The incidence of hematuria (any degree or only macroscopic), polycythemia, and hypeension was similar in patients with and without metastasis regardless of tumor thrombus status. In patients without tumor thrombus, anemia and pleural effusion occurred considerably more often when metastatic disease was present, whereas in patients with tumor thrombus, hypercalcemia was more common when metastatic disease was present ($P = .01$).

Patients with metastatic RCC may present with symptoms secondary to the growth and to the extension of the primary tumor or the metastatic deposit. In a review of the UCLA study results, 61% of patients with metastatic RCC presented with involvement of the lungs (Table 42.3). Other frequent sites of metastatic involvement included lymph nodes in 35% of patients and bone in 27%. As expected, these same organ systems are also the most frequent sites of disease recurrence following nephrectomy for clinically localized disease (Table 42.4). The specific site of metastasis is not prognostically significant (15). When disease-specific survival was stratified by metastatic site, there was no survival difference for patients with involvement of the three most common sites (Fig. 42.1). However, the number of organ systems involved in metastatic RCC was a major predictor of survival (Fig. 42.2). Half of the number of patients presenting with metastatic disease had involvement of multiple organ systems (Table 42.5).

Patients newly diagnosed with RCC should undergo a metastatic workup that includes an abdominal CT scan or magnetic resonance imaging (MRI), chest radiograph, serum chemistries, and liver function tests. Any patient with hypercalcemia, bone pain, or poor performance status should also receive a bone scan. In one study, the frequency of bone metastasis was as high as 19% and 41% for patients with Eastern Cooperative Oncology Group (ECOG) performance status of 1 and ≥2, respectively (16). The initial workup should also include a careful and thorough neurologic evaluation, and any positive neurologic findings should prompt a brain MRI.

TABLE 42.2

PRESENTATION OF RENAL CELL CARCINOMA (LOCALIZED AND METASTATIC) WITH AND WITHOUT TUMOR THROMBUS IN PATIENTS UNDERGOING NEPHRECTOMY

	No tumor thrombus	Renal vein	Inferior vena cava	*P* value
Number of patients	607	107	100	
Number presenting with signs/symptoms (%)				
Incidental asymptomatic	128 (21%)	3 (3%)	2 (2%)	.002
Incidental symptomatic	96 (16%)	4 (4%)	3 (3%)	.001
Nonincidental symptomatic	383 (63%)	100 (94%)	95 (95%)	.002
Hematuria, flank mass + flank pain	4 (0.7%)	1	2 (2%)	NS
Macroscopic hematuria	126 (21%)	46 (43%)	35 (36%)	NS
Hypercalcemia	8 (1.3%)	4 (3.7%)	3 (3%)	.008
Polycythemia	3 (.5%)	2 (1.9%)	0	NS
Pleural effusion	15 (2.5%)	1 (.9%)	2 (2%)	NS
Anemia	36 (5.9%)	16 (15%)	20 (20%)	.0001
Mean number of symptoms/pt. ± SD:				
Renal cell carcinoma associated	.58 ± .69	.83 ± .73	2.43 ± 1.15	.1810
Nonspecific symptoms	.28 ± .53	.36 ± .57	.25 ± .46	.0457
Systemic symptoms	.70 ± 1.22	1.16 ± 1.53	1.51 ± 1.47	.0064

pt., patient; SD, standard deviation.

Although the brain is a relatively rare site for metastasis, the management of brain metastasis should receive the highest priority. The slightest growth in the metastatic deposit can result in significant functional consequences. Patients with brain metastasis should be urgently referred to neurosurgery and radiation oncology before further system therapy or cytoreductive nephrectomy is considered for them.

PROGNOSTIC IMPLICATIONS OF PARANEOPLASTIC SYNDROMES

Localized RCC rarely causes symptoms, and metastatic RCC may result in signs and symptoms specific to the site of metastatic disease. However, it is reported that approximately 20% of all patients diagnosed with RCC present with paraneoplastic symptoms (17). Another 10% to 40% of patients will develop paraneoplastic symptoms during the course of their disease. Paraneoplastic findings are distinct from the sequelae of local or distant invasion by RCC. These findings represent a constellation of signs and symptoms that result from the humoral release of various tumor-associated proteins. The proteins responsible for the paraneoplastic effects may be elaborated directly by the tumor cells or by the immune system in response to the tumor. As a rule, paraneoplastic effects resolve following complete surgical resection of the tumor.

Paraneoplastic syndromes include a long list of varied signs and symptoms. In a modern series of patients with RCC, the most common findings at the time of presentation were anemia, hepatic dysfunction, unintended weight loss, malaise, hypoalbuminemia, and hypercalcemia (Table 42.6) (7). These findings likely represent paraneoplastic effects; however, confirmation of a paraneoplastic effect requires the documentation of resolution of the sign or symptom following complete resection. Most findings listed in Table 42.6 occurred more

TABLE 42.3

SITES OF METASTATIC INVOLVEMENT IN PATIENTS PRESENTING WITH METASTATIC RENAL CELL CARCINOMA

Site	%
Lung	61
Lymph nodes	35
Bone	27
Adrenal	16
Liver	13
Contralateral kidney	10
Brain	6
Soft tissue	4

TABLE 42.4

SITES OF RECURRENCE AFTER NEPHRECTOMY FOR LOCALIZED RENAL CELL CARCINOMA

Site	%
Lung	50
Lymph nodes	15
Bone	10
Local	7
Adrenal	5
Liver	5
Brain	4
Soft tissue	2
Contralateral kidney	2

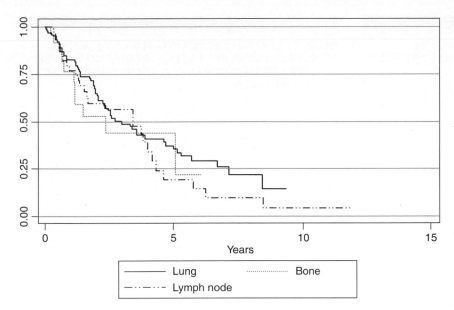

FIGURE 42.1. Site of solitary metastasis. Disease-specific survival.

frequently in patients with localized rather than metastatic RCC, suggesting that these findings reflect tumor biology rather than simply the local or distal extent of the tumor. In a univariate analysis, all but the rarest findings portended a significantly worse prognosis. The highest hazard scores were associated with anorexia, unintended weight loss, malaise, thrombocytosis, and night sweats.

Of the paraneoplastic effects examined in the UCLA series, hypoalbuminemia, weight loss, anorexia, and malaise were the predictors of poor survival that were independent of stage, grade, and performance status (Table 42.7) (7). All four independent predictors of survival are also signs and symptoms associated with tumor cachexia; therefore, the term *cachexia-related finding* was coined in the study. Although there was a trend toward worse survival with increasing numbers of cachexia-related findings, the difference in survival between patients with one versus all four cachexia-related findings was not statistically different (Fig. 42.3). In patients with localized RCC, the 2-year survival rate was 95% in patients without cachexia compared with 79% in patients with at least one cachexia-related finding (P <.0001). In patients

with metastatic RCC, the median survival was 12 months in patients with cachexia compared with 31 months in patients without cachexia (P <.001).

Cachexia is a universal finding in patients with widely metastatic and advanced malignancies. Therefore, in order to better assess whether cachexia reflects tumor biology in addition to tumor burden, patients with localized T1 RCC were evaluated in a separate study (18). In this subgroup, at least one of the cachexia-related findings was found in approximately 15% of the patients. Cachexia was an independent predictor for both tumor recurrence following nephrectomy and poor survival. The effect of cachexia on survival rates was most pronounced for patients with high-grade RCC where the presence and absence of cachexia were associated with 5-year survival rates of 55% and 75%, respectively.

Several studies have compared the prognostic significance of symptomatic presentation of RCC. In these studies, all patients with a variety of symptoms were grouped together. Two previous reports concluded that there was no difference in prognosis for patients with RCC presenting with symptoms or without symptoms (19,20). However, others have reported that symptomatic

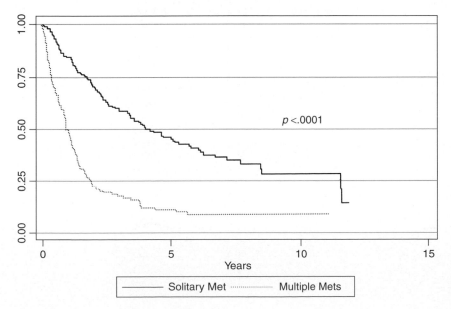

FIGURE 42.2. Number of organ systems involved. Disease-specific survival.

TABLE 42.5

NUMBER OF ORGAN SYSTEMS INVOLVED IN PATIENTS PRESENTING WITH METASTATIC RENAL CELL CARCINOMA

Number of organ systems	%
1	50
2	33
3	12
≥4	5

presentation portends a worse prognosis (8,21,22). These conflicting results suggest that specific signs and symptoms (i.e., cachexia-related findings), and not simply the presence or absence of symptoms, have a prognostic significance.

METABOLIC SYNDROMES

Paraneoplastic effects result from elaboration of various proteins by the tumor or by normal cells in response to the tumor. Hypercalcemia affects 10% to 20% of patients with cancer and has been reported in up to 20% of patients with RCC (23,24). Hypercalcemia in patients with solid tumors and no bone metastases ("humoral hypercalcemia") is a phenomenon that has undergone considerable research over the past 20 years. Several humoral mediators of bone resorption have been identified. Secretion of parathyroid hormone (PTH)–like peptide as well as PTH by the tumor has been implicated as the cause of hypercalcemia (25). Recent studies have examined a possible contribution of interleukin-6 (IL-6), known to stimulate osteoclastic bone resorption, to the hypercalcemia of RCC (24). Other humoral factors described as contributing to the humoral hypercalcemia of malignancy include osteoclast-activating factor (OAF), transforming growth factor-α (TGF-α), interleukin-1 (IL-1), and tumor necrosis factor-α (TNF-α) (23). The clinical

TABLE 42.7

PRESENTATIONS PREDICTING SURVIVAL AFTER CONTROLLING FOR STAGE[a], GRADE AND EASTERN COOPERATIVE ONCOLOGY GROUP–PEFORMANCE STATUS (ECOG-PS)

	Hazard ratio	95% CI	P value
Hypoalbuminemia	1.4	1.0–2.1	.0402
Weight loss	1.4	1.1–1.8	.0079
Anorexia	1.5	1.1–2.0	.0193
Malaise	1.6	1.2–2.1	.0005
At least one of the above (Cachexia)	2.8	2.1–3.8	<.0001

[a]TNM stage was controlled as T category, N category, and M category presence of hypoalbuminemia (<3.6 g/dL), Weight loss (>5 lb), anorexia or malaise.

manifestations of hypercalcemia are influenced by many factors that include the duration of hypercalcemia, performance status, age, prior chemotherapy, hepatic or renal dysfunction, as well as sites of metastatic disease (26).

Initial therapy for patients with symptomatic hypercalcemia is aggressive intravascular volume replacement with normal saline. Once intravascular volume has been replaced, loop diuretics can be added to promote urinary calcium excretion. Following initial fluid replacement, therapy is directed at normalizing calcium homeostasis by inhibiting osteoclastic bone resorption. The bisphosphonates are the most effective agents, and these drugs are thought to work by several mechanisms, including inhibition of hydroxyapatite crystal growth and direct osteoclast cytotoxic effects (27).

Hypercalcemia may also be secondary to stimulation of osteoclasts by metastatic deposits in the bone (28). The etiology of metastatic hypercalcemia has not been completely defined, but

TABLE 42.6

PRESENTATION OF RENAL CELL CARCINOMA (LOCALIZED AND METASTATIC) AND EFFECT ON DISEASE-SPECIFIC SURVIVAL

	Percent (n)	Localized/ metastatic	Hazard ratio	P Value (Univariate)
Paraneoplastic				
Anemia	52	.7	2.0	<.0001
Hepatic dysfunction	32	.6	2.1	<.0001
Weight loss	23	.3	3.0	<.0001
Malaise	19	.6	2.9	<.0001
Hypoalbuminemia	20	.6	2.3	<.0001
Hypercalcemia	13	.6	1.8	.0223
Anorexia	11	.4	3.1	<.0001
Thrombocytosis	9	.6	2.6	<.0001
Night sweats	8	.6	2.5	<.0001
Fever	8	.5	2.0	<.0001
Hypertension	3	.6	1.4	.3945
Erythrocytosis	4	.47	1.4	.1810
Chills	3	.6	1.7	.0457
Classic Triad				
Gross hematuria	24	.7	1.2	.0744
Flank pain	20	.6	1.3	.0631
Flank/abdominal mass	4	.4	1.8	.0064

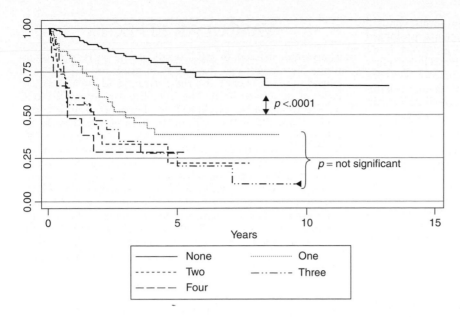

FIGURE 42.3. Number of cachexia-related symptoms. Disease-specific survival.

prostaglandin secretion by tumor cells has been linked to bone resorption. Local and systemic factors mediating bone resorption have also been described (28). The presentation, clinical course, and therapy for metastatic hypercalcemia are similar to those of humoral hypercalcemia of malignancy. However, patients with metastatic hypercalcemia may not respond to nephrectomy, in contrast to patients with nonmetastatic hypercalcemia. In addition, hypercalcemia associated with bone disease may be improved with radiotherapy (RT).

Hypertension is present in up to 25% of patients with RCC, and renin production by the tumor has been documented in 37% of patients (17). Hypertension may result from the secretion of renin by the tumor itself or by the juxtaglomerular apparatus in response to the local extension of the tumor. The excess renin and hypertension associated with RCC is generally refractory to antihypertensive therapy but may respond to nephrectomy. Other potential mechanisms for hypertension in RCC include polycythemia, compression of the renal artery, or arteriovenous shunting secondary to tumor vascularity because renin levels may rise when tumor growth exceeds blood supply.

The list of potential paraneoplastic findings with less-established association with RCC is long. Endocrine disorders that may represent paraneoplastic effects include Cushing syndrome (29), hyperprolactinemia (30), and abnormalities in glucose metabolism that may result in hyperglycemia or hypoglycemia (31,32).

HEMATOLOGIC SYNDROMES

Erythrocytosis is thought to result from ectopic production of erythropoietin by RCC and may even predict response to immunotherapy (33). The etiology for erythrocytosis is felt to be increased erythropoietin production or production of a biologically analogous substance by the tumor (34). Local tissue hypoxia resulting from the presence of the tumor was postulated as a possible cause of erythrocytosis in some patients (35,36). Erythrocytosis typically resolves following nephrectomy or resection of metastases, but it may reappear with disease recurrence (37).

Only 1% to 8% of patients with RCC manifest erythrocytosis (35,36). Anemia is much more common, and, at the time of diagnosis, 16% to 40% of patients are anemic (35,36). The anemia generally is normocytic or microcytic and hypochromic. Autoimmune hemolytic anemia has been reported in a few patients

in association with RCC (38). Although the anemia generally is consistent with that of chronic disease, there sometimes is a severe anemia, with hematocrit levels from 15% to 25% without evidence of bleeding or hemolysis. Suppression of erythropoietin production by the tumor that is capable of secreting an "antierythropoietin" is a possible mechanism.

Leukocytosis and thrombocytosis also are observed occasionally in patients with RCC. Some correlation of platelet levels with IL-6 levels has been shown (39). Some patients with metastatic RCC have been reported to have elevated levels of IL-6 (40). In a subsequent report, normalization of platelet counts occurred following the administration of anti-IL-6 to 12 patients with RCC, elevated IL-6 levels, and thrombocytosis (41). After withdrawal of anti-IL-6, platelet counts returned to pretreatment levels at 19 days. This observation suggests that the paraneoplastic thrombocytosis may be mediated by IL-6, either directly or indirectly, by stimulating other cytokines. Leukocytosis could be related to tumor necrosis or could be cytokine mediated. Leukemoid reactions are known to occur with RCC, although it is not clear whether an associated myeloproliferative disease was entirely excluded in some patients (42). Eosinophilia has also been noted in RCC, but this is infrequent (43). Pancytopenia has occurred occasionally in patients with RCC, and it almost invariably has been associated with involvement of the bone marrow by the tumor. Disorders of coagulation are observed occasionally in RCC, and such disorders appear to be part of the spectrum of malignancy-associated coagulopathy.

Amyloidosis is characterized by abnormal protein deposition in the extracellular spaces of various organs and has been reported in 3% to 8% of patients with RCC (17). The pathogenesis of the amyloidosis is poorly understood, but its disappearance after nephrectomy clearly indicates it is paraneoplastic. The amyloid has been characterized as AA protein (44).

HEPATIC SYNDROMES

For most paraneoplastic findings, the precise etiology is poorly understood. Stauffer (45) first described a patient with RCC with hepatic dysfunction in the absence of hepatic metastasis. Following nephrectomy, the hepatic dysfunction resolved. The incidence of Stauffer syndrome varies from 3% to 20% (37). Patients classically present with hepatosplenomegaly, fever, fatigue, and weight loss. Several biochemical abnormalities are present, which include elevated transaminases levels, elevated alkaline phosphatase levels, hypoprothrombinemia, prolonged partial thromboplastin time, and elevated α_2-globulin levels (34,37,46). A variety of mechanisms for hepatocellular injury have been proposed, including secretion of hepatotoxins by the tumor and activation of the immune system against hepatocytes (47). However, the exact nature of the hepatotoxin thought to cause Stauffer syndrome has yet to be characterized.

RENAL SYNDROMES

Paraneoplastic glomerulopathies are recognized in association with RCC, although they are considered to be rare (48). These renal syndromes are attributed to the formation of immune complexes. The glomerulopathies associated with RCC are described as membranous glomerulonephritis and minimal-change glomerulonephritis. The nephrotic syndrome may be the presenting clinical finding.

NEUROMUSCULAR SYNDROMES

Rare cases of neuromyopathies, such as polyneuromyopathy, polymyositis, and myopathy, have been reported in patients with RCC that has resolved following nephrectomy (49,50). With the development of metastatic disease, polymyositis and polyneuromyopathy have recurred. The myopathy is characterized as involving proximal muscles and is associated with elevated serum levels of creatine kinase and aldolase. Approximately 4% of patients are observed to have paraneoplastic polyneuropathy. Paraneoplastic neurologic syndromes sometimes are attributed to autoimmune mechanisms (51).

PARANEOPLASTIC SKIN CONDITIONS

Several cutaneous markers of malignancy may be associated with RCC (52–54). Dermatitis herpetiformis and cutaneous leukocytoclastic vasculitis are reported (52,53). In some patients, the cutaneous lesions antedated the diagnosis of the disease and may completely clear after nephrectomy. Hypertrichosis lanuginosa acquisita has been reported in one patient with RCC (54). After nephrectomy, no further hair growth developed, but the existing hair pattern did not change. Levels of testosterone, follicle-stimulating hormone, luteinizing hormone, and serum dehydroepiandrosterone were normal.

CONSTITUTIONAL SYMPTOMS

Nonspecific symptoms such as cachexia and malaise are common presenting features in up to one-third of patients with RCC (17). It has been suggested that cachexia and malaise may be due to the secretion of TNF-α, IL-1, IL-6, γ-interferon by the tumor or by the infiltrating immune cells (34,55). The cachexia may improve after resection of the tumor, but it typically represents widespread disease. Fever has been reported in 15% to 80% of patients with RCC and is the presenting sign of malignancy in approximately 2% to 12% of patients (34,56,57). The fever disappears after nephrectomy and may recur when metastases develop. IL-6 has been identified as a cytokine that may stimulate acute-phase reactants in patients with RCC (58,59). The reactants may, in turn, cause paraneoplastic syndromes such as fever and hepatic dysfunction.

VASCULAR EFFECTS

The vascular effects of RCC occur on the basis of two features: the tendency of the tumor to grow into the RV and extend to the vena cava and right atrium, and the high vascularity of the tumor itself. The intravascular growth of RCC has led to a number of clinical developments. Tumor extension into the RV or IVC with obstruction may lead to the development of a right- or left-sided varicocele, which sometimes has been a presenting sign of RCC (3). Hepatic vein occlusion with Budd-Chiari syndrome also is recognized (60). Tumor emboli to the lung also occur as a direct consequence of the intravascular growth of RCC (61). The vascular effects of RCC related to the vascularity of the tumor are less varied but are clinically significant. There may be an audible bruit over the tumor or its metastases (57). Renal arteriovenous fistula may occur with growth into the RV and erosion into the renal artery (62,63). Cardiomegaly or congestive failure may develop as a consequence of arteriovenous fistulas involving the primary tumor or highly vascular metastatic deposits (62,63). When the primary tumor functions as an arteriovenous fistula, nephrectomy has been followed by a decrease in cardiomegaly and a reversal of congestive heart failure (64).

CONCLUSION

Given the wide range of signs and symptoms associated with RCC, a thorough evaluation at the time of presentation is crucial. In general, paraneoplastic findings imply a worse prognosis. Paraneoplastic findings that independently predict poor prognosis include hypoalbuminemia, weight loss, anorexia, and malaise. Although symptomatic treatment may be indicated, the most effective treatment of paraneoplastic findings in patients with localized disease is a nephrectomy.

References

1. Jemal A, Tiwari RC, Murray T, et al. Cancer statistics, 2004. *CA Cancer J Clin* 2004;54:8–29.
2. Rabinovitch RA, Zelefsky MJ, Gaynor JJ, et al. Patterns of failure following surgical resection of renal cell carcinoma: implications for adjuvant local and systemic therapy. *J Clin Oncol* 1994;12:206–212.
3. Skinner DG, Colvin RB, Vermillion CD, et al. Diagnosis and management of renal cell carcinoma. A clinical and pathologic study of 309 cases. *Cancer* 1971;28:1165–1177.
4. Hock LM, Lynch J, Balaji KC. Increasing incidence of all stages of kidney cancer in the last 2 decades in the United States: an analysis of surveillance, epidemiology and end results program data. *J Urol* 2002;167:57–60.
5. deKernion JB. Treatment of advanced renal cell carcinoma—traditional methods and innovative approaches. *J Urol* 1983;130:2–7.
6. deKernion JB, Lowitz B, Casciato D. Urinary tract cancers. In: Casciato D, Lowitz B, eds. *Manual of clinical oncology.* Boston, MA: Little, Brown and Company, 1998:198–219.
7. Kim HL, Belldegrun AS, Freitas DG, et al. Paraneoplastic signs and symptoms of renal cell carcinoma: implications for prognosis. *J Urol* 2003;170: 1742–1746.
8. Tsui KH, Shvarts O, Smith RB, et al. Renal cell carcinoma: prognostic significance of incidentally detected tumors. *J Urol* 2000;163:426–430.
9. Konnak JW, Grossman HB. Renal cell carcinoma as an incidental finding. *J Urol* 1985;134:1094–1096.
10. Zisman A, Pantuck AJ, Dorey F, et al. Improved prognostication of renal cell carcinoma using an integrated staging system. *J Clin Oncol* 2001;19: 1649–1657.
11. Ljungberg B, Stenling R, Osterdahl B, et al. Vein invasion in renal cell carcinoma: impact on metastatic behavior and survival. *J Urol* 1995;154: 1681–1684.
12. Naitoh J, Kaplan A, Dorey F, et al. Metastatic renal cell carcinoma with concurrent inferior vena caval invasion: long-term survival after combination therapy with radical nephrectomy, vena caval thrombectomy and postoperative immunotherapy. *J Urol* 1999;162:46–50.
13. Pagano F, Dal Bianco M, Artibani W, et al. Renal cell carcinoma with extension into the inferior vena cava: problems in diagnosis, staging and treatment. *Eur Urol* 1992;22:200–203.

14. Zisman A, Pantuck AJ, Chao DH, et al. Renal cell carcinoma with tumor thrombus: is cytoreductive nephrectomy for advanced disease associated with an increased complication rate? *J Urol* 2002;168:962–967.

15. Han KR, Pantuck AJ, Bui MH, et al. Number of metastatic sites rather than location dictates overall survival of patients with node-negative metastatic renal cell carcinoma. *Urology* 2003;61:314–319.

16. Shvarts O, Lam JS, Kim HL, et al. Eastern Cooperative Oncology Group performance status predicts bone metastasis in patients presenting with renal cell carcinoma: implication for preoperative bone scans. *J Urol* 2004; 172:867–870.

17. McDougal SW, Garnick MB. Clinical signs and symptoms of renal cell carcinoma. In: Vogelzang NJ, Scardino PT, Shipley WU, et al. *Comprehensive textbook of genitourinary oncology*, 2nd ed. Philadelphia, PA: Lippincott Williams & Wilkins, 2000:111–115.

18. Kim HL, Han KR, Zisman A, et al. Cachexia-like symptoms predict a worse prognosis in localized t1 renal cell carcinoma. *J Urol* 2004;171: 1810–1813.

19. Jayson M, Sanders H. Increased incidence of serendipitously discovered renal cell carcinoma. *Urology* 1998;51:203–205.

20. Mevorach RA, Segal AJ, Tersegno ME, et al. Renal cell carcinoma: incidental diagnosis and natural history: review of 235 cases. *Urology* 1992; 39:519–522.

21. Kattan MW, Reuter V, Motzer RJ, et al. A postoperative prognostic nomogram for renal cell carcinoma. *J Urol* 2001;166:63–67.

22. Thompson IM, Peek M. Improvement in survival of patients with renal cell carcinoma—the role of the serendipitously detected tumor. *J Urol* 1988;140:487–490.

23. Muggia FM. Overview of cancer-related hypercalcemia: epidemiology and etiology. *Semin Oncol* 1990;17:3–9.

24. Weissglas M, Schamhart D, Lowik C, et al. Hypercalcemia and cosecretion of interleukin-6 and parathyroid hormone related peptide by a human renal cell carcinoma implanted into nude mice. *J Urol* 1995;153: 854–857.

25. Mangin M, Webb AC, Dreyer BE, et al. Identification of a cDNA encoding a parathyroid hormone-like peptide from a human tumor associated with humoral hypercalcemia of malignancy. *Proc Natl Acad Sci U S A* 1988; 85:597–601.

26. Warrell RP Jr. Metabolic emergencies. In: DeVita JVT, Hellman S, Rosenberg SA, eds. *Cancer principles and practices of oncology*, 6th ed., Vol. 2. Philadelphia, PA: Lippincott Williams & Wilkens, 2001:2633–2644.

27. Berenson JR, Lichtenstein A, Porter L, et al, Myeloma Aredia Study Group. Efficacy of pamidronate in reducing skeletal events in patients with advanced multiple myeloma. *N Engl J Med* 1996;334:488–493.

28. Mundy GR. Pathophysiology of cancer-associated hypercalcemia. *Semin Oncol* 1990;17:10–15.

29. Riggs BL Jr, Sprague RG. Association of Cushing's syndrome and neoplastic disease: observations in 232 cases of Cushing's syndrome and review of the literature. *Arch Intern Med* 1961;108:841–849.

30. Turkington RW. Ectopic production of prolactin. *N Engl J Med* 1971;285: 1455–1458.

31. Gleeson MH, Bloom SR, Polak JM, et al. Endocrine tumour in kidney affecting small bowel structure, motility, and absorptive function. *Gut* 1971; 12:773–782.

32. Pavelic K, Popovic M. Insulin and glucagon secretion by renal adenocarcinoma. *Cancer* 1981;48:98–100.

33. Janik JE, Sznol M, Urba WJ, et al. Erythropoietin production. A potential marker for interleukin-2/interferon-responsive tumors. *Cancer* 1993;72: 2656–2659.

34. Laski ME, Vugrin D. Paraneoplastic syndromes in hypernephroma. *Semin Nephrol* 1987;7:123–130.

35. Kvarstein B, Lindemann R, Mathisen W. Renal carcinoma with increased erythropoietin production and secondary polycythemia. *Scand J Urol Nephrol* 1973;7:178–180.

36. von Knorring J, Selroos O, Scheinin TM. Haematologic findings in patients with renal carcinoma. *Scand J Urol Nephrol* 1981;15:279–283.

37. Rosenblum SL. Paraneoplastic syndromes associated with renal cell carcinoma. *J S C Med Assoc* 1987;83:375–378.

38. Bradley GW, Harvey M. Haemolytic anaemia with hypernephroma. *Postgrad Med J* 1981;57:46–47.

39. Ishibashi T, Kimura H, Shikama Y, et al. Interleukin-6 is a potent thrombopoietic factor in vivo in mice. *Blood* 1989;74:1241–1244.

40. Blay JY, Negrier S, Combaret V, et al. Serum level of interleukin 6 as a prognosis factor in metastatic renal cell carcinoma. *Cancer Res* 1992;52: 3317–3322.

41. Blay JY, Favrot M, Rossi JF, et al. Role of interleukin-6 in paraneoplastic thrombocytosis. *Blood* 1993;82:2261–2262.

42. Reiss O. Leukemoid reaction due to hypernephroma. *JAMA* 1962;180: 1126–1127.

43. Bauke J, Rottger P. Intense eosinophilic reaction in hypernephroma. *Med Welt* 1966;16:865–874.

44. Vanatta PR, Silva FG, Taylor WE, et al. Renal cell carcinoma and systemic amyloidosis: demonstration of AA protein and review of the literature. *Hum Pathol* 1983;14:195–201.

45. Stauffer MH. Nephrogenic hepatosplenomegaly. *Gastroenterology* 1961; 40:694.

46. Hanash KA. The nonmetastatic hepatic dysfunction syndrome associated with renal cell carcinoma (hypernephroma): Stauffer's syndrome. *Prog Clin Biol Res* 1982;100:301–316.

47. Eddleston AL. Immunology and the liver. In: Parker CW, ed. *Clinical immunology*. Philadelphia, PA: Saunders, 1980:1009.

48. Norris SH. Paraneoplastic glomerulopathies. *Semin Nephrol* 1993;13: 258–272.

49. Evans BK, Fagan C, Arnold T, et al. Paraneoplastic motor neuron disease and renal cell carcinoma: improvement after nephrectomy. *Neurology* 1990;40:960–962.

50. Thomas NE, Passamonte PM, Sunderrajan EV, et al. Bilateral diaphragmatic paralysis as a possible paraneoplastic syndrome from renal cell carcinoma. *Am Rev Respir Dis* 1984;129:507–509.

51. Darnell RB. Onconeural antigens and the paraneoplastic neurologic disorders: at the intersection of cancer, immunity, and the brain. *Proc Natl Acad Sci U S A* 1996;93:4529–4536.

52. Gjone E, Nordoy A. Dermatitis herpetiformis, steatorrhoea, and malignancy. *Br Med J* 1970;1:610.

53. Lacour JP, Castanet J, Perrin C, et al. Cutaneous leukocytoclastic vasculitis and renal cancer: two cases *Am J Med* 1993;94:104–108

54. Duncan LE, Hemming JD. Renal cell carcinoma of the kidney and hypertrichosis lanuginosa acquisita. *Br J Urol* 1994;74:678–679.

55. Sufrin G, Mirand EA, Moore RH, et al. Hormones in renal cancer. *J Urol* 1977;117:433–438.

56. Gordon DA. The extrarenal manifestations of hypernephroma. *Can Med Assoc J* 1963;88:61–67.

57. Cronin RE, Kaehny WD, Miller PD, et al. Renal cell carcinoma: unusual systemic manifestations. *Medicine (Baltimore)* 1976;55:291–311.

58. Tsukamoto T, Kumamoto Y, Miyao N, et al. Interleukin-6 in renal cell carcinoma. *J Urol* 1992;148:1778–1781; discussion 1781–1772.

59. Jobe BA, Bierman MH, Mezzacappa FJ. Hyperglycemia as a paraneoplastic endocrinopathy in renal cell carcinoma: a case report and review of the literature. *Nebr Med J* 1993;78:349–351.

60. Schwerk WB, Schwerk WN, Rodeck G. Venous renal tumor extension: a prospective US evaluation. *Radiology* 1985;156:491–495.

61. Greenberg RE, Charles RS, Samaha AM, et al. Surgical management of recurrent genitourinary malignancies. *Semin Oncol* 1993;20:473–492.

62. Wise GJ, Bosniak MA, Hudson PB. Arteriovenous fistula associated with renal cell carcinoma of the kidney. Report of three cases with cardiovascular findings. *Br J Urol* 1967;39:170–177.

63. Sondag TJ, Patel SK, Petasnick JP, et al. Hypernephromas with massive arteriovenous fistulas. *Am J Roentgenol Radium Ther Nucl Med* 1973;117: 97–103.

64. Pickens S. Hypernephroma presenting as cardiomegaly. *Br Med J* 1973;3: 678–679.

CHAPTER 43 ■ EPIDEMIOLOGY OF RENAL CELL CARCINOMA

WONG-HO CHOW, SUSAN S. DEVESA, AND LEE E. MOORE

Malignant tumors of the kidney account for more than 2% of cancer incidence and mortality in the United States, with over 36,000 new cases and 12,000 deaths having been estimated for 2005 (1). More than 85% of kidney cancers arise in the renal parenchyma, with the remainder arising in the renal pelvis (2). Nearly all kidney cancers originating in the renal parenchyma are adenocarcinomas [renal cell carcinoma (RCC)], whereas most of the renal pelvis cancers are transitional cell carcinomas. It is estimated that 80% to 85% of the RCCs are of the clear cell type, whereas approximately 10% are of the papillary type, with the remainder made up of rare histologic types such as oncocytomas and chromophobe carcinomas (3,4).

The etiology of renal carcinomas varies by subsite of origin. Cigarette smoking and phenacetin-containing analgesics, now withdrawn from most markets worldwide, are the major determinants of renal pelvis cancer (5,6), whereas the risk factors for RCC are more diverse. This chapter focuses on RCC.

DESCRIPTIVE EPIDEMIOLOGY

Incidence Patterns

On the basis of data from nine registries, the U.S. Surveillance, Epidemiology, and End Results (SEER) program (7,8) reported that the age-adjusted (2000 US standard) incidence rates of RCC during 1996 to 2000 for white men, white women, African-American men, and African American women were 12.6, 5.9, 14.3, and 7.6 per 100,000 person-years, respectively.

Incidence rates during 1988 to 2000 increased consistently with age, before plateauing around the age of 70 years (Fig. 43.1). Overall, rates for men were approximately twice those for women, with the excesses most prominent after the age of 45 years. In both men and women, rates were higher among blacks than whites across almost all ages.

Incidence rates of kidney cancer vary substantially worldwide, driven predominantly by renal cell cancer rates (Fig. 43.2) (9). The highest rates were reported in several Central European and Scandinavian countries, whereas intermediate rates were observed in North America. There were greater variations in incidence rates across countries in Europe than across racial/ethnic subgroups in the United States and Canada. A notable exception was the low rates among Asians in the United States (exemplified by Japanese in Hawaii in Fig. 43.2), which is consistent with the low rates among Asians in their countries of origin (9,10). In contrast, despite the relatively

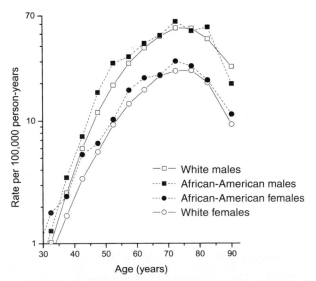

FIGURE 43.1. Age-specific renal cell carcinoma incidence rates by race and gender, SEER 9, 1988–2000.

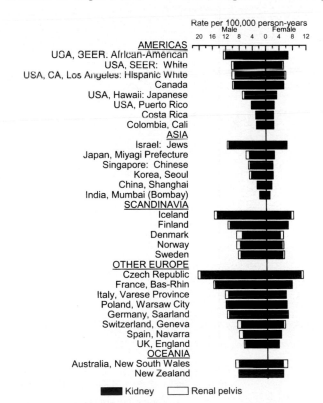

FIGURE 43.2. International variation in total kidney cancer, renal cell cancer, and renal pelvis cancer; age-adjusted (world standard) incidence by continent, registry, and gender, 1993–1997. (Source: from Parkin DM, Whelan SL, Ferlay J, et al. *Cancer incidence in five continents, volume VIII,* IARC Scientific Publications No. 155, Lyon: International Agency for Research on Cancer, 2002.)

high incidence of this cancer among Hispanics in the United States, low rates were reported in Central and South America.

Recent geographic patterns of incidence (7) and mortality rates (11) have not revealed evidence of an urban/rural gradient, as suggested in some earlier studies (6,12). Studies examining education level, income, or social class have shown no consistent relation to renal cancer (13–18).

Time Trends

RCC incidence rates have increased steadily in the United States over time (Fig. 43.3) (8). Between 1975 and 2000, the incidence rates were increasing annually by 2.3% among white men, 2.8% among white women, 3.1% among black men, and 4.1% among black women. Since the mid-1980s, the incidence rates among blacks have exceeded those among whites in both sexes. Renal cell cancer incidence rates rose across all ages among all race/gender groups (Fig. 43.4). The increases were most rapid among persons aged 65 to 84 years and were generally least pronounced among individuals aged 85 and older. Rapid increases in kidney cancer incidence also have been observed in other countries (9,19–22). In addition, kidney cancer mortality rates in the United States increased until the early 1990s, especially among blacks, when rates leveled among the four major race and gender groups (Fig. 43.3).

Clinical surveys of patients with RCC have revealed that the incidental detection of renal tumors is rising, at least partly because of increased use of imaging procedures such as computerized axial tomography (CAT) scan and magnetic resonance imaging (MRI) (23–25). The incidentally detected renal cell cancers tend to be smaller in size and have an improved prognosis. The leveling of kidney cancer mortality trends since the early 1990s, along with the more rapid increases in incidence trends for tumors diagnosed at localized stage (Fig. 43.5), supports this clinical observation. However, upward trends are also observed for tumors diagnosed at more advanced stages, particularly among African-American women. These patterns suggest that the incidental diagnosis of preclinical tumors is not likely to fully explain the upward trends of RCC.

Stage at Diagnosis and Survival

Consistent with the temporal incidence trends, the proportion of renal cell cancers that are diagnosed at localized stage has increased. Overall, 56% of the RCCs reported to the SEER program from 1990 to 1999 were localized tumors, compared with 45% of those diagnosed during 1975 to 1984. Improvement in stage at diagnosis is seen across all racial and gender groups, although African-Americans tend to have a higher proportion of localized tumors than whites (Table 43.1).

The overall 5-year relative survival rate, which is the percentage of patients diagnosed with renal cell cancer who survived 5 years after diagnosis, adjusting for the expected survival experience of the general population, has improved over time (Table 43.2). For patients diagnosed from 1990 to 1999, the overall 5-year relative survival rates were 67%, 69%, 64%, and 66% for white men, white women, black men, and black women, respectively. Compared to whites, the

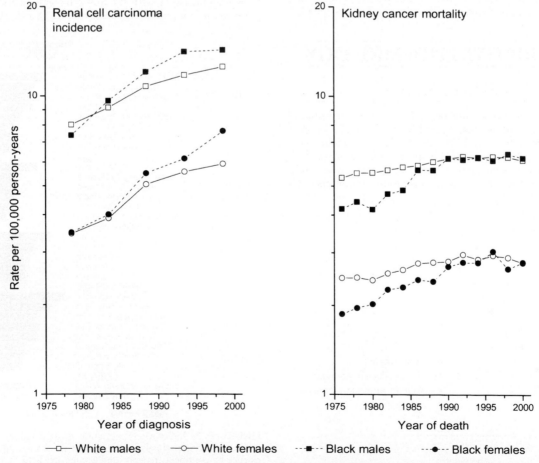

FIGURE 43.3. Age-adjusted (2000 US standard) trends in SEER 9 incidence rates for renal cell carcinoma 1976–1980 to 1996–2000 and US mortality rates for total kidney cancer 1975–1976 to 1999–2000 by race and gender.

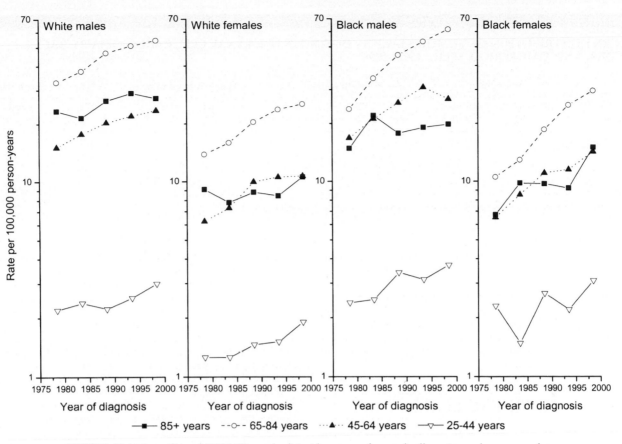

FIGURE 43.4. Age-adjusted (2000 US standard) incidence rates for renal cell carcinoma by race, gender, and age group at iagnosis, SEER 9, 1976–1980 to 1996–2000.

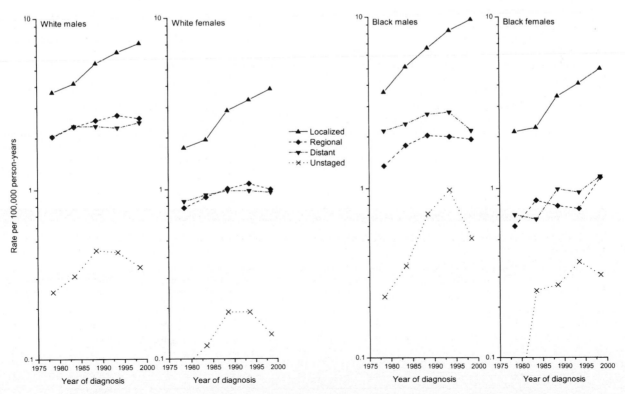

FIGURE 43.5. Age-adjusted (2000 US standard) incidence rates for renal cell carcinoma by race, gender, and tumor stage at diagnosis, SEER 9, 1976–1980 to 1996–2000.

TABLE 43.1

PERCENT DISTRIBUTION OF TUMOR STAGE AT DIAGNOSIS FOR RENAL CELL CARCINOMA BY RACE, GENDER, AND TIME PERIOD, SEER,[a] 1975–1999

Stage at diagnosis	White men		White women		African-American men		African-American women	
	1975–84 N = 5,234	1990–99 N = 8,427	1975–84 N = 2,740	1990–99 N = 4,880	1975–84 N = 438	1990–99 N = 930	1975–84 N = 242	1990–99 N = 623
Localized	43	54	48	60	46	60	56	64
Regional	27	23	24	19	23	15	22	14
Distant	27	21	26	19	28	20	19	17
Unstaged	3	3	3	3	3	5	4	5

[a]Surveillance, Epidemiology, and End Results program supported by the National Cancer Institute.

improvement in survival for black patients with localized tumors was more modest, whereas survival from distant and unstaged tumors declined over time. The racial disparities in survival across tumor stages explain, to some extent, the overall lower relative survival rates among blacks than among whites, despite the higher percentage of blacks with localized tumors. These survival patterns also argue against early detection of preclinical tumors as the sole explanation for the upward incidence trends of RCC.

RISK FACTORS

Several risk factors have been implicated in the development of RCC, including environmental and lifestyle factors such as smoking and certain medications, preexistent conditions such as obesity and hypertension, and genetic predispositions. Most of the information on risk factors has come from case-control studies, although cohort studies and family-based investigations have also contributed new insights.

Cigarette Smoking

Although the findings are not entirely consistent, most case–control studies have reported significantly elevated risks of RCC among cigarette smokers (12,14–17,26–36). The absence of significant associations in a few studies may be explained partly by small sample sizes and by the use of hospital controls with a high prevalence of smoking (13,37–41). Cohort studies with sufficient sample size have been generally positive, with a follow-up of US veterans showing a clear dose-response relation (42–44).

The relative risks associated with cigarette smoking are moderately elevated, ranging from 30% to 100%. A dose-response of risk with increasing amount or duration of smoking has been observed in both men and women (15,32–35,45). Among former smokers, the risk decreases with increasing years of smoking cessation, but the reduction in risk is generally small until at least 20 years after smoking cessation (34,35,45). An association with other tobacco products, including cigars, pipes, and chewing tobacco, has not been consistently observed (12,16,26,27,29,33–35,37).

Population-based attributable risks indicate that between approximately 27% to 37% of the incidences of renal cell cancers among men and 10% to 24% among women may be caused by cigarette smoking (26,31,46). However, it is unlikely that cigarette smoking has contributed to the recent upward trends of renal cell cancer because the prevalence of smoking in the United States has declined for over four decades (47).

Obesity

With a few exceptions (39,48,49), nearly all studies examining the relation of body weight and RCC have found a positive association. Obese persons have experienced elevated risks of 20% to more than 200%, and risks tend to rise with increasing levels of body mass index. The range of risks found in case-control studies (12,14,26,27,30,32,33,37,38,40,50–57) are comparable to those reported in several cohort studies (44,58–65), adding credence to the validity of this association. Weight fluctuation (52) and weight gain during adulthood (26,63) have been suggested as independent risk factors but have not been consistently observed in case-control studies (38,53,54). However, in a large cohort study of Swedish men

TABLE 43.2

RELATIVE 5-YEAR SURVIVAL RATE (%) FOR RENAL CELL CARCINOMA BY RACE, GENDER, AND TIME PERIOD, SEER,[a] 1975–1999

Stage at diagnosis	White men		White women		African-American men		African-American women	
	1975–84	1990–99	1975–84	1990–99	1975–84	1990–99	1975–84	1990–99
Total Invasive	55	67	55	69	55	64	61	66
Localized	84	93	84	92	82	86	86	87
Regional	55	63	54	62	55	65	47	55
Distant	8	9	5	8	11	4	5	4
Unstaged	48	50	44	34	43	32	60	41

[a]Surveillance, Epidemiology, and End Results program supported by the National Cancer Institute.

in which multiple measurements of height and weight were taken during a succession of health examinations, the risk increased further with increasing body mass index over time. Compared to men whose weight remained stable, the risk was doubled for men whose body mass index had increased by more than 14% over a 6-year period (64). Elevated kidney cancer mortality also has been linked to obesity in a large US cohort study (66).

In a case-control study conducted in Minnesota, it was estimated that approximately 20% of renal cell cancer cases are attributable to excess weight (46). Therefore, the marked increases in the prevalence of obesity in the United States during the last few decades (67,68) likely have contributed to the rising incidence of this cancer. The mechanism by which obesity predisposes to renal cell cancer is unclear. Obesity may influence risk by increasing the levels of endogenous estrogens (69) because estrogenic compounds have been shown to induce renal carcinomas in hamsters (70). Obesity also may increase the bioavailability of free insulinlike growth factors (71) that may be involved in renal carcinogenesis (72,73). In addition, obesity predisposes to hypertension, arterionephrosclerosis, and metabolic changes that may render the kidney more susceptible to tumor induction (74,75). Damage to the proximal renal tubules due to lipid peroxidation, which is increased in obese individuals, has also been suggested to be a mechanism leading to elevated risk of renal cell cancer (76).

Hypertension

Most epidemiologic studies that have examined the relation between hypertension and RCC have found excess risks ranging from 20% to nearly 200%. Although earlier epidemiologic studies were inconclusive about whether hypertension or its treatment is the main risk factor, recent studies have provided convincing evidence that hypertension per se plays a role in renal carcinogenesis. After adjustment for use of diuretics and/or other antihypertensive medications, some studies have found that the hypertension-related risk remains elevated (50, 77–80), whereas others have found that the risk is attenuated to insignificant levels (27,32,49,81–83). Some other studies did not adjust for medications as their use is highly correlated with hypertension (26,30,43,48,55,62,84–86). Although some investigations have found an excess risk only among hypertensive subjects who were medically treated (44,63,87), it is possible that treatment reflects the severity of the underlying disease and a prolonged course of hypertension and associated renovascular and other changes that may promote the development of cancer. In the Swedish cohort study, renal cell cancer risk was elevated with hypertension in a dose-response manner (64). Moreover, regardless of the baseline blood pressure levels, the risk further increased among those whose blood pressure increased above the baseline measurement and reduced among those whose blood pressure declined over time. The effect of hypertension on renal cell cancer risk was found to be independent of the effect of obesity. These data suggest that hypertension is a promoting factor in renal cell cancer development, and the risk can be modified with better control of blood pressure.

Because certain types of RCC can cause hypertension (88), several studies have focused on the risks among patients with long-term hypertension. Similar or greater excess risks were reported among patients with hypertension diagnosed 5 to more than 20 years previously (30,43,50,55,64,87), suggesting that the association with hypertension is unlikely to be an early manifestation of renal tumors.

In the United States, the prevalence of hypertension is highest among African-Americans, although it is increasing across all racial and gender groups (89). The increases in hypertension prevalence likely have contributed to the upward trends of RCC and perhaps also to the higher incidence of this cancer among African-Americans. The mechanism by which hypertension may increase renal cell cancer risk is still unclear. Increased levels of angiogenic and other growth factors in persons with hypertension may play a role in renal carcinogenesis (90,91). Lipid peroxidation of the proximal renal tubules also is increased in individuals with hypertension (76). In addition, subtle acquired microvascular and tubulointerstitial injury preceding clinical hypertension may increase proximal tubular cell proliferation and render the kidney susceptible to carcinogens (92,93). It has been shown that the risk of renal cell cancer was tripled among men who were found to have proteinuria during health examinations at college entrance decades earlier (59).

Medications

Diuretics have been linked to RCC in several epidemiologic studies, including follow-up of cohorts of patients hospitalized for conditions requiring treatment with diuretics (94,95). The elevated risk has varied from 30% to 300% (27,30,32,44, 48–50,55,63,79–83,86,87,96,97), with a dose-response relation suggested in a few studies (49,80,83,87,97). It has been reported in some studies that the elevated risk is mainly among women (27,30,32,49,82,96,97) and that the risks associated with various classes of diuretics are generally similar (55,80,82,83,87). In some studies, the excess risk associated with diuretics has been mainly among patients with hypertension (55,87). The findings for diuretics, however, are not consistent, and it has been difficult to disentangle the effects of diuretics from hypertension per se or from other antihypertensive drugs.

In studies of renal cell cancer, the risks reported for other antihypertensive medications have varied from unity to increases greater than twofold, but no particular class of drugs has been singled out in the positive studies (28,30,50,55,79, 80,82,83,86,87,98).

As with diuretics, it has been difficult to distinguish treatment effects of antihypertensive medications from the underlying disease. The problem is complicated by the insidious nature and inconsistent definition of hypertension (99), the potential for misclassification of highly correlated events, and possible confounding by factors that influence the development and course of hypertension and of renal cell cancer, such as obesity (75). Although the link between antihypertensive medication use and risk of renal cell cancer is inconclusive, there is evidence to suggest that effective control of hypertension may reduce risk (64). Advances in molecular genetics may help further delineate the effects of hypertension from its treatment by incorporating genetic polymorphisms in drug metabolism in epidemiologic studies of gene-environment interactions in renal cell cancer.

After attempts to adjust for the effect of obesity, the use of diet pills, including those containing amphetamine, has been associated with renal cell cancer risk, but it has been difficult to truly control for the independent effect of obesity (27,50–55).

Analgesics have been related to renal cell cancer in some studies, but the epidemiologic evidence is not conclusive. Major suspicion from case-control and cohort studies has centered on phenacetin-containing analgesics, although the data are less persuasive than for renal pelvis cancer (26,28,30,32,82, 100–103). Although a link with aspirin products and acetaminophen has been reported (103–106), the evidence is not convincing, and it has been difficult to separate the effects of various types of analgesics (107–109). Because phenacetin products have been generally unavailable in the United States and elsewhere since the 1970s and were withdrawn from the US market in 1983 (110), any effect of phenacetin on renal cell cancer risk should diminish over time. Furthermore, because acetaminophen is a major metabolite of phenacetin (111) and its use in the United States did not become widespread until the mid-1970s, continued monitoring of risks associated with acetaminophen use would be prudent.

Preexisting Renal Conditions

Increased incidence of RCC has been observed among patients with uremia undergoing hemodialysis and renal transplantation, particularly among those with acquired cystic kidney disease (112–114). The prevalence of acquired cystic disease has been shown to increase with years on dialysis (114) and may represent a precursor state to renal cell cancer.

An elevated risk of RCC has been associated in some studies with a number of kidney diseases, including stones, cysts, and infection (14,26,39,50,79,82,115). However, the findings have not been consistent (26–28,32,33,55), suggesting that recall bias and unstable risk estimates due to a small number of affected cases may have contributed to the reported associations. In a cohort study with long-term follow-up of patients hospitalized for kidney or ureter stones, no excess risk of renal cell cancer was found (116).

The role of developmental defects in renal cell cancer has been suggested by reports of associated renal anomalies, including polycystic kidneys (117), horseshoe kidneys (118), and familial glomerulopathy (119).

Diabetes Mellitus

An elevated incidence of RCC has been observed during long-term follow-up of patients hospitalized for diabetes mellitus (120–122), although mortality from renal cancer was not increased in an earlier cohort of patients with diabetes mellitus (123). Increased risk of kidney cancer was also found in a cohort study of patients hospitalized for acromegaly, an overgrowth syndrome with a high risk of impaired glucose tolerance and diabetes mellitus, as well as for obesity and hypertension (124,125). Cohort studies involving the general population have shown little evidence of an association, although usually based on small numbers of cases with both conditions (43,63). Several case-control studies reported a positive association of borderline significance (55,79,115,126), whereas others found no significant relation (30,32,33,37,50,82,126). Given the strong correlation between diabetes and the risk factors of obesity and hypertension, a detailed assessment of potential confounding by associated conditions is needed before a causal link between diabetes mellitus and RCC can be accepted.

Reproductive and Hormonal Factors

A potential hormonal mechanism for RCC is suggested by laboratory studies showing estrogen-induced renal adenomas and carcinomas in hamsters (70), as well as receptors for sex hormones in renal tumors and certain growth factors in laboratory studies (127,128). However, evidence from epidemiologic studies linking renal cell cancer to a history of hysterectomy and use of oral contraceptives and hormone replacement therapy has been inconclusive (129–131). A few case-control studies have suggested an increased risk associated with number of births, particularly among women with a history of hypertension or high body mass index (32,129,132). After controlling for age at first birth, a Swedish nationwide record-linkage study found a significant 15% increase in risk of renal cell cancer with each additional birth (133). If this observation is confirmed, it may provide clues to hormonal mechanisms in human renal cell carcinoma.

Diet and Beverages

Epidemiologic studies of renal cell cancer have linked excess risks with intake of certain meats (13,14,26,30,32, 134–137), dairy products (26,28,138,139), and margarine and oils (39), but associations with specific food items have not been consistently observed. In a large international study, excess risk was related to consumption of fried/sautéed and well-done/charred/burnt meat but not to meat in general (140), suggesting an effect of the pyrolysis compounds that were produced during high-temperature cooking of meat (141). It is still unclear whether any specific macronutrient, such as protein or fat, or total caloric intake elevates risk (14,134,140).

Most studies of RCC evaluating the association with consumption of fruits and vegetables have found a reduced risk with selected foods (14,30,39,48,135,137–140), although micronutrients that are common in plant sources, such as vitamins C and E and carotenoids, have not been consistently implicated (14,63,134,138–140,142). Overall, the limited evidence to date suggests that a prudent diet low in animal protein and fat and high in fruits and vegetables may protect against renal cell cancer.

A relation between renal cell cancer and consumption of alcohol, coffee, tea, and juices has been suggested in some studies, but the overall epidemiologic evidence suggests no clear association with these beverages (135,137,143–145).

Physical Activity

The relation between physical activity and renal cell cancer risk is unclear. A few recent studies have reported a reduction in risk with high levels of recreational activities (146,147) or occupational activities among men (148). These associations, however, have not been consistently observed among the studies (37,53,146,147,149,150). Because physical activity levels are highly correlated with dietary intake of calories and body mass index, possible risk factors for renal cell cancer, further evaluation of the role of physical activity and energy balance in renal cancer development is warranted.

Occupation

Renal cell cancer is generally not considered an occupational cancer, but there are reports of excess risk among several occupational groups, including insulators; shipyard and railway workers exposed to asbestos (151–154); coke-oven workers exposed to polycyclic aromatic hydrocarbons (153,155); dry cleaners and other workers exposed to a variety of solvents (153,156,157); oil-refinery workers and service station attendants exposed to gasoline and other petroleum products (153, 158,159); and workers exposed to lead, cadmium, and other metals (153,154,157,160). Increased risk with exposures to other chemicals, such as vinyl chloride and pesticides, also has been reported (18). In addition, excess risk has been reported among pulp and paper mill workers (161), paperboard printing workers (162), cardboard workers (163), and architects (164). However, none of these occupations or exposures have been conclusively related to risk in epidemiologic studies. The lack of consistency in occupational findings in part may be explained by small sample size, recall bias, misclassification and low levels of exposures, inadequate adjustment for confounding factors, and short duration of follow-up in some studies.

Perhaps the strongest evidence suggesting a potential occupational etiology for renal cell cancer was reported in a German study that found a mutational hot spot in the von Hippel Lindau

(*VHL*) gene in tumor DNA from patients with heavy exposures to trichloroethylene (TCE) but not in the tumor DNA from unexposed patients (165). This finding, however, has yet to be replicated in interdisciplinary studies among other populations with well-documented range of exposures to TCE. In a recent record-linkage cohort study in Denmark, a 40% excess risk of renal cell cancer with borderline statistical significance was observed among TCE-exposed workers (166). These findings, along with results from a few other studies linking TCE exposure to renal cell cancer (167,168) and experimental studies suggesting plausible biologic mechanisms for TCE-induced renal toxicity and carcinogenesis (169,170), underscore the need for continuing monitoring of renal cell cancer risk among TCE-exposed workers.

Genetic Susceptibility

Increased risk of renal cell cancer among individuals with a family history of kidney cancer has been observed in epidemiologic studies (115,171). Using an extensive genealogy database in Iceland, Gudbjartsson et al. (172) found that patients with renal cell cancer diagnosed over a 45-year period were significantly more related to each other than a randomly selected control group with similar distributions in year of birth, sex, and number of ancestors from the database. The excess risk of renal cell cancer was found not only in first-degree relatives, but also in second- and third-degree relatives, suggesting that perhaps a multigenic inheritance pattern of less penetrant genes may play a role in susceptibility to sporadic cancer. In addition, strong evidence for the role of genetic susceptibility is provided by numerous reports of familial renal cell cancer. These studies have thus far identified at least four genes that are associated with the inherited forms of kidney cancer (173,174). Tumors associated with the Von Hippel Lindau (VHL) syndrome are primarily of the clear cell type and are associated with germline mutations of the *VHL* gene located on chromosome 3p (174,175). Familial occurrence of clear cell renal cancer also has been described in the absence of VHL syndrome and has featured constitutional balanced translocations involving chromosome 3p (176). In sporadic cases, somatic *VHL* mutations have been observed in approximately 50% of tumors (177,178). Epigenetic gene silencing through promoter methylation has been observed in an additional 20% of sporadic tumors, suggesting that the *VHL* gene may be inactivated in as many as 70% of sporadic RCC tumors (179,180).

Hereditary papillary renal cancer is related to germline mutations and activation of the *MET* proto-oncogene located on chromosome 7p (181). Kidney cells with *MET* gene mutations have aberrant hepatocyte growth factor (HGF) receptors. Unlike cells with normal receptors, these cells are unable to deactivate after HGF binding. HGF is expressed in many tissues and appears to be a cellular mitogen (182). Somatic *MET* gene mutations have also been described in some sporadic cases of papillary renal cell cancers

Recent reports have identified additional genes involved in two rare, dominantly inherited forms of renal cancer. The *fumarate hydratease (FH)* gene located on chromosome 1q42.3-q43 was recently observed to be associated with hereditary leiomyomatosis and papillary renal cell cancers (HRCC) (183–185). Birt-Hogg-Dube (BHD) syndrome, another inherited cancer syndrome, is primarily associated with chromophobe renal cell cancer, although clear cell tumors and hybrid chromophobe/oncocytic tumors are also found (173). The gene associated with BHD syndrome has been mapped to chromosome 17p11.2 and expresses a novel protein, folliculin, the function of which is not yet known (186,187).

Tumor Markers

The presence of somatic mutations in *VHL* and *MET* in sporadic renal cell cancers suggests that these genes could play an important role in renal cancer development in the general population. Limited epidemiologic studies have examined environmental, occupational, and other risk factors in renal cancer and associated *VHL* gene mutation patterns in tumor DNA. A high prevalence of *VHL* gene mutation was reported in tumor DNA from patients with renal cell cancer with excessive cumulative exposure to trichloroethylene but not among unexposed patients (165). More recent investigations have proposed additional types of mutation patterns in this gene (178,188). In another study of a renal cell cancer series from a case-control study, consumption of vegetables, citrus fruits, and selenium was associated with a decrease in specific types of *VHL* mutations (189). Specific types of *VHL* mutations have also been shown to differ among patients carrying polymorphisms in genes encoding certain metabolic enzymes (177).

Radiation-induced renal cell cancer has been reported in a clinical series of patients who received radiation therapy (190). Following the 1986 accident at the Chernobyl power plant in Ukraine, the molecular profiles of renal tumors from individuals environmentally exposed to cesium-137 (^{137}Cs) were examined. Strong proliferating cell nuclear antigen and K-*ras* protein expression were observed in the tumor tissues of the exposed Ukrainian patients but not in a control group of unexposed Spanish patients (191). These changes, along with an increase in proliferative atypical nephropathy, tubular epithelial nuclear atypia, and carcinoma *in situ* (CIS) in tissues adjacent to tumors, are postulated to be precursors of malignancy resulting from chronic low-level radiation exposure as ^{137}Cs is excreted by the kidneys (192).

Genetic Polymorphisms

In the last few years, a few studies of renal cell cancer risk among subgroups of individuals carrying polymorphic genes encoding phase I and II metabolic enzymes have been conducted. The studies published to date have examined a variety of polymorphisms in relation to exposures, but most findings have not been confirmed. Moreover, the studies have been small (ranging from 50 to 300 cases) and lack sufficient power to detect main effects of polymorphic variants or evidence of gene-environment interactions (193). Although results from these studies should be interpreted with caution, they provide some evidence that cancer risk may differ among genetically determined subgroups.

Polymorphisms in the *glutathione S-transferase M1 (GSTM1)* and *GSTT1* genes are frequently studied because they are important in phase II detoxification of tobacco and other smoke, ethylene oxide, and some solvents. Several studies of renal cell cancer observed considerably elevated risks in individuals carrying the active variants of these genes who were exposed to occupational carcinogens, including exposures to trichloroethylene (194), metals, pesticides, and solvents (195). In another study (196), elevated renal cell cancer risk was found in those carrying the variant cytochrome *P-450 1A1* gene (*CYP1A1*) allele alone and in combination with the active *GSTT1* polymorphism and the *N*-acetyltransferase (*NAT2*) slow acetylator polymorphism. Only one study reported a significant excess risk of renal cell cancer in individuals carrying the inactive *GSTT1* (null) polymorphism, particularly among those with low body mass index (197). The *NAT2* polymorphism also has been shown to modify tobacco-related renal cell cancer risk. Risk was considerably elevated only among smokers carrying the slow acetylator variant but not among those carrying the fast acetylator variant (198). Although these studies provide promising leads, larger well-designed studies with sufficient power to examine gene–gene and gene-environment interactions are needed to confirm these findings.

CONCLUSION

There is convincing epidemiologic evidence linking cigarette smoking, obesity, and hypertension to an elevated risk of RCC. In combination, these three factors are estimated to account for nearly 50% of cases in the US population (46) and may have contributed to the upward incidence trends as well as to the racial disparities. Preventive measures aimed at reducing these risk factors will help lower incidence rates. However, the 50% of unexplained cases underscores the need for further research into the environmental and genetic determinants of this increasingly common cancer. In particular, work is needed to examine mechanisms by which hypertension may increase renal cell cancer risk and to identify factors that may affect early detection and successful treatment of hypertension. The role of obesity also warrants further clarification, including its mechanisms of action and its determinants, such as dietary factors and physical activity, that may also affect the risk of renal cell cancer. In view of recent findings implicating trichloroethylene exposure in renal carcinogenesis, occupational risk factors for renal cell cancer also warrant further evaluation. The recent discoveries in the molecular genetics of RCC provide new opportunities to clarify the multifactorial origins of this tumor, including gene-environment interactions that may be unraveled by epidemiologic studies that incorporate biochemical and molecular biomarkers. Finally, the high survival rates for patients diagnosed with localized tumors indicate the importance of early detection, particularly among high-risk individuals, to reduce mortality from renal cell cancer. Long-term follow-up of patients also will help identify additional factors that may influence survival, including histologic and genetic subtypes of tumor, targeted therapy, and modification of lifestyle and other exposure factors.

References

1. Jemal A, Murray T, Ward E, et al. Cancer statistics, 2005. *CA Cancer J Clin* 2005;55:10–30.
2. Chow WH, Devesa SS, Warren J, et al. Kidney cancer incidence trends in the United States. *JAMA* 1999;281:1628–1631.
3. Linehan WM, Lerman MI, Zbar B. Identification of the von Hippel-Lindau (VHL) gene. *JAMA* 1995;273:564–570.
4. Zbar B, Lerman M. Inherited carcinomas of the kidney. *Adv Cancer Res* 1998;75:163–201.
5. McCredie M, Stewart JH, Ford JM. Analgesics and tobacco as risk factors for cancer of the ureter and renal pelvis. *J Urol* 1983;130:28–30.
6. McLaughlin JK, Blot WJ, Devesa SS, et al. Renal cancer. In: Schottenfeld D, Fraumeni JF Jr, eds. *Cancer epidemiology and prevention*, 2nd ed. New York: Oxford University Press, 1996:1142–1155.
7. Ries LAG, Eisner MP, Kosary CL et al., eds. SEER cancer statistics review, 1975-2000. Bethesda, MD: National Cancer Institute, 2003. http://seer.cancer.gov/csr/1975_2000
8. Surveillance, Epidemiology, and End Results (SEER) Program (www.seer.cancer.gov) SEER*Stat Database: Incidence—SEER 9 Regs Public-Use, November 2002 Sub (1973–2000), National Cancer Institute, DCCPS, Surveillance Research Program, Cancer Statistics Branch, released April 2003, based on the November 2002 submission.
9. Parkin DM, Whelan SL, Ferlay J, et al. *Cancer incidence in five continents, volume VIII*, IARC Scientific Publications No. 155, Lyon: International Agency for Research on Cancer, 2002.
10. Miller BA, ed. *Racial/ethnic patterns of cancer in the United States 1988-1992*. Bethesda, MD, NIH Publication No. 96-4104: National Cancer Institute, 1996:1–A9.
11. Devesa SS, Grauman DG, Blot WJ, et al. *Atlas of cancer mortality in the United States, 1950-94*. Bethesda, MD, NIH Publication No. 99-4564: National Cancer Institute, 1999.
12. Wynder EL, Mabuchi K, Whitmore WF Jr. Epidemiology of adenocarcinoma of the kidney. *J Natl Cancer Inst* 1974;53:1619–1634.
13. Armstrong B, Garrod A, Doll R. A retrospective study of renal cancer with special reference to coffee and animal protein consumption. *Br J Cancer* 1976;33:127–136.
14. Maclure M, Willett W. A case-control study of diet and risk of renal adenocarcinoma. *Epidemiology* 1990;1:430–440.
15. La Vecchia C, Negri E, D'Avanzo B, et al. Smoking and renal cell carcinoma. *Cancer Res* 1990;50:5231–5233.
16. Mellemgaard A, Engholm G, McLaughlin JK, et al. Risk factors for renal cell carcinoma in Denmark. I. Role of socioeconomic status, tobacco use, beverages, and family history. *Cancer Causes Control* 1994;5:105–113.
17. Schlehofer B, Heuer C, Blettner M, et al. Occupation, smoking and demographic factors, and renal cell carcinoma in Germany. *Int J Epidemiol* 1995;24:51–57.
18. Hu J, Mao Y, White K, et al. Renal cell carcinoma and occupational exposure to chemicals in Canada. *Occup Med* 2002;52:157–164.
19. Jin F, Devesa SS, Zheng W, et al. Cancer incidence trends in urban Shanghai, 1972-1989. *Int J Cancer* 1993;53:764–770.
20. Liu S, Semenciw R, Morrison H, et al. Kidney cancer in Canada: the rapidly increasing incidence of adenocarcinoma in adults and seniors. *Can J Public Health* 1997;88:99–104.
21. McCredie M. Bladder and kidney cancers. In: Doll R, Fraumeni JF Jr, Muir CS, eds. *Cancer surveys: trends in cancer incidence and mortality*. Vol. 19/20. Plainview, NY: Cold Spring Harbor Laboratory Press; 1994:343–368.
22. Mathew A, Devesa SS, Fraumeni JF Jr, et al. Global increases in kidney cancer incidence, 1973-1992. *Eur J Cancer Prev* 2002;11:171–178.
23. Jayson M, Sanders H. Increased incidence of serendipitously discovered renal cell carcinoma. *Urology* 1998;51:203–205.
24. Bos SD, Mellema CT, Mensink HJ. Increase in incidental renal cell carcinoma in the northern part of the Netherlands. *Eur Urol* 2000;37:267–270.
25. Beisland C, Medby PC, Beisland HO. Renal cell carcinoma: gender difference in incidental detection and cancer-specific survival. *Scand J Urol Nephrol* 2002;36:414–418.
26. McLaughlin JK, Mandel JS, Blot WJ, et al. A population-based case-control study of renal cell carcinoma. *J Nat Cancer Inst* 1984;72:275–284.
27. Yu MC, Mack TM, Hanisch R, et al. Cigarette smoking, obesity, diuretic use, and coffee consumption as risk factors for renal cell carcinoma. *J Natl Cancer Inst* 1986;77:351–356.
28. McCredie M, Ford JM, Stewart JH. Risk factors for cancer of the renal parenchyma. *Int J Cancer* 1988;42:13–16.
29. Brownson RC. A case-control study of renal cell carcinoma in relation to occupation, smoking, and alcohol consumption. *Arch Environ Health* 1988;43:238–241.
30. McLaughlin JK, Gao Y-T, Gao R-N, et al. Risk factors for renal-cell cancer in Shanghai, China. *Int J Cancer* 1992;52:562–565.
31. McCredie M, Stewart JH. Risk factors for kidney cancer in New South Wales – I. Cigarette smoking. *Eur J Cancer* 1992;28A:2050–2054.
32. Kreiger N, Marrett LD, Dodds L, et al. Risk factors for renal cell carcinoma: results of a population-based case-control study. *Cancer Causes Control* 1993;4:101–110.
33. Muscat JE, Hoffmann D, Wynder EL. The epidemiology of renal cell carcinoma: a second look. *Cancer* 1995;75:2552–2557.
34. McLaughlin JK, Lindblad P, Mellemgaard A, et al. International renal-cell cancer study. I. Tobacco use. *Int J Cancer* 1995;60:194–198.
35. Yuan J-M, Castelao JE, Gago-Dominguez M, et al. Tobacco use in relation to renal cell carcinoma. *Cancer Epidemiol Biomarkers Prev* 1998;7:429–433.
36. Chiu BC-H, Lynch CF, Cerhan JR, et al. Cigarette smoking and risk of bladder, pancreas, kidney and colorectal cancers in Iowa. *Ann Epidemiol* 2001;11:28–37.
37. Goodman MT, Morgenstern H, et al. A case-control study of factors affecting the development of renal cell cancer. *Am J Epidemiol* 1986;124:926–941.
38. Asal NR, Geyer JR, Risser DR, et al. Risk factors in renal cell carcinoma: I. Methodology, demographics, tobacco, beverage use, and obesity. *Cancer Detect Prev* 1988;11:359–377.
39. Talamini R, Barón AE, Barra S, et al. A case-control study of risk factor for renal cell cancer in northern Italy. *Cancer Causes Control* 1990;1: 125–131.
40. Benhamou S, Lenfant M-H, Ory-Paoletti C, et al. Risk factors for renal-cell carcinoma in a French case-control study. *Int J Cancer* 1993;55:32–36.
41. Siemiatycki J, Krewski D, Franco E, et al. Associations between cigarette smoking and each of 21 types of cancer: a multi-site case-control study. *Int J Epidemiol* 1995;24:504–514.
42. McLaughlin JK, Hrubec Z, Blot WJ, et al. Smoking and cancer mortality among US veterans: a 26-year follow-up. *Int J Cancer* 1995;60:190–193.
43. Coughlin SS, Neaton JD, Randall B, et al. Predictors of mortality from kidney cancer in 332,547 men screened for the Multiple Risk Factor Intervention Trial. *Cancer* 1997;79:2171–2177.
44. Heath CW Jr, Lally CA, Calle EE, et al. Hypertension, diuretics, and antihypertensive medications as possible risk factors for renal cell cancer. *Am J Epidemiol* 1997;145:607–613.
45. Parker AS, Cerhan JR, Janney CA, et al. Smoking cessation and renal cell carcinoma. *Ann Epidemiol* 2003;13:245–251.
46. Benichou J, Chow WH, McLaughlin JK, et al. Population attributable risk of renal cell cancer in Minnesota. *Am J Epidemiol* 1998;148:424–430.
47. National Center for Health Statistics. *Health, United States, 2003*. With Chartbook on Trends in the Health of Americans. Tables 60-61. Hyattsville, MD: NCHS, CDC, 2003. http://www.cdc.gov/nchs

48. Fraser GE, Phillips R, Beeson WL. Hypertension, antihypertensive medication and risk of renal carcinoma in California Seventh-Day Adentists. *Int J Epidemiol* 1990;19:832–838.

49. Hiatt RA, Tolan K, Quesenberry CP Jr. Renal cell carcinoma and thiazide use: a historical, case-control study (California, USA). *Cancer Causes Control* 1994;5:319–325.

50. McCredie M, Stewart JH. Risk factors for kidney cancer in New South Wales, Australia. II. Urologic disease, hypertension, obesity, and hormonal factors. *Cancer Causes Control* 1992;3:323–331.

51. Mellemgaard A, Engholm G, McLaughlin JK, et al. Risk factors for renal-cell carcinoma in Denmark. III. Role of weight, physical activity and reproductive factors. *Int J Cancer* 1994;56:66–71.

52. Lindblad P, Wolk A, Bergström R, et al. The role of obesity and weight fluctuations in the etiology of renal cell cancer: a population-based case-control study. *Cancer Epidemiol Biomarkers Prev* 1994;3:631–639.

53. Mellemgaard A, Lindblad P, Schlehofer B, et al. International renal-cell cancer study. III. Role of weight, height, physical activity, and use of amphetamines. *Int J Cancer* 1995;60:350–354.

54. Chow WH, McLaughlin JK, Mandel JS, et al. Obesity and risk of renal cell cancer. *Cancer Epidemiol Biomarkers Prev* 1996;5:17–21.

55. Yuan J-M, Castelao JE, Gago-Dominguez M, et al. Hypertension, obesity and their medications in relation to renal cell carcinoma. *Br J Cancer* 1998;77:1508–1513.

56. Shapiro JA, Williams MA, Weiss NS. Body mass index and risk of renal cell carcinoma. *Epidemiology* 1999;10:188–191.

57. Hu J, Mao Y, White K. Overweight and obesity in adults and risk of renal cell carcinoma in Canada. *Soz Praventivmed* 2003;48:178–185.

58. Lew EA, Garfinkel L. Variations in mortality by weight among 750,000 men and women. *J Chronic Dis* 1979;32:563–576.

59. Whittemore AS, Paffenbarger RS Jr, Anderson K, et al. Early precursors of urogenital cancers in former college men. *J Urol* 1984;132:1256–1261.

60. Mellemgaard A, Møller H, Olsen JH, et al. Increased risk of renal carcinoma among obese women. *J Natl Cancer Inst* 1991;83:1581–1582.

61. Møller H, Mellemgaard A, Lindvig K, et al. Obesity and cancer risk: a Danish record-linkage study. *Eur J Cancer* 1994;30A:344–350.

62. Tulinius H, Sigfússon N, Sigvaldason H, et al. Risk factors for malignant diseases: a cohort study on a population of 22,946 Icelanders. *Cancer Epidemiol Biomarkers Prev* 1997;6:863–873.

63. Prineas RJ, Folsom AR, Zhang ZM, et al. Nutrition and other risk factors for renal cell carcinoma in postmenopausal women. *Epidemiology* 1997; 8:31–36.

64. Chow WH, Gridley G, Fraumeni JF Jr, et al. Obesity, hypertension, and the risk of kidney cancer in men. *N Engl J Med* 2000;343:1305–1311.

65. Samanic C, Gridley G, Chow WH, et al. Obesity and cancer risk among white and black United States veterans. *Cancer Causes Control* 2004; 15:35–43.

66. Calle EE, Rodriguez C, Walker-Thurmond K, et al. Overweight, obesity, and mortality from cancer in a prospectively studied cohort of US adults. *N Engl J Med* 2003;348:1625–1638.

67. Legal KM, Carroll MD, Kuczmarski RJ, et al. Overweight and obesity in the United States: prevalence and trends, 1960–1994. *Int J Obes* 1998;22: 39–47.

68. Freedman DS, Khan LK, Serdula MK, et al. Trends and correlates of class 3 obesity in the United States from 1990 through 2000. *JAMA* 2002;288: 1758–1761.

69. Kumar A, Mittal S, Buckshee K, et al. Reproductive functions in obese women. *Prog Food Nutr Sci* 1993;17:89–98.

70. Weisz J, Fritz-Wolz G, Clawson GA, et al. Induction of nuclear catechol-O-methyltransferase by estrogens in hamster kidney: Implications for estrogen-induced renal cancer. *Carcinogenesis* 1998;19:1307–1312.

71. Attia N, Tamborlane WV, Heptulla R, et al. The metabolic syndrome and insulin-like growth factor I regulation in adolescent obesity. *J Clin Endocrinol Metab* 1998;83:1467–1471.

72. Narayan S, Roy D. Insuline-like growth factor I receptors are increased in estrogen-induced kidney tumors. *Cancer Res* 1993;53:2256–2259.

73. Jungwirth A, Schally AV, Pinski J, et al. Growth hormone-releasing hormone antagonist MZ-4-71 inhibits in vivo proliferation of Caki-I renal adenocarcinoma. *Proc Natl Acad Sci USA* 1997;94:5810–5813.

74. Kasiske BL, O'Donnell MP, Keane WF. The Zucker rat model of obesity, insulin resistance, hyperlipidemia, and renal injury. *Hypertension* 1992; 19:I110–I115.

75. Huang Z, Willett WC, Manson JE, et al. Body weight, weight change, and risk for hypertension in women. *Ann Intern Med* 1998;128:81–88.

76. Gago-Dominguez M, Castelao E, Yuan JM, et al. Lipid peroxidation: a novel and unifying concept of the etiology of renal cell carcinoma (United States). *Cancer Causes Control* 2002;13:287–293.

77. Raynor WJ Jr, Shekelle RB, Rossof AH, et al. High blood pressure and 17-year cancer mortality in the Western Electric Health Study. *Am J Epidemiol* 1981;113:371–377.

78. Goldbourt U, Holtzman E, Yaari S, et al. Elevated systolic blood pressure as a predictor of long-term cancer mortality: analysis by site and histologic subtype in 10,000 middle-aged and elderly men. *J Natl Cancer Inst* 1986; 77:63–70.

79. Asal NR, Lee ET, Geyer JR, et al. Risk factors in renal cell carcinoma. II. Medical history, occupation, multivariate analysis, and conclusions. *Cancer Detect Prev* 1988b;13:263–279.

80. Chow WH, McLaughlin JK, Mandel JS, et al. Risk of renal cell carcinoma in relation to diuretics, antihypertensive drugs, and hypertension. *Cancer Epidemiol Biomarkers Prev* 1995;4:327–331.

81. Grove JS, Nomura A, Severson RK, et al. The association of blood pressure with cancer incidence in a prospective study. *Am J Epidemiol* 1991; 134:942–947.

82. Mellemgaard A, Niwa S, Mehl ES, et al. Risk factors for renal cell carcinoma in Denmark: role of medication and medical history. *Int J Epidemiol* 1994;23:923–930.

83. McLaughlin JK, Chow WH, Mandel JS, et al. International renal-cell cancer study. VIII. Role of diuretics, other anti-hypertensive medications and hypertension. *Int J Cancer* 1995;63:216–221.

84. Buck C, Donner A. Cancer incidence in hypertensives. *Cancer* 1987;59: 1386–1390.

85. Hole DJ, Hawthorne VM, Isles CG, et al. Incidence of and mortality from cancer in hypertensive patients. *Br Med J* 1993;306:609–611.

86. Shapiro JA, Williams MA, Weiss NS, et al. Hypertension, antihypertensive medication use, and risk of renal cell carcinoma. *Am J Epidemiol* 1999; 149:521–530.

87. Weinmann S, Glass AG, Weiss NS, et al. Use of diuretics and other antihypertensive medications in relation to the risk of renal cell cancer. *Am J Epidemiol* 1994;140:792–804.

88. Steffens J, Bock R, Braedel HU, et al. Renin-producing renal cell carcinomas—clinical and experimental investigations on a special form of renal hypertension. *Urol Res* 1992;20:111–115.

89. Hajjar I, Kotchen TA. Trends in prevalence, awareness, treatment, and control of hypertension in the United States, 1988-2000. *JAMA* 2003;290: 199–206.

90. Scaglione R, Argano C, Parrinello G, et al. Relationship between transforming growth factor β1 and progression of hypertensive renal disease. *J Hum Hypertens* 2002;16:641–645.

91. Shimabukuro T, Ohmoto Y, Naito K. Transforming growth factor-beta1 and renal cell cancer: cell growth, mRNA expression and protein production of cytokines. *J Urol* 2003;169:1865–1869.

92. Johnson RJ, Herrera-Acosta J, Schreiner GF, et al. Subtle acquired renal injury as a mechanism of salt-sensitive hypertension. *N Engl J Med* 2002; 346:913–923.

93. Mazzali M, Jefferson JA, Ni Z, et al. Microvascular and tubulointerstitial injury associated with chronic hypoxia-induced hypertension. *Kidney Int* 2003;63:2088–2093.

94. Mellemgaard A, Møller H, Olsen JH. Diuretics may increase risk of renal cell carcinoma. *Cancer Causes Control* 1992;3:309–312.

95. Lindblad P, McLaughlin JK, Mellemgaard A, et al. Risk of kidney cancer among patients using analgesics and diuretics: a population-based cohort study. *Int J Cancer* 1993;55:5–9.

96. McLaughlin JK, Blot WJ, Fraumeni JF Jr. Diuretics and renal cell cancer. *J Natl Cancer Inst* 1988;80:378.

97. Finkle WD, McLaughlin JK, Rasgon SA, et al. Increased risk of renal cell cancer among women using diuretics in the United States. *Cancer Causes Control* 1993;4:555–558.

98. Rosenberg L, Rao S, Palmer JR, et al. Calcium channel blockers and the risk of cancer. *JAMA* 1998;279:1000–1004.

99. Fahey TP, Peters TJ. What constitutes controlled hypertension? Patient based comparison of hypertension guidelines. *Br Med J* 1996;313:93–96.

100. McLaughlin JK, Blot WJ, Mehl ES, et al. Relation of analgesic use to renal cancer: population-based findings. *Natl Cancer Inst Monogr* 1985;69: 217–222.

101. Maclure M, MacMahon B. Phenacetin and cancers of the urinary tract. *Lancet* 1985;313:1479.

102. McCredie M, Stewart JH, Carter JJ, et al. Phenacetin and papillary necrosis: independent risk factors for renal pelvis cancer. *Kidney Int* 1986;30: 81–84.

103. Gago-Dominguez M, Yuan JM, Castelao JE, et al. Regular use of analgesics is a risk factor for renal cell carcinoma. *Br J Cancer* 1999;81:542–548.

104. Paganini-Hill A, Chao A, Ross RK, et al. Aspirin use and chronic diseases: a cohort study of the elderly. *Br Med J* 1989;299:1247–1250.

105. Derby LE, Jick H. Acetaminophen and renal and bladder cancer. *Epidemiology* 1996;7:358–362.

106. McCredie M, Stewart JH, Day NE. Different roles for phenacetin and paracetamol in cancer of the kidney and renal pelvis. *Int J Cancer* 1993; 53:245–249.

107. Chow WH, McLaughlin JK, Linet MS, et al. Use of analgesics and risk of renal cell cancer. *Int J Cancer* 1994;59:467–470.

108. McCredie M, Pommer W, McLaughlin JK, et al. International renal-cell cancer study. II. Analgesics. *Int J Cancer* 1995;60:345–349.

109. Rosenberg L, Rao RS, Palmer JR, et al. Transitional cell cancer of the urinary tract and renal cell cancer in relation to acetaminophen use (United States). *Cancer Causes Control* 1998;9:83–88.

110. US Congress. *Federal Registry*. Washington, DC, October 5, 1983.

111. Hinson JA. Reactive metabolites of phenacetin and acetaminophen: a review. *Environ Health Perspect* 1983;50:37–49.

112. Kliem V, Kolditz M, Behrend M, et al. Risk of renal cell carcinoma after kidney transplantation. *Clin Transplant* 1997;11:255–258.

113. Ishikawa N, Tanabe K, Tokumoto T, et al. Clinical study of malignancies after renal transplantation and impact of routine screening for early detection: a single-center experience. *Transplant Proc* 2000;32:1907–1910.

114. Denton MD, Magee CC, Ovuworie C, et al. Prevalence of renal cell carcinoma in patients with ESRD pre-transplantation: a pathologic analysis. *Kidney Int* 2002;61:2201–2209.

115. Schlehofer B, Pommer W, Mellemgaard A, et al. International renal-cell-cancer study. VI. The role of medical and family history. *Int J Cancer* 1996;66:723–726.

116. Chow WH, Lindblad P, Gridley G, et al. Risk of urinary tract cancers following kidney or ureter stones. *J Natl Cancer Inst* 1997;89:1453–1457.

117. Hayakawa M, Hatano T, Tsuji A, et al. Patients with renal cysts associated with renal cell carcinoma and the clinical implications of cyst puncture: a study of 223 cases. *Urology* 1996;47:643–646.

118. Hohenfellner M, Schultz-Lampel D, Lampel A, et al. Tumor in the horseshoe kidney: clinical implications and review of embryogenesis. *J Urol* 1992; 147:1098–1102.

119. Gemperle O, Neuweiler J, Reutter FW, et al. Familial glomerulopathy with giant fibrillar (fibronectin-positive) deposits: 15-year follow-up in a large kindred. *Am J Kidney Dis* 1996;28:668–675.

120. Adami H-O, McLaughlin J, Ekbom A, et al. Cancer risk in patients with diabetes mellitus. *Cancer Causes Control* 1991;2:307–314.

121. Wideroff L, Gridley G, Mellemkjær L, et al. Cancer incidence in a population-based cohort of patients hospitalized with diabetes mellitus in Denmark. *J Natl Cancer Inst* 1997;89:1360–1365.

122. Lindblad P, Chow WH, Chan J, et al. The role of diabetes mellitus in the etiology of renal cell cancer. *Diabetologia* 1999;42:107–112.

123. Kessler II. Cancer mortality among diabetics. *J Natl Cancer Inst* 1970;44: 673–686.

124. Baris D, Gridley G, Ron E, et al. Acromegaly and cancer risk: a cohort study in Sweden and Denmark. *Cancer Causes Control* 2002;13:395–400.

125. Baldelli R, Battista C, Leonetti F, et al. Glucose homeostasis in acromegaly: effects of long-acting somatostatin analogues treatment. *Clin Endocrinol* 2003;59:492–499.

126. La Vecchia C, Negri E, Franceschi S, et al. A case-control study of diabetes mellitus and cancer risk. *Br J Cancer* 1994;70:950–953.

127. Corté-vizcaíno V, Llombart-Bosch A. Estrogen and progesterone receptors in the diethylstilbestrol-induced kidney neoplasms of the Syrian golden hamster: correlation with histopathology and tumoral stages. *Carcinogenesis* 1993;14:1215–1219.

128. Halmos G, Schally AV, Varga J, et al. Human renal cell carcinoma expresses distinct binding sites for growth hormone-releasing hormone. *Proc Natl Acad Sci USA* 2000;97:10555–10560.

129. Lindblad P, Mellemgaard A, Schlehofer B, et al. International renal-cell cancer study. V. Reproductive factors, gynecologic operations and exogenous hormones. *Int J Cancer* 1995;61:192–198.

130. Gago-Dominguez M, Castelao JE, Yuan JM, et al. Increased risk of renal cell carcinoma subsequent to hysterectomy. *Cancer Epidemiol Biomarkers Prev* 1999;8:999–1003.

131. Adami H-O, Persson I, Hoover R, et al. Risk of cancer in women receiving hormone replacement therapy. *Int J Cancer* 1989;44:833–839.

132. Chow WH, McLaughlin JK, Mandel JS, et al. Reproductive factors and the risk of renal cell cancer among women. *Int J Cancer* 1995;60: 321–324.

133. Lambe M, Lindblad P, Wuu J, et al. Pregnancy and risk of renal cell cancer: a population-based study in Sweden. *Br J Cancer* 2002;86:1425–1429.

134. Chow WH, Gridley G, McLaughlin JK, et al. Protein intake and risk of renal cell cancer. *J Natl Cancer Inst* 1994;86:1131–1139.

135. Boeing H, Schlehofer B, Wahrendorf J. Diet, obesity and risk for renal cell carcinoma: results from a case control study in Germany. *Z Ernahrungswiss* 1997;36:3–11.

136. De Stefani E, Fierro L, Mendilaharsu M, et al. Meat intake, 'mate' drinking and renal cell cancer in Uruguay: a case-control study. *Br J Cancer* 1998;78:1239–1243.

137. Handa K, Kreiger N. Diet patterns and the risk of renal cell carcinoma. *Public Health Nutr* 2002;5:757–767.

138. Mellemgaard A, McLaughlin JK, Overvad K, et al. Dietary risk factors for renal cell carcinoma in Denmark. *Eur J Cancer* 1996;32A:673–682.

139. Yuan J-M, Gago-Dominguez M, Castelao JE, et al. Cruciferous vegetables in relation to renal cell carcinoma. *Int J Cancer* 1998;77:211–216.

140. Wolk A, Gridley G, Niwa S, et al. International renal cell cancer study. VII. Role of diet. *Int J Cancer* 1996;65:67–73.

141. Wakabayashi K, Totsuka Y, Fukutome K, et al. Human exposure to mutagenic/carcinogenic heterocyclic amines and comutagenic betacarbolines. *Mutat Res* 1997;376:499–503.

142. Virtamo J, Edwards BK, Virtanen M, et al. Effects of supplemental alpha-tocopherol and beta-carotene on urinary tract cancer: incidence and mortality in a controlled trial (Finland). *Cancer Causes Control* 2000;11: 933–939.

143. Wolk A, Lindblad P, Adami H-O. Nutrition and renal cell cancer. *Cancer Causes Control* 1996;7:5–18.

144. Blot WJ, Chow WH, McLaughlin JK. Tea and cancer: a review of the epidemiologic evidence. *Eur J Cancer Prev* 1996;5:425–438.

145. Parker AS, Cerhan JR, Lynch CF, et al. Gender, alcohol consumption, and renal cell carcinoma. *Am J Epidemiol* 2002;155:455–462.

146. Menezes RJ, Tomlinson G, Kreiger N. Physical activity and risk of renal cell carcinoma. *Int J Cancer* 2004;107:642–646.

147. Mahabir S, Leitzmann MF, Pietinen P, et al. Physical activity and renal cell cancer risk in a cohort of male smokers. *Int J Cancer* 2004;108: 600–605.

148. Bergström A, Moradi T, Lindblad P, et al. Occupational physical activity and renal cell cancer: a nationwide cohort study in Sweden. *Int J Cancer* 1999;83:186–191.

149. Paffenbarger RS Jr, Hyde RT, Wing AL, et al. Physical activity and incidence of cancer in diverse populations: a preliminary report. *Am J Clin Nutr* 1987;45:312–317.

150. Bergström A, Terry P, Lindblad P, et al. Physical activity and risk of renal cell cancer. *Int J Cancer* 2001;92:155–157.

151. Selikoff IJ, Hammond EC, Seidman H. Mortality experience of insulation workers in the United States and Canada, 1943-1976. *Ann N Y Acad Sci* 1979;330:91–116.

152. Enterline PE, Hartley J, Henderson V. Asbestos and cancer: a cohort followup to death. *Am J Ind Med* 1987;44:396–401.

153. Mandel JS, McLaughlin JK, Schlehofer B, et al. International renal-cell cancer study. IV. Occupation. *Int J Cancer* 1995;61:601–605.

154. Mattioli S, Truffelli D, Baldasseroni A, et al. Occupational risk factors for renal cell cancer: a case-control study in Northern Italy. *J Occup Environ Med* 2002;44:1028–1036.

155. Redmond CK. Cancer mortality among coke oven workers. *Environ Health Perspect* 1983;52:67–73.

156. Brown DP, Kaplan SD. Retrospective cohort mortality study of dry cleaning workers using perchloroethylene. *J Occup Med* 1987;29:535–541.

157. Pesch B, Haerting J, Ranft U, et al. Occupational risk factors for renal cell carcinoma: agent-specific results from a case-control study in Germany. *Int J Epidemiol* 2000;29:1014–1024.

158. McLaughlin JK, Blot WJ, Mehl ES, et al. Petroleum-related employment and renal cell cancer. *J Occup Med* 1985;27:672–674.

159. Partanen T, Heikkilä P, Hernberg S, et al. Renal cell cancer and occupational exposure to chemical agents. *Scand J Work Environ Health* 1991; 17:231–239.

160. Cocco P, Hua F, Boffetta P, et al. Mortality of Italian lead smelter workers. *Scand J Work Environ Health* 1997;23:15–23.

161. Band PR, Nhu DL, Fang R, et al. Cohort mortality study of pulp and paper mill workers in British Columbia, Canada. *Am J Epidemiol* 1997; 146:186–194.

162. Sinks T, Lushniak B, Haussler BJ, et al. Renal cell cancer among paperboard printing workers. *Epidemiology* 1992;3:483–489.

163. Henschler D, Vamvakas S, Lammert M, et al. Increased incidence of renal cell tumors in a cohort of cardboard workers exposed to trichloroethene. *Arch Toxicol* 1995;69:291–299.

164. Lowery JT, Peters JM, Deapen D, et al. Renal cell carcinoma among architects. *Am J Ind Med* 1991;20:123–125.

165. Brauch H, Weirich G, Hornauer MA, et al. Trichloroethylene exposure and specific somatic mutations in patients with renal cell carcinoma. *J Natl Cancer Inst* 1999;91:854–861.

166. Raaschou-Nielsen O, Hansen J, McLaughlin JK, et al. Cancer risk among workers at Danish companies using trichloroethylene: a cohort study. *Am J Epidemiol* 2003;158:1182–1192.

167. Dosemeci M, Cocco P, Chow WH. Gender differences in risk of renal cell carcinoma and occupational exposures to chlorinated aliphatic hydrocarbons. *Am J Ind Med* 1999;36:54–59.

168. Brüning T, Pesch B, Wiesenhütter B, et al. Renal cell cancer risk and occupational exposure to trichloroethylene: results of a consecutive case-control study in Arnsberg, Germany. *Am J Ind Med* 2003;43:274–285.

169. National Toxicology Program. NTP toxicology and carcinogenesis studies of trichloroethylene (CAS No. 79-01-6) in four strains of rats (ACI, August, Marshall, Osborne-Mendel) (Gavage Studies). *Natl Toxicol Program Tech Rep Ser* 1988;273:1–299.

170. Cummings BS, Lash LH. Metabolism and toxicity of trichloroethylene and S-(1,2-Dichlorovinvl)-L-Cysteine in freshly isolated human proximal tubular cells. *Toxicol Sci* 2000;53:458–466.

171. Gago-Dominguez M, Yuan JM, Castelao JE, et al. Family history and risk of renal cell carcinoma. *Cancer Epidemiol Biomarkers Prev* 2001;10: 1001–1004.

172. Gudbjartsson T, Jonasdottir TJ, Thoroddsen A, et al. A population–based familial aggregation analysis indicates genetic contribution in most renal cell carcinomas. *Int J Cancer* 2002;100:476–479.

173. Phillips JL, Pavlovich CP, Walther M, et al. The genetic basis of renal epithelial tumors: advances in research and its impact on prognosis and therapy. *Curr Opin Urol* 2001;11:463–469.

174. Zbar B, Klausner R, Linehan WM. Studying cancer families to identify kidney cancer genes. *Annu Rev Med* 2003;54:217–233.

175. Latif F, Tory K, Gnarra J, et al. Identification of the von Hippel-Lindau disease tumor suppressor gene. *Science* 1993;260:1317–1320.

176. Gemmill RM, West JD, Boldog F, et al. The hereditary renal cell carcinoma 3;8 translocation fuses *FHIT* to a *patched*-related gene, *TRC8*. *Proc Natl Acad Sci USA* 1998;95:9572–9577.

177. Gallou C, Longuemaux S, Delomenie C, et al. Association of GSTT1 non-null and NAT1 slow/rapid genotypes with von Hippel-Lindau tumour suppressor gene transversions in sporadic renal cell carcinoma. *Pharmacogenetics* 2001;11:521–535.

178. Ma X, Yang K, Lindblad P, et al. VHL gene alterations in renal cell carcinoma patients: novel hotspot or founder mutations and linkage disequilibrium. *Oncogene* 2001;20:5393–5400.

179. Foster K, Prowse A, van Den BA, et al. Somatic mutations of the von Hippel-Lindau disease tumour suppressor gene in non-familial clear cell renal carcinoma. *Hum Mol Genet* 1994;3:2169–2173.

180. Clifford SC, Prowse AH, Affara NA, et al. Inactivation of the von Hippel-Lindau (VHL) tumour suppressor gene and allelic losses at chromosome arm 3p in primary renal cell carcinoma: evidence for a VHL-independent pathway in clear cell renal tumourigenesis. *Genes Chromosomes Cancer* 1998;22:200–209.

181. Fischer J, Palmedo G, von Knobloch R, et al. Duplication and overexpression of the mutant allele of the MET proto-oncogene in multiple hereditary papillary renal cell tumours. *Oncogene* 1998;17:733–739.

182. Johnson M, Koukoulis G, Matsumoto K, et al. Hepatocyte growth factor induces proliferation and morphogenesis in nonparenchymal epithelial liver cells. *Hepatology* 1993;17:1052–1061.

183. Tomlinson IP, Alam NA, Rowan AJ, et al. Germline mutations in FH predispose to dominantly inherited uterine fibroids, skin leiomyomata and papillary renal cell cancer. *Nat Genet* 2002;30:406–410.

184. Choyke PL, Glenn GM, Walther MM, et al. Hereditary renal cancers. *Radiology* 2003;226:33–46.

185. Toro JR, Nickerson ML, Wei M-H, et al. Mutations in the *fumarate hydratase* gene cause hereditary leiomyomatosis and renal cell cancer in families in North America. *Am J Hum Genet* 2003;73:95–106.

186. Nickerson ML, Warren MB, Toro JR, et al. Mutations in a novel gene lead to kidney tumors, lung wall defects, and benign tumors of the hair follicle in patients with the Birt-Hogg-Dube syndrome. *Cancer Cell* 2002;2:157–164.

187. Khoo SK, Giraud S, Kahnoski K, et al. Clinical and genetic studies of Birt-Hogg Dube syndrome. *J Med Genet* 2002;39:906–912.

188. Brauch H, Weirich G, Brieger J, et al. VHL alterations in human clear cell renal carcinoma: association with advanced tumor stage and a novel hot spot mutation. *Cancer Res* 2000;60:1942–1948.

189. Hemminki K, Jiang Y, Ma X, et al. Molecular epidemilogy of VHL gene mutations in renal cell carcinoma patients: relation to dietary and other factors. *Carcinogenesis* 2002;23:809–815.

190. Vogelzang NJ, Yang X, Goldman S, et al. Radiation induced renal cell cancer: a report of 4 cases and review of the literature. *J Urol* 1998;160:1987–1990.

191. Romanenko A, Morell-Quadreny L, Nepomnyaschy V, et al. Pathology and proliferative activity of renal-cell carcinomas (RCCS) and renal oncocytomas in patients with different radiation exposure after the Chernobyl accident in Ukraine. *Int J Cancer* 2000;87:880–883.

192. Romanenko A, Morell-Quadreny L, Nepomnyaschy V, et al. Radiation sclerosing proliferative atypical nephropathy of peritoumoral tissue of renal-cell carcinomas after the Chernobyl accident in Ukraine. *Virchows Arch* 2001;438:146–153.

193. Garcia-Closas M, Lubin JH. Power and sample size calculations in case-control studies of gene-environment interactions: comments on different approaches. *Am J Epidemiol* 1999;49:689–692.

194. Bruning T, Lammert M, Kempkes M, et al. Influence of polymorphisms of GSTM1 and GSTT1 for risk of renal cell cancer in workers with long-term high occupational exposure to trichloroethene. *Arch Toxicol* 1997;71:596–599.

195. Buzio L, DePalma G, Mozzoni P, et al. Glutathione S-transferases M1-1 and T1-1 as risk modifiers for renal cell cancer associated with occupational exposure to chemicals. *Occup Environ Med* 2003;60:789–793.

196. Longuemaux S, Delomenie C, Gallou C, et al. Candidate genetic modifiers of individuals susceptibility to renal cell carcinoma: a study of polymorphic human xenobiotic-metabolizing enzymes. *Cancer Res* 1999;59:2903–2908.

197. Sweeney C, Farrow DC, Schwartz SM, et al. Glutathione S-transferase M1, T1, and P1 polymorphisms as risk factors for renal cell carcinoma: a case-control study. *Cancer Epidemiol Biomarkers Prev* 2000;9:449–454.

198. Semenza JC, Ziogas A, Largent J, et al. Gene-environment interactions in renal cell carcinoma. *Am J Epidemiol* 2001;153:851–859.

CHAPTER 44 ■ PATHOLOGY OF RENAL CELL CARCINOMA

CHAPTER 44A
Renal Cancer Pathology and Prognostic Factors

Victor E. Reuter, Paul Russo, and Robert J. Motzer

INTRODUCTION

Most renal neoplasms are of epithelial origin and are malignant. Renal cell carcinomas (RCCs) have been regarded as single entities until recently; however, studies now have proven conclusively that renal epithelial neoplasms are not single tumors but are rather a group of distinguishable entities (1,2). This understanding is based on histologic (3), as well as cytogenetic and molecular, studies (4–15). This newly found knowledge led to a meeting of experts in the field of renal cancer, organized by Guyla Kovacs at the University of Heidelberg in Germany, and was quickly followed by a consensus conference sponsored by the Mayo Clinic, the American Cancer Society, Union Internationale Contre le Cancer (UICC), and the American Joint Committee on Cancer (AJCC). The result was a new classification for renal neoplasms (16,17) (Table 44A.1). It is very satisfying to know that the morphologic and genetic features of most of these tumors are tightly related and that this classification has been adopted virtually verbatim by the World Health Organization (18) (Table 44A.2). Just as rewarding is the recent evidence that this new classification defines the distinct clinical entities as well (19) (Table 44A.3). Unfortunately, our newly found knowledge renders much of the old literature on renal carcinomas obsolete, especially those writings that deal with clear cell, granular cell, or sarcomatoid tumors, all of which include a mixture of entities with diverse natural histories. In this chapter we discuss the more common variants of renal epithelial tumors because they constitute the entities a clinician is likely to encounter in the clinic.

GRADING AND STAGING OF RENAL TUMORS

Several systems have been proposed over the years for the grading of renal tumors. Of these, the one proposed by Fuhrman et al. is the most widely used (20–25). This system uses nuclear grades based on nuclear size, irregularity of the nuclear membrane, and nucleolar prominence. Although we and others have demonstrated good correlation between Fuhrman nuclear grade and survival in clear cell (conventional) carcinomas, application may be cumbersome because it requires the pathologist to measure nuclear size and poor interobserver reproducibility (24).

Although some of us believe a different grading system with a better discriminatory power is necessary (25), we recommend that the Fuhrman grading system be used until a more reproducible and clinically relevant classification emerges. The utility of the Fuhrman or any other grading scheme in papillary and chromophobe cell carcinomas remains controversial. Amin et al. (26) report a strong correlation within papillary renal cell carcinoma (PRCC) on univariate analysis. We and others have not found any significant correlation between the nuclear grade and survival (27,28) nor did Amin et al. find the same on multivariate analysis (26). Similarly, chromophobe renal cell carcinoma very frequently shows marked nuclear irregularities (grade 3 nuclei) in spite of the overall excellent survivals. There is no reason to grade renal oncocytomas since they are benign tumors.

In 1969, Robson et al. published a staging scheme that was adopted by most clinicians and pathologists and has been shown to correlate well with survival (29). During the ensuing years, the AJCC, in collaboration with the UICC, published the Tumor, Nodes, and Metastases (TNM) classification in which stage I and II tumors were confined to the kidney, but the former measured 2.5 cm or less (30). This classification was modified in 1997, and even further modifications were made in 2002 (31) (Table 44A.4). Undoubtedly, any of these classifications offer valuable prognostic information, but only within specific tumor types. For example, large size and extra capsular extension do not have the same prognostic significance in cases of oncocytoma or even chromophobe carcinomas as they have in clear cell (conventional) tumors. Up to 20% of renal oncocytomas may present with pT3 disease even though they are benign tumors (Table 44A.3). The mean tumor size of chromophobe carcinomas is approximately 8.0 to 9.0 cm, the largest of all renal cortical neoplasms, and yet the disease-free survival in virtually all published series is more than 90% (32). We recommend that tumors be classified using the latest TNM classification in an attempt to establish uniformity in reporting, although future editions will surely correct deficiencies in the present system (31,33).

CLEAR CELL (CONVENTIONAL) RENAL CELL CARCINOMA

Clear cell (conventional) carcinomas comprise approximately 60% to 65% of renal tumors. The mean age at diagnosis is in the sixth to seventh decade of life. Although they are the most common of all renal cancers, the full spectrum of their pathologic and clinical features are only now being understood. Almost all studies dealing with this tumor type and those published before 1995 are flawed because of errors in classification. Because clear cell tumors may exhibit few or no cells with clear cytoplasm, some authors have used the term *conventional* to describe this entity. However, the new World Health Organization (WHO) classification published in 2004 retains the term *clear cell* as the preferred nomenclature (18).

TABLE 44A.1

RENAL CELL NEOPLASMS CLASSIFICATION[a]

Benign	Malignant
Oncocytoma	Clear cell (conventional) renal cell carcinoma
Papillary (chromophil) adenoma	Papillary (chromophil) renal cell carcinoma
Metanephric adenoma	Chromophobe renal cell carcinoma
Nephrogenic adenofibroma	Collecting duct carcinoma
	Medullary carcinoma
	Mixed tubular and spindle cell carcinoma
	Renal cell carcinoma, unclassified
Tumor of undetermined malignant potential	
Multilocular cystic renal cell carcinoma	

[a]Does not include several types, including some seen particularly in the pediatric age group.

TABLE 44A.2

RENAL CELL NEOPLASMS PUTATIVE CELL OF ORIGIN, CLASSIFICATION, AND GENETIC CORRELATES

Proximal nephron	Cells of the proximal convoluted tubule	Conventional RCC • 3p− • other losses/gains
	? Cells of the distal convoluted tubule	Papillary RCC • 7+, 17+, 3+, Y− • other losses/gains
	Loop of Henle or collecting ducts	Tubular and spindle cell TM Oncocytoma • Y−, 1−
	Intercalated cells of the renal cortex	Chromophobe RCC • Y−, 1−
Distal Nephron	Collecting ducts of the renal medulla	Collecting duct carcinoma • 1−, 6−, 14−, 15−, 22− Medullary carcinoma • unknown (sickle trait)

RCC, renal cell carcinoma; TM, thrombomodulin.

TABLE 44A.3

RENAL EPITHELIAL NEOPLASMS CLINICOPATHOLOGIC FEATURES AND SURVIVAL

	CRCC	Papillary	Chromophobe	Oncocytoma
Cases studied	410	156	84	97
Men:Women	1.3:1	2.4:1	1.2:1	1.5:1
Multifocal	9.5%	35.2%	10.7%	14.4%
Age	61	60	59	66
Size (cm)	7.1	6.3	8.3	5.1
pT1–pT2	57.1%	81.4%	70.2%	80%
Outcome (DOD)	29.3%	12.2%	5.5%	0%
Disease-specific survival (5/10 yr)[a,b]	76%/70%	86%/82%	100%/90%	100%/100%

CRCC, clear cell (conventional) renal cell carcinoma; DOD, dead of disease.
[a]CRCC were consecutively resected between 1985 and 1988.
[b]Papillary, chromophobe, and oncocytic tumors were consecutively resected between 1980 and 1995.

TABLE 44A.4

TUMOR, NODES, AND METASTASES CLINICAL CLASSIFICATION (2002)

pT—Primary Tumor

pTx	Primary tumor cannot be assessed
pT0	No evidence of primary tumor
pT1a	<4.0 cm; limited to kidney
pT1b	4–7 cm; limited to kidney
pT2	>7.0 cm; limited to the kidney
pT3	Tumor extends into major veins or invades adrenal gland or perinephric tissues but not beyond Gerota fascia
pT3a	Tumor invades adrenal gland or perinephric tissues but not beyond Gerota fascia
pT3b	Tumor grossly extends into renal vein(s) or vena cava below diaphragm
pT3c	Tumor grossly extends into vena cava above diaphragm
pT4	Tumor invades beyond Gerota fascia

N—Regional Lymph Nodes

NX	Regional lymph nodes cannot be assessed
N0	No regional lymph node metastasis
N1	Metastasis in a single regional lymph node
N2	Metastasis in more than one regional lymph node

M—Distant Metastasis

Mx	Distant metastasis cannot be assessed
M0	No distant metastasis
M1	Distant metastasis

Clear cell RCCs are characterized by the loss of genetic material of the short arm of chromosome 3 (3p) and mutations in the *von Hippel-Lindau (VHL)* gene (5,15,34–36). In patients with VHL disease, such losses and mutations are described in almost all cases. Interestingly, somatic mutations and/or hypermethylations in the same region can be found in 75% to 80% of the more common sporadic, unilateral, and unifocal tumors as well (37).

Gross and Microscopic Features

The classic case is solitary, well circumscribed, and has a golden yellow color because of abundant intracytoplasmic lipid. Higher-grade tumors contain less lipid and glycogen and have a more varied appearance. Tumor size may range from microscopic to more than 20 cm. We have experienced a dramatic stage and size migration over the last two decades. A consecutive series of clear cell tumors resected at our institution between 1983 and 1985 had a mean tumor size of 8.0 cm, whereas a similar group of tumors resected between 1995 and 1997 had a mean tumor size of 5.5 cm (38). The minority of cases may show cystic degeneration or gross invasion of the renal vein.

Approximately 50% of cases exhibit either a solid or an acinar growth pattern exclusively. They are characterized by solid sheets of tumor cells, compartmentalized into solid acinar structures by delicate, richly vascularized fibrous septa (Fig. 44A.1). In some cases, the acinar pattern is less well defined, yet the prominent vascularity is retained. In the remaining cases, these tumors contain a mixture of growth patterns, including cystic, papillary, pseudopapillary, tubular, and sarcomatoid. A rich capillary network is prominent in all but the sarcomatoid areas. Growth pattern is loosely associated with grade because most low-grade lesions have an acinar growth,

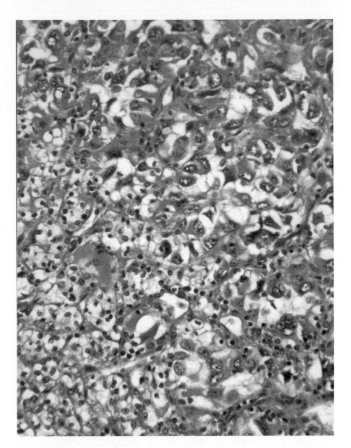

FIGURE 44A.1. Clear cell carcinoma, Fuhrman grade 1. Tumor cells are arranged in nests and have small dark nuclei with inconspicuous nucleoli (original magnification ×100). (From Lee CT, Katz J, Fearn PA, Russo P. Mode of presentation of renal cell carcinoma provides prognostic information. *Urol Oncol* 2002;7:135–140, with permission.)

whereas higher-grade areas are more likely to exhibit solid, pseudopapillary, or sarcomatoid features. Tumors exhibiting a pseudopapillary growth pattern, which must not be mistaken for the true papillary growth pattern seen typically in PRCCs, are characterized by pseudopapillae lacking a true fibrovascular core. These tumors are often due to degenerative changes in areas of solid and/or acinar growth. Focal fibrosis or hyalinization due to degenerative changes is seen in more than 75% of cases; however, true desmoplasia is absent or minimal. Geographic necrosis and focal hemorrhage are common histologic findings as well. These tumors may contain an inflammatory infiltrate, which is predominantly lymphocytic. Calcifications and osseous metaplasia are rare findings, seen in less than 10% and 4% of cases, respectively.

In most cases, tumor cells are either polygonal or cuboidal in shape. Cell shape is more variable in higher-grade lesions. Fuhrman grade 4 lesions contain bizarre, pleomorphic cells, some of which mimic the giant cells seen in some chromophobe cell tumors and angiomyolipomas. The spindle cells seen in sarcomatoid areas should be considered as evidence of high-grade disease. Most tumors show a mixture of cytoplasmic features, namely clear or granular–eosinophilic cytoplasm. The cytoplasmic features can be correlated with tumor grade because grade 1 lesions invariably contain clear cytoplasm, whereas the cytoplasm of higher-grade lesions is more likely to be variably eosinophilic and granular (Figs. 44A.1, 44A.2). Some grades 3 and 4 lesions may lack clear cytoplasm altogether. These tumors should be classified as clear cell RCC rather than being lumped into the category of granular cell

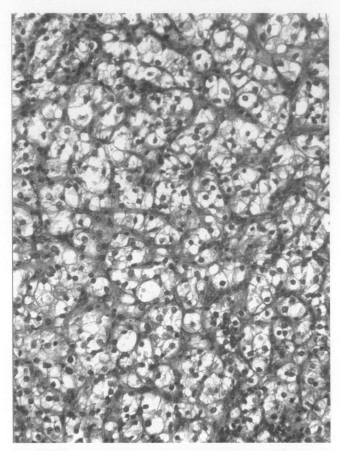

FIGURE 44A.2. Clear cell carcinoma, Fuhrman grade 4. High-grade areas have larger, pleomorphic nuclei and the cytoplasm is no longer clear (original magnification ×100). (From Russo P, Snyder ME, Di Blasio CJ, Sorbellini M, Kattan M, Motzer RJ, Reuter VE. Changing demographics and the contemporary surgical management of renal cortical tumors. *J Urol* 2003;69:347A, with permission.)

renal carcinomas, a term that should be discarded because of its lack of specificity.

MULTILOCULAR CYSTIC RENAL CELL CARCINOMA

Multilocular cystic renal cell carcinoma represents a rare variant of clear cell RCC, constituting between 3.1% and 6% of this tumor type (39–44). They have been described in adult patients with a mean age of 51 at diagnosis. The follow-up information available is limited. Nevertheless, none of the reported cases have progressed (45). The gross appearance is that of a well-circumscribed, multicystic mass that is separated from the adjacent renal parenchyma by a fibrous pseudocapsule. The size can vary but may reach 13 cm in greatest dimension. The cysts are lined by thin fibrous septa, are variable in size, and may contain serous or bloody fluid or clot. No solid or expansile masses of tumor are present. One might question why they are regarded as carcinoma, considering that none have demonstrated malignant behavior.

PAPILLARY (CHROMOPHIL) RENAL CELL CARCINOMA

PRCCs comprise from 7% to 14% of primary epithelial renal neoplasms (39,46). They received little attention as a distinct

clinical entity until Mancilla-Jimenez et al. published a study of 34 cases of PRCC in 1976 (47), although earlier clinical studies had suggested specific clinical characteristics for these tumors (48). The term *chromophil renal carcinoma* has been used to describe these tumors (2), but we have chosen to retain the term papillary RCC because it is more widely accepted and describes the growth pattern of most tumors. Age at presentation ranges from the third to eighth decade of life, with peak incidence in the sixth and seventh decades, similar to other tumor types. An increasing number of cases present as incidental masses discovered during workup for unrelated causes, with more than 60% of our cases presenting in this fashion. The men-to-women ratio ranges from 2:1 to 3.9:1 (49–51). Most patients present with unilateral tumors, although patients with PRCC are more likely to have bilateral as well as multifocal disease, the latter being reported in up to 49% of cases (50,51).

Cytogenetic and molecular studies have revealed distinct findings in PRCC that distinguish them from other renal epithelial tumors (11,14). Most sporadic PRCC are characterized by trisomy of chromosomes 7 and 17, as well as by loss of chromosome Y (1,4,8,11,51–53). In a subgroup of PRCC (54–56), t(X;1)(p11;q21) has been encountered. This translocation results in the fusion of the TFE3 gene on chromosome X to a novel gene, PRCC, on chromosome 1 (55–57). The gene product is believed to play a role in disrupting normal mitotic spindle checkpoints, with resultant tumorigenesis (58). Interestingly, the TFE3 gene at Xp11.2 has been shown recently to be involved in translocations with the ASPL gene at 17q25 in a group of renal tumors in young people, a translocation also seen in alveolar soft part sarcoma (59,60). Approximately 10% of the sporadic PRCC have also been reported to show somatic mutations in c-MET gene, a genetic abnormality that is commonly seen as a germline mutation in familial cases (61).

Gross and Microscopic Features

A PRCC tumor appears as a discrete mass within the renal cortex. Size can be quite variable, ranging in our series from 1 cm to 18 cm or greater. Less than one third of cases are surrounded by a fibrous pseudocapsule. Multifocality is present in over 45% of cases, in some instances reported to be a microscopic finding only. Most tumors exhibit a variegated appearance. We have found that the color of the tumor is in great part related to the microscopic findings; tumors containing abundant foamy macrophages are tan-to-yellow, whereas those with intratumoral hemorrhage are dark tan-to-brown. Some lesions may be frankly necrotic.

The majority of PRCCs exhibit a broad morphologic spectrum, including papillary, papillary-trabecular, and papillary-solid areas (28,50,62–66). The classic papillary pattern is characterized by discrete papillary fronds lined by neoplastic epithelial cells and containing a central fibrovascular core, easily recognized on low magnification. (Fig. 44A.3).

Areas containing classic papillary, papillary-trabecular, and/or papillary-solid patterns of growth are seen in almost all cases. However, more than half the cases can exhibit other morphologies, including truly solid, tubular, and/or glomeruloid growth patterns, and 20% to 25% of cases exhibit less than 50% papillary growth (2). In isolated cases, papillary growth comprises a very minor component of the tumor. For this reason, the percentage of papillary growth should not be used to determine whether a tumor should be classified as a PRCC. Renshaw et al. have shown that solid variants of PRCC contain the same genetic alterations as other classic papillary tumors (62).

Geographic necrosis is a common finding, as is the presence of psammoma bodies and foamy macrophages within

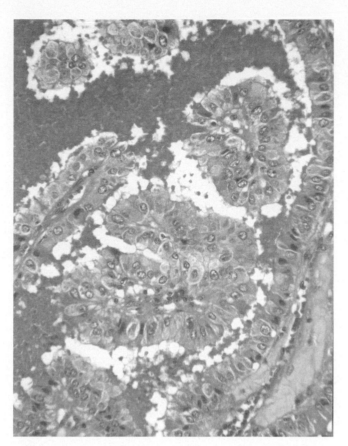

FIGURE 44A.3. Papillary carcinoma, low grade (type 1). There is a single layer of epithelial cells with small nuclei and basophilic/amphophilic cytoplasm (original magnification ×100). (From Kattan MW, Reuter V, Motzer RJ, Katz J, Russo P: A postoperative prognostic nomogram for renal cell. *J Urol* 2001;166:63–67, with permission.)

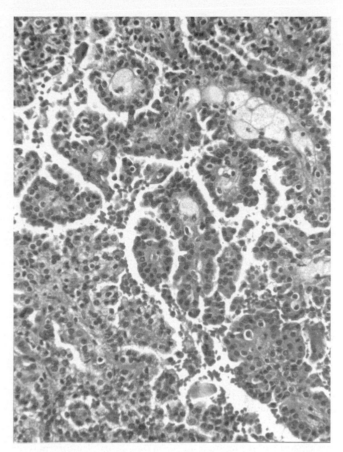

FIGURE 44A.4. Papillary carcinoma, high grade (type 2). Tumor cells have large nuclei with prominent nucleoli and abundant eosinophilic cytoplasm (original magnification ×100).

the fibrovascular stalk. At times, the fibrovascular stalk becomes hyalinized or fibrotic, masking the papillary nature of the lesion. Hemosiderin pigment may be present in the cytoplasm of the tumor cells in a patchy distribution. It is common for these tumors to be surrounded by a thick fibrous pseudocapsule.

The prognosis of PRCC is more favorable than clear cell RCC and less so than chromophobe RCC. The reported 5-year disease-free survival varies from 79% to 92% (47,66). Grading remains controversial. Amin et al. (26) found that it was a strong predictor of survival on univariate analysis but not on multivariate analysis. They also found that tumors with eosinophilic cytoplasm were likely to be high grade, whereas basophilic tumors were low grade. Delahunt and Eble divided their cases into type 1 and type 2 lesions according to architectural and cytologic features (63), with some genetic differences reported between them (Fig. 44A.4) (64,67). Subsequently, Delahunt et al. reported major differences in overall survival between the two groups (28). On the basis of a study of 103 cases of PRCC, we have not been able to confirm these results (27). One of the reasons for these differences in results may be the small number of events that occur in PRCC (e.g., progression, or deaths due to disease), as reported in both our series (27) and that reported by Amin et al. (26). Surprisingly, and contrary to the known behavior of PRCC, Delahunt et al. (28) have reported a very high rate of death in their series (27 deaths in 66 patients). The utility of grading of PRCC and the system by which it should be performed is therefore controversial and remains to be validated clinically.

PAPILLARY/TUBULOPAPILLARY (CHROMOPHIL) "ADENOMA"

Although size often correlates well with clinical outcome, characterizing a tumor as carcinoma or adenoma solely on the basis of size is scientifically unsound. Despite the fact that these lesions are architecturally and cytologically identical to larger lesions, it is a common practice among pathologists to use the term *papillary/tubulopapillary (chromophil) adenoma* for small (<5 mm) papillary lesions in which common sense tells us that the likelihood of metastasis is minimal. Empirical data available have taught us that metastatic potential for lesions measuring even up to 1 cm and containing small, regular nuclei with compact chromatin and small or absent nucleoli is also virtually nil.

CHROMOPHOBE RENAL CELL CARCINOMA

Chromophobe renal cell carcinoma (CRCC) comprises 6% to 11% of renal epithelial tumors. The age and sex distribution is virtually identical to that seen in clear cell RCC. Bannasch et al. were first to report the occurrence of chromophobe cell tumors in kidneys of animals exposed to nitrosomorpholine. In 1985, Thoenes et al. recognized this variant in human renal epithelial tumors and illustrated its morphologic, histochemical, and ultrastructural findings (68). Over the ensuing years, our awareness of CRCC has increased dramatically, as evidenced by the increasing number of studies published on this subject (32,69–74). It is important to recognize this variant of RCC for two reasons. First, stage for stage, CRCC has a considerably better prognosis than conventional (clear cell) RCCs (Table 44A.3) (32,69,70). Interestingly, a recent study of metastatic nonclear cell RCC showed a longer survival in patients with metastatic CRCC than in those with RCCs of other morphologic subtypes (75). These findings further support the indolent nature of these tumors. Second, the morphologic features may overlap somewhat with oncocytomas, benign tumors with which CRCC may be confused.

CRCC is characterized genetically by loss of chromosomes 1 and Y, as well as by combined chromosomal losses, usually affecting chromosomes 1, 6, 10, 13, 17, and 21 (2,76–78). Loss of multiple chromosomes leads to hypodiploid tumor cells, a unique feature seen in many of these tumors (79). Abnormalities in mitochondrial DNA may be observed, but their specificity remains controversial (80).

CRCC is thought to arise from intercalated cells of the renal cortex, similar to oncocytomas. In recent years, several investigators have drawn attention to the possible link between chromophobe and oncocytic tumors, suggesting that "hybrid" tumors may exist. This issue is discussed in greater length in the section entitled "Oncocytosis" later in this chapter.

Gross and Microscopic Features

The gross appearance is very helpful in the diagnosis of CRCC. Characteristically, these tumors are solitary and discrete, but not encapsulated, and show a homogenous beige or pale-tan cut surface. Nonetheless, we and others have observed rare tumors with dark brown and mahogany color. A central scar is present in approximately 15% of our cases. Tumors may be quite large, ranging in size from 2.0 cm to 23.0 cm. In our series, the mean size was 9.0 cm. Tumors commonly have a lobulated appearance and roughly one-fourth to one-third of cases exhibit gross areas of hemorrhage or necrosis.

Virtually all tumors are nonencapsulated microscopically. The pattern of growth is predominantly solid, separated by thin, incomplete fibrovascular septa, but may be focally admixed with tubular, trabecular, and cystic patterns. A small percentage of cases may exhibit a sarcomatoid pattern of growth. In fact, Akhtar et al. state that CRCC may be the renal epithelial tumor most frequently associated with a sarcomatoid growth pattern (81).

The typical histology of CRCC consists of large round-to-polygonal cells with well-defined cell borders and amphophilic-to-pale basophilic cytoplasm admixed with a smaller population of polygonal cells with eosinophilic cytoplasm. (Fig. 44A.5) A predominance of tumor cells with more densely eosinophilic "oncocytic" cytoplasm is seen in 30% of cases. This latter group of tumors constitutes what has been called the "eosinophilic variant" of CRCC. Although the distinction between the "typical" and the eosinophilic variants of CRCC is clinically unimportant, its introduction was necessary to alert pathologists to the wide spectrum of morphologic changes seen in CRCC and to avoid misinterpreting the tumor as an oncocytoma (69). Perinuclear halos are seen invariably, and the nuclei are typically hyperchromatic with irregular nuclear membranes. Focal cytologic atypia with bizarre nuclei are seen in half the cases but are prominent in only a small minority of tumors. Mitotic activity is very low, except in sarcomatoid areas.

ONCOCYTOMA

Oncocytoma is a benign renal epithelial neoplasm first described by Zippel in 1942 (82), then largely ignored until the publication of 13 additional cases by Klein and Valensi (83). It

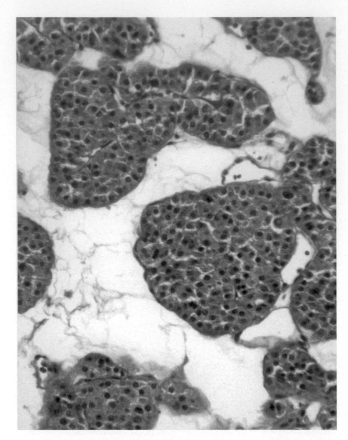

FIGURE 44A.5. Chromophobe carcinoma. Tumor cells have irregular nuclei and perinuclear cytoplasmic clearing. Cytologic atypia may be extreme (original magnification ×100).

is estimated that oncocytomas comprise from 3.2% to 7% of all primary renal neoplasms (84–87). Most series show a wide age distribution at presentation with a peak incidence in the seventh decade of life. Men are affected nearly twice as often as women (85,87). Most patients are asymptomatic at presentation and uncovered during the workup of other unrelated, nonurologic conditions. A minority of the patients present with hematuria, flank pain, or a palpable mass.

Unlike other renal epithelial neoplasms, no consistent unique genetic abnormality characterizes oncocytoma. However, the most frequent genetic change is loss of chromosomes 1 and Y (88). Less common are translocations involving chromosomes 9 and 11 [t(9;11)(p23;q13)] (89–91) and chromosomes 5 and 11 [t(5;11)(q35;q13)] (92). It is of interest that genes encoding mitochondrial DNA are found in the translocation region of chromosome 11. Familial cases have been described but are uncommon (93).

Gross and Microscopic Features

Oncocytomas are well-circumscribed, nonencapsulated neoplasms that are classically mahogany brown and less often tan to pale yellow. The presence of a central, stellate, radiating scar is seen in roughly 33% of cases and is related to size (87). One should bear in mind that low-grade clear cell renal cell carcinoma and chromophobe renal cell carcinoma may also contain a central scar. Gross hemorrhage is present in 20% of cases, but necrosis is rare (87). Cysts and gross extension into perinephric adipose tissue may be seen but are unusual. Multifocal tumors are seen in up to 17% of cases and bilateral tumors in 4% (85,87). Microscopically the appearance is variable and consists

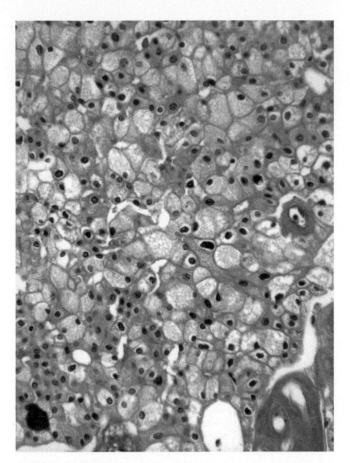

FIGURE 44A.6. Renal oncocytoma. Tumor cells are arranged in nests and have densely eosinophilic cytoplasm. Focal cytologic atypia may be present (original magnification ×100).

of solid, compact nests, acini, tubules, or microcysts embedded within a hypocellular, often hyalinized stroma (Fig. 44A.6). The predominant cell type (so-called "oncocyte") is round to polygonal with granular–eosinophilic cytoplasm, round and regular nuclei with evenly dispersed chromatin, and a centrally placed nucleolus. Occasional clusters of cells with pleomorphic and hyperchromatic nuclei are common. Mitotic activity is rare; necrosis and atypical mitotic figures are not seen. Extension into perinephric adipose tissue is seen in up to 20% of cases (87,94) and vascular invasion in as many as 5% (86,87,94). Because oncocytomas are benign neoplasms, nuclear grading using the criteria of Fuhrman et al. (20) is not clinically useful and should not be performed.

Oncocytosis

Rarely, kidneys with oncocytic tumors may present a spectrum of morphologic features besides the dominant mass. These features include extreme multifocality, oncocytic change in benign tubules, microcysts lined by oncocytic cells, and neoplastic oncocytes infiltrating between benign tubules. The macro- and microscopic oncocytic nodules usually have the morphologic and ultrastructural features of oncocytoma, although some may have either chromophobe or hybrid features. We have chosen the term *oncocytosis* to describe the entire spectrum of morphologic changes present (95). Until the clinical behavior of such hybrid tumors has been better defined, we regard them as low-grade malignant neoplasms much like pure chromophobe renal cell carcinoma. These rare lesions are further evidence of the possible relationship between oncocytoma and chromophobe renal cell carcinoma.

COLLECTING DUCT CARCINOMA

Collecting duct carcinoma (CDC), also known as Bellini duct carcinoma, is rare, comprising less than 1% of renal epithelial tumors. CDC may occur at any age, the mean age at presentation approximating 53 years, with a range of 13 to 83 years. Nevertheless, the overall impression of most experts is that such carcinomas tend to present in younger patients. In the series of six cases reported by Kennedy et al. the mean age was 34 years (96). Although earlier cases had been reported, CDC was not recognized as a clinicopathologic entity until 1986, when Fleming and Lewi described the clinical and morphologic features of six cases (97). CDC is thought to arise within the collecting ducts of the renal medulla, and its rarity is evidenced by the fact that the largest series in the literature includes a mere 12 cases (96–101). The aggressive nature of most of these tumors is evidenced by the fact that more than 50% present with metastatic disease. Although most authors suggest that these aggressive tumors have very distinctive morphologic features, we feel that the true spectrum of the disease remains to be defined. Many high-grade renal epithelial tumors with a papillary or papillary/tubular pattern of growth are placed in this category by default. It is hoped that in the near future this entity will be better defined morphologically, clinically, and genetically. In fact, the genetic and molecular genetic findings of fewer than 25 cases of CDC have been reported (102–106). Fuzesi et al. studied three cases and found consistent monosomy of chromosomes 1, 6, 14, 15, and 22 (106). Polascik et al. found loss of heterozygosity of chromosomal arm 1q in 10 out of 18 cases (102). The latter group subsequently reported that the minimal area of deletion is located at 1q32.1-32.2 (104). Importantly, of all the tumors studied, none has shown trisomy 7/17 or losses of chromosome 3, features seen in PRCC and clear cell RCC, respectively.

Gross and Microscopic Features

CDCs are centered in the medulla, although large tumors may occupy the cortex as well. They are unifocal, solid, tan-white, and firm but may contain cysts as well as gross evidence of hemorrhage and necrosis. Most lesions are poorly circumscribed and often extend into renal sinus and hilar fat.

The histologic features of classic tumors are neoplastic ducts, tubules, and papillae in a fibrotic or desmoplastic stroma (Fig. 44A.7) (96,98,99). Focal spindle cell differentiation is not unusual, and rare cases may be frankly sarcomatoid (107). Distinguishing high-grade urothelial carcinoma from CDC may present a more formidable problem because both may be associated with an inflamed, fibrotic, or desmoplastic stroma and may contain neoplastic cells within renal tubules. In addition, both may have a tubular or tubulopapillary pattern of growth and a similar immunophenotype. Intracytoplasmic mucin may be seen in urothelial tumors, as well. In our experience, the best way to resolve this differential diagnosis is by sampling the renal pelvis well, looking for in situ urothelial carcinoma. Molecular studies also may be of diagnostic utility.

MEDULLARY CARCINOMA

In 1995, Davis et al. from the Armed Forces Institute of Pathology reported a unique group of tumors affecting predominantly young patients of African American descent (108). These tumors appear to be centered in the medulla of the kidney, had distinctive morphologic features, and followed a very aggressive clinical course. Most reported cases had metastatic disease at the time of presentation. They are believed to arise from the

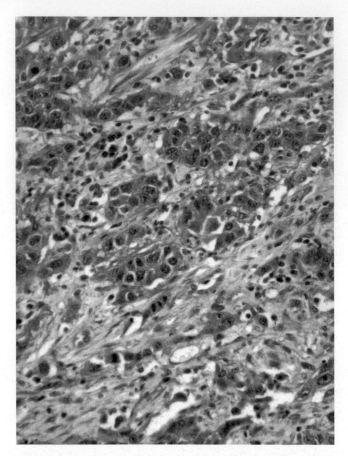

FIGURE 44A.7. Collecting duct carcinoma. Tumor cells are arranged in nests, and tubules have high nuclear grade and are associated with stromal desmoplasia. These tumors may be very difficult to differentiate from urothelial carcinoma, which shares many morphologic and immunohistochemical features (original magnification ×100).

distal portions of the collecting ducts. Patients ranged in age from 11 to 39 years, with a mean of 22 years. Men predominated, especially in patients below the age of 25 years. Mean size of the tumor was 7.0 cm and ranged from 4.0 to 12.0 cm. Interestingly, all patients were believed to have sickle cell trait except for one who had hemoglobin sickle cell disease. Its association with young patients with sickle cell trait, whether of African American, Mediterranean, or other ancestry, has been confirmed in other reports (109–113). Morphologically, these tumors share many features with CDC and, in fact, are believed to be a particularly virulent variant of that entity (98). Tumors are composed of cells with high-grade nuclei and prominent nucleoli arranged in solid nests or irregular tubules. The surrounding stroma is usually fibrotic or desmoplastic and infiltrated by abundant inflammatory cells, mostly polymorphonuclear cells. Sickled and deformed red blood cells are easily identified within the vessels.

RENAL CELL CARCINOMA, UNCLASSIFIED

This diagnostic category includes the renal carcinomas that do not fit into any of the previously described categories, even after genetic analysis (17). Therefore, tumors of unrecognizable cell or architectural types, or those with apparent composites of the recognized types, are all included in this category. These form up to 6% of all renal epithelial tumors (39). Although many of the tumors from this category are of

high cytomorphological grade and aggressive clinical behavior (114), by definition they are not pure entities and include highly aggressive and less aggressive tumor types. An example of the latter group would be those cases that are difficult to classify as oncocytoma or an eosinophilic variant of CRCC.

OTHER EPITHELIAL RENAL NEOPLASMS

Other types of renal neoplasms have been described, some of which are clinically and genetically distinct. Nevertheless, they comprise a small fraction of renal neoplasms and are beyond the scope of this chapter. The authors encourage readers interested in learning more about these entities to go to other sources in the literature (115).

CLINICAL PROGNOSTIC FACTORS IN LOCALIZED RENAL CORTICAL TUMORS

Introduction

A rational means of predicting outcome following definitive surgical treatment, whether by partial or radical nephrectomy, is important for clinicians caring for patients with nonmetastatic renal cortical tumors (Table 44A.5). Historically, prognostic factors focused on pathologic features of the tumor (e.g., nuclear grade, cell morphology), tumor size and stage, local tumor extension, lymph node and adrenal involvement, and presence of metastatic disease (116). In the last decade, however, advances in cytogenetics and histopathologic reclassification have changed our understanding of renal cortical tumors, dramatically necessitating the incorporation of new and important prognostic factors into predictive models. It is now known that renal cortical tumors, viewed previously as a single cancer (i.e., "hypernephroma or renal cell carcinoma) are, instead, a complex family of renal cortical neoplasms with distinct histologic subtypes with unique cytogenetic and molecular defects (117–120). Metastatic potential, once thought to be strictly dependent on tumor size, grade, and stage, is now understood to vary also according to tumor histologic subtype. Rates of metastases range from the most potentially malignant conventional clear cell carcinoma to the more indolent papillary and chromophobe carcinomas to the virtually benign renal oncocytoma (121). In 1997, international investigators defined the Heidelberg classification of renal cortical tumors as follows: *benign* oncocytoma, metanephric adenoma, papillary adenoma; *malignant* conventional clear cell, papillary, chromophobe, collecting duct, and unclassified (Table 44A.1) (16). Also in 1997, the UICC staging system changed the classification of T1 tumors from 2.5 cm or less to 7 cm or less (122). The rise of the incidentally detected renal tumors has also created a tumor stage and size migration that also affects prognosis. The contemporary literature concerning prognostic factors in renal cortical tumors has now moved to incorporate this new information concerning mode of presentation, pathologic staging, and tumor histologic subtypes into predictive models to estimate outcome.

PROGNOSTIC IMPACT OF CLINICAL PRESENTATION

The historic presentation of renal cancer in patients with flank pain, abdominal or flank mass, and hematuria is distinctly uncommon today (<5% of cases) and has been replaced largely by the incidentally discovered solid renal mass (2003, 70% T1, median tumor size 4.5 cm) discovered when abdominal imaging with computerized tomography, magnetic resonance imaging, or ultrasonography is performed for nonspecific abdominal or musculoskeletal complaints or during follow-up of other malignancies (123,124). The ensuing tumor size and stage migration have lead to improved survival following definitive surgical treatment, whether by partial or radical nephrectomy, and is particularly important to recognize when evaluating historical series that may be subjected to reassignment of pathologic subtype or tumor stage using contemporary renal tumor or classification systems (121).

Lee et al. from Memorial Sloan-Kettering Cancer Center (MSKCC) analyzed a large cohort of patients ($n = 718$) who were operated on between 1989 and 1997 and correlated survival to mode of presentation. Symptomatic presentation was defined as a renal tumor detected during evaluation hematuria, flank or abdominal pain, mass, or systemic manifestations such as paraneoplastic syndrome or chronic fatigue (125). In this cohort, 57% of patients had incidental detection and 43% were symptomatic. When compared to incidental cases, symptomatic cases were detected significantly in younger patients (mean age 59 vs. 63), in men, in tumors of conventional clear cell histology, in larger tumors (mean 8.1 cm vs. 4.8 cm), and in tumors that ultimately were nonorgan confined. In multivariate analysis, symptomatic presentation was an independent predictor of disease-free and disease-specific survival, with patients with incidental detected renal tumor living significantly longer than local symptom patients who in turn lived longer than those presenting with systemic symptoms (Fig. 44A.8).

PROGNOSTIC IMPORTANCE OF P-STAGE

Robson et al. initially established the association between renal tumor stages and survival in their initial reports describing the radical nephrectomy (29). Robson et al. described a 65% survival rate for patients with tumors confined within Gerota fascia (Robson 1 and 2), but the finding of metastatic regional nodes was associated with a <30% 5-year survival. Because of descriptive limitations in the Robson system relative to regional node involvement and renal vein or inferior vena cava involvement, most clinical investigators utilize the TNM staging system, which more accurately describes the extent of the local and regional disease (126). Modifications in the TNM classification were made in 1997 that described P1 as 7 cm or less instead of 2.5 cm or less. Another modification in 2002 divided T1 into T1a (<4 cm) and T1b (4–7 cm) (127) (Table 44A.4).

Moch et al. from Switzerland confirmed the prognostic validity of the 1997 TNM staging system in a series of 588 patients dating from 1970 to 1994 with significant differences in overall median survival between pT1 (125 months) and pT2 (90 months) and between pT2 and pT3 (45 months) (128). The Mayo Clinic group also confirmed the validity of the 1997 staging system in a series of 1,547 patients with renal cell carcinoma operated upon between 1970 and 1988 (histologic subtypes not specified) (129).

The impact of modern imaging and changes in the mode of presentation, tumor size, and stage of renal cortical tumors was observed in a 13-year study from the MSKCC, which prospectively tracked 1,378 patients operated upon from 1989 to 2003. Significant trends were observed in incidental presentation (1989: 56%; 2001: 73%) and mean tumor size (1989: 7.9 cm; 2002: 5.15 cm). The percentage of patients with a P1a tumor rose from 8% in 1989 to 43% in 2002, while patients presenting with N+/M+ disease decreased 36% to 8%. Prognostic stratification was achieved with 5-year progression-free probability for P1a/P1b of 96%; P2/3a of 82%; P3b/P3c of 65%; and N1/M1 of 13% (121). Metastatic disease at any site, whether of regional nodal, ipsilateral adrenal, or distant metastases, carried an equally bleak prognosis (130). There is little question that future staging systems will need to incorporate important histologic tumor subtypes to account for stage and size independent differences in metastatic potential.

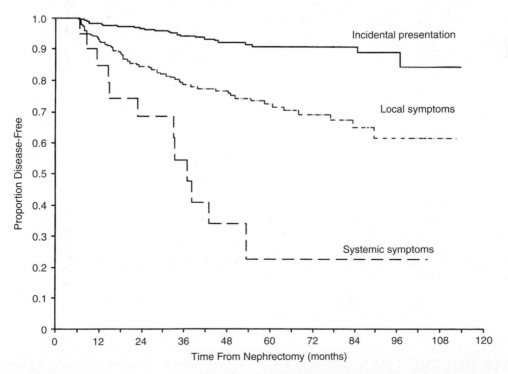

FIGURE 44A.8. Disease-free survival as a function of incidental, local, or systemic presentation. (Source: Lee C.T., Katz J., Fearn P.A., Russo P: Mode of presentation of renal cell carcinoma provides prognostic information. *Urol Oncol* 2002;7:135–140.)

PROGNOSTIC IMPORTANCE OF RENAL CORTICAL TUMOR HISTOLOGY

The pathologic distinctions between tumors of the renal cortex have been realized largely only in the last 25 years. Renal tumor histologic subtypes were previously described by terms such as *granular, clear cell,* and *sarcomatoid,* and recognized differences in tumor growth pattern were not thought to represent distinct histologic entities (131). In 1976, renal oncocytoma was described as a distinct subtype of renal cortical tumor with a lack of metastatic potential (83), although a later report from the MSKCC demonstrated a small but real metastatic potential for these tumors (87). Also in 1976, Mancilla-Jimenez et al. demonstrated a better survival for patients with papillary renal carcinomas (47). The pathologic features of chromophobe renal cell carcinoma were described in 1985 by Thoenes et al. (69). The creation of the Heidelberg renal tumor classification (16) led a number of investigators to incorporate tumor histology into outcome analyses. Moch et al. from Switzerland reviewed 588 nephrectomy specimens accumulated at the University of Basel from 1970 to 1994 and reassigned the histopathology according to the Heidelberg classification and the 1997 TNM classification (P1 <7 cm). In this series, 83% ($n = 487$) were conventional clear cell, 11% ($n = 64$) were papillary, and 5% ($n = 31$) were chromophobe. Survival was significantly associated with pathologic (P) stage. Chromophobe tumors, compared with papillary carcinoma, had a significantly better 5-year survival than conventional clear cell (78% vs. 50%) and tended toward, but did not reach significance. Histologic grade, presence of necrosis, and sarcomatoid differentiation provided independent prognostic information on the conventional clear cell type, but only sarcomatoid differentiation did in the papillary tumors (128). Amin et al. from Henry Ford Hospital in Detroit, Michigan, found similar results in their review of 405 cases of renal cortical tumors of which 63% ($n = 255$) were the conventional clear cell carcinomas, 18.5% ($n = 75$) were papillary carcinomas, 5.7% ($n = 23$) were unclassified, and 7% were benign tumors ($n = 27$ oncocytomas, and $n = 1$ metanephric adenoma). Five-year survival was directly correlated to histologic subtype and was 100% for benign tumors and chromophobe, 86% for papillary, 76% for conventional clear cell, and 24% for unclassified. Other adverse prognosticators in this series included Fuhrman grade, advanced P-stage, vascular invasion, and necrosis (39). In a large, contemporary series of 1,057 patients with nonmetastatic renal cortical malignancies (excluding oncocytoma, unclassified, collecting duct, and medullary types) operated upon between 1989 and 2002 at the MSKCC, Beck et al. confirmed the decreased metastatic potential of chromophobe and papillary carcinoma when compared to conventional clear cell. With a follow-up ranging from 33.2 to 43 months, metastases occurred in 11.9% of 794 conventional clear cell patients, as opposed to 5.7% of 157 and 5.7% of 106 patients with papillary and chromophobe carcinomas, respectively. Multivariate analysis revealed tumor size, tumor stage, and chromophobe histology to be significant variables for disease progression. For tumors of 7 cm or less (P1), eventual metastatic disease occurred in 1.8% of papillary carcinoma and 11.8% of conventional clear cell carcinoma. No patient with a chromophobe carcinoma metastasized less than 7 cm. These studies clearly established the important link between tumor histology and metastatic disease (132).

OUTCOME PREDICTION MODELS

Several groups have worked diligently to create prediction models for renal cortical carcinomas that incorporate multiple variables that separately provide important prognostic information but taken together give a more accurate assessment of the risk of disease progression than the individual variable. Accurate prediction of long-term disease-free survival following resection of a localized renal cortical tumor is a valuable tool for use in patient counseling, planning cost-effective follow-up studies, and identifying poor-risk patients who could be enrolled in adjuvant therapy clinical trials. In addition, because a specific tracking serum or urine biologic marker predictive of systemic relapse in renal cortical tumors has yet to be identified, these predictive models are extremely important tools.

In 1997, investigators from the University of California at Los Angeles (UCLA) described the first such novel staging system—the UCLA Integrated Staging System (UISS)—which incorporated the 1997 TNM stage, Fuhrman grade, and Eastern Cooperative Oncology Group (ECOG) performance status (PS), which, using a multivariate analysis, were effective in stratifying patients into five categories of risk as follows: *UISS 1, low risk patients;* P1, Fuhrman grade 1,2, PS 0. *UISS 2, intermediate-risk patients;* P1, Fuhrman 1,2 PS equal to or greater than 1; P1, Fuhrman 3,4 any PS; P2 with any Fuhrman grade or PS; P3 with any Fuhrman grade and PS 0; or P3, Fuhrman grade 1, PS equal to or greater than 1. *UISS 3–5, high-risk patients;* P3-4, Fuhrman 2-4, PS 0 or equal to or greater than 1 (133). This same group subsequently designed mathematical formulas for both nonmetastatic and metastatic presentation that synthesized the risk of multiple variables to form a single probability of survival. They performed internal validation by comparing the survival curves predicted by their formula to Kaplan Meier survival distributions and found close correlation (134). The UCLA investigators subsequently created comprehensive algorithms in the form of decision boxes utilizing T stage, Fuhrman grade, and PS to allow rapid assignment of risk groups for patients with both clinically localized and metastatic disease, and they were effective in distinguishing outcome relative to risk category. For example, nonmetastatic low-risk patients had 91% disease-specific survival at 5 years, lower recurrence rate, and better disease-free survival compared with nonmetastatic intermediate-risk and high-risk patients (50% progression rate). The investigators also factored immunotherapy into the algorithms for high-risk patients to account for the fact that nonmetastatic high-risk patients had the same survival as metastatic low-risk patients treated with cytoreductive nephrectomy and adjuvant immunotherapy. After immunotherapy, 25% of the metastatic low-risk patients had longer survivals (11 months) than did high-risk metastatic patients (<6 months). The patient population studied at UCLA was skewed toward the metastatic (43%) because of active cytokine-based protocols and does not reflect the current distribution of patients seen with renal cortical tumors in most centers (135). In addition, none of the UCLA studies discussed the important histologic subtypes of renal cortical tumors. This point is important because metastatic nonconventional clear cell tumors, which comprise approximately 10% of the total patients that present with or develop metastases, are refractory to standard cytokine therapies (75). The UCLA investigators recently collaborated with colleagues at the University of Nijmegen, the Netherlands, and the M.D. Anderson Cancer Center to effectively stratify 1,060 patients into low risk (92%–94% 5-year survival), intermediate risk (65%–78% 5-year survival), and high risk (30%–48% 5-year survival), thereby validating their predictive model (136).

With the intent to develop an algorithm to predict progression to metastases after radical nephrectomy and to allow stratification of patients for potential adjuvant therapy trials, Mayo Clinic investigators between 1970 and 2000 evaluated 1,671 patients undergoing radical nephrectomy at their institution for conventional clear cell carcinoma. Tumors of nonclear cell histology were excluded from this study. Clinical features examined included age, gender, smoking history, hypertension, PS, and presenting symptoms. The pathologic features include surgical margins, P stage, regional lymph node status, tumor size, nuclear grade, tumor necrosis, cystic architecture, and tumor multifocality. A multivariate Cox proportional hazards regression model was used to determine associations between the clinical and pathologic features and distant metastases. The investigators found that the most important features associated with progression to metastases were P stage, nodal status, tumor size, nuclear grade, and histologic tumor necrosis. Using the regression coefficients from the multivariate model, they developed a scoring algorithm. The coefficient for each feature was divided by the coefficient for primary tumor stage, multiplied by 4, and rounded to the nearest whole number. The median score was 3 (range 0–11), and this method led to effective stratification of metastases-free survival with an internal validation from bootstrapping of .819 (.5 being chance, 1.0 being a perfect prediction). In this study, patients with scores of 0 to 2 did not reach a median survival, whereas median survivals were 12.1 years for a score of 5, 2.2 years for a score of 6, 1.5 years for a score of 7, and 0.5 years for a score greater than 8 (137).

In an effort to determine the factors associated with site-specific metastases, in a recent study the Mayo Clinic investigators designed scoring algorithms based on 1,864 patients operated upon for conventional clear cell carcinoma. The most common sites of metastatic disease were the thorax (16%), abdomen (10%), bone (7%), and brain (4%). Positive surgical margins, TNM stage, size, grade, and necrosis were significantly associated with abdominal recurrence, whereas all of these factors except the positive margins were associated with thoracic recurrence. TMN stage, grade, and necrosis were most predictive of bone metastases. The investigators argued that follow-up scans can be tailored to the most likely sites of eventual metastases (138).

Investigators from the MSKCC created a postoperative nomogram using Cox proportional hazards regression analysis and modeled pathologic data and clinical follow-up in 601 patients treated July 1, 1989, through December 31, 1998. Factors incorporated into the nomogram included the major malignant tumor histologic subtypes (conventional clear cell, papillary, chromophobe), the mode of presentation (incidental, local, or systemic), tumor size, and pathologic stage. More precise pathologic features that did not apply across all histologic subtypes were not included. In this cohort, disease recurrence was noted in 66 of 601 patients, and the 5-year probability of freedom of recurrence was 86% (95% confidence interval of 82%–89%). Using internal validation techniques, predictions by the nomogram appeared accurate and discriminating with an area under the operating curve—that is, the comparison of the predicted probability with actual outcome of 0.74 (Fig. 44A.9) (139).

This postoperative nomogram has proven highly effective in clinical practice for use in patient teaching and counseling, designing more cost-effective and less-intense patient follow schemes (particularly in good prognostic patients), and has the potential to play a role in clinical trial design. The MSKCC postoperative renal cancer nomogram is currently available for use with handheld personal digital assistants and can be viewed on the MSKCC Web site. This group is currently designing a postoperative nomogram specifically for conventional clear cell carcinoma utilizing pathologic stage, Fuhrman grade, tumor size, necrosis, vascular invasion, and clinical presentation. As important prognostic factors are discovered (i.e., tumor specific markers), they can be added to nomograms in order to improve their predictive value.

PROGNOSTIC FACTORS FOR METASTATIC RENAL CORTICAL TUMORS

Introduction

Metastatic renal cell carcinoma is generally associated with a poor prognosis, since RCC is highly resistant to chemotherapy (140). Immunotherapy with interleukin-2 and/or interferon-α achieves clinical responses in 10% to 20% of patients (140). The identification of prognostic factors is helpful in assessing treatment outcome of new therapies studied in phase II and III trials and may potentially be applied to risk-directed therapy.

Early experience showed that patients most likely to respond to interferon-α had undergone a prior nephrectomy and had small-volume lung-only metastasis (141). In a randomized phase III trial conducted by the ECOG, a major response proportion (complete plus partial response) of 30% was reported for patients with these clinical features (142). Univariate analyses showed that longer survival following treatment with immunotherapy was associated with high PS, prior nephrectomy, and lung-predominant metastases (143,144). Prognostic factors varied to some degree between studies but consistently included PS, nephrectomy, and a measure of extent of disease (145–150).

MODELS FROM MULTIVARIATE ANALYSIS

A selection of multivariate analyses that resulted in criteria for risk stratification is shown in Table 44A.1 (145–150). The first comprehensive analysis was reported by Elson et al. in 610 patients treated with chemotherapy on phase II trials prior to 1984 (145). The patient population (145) differs from that of the present era, since imaging techniques have improved and patients were selected for phase II trials of cytotoxic agents. The median survival for patients treated in that series was 5.6 months (145) compared to 10 months in a recent series (151). Efforts now include models for predicting survival following treatment with interferon-α or interleukin-2 (152) and a model for predicting survival in patients with localized and metastatic RCC at initial diagnosis (135). The experiences of the MSKCC, the Groupe Francais d'Immunotherapie, and UCLA are highlighted.

MSKCC MODELS

Factors related to survival in 670 patients with advanced RCC treated in 24 consecutive clinical trials from September 1975 to July 1996 were studied. Treatment on the clinical trial was classified as an immunotherapy (interferon-α, interleukin-2) or chemotherapy (151). The median overall survival time was 10 months. The proportion of patients surviving at 1 year was 42%; the 2- to 3-year survival proportions were 20% and 11%, respectively.

Seven variables identified in the univariate analysis were analyzed according to multivariate analysis to determine whether they had an independent relation to survival. These included hemoglobin, serum lactate dehydrogenase, corrected calcium, prior nephrectomy, Karnofsky PS, hepatic metastases, and the interval from diagnosis to treatment. Pretreatment features associated with a shorter survival that maintained independent significance after the multivariate analysis were low Karnofsky PS (<80%), High

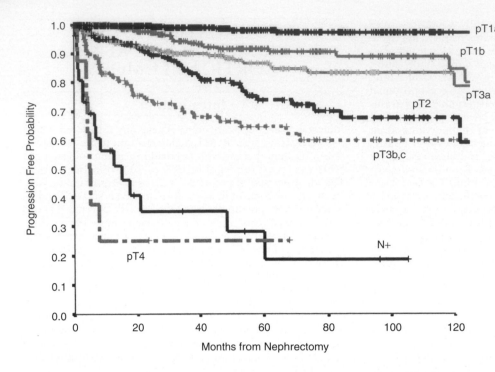

FIGURE 44A.9. Progression-free survival as a function of pathologic (P) stage. (Source: Russo P., Snyder M.E., Di Blasio C.J., Sorbellini M., Kattan M., Motzer R.J., Reuter V.E., Changing demographics and the contemporary surgicall management of renal cortical tumors. *J Urol* 2003;169: 347A.)

serum lactate dehydrogenase (>1.5 times upper limit of normal), low hemoglobin (< lower limit of normal), high "corrected" serum calcium (>10 mg per dL), and the absence of a prior nephrectomy.

These five prognostic factors were used to assign patients by risk into three different groups (Table 44A.6). The median time to death in the 25% of patients with zero risk factors (favorable risk) was 20 months. Of the patients, 53% had one or two of these prognostic features (intermediate risk), and the median survival in this group was 10 months. Patients with three or more risk factors (poor risk), comprising 22% of the patients, had a median survival of only 4 months.

The predictive performance of the model was internally validated through a two-step nonparametric bootstrapping process. The model was also applied to an external data set from ECOG composed of 175 patients treated with of interferon-α therapy on a phase III randomized trial. In this cohort, the median survival times of favorable-, intermediate-, and poor-risk patients were 29, 14, and 4 months, respectively.

Reducing heterogeneity due to varied therapies and assessing the role of nephrectomy as a risk factor in light of a randomized trial (153) prompted an analysis on prognostic factors for survival following interferon-α therapy for 463 previously untreated patients (154). The median overall survival time was

TABLE 44A.5

SELECTED SERIES OF PROGNOSTIC FACTORS FOR SURVIVAL

Author	Yr	Patients	Treatment	Independent pretreatment prognostic factors used in model
Elson et al. {4496}	1988	610	Chemotherapy	Performance status, time from initial diagnosis, number of metastatic sites, prior chemotherapy, and prior weight loss
DeForges {4495}	1988	134	Chemotherapy and interferon	Hepatic metastasis, lung metastasis, time from initial diagnosis, sedimentation rate, weight loss
Palmer et al. {3571}	1992	327	Interleukin-2	Performance status, time from initial diagnosis, number of metastatic sites
Jones et al. {4494}	1993	387	Interleukin-2	Performance status, number of metastatic sites, time from initial diagnosis
Fossa et al. {4531}	1994	295	Interferon + chemotherapy	Performance status, sedimentation rate, weight loss
Lopez-Hannineh et al. {4080}	1996	215	Interleukin-2 with/without interferon, FU	Erythrocyte sedimentation rate, lactate dehydrogenase concentration, neutrophil count, hemoglobin, extrapulmonary metastases
Motzer et al. {4709}	1998	670	Interferon, interleukin-2, chemotherapy	Nephrectomy, Karnofsky performance status, hemoglobin, adjusted calcium, lactate dehydrogenase
Negrier et al. {4967}	2002		Interferon, interleukin-2	Neutrophil count, time from initial diagnosis, number of metastatic sites, liver metastases

TABLE 44A.6

PATIENT SURVIVAL ACCORDING TO RISK GROUP

Number of risk factors	%	% alive	Median survival (95% CI)	1-yr survival (%)	3-yr survival (%)
0	25	18	19.9 (17.1, 27.9)	71	31
1 or 2	53	7	10.3 (8.9, 11.4)	42	7
3, 4, or 5	22	0.7	3.9 (3.4, 5.0)	12	0

CI, confidence interval.

POSTOPERATIVE PROGNOSTIC NOMOGRAM FOR RCC

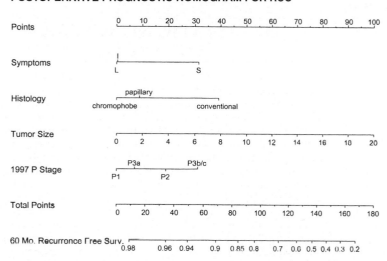

Instructions for Physician: Locate the patient's symptoms (I = incidental, L = local, S = systemic) on the Symptoms axis. Draw a line straight upwards to the **Points** axis to determine how many points towards recurrence the patient receives for his symptoms. Repeat this process for the other axes, each time drawing straight upward to the **Points** axis. Sum the points achieved for each predictor and locate this sum on the **Total Points** axis. Draw a line straight down to find the patient's probability of remaining recurrence free for 5 years assuming he or she does not die of another cause first.

Instruction to Patient. "Mr. X, if we had 100 men or women exactly like you, we would expect between <predicted percentage from nomogram – 10%> and <predicted percentage + 10%> to remain free of their disease at 5 years following surgery, though recurrence after 5 years is still possible."

FIGURE 44.10.

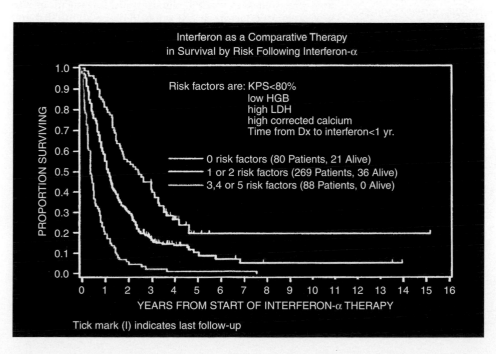

FIGURE 44.11.

13 months (95% CI: 12–15 months). The proportion of patients surviving at 1 and 3 years was 54% and 19%, respectively. The median time to progression was 4.7 months (95% CI: 4.1–5.3 months) (154).

Five variables were selected by univariate and multivariate analysis as prognostic and were used as risk factors for short survival: low Karnofsky PS (<80%), high lactate dehydrogenase (>1.5 × times limit of normal), low serum hemoglobin (< lower limit of normal), high "corrected" serum calcium (>10 mg per dL) and time from initial RCC diagnosis to start of interferon-α therapy for less than 1 year (154). Each patient was assigned to one of three risk groups: those with zero (favorable), one or two (intermediate), and three or more (poor) risk factors. There was a significant difference in survival distributions of the three risk groups (P <.0001). The median time to death of patients deemed favorable risk was 30 months (154). Median survival in the intermediate-risk group was 14 months (154). In contrast, the poor-risk group had a median survival of 5 months. Recently, the model was found to be predictive when applied to an independent data set from the Cleveland Clinic (155).

GROUP FRANCAIS D'IMMUNOTHERAPIE EXPERIENCE

The Group Francais d'Immunotherapie examined prognostic factors associated with survival and rapid progression in patients with metastatic RCC treated by cytokines (152). The population consisted of 782 patients treated on five multicenter trials using cytokine combinations of interferon-α, interleukin-2, or both. Nine parameters were identified as independent prognostic factors: signs of inflammation as detected by sedimentation rate or C-reactive protein, time interval from renal tumor to metastases, number of circulating neutrophils, presence of liver metastases, presence of bone metastases, ECOG PS, number of metastatic sites, elevated level of alkaline phosphatase, and hemoglobin level. The researchers highlighted five parameters: PS, number of metastatic sites, disease-free interval, signs of inflammation, and hemoglobin level. Also, they identified four independent factors predictive of rapid disease progression during cytokine therapy: presence of hepatic metastases, less than 1-year interval from renal tumor to metastases, more than one site of metastases, and elevated neutrophil count. Patients who had three or more of these factors had >80% probability of rapid progression within 3 months despite treatment. The authors recommended that these patients be considered for novel therapies rather than treatment with a cytokine.

UNIVERSITY OF CALIFORNIA AT LOS ANGELES MODEL

Prognostic indicators were analyzed for patients at initial diagnosis by nephrectomy (156). The 643 patients mostly had tumors localized to the kidney, but some had clinical evidence of metastases. Patients were evaluated for preoperative functional status; tumor, nodes, and metastases (TNM) stage; and disease grade. The 5-year cancer-specific survival rate based on TNM stage was 91%, 74%, 67%, and 32% for stages I, II, III, and IV tumors, respectively. Tumor grade strongly correlated with survival. Multivariate analysis revealed that the overall TNM stage and grade of disease were most important prognostic indicators, with ECOG classification prior to surgery and tumor stage less predictive.

Data from the 477 patients undergoing nephrectomy were used to derive a mathematical model to predict individual survival and thus guide decisions regarding surgery (156). A population of 292 nonmetastatic RCC patients and 262 metastatic RCC patients who underwent nephrectomy was evaluated for survival. Metastatic and nonmetastatic patients were analyzed separately. For nonmetastatic patients, the significant factors predicting survival were Fuhrman grade and ECOG PS. For metastatic patients, the significant factors predicting survival were classification of T stage, number of symptoms, nodal involvement, and immunotherapy. These variables were then implanted into an exponential Nadas equation to derive a mathematical model to predict survival, with separate equations for nonmetastatic and metastatic patients (134).

METASTATIC NONCLEAR CELL TYPES

Progress in understanding the genetic features of RCC has facilitated classification into clear cell and nonclear cell subtypes such as papillary, chromophobe, and collecting duct histology. The responsiveness of the nonclear cell types to immunotherapy remains to be determined. More than 90% of patients with metastatic RCC have clear cell histology. The outcome data for 64 patients with histologies other than clear cell type was reviewed (75). Histologies were collecting duct tumors in 26 patients, chromophobe tumors in 12 patients, papillary histology in 19 patients, and unclassifiable tumors in 7 patients. The median overall survival time was 9.4 months. The survival was longer for patients with chromophobe tumors compared to collecting duct or papillary histology, and this group included patients with survival >3 years. In contrast, patients with metastatic papillary and collecting duct cell types had a shorter survival.

CONCLUSION

Prognostic models based on pretreatment clinical and laboratory variables can help define patients more likely to benefit from standard therapies and can assist in the interpretation of drug effectiveness in Phase II clinical trials. Investigations into new prognostic factors–based tumor biology are needed and are of the highest priority.

References

1. van den Berg E, van der Hout AH, Oosterhuis JW, et al. Cytogenetic analysis of epithelial renal-cell tumors: Relationship with a new histopathological classification. *Int J Cancer* 1993;55:223–227.
2. Weiss LM, Gelb AB, Medeiros LJ. Adult renal epithelial neoplasms. *Am J Clin Pathol* 1995;103:624–635.
3. Thoenes W, Storkel S, Rumpelt HJ. Histopathology and classification of renal cell tumors (adenomas, oncocytomas and carcinomas): The basic cytological and histopathological elements and their use for diagnostics. *Pathol Res Pract* 1986;181:125–143.
4. Dal Cin P, Gaeta J, Huben R, et al. Renal cortical tumors. Cytogenetic characterization. *Am J Clin Pathol* 1989;92:408–414.
5. Kovacs G, Erlandsson R, Boldog F, et al. Consistent chromosome 3p deletion and loss of heterozygosity in renal cell carcinoma. *Proc Natl Acad Sci U S A* 1988;85:1571–1575.
6. Kovacs G, Frisch S. Clonal chromosome abnormalities in tumor cells from patients with sporadic renal cell carcinomas. *Cancer Res* 1989;49:651–659.
7. Fleming S. The impact of genetics on the classification of renal carcinoma. *Histopathology* 1993;22:89–92.
8. Kovacs G, Wilkens L, Papp T, et al. Differentiation between papillary and nonpapillary renal cell carcinomas by DNA analysis. *J Natl Cancer Inst* 1989;81:527–530.
9. Kovacs G, Fuzesi L, Emanual A, et al. Cytogenetics of papillary renal cell tumors. *Genes Chromosomes Cancer* 1991;3:249–255.

10. Kovacs G. Molecular differential pathology of renal cell tumours. *Histopathology* 1993;22:1–8.
11. Presti JC, Rao PH, Chen Q, et al. Histopathological, cytogenetic, and molecular characterization of renal cortical tumors. *Cancer Res* 1991;51: 1544–1552.
12. Hughson MD, Johnson LD, Silva FG, et al. Nonpapillary and papillary renal cell carcinoma: A cytogenetic and phenotypic study. *Mod Pathol* 1993;6:449–456.
13. Presti JC Jr, Reuter VE, Cordon-Cardo C, et al. Allelic deletions in renal tumors: Histopathological correlations. *Cancer Res* 1993;53:5780–5783.
14. Yoshida MA, Ohyashiki K, Ochi H, et al. Cytogenetic studies of tumor tissue from patients with nonfamilial renal cell carcinoma. *Cancer Res* 1986; 46:2139–2147.
15. Carroll PR, Murty VV, Reuter V, et al. Abnormalities at chromosome region 3p12–14 characterize clear cell renal carcinoma. *Cancer Genet Cytogenet* 1987;26:253–259.
16. Kovacs G, Akhtar M, Beckwith BJ, et al. The Heidelberg classification of renal cell tumours. *J Pathol* 1997;183:131–133.
17. Storkel S, Eble JN, Adlakha K, et al. Classification of renal cell carcinoma: Workgroup No. 1. Union Internationale Contre le Cancer (UICC) and the American Joint Committee on Cancer (AJCC). *Cancer* 1997;80:987–989.
18. Eble J, Sauter G, Epstein J, et al. *Pathology and genetics of tumours of the urinary system and male genital organs.* Lyon: IARC Press, 2004.
19. Motzer RJ, Bander NH, Nanus DM. Renal-cell carcinoma. *N Engl J Med* 1996;335:865–875.
20. Fuhrman SA, Lasky LC, Limas C. Prognostic significance of morphologic parameters in renal cell carcinoma. *Am J Surg Pathol* 1982;6:655–663.
21. Schouman M, Warter A, Ross M, et al. Renal cell carcinoma. Statistical study of survival based on pathological criteria. *World J Urol* 1984;2:109–113.
22. Medeiros LJ, Jones EC, Aizawa S, et al. Grading of renal cell carcinoma: Workgroup No. 2. Union Internationale Contre le Cancer and the American Joint Committee on Cancer (AJCC). *Cancer* 1997;80:990–991.
23. Goldstein NS. The current state of renal cell carcinoma grading. Union Internationale Contre le Cancer (UICC) and the American Joint Committee on Cancer (AJCC). *Cancer* 1997;80:977–980.
24. Lanigan D, Conroy R, Barry-Walsh C, et al. A comparative analysis of grading systems in renal adenocarcinoma. *Histopathology* 1994;24:473–476.
25. Storkel S, Thoenes W, Jacobi GH, et al. Prognostic parameters in renal cell carcinoma: A new approach. *Eur Urol* 1989;16:416–422.
26. Amin MB, Corless CL, Renshaw AA, et al. Papillary (chromophil) renal cell carcinoma: Histomorphologic characteristics and evaluation of conventional pathologic prognostic parameters in 62 cases. *Am J Surg Pathol* 1997;21:621–635.
27. Tickoo S, Reuter V. Subtyping papillary renal cell carcinoma: A clinicopathologic study of 103 cases. *Mod Pathol* 2001;14:124A.
28. Delahunt B, Eble JN, McCredie MR, et al. Morphologic typing of papillary renal cell carcinoma: Comparison of growth kinetics and patient survival in 66 cases. *Hum Pathol* 2001;32:590–595.
29. Robson CJ, Churchill BM, Anderson W. The results of radical nephrectomy for renal cell carcinoma. *J Urol* 1969;101:297–301.
30. Beahrs OH, Henson DE, Hutter RV, et al. *Handbook for staging of cancer.* Philadelphia, PA: Lippincott, 1993.
31. Green F, Page D, Fleming I, et al. *AJCC cancer staging manual.* Springer, 2002.
32. Crotty TB, Farrow GM, Lieber MM. Chromophobe cell renal carcinoma: Clinicopathological features of 50 cases. *J Urol* 1995;154:964–967.
33. Guinan P, Sobin LH, Algaba F, et al. TNM staging of renal cell carcinoma: Workgroup No. 3. Union International Contre le Cancer (UICC) and the American Joint Committee on Cancer (AJCC). *Cancer* 1997;80:992–993.
34. Nordenson I, Ljungberg B, Roos G. Chromosomes in renal carcinoma with reference to intratumor heterogeneity. *Cancer Genet Cytogenet* 1988; 32:35–41.
35. Walter TA, Berger CS, Sandberg AA. The cytogenetics of renal tumors: Where do we stand, where do we go? *Cancer Genet Cytogenet* 1989;43: 15–34.
36. Teyssier JR, Ferre D. Chromosomal changes in renal cell carcinoma. No evidence for correlation with clinical stage. *Cancer Genet Cytogenet* 1990; 45:197–205.
37. Zbar B. Von Hippel-Lindau disease and sporadic renal cell carcinoma. *Cancer Surv* 1995;25:219–232.
38. Bryant D, Scheinfeld A, Russo P, et al. Conventional renal cell carcinomas: A clinicopathologic study of 183 cases from 1991 to 1994. *Mod Pathol* 1998;11:77A.
39. Amin MB, Tamboli P, Javidan J, et al. Prognostic impact of histologic subtyping of adult renal epithelial neoplasms: An experience of 405 cases. *Am J Surg Pathol* 2002;26:281–291.
40. Eble JN, Bonsib SM. Extensively cystic renal neoplasms: Cystic nephroma, cystic partially differentiated nephroblastoma, multilocular cystic renal cell carcinoma, and cystic hamartoma of renal pelvis. *Semin Diagn Pathol* 1998;15:2–20.
41. Murad T, Komaiko W, Oyasu R, et al. Multilocular cystic renal cell carcinoma. *Am J Clin Pathol* 1991;95:633–637.
42. Taxy JB, Marshall FF. Multilocular renal cysts in adults. Possible relationship to renal adenocarcinoma. *Arch Pathol Lab Med* 1983;107:633–637.
43. Tamura Y, Okamura K, Ogura H, et al. Multilocular cystic renal cell carcinoma: A report of 2 cases. *Hinyokika Kiyo* 1990;36:437–441.
44. Sakurai M, Sugimura Y, Satani H, et al. Multilocular cystic renal cell carcinoma: A report of two cases. *Hinyokika Kiyo* 1993;39:45–49.
45. Nassir A, Jollimore J, Gupta R, et al. Multilocular cystic renal cell carcinoma: A series of 12 cases and review of the literature. *Urology* 2002;60: 421–427.
46. Cheville JC, Lohse CM, Zincke H, et al. Comparisons of outcome and prognostic features among histologic subtypes of renal cell carcinoma. *Am J Surg Pathol* 2003;27:612–624.
47. Mancilla-Jimenez R, Stanley RJ, Blath RA. Papillary renal cell carcinoma: A clinical, radiologic, and pathologic study of 34 cases. *Cancer* 1976;38: 2469–2480.
48. Skinner DG, Colvin RB, Vermillion CD, et al. Diagnosis and management of renal cell carcinoma. A clinical and pathologic study of 309 cases. *Cancer* 1971;28:1165–1177.
49. El-Naggar AK, Ro JY, Ensign LG. Papillary renal cell carcinoma: Clinical implication of DNA content analysis. *Hum Pathol* 1993;24:316–321.
50. Kovacs G. Papillary renal cell carcinoma. A morphologic and cytogenetic study of 11 cases. *Am J Pathol* 1989;134:27–34.
51. Henn W, Zwergel T, Wullich B, et al. Bilateral multicentric papillary renal tumors with heteroclonal origin based on tissue-specific karyotype instability. *Cancer* 1993;72:1315–1318.
52. Ishikawa I, Shikura N, Ozaki M. Papillary renal cell carcinoma with numeric changes of chromosomes in a long-term hemodialysis patient: A karyotype analysis. *Am J Kidney Dis* 1993;21:553–556.
53. De Jong B, Molenaar IM, Leeuw JA, et al. Cytogenetics of a renal adenocarcinoma in a 2-year-old child. *Cancer Genet Cytogenet* 1986;21:165–169.
54. Shipley JM, Birdsall S, Clark J, et al. Mapping the X chromosome breakpoint in two papillary renal cell carcinoma cell lines with a t(X;1)(p11.2;q21.2) and the first report of a female case. *Cytogenet Cell Genet* 1995;71:280–284.
55. Sidhar SK, Clark J, Gill S, et al. The t(X;1)(p11.2;q21.2) translocation in papillary renal cell carcinoma fuses a novel gene PRCC to the TFE3 transcription factor gene. *Hum Mol Genet* 1996;5:1333–1338.
56. Takahashi M, Kahnoski R, Gross D, et al. Familial adult renal neoplasia. *J Med Genet* 2002;39:1–5.
57. Weterman MA, van Groningen JJ, den Hartog A, et al. Transformation capacities of the papillary renal cell carcinoma-associated PRCCTFE3 and TFE3PRCC fusion genes. *Oncogene* 2001;20:1414–1424.
58. Weterman MA, van Groningen JJ, Tertoolen L, et al. Impairment of MAD2B–PRCC interaction in mitotic checkpoint defective t(X;1)-positive renal cell carcinomas. *Proc Natl Acad Sci U S A* 2001;98:13,808–13,813.
59. Ladanyi M, Lui MY, Antonescu CR, et al. The der(17)(X;17)(p11;q25) of human alveolar soft part sarcoma fuses the TFE3 transcription factor gene to ASPL, a novel gene at 17q25. *Oncogene* 2001;20:48–57.
60. Argani P, Antonescu CR, Illei PB, et al. Primary renal neoplasms with the ASPL-TFE3 gene fusion of alveolar soft part sarcoma: A distinctive tumor entity previously included among renal cell carcinomas of children and adolescents. *Am J Pathol* 2001;159:179–192.
61. Schmidt L, Junker K, Nakaigawa N, et al. Novel mutations of the MET proto-oncogene in papillary renal carcinomas. *Oncogene* 1999;18: 2343–2350.
62. Renshaw AA, Zhang H, Corless CL, et al. Solid variants of papillary (chromophil) renal cell carcinoma: Clinicopathologic and genetic features. *Am J Surg Pathol* 1997;21:1203–1209.
63. Delahunt B, Eble JN. Papillary renal cell carcinoma: A clinicopathologic and immunohistochemical study of 105 tumors. *Mod Pathol* 1997;10:537–544.
64. Jiang F, Richter J, Schraml P, et al. Chromosomal imbalances in papillary renal cell carcinoma: Genetic differences between histological subtypes. *Am J Pathol* 1998;153:1467–1473.
65. Renshaw AA, Corless CL. Papillary renal cell carcinoma. Histology and immunohistochemistry. *Am J Surg Pathol* 1995;19:842–849.
66. Lager DJ, Huston BJ, Timmerman TG, et al. Papillary renal tumors: Morphologic, cytochemical, and genotypic features. *Cancer* 1995;76:669–673.
67. Sanders ME, Mick R, Tomaszewski JE, et al. Unique patterns of allelic imbalance distinguish type 1 from type 2 sporadic papillary renal cell carcinoma. *Am J Pathol* 2002;161:997–1005.
68. Thoenes W, Storkel S, Rumpelt HJ. Human chromophobe cell renal carcinoma. *Virchows Arch B Cell Pathol Incl Mol Pathol* 1985;48:207–217.
69. Thoenes W, Storkel S, Rumpelt HJ, et al. Chromophobe cell renal carcinoma and its variants: A report on 32 cases. *J Pathol* 1988;155:277–287.
70. Akhtar M, Kardar H, Linjawi T, et al. Chromophobe cell carcinoma of the kidney: A clinicopathologic study of 21 cases. *Am J Surg Pathol* 1995;19: 1245–1256.
71. Cochand-Priollet B, Molinie V, Bougaran J, et al. Renal chromophobe cell carcinoma and oncocytoma: A comparative morphologic, histochemical, and immunohistochemical study of 124 cases. *Arch Pathol Lab Med* 1997;121:1081–1086.
72. DeLong WH, Sakr W, Grignon DG. Chromophobe renal cell carcinoma. A comparative histochemical and immunohistochemical study. *J Urol Pathol* 1996;4:1–8.
73. Renshaw AA, Henske EP, Loughlin KR, et al. Aggressive variants of chromophobe renal cell carcinoma. *Cancer* 1996;78:1756–1761.
74. Bonsib SM, Lager DJ. Chromophobe cell carcinoma: Analysis of five cases. *Am J Surg Pathol* 1990;14:260–267.
75. Motzer RJ, Bacik J, Mariani T, et al. Treatment outcome and survival associated with metastatic renal cell carcinoma of non-clear-cell histology. *J Clin Oncol* 2002;20:2376–2381.

76. Bugert P, Gaul C, Weber K, et al. Specific genetic changes of diagnostic importance in chromophobe renal cell carcinomas. *Lab Invest* 1997;76: 203–208.

77. Schwerdtle RF, Storkel S, Neuhaus C, et al. Allelic losses at chromosomes 1p, 2p, 6p, 10p, 13q, 17p, and 21q significantly correlate with the chromophobe subtype of renal cell carcinoma. *Cancer Res* 1996;56:2927–2930.

78. Kovacs A, Kovacs G. Low chromosome number in chromophobe renal cell carcinomas. *Genes Chromosomes Cancer* 1992;4:267–268.

79. Akhtar M, Al-Sohaibani MO, Haleem A, et al. Flow cytometric DNA analysis of chrmophobe cell carcinoma of the kidney. *J Urol Pathol* 1996; 4:15–23.

80. Kovacs A, Storkel S, Thoenes W, et al. Mitochondrial and chromosomal DNA alterations in human chromophobe renal cell carcinomas. *J Pathol* 1992;167:273–277.

81. Akhtar M, Tulbah A, Kardar AH, et al. Sarcomatoid renal cell carcinoma: The chromophobe connection. *Am J Surg Pathol* 1997;21:1188–1195.

82. Zippel L. Zur kenntnis der onkocytonen. *Virchows Arch Pathol Anat* 1942;308:360–382.

83. Klein MJ, Valensi QJ. Proximal tubular adenomas of kidney with so-called oncocytic features: A clinicopathologic study of 13 cases of a rarely reported neoplasm. *Cancer* 1976;38:906–914.

84. Frydenberg M, Eckstein RP, Saalfield JA, et al. Renal oncocytomas: An Australian experience. *Br J Urol* 1991;67:352–357.

85. Amin MB, Crotty TB, Tickoo SK, et al. Renal oncocytoma: A reappraisal of morphologic features with clinicopathologic findings in 80 cases. *Am J Surg Pathol* 1997;21:1–12.

86. Lieber MM, Tomera KM, Farrow GM. Renal oncocytoma. *J Urol* 1981; 125:481–485.

87. Perez-Ordonez B, Hamed G, Campbell S, et al. Renal oncocytoma: A clinicopathologic study of 70 cases. *Am J Surg Pathol* 1997;21:871–883.

88. Crotty TB, Lawrence KM, Moertel CA, et al. Cytogenetic analysis of six renal oncocytomas and a chromophobe cell renal carcinoma: Evidence that -Y, -1 may be a characteristic anomaly in renal oncocytomas. *Cancer Genet Cytogenet* 1992;61:61–66.

89. Fuzesi L, Gunawan B, Braun S, et al. Renal oncocytoma with a translocation t(9;11)(p23;q13). *J Urol* 1994;152:471–472.

90. Neuhaus C, Dijkhuizen T, van den Berg E, et al. Involvement of the chromosomal region 11q13 in renal oncocytoma: Case report and literature review. *Cancer Genet Cytogenet* 1997;94:95–98.

91. Walter TA, Pennington RD, Decker HJ, et al. Translocation t(9;11) (p23;q12): A primary chromosomal change in renal oncocytoma. *J Urol* 1989;142:117–119.

92. Van den Berg E, Dijkhuizen T, Storkel S, et al. Chromosomal changes in renal oncocytomas: Evidence that t(5;11)(q35;q13) may characterize a second subgroup of oncocytomas. *Cancer Genet Cytogenet* 1995;79:164–168.

93. Weirich G, Glenn G, Junker K, et al. Familial renal oncocytoma: Clinicopathological study of 5 families. *J Urol* 1998;160:335–340.

94. Davis CJ Jr, Mostofi FK, Sesterhenn I, et al. Renal oncocytoma: Clinicopathological study of 166 patients. *J Urogen Pathol* 1991;1:41–52.

95. Tickoo SK, Reuter VE, Amin MB, et al. Renal oncocytosis: A morphologic study of fourteen cases. *Am J Surg Pathol* 1999;23:1094–1101.

96. Kennedy SM, Merino MJ, Linehan WM, et al. Collecting duct carcinoma of the kidney. *Hum Pathol* 1990;21:449–456.

97. Fleming S, Lewi HJ. Collecting duct carcinoma of the kidney. *Histopathology* 1986;10:1131–1141.

98. Amin MB, Varma MD, Tickoo SK, et al. Collecting duct carcinoma of the kidney. *Adv Anat Pathol* 1997;4:85–94.

99. Srigley JR, Eble JN. Collecting duct carcinoma of kidney. *Semin Diagn Pathol* 1998;15:54–67.

100. Rumpelt HJ, Storkel S, Moll R, et al. Bellini duct carcinoma: Further evidence for this rare variant of renal cell carcinoma. *Histopathology* 1991; 18:115–122.

101. Dimopoulos MA, Logothetis CJ, Markowitz A, et al. Collecting duct carcinoma of the kidney. *Br J Urol* 1993;71:388–391.

102. Polascik TJ, Cairns P, Epstein JI, et al. Distal nephron renal tumors: Microsatellite allelotype. *Cancer Res* 1996;56:1892–1895.

103. Schoenberg M, Cairns P, Brooks JD, et al. Frequent loss of chromosome arms 8p and 13q in collecting duct carcinoma (CDC) of the kidney. *Genes Chromosomes Cancer* 1995;12:76–80.

104. Steiner G, Cairns P, Polascik TJ, et al. High-density mapping of chromosomal arm 1q in renal collecting duct carcinoma: Region of minimal deletion at 1q32.1-32.2. *Cancer Res* 1996;56:5044–5046.

105. Gregori-Romero MA, Morell-Quadreny L, Llombart-Bosch A. Cytogenetic analysis of three primary Bellini duct carcinomas. *Genes Chromosomes Cancer* 1996;15:170–172.

106. Fuzesi L, Cober M, Mittermayer C. Collecting duct carcinoma: Cytogenetic characterization. *Histopathology* 1992;21:155–160.

107. Baer SC, Ro JY, Ordonez NG, et al. Sarcomatoid collecting duct carcinoma: a clinicopathologic and immunohistochemical study of five cases. *Hum Pathol* 1993;24:1017–1022.

108. Davis CJ, Mostofi FK, Sesterhenn IA. Renal medullary carcinoma: The seventh sickle cell nephropathy. *Am J Surg Pathol* 1995;19:1–11.

109. Figenshau RS, Basler JW, Ritter JH, et al. Renal medullary carcinoma. *J Urol* 1998;159:711–713.

110. Avery RA, Harris JE, Davis CJ, et al. Renal medullary carcinoma: Clinical and therapeutic aspects of a newly described tumor. *Cancer* 1996;78: 128–132.

111. Rodriquez-Jurado R, Gonzalez-Crussi F. Renal medullary carcinoma. Immunohistochemical and ultrastructural observations. *J Urol Pathol* 1996; 4:191–203.

112. Friedrichs P, Lassen P, Canby E, et al. Renal medullary carcinoma and sickle cell trait. *J Urol* 1997;157:1349.

113. Herring JC, Schmetz MA, Digan AB, et al. Renal medullary carcinoma: A recently described highly aggressive renal tumor in young black patients. *J Urol* 1997;157:2246–2247.

114. Zisman A, Chao DH, Pantuck AJ, et al. Unclassified renal cell carcinoma: Clinical features and prognostic impact of a new histological subtype. *J Urol* 2002;168:950–955.

115. Reuter V, Tickoo SK. Adult renal tumors. In: Reuter V, ed. *Sternberg's diagnostic surgical pathology*. Philadelphia, PA: Lippincott Williams & Wilkins, 2004.

116. Thrasher JB, Paulson DF. Prognostic factors in renal cancer. *Urol Clin North Am* 1993;20:247–262.

117. Zambrano NR, Lubensky IA, Merino MJ, et al. Histopathology and molecular genetics of renal tumors toward unification of a classification system. *J Urol* 1999;162:1246–1258.

118. Gnarra JR, Glenn GM, Latif F, et al. Molecular genetic studies of sporadic and familial renal cell carcinoma. *Urol Clin North Am* 1993;20:207–216.

119. Linehan WM, Lerman MI, Zbar B. Identification of the von Hippel-Lindau (VHL) gene: Its role in renal cancer. *JAMA* 1995;273:564–570.

120. Linehan WM, Walther MM, Zbar B. The genetic basis of cancer of the kidney. *J Urol* 2003;170:2163–2172.

121. Russo P, Snyder ME, DiBlasio CJ, et al. Changing demographics and the contemporary surgical management of renal cortical tumors. *J Urol* 2003; 169:347A.

122. Sobin LH, Wittekind C. International Union against Cancer. *TNM classification of malignant tumours*. New York: John Wiley and Sons, 1997.

123. Russo P. Renal cell carcinoma: Presentation, staging, and surgical treatment. *Semin Oncol* 2000;27:160–176.

124. Rabbani F, Grimaldi G, Russo P. Multiple primary malignancies in renal cell carcinoma. *J Urol* 1998;160:1255–1259.

125. Lee CT, Katz J, Fearn PA, et al. Mode of presentation of renal cell carcinoma provides prognostic information. *Urol Oncol* 2002;7:135–140.

126. Fleming ID, Cooper JS, Henson DE. *AJCC cancer staging manual*. Philadelphia, PA: Lippincott, 1997.

127. Greene FL, American Joint Committee on Cancer, American Cancer Society. *AJCC cancer staging manual*. New York: Springer-Verlag, 2002.

128. Moch H, Gasser T, Amin MB, et al. Prognostic utility of the recently recommended histologic classification and revised TNM staging system of renal cell carcinoma: A Swiss experience with 588 tumors. *Cancer* 2000; 89:604–614.

129. Gettman MT, Blute ML, Spotts B, et al. Pathologic staging of renal cell carcinoma: Significance of tumor classification with the 1997 TNM staging system. *Cancer* 2001;91:354–361.

130. Patel MI, Beck SD, Simmons R, et al. Adrenal and nodal status are indicators of metastatic disease: Time to change the TNM classification for kidney cancer. *J Urol* 2003;169:1A.

131. Bennington JL, Beckwith JB. *Tumors of the kidney, renal pelvis, and ureter*. Washington, DC: Armed Forces Institute of Pathology, 1975.

132. Beck SD, Patel MI, Snyder ME, et al. Effect of papillary and chromophobe cell type on disease-free survival after nephrectomy for renal cell carcinoma. *Ann Surg Oncol* 2004;11:71–77.

133. Zisman A, Pantuck AJ, Dorey F, et al. Improved prognostication of renal cell carcinoma using an integrated staging system. *J Clin Oncol* 2001;19: 1649–1657.

134. Zisman A, Pantuck AJ, Dorey F, et al. Mathematical model to predict individual survival for patients with renal cell carcinoma. *J Clin Oncol* 2002;20:1368–1374.

135. Zisman A, Pantuck AJ, Wieder J, et al. Risk group assessment and clinical outcome algorithm to predict the natural history of patients with surgically resected renal cell carcinoma. *J Clin Oncol* 2002;20:4559–4566.

136. Han KR, Bleumer I, Pantuck AJ, et al. Validation of an integrated staging system toward improved prognostication of patients with localized renal cell carcinoma in an international population. *J Urol* 2003;170: 2221–2224.

137. Leibovich BC, Blute ML, Cheville JC, et al. Prediction of progression after radical nephrectomy for patients with clear cell renal cell carcinoma: A stratification tool for prospective clinical trials. *Cancer* 2003;97:1663–1671.

138. Frank I, Blute ML, Cheville JC, et al. A multifactorial postoperative surveillance model for patients with surgically treated clear cell renal cell carcinoma. *J Urol* 2003;170:2225–2232.

139. Kattan MW, Reuter V, Motzer RJ, et al. A postoperative prognostic nomogram for renal cell carcinoma. *J Urol* 2001;166:63–67.

140. Motzer RJ, Russo P. Systemic therapy for renal cell carcinoma. *J Urol* 2000;163:408–417.

141. Krown SE. Interferon treatment of renal cell carcinoma. Current status and future prospects. *Cancer* 1987;59:647–651.

142. Neidhart JA, Anderson SA, Harris JE, et al. Vinblastine fails to improve response of renal cancer to interferon alfa-n1: High response rate in patients with pulmonary metastases. *J Clin Oncol* 1991;9:832–836.

143. Minasian LM, Motzer RJ, Gluck L, et al. Interferon alfa-2a in advanced renal cell carcinoma: Treatment results and survival in 159 patients with long-term follow-up. *J Clin Oncol* 1993;11:1368–1375.

144. Fossa SD, Martinelli G, Otto U, et al. Recombinant interferon alfa-2a with or without vinblastine in metastatic renal cell carcinoma: Results of a European multi-center phase III study. *Ann Oncol* 1992;3:301–305.

145. Elson PJ, Witte RS, Trump DL. Prognostic factors for survival in patients with recurrent or metastatic renal cell carcinoma. *Cancer Res* 1988;48: 7310–7313.

146. De Forges A, Rey A, Klink M, et al. Prognostic factors of adult metastatic renal carcinoma: A multivariate analysis. *Semin Surg Oncol* 1988;4: 149–154.

147. Palmer PA, Vinke J, Philip T, et al. Prognostic factors for survival in patients with advanced renal cell carcinoma treated with recombinant interleukin-2. *Ann Oncol* 1992;3:475–480.

148. Jones M, Philip T, Palmer P, et al. The impact of interleukin-2 on survival in renal cancer: A multivariate analysis. *Cancer Biother* 1993;8:275–288.

149. Fossa SD, Kramar A, Droz JP. Prognostic factors and survival in patients with metastatic renal cell carcinoma treated with chemotherapy or interferon-alpha. *Eur J Cancer* 1994;30A:1310–1314.

150. Lopez Hanninen E, Kirchner H, Atzpodien J. Interleukin-2 based home therapy of metastatic renal cell carcinoma: Risks and benefits in 215 consecutive single institution patients. *J Urol* 1996;155:19–25.

151. Motzer RJ, Mazumdar M, Bacik J, et al. Survival and prognostic stratification of 670 patients with advanced renal cell carcinoma. *J Clin Oncol* 1999;17:2530–2540.

152. Negrier S, Escudier B, Gomez F, et al. Prognostic factors of survival and rapid progression in 782 patients with metastatic renal carcinomas treated by cytokines: A report from the Groupe Francais d'Immunotherapie. *Ann Oncol* 2002;13:1460–1468.

153. Flanigan RC, Blumenstein BA, Salmon S, et al. Cytoreduction nephrectomy in metastatic renal cancer: The results of the Southwest Oncology Group trial 8949. *Proc Amer Soc Clin Oncol* 2000;19:2a.

154. Motzer RJ, Bacik J, Murphy BA, et al. Interferon-alfa as a comparative treatment for clinical trials of new therapies against advanced renal cell carcinoma. *J Clin Oncol* 2002;20:289–296.

155. Abou-Jawde R, Mekhail G, Merhi B, et al. Prognostic factors for survival in previously untreated metastatic renal cell cancer: A comprehensive evaluation and validation of established risk groups. *Proc Amer Soc Clin Oncol* 2003;22:385.

156. Tsui KH, Shvarts O, Smith RB, et al. Prognostic indicators for renal cell carcinoma: A multivariate analysis of 643 patients using the revised 1997 TNM staging criteria. *J Urol* 2000;163:1090–1095; quiz 1295.

CHAPTER 44B
Pathology of Inherited Forms of Renal Carcinoma

Maria J. Merino and Carlos A. Torres-Cabala

Renal cell carcinoma (RCC) affects approximately 30,000 individuals per year in the United States and is responsible for close to 12,000 annual deaths. Kidney cancer is a tumor comprising several histologic subtypes, the molecular hallmarks of which support their classification as distinct entities. Although most renal tumors occur sporadically, approximately 5% are found in association with syndromes of a heritable nature. Identification of genes involved in the hereditary forms of RCC has provided significant information about the genes involved in the common, sporadic (nonhereditary) forms of the disease.

Recognition of this group of tumors is, however, rather important both clinically and scientifically because it is now recognized that kidney tumors may occur in familial settings more frequently than previously contemplated. Early detection and diagnosis of these tumors, identification of specific genes that characterize each syndrome, and elucidation of mechanisms responsible for the development of tumors are important in establishing appropriate therapies, as well as for genetic counseling. At the moment, only morphology can assist in identifying and diagnosing some of the newly recognized syndromes.

Hereditary renal syndromes include the following:

> von Hippel-Lindau (VHL)
> hereditary papillary renal cell carcinoma (HPRC)
> Birt-Hogg-Dubé (BHD)
> hereditary leiomyomatosis and renal cell carcinoma (HLRCC)
> tuberous sclerosis (TS)
> familial renal oncocytoma
> syndromes associated with Wilms tumor

Each syndrome is associated with a specific renal pathology. Clinically, the tumors are more likely to be multifocal and bilateral and with early or incipient lesions scattered throughout the adjacent renal parenchyma. The most common form of hereditary kidney cancer is VHL, which is associated with clear cell or conventional renal carcinoma (approximately 75%). This disease has been associated with mutations in the *VHL* gene (at 3p25) and loss of heterozygosity at chromosome 3p. Next in frequency is papillary renal cell carcinoma (approximately 10%), associated with trisomies of chromosomes 7 and 17 and losses of chromosome Y. Chromophobe renal cell carcinoma is even more rare (approximately 5%), is associated with numerous specific chromosomal losses (-1, -2, -6, -10, -13, -17, -21), and is seen in patients with BHD syndrome. Renal oncocytoma, a benign neoplasm most often without any chromosomal abnormalities, is represented at a frequency of approximately 3% to 5%.

VON HIPPEL-LINDAU: THE VHL KIDNEY CANCER TUMOR SUPPRESSOR GENE

VHL is an autosomal dominant cancer syndrome in which affected individuals are at risk to develop tumors in a number of organs. The most frequent clinical manifestations are the following:

> Bilateral, multifocal clear cell renal carcinoma
> Central nervous system hemangioblastomas (cerebellum, spine)
> Pancreatic neuroendocrine tumors
> Pheochromocytomas
> Retinal angiomas
> Endolymphatic sac tumors
> Epididymal cystadenomas

The tumors identified in patients with VHL are frequently bilateral and multifocal.

Morphologically, they are similar to sporadic RCC. Grossly, the tumors vary in size and have a characteristic yellow color with extensive areas of hemorrhage and necrosis. The tumor cells are large with clear cytoplasm, although occasional eosinophilic cells may be identified (Fig. 44B.1). A variety of growth patterns—solid, tubular, and papillary—can be found.

Cysts are frequently present in VHL. They vary in size and are separated by dense fibrous/hyalinized septa. The cysts are usually lined by a single row of low nuclear-grade tumor cells (Fig. 44B.2).

The VHL gene is known to be located in 3p25 to 3p26, but changes have been reported in 5q21+ (70%) and 14q− (41%). The allele of the *VHL* gene that is not deleted shows somatic mutations or hypermethylation-induced inactivation in 80% of cases. *VHL* is a tumor suppressor gene that encodes for a protein that binds to Elongin C/B, Cul 2, and Rbx-1. This complex ubiquitinylates—and degrades—proteins such as hypoxia-inducible factor (HIF). HIF stimulates the transcription of a series of genes, including vascular endothelial growth factor (VEGF). Therefore, loss of VHL causes an increase in VEGF, which may cause the increased vascularity of these tumors.

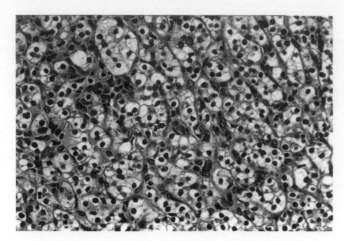

FIGURE 44B.1. Clear cell renal cell carcinoma (hematoxylin and eosin, original magnification ×100). (See color insert.)

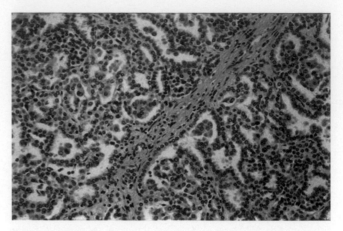

FIGURE 44B.3. Papillary renal cell carcinoma type I (hematoxylin and eosin, original magnification ×100). (See color insert.)

Patients with VHL-associated tumors have a better prognosis and longer survivals than those with sporadic RCC. In sporadic cases, 38% of patients die from disease, and metastases develop in 27% to 37% of patients. Metastases occur frequently to lung, liver, and bone, and they have a morphology similar to that of the primary tumor.

HEREDITARY PAPILLARY RENAL CELL CARCINOMA

HPRC is an autosomal dominant disease characterized by the development of multifocal papillary (chromophil) type I renal cell tumors.

Type I papillary RCC is recognized by the formation of papillary structures lined by small cuboidal cells with scanty basophilic cytoplasm and small indolent nuclei (Fig. 44B.3). The tumors can also exhibit focal tubular or solid patterns of growth. The papillae may be filled with foamy macrophages, and psammoma bodies are common (type I). Marked nuclear atypia is rare. Type I papillary RCC derive from the proximal tubule, as do clear cell tumors. The tumors are multifocal in more that 80% of cases, and incipient lesions can be found scattered throughout the adjacent renal parenchyma. Tumors stain positive for CK7 and negative for CK20.

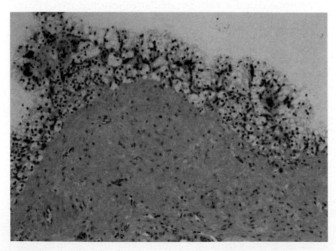

FIGURE 44B.2. Simple renal cyst (hematoxylin and eosin, original magnification ×100). (See color insert.)

HPRC is a rare condition characterized by mutations in the tyrosine-kinase domain of the *c-MET* proto-oncogene on 7q34. Trisomy of chromosome 7 is thought to be the initiating event along with the loss of a sex chromosome.

It is estimated that approximately half the members of affected families will develop tumors by the age of 50. The 5-year survival for patients with this type of tumor is approximately 82% to 90%, much better than for clear cell carcinomas regardless of stage. Metastases can occur to regional lymph nodes and lung.

BIRT-HOGG-DUBÉ SYNDROME

BHD syndrome, first described in 1977 by Drs. Birt, Hogg, and Dubé, was initially characterized by a predisposition to develop multiple small papules on the head and neck. These papules are benign tumors of the hair follicles (fibrofolliculomas). It is now known that this syndrome is associated with such other conditions as lung cysts and renal carcinoma. Of affected BHD individuals, 15% to 35% develop renal carcinoma. The histologic type of BHD-associated renal carcinoma is markedly different from that of either VHL (clear cell RCC) or HPRC (type I papillary RCC). Patients with BHD are at risk to develop chromophobe RCC, oncocytic RCC, and oncocytoma. The hybrid and chromophobe RCC are the predominant types.

The size of tumors at presentation is variable. In diameter, the hybrid tumors average 2.2 cm, the chromophobe RCCs 3.0 cm, and the clear cell RCCs 4.7 cm.

Morphologically, these hybrid oncocytic tumors have zones classic for oncocytoma (large cells, poorly defined cell borders, finely granular eosinophilic cytoplasm throughout, and large nuclei with homogenous basophilic chromatin) as well as other zones consistent with chromophobe RCC (well-defined cell borders, "fluffy" eosinophilic cytoplasm, pyknotic nuclei, and perinuclear halos) (Fig. 44B.4). Cells in the chromophobe zones of these tumors were arranged in the characteristic plantlike distribution of chromophobe RCC. Incipient lesions, or oncocytosis, were widespread throughout the renal parenchyma in almost all cases (Fig. 44B.5).

The BHD gene has been localized to 17p11.2. The prognosis of patients with these tumors is similar to that of papillary type I unless clear cell cancers develop. The morphology of clear cell tumors associated with BHD is similar to sporadic RCC.

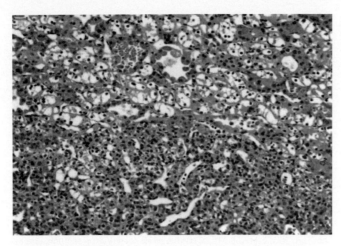

FIGURE 44B.4. Hybrid tumor composed of oncocytic and chromophobe cells (hematoxylin and eosin, original magnification ×100). (See color insert.)

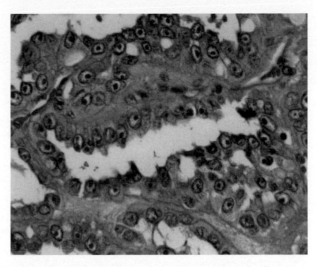

FIGURE 44B.6. Hereditary leiomyomatosis and renal cell carcinoma with papillary configuration (hematoxylin and eosin, original magnification ×100). (See color insert.)

HEREDITARY LEIOMYOMATOSIS RENAL CELL CARCINOMA

In 2001, an autosomal dominant hereditary syndrome involving cutaneous and uterine leiomyomas was reported to be associated with renal cancer in two families. A familial autosomal dominant predisposition to multiple cutaneous leiomyomas (MCLs) was noted in the 1950s. In 1965, Mezzadra suggested the association of uterine leiomyomas with cutaneous leiomyomas. Subsequent reports have confirmed a dominant familial predisposition to cutaneous and uterine leiomyomas and to MCL.

Alam et al. performed a genome-wide screening of 11 families with this disorder and found linkage to 1q42.3-q43. They reduced the critical region to 14cM, naming the locus as MCUL1 (multiple cutaneous and uterine leiomyomata).

In 2001, Lanonen et al. reported the clinical, histopathologic, and molecular features of a cancer syndrome with predisposition to uterine leiomyomas and papillary renal cancer. The four kidney cancer cases occurred in young women (33 to 48 years old) and displayed a unique natural history. All these renal tumors were of papillary histology and presented as unilateral solitary lesions that had metastasized at the time of diagnosis. A second, smaller family was studied also. Linkage analysis mapped the predisposition gene to chromosome 1q.

Losses of the normal chromosome 1q were observed in tumors that had occurred in the kindred displaying the phenotype. The Finnish group recently reported the finding of mutation of fumarate hydratase (fumarase) in the germline of some of the HLRCC and MCL kindreds. It is now believed that MCL and HLRCC are the same disorder.

Although the original description of these tumors was that of papillary type II, we have recently described a variety of patterns, including tubular, solid, papillary, and mixed (Fig. 44B.6). The hallmark of these neoplasms is the presence of large nuclei with prominent orangiophilic nucleoli (Fig. 44B.7).

TUBEROUS SCLEROSIS

Tuberous sclerosis (TS) is an autosomal dominant disease characterized by cortical tubers, giant cell astrocytomas, retinal hamartomas, and cardiac and renal tumors. The disease is associated with two predisposing genes: TSC1 at 9q34 and TSC2 at 16p13. Renal tumors are most frequently angiomyolipomas, but clear cell RCC has also been described.

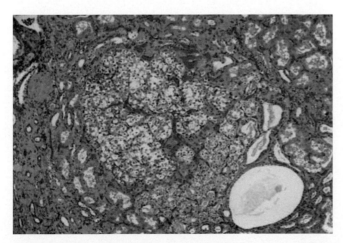

FIGURE 44B.5. Oncocytosis (hematoxylin and eosin, original magnification ×100). (See color insert.)

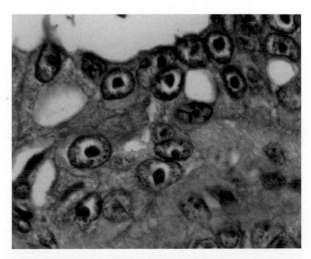

FIGURE 44B.7. Characteristic prominent nucleoli (hematoxylin and eosin, original magnification ×100). (See color insert.)

References

1. Barker KT, Bevan S, Wang R, et al. Low frequency of somatic mutations in the FH/multiple cutaneous leiomyomatosis gene in sporadic leiomyosarcomas and uterine leiomyomas. *Br J Cancer* 2002;87:446–448.

2. Choyke PL, Glenn GM, Walther MM, et al. Hereditary renal cancers. *Radiology* 2003;226:33–46.

3. Cohen AJ, Li FP, Berg S, et al. Hereditary renal-cell carcinoma associated with a chromosomal translocation. *N Engl J Med* 1979;301:592–595.

4. Delahunt B, Eble JN. Papillary renal cell carcinoma: A clinicopathologic and immunohistochemical study of 105 tumors. *Mod Pathol* 1997;10:537–544.

5. Fryer AE, Chalmers A, Connor JM, et al. Evidence that the gene for tuberous sclerosis is on chromosome 9. *Lancet* 1987;1:659–661.

6. Gatalica Z, Kovatich A, Miettinen M. Consistent expression of cytokeratin 7 in papillary renal-cell carcinoma: An immunohistochemical study in formalin-fixed, paraffin embedded tissues. *J Urol Pathol* 1995;3:205–211.

7. Kandt RS, Haines JL, Smith M, et al. Linkage of an important gene locus for tuberous sclerosis to a chromosome 16 marker for polycystic kidney disease. *Nat Genet* 1992;2:37.

8. Kennedy SM, Merino MJ, Linehan WM, et al. Collecting duct carcinoma of the kidney. *Hum Pathol* 1990;21:449–456.

9. Kiuru M, Launonen V, Hietala M, et al. Familial cutaneous leiomyomatosis is a two-hit condition associated with renal cell cancer of characteristic histopathology. *Am J Pathol* 2001;159:825–829.

10. Kiuru M, Lehtonen R, Arola J, et al. Few FH mutations in sporadic counterparts of tumor types observed in hereditary leiomyomatosis and renal cell cancer families. *Cancer Res* 2002;62:4554–4557.

11. Kovacs G, Akhtar M, Beckwith BJ, et al. The Heidelberg classification of renal cell tumours. *J Pathol* 1997;183:131–133.

12. Latif F, Tory K, Gnarra J, et al. Identification of the von Hippel-Lindau disease tumor suppressor gene. *Science* 1993;260:1317–1320.

13. Launonen V, Vierimaa O, Kiuru M, et al. Inherited susceptibility to uterine leiomyomas and renal cell cancer. *Proc Natl Acad Sci USA* 2001;98:3387–3392.

14. Nickerson ML, Warren MB, Toro JR, et al. Mutations in a novel gene lead to kidney tumors, lung wall defects, and benign tumors of the hair follicle in patients with the Birt Hogg-Dube syndrome. *Cancer Cell* 2002;2:157–164.

15. Pavlovich CP, Walther MM, Eyler RA, et al. Renal tumors in the Birt-Hogg-Dube syndrome. *Am J Surg Pathol* 2002;26:1542–1552.

16. Schmidt L, Duh FM, Chen F, et al. Germline and somatic mutations in the tyrosine kinase domain of the MET proto-oncogene in papillary renal carcinomas. *Nat Genet* 1997;16:68–73.

17. Storkel S, Eble JN, Adlakha K, et al. Classification of renal cell carcinoma: workgroup No. 1. Union Internationale Contre le Cancer (UICC) and the American Joint Committee on Cancer (AJCC). *Cancer* 1997;80:987–989.

18. Toro JR, Glenn G, Duray P, et al. Birt-Hogg-Dube syndrome: A novel marker of kidney neoplasia. *Arch Dermatol* 1999;135:1195–1202.

19. Toro JR, Nickerson ML, Wei MH, et al. Mutations in the fumarate hydratase gene cause hereditary leiomyomatosis and renal cell cancer in families in North America. *Am J Hum Genet* 2003;73:95–106

20. Weirich G, Glenn G, Junker K, et al. Familial renal oncocytoma: Clinicopathological study of 5 families. *J Urol* 1998;160:335–334.

21. Zbar B, Tory K, Merino MJ, et al. Hereditary papillary renal cell carcinoma. *J Urol* 1994;151:561–566.

CHAPTER 45 ■ GENETIC BASIS OF KIDNEY CANCER

W. MARSTON LINEHAN, JONATHAN A. COLEMAN, MCCLELLAN M. WALTHER, AND BERTON ZBAR

BACKGROUND

Kidney cancer affects more than 32,000 individuals annually in the United States and is responsible for more than 12,000 deaths per year. Patients who are found to have localized renal tumors, T1-T2, can have a 95% chance of surviving 5 or 10 years (1). Those who present with metastatic disease have an 18% chance of surviving 2 years. Kidney cancer is not a single disease; it is made up of a number of different types of cancer that occur in the kidney, each with a different histology, a different clinical course, and caused by alteration of different genes (2). Kidney tumors occur as clear cell (75%), type 1 or type 2 papillary renal carcinoma (15%), chromophobe renal carcinoma (5%), in collecting duct carcinoma, medullary renal carcinoma, and oncocytoma (5%) (Fig. 45.1).

HEREDITARY FORMS OF KIDNEY CANCER

Kidney cancer, like prostate cancer, breast cancer, and colon cancer, occurs in both a familial (inherited) and a nonfamilial (sporadic) form. There are four types of inherited epithelial kidney cancer: von Hippel-Lindau (VHL) (clear cell renal carcinoma), hereditary papillary renal carcinoma (HPRC) (type 1 papillary renal carcinoma), the Birt-Hogg-Dubé (BHD) syndrome (chromophobe renal carcinoma and oncocytoma), and hereditary leiomyomatosis renal cell carcinoma (HLRCC) (type 2 papillary renal carcinoma, and others) (Fig. 45.2; Table 45.1).

Von Hippel-Lindau: Clear Cell Renal Carcinoma

VHL is an inherited form of renal carcinoma in which affected individuals are at risk for the development of tumors in a number of organs, including the kidneys. Patients with VHL are at risk for the development of early onset, bilateral, multifocal renal tumors, and cysts. The renal tumors are uniformly of clear cell type. It has been estimated that these patients may develop up to 600 tumors and 1,100 cysts per kidney. These tumors tend to occur early in life, sometimes as early as the second decade. VHL-associated renal carcinomas can metastasize if not detected and treated. Historically, 35% to 45% of patients with VHL died of renal carcinoma. The surgical management of renal carcinoma in patients with VHL is discussed in Chapter 47E. Because of the multifocal nature of VHL-associated renal carcinoma and the need for repeat surgery for recurrent lesions, the current recommendation is for management of small renal tumors with observation until the largest tumor reaches 3 cm. Nephron-sparing surgery is then recommended (Fig. 45.3; Table 45.2).

Patients with VHL are also at risk for the development of pheochromocytomas. These may occur in children before the age of 10 and may be bilateral, multifocal, and extra-adrenal (4,5). These patients also may develop pancreatic islet cell tumors and cysts. The islet cell tumors are malignant and can metastasize (6). Affected patients with VHL are also at risk for the development of central nervous system (CNS) and spinal hemangioblastomas, endolymphatic sac tumors, and retinal angioma. Neither the CNS

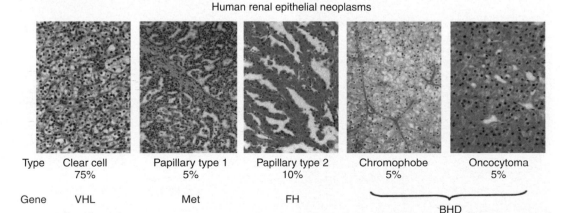

Human renal epithelial neoplasms

Type	Clear cell 75%	Papillary type 1 5%	Papillary type 2 10%	Chromophobe 5%	Oncocytoma 5%
Gene	VHL	Met	FH		BHD

FIGURE 45.1. Kidney cancer is made up of a number of different types of cancer, each with a different histology, a different course, a different response to therapy, and caused by alteration of a different gene. (From Linehan WM, Walther MM, Zbar B. The genetic basis of cancer of the kidney. *J Urol* 2003; 170:2163, with permission.) (See color insert.)

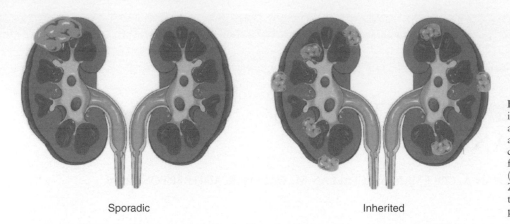

Sporadic

Inherited

FIGURE 45.2. Kidney cancer occurs in both a sporadic (noninherited) and a hereditary (inherited) form. Patients at risk for inherited forms of renal carcinoma may develop bilateral, multifocal renal tumors at an early age. (From Linehan WM, Walther MM, Zbar B. The genetic basis of cancer of the kidney. *J Urol* 2003;170:2163, with permission.)

TABLE 45.1

INHERITED FORMS OF RENAL CARCINOMA

1. Von Hippel-Lindau (VHL)
   Clear cell RCC
2. Hereditary papillary renal carcinoma (HPRC)
   Papillary type 1 RCC
3. Birt-Hogg-Dubé (BHD)
   Chromophobe RCC/oncocytoma
4. Hereditary leiomyomatosis RCC (HLRCC)
   Papillary type 2 RCC

RCC, renal cell carcinoma.

TABLE 45.2

CLINICAL FEATURES OF VON HIPPEL-LINDAU

Kidney tumors (clear cell RCC)
Adrenal tumors (pheochromocytoma)
Pancreatic tumors (islet tumors)
CNS tumors (hemangioblastoma)
Retinal tumors (angioma)
Endolymphatic sac tumors (inner ear)
Epididymal cystadenoma

RCC, renal cell carcinoma; CNS, central nervous system.

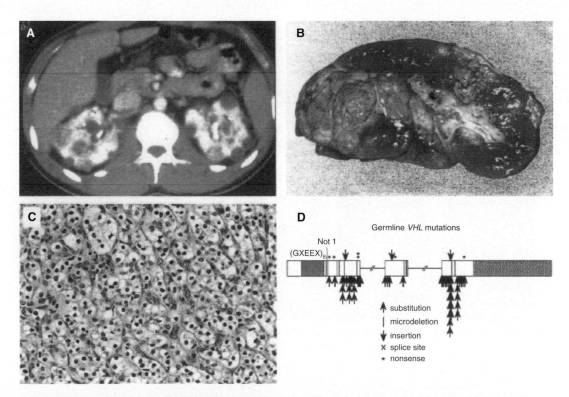

FIGURE 45.3. von Hippel-Lindau (VHL)–associated renal carcinoma may be bilateral and multifocal and may appear as early as the second decade. Affected individuals in VHL kindreds are characterized by germline mutation of the *VHL* gene (3). (From Linehan WM, Walther MM, Zbar B. The genetic basis of cancer of the kidney. *J Urol* 2003;170:2163, with permission.) (See color insert.)

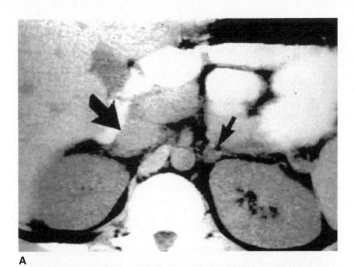

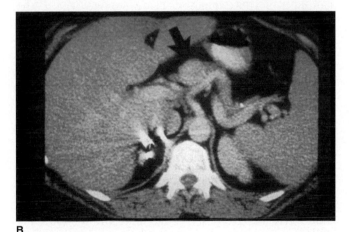

FIGURE 45.4. Patients affected with Von Hippel-Lindau (VHL) are at risk for the development of pheochromocytoma (**A**) and pancreatic islet cell tumors (**B**) (7). (From Linehan WM, Zbar B, Klausner RD. Renal carcinoma. In: Scriver CR, Beaudet AL, Sly WS et al., eds. *The metabolic and molecular bases of inherited disease*, 8th ed., Chap. 41. New York: McGraw-Hill, 2001:907, with permission.)

hemangioblastoma nor the retinal angioma are malignant; however, both can be associated with significant morbidity (Fig. 45.4; Table 45.3).

Identification of the *VHL* Gene

In order to identify the *VHL* gene, investigators conducted genetic linkage analysis in VHL families. The *VHL* gene was

TABLE 45.3

CLINICAL EVALUATION: VON HIPPEL-LINDAU

VHL gene germline mutation testing
MRI of the brain and spine
Abdominal CT scan and ultrasound
Ophthalmologic evaluation
Audiometric and ENT evaluation
Testicular ultrasound
Metabolic evaluation (catechols)

VHL, von Hippel-Lindau; MRI, magnetic resonance imaging; CT, computerized tomography; ENT, ear, nose, throat.

TABLE 45.4

MOLECULAR GENETIC CLASSIFICATION OF SPORADIC (NONHEREDITARY) RENAL CARCINOMA

Gene	Histology
VHL	Clear cell/compact growth
Met	Papillary type 1 (granular cells, papillary growth pattern)
To be determined	Papillary type 2 RCC
To be determined	Chromophobe RCC/oncocytoma

VHL, von Hippel-Lindau; RCC, renal cell carcinoma.

identified on the short arm of chromosome 3 (3). The *VHL* gene was found to be mutated in the germline of patients affected by VHL (8). This provided a clinical test to make the diagnosis of VHL in at-risk individuals in VHL kindreds.

von Hippel-Lindau: Clear Cell Kidney Cancer Gene

When tumor tissue from patients with sporadic (noninherited) kidney cancer was evaluated for alteration of the *VHL* gene, mutation of this gene was found in a high percentage of tumors from patients with clear cell renal carcinoma (9,10). *VHL* gene mutations were not found in tumors from patients with papillary renal carcinoma, chromophobe renal carcinoma, or oncocytoma. The *VHL* gene is responsible for the common form of sporadic clear cell renal carcinoma (Fig. 45.5; Tables 45.4, 45.5).

Clinical Implications

Understanding the genetic basis of cancer of the kidney provides a method for molecular classification of the cancer and could provide enhanced methods for diagnosis of this disease. Yao et al. have shown that there is an improved survival rate in patients with sporadic clear cell renal carcinoma with *VHL* mutation (12). *VHL* mutations have been detected in circulating cells, lymph nodes, and urine of patients with clear cell renal carcinoma, providing possible approaches for early diagnosis of this disease. Clear cell kidney cancer is the only histology to date that has been shown to be responsive to IL-2-based systemic immunotherapies. Studies are currently underway to determine if there is a relation between *VHL* gene mutation and response to immunotherapy.

VHL Gene Pathway: The VHL Complex Targets Hypoxia-inducible Factors for Degradation

The VHL protein forms a multiprotein complex with proteins such as elongin c and b and Cul2 to target the α subunits of

TABLE 45.5

SOMATIC VON HIPPEL-LINDAU GENE MUTATION ANALYSIS: POTENTIAL CLINICAL APPLICATIONS

Detection of VHL Gene Abnormalities in

- Formalin-fixed tissues
- Tissue aspirates
- Early diagnosis
  - Circulating cells
  - Urine

VHL, von Hippel-Lindau.

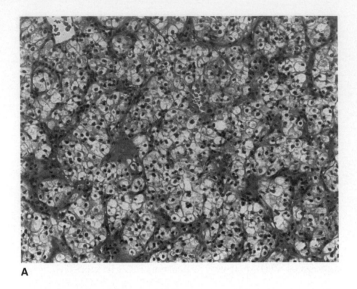

A

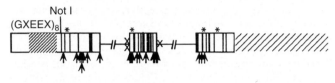

Sporadic renal carcinoma *VHL* mutations

↑ substitution

| microdeletion

↓ insertion

X splice site

* nonsense

B

FIGURE 45.5. *von Hippel-Lindau (VHL)* gene: clear cell renal carcinoma. *VHL* gene mutations (**B**) have been found in a high percentage of tumors from patients with sporadic, nonhereditary clear cell renal carcinoma (**A**) (10,11) (see color insert). *VHL* gene mutations have not been found in type 1 or type 2 papillary renal carcinoma, chromophobe renal carcinoma, or oncocytoma. (From Gnarra JR, Tory K, Weng YW, et al. Mutation of the VHL tumour suppressor gene in renal carcinoma. *Nat Genet* 1994;7:85, with permission.)

the hypoxia-inducible factors (HIFs), HIF1α and HIF2α, for ubiquitin-mediated degradation (13–15). This is a hypoxia-mediated process. When there is normoxia, the VHL complex targets HIF and degrades it. When there is hypoxia, the complex cannot degrade HIF, and HIF overaccumulates in the cell. HIF is a transcription factor that regulates the transcription of a number of genes important in cancer, such as vascular endothelial growth factor (VEGF), transforming growth factor α (TGFα), platelet derived growth factor (PDGF), and the epidermal growth factor receptor (EGFR) (16,17).

VHL Gene Pathway: Opportunity for Disease-specific Therapy for Clear Cell RCC

One potential approach to the development of effective forms of therapy for patients with advanced clear cell renal carcinoma is to develop agents that block the VHL pathway. Clinical trials are underway to evaluate the role of agents that block VEGF, EGFR, and other downstream targets of the VHL/HIF pathway. The initial study by Yang et al. demonstrated an increase in progression-free survival in patients with advanced clear cell renal carcinoma treated with anti-VEGF antibody

therapy (18). Further studies are underway to evaluate the role of single agents and combination agents that target VEGF, EGFr, and c-Raf in patients with advanced clear cell renal carcinoma (Fig. 45.6).

Hereditary Papillary Renal Carcinoma: Type 1 Papillary Renal Carcinoma

HPRC is a hereditary cancer syndrome in which affected individuals are at risk for the development of bilateral, multifocal papillary renal carcinoma. HPRC is inherited in an autosomal dominant fashion. Patients with HPRC are at risk for developing bilateral, multifocal type 1 papillary renal carcinoma (19). It has been estimated that these patients are at risk for the development of up to 3,000 tumors per kidney (20).

In order to identify the gene for the hereditary form of type 1 papillary renal carcinoma, genetic linkage analysis was performed in HPRC families. The proto-oncogene, c-Met, was found to be the gene for HPRC (21). Met is a proto-oncogene; it is the cell surface receptor for the ligand hepatocyte growth factor (HGF). Activating mutations of Met are found in the germline of patients affected with HPRC (22) and have been found in tumors in a subset of patients with noninherited, sporadic type 1 papillary renal carcinoma (23) (Table 45.6).

Germline testing of the *c-Met* gene is available for patients suspected of being at risk for HPRC and can aid in making the diagnosis of HPRC and determining which individuals are affected with this hereditary cancer syndrome. Because of the multifocal and bilateral nature of HPRC-associated renal tumors, nephron-sparing surgery is generally recommended when the largest tumor reaches the 3-cm size (see Chapter 47E). Although HPRC-associated renal carcinomas may be late onset, a recent report indicates that HPRC can occur as early as the third decade (24) (Fig. 45.7).

Hereditary Leiomyomatosis Renal Cell Carcinoma: Type 2 Papillary Renal Carcinoma

HLRCC is an inherited cancer syndrome in which affected individuals are at risk for the development of cutaneous and uterine leiomyoma and type 2 papillary renal carcinoma (26). HLRCC is characterized by germline mutations of the Krebs cycle enzyme, fumarate hydratase (FH) (27,28) (Table 45.7).

The cutaneous manifestations of HLRCC consist of multiple cutaneous leiomyomas. These typically occur on the arms or chest and are often unilateral and segmental, and they may be painful. Women affected with HLRCC are at risk for the development of multiple uterine leiomyomas (fibroids). These often occur during the second decade and may result in hysterectomy (Table 45.8).

The gene for HLRCC is the Krebs cycle enzyme, *FH* (27,28). Mutations of this gene are found in the germline of patients with HLRCC. This gene has the characteristics of a tumor suppressor gene; that is, mutation of the gene and loss of the second copy of the gene have been found in type 2 papillary renal tumors from patients with HLRCC (29). In patients with multiple cutaneous leiomyomas and renal tumors, FH germline mutation testing can aid in making the diagnosis of HLRCC.

Patients with HLRCC are at risk for the development of an aggressive form of type 2 papillary renal carcinoma or collecting duct carcinoma. These tumors can be aggressive and may

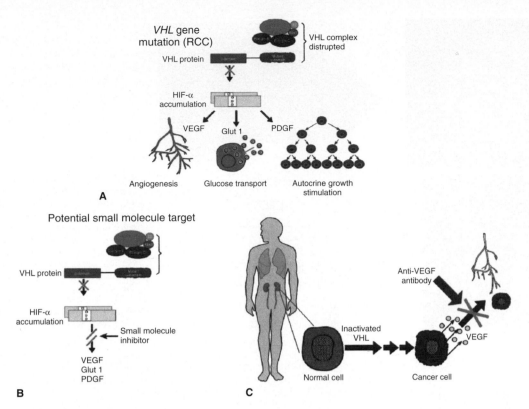

FIGURE 45.6. The *von Hippel-Lindau (VHL)* gene pathway. *VHL* is the gene for clear cell renal carcinoma. The VHL protein forms a complex that targets the hypoxia-inducible factors (HIFs) for ubiquitin-mediated degradation. HIF is a transcription factor that regulates transcription of a number of genes, such as vascular endothelial growth factor (VEGF), platelet derived growth factor (PDGF), and epidermal growth factor receptor (EGFR), thought to be important in kidney cancer tumorigenesis. Potential targeted molecular therapeutic approaches include blocking the effect of HIF or VEGF. (From Linehan WM, Walther MM, Zbar B. The genetic basis of cancer of the kidney. *J Urol* 2003;170:2163, with permission.)

metastasize early. Observation of HLRCC tumors is not recommended (see Chapter 47E) (Fig. 45.8).

Birt-Hogg-Dubé: Chromophobe and Oncocytic Renal Carcinoma and Oncocytoma

Birt-Hogg-Dubé (BHD) is a hereditary cancer syndrome in which affected individuals are at risk for the development of cutaneous fibrofolliculomas, pulmonary cysts and pneumothorax, and renal tumors (30,31). BHD was initially described in a Canadian kindred in which family members were found to have cutaneous fibrofolliculoma (30). Patients affected with BHD are at risk for the development of bilateral, multifocal pulmonary cysts and pneumothorax. In a

---

TABLE 45.6

HEREDITARY PAPILLARY RENAL CARCINOMA (HPRC)

Clinical features
Bilateral, multifocal papillary renal cell carcinoma
Type I papillary renal carcinoma
Clinical evaluation
C-Met gene germline mutation testing
Abdominal CT scan and ultrasound

CT, computerized tomography.

TABLE 45.7

CLINICAL FEATURES OF HEREDITARY LEIOMYOMATOSIS RENAL CELL CARCINOMA (HLRCC)

Cutaneous nodules (leiomyomas)
Uterine leiomyoma (fibroids)
Uterine leiomyosarcoma
Renal tumor (type 2 papillary RCC)
• Often solitary
• Aggressive, early to metastasize

RCC, renal cell carcinoma.

TABLE 45.8

CLINICAL EVALUATION: HLRCC

FH gene germline mutation testing
Dermatologic evaluation—skin biopsy
Abdominal CT scan/ultrasound
Pelvic CT scan/uterine ultrasound

CT, computerized tomography; FH, fumarate hydratase.

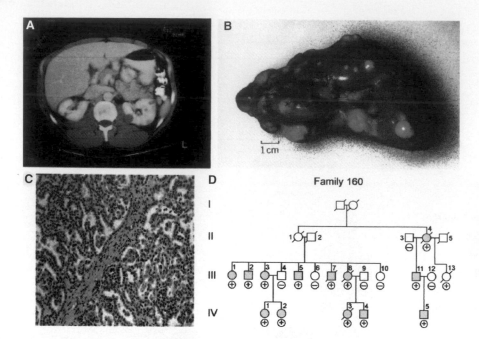

FIGURE 45.7. Hereditary papillary renal carcinoma (HPRC) is an inherited cancer syndrome in which affected individuals are at risk for the development of bilateral, multifocal papillary renal carcinoma (**A, B**) (25). The kidney cancer in HPRC is uniformly type 1 papillary renal carcinoma (**C**). HPRC is inherited in an autosomal dominant fashion (**D**) and is caused by germline mutation of the c-Met oncogene (21). (From Linehan WM, Walther MM, Zbar B. The genetic basis of cancer of the kidney. *J Urol* 2003; 170:2163, with permission.)

study of nearly 100 patients with BHD, Zbar et al. found pulmonary cysts in over 80% of affected individuals. Twenty percent of patients had a history of pneumothorax (31) (Fig. 45.9; Tables 45.8, 45.9).

Patients with BHD are at risk for the development of kidney tumors. These may occur in 15% to 25% of patients (31,32). The renal tumors are chromophobe renal carcinoma (33%), hybrid-oncocytic renal carcinoma (50%), clear cell renal carcinoma (9%), and oncocytoma (4%) (33). BHD-associated kidney tumors can be solitary or bilateral and multifocal. These tumors are most often malignant and can metastasize. Because BHD-associated renal tumors can frequently be recurrent, and repeated surgical treatment may be necessary, the current

recommendation for BHD-associated renal tumors is partial nephrectomy when the largest tumor reaches the 3-cm threshold (see Chapter 47E).

DEOXYRIBONUCLEIC ACID DIAGNOSIS OF HEREDITARY RENAL CARCINOMA

DNA tests are now available for each of the four types of inherited epithelial renal carcinoma. By a study of DNA extracted from a sample of peripheral blood, it is possible to establish

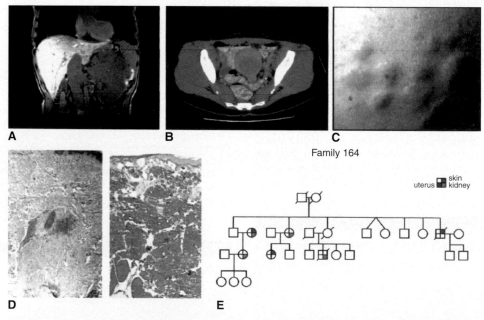

FIGURE 45.8. Hereditary leiomyomatosis renal cell carcinoma (HLRCC) is an inherited cancer syndrome in which affected individuals are at risk for the development of cutaneous (**C** and **D**) and uterine (**B**) leiomyomas and type 2 papillary renal carcinoma (**A**). HLRCC has an autosomal dominant inheritance pattern (**E**) and is characterized by germline mutation of the *FH* gene (27,28). (From Linehan WM, Walther MM, Zbar B. The genetic basis of cancer of the kidney. *J Urol* 2003;170:2163, with permission.)

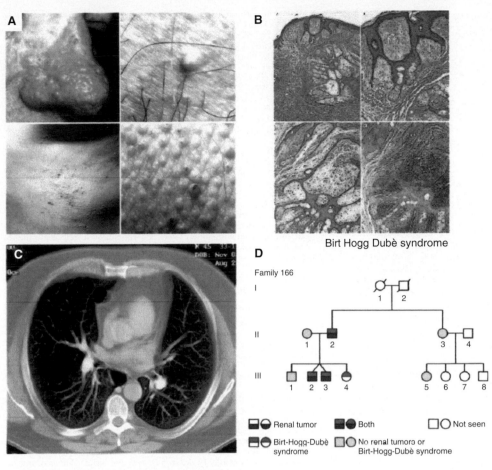

Birt Hogg Dubè syndrome

FIGURE 45.9. Birt-Hogg-Dubé (BHD) is a hereditary cancer syndrome in which affected individuals are at risk for the development of cutaneous fibrofolliculomas (A, B), pulmonary cysts (C), and renal tumors. BHD is inherited in an autosomal dominant fashion (D); that is, offspring have a 50/50 chance of carrying the gene. (From Linehan WM, Walther MM, Zbar B. The genetic basis of cancer of the kidney. *J Urol* 2003;170:2163; and Toro J, Duray PH, Glenn GM, et al. Birt-Hogg-Dubé syndrome: a novel marker of kidney neoplasia. *Arch Dermatol* 1999;135:1195, with permission.) (See color insert.)

unequivocally that a patient has a genetic change that produces an increased risk for development of renal carcinoma. The presence of a kidney cancer germline mutation means that other family members are at increased risk for developing renal carcinoma and would benefit from a combination of genetic counseling, DNA diagnosis, and screening tests.

DNA tests for hereditary renal carcinoma can be useful to the clinicians in a variety of clinical settings. (i) DNA tests can be used to confirm the clinical diagnosis of VHL, HPRC, BHD, and HLRCC. (ii) DNA tests can be used to establish a diagnosis in families with multiple members with kidney cancer where the clinical diagnosis is uncertain. (iii) DNA tests can be useful in establishing a diagnosis in patients with bilateral renal carcinoma where the clinical diagnosis is uncertain (Table 45.10).

FAMILIAL RENAL CARCINOMA

Studies in families in which multiple members have been found to have kidney cancer, but who do not appear to be affected with known kidney cancer syndromes (VHL, HPRC, HLRCC, or BHD), have raised the possibility that there is more of an inherited basis to sporadic kidney cancer than was previously appreciated (34). Hereditary cancer syndromes such as VHL, HPRC, HLRCC, and BHD have an autosomal inheritance pattern and are characterized by high penetrance. In these well-described syndromes, individuals who inherit an altered disease gene (*VHL, Met, FH,* or *BHD*) are highly likely to develop the clinical manifestations of the syndrome.

In order to determine whether or not there is an inherited predisposition to sporadic kidney cancer, Gudbjartsson et al. studied all patients in Iceland who had had kidney cancer since 1954 (35). In this remarkable study, they found that nearly 60% of patients with kidney cancer had a relative (as far removed as a second cousin) with kidney cancer. This

TABLE 45.9

CLINICAL FEATURES OF BIRT-HOGG-DUBÉ (BHD)

Cutaneous nodules (hair follicle tumors, fibrofolliculoma) on the face and neck
Pulmonary cysts
Renal tumors
- Chromophobe RCC
- Oncocytic hybrid RCC
- Clear cell RCC
- Oncocytoma

RCC, renal cell carcinoma.

TABLE 45.10

CLINICAL EVALUATION: BHD

BHD gene germline mutation testing
Dermatologic evaluation: skin biopsy
Lung CT scan
Abdominal CT scan/ultrasound

BHD, Birt-Hogg-Dubé; CT, computerized tomography.

Kidney Cancer in Families

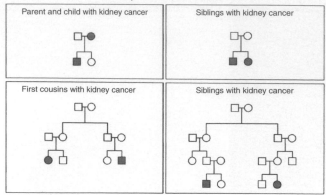

FIGURE 45.10. Familial renal carcinoma (FRC) is a condition in which multiple members of a family develop cancer of the kidney. Investigators in Iceland have demonstrated that nearly 60% of patients in that country who have developed kidney cancer since 1954 have up to a second cousin with kidney cancer (35). This study suggests that there is an inherited feature in a significant number of sporadic kidney cancers. (From Linehan WM, Walther MM, Zbar B. The genetic basis of cancer of the kidney. *J Urol* 2003;170:2163, with permission.)

study suggests that there is far more of an inherited basis to kidney cancer than was previously recognized, that is, that low penetrance "susceptibility genes" may predispose individuals to develop cancer of the kidney. Studies are currently underway to identify families in which multiple members develop kidney cancer [familial renal carcinoma, (FRC)] in order to identify these genes (Fig. 45.10).

CONCLUSION

Kidney cancer is not a single cancer but is made up of a number of different types of cancers occurring in the kidney, each with a different histology, a different clinical course, responding differently to therapy, and caused by alteration of different genes. Inherited kidney cancer is caused by alteration of different genes. Mutations in the *VHL* gene are found in most sporadic clear cell renal carcinomas. However, mutations in the *MET* gene, the *BHD* gene, and the *FH* genes are not found in most sporadic tumors of papillary type 1, papillary type 2, and oncocytic histology. The genes that cause sporadic papillary type 1, sporadic papillary type 2, and oncocytic tumors remain to be identified. Kidney cancer occurs in both an inherited (familial) and a sporadic (noninherited) form. Study of the hereditary forms of kidney cancer has led to the identification of genes important for understanding noninherited kidney cancer. It is hoped that understanding the pathways of these cancer genes will lead to the development of effective forms of therapy for patients with each of these forms of kidney cancer.

References

1. Linehan WM, Yang JC, Bates SE. Cancer of the kidney. In: DeVita SE, Hellman S, Rosenberg SA, eds. *Cancer principles and practice of oncology*, 7th ed. Philadelphia, PA: Lippincott Williams & Wilkins, 2004 (in press).
2. Linehan WM, Walther MM, Zbar B. The genetic basis of cancer of the kidney. *J Urol* 2003;170:2163.
3. Latif F, Tory K, Gnarra JR, et al. Identification of the von Hippel-Lindau disease tumor suppressor gene. *Science* 1993;260:1317.
4. Eisenhofer G, Walther MM, Huynh T, et al. Pheochromocytomas in von Hippel-Lindau syndrome and multiple endocrine neoplasia type 2 display distinct biochemical and chemical phenotypes. *J Clin Endocrinol Metab* 2001;86:1999.
5. Choyke PL, Glenn GM, Walther MM, et al. Hereditary renal cancers in adults. *Radiology* 2003;226:33.
6. Libutti SK, Linehan WM, Choyke PL, et al. Clinical and genetic analysis of patients with pancreatic neuroendocrine tumors associated with von Hippel-Lindau. *Surgery* 2000;128:1022.
7. Linehan WM, Zbar B, Klausner RD. Renal carcinoma. In: Scriver CR, Beaudet AL, Sly WS et al., eds. *The metabolic and molecular bases of inherited disease*, 8th ed., Chap. 41. New York: McGraw-Hill, 2001:907.
8. Stolle C, Glenn G, Zbar B, et al. Improved detection of germline mutations in the von Hippel-Lindau disease tumor suppressor gene. *Hum Mutat* 1998; 12:417.
9. Gnarra JR, Tory K, Weng Y, et al. Mutation of the VHL tumour suppressor gene in renal carcinoma. *Nat Genet* 1994;7:85.
10. Shuin T, Kondo K, Torigoe S, et al. Frequent somatic mutations and loss of heterozygosity of the von Hippel-Lindau tumor suppressor gene in primary human renal cell carcinomas. *Cancer Res* 1994;54:2852.
11. Gnarra JR, Tory K, Weng Y, et al. Mutations of the VHL tumor suppressor gene in renal carcinoma. *Nat Genet* 1994;7:85.
12. Yao M, Yoshida M, Kishida T, et al. VHL tumor suppressor gene alterations associated with good prognosis in sporadic clear-cell renal carcinoma. *J Natl Cancer Inst* 2002;94:1569.
13. Duan DR, Pause A, Burgess WH, et al. Inhibition of transcription elongation by the VHL tumor suppressor protein. *Science* 1995;269:1402.
14. Pause A, Lee S, Worrell RA, et al. The von Hippel-Lindau tumor-suppressor gene product forms a stable complex with human CUL-2, a member of the Cdc53 family of proteins. *Proc Natl Acad Sci U S A* 1997;94:2156.
15. Lonergan KM, Iliopoulos O, Ohh M, et al. Regulation of hypoxia-inducible mRNAs by the von Hippel-Lindau tumor suppressor protein requires binding to complexes containing elongins B/C and Cul2. *Mol Cell Biol* 1998;18:732.
16. Tyers M, Rottapel R. VHL: a very hip ligase. *Proc Natl Acad Sci U S A* 1999;96:12230.
17. Seagroves T, Johnson RS. Two HIFs may be better than one. *Cancer Cell* 2002;1:211.
18. Yang JC, Haworth L, Sherry RM, et al. A randomized trial of bevacizumab, an anti-vascular endothelial growth factor antibody, for metastatic renal cancer. *N Engl J Med* 2003;349:427.
19. Lubensky IA, Schmidt L, Zhuang Z, et al. Hereditary and sporadic papillary renal carcinomas with c-met mutations share a distinct morphological phenotype. *Am J Pathol* 1999;155:517.
20. Ornstein DK, Lubensky IA, Venzon D, et al. Prevalence of microscopic tumors in normal appearing renal parenchyma from patients with hereditary papillary renal cancer. *J Urol* 2000;163:431.
21. Schmidt L, Duh F-M, Chen F, et al. Germline and somatic mutations in the tyrosine kinase domain of the MET proto-oncogene in papillary renal carcinomas. *Nat Genet* 1997;16:68.
22. Schmidt L, Junker K, Weirich G, et al. Two North American families with hereditary papillary renal carcinoma and identical novel mutations in the MET proto-oncogene. *Cancer Res* 1998;58:1719.
23. Schmidt L, Junker K, Kinjerski T, et al. Novel mutations of the MET proto-oncogene in papillary renal carcinomas. *Oncogene* 1999;18:2343.
24. Schmidt LS, Nickerson ML, Angeloni D, et al. Early onset hereditary papillary renal carcinoma: germline missense mutations in the tyrosine kinase domain of the MET proto-oncogene. *J Urol* 2004;172:1256.
25. Zbar B, Tory K, Merino M, et al. Hereditary papillary renal cell carcinoma. *J Urol* 1994;151:561.
26. Launonen V, Vierimaa O, Kiuru M, et al. Inherited susceptibility to uterine leiomyomas and renal cell cancer. *Proc Natl Acad Sci U S A* 2001;98:3387.
27. The Multiple Leiomyoma Consortium. Germline mutations in FH predispose to dominantly inherited uterine fibroids, skin leiomyomata and papillary renal cell cancer. *Nat Genet* 2002;30:1.
28. Toro JR, Nickerson ML, Wei MH, et al. Mutations in the fumarate hydratase gene cause hereditary leiomyomatosis and renal cell cancer in families in North America. *Am J Hum Genet* 2003;73:95.
29. Kiuru M, Launonen V, Hietala M, et al. Familial cutaneous leiomyomatosis is a two-hit condition associated with renal cell cancer of characteristic histopathology. *Am J Pathol* 2001;159:825.
30. Birt AR, Hogg GR, Dubé WJ. Hereditary multiple fibrofolliculomas with trichodiscomas and acrochordons. *Arch Dermatol* 1977;113:1674.
31. Zbar B, Alvord G, Glenn G, et al. Risk of renal and colon neoplasms and spontaneous pneumothorax in the Birt Hogg Dubé syndrome. *Cancer Epidemiol Biomarkers Prev* 2002;11:393.
32. Toro J, Duray PH, Glenn GM, et al. Birt-Hogg-Dubé syndrome: a novel marker of kidney neoplasia. *Arch Dermatol* 1999;135:1195.
33. Pavlovich CP, Hewitt S, Walther MM, et al. Renal tumors in the Birt-Hogg-Dubé syndrome. *Am J Surg Pathol* 2002;26:1542.
34. Teh BT, Giraud S, Sari NF, et al. Familial non-VHL non-papillary clear-cell renal cancer. *Lancet* 1997;349:848.
35. Gudbjartsson T, Jonasdottir TJ, Thoroddsen A, et al. A population-based familial aggregation analysis indicates genetic contribution in a majority of renal cell carcinomas. *Int J Cancer* 2002;100:476.

CHAPTER 46 ■ RADIOLOGIC IMAGING OF RENAL CELL CARCINOMA: ITS ROLE IN DIAGNOSIS

PETER L. CHOYKE

INTRODUCTION

Imaging plays a major role in the diagnosis and management of renal cancer. Advances in imaging technology have resulted in uniformly high-quality scans, which, in turn, result in the detection of small renal masses hitherto unrecognized. Because these tumors tend to be low grade, their detection has improved the overall outcome from renal cancer. It has also added to the burden of deciding whether particular lesions require follow-up or intervention. This chapter reviews the technical aspects of current imaging modalities: computed tomography (CT), magnetic resonance imaging (MRI), ultrasound, and positron emission tomography (PET). The chapter also discusses the role of imaging in detecting and classifying cystic and solid lesions, as well as approaches to small renal masses. Finally, percutaneous image-guided therapies, radiofrequency ablation (RFA), and cryotherapy are also discussed.

IMAGING MODALITIES

Computed Tomography

Among the imaging modalities in clinical use, CT scan ranks as the most reliable method for detecting and staging renal cancers. In the United States, practically all CT scans are now performed in the helical or spiral mode instead of the older slice-by-slice mode. In the helical mode, the patient moves continuously, while the x-ray tube subtends a circle around the patient. Because of these two motions, the actual scanning path is a helix. The major implication of this is increased speed of scanning; another is that the data is no longer in a two-dimensional format, but rather can be considered a three-dimensional data set (Fig. 46.1). This means that it is more readily reformatted in the coronal or sagittal planes without the jagged edges that accompanied two-dimensional acquisitions (Fig. 46.2). Modern scanners also have multiple detectors so that each full rotation of the x-ray tube produces multiple helices, thereby further improving speed. The development of multiple-detector CT scanners with 4, 8, 16, or 32 rows of detectors has dramatically increased the speed of CT scanning.

Contrast media is a vital part of the CT scan. Typically, a nonionic iodinated contrast media is given to the patient through a 20-G intravenous line at 3 mL/sec using a mechanical injector. Nonionic contrast has fewer side effects (nausea, vomiting, and anaphylactoid reactions) than ionic contrast media (1). It is also less nephrotoxic (2). Indeed, recent evidence suggests that iso-osmolar (e.g., iodixanol) contrast media may be preferred over low-osmolar contrast media for preventing contrast nephrotoxicity (3). Patients with prior history of allergy to contrast media should be given prophylaxis consisting of a steroid preparation and antihistamine before injection (4). Patients with compromised renal function should be well hydrated and any nephrotoxic drugs should be discontinued (2,5). There is some evidence that N-acetyl cysteine given orally before and after contrast administration reduces contrast-induced nephrotoxicity (6,7). It is unclear what the cutoff value of serum creatinine for administering intravenous iodinated contrast should be, but most centers use a value between 1.7 and 2.0 mg/dL. Creatinine clearance or calculated clearance based on race, body weight, and gender (e.g., Cockroft-Gault) may be a superior method of determining a cutoff for administering contrast media. It should be emphasized, however, that all patients should be well hydrated before receiving intravenous iodinated contrast media and that persons with diabetes are at especially increased risk of contrast nephrotoxicity. Contrast nephrotoxicity generally occurs within 48 hours of the injection and resolves with conservative measures within 7 to 10 days, although a small fraction of patients have permanent damage to their renal function.

The ideal CT scan for renal masses begins with a noncontrast-enhanced ("precontrast") series of images through the kidney with 2.5 to 5 mm thick slices. It is very important that the same technical factors (i.e., slice thickness, milliampere-seconds, kilovoltage, and field of view) be used on all images so that changes in density within a lesion can be attributed only to the characteristics of the lesion and not to the technique. This allows the reliable detection and characterization of renal masses down to approximately 1 cm in diameter. Below this diameter it is still possible to characterize lesions as cysts but not unequivocally detect enhancement within a lesion. This is caused by a fundamental limitation of CT scan known as *partial volume averaging*. If the slice thickness includes both the lesion and part of the normal renal parenchyma, then the CT scan density reading is a weighted average of both. In the case of a cyst, this could lead to a falsely high density reading implying that the lesion is enhancing and therefore not a cyst. To avoid this, thin slices can be used; however, there are several problems with this approach. First, as the slice thickness decreases, the relative noise increases, making the images grainy and causing a wider spread of density measurements. Also, as slice thickness decreases, the radiation dose to the patient (to maintain signal to noise ratios) increases, and the number of slices increase, making data management more difficult. Therefore, 2.5 to 5 mm is a reasonable compromise for renal imaging, although thinner slices are needed for three-dimensional reconstructions (Fig. 46.1).

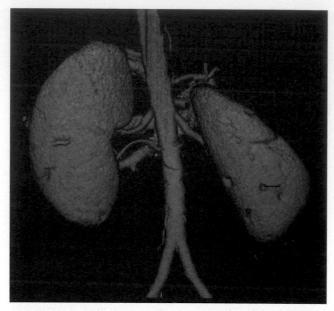

FIGURE 46.1. Three-dimensional volume rendering of the kidneys from a high resolution computed tomography (CT) scan of the kidneys made possible by helical acquisition of the data. Note that an accessory right renal artery is seen (see color insert).

The ideal CT scan for renal masses can be divided into four phases: precontrast, arterial phase (approximately 25 seconds postinjection), nephrographic (approximately 90 seconds postinjection), and excretory phase (approximately 5 to 7 minutes postinjection). Not all of these phases are necessary in all cases. Indeed, concerns about radiation exposure may lead to limited scanning to just the most informative phases. Among these the more important are the precontrast and nephrographic phases.

During the arterial phase the cortex brightly enhances compared to the medulla (Fig. 46.3). This phase is most useful for identifying the renal arteries and for hypervascular masses, especially small ones that may be more difficult to see on later images (8). A limitation of the arterial phase image, however, is that hyperenhancing lesions may be lost in the bright background of the hyperenhancing cortex (8) (Fig. 46.4).

The nephrographic phase is generally the most useful for detecting renal lesions because the normal renal parenchyma is uniformly enhanced, yet there is still no excretion of contrast to interfere with the image. As a consequence, tumors generally appear as low in density compared to the normal

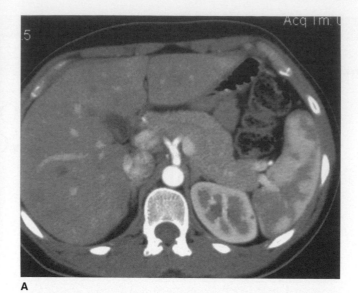

A

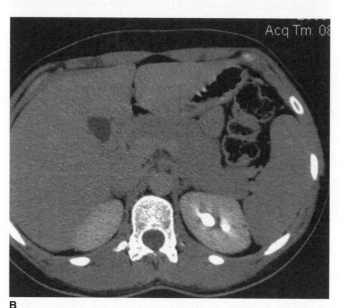

B

FIGURE 46.3. Value of arterial phase images. **A:** The arterial phase computed tomography (CT) image of the left kidney depicts a small cortical cyst relatively easily, whereas (**B**) the lesion is obscured on delayed-phase images.

parenchyma. Highly vascular tumors, however, may be masked by the relatively high-density normal parenchyma. This phase also offers uniform enhancement of the veins, making it the best time-point for assessing renal vein and inferior vena cava (IVC) thrombus arising from a tumor (Fig. 46.5). This phase has the highest sensitivity and specificity for renal masses (Fig. 46.6).

The excretory phase is obtained approximately 5 to 7 minutes after injection at a time when the kidney has excreted a large amount of the contrast into the urinary tract. As a consequence, assessment of collecting system and renal pelvic involvement by a tumor can be made most easily (9,10) (Fig. 46.7). For hematuria work-ups this phase offers the possibility of examining the urothelial tract for tumors as well. In fact, a technique known as "CT urography" is becoming more widely used for hematuria work-ups. In CT urography a precontrast scan is obtained from above the kidneys to below the bladder to evaluate for stones. Following this, a nephrographic phase CT scan is obtained through the kidneys. Finally, the

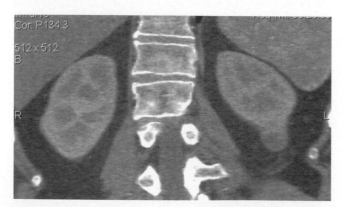

FIGURE 46.2. Coronal reformat of a computed tomography (CT) scan. Note that the coronal reformat demonstrates a left lower pole renal cancer without loss of resolution and with no "stair step" artifacts.

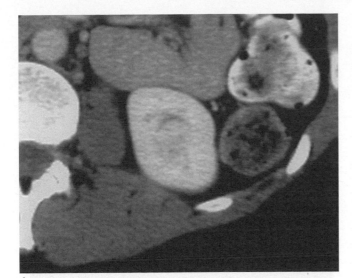

A

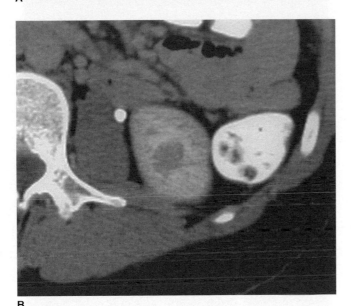

B

FIGURE 46.4. Value of delayed-phase images. **A:** The arterial phase computed tomography (CT) scan demonstrates a hyperenhancing renal cancer in the lower pole of the left kidney, which is isodense with the renal parenchyma. **B:** Delayed-phase image demonstrates the tumor to better advantage as a low density lesion near the lower pole renal sinus.

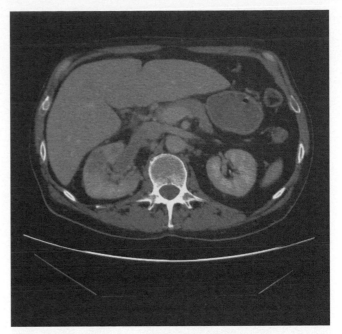

FIGURE 46.5. Right renal vein tumor thrombus depicted on computed tomography (CT) scan. This early-phase CT scan demonstrates part of a right renal tumor and a filling defect within the right renal vein extending into the inferior vena cava (IVC). The nephrographic phases of CT scan are better suited to the task of detecting venous thrombus than are later phases when the intensity of contrast within the veins is diminished.

patient is turned prone (or given low doses of Lasix) and thin section CT scan is obtained at 5 to 7 minutes from above the kidney to below the bladder to evaluate the ureters and bladder. If the patient is well hydrated, excellent opacification of the ureters is seen and small filling defects indicative of urothelial tumors can be readily detected.

The unit of density measurement in CT scan is named the *Hounsfield unit* (HU) in honor of Sir Godfrey Hounsfield, the inventor of the first CT scan device. The Hounsfield scale runs from −1,000 to +1,000. Zero HU corresponds to pure water. Fat ranges from −100 to −20 HU, whereas the normal unenhanced renal parenchyma ranges from 25 to 35 HU (Fig. 46.5). Renal stones are usually greater than 100 HU and air usually is less than −500 HU. The Hounsfield unit scale is clinically important because it is used to judge the degree of enhancement, a surrogate for the presence of tumor. Changes of less than 10 HU are not considered significant and indicate that

the lesion is a cyst. Changes in density greater than 20 HU are invariably caused by tumors. Changes in density between 10 and 20 HU must be considered on an individual basis. If the scan is technically optimal and there are no focal morphologic abnormalities within the lesion, the change may be considered abnormal. However, technical artifacts may also be responsible for this apparent enhancement. It should be noted that just as tumors enhance, they also de-enhance. A drop in density on two scans taken at two different times after the same injection (e.g., 1 minute and 2 minutes after intravenous contrast) has the same importance as enhancement, indicating the presence of a tumor. Therefore, lesions measuring 0 to 20 HU that do not change density after intravenous contrast are generally considered cysts. After intravenous contrast the density measurements of cysts may rise slightly but usually less than 10 HU. Why do the values change at all if the cyst is avascular? There are several reasons. First, the surrounding parenchyma usually increases from 25 to 35 HU to well over 150 HU. Even subtle partial-volume effects will cause a rise in the apparent density of a cyst. Moreover, because the kidneys and other organs of the body are higher in density after contrast media, the x-ray beam tends to "harden," that is, the lower energy x-rays are preferentially absorbed by the higher density tissue leaving only the higher energy x-rays to form the image. This shift in x-ray energy distribution, or "beam hardening," can cause a slight increase in the density of nonenhancing lesions such as cysts, which is known as "pseudoenhancement" (11–14). Streak artifacts arising from very dense contrast in the renal collecting system can also artifactually increase the apparent density of a lesion (Fig. 46.3b).

Three-dimensional imaging of the kidneys is now possible on most CT scanners. Instead of 5-mm collimation, however, 1- to 3-mm overlapping slices are obtained. Overlapping sections allow the computer algorithm to select thin slices that overlap each other by 50%, which in turn allows the creation

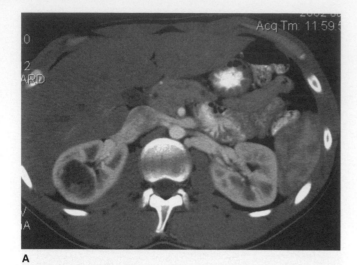

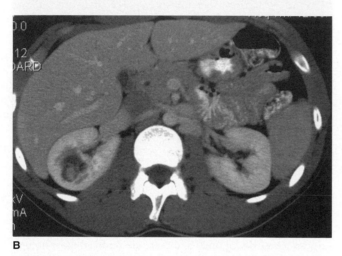

FIGURE 46.6. Complex cystic renal cancer depicted on nephrographic phase computed tomography (CT) scan. **A:** Early-phase CT scan demonstrates a cystic lesion in the right kidney with minimal enhancement. **B:** Nephrographic-phase CT scan demonstrates clear filling in of the lesion with central and mural enhancement, which is indicative of a cystic renal cancer.

of very smooth three-dimensional volume renderings of the kidney. A three-dimensional rendering obtained during the arterial phase will create a CT angiogram (CTA), which can be used to determine the number and location of renal arteries (15) (Fig. 46.8). Renderings from the nephrographic phase can be used to identify a renal mass within the kidney and display it because it would be seen intraoperatively. This can be useful for planning nephron-sparing surgery (16,17). Finally, three-dimensional renderings during the excretory phase, known as *CT urography* or CTU, can display the ureters and collecting system in a manner analogous to the intravenous urogram (10) (Fig. 46.9). It should be noted that CTA, nephrographic phase reconstructions, and CTU studies require additional time and expertise to process, and therefore are more expensive than conventional CT scans. The ultimate role of these three-dimensional methods, which add some radiation exposure and expense, remains to be determined.

Magnetic Resonance Imaging

MRI has evolved to the point where it can easily substitute for CT scanning when the latter cannot be performed. MRI can

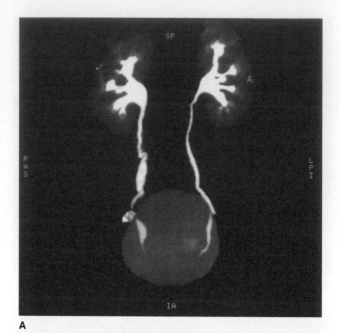

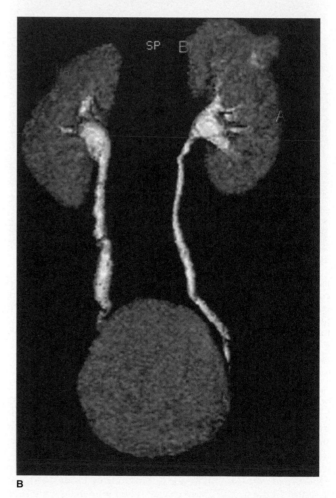

FIGURE 46.7. Excretory phase images obtained 5 minutes after contrast administration. **A:** Patient undergoing work-up for hematuria demonstrates no filling defects within the collecting system on this coronal reformatted projection image of the ureters. The outpouching in the distal right ureters is due to a sharp turn in the course of the ureters. **B:** Patient with upper pole tumor in the left kidney obtained with volume rendering demonstrates that the small tumor has no connection with the collecting system.

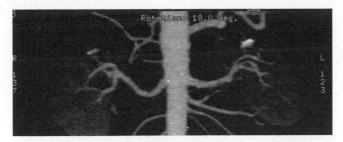

FIGURE 46.8. Maximum intensity projection image (MIP) of the kidneys obtained during the arterial phase demonstrates a normal CT angiogram (CTA). Note both main renal arteries are easily detected. Other branches arise from the superior mesenteric artery or lumbar arteries and are unrelated to the kidney.

be performed even when renal function is very poor because the gadolinium-chelates used in MRI are not nephrotoxic (18). Moreover, patients with severe allergies to iodinated contrast agents may safely have a contrast-enhanced MRI.

The MRI of the kidney consists of several parts. T1 axial scans are obtained to look for areas of hemorrhage or fat within the kidney, both of which are high in signal on T1-weighted images (Fig. 46.9). Slice thickness is generally 5 to

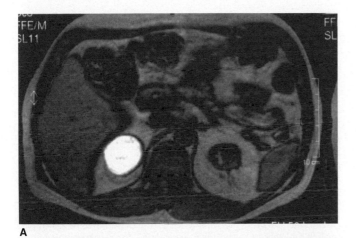

A

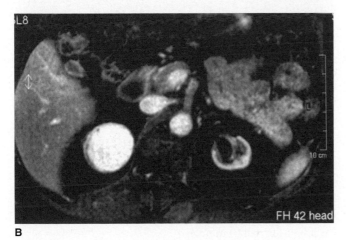

B

FIGURE 46.9. Pre- and postcontrast magnetic resonance imaging (MRI) of the kidney. **A:** Precontrast T1-weighted MRI depicts a high signal intensity lesion in the right kidney. This could represent either a hemorrhagic cyst or lipid within an angiomyolipoma. **B:** Post gadolinium-enhanced T1-weighted MR with fat saturation demonstrates that the lesion does not enhance and that it does not suppress with fat saturation excluding an angiomyolipoma and confirming a hemorrhagic cyst.

7 mm. T2-weighted axial or coronal images are highly sensitive for fluid within renal cysts (19). Cysts are typically very high in signal intensity unless they contain hemorrhage or high protein content (Fig. 46.10). Therefore, T2-weighted imaging can help identify cysts (Fig. 46.11). However, the most useful of the types of scans used in MRI is the pre- and postcontrast T1-weighted MRI scans. Precontrast scans and postcontrast scans must be obtained within the same series in MRI, otherwise the MR unit may reset the gain values on the receiver (20). If this happens it may be impossible to compare the signal obtained from a lesion before and after intravenous contrast. During a typical MR, a low-molecular-weight gadolinium-chelate (Gd) is injected (0.1 mmol/kg) intravenously. This can usually be accomplished quickly because of the small volumes of gadolinium-chelates that are required for MRI (10 to 20 cc). Serial T1-weighted images in the coronal or axial planes are typically obtained during breath-holding (Fig. 46.11). Because there is no ionizing radiation with MRI the acquisitions can be performed over and over without penalty. For practical reasons we usually scan immediately before, immediately after, and at four additional times at 1-minute intervals (Fig. 46.11). A lesion can then be measured serially at five time-points to determine whether it changes in enhancement. A "noise floor" of approximately 15% is accepted, meaning that signal changes within 15% of baseline are considered noise (20). It is also useful to evaluate the pattern of enhancement. A pattern characterized by an immediate increase in intensity followed by a slow decline in intensity is highly suggestive of an enhancing neoplasm, whereas a pattern characterized by unpredictable increases and decreases in signal is most likely related to a motion artifact. Subtraction can also be performed (the postcontrast image is subtracted from the precontrast image) to obtain a net enhancement image. In theory, nonenhancing structures should be black on the subtraction image, whereas in fact, changes in position at different times may create registration artifacts on the subtracted image.

A unique feature of MRI that can be exploited in urologic imaging is its sensitivity for blood flow. A family of techniques, known as "bright blood" methods, depicts normally flowing blood as high in signal. Therefore, thrombi within the vein, for instance, will appear as defects within the lumen of the vessel. This technique is very useful for staging renal cancers (Fig. 46.12).

Like CT scan, MR images can be rendered in three-dimensional view. Therefore, MR angiography (MRA) can be used to determine the number and location of renal arteries. MR venography (MRV) can assist in localizing the extent of renal vein thrombus, and MR urography (MRU) can be used to assess the collecting system and ureters. All these techniques require the administration of intravenous Gd and delays of varying times. It has been found that the addition of a small amount of Lasix (<20 mg) intravenously results in improved distention of the urothelial tract and therefore improved diagnosis when employing MRU (21–23).

Ultrasound

Ultrasound is an important and easily performed diagnostic method that is sometimes overlooked in the work-up of renal masses. Ultrasound imaging is based on the reflection of sound from tissue interfaces. Cysts, having no internal interfaces, do not reflect sound and therefore, are black on ultrasound. Additionally, "enhancement of the back wall," a brightening of the tissues deep in the cyst, occurs because the sound wave is unattenuated through the cyst. Solid lesions, however, have internal specular reflectors, which reflect sound back to the transducer, and therefore tumors have internal echoes (Fig. 46.13). Moreover, because these tumors attenuate sound, there is no "back wall

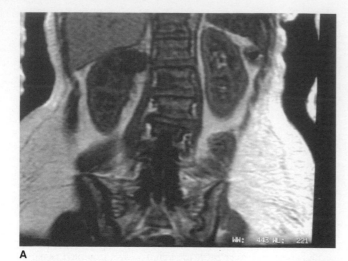

A

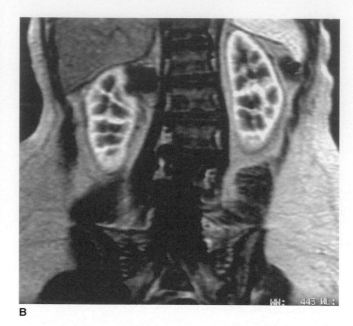

B

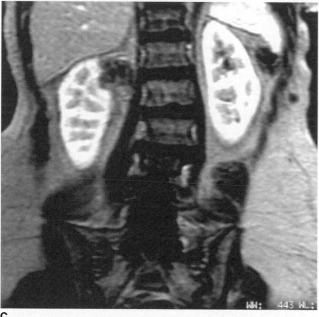

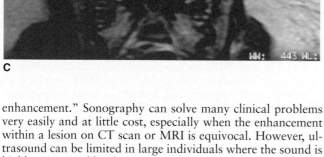

C

FIGURE 46.10. Serial dynamic enhanced magnetic resonance imaging (MRI) of an upper-pole renal tumor (clear cell carcinoma). A: Precontrast scan demonstrates no specific findings except for a mass in the right upper pole. B: Early dynamic enhanced MRI approximately 1 minute after intravenous contrast administration demonstrates minimal visible enhancement. C: Delayed dynamic enhanced MRI approximately 2 minutes after intravenous contrast demonstrates enhancement within the tumor. Serial dynamic MRI is easily performed and there is no "radiation penalty" for repeated imaging. In this case the tumor enhanced 25% over baseline.

enhancement." Sonography can solve many clinical problems very easily and at little cost, especially when the enhancement within a lesion on CT scan or MRI is equivocal. However, ultrasound can be limited in large individuals where the sound is highly attenuated by the excess body tissue.

Depending on the patient size, 3 to 7 MHz transducers are used to identify lesions within the kidney. The best imaging window is usually found with the patient on his or her side; the kidney is often obscured anteriorly by bowel gas, and the decubitus position helps move bowel gas away from the kidney. Conventional imaging usually suffices with modern equipment; however, harmonic imaging is especially important in imaging large individuals. Harmonic imaging involves the sampling of multiples of the insonating frequency. For example, the first harmonic of an insonating frequency of 3 MHz is 6 MHz. Harmonic imaging reduces overall signal; however, it also decreases background noise and can clarify scans (24,25) (Fig. 46.14).

There is no intravenous contrast agent in routine use for ultrasound. Ultrasonic microbubbles have been approved for use in echocardiography and have been applied to renal masses (26,27). In general, the renal mass becomes hyperechogenic soon after the administration of intravenous ultrasound microbubbles (26).

Unfortunately, the microbubbles are also destroyed by the insonating ultrasound beam so that intermittent and low mechanical index imaging is necessary. The role of ultrasound microbubbles in the diagnosis of renal cancer remains to be determined.

Positron Emission Tomography

PET has become an increasingly popular method of imaging cancers in the last 5 years. The agent most commonly employed in the clinic is called fluorodeoxyglucose (FDG). FDG is available commercially although it has a very limited shelf-life (a few hours) because of the radioactive decay of ^{18}F, which has a half-life of 110 minutes.

The principles underlying PET differ from conventional radionuclide methods. In a conventional radionuclide study the radiopharmaceutical distributes to its physiologic target (think of the bone scan) and emits γ-rays as a consequence of radioactive decay. The emissions are single, random in direction, and distributed in energy.

In PET imaging, the radionuclide (e.g., ^{18}F) emits a positron, a positively charged particle that has approximately the same

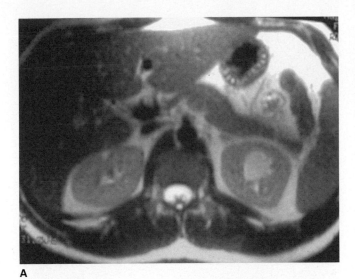

A

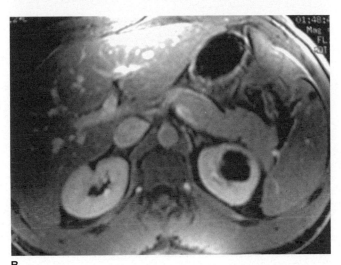

B

FIGURE 46.11. Benign complex cyst. **A:** T2-weighted magnetic resonance imaging (MRI) demonstrates a high-signal-intensity lesion within the left kidney with a small internal defect. Although not quite as bright as the cerebrospinal fluid seen in the spinal canal, the lesion is nonetheless most consistent with a cyst. **B:** Postcontrast enhanced T1-weighted scan demonstrates no enhancement within the cyst except at two small projections at opposite sides of the lesion. These represent the insertion sites of a septum crossing the lesion, which is not visible on the MRI due to lack of enhancement. These findings suggest that this is a simple septated cyst (Bosniak Type II).

mass as an electron. The positron wanders a short distance from its source before colliding with an electron. The result is annihilation and two γ-rays are emitted in diametrically opposite directions and at a characteristic energy, 511 keV. A ring of photomultipliers detects the coincident and opposite emission of the two γ-rays and then traces the two γ-rays to their source within the body. The advantages are high sensitivity and relatively good resolution (compared to other radionuclide methods but not compared to CT scan or MRI). The value of PET can be substantially improved by combining it with a CT scanner (Fig. 46.15). Positron emission tomography-computerized tomography (PET-CT) scanners are now in widespread use and combine the sensitivity of PET with the resolution of a CT scan.

Early results with FDG PET in renal cancer suggests that it is insensitive for low-grade tumors in the renal parenchyma (28,29). This is likely due to a combination of relatively low

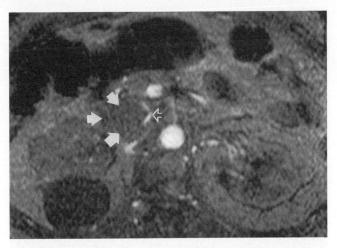

FIGURE 46.12. Tumor thrombus within the inferior vena cava (IVC) depicted on a "bright blood" technique. The IVC should have a high signal on this sequence, but in this case it is filled with a tumor thrombus (*arrows*) that decreases the signal except for a small medial portion of the IVC where blood still flows (*open arrow*). There is a large right-sided renal cancer partly demonstrated on this sequence.

uptake by the tumor and the relatively high but heterogenous uptake by the kidney (30). FDG is excreted by the kidneys; therefore, the kidneys, ureters, and bladder generally have intense activity. However, in metastatic work-ups or when searching for sites of recurrence after nephrectomy, the uptake of FDG is relatively high, and it has already proven to be a useful tool (Fig. 46.15). FDG represents only one of many different PET agents that have been developed, and it is quite likely that other PET agents will be very useful for localized renal tumors in the future.

SYMPTOMATIC RENAL MASSES

Patients presenting with symptoms generally have large and/or central renal tumors. Asymptomatic tumors or incidental tumors will be considered separately. The patient may present with flank pain or hematuria. Metastatic disease may present as cough, hemoptysis, headache, seizure, or bone and/or muscle pain. Generally, tumors are larger than 3 cm at presentation. It should be noted that tumors less than 3 cm in diameter can metastasize but usually present with metastases rather than developing them later (31).

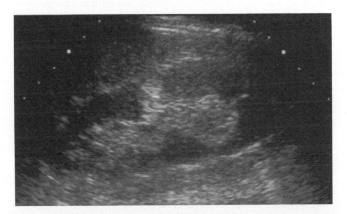

FIGURE 46.13. Echogenic mass in the kidney depicted by ultrasound. Such masses can represent renal tumors or angiomyolipomas. Computed tomography (CT) scan may be necessary to distinguish the two entities.

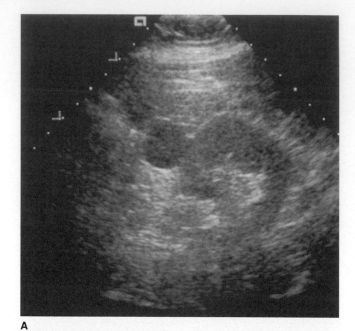

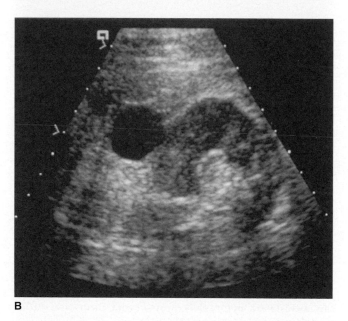

FIGURE 46.14. Value of harmonic imaging in a large patient. **A:** Conventional sonogram at the native frequency demonstrates a lesion with internal echoes suggestive of a solid mass. **B:** First harmonic sonogram demonstrates that the lesion is a cyst, with few internal echoes and good through-transmission of sound (back wall enhancement).

The imaging method of choice is CT scan for a suspected renal mass. Scans should be obtained before and after intravenous contrast. If CT scan is not feasible, MRI is a suitable substitute. Ultrasound can be used as a problem-solving tool when the CT scan or MRI are inconclusive for a tumor. The intravenous urogram is no longer considered an appropriate method of diagnosing a renal mass.

Solid masses of the kidney can represent one of several histologies including clear cell (including granular), papillary, chromophobe, oncocytomas, nonfatty angiomyolipomas, leiomyomas (capsulomas), and other cell types (32). Histology cannot be determined by imaging alone but there are clues. For instance, clear cell carcinomas tend to become heterogeneous as they grow beyond 4 cm, with a highly vascular component

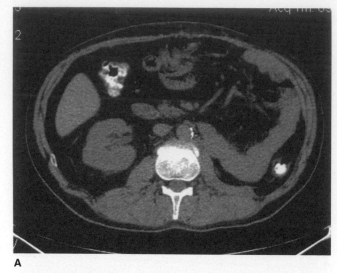

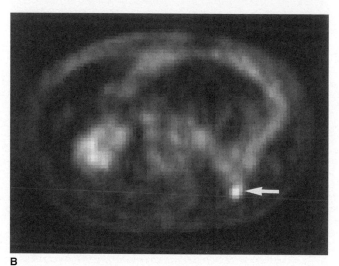

FIGURE 46.15. Positron emission tomography (PET) for recurrent renal cancer. **A:** CT scan of patient after left radical nephrectomy demonstrates nonspecific findings in the left renal fossa. **B:** Fluorodeoxyglucose (FDG) PET scan, although substantially lower in resolution, demonstrates increased activity in the renal fossa (*arrow*) from residual renal cancer.

and necrotic regions (Fig. 46.16). Papillary tumors tend to be poorly enhancing even early after contrast media and remain homogeneous when small (Fig. 46.17). They tend to slowly accumulate contrast within them as opposed to clear cell carcinomas where the contrast rapidly washes out. Larger tumors have poorly enhancing mural nodules but are heterogeneous (33–36). Chromophobe and oncocytomas tend to be homogeneously hyperenhancing. Transitional cell carcinomas invading the kidney typically are infiltrative rather than nodular. Nonfatty angiomyolipomas are hyperdense before contrast and enhance uniformly and intensely (36) (Fig. 46.18). Leiomyomas tend to be superficial because they arise from the renal capsule. These "rules of thumb" can be helpful in guiding clinical decision-making, but do not substitute for histologic specimens.

An important differential consideration is renal lymphoma. Most renal lymphoma is multifocal within the kidney and is associated with retroperitoneal adenopathy (37,38) (Fig. 46.19). However, occasionally a single large mass arising from the kidney can mimic a primary renal tumor. Clues to the diagnosis of lymphoma include disproportionate adenopathy in

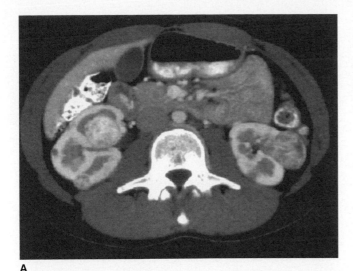

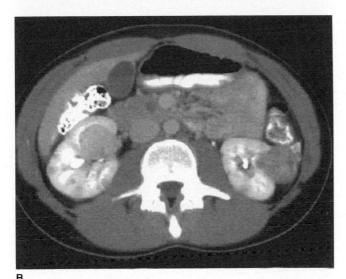

FIGURE 46.16. Hyperenhancing bilateral clear cell carcinomas in a patient with von Hippel-Lindau (VHL) syndrome. A: Arterial-phase computed tomography (CT) scan demonstrates hypervascular tumors that are brighter than the surrounding renal cortex. B: Venous-phase CT scan demonstrates the tumors to be less dense than the adjacent renal parenchyma. This pattern is typical of small clear cell carcinomas.

atypical locations, extensive invasion of adjacent organs, particularly bowel, absence of venous invasion, and infiltrative appearance. Renal mass biopsy is indicated in cases where there is a question about whether the lesion is lymphomatous, metastatic disease, or other atypical pathology. It is important to remember that renal lymphoma may not be accompanied by retroperitoneal adenopathy.

Having established that a solid mass is present, the tumor must be staged. For renal cancers, this includes a CT scan of the chest, abdomen, and pelvis, a bone scan, and an MRI of the brain.

STAGING

Local Staging

When staging a renal cancer, the tumor should be systematically evaluated for (i) capsular or renal sinus invasion, (ii)

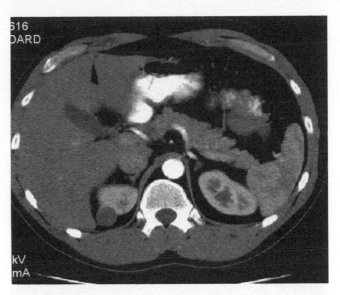

FIGURE 46.17. Hypoenhancing papillary renal tumor. This tumor in the upper pole of the right kidney is poorly enhancing and appears cystic, yet was proven to be solid by sonography (not shown). Papillary renal cancers tend to be hypoenhancing compared with other cell types.

perirenal extension and collateral vessels, (iii) regional lymphadenopathy, (iv) renal venous and inferior vena caval (IVC) thrombus, (v) psoas or abdominal muscle invasion, and (vi) adjacent organ invasion (bowel, pancreas, liver, abdominal) (39). CT scan with intravenous contrast performs well for these tasks; however, MRI is superior for detecting renal venous and IVC thrombus (Fig. 46.20). Bright blood and gadolinium-enhanced three-dimensional MRI images can better identify the superior extent of thrombus and identify retrograde thrombus propagation (40). CT scan is limited by mixing artifacts wherein unopacified blood from the lower extremities mixes with opacified blood from the kidneys causing artifactual filling defects near the renal vein ostia (Fig. 46.21) Previous reports stating that renal vein enlargement alone is a finding of renal vein thrombosis have proven unreliable (17).

Chest CT scan and bone scan remain important components of the work-up of renal cancer. Recently, FDG PET scanning has generated much interest because it appears quite sensitive for both bony and nodal metastases throughout the body. As mentioned previously, FDG PET is of limited value in non-metastatic early renal cancer but appears quite useful both in initial staging and in monitoring patients for recurrence after nephrectomy (28,41,42). Experience is still limited with regard to using FDG PET to judge the response of metastatic disease to systemic therapy.

Follow-up Imaging

The frequency and duration of follow-up imaging after renal cancer surgery remains controversial. This, of course, is not simply a medical issue but is a societal one, and policy makers seek methods of reducing costs. It is accepted that annual CT scans should be obtained for several years after surgery and bone scans or brain MRIs should be obtained on the basis of new symptoms, but the benefits of long-term CT scanning and bone scanning has been questioned (43). It is well known that renal cancers can present with metastases 10 years or more after surgery; however, it is currently believed that there is little benefit to the early detection of metastatic disease so that routine monitoring of patients is not routinely warranted. Of course, in individual cases closer monitoring may be justified by particular clinical concerns or in research settings.

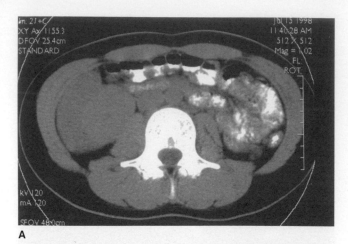

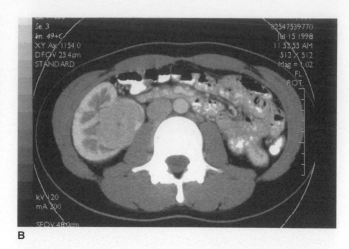

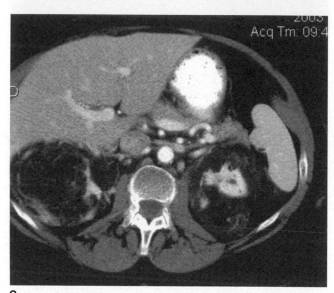

FIGURE 46.18. Nonfatty angiomyolipoma. **A:** Precontrast computed tomography (CT) scan demonstrates slightly hyperdense solid lesion in the left kidney. **B:** Postcontrast CT scan demonstrates a uniformly enhancing solid lesion except in the center. This lesion is indistinguishable from a solid renal cancer except for the hyperdensity before contrast and the uniformity of enhancement after contrast administration, which is atypical for renal cancers. **C:** For comparison, bilateral fat containing angiomyolipomas is demonstrated in a patient with tuberous sclerosis.

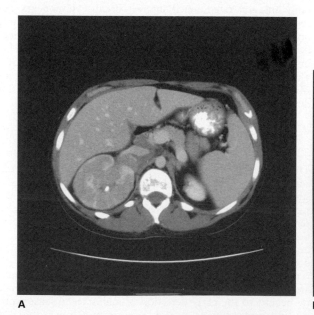

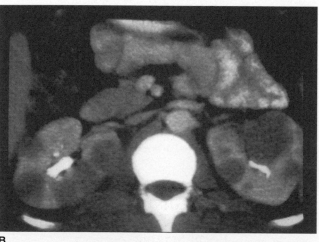

FIGURE 46.19. Two cases of renal lymphoma. **A:** Unilateral renal lymphoma with adenopathy behind the inferior vena cava (IVC). **B:** Bilateral renal lymphoma with no retroperitoneal adenopathy.

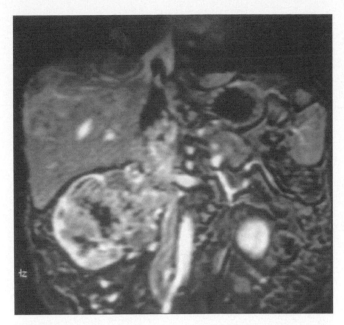

FIGURE 46.20. Intrahepatic inferior vena caval thrombus from a primary renal cancer in the right kidney. This coronal gadolinium-enhanced T1-weighted magnetic resonance imaging (MRI) demonstrates a large tumor thrombus extending to the level of the right atrium. The lower portions of the thrombus are enhancing, indicative of active tumor, whereas the superior portions are nonenhancing, typical of bland thrombus.

ASYMPTOMATIC OR INCIDENTAL RENAL MASSES

With the widespread use of cross-sectional imaging, a large number of patients are discovered with incidental masses. In this section we will discuss the incidental cystic lesion and the small renal mass.

Cystic Renal Lesions: The Bosniak Classification

In the early 1980s it became apparent that CT scan was disclosing many more renal lesions than were previously recognized clinically. Most of these, more than 90%, were simple renal cysts that were easily recognized by their uniform, low-density appearance. However, at the same time more complex cystic lesions were also being identified. In 1986, Dr. Morton Bosniak from New York University described a classification system of renal cysts now known as the *Bosniak Classification* (44).

In the original classification there were four categories of renal cystic lesions. Type I lesions were simple renal cysts; the cyst wall was thin and regular, there were no calcifications or septa, and there was no enhancement. On ultrasound, these lesions had all the features of a simple renal cyst: smooth wall, no internal echoes, backwall enhancement, and refraction artifacts laterally. These lesions carried no risk of malignancy and could be safely ignored.

Type II lesions demonstrated some level of complexity. For instance, they might have a slightly thickened (1 to 2 mm) wall, still smooth in contour. Several thin septa (again, 1 to 2 mm) might be observed or thin curvilinear calcification might be present. These lesions did not enhance. The risk of malignancy was considered very low and these lesions were generally dismissed. It should be noted that the type of calcification (curvilinear, thick, chunky) seems to have little

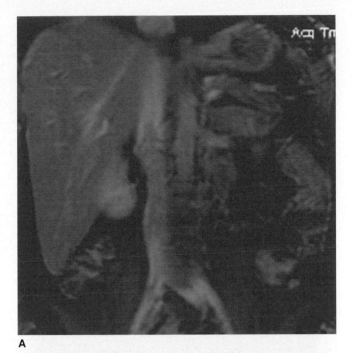

A

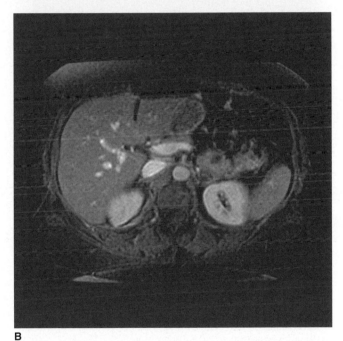

B

FIGURE 46.21. False-positive coronal magnetic resonance imaging (MRI) for inferior vena caval (IVC) thrombus. **A:** Coronal T1-weighted MRI demonstrates a long filling defect within the IVC suggestive of thrombus. **B:** Axial gadolinium-enhanced T1-weighted scan demonstrates no filling defect. The original defect is due to flow artifacts and should not be misinterpreted as an IVC thrombus.

bearing on the ultimate histology (45) (Fig. 46.22). In the absence of enhancement or nodularity, calcification alone carries no increased risk of malignancy. Another Type II lesion is the hemorrhagic cyst. Without precontrast scans, hemorrhagic cysts can mimic solid tumors. However, the absence of change in density or signal before and after intravenous contrast media indicates that the lesion is simply a hemorrhagic cyst (Fig. 46.23).

Type III lesions demonstrated increasing complexity including nodularity or increased thickening of the wall (>2 mm),

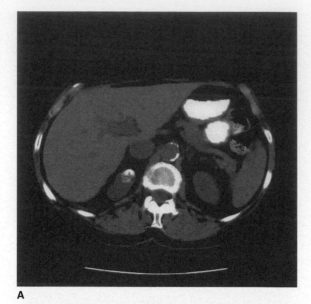

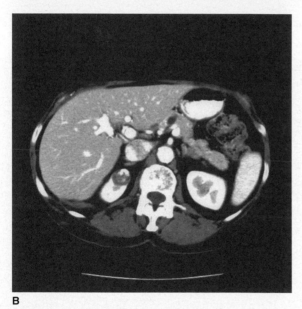

FIGURE 46.22. Nonenhancing calcified benign cyst of the right upper pole. **A:** Precontrast computed tomography (CT) scan demonstrates dense chunky calcification. **B:** After intravenous iodinated contrast media the lesion fails to enhance indicating its benign nature. Failure to enhance is a reliable finding of a benign renal lesion despite the complex appearance of the calcification.

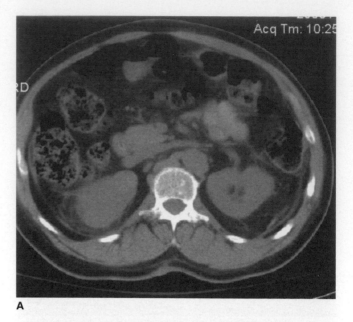

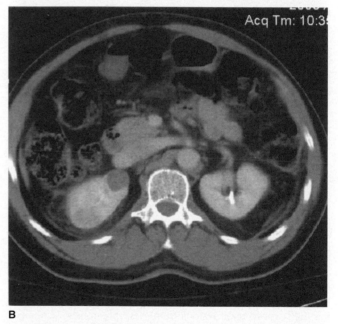

FIGURE 46.23. Nonenhancing hemorrhagic cyst. **A:** Precontrast computed tomography (CT) scan demonstrates a slightly hyperdense [40 Hounsfield units (HU)] renal lesion in the lower pole of the right kidney. **B:** Postcontrast CT scan demonstrates no change in density measurements (42 HU) indicative of a hemorrhagic cyst. There is a patchy heterogenous enhancement in the lower pole parenchyma because of a renal infection in this patient.

multiple septa (which enhanced with intravenous contrast), chunky calcification, and partial enhancement. A prototypical Type III lesion is a cystic renal cancer with a nodular or septal-enhancing component (Fig. 46.24). Of course, it is acknowledged that the multilocular cystic nephroma (MLCN), a benign lesion found in young boys and middle-aged women, has all the characteristics of a Type III lesion as well (Fig. 46.24). In general, Type III lesions are considered suspicious for malignancy and several studies have shown that 40% to 60% of them harbor cancers. Therefore, all Type III lesions are considered as surgical lesions. Because imaging has improved, the percentage of false-positive Type III lesions (benign at histology) is decreasing.

Type IV lesions have significant solid portions that unequivocally enhance. Most of these lesions are malignant and should be removed.

A major criticism of the original Bosniak classification is that different observers often differ in classifying lesions, especially Type II and Type III lesions. Inconsistencies in classification are largely due to lack of familiarity with the classification. However, it was acknowledged several years after its introduction that there were lesions for which there was a low level of suspicion but nonetheless had one or more suspicious features that warranted follow-up. Bosniak termed these lesions *Type IIF* (F for follow-up) and recommended follow-up at 6-month and then yearly intervals (46,47). In a review of this strategy, Bosniak et al. evaluated 42 patients with Type IIF lesions who were followed for a median of 5 years. Thirty-nine of them

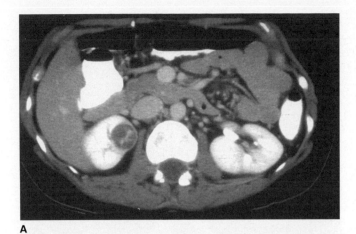

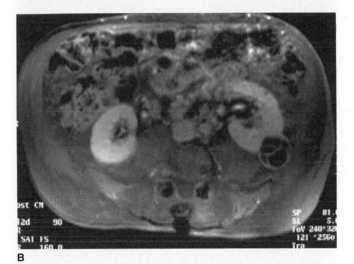

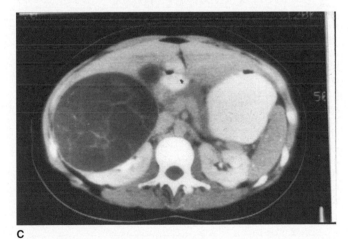

FIGURE 46.24. Several different Type III Bosniak lesions. **A:** Small cystic renal tumor with enhancing septum. **B:** Gadolinium-enhanced T1 weighted magnetic resonance imaging (MRI) demonstrated a multiseptated enhancing cystic lesion that proved to be a renal cell carcinoma. **C:** Computed tomography (CT) scan demonstrated a multiseptated renal mass with enhancement, which proved to be a multiloculated cystic nephroma at surgery.

remained stable (46). Three, however, enlarged and began to demonstrate enhancement. These proved to be cystic renal carcinomas at pathology. Therefore, IIF lesions are mostly benign but can "migrate" to Type III lesions over time with a frequency of approximately 10%.

Small Renal Masses

The widespread use of abdominal CT scan, MRI, and ultrasound has resulted in the incidental detection of small renal masses (Fig. 46.25). When these lesions are >1 cm in diameter they can generally be accurately characterized as solid or cystic. They carry a very low risk of metastatic disease when they are detected at this size, unless they present with metastases (31,48). As a consequence of their increased detection, both the prevalence and the survival rates for renal cancer have improved over the last 15 years. However, it has also become clear that the traditional radical nephrectomy may not always be warranted for these small lesions and nephron-sparing approaches are gaining popularity.

Many small renal masses are amenable to nephron-sparing surgery. Three-dimensional CT scan or MR evaluation can be helpful in determining the number and location of renal arteries, the status of the renal veins and IVC, and the location of the renal mass and its proximity to the central sinus structures and venous collaterals. It is sometimes helpful, especially when dealing with more than one solid renal mass, to employ intraoperative ultrasound to identify the renal mass and minimize damage to the remainder of the kidney (49). A small ultrasound unit is placed next to the operating table and the transducer is draped and covered in a sterile sheath with sterile gel inside the sheath. Water is used as a coupling medium in the surgical bed. Real-time ultrasound with color Doppler is used to identify the tumors and identify large vessels in the vicinity.

Very Small Renal Lesions

Although modern imaging brings many blessings it also brings a curse, the tiny indeterminate renal lesion. Statistically, these lesions will prove to be small cysts in most cases (Fig. 46.25). It is difficult to justify following every <1-cm lesion identified on routine CT scan or MRI scans. In patients with a hereditary predisposition to renal cancer or in patients who have already had a primary renal cancer removed, follow-up of such

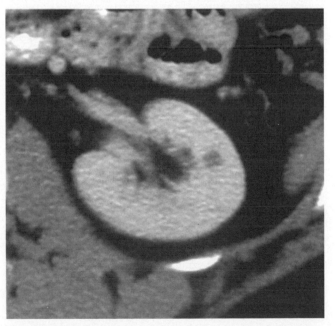

FIGURE 46.25. Contrast enhanced CT scan demonstrating a small low density lesion in the kidney. Statistically, this lesion is a simple renal cyst, however, it is not possible to be certain on the basis of a CT alone. T2 weighted MRI scans can be helpful when doubt exists about whether the lesion is a cyst.

lesions may be warranted. However, in a patient with only general-population risk of renal cancer, these lesions are generally dismissed as cysts. Naturally, this policy carries some small risk of being incorrect but serves most patients well. To some extent, the decision to follow can be guided by the wishes of an informed patient after discussions of the risks and benefits.

Screening

In the general population screening for renal cancer with imaging is not cost effective. A large study conducted in Japan using ultrasound as the screening technique detected only 0.1% to 0.3% with tumors of the kidney (50,51). Moreover, screening disclosed a number of nonmalignant conditions requiring work-up, which had minimal or no clinical significance. However, screening may very well become justified in high-risk groups identified either by family history or, in the future, by serum or genomic assays (52–54).

Disease entities now understood to carry an increased risk of malignancy for which screening is justified include Von Hippel-Lindau (VHL) (clear cell carcinoma), Birt-Hogg-Dubé (chromophobe, oncocytic neoplasm), hereditary papillary renal cancer (type I papillary tumors), and hereditary leiomyoma renal cell carcinoma (type II papillary tumors). Computerized tomography is considered the best method of screening based on the insensitivity of ultrasound for small renal masses and the added expense of MRI (55). The interval needs to be based on the patient's prior history of disease as well as the behavior of tumors within the family. Note that not all solid tumors are immediately removed in hereditary cancer syndromes. In fact, many tumors are observed until they reach 3 cm before they are removed in a conscious strategy to preserve renal function and minimize the total number of surgeries, while the tumors remain localized to the kidney.

IMAGE-GUIDED THERAPY

An alternative to surgery in some cases is the use of percutaneous or laparoscopic-assisted procedures. These include radiofrequency ablation (RFA) and cryoablation. These procedures are generally reserved for higher-risk patients, patients with compromised renal function, or patients with recurrent or hereditary forms of renal cancer.

RFA involves the placement of a high-energy probe within the tumor. Once the generator is turned on the tissue heats rapidly causing microbubbles to form within the tissue. The tumor can therefore be ablated by this method (Fig. 46.26). Tumors adjacent to large vessels may be difficult to treat because the vessel will act as a heat sink and draw heat away from the tumor (56,57). Tumors close to bowel or other vital structures may also be difficult to treat in this manner and may require laparoscopic guidance to keep the normal tissue away from the treatment probe (58,59). Typically, the original lesion involutes and fails to enhance after RFA. A halo of fat necrosis is commonly seen (Fig. 46.26).

Cryotherapy is based on the killing properties of the freeze-thaw cycle. During freezing, ice crystals form within cells (60–63). During thaw these crystals burst the cell membranes leading to cell death. Liquid nitrogen is introduced into a probe, which is insulated except at the tip. A series of freeze-thaw cycles are completed to ablate the tumor.

Both RFA and cryotherapy are limited by the lack of good real time monitoring of the process. Therefore, the lesions are generally overtreated in order to assure that the target lesion is completely ablated. Once the lesion is felt to be ablated it can be followed at 6-month intervals. It is critical that lesions be

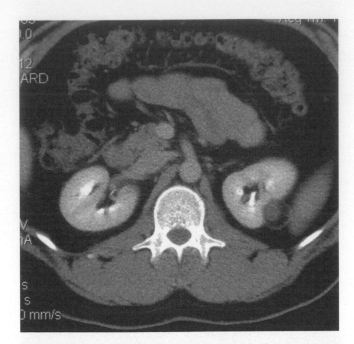

FIGURE 46.26. The appearance of an RFA-treated lesion 9 months after therapy. This contrast enhanced CT demonstrates a fat density defect in the kidney surrounded by a halo of fat necrosis. This pattern is commonly seen in successfully treated lesions.

followed because remnant tumor can be considered part of a much larger lesion. Moreover, the full effects of partial heating or cooling of a tumor are not yet well understood. For this reason, careful monitoring of patients after these minimally invasive procedures is mandatory.

CONCLUSION

Imaging of renal cancers has undergone a remarkable set of advances in the last decade. Helical CT scan is the primary imaging modality of choice, but MRI and ultrasound can play important roles. The role of FDG PET imaging remains to be completely defined, but its use in evaluating metastatic disease or disease recurrence seems warranted. The combined use of CT scan and PET makes localization of abnormalities even more straightforward. Advances in imaging have meant that smaller tumors can be detected. These tumors are amenable to nephron-sparing procedures. Screening for renal cancer with imaging is not yet practical, but the development of genetic or proteomic assays may soon propel imaging into an early detection mode that promises new opportunities for the cure of renal cancer.

References

1. Cohan RH, Bullard MA, Ellis JH, et al. Local reactions after injection of iodinated contrast material: detection, management, and outcome. *Acad Radiol* 1997;4:711–718.
2. Thomsen HS, Morcos SK. Contrast media and the kidney: European Society of Urogenital Radiology (ESUR) guidelines. *Br J Radiol* 2003;76: 513–518.
3. Aspelin P, Aubry P, Fransson SG, et al. Nephrotoxic effects in high-risk patients undergoing angiography. *N Engl J Med* 2003;348:491–499.
4. Cohan RH, Ellis JH. Iodinated contrast material in uroradiology. Choice of agent and management of complications. *Urol Clin North Am* 1997; 24:471–491.
5. Mueller C, Buerkle G, Buettner HJ, et al. Prevention of contrast media-associated nephropathy: randomized comparison of 2 hydration regimens in 1620 patients undergoing coronary angioplasty. *Arch Intern Med* 2002;162: 329–336.

6. Briguori C, Manganelli F, Scarpato P, et al. Acetylcysteine and contrast agent-associated nephrotoxicity. *J Am Coll Cardiol* 2002;40:298–303.

7. Shyu KG, Cheng JJ, Kuan P. Acetylcysteine protects against acute renal damage in patients with abnormal renal function undergoing a coronary procedure. *J Am Coll Cardiol* 2002;40:1383–1388.

8. Cohan RH, Sherman LS, Korobkin M, et al. Renal masses: assessment of corticomedullary-phase and nephrographic-phase CT scans. *Radiology* 1995;196:445–451.

9. Herts BR. Imaging for renal tumors. *Curr Opin Urol* 2003;13:181–186.

10. Caoili EM, Cohan RH, Korobkin M, et al. Urinary tract abnormalities: initial experience with multi-detector row CT urography. *Radiology* 2002; 222:353–360.

11. Abdulla C, Kalra MK, Saini S, et al. Pseudoenhancement of simulated renal cysts in a phantom using different multidetector CT scanners. *AJR Am J Roentgenol* 2002;179:1473–1476.

12. Birnbaum BA, Maki DD, Chakraborty DP, et al. Renal cyst pseudoenhancement: evaluation with an anthropomorphic body CT phantom. *Radiology* 2002;225:83–90.

13. Bae KT, Heiken JP, Siegel CL, et al. Renal cysts: is attenuation artifactually increased on contrast-enhanced CT images? *Radiology* 2000;216:792–796.

14. Coulam CH, Sheafor DH, Leder RA, et al. Evaluation of pseudoenhancement of renal cysts during contrast-enhanced CT. *AJR Am J Roentgenol* 2000;174:493–498.

15. Pozniak MA, Balison DJ, Lee FT Jr, et al. CT angiography of potential renal transplant donors. *Radiographics* 1998;18:565–587.

16. Coll DM, Uzzo RG, Herts BR, et al. 3-dimensional volume rendered computerized tomography for preoperative evaluation and intraoperative treatment of patients undergoing nephron sparing surgery. *J Urol* 1999; 161:1097–1102.

17. Oto A, Herts BR, Remer EM, et al. Inferior vena cava tumor thrombus in renal cell carcinoma: staging by MR imaging and impact on surgical treatment. *AJR Am J Roentgenol* 1998;171:1619–1624.

18. Prince MR, Arnoldus C, Frisoli JK. Nephrotoxicity of high-dose gadolinium compared with iodinated contrast. *J Magn Reson Imaging* 1996;6:162–166.

19. Tello R, Davison BD, O'Malley M, et al. MR imaging of renal masses interpreted on CT to be suspicious. *AJR Am J Roentgenol* 2000;174:1017–1022.

20. Ho VB, Allen SF, Hood MN, et al. Renal masses: quantitative assessment of enhancement with dynamic MR imaging. *Radiology* 2002;224:695–700.

21. Schad LR, Semmler W, Knopp MV, et al. Preliminary evaluation: magnetic resonance of urography using a saturation inversion projection spin-echo sequence. *Magn Reson Imaging* 1993;11:319–327.

22. Roy C, Saussine C, Jacqmin D. Magnetic resonance urography. *BJU Int* 2000;86(Suppl. 1):42–47.

23. Wille S, von Knobloch R, Klose KJ, et al. Magnetic resonance urography in pediatric urology. *Scand J Urol Nephrol* 2003;37:16–21.

24. Desser TS, Jeffrey RB Jr, Lane MJ, et al. Tissue harmonic imaging: utility in abdominal and pelvic sonography. *J Clin Ultrasound* 1999;27:135–142.

25. Choudhry S, Gorman B, Charboneau JW, et al. Comparison of tissue harmonic imaging with conventional US in abdominal disease. *Radiographics* 2000;20:1127–1135.

26. Quaia E, Siracusano S, Bertolotto M, et al. Characterization of renal tumours with pulse inversion harmonic imaging by intermittent high mechanical index technique: initial results. *Eur Radiol* 2003;13:1402–1412.

27. Forsberg F, Shi WT, Goldberg BB. Subharmonic imaging of contrast agents. *Ultrasonics* 2000;38:93–98.

28. Majhail NS, Urbain JL, Albani JM, et al. F-18 fluorodeoxyglucose positron emission tomography in the evaluation of distant metastases from renal cell carcinoma. *J Clin Oncol* 2003;21:3995–4000.

29. Miyakita H, Tokunaga M, Onda H, et al. Significance of 18F-fluorodeoxyglucose positron emission tomography (FDG-PET) for detection of renal cell carcinoma and immunohistochemical glucose transporter 1 (GLUT-1) expression in the cancer. *Int J Urol* 2002;9:15–18.

30. Mathews D, Oz OK. Positron emission tomography in prostate and renal cell carcinoma. *Curr Opin Urol* 2002;12:381–385.

31. Bosniak MA. The small (less than or equal to 3.0 cm) renal parenchymal tumor: detection, diagnosis, and controversies [published erratum appears in *Radiology* 1991 Oct;181(1):289]. *Radiology* 1991;179:307–317.

32. Choyke PL, Glenn GM, Walther MM, et al. Hereditary renal cancers. *Radiology* 2003;226:33–46.

33. Herts BR, Coll DM, Novick AC, et al. Enhancement characteristics of papillary renal neoplasms revealed on triphasic helical CT of the kidneys. *AJR Am J Roentgenol* 2002;178:367–372.

34. Jinzaki M, Tanimoto A, Mukai M, et al. Double-phase helical CT of small renal parenchymal neoplasms: correlation with pathologic findings and tumor angiogenesis. *J Comput Assist Tomogr* 2000;24:835–842.

35. Choyke PL, Walther MM, Glenn GM, et al. Imaging features of hereditary papillary renal cancers. *J Comput Assist Tomogr* 1997;21:737–741.

36. Lemaitre L, Claudon M, Dubrulle F, et al. Imaging of angiomyolipomas. *Semin Ultrasound CT MR* 1997;18:100–114.

37. Eisenberg PJ, Papanicolaou N, Lee MJ, et al. Diagnostic imaging in the evaluation of renal lymphoma. *Leuk Lymphoma* 1994;16:37–50.

38. Porcaro AB, D'Amico A, Novella G, et al. Primary lymphoma of the kidney. Report of a case and update of the literature. *Arch Ital Urol Androl* 2002;74:44–47.

39. Israel GM, Bosniak MA. Renal imaging for diagnosis and staging of renal cell carcinoma. *Urol Clin North Am* 2003;30:499–514.

40. Choyke PL, Walther MM, Wagner JR, et al. Renal cancer: preoperative evaluation with dual-phase three-dimensional MR angiography. *Radiology* 1997;205:767–771.

41. Hain SF, Maisey MN. Positron emission tomography for urological tumours. *BJU Int* 2003;92:159–164.

42. Jadvar H, Kherbache HM, Pinski JK, et al. Diagnostic role of [F-18]-FDG positron emission tomography in restaging renal cell carcinoma. *Clin Nephrol* 2003;60:395–400.

43. Sandock DS, Seftel AD, Resnick MI. A new protocol for the followup of renal cell carcinoma based on pathological stage. *J Urol* 1995;154:28–31.

44. Bosniak M. The current radiological approach to renal cysts. *Radiology* 1986;158:1.

45. Israel GM, Bosniak MA. Calcification in cystic renal masses: is it important in diagnosis? *Radiology* 2003;226:47–52.

46. Israel GM, Bosniak MA. Follow-up CT of moderately complex cystic lesions of the kidney (Bosniak category IIF). *AJR Am J Roentgenol* 2003; 181:627–633.

47. Bosniak MA. Should we biopsy complex cystic renal masses (Bosniak category III)? *AJR Am J Roentgenol* 2003;181:1425–1426; author reply 1426.

48. Bosniak MA, Rofsky NM. Problems in the detection and characterization of small renal masses. *Radiology* 1996;198:638–641.

49. Choyke PL, Pavlovich CP, Daryanani KD, et al. Intraoperative ultrasound during renal parenchymal sparing surgery for hereditary renal cancers: a 10-year experience. *J Urol* 2001;165:397–400.

50. Yamashita Y, Takahashi M, Watanabe O, et al. Small renal cell carcinoma: pathologic and radiologic correlation [published erratum appears in *Radiology* 1993 Dec;189(3):925]. *Radiology* 1992;184:493–498.

51. Filipas D, Spix C, Schulz-Lampel D, et al. Screening for renal cell carcinoma using ultrasonography: a feasibility study. *BJU Int* 2003;91:595–599.

52. Unwin RD, Knowles MA, Selby PJ, et al. Urological malignancies and the proteomic genomic interface. *Electrophoresis* 1999;20:3629–3637.

53. Klade CS, Voss T, Krystek E, et al. Identification of tumor antigens in renal cell carcinoma by serological proteome analysis. *Proteomics* 2001;1: 890–898.

54. Rogers MA, Clarke P, Noble J, et al. Proteomic profiling of urinary proteins in renal cancer by surface enhanced laser desorption ionization and neural-network analysis: identification of key issues affecting potential clinical utility. *Cancer Res* 2003;63:6971–6983.

55. Jamis-Dow CA, Choyke PL, Jennings SB, et al. Small (< or = 3-cm) renal masses: detection with CT versus US and pathologic correlation. *Radiology* 1996;198:785–788.

56. Zagoria RJ. Percutaneous image-guided radiofrequency ablation of renal malignancies. *Radiol Clin North Am* 2003;41:1067–1075.

57. Mayo-Smith WW, Dupuy DE, Parikh PM, et al. Imaging-guided percutaneous radiofrequency ablation of solid renal masses: techniques and outcomes of 38 treatment sessions in 32 consecutive patients. *AJR Am J Roentgenol* 2003;180:1503–1508.

58. Pautler SE, Pavlovich CP, Mikityansky I, et al. Retroperitoneoscopic-guided radiofrequency ablation of renal tumors. *Can J Urol* 2001;8:1330–1333.

59. Wood BJ, Ramkaransingh JR, Fojo T, et al. Percutaneous tumor ablation with radiofrequency. *Cancer* 2002;94:443–451.

60. Sewell PE, Howard JC, Shingleton WB, et al. Interventional magnetic resonance image-guided percutaneous cryoablation of renal tumors. *South Med J* 2003;96:708–710.

61. Shingleton WB, Sewell PE Jr. Cryoablation of renal tumours in patients with solitary kidneys. *BJU Int* 2003;92:237–239.

62. Lowry PS, Nakada SY. Renal cryotherapy: 2003 clinical status. *Curr Opin Urol* 2003;13:193–197.

63. Finelli A, Rewcastle JC, Jewett MA. Cryotherapy and radiofrequency ablation: pathophysiologic basis and laboratory studies. *Curr Opin Urol* 2003;13:187–191.

CHAPTER 47 ■ SURGICAL MANAGEMENT OF LOCALIZED RENAL CELL CARCINOMA

CHAPTER 47A
Open Radical Nephrectomy for Localized Renal Cell Carcinoma

Paul Russo

INTRODUCTION

The last decade has brought an immense expansion in the understanding of the cytogenetics, histopathology, epidemiology, and clinical surgery of renal cortical tumors. The translation of this new information into clinical practice has also been effective in changing surgical practice with contemporary concerns for the effective local control over the tumor by either radical or partial nephrectomy coupled with long-term concerns for the renal health of the patient and the small but real risk of contralateral kidney tumor formation. Radical nephrectomy remains an integral part of the surgical management of renal cortical tumors but is now one of several appropriate surgical options as opposed to the "gold standard" at our institution. This chapter discusses the historical and contemporary view of radical nephrectomy, important surgical anatomy and technical considerations, and the surgical complications associated with this operation.

RADICAL NEPHRECTOMY: HISTORICAL CONTEXT

Successful attempts to surgically cure renal tumors were reported largely after World War II with strategies designed to address renal capsular and perinephric fat infiltration that was observed in up to 70% of the tumors at that time (1). Using a thoracoabdominal incision, Mortensen (1948) reported the first radical nephrectomy, an operation that removed all of the contents of the Gerota fascia (2). Radical nephrectomy was popularized in the 1960s by Robson, who described this operation as the perifascial resection of the tumor-bearing kidney, along with perirenal fat, regional lymph nodes, and the ipsilateral adrenal gland (3). In 1969, Robson reported the results of a radical nephrectomy series of 88 patients and described a 65% survival for tumors confined within the Gerota fascia (Robson stage 1 and 2). However, the finding of regional nodal metastases led to less than a 30% 5-year survival rate (4). *En bloc* radical nephrectomy, ipsilateral adrenalectomy, and extensive regional lymphadenectomy, usually through large abdominal or transthoracic incisions, became the standard approach to the renal tumors for the next 20 years as major centers began reporting favorable results (5,6). In this era, imaging studies used to diagnose a patient, who was generally symptomatic with a large renal tumor, were intravenous urograms and arteriograms.

These techniques were unable to detect small tumors, and the incidental tumor detection rate was less than 5%. Despite the wide acceptance of radical nephrectomy by urologic surgeons, convincing data did not exist establishing the therapeutic impact of the component parts of the operation (i.e., the need for adrenalectomy (7) or the need for and extent of lymph node dissection (8,9). Historical series were subjected to selection biases, and the virtues of randomized trials in clinical investigation to address the many questions in kidney tumor surgery were not yet realized. Although a subsequent report with longer follow-up by Robson in 1982 projected declining long-term survival rates in the range of 40% (10), there was no doubt that the surgical techniques associated with the safe removal of large renal tumors were established, well described, and reproducible, making radical nephrectomy the only effective treatment of renal cortical tumors.

RADICAL NEPHRECTOMY: CONTEMPORARY PERSPECTIVE

In 2003, it was estimated that 31,900 new cases and 11,900 deaths would occur from kidney cancer in the United States (1). Since 1950, there has been a 126% increase in the incidence of renal cancer and a 36.5% increase in annual mortality (11,12). In the last decade, our understanding of tumors arising from the renal cortex has dramatically expanded because of advances in cytogenetics, histopathologic reclassification, and improved abdominal imaging technology leading to a tumor size and stage migration, and changing surgical strategies. Renal cortical tumors, viewed previously as a single cancer [i.e., hypernephroma, renal cell carcinoma (RCC), or kidney cancer] with a uniform metastatic potential, are instead a complex family of renal cortical neoplasms with distinct histologic subtypes (13,14) and unique cytogenetic and molecular defects (15,16). Metastatic potential, once thought to be strictly dependent on tumor size, grade, and stage, is currently understood to vary also according to tumor histologic subtype. Rates of metastases range from the most potentially malignant conventional clear cell carcinoma (65%) to the indolent papillary and chromophobe carcinomas (25%) to the virtually benign renal oncocytoma (10%). The historical presentation of renal cancer in patients with flank pain, abdominal or flank mass, and hematuria is distinctly uncommon today (<5% of cases) and has largely been replaced by the incidentally discovered solid renal mass (70% T1a or T1b, median tumor size 4.5 cm) discovered when abdominal imaging studies are performed for nonspecific abdominal or musculoskeletal complaints or during follow-up of other malignancies (17,18). Unfortunately, as of now, there is no preoperative imaging study or biopsy method with sufficient accuracy to diagnose the histologic subtypes of renal cortical tumors short of operative resection. Despite the clarity of modern imaging techniques, approximately 20% of resected renal cortical tumors represent a benign process or oncocytoma (19).

725

As the described tumor stage and size migration has progressed, the deleterious impact of radical nephrectomy compared to partial nephrectomy on renal function has recently been well documented by investigators at the Mayo Clinic and Memorial Sloan-Kettering Cancer Center (MSKCC) (20,21). Although data does not exist indicating that the risk of dialysis is greater with radical nephrectomy than with partial nephrectomy, these studies raise concerns for the overall renal health of the patient, who, as time goes on, can also experience renal damage from common medical conditions such as diabetes or hypertension, which can equal or surpass the oncological risk imparted by the resection of a small renal tumor. As patients are expected to live longer following the resection of smaller renal tumors, lifetime surveillance of the tumor-bearing kidney (in the case of patients treated by partial nephrectomy) and contralateral kidney (in patients treated by either partial or radical nephrectomy) leaves a risk of approximately 5% rate of recurrence (22). Once tumor resection is accomplished, postoperative nomograms now are available that incorporate clinical presentation, tumor histologic subtype, size, and stage to provide an accurate prediction of outcome that more accurately reflects the biology of the tumor. Results for our center indicate 5-year survival rates following resection of nonmetastatic tumors ranging from 70% to 98% depending on the clinical and pathologic features mentioned previously. This postoperative nomogram has been essential for patient counseling, tailoring cost-effective follow strategies, and designing clinical trials (23). Although numerous studies have supported the use of partial nephrectomy (i.e., nephron sparing, kidney sparing) for T1a (<4 cm) renal tumors (24), the rationale now exists to extend the partial nephrectomy to larger tumors, particularly if they are exophytic and polar in location (25).

RADICAL NEPHRECTOMY: PATIENT SELECTION AND PREOPERATIVE EVALUATION

To a large extent, the modern imaging studies of CT scan, ultrasound, and magnetic resonance imaging (MRI), which have been so effective in creating the era of the "incidentaloma" and the associated tumor size and stage migration, also provide the surgeon with an accurate description of the extent of disease before operation. At MSKCC, tumors routinely selected for radical nephrectomy include those large and centrally localized tumors that have effectively replaced most of the normal renal parenchyma, those large tumors associated with regional adenopathy (of benign or malignant etiology), those with inferior vena cava (IVC) or right atrial extension, and those in patients with metastatic disease referred by medical oncology for cytoreductive nephrectomy before the initiation of systemic therapy (26).

Patients with extensive metastatic disease and a poor Karnofsky performance status are advised to undergo percutaneous needle biopsy of the primary tumor or a metastatic site and subsequently referred for systemic therapy. Patients with small incidentally discovered or exophytic tumors amenable to partial nephrectomy are asked to also sign consent for radical nephrectomy if observed operative findings or technical problems arise making partial nephrectomy unsafe or unwise. Partial and radical nephrectomies are currently done with equal frequency at our center.

Before the operation, routine serum chemistries, coagulation profile, type and cross match (or autologous blood donation), and chest x-ray are obtained. Routine brain and bone scanning is not performed unless abnormalities in the history and physical examination are discovered. For patients with significant comorbid conditions, particularly cardiac and pulmonary related, appropriate consultations are obtained in order to optimize patients before their operation. Patients with significant coronary or carotid artery disease may require revascularization before radical nephrectomy. For patients with compromised pulmonary status, consultation with anesthesiology is requested for consideration of epidural postoperative analgesia.

RADICAL NEPHRECTOMY: SURGICAL ANATOMY, CHOICE OF INCISIONS, AND OPERATIVE CONSIDERATIONS

The kidneys are retroperitoneal organs located in the lumbar fossa. They are covered with a variable amount of perinephric

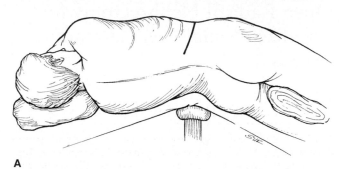

A

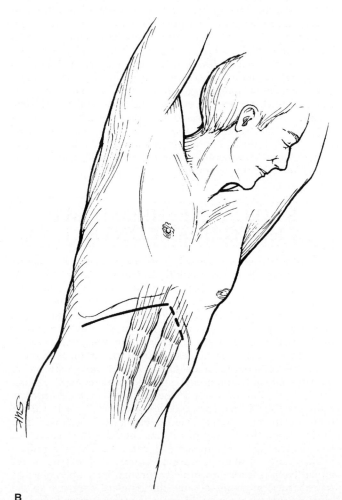

B

FIGURE 47A.1. Incisions for radical nephrectomy. Dashed lines represent potential extensions of the basic incision. Flank (**A**); subcostal (**B**); midline upper abdominal (**C**); chevron (**D**); thoracoabdominal.

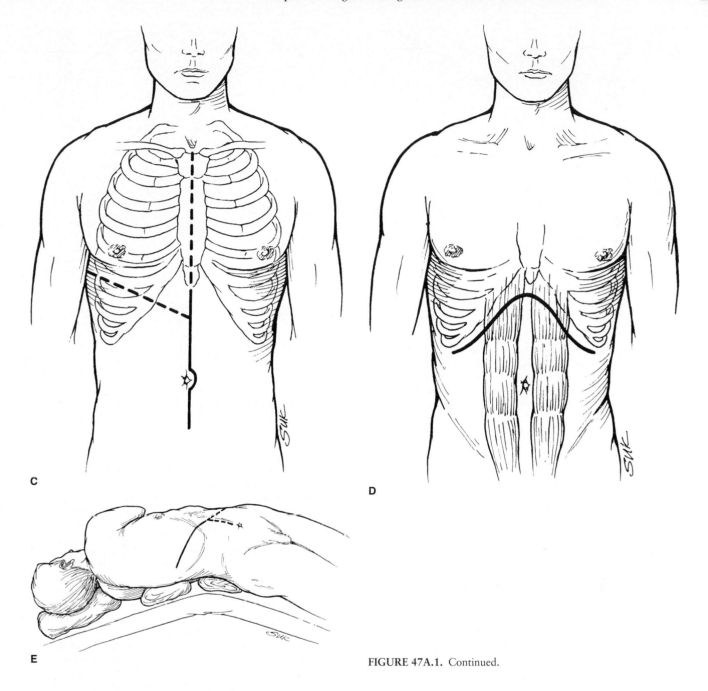

FIGURE 47A.1. Continued.

fat and a fascial layer, called *Gerota fascia*, and lay in proximity to the psoas major and quadratus lumborum muscles and diaphragm. The right kidney abuts the right adrenal gland; the liver, the hepatic flexure of the colon, and the second portion of the duodenum covers the renal hilum. The left kidney is in proximity to the left adrenal, pancreatic tail, and spleen superiorly and the left colon medially. Depending on the surgeon's preference, relating mainly to the patient's body habitus, the tumor size, and tumor location, the radical nephrectomy can be performed through an 11th rib flank incision, a transperitoneal midline or subcostal incision, or a transthoracic incision. We have recently employed a supra-11th rib "mini flank incision," which has the advantage of speedy entry into the retroperitoneum and avoidance of the rib resection with subsequent atony of the flank muscles and bulge (Fig. 47A.1). For large tumors with any question of liver, pancreatic, splenic, or IVC extension, optimum exposure with bilateral subcostal (chevron) or thoracoabdominal incision is preferred. In the

retroperitoneal approach to radical nephrectomy, the peritoneum and pleura are dissected off the Gerota fascia, exposing the kidney. In transabdominal approaches to the kidney, the colon, small intestine, liver, pancreas, and spleen (for left-sided tumors) are mobilized, exposing the great vessels and the kidney within the Gerota fascia. For left-sided tumors, splenorenal ligaments are carefully divided and care is taken not to avulse the ligaments from the splenic capsule, which may lead to capsular tear and or subcapsular hematoma. We commonly employ self-retaining retractors to provide maximum exposure with care taken to pad organs prone to iatrogenic injury such as the spleen and pancreas. During the radical nephrectomy, the surgeon gains early control of the renal hilum and ligates and divides the renal artery and then the renal vein (Fig. 47A.2). Approximately 20% of people have multiple renal arteries, leading the surgeon to take care to identify, ligate, and divide any aberrant renal, lumbar, or tumor vessels that may supply the kidney. The classic radical

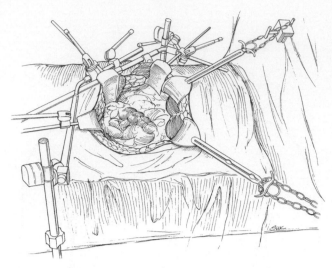

FIGURE 47A.2. Exposures of the operative field obtained by use of the Goligher and Thompson retractors.

nephrectomy is completed with an ipsilateral adrenalectomy and regional lymph node dissection typically skeletonizing the ipsilateral great vessel (vena cava or aorta). A more complete retroperitoneal lymph node dissection is performed if enlarged (hyperplastic or metastatic) lymph nodes are encountered at the time of radical nephrectomy. Although the therapeutic impact of resecting metastatic regional nodes is likely minimal, the finding of metastatic nodes provides important staging information, may intensify follow-up studies, and may make patients eligible for earlier adjuvant therapy protocols (27).

During left radical nephrectomy, the left colon is mobilized along the white line of Toldt and reflected medially. With gentle downward traction on the kidney, the splenic flexure of the colon is also reflected medially (Fig. 47A.3). Splenorenal ligamentous attachments are carefully divided with care taken not

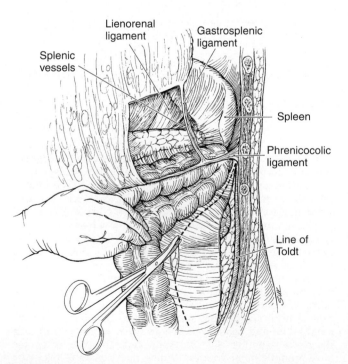

FIGURE 47A.3. Anatomic basis for safe dissection of the splenic flexure of the colon.

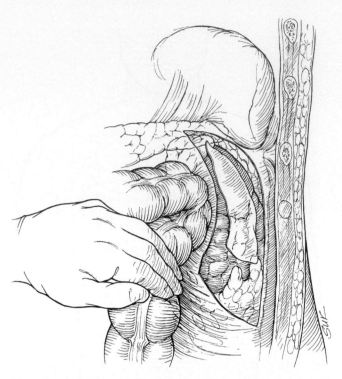

FIGURE 47A.4. Two parallel incisions in the posterior peritoneum, the first in the white line of Toldt and the second just lateral to the colon, leave a strip of peritoneum attached to the tumor when it is removed.

to cause a splenic capsular tear (Fig. 47A.4). Inferiorly, the ureter is identified and divided. The gonadal vessels are identified coursing through the retroperitoneal soft tissues entering the left renal vein, where it is ligated and divided. Next, medial dissection along the aorta is carried out to the level of the renal vein, and a nodal package is dissected off the aorta. At the level of the renal vein, a usually present and sizable lumbar vein is identified, ligated, and divided. With gentle upward traction on the kidney the renal artery is identified beneath the renal vein at its aortic ostium, then ligated, suture ligated, and divided. The arterial decompression that ensues renders the kidney more mobile and deflates any fragile and distended parasitic vessels along the surface of the kidney that often bleed during this mobilization process (Fig. 47A.5). At this point, attention is turned to the superior aspect of the renal vein, where the adrenal vein is identified, ligated, and divided. Once this is done, a vessel loop is carefully placed around the renal vein, and the vein is palpated to determine if there is a clinically occult vein thrombus and to be certain that it too is decompressed. Lack of renal vein decompression indicates an accessory renal artery often emanating from the aorta superior to the level of the renal vein. If the renal vein is ligated before complete arterial decompression, marked venous congestion and hemorrhage from the tumor and parasitic vessels will occur. Once the renal vein is controlled, dissection continues along the aorta, clipping and ligating arterial and venous supply to the adrenal. Care is taken not to traumatize the tail of the pancreas or the splenic vein during this portion of the dissection. Following removal of the kidney and surrounding perinephric soft tissues and adrenal glands, the operative bed is thoroughly irrigated and inspected for any bleeding vessels. The spleen and pancreas are thoroughly reinspected. Drains are not used unless a laceration of the pancreas is suspected or documented.

During right radical nephrectomy, soft tissues lateral to the kidney are incised and, using blunt dissection, the kidney and surrounding perinephric soft tissues are mobilized, exposing

of nodes harvested from the right side is generally less than the paraaortic node dissection. Drains are not used.

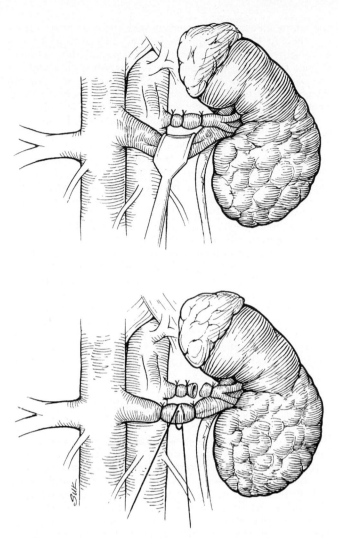

FIGURE 47A.5. Ligation (**A**) and transection (**B**) of the left renal artery and vein.

RADICAL NEPHRECTOMY: INTERPRETATION OF CONTEMPORARY RESULTS

The contemporary results of the surgical resection of renal cortical tumors as a treatment of renal cortical tumors must now be interpreted in the current context of the tumor stage and size migration induced by modern imaging devices and described using the most recent tumor histologic classification and our current knowledge of tumor histology and the prognosis inferred by mode of presentation (incidental, local, systemic), P-stage, tumor size, and tumor histologic subtype (chromophobe, papillary, conventional clear cell) (28). In addition, evaluation of surgical results relative to perioperative perimeters should be described in a contemporary and not a historical light because improvements in perioperative care and use of clinical pathways has improved the rates postoperative recovery and decreased hospital length of stay (LOS). In a series from our institution of 688 radical nephrectomies performed between 1995 and 2002, mean operative time was 3.3 hours, mean hospital LOS was 6.2 days, median estimated blood loss was 300 mL, and mean number of units of blood transfused was 0.4, with 15% of patients requiring a transfusion of either autologous or nonautologous blood (29). Depending on the combination of clinical and pathologic factors, the complete resection of clinically localized tumors can lead to 5-year survival rates of 70% to 98%. The presence of metastatic regional lymph nodes, metastatic involvement of the adrenal, adjacent organ invasion, or distant metastatic disease all confer equally poor prognosis with 5-year survival rates in the range of 5% to 15% (30). Contemporary articles describing new methods or techniques to treat renal cortical tumors (e.g., minimally invasive surgery) must describe their results in contemporary terms if meaningful comparisons between treatment approaches are to be made (31).

SURGICAL COMPLICATIONS

In a recent review of 688 radical nephrectomies performed at MSKCC between 1995 and 2002, 112 patients (16%) experienced a perioperative complication (29). Complications were graded using a five-tiered scale based on the severity of impact or the intensity of treatment required to address the complication (32). There were 21 (3%) complications that were directly attributed to the procedure (procedure-related), including three patients with acute renal failure, one patient with a retroperitoneal hemorrhage, seven patients with an adjacent organ injury, four patients with a bowel obstruction, and six patients with a pneumothorax. Four patients required surgical reexploration, three for decompression of bowel obstruction, and one for delayed splenic rupture (grade 4, N = 3). There were three postoperative deaths (grade 5), two due to myocardial infarction and one due to pulmonary embolism. The remainder of the complications were grade 1 to 3 and were managed by oral medication or bedside care (grade 1, N = 78), intravenous therapy or thoracostomy tube (grade 2, N = 43), or intubation, interventional radiology, endoscopy, or reoperation (grade 3, N = 11). The grading scale employed correlated with mean hospital LOS as follows: no complications, 5.2 days; grade 1 complications, 6.8 days; grade 2 complications, 7.4 days; and grade 3 to 5 complications, 9.3 days. We have found that grading complications provides an effective means of describing the severity of complications and feel that this method

the psoas muscle. First the right colon and then the duodenum are mobilized medially (Kocher maneuver), exposing the IVC. Inferiorly, the ureter is identified, ligated, and divided. The dissection then proceeds along the lateral aspect of the IVC to the level of the renal vein. On the right side, the gonadal vein drains directly into the vena cava, and its division is usually not required. With upward traction on the kidney, the renal artery can be identified coursing beneath the vena cava. For large tumors obscuring the vena cava, dissection between the aorta and vena cava (interaortacaval) can identify the right renal artery and its origin. Decompression of the kidney following arterial ligation allows for more mobility as the nephrectomy is completely mobilized along the paracolic gutter. Superiorly, retroperitoneal attachments to the liver are incised with care taken not to exert too much traction, leading to a tear in the liver capsule. The renal vein is isolated with a vessel loop, and dissection proceeds superiorly along the vena cava, ligating and dividing short adrenal attachments to the vena cava. Care must be taken not to exert too much traction on the adrenal, leading to an avulsion of short adrenal veins and extremely troublesome bleeding from the vena cava as it travels beneath the right lobe of the liver. Following the final ligation and division of the renal vein, the specimen is delivered and the operative bed is thoroughly irrigated and inspected for any bleeding. A pericaval and precaval lymph node dissection (regional) is performed, although the number

should be also used for describing complications in developing alternative surgical treatments of renal cortical tumors (i.e., laparoscopic or percutaneous ablative treatments).

FOLLOW-UP STRATEGIES FOLLOWING RADICAL NEPHRECTOMY

No uniform guidelines have been established for the follow-up of patients who have undergone surgical treatment of RCC. Despite emerging evidence that some patients can benefit from aggressive surgical treatment of limited metastatic disease, different practices exist among urologic surgeons regarding the search for and management of recurrent disease. The intensity of follow-up and the tests ordered during follow-up also vary among centers (32,33). In the absence of effective systemic therapy for metastatic disease, overly compulsive follow-up may diagnose asymptomatic metastatic disease earlier but not necessarily provide a therapeutic advantage. Excessive costs and patient anxiety may also occur unnecessarily during this follow-up. In addition, emerging evidence that radical nephrectomy can have a deleterious impact on renal function (20,21) requires strict surveillance over renal function as well surveillance over the contralateral kidney that has a small but real chance of developing an asynchronous renal cortical tumor (22).

Follow-up strategies were proposed from a nephrectomy series by Sandock et al. after a detailed analysis of the pattern of metastatic disease progression, sites of metastatic failure, and the efficacy of tests required to diagnose recurrence (34). These investigators reviewed 137 patients with node-negative, nonmetastatic RCC who underwent radical nephrectomy between 1979 and 1993 at the Case Western affiliated hospitals. Recurrence correlated closely with the clinical stage of the tumor at the time of diagnosis. Using the older American Joint Committee on Cancer (AJCC) classification (T1 <2.5 cm), no patients with T1 disease relapsed, 15% of patients with T2 relapsed, and 53% of patients with T3 tumors relapsed. Of the 19 patients in whom pulmonary metastases developed, 14 (74%) had cough, dyspnea, pleuritic chest pain, or hemoptysis. In all patients with pulmonary metastases, the metastatic disease was diagnosed by a plain chest x-ray. Of the 13 patients in this series who developed intraabdominal metastatic disease, 12 (92%) complained of abdominal symptoms or had abnormal liver function studies that led to the diagnosis. All 10 patients who developed bone metastases complained of new bone pain that directed the diagnosis by plain film and bone scan. Only one patient had an isolated brain metastasis, which was associated with central nervous system (CNS) symptoms and was confirmed by brain CT scan. Two patients developed cutaneous metastases that were detected on physical examination. In this series, 85% of patients who experienced a recurrence of their disease did so during the first 3 years after nephrectomy; the remaining relapses occurred between 3.4 and 11.4 years.

Levy et al. from M.D. Anderson Cancer Center tracked the pattern of recurrence in 286 patients with P1-3N0 or Nx RCC operated upon between 1985 and 1995. Perhaps reflecting the previously described stage migration that has occurred in RCC over the last 10 years, 59 of 92 (62%) patients diagnosed with metastatic disease were asymptomatic, including 32 detected by routine chest x-ray and 12 detected by routine blood work. Isolated asymptomatic intraabdominal metastases were diagnosed by surveillance CT scan in only 6 patients (9%) (35). As in the Sandock study, as the P-stage increased the likelihood of recurrence increased from 7% for P1, 27% for P2, and 39% for P3, leading the authors to conclude that a stage-specific surveillance protocol would tailor the follow-up evaluation intensity with the relative risk of recurrence. At MSKCC, we have incorporated the tumor histologic subtype, tumor size, and mode of presentation with the P-stage to create a postoperative nomogram (23). Following the postoperative recovery, we generally see P1 (<7 cm) and P2 nonclear cell histology (papillary, chromophobe) patients back every 6 months with renal function studies and yearly with an imaging study of the remaining kidney (CT scan or ultrasonography (USG)), chest x-ray, and renal function studies for a total of 3 years, and then a yearly visit usually with CT scan of the chest, abdomen, and pelvis or renal ultrasound and chest x-ray. For tumors above P2 (P3a–c, P4) particularly with conventional clear cell histology, we perform biannual chest x-ray and annual CT scan of the chest, abdomen, and pelvis coupled with renal function studies at each visit. Routine brain or bone scans are not performed unless the patient reports symptoms referable to those sites. RCC is notorious for unusual, late, symptomatic, metastatic recurrences in organs such as the pancreas, thyroid, skin, duodenum, and adrenal glands. These recurrences are often mistaken for new primary tumors, and aggressive surgical resection is undertaken and can be associated with long-term survival depending on the patient age, the number of sites of metastases, and disease-free interval (36). Whether such metastectomy procedures are truly therapeutic or patient survival is within the confines of the often long and unpredictable natural history of RCC is not known.

CONCLUSION

The last decade has brought an immense expansion in our knowledge of renal cortical tumors that has inspired changing surgical strategies. These tumors are now recognized to be a family of neoplasms with distinct histopathologic and cytogenetic features and variable metastatic potential. Approximately 70% of patients with operable tumors today are detected incidentally during abdominal or musculoskeletal imaging, leading to a tumor stage and size migration. New concerns for the overall renal health of a patient otherwise likely destined to do well following tumor resection as well as the small but real possibility of a contralateral tumor has led to an expansion of kidney-sparing operations.

Radical nephrectomy remains a critical tool in the treatment of renal cortical tumors. Patients with large tumors not amenable to partial nephrectomy or associated with regional adenopathy or renal vein or vena caval extension should undergo radical nephrectomy. Although commonly performed with radical nephrectomy, the role for regional lymph node dissection or ipsilateral adrenalectomy is likely limited to pathologic staging because metastatic disease in those sites portends a prognosis as poor as overtly metastatic disease. Open radical nephrectomy is associated with low rates of procedure-related morbidity, major perioperative complications, and death. Patient follow-up strategies should be tailored with knowledge of tumor histology, mode of presentation, tumor size and stage, and with increasing intensity for large conventional clear cell tumors.

References

1. Beare JB, McDonald JR. Involvement of renal capsule in surgically removed hypernephroma: gross and histopathological study. *J Urol* 1949;61: 857–861.
2. Mortensen H. Transthoracic nephrectomy. *J Urol* 1948;60:855.
3. Robson CJ. Radical nephrectomy for renal cell carcinoma. *J Urol* 1963; 89:37.
4. Robson CJ, Churchill BM, Andersen W. The results of radical nephrectomy for renal cell carcinoma. *J Urol* 1969;101:297.

5. Skinner DG, Colvin RB, Vermillion CD, et al. Diagnosis and management of renal cell carcinoma: a clinical and pathological study of 309 cases. *Cancer* 1971;28:1165–1177.

6. Patel NP, Lavengood RW. Renal cell carcinoma: natural history and results of treatment. *J Urol* 1978;119:722.

7. Sagalowsky AI, Kadesky KT, Ewalt DM, et al. Factors influencing adrenal metastases in renal cell carcinoma. *J Urol* 1994;151:1181–1184.

8. Herrlinger JA, Schrott KM, Schott G, et al. What are the benefits of extended dissection of the regional lymph nodes in the therapy of renal cell carcinoma. *J Urol* 1991;146:1224.

9. Ditonno P, Traficante A, Battaglia M, et al. Role of lymphadenectomy in renal cell carcinoma. *Prog Clin Biol Res* 1992;378:169.

10. Robson CJ. Results of radical thoraco-abdominal nephrectomy in the treatment of renal cell carcinoma. *Proc Clin Biol Res* 1982;100:481–488.

11. Jemal A, Murray T, Samuels A, et al. Cancer statistics 2003. *CA Cancer J Clin* 2003;53:5–43.

12. Pantuck AJ, Zisman A, Belldegrun AS. The changing natural history of renal cell carcinoma. *J Urol* 2001;166:1611–1623.

13. Kovacs G, Akhtar M, Beckwith BJ, et al. The Heidelberg classification of renal cell tumours. *J Pathol* 1997;183:131–133.

14. Zambrano NR, Lubensky IA, Merino MJ, et al. Histolopathology and molecular genetics of renal tumors toward unification of a classification system. *J Urol* 1999;162:1246–1258.

15. Linehan WM, Lerman MI, Zbar B. Identification of the von Hippel-Lindau (VHL) gene. Its role in renal cancer. *JAMA* 1995;273:564–570.

16. Gnarra JR, Glenn GM, Latif F, et al. Molecular genetic studies of sporadic and familial renal cell carcinoma. *Urol Clin North Am* 1993;20:207–216.

17. McKiernan JM, Yossepowitch O, Kattan MW, et al. Partial nephrectomy for renal cortical tumors: pathological findings and impact on outcome. *Urology* 2002;60:1003–1009.

18. Russo P. Renal cell carcinoma: presentation, staging, and surgical treatment. *Semin Oncol* 2000;27:160–176.

19. Rabbani F, Grimaldi G, Russo P. Multiple primary malignancies in renal cell carcinoma. *J Urol* 1998;160:1255–1259.

20. Lau WK, Blute ML, Weaver AL, et al. Matched comparison of radical nephrectomy vs. nephron-sparing surgery in patients with unilateral renal cell carcinoma and a normal contralateral kidney. *Mayo Clin Proc* 2000;75:1236–1242.

21. McKiernan J, Simmons R, Katz J, et al. Natural history of chronic renal insufficiency after partial and radical nephrectomy. *Urology* 2002;59:816–820.

22. Patel MI, Simmons R, Kattan MW, et al. Long term follow up of bilateral sporadic renal tumors. *Urology* 2003;61:921–925.

23. Kattan MW, Reuter VE, Motzer RJ, et al. A postoperative prognostic nomogram for renal cell carcinoma. *J Urol* 2001;166:63.

24. Lee CT, Katz J, Shi W, et al. Surgical management of renal tumors 4 cm or less in a contemporary cohort. *J Urol* 2000;163:730–736.

25. Russo P, Goetzl M, Simmons R, et al. Partial nephrectomy: the rationale for expanding the indications. *Ann Surg Oncol* 2002;9:680–687.

26. Flanigan RC, Salmon SE, Blumenstein BA, et al. Nephrectomy followed by interferon alfa-2b compared with interferon alfa-2b alone for metastatic renal-cell cancer. *N Engl J Med* 2001;23:1655–1659.

27. Vasselli JR, Yang JC, Linehan WM, et al. Lack of retroperitoneal lymphadenopathy predicts survival of patients with metastatic renal cell carcinoma. *J Urol* 2001;166:68.

28. Russo P, Snyder ME, DiBlasio CJ, et al. Changing demographics and the contemporary surgical management of renal cortical tumors. *J Urol* 2003;169:346A.

29. Stephenson AJ, Hakimi A, Snyder ME, et al. Complications of radical and partial nephrectomy in a large contemporary cohort based on a five-tiered complications grading scale. *J Urol* 2003;171:130–134.

30. Patel MI, Beck S, Simmons R, et al. Adrenal and nodal status are indicators of metastatic disease. Time to change the TNM classification for kidney cancer. *J Urol* 2003;169:1A.

31. Russo P. Laparoscopic radical nephrectomy: cancer control for renal cell carcinoma. *J Urol* 2002;168:1109.

32. Martin RC, Brennan MF, Jaques DP. Quality of complication reporting in the surgical literature. *Ann Surg* 2002;235:803.

33. Montie JE. Follow-up after partial or total nephrectomy for renal cell carcinoma. *Urol Clin North Am* 1994;21:589.

34. Sandock DS, Seftel AD, Resnick MI. A new protocol for the follow-up of renal cell carcinoma based on pathological stage. *J Urol* 1995;154:28–31.

35. Levy DA, Slaton JW, Swanson DA, et al. Stage specific guidelines for surveillance after radical nephrectomy for local renal cell carcinoma. *J Urol* 1998;159:1163–1167.

36. Kavolius JP, Mastorakos DP, Pavolvich C, et al. Resection of metastatic renal cell carcinoma. *J Clin Oncol* 1998;16:2261.

CHAPTER 47B
Laparoscopic Radical Nephrectomy

Isaac Yi Kim and Ralph V. Clayman

INTRODUCTION

The first laparoscopic nephrectomy was performed at Washington University, St. Louis, Missouri, in 1990 (1). The procedure was carried out in an 85-year-old woman with a 3-cm solid renal mass. Using five ports, the specimen was removed by morcellation after 6 hours and 45 minutes in the operating room. The final diagnosis was oncocytoma. Since then, laparoscopic radical nephrectomy for renal cell carcinoma (RCC) has become widely accepted by the urologic community. The technique itself has evolved into three categories—a pure transperitoneal laparoscopic procedure, a hand-assisted laparoscopic procedure, and a retroperitoneal procedure. In this chapter, these three basic approaches of laparoscopic radical nephrectomy are described, followed by a discussion on benefits, effectiveness, efficiency, and complications.

INDICATIONS AND CONTRAINDICATIONS

Laparoscopic radical nephrectomy is classically indicated for T1–T2 tumors with size less than 10 cm. However, the procedure has been completed successfully in tumors ranging in size from 12 to 18 cm and in T3a disease as long as the size of the tumor permits a safe completion of the surgery. In addition, laparoscopic radical nephrectomy has been used to treat T3b tumors with renal vein involvement and rarely for tumors just barely extending into the inferior vena cava (2). Laparoscopic radical nephrectomy is contraindicated in tumors with large, localized vena caval thrombi or those in which the thrombus extends to the level of the hepatic veins or higher. Likewise, laparoscopic radical nephrectomy is also contraindicated among patients with extensive nodal involvement. Relative contraindications include prior history of ipsilateral renal surgery, multiple abdominal procedures, and perinephric inflammation. The general *caveat*s for laparoscopy, such as severe chronic obstructive pulmonary disease and morbid obesity, also apply.

PREOPERATIVE EVALUATION AND PREPARATION

Preoperative evaluation and patient preparation for laparoscopic radical nephrectomy are the same as those for open radical nephrectomy. Routine laboratory tests include complete blood count; serum electrolytes, blood; urea; nitrogen, creatinine, calcium levels; basic liver function tests; and urinalysis. Urine culture and sensitivity should be performed selectively on the basis of the result of the urinalysis. In patients with a history of a bleeding diathesis, a coagulation profile is obtained. Type and screen for blood products must be done, although autologous or cross-matched blood products can be made available in select cases on the basis of the surgeon's experience and the patient's preference. In addition to being NPO (*nulla per os*, Latin for "nothing by mouth") after midnight, many laparoscopic surgeons recommend that a patient adhere to a clear-liquid diet and take a laxative (e.g., Dulcolax suppository, Dulcolax tablets, or half a bottle of magnesium citrate) the day prior to the procedure in order to empty the bowels as much as possible. A complete mechanical and antibiotic bowel preparation should be considered only in patients with a history of extensive abdominal surgery.

Recommended preoperative imaging studies include chest radiograph or chest computed tomography (CT) scan and abdominal CT scan. Bone scan should be performed if patients have symptomatic bone pain or elevation of serum calcium or alkaline phosphatase. A head CT scan is performed only in the rare case of neurologic findings. Magnetic resonance imaging (MRI), sonogram, or three-dimensional reconstruction CT scan should be sufficient to delineate the renal vascular supply and to assess for renal vein or vena caval thrombi. The function of the contralateral kidney should be assessed with abdominal CT scan with contrast and serum creatinine. If the function of the contralateral kidney is uncertain, 24-hour urine collection and a renal scan may be necessary.

SURGICAL APPROACHES

Table 47B.1 shows the results comparing standard laparoscopy, hand-assisted laparoscopy, and retroperitoneoscopy. Transperitoneal laparoscopic radical nephrectomy is the most widely used approach because it optimizes movements of instruments by offering a wide working space and providing maximum distance between working ports. This approach is most useful when the specimen size is large and entrapment is desired before removal. The advantages of the transperitoneal approach are most obvious in standard laparoscopic cases where specimen entrapment with tissue morcellation is used to minimize the incision length. The main disadvantage of the standard transperitoneal laparoscopic radical nephrectomy is the longer operative time (up to 56 minutes longer) compared to the retroperitoneal and hand-assisted approaches (3). In circumstances where the plan is to remove the specimen intact, some authors have argued that either a hand-assisted transperitoneal or a retroperitoneal approach is more practical; however, with the latter, specimen entrapment before removal is more difficult.

In hand-assisted laparoscopic radical nephrectomy, an incision large enough to accommodate the surgeon's hand (usually 7 to 8 cm) is required. The hand-assist devices have acted as a bridge between open and purely laparoscopic surgery for the novice laparoscopic surgeon and have in most circumstances reduced operating room time compared to standard or even retroperitoneal laparoscopic approaches (3,7,8). Major disadvantages of the hand-assisted approach include hand fatigue, difficult placements of working ports in small patients, larger incisional scar, and increased frequency of wound complications (9,10). Nevertheless, comparison with the standard laparoscopic approach has demonstrated that the use of the larger incision for the hand-port does not meaningfully increase the postoperative convalescence time (3,7,8,11). Currently, there are six types of commercially available hand-ports. Although each device has its own merits, a recent study by Stifelman et al. reported that novice laparoscopists perceived little difference among the three most commonly used hand-ports (12). In general, a device that self-coapts is preferred because it allows the surgeon to use either hand, eliminates the use of cuffs or sleeves, and provides rapid entry and exit.

The retroperitoneoscopic radical nephrectomy avoids the peritoneal cavity and therefore the need to mobilize the colon and the surrounding organs in gaining access to the kidney. Another advantage of this approach is that the renal artery is encountered early during the procedure. Operative times have been reported to be faster than the standard transperitoneal approach by as much as 30% (13), although hospital stay and convalescence are similar. Retroperitoneal radical nephrectomy is the surgical approach of choice in patients who need peritoneal dialysis or have a history of multiple abdominal procedures. The main disadvantage of the retroperitoneal approach is the small working space that largely precludes specimen entrapment and morcellation. As a result, the specimen is removed either transvaginally or with a muscle-splitting flank or a Pfannenstiel incision (14,15). Also, most of these specimens are removed without first being entrapped in an impermeable sack; this practice risks possible wound contamination as the specimen is manipulated and pulled through a "tight" skin incision (16).

TABLE 47B.1

COMPARISON OF OPERATIVE RESULTS AMONG STANDARD TRANSPERITONEAL LAPAROSCOPY, HAND-ASSISTED TRANSPERITONEAL LAPAROSCOPY, AND RETROPERITONEOSCOPY

	Transperitoneal laparoscopy	Hand-assisted transperitoneal llaparoscopy	Retroperitoneoscopy
Patients	$16^b/43^c$	$12^a/22^b$	$12^a/45^c$
OR time (hr)	$4.5^b/3.4^c$	$4.0^a/3.4^b$	$4.3^a/2.6^c$
EBL (mL)	$289^b/190^c$	$293^a/191^b$	$142^a/233^c$
Mean morphine sulfate equivalent (mg)	$30^b/26^c$	$35.7^a/31^b$	$24.5^a/21^c$
Hospital stay	$2.4^b/1.7^c$	$4.4^a/2.7^b$	$3.6^a/1.6^c$
Convalescence		$75\%^a$ (at 2 wk)	$77\%^a$ (at 2 wk)
Complications (major)	$13\%^b/16\%^c$	$8\%^a/23\%^b$	$8\%^a/12\%^c$
Complications (minor)	$45\%^b/12\%^c$	$25\%^b$	$4\%^c$

OR, operation room; EBL, estimated blood loss.
[a] Batler RA, Campbell SC, Funk JT, et al. Hand-assisted vs. retroperitoneal laparoscopic nephrectomy. *J Endourol* 2001;15:899–902.
[b] From Nelson CP, Wolf JS. Comparison of hand-assisted versus standard laparoscopic radical nephrectomy for suspected renal cell carcinoma. *J Urol* 2002;167:1989–1994.
[c] From Gill I, Strzempkowski B, Kaouk J, et al. Prospective randomized comparison: transperitoneal vs retroperitoneal laparoscopic radical nephrectomy. *J Urol* 2002;167:19, Abstract 78.

Transperitoneal Standard Laparoscopic Total/Radical Nephrectomy

Patient Positioning and Trocar Placement

In the operating room, two monitors are required. The primary monitor should be placed on the patient's ipsilateral side at the chest level while the surgeon and the assistant stand on the patient's contralateral side. After general anesthesia is induced, either a nasogastric or an orogastric tube and Foley catheter are placed. Subsequently, the patient is placed in a modified flank position with approximately 30- to 50-degree elevation of the ipsilateral side. It is helpful to use gel pads on the table to cushion the patient; in our experience, these provide far better distribution of pressure than foam (e.g., "egg crate") or a bean bag. A gel pad that literally extends the length of the table is recommended. The posterior iliac crest should overlie the kidney rest, and arms should be flexed either in a prayer position or outstretched on an arm rest (contralateral arm) and a parallel elevated arm rest (ipsilateral arm). Next, all potential pressure points, including ipsilateral arm, contralateral elbow, both legs, and ankles, are further padded. The patient should have an axillary role for the brachial plexus. Subsequently, the table is flexed 30 to 45 degrees to provide additional working space between the ipsilateral costal margin and iliac crest; the kidney rest may be raised, but if this is done, it is recommended that it be reduced to its resting position after approximately 2 hours in order to reduce any prolonged pressure on the muscles of the contralateral hip and buttock. Once the patient is positioned appropriately, wide tape for security should be placed over the ipsilateral leg, hip, and shoulder, with padding placed between the tape and any pressure point (e.g., elbow and knee). Before starting the procedure, rotate the bed to ensure that the patient is completely secured. The nursing staff should scrub and drape the patient from nipple to pubis and from contralateral rectus to the paraspinous muscles.

For peritoneal insufflation, the Veress needle can be inserted in the lower abdominal quadrant 2 finger breadths above and 3 to 4 finger breadths medial to the superior iliac crest. Alternative sites include the umbilicus (with the patient rolled almost flat) or the midclavicular line subcostal. When the site for needle placement is selected, it is helpful to make a 10- to 12-mm incision, spread the fat, and grasp the anterior abdominal wall fascia with an Allis clamp to stabilize the abdominal wall during needle passage. Once the needle is placed, it must be confirmed that the tip of the needle is in the peritoneal cavity by sequentially aspirating and injecting 1 to 2 cc of normal saline without any return of blood or bowel contents; the remaining portion of the fluid in the bevel of the needle should drop readily into the abdominal cavity. After connecting the carbon dioxide insufflation tubing to the Veress needle and instilling 1 L of carbon dioxide at low pressure (i.e., <15 mm Hg), the insufflation pressure is raised to 20 to 25 mm Hg. Once this level is reached, the initial blunt-tipped trocar may be placed; bladed trocars are no longer used in our operating rooms. The blunt-tipped trocar, when it is of the 10- or 12-mm size, is affixed to a zero-degree laparoscope so that the advance of the trocar into the peritoneal cavity can be endoscopically monitored. Alternatively, initial access to the peritoneal cavity can be obtained using the Hasson open technique (17). Although some surgeons have suggested that the rate of complication of the closed access technique described herein is significantly higher than the Hasson approach (18), a more recently published study by Merlin et al. demonstrated no significant difference between the two access techniques (19).

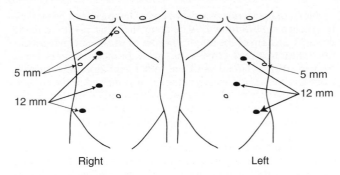

FIGURE 47B.1. Port placements for transperitoneal "standard" laparoscopic radical nephrectomy.

Figure 47B.1 shows the recommended port placements for a transperitoneal laparoscopic radical nephrectomy. Although three ports are usually sufficient to complete the procedure, a fourth port is often used for specimen entrapment and/or retraction. The first trocar, usually 12 mm, is placed at the site of insufflation in the lower abdomen off the iliac crest area, in the subcostal midclavicular line, or at the umbilicus using endoscopic visualization (e.g., Optiview, Ethicon Endo-Surgery, Cincinnati, OH). Once the first port is placed successfully in the lower abdomen, the abdominal pressure is decreased to 15 mm Hg. The second trocar is placed in the midclavicular line 2 to 3 finger breadths above the umbilicus, and the third port is usually placed subcostal in the midclavicular line; both the second and third ports should be 12 mm. If necessary, the accessory 5-mm fourth port is placed at the anterior axillary line below the costal margin. On the right side, a 5-mm fifth port may be placed, midline below the xiphoid process for a right nephrectomy to aid with retraction of the liver. The midclavicular line supraumbilical port should be used for the camera, and the remaining two 12-mm ports should be used by the surgeon.

Procedure

The approach to the kidney depends upon whether the right or left kidney is to be removed. Laparoscopic right radical nephrectomy is first started by incising the line of Toldt from the level of the right common iliac artery to the lower pole of the kidney; this line of dissection is then carried cephalad alongside the kidney to the level of the diaphragm. In doing this, the triangular ligament of the liver is also divided. The surgeon must be cognizant that the right colon lies medial to the anterolateral renal surface and below the upper pole of the right kidney. Therefore, only the colon should be mobilized, and the peritoneum over the lateral and upper pole is left intact. To completely mobilize the ascending colon, the surgeon "T"s off the cephalocaudal incision at the level of the lower pole of the kidney approximately 2 to 3 cm above the colon; the peritoneal reflection on the kidney is thereby incised along the medial border of the kidney, thereby freeing the colon so it can be moved medially and caudal. After mobilizing the ascending colon, the duodenum can be identified and mobilized medially (Kocher maneuver) to expose the inferior vena cava clearly. The anterior surface of the inferior vena cava can then be dissected cephalad, thereby exposing the renal vein and the adrenal vein; it can then be dissected caudal, revealing the right gonadal vein, which can be secured with a pair of clips or a bipolar device, and divided. The ureter lies just lateral and posterior to the gonadal vein and can be dissected and secured at this time. It is our practice to divide the ureter at the very end of the procedure so it can serve as a "handle" to facilitate specimen entrapment.

Next, the posterior coronary hepatic ligament can be incised. If a radical nephrectomy is to be done, then this incision is made within 1 to 2 cm of the inferior border of the liver. Having identified the inferior vena cava in this area, the incision can be made from medial to lateral until the initial cephalocaudal incision from iliac vessels to the diaphragm is encountered. If the adrenal is to be spared, then the surgeon makes a lateral incision in the posterior coronary hepatic ligament in order to enter the Gerota fascia and identify the upper pole of the kidney. Dissection continues cephalad and medial along the upper pole, thereby separating the adrenal gland cephalad from the renal surface.

This dissection of the right kidney creates a "wedge" around the kidney; the edge of the wedge is positioned lateral; it is formed by the initial cephalocaudal incision from the iliac vessels to the diaphragm, incorporating the lowermost portion of the line of Toldt, the retroperitoneum along the lateral border of the kidney, and the hepatic triangular ligament. The sides of the wedge are the incisions to mobilize the colon off the lower pole of the kidney and the incision in the posterior coronary hepatic ligament. The broad, medially directed surface of the wedge consists of the three planes of dissection: mobilization of the colon along the medial border of the kidney, reflection of the duodenum, and dissection of the anterior surface of the inferior vena cava.

For a left radical nephrectomy, the line of Toldt is incised from the left common iliac artery to the splenic flexure; this incision is continued cephalad in order to also divide the splenophrenic attachments, thereby releasing the spleen laterally. Unlike the right kidney, the entire anterior surface of the left kidney is covered by the descending colon so that little or no peritoneum is left on the specimen. To permit a satisfactory mobilization of the descending colon, the incision should be carried medially around the splenic flexure and the splenocolic, and, if possible, the deeper-lying splenorenal ligaments are divided completely. Often, the latter is divided more completely at the end of the procedure after the hilar dissection has been completed. Next, the mesentery of the descending colon and the splenic flexure are dissected from the Gerota fascia, and the entire descending colon is thereby moved medially; in doing this, it is important for the surgeon to clearly identify the colonic mesentery and avoid "buttonholing," which may result in a mesenteric hematoma.

Once the colon is mobilized medially, the midureter is located in the retroperitoneal fat medial to the psoas muscle. Typically the gonadal vein, lying more superficial than the ureter, is encountered first. The gonadal vein should be gently elevated and the dissection carried cephalad toward the hilum. By following the gonadal vein cephalad, its juncture with the main renal vein can be clearly seen. All tissues, including the medial extension of the Gerota fascia, lying directly anterior (i.e., overlying) to the gonadal and renal vein, can be incised. The gonadal vein is divided followed by dissection and division of the ascending lumbar vein. The ascending lumbar vein may be absent; however, this vein has a tremendous variability and may be found inserting into the gonadal vein, the posterior surface of the renal vein lateral to the gonadal vein, or the renal vein medial to the gonadal vein. Once the inferior surface of the renal vein is cleared, then attention is turned to the superior surface of the left renal vein. The adrenal vein, usually lying directly cephalad to or just medial to the insertion of the gonadal vein, is dissected and secured. Once the renal vein is freed, it can be manipulated to aid in the subsequent identification and dissection of the left renal artery. When dissecting the hilum, particularly the renal artery, it is helpful to divide the dense lymphatic and neural tissues with a fine electrosurgical instrumentation (e.g., a hook electrode) or the ultrasonic shears rather than using surgical clips; clips are associated with a failure of the endovascular stapler when it is fired across the renal vein later in the case (20).

If during this part of the dissection, the surgeon sees the "renal" artery before clearly dissecting the renal vein, there is a strong possibility that this "renal" artery is in actuality the superior mesenteric artery. The renal artery is invariably located behind the renal vein; any other arrangement must raise the suspicion in the surgeon's mind that what is being dissected is either a superior mesenteric artery or an artery within the colonic mesentery. Similarly, if arteries are seen that appear to be running cephalocaudal, the surgeon may well have entered into the colonic mesentery and needs to move more laterally and find the true plane between the colonic mesentery and Gerota fascia.

This dissection of the left kidney in essence forms an inverted cone or "water scooper" that encompasses the specimen. The long limb of the water scooper is the initial incision in the line of Toldt carried upward to include the lienophrenic attachments. The medial edge of the cone is the dissection of the colonic mesentery from the Gerota fascia. The opening in the cone is formed anteriorly by the incision in the lienocolic ligament, and the posterior opening in the cone is formed by the splenorenal ligament.

In general, the remainder of the procedure is similar for both the right and left kidney. Once the renal vein is dissected adequately, the renal artery is identified and controlled with either an endovascular stapler or endoclips; for the former, 2-mm size staples are recommended because there have been two case reports of bleeding through a splenic artery stump when 2.5-mm staples were used (21). If clips are used, five large metal clips or three Hemolok clips should be placed on the artery; the artery should be divided such that a 1-mm cuff is left on the stump, which should also have either three metal or two Hemolok clips remaining. Once the renal artery has been divided, the renal vein is transected with an endovascular stapler. As stated earlier, the surgeon must ensure that no clip lies within the jaws of the endovascular stapler, or else it may misfire (20). In cases where the renal artery cannot be dissected safely from the renal vein, the hilar vessels may be controlled *en bloc* with a single endovascular stapler rather than converting to an open procedure. However, these patients should be followed closely postoperatively because of the theoretical risk of arteriovenous fistula formation (22).

Once the hilum is controlled, the dissection should be carried to the upper and lateral renal attachments. The decision to spare or remove the adrenal gland will dictate the superior margin of dissection. To spare the ipsilateral adrenal gland, the Gerota fascia should be entered to separate the adrenal gland from the upper pole; on the right side, the adrenal vein is spared, whereas on the left side it is divided. To remove the right adrenal gland *en bloc*, the surgeon should dissect along the vena cava to identify the adrenal vein on the right side. This right adrenal vein is short, and usually only three clips can be placed (i.e., two are left on the stump side); alternatively, it can be divided with the 10-mm Ligasure device. As previously stated, the left adrenal vein is always divided during the dissection. Once the adrenal vein is controlled, the adrenal attachments should be divided superiorly, medially, and posteriorly. Because the adrenal gland often has accessory vessels, the surgeon should clip or coagulate all tissues in this area; for this purpose, the harmonic shears or bipolar feedback instrumentations work well. During the dissection of the left adrenal gland medially and posteriorly, the splenic hilum and the tail of pancreas must not be injured. Once the upper pole of the kidney is mobilized, the kidney is then completely dissected from the retroperitoneum; next, the ureter is divided between clips or with the harmonic shears or the bipolar device.

The specimen should be entrapped in an impermeable bag. If intact removal is planned, then the 15-mm Endocatch bag (US Surgical Norwalk, Connecticut) can be substituted for one of the 12-mm ports. This bag consists of a plastic sack attached to a self-opening, flexible metal ring; this design allows the specimen to be easily manipulated into the opening of the bag. Usually, the skin incision for the 12-mm port does not have to be widened to pass this 15-mm device; the port is removed, and the 15-mm device is passed through the skin incision and endoscopically guided into the abdominal cavity. Using the ureter as a "handle," the surgeon can suspend the kidney onto the surface of the liver (right nephrectomy) or spleen (left nephrectomy). This is done by securing the ureter with a locking grasping forceps passed via the lateralmost cephalad port; a retractor can be used via a lower port site to help elevate the specimen onto the anterior surface of the ipsilateral organ. The plastic sack is then opened just below the edge of the liver or spleen; the specimen is then moved into the sack with the grasper that is affixed to the ureter. The device is closed and the drawstring is cut. Now, via a 7- to 8-cm incision, the intact specimen can be removed.

Alternatively, the specimen can be morcellated; it has been demonstrated that this does not alter patient treatment decisions after laparoscopic radical nephrectomies (23). To morcellate in the plastic sack, a 4-cm incision is made, and the neck of the sack is triply draped (e.g., towel drape, sticky drape, and nephrostomy drape). Through this 3- to 4-cm incision, the specimen can be delivered piecemeal from the entrapment sack using a ring forceps under direct vision. This entire maneuver is done under direct visual control because the morcellation process must be done above the abdominal wall.

If the surgeon wishes to morcellate the specimen as originally described, then an 8- by 10-inch LapSac (Cook Urological Spencer, Indiana) is passed via a bare 12-mm port site; the LapSac is a double layer of plastic and nondistensible nylon that is impermeable to bacteria and cells (24). Prior to its passage, the neck of the sack is twice looped with a nitinol guidewire by passing the tip of the guidewire in and out of every other hole through which the drawstring has been passed. As such, when the sack is passed into the abdomen via the uppermost medial 12-mm port site, the mouth of the sack springs open within the abdomen. The original 12-mm port is replaced. With the mouth of the sack open, the rest of the sack is bluntly unfurled using atraumatic graspers. Now the laparoscope is moved to the upper medial 12-mm port, where it is used to further open the sack by passing it deep into the sack. The upper and lower edge of the sack is secured with two or, if necessary, three separate grasping forceps; the third forceps can be a 3-mm instrument passed via a separate incision. With the sack stabilized, the specimen is moved off the liver or the spleen and into the sack. The drawstring is grasped and closed,

and the neck of the sack is delivered via the lowermost 12-mm port; this port is removed, and the port site is extended to 2 cm. The neck of the sack is triply draped, as previously described, and the morcellation process proceeds under laparoscopic control within the intra-abdominal sack. Once the sack is removed, the three protective drapes are likewise removed, and the morcellation team regowns and regloves. The morcellation port site is bathed in Betadine; it is the only port site that requires a fascial closure at the end of the procedure.

Hand-Assisted Transperitoneal Laparoscopic Total/Radical Nephrectomy

As with the standard transperitoneal laparoscopic radical nephrectomy, the patient is placed in the modified flank position with the ipsilateral side elevated approximately 30 degrees. To avoid a blind and unmonitored passage of the trocars, the hand-assist device is placed at the outset of the procedure by entering the peritoneal cavity via a 7- to 8-cm incision under direct vision through the planned hand-port site. Following the placement of the hand port, the peritoneal cavity is insufflated to 15 mm Hg. The ports for instruments and the laparoscope are placed under endoscopic vision or via manual guidance through the hand port.

Figure 47B.2 shows the port placements recommended for the hand-assisted laparoscopic radical nephrectomy. In general, the surgeon's nondominant hand uses the hand port. For a right nephrectomy by a right-hand dominant surgeon, the hand port can be placed through a 7- to 8-cm vertical incision around the umbilicus (25,26); additional ports can be placed in the midline above the hand port and midclavicular line subcostal or above the umbilicus, pararectus line, and midclavicular line subcostal. For a left-sided procedure performed by a right-handed surgeon, a 12-mm camera port is placed in the midclavicular line just lateral to the rectus at or just below the level of umbilicus. The 12-mm working port should be placed in the midclavicular line just below the costal margin or in the anterior axillary line on a level with the umbilicus. For a left-handed surgeon, the set-up on the right and left side are reversed (e.g., right side would be the same as the set-up for the left side for a right-handed surgeon).

The procedure with the hand-assisted approach is identical to standard laparoscopy except for a few nuances in technique. During the hilar dissection, it is helpful for the surgeon to create a "C" with his or her thumb and index finger; dissection of

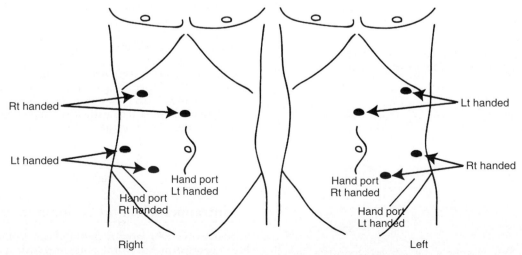

FIGURE 47B.2. Port placements for hand-assisted laparoscopic radical nephrectomy.

the hilum then proceeds within the "C"; the two digits provide excellent traction and countertraction to expose the hilar vessels. Also, when using the hand to dissect bluntly, it is helpful for the surgeon to always show the palm side of the hand to the laparoscope so that tissue is always being moved toward rather than away from the laparoscope.

At the end of the procedure, the specimen can be easily entrapped in a 15-mm Endocatch device and removed via the hand-port, usually without the need to enlarge the incision. Again, the authors caution against unentrapped intact removal, which could potentially lead to wound seeding (16).

Retroperitoneal Laparoscopic Total/Radical Nephectomy

For the retroperitoneoscopic radical nephrectomy, the patient should be positioned in the full flank position and the table extended to accentuate the ipsilateral flank. Initially, it may be helpful to have the kidney rest elevated; however, usually within 2 hours of starting the case, the kidney rest can be lowered. Initial access to the retroperitoneum is obtained through an incision made at the tip of the 12th rib and carried posteriorly for 2 cm. The anterior fascia is exposed by blunt dissection and incised. The underlying muscle layers are separated, and the lumbodorsal fascia is encountered and incised under direct vision; "S" retractors are helpful to expose the various planes to the surgeon. At this point, the pararenal fat should be clearly visible. Subsequently, the surgeon places the index finger into the retroperitoneal space; the psoas muscle should be clearly palpated. The surgeon can now insert a balloon dilator (US Surgical). To ensure an optimal use of the balloon dilator, it should be placed somewhat cephalad and inflated to 800 cc using 40 pumps on the rubber inflator bulb. During the inflation, the camera may be placed within the clear balloon to monitor the dissection. The balloon is deflated, and a second inflation may be completed caudal to establish the largest possible working space. Following this, two additional ports are placed in an "I" configuration with the aid of finger palpation along the costal margin: a 12-mm port just lateral to the paraspinous muscles just under the margin of the 12th rib and just above the psoas muscle and a 5-mm port on the midaxillary line, subcostal. If a four-port "T" approach is used, then an additional 12-mm port can be placed just above the anterior superior iliac crest at the midaxillary line (Petit triangle). Some surgeons prefer a "W" port arrangement and therefore will introduce a fifth port (i.e., 5 mm) just medial to the port at the Petit triangle (Fig. 47B.3). The original 2-cm access site is cannulated with a 10-mm balloon-type blunt trocar to prevent a CO$_2$ leak (Bluntport, US Surgical Norwalk, Connecticut) (27). The auxiliary ports can be placed under direct digital or endoscopic guidance.

In the retroperitoneal approach, the dissection begins by fully mobilizing all tissue off of the psoas margin until its medial border is clearly delineated. This is a crucial step in the procedure; failure to clearly see the medial border of the psoas can result in the surgeon beginning dissection of the kidney prematurely, in which case the kidney passes posterior to the surgeon's plane, making subsequent hilar identification nearly impossible. Once the medial border of the psoas can be clearly seen, a retractor is passed via the medialmost port, and the retroperitoneal tissues are retracted medial and anterior, thereby putting the renal hilum "on stretch." The pulsations of the renal artery can usually be seen. The thin posterior veil of Gerota fascia is incised overlaying the renal artery. The remainder of the hilar dissection is as described for the transperitoneal approach except that the renal vein is not dissected until the renal artery has been divided. In doing this part of the procedure, it is essential for the surgeon to remain spatially oriented at all times. The renal artery must be taken only after it is clearly seen to be traveling in a medial to lateral, never cephalocaudal, direction. As such, in the retroperitoneal approach, the hilar dissection is completed at the outset. At this point, the kidney is mobilized from the retroperitoneum. The fate of the adrenal is dependent upon the tumor's location. The ureter is taken at the end of the procedure between pairs of clips.

To remove the kidney, the specimen should be placed in an entrapment bag. If an intact specimen is desired, the 15-mm Endocatch retrieval device and bag should be placed directly through the skin after the removal of the 12-mm trocar. The specimen is removed by extending the original 2-cm flank incision. Alternatively, the surgeon may use a vaginal or a Pfannenstiel incision to remove the specimen (14,15). To entrap the specimen in the retroperitoneum, it is helpful to move the specimen as far cephalad as possible and then introduce the Endocatch bag via the lowermost 12-mm port site. The sack is then opened directly beneath the inferior border of the specimen. The specimen is moved until it completely overlies the opened sack, and then, using a "jiggling" action (similar to movements used with a popcorn popper), the Endocatch device is moved upward, thereby allowing the specimen to settle ever more deeply into the sack. Also during this process, the surgeon can use two graspers to move along the edge of the sack and to pull it up and over the specimen. Once the specimen is entrapped, the metal delivery device is removed and the drawstring is pulled closed.

Postoperative Management

Postoperatively, the patient is maintained on IV fluids and pain is controlled with a patient-controlled analgesia (PCA) device. Routine blood work, including complete blood count, electrolytes, and serum creatinine, is performed. In addition, a chest radiograph is usually recommended to rule out pneumothorax from an inadvertent diaphragmatic injury. A clear-liquid diet is begun the same day of surgery. The following day, the bladder catheter is removed, ambulation is initiated, and diet is advanced to regular. Once the patient tolerates oral intake, the PCA device is discontinued and oral analgesic medication is started. Postoperative antibiotics are usually discontinued after 24 hours. The patient is usually discharged on the evening of the second or the morning of the third postoperative day.

Results

Intraoperative and Perioperative Results

To date, over 640 laparoscopic radical nephrectomies have been reported in the world's literature. Most of these cases have been done in a standard transperitoneal fashion, followed

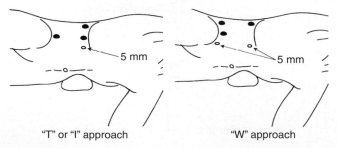

FIGURE 47B.3. Port placements for retroperitoneoscopic radical nephrectomy.

TABLE 47B.2

COMPARISON OF OPERATIVE RESULTS BETWEEN LAPAROSCOPIC RADICAL NEPHRECTOMY AND OPEN RADICAL NEPHRECTOMY

Procedure	Dunn et al. 2000 (28) Lap[a]	Dunn et al. 2000 (28) Open	Portis et al. 2002 (29) Lap[b]	Portis et al. 2002 (29) Open	Chan et al. 2001 (30) Lap[c]	Chan et al. 2001 (30) Open	Saika et al. 2003 (31) Lap[d]	Saika et al. 2003 (31) Open
Number	61	33	64	69	67	54	195	68
OR time (min)	330	168	287	128	256	193	275.7	203.1
EBL (mL)	172	451	219	354	289	309	248.5	482.0
Hospital stay (d)	3.4	5.2	4.8	7.4	3.8	7.2	—	—
Time to full convalescence (d)	25.2	56.7	—	—	—	—	22.7	58.7
Conversion rate	1.6%	—	—	—	1.5%	—	3.6%	—
Tumor size (cm)	5.3	7.4	4.3	6.2	5.1	5.4	3.7	4.4
Stage	T1	pT1	T1	pT1	T1	pT1	pT1	pT1
	T2	pT2	T2	pT2	T2	pT2		
	T3	pT3			T3			

OR, operating room; EBL, estimated blood loss.
[a] 55 transperitoneal, 3 retroperitoneal, and 3 combined transperitoneal and retroperitoneal laparoscopic radical nephrectomies.
[b] 52 transperitoneal and 12 retroperitoneal laparoscopic radical nephrectomies.
[c] 66 transperitoneal and 1 retroperitoneal laparoscopic radical nephrectomies.
[d] 177 transperitoneal and 18 retroperitoneal laparoscopic radical nephrectomies.

by hand-assisted, and, finally, by the retroperitoneoscopic method. Multiple studies are available that have analyzed the operative results of laparoscopic radical nephrectomy (28–35). Four studies that compared the results of laparoscopic radical nephrectomy with those of contemporary series of open radical nephrectomy are summarized in Table 47B.2. Overall, laparoscopic radical nephrectomy takes longer than open radical nephrectomy to complete. However, estimated blood loss (EBL) tended to be smaller, and the length of hospital stay was shorter. The use of analgesics was also much less. The time to convalescence for laparoscopy ranged from 23 to 25 days, whereas that of the open procedure ranged from 57 to 59 days. The conversion rate to an open procedure was 1.5% to 3.6%.

Oncologic Outcome

The long-term follow-up data have clearly demonstrated that laparoscopic radical nephrectomy is comparable to open radical nephrectomy (Table 47B.3). The largest series was published by Saika et al. and showed that the 5-year disease-specific survival rate was 94% in 195 patients treated with either a transperitoneal or a retroperitoneal laparoscopic radical nephrectomy for pathologic T1 RCC (31). In addition, smaller studies by Portis et al. and Chan et al. reported the 5-year cancer-specific survival rate to be 98% and 86%, respectively (29,30). The two

contemporary studies that examined the oncologic outcome after the traditional open nephrectomy reported the 5-year disease-specific survival rate to be 83% to 94% (36,37). These results reveal that laparoscopy does not compromise oncologic outcome so long as the principles of surgical oncology are strictly followed.

To date, four cases of port site seeding have been reported after a laparoscopic radical nephrectomy for RCC; three cases involve morcellation of specimens and one case involves a recurrence of hand-port site. The first recurrence was reported by Fentie et al. in 2000 (38) in which the patient had a large Fuhrman grade IV/IV tumor, with sarcomatoid features; the specimen was morcellated in a LapSac, and no leakage of contents from the sack was noted during the fragmentation procedure. The second case was reported by Castilho et al. in 2001 (39) in which the surgical team used a plastic entrapment device for intra-abdominal morcellation in a patient with ascites. These same authors also reported the third incidence in a letter to the editor, again in a patient with low-grade T1 (40). These last two cases demonstrate the dangers of morcellation among patients with ascites and of intra-abdominal morcellation in a nonnylon reinforced plastic sack. Of note is that there has been not a single case of seeding noted in the Johns Hopkins, Washington University, or Nagoya experience despite more than a decade of laparoscopic radical nephrectomy at all three institutions in more than 300 patients. To minimize the risk of tumor seeding and spillage during the morcellation process, various

TABLE 47B.3

COMPARISON OF CONTEMPORARY ONCOLOGICAL OUTCOME DATA AFTER LAPAROSCOPIC VERSUS OPEN RADICAL NEPHRECTOMY

Authors	Approach	Sample size	Mean F/U, m	T stage	5-year cancer-specific survival (%)
Portis et al. 2002 (29)	Lap	64	54	T1, T2	98
Saika et al. 2003 (31)	Lap	188	40	T1	94
Chan et al. 2001 (30)	Lap	67	35.6	T1, T2	86
Tsui et al. 2000 (37)	Open	227	47	T1	83
Javidan et al. 1999 (36)	Open	205	—	T1	95

F/U, follow-up.

TABLE 47B.4

MAJOR COMPLICATION RATES AFTER LAPAROSCOPIC RADICAL NEPHRECTOMY

Authors	Number	Procedure	Major complications (%)
Dunn et al. 2000 (28)	61	Transperitoneal	3 (10)
Siqueira et al. 2002 (44)	213	Transperitoneal	16 (7.5)
Chan et al. 2001 (30)	67	Transperitoneal	10 (15)
Patel and Leveillee, 2003 (45)	60	Hand-assisted	3 (5)
Lee et al. 2003 (13)	54	Hand-assisted	7.4 (4)
Cicco et al. 2001 (46)	50	Retroperitoneal	2 (4)

authors have made the following recommendations (41). First, only a LapSac should be used, especially for intra-abdominal morcellation. Second, morcellation should not be used if the patient has ascites. Third, the surgical team must be vigilant in monitoring the pneumoperitoneum and LapSac during morcellation; the entire process must be done under endoscopic control, and any leakage seen from the sack should prompt immediate enlargement of the incision and intact removal. Fourth, the neck of the sack should be triply draped. Fifth, after morcellation, the surgeon and the assistant should change gloves and gowns and remove the three drapes that came into contact with the neck of the sack. Sixth, the site of morcellation can be swabbed with Betadine after removal of the LapSac.

The lone case of hand-port site metastasis occurred in a patient with 10-cm by 7-cm pT2 RCC (16). The authors extracted the specimen without entrapment through an 8-cm midline incision. This report shows the potential danger of extracting unentrapped specimens. Indeed, in the editorial comment immediately following the aforementioned report, Nakada suggested that LapSac be used to extract all specimens after hand-assisted laparoscopic radical nephrectomies (42).

Complications

At the beginning of the surgery, the surgical team must be cognizant of the possibility that an emergent open conversion may be necessary at any point during the procedure. Therefore, a general laparotomy set with vascular clamps must be available during the entire operation. Complications associated with laparoscopic radical nephrectomy may be divided into three categories: access-related, intraoperative, and postoperative. As with any novel surgical technique, laparoscopic radical nephrectomy is associated with a significant learning curve. In a multi-institutional review involving 185 patients, it was noted that 71% of complications occurred during the initial 20 cases at each institution (43). More recently, Siqueira et al. reported on the experience at Indiana University with 213 laparoscopic nephrectomy cases (44). In this study, access-related complications included bowel herniation, abdominal wall hematoma, bowel or solid organ injury, and vascular injury; intraoperative complications were composed of uncontrollable bleeding and injuries to liver, spleen, and bowel. Postoperatively, the authors noted respiratory and gastrointestinal bleeding. Overall, the rate of major complications was 7.5%. Other authors have reported similar rates of major complications following laparoscopic nephrectomy (13,28,30,44–46) (Table 47B.4).

Futures

Laparoscopic radical nephrectomy is being applied in two new areas: cytoreductive surgery and tumors with renal vein and small inferior vena caval thrombi. Walther et al. first noted that patients undergoing laparoscopic cytoreductive surgery for RCC came to be treated approximately 30 days earlier than patients who had traditional open procedures (47). Mosharafa et al. also reported similar findings (48).

To date, eight cases of laparoscopic treatment of patients with T3b (renal vein involvement) have been successfully undertaken; blood loss has averaged 350 cc with a 3.3-hour operative time and a 2.3-day hospital stay (49–51). Indeed, Sundaram et al. have recently reported treating a small inferior venal caval thrombus laparoscopically (52). However, to date a subhepatic thrombus with cavotomy has not been done laparoscopically; but it is likely only a matter of time before the procedure is performed.

CONCLUSION

Since the first case of laparoscopic nephrectomy nearly 13 years ago, tremendous strides have been made. Numerous studies have demonstrated that laparoscopic radical nephrectomy has fulfilled its initial promise of decreased patient morbidity while maintaining the high standard of oncologic outcome established by the open procedure. The development of hand-assisted techniques along with better modalities for achieving hemostasis (Hemolok clips, bipolar device, harmonic shears, argon beam coagulation, etc.) have fostered the spread of laparoscopic renal surgery among many urologic surgeons. At this time, laparoscopic radical nephrectomy has become a "new" standard surgical technique for treating patients with localized RCC. In this regard, it is applicable to T1a (i.e., not amenable to a partial nephrectomy), all T1b, most T2 (i.e., <15 cm tumor), and T3a stages of RCC.

References

1. Clayman RV, Kavoussi LR, Soper NJ, et al. Laparoscopic nephrectomy: initial case report. J Urol 1991;146:278–282.
2. Hsu T, Jeffrey RB, Chon C, et al. Laparoscopic radical nephrectomy incorporating ultrasonography for renal cell carcinoma with renal vein tumor thrombus. Urology 2003;61:1246–1248.
3. Kercher KW, Joels CS, Matthews BD, et al. Hand-assisted surgery improves outcome for laparoscopic nephrectomy. Am Surg 2003;69:1061–1066.
4. Batler RA, Campbell SC, Funk JT, et al. Hand-assisted vs. retroperitoneal laparoscopic nephrectomy. J Endourol 2001;15:899–902.
5. Nelson CP, Wolf JS. Comparison of hand-assisted versus standard laparoscopic radical nephrectomy for suspected renal cell carcinoma. J Urol 2002;167:1989–1994.
6. Gill I, Strzempkowski B, Kaouk J, et al. Prospective randomized comparison: transperitoneal vs retroperitoneal laparoscopic radical nephrectomy. J Urol 2002;167:19, Abstract 78.
7. Wolf JS Jr. Hand-assisted laparoscopy: pro. Urology 2001;58:310–312.
8. Nelson CP, Wolf JS Jr. Comparison of hand-assisted versus standard laparoscopic radical nephrectomy for suspected renal cell carcinoma. J Urol 2002;167:1989–1994.

9. Okeke AA, Timoney AG, Keeley FX Jr. Hand-assisted laparoscopic nephrectomy: complications related to the hand-port site. *BJU Int* 2002; 90:364–367.

10. Gill IS. Hand-assisted laparoscopy: con. *Urology* 2001;58:313–317.

11. Wolf JS, Moon TD, Nakada SY Jr. Hand-assisted laparoscopic nephrectomy: comparison to standard laparoscopic nephrectomy. *J Urol* 1998;160:22–27.

12. Stifelman M, Nieder AM. Prospective comparison of hand-assisted laparoscopic devices. *Urology* 2002;59:668–672.

13. Lee SE, Ku JH, Kwak C, et al. Hand-assisted laparoscopic radical nephrectomy: comparison with open radical nephrectomy. *J Urol* 2003;170:756–759.

14. Gill IS, Cherullo EE, Meraney AM, et al. Vaginal extraction of the intact specimen following laparoscopic radical nephrectomy. *J Urol* 2002;167: 238–241.

15. Matin SR, Gill IS. Modified Pfannenstiel incision for intact specimen extraction after retroperitoneoscopic renal surgery. *Urology* 2003;61:830–832.

16. Chen YT, Yang SSD, Hsieh CH, et al. Hand port-site metastasis of renal-cell carcinoma following hand-assisted laparoscopic radical nephrectomy: case report. *J Endourol* 2003;17:771–773.

17. Hasson HM, Rotman C, Rana N, et al. Open laparoscopy: 29-year experience. *Obstet Gynecol* 2000;96:763–766.

18. Bonjer HJ, Hazebroek EJ, Kazemier G, et al. Open versus close establishment of pneumoperitoneum in laparoscopic surgery. *Br J Surg* 1997;84:599–602.

19. Merlin TL, Hiller JE, Maddern GJ, et al. Systemic review of the safety and effectiveness of methods used to establish pneumoperitoneum in laparoscopic surgery. *Br J Surg* 2003;90:668–679.

20. Chan D, Bishoff JT, Ratner L, et al. Endovascular gastrointestinal stapler device malfunction during laparoscopic nephrectomy: early recognition and management. *J Urol* 2000;164:319–321.

21. Kercher KW, Novitsky YW, Czerniach DR, et al. Staple line bleeding following laparoscopic splenectomy: intraoperative prevention and postoperative management with splenic artery embolization. *Surg Laparosc Endosc Percutan Tech* 2003;15:353–356.

22. Kerbl K, Chandhoke PS, Clayman RV, et al. Ligation of the renal pedicle during laparoscopic nephrectomy: a comparison of staples, clips, and sutures. *J Laparoendosc Surg* 1993;3:9–12.

23. Hernandez F, Rha KH, Pinto PA, et al. Laparoscopic nephrectomy: assessment of morcellation versus intact specimen extraction on postoperative status. *J Urol* 2003;170:412–415.

24. Urban DA, Kerbl K, McDougall EM, et al. Organ entrapment and renal morcellation: permeability studies. *J Urol* 1993;150:1792–1794

25. Fadden PT, Nakada SY. Hand-assisted laparoscopic renal surgery. *Urol Clin North Am* 2001;28:167–176.

26. Stifelman M, Andrade A, Sosa RE, et al. Simple nephrectomy: hand-assisted technique. *J Endourol* 2000;14:793–798.

27. McDougall E. Simple nephrectomy: transperitoneal and retroperitoneal: which, when, and why? In: Clayman RV, ed. *AUA 96th annual meeting course handout: H0019-PG laparoscopic organ ablative urology.* Anaheim, CA: 2001:1–9

28. Dunn MD, Portis AJ, Shalhav AL, et al. Laparoscopic versus open radical nephrectomy: a 9-year experience. *J Urol* 2000;164:1153–1159.

29. Portis AJ, Yan Y, Landman J, et al. Long-term followup after laparoscopic radical nephrectomy. *J Urol* 2002;167:1257–1262.

30. Chan DY, Cadeddu JA, Jarret TW, et al. Laparoscopic radical nephrectomy: cancer control for renal cell carcinoma. *J Urol* 2001;166: 2095–2100.

31. Saika T, Ono Y, Hattori R, et al. Long-term outcome of laparoscopic radical nephrectomy for pathologic T1 renal cell carcinoma. *Urology* 2003;62: 1018–1023.

32. Cadeddu JA, Ono Y, Clayman RV, et al. Laparoscopic nephrectomy for renal cell cancer: evaluation of efficacy and safety: a multicenter experience. *Urology* 1998;52:773–777.

33. Ono Y, Kinukawa T, Hattori R, et al. Laparoscopic radical nephrectomy for renal cell carcinoma: a five year experience. *Urology* 1999;53:280–286.

34. Barrett PH, Fentie DD, Taranger LA. Laparoscopic radical nephrectomy with morcellation for renal cell carcinoma: the Saskatoon experience. *Urology* 1998;52:23–28.

35. Janetschek G, Jeschke K, Peschel R, et al. Laparoscopic surgery for renal cell carcinoma: radical and partial nephrectomy. *J Endourol* 2000;14(Suppl. 7):A45.

36. Javidan J, Stricker HJ, Tamboli P, et al. Prognostic significance of the 1997 TNM classification of renal cell carcinoma. *J Urol* 1999;162:1277–1281.

37. Tsui K-H, Shvarts O, Smith RB, et al. Prognostic indicators for renal cell carcinoma: a multivariate analysis of 643 patients using the revised 1997 TNM staging criteria. *J Urol* 2000;163:1090–1095.

38. Fentie DD, Barrett PH, Taranger LA. Metastatic renal cell cancer after laparoscopic radical nephrectomy: long-term follow-up. *J Endourol* 2000;14: 407–411.

39. Castilho LN, Fugita OEH, Mitre AI, et al. Port site tumor recurrences of renal cell carcinoma after videolaparoscopic radical nephrectomy. *J Urol* 2001;165:519.

40. Castilho LN, Fugita OEH, Mitre AI, et al. Re: port site recurrences of renal cell carcinoma after videolaparoscopic radical nephrectomy. *J Urol* 2001;166:629–630.

41. Landman J, Clayman RV. Re: port site tumor recurrences of renal cell carcinoma after videolaparoscopic radical nephrectomy. *J Urol* 2001;166: 629–630.

42. Nakada SY. Editorial comment for: hand port-site metastasis of renal-cell carcinoma following hand-assisted laparoscopic radical nephrectomy: case report. *J Endourol* 2003;17:774.

43. Gill IS, Kavoussi LR, Clayman RV, et al. Complications of laparoscopic nephrectomy in 185 patients: a multi-institutional review. *J Urol* 1995; 154:479–483.

44. Siqueira TM Jr, Kuo RL, Gardner TA, et al. Major complications in 213 laparoscopic nephrectomy cases: the Indianapolis experience. *J Urol* 2002; 168:1361–1365.

45. Patel VR, Leveillee RJ. Hand-assisted laparoscopic nephrectomy for stage T1 and large stage T2 renal tumors. *J Endourol* 2002;17:379–383.

46. Cicco A, Salomon L, Hoznek A, et al. Results of retroperitoneal laparoscopic radical nephrectomy. *J Endourol* 2001;15:355–359.

47. Walther MM, Lyne JC, Libutti SK, et al. Laparoscopic cytoreductive nephrectomy as preparation for administration of systemic interleukin-2 in the treatment of metastatic renal cell carcinoma: a pilot study. *Urology* 1999; 53:496–501.

48. Mosharafa A, Koch M, Shalhav A, et al. Nephrectomy for metastatic renal cell carcinoma: Indiana University experience. *Urology* 2003;62:636–640.

49. Desai MM, Gill IS, Ramani AP, et al. Laparoscopic radical nephrectomy for cancer with level I renal vein involvement. *J Urol* 2003;169:487–491.

50. Savage SJ, Gill IS. Laparoscopic radical nephrectomy for renal cell carcinoma in a patient with level I renal vein tumor thrombus. *J Urol* 2000; 163:1243–1244.

51. McDougall EM, Clayman RV, Elashry OM. Laparoscopic radical nephrectomy for renal tumor: the Washington University experience. *J Urol* 1996; 155:1180–1185.

52. Sundaram CP, Rehman J, Landman J, et al. Hand assisted laparoscopic radical nephrectomy for renal cell carcinoma with inferior vena caval thrombus. *J Urol* 2002;168:176–179.

CHAPTER 47C
Surgical Management of Renal Cell Carcinoma: Role of Lymphadenectomy in Renal Cell Carcinoma Surgery

Hyung L. Kim, John S. Lam, and Arie S. Belldegrun

Each year, more than 30,000 new cases of renal cell carcinoma (RCC) are diagnosed in the United States (1). With increased use of ultrasounds and computed tomography (CT) scans in medicine, incidental detection of early RCC has at least in part accounted for a 3% increase in incidence each year since the 1970s (2,3). Currently, RCC represents approximately 3% of all malignancies.

The standard of care for both localized and metastatic RCC includes a nephrectomy. The goal of surgical resection for a localized renal cancer is cure. Approximately one third of patients newly diagnosed with RCC have metastatic disease. For metastatic RCC, a radical nephrectomy may be an effective neoadjuvant therapy before administering immunotherapy. In two separate randomized clinical trials, patients with metastatic RCC treated with cytoreductive nephrectomy and immunotherapy had longer survival than patients treated with immunotherapy alone (4,5).

At the time of nephrectomy, a retroperitoneal lymph node dissection (LND) can be performed. The role of LND for RCC has been actively debated for over half a century (6–9). Potential benefits include more accurate staging, decreased risk of local recurrence, and improved survival. However, the true benefits of lymph dissection remain unproven, and there is currently no consensus on the role for an LND.

A recent survey of practice patterns among academic urologists illustrates this lack of consensus. We surveyed members of the Society of Urologic Oncology and urologic oncologists in the American Association of Genitourinary Surgeons. For localized RCC, 26% of urologists do not perform a formal LND, whereas 41% perform a limited node dissection, and 33% perform a full retroperitoneal LND that extends from the crus of the diaphragm to the bifurcation of the aorta or vena cava. For metastatic disease, 21% of surveyed urologists do not perform a formal node dissection, and 43% and 36% perform a limited or a full retroperitoneal LND, respectively.

ANATOMY

The current understanding of the lymphatic drainage of the kidneys is based on anatomic studies performed in the early part of the 20th century (Fig. 47C.1). Poirier et al. performed cadaveric studies and provided some of the earliest anatomic descriptions of the renal lymphatics (10). A classic study by Alice Parker provides much of our understanding of the sequential drainage pattern of the kidney (11). Using 65 stillborn infants and seven adult cadavers, she mapped the lymphatic drainage pattern of the kidney by injecting Prussian blue dye into the kidney and lymphatics.

Parker's study demonstrates that the primary, regional drainage of the kidney is predictable. On the right, the regional nodal drainage includes the lateral caval nodes, the postcaval nodes, precaval nodes, and the interaortocaval nodes. The regional drainage for the left kidney includes the left lateral lumbar nodes, preaortic nodes, and postaortic nodes. However, secondary drainage varies and is unpredictable. The secondary lymphatic drainage often crosses the great vessels into the contralateral retroperitoneum or passes through the diaphragm into the thoracic duct.

STAGING

It is well established that the extent of lymph node involvement significantly affects prognosis in RCC (12–14). Furthermore,

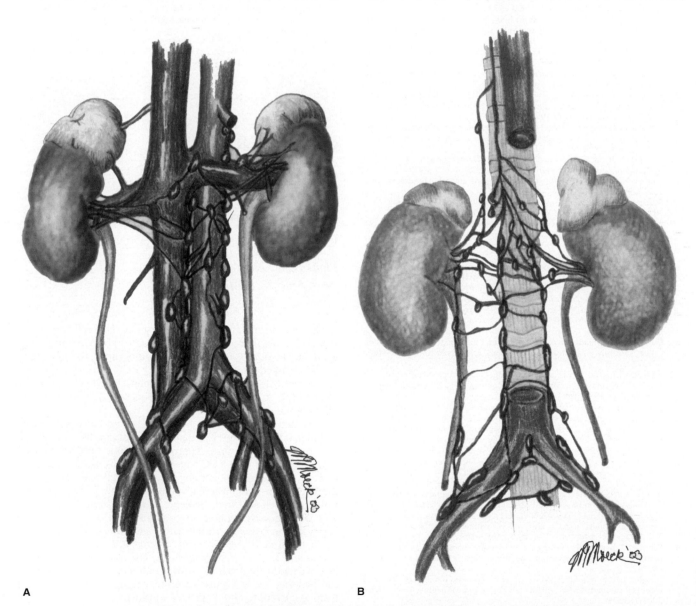

A   **B**

FIGURE 47C.1. The regional nodal drainage for the right kidney includes the lateral caval nodes, the postcaval nodes, the precaval nodes, and the interaortocaval nodes. The regional drainage for the left kidney includes the left lateral lumbar nodes, the preaortic nodes, and the postaortic nodes. **A:** Retroperitoneal lymph nodes anterior to the great vessels draining the kidneys. **B:** Retroperitoneal lymph nodes posterior to the great vessels draining the kidneys.

the number of organ systems involved in metastatic RCC has important prognostic implications (15,16). However, currently no imaging study can accurately identify positive lymph nodes preoperatively. Studer et al. reported that lymph node involvement was histologically confirmed in only 42% of patients with nodal enlargement on preoperative CT scan (17).

A recent retrospective analysis by Terrone et al. of 725 patients with RCC suggests that performing an LND results in more accurate staging (18). In this study, the number of lymph nodes removed during radical nephrectomy correlated with the percentage of patients with pathologically positive lymph nodes. This relationship existed even after controlling for the local extent of the disease, tumor grade, and metastasis status. The authors report that at least 13 lymph nodes must be removed and examined for accurate staging. For patients with less than 13 nodes examined, 10.2% had positive nodes, and for patients with at least 13 nodes examined, 20.8% had positive nodes.

This is consistent with similar observations for other urologic malignancies. For example, in bladder cancer, Herr reported that at least 11 to 14 pelvic lymph nodes should be removed for accurate staging (19). The number of nodes examined was related directly to lymph node density, defined as the ratio of positive-to-total number of nodes removed. For patients undergoing radical prostatectomy, Barth et al. reported that if more than 12 lymph nodes are examined, the likelihood of finding positive lymph nodes is increased twofold (20).

For other urologic malignancies, the experience of the surgeon and variations in patient anatomy affect the number of lymph nodes removed (21,22). However, for RCC, the primary factor determining the number of lymph nodes removed at the time of a radical nephrectomy is the preferred technique of the surgeon (18). This observation reflects the lack of consensus for the role of LND and the various surgical approaches applied. If all surgeons performed the operation using the same technique, it would be expected that the outcome would reflect the experience of the surgeons rather than variations in surgical approach.

The pathologist also represents a potential variable in nodal staging of RCC. There is no standard among pathologists for counting nodes in lymphatic specimens. Bochner et al. found that an average of 2.4 nodes were identified by the pathologist for pelvic lymph tissue when the nodal tissue was submitted *en bloc*; however, on average 9 nodes were identified when the tissue was submitted in two or three smaller packets (23). In addition, the technique used to process lymphatic tissue affects staging. Identification of lymph nodes can be enhanced by using fat-dissolving solutions (24) and staining the nodal tissue immunohistochemically for cytokeratin (25,26).

IS ACCURATE NODAL STAGING NECESSARY?

For RCC, the axiom "The more you look, the more you find" appears to hold true for both the surgeon and the pathologist. However, an important question is whether accurate nodal staging is clinically important. Given a false-positive rate of 58% to 75% (17,27) for preoperative imaging, a limited LND may be useful for patients with bulky lymphadenopathy noted on preoperative CT scan or magnetic resonance imaging (MRI). The risk of having a positive lymph node is significant in this group, and an LND will provide accurate staging information.

However, for patients with clinically localized RCC and no evidence preoperatively of lymph node involvement, a compelling argument can be made that an LND is unnecessary. The false-negative rate for modern imaging studies such as CT scans and MRIs is low, at approximately 4% (17,28). For patients with tumors <7 cm and clinically localized disease,

<0.5% of patients have clinically unsuspected lymph node involvement detected histologically by performing a lymphadenectomy (15).

Patients with lymph node involvement have a poor prognosis. However, no effective adjuvant therapy has been identified for patients with node-positive disease. Adjuvant therapies that have been shown to be ineffective in randomized clinical trials include radiation therapy (29), medroxyprogesterone (30), tumor vaccine (31), interferon (32), and interleukin-2 (33). The low incidence of unsuspected lymph node involvement in patients with clinically localized RCC, as well as the lack of effective adjuvant therapy, argue against performing routine LND in patients with localized disease.

Although no consensus exists regarding the role of lymphadenectomy, a standardized approach for managing the lymph nodes may be useful in the context of a clinical trial. Accurate staging and prediction of baseline prognosis are important in assessing the effectiveness of a new therapy. For clinical trials with multiple treatment groups, accurate nodal staging, especially in patients with enlarged nodes on preoperative imaging, will ensure that comparable groups are being assessed.

DECREASED RISK OF LOCAL RECURRENCE

It has been proposed that performing a formal LND at the time of radical nephrectomy may decrease the risk of local recurrence. Removing the retroperitoneal lymphatic tissue effectively results in resection of a larger margin of tissue surrounding the nephrectomy specimen and may, in theory, decrease the risk of positive margins (34). Some of the older nephrectomy series seem to support this. In series where a nephrectomy and LND were performed, the local recurrence rates were 2.5% to 8% (35–37), whereas the local recurrence rates in nephrectomy series without LND were approximately 11% (38,39).

However, in more modern series, local recurrences are very rare even when LNDs are not performed. Itano et al. reported that isolated local recurrence occurred in 1.8% of 1,737 patients who underwent radical nephrectomy for T1-3 N0M0 RCC (40). Rassweiler et al. reported a local recurrence rate of 2.2% following laparoscopic radical nephrectomy for localized RCC (41). At the University of California at Los Angeles (UCLA), the local recurrence rate is approximately 2.8% following radical nephrectomy, and there is no significant difference in local recurrence rate when patients with and without LND are compared (15).

The low rate of local recurrences in modern series reflects the widespread use of imaging studies in medicine. As most renal tumors are now being detected incidentally on imaging studies performed for unrelated indications, RCCs are being detected earlier and at lower stages. Therefore, it is unlikely that any modification in surgical technique will significantly lower the risk of local recurrence, and an LND will result in "overtreatment" of most patients with clinically localized disease.

IMPROVED SURVIVAL

Localized Renal Cell Carcinoma

An improved survival associated with removal of lymph nodes at the time of nephrectomy would provide the best argument for performing LNDs. However, for localized RCC, no studies clearly document a survival advantage. Herrlinger et al. initially reported a statistically significant survival advantage for patients undergoing lymphadenectomy for Robson stage I, II,

IIIb, and IIIc tumors (42). They assessed outcomes retrospectively in 511 patients who underwent surgery for RCC at the University of Erlangen–Nurnberg. The 5- and 10-year survival rates were 66% and 56.1%, respectively, for patients who underwent extended lymphadenectomy, compared to 58% and 40.9%, respectively, for patients who did not undergo formal LND. However, this study did not provide any information to show that the two groups were comparable with respect to patient age, tumor stage, and tumor grade; and a multivariable analysis was not performed.

In a second retrospective analysis of an expanded series that included 1,320 patients from the same institution, the University of Erlangen–Nurnberg, the authors again reported a statistically significant survival advantage for patients undergoing a systematic LND when compared to patients who did not undergo lymphadenectomy (43). However, the group undergoing LND had a lower mean age of 55.5 years when compared to the group that did not undergo LND, which had a mean age of 64.1 years. When these groups were subjected to population-based age correction, there was no difference in survival between the two groups. These two studies from the same institution highlight the potential pitfalls of retrospective analyses.

Other authors have reported that LND for localized RCC does not affect survival. Siminovitch et al. reviewed the results of 102 patients treated with a radical nephrectomy and LND at the Cleveland Clinic (44). The 5-year survival rate for patients with localized RCC was 58% if they underwent an extended lymphadenectomy and was 69% if only a regional lymphadenectomy was performed. Of the 102 patients, 9 patients had positive lymph nodes and only 1 patient remained disease-free 7 years following surgery. Minervini et al. compared 108 patients who underwent radical nephrectomy alone with 59 patients who underwent radical nephrectomy and LND (27). The 5-year survival rates for these two groups were similar: 79% and 78%. A retrospective analysis of 495 N0M0 patients undergoing nephrectomy at UCLA revealed no difference in survival whether an LND was performed or not (15) (Fig. 47C.2).

The only prospective, randomized study to assess the role of LND for localized RCC was performed by the EORTC Genitourinary group (28). A total of 772 patients were randomized to undergo radical nephrectomy alone or radical nephrectomy and complete LND. For patients randomized to undergo LND, the dissection extended from the crus of the diaphragm to the bifurcation of the aorta or vena cava. On the right, lateral caval, precaval, postcaval, and interaortocaval nodes were removed. On the left, left lateral lumbar, left diaphragmatic, and preaortic nodes were removed.

The preliminary results of the EORTC trial have been published (28). With a median follow-up of 5 years, 17% of the patients have died or have had recurrence of disease. Although the study was powered to detect a 10% difference in survival between the two groups, these data are not yet mature enough to make survival comparisons. The incidence of unsuspected lymph node metastasis was 3.3%. These patients with lymph node involvement are most likely to benefit from an LND. However, given the infrequent occurrence of unsuspected lymph node metastasis, this study may never reveal a difference in survival between patients randomized to the two groups.

In patients undergoing an LND, the most frequent complication was bleeding (>1 L), which occurred in 9.8% of patients. Other complications included pleural damage in 4.6%, infection in 5.5%, and lymph leakage in 2.6%. The overall complication rate was 25.7%. The overall complication rate for patients undergoing nephrectomy alone was 22.2%, and the difference in complication rates between the two groups was not statistically significant, suggesting that formal lymphadenectomy does not increase morbidity.

Renal Cell Carcinoma with Lymphatic Involvement

Patients with lymphatic metastasis of RCC may benefit from an LND. For patients with lymph node metastasis treated at UCLA, the median survival was approximately 5 months longer for patients who underwent LND than for patients who did not (15) (Fig. 47C.3). The difference in survival between these two groups was statistically significant. This difference may be partly explained by the observation that positive lymph nodes rarely respond to immunotherapy (45). Therefore, surgical resection of involved lymph nodes may offer the best chance for a complete response.

Others have also reported improved survival associated with an LND for patients with more advanced RCC (46,47). Peters and Brown reported that in a review of 356 patients undergoing nephrectomy, there was no difference in 5-year survival when

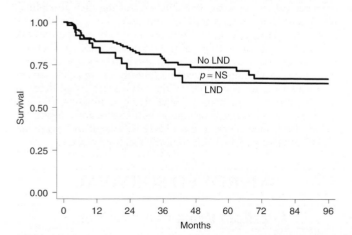

FIGURE 47C.2. Lymph node dissection (LND) at the time of nephrectomy for localized renal cell carcinoma (RCC) did not affect survival in 495 patients treated at the University of California at Los Angeles. [Reproduced with permission from Pantuck AJ, Zisman A, Dorey F, et al. Renal cell carcinoma with retroperitoneal lymph nodes: Role of lymph node dissection. *J Urol* 2003;169:2076–2083 (15).]

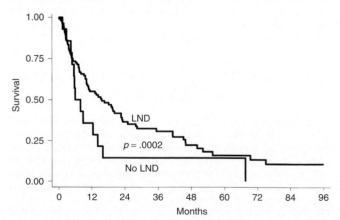

FIGURE 47C.3. Survival of patients with lymphatic involvement undergoing cytoreductive nephrectomy before planned systemic immunotherapy was significantly better in those undergoing lymph node dissection (LND) as part of nephrectomy. [Reproduced with permission from Pantuck AJ, Zisman A, Dorey F, et al. Renal cell carcinoma with retroperitoneal lymph nodes: role of lymph node dissection. *J Urol* 2003;169: 2076–2083 (15).]

patients with Robson stage A and stage B disease treated with and without LND were compared (46). However, for stage C disease, patients undergoing LND had a statistically higher 5-year survival (44%) when compared to patients undergoing nephrectomy alone (26%).

Although these findings suggest a role for LND in patients with more advanced disease, these findings should be cautiously applied in clinical practice. These studies were performed retrospectively; patients who did not undergo LND may represent a selected group with the most extensive disease. For example, patients who did not undergo a complete lymphadenectomy in the presence of lymphatic involvement may have had unresectable disease. A study from the National Cancer Institute documented that patients with minimal or extensive LND had better survival rates than patients who were considered to have unresectable disease (48).

CONCLUSION

There is currently no accepted standard for managing the lymph nodes at the time of nephrectomy. In the era of modern preoperative imaging, the occurrence of unsuspected lymph node involvement is rare. Therefore, staging accuracy is unlikely to be significantly improved by a formal node dissection when preoperative imaging is negative. However, given the high false-positive rate associated with CT scans and MRI, an LND may be useful for accurately staging patients when the lymph nodes are noted to be enlarged preoperatively.

For patients with localized RCC, a lymphadenectomy at the time of radical nephrectomy is unlikely to lead to a lower risk of local recurrence or improved survival. For patients with lymphatic involvement, several retrospective studies suggest that a formal LND may improve survival. However, in the absence of a randomized, prospective study, strong recommendations cannot be made regarding the role of lymphadenectomy in this population.

References

1. Jemal A, Murray T, Samuels A, et al. Cancer statistics, 2003. *CA Cancer J Clin* 2003;53:5–26.
2. Pantuck AJ, Zisman A, Belldegrun AS. The changing natural history of renal cell carcinoma. *J Urol* 2001;166:1611–1623.
3. Tsui KH, Shvarts O, Smith RB, et al. Renal cell carcinoma: prognostic significance of incidentally detected tumors. *J Urol* 2000;163:426–430.
4. Flanigan RC, Salmon SE, Blumenstein BA, et al. Nephrectomy followed by interferon alfa-2b compared with interferon alfa-2b alone for metastatic renal-cell cancer. *N Engl J Med* 2001;345:1655–1659.
5. Mickisch GH, Garin A, van Poppel H, et al. Radical nephrectomy plus interferon-alfa-based immunotherapy compared with interferon alfa alone in metastatic renal-cell carcinoma: a randomised trial. *Lancet* 2001;358:966–970.
6. Flocks RH, Kadesky MC. Malignant neoplasms of the kidney: an analysis of 353 patients followed five years or more. *J Urol* 1958;79:196.
7. Foley FEB, Mulvaney WP, Richardson EJ, et al. Radical nephrectomy for neoplasm. *J Urol* 1952;68:39.
8. Foot NC, Humphreys GA, Whitmore WF. Renal tumors: pathology and prognosis in 295 cases. *J Urol* 1951;66:190.
9. Mintz ER, Gaul EA. Kidney tumors: some causes of poor end results. *N Y State J Med* 1939;39:1405.
10. Poirier P, Cuneo B, Delamere G. *The Lymphatics.* London: Archibald Constable & Co., Ltd, 1903.
11. Parker AE. Studies on the main posterior lymph channels of the abdomen and their connections with the lymphatics of the genitourinary system. *Amer J Anat* 1935;56:409.
12. Zisman A, Pantuck AJ, Dorey F, et al. Improved prognostication of renal cell carcinoma using an integrated staging system. *J Clin Oncol* 2001;19:1649–1657.
13. Skinner DG, Vermillion CD, Colvin RB. The surgical management of renal cell carcinoma. *J Urol* 1972;107:705–710.
14. Robson CJ, Churchill BM, Anderson W. The results of radical nephrectomy for renal cell carcinoma. *J Urol* 1969;101:297–301.
15. Pantuck AJ, Zisman A, Dorey F, et al. Renal cell carcinoma with retroperitoneal lymph nodes: Role of lymph node dissection. *J Urol* 2003;169:2076–2083.
16. Han KR, Pantuck AJ, Bui MH, et al. Number of metastatic sites rather than location dictates overall survival of patients with node-negative metastatic renal cell carcinoma. *Urology* 2003;61:314–319.
17. Studer UE, Scherz S, Scheidegger J, et al. Enlargement of regional lymph nodes in renal cell carcinoma is often not due to metastases. *J Urol* 1990;144:243–245.
18. Terrone C, Guercio S, De Luca S, et al. The number of lymph nodes examined and staging accuracy in renal cell carcinoma. *BJU Int* 2003;91:37–40.
19. Herr HW. Extent of surgery and pathology evaluation has an impact on bladder cancer outcomes after radical cystectomy. *Urology* 2003;61:105–108.
20. Barth PJ, Gerharz EW, Ramaswamy A, et al. The influence of lymph node counts on the detection of pelvic lymph node metastasis in prostate cancer. *Pathol Res Pract* 1999;195:633–636.
21. Leissner J, Allhoff EP, Hohenfellner R, et al. Significance of pelvic lymphadenectomy for the prognosis after radical cystectomy. *Zentralbl Chir* 2002;127:315–321.
22. Weingartner K, Ramaswamy A, Bittinger A, et al. Anatomical basis for pelvic lymphadenectomy in prostate cancer: results of an autopsy study and implications for the clinic. *J Urol* 1996;156:1969–1971.
23. Bochner BH, Herr HW, Reuter VE. Impact of separate versus en bloc pelvic lymph node dissection on the number of lymph nodes retrieved in cystectomy specimens. *J Urol* 2001;166:2295–2296.
24. Koren R, Paz A, Lask D, et al. Lymph-node revealing solution: a new method for detecting minute lymph nodes in cystectomy specimens. *Br J Urol* 1997;80:40–43.
25. Herr HW. Pathologic evaluation of radical cystectomy specimens. *Cancer* 2002;95:668–669.
26. Jeffers MD, O'Dowd GM, Mulcahy H, et al. The prognostic significance of immunohistochemically detected lymph node micrometastases in colorectal carcinoma. *J Pathol* 1994;172:183–187.
27. Minervini A, Lilas L, Morelli G, et al. Regional lymph node dissection in the treatment of renal cell carcinoma: is it useful in patients with no suspected adenopathy before or during surgery? *BJU Int* 2001;88:169–172.
28. Blom JH, van Poppel H, Marechal JM, et al. EORTC Genitourinary Group. Radical nephrectomy with and without lymph node dissection: preliminary results of the EORTC randomized phase III protocol 30881. *Eur Urol* 1999;36:570–575.
29. Kjaer M, Iversen P, Hvidt V, et al. A randomized trial of postoperative radiotherapy versus observation in stage II and III renal adenocarcinoma: a study by the Copenhagen Renal Cancer Study Group. *Scand J Urol Nephrol* 1987;21:285–289.
30. Pizzocaro G, Piva L, Di Fronzo G, et al. Adjuvant medroxyprogesterone acetate to radical nephrectomy in renal cancer: 5-year results of a prospective randomized study. *J Urol* 1987;138:1379–1381.
31. Galligioni E, Quaia M, Merlo A, et al. Adjuvant immunotherapy treatment of renal carcinoma patients with autologous tumor cells and bacillus Calmette-Guerin: five-year results of a prospective randomized study. *Cancer* 1996;77:2560–2566.
32. Pizzocaro G, Piva L, Colavita M, et al. Interferon adjuvant to radical nephrectomy in Robson stages II and III renal cell carcinoma: a multicentric randomized study. *J Clin Oncol* 2001;19:425–431.
33. Clark J, Atkins MB, Urba W, et al. Adjuvant high-dose bolus interleukin-2 (HD IL-2) for patients (pts) with high-risk renal cell carcinoma (RCC): a Cytokine Working Group randomized trial. *Proc Am Soc Clin Oncol* 2003;22:164.
34. DeKernion JB. Lymphadenectomy for renal cell carcinoma: therapeutic implications. *Urol Clin North Am* 1980;7:697–703.
35. Giuliani L, Martorana G, Giberti C, et al. Results of radical nephrectomy with extensive lymphadenectomy for renal cell carcinoma. *J Urol* 1983;130:664–668.
36. Skinner DG, Colvin RB, Vermillion CD, et al. Diagnosis and management of renal cell carcinoma: a clinical and pathologic study of 309 cases. *Cancer* 1971;28:1165–1177.
37. Bassil B, Dosoretz DE, Prout GR Jr. Validation of the tumor, nodes and metastasis classification of renal cell carcinoma. *J Urol* 1985;134:450–454.
38. Parienty RA, Richard F, Pradel J, et al. Local recurrence after nephrectomy for primary renal cancer: computerized tomography recognition. *J Urol* 1984;132:246–249.
39. Phillips E, Messing EM. Role of lymphadenectomy in the treatment of renal cell carcinoma. *Urology* 1993;41:9–15.
40. Itano NB, Blute ML, Spotts B, et al. Outcome of isolated renal cell carcinoma fossa recurrence after nephrectomy. *J Urol* 2000;164:322–325.
41. Rassweiler J, Tsivian A, Kumar AV, et al. Oncological safety of laparoscopic surgery for urological malignancy: experience with more than 1,000 operations. *J Urol* 2003;169:2072–2075.
42. Herrlinger A, Schrott KM, Schott G, et al. What are the benefits of extended dissection of the regional renal lymph nodes in the therapy of renal cell carcinoma? *J Urol* 1991;146:1224–1227.
43. Schafhauser W, Ebert A, Brod J, et al. Lymph node involvement in renal cell carcinoma and survival chance by systematic lymphadenectomy. *Anticancer Res* 1999;19:1573–1578.

44. Siminovitch JP, Montie JE, Straffon RA. Lymphadenectomy in renal adenocarcinoma. *J Urol* 1982;127:1090–1091.
45. Pantuck AJ, Zisman A, Dorey F, et al. Renal cell carcinoma with retroperitoneal lymph nodes: impact on survival and benefits of immunotherapy. *Cancer* 2003;97:2995–3002.
46. Peters PC, Brown GL. The role of lymphadenectomy in the management of renal cell carcinoma. *Urol Clin North Am* 1980;7:705–709.
47. Golimbu M, Joshi P, Sperber A, et al. Renal cell carcinoma: survival and prognostic factors. *Urology* 1986;27:291–301.
48. Vasselli JR, Yang JC, Linehan WM, et al. Lack of retroperitoneal lymphadenopathy predicts survival of patients with metastatic renal cell carcinoma. *J Urol* 2001;166:68–72.

CHAPTER 47D
Open Nephron-Sparing Surgery for Renal Cell Carcinoma

Andrew C. Novick

Nephron-sparing surgery (NSS) has become a successful form of treatment for patients with localized renal cell carcinoma (RCC) when there is a need to preserve the functioning renal parenchyma (1). This need is present in patients with bilateral RCC, RCC involving a solitary functioning kidney, chronic renal failure, or in those with unilateral RCC and a functioning opposite kidney that is at risk for future impairment from an intercurrent disorder. The technical success rate with NSS is excellent, and long-term, cancer-free patient survival rates are comparable with those obtained after radical nephrectomy, particularly for low-stage RCC. The major disadvantage of NSS for RCC is the risk of postoperative local tumor recurrence in the operated kidney, which has occurred in 5% to 6% of patients. These local recurrences are most likely a manifestation of undetected, microscopic, multifocal RCC in the remnant kidney. The risk of local tumor recurrence after radical nephrectomy has not been studied, but it is presumably very low.

INDICATIONS FOR NEPHRON-SPARING SURGERY

Standard indications for NSS fall into three categories: absolute, relative, and elective. Absolute indications for NSS include circumstances in which radical nephrectomy would render the patient anephric, with subsequent immediate need for dialysis. These circumstances encompass patients with bilateral RCC or RCC involving a solitary functioning kidney, whether resulting from unilateral renal agenesis, prior removal of the contralateral kidney, or irreversible impairment of contralateral renal function. Patients with bilateral synchronous renal tumors also have an absolute indication for NSS, and an attempt should be made to preserve as much functioning parenchyma as possible. Preservation involves performing bilateral partial nephrectomy when feasible, usually as a staged procedure with the less involved side done first. When partial nephrectomy is not indicated on one side because of tumor size or anatomy, initial partial nephrectomy is performed as a separate procedure on the less involved side, followed by contralateral radical nephrectomy. Such an ordering precludes the need for temporary dialysis in the immediate postoperative period should acute tubular necrosis arise following partial nephrectomy, and it also affords flexibility when preparing the contralateral operation (1).

Relative indications for NSS include patients with unilateral RCC and a functioning opposite kidney, when the opposite kidney is affected by a condition that might threaten its future function, such as calculus disease, chronic pyelonephritis, renal artery stenosis (RAS), ureteral reflux, or systemic diseases such as diabetes and nephrosclerosis. In such patients, the risks and benefits of NSS must be considered in the context of the general clinical status, including age, comorbidities, risk of disease progression, and the possibility that these conditions will negatively affect remaining renal function (1).

Relative indications for NSS also include patients with hereditary forms of RCC such as von Hippel-Lindau (VHL) disease, where there is a high likelihood of subsequent lesions developing in the remaining renal parenchyma. The natural history of RCC in patients with VHL differs from sporadic RCC in that the diagnosis is made at a younger age, and there usually are multiple bilateral renal tumors (2). In patients with VHL or other hereditary renal malignancies, NSS is offered on the basis of the genetic predisposition to recurrence. Furthermore, preservation of renal function in young patients often poses an important clinical concern.

Elective indications for NSS include patients with localized unilateral RCC and a healthy contralateral kidney. Recent studies have clarified the role of NSS in such patients (3–7). With evolving longer-term data, a size criterion has gained gradual acceptance for elective NSS. Data from our institution (8) as well as from the Mayo Clinic (9) and Memorial Sloan-Kettering Cancer Center (MSKCC) (10) indicate that radical nephrectomy and NSS provide equally effective curative treatment of such patients who present with a single, small (<4 cm), and clearly localized RCC. The results of NSS are less satisfactory in patients with larger (>4 cm) or multiple localized RCCs, and radical nephrectomy should remain the treatment of choice in such cases when the opposite kidney is healthy.

Except in exceptional circumstances, NSS is contraindicated in the presence of lymph node metastasis because the prognosis for these patients is poor. A biopsy should be performed on enlarged or suspicious-looking lymph nodes before initiating the renal resection.

PREOPERATIVE EVALUATION

Evaluation of patients with RCC before NSS must include a detailed history and physical examination, a laboratory evaluation including serum creatinine, liver function tests, and urinalysis or urine dipstick check to screen for preoperative proteinuria. Radiographic testing is used to rule out locally extensive or metastatic disease, including chest x-ray and abdominal computed tomography (CT) scan, as well as possible bone scan and chest or head CT scan depending on the clinical circumstances.

However, NSS is technically challenging and requires a more detailed understanding of renal anatomy than *en bloc* removal of the kidney by radical nephrectomy (11). Knowledge of the relation of the tumors to the collecting system and adjacent normal parenchyma, and of the renal and tumor vascular supply, is essential for preoperative planning. Therefore, more extensive and invasive preoperative imaging studies are often necessary before NSS. These include renal CT scan, arteriography, and, occasionally, venography. Arteriography has been used to delineate the intrarenal vasculature and may aid in excision of the tumor while minimizing blood loss and injury to normal adjacent parenchyma. It is most useful for nonperipheral tumors encompassing two or more renal arterial segments. Selective renal venography is performed in patients with large or centrally located tumors to evaluate for the presence of intrarenal venous thrombosis and assess adequacy of venous drainage of the planned renal remnant. These studies provide a 2D map to aid complete excision of tumors, assess arterial and venous involvement, and plan complex reconstruction of the renal remnant. However, these studies yield only limited information on the anatomical spatial relations among the tumor, normal renal parenchyma, collecting system, and vascular supply. Furthermore, the risks and costs of conventional arteriography or venography are substantial.

CT scan is widely accepted as the preferred imaging technique for detecting and staging RCC because of the low cost, high accuracy, and ready accessibility. Advances in helical CT scan image acquisition and computer technology allow production of high-quality three-dimensional (3D) images of the renal vasculature and soft tissue anatomy. The latest development in 3D imaging is volume rendering, which allows real-time interactive stereoscopic viewing and presents complex anatomy not possible with conventional axial CT scan. By combining helical CT scan and 3D volume rendering, a single noninvasive preoperative test has the potential to provide all of the critical information needed for planning and intraoperative management of renal mass lesions. New volume-rendering software allows real-time interactive stereoscopic viewing of these images and provides a topographic map of the renal surface and multiplanar views of the intrarenal anatomy. This permits evaluation of the complex renal anatomy using a single, unified study in a format that is familiar to the surgeon and consistent with intraoperative findings, thereby obviating the need for mental reconstruction of several two-dimensional (2D) imaging studies. A detailed prospective study at the Cleveland Clinic demonstrated the utility of 3D volume rendering CT scan in accurately depicting the renal parenchyma and vascular anatomy necessary for the performance of NSS (12). The data from 3D CT scan integrate essential information from angiography, venography, excretory urography, and conventional 2D CT scan into a single preoperative staging test that diminishes the need for more invasive imaging. The use of a 3- to 5-minute videotape in the operating room provides concise, accurate, and immediate 3D information to the surgeon during the dissection, allowing him or her to anticipate the subtleties of the anatomy. 3D volume-rendered CT scan has become the imaging modality of choice prior to NSS, allowing hilar dissection, tumor removal, and reconstruction to proceed quickly and confidently.

SURGICAL TECHNIQUE

It is usually possible to perform open NSS for malignancy *in situ* by using an operative approach that optimizes exposure of the kidney and by combining meticulous surgical technique with an understanding of the renal vascular anatomy in relation to the tumor. We use an extraperitoneal flank incision through the bed of the 11th or 12th rib for almost all of these operations; we occasionally use a thoracoabdominal incision for very large tumors involving the upper portion of the kidney. These incisions allow the surgeon to operate on the mobilized kidney almost at skin level and provide excellent exposure of the peripheral renal vessels (Fig. 47D.1). With an anterior, subcostal, transperitoneal incision, the kidney is invariably located in the depth of the wound, and the surgical exposure is simply not as good. Extracorporeal surgery is rarely necessary in these patients.

When performing *in situ* nephron-sparing tumor excision, the kidney is mobilized within the Gerota fascia, while the perirenal fat around the tumor is left intact. For small, peripheral renal tumors, it is not necessary to control the renal artery. In most other cases, however, NSS is most effectively performed after temporary renal arterial occlusion. This measure not only limits intraoperative bleeding but also improves access to intrarenal structures by reducing renal tissue turgor.

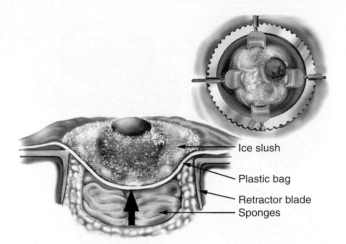

Ice slush
Plastic bag
Retractor blade
Sponges

FIGURE 47D.1. Sketch illustrating elevation of the mobilized kidney to skin level by placing sponges under the plastic bag containing the kidney and ice slush. (From Novick AC. Anatomic approaches in nephron-sparing surgery for renal cell carcinoma. *Atlas urol Clin North Am* 1998;6:39, with permission.)

When possible, it is helpful to leave the renal vein patent throughout the operation. This measure decreases intraoperative renal ischemia and, by allowing venous backbleeding, facilitates hemostasis by enabling identification of small, transected renal veins. In patients with centrally located tumors, it is necessary to occlude the renal vein temporarily to minimize intraoperative bleeding from transected major venous branches.

When the renal circulation is temporarily interrupted, *in situ* renal hypothermia is used to protect against postischemic renal injury. Surface cooling of the kidney with ice slush allows up to 3 hours of safe ischemia without permanent renal injury. An important caveat with this method is to keep the entire kidney covered with ice slush for 10 to 15 minutes immediately after occluding the renal artery and before commencing the NSS (Fig. 47D.1). This amount of time is needed to obtain core renal cooling to a temperature (approximately 20°C) that optimizes *in situ* renal preservation. During excision of the tumor, large portions of the kidney invariably are no longer covered with ice slush and, in the absence of adequate prior renal cooling, rapid rewarming and ischemic renal injury can occur. Cooling by perfusion of the kidney with a cold solution instilled via the renal artery is not recommended because of the theoretic risk of tumor dissemination. Mannitol is given intravenously 5 to 10 minutes before temporary renal arterial occlusion. Systemic or regional anticoagulation to prevent intrarenal vascular thrombosis is not necessary.

A variety of surgical techniques are available for performing partial nephrectomy in patients with malignancy. These include polar (apical or basilar) segmental nephrectomy, wedge resection, and transverse resection (Fig. 47D.2). All of these techniques require adherence to basic principles of early vascular control, avoidance of ischemic renal damage with complete tumor excision with free margins, precise closure of the collecting system, careful hemostasis, and closure or coverage of the renal defect with adjacent fat, fascia, peritoneum, or Oxycel. With each technique, the tumor is removed with a small, surrounding margin of grossly normal renal parenchyma. Intraoperative ultrasound helps in achieving accurate tumor localization, particularly for intrarenal lesions that are not visible or palpable from the external surface of the kidney (13).

When performing a transverse resection of the upper part of the kidney, care must be taken to avoid injury to the posterior segmental renal arterial branch, which may also occasionally

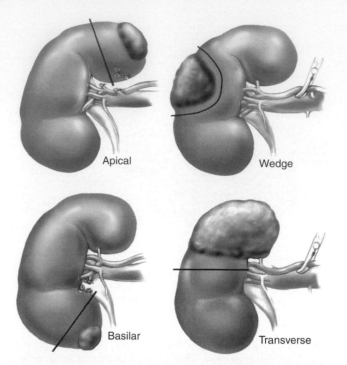

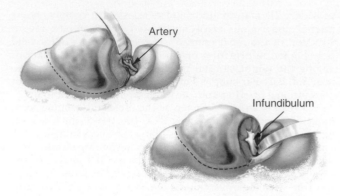

FIGURE 47D.2. Techniques of apical or basilar segmental nephrectomy, wedge resection, and transverse resection for renal malignancy. The latter two techniques are generally performed with temporary renal arterial occlusion. (From Novick AC. Anatomic approaches in nephron-sparing surgery for renal cell carcinoma. *Atlas Urol Clin North Am* 1998;6:39, with permission.)

FIGURE 47D.3. As the parenchyma around the tumor is incised, major vessels supplying the tumor are identified and secured. Similarly, infundibulum draining the tumor-bearing position of the kidney are also identified and secured. (From Novick AC. Anatomic approaches in nephron-sparing surgery for renal cell carcinoma. *Atlas Urol Clin North Am* 1998;6:39.)

supply the basilar renal segment. Preoperative vascular imaging is integral to identifying and preserving the posterior segmental artery at surgery, thereby avoiding devascularization of a major portion of the healthy remnant kidney. Midrenal resections may also be particularly complicated because the arterial supply comprises branches of anterior and posterior renal artery divisions, and the calices often enter the same infundibula as those draining the upper and lower poles.

With each nephron-sparing technique, the parenchyma around the tumor is divided with a combination of sharp and blunt dissection. In many cases, the tumor extends deeply into the kidney, and the collecting system is entered. Often, renal arterial and venous branches supplying the tumor can be identified as the parenchyma is being incised, and these should be directly suture ligated when they are most visible (Fig. 47D.3). Similarly, in many cases, direct entry into the collecting system may be avoided by isolating and ligating major infundibula draining the tumor-bearing renal segment as the incision into the parenchyma is developed (Fig. 47D.3).

After the excision of the tumor, remaining transected blood vessels on the renal surface are secured with figure-of-eight 4-0 chromic sutures. Bleeding at this point is usually minimal, and the operative field can be kept satisfactorily clear by gentle suction during placement of hemostatic sutures. Residual collecting system defects are similarly closed with interrupted or continuous 4-0 chromic sutures. At this point, with the renal artery still clamped but with the renal vein open, the anesthesiologist is asked to hyperinflate the lungs and, thereby, raise the central and renal venous pressure, which forces blood out through residual, unsecured, transected veins on the renal surface and facilitates their detection (Fig. 47D.4). Once identified, these veins are secured with interrupted figure-of-eight 4-0 chromic sutures. The argon beam coagulator is a useful adjunct for achieving hemostasis on the transected peripheral renal surface.

In most cases, after securing the renal vasculature and collecting system, the kidney is closed on itself by approximating the transected cortical margins with simple, interrupted 3-0 chromic sutures after placing a small piece of Oxycel at the base of the defect (Fig. 47D.5). This is an important additional hemostatic measure. When this step is done, there must be no tension on the suture line and no significant angulation or kinking of blood vessels supplying the kidney. After closure of the renal defect, the renal artery is unclamped and circulation to the kidney is restored. When the remnant kidney resides within a large retroperitoneal fossa, the kidney is fixed to the posterior musculature with interrupted 3-0 chromic sutures to prevent postoperative movement or rotation of the kidney, which may compromise the blood supply (Fig. 47D.6). A retroperitoneal drain is always left in place for at least 7 days, and an intraoperative ureteral stent is placed only when major reconstruction of the intrarenal collecting system has been performed.

When NSS is performed, after excision of all gross tumor, absence of malignancy in the remaining portion of the kidney

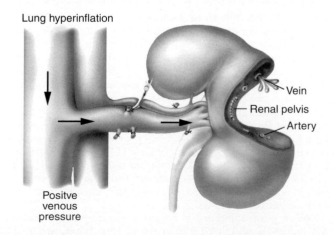

FIGURE 47D.4. Identification of residual, unsecured, transected vessels (particularly veins) on the renal surface is facilitated by increasing the renal venous pressure through hyperinflation of the lungs. (From Novick AC. Anatomic approaches in nephron-sparing surgery for renal cell carcinoma. *Atlas Urol Clin North Am* 1998;6:39, with permission.)

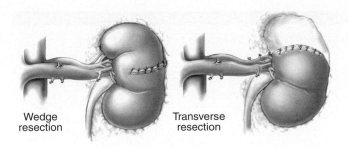

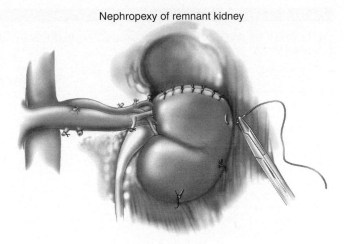

Nephropexy of remnant kidney

FIGURE 47D.5. The defect created by nephron-sparing tumor excision is closed by suturing the kidney on itself. (From Novick AC. Anatomic approaches in nephron-sparing surgery for renal cell carcinoma. *Atlas Urol Clin North Am* 1998;6:39, with permission.)

FIGURE 47D.6. Nephropexy of the remnant kidney to the retroperitoneum is achieved with several interrupted sutures. (From Novick AC. Anatomic approaches in nephron-sparing surgery for renal cell carcinoma. *Atlas Urol Clin Am* 1998;6:39, with permission.)

should be verified intraoperatively by frozen-section examinations of biopsy specimens obtained at random from the renal margin of excision. It is unusual for such biopsies to demonstrate residual tumor, but, if they do, additional renal tissue must be excised.

Some RCCs are surrounded by a distinct pseudocapsule of fibrous tissue, and the technique of simple enucleation has been used in such cases to achieve tumor removal. Initial reports indicated satisfactory short-term clinical results after enucleation with good patient survival rates and a low rate of local tumor recurrence. However, most studies have suggested a higher risk of leaving residual malignancy in the kidney when enucleation is performed. These reports include several careful histopathologic studies that have demonstrated frequent microscopic tumor penetration of the pseudocapsule that surrounds the neoplasm. These data indicate that it is not always possible to be assured of complete tumor encapsulation before surgery. Local recurrence of tumor in the treated kidney is a grave complication of partial nephrectomy for RCC, and every attempt should be made to prevent it. Therefore, it is my view that a surrounding margin of normal parenchyma should be removed with the tumor whenever possible. This provides an added margin of safety against the development of local tumor recurrence and, in most cases, does not appreciably increase the technical difficulty of the operation. The technique of enucleation is currently used only in occasional patients with VHL disease who have multiple low-stage encapsulated tumors involving both kidneys.

Postoperative follow-up after NSS surgery involves serum creatinine measurement and excretory urography at 4 to 6 weeks to document renal function and anatomy. Subsequent surveillance strategies (Table 47D.1) follow stage-specific guidelines (14) and are no more extensive or expensive than surveillance after radical nephrectomy for low-stage pT1 or pT2 disease. Locally recurrent disease may be treated with repeat partial or complete nephrectomy depending on the clinical circumstances and the anatomy of the remnant kidney (15).

CLINICAL RESULTS OF NEPHRON-SPARING SURGERY FOR RENAL CELL CARCINOMA

The technical success rate with NSS for RCC is excellent, and long-term patient survival free of cancer is comparable with that obtained after radical nephrectomy. Table 47D.2 lists results of NSS for RCC in more than 1,262 patients reported in the literature since 1990. The reported mean cancer-specific survival for all patients undergoing NSS for localized RCC is 88% to 97.5%. Mean follow-up for these studies ranged between 3 and 6 years.

Recently, Fergany et al. (20) reviewed the results of NSS in 107 patients with localized sporadic RCC who were treated before 1988 and were followed up for a minimum of 10 years at the Cleveland Clinic. Tumors were symptomatic in 73 patients

---

TABLE 47D.1

RECOMMENDED POSTOPERATIVE SURVEILLANCE AFTER NEPHRON-SPARING SURGERY FOR SPORADIC LOCALIZED RENAL CELL CARCINOMA

Pathologic tumor stage	History, examination, blood test[a]	Chest x-ray	Abdominal CT scan
T1	Yearly	—	—
T2	Yearly	Yearly	Every 2 yr
T3	Yearly	Yearly	Every 6 mo for 2 yr, then every 2 yr

CT, computed tomography.
[a]Medical history, physical examination, and measurement of serum calcium, alkaline phosphatase, liver function, and renal function.
The need for postoperative radiographic surveillance studies varies according to the initial pathologic tumor (pT) stage (Table 47D.1). Patients who undergo NSS for pT1 RCC do not require radiographic imaging postoperatively in view of the very low risk of recurrent malignancy. A yearly chest radiograph is recommended after NSS for pT2 or pT3 RCC because the lung is the most common site of postoperative metastasis in both groups. Abdominal or retroperitoneal tumor recurrence is uncommon in pT2 patients, particularly early after NSS, and these patients require only occasional follow-up abdominal CT scanning. Patients with pT3 RCC have a higher risk of developing local tumor recurrence, particularly during the first 2 years after NSS, and they may benefit from more frequent follow-up abdominal CT scanning initially.

TABLE 47D.2

OUTCOME IN PATIENTS UNDERGOING NEPHRON-SPARING SURGERY FOR LOCALIZED RENAL CELL CARCINOMA

Study	n	% Disease-specific survival	Number of local recurrences	Mean follow-up (mo)
Moll et al. (7)	142	98	1.4	34.8
Provert et al. (5)	44	88	2	36
Lee et al. (10)	79	96	0	40
Lerner et al. (16)	185	89	5.9	44
Steinbach et al. (4)	121	90	4.1	47
Hafez et al. (8)	485	92	3.2	7
Babalias et al. (17)	41	97.5	7.3	59
D'Armiento et al. (18)	19	95	0	70
Belldegrun et al. (19)	146	93	2.7	74

(68%), and indications for surgery were imperative in 96 (90%). All patients were followed up for at least 10 years or until death. Cancer-specific survival was 88.2% at 5 years and 73% at 10 years, and 26% of the patients died of metastatic disease. Long-term preservation of renal function was achieved in 93% of patients. Cancer-specific survival for tumors ≤4 cm was 98% at 5 years and 92% at 10 years regardless of the indication for partial nephrectomy. Important negative predictors of survival included high tumor grade, high tumor stage, bilateral disease, and tumors >4 cm. These data are consistent with other shorter-term previously published series that confirmed that tumor stage, grade, and size remain the most important prognostic indicators determining outcome after NSS (21). On the other hand, there are no significant biologic differences between centrally located and peripherally located small, solitary, unilateral RCCs, and treatment with NSS or radical nephrectomy is equally effective regardless of tumor location in these patients (22).

NEPHRON-SPARING SURGERY WITH A NORMAL CONTRALATERAL KIDNEY

Although radical nephrectomy remains the standard treatment for localized RCC in patients with an anatomically and functionally healthy opposite kidney, a growing number of authors are reporting excellent results with NSS in this setting. Disease-specific survival in this setting is 90% to 100%, with extended follow-up in several series. In a recent study from MSKCC, Herr (23) reported the 10-year results of elective NSS in the setting of a healthy contralateral kidney. Of the 70 patients with an average tumor size of 3 cm with predominantly low-grade, low-stage tumors, 69 patients (98.5%) had no local recurrence, and 68 (97%) survived free of metastasis (23).

Although the long-term functional advantage of NSS when there is a healthy opposite kidney remains to be definitely demonstrated, the benefit of maximal nephron preservation may include a decreased risk of progression to chronic renal insufficiency and end-stage renal disease. In recent studies by McKiernan et al. from MSKCC (24) and by Lau et al. from the Mayo Clinic (25), patients who underwent radical nephrectomy were compared with patients who underwent elective NSS. Each institution's groups were well matched for age, grade, stage, tumor size, preoperative creatinine, and year of surgery. Although they identified no significant difference in cancer-free survival, Lau et al. demonstrated that at 10 years, renal insufficiency (defined as an increase in serum creatinine to >2 mg/dL)

was significantly different between the groups, occurring in 12.4% of radical nephrectomy cases compared with only 2.3% of NSS cases. Similarly, McKiernan et al. found that the chance of progression to renal insufficiency was significantly higher in the radical nephrectomy group. In both groups, differences in functional renal reserve were thought to be responsible for these findings. Therefore, given the excellent short-term and long-term results of elective NSS for cancer control and the increasingly recognized functional benefits of this approach, patients with a single, small, unilateral, localized RCC may now be considered suitable candidates for NSS even when the opposite kidney is completely healthy.

INDICATIONS AND OUTCOMES FOR NEPHRON-SPARING SURGERY IN SPECIAL CIRCUMSTANCES

Hereditary Renal Tumors and Nephron-Sparing Surgery

Hereditary conditions that predispose patients to renal tumors include VHL disease associated with clear cell RCC, hereditary papillary RCC, hereditary oncocytoma, and the Birt-Hogg-Dubé (BHD) syndrome. Considerations regarding the treatment of solid renal malignancies in these patients differ significantly from those with sporadic renal neoplasms, primarily because of the propensity for hereditary lesions to be bilateral, multifocal, and often microscopic. Treatment of RCC in patients with VHL disease differs significantly from that of patients with sporadic renal neoplasms primarily because the tendency of lesions in VHL to be bilateral, multifocal, and often microscopic. This reflects the changes in the germline of the VHL gene located on the short arm of chromosome 3 (3p25-26). For this reason, RCC occurs at a much younger age in patients with hereditary renal tumors such as VHL, and the entire renal parenchyma has a higher lifetime risk for developing subsequent tumors. Additionally, the malignant potential of cysts is often underappreciated on ultrasound or CT scan in such patients, and, histologically, these cysts frequently contain either frank carcinoma or a hyperplastic clear cell lining that may represent incipient tumor (26). For instance, adequate surgical treatment of localized RCC in VHL, therefore, requires complete excision of all solid and cystic renal lesions. Available options include observation of lesions <3 cm, NSS with close surveillance, and subsequent resection of recurrent disease or bilateral radical nephrectomy, thereby rendering the patient anephric with the potential for subsequent transplantation (27,28). Walther et al. evaluated a 3-cm surgical threshold for performing NSS in 52 patients with VHL and hereditary papillary renal carcinoma (29). No patient was noted to have metastatic disease during observation with a dominant tumor of <3 cm during a median follow-up of 60 months. Regardless of the treatment course elected, the patient must be advised of the need for strict lifelong follow-up, the possible need for resection of recurrent disease in the setting of NSS, and the risks of immune suppression in the setting of previous RCC if transplantation is elected.

The role of NSS in preserving renal function and avoiding or postponing dialysis in patients with VHL disease was examined in a multicenter study of 49 patients who underwent NSS for RCC; the 5- and 10-year cancer-specific survival rates were 100% and 81%, respectively. At a mean follow-up of 68 months, 51% of the patients treated with NSS had local recurrence, most of whom underwent salvage by repeat NSS or removal of the renal remnant. Whether these recurrences represent *de novo* tumors or microscopic, clinically undetected foci present at the time of the original surgery is not known. Survival free of local recurrence was 71% at 5 years, but only 15% at 10 years. These data underscore the need for diligent surveillance in these patients. NSS is therefore feasible in well-selected patients with VHL and can preserve renal function without compromising cancer-free survival in most patients.

Nephron-Sparing Surgery with Coexistent Renal Artery Disease

Occasionally, preoperative history and radiographic imaging reveal both RCC and RAS in the same patient. This can complicate the clinical picture. When RCC and RAS are found in the same kidney and a healthy contralateral kidney is present, the treatment of choice is radical nephrectomy. Involvement of all functional renal parenchyma by either or both of these processes poses a more difficult therapeutic dilemma. Management of such cases must be individualized to achieve maximal cancer control while balancing the need to preserve overall renal function.

Campbell et al. reviewed their experience in the management of 34 patients with concurrent RCC and RAS affecting all of the functioning renal parenchyma (30). The mean patient age was 67, and 88% of cases of RAS were due to atherosclerotic disease. Patients were divided into four groups: patients with a solitary kidney with RCC and RAS, patients with bilateral RCC and bilateral RAS, patients with unilateral RCC and contralateral RAS, and patients with unilateral RCC and bilateral RAS. All patients underwent complete surgical excision of their tumor, and a nephron-sparing approach was utilized in 88%. Eight patients underwent simultaneous partial or radical nephrectomy and surgical renal revascularization with excellent cancer-free survival and maintenance of renal function in all but one patient, who ultimately required dialysis. In recent years, improved endovascular management of RAS has increased the number of therapeutic options available for the management of patients with RCC and coexisting renal artery disease (31).

Nephron-Sparing Surgery for Advanced Renal Cell Carcinoma

NSS in patients with locally advanced or metastatic disease is primarily indicated to avoid rendering the patient anephric and in need of renal replacement therapy, and to obtain tissue for adoptive immunotherapy protocols. Under these circumstances, it is possible to provide symptomatic relief for locally advanced disease and, in some cases, to aggressively resect all clinically evident tumor while maintaining acceptable renal function. Few studies have examined the role of partial nephrectomy in these selected circumstances. Angermeier et al. reviewed 9 patients who underwent partial nephrectomy for tumor with venous involvement in a solitary kidney (32). Although all cases were technically successful and renal function was preserved, many patients developed local or distant metastasis. Krishnamurthi et al. reviewed the clinical outcome of 15 patients with metastatic RCC who underwent NSS and surgical or systemic treatment of metastases (33). All cases were technically successful, and the need for renal replacement therapy was obviated in all but 1 patient. In patients with metachronous metastases in a solitary kidney, death from disease occurred later than in patients with synchronous lesions resected from the kidney and other soft tissues. Although these preliminary data are from highly selected patient populations, they suggest that partial nephrectomy can occasionally provide effective treatment of patients with locally advanced or completely resected metastatic RCC.

References

1. Licht MR, Novick AC. Nephron-sparing surgery for renal cell carcinoma. *J Urol* 1993;149:1–7.
2. Spencer WF, Novick AC, Montie JE, et al. Surgical treatment of localized renal cell carcinoma in von Hippel-Lindau's disease. *J Urol* 1988;139:507–509.
3. Pertritsch PH, Rauchenwald M, Zechner O, et al. An Austrian Multicenter Study. Results after organ-preserving surgery for renal cell carcinoma. *Eur Urol* 1990;18:84–87.
4. Steinbach F, Stockle M, Hohenfellner R. Clinical experience with nephron-sparing surgery in the presence of a normal contralateral kidney. *Semin Urol Oncol* 1995;13:288–291.
5. Provert J, Tessler A, Brown J, et al. Partial nephrectomy for renal cell carcinoma indications, results and implications. *J Urol* 1991;145:472–476.
6. Butler BP, Novick AC, Miller DP, et al. Management of small unilateral renal cell carcinomas: radical versus nephron-sparing surgery. *Urology* 1995;45:34–40.
7. Moll V, Becht E, Ziegler M. Kidney preserving surgery in renal cell tumors: indications, techniques and results in 152 patients. *J Urol* 1993;150:319–323.
8. Hafez KS, Fergany AF, Novick AC. Nephron sparing surgery for localized renal cell carcinoma: impact of tumor size on patient survival, tumor recurrence and TNM staging. *J Urol* 1999;162:1930–1933.
9. Lerner SE, Hawkins CA, Blute ML, et al. Disease outcome in patients with low stage renal cell carcinoma treated with nephron sparing or radial surgery. *J Urol* 2002;167:884–889.
10. Lee CT, Katz J, Shi W, et al. Surgical management of renal tumors 4 cm or less in a contemporary cohort. *J Urol* 2000;163:730–736.
11. Campbell SC, Novick AC. Surgical technique and morbidity of elective partial nephrectomy. *Semin Urol Oncol* 1995;13:281–287.
12. Coll DM, Uzzo RG, Herts BB, et al. 3-Dimensional volume-rendered computerized tomography for preoperative evaluation and intraoperative management of patients undergoing nephron-sparing surgery. *J Urol* 1999;161:1097.
13. Campbell SC, Fichtner J, Novick AC, et al. Intraoperative evaluation of renal cell carcinoma: a prospective study of the role of ultrasonography and histopathological frozen sections. *J Urol* 1996;155:1191–1195.
14. Hafez KS, Novick AC, Campbell SC. Patterns of tumor recurrence and guidelines for follow-up after nephron-sparing surgery for sporadic renal cell carcinoma. *J Urol* 1997;157:2067–2070.
15. Campbell SC, Novick AC. Management of local recurrence following radical nephrectomy or partial nephrectomy. *Urol Clin North Am* 1994;21:593–599.
16. Lerner SE, Hawkins CA, Blute ML, et al. Disease outcome in patients with low stage renal cell carcinoma treated with nephron sparing or radical surgery. *J Urol* 1996;155:1868–1873.
17. Babalias GA, Liatsikos EN, Tsintayis A, et al. Adenocarcinoma of the kidney: nephron-sparing surgical approach vs radical nephrectomy. *J Surg Oncol* 1999;72:156–161.
18. D'Armiento M, Damiano R, Felepa B, et al. Elective conservative surgery for renal carcinoma vs radical nephrectomy: a prospective study. *Br J Urol* 1997;79:15–19.
19. Belldegrun A, Tsui KH, deKernion JB, et al. Efficacy of nephron-sparing surgery for renal cell carcinoma: analysis based on the new 1997 tumor-node metastasis staging system. *J Clin Oncol* 1999;17:2868–2875.

20. Fergany AF, Hafez KS, Novick AC. Long-term results of nephron-sparing surgery for localized renal cell carcinoma: 10-year follow-up. *J Urol* 2000; 163:442–445.

21. Bostwick DG, Murphy GP. Diagnosis and prognosis of renal cell carcinoma: highlights from an international consensus workshop. *Semin Urol Oncol* 1998;16:46–52.

22. Hafez KS, Novick AC, Butler BP. Management of small solitary unilateral renal cell carcinomas: impact of central versus peripheral tumor location. *J Urol* 1998;159:1156–1160.

23. Herr HW. Partial nephrectomy for unilateral renal carcinoma and a normal contralateral kidney: 10-year follow-up. *J Urol* 1999;161:33–34.

24. McKiernan J, Simmons R, Katz J, et al. Natural history of chronic renal insufficiency after partial and radical nephrectomy. *Urology* 2002;59: 816–820.

25. Lau WK, Blute ML, Weaver AL, et al. Matched comparison of radical nephrectomy vs nephron-sparing surgery in patients with unilateral renal cell carcinoma and a normal contralateral kidney. *Mayo Clin Proc* 2000; 75:1236–1242.

26. Christenson PJ, Craig JP, Bibro MC, et al. Cysts containing renal cell carcinoma in von Hippel-Lindau disease. *J Urol* 1982;128:798–800.

27. Goldfarb DA, Neumann HP, Penn I, et al. Results of renal transplantation in patients with renal cell carcinoma and von Hippel-Lindau disease. *Transplant* 1997;64:1726–1729.

28. Steinbach F, Novick AC, Zincke H et al, A Multicenter Study. Treatment of renal cell carcinoma in von Hippel-Lindau disease. *J Urol* 1995;153: 1812–1816.

29. Walther MM, Choyke PL, Glenn G, et al. Renal cancer in families with hereditary renal cancer: prospective analysis of a tumor size threshold for renal parenchymal sparing surgery. *J Urol* 1999;161:1475–1479.

30. Campbell SC, Novick AC, Streem SB, et al. Management of renal cell carcinoma with coexistent renal artery disease. *J Urol* 1993;150:808–813.

31. Hafez KS, Krishnamurthi V, Campbell SC, et al. Contemporary management of renal cell carcinoma with coexistent renal artery disease: update of the Cleveland clinic experience. *Urology* 2000;56:382–386.

32. Angermeier KW, Novick AC, Streem SB, et al. Nephron-sparing surgery for renal cell carcinoma with venous involvement. *J Urol* 1990;144:1352–1355.

33. Krishnamurthi V, Novick AC, Bukowski R. Nephron-sparing surgery in patients with metastatic renal cell carcinoma. *J Urol* 1996;156:36–39.

CHAPTER 47E
Management of Inherited Forms of Renal Cancer

Robert L. Grubb III, W. Marston Linehan, and McClellan M. Walther

INTRODUCTION

Renal cell carcinoma incidence has increased during the past two decades, according to Surveillance, Epidemiology and End Results data (1). Study of the molecular mechanisms of hereditary forms of renal cancer has contributed greatly to the understanding of sporadic renal cancer, as many of the molecular mechanisms in both tumor types are thought to be similar. Known hereditary renal cancer syndromes include von Hippel-Lindau (VHL), hereditary papillary renal cancer (HPRC), Birt-Hogg-Dubé (BHD), and hereditary leiomyomatosis and renal cell cancer (HLRCC). Each of these syndromes carries a varying risk of renal cancer, and most are associated with characteristic tumor histology and associated clinical abnormalities. Effective urologic management of these patients requires an understanding of the unique renal tumor biology and the extrarenal manifestations of the syndromes.

HEREDITARY RENAL CANCER

It is estimated that 4% of renal cancer cases are attributable to hereditary causes (2). Hereditary renal cancer is characterized by

several important differences from sporadic renal cancer (3,4). Whereas sporadic renal cancers occur most frequently in the 6th and 7th decades (5), hereditary renal cancers may develop as early as the 2nd decade (2). In contradistinction to sporadic tumors, hereditary tumors are frequently multifocal and bilateral (2). The distribution of hereditary tumors among the sexes tends to be more equal than in the case of sporadic renal cancer.

Study of the molecular genetics of renal cell cancer during the last decade has led to the identification of genes for several of the hereditary renal cancer syndromes. VHL is characterized by a mutation in the *VHL* gene, found on chromosome 3p25. HPRC is caused by a mutation in the *c-MET* oncogene on chromosome 7q31 (6). The gene for Birt-Hogg-Dubé, *BHD*, recently has been located on chromosome 17p11.2 (7). HLRCC is associated with mutation in the gene for the Krebs cycle enzyme, fumarate hydratase (*FH*) (8). Blood tests for germline mutations make possible presymptomatic screening of at-risk individuals.

VON HIPPEL-LINDAU

VHL is an autosomal dominantly inherited disorder that leads to the development of hemangioblastomas of the central nervous system (CNS), endolymphatic sac tumors (ELST), pancreatic cysts and tumors, pheochromocytoma, renal cysts and cancers, and cystadenomas of the epididymis and broad ligament. Renal tumors and cysts occur in 25% to 60% of patients and can be detected in patients as early as the second decade of life, although the average age of onset is 39 years (range 16–67 years) (Fig. 47E.1) (9,10). Renal cancer was historically a major cause of mortality for patients with VHL, whose life expectancy prior to widespread screening was <50 years (11). Renal cancers in VHL are uniformly of clear cell histology, usually of a low Fuhrman grade. It has been estimated that a VHL kidney involved could harbor as many as 600 microscopic clear cell renal cell cancers and up to 1,100 clear cell cystic lesions (12).

Genetic testing is available for VHL with accuracy as high as 100% in experienced labs (13). Screening for visceral manifestations (i.e., pheochromocytoma, pancreatic cysts and tumors, and renal cysts and tumors) of VHL with a computed

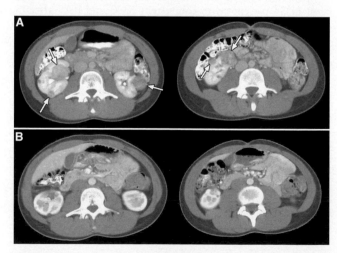

FIGURE 47E.1. von Hippel-Lindau (VHL) renal tumors before (**A**) and after partial nephrectomy (**B**). Patients affected with VHL are at risk for the development of bilateral, multifocal, multiple renal tumors (*arrows*) and cysts (**A**). Nephron-sparing surgical approaches are recommended, when technically feasible, because patients with VHL are at risk for recurrent tumor formation. Computed tomography (CT) scan of patient after undergoing staged bilateral partial nephrectomies (**B**).

tomography (CT) scan of the abdomen and pelvis often commences at the age of 18 years and may be performed annually (10). Screening intervals may be lengthened for patients with minimal disease manifestations or can be shortened in patients with active intra-abdominal lesions. Ultrasound may be used as an adjunct to CT scan or magnetic resonance imaging (MRI) of the abdomen, but does not possess adequate resolution to be relied upon as the primary screening modality. Early arterial phase contrast CT scan images have greater sensitivity for pancreatic lesions (14). Delayed cortimedullary images may help increase the number of renal tumors seen.

Management of Renal Cysts and Tumors in von Hippel-Lindau

Because of the diverse manifestations of VHL and the presence of neoplasms in multiple organ systems, multidisciplinary involvement is needed to optimize management of patients with VHL. Ideally, patients are managed by a team of ophthalmologists, otolaryngologists, neurosurgeons, urologists, and genetic counselors. Because renal cysts and tumors are the most common tumors in VHL, urologists should be aware of issues in screening for and managing extrarenal manifestations of the syndrome.

Goals of treatment of patients with VHL or other hereditary cancer syndromes should be prevention of metastatic disease, preservation of renal function, and minimization of the number of operative procedures that patients must undergo (15,16). Renal tumors in VHL, as in other hereditary renal cancer syndromes, are bilateral and multiple and can be recurrent.

Before the wide availability of CT scan, 13% to 42% of patients with VHL died of metastatic renal cell carcinoma (RCC) (16). Although VHL tumors tend to be low grade, the high historical rate of metastasis in poorly screened patients makes watchful waiting an unappealing management option. The treatment strategy of bilateral nephrectomy was developed to pre-emptively remove all tissue at risk for renal cancer. This strategy necessitates renal replacement therapy, and the 5-year survival for patients demographically similar to patients with VHL is 71% on hemodialysis and 86% with renal transplantation (17). Goldfarb et al. reviewed a multicenter experience with renal transplantation in patients with VHL; the 5-year survival in this cohort was 65% (18). Three of 32 patients in the study cohort died of metastatic disease, and two had non-cancer-related deaths.

Because of the high morbidity and mortality associated with renal replacement therapy, a strategy has been developed for following patients closely with serial imaging until the largest tumor is 3 cm in diameter before recommending intervention, regardless of the number or pattern of tumors (15,16). The 3-cm size threshold was selected because of the low reported occurrence of metastases in patients with sporadic renal tumors <3 cm (19,20).

At-risk patients are screened with serial abdominal CT scans and are advised to undergo nephron-sparing surgery when the largest tumor reaches 3 cm. The efficacy of nephron-sparing approaches has been demonstrated for sporadic tumors <4 cm (20). Nephron-sparing approaches for patients with VHL have also been advocated by multiple authors (21–23). Novick and Streem reported long-term follow-up of 9 patients with VHL with bilateral renal involvement (24). One patient died of metastatic disease at 43 months. One patient had not experienced a recurrence at >5 years of follow-up. Of the remaining 7 patients (mean follow-up of 88 months), 6 had required reoperation for local tumor recurrence, but only 3 retained native functioning renal parenchyma (24). Because of the high rate of local recurrence and because only 3 out of 9 patients retained native renal function,

the authors concluded that the results of nephron-sparing approaches were less satisfactory in patients with VHL than in patients with sporadic RCC. The high local recurrence rate found by these researchers may be explained by studies predicting as many as 600 microscopic renal cell tumors in VHL kidneys (12). Other groups have recommended conservative treatment of patients with VHL with low-stage bilateral RCC, while noting that patients with VHL with bilateral higher stage disease may be better served with bilateral radical nephrectomy and subsequent renal replacement therapy (25). In addition to higher local recurrence rates, patients with VHL undergoing nephron-sparing surgery had lower disease-specific survival rates when compared with patients with sporadic renal cell cancer (24–27). Many of the patients in these studies had larger tumors and tumors of higher grade.

More recently, there have been reports of the results of managing a cohort of patients with VHL using the strategy of waiting until the largest tumor in a renal unit reached 3 cm in CT scan diameter before recommending intervention (16,28). Outcomes of 108 patients with VHL and whose renal tumors were <3 cm at the time of diagnosis were compared with outcomes of a group of 73 patients with VHL and tumors >3 cm at the time of diagnosis. Median follow-up for both groups was >3 years. In the group of patients with tumors <3 cm at diagnosis, no patients developed metastatic disease and no patients required hemodialysis or transplantation. Thirty-four percent of these patients (37/108) were managed with observation alone, because they did not develop tumors >3 cm during the study period. Metastatic renal cancer developed in 27% (20/73) of patients with renal tumors >3 cm at the time of presentation. Patients whose renal tumors were <3 cm at presentation who subsequently required surgery because their tumors grew >3 cm were managed more frequently with nephron-sparing surgery than were those whose tumors were >3 cm at presentation (16,28). The authors concluded that the strategy of observing tumors until they reached a 3-cm threshold provided good cancer control (the patients were not necessarily cured of cancer, but metastatic disease was prevented), while preserving renal function and minimizing the number of operative procedures for each patient.

Because hereditary renal cancers tend to be bilateral, multifocal, and recurring, techniques for nephron-sparing surgery in VHL and other hereditary renal cancer syndromes are different than nephron-sparing surgery for patients with sporadic renal cancers. A technique of enucleation for hereditary renal tumors has been described (29). VHL tumors tend to have a surrounding pseudocapsule that facilitates enucleation with a negative margin. Gerotas fascia is opened, but preserved; closing Gerotas fascia and the perirenal fat around the remaining renal unit may make subsequent renal explorations less difficult. Hilar dissection should be minimized to prevent scarring that could complicate future operations unless there are deep central lesions that may require cold ischemia for resection. Once the kidney has been completely exposed, the renal capsule is incised, circumscribing the lesion. Penfield neurodissectors can be used to bluntly enucleate the lesion. Vessels can be dissected with an Adson clamp and suture ligated as they are encountered. Thrombin-soaked gelfoam can be placed into the defect and pressure held to control any venous oozing (30). Cystic lesions can be unroofed and the base fulgurated, as these may harbor RCC (31). Deep intraparenchymal simple-appearing cystic lesions are not resected.

After resection of all visible tumors and cysts, intraoperative ultrasound with color Doppler can be used to identify deep intraparenchymal solid lesions not visible on the surface and lesions that may not have been apparent on preoperative imaging (Fig. 47E.2) (32,33). The ability to remove all lesions in a renal unit is paramount to the ability to "reset the clock" for patients with hereditary cancer syndromes by finding incipient

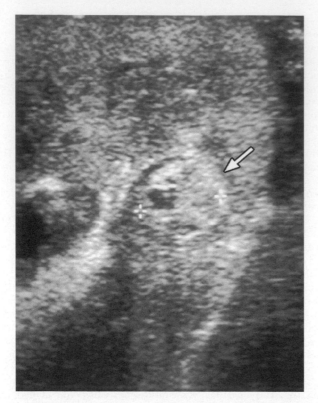

FIGURE 47E.2. Intraoperative Ultrasound during von Hippel-Lindau (VHL) kidney cancer surgery intraoperative ultrasound is an invaluable adjunct for localizing deep tumors and visualizing small tumors not seen on preoperative imaging. Tumor is shown by the arrow. Surface of the kidney is at the top of the figure.

tumors not otherwise detectable. Intraoperative ultrasound identified small [i.e., mean 1.0 cm (2 mm–4 cm)] renal cancers that were not identified by the surgeon in 25% of procedures where the technique was used (33).

Lesions that are not amenable to nephron-sparing surgery may require radical nephrectomy. In one series of 71 operations with the intent of performing nephron-sparing surgery on patients with hereditary renal cancers, 64 patients (90%) underwent partial nephrectomy and 7 (10%) required radical nephrectomy (30). To date, experience with laparoscopic techniques for nephron-sparing surgery for patients with hereditary renal cancer syndromes with multiple renal masses is limited, but the evolution of laparoscopic skills and improved equipment and hemostatic agents may make this more feasible in the near future (34).

Ablative technologies such as cryotherapy and radiofrequency ablation (RFA) have been explored as alternatives to extirpative surgery to minimize the morbidity of managing patients with hereditary renal cancer syndromes. Percutaneous cryoablation with MRI guidance has been used to treat renal tumors in 5 patients with VHL (35). Shingleton et al. concluded that initial success with percutaneous cryoablation may allow patients with VHL to avoid multiple open surgical procedures. No comment was made on size criterion, but 50% of tumors >3 cm required retreatment (35).

RFA is another minimally invasive technique that has been used to treat patients with VHL with renal tumors. Procedures have been performed both percutaneously and with laparoscopic assistance (36,37). Hwang et al. described a series of 24 lesions in patients with VHL and HPRC treated with percutaneous RFA (37). The median size of the treated lesions was 2.26 cm. Ninety-six percent (23 out of 24) of tumors were successfully treated on the basis of change in lesion size and

CT scan enhancement characteristics. Complications included gross hematuria and the development of a ureteropelvic junction obstruction after ablation of a tumor, requiring open surgical repair (37). Other institutions have reported similar success rates in treating patients with VHL and renal masses. Farrell et al. also have reported excellent initial results of RFA treatment of patients with small renal masses, including several patients with VHL. The authors reported intraoperative sonographically guided RFA treatment of four tumors in a single renal unit in one patient with VHL (38). More experience and longer-term follow-up is needed to determine the role of ablative therapies such as cryoablation and RFA in the management of patients with VHL and other hereditary renal cancer syndromes.

HEREDITARY PAPILLARY RENAL CELL CANCER

HPRC was initially described by Zbar et al. in 1994 (6). The clinical syndrome is marked by the predisposition of patients to form multifocal, bilateral renal tumors of papillary type I pathology (Fig. 47E.3) (39). The tumors may occur later than in other hereditary renal cancer syndromes, with onset in the 4th, 5th and 6th decades of life; however, HPRC renal tumors have been detected in the 2nd decade (16,40). There does not appear to be associated nonrenal manifestations of HPRC, unlike there are for other hereditary renal cancer syndromes.

It is recommended that patients with HRPC be screened at regular intervals with contrast-enhanced abdominal CT scan. The renal tumors in HPRC tend to be *hypo*vascular and, as a result, may have minimal CT scan enhancement [10 to 15 Hounsfield units (HU)] after contrast administration (Fig. 47E.4A, 47E.4B) (14,41). Ultrasound, which can be useful in further characterizing renal masses in other hereditary renal cancer syndromes, may miss small (<3 cm) HPRC renal lesions because they are often isoechoic (41).

Managing Renal Tumors in Hereditary Papillary Renal Cancer

Because renal tumors in HPRC are multifocal and bilateral like renal tumors in VHL, similar management strategies are

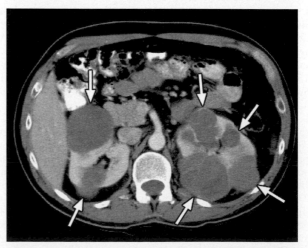

FIGURE 47E.3. Hereditary papillary renal carcinoma (HPRC): Patients with type I HPRC are at risk for the development of bilateral, multifocal type I papillary renal carcinoma (*shown by arrows*). Nephron-sparing surgery is recommended when the tumors reach the 3-cm threshold.

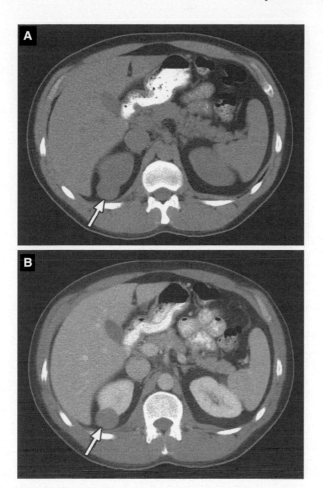

FIGURE 47E.4. Hereditary papillary renal cancer tumors characteristically demonstrate hypoenhancement on computed tomography (CT) scan. Precontrast images of an HPRC tumor (*shown by arrows*) measure 31 Hounsfield units (HU) (**A**); after contrast administration, the lesion enhances only to 43 HU (**B**). These hypoenhancing lesions can be mistakenly interpreted as renal cysts.

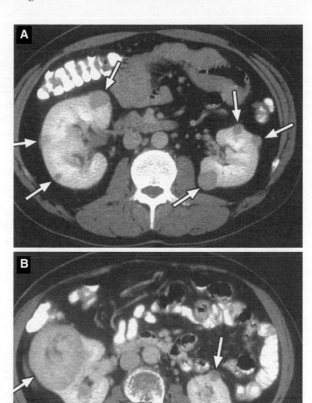

FIGURE 47E.5. Birt-Hogg-Dubé (BHD)–associated renal tumors: Patients with chromophobe renal carcinoma and oncocytoma who have BHD are at risk to develop bilateral, multifocal renal chromophobe and oncocytic renal carcinoma and oncocytoma (**A,B**). Renal tumors (*shown by arrows*) may develop in 15% to 30% of patients with BHD. Partial nephrectomy is recommended, when possible, in the management of BHD renal tumors.

applied. The strategy of observation until the largest tumor in any renal unit reaches 3 cm, at which stage patients are recommended to undergo surgery, has been reported for patients with HPRC (16). Forty-three percent of patients had tumors <3 cm at initial presentation. Two of these patients had undergone previous renal surgery. In 14 patients in the study who underwent surgery, 6 partial and 15 radical nephrectomies were performed. Fifteen percent (2 out of 13) of the patients who presented with tumors >3 cm presented with metastatic disease (tumor sizes 7 and 15 cm). No patients managed under this strategy with tumors <3 cm at presentation had metastatic disease in the follow-up period (16).

BIRT-HOGG-DUBÉ

BHD is an autosomal dominant disorder initially characterized by its characteristic cutaneous lesion, the fibrofolliculoma. Reported internal manifestations of BHD include air-filled lung cysts, spontaneous pneumothorax (42), and renal tumors (43,44).

Zbar et al. reported on the findings of families identified as having BHD by dermatologic criteria. Lung cysts, spontaneous pneumothorax, and solid renal tumors were associated with BHD (45). Renal tumors were found in 15% of patients with BHD (Fig. 47E.5).

VHL and HPRC are hereditary syndromes associated with renal cancers of specific histologies. In contrast, BHD predisposes to a variety of renal tumor histologic types (46). The predominant renal lesion found in a review of 130 tumors from 30 patients with BHD was the hybrid oncocytic tumor, which contains a mixture of oncocytes and chromophobe cells arranged in patterns reminiscent of oncocytoma in some parts and chromophobe RCC in others. Other tumors found in patients with BHD include chromophobe (34%), clear cell (9%), oncocytoma (5%), and papillary (2%) types (46).

Patients with the clinical features of BHD (i.e., characteristic skin lesions, history of spontaneous pneumothorax or pulmonary cysts, and multiple bilateral renal tumors) and at-risk patients can now be diagnosed by germline genetic testing. Renal tumors can be seen as early as the 4th decade; annual renal screening of affected or at-risk patients often begins at the age of 20 with ultrasound or contrast-enhanced CT scan (44). Because of the risk of lung cysts and spontaneous pneumothorax, a baseline high-resolution CT scan of the chest is obtained in affected or at-risk patients, and screening chest CT scan is obtained at regular intervals. Renal tumors are typically solid and are uniformly enhancing; cysts are rare, which may help differentiate BHD from VHL (14). Imaging cannot reliably distinguish the differing histologic types of RCC in the BHD spectrum; therefore, all tumors must be presupposed to be potentially malignant.

Management of Renal Tumors in Birt-Hogg-Dubé

Because BHD is a newly described syndrome, little has been written about the management of these patients. Several case reports have described renal tumors in patients with BHD (43,47). Toro et al. screened 152 patients at risk for BHD and found renal tumors in 7 of 13 BHD-affected patients (44). Published data concerning the strategy of observing renal tumors until the largest tumor reaches 3 cm in size in BHD is limited. Early results, however, suggest that this strategy may be efficacious for tumors in BHD (30,48).

HEREDITARY LEIOMYOMATOSIS RENAL CELL CARCINOMA

Individuals affected with hereditary leiomyomatosis renal cell carcinoma (HLRCC) are at risk to develop multiple cutaneous leiomyomas (occasionally painful, firm, skin-colored to light brown papules found on the trunk and extremities), uterine leiomyomas (women), and type II papillary renal cancer (49–51).

Imaging patients at risk for HLRCC focuses on the kidneys and uterus. CT scanning is considered the first-line imaging modality (14). Renal tumors in HLRCC, as in HPRC, may be hypovascular with subtle CT scan contrast enhancement. Close attention is paid to potential sites of metastatic disease, even with small tumors. Multidisciplinary management between medical geneticists, urologists, dermatologists, and gynecologic surgeons can be helpful in accurately cataloging the manifestations of the syndrome.

Managing Renal Tumors in Hereditary Leiomyomatosis and Renal Cell Cancer

Kiuru et al. first reported the link between cutaneous and uterine leiomyomas and renal cancer (49). Launonen et al. found renal tumors in 31% (6 out of 19) of patients in two families with HLRCC (50). Toro et al. found 13 patients with renal tumors from 95 mutational carriers evaluated (14%) (51). Median ages of onset in the two series were 36 and 44 years, with tumors presenting as early as 23 years (50,51). HLRCC renal pathology has most commonly been classified as papillary, type II. Tumors with features of collecting duct carcinoma have been seen in a few patients (51). These tumors have been high grade, in contrast to VHL, HPRC, and BHD, in which lower nuclear grades are the norm.

In the report of Launonen et al. all 6 patients with renal tumors had metastatic disease at presentation and all of the patients had died of the disease at the time of the study (50). Other researchers have reported similarly aggressive behavior (51). Thirty-one percent (4 out of 13) of patients were diagnosed with renal tumors before the age of 30. Seventy percent (9 out of 13) of patients died of metastatic disease within 5 years of diagnosis (51). HLRCC renal tumors may represent a potentially much more aggressive type of hereditary renal cancer than VHL, HPRC, or BHD (Fig. 47E.6). Conservative management strategies that have been utilized for other forms of hereditary renal cancer may not be prudent for HLRCC. Early surgical intervention is recommended when HLRCC-associated renal tumors are detected, but longer-term follow-up and prospective analysis is required before a definitive management strategy is developed.

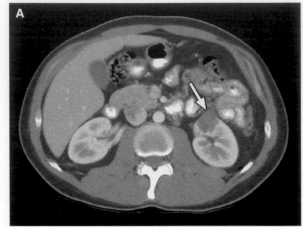

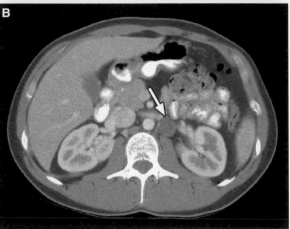

FIGURE 47E.6. Hereditary leiomyomatosis renal cell carcinoma (HLRCC): Patients with type II papillary renal carcinoma who have HLRCC are at risk for the development of an aggressive form of type 2 papillary renal carcinoma. Pictured here is the computed tomography (CT) scan of a 32-year-old man affected with HLRCC who was found on preclinical screening to have a small (2.3 cm) renal tumor (*shown by arrow*) (**A**). Nodal metastasis (*shown by arrow*) was detected at presentation in the same patient (**B**). Early surgical intervention is recommended for kidney cancer in patients with HLRCC.

CONCLUSION

Advances in the last two decades have expanded our understanding of the role of genetics in renal cancer. At least four distinct syndromes associated with increased risk of renal cancer have been identified, including VHL, HPRC, BHD, and HLRCC. Multidisciplinary teams can aid in managing the extrarenal manifestations of the syndromes. By establishing a 3-cm size threshold for recommending intervention in patients with VHL, HPRC, and BHD, the number of renal surgeries can be minimized and the need for renal replacement obviated, with good cancer control. The success of this type of strategy is predicated on effective diagnosis and diligent screening. More experience with minimally invasive modalities such as laparoscopic partial nephrectomy and tissue ablative procedures such as cryotherapy or RFA is needed before definitive recommendations can be made regarding their role in managing patients with hereditary renal cancer syndromes. Because of the potentially more aggressive biologic behavior of HLRCC renal tumors, early surgical treatment of HLRCC-associated renal tumors is recommended.

References

1. Chow WH, Devesa SS, Warren JL, et al. Rising incidence of renal cell cancer in the United States. *JAMA* 1999;281:1628–1631.
2. Choyke PL, Glenn GM, Walther MM, et al. Hereditary renal cancers. *Radiology* 2003;226:33–46.
3. Zbar B. Inherited epithelial tumors of the kidney: old and new diseases. *Semin Cancer Biol* 2000;10:313–318.
4. Phillips JL, Pavlovich CP, Walther M, et al. The genetic basis of renal epithelial tumors: advances in research and its impact on prognosis and therapy. *Curr Opin Urol* 2001;11:463–469.
5. Motzer RJ, Bander NH, Nanus DM. Renal-cell carcinoma. *N Engl J Med* 1996;335:865–875.
6. Zbar B, Tory K, Merino M, et al. Hereditary papillary renal cell carcinoma. *J Urol* 1994;151:561–566.
7. Nickerson ML, Warren MB, Toro JR, et al. Mutations in a novel gene lead to kidney tumors, lung wall defects, and benign tumors of the hair follicle in patients with the Birt-Hogg-Dubé syndrome. *Cancer Cell* 2002;2:157–164.
8. Tomlinson IP, Alam NA, Rowan AJ, et al. Germline mutations in FH predispose to dominantly inherited uterine fibroids, skin leiomyomata and papillary renal cell cancer. *Nat Genet* 2002;30:406–410.
9. Maher ER, Yates JR, Harries R, et al. Clinical features and natural history of von Hippel-Lindau disease. *Q J Med* 1990;77:1151–1163.
10. Choyke PL, Glenn GM, Walther MM, et al. von Hippel-Lindau disease: genetic, clinical, and imaging features. *Radiology* 1995;194:629–642.
11. Lonser RR, Glenn GM, Walther MM, et al. von Hippel-Lindau disease. *Lancet* 2003;361:2059–2067.
12. Walther MM, Lubensky IA, Venzon D, et al. Prevalence of microscopic lesions in grossly normal renal parenchyma from patients with von Hippel-Lindau disease, sporadic renal cell carcinoma and no renal disease: clinical implications. *J Urol* 1995;154:2010–2014.
13. Stolle C, Glenn G, Zbar B, et al. Improved detection of germline mutations in the von Hippel-Lindau disease tumor suppressor gene. *Hum Mutat* 1998;12:417–423.
14. Choyke PL. Imaging of hereditary renal cancer. *Radiol Clin North Am* 2003;41:1037–1051.
15. Walther MM, Choyke PL, Weiss G, et al. Parenchymal sparing surgery in patients with hereditary renal cell carcinoma. *J Urol* 1995;153:913–916.
16. Walther MM, Choyke PL, Glenn G, et al. Renal cancer in families with hereditary renal cancer: prospective analysis of a tumor size threshold for renal parenchymal sparing surgery. *J Urol* 1999;161:1475–1479.
17. United States Renal Data System: *1997 Annual data report.* Washington, DC: U.S. Department of Health and Human Services, 1997.
18. Goldfarb DA, Neumann HP, Penn I, et al. Results of renal transplantation in patients with renal cell carcinoma and von Hippel-Lindau disease. *Transplantation* 1997;64:1726–1729.
19. Butler BP, Novick AC, Miller DP, et al. Management of small unilateral renal cell carcinomas: radical versus nephron-sparing surgery. *Urology* 1995;45:34–40.
20. Lerner SE, Hawkins CA, Blute ML, et al. Disease outcome in patients with low stage renal cell carcinoma treated with nephron sparing or radical surgery. *J Urol* 1996;155:1868–1873.
21. Levine E, Weigel JW. Collins DL diagnosis and management of asymptomatic renal cell carcinomas in von Hippel-Lindau syndrome. *Urology* 1983;21:146–150.
22. Loughlin KR, Gittes RF. Urological management of patients with von Hippel-Lindau's disease. *J Urol* 1986;136:789–791.
23. Spencer WF, Novick AC, Montie JE, et al. Surgical treatment of localized renal cell carcinoma in von Hippel-Lindau's disease. *J Urol* 1988;139:507–509.
24. Novick AC, Streem SB. Long-term follow-up after nephron sparing surgery for renal cell carcinoma in von Hippel-Lindau disease. *J Urol* 1992;147:1488–1490.
25. Frydenberg M, Malek RS, Zincke H. Conservative renal surgery for renal cell carcinoma in von Hippel-Lindau's disease. *J Urol* 1993;149:461–464.
26. Lund GO, Fallon B, Curtis MA, et al. Conservative surgical therapy of localized renal cell carcinoma in von Hippel-Lindau disease. *Cancer* 1994;74:2541–2545.
27. Steinbach F, Novick AC, Zincke H, et al. Treatment of renal cell carcinoma in von Hippel-Lindau disease: a multicenter study. *J Urol* 1995;153:1812–1816.
28. Duffey BG, Choyke PL, Glenn G, et al. The relationship between renal tumor size and metastases in patients with von Hippel-Lindau disease. *J Urol* 2004;172:63–65.
29. Walther MM, Thompson N, Linehan W. Enucleation procedures in patients with multiple hereditary renal tumors. *World J Urol* 1995;13:248–250.
30. Herring JC, Enquist EG, Chernoff A, et al. Parenchymal sparing surgery in patients with hereditary renal cell carcinoma: 10-year experience. *J Urol* 2001;165:777–781.
31. Poston CD, Jaffe GS, Lubensky IA, et al. Characterization of the renal pathology of a familial form of renal cell carcinoma associated with von Hippel-Lindau disease: clinical and molecular genetic implications. *J Urol* 1995;153:22–26.
32. Walther MM, Choyke PL, Hayes W, et al. Evaluation of color Doppler intraoperative ultrasound in parenchymal sparing renal surgery. *J Urol* 1994;152:1984–1987.
33. Choyke PL, Pavlovich CP, Daryanani KD, et al. Intraoperative ultrasound during renal parenchymal sparing surgery for hereditary renal cancers: a 10-year experience. *J Urol* 2001;165:397–400.
34. Lee Christopher S, Grubb R, Franks ME, et al. Analysis of laparoscopic partial nephrectomy outcomes for patients with familial renal cell carcinoma versus sporadic renal tumors. *J Urol* 2004;171:A1303, 343.
35. Shingleton WB, Sewell PE Jr. Percutaneous renal cryoablation of renal tumors in patients with von Hippel-Lindau disease. *J Urol* 2002;167:1268–1270.
36. Pavlovich CP, Walther MM, Choyke PL, et al. Percutaneous radio frequency ablation of small renal tumors: initial results. *J Urol* 2002;167:10–15.
37. Hwang JJ, Walther MM, Pautler SE, et al. Radio frequency ablation of small renal tumors: intermediate results. *J Urol* 2004;171:1814–1818.
38. Farrell MA, Charboneau WJ, DiMarco DS, et al. Imaging-guided radiofrequency ablation of solid renal tumors. *AJR Am J Roentgenol* 2003;180:1509–1513.
39. Schmidt L, Junker K, Weirich G, et al. Two North American families with hereditary papillary renal carcinoma and identical novel mutations in the MET proto-oncogene. *Cancer Res* 1998;58:1719–1722.
40. Linehan WM, Walther MM, Zbar B. The genetic basis of cancer of the kidney. *J Urol* 2003;170:2163–2172.
41. Choyke PL, Walther MM, Glenn GM, et al. Imaging features of hereditary papillary renal cancers. *J Comput Assist Tomogr* 1997;21:737–741.
42. Binet O, Robin J, Vicart M, et al. Fibromes perifolliculaires, polypose coliqe familiale, pneumothorax spontanes familiaux. *Ann Dermatol Venereol* 1986;113:928–930.
43. Roth JS, Rabinowitz AD, Benson M, et al. Bilateral renal cell carcinoma in the Birt-Hogg-Dubé syndrome. *J Am Acad Dermatol* 1993;29:1055–1056.
44. Toro JR, Glenn G, Duray P, et al. Birt-Hogg-Dubé syndrome: a novel marker of kidney neoplasia. *Arch Dermatol* 1999;135:1195–1202.
45. Zbar B, Alvord WG, Glenn G, et al. Risk of renal and colonic neoplasms and spontaneous pneumothorax in the Birt-Hogg-Dubé syndrome. *Cancer Epidemiol Biomarkers Prev* 2002;11:393–400.
46. Pavlovich CP, Walther MM, Eyler RA, et al. Renal tumors in the Birt-Hogg-Dubé syndrome. *Am J Surg Pathol* 2002;26:1542–1552.
47. Durrani OH, Ng L, Bihrle W III. Chromophobe renal cell carcinoma in a patient with the Birt-Hogg-Dubé syndrome. *J Urol* 2002;168:1484, 1485.
48. Grubb R, Perlmutter M, Pavlovich CP, et al. Analysis of 3 cm tumor size threshold for renal parenchymal-sparing surgery in Birt-Hogg-Dubé syndrome. *J Urol* 2003;169:ADP34, 347.
49. Kiuru M, Launonen V, Hietala M, et al. Familial cutaneous leiomyomatosis is a two-hit condition associated with renal cell cancer of characteristic histopathology. *Am J Pathol* 2001;159:825–829.
50. Launonen V, Vierimaa O, Kiuru M, et al. Inherited susceptibility to uterine leiomyomas and renal cell cancer. *Proc Natl Acad Sci U S A* 2001;98:3387–3392.
51. Toro JR, Nickerson ML, Wei MH, et al. Mutations in the fumarate hydratase gene cause hereditary leiomyomatosis and renal cell cancer in families in North America. *Am J Hum Genet* 2003;73:95–106.

CHAPTER 47F

Management of Localized Renal Cell Carcinoma: Minimally Invasive Nephron-Sparing Treatment Options

Sidney C. Abreu, Antonio Finelli, and Inderbir S. Gill

INTRODUCTION

The widespread use of modern imaging techniques has resulted in an increased detection of incidental renal tumors. These tumors are usually small and generally have a favorable biologic behavior, including a slow growth rate and a low incidence of local recurrence and metastasis. Moreover, these incidental renal tumors have a 22% chance of being benign on final

TABLE 47F.1

PUBLISHED SERIES OF LAPAROSCOPIC PARTIAL NEPHRECTOMY WITH AT LEAST 10 PATIENTS TREATED

Reference	Number of pts.	Mean tumor size	Hilar control	Number of pelvicalyceal repairs	Hemostasis	Mean EBL (mL)	Mean O.R. time (hr)	Mean hospital stay	Number of urine leak cases (%)	Number of complications (%)	Follow-up (mo)
Janetschek et al. (3)	25	1.9	No	0	Bipolar, argon beam, glue	287	2.7	5.8	0	3 (12)	22.2
Harmon et al. (4)[a]	15	2.3	No	3	Argon beam, bolster	368	2.8	2.6	0	0	8
Rassweiler et al. (5)[a]	53	2.3	—	—	Harmonic, bipolar, argon beam, Nd:YAG	725	3.2	5.4	5 (9.4)	10 (19)	24
Gill et al. (9)	100	2.8	Yes (91)	64	Suture over bolsters	125	3	2.0	3 (3)	21 (21)	18
Guillonneau et al. (6)	28	1.9 / 2.5	No (12) / Yes (16)	0 / 11	Bipolar, harmonic Suture over bolsters	708 / 270	3.0 / 2.0	4.7 / 4.7	0 / 0	3 (25) / 3 (19)	12.2 / 1.2
Kim et al. (7)	79	2.5	Yes (52)	—	Suture over bolsters	391	3.0	2.8	2 (2.5)	12 (15)	—
Simon et al. (8)	19	2.1	No	0	Harmonic, Tissue Link	120	2.2	2.2	0	4 (21)	8.2

pts, patients; EBL, estimated blood loss; O.R., operation room; Nd: Yag, Neodinium: yttrium aluminum garnate.
[a]Multi-institutional reports.
From: Gill IS. Minimally invasive nephron-sparing surgery. *Urol Clin North Am* 2003;30:551–579, with permission.

pathologic analysis (1). On the basis of these characteristics, there has been a change in the management of these small tumors, with a definite trend away from radical nephrectomy toward nephron-conserving surgery.

In the last decade, several minimally invasive therapy options for nephron-sparing surgery have been devised in an attempt to minimize operative morbidity while achieving comparable cancer control and preserving kidney function. These minimally invasive procedures comprise (a) tumor excision (laparoscopic partial nephrectomy), which aims to duplicate established open partial nephrectomy; (b) probe-ablative techniques [cryoablation, radiofrequency ablation (RFA)]; and (c) extracorporeal techniques [high-intensity focused ultrasound (HIFU), photon irradiation], which employ noninvasive energy sources. In this chapter, we discuss the current status of minimally invasive nephron-sparing surgery (NSS).

LAPAROSCOPIC PARTIAL NEPHRECTOMY

Compared to radical nephrectomy, laparoscopic partial nephrectomy is a considerably more technically challenging procedure mainly because of the technical difficulty in securing renal hypothermia, renal parenchymal hemostasis, pelvicalyceal reconstruction, and parenchymal renorrhaphy by pure laparoscopic techniques. However, ongoing advances in laparoscopic techniques and operator skills have allowed the development of a reliable technique of laparoscopic partial nephrectomy, which aims to replicate the technical steps established for open partial nephrectomy (2). As a result, laparoscopic partial nephrectomy is emerging as an attractive, minimally invasive nephron-sparing option at select institutions. The worldwide experience with laparoscopic partial nephrectomy is summarized in Table 47F.1 (3–9).

Indications and Contraindications

Initially, laparoscopic partial nephrectomy was reserved for only the select patient with favorably located, small, peripheral, superficial, and exophytic tumor (10–12). With experience, we are carefully expanding the indications to select patients with more complex tumors: tumor invading deeply into the parenchyma up to the collecting system or renal sinus, completely intrarenal tumor, tumor abutting the renal hilum, tumor in a solitary kidney, or tumor that is substantial enough to require heminephrectomy. Laparoscopic partial nephrectomy for these complex tumors is indicated in the setting of compromised or threatened global nephron mass wherein nephron preservation is an important concern. In 2004, our absolute contraindications for laparoscopic partial nephrectomy included renal vein thrombus, or a midpolar to interpolar completely intrarenal central tumor (13). Morbid obesity and a history of prior ipsilateral renal surgery may prohibitively increase the technical complexity of the procedure and should be considered a relative contraindication for laparoscopic partial nephrectomy at this time. The patient should not be on any anticoagulant medications.

Surgical Technique

Laparoscopic partial nephrectomy is preferably performed transperitoneally. However, posterior or posteromedially located tumors may be better approached retroperitoneoscopically. Three-dimensional computed tomography (CT) scan is the preferred preoperative imaging study, which provides the

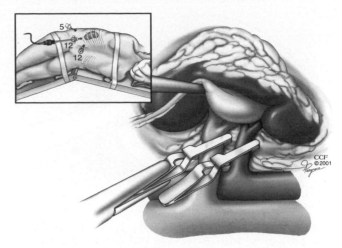

FIGURE 47F.1. Retroperitoneal laparoscopic partial nephrectomy. Because of the limited working space, the renal vein and artery were initially isolated and controlled with laparoscopic bulldog clamps. (From Gill IS, Desai MM, Kaouk JH, et al. Laparoscopic partial nephrectomy for renal tumor: Duplicating open surgical techniques. *J Urol* 2002;167:469–475, with permission.)

necessary information about tumor size, location, parenchymal infiltration, proximity to renal sinus and renal hilum, and the number and location of renal vessels. An open-ended 5 French (F) ureteral catheter is inserted cystoscopically up to the renal pelvis.

The basic operative strategy involves preparation of the renal hilum for cross-clamping, followed by mobilization of the kidney and isolation of the tumor (2). In our early experience, laparoscopic bulldog clamps were used to individually occlude the renal artery and vein (Fig. 47F.1). However, it soon became obvious that current laparoscopic bulldog clamps have somewhat suboptimal and inconsistent occlusive strength and may result in intraoperative hemorrhage caused by inadequate occlusion, especially in the setting of atherosclerotic disease in the renal artery. In contrast, the laparoscopic Satinsky clamp is inherently more reliable for renal hilum clamping (Fig. 47F.2). As such, our current routine is to employ a Satinsky clamp to occlude the renal hilum *en bloc* for either the transperitoneal or retroperitoneal approach. On occasion, the restricted working space in the retroperitoneum

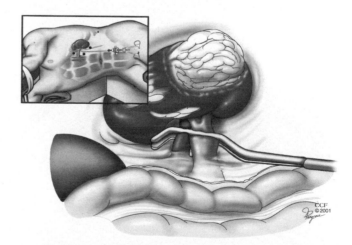

FIGURE 47F.2. Transperitoneal laparoscopic partial nephrectomy: A laparoscopic Satinsky clamp is used to clamp the hilum en bloc. (From Gill IS, Desai MM, Kaouk JH, et al. Laparoscopic partial nephrectomy for renal tumor: Duplicating open surgical techniques. *J Urol* 2002;167:469–475, with permission.)

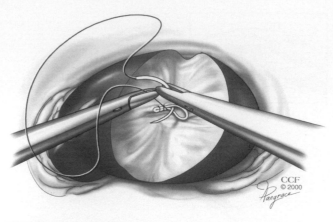

FIGURE 47F.3. Free-hand intracorporeal laparoscopic suture repair of the pelvicalyceal defect. (From Desai MM, Gill IS, Kaouk JH, et al. Laparoscopic partial nephrectomy with suture repair of the pelvicaliceal system. *Urology* 2003;61:99–104, with permission.)

may make the use of a Satinsky clamp somewhat awkward. Development of more reliable bulldog clamps similar to those available for open surgery would help avoid this problem. Laparoscopic ultrasonography (US) precisely delineates tumor size, intraparenchymal extension, and distance from renal sinus, and it also evaluates any preoperatively unsuspected secondary satellite renal masses. An adequate margin of normal renal parenchyma is scored circumferentially around the tumor under sonographic guidance. The hilum is clamped, and the tumor is excised with cold scissors in a clear, bloodless field. Retrograde injection of dilute indigo carmine through the preoperatively placed ureteral catheter identifies any pelvicalyceal entry, which is precisely suture-repaired by intracorporeal laparoscopic techniques (Fig. 47F.3) (14). Polascik et al. (15) compared the incidence of urinary fistulae with and without using a ureteral catheter for retrograde injection of methylene blue during open partial nephrectomy. Urinary fistula occurred in 21% of patients in whom methylene blue was not used compared to 0% in patients in whom retrograde methylene blue injection was employed routinely. Figure-of-eight sutures are specifically placed at the site of visible transected intrarenal vessels in the partial nephrectomy bed. Finally, the renal parenchyma is reconstructed using Vicryl suture over a prefashioned Surgicel bolster to complete a hemostatic renorrhaphy (Fig. 47F.4). We use Hem-o-Lok clips (Weck Closure

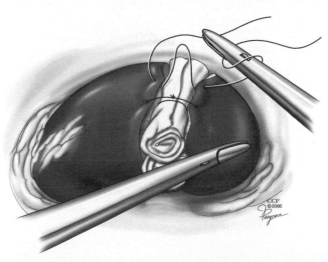

FIGURE 47F.4. Renal parenchymal repair over bolsters. (From Gill IS, Desai MM, Kaouk JH, et al. Laparoscopic partial nephrectomy for renal tumor: duplicating open surgical techniques. *J Urol* 2002;167: 469–475, with permission.)

System, research triangle park, NC) to secure the suture on either side of the renal parenchyma and employ simple interrupted stitches. Recently, the biologic hemostatic gelatin matrix-thrombin tissue sealant FloSeal (Baxter, Deerfield, IL) has been incorporated as an important hemostatic adjunct during renorrhaphy. A Jackson-Pratt drain is placed in all patients undergoing pelvicalyceal repair or if there is any concern of hemostasis.

Renal Hilar Clamping

Transient hilar clamping is an important prerequisite for a technically superior laparoscopic partial nephrectomy. Nonetheless, a small, completely exophytic tumor may be resected without hilar control. Recently, Guillonneau et al. compared the outcomes of laparoscopic partial nephrectomy with hilar clamping (group I, 12 patients) and without hilar clamping (group II, 16 patients) (6). Mean laparoscopic operating time was 179 minutes in group I compared to 121 minutes in group II ($P = .004$). A significantly higher intraoperative blood loss was reported in the patients without hilar clamping (708 ± 569 mL vs. 270 ± 281 mL, $P = .014$). Three patients in group I and two patients in group II required blood transfusion. Surgical margins were negative in all specimens. The authors acknowledge that bipolar cautery or ultrasonic shears may provide hemostasis without renal vascular control. However, these modalities of hemostasis char the tissue, resulting in poor visualization of tumor margins. The authors highlighted that the main advantage of renal vascular clamping is the quality of visualization of the renal parenchyma that facilitates accurate tumor excision.

Laparoscopic Renal Hypothermia

Target hypothermic temperature of 15°C or less offers adequate renoprotection from ischemic insult. During open partial nephrectomy, surface cooling of the kidney with iceslush is the technique of choice for achieving the desired core hypothermia. In the minimally invasive realm, three techniques of achieving renal hypothermia have been described: surface cooling with ice slush, intraarterial perfusion, and retrograde perfusion of the calyceal system. We recently described the technique of intracorporeal ice slush renal hypothermia for laparoscopic partial nephrectomy, which mirrors the open approach of using ice slush. Twelve selected patients with an infiltrating renal tumor underwent transperitoneal laparoscopic partial nephrectomy with hypothermia (16). Median tumor size was 3.2 cm (range, 1.5–5.5 cm), and an imperative indication for partial nephrectomy existed in 7 patients (58%), including 2 patients (17%) with a tumor in a solitary kidney. An Endocatch-II bag (US Surgical, Norwalk, CT) was placed around the mobilized kidney, and its drawstring was cinched around the intact renal hilum. The renal artery and vein were occluded *en bloc* with the Satinsky clamp. The bottom of the engaged bag was retrieved through a 12-mm port site and was opened, and then ice slush was introduced into the bag through modified 30 mL syringes whose nozzles had been cut off previously. Therefore, the entrapped kidney was completely surrounded by ice slush within the bag. After renal hypothermia was achieved, laparoscopic partial nephrectomy was performed using our standard technique. All procedures were successfully completed laparoscopically without open conversion. Median time to deploy the bag around the kidney was 7 minutes (range, 5–20 minutes), median volume of ice slush introduced was 600 mL (range, 30–750 mL), and time taken to insert the ice-slush was 4 minutes (range, 3–10 minutes). Nadir renal parenchymal temperature ranging from 5°C to 19.1°C was achieved in the

5 patients in whom thermocouple measurements were performed. Terminal renal parenchymal temperatures upon completion of partial nephrectomy, just before hilar unclamping, ranged from 19°C to 23.8°C following 43 to 48 minutes of ischemia.

Janetsheck et al. described laparoscopic partial nephrectomy in cold ischemia achieved by renal artery perfusion in 15 patients (17). The mean tumor size was 2.7 cm (range, 1.5–4 cm). Cold ischemia was achieved by continuous perfusion of Ringer lactate solution at 4°C at a rate of 50 mL/min though an angiocatheter that was passed into the main renal artery through a percutaneous femoral puncture. The procedure was performed in the operating room by an interventional radiologist to diminish the risk of catheter dislodgement. Using laparoscopic techniques, the renal hilum was dissected and the renal artery was occluded with a tourniquet, allowing tumor excision in a bloodless field. Mean operative time was 185 minutes (range 135–220 minutes). Mean ischemia time was 40 minutes (range 27–101 minutes), and renal parenchymal temperatures were 25°C. Although feasible, this technique has limitations, such as the potential for renal artery injury and thrombosis, femoral artery puncture site sequelae, catheter slippage, the need to involve an interventional radiologist, and the inability to use this technique in the presence of atherosclerotic, multiple, aberrant, or small-diameter renal arteries.

Landman et al. described renal parenchymal hypothermia using retrograde ureteral access during laparoscopic partial nephrectomy in a pig model (18). A 12/14 ureteral access sheath was advanced to the ureteropelvic junction under fluoroscopic guidance; through the access sheath, a 7.1-F pigtail catheter was also inserted. After clamping the renal artery and vein, ice-cold saline was circulated through the access sheath and drained via the 7.1-F pigtail catheter. Renal cortical and medullary parenchymal temperatures, measured using thermocouples, were noted to be 27.3°C and 21.3°C, respectively. Inadequate cortical cooling of the human kidney, which is considerably larger than the porcine kidney, is a potential drawback of this technique. Further, during laparoscopic partial nephrectomy for an infiltrating tumor, incisional entry into the collecting system occurs early on within 1 to 2 minutes of initiating tumor resection, which would lead to leakage of the transureteral cold perfusate, potentially compromising continued core hypothermia for most of the duration of surgery.

Complications of Laparoscopic Partial Nephrectomy

Ramani et al. (19) performed a thorough review of the incidence and nature of complications following laparoscopic partial nephrectomy in our first 200 patients (Ramani AP et al. submitted). The transperitoneal approach was employed in 122 patients (61%) and the retroperitoneal approach in 76 (38%). Mean tumor size on preoperative CT scan was 2.9 cm (range 0.9–10 cm). Mean depth of parenchymal invasion on intraoperative US was 1.5 cm (range 0.2–5 cm). Of the procedures, 198 (99%) were completed laparoscopically with two open conversions. Mean operation room time was 199 minutes (range 45–360 mins.), with a mean blood loss of 247 mL (range 25–1,500 mL). Blood transfusion was required in 18 patients (9%).

Thirty-nine (19.5%) patients developed urologic complications, which included renal hemorrhage (21; 10.5%), urinary leak (9 patients), inferior epigastric injury (1 patient), epididymitis (1 patient), and hematuria (1 patient). Renal parenchymal hemorrhage occurred in 21 patients (10.5%): intraoperative in 8 (4%), postoperative in 5 (2.5%), and delayed in 8 (4%). Intraoperative hemorrhage in 7 of 8 patients was due to inadequate clamping of the renal hilum: laparoscopic

bulldog clamp malfunction (four patients), laparoscopic Satinsky clamp malfunction (1 patient), unrecognized accessory renal artery that was missed intraoperatively and on preoperative 3D CT scan (2 patients). Postoperative hemorrhage before discharge occurred in 5 patients, ostensibly from the partial nephrectomy bed. In all 5 patients, complete hemostasis was achieved to the surgeon's satisfaction intraoperatively. Four of these patients had no obvious precipitating cause for the postoperative bleed and responded to conservative management and transfusions. The fifth patient was therapeutically heparinized for a pulmonary embolism, which elevated the coagulation parameters, with resultant renal bleeding. This patient underwent successful exploratory laparotomy for control of renal "oozing" on postoperative day 7. Delayed bleeding after discharge (day 6 to day 30) occurred in 8 patients. A possible precipitating cause could be identified in 3 patients: vigorous exercise (1 patient), fall (1 patient), and coagulopathy (1 patient). Treatment included transfusion in 5 patients, percutaneous selective angioembolization in 2 patients, and delayed nephrectomy in 1 patient. One patient presented with delayed hematuria and was managed with bed rest and bladder irrigation.

Nine patients developed a urine leak. Of these, 6 required placement of a double J-stent, 2 required a double J-stent plus CT scan–guided drainage of urine collection, and 1 resolved spontaneously with observation. No patient with a urine leak required operative reexploration. A total of 4 patients (2%) required at least one session of hemodialysis following surgery. One patient undergoing 65% resection of a solitary kidney for a 6.5-cm tumor developed acute renal failure postoperatively, requiring transient dialysis for 3 weeks. Two patients required transient dialysis to manage acute tubular necrosis (ATN) at days 8 and 30 following surgery.

Nonurologic complications occurred in 29 patients (14.5%). A small (<1 cm), superficial, serosal bowel incision with the port site closure needle was expeditiously repaired with a single figure-of-eight serosal stitch. A pleural injury, recognized intraoperatively, was suture repaired. Segmental ischemia of the colon occurred in one patient for unclear reasons, perhaps thromboembolic, and required exploratory laparotomy and colon resection. Other nonurologic complications included deep venous thrombosis (4 patients), wound-related complications (4 patients), atelectasis (3 patients), pneumonia (3 patients), atrial fibrillation (2 patients), pleural effusion (2 patients), gluteal compartment syndrome (1 patient), pulmonary embolism (1 patient), congestive cardiac failure (2 patients), prolonged ileus (1 patient), sepsis (2 patients), and a small splenic capsular tear managed by argon beam coagulation (1 patient).

These data attest that laparoscopic partial nephrectomy is indeed a technically complex operation that requires advanced laparoscopic skills and has potential for serious complications. Other groups have reported their experiences with laparoscopic partial nephrectomy (Table 47F.1). A multiinstitutional series from Europe of 53 patients undergoing laparoscopic partial nephrectomy reported an overall urologic complication rate of 23% (5). Hemorrhage occurred in 5 patients (10%): intraoperative (5 patients; 8%) and postoperative (1 patient; 2%). Issues of hemostasis required emergent open conversion in 2 patients (4%) and secondary radical nephrectomy in 1 patient. Urine leak occurred in 5 patients (10%), requiring J-stenting (3 patients), percutaneous nephrostomy (1 patient), and nephrectomy (1 patient). Overall, 2 kidneys (4%) were lost. In a recent review, Kim et al. (7) compared complications occurring during 35 laparoscopic radical nephrectomies and 79 laparoscopic partial nephrectomies. In the partial nephrectomy group, complications included intraoperative hemorrhage (6 patients; 7.5%), urine leak (2 patients; 2.4%), ureteral injury (1 patient), acute renal failure (1 patient), postoperative atelectasis (1 patient), and clot retention

(1 patient). One case in each group required open conversion to achieve hemostasis.

Comparison of Open and Laparoscopic Partial Nephrectomy

A recent retrospective review compared 200 patients undergoing partial nephrectomy at the Cleveland Clinic either by the laparoscopic ($n = 100$) or by the open ($n = 100$) approach (9). Median tumor size was 2.8 cm in the laparoscopic group and 3.3 cm in the open group ($P = .005$), and a solitary kidney was present in 7 and 28 patients, respectively ($P = .001$). The tumor was located centrally in 35% and 33% of cases ($P = .83$), respectively, and the indication for a partial nephrectomy was imperative in 41% and 54% of cases, respectively ($P = .001$). Comparing the laparoscopic with open groups, median surgical time was 3 hours versus 3.9 hours ($P <.001$), blood loss was 125 mL versus 250 mL ($P <.001$), and warm ischemia time was 28 minutes versus 18 minutes ($P <.001$). In the laparoscopic and open groups, the analgesic requirement was 20.2 mg morphine sulfate equivalent versus 252.5 mg ($P <.001$), hospital stay was 2 days versus 5 days ($P <.001$), and convalescence averaged 4 weeks versus 6 weeks ($P <.001$). None of the patients who were to undergo laparoscopic surgery were subjected to open surgery. The laparoscopic group had a higher incidence of intraoperative complications (5% vs. 0%; $P = .02$), including hemorrhage ($n = 3$), ureteral injury ($n = 1$), and bowel serosal injury ($n = 1$). The rate of postoperative complications was similar (9% vs. 14%; $P = .27$). Renal/urologic complications occurred in 7 patients in the laparoscopic group and 2 patients in the open group. Median preoperative serum creatinine (1.0 mg/dL vs. 1.0 mg/dL) and postoperative serum creatinine (1.0 mg/dL vs. 1.1 mg/dL) were similar ($P = .99$). Pathology confirmed renal cell carcinoma (RCC) in 75% of patients in the laparoscopic group and in 85% in the open group ($P = .003$). Parenchymal margin of resection was positive in three laparoscopic cases and in none of the open cases ($P = .11$); median width of margin was 4 mm in each group ($P = .11$). No patient in the laparoscopic group developed a local or port-site recurrence. No kidney was lost because of warm ischemic injury in this study of 200 patients.

Unique Applications of Laparoscopic Partial Nephrectomy

Laparoscopic partial nephrectomy has been applied in the setting of two or more ipsilateral synchronous tumors (20), coexisting renal artery disease (21), and concomitant *en bloc* adrenalectomy (22).

Hemostatic Aids

Although various techniques of parenchymal hemostasis have been reported (23–25), these techniques are not routinely reliable, thereby prompting us to employ intracorporeal suturing exclusively. Physical means of compressing the kidney to achieve polar hemostasis include renal parenchymal tourniquets and cable tie devices. They have been tested to achieve vascular control by circumferential compression of the renal parenchyma during a polar partial nephrectomy (26–28). Although effective in the experimental setting of a smaller porcine kidney, these devices are clinically unreliable in the larger human kidney.

Fibrin sealants have been studied for a variety of urologic applications (29). The basic mechanism of action is to facilitate the conversion of fibrinogen to fibrin, and, thereafter, the soluble fibrin monomers are cross-linked to form insoluble fibrin, which acts as a vessel sealant. Concerns with this technology include single-donor cryoprecipitate-derived fibrinogen, which does not entirely eliminate the risk of viral disease transmission, and bovine-derived thrombin (allergic reaction and potential transmission of prion diseases); these products often require two components to be mixed and/or sequentially applied, placing further demands on the surgeon in a laparoscopic forum.

A more readily applicable and user-friendly sealant, FloSeal, has been incorporated into our current technique and applied in the most recent 50 patients. It is a highly effective adjunct in maintaining hemostasis. It is easily prepared within minutes and immediately effective in the setting of an incompletely dry field. The gelatin matrix–thrombin composite in FloSeal mechanically slows down bleeding and provides exposure to a high thrombin concentration, which accelerates long-term hemostasis by clot formation (30). In the future, we believe that potent bioadhesives may assume a primary rather than an adjunctive role in obtaining renal parenchymal hemostasis during laparoscopic partial nephrectomy.

Experience with laparoscopic partial nephrectomy continues to grow, and issues of hemostasis and renal ischemia are being further addressed in the laboratory. Laparoscopic partial nephrectomy is a technically advanced procedure that requires the complete laparoscopic skill set applied in a time-sensitive environment. However, it is the only form of minimally invasive treatment of localized RCC that replicates the steps of open partial nephrectomy, the current gold standard of care. Therefore, until the true oncologic efficacy of energy ablative techniques is demonstrated, this should be considered the primary form of minimally invasive NSS for localized RCC.

CRYOTHERAPY

Introduction

Percutaneous cryoablation of renal tissue was first described in 1995 (31), with the initial clinical laparoscopic series reported in 1998 (32). Cryoenergy is the most studied and clinically used modality for targeted ablation of renal tumors. During cryoablation, heat is removed from the target tissue, freezing the renal parenchyma incorporated in the expanding cryoprobe iceball and resulting in cell death.

Pathophysiology

Cryoablation causes cell death by direct and indirect mechanisms. Direct cellular injury can result from intracellular ice formation or from solution effects secondary to osmotic imbalance. Intracellular ice formation only occurs within a few millimeters of the cryoprobe but is usually universally lethal because of irreversible cell membrane damage (33,34). During cryotherapy, the ice forming outside the cell increases the extracellular osmotic concentration, which in turn draws water out into the extracellular space, producing a state of relative intracellular dehydration. This state results in pH changes and protein denaturation that lead to cell death. Direct injury does not completely kill all cells. Indirect damage occurs hours to days after the initial cellular insult. Endothelial cells damaged by freezing result in thrombosis, vascular occlusion, regional tissue ischemia, and, ultimately, delayed cell death (35). This may be the dominant mechanism of cell death. There is also some evidence of an immunologic response to cryoablation, but experimental results have been inconsistent, and its existence, let alone significance, remains controversial (35).

Freezing and thawing tissue results in necrosis. Cellular survival during cryoablation depends not only on the freezing and thawing rates but also, most importantly, on the lowest temperature reached and the hold time at subzero temperatures (36). The critical temperature required to produce complete necrosis is highly dependent on the cell type. Although initial reports indicated that the critical temperature to ensure cell death was −40°C (37), the minimal temperature required for renal tissue necrosis was determined to be −19.4°C (38). Other reports have studied the relation of the tissue margin distance from the iceball and completeness of cell death (39). Complete necrosis begins 3.1 mm inside the visible edge of the iceball, and this physical location corresponds to a temperature of −19.4°C (39). Clinically, the target temperature for achieving reliable deaths of normal and cancerous renal cells is usually set at −40°C. Although repetition of the freeze–thaw cycle exacerbates cell damage, the optimal parameters (i.e., number of cycles, length of freeze time, and type of thaw) are yet to be determined. Single and double freeze–thaw cycles with active and passive thaws have been compared (40). A double freeze–thaw cycle produced considerably larger areas of liquefaction necrosis than a single freeze–thaw cycle, with no difference between an active or passive thaw. However, other studies have found enhanced cell death with passive thawing (41); therefore, a slow thaw is recommended (42).

Theoretically, renal blood flow could retard the rate of cooling; however, renal artery clamping would require further surgical dissection with its inherent risks and expose the entire kidney to an ischemic insult. Furthermore, in the canine model, renal arterial occlusion resulted in no differences in the rate of cooling, nadir temperature achieved, or mean diameter of the cryoinfarcted zone (39). Although adjacent structures may be injured during cryoablation, studies of intentional collecting system freezing have shown no adverse sequelae unless the pelvicalyceal system is punctured with the probe (43). Therefore, more centrally located tumors can be safely treated. Renal cryoablation does not lead to any clinically significant systemic hypothermia. The ischemic necrotic renal cryolesion does not trigger renin-angiotensin–mediated hypertension or have deleterious effects on renal function over a follow-up period of up to 20 months (44).

Technique

Various clinically relevant cryogens are available, the boiling point of each determining the nadir temperature that the specific cryoprobe can produce. Liquid argon and liquid nitrogen, the two most commonly used cryogens, have boiling points of −185.9°C and −195.8°C, respectively. The size and efficiency of a cryolesion are influenced by the physical characteristics of the cryoprobe, such as the nadir temperature and diameter. At the author's center, the 4.8-mm-diameter argon-based probe has routinely been employed for clinical renal cryotherapy. Although exposure may be obtained with an open approach, laparoscopic and percutaneous techniques offer the advantages of minimally invasive surgery with nephron-sparing ablation. Regardless of whether it is performed laparoscopically or percutaneously, the essential technical requirements of renal cryotherapy are the same. The

procedure involves real-time imaging of the tumor; preplanning the precise angle and depth of cryoprobe entry; precryoablation needle biopsy of the tumor for histologic tissue diagnosis; insertion of the cryoprobe perpendicularly through the center of the tumor and advancement up to, or just beyond, the inner (deep) margin of the tumor; creation of a cryolesion approximately 1 cm larger than the size of the tumor under real-time radiologic monitoring; and confirmation of postcryoablation renal hemostasis.

Laparoscopic renal cryoablation is performed under ultrasound guidance (32), whereas percutaneous cryoablation is performed with a magnetic resonance–compatible cryosystem (Galil Medical Systems, Yokneam, Israel) (45). The laparoscopic approach offers distinct delivery advantages, which are particularly beneficial for anteromedially located tumors. The colon can be reflected and the entire kidney mobilized, allowing direct visual access to the tumor while minimizing injury to adjacent organs. Also, this approach permits the dual control of direct laparoscopic visualization and ultrasound monitoring to ensure the creation of a technically adequate iceball.

Results

Renal cryoablation has been performed by percutaneous (31,45), laparoscopic (31,45–49), and open techniques (50,51) (Table 47F.2). In one of the largest clinical reports to date, laparoscopic cryoablation was carried out in 32 patients with a mean tumor size of 2.3 cm (47). More clinical experience has been documented, and since September 1997, 100 patients have undergone laparoscopic renal cryoablation at the Cleveland Clinic. Of these, 56 patients have each completed a 3-year follow-up (Gill IS, et al.) (52). All 56 procedures were completed successfully, and no kidney was lost. For a mean renal tumor size of 2.3 cm, the mean intraoperative size of the created cryolesion was 3.6 cm. Intraoperative precryoablation needle biopsy confirmed RCC in 36 patients (60%). Sequential mean cryolesion size on magnetic resonance imaging (MRI) scanning at postoperative day 1, 3 months, 6 months, 1 year, 2 years, and 3 years was 3.7 cm, 2.8 cm, 2.3 cm, 1.7 cm, 1.2 cm, and 0.9 cm, respectively. These values represent a percentage reduction in cryolesion size of 26%, 39%, 56%, 69%, and 75% at 3 months, 6 months, 1 year, 2 years, and 3 years, respectively. At 3 years, 17 cryolesions (38%) had completely disappeared on MRI scanning. Postoperative needle biopsy identified locally persistent/recurrent renal tumor in 2 patients (3.6%). New de novo renal lesions at a location remote from the cryoablated site developed in 3 patients (5.4%). Six patients (11%) have died from various causes: preexisting metastatic disease (4 patients), myocardial infarction (1 patient), and bilateral renal cancer (1 patient). Cryoablation had minimal impact on renal function status: preoperative serum creatinine 1.2 mg/dL, postoperative serum creatinine 1.4 mg/dL at mean follow-up of 43 months. In none of the patients was surgery converted to open surgery, none of the patients developed a urinary fistula or required dialysis, and none of the patients developed a perirenal or port-site recurrence.

Cryotherapy for localized RCC is the most studied of the probe-ablative techniques. Advantages of cryotherapy include predictable, clearly necrotic lesions that can be monitored reliably with real-time imaging. Intermediate-term oncologic data support the continued use of renal cryoablation in carefully selected patients in the controlled setting of a clinical trial. Five-year data are necessary to determine the proper place of renal cryotherapy in the evolving menu of minimally invasive nephron-sparing options.

TABLE 47F.2

RENAL CRYOSURGERY: CLINICAL SERIES

Study	Approach	Number of pts.	Stage	Tumor size (cm)	EBL (mL)	Operative time (min)	Complication	Hospital stay (d)	Follow-up (mo)
Uchida et al. (31)	Percutaneous	2	Metastatic RCC	NA	NA	NA	0	NA	5 and 10
Delworth et al. (50)	Open	2	T1N0M0	RCC (3) AML (7)	450	240	0	5	RCC (1) AML (3)
Gill et al. (47)	Laparoscopic	32	T1N0M0	2.3	66.8	174	2	1.8	16.2
Bishoff et al. (46)	Laparoscopic	8	T1N0M0	2	140		0	3.5	7.7
Rukstalis et al. (51)	Open	29	T1N0M0	2.2	200	NA	Parenchymal tear 5 (major 1, minor 4)	3.4	16
Shingelton and Sewell (45)	Percutaneous	20	T1N0M0	3.2	NA	97	1	1	9.1
Lee et al. (48)	Laparoscopic	20	T1N0M0	2.6	93	306	5 minor, 1 major	2.6	14.2
Nadler et al. (49)	Laparoscopic	15	T1N0M0	2.2	67	260	2	3.5	15

AML, angiomyolipoma; EBL, estimated blood loss; NA, not applicable; RCC, renal cell carcinoma Reproduced with permission from Gill IS. Minimally invasive nephron-sparing surgery. *Urol Clin North Am* 2003;30:551–579.

RADIOFREQUENCY ABLATION

Introduction

Zlotta et al. (53) performed the first radiofrequency ablation (RFA) of a renal tumor in 1997. Since this initial report, RFA has gained considerable attention. The benefits of this technique include percutaneous delivery and treatment under intravenous sedation without the need for general anesthesia. These features are particularly advantageous in patients with significant medical comorbidities. In contrast to cryotherapy, RFA involves the delivery of high-frequency electrical current, causing heat-based tissue destruction.

Pathophysiology

As tissue temperatures increase to between 60° and 100°C, there is an instantaneous induction of irreversible cellular damage referred to as coagulation necrosis (54). RFA also causes vascular thrombosis within the treatment zone (55,56). Porcine kidneys treated with RFA and analyzed at 7 days demonstrated central residual thermal effects and vascular thrombosis causing an ischemic lesion with a peripheral collar zone of necrosis and small-vessel thrombosis (56). Segmental arterial thrombosis was consistent with the finding of wedge-shaped RFA lesions (56).

Technique

Although open and laparoscopic approaches can be used, percutaneous access is most commonly employed. Grounding electrode pads are applied to the patient's skin surface to complete the electric circuit to the RFA generator. The electrode delivers alternating current to the tissue, causing ionic agitation in the cells. The electrical impedance of the tissue (resistance to RF current flow) produces local heating and, provided that tissue impedance remains low, a dynamically expanding sphere of tissue damage is created. Temperature or impedance-based systems can be used during RFA. With temperature-based systems, the electrode tips sense tissue temperature, and treatment is completed when a preset temperature (usually 60°C–100°C) is maintained for a predetermined time (usually 5–12 minutes). With impedance-based systems, the ablative process stops when electrical impedance rises to a point that resists the flow of any current. This effect may limit the size of the treatment zone.

RFA via a dry probe can lead to a rapid increase in temperature that results in tissue desiccation and charring, which may interfere with expansion of the ablative perimeter, ultimately limiting the size of the radiofrequency-induced lesion. Saline-enhanced RFA involves the introduction of normal or hypertonic saline into the target tissue via a cannula in order to amplify the ablative sphere (57). The infused saline solution either facilitates the conduction of energy or improves thermal transmission away from the RFA needle, expanding the thermal zone. However, saline injection may sacrifice uniformity or predictability because the solution may diffuse in an irregular fashion. An additional barrier to successful RFA is the "heat sink" effect during treatment of tumors in well-vascularized tissues or those adjacent to blood vessels. Adjacent vasculature conducts thermal energy away from the target tissue and into the relatively cooler blood. This effect may spare tumor cells nearest to blood vessels, ultimately compromising therapeutic success.

While US can be used to monitor iceball formation during cryotherapy, its use with RFA is limited to monitoring needle placement and the initiation of ablation. Gas bubbles produced during heating hinder visualization. In 2003, Ogan et al. (58) reported the use of laparoscopic thermography to monitor

RFA lesions in real time. During RFA, a laparoscopic infrared (IR) camera was used to measure surface parenchymal temperatures in conjunction with thermocouples. The IR camera was able to predict the region of necrosis of the renal parenchyma during RFA. Although promising, shallow tissue penetration may limit its clinical use to exophytic tumors (58).

Results

Although several centers have reported their experiences with RFA of renal tumors, long-term data are lacking (59–65). While easily performed percutaneously under intravenous sedation as an outpatient procedure, the therapeutic efficacy of RFA has been called into question. A study by Rendon et al. (59) triggered discussion of the histologic assessment of renal tumors post-RF ablation (66). Impedance-based dry RFA was used in 5 patients who then immediately underwent partial or radical nephrectomy. Another 5 patients were treated percutaneously with US or CT scan–guided RFA 7 days before partial or radical nephrectomy. Hematoxylin and eosin (H&E) staining demonstrated residual viable tumor in approximately 5% of the volume in 4 of the 5 tumors in the acute group and in 3 of the 6 masses in the delayed group. Persistent tumor cells were invariably present at the margins of the treated zones.

Although some of the earlier reports of RFA failures may have been a consequence of histologic interpretation, other treatment failures have now been reported (60–63,65). Matlaga et al. (60) utilized intraoperative saline-cooled RFA to treat renal tumors immediately before partial or radical nephrectomy. On the basis of H&E and NADH staining, 2 of 10 tumors were incompletely ablated. Michaels et al. (62) treated 15 patients with a total of 20 tumors. RFA with an open surgical approach was immediately followed by partial nephrectomy. The 5 most recent tumors were stained with H&E and NADH (nicotinamide adenine dinucleotide, reduced form). Of the 5 specimens, 4 stained positively with NADH in areas confirmed to be tumor with H&E.

In the National Institutes of Health experience, 21 patients underwent 24 percutaneous renal RFAs for a tumor 3 cm or less in size (64). Nineteen patients had von Hippel-Lindau (VHL) syndrome. At 2-month follow-up, tumor size decreased from 2.4 cm to 2 cm, and 79% of tumors ceased to enhance on contrast CT scan. Five renal tumors continued to have persistent enhancement on CT scan, raising concerns regarding residual malignancy. No postoperative biopsy data were reported (64). In the Massachusetts General Hospital experience, 24 percutaneous RFA treatments were performed for 9 RCCs in 8 patients (63). Of the 9 tumors, 3 (33%) demonstrated continued enhancement that required repeat treatment (63). Su et al. reported the Johns Hopkins experience with 37 CT scan-guided percutaneous RFAs of 35 renal tumors in 29 patients (65). The mean tumor size was 2.2 cm, and a 2- to 3.5-cm probe was employed. Two patients required repeat ablation because of the presence of a small area of enhancement following treatment. The remaining 33 lesions demonstrated no evidence of enhancement at a mean radiographic follow-up of 8.4 months (65). In 2003 Mayo-Smith et al. (61) reported their experiences with RFA of renal tumors in 32 patients. The average tumor size was 2.6 cm. With a mean follow-up of 9 months, 6 patients (19%) had persistent contrast enhancement in the treated region. Of the 6 retreatments, 5 were successful. Notably, 1 patient developed a 5-mm skin metastasis at the electrode insertion site. This was resected without recurrence.

Although it is unlikely, tumors with persistent enhancement may regress over time. In the absence of posttreatment biopsies, one must rely on follow-up imaging to assess treatment success. However, the lack of contrast enhancement does not ensure absence of viable tumor cells. In the study by Rendon et al. (59), only one of the three patients in the delayed group with remaining viable tumor demonstrated contrast enhancement after RFA. Consequently, the current rate of residual contrast enhancement is an underestimation of the true incidence of treatment failure.

The advantage of RFA lies in its percutaneous delivery, potentially under intravenous sedation as an outpatient. Currently, short-term data continue to reveal treatment failures. As is the case with all probe-ablative techniques, the treated tumor is left *in situ*. Perhaps better intraoperative monitoring and refinement of technique may resolve the issue of incomplete cell kill.

HIGH-INTENSITY FOCUSED ULTRASOUND

HIFU has the potential to be the least invasive of tumor ablative techniques. HIFU employs beams of ablative ultrasound frequency generated by a cylindrical piezoelectric element focused by a paraboloid reflector. Similar to extracorporeal shock wave lithotripsy, this beam is then focused on the lesion. Most of the literature related to HIFU performed for renal tumors has been only experimental in nature, with the first report of treatment with curative intent published in 2002 (67). In 2003, Wu et al. performed HIFU in 12 patients with advanced stage RCC and 1 patient with colon cancer metastasized to kidney (68). Ten patients received partial HIFU ablation as palliative treatment to impede tumor growth and improve quality of life. The remaining 3 patients had organ-confined disease and underwent complete HIFU treatment with a 1-cm margin of tissue for curative intent. The first 6 patients received epidural anesthesia, and the remaining 7 patients received general anesthesia. Real-time US was used to target the tumor, guide US energy deposition, and assess the extent of coagulation necrosis during the procedure.

HIFU treatment was successfully performed in all patients. The ablative extent ranged from 40% to 90% of target tumor volume. The number of HIFU sessions ranged from 1 to 2 (median 1.3), and the treatment time ranged from 1.5 to 9 hours (median 5.4). The percentage of change in tumor size was assessed according to the largest and the perpendicular diameters of the tumor measured on US before and after HIFU ablation. On this basis, tumor size decreased by 23.1%, 48.7%, and 58.3% at 3, 6, and 12 months, respectively. After HIFU, hematuria resolved in 7 of 8 patients and flank pain, presumed to be of malignant origin, disappeared in 9 of 10 patients. Each patient underwent at least one MRI study after HIFU treatment, and it was common to observe the absence of contrast enhancement in the treated region.

The only complication related to the procedure was a minor skin burn in the first treated patient, which was observed and healed over 2 weeks. There was no tumor hemorrhage, no large blood vessel rupture, and no evidence of postoperative urine extravasation or renal dysfunction in any patients during follow-up. After a median follow-up of 14.1 months (range 2–27), 6 of the 13 patients were alive. The tumors of 2 patients, which had previously been considered unresectable because of proximity to the abdominal aorta, sufficiently decreased in size after HIFU to allow radical nephrectomy after 8 and 11 months, respectively. One patient with bilateral RCC had local recurrence proven by needle biopsy on the left diseased kidney 18 months after HIFU, and partial nephrectomy was immediately performed. Partial coagulation necrosis in the treated region was observed in these surgical specimens. Lung metastases were stable after treatment, and no new lung metastasis was seen. Although the mechanism remains unclear, an immunologic effect from the thermal ablation could be responsible for the temporary stability.

HIFU represents the least invasive form of treatment of RCC. Preliminary evidence suggests therapeutic potential for this extracorporeal modality of energy ablation. However, this procedure is currently experimental and requires refinement in technique. Furthermore, as with the probe-ablative strategies, additional research and investigation with long-term follow-up are required before considering this mode of therapy for curative treatment of RCC.

Conclusion

Laparoscopic partial nephrectomy is an evolving technique for select patients who are candidates for NSS. Open partial nephrectomy continues to be the gold standard of NSS. Laparoscopic partial nephrectomy duplicates the steps of open partial nephrectomy in a less invasive manner. The short-term oncologic adequacy of laparoscopic partial nephrectomy is equivalent to open partial nephrectomy. However, long-term data are required. Emerging techniques involving energy ablation include cryotherapy, RFA, and HIFU. HIFU is in the earliest phase of development and clearly experimental. The greatest experience is with cryotherapy, and the short-term data are encouraging. Although RFA can be performed percutaneously under intravenous sedation, incomplete tumor ablation accounts for ongoing concern. Careful long-term clinical and radiologic follow-up with sequential MRI and/or CT scanning complemented by needle biopsy evaluation are important to monitor progress and to allow early detection of any local or systemic recurrence. Until 5-year oncologic data are available, probe-ablative strategies must be considered developmental in nature and limited to the select patient with a small exophytic renal mass.

References

1. Herts BR. Imaging for renal tumors. *Curr Opin Urol* 2003;13:181–186.
2. Gill IS, Desai MM, Kaouk JH, et al. Laparoscopic partial nephrectomy for renal tumor: Duplicating open surgical techniques. *J Urol* 2002;167:469–475.
3. Janetschek G, Jeschke K, Peschel R, et al. Laparoscopic surgery for stage T1 renal cell carcinoma: Radical nephrectomy and wedge resection. *Eur Urol* 2000;38:131–138.
4. Harmon WJ, Kavoussi LR, Bishoff JT. Laparoscopic nephron-sparing surgery for solid renal masses using the ultrasonic shears. *Urology* 2000;56:754–759.
5. Rassweiler JJ, Abbou C, Janetschek G, et al. Laparoscopic partial nephrectomy. The European experience. *Urol Clin North Am* 2000;27:721–736.
6. Guillonneau B, Bermudez H, Gholami S, et al. Laparoscopic partial nephrectomy for renal tumor: Single center experience comparing clamping and no clamping techniques of the renal vasculature. *J Urol* 2003;169:483–486.
7. Kim FJ, Rha KH, Hernandez F, et al. Laparoscopic radical versus partial nephrectomy: Assessment of complications. *J Urol* 2003;170:408–411.
8. Simon SD, Ferrigni RG, Novicki DE, et al. Mayo Clinic Scottsdale experience with laparoscopic nephron sparing surgery for renal tumors. *J Urol* 2003;169:2059–2062.
9. Gill IS, Matin SF, Desai MM, et al. Comparative analysis of laparoscopic versus open partial nephrectomy for renal tumors in 200 patients. *J Urol* 2003;170:64–68.
10. Gill IS. Minimally invasive nephron-sparing surgery. *Urol Clin North Am* 2003;30:551–579.
11. Winfield HN, Donovan JF, Godet AS, et al. Laparoscopic partial nephrectomy: Initial case report for benign disease. *J Endourol* 1993;7:521–526.
12. McDougall EM, Elbahnasy AM, Clayman RV. Laparoscopic wedge resection and partial nephrectomy: The Washington University experience and review of the literature. *JSLS* 1998;2:15–23.
13. Gill IS, Delworth MG, Munch LC. Laparoscopic retroperitoneal partial nephrectomy. *J Urol* 1994;152:1539–1542.
14. Desai MM, Gill IS, Kaouk JH, et al. Laparoscopic partial nephrectomy with suture repair of the pelvicaliceal system. *Urology* 2003;61:99–104.
15. Polascik TJ, Pound CR, Meng MV, et al. Partial nephrectomy: Technique, complications and pathological findings. *J Urol* 1995;154:1312–1318.
16. Gill IS, Abreu SC, Desai MM, et al. Laparoscopic ice slush renal hypothermia for partial nephrectomy: The initial experience. *J Urol* 2003;170:52–56.
17. Janetschek G, Abdelmaksoud A, Bagheri F, et al. Laparoscopic partial nephrectomy in cold ischemia: Renal artery perfusion. *J Endourol* 2003;17:A104.
18. Landman J, Rehman J, Sundaram CP, et al. Renal hypothermia achieved by retrograde intracavitary saline perfusion. *J Endourol* 2002;16:445–449.
19. Ramani AP, Desai MM, Steinberg AP, et al. Complications of laparoscopic partial nephrectomy in 200 cases. *J Urol* 2005;173(1):42–47.
20. Steinberg AP, Kilciler M, Abreu SC, et al. Laparoscopic nephron-sparing surgery for 2 or more ipsilateral renal tumors. *Urology* 2004;64(2):225–228.
21. Steinberg AP, Abreu SC, Desai MM, et al. Laparoscopic nephron-sparing surgery in the presence of renal artery disease. *Urology* 2003;62:935–939.
22. Ramani AP, Abreu SC, Desai MM, et al. Laparoscopic upper pole partial nephrectomy with concomitant en bloc adrenalectomy. *Urology* 2003;62:223–226.
23. Hayakawa K, Baba S, Aoyagi T, et al. Laparoscopic heminephrectomy of a horseshoe kidney using microwave coagulator. *J Urol* 1999;161:1559.
24. Jackman SV, Cadeddu JA, Chen RN, et al. Utility of the harmonic scalpel for laparoscopic partial nephrectomy. *J Endourol* 1998;12:441–444.
25. Elashry OM, Wolf JS Jr, Rayala HJ, et al. Recent advances in laparoscopic partial nephrectomy: Comparative study of electrosurgical snare electrode and ultrasound dissection. *J Endourol* 1997;11:15–22.
26. McDougall EM, Clayman RV, Chandhoke PS, et al. Laparoscopic partial nephrectomy in the pig model. *J Urol* 1993;149:1633–1636.
27. Gill IS, Munch LC, Clayman RV, et al. A new renal tourniquet for open and laparoscopic partial nephrectomy. *J Urol* 1995;154:1113–1116.
28. Cadeddu JA, Corwin TS. Cable tie compression to facilitate laparoscopic partial nephrectomy. *J Urol* 2001;165:177–178.
29. Shekarriz B, Stoller ML. The use of fibrin sealant in urology. *J Urol* 2002;167:1218–1225.
30. Richter F, Schnorr D, Deger S, et al. Improvement of hemostasis in open and laparoscopically performed partial nephrectomy using a gelatin matrix–thrombin tissue sealant (FloSeal). *Urology* 2003;61:73–77.
31. Uchida M, Imaide Y, Sugimoto K, et al. Percutaneous cryosurgery for renal tumours. *Br J Urol* 1995;75:132–136; discussion 136–137.
32. Gill IS, Novick AC, Soble JJ, et al. Laparoscopic renal cryoablation: Initial clinical series. *Urology* 1998;52:543–551.
33. Bischof JC, Smith D, Pazhayannur PV, et al. Cryosurgery of dunning AT-1 rat prostate tumor: Thermal, biophysical, and viability response at the cellular and tissue level. *Cryobiology* 1997;34:42–69.
34. Rewcastle JC, Muldrew K, Sandison GA. In vitro injury mapping for single cryoprobe cryosurgery. *Cryobiology* 2001;43:322.
35. Hoffmann NE, Bischof JC. The cryobiology of cryosurgical injury. *Urology* 2002;60:40–49.
36. Smith DJ, Fahssi WM, Swanlund DJ, et al. A parametric study of freezing injury in AT-1 rat prostate tumor cells. *Cryobiology* 1999;39:13–28.
37. Baust J, Gage AA, Ma H, et al. Minimally invasive cryosurgery: Technological advances. *Cryobiology* 1997;34:373–384.
38. Chosy SG, Nakada SY, Lee FT Jr, et al. Monitoring renal cryosurgery: Predictors of tissue necrosis in swine. *J Urol* 1998;159:1370–1374.
39. Campbell SC, Krishnamurthi V, Chow G, et al. Renal cryosurgery: Experimental evaluation of treatment parameters. *Urology* 1998;52:29–33; discussion 33–24.
40. Woolley ML, Schulsinger DA, Durand DB, et al. Effect of freezing parameters (freeze cycle and thaw process) on tissue destruction following renal cryoablation. *J Endourol* 2002;16:519–522.
41. Gage AA, Baust J. Mechanisms of tissue injury in cryosurgery. *Cryobiology* 1998;37:171–186.
42. Desai MM, Gill IS. Current status of cryoablation and radiofrequency ablation in the management of renal tumors. *Curr Opin Urol* 2002;12:387–393.
43. Sung GT, Gill IS, Meraney AM. Effect of intentional cryoinjury to the renal collection system (abstract). *J Urol* 2000;163:113.
44. Carvalhal EF, Gill IS, Meraney AM, et al. Laparoscopic renal cryoablation: Impact on renal function and blood pressure. *Urology* 2001;58:357–361.
45. Shingleton WB, Sewell PE, Jr. Percutaneous renal tumor cryoablation with magnetic resonance imaging guidance. *J Urol* 2001;165:773–776.
46. Bishoff JT, Chen RB, Lee BR, et al. Laparoscopic renal cryoablation: Acute and long-term clinical, radiographic, and pathologic effects in an animal model and application in a clinical trial. *J Endourol* 1999;13:233–239.
47. Gill IS, Novick AC, Meraney AM, et al. Laparoscopic renal cryoablation in 32 patients. *Urology* 2000;56:748–753.
48. Lee DI, McGinnis DE, Feld R, et al. Retroperitoneal laparoscopic cryoablation of small renal tumors: Intermediate results. *Urology* 2003;61:83–88.
49. Nadler RB, Kim SC, Rubenstein JN, et al. Laparoscopic renal cryosurgery: The Northwestern experience. *J Urol* 2003;170:1121–1125.
50. Delworth MG, Pisters LL, Fornage BD, et al. Cryotherapy for renal cell carcinoma and angiomyolipoma. *J Urol* 1996;155:252–254; discussion 254–255.
51. Rukstalis DB, Khorsandi M, Garcia FU, et al. Clinical experience with open renal cryoablation. *Urology* 2001;57:34–39.
52. Gill IS, Remer EM, Hasan WA, et al. Renal cryoablation: outcome at 3 years. *J Urol* 2005;173(6):1903–1907.

53. Zlotta AR, Wildschutz T, Raviv G, et al. Radiofrequency interstitial tumor ablation (RITA) is a possible new modality for treatment of renal cancer: Ex vivo and in vivo experience. *J Endourol* 1997;11:251–258.

54. Solbiati L, Goldberg SN, Ierace T, et al. Hepatic metastases: Percutaneous radio-frequency ablation with cooled-tip electrodes. *Radiology* 1997;205: 367–373.

55. Gill IS, Hsu TH, Fox RL, et al. Laparoscopic and percutaneous radiofrequency ablation of the kidney: Acute and chronic porcine study. *Urology* 2000;56:197–200.

56. Rendon RA, Gertner MR, Sherar MD, et al. Development of a radiofrequency based thermal therapy technique in an in vivo porcine model for the treatment of small renal masses. *J Urol* 2001;166:292–298.

57. Leveillee RJ, Hoey MF, Hulbert JC, et al. Enhanced radiofrequency ablation of canine prostate utilizing a liquid conductor: The virtual electrode. *J Endourol* 1996;10:5–11.

58. Ogan K, Roberts WW, Wilhelm DM, et al. Infrared thermography and thermocouple mapping of radiofrequency renal ablation to assess treatment adequacy and ablation margins. *Urology* 2003;62:146–151.

59. Rendon RA, Kachura JR, Sweet JM, et al. The uncertainty of radio frequency treatment of renal cell carcinoma: Findings at immediate and delayed nephrectomy. *J Urol* 2002;167:1587–1592.

60. Matlaga BR, Zagoria RJ, Woodruff RD, et al. Phase II trial of radio frequency ablation of renal cancer: Evaluation of the kill zone. *J Urol* 2002; 168:2401–2405.

61. Mayo-Smith WW, Dupuy DE, Parikh PM, et al. Imaging-guided percutaneous radiofrequency ablation of solid renal masses: Techniques and outcomes of 38 treatment sessions in 32 consecutive patients. *AJR Am J Roentgenol* 2003;180:1503–1508.

62. Michaels MJ, Rhee HK, Mourtzinos AP, et al. Incomplete renal tumor destruction using radio frequency interstitial ablation. *J Urol* 2002;168: 2406–2409; discussion 2409–2410.

63. Gervais DA, McGovern FJ, Wood BJ, et al. Radio-frequency ablation of renal cell carcinoma: Early clinical experience. *Radiology* 2000;217:665–672.

64. Pavlovich CP, Walther MM, Choyke PL, et al. Percutaneous radio frequency ablation of small renal tumors: Initial results. *J Urol* 2002;167: 10–15.

65. Su LM, Jarrett TW, Chan DY, et al. Percutaneous computed tomography-guided radiofrequency ablation of renal masses in high surgical risk patients: Preliminary results. *Urology* 2003;61:26–33.

66. Ogan K, Cadeddu JA. Re: The uncertainty of radio frequency treatment of renal cell carcinoma: Findings at immediate and delayed nephrectomy. *J Urol* 2002;168:2128; discussion 2129–2130.

67. Kohrmann KU, Michel MS, Gaa J, et al. High intensity focused ultrasound as noninvasive therapy for multilocal renal cell carcinoma: Case study and review of the literature. *J Urol* 2002;167:2397–2403.

68. Wu F, Wang ZB, Chen WZ, et al. Preliminary experience using high intensity focused ultrasound for the treatment of patients with advanced stage renal malignancy. *J Urol* 2003;170:2237–2240.

CHAPTER 48 ■ MANAGEMENT OF METASTATIC RENAL CELL CARCINOMA

CHAPTER 48A
Management of Metastatic Renal Cell Carcinoma: The Role of Surgery

Robert C. Flanigan and Bradley G. Orris

Up to one third of patients with renal cell carcinoma (RCC) will present with metastatic disease, and 20% to 40% of those with clinically localized disease will eventually be found to have metastatic involvement. Prognosis continues to be guarded for this population, with a 2-year survival rate of only 10% to 30%. While advancements are being made in the medical management of RCC, the role of surgery in the treatment algorithm is also being further refined. Palliative surgery, either via nephrectomy or at the site of metastasis, has a role in certain very well-selected patients. Some data support total metastectomy either at the time of nephrectomy or at the time of recurrence in a small, well-selected group of patients with minimal, resectable metastases. More controversial is the idea of cytoreductive nephrectomy as an adjunct to immunotherapy. Recent Phase III trials indicate that nephrectomy may actually play an important role in management of metastatic RCC in conjunction with cytokine-based immunotherapy. Nephrectomy is also an essential component of adoptive immunotherapy protocols and may play a role in other novel therapies.

PALLIATIVE SURGERY

Patients with metastatic RCC may be debilitated with symptoms directly related to their primary tumor (1). Flank pain, persistent hemorrhage, and large arteriovenous malformations leading to high-output heart failure and hypertension have all been reported but are, fortunately, uncommon manifestations of advanced local disease. Although nephrectomy has been advocated as a treatment of all these conditions, it is rarely necessary, considering the effectiveness of less invasive treatments. Most patients with hematuria can be managed by angioembolization, and intractable flank pain can often be managed by more intensive efforts in pain management in coordination with pain specialists. It is important to remember the poor overall survival of patients in this group when considering the morbidity of a surgical procedure simply for palliation.

RCC is also known to cause a number of potentially debilitating paraneoplastic syndromes such as hypercalcemia, fever, hepatic dysfunction, and erythrocytosis. While nephrectomy may occasionally be necessary in treatment of these conditions, it is important to remember that paraneoplastic symptoms may not be produced only by the primary tumor (2). Walther et al. reported that nephrectomy for hypercalcemia in advanced RCC caused reduction of calcium levels in only 7 of 12 patients, with median survival being unaffected in either group and limited to only 6 months (3).

In general, palliative nephrectomy alone for metastatic disease, without adjuvant therapy, is not felt to improve survival and has a significant chance to cause morbidity or death. It should be undertaken only in the rare patient for whom more conservative measures have been unable to adequately control symptoms from the primary tumor.

Palliative surgery for metastatic lesions also has a role in select patients. Operative repair of impending bony fractures, pathologic fractures, or spinal cord compression caused by metastatic RCC is effective and occasionally necessary (4). Preoperative embolization of bony metastases is sometimes used to assist in hemostasis, and postoperative radiation therapy is commonly given. Brain metastases also can cause severe symptoms requiring palliative intervention (5). Brain metastases can be managed with corticosteroids and whole brain irradiation. More aggressive therapy can include surgical resection of solitary or limited brain lesions. Stereotactic radiosurgery often plays a role now in the management of select brain metastases.

METASTECTOMY DURING OR AFTER NEPHRECTOMY

Several reports describe the potential benefit of nephrectomy with simultaneous or subsequent resection of all identifiable metastatic disease when solitary or low-volume metastatic disease is present. Unfortunately, these potentially curable patients represent only an estimated 1.6% to 3.6% of patients diagnosed with metastatic RCC (6,7). Kierney et al. reported on 41 well-selected patients undergoing metastectomy after previous nephrectomy done with curative intent (8). Complete surgical excision was achieved in 88% of patients and the 3- and 5-year survival rates were 59% and 31%, respectively. Tolia and Whitmore reported on 17 patients undergoing aggressive therapy for solitary metastatic disease including 12 with bony metastases (9). Overall 5-year survival rate was 35%. O'Dea et al. reported on 44 patients with solitary metastases (10). Of 18 patients with synchronous metastases, there was only 1 survivor at 5 years compared to 26 patients with metachronous metastases who had a 50% 5-year survival rate. A more recent report by Kavolius et al. consisted of 141 patients undergoing curative metastectomy for a first recurrence after nephrectomy and showed a 44% 5-year overall survival rate (11). In a subgroup of the 94 patients with solitary recurrences, 5-year overall survival was 52% including 54% in the pulmonary metastases-only group (50 patients), 18% for patients with solitary brain metastases (11 patients) and 40% for those with solitary bony metastases (5 patients). For patients undergoing second and third resections of metastatic disease recurrence, the 5-year overall survival rate was 46% and 44%, respectively.

These patients are uncommon, and patient selection is paramount in achieving the desired outcome. Patients most likely to benefit are those with solitary or pulmonary-only metastatic foci, long disease-free interval after nephrectomy, and good performance status (PS). Most studies indicate that resection of metachronous rather than synchronous metastases leads to improved survival with a disease-free interval greater than 1 year indicative of better outcome (6,9,11). Recurrences after initial metastectomy should not preclude further attempts at curative resection if the surgeon feels that complete resection is possible and PS remains good.

EMBOLIZATION PLUS NEPHRECTOMY

The combination of nephrectomy with preoperative embolization has also been reported. The speculation is that tumor antigens released from the tumor may provide a powerful stimulus to host immune responses. An early report of 100 patients followed for at least 12 months showed a 28% overall response (OR) rate, complete response (CR) in 7 patients, >50% regression in 8 patients, and prolonged disease stabilization in 13 (12). Unfortunately, a multiinstitutional Southwest Oncology Group (SWOG) study failed to validate these results (13). Thirty patients were followed up for 1 year or more. There were no complete responders and only 1 partial response (PR) that lasted 21 months. The overall 1-year survival rate was 28%, and median survival was 7 months. Significant side effects associated with renal embolization include pain, nausea, vomiting, diarrhea, fever, ileus, and inadvertent embolization of other peripheral vessels. In general, therefore, embolization should be reserved for palliative efforts, and in patients with very large tumors or potentially difficult hilar dissections as an aid to nephrectomy.

SPONTANEOUS REGRESSION

One of the more fascinating aspects of RCC is the occasional occurrence of spontaneous regression of metastatic lesions that is believed to be due to host-mediated cytotoxicity. Spontaneous regression of distant metastases in RCC has been estimated to occur in 0.4% to 0.8% of patients (14). Of 51 cases of spontaneous regression reviewed by Freed et al. (15), 45 involved pulmonary lesions. The National Cancer Institute (NCI) found 4 out of 91 total patients who experienced complete regression of metastatic disease after nephrectomy. The mean time of regression was 24.3 months, and pulmonary-only metastases were present in all 4 patients (16). It is important to note that regression of RCC metastases is a real phenomenon, but most reported cases have not involved biopsy-proven lesions and may instead have been old granulomas, fungal lesions, or pulmonary infarcts. Spontaneous regression of metastases is a rare and unpredictable event and is not considered an indication for nephrectomy outside the setting of further adjuvant therapies.

CYTOREDUCTIVE NEPHRECTOMY

To date, the most effective systemic treatment of metastatic RCC is cytokine-based immunotherapy. The role of nephrectomy in this treatment paradigm, either before or after the immunotherapy, remains a controversial topic. We now have two randomized prospective trials that suggest an advantage to preimmunotherapy cytoreductive nephrectomy in appropriately selected patients.

Biological Rationale

The rationale for cytoreduction can be better understood by examining the tumor biology of RCC. The ability of RCC to manipulate and suppress the body's natural immunity has been recognized for many years and studied extensively. The phenomenon of spontaneous regression of metastatic RCC is the strongest evidence that immunologic methods can eradicate RCC. Since nearly all foci of spontaneous metastatic regression occur in the lung and only after the primary tumor has been extirpated, Freed speculated that the lung, with its rich supply of macrophages, lymphocytes, and immunoglobulin, might suppress the metastases through host immune mechanisms and that the primary tumor suppresses this antitumor effect (17). He cited animal data revealing that cell-mediated cytotoxicity is diminished with continuing growth of the primary tumor. In a sense, the primary tumor may act as an "immunologic sink" by diverting circulating antibodies and lymphocytes away from distant metastases (18). Robertson et al. from the NCI, quote animal data that also suggest greater effectiveness of adoptive immunotherapy with decreased tumor bulk (19).

Our knowledge of lymphocyte cellular signaling and regulation pathways has continued to advance, resulting in a much greater appreciation of the immune dysfunction caused by RCC. RCC (along with some other solid malignancies) continues to progress despite significant tumor-infiltrating lymphocytes (TILs), implying that host immune dysfunction and poor tumor antigen recognition and/or presentation may be taking place (20). Lymphocytes from patients with metastatic RCC have been shown to have defective T-cell receptors (21), increased apoptosis (22,23), and defective signal transduction (20,24) with TILs often showing greater dysfunction than peripheral blood lymphocytes. RCC has also been shown to produce high levels of proinflammatory and T-cell-inhibitory cytokines such as interleukin (IL)-8, IL-6, granulocyte–macrophage colony-stimulating factor (GM-CSF), tumor necrosis factor (TNF)a-α, IL-10 and transforming growth factor (TG)b-1, which also may actively suppress immunologic responses (25,26).

It has also been documented that the primary lesion in metastatic RCC rarely responds to systemic immunotherapy, even when significant regression of metastases occurs. The NCI reported on a series of 51 patients who were not candidates for nephrectomy prior to the initiation of IL-2–based systemic therapy and noted a response rate of only 6% with no significant responses seen in the primary tumor (27). In a report by Sella et al. of 17 patients undergoing nephrectomy after response to interferon-α–based immunotherapy, 15 patients (88%) had viable tumor present in the nephrectomy specimens (28). Rackley et al. reported on 25 patients treated with initial biologic response modifier (BRM) therapy and reported a response in 3 patients (12%) (29). Those 3 patients underwent subsequent nephrectomy, and significant residual tumor burden was demonstrated in the kidneys of all patients. The primary tumor's lack of response to immunotherapy is further evidence that the primary tumor causes immune dysfunction, and this implies a benefit to preimmunotherapy cytoreductive nephrectomy.

Other potential benefits of nephrectomy prior to BRM therapy include the prevention of further shedding of tumor cells into the blood supply, possibly leading to slower progression of disease, and palliation of complications of locally advanced disease or paraneoplastic syndromes during immunotherapy.

Multiple retrospective reports of immunotherapy for RCC have shown prior nephrectomy to be a positive prognostic factor independent of other well-recognized factors such as PS and site or burden of disease (30–35). In 670 patients, reported by Motzer et al. treated with immunotherapy and chemotherapy, median survival was 10 months. Pretreatment features associated with shorter survival in the multivariate analysis were absence of nephrectomy, low Karnofsky PS (<80%), lactate dehydrogenase >1.5 times normal, hemoglobin lower than normal, and corrected serum calcium >10 mg/dL.

Retrospective Studies

A number of retrospective series have examined preimmunotherapy cytoreductive nephrectomy (Table 48A.1). Unfortunately, all these studies are subject to the selection bias inherent in retrospective reviews, making analysis of their conclusions difficult. The largest series reported is from the NCI and included 195 patients who underwent nephrectomy with resection of adjacent or contiguous metastases prior to undergoing IL-2 therapy (36). The OR rate in this series was 18%, including 4% CRs and 14% PRs, which is similar to what one would expect from immunotherapy alone. In this series, 38% of patients were unable to undergo treatment with IL-2 secondary to progression of tumor, postoperative complications, or a debilitated state. A 1% mortality rate was seen in this series. Smaller series have reported mixed results with cytoreductive nephrectomy (Table 48A.1), with response rates varying between 8% and 35%. The number of patients unable to receive systemic therapy after nephrectomy varies as well from 7% to 77%, and mortality rates are 0% to 17%. Variability in patient selection, including the distribution of those with good versus poor PS, limited versus extensive metastases, location of metastases, and long versus short metastasis-free interval most likely accounts for these conflicting results.

Bennett et al. represents the poorest outcomes as regards surgical morbidity, mortality, and the inability to receive postoperative systemic therapy (38). There was a 17% mortality rate, and 77% of patients were unable to receive systemic immunotherapy after surgery. Certainly, patient selection was at least partially the cause of these poor outcomes. In this series, almost one third of patients had brain metastases, 43% had bony metastases, and 37% had hepatic metastases. Of the 30 patients only 2 were Eastern Cooperative Oncology Group (ECOG) status 0, 24 were ECOG status 1, and 4 were ECOG status 2. This study reinforces the dangers of poor patient selection when considering cytoreductive nephrectomy.

In 1997 Fallick et al. identified several criteria felt to be predictive of good outcome after cytoreductive nephrectomy and applied these to all patients in their series with metastatic RCC (39). The criteria included the absence of central nervous system, bone, or liver metastases, an ECOG PS of 0 or 1, the possibility of >75% tumor debulking, and predominantly clear cell histology on any biopsies of the tumor. Using these criteria, only 28 patients out of a total of 85 were felt to be candidates for cytoreductive nephrectomy. There were, however, no perioperative deaths or complications that prevented further systemic therapy, and only a single patient had progression of disease requiring withholding of systemic therapy in this series. The OR rate was 39%, including 5 CRs and 6 PRs, with a median survival of 20.5 months in the entire group.

Because of the morbidity involved with nephrectomy, and the possibility of disease progression while recovering, some groups have investigated combining cytoreductive nephrectomy with laparoscopic techniques. In one report, Walther et al. compared treatment groups of open nephrectomy, hand-assisted laparoscopic nephrectomy (performed with a small incision for completing dissection and specimen delivery), and pure laparoscopic nephrectomy with tissue morcellation (42). The median number of days required before onset of immunotherapy in the 19 patients undergoing open nephrectomy was 67 days (range 50 to 151 days), in the 5 hand-assisted laparoscopic patients 60 days (range 47 to 63 days), and in the 6 pure laparoscopic patients only 37 days (range 34 to 57 days). The morbidity of laparoscopic nephrectomy was comparable to traditional open nephrectomy, and the procedure, including tissue morcellation, was feasible even for large tumors. In a larger subsequent report of 31 patients undergoing attempted laparoscopic nephrectomy, however, the same group showed the potential difficulties of this operation (43). Eleven cases required open conversion, and blood loss was much higher (750–3,000 mL) than is typically expected from laparoscopic nephrectomy. Only 18 patients proceeded to immunotherapy postoperatively. Local invasion, obliteration of tissue planes, and enhanced vascularity increase the difficulty of this procedure. While the role of laparoscopy is still being refined in cytoreductive nephrectomy, it seems clear that this will be reserved for centers with extensive laparoscopic experience and for patients who are properly selected and counseled.

Cytoreductive nephrectomy has also been studied in the setting of locally advanced RCC, including extension to the renal vein and inferior vena cava (IVC). Slaton et al. retrospectively reviewed 15 patients who underwent nephrectomy and caval thrombectomy with concurrent metastases (44). There were 2 reexplorations for postoperative hemorrhage, but no perioperative deaths were reported. Median time to initiation of postoperative immunotherapy was 48 days for the 6 patients in which it was planned (other patients had pre- and postoperative immunotherapy, or resection of metastases only as adjuvant therapy). In another series, 105 patients were reported with metastatic RCC and renal vein thrombus (51 patients) or IVC thrombus (54 patients) undergoing nephrectomy (45). Comparison was made to a group of nonmetastatic RCC patients with

TABLE 48A.1

CYTOREDUCTIVE NEPHRECTOMY IN PREPARATION FOR IMMUNOTHERAPY: RETROSPECTIVE STUDIES

Author	Number of Pts	Surgical mortality (%)	Unable to receive postoperative BRM therapy	OR (%)	CR (%)	PR (%)
Rackley et al. (1994) (29)	37	1 (2.7%)	8 (21.6%)	3 (8.1%)	0 (0.0)	3 (8.1)
Wolf et al. (1994) 37)	23	0 (0.0%)	6 (26.1%)	3 (13.0%)	2 (8.7)	1 (4.3)
Bennett et al. (1995) 38)	30	5 (17%)	23 (76.6%)	4 (13.3%)	3 (10.0)	1 (3.3)
Fallick et al. (1997) 39)	28	1 (3.6%)	2 (7.1%)	11 (39.3%)	5 (17.9)	6 (21.4)
Walther et al. (1997) 36)	195	2 (1.0%)	74 (37.9%)	19 (17.8%)	4 (3.7)	15 (14.0)
Figlin et al. (1997) (40)	62	0 (0.0%)	7 (11.3%)	19 (34.5%)	5 (9.1)	14 (25.5)
Levy et al. (1998) (41)	66	2 (3.0%)	12 (18.1%)	—	—	—
Total	441	11/441 (2.5%)	132/441 (29.9%)	59/375 (15.7%)	19/375 (5.1)	40/375 (10.7)

BRM, biologic response modifier; pts, patients; OR, overall response; CR, complete response; PR, partial response.

renal vein or IVC involvement. Early postoperative complications and mortality were not significantly different in patients undergoing thrombectomy with or without the presence of metastases. Patients with metastases undergoing nephrectomy with thrombectomy were also able to complete timely immunotherapy as often as those undergoing nephrectomy without thrombectomy. Excellent PS is critical for success with these extensive resections. Careful screening for cardiovascular and cerebrovascular disease is recommended, particularly if cardiopulmonary bypass and hypothermic circulatory arrest will be required for the operation.

Prognostic Factors for Cytoreductive Nephrectomy

Due to the variable response to cytoreductive nephrectomy and immunotherapy, several investigators have tried to identify pretherapy characteristics that predict good response to therapy. Wood et al. evaluated 126 consecutive patients undergoing cytoreductive nephrectomy and found that length of stay (LOS) after nephrectomy, tumor grade, preoperative white blood cell (WBC) count, and partial thromboplastin time (PTT) were significant predictors of survival after cytoreductive nephrectomy (46). The conclusion was that pretherapy biopsy may be warranted to rule out high-grade tumors such as sarcomatoid variants that may exclude a patient from nephrectomy. If radiologic findings suggest the possibility of a collecting duct carcinoma with metastases, a preoperative biopsy also may be useful, as these patients have very poor prognosis regardless of nephrectomy (47). Slaton et al. have reported that patients with metastatic RCC involving multiple organs, particularly the liver or central nervous system, are at high risk for death during the first 6 months following nephrectomy and are less likely to be palliated by the surgery (48). Han et al. also retrospectively analyzed factors that predict response to cytoreductive nephrectomy and found that patients with lung-only or bone-only metastases who underwent cytoreductive nephrectomy followed by immunotherapy had a median survival of 31 months, compared with a 13-month median survival ($P = .001$) in patients with multiple metastatic sites undergoing nephrectomy and immunotherapy (49). They concluded that patients with bone-only metastases, while less common than those with lung-only or multiple metastatic sites, fare relatively well with cytoreductive nephrectomy followed by immunotherapy and that those with multiple metastatic sites do poorly overall. Interestingly, only 30% of patients with bone-only metastases (10 of 33 patients) underwent cytoreductive nephrectomy followed by immunotherapy compared to 68% of patients who had lung-only metastases. This likely reflects the bias of medical oncologists and urologists, and introduces significant selection bias into their review.

In another analysis of the same database at the University of California at Los Angeles (UCLA), 236 patients with metastatic disease and no lymphadenopathy (N0M1) were compared to 86 patients with distant metastases and concomitant regional lymph node disease (N+M1) (50). Of those who underwent postnephrectomy immunotherapy, objective response rates were 30% for the N0M1 group and only 11% for the N+M1 group. N+M1patients not undergoing immunotherapy had the worst prognosis, with an overall median survival of 4.5 months, which was not significantly different ($P = .18$) than N+M1patients who did undergo immunotherapy (overall median survival of 10.8 months). In an analysis of 154 patients with metastatic RCC at the NCI undergoing nephrectomy prior to IL-2–based therapy, median survival in lymph-node–positive patients (8.5 months) was also found to be significantly inferior to that of lymph-node–negative patients (15 months) (51).

Others have analyzed serum immunologic markers such as C-reactive protein (CRP) to try to predict response to cytoreductive nephrectomy (52). They found that in patients with a normal preoperative CRP, the levels of serum immunosuppressive acidic protein and natural killer cell activity did not differ significantly before and after nephrectomy. In contrast, those with an elevated CRP preoperatively had significantly elevated serum immunosuppressive acidic protein, which dropped significantly postoperatively, and also significantly decreased preoperative natural killer cell activity that increased significantly postoperatively. They concluded that those patients with elevated CRP preoperatively may benefit the most from cytoreductive nephrectomy followed by immunotherapy.

Prospective Phase III Trials

The variable results found from multiple retrospective trials of cytoreductive nephrectomy made a randomized prospective trial vital to advancing our knowledge of treatment of metastatic RCC. Recently, SWOG Trial 8949 and European Organization for Research and Treatment of Cancer (EORTC) Trial 30947 were reported (53–55). They used a treatment protocol identical to the one designed by SWOG. These trials provide the best information to date regarding the utility of cytoreductive nephrectomy. The eligibility criteria for these trials included a histologically confirmed diagnosis of metastatic renal cancer (biopsy of the primary tumor or metastatic foci was allowed), a primary tumor that was considered resectable by the attending physician (IVC thrombus below the hepatic veins and regional lymphadenopathy were allowed), an ECOG PS of 0 or 1, and no history of prior treatment with chemotherapy, hormonal therapy, IL-2, interferon, lymphokine-activated killer (LAK) cells, or other BRMs. In addition, prior or concomitant radiation therapy to the primary tumor or to metastatic sites was not allowed, and serum bilirubin level no higher than three times the upper limit of normal at each institution and a serum creatinine no higher than 3.0 mg per dL were required. Patients were randomly assigned to nephrectomy followed by interferon-α-2b, or interferon-α-2b alone. The results for the two trials and a combined analysis are shown in Table 48A.2. Both trials demonstrated significantly longer overall survival in the groups randomized to nephrectomy prior to immunotherapy, and this benefit persisted across all study stratifications, including PS, site of metastasis, and measurable versus nonmeasurable disease. There was a single perioperative death in each of the series after nephrectomy, and overall less than 6% of patients did not receive immunotherapy in the group randomized to nephrectomy plus interferon. Despite the increased survival seen with nephrectomy, there were no differences in response rates between the study and control groups, and there was also a large discrepancy in response rates between the two studies. Patients with a PS of 0 had a significantly longer survival than patients with a PS of 1. Both studies demonstrated that nephrectomy can be performed safely with little chance of interfering with the subsequent ability to receive immunotherapy. Unfortunately, the overall median survival was only 13.6 months, with a benefit of only 5.8 months for the nephrectomy group. While it seems likely based on retrospective studies that the use of IL-2 over interferon alone will enhance survival in this population, we will have to wait for prospective studies to answer this question definitively (56).

As stated previously, an improved response rate in the nephrectomy arms of these two trials was not found, while a survival advantage was demonstrated. How might this be explained? One interesting theory put forth recently is that the enhanced survival of patients after cytoreductive nephrectomy could be due to postoperative azotemia from resection of the kidney, and not through any immune system basis at all (57). Mathematical models of malignant invasion based on tumor-induced toxicity in adjacent normal tissue have been proposed. These models suggest that mild systemic acidosis caused

TABLE 48A.2

PHASE III TRIALS OF INTERFERON-α-2B VERSUS INTERFERON-α-2B WITH NEPHRECTOMY

	Number of Pts	Median survival (mo)			Response to therapy (%)			Unable to receive postsurgery immuno therapy (%)	Operative mortality (%)
		Interferon	Surgery + interferon	P	Interferon	Surgery + interferon	P		
SWOG 8949 (2001) (53)	241	8.1	11.1	0.05	3.3	3.6	NS	NR	1 (0.8)
EORTC 30947 (2001) (54)	85	7	17	0.03	12	19	0.38	NR	1 (2.4)
Combined analysis (55)	331	7.8	13.6	0.002	5.7	6.9	0.60	9 (5.6)	2 (1.4)

NS, not significant; NR, not reported; pts, patients.

by resection of functioning nephrons can alter the microenvironment in the tumor and peritumoral normal tissue sufficiently to reduce tumor growth rate and prolong survival. This hypothesis was tested retrospectively by reviewing the patient data from the SWOG 8949 trial. In patients with no postoperative renal dysfunction, the median survival was only 4 months compared to 17 months in those with a postoperative elevation of blood urea nitrogen (BUN) and creatinine. Unfortunately, information regarding systemic pH, serum electrolytes, and other clinical data was unavailable due to the retrospective nature of the review. This fact limits the conclusions that can be drawn. Obviously if these results can be confirmed, they suggest a broad new range of therapies for tumors beyond only RCC.

NEPHRECTOMY OR METASTECTOMY AFTER RESPONSE TO SYSTEMIC IMMUNOTHERAPY

In contrast to nephrectomy prior to initiation of BRM therapy, many clinicians feel that surgery should be reserved for those who demonstrate a significant response to immunotherapy. The advantage to this strategy is the avoidance of the morbidity, mortality, and cost associated with nephrectomy. Experimental evidence also suggests that surgery in itself can cause immunosuppression and decreased response to adjuvant immunotherapy. In 1987 Eggermont et al. demonstrated that surgical trauma could augment tumor growth and inhibit the effects of IL-2 and LAK cells on the tumor cells (58). It was theorized that this phenomenon was caused by peptide growth factors, such as platelet-derived growth factor (PDGF) and TGFα and β, that are released during surgery. Certainly, rapid tumor progression at metastatic sites after removal of the primary tumor, which has been reported in up to 33% of patients, is a common cause of inability to proceed to immunotherapy after nephrectomy (36,38).

To elucidate whether there is benefit to surgical resection of disease after response to systemic therapies, several studies have been undertaken. One of the first reports was by Fleischmann and Kim in 1991 (59). Ten patients with metastatic RCC were given IL-2–based immunotherapy, and 3 had complete regression of disease outside the abdomen. Two of these patients were subsequently rendered disease-free after surgical resection of the renal primary or a retroperitoneal recurrence, and they remained disease free after surgery for 9 and

18 months, respectively. Surgical specimens revealed less than 1% viable tumor. Another multiinstitution study reviewed 399 patients from 14 institutions who underwent IL-2 therapy, with or without LAK cell therapy (60). Sixty-two patients (15.5%) demonstrated either a CR (18 patients, 4.5%) or a PR (44 patients, 11.0%). Of these, 11 patients underwent resection of residual tumor in the lung, kidney, retroperitoneum, or pelvis. At a median follow-up of 21 months, all 11 patients remained alive without evidence of disease. In contrast, among patients who did not receive surgery after immunotherapy, only 14 patients (76%) with a CR and 15 (35%) of those with a PR remained free of disease progression.

Rackley et al. reported on 62 patients, 37 of whom underwent nephrectomy prior to immunotherapy and 25 of whom were enrolled for adjuvant nephrectomy if a response to immunotherapy was seen (Table 48A.1) (29). Although only 3 of the 25 responded to immunotherapy and underwent nephrectomy, two of those patients remained alive after 18 and 42 months, respectively, of follow-up. In this series, the initial nephrectomy group had an 8% response rate and a 12-month median survival, whereas the initial immunotherapy followed by nephrectomy group had a 12% response rate and a 14-month median survival. The paucity of responders in either group and the retrospective nature of the review, however, make comparisons between groups meaningless. Another review included 14 highly selected patients who had received initial immunotherapy with an objective response or stable disease who underwent subsequent surgical resection of all metastatic disease sites and the primary tumor (if not already removed) (61). The cancer-specific survival rate for this group was 81.5% at 3 years.

As previously discussed, NCI investigators reported on 51 highly selected patients who underwent immunotherapy with the primary tumor in place (27). A total of 3 patients (6%) had objective responses at extrarenal sites and underwent nephrectomy. The duration of the responses were 11 months, 4 months, and >88 months. Median survival in all patients was 13 months. The 6% objective response rate compares poorly with the 18% response seen in 195 patients who underwent preimmunotherapy cytoreductive nephrectomy at the NCI.

No randomized prospective trial has compared cytoreductive nephrectomy before immunotherapy to nephrectomy after a response to immunotherapy. Until that study is done, it is not clear whether the seemingly better response to immunotherapy after cytoreductive nephrectomy offsets the number of patients who fail to reach systemic immunotherapy due to complications of nephrectomy or rapid tumor progression.

NEPHRECTOMY AS A COMPONENT OF ADOPTIVE IMMUNOTHERAPY

Adoptive immunotherapy is treatment involving transfer of anti-tumor cells into the host to mediate tumor regression. Nephrectomy is typically a requirement for these protocols as a source for tumor antigens or TILs. The group from UCLA has reported perhaps the most encouraging results with this therapy (40). In this protocol, TIL cells were harvested from the nephrectomy specimens, expanded *ex vivo*, and reinfused along with IL-2. Many patients also received preoperative cytokines to improve the yield of TILs, and in some cases CD8+ cytotoxic lymphocytes were enriched to enhance responses. Sixty-two patients were enrolled, and 55 eventually underwent treatment after nephrectomy. A 25.5% overall PR rate with a 9.1% CR rate was reported. On the basis of these encouraging results a prospective, randomized trial comparing standard low-dose IL-2 therapy given with and without TIL cells was undertaken (62). OR rate was 9.9% in the IL-2 + TIL group and 11.4% in the IL-2–only group ($P = .753$). Median survival was 12.8 months for the TIL + IL-2 group and 11.5 months in the IL-2–alone group. While these results are disappointing, nephrectomy may continue to be a part of adoptive immunotherapy protocols in the context of informed consent at tertiary-care facilities that can support these highly technical procedures.

CONCLUSION

The role of surgery in the management of metastatic RCC is still being defined, but certain conclusions can be made. Surgery for palliation of symptoms related to the primary tumor or metastases is justified, but only in rare circumstances when angioinfarction or other strategies cannot adequately control the symptoms. Resection of the primary tumor along with complete resection of solitary or limited metastases can often lead to long-term survival, but it is an unusual patient who satisfies the criteria for this type of surgery. Nephrectomy prior to immunotherapy has been shown in phase III trials to result in a survival benefit in patients with good PS and limited burden of disease, although the overall improvement in survival is modest. Whether nephrectomy performed after a response to immunotherapy will provide as significant a benefit as preimmunotherapy nephrectomy remains to be seen. Clearly, additional randomized, prospective trials must be completed to further elucidate the role for nephrectomy in metastatic RCC. Nephrectomy will continue to play a role in adoptive immunotherapy strategies. Hopefully, further research into novel therapies such as dendritic cell therapy, gene therapy, and tumor vaccines will lead to the breakthrough that is so greatly needed for the management of patients with metastatic RCC.

References

1. Johnson DE, Kaesler KE, Samuels ML. Is nephrectomy justified in patients with metastatic renal carcinoma? *J Urol* 1975;114:27–29.
2. Montie JE, Stewart BH, Straffon RA, et al. The role of adjunctive nephrectomy in patients with metastatic renal cell carcinoma. *J Urol* 1977;117: 272–274.
3. Walther MM, Patel B, Choyke PL, et al. Hypercalcemia in patients with metastatic renal cell carcinoma. Effect of nephrectomy and metabolic evaluation. *J Urol* 1997;158(3 Pt 1):733–739.
4. Kollender Y, Bickels J, Price WM, et al. Metastatic renal cell carcinoma of bone: indications and technique of surgical intervention. *J Urol* 2000; 164 (5):1505–1508.
5. Sheehan JP, Sun MH, Kondziolka D, et al. Radiosurgery in patients with renal cell carcinoma metastasis to the brain: long-term outcomes and prognostic factors influencing survival and local tumor control. *J Neurosurg* 2003; 98(2): 342–349.
6. Skinner DG, Colvin RB, Vermillon CD, et al. Diagnosis and management of renal cell carcinoma: a clinical and pathologic study of 309 cases. *Cancer* 1971;28:1165.
7. Middleton RG. Surgery for metastatic renal cell carcinoma. *J Urol* 1967; 97:973.
8. Kierney PC, van Heerden JA, Segura JW, et al. Surgeon's role in the management of solitary renal cell carcinoma metastases occurring subsequent to initial curative nephrectomy: an institutional review. *Ann Surg Oncol* 1994;1:345–352.
9. Tolia BM, Whitmore WF Jr. Solitary metastasis from renal cell carcinoma. *J Urol* 1975;114:836–838.
10. O'Dea MJ, Zincke H, Utz DC, et al. The treatment of renal cell carcinoma with solitary metastasis. *J Urol* 1978;120:540–542.
11. Kavolius JP, Mastorakos DP, Pavlovich C, et al. Resection of metastatic renal cell carcinoma. *J Clin Oncol* 1998;16(6):2261–2266.
12. Swanson D, Johnson D, von Eschenbach AD. Angioinfarction plus nephrectomy for metastatic renal cell carcinoma: an update. *J Urol* 1983;130: 449.
13. Gottesman JE, Crawford ED, Grossman HB, et al. Infarction-nephrectomy for metastatic renal carcinoma: Southwest Oncology Group study. *Urology* 1985;25(3):248–250.
14. Couillard DR, de Vere White RW. Surgery of renal cell carcinoma. *Urol Clin North Am* 1993;20(2):263–275.
15. Freed SZ, Halperin JP, Gordon M. Idiopathic regression of metastases from renal cell carcinoma. *J Urol* 1977;118:538–542.
16. Marcus SG, Choyke PL, Reiter R. Regression of metastatic renal cell carcinoma after cytoreductive nephrectomy. *J Urol* 1993;150:463–466.
17. Freed SZ. Nephrectomy for renal cell carcinoma with metastases. *Urology* 1977;9(6):613–616.
18. Spencer WF, Linehan WM, McClellan MW. Immunotherapy with interleukin-2 and interferon in patients with metastatic renal cell cancer in situ primary cancers: a pilot study. *J Urol* 1992;147:24–30.
19. Robertson CN, Linehan WM, Pass HI. Preparative cytoreductive surgery in patients with metastatic renal cell carcinoma treated with adoptive immunotherapy with interleukin-2 or interleukin-2 plus lymphokine activated killer cells. *J Urol* 1990;144:614.
20. Ng CS, Novick AC, Tannenbaum CS, et al. Mechanisms of immune evasion by renal cell carinoma: tumor-induced T-Lymphocyte apoptosis and NFκB suppression. *Urology* 2002;59:9–14.
21. Finke JH, Zea AH, Stanly J, et al. Loss of T-cell receptor zeta chain and p561ck in T-cells infiltrating human renal cell carcinoma. *Cancer Res* 1993;53:5613–5616.
22. Uzzo RG, Rayman P, Kolenko V, et al. Mechanisms of apoptosis in T cells from patients with renal cell carcinoma. *Clin Cancer Res* 1999;5: 1219–1229.
23. Cardi G, Heaney JA, Schned AR, et al. Expression of Fas (APO-1/CD95) in tumor infiltrating and peripheral blood lymphocytes in patients with renal cell carcinoma. *Cancer Res* 1998;58(10):2078–2080.
24. Li X, Liu J, Park JK, et al. T cells from renal cell carcinoma patients exhibit an abnormal pattern of kappa B-specific DNA-binding activity: a preliminary report. *Cancer Res* 1994;54:5424–5429.
25. Figlin RA. Renal cell carcinoma: management of advanced disease . *J Urol* 1999;161(2):381–387.
26. Lahn M, Fisch P, Kohler G, et al. Pro-inflammatory and T cell inhibitory cytokines are secreted at high levels in tumor cell cultures of human renal cell carcinoma. *Eur Urol* 1999;35(1):70–80.
27. Wagner JR, Walther MM, Linehan WM, et al. Interleukin-2 based immunotherapy for metastatic renal cell carcinoma with the kidney in place. *J Urol* 1999;162:43–45.
28. Sella A, Swanson DA, Ro JY, et al. Surgery following response to interferon-alpha–based therapy for residual renal cell carcinoma. *J Urol* 1993;149: 19–22.
29. Rackley R, Novick A, Klein E. The impact of adjuvant nephrectomy on multimodality treatment of metastatic renal cell carcinoma. *J Urol* 1994; 152:1399.
30. Motzer RJ, Mazumdar M, Bacik J, et al. Survival and prognostic stratification of 670 patients with advanced renal cell carcinoma. *J Clin Oncol* 1999;17:2530.
31. Motzer RJ, Russo P. Systemic therapy for renal cell carcinoma. *J Urol* 2000;163:408–417.
32. Muss H, Constanzi JJ, Leavit R, et al. Recombinant alpha interferon in renal cell carcinoma: randomized trial of two routes of administration. *J Clin Oncol* 1987;5:286–291.
33. Umeda T, Niijima T. Phase II study of alpha interferon on renal cell carcinoma. *Cancer* 1986;58:1231–1235.
34. Fisher RI, Coltman CA, Doroshaw JH, et al. Metastatic renal cancer treated with interleukin-2 and lymphokine-activated killer cells. *Ann Intern Med* 1988;108:518–523.
35. Mani S, Todd MB, Katz K, et al. Prognostic factors for survival in patients with metastatic renal cancer treated with biological response modifiers. *J Urol* 1995;154(1):35–40.
36. Walther MM, Yang JC, Pass HI. Cytoreductive surgery before high dose interleukin-2 based therapy in patients with metastatic renal cell carcinoma. *J Urol* 1997;158:1675–1678.

37. Wolf JS, Aronson FR, Small EJ, et al. Nephrectomy for metastatic renal cell carcinoma: a component of systemic treatment regimens. *J Surg Oncol* 1994;55:7–13.
38. Bennett RT, Lerner SE, Taub HC, et al. Cytoreductive surgery for stage IV renal cell carcinoma. *J Urol* 1995;154(1):32–34.
39. Fallick ML, McDermott DF. Nephrectomy before interleukin-2 therapy for patients with metastatic renal cell carcinoma. *J Urol* 1997; 158(5):1691.
40. Figlin RA, Pierce WC, Kaboo R, et al. Treatment of metastatic renal cell carcinoma with nephrectomy, interleukin-2 and cytokine-primed or CD8(+) selected tumor infiltrating lymphocytes from primary tumor. *J Urol* 1997; 158(3):740–745.
41. Levy DA, Swanson DA, Slaton JW, et al. Timely delivery of biological therapy after cytoreductive nephrectomy in carefully selected patients with metastatic renal cell carcinoma. *J Urol* 1998;159(4):1168–1172.
42. Walther MM, Lyne JC, Libutti SK, et al. Laparoscopic cytoreductive nephrectomy as preparation for administration of systemic interleukin-2 in the treatment of metastatic renal cell carcinoma: a pilot study. *Urology* 1999;53(3):496–500.
43. Pautler SE, Choyke PL, Phillips JL, et al. Laparoscopic cytoreductive radical nephrectomy for metastatic renal cell carcinoma: a feasibility study. *J Urol* 2001;165(Suppl. 1):185A.
44. Slaton JW, Balbay MD, Levy DA, et al. Nephrectomy and vena caval thrombectomy in patients with metastatic renal cell carcinoma. *Urology* 1997;50(5):673–677.
45. Zisman A, Pantuck AJ, Chao DH, et al. Renal cell carcinoma with tumor thrombus: is cytoreductive nephrectomy for advanced disease associated with an increased complication rate? *J Urol* 2002;168:962–967.
46. Wood CG, Huber N, Madsen L, et al. Clinical variables that predict survival following cytoreductive nephrectomy for metastatic renal cell carcinoma. *J Urol* 2001;165(5):184A.
47. Méjean A, Rouprêt M, Larousserie F, et al. Is there a place for radical nephrectomy in the presence of metastatic collecting duct carcinoma? *J Urol* 2003;169:1287–1290.
48. Slaton JW, Perrotte P, Balbay MD, et al. Reassessment of the selection criteria for cytoreductive nephrectomy in patients with metastatic renal cell carcinoma. *J Urol* 2000;163(Suppl. 4):79.
49. Han K, Pantuck AJ, Bui MHT, et al. Number of metastatic sites rather than location dictates overall survival of patients with node-negative metastatic renal cell carcinoma. *Urology* 2003;61(2):314–319.
50. Pantuck AJ, Zisman A, Dorey F, et al. Renal cell carcinoma with retroperitoneal lymph nodes: impact on survival and benefits of immunotherapy. *Cancer* 2003;97(12):2995–3002.
51. Vasselli JR, Yang JC, Linehan WM, et al. Lack of retroperitoneal lymphadenopathy predicts survival of patients with metastatic renal cell carcinoma. *J Urol* 2001;166(1):68–72.
52. Fujikawa K, Matsui Y, Miura K, et al. Serum immunosuppressive acidic protein and natural killer cell activity in patients with metastatic renal cell carcinoma before and after nephrectomy. *J Urol* 2000;164: 673–675.
53. Flanigan RC, Salmon SE, Blumenstein BA, et al. Nephrectomy followed by interferon-alfa-2b compared with interferon-alfa-2b alone for metastatic renal-cell cancer. *N Engl J Med* 2001;345(23):1655–1659.
54. Mickisch GHJ, Garin A, van Poppell H, et al. Radical nephrectomy plus interferon-alfa-based immunotherapy compared with interferon alfa alone in metastatic renal-cell carcinoma: a randomised trial. *Lancet* 2001;358: 966–970.
55. Flanigan RC, Mickisch GHJ, Sylvester R, et al. Cytoreductive nephrectomy in patients with metastatic renal cancer: a combined analysis *J Urol* 2004;171(3):1071–1076.
56. Pantuck AJ, Belldegrun AS, Figlin RA. Nephrectomy and interleukin-2 for metastatic renal-cell carcinoma. *N Engl J Med* 2001;345(23): 1711–1712.
57. Gatenby RA, Gawlinski ET, Tangen CM, et al. The possible role of postoperative azotemia in enhanced survival of patients with metastatic renal cancer after cytoreductive nephrectomy. *Cancer Res* 2002;62: 5218.
58. Eggermont AMM, Steller EP, Sugarbaker PH. Laparotomy enhances intraperitoneal tumor growth and abrogates the antitumor effects of interleukin-2 and lymphokine activated killer cells. *Surgery* 1987;123: 71–78.
59. Fleischmann JD, Kim B. Interleukin-2 immunotherapy followed by resection of residual renal cell carcinoma. *J Urol* 1991;145:938–941.
60. Kim B, Louie AC. Surgical resection following interleukin 2 therapy for metastatic renal cell carcinoma prolongs remission. *Arch Surg* 1992;127: 1343–1349.
61. Krishnamurthi V, Novick AC, Bukowski RM, et al. Efficacy of multimodality therapy in advanced renal cell carcinoma. *Urology* 1998;51(6): 933–937.
62. Figlin RA, Thompson JA, Bukowski RM, et al. Multicenter, randomized, phase III trial of CD8+ tumor-infiltrating lymphocytes in combination with recombinant interleukin-2 in metastatic renal cell carcinoma. *J Clin Oncol* 1999;17(8):2521–2529.

CHAPTER 48B
Management of Metastatic Renal Cell Carcinoma: Interleukin-2

David F. McDermott and Micheal B. Atkins

BACKGROUND

The prognosis for patients with recurrent and/or metastatic renal cell carcinoma is poor because median survival is 10 to 13 months and 5-year survival is less than 5% (1–4). These figures underscore the need for effective systemic therapy in this disease. Chemotherapy has limited activity and although interferon-α (IFN-α) can produce marginal survival benefits, response rates (RR) are 5% to 15%, and most of these responses are partial and short lived (5–8). In contrast, the administration of high-dose (HD) bolus interleukin-2 (IL-2) has consistently produced durable responses in a modest percentage of patients with advanced renal cell cancer (9), leading to its approval by the U.S. Food and Drug Administration (FDA) in 1992 for the treatment of metastatic renal cell cancer. This chapter examines the efficacy and toxicity of IL-2 in patients with renal cell cancer and focuses on factors that are predictive of response to IL-2 and that might allow this therapy to be applied more selectively to patients who are most likely to benefit.

EFFICACY OF INTERLEUKIN-2 REGIMENS

Interleukin-2 Plus Lymphokine-Activated Killer Cells

Investigations of IL-2 (Aldesleukin, Chiron) in patients with renal cell carcinoma began in the mid-1980s. Initial studies evaluated HD bolus IL-2 therapy in combination with the infusion of autologous lymphocytes activated *ex vivo* in IL-2 (lymphokine-activated killer or LAK cells) (10). Although dramatic and durable responses were reported in some patients (11,12), subsequent studies found the efficacy of HD bolus IL-2 alone to be equivalent to that of the combination of IL-2 and LAK cells, prompting the abandonment of this more complex cellular therapy component (13,14).

High-dose Interleukin-2

In 1992, HD bolus IL-2 was approved by the FDA for the treatment of patients with metastatic renal cell cancer on the basis of the data presented on 255 patients entered onto seven phase II clinical trials (9). In these studies, 600,000 to 720,000 IU/kg of recombinant human IL-2 was administered by 15-minute infusion every 8 hours; this was done for 14 dosages, thereby constituting a cycle of therapy. Patients received a course of therapy, consisting of two cycles separated by 5 to 9 days of rest (maximum of 28 doses), and courses were repeated every 8 to 12 weeks in stable or responding patients. Although 35% of patients received 720,000 IU/kg of IL-2 per dose and the remainder received 600,000 IU/kg/dose, the median cumulative amount of IL-2 administered was the same in both groups because patients receiving 720,000 IU/kg/dose tolerated fewer IL-2 doses. Ninety-six percent of these patients had an Eastern Cooperative Oncology Group (ECOG) performance status of 0 or 1, 85% had undergone a nephrectomy before starting IL-2 therapy, none had received prior immunotherapy, and the median time from diagnosis to treatment was 8.5 months.

Objective responses were seen in 37 of the 255 patients (RR 15%). There were 17 (7%) complete responses (CRs) and 20 (8%) partial responses (PRs). Fourteen of the responding patients (38%) began therapy with tumor burdens greater than 50 cm² on pretreatment scans and 60% of patients with PRs had greater than 90% regression of all measurable disease. The median duration of response was 54 months for all responders, 20 months for patients with PRs, and CR has not yet been reached. The median survival was 16 months for all 255 patients.

Follow-up data on these patients has now been accumulated through June 2002, with a median follow-up of over 10 years (15,16). Although some late relapses are still being observed, the response duration curve appears to have leveled off after the 30-month time point and 60% of patients with CRs remain in remission. In addition, four patients with PRs who underwent surgical resection of residual disease while still in response remain alive and disease-free at a minimum of 65+ months. Therefore, many patients with CRs remaining free from progression for more than 30 months and those patients with PRs resected to no evidence of disease (NED) after a response to HD IL-2 are unlikely to progress and may actually be cured. Therefore, although the response rate to HD bolus IL-2 is modest, the quality and durability of the responses with this treatment appears to be superior to that typically seen with IFN-α or chemotherapy (Fig. 48B.1).

Alternative Interleukin-2-based Regimens

Efforts to enhance the therapeutic index of IL-2 have led to the investigation of regimens involving lower doses of IL-2 and different routes of administration. Approaches have included continuous intravenous infusion, outpatient subcutaneous (SC) therapy, and low/intermediate-dose intravenous therapy. Although many initial reports were encouraging, long-term follow-up data and expanded phase II data has generally been lacking.

Continuous Intravenous Infusion

Although antitumor activity similar to HD bolus IL-2 has been seen with continuous IV infusion regimens, this approach has also produced at least equivalent toxicity (17,18), for example, one study randomly assigned 94 patients with advanced renal cell carcinoma to either HD bolus or continuous infusion IL-2 each together with LAK cells (18). Objective responses were observed in 20% and 15% of patients in the bolus and continuous infusion groups, respectively. Despite the fact that patients treated by continuous infusion received one-third the amount of IL-2, there was no difference in the incidence of life-threatening toxic side effects (such as hypotension and/or oliguria) between the two groups. Furthermore, fever, infection, and elevated serum levels of alkaline phosphatase were more common in the continuous infusion group. In subsequent studies that omitted the LAK cells and/or lowered the IL-2 dose further to enable more prolonged administration, the antitumor activity appeared to be compromised (19–21).

Outpatient Subcutaneous Administration

Multiple studies have examined the effectiveness and toxicity of subcutaneously administered IL-2 in outpatients (22–24). In one series of 27 outpatients, the daily subcutaneous administration of IL-2 resulted in a 22% response rate (two CRs and four PRs) (22). Two patients had ongoing CRs of 19 and 17 months at the time of publication in 1992; however, no additional information has been reported. In another report describing results of subcutaneous IL-2 therapy, only one of 16 patients (6%) exhibited a partial remission (24).

Lower-Dose Intravenous Therapy

Investigators at the National Cancer Institute (NCI) Surgery Branch have extensively studied a regimen in which each dose is 10% (72,000 IU/kg) of the standard HD intravenous dose. The initial report on the first 65 patients described a 15% response rate in patients with metastatic renal cell carcinoma (25). A randomized phase III trial that compared this regimen with HD IL-2 and a daily subcutaneous regimen will be discussed in subsequent text (26).

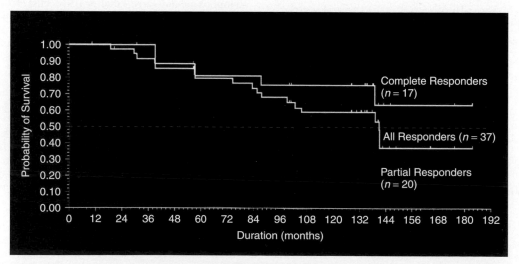

FIGURE 48B.1. The Kaplan-Meier projection response duration curves for the 37 responding patients with renal cancer who were in the initial cohort of 255 patients treated with high-dose IV bolus rIL-2 presented to the U.S. Food and Drug Administration (FDA) in 1992. (From McDermott DM, Atkins MB. Application of IL-2 and other cytokines in renal cancer, *Expert Opinion Biologic Therapy.* 2004;4:455–468, with permission.)

Interleukin-2 Plus Interferon-α

Combinations of IL-2 and IFN-α have been extensively studied in patients with metastatic renal cell carcinoma with largely mixed results. IFN-α upregulates the expression of HLA class I and tumor-associated antigens, thereby possibly increasing the immunogenicity of tumor cells, and increasing their susceptibility to IL-2-mediated cytolysis. Several animal experiments showed that the combination of IL-2 and type I IFNs enhanced effector cell activation and produced antitumor effects superior to that seen with the maximum tolerated doses of the single agents in the same tumor models (27–30). Although the initial phase I study of HD intravenous IL-2 and IFN-α produced a 31% (11 of 35) response rate in patients with renal cell carcinoma (31), subsequent studies showed that the combination produced what appeared to be more neurologic and cardiac toxicity without enhancing the antitumor activity seen with HD IL-2 alone (32–36).

Many regimens that combined lower doses of IFN-α and IL-2 were found to be suitable for administration in an outpatient setting. Response rates for these approaches ranged from 22% to 39% (32,37–55). Atzpodien et al. (43) noted responses in 25% of patients who received subcutaneous IL-2 and IFN-α. Subsequently, they developed a regimen that alternated 4 weeks of subcutaneously administered IL-2 and IFN-α with 4 weeks of combined 5-FU and IFN-α and reported a response rate of 39% in 120 patients (48). Response durations and numbers of durable CRs (CRs lasting >2 yr) were not fully reported; however, the median response duration was approximately 12 months for each regimen.

In an effort to confirm and to extend the results of several of the more promising outpatient IL-2-based regimens, the Cytokine Working Group conducted two phase II trials that evaluated the administration of subcutaneous IL-2 and IFN-α in the outpatients and the combination of subcutaneous IL-2 and IFN-α alternating with 5-fluorouracil (5FU) and IFN-α in patients with metastatic renal cell carcinoma (32,54,55). All patients in these studies met the eligibility criteria for the HD inpatient regimen. The addition of 5FU to outpatient IL-2 and IFN-α did not substantially improve efficacy but it did increase toxicity. Response rates (17% and 18%) and median survival (20.4 and 17.5 months) in both trials were similar to those seen with HD IL-2. Although acute toxicity was less common in the outpatient regimens than with HD IL-2, durable responses appeared to be less frequent (median response duration 12 and 8 months, respectively, versus 53 months for HD IL-2) and fewer patients were progression free at 3 years (2% for both trials vs. 9% for HD IL-2). Given that these studies were conducted sequentially, it was impossible to exclude selection bias over time as the reason for the discrepancy in response quality.

Randomized Trials with Interleukin-2 +/– Interferon

Given that HD bolus IL-2 was approved by the FDA for its ability to produce durable tumor responses, before accepting lower-dose regimens as equivalent, it was imperative to establish that the quality of the tumor responses with these lower-dose regimens were not inferior to the HD bolus IL-2 regimen. Three large-scale randomized trials have now been completed that provide clinicians with useful insights into the relative merits of these various regimens and therefore into the optimal management of patients with metastatic renal cell carcinoma (Table 48B.1).

Investigators in France conducted a large-scale, phase III randomized trial comparing intermediate-dose IL-2 administered by continuous intravenous infusion plus subcutaneous IFN-α with either IL-2 or IFN-α administered alone (42); 425 patients were enrolled. The three treatment groups were well-balanced for age and gender, as well as for known predictors of response and survival. The response rate and 1-year event-free survival were significantly greater for the combined IL-2 and IFN-α arm than for either of the single-agent arms, although there was no significant difference in overall survival among the three groups. Of note, responses were seen in only 6.5% and 7.5% of patients receiving IL-2 or IFN-α alone, respectively, with only 2.9% and 6.1% of these patients still responding at the week 25 evaluation. Although more antitumor activity was seen with the combination arm, this was largely due to the rather limited activity of the single-agent regimens. How an intermediate-dose combination of IL-2 and IFN-α would compare with HD IL-2 alone remained to be established.

The NCI Surgery Branch investigators performed a randomized trial comparing standard HD IL-2 and the intermediate-dose intravenous bolus IL-2 regimen (LD IV IL-2) developed by Yang et al. (26) After randomizing 117 patients, a third arm was added involving subcutaneously IL-2 administered in a fashion similar to that previously described by Sleijfer et al. (22). Results were analyzed and reported according to groups that were concurrently randomized. Among the 306 patients concurrently assigned to either HD or LD IV IL-2, the response rate was significantly higher with HD therapy (21% vs. 13%), with a trend toward more durable responses. Duration of response was superior in patients who received the HD intravenous IL-2 compared to those who received the LD IV IL-2. There were no differences in overall survival. Although toxicities were also significantly greater in the HD group (particularly hypotension), there were no deaths attributable to IL-2 in either arm, and patient assessments of quality of life were found to be roughly equivalent. Among the patients concurrently assigned to either subcutaneous IL-2 or HD intravenous bolus IL-2, a higher response rate was seen with HD IL-2 (21% vs. 10%), but the difference was of borderline statistical significance. Once again there were no differences in overall survival.

In an effort to determine the value of outpatient subcutaneous IL-2 and IFN-α relative to HD IL-2 the Cytokine Working Group performed a phase III trial in which patients were randomized to receive either outpatient IL-2 (5 MIU/m^2 subcutaneously every 8 hours for 3 dosages on day 1, then daily 5 days/week for 4 weeks) and IFNα (5 MIU/m^2 subcutaneously 3 days/week for 4 weeks) every 6 weeks or standard HD inpatient IL-2 [600,000 IU/kg/dose every 8 hours intravenously, days 1 to 5 and 15 to 19 (max 28 doses)] every 12 weeks (56). Of the 193 patients enrolled, 186 were evaluable. Patients were stratified for bone or liver metastases, primary in place and performance status 0/1, and the treatment arms were evenly balanced for these characteristics, as well as for other factors: 44% patients had bone or liver metastases; 31% had primary in place; and 60% were PS 0, respectively. Toxicities seen were typical for these regimens, including one treatment-related death from progressive disease and acute respiratory distress syndrome (ARDS) on IL-2 and IFN-α arm and one death from capillary leak syndrome on HD IL-2.

The response rate for dose IL-2 was 23% (22/95) versus 10% (9/91) for IL-2/IFN-α ($P = .018$). Eight patients achieved a CR on HD IL-2 versus only three on low-dose (LD) IL-2/IFN-α (56). The median response durations were 24 months for HD IL-2 and 15 months for IL-2/IFN-α ($P = .18$). Median overall survivals were 17.5 and 13 months ($P = .24$), favoring HD IL-2. Ten patients on HD IL-2 were progression free at 3 years, compared to three on IL-2/IFN-α ($P = .08$). Of note, responses to HD IL-2 were seen with equal frequency across the stratification criteria, whereas LD IL-2/IFN-α appeared to produce less responses in patients with liver and/or bone metastases and in those who had not undergone prior nephrectomy to remove the

TABLE 48B.1

RANDOMIZED TRIALS OF INTERLEUKIN-2 IN THE TREATMENT OF METASTATIC RENAL CELL CANCER

Investigators	Number of Pts.	Dose of IL-2	Dose of interferon (schedule)	CR	PR	RR (%)	Comments
Negrier et al. (1998)	138	18 (IU/m^2/d × 10^6)	—	2	7	6.5	P <.01 for RR in IL-2 plus IFN versus IL-2 alone: survival not different
	140	18 (IU/m^2/d × 10^6)	6 × 10^6 IU (s.c. 3d/wk)	1	25	18.6	
Yang et al. (2003) (26)	155	720 (IU/kg × 10^3 q8h)	—	11	22	21	P = .048 for RR in HD IL-2 versus LD IL-2, survival not different RR for s.c. IL-2 was similar to LD IL-2 and different from HD IL-2 P = .033
	149	72 (IU/kg × 10^3)	—	6	13	13	
	93	250 (IU/kg × 10^3) s.c. QD × 5d wk 1, then 125 (IU/kg × 10^3) s.c. QD × 5d wks 2–6	—	2	7	10	
Atkins (2003) (57)	96	5 MIU/m2 s.c. q8 × 3 day one then QD 5d/wk for 4 wks	5 MIU/m^2 s.c. 3d/wk	8	14	23	P = .018 for RR in HD IL2 versus LD IL-2/ IFN, survival not different, 3 yr PFS favored HD IL-2 P = .08
	96	600 (IU/kg × 10^3 q8h)	—	3	6	9	

CR, complete response; PR, partial response; pts, patients ; RR, response rate (CR + PR).
From McDermott DM, Atkins MB. Application of IL-2 and other cytokines in renal cancer, *Expert Opinion Biologic Therapy*. 2004;4:455–468, with permission.

primary tumor. For patients with bone or liver metastases (P = .001) or primary in place (P = .04), survival was superior with HD IL-2 compared to IL-2/IFN-α, whereas no significant survival differences between the two treatments were noted for patients who had undergone prior nephrectomy or who were without bone or liver metastases. Moreover, patients who had undergone a recent nephrectomy (debulking nephrectomy in the setting of stage IV disease) appeared to fare as well with IL-2/IFN-α as with HD IL-2 (58).

Taken together, these studies suggest that HD bolus IL-2 is superior in terms of response rate and, possibly, response quality when compared to regimens involving LD IL-2 and IFN-α, intermediate or LD IL-2, or LD IFN-α. Furthermore, the benefit of HD IL-2 relative to the lower-dose regimens may be most pronounced in patients with unresected primary tumors or with bone and/or liver metastases. Consequently, we must conclude that HD IL-2 should remain the preferred therapy for appropriately selected patients with access to such therapy. However, given the toxicity and limited efficacy of HD IL-2 therapy, additional effort should be directed at better defining the patient population for whom this therapy is appropriate.

Toxicity of Interleukin-2

While HD bolus IL-2 is active in metastatic renal cell cancer and can produce durable CRs in a small number of patients, its widespread use is limited by the considerable toxicity associated with its administration. The toxicity of HD IL-2 not only limits the number of centers with the appropriate clinical expertise to provide this treatment modality but also limits therapy to those patients with adequate organ function. Even with experienced clinicians and optimal patient selection, only rarely will patients receive all of the proposed therapy (59–61).

Two of the most problematic toxicities are hypotension and capillary leak syndrome. Grade 3 to Grade 4 hypotension requiring both fluid resuscitation and pressor support occurs in 50% to 75% of patients treated with HD bolus IL-2 (9,60). This toxicity usually appears earlier and is more marked during the second week of a standard 2-week course of therapy. Capillary leak syndrome is manifested by weight gain secondary to fluid retention, edema of the face and extremities, and, in some cases, ascites, and respiratory distress due to pulmonary edema and/or pleural effusion. The pulmonary symptoms from capillary leak have been observed in 10% to 20% of patients treated with HD IL-2 and can range from dyspnea with exertion to dyspnea at rest to, rarely, respiratory failure requiring intubation and mechanical ventilation. Edema and weight gain greater than 5% of baseline is observed in 50% to 60% of patients (61,62). Overall, complications from capillary leak have been considerably diminished in recent years when compared with the earliest trials of HD IL-2 because of the more judicious use of fluids and the early application of pressors to treat IL-2-induced hypotension.

Interleukin-2 is a potent inducer of proinflammatory cytokines, such as IL-1, tumor necrosis factor-α (TNF-α), and IFN-γ (63–66). These substances and others, including nitric oxide (67), are likely to play a major role in IL-2 toxicity. Tumor responses, on the other hand, are thought to be mediated through cellular immune mechanisms, raising the possibility of dissociating the toxicity of IL-2 from its antitumor effect by combining IL-2 with various inhibitors of secondary cytokine function. The addition of dexamethasone was shown to prevent the usual induction of TNF-α by IL-2 and to significantly reduce treatment-related toxicity. However, potential interference with antitumor effects limited this approach (68,69). The use of more selective inhibitors of secondary cytokine function (e.g., CT1501R, CNI-1493 or soluble TNF-α or IL-1 receptors), despite promise in animal models have not been able to significantly block IL-2 toxicity clinically (70–73). Future exploration of this approach is likely to require combinations of cytokine antagonists, or the use of novel antagonists of secondary cytokines with more pluripotent inhibitory effects.

Adjuvant Therapy

In an effort to apply the clinical activity observed with cytokines to patients with earlier stages of disease, a variety of adjuvant trials have been performed (74,75). The Cytokine Working Group performed a trial randomly assigning patients who satisfied these high-risk staging criteria (Stage T3b-4, N1–3 or resected metastatic disease) to either a single cycle of HD IL-2 or observation (with IL-2-based therapy at the time of recurrence) (76). This study took several years to accrue 69 patients and ultimately was closed early after an interim analysis determined that the anticipated 30% improvement in disease-free survival for the patients receiving HD IL-2 could not be achieved.

Therefore, there is currently no evidence to support the use of IL-2 in the adjuvant setting in patients with high-risk renal cancer. Adjuvant studies have been compromised by the inability to clearly define a population at high risk of recurrence and by the increasing lack of availability of such high-risk patients. Furthermore, there is a growing uncertainty as to whether the biology (in particular, susceptibility to cytokine-based therapy) of tumors metastasizing to regional nodes is identical to that of tumors that metastasize systemically (77). Until this crucial issue can be sorted out, it will remain difficult to translate advances in the treatment of patients with stage IV disease to the adjuvant setting.

Predictors of Clinical Benefit from Cytokine-based Therapy

Many groups have attempted to determine reliable predictors of response and survival for patients with metastatic renal cell carcinoma who were receiving immunotherapy. Factors that have been variably associated with response to IL-2 include performance status (9), number of organs with metastases (one vs. two or more) (41), absence of bone metastases (31),

prior nephrectomy (78), degree of treatment-related thrombocytopenia, absence of prior interferon therapy (79), thyroid dysfunction (80), lymphocyte count (81), rebound lymphocytosis (82), erythropoietin production (83), and posttreatment elevations of blood TNF-α and IL-1 levels.

Negrier et al. identified independent predictors of rapid disease progression, defined as progression within 10 weeks of initiation of therapy (84). These predictors included more than one metastatic site, disease-free interval of less than 1 year, and presence of liver metastases or mediastinal nodes, as well as the type of immunotherapy used. Patients with liver metastases, more than one site of disease, and disease-free interval of less than 1 year had a lower response rate and a median survival of only 6 months, even while receiving combination IL-2 and IFN-α therapy. Figlin et al. identified prior nephrectomy and time after nephrectomy to relapse as important predictors of survival in patients receiving IL-2-based therapy (78). In their series, patients who received systemic immunotherapy for metastatic disease for more than 6 months after nephrectomy had the best median survival and had a 3-year survival rate of 46%. A recent multivariate analysis by the same group of investigators, which was confined to patients who received IL-2 after nephrectomy, revealed survival to be inversely associated with lymph node involvement, constitutional symptoms, sarcomatoid histology, metastases involving sites other than bone or lung or multiple sites, and a thyroid stimulating hormone (TSH) level >2.0 mIU/L (85). They proposed a scoring algorithm based on these features in which survival at 1-year was predicted to vary from 1% to 92%.

Recent data from the Cytokine Working Group phase III trial, mentioned previously, suggested that disease site factors such as primary in place, or hepatic or bone metastases, may be more predictive of a poor response to LD IL-2 and IFN-α regimens than to HD IL-2 (56,57). Furthermore, this study suggested that the greatest benefit from HD IL-2, relative to lower-dose regimens, might be seen in patients with primaries in place and/or liver and bone metastases. This data calls into question some of the prior studies and suggests that additional predictors of response and survival in patients receiving cytokine-based immunotherapy are necessary.

Pathologic and Molecular Predictors of Response to Interleukin-2

Influence of Histologic Subtype

Responses to immunotherapy are most frequently seen in patients with renal cell carcinoma of the clear cell histology (86–88). This observation was recently detailed in a retrospective analysis of pathology specimens obtained from 236 patients who had received IL-2 therapy on Cytokine Working Group clinical trials (88). Among patients with tumor specimens available for review, the response rate to IL-2 was 20% (30 of 148 patients) for patients with clear cell histology primary tumors, compared to 6% for patients with non-clear cell histology (one responder in 17 patients). Among the patients with clear cell cancer, response to IL-2 was also associated with the presence of alveolar features, no papillary features, granular features in less than 50% of the pathologic material, and major renal vein involvement. The response rate was 41% (16 responders of 39 patients) in patients with all these features. In addition, patients with primary tumors of clear cell histology, alveolar but not papillary features, and 50% granular features had a response rate of 25% (29 responders of 115 patients) compared to 4% (two responders of 50 patients) in the other patients. When this model was then applied to the 71 patients with specimens from other metastatic sites, all seven tumor responses were seen in the 38 patients with clear cell cancer and all the good prognostic features, thereby confirming the validity of the model developed from the primary kidney tumor specimens. As a result of these data, it is likely appropriate to offer patients with nonclear cell histology and those with clear cell histology but adverse pathologic features (i.e., papillary and/or no alveolar features, and/or >50% granular features) alternative, nonimmunotherapy-based treatments. However, given that even in the most favorable prognostic group, more than 50% of patients failed to respond to IL-2 therapy, additional investigations into tumor-associated predictors of responsiveness to IL-2 are still necessary.

Molecular Markers

Some investigators have begun to examine tumor tissue to identify molecular markers that might predict the outcome of patients with renal cell carcinoma. Recently, carbonic anhydrase IX (CAIX) has been identified as one potential marker. CAIX is thought to play a role in cell proliferation in response to hypoxic conditions. CAIX expression is mediated by the HIF-1 α-transcriptional complex and is induced in many tumors types but is absent in most normal tissue, with the exception of epithelial cells of the gastric mucosa. Bui et al. used a monoclonal antibody designed to detect CAIX expression to perform an immunohistochemical analysis of paraffin-embedded renal cell carcinoma specimens. They showed that >90% of renal cell carcinoma express CAIX and that its expression decreases with the advancing stage of the disease (89). In their analysis, high CAIX expression in primary tumors was seen in 79% of patients and was associated with improved survival and, possibly, with response to IL-2-based therapy. In addition, all long-term responders to IL-2-based treatment had high CAIX expression. In this study, low CAIX expression was associated with a worse outcome for patients with localized, advanced renal cell carcinoma and was an independent predictor of outcome in patients with metastatic disease.

Building on this work, Atkins et al. performed a nested case–control study within the larger cohort of patients whose pathology was analyzed (90). CAIX expression levels were correlated with response to IL-2, pathologic risk categorization and survival. As in the report by Bui et al. the percentage of CAIX-positive tumor cells was utilized to separate high (>85%) and low (≤85%) expressors. Twenty-seven of 66 selected patients (41%) had responded to IL2-based regimens, with 20 (30%) remaining alive at a median follow-up of 2.6 years. Twenty-four (36%), 31 (47%), and 11 (17%) patients were classified into good, intermediate, or high-risk groups according to the pathology model described above. Forty-one specimens (62%) had high CAIX expression. Twenty-one of 27 (78%) responding patients had high CAIX expression compared to 20 of 39 (51%) of nonresponders (Odds Ratio = 3.3, P = .04). Median survivals were 3 years and 1 year for high- and low-CAIX expressors, respectively (P = .04). Survival greater than 5 years was only seen in the high CAIX-expressing group. High CAIX staining was associated with better pathologic features but remained an independent predictor of response. For example, in patients within the intermediate pathology group, 9 of 9 responders, as compared to 11 of 22 nonresponders had high CAIX expression. A two-compartment model was proposed in which one group of patients with either good pathology or intermediate pathology and high CAIX expression contained 26 of 27 (96%) responders compared to only 18 of 39 (46%) nonresponders (Odds Ratio = 30; P <.01). Significant survival benefit was also seen for this group (P <.01).

Although this model requires prospective validation, it highlights the potential for using pathologic and molecular features of the tumor to identify the optimal patients to receive IL-2 therapy. Additional studies to explain these preliminary observations and to correlate results with previously described clinical features are necessary. In addition, gene-expression profiling of tumor specimens to identify new proteins or patterns of gene expression that might be associated with IL-2 responsiveness may eventually help further narrow the application of IL-2 therapy to those who will benefit the most from it.

CONCLUSION

High-dose bolus IL-2 remains the gold standard and should be considered for appropriately selected patients with access to such treatment (91). Given the toxicity, expense, and limited availability of this treatment, appropriate selection criteria need to be reevaluated and further investigated. Lowering the dose of IL-2 or combining it with other cytokines appears to reduce its ability to produce durable responses. Patients with nonclear cell histology and with papillary or extensive granular features within their cancer specimen respond poorly to IL-2 and should be considered for nonimmunotherapeutic approaches. Those patients who fail IL-2 therapy should be considered for experimental therapies that focus on new targets (e.g., angiogenesis and signal transduction) that are showing great promise. Careful investigation of IL-2 in combination with novel agents (e.g., Bevacizumab) will be critical to the future application of this cytokine.

References

1. Linehan WM, Shipley WU, Parkinson DR. Cancer of the kidney and ureter. In: DeVita VT Jr, (Ed.) *Cancer: principles and practice of oncology*, 4th ed. Philadelphia, PA: JB Lippincott Co, 1993.
2. Motzer RJ, Bander NH, Nanus DM. Renal-cell carcinoma. *N Engl J Med* 1996;335:865.
3. Motzer RJ, Mazumdar M, Bacik J, et al. Survival and prognostic stratification of 670 patients with advanced renal cell carcinoma. *J Clin Oncol* 1999;17(8):2530.
4. Motzer RJ, Bacik J, Murphy BA, et al. Interferon-alfa as a comparative treatment for clinical trials of new therapies against advanced renal cell carcinoma. *J Clin Oncol* 2002;20(1):289–296.
5. Yagoda A, Petrylak D, Thompson S. Cytotoxic chemotherapy for advanced renal cell carcinoma. *Urol Clin North Am* 1993;20:303–314.
6. Pyrhonen S, Salminen E, Lehtonen T, et al. Recombinant interferon alfa-2a with vinblastine vs. vinblastine alone in advanced renal cell carcinoma: a phase II study. *Proc Am Soc Clin Oncol* 1996;15:244.
7. Muss HB. Interferon therapy for renal cell carcinoma. *Semin Oncol* 1987;14:36–42.
8. Muss HB, Costanzi JJ, Leavitt R, et al. Recombinant alfa interferon in renal cell carcinoma: a randomized trial of two routes of administration. *J Clin Oncol* 1987;5:286–291.
9. Fyfe G, Fisher RI, Rosenberg SA, et al. Results of treatment of 255 patients with metastatic renal cell carcinoma who received high-dose recombinant interleukin-2 therapy. *J Clin Oncol* 1995;13:688–696.
10. Mazumber A, Rosenberg SA. Successful immunotherapy of natural killer-resistant established pulmonary melanoma metastases by the intravenous adaptive transfer of syngeneic lymphocytes activated in vitro by interleukin 2. *J Exp Med* 1984;159:495.
11. Fisher RI, Coltman CA, Doroshow JH, et al. Metastatic renal cancer treated with interleukin-2 and lymphokine-activated killer cells: a phase II clinical trial. *Ann Intern Med* 1988;108:518.
12. Rosenberg SA, Lotze MR, Muul LM, et al. A progress report on the treatment of 157 patients with advanced cancer using lymphokine-activated killer cells and interleukin-2 or high-dose interleukin-2 alone. *N Engl J Med* 1987;316:889.
13. Sunderland MC. Weiss GRl: high dose IL-2 treatment of renal cell carcinoma. In: Atkins MB, Mier JW, eds. *Therapeutic applications of interleukin-2*, New York: Marcel Dekker Inc, 1993:119.
14. Rosenberg SA, Lotze MT, Yang JC, et al. Prospective randomized trial of high-dose interleukin-2 alone or in conjunction with lymphokine-activated killer cells for the treatment of patients with advanced cancer. *J Natl Cancer Inst* 1993;85:622.
15. Fisher RI, Rosenberg SA, Fyfe G. Long-term survival update for high-dose recombinant interleukin-2 in patients with renal cell carcinoma. *Cancer J Sci Am* 2000;6:S55–S57.
16. Rosenberg SA, Yang JC, White DE, et al. Durability of complete responses in patients with metastatic cancer treated with high-dose interleukin-2. Identification of the antigens mediating response. *Ann Surg* 1998;228: 307–319.
17. Dillman RO, Oldman RK, Tauer KW, et al. Continuous interleukin-2 and lymphokine-activated killer cells for advanced cancer: a National Biotherapy Study Group trial. *J Clin Oncol* 1991;9:1223.

18. Weiss GR, Margolin KA, Aronson FR. A randomized phase II trial of continuous infusion interleukin-2 or bolus injection interleukin-2 plus lymphokine-activated killer cells for advanced renal cell carcinoma. *J Clin Oncol* 1992;10:275.

19. Gold PJ, Thompson JA, Markowitz DR, et al. Metastatic renal cell carcinoma: long-term survival after therapy with high-dose continuous-infusion interleukin-2. *Cancer J Sci Am* 1997;3:S85.

20. Sosman JA, Kohler PC, Hank J, et al. Repetitive weekly cycles of recombinant human interleukin-2: responses of renal carcinoma with acceptable toxicity. *J Natl Cancer Inst* 1988;80:60.

21. Caligiuri MA, Murray C, Robertson MJ, et al. Selective modulation of human natural killer cells in vivo after prolonged infusion of low dose recombinant interleukin 2. *J Clin Invest* 1993;91:123.

22. Sleijfer DT, Janssen RAJ, Buter J, et al. Phase II study of subcutaneous interleukin-2 in unselected patients with advanced renal cell cancer on a outpatient basis. *J Clin Oncol* 1992;10:1119.

23. Lissoni P, Bordin V, Vaghi M, et al. Ten-year survival results in metastatic renal cell cancer patients treated with monoimmunotherapy with subcutaneous low-dose interleukin-2. *Anticancer Res* 2002;22:1061–1064.

24. Lopen Hanninen E, Kirchner H, Atzpodien J, et al. Interleukin-2 based home therapy of metastatic renal cell carcinoma: risk and benefits in 215 consecutive single institution patients. *J Urol* 1996;155:19.

25. Yang JC, Toplalian SL, Parkinson D, et al. Randomized comparison of high-dose intravenous interleukin-2 for the therapy of metastatic renal cell carcinoma: an interim report. *J Clin Oncol* 1994;12:1572.

26. Yang JC, Sherry RM, Stienberg SM, et al. A three-arm randomized comparison of high and low dose intravenous and subcutaneous interleukin-2 in the treatment of metastatic renal cancer. *J Clin Oncol* 2003;21:3127.

27. Cameron RB, McIntosh JK, Rosenberg SA. Synergistic anti-tumor effects of combinations immunotherapy with recombinant interleukin-2 and a recombinant hybrid alpha-interferon in the treatment of established murine hepatic metastases. *Cancer Res* 1988;48:5810.

28. Igo M, Sakurai M, Tamura T, et al. In vivo anti-tumor activity of multiple injections of recombinant interleukin 2, alone and in combination with three different types of recombinant interferon, on various syngeneic murine tumors. *Cancer Res* 1988;48:260.

29. Cameron RB, McIntosh JK, Rosenberg SA. Synergistic anti-tumor effects of combination immunotherapy with recombinant interleukin-2 and a recombinant hybrid alpha-interferon in the treatment of established murine hepatic metastases. *Cancer Res* 1988;48(20):5810–5817.

30. Igo M, Sakurai J, Tamura T, et al. In vivo anti-tumor activity of multiple injections of recombinant interleukin-2 alone and in combination with three different types of recombinant interferon, on various syngeneic murine tumors. *Cancer Res* 1988;48:260–264.

31. Rosenberg SA, Lotze MT, Yang JC, et al. Combination therapy with interleukin-2 and alpha-interferon for the treatment of patients with advanced cancer. *J Clin Oncol* 1989;7:1863.

32. Dutcher JP, Fisher R, Weiss G, et al. Interleukin-2-based therapy for metastatic renal cell cancer: the cytokine working group experience, 1989-1997. *Cancer J Sci Am* 1997;3:S73–S78.

33. Sznol M, Mier J, Sparano J, et al. A phase I study of high-dose interleukin-2 combination with interferon-alfa 2B. *J Biol Response Mod* 1990;9:529–537.

34. Bergman L, Fenchel K, Weidmann E, et al. Daily alternating administration of high-dose alfa-2b-interferon and interleukin-2 bolus infusion in metastatic renal cell carcinoma. *Cancer* 1993;72:1733–1742.

35. Spencer WF, Linehan WM, Walther HM, et al. Immunotherapy with interleukin-2 and alpha-interferon in patients with metastatic renal cell cancer with in situ primary cancer. A pilot study. *J Urol* 1992;147:24–30.

36. Budd GT, Murhty S, Finke J, et al. Phase I trial of high-dose bolus interleukin-2 and interferon alfa-2a in patients with metastatic malignancy. *J Clin Oncol* 1992;10:804–809.

37. Figlin RA, Bellegrun A, Moldawer N, et al. Concomitant administration of recombinant human interleukin-2 and recombinant interferon alfa-2A: an active outpatient regimen in metastatic renal cell carcinoma. *J Clin Oncol* 1992;10:414–421.

38. Lipton A, Harvey H, Givant E, et al. Interleukin-2 and interferon-a-2a outpatient therapy for metastatic renal cell carcinoma. *J Immunother* 1993;13:122–129.

39. Dillman RO, Church C, Oldham RK, et al. Inpatient continuous-infusion interleukin-2 in 788 patients with cancer. The National Biotherapy Study Group Experience. *Cancer* 1993;71:2358–2370.

40. Beldgrun A, Pierce W, Kaboo R, et al. Interferon-alpha primed tumor-infiltrating lymphocytes with Interleukin-2 and interferon-alpha as therapy for metastatic renal cell carcinoma. *J Urol* 1993;150:1384–1390.

41. Besana C, Borri A, Bucci E, et al. Treatment of advanced renal cell cancer with sequential intravenous recombinant interleukin-2 and subcutaneous α-interferon. *Eur J Cancer* 1994;9:1292–1298.

42. Negrier S, Lasset C, Douillard J-Y, et al. Recombinant human interleukin-2, recombinant human interferon alfa-2a, or both in metastatic renal-cell carcinoma. *N Engl J Med* 1998;338:1272–1278.

43. Atzpodien J, Poliwoda H, Kirchner H, et al. Alfa-interferon and interleukin-2 in RENAL CELL CARCINOMA: studies in non-hospitalized patients. *Semin Oncol* 1991;18:S108–S112.

44. Palmer PA, Atzpodien J, Philip T, et al. A comparison of 2 modes of administration of recombinant interleukin-2: continuous intravenous infusion alone

45. Atzpodien J, Lopez Hanninen E, Kirchner H, et al. Multi-institutional home therapy trial of recombinant human interleukin-2 and interferon alfa-2 in progressive metastatic renal cell carcinoma. *J Clin Oncol* 1995; 13:497–501.

46. Vogelzang N, Lipton A, Figlin RA. Subcutaneous interleukin-2 plus interferon alfa-2a in metastatic renal cancer: an outpatient multicenter trial. *J Clin Oncol* 1993;11:1809–1816.

47. Lummen G, Goeppel M, Mollhoff S, et al. Phase II study of interferon gamma versus interleukin-2 and interfereon a2b in metastatic RENAL CELL CARCINOMA. *J Urol* 1996;155:455–458.

48. Atzpodien J, Kirchner H, Hanninen EL, et al. Interleukin-2 in combination with interferon-alpha and 5-fluorouracil for metastatic renal cell cancer. *Eur J Cancer* 1993;29A:S6–S8.

49. Aztpodien J, Krchner H, Jonas U, et al. Interleukin-2 and interferon alfa-2a-based immunochemotherapy in advanced renal cell carcinoma: a prospectively randomized trial of the chemoimmunotherapy group (DGCIN). *J Clin Oncol* 2004;22:1188–1194.

50. Hofmockel G, Langer W, Theiss M, et al. Immunochemotherapy for metastatic renal cell carcinoma using a regimen of interleukin-2, interferon-alpha and 5-fluorouracil. *J Urol* 1996;156:18–21.

51. Dutcher JP, Fisher RI, Weiss G, et al. Outpatient subcutaneous interleukin-2 plus alpha interferon in metastatic renal cell cancer three year follow-up of the Cytokine Working Group Study. *Cancer J Sc Amer* 1997;3: 157–162.

52. Clark JI, Kuzel TM, Lestingi TM, et al. A multi-institutional phase II trial of a novel inpatient schedule of continuous interleukin-2 with interferon alpha-2b in advanced renal cell carcinoma: major durable responses in a less highly selected patient population. *Ann Oncol* 2002;13:606–613.

53. Tourani JM, Pfister C, Tubiana N, et al. Subcutaneouos interleukin-2 and interferon alfa administration in patients with metastatic renal cell carcinoma: final results of SCAPP III, a large, multicenter, phase II, nonrandomized study with sequential analysis design—the Subcutaneous Administration Propeukin Program Cooperative Group. *J Clin Oncol* 2003;21:3987–3994.

54. Dutcher JP, Atkins MB, Fisher R, et al. Interleukin-2 based therapy for metastatic renal cell cancer: the Cytokine Working Group Experience, 1989-1997. *Cancer J Sci Am* 1997;3:S73–S78.

55. Dutcher JP, Logan T, Gordon M, et al. Phase II trial of interleukin-2, interferon-alpha, and 5-fluorouracil in metastatic renal cell cancer: A Cytokine Working Group Study. *Clin Cancer Res* 2000;6:3442–3450.

56. McDermott DF, Regan MM, Clark JL, et al. A randomized phase III trial of high-dose interleukin-2 (HD IL2) versus subcutaneous (SC) IL2/Interferon (IFN) in patients with metastatic renal cell carcinoma. *J Clin Oncol* 2005;23(1):133–141.

57. Atkins MB, McDermott DF. Results of the Cytokine Working Group phase III trial of high dose IL-2 vs. low dose IL-2 and IFN therapy in patients with metastatic renal cell carcinoma. *Ortho Biotech Oncology, Chemotherapy Foundation Symposium XX Innovative Cancer Therapy for Tomorrow* 2003;72:87–88.

58. McDermott D, Parker R, Youmans A, et al. The effect of recent nephrectomy on treatment with high-dose interleukin-2 (HD IL-2) or subcutaneous (SC) IL-2/Interferon alfa-2b (IFN) in patients with metastatic renal cell carcinoma (RENAL CELL CARCINOMA). *Proc Am Soc Clin Oncol* 2003;22:1547.

59. Margolin KA, Rayner AA, Hawkins MJ, et al. Interleukin-2 and lymphokine-activated killer cell therapy of solid tumors: analysis of toxicity and management guidelines. *J Clin Oncol* 1989;7:486–498.

60. Rosenberg SA, Yang JC, Topalian SL, et al. Treatment of 283 consecutive patients with metastatic melanoma or renal cell cancer using high-dose bolus interleukin-2. *JAMA* 1994;271:907–913.

61. Rosenberg SA, Lotze MT, Yang JC, et al. Prospective randomized trial of high-dose interleukin-2 alone or in conjunction with lymphokine-activated killer cells for the treatment of patients with advanced cancer. *J Natl Cancer Inst* 1993;85:622–632.

62. Atkins MB, Sparano J, Fisher RI, et al. A randomized phase II trial of high dose IL-2 either alone or in combination with interferon alpha 2B in advanced renal cell carcinoma. *J Clin Oncol* 1993;11:661–670.

63. Mier JW. Pathogenesis of the interleukin-2-induced vascular leak syndrome. In: Atkins MB, ed. *Therapeutic applications of interelukin-2*, 1st ed. New York: Marcel Dekker Inc, 1993.

64. Numerof RP, Aronson FR, Mier JW. IL-2 stimulates the production of IL-1 alpha and IL-1 beta by human peripheral blood mononuclear cells. *J Immunol* 1988;141(12):4250–4257.

65. Mier JW, Vachino G, Van Der Meer JW, et al. Induction of circulating tumor necrosis factor (TNF alpha) as the mechanism for the febrile response to interleukin-2 (IL-2) in cancer patients. *J Clin Immunol* 1988;8:426–436.

66. Lotze MT, Matory YL, Ettinghausen SE, et al. In vivo administration of purified human interleukin 2. II. Half life, immunologic effects, and expansion of peripheral lymphoid cells in vivo with recombinant IL 2. *J Immunol* 1985;135:2865–2875.

67. Hibbs JB Jr, Westenfelder C, Taintor R, et al. Evidence for cytokine-inducible nitric oxide synthesis from L-arginine in patients receiving interleukin-2 therapy. *J Clin Invest* 1992;89:867–877.

68. Mier JW, Vachino G, Klempner MS, et al. Inhibition of interleukin-2-induced tumor necrosis factor release by dexamethasone: prevention of an acquired neutrophil chemotaxis defect and differential suppression of interleukin-2-associated side effects. *Blood* 1990;76:1933–1940.

versus subcutaneous administration plus interferon alfa in patients with advanced renal cell carcinoma. *Cancer Biother* 1993;8:123–126.

69. Vetto JT, Papa MZ, Lotze MT, et al. Reduction of toxicity of interleukin-2 and lymphokine-activated killer cells in humans by the administration of corticosteroids. *J Clin Oncol* 1987;5:496–503.

70. Trehu EG, Mier JW, Dubois JS, et al. A phase I trail of interleukin-2 in combination with the soluble tumor necrosis factor receptor p75 IgG chimera (TNFR:Fc). *J Clin Oncol* 1996;15:1052–1062.

71. Dubois JS, Trehu EG, Mier JW, et al. Randomized placebo-controlled clinical trial of high-dose interleukin-2 in combination with a soluble p75 tumor necrosis factor receptor immunoglobulin G chimera in patients with advanced melanoma and renal cell carcinoma. *J Clin Oncol* 1997; 5: 1052–1062.

72. Margolin K, Atkins M, Sparano J, et al. Prospective randomized trial of lisofylline for the prevention of toxicities of high-dose interleukin 2 therapy in advanced renal cancer and malignant melanoma. *Clin Cancer Res* 1997;3:565–572.

73. McDermott D, Trehu EG, Dubois J, et al. Phase I clinical trial of the soluable IL-1 receptor either alone or in combination with high-dose IL-2 in patients with advanced malignancies. *Clin Cancer Res* 1966;5: 1203–1213.

74. Messing EM, Manola J, Wilding G, et al. Phase III study of interferon alfa-NL as adjuvant treatment for respectable renal cell carcinoma: an Eastern Cooperative Oncology Group/Intergroup trial. *J Clin Oncol* 2003;21: 1214–1222.

75. Porzsolt F. Adjuvant therapy of renal cell cancer with interferon alfa-2a. *Proc Am Soc Clin Oncol* 1992;11:202.

76. Clark JI, Atkins MB, Urba WJ, et al. Adjuvant high-dose bolus inter-luekin-2 in patients with high-risk renal cell carcinoma—a Cytokine Working Group Phase III trial. *J Clin Oncol* 2003;21:3133.

77. Pantuck AJ, Zisman A, Dorey F, et al. Renal cll carcinoma with retroperi-toneal lymph nodes. Impact on survival and benefits of immunotherapy. *Cancer* 2003;97:2995–3002.

78. Figlin R, Gitlitz B, Franklin J, et al. Interleukin-2-based immunotherapy for the treatment of metastatic renal cell carcinoma: an analysis of 203 consecutively treated patients. *Cancer J Sci Am* 1997;3:S92.

79. Royal RE, Steinberg SM, Krouse RS, et al. Correlates of response to IL-2 therapy in patients treated for metastatic renal cancer and melanoma. *Cancer J Sci Am* 1996;2:91.

80. Atkins MB, Mier JW, Parkinson DR, et al. Hypothyroidism after treatment with interleukin-2 and lymphokine-activated killer cells. *N Engl J Med* 1988;318:1557–1563.

81. Fumagalli LA, Vinke J, Hoff W, et al. Lymphocyte counts independently predict overall survival in advanced cancer patients: a biomarker for IL-2 immunotherapy. *J Immunother* 2003;26:394–402.

82. West WH, Tauer KW, Yanelli JR, et al. Constant-infusion recombinant in-terleukin-2 in adoptive immunotherapy of advanced cancer. *N Engl J Med* 1987;316:898–905.

83. Janik JE, Sznol M, Urba WJ, et al. Erythropoietin production. A potential marker for interleukin-2/interferon-responsive tumors. *Cancer* 1993;72: 2656–2659.

84. Negrier S, Caty A, Lesimpl T, et al. Treatment of patients with metastatic renal carcinoma with a combination of subcutaneous interleukin-2 and inter-feron alfa with or without fluorouracil. *J Clin Oncol* 2000;18: 4009–4015.

85. Leibovich BC, Han KR, Bui MH, et al. Scoring algorithm to predict survival after nephrectomy and immunotherapy in patients with metastatic renal cell carcinoma: a stratification tool for prospective clinical trials. *Cancer* 2003;98(12):2566–2575.

86. Cangiano T, Liao J, Naitoh J, et al. Sarcomatoid renal cell carcinoma: bio-logic behavior, prognosis, and response to combined surgical resection and immunotherapy. *J Clin Oncol* 1999;17:523.

87. Motzer RJ, Bacil J, Mariani T, et al. Treatment outcome and survival associated with metastatic renal cell carcinoma of non-clear-cell histology. *J Clin Oncol* 2002;20:2376.

88. Upton MP, Parker RA, Youmans A, et al. Renal Cell Carcinoma: Histo-logic predictors of cytokine response. *J Immunotherapy* 2005 (in press).

89. Bui MHT, Seligson D, Han K, et al. Carbonic anhydrase IX is an inde-pendent predictor of survival in advanced renal cell carcinoma:implica-tions for prognosis and therapy. *Clin Cancer Res* 2003;9:802–811.

90. Atkins M, McDermott D, Regan M, et al. Carbonic anhydrase IX expres-sion predicts outcome of Interlukin-2 therapy for renal cancer. *Clin Cancer Res* 2005;11(10):3714–3721.

91. Dutcher J. Current status of interleukin-2 therapy for metastatic renal cell carcinoma and metastatic melanoma. *Oncology* 2002;16:4.

CHAPTER 48C
Cytokines
Thomas E. Hutson and Ronald M. Bukowski

INTRODUCTION

The systemic therapy for metastatic renal cell carcinoma (RCC) remains a challenge for the medical oncologist and urologist. RCC is highly resistant to chemotherapy, with no single agent showing major antitumor activity (1,2). The reports of spontaneous regression of metastatic lesions (3), the presence of cytotoxic T lymphocytes in renal tumors (4), the reports of prolonged stable disease in the absence of systemic therapy (5), and the recent descriptions of tumor-associated and HLA-restricted antigens on renal cancer cells suggest that immunologic approaches to the therapy for this tumor are reasonable. Spontaneous regression of metastatic lesions has been noted in two circumstances. First, in patients with synchronous metastatic disease, adjunctive nephrectomy is rarely (<1% of patients) associated with tumor regression (6). In patients with metachronous pulmonary metastasis, two reports have noted partial regression of lesions in up to 6% of patients (4,7). In the report by Gleave et al. (7), a randomized trial of interferon-γ (IFN-γ) compared with a placebo was conducted, in which 6% of patients receiving the placebo had tumor regression. These reports are generally short, but the mention of tumor regression in the placebo group is of biologic interest.

These findings have provided a strong rationale to pursue immunotherapy in patients with this tumor. The major approaches used have included cytokines as single agents or in combination with chemotherapy and adaptive therapy. The interleukins (IL), interferons (IFN), hematopoietic growth factors, and chemokines represent varieties of cytokines, and agents from the first three categories have been used in patients with renal cancer as therapy for metastatic disease.

The therapeutic effects of natural and recombinant cytokines have been investigated over the past two decades. Two agents, interleukin 2 (IL-2) and interferon α (IFN-α), appear to produce tumor regressions in 10% to 15% of patients in a reproducible manner. Other cytokines have been investigated in metastatic RCC; however, their antitumor activity has not been consistently demonstrated. Several clinical factors have recently been described in patients with RCC receiving cytokine-based therapy (8,9). Factors predictive of rapid progression under cytokine treatment include the presence of hepatic metastases, a short interval from renal tumor to metastases (<1 year), the presence of more than one metastatic site, and elevated neutrophil counts (8,9). Additionally, patients with clear cell cancer (classical histology) appear to derive the most benefit from cytokine-based treatment (10). In this chapter, we review the current status of cytokine therapy for metastatic RCC, focusing on the IFN, novel cytokines, and combinations, as well as biochemotherapy. The role of IL-2 as therapy for metastatic RCC is reviewed in the preceding chapter (Chapter 48B).

INTERFERONS

Historical Perspective and Background

IFNs are natural proteins produced by eukaryotic cells in response to viral infections and to different types of biologic or synthetic stimuli (11). First described by Nagano and Kojima in 1954 (12) and by Isaacs and Linderman in 1957 (13), the name, interferons, was taken from their ability to mediate viral interference, where one virus interferes with the replication of a second (13). Since then, more than 20 homologous proteins have been identified with distinct antigenic, biologic, and chemical properties. Three subtypes of IFN (-α, -β, and -γ) were described in humans, cloned, and made commercially available (14). IFN-α and -β are encoded on chromosome 9, share 45% structural homology, bind to the same cell surface receptor, and are referred to as Type I IFN (14,15). IFN-γ is encoded on chromosome 12, shares little sequence similarities with IFN-α and -β, binds to a distinct cell membrane receptor, and is referred to as type II interferon (15).

The most studied IFNs in the treatment of metastatic RCC are IFN-α, -β, and -γ, which are derived from leukocytes, fibroblasts, and lymphocytes, respectively. The original leukocyte-derived IFN was a mixture of IFN-α species produced by lymphocytes, lymphoblasts, and macrophages in response to viruses, foreign cells, and certain mitogens (16,17). Whereas IFN-β derives from fibroblasts or epithelial cells stimulated with natural or synthetic double-stranded ribonucleic acid (RNA), IFN-γ is produced by T lymphocytes following their activation by a variety of antigens or cytokines (17). *In vitro* studies of nonrecombinant IFN-α and -β and recombinant subtypes of IFN-α_2, -β, and -γ have demonstrated comparable growth-inhibitory activity, a direct dose-response tumor-inhibiting relation, and heterogeneity of activity in different tumor types (18).

The actual mechanisms responsible for the antitumor activity of IFNs in human cancer remain uncertain. Possible mechanisms may include inhibition of oncogene function (19) and enhancement of immune regulatory actions including effector cell cytolytic activity and expression of class II major histocompatability complex (MHC) proteins on cell surfaces (19). *In vitro* and *in vivo* studies utilizing both physiologic and pharmacologic doses of IFN demonstrate potent immune stimulatory activity that includes activation of cytotoxic T lymphocytes (20,21), augmentation of antibody-dependent cellular cytotoxicity (22–24), and activation of natural killer (NK) cells (25–27). In addition to its immune regulatory actions, IFN also has its direct effects on tumor cell proliferation and angiogenesis (28–33), the former being demonstrated in a range of tumor cells, including RCC *in vitro* (34,35).

Interferon Monotherapy

The antitumor activity of IFN in patients with RCC was first reported in 1983 by two groups of investigators. Quesada et al.

(36) treated 19 patients with leukocyte IFN-α on a schedule of 3 MU intramuscularly daily and reported a 26% objective response rate. In a similarly designed, but larger study, deKernion et al. (37) achieved a 16.5% objective response in 48 patients with advanced disease. These studies demonstrated, for the first time, that cytokine therapy could affect tumor regression and heralded the modern era of immunotherapy in RCC.

Interferon α

The first cytokine investigated in patients with advanced RCC was IFN-α (36,37). The combined clinical response rates (complete plus partial) from these early trials were documented in up to 26% of patients and provided a basis for multiple phase II trials of IFN-α in the treatment of RCC. Since then, various IFN-α preparations have been used, including both natural and recombinant formulations, and an overview (17,38) of more than 1,300 patients suggests that response rates vary from 12% to >18% (Table 48C.1). In a recent meta-analysis by Coppin et al. (39), results from six randomized trials using subcutaneous (SC) IFN-α, involving 963 patients with metastatic RCC, indicate that IFN-α is superior to controls [odds ratio (OR) for death at 1 year = .67, 95% confidence interval (CI) .50% to .89%]. The pooled hazard ratio (HR) for survival from this analysis was .78 (.67 to .90) and the weighted average median improvement in survival was 2.6 months. Additionally, there was no statistically significant difference when IFN-α was compared with subcutaneous IL-2, and there was no difference between various IFN-α subtypes.

Various dosing schedules, such as subcutaneous, intravenous, intramuscular, or oral administration, daily to three times weekly, and dose levels from 1.0 to 50 MU/m^2 have been used. Optimal results appear to be associated with doses from 5 to 10 MU/m^2 (17). Responses occur most frequently in patients with pulmonary metastases and good performance status (17,40). Median response duration is generally between 6 and 10 months, but occasionally durable complete regressions over 2 years are seen (40). Pharmacokinetic trials using different routes of administration of IFN-α demonstrate higher peak levels with intravenous administration but a considerably shorter half-life when compared with either subcutaneous or intramuscular injection (41). In a phase II study of weekly bolus intravenous IFN by Eisenhauer et al. (42), there was no apparent advantage of this administration over subcutaneous administration. A randomized trial comparing intravenous and subcutaneous IFN demonstrated no significant difference in clinical activity (43).

The most commonly used preparations in clinical practice are recombinant IFN-α_{2a} (Roferon A, Hoffman-LaRoche,

---

TABLE 48C.1

SUMMARY OF SINGLE-AGENT INTERFERON α IN METASTATIC RENAL CELL CARCINOMA

Preparation	Number of pts.	% CR	PR	ORR
Partially purified human leukocyte IFN-α	141	4.3	14.2	18.5
Human lymphoblastoid IFN-α	398	1.0	14.3	15.3
Recombinant IFN-α	767	1.8	10.2	12.0
Total	1,306	1.8	11.8	13.7

IFN-α, interferon α; pts, patients; CR, complete response; PR, partial response; ORR, overall response rate
Adapted from Bukowski RM, Novick AC. Clinical practice guidelines: renal cell carcinoma. *Cleve Clin J Med* 1997;64:S1–48, with permission; and Bukowski RM. Cytokine therapy for metastatic renal cell carcinoma. *Semin Urol Oncol* 2001;19(2):148–154.

TABLE 48C.2

SELECTED CLINICAL TRIALS OF RECOMBINANT INTERFERON α IN PATIENTS WITH ADVANCED RENAL CELL CARCINOMA

Author	n	Dose schedule ($\times 10^6$ IU)	IFN type	CR	PR	ORR%
Minassian et al. (40)	39	59 TIW i.m.	2a	0	7	18
	59	3–36 daily i.m.	2a	2	5	11
Quesada et al. (44)	41	$20/m^2$ daily i.m.	2a	1	11	29
	15	$2/m^2$ daily i.m.	2a	0	0	0
Umeda et al. (45)	108	$3–36/m^2$ daily i.m.	2a	2	13	14
Schnall et al. (46)	22	$3–36/m^2$ daily i.m.	2a	0	1	5
Kempf et al. (47)	10	$2/m^2$ TIW i.m.	2a	0	0	0
	10	$30/m^2$ TIW i.m.	2a	0	1	10
Fossa et al. (48)	17	$18–36/m^2$ TIW i.m.	2a	0	2	11
Foon et al. (49)	21	$2/m^2$ TIW i.m.	2b	0	1	5
Steineck et al. (50)	30	$10–20/m^2$ TIW i.m.	2a	1	1	6
Marshall et al. (51)	17	$1/m^2$ aily s.c.	2a	0	4	24
Umeda et al. (45)	45	$3–36/m^2$ daily i.m.	2b	1	7	18
Muss et al. (43)	46	$30–50/m^2$ daily i.v. $5\times$/week q3wk	2b	1	2	7
Levens et al. (52)	15	$10/m^2$ daily s.c.	2b	1	3	27
Bono et al. (53)	61	$3/m^2$ TIW s.c.	2b	2	3	8
Buzaid et al. (54)	22	$3–36/m^2$ daily i.m.	2a	0	5	23
Figlin et al. (131)	19	$3–36/m^2$ daily i.m.	2a	1	4	26

TIW, three times weekly; i.m., intramuscular; s.c., subcutaneous; i.v., intravenous; CR, complete response; PR, partial response; ORR%, overall response rate %.
Adapted from Motzer RJ, Berg WJ. Role of interferon in metastatic renal cell carcinoma. In: Bukowski RM, Novick AC, eds. *Current clinical oncology: renal cell carcinoma*. Totowa, NJ: Humana Press, 2001:319–329, with permission.

Nutley, NJ) and recombinant IFN-α_{2b} (Intron A, Schering-Plough Laboratories, Kenilworth, NJ). Both preparations have been studied extensively in patients with metastatic RCC in dosages ranging from 3 MU to 50 MU per day (Table 48C.2). Response rates range from 0% to 30% (40,43–54) and the overall response rate is 14.5% (13 complete responses and 81 partial responses, 95% CI 12% to 17%) in 648 patients (14). Recently, several randomized trials have been conducted in which IFN-α has been compared with other therapeutic approaches. These trials include comparisons with either a non-cytokine regimen or

with other cytokines. The studies of greatest interest are summarized in Table 48C.3. Pyrhonen et al. (55) reported a trial in which 160 patients received either the combination of IFN-α and vinblastine (VBL) or vinblastine alone. Improvement in both response rates and median survivals in patients treated with IFN-α were detected. The response rates were 16.5% and 2.5%, respectively, and median survivals were 15.8 months and 8.8 months. These findings suggest that interferon as a single agent may enhance survival because the clinical activity of vinblastine is minimal (55). A second trial reported by Ritchie et al. (56)

TABLE 48C.3

SELECTED RANDOMIZED TRIALS OF INTERFERON α IN METASTATIC RENAL CELL CARCINOMA

Author	Treatment	n	RR	m^a
Pyrhonen et al. (55)	IFN-α 18 MU s.c. TIW plus VBL .1 mg/kg IVB q3wk	79	16%	15.8
	vs.			
	VBL .1 mg/kg IVB q3wk	81	2.5%	8.8
Ritchie et al. (56)	IFN-α 10 MU s.c. TIW for 12 wk	167	NS	8.5
	vs.			
	MPA 300 mg/d	168	NS	6.0

MPA, medroxyprogesterone; NS, not stated; RR, response rate; s.c., subcutaneous; MU, million units; VBL, vinblastine; IVB, intravenous bolus; TIW, three times weekly; m, median survival.
$^a P < .01$.
Adapted from Bukowski RM. Cytokine therapy for metastatic renal cell carcinoma. *Semin Urol Oncol* 2001;19(2):148–154, with permission.

compared IFN-α (10 MU subcutaneous three times weekly) with medroxyprogesterone (MPA) (300 mg daily) in 335 patients. Results with IFN-α were significantly better than those with medroxyprogesterone. In the group with measurable disease, IFN-α produced responses in 13% of patients compared with 7% in patients treated with medroxyprogesterone. These results suggest that IFN-α significantly enhanced survival in patients with metastatic RCC (8.5 months vs. 6 months), although the effect is modest.

Recently, two randomized trials demonstrated a statistically significant survival advantage in patients with RCC with synchronous metastatic disease who received cytoreductive nephrectomy followed by IFN-α (57,58). The first trial reported by the Southwest Oncology Group (57) randomized 246 patients to nephrectomy, followed by IFN-α compared with single-agent IFN-α without surgery. In the 120 eligible patients undergoing adjunctive nephrectomy followed by IFN-α, improvement in survival was noted (11.1 months vs. 8.1 months; $P = .05$). In the second trial, Mickisch et al. (58) randomized 85 patients to nephrectomy followed by IFN-α or single-agent IFN-α without surgery. Both time to progression (5 months vs. 3 months, hazard ratio .60, 95% CI .36% to .97%) and median duration of survival were significantly better in the patients receiving nephrectomy and IFN-α (17 months vs. 7 months, hazard ratio .54, 95% CI .31% to .94%). These trials suggest that patients with primary tumors in place and those with metastatic disease should be considered for nephrectomy (if medically possible) before IFN-α therapy. Retrospective reviews of data also suggest this approach can be considered in patients receiving other cytokines, such as IL-2 (38).

IFN-α therapy requires frequent injections and generally has constitutional side effects. Acute toxicity may be severe, with chills, fever, hypotension, and renal abnormalities predominating. Chronic side effects may include neuropathy, depression, hematologic abnormalities, and dermatologic findings. Therefore, the choice of treatment regimen should be guided by patient status, comorbid factors, and the degree and severity of side effects that are acceptable. Several attempts have been undertaken to ameliorate the toxicity profile of IFN-α. In a study by Creagan et al. (59), patients were treated with recombinant IFN-α_{2a} and aspirin in an attempt to affect the degree of constitutional symptoms. However, the constitutional symptoms reported in the patients treated with aspirin were similar to historical controls. Acetaminophen is effective in the treatment and prophylaxis of IFN-induced constitutional symptoms and is the preferred standard therapy.

Interferon β and Interferon γ

In comparison with the clinical experience with IFN-α, there is only limited data on the use of IFN-β and IFN-γ in the treatment of metastatic RCC (60–75). Few studies with IFN-β and IFN-γ have been published (Table 48C.4). The overall response rate with IFN-β was 11% in four trials composed of 71 patients (60–63). Clinical response rates of patients treated with IFN-γ ranged from 0% to 33% in 11 trials of 570 patients (64–75). In total, the combined response rates (complete plus partial) range from 6% to 33% and are similar to those obtained in studies using IFN-α.

Interferon and Interleukin-2 Combination Therapy

Several preclinical tumor models suggest synergistic antitumor activity when IFN-α is combined with IL-2 (76). A series of phase I and II trials were conducted to investigate the clinical activity of this combination of IFN-α and IL-2. A recent

---

TABLE 48C.4

SINGLE AGENT TRIALS OF RECOMBINANT INTERFERON β AND RECOMBINANT INTERFERON-γ IN METASTATIC RENAL CELL CARCINOMA.

Author (Ref.)	N	Dose schedule ($\times 10^6$ IU)	CR	PR	ORR%
		IFN-β			
Rinehart et al. (60)	15	—	0	2	13
Kish et al. (61)	16	—	0	1	6
Nelson et al. (62)	15	—	0	0	0
Kinney et al. (63)	25	—	1	4	20
		IFN-γ			
Quesada et al. (64)	14	5–20/m^2 i.m.	0	1	7
	16	.2–1/m^2 i.v.	0	1	6
Koiso et al. (65)	32	8–12/m^2 daily i.v. or i.m.	0	2	6
	39	40/m^2 IV	1	5	20
Takaku et al. (66)	32	8–12/m^2 daily i.v. or i.m.	0	2	6
	30	40/m^2 daily × 5 q2wk i.v.	1	5	20
Rinehart et al. (67)	13	.01–75/m^2 twice weekly i.v.	0	0	0
Garnick et al. (68)	41	.2–60/m^2 daily i.v.	1	3	10
Kuebler et al. (69)	27	.25/m^2 daily q4wk CIV	0	0	0
Aulitzky et al. (70)	20	2/m^2 TIW q2wk s.c.	2	4	30
Grups et al. (71)	9	5/m^2 daily × 8 q4wk i.m.	0	3	33
Bruntsch et al. (72)	40	2/m^2 TIW q2wk i.v.	0	1	2
Foon et al. (73)	21	1/m^2 TIW s.c.	0	1	5
Ellerhost et al. (74)	34	100 μg/m^2 weekly s.c.	1	3	15
Small et al. (75)	202	60 μg/m^2 weekly s.c.	3	3	3

CR, complete response; PR, partial response; ORR%, overall response rate %; i.m., intramuscular; i.v., intravenous; s.c., subcutaneous; TIW, three times weekly; N, number of patients.
Adapted from Motzer RJ, Berg WJ. Role of interferon in metastatic renal cell carcinoma. In: Bukowski RM, Novick AC, eds. *Current clinical oncology: renal cell carcinoma.* Totowa, NJ: Humana Press, 2001:319–329, with permission.

TABLE 48C.5

SUMMARY OF CLINICAL TRIALS OF INTERLEUKIN-2 AND INTERFERON α IN PATIENTS WITH METASTATIC RENAL CELL CARCINOMA

Route of administration			%		
IL-2	IFN-α	N	CR	PR	ORR
SC	s.c.	675	5	16.1	21.2
CIV	s.c.	556	3.4	16.6	20.0
IVB	s.c.	180	5	15.6	20.5
	Totals	1411	4.4	16.2	20.6

CR, complete response; PR, partial response; ORR, overall response rate; s.c., subcutaneous; CIV, continuous intravenous infusion; IVB, intravenous bolus; N, number of patients.
Adapted from Bukowski RM. Natural history and therapy of metastatic renal cell carcinoma: role of interleukin-2. *Cancer* 1997;80: 1198–1220, with permission; and Bukowski RM, Dutcher JP. Low dose interleukin-2. In: Voglezang NJ, Scardino PT, Shipley WW et al., eds. *Genitourinary oncology.* Philadelphia, PA: Lippincott William & Wilkins, 2000:218–233.

review of the results in more than 1,400 patients has been published (77). Regardless of the route of administration or the dose of IL-2 or IFN-α used, response rates of approximately 20% have been noted (Table 48C.5). As with single agent IL-2, complete responses have been noted in up to 5% of patients.

Several randomized trials comparing the combination of IL-2 and IFN-α have been completed (79–82). In one trial by Negrier et al. (80) the combination resulted in a greater overall response rate when compared with either IL-2 or IFN-α monotherapy. This finding has been suggested in the two largest randomized trials of IL-2 and IFN-α (79,80). Results reported by Negrier et al. (80) suggest that the overall regression rates and 1-year event-free survival in patients receiving IL-2 and IFN-α are statistically superior compared with monotherapy with either agent (18.6% ORR combination, 6.5% ORR CIV IL-2, 7.5% ORR SC IFN-α; P <.04). However, in this trial, patients were allowed to crossover to either IL-2 or IFN-α after failing to respond, and therefore comparisons of survival are difficult and no significant differences in survival were noted. The available data suggest this combination of cytokines may increase response rates, but improvement in survival has not been demonstrated. To date, there has been no sufficiently powered randomized phase III trial showing a survival benefit for combination therapy compared with IFN-α monotherapy. Therefore, given the lack of significant clinical research data regarding improvement in response rate and survival, the added toxicity associated with combination therapy with IL-2 and IFN-α in routine clinical use is difficult to justify.

Pegylated Interferon

Given the requirements for frequent injections and underlying toxicity of chronic treatment with IFN-α, alternative formulations with the potential for greater efficacy and less toxicity have been investigated. The most studied has been the conjugation of the IFN-α molecule with polyethylene glycol (PEG), a process known as pegylation. The two commercially available pegylated IFNs (PEG IFN-α$_{2a}$, PEGASYS, Hoffman-La Roche, Nutley, NJ; PEG IFN-α$_{2b}$, PEG Intron, Schering-Plough Laboratories, Kenilworth, NJ) are modified forms of recombinant human IFN-α with sustained absorption and prolonged half-life when administered subcutaneously or intramuscularly (83,84).

PEG IFN-α$_{2a}$ and PEG IFN-α$_{2b}$ have been evaluated as single agents in metastatic RCC demonstrating similar efficacy and toxicity to non-pegylated IFN with the advantage of less frequent dosing (84). In a phase I trial by Motzer et al. (85), 27 previously untreated patients with metastatic RCC were treated with PEG IFN-α$_{2a}$ in doses ranging from 180 to 540 μg subcutaneous once weekly. After 12 months of therapy, five patients (19%) had achieved a partial response (50% tumor shrinkage) with three patients remaining progression-free for >13 months. In a recently reported phase II trial, 40 previously untreated patients with metastatic RCC received 450 μg of PEG IFNα$_{2a}$ subcutaneous weekly (86). Five (13%) of the 38 evaluable patients achieved a major response (4 partial and 1 complete) and 72% of patients were alive at 13-month follow-up. Toxicities from this study were similar to previous studies with fatigue, neutropenia, and elevated liver enzymes being most common. Bukowski et al. (87) recently reported the results of a phase I/II study of PEG IFNα$_{2b}$ in 35 previously treated patients with advanced solid tumors, including 22 patients with metastatic RCC. The most commonly reported adverse events were nausea, anorexia, fatigue, and rigors. In the phase II portion of this trial, 35 previously untreated patients with metastatic RCC were treated with 6.0 and 7.5 μg/kg/wk for up to 12 weeks and continued to receive treatment for up to 1 year in the presence of response or stable disease. Among the 57 total patients with metastatic RCC including 44 with no prior therapy, 23 patients had a response or stable disease at 12 weeks and continued therapy for 1 year. Overall, 6 patients (11%) with metastatic RCC had a response (2 complete and 4 partial) with continued treatment. All of the responses occurred in patients without previous treatment. The median survival was 13.2 months. The pharmacokinetic profile of PEG IFN-α$_{2b}$ from this trial, demonstrates that prolonged serum concentrations are maintained for up to 7 days after a single SC dose and supports once-weekly administration. Although there is no direct pharmacokinetic comparison between PEG IFNα$_{2b}$ and IFN-α$_{2b}$, the 6.0 μg/kg/wk dose may achieve exposure comparable with 180 MIU/wk of IFN-α$_{2b}$.

The initial trials of PEG IFN-α$_{2a}$ (85,86) and PEG IFN-α$_{2b}$ (87) in patients with metastatic RCC demonstrate similar efficacy in untreated patients (13% and 14%, respectively) to non-pegylated IFN (7.5% to 14%;(56,80)), as well as comparable safety with the advantage of weekly administration. The toxicity profiles between the pegylated IFNs were also similar. However, three patients treated with PEG IFN-α$_{2a}$ developed grade 3 [National Cancer Institute (NCI) Common Toxicity Criteria, version 2.0] hepatotoxicity. One possible explanation for this unexpected toxicity may be the higher molecular weight (40 kDa) of PEG IFN-α$_{2a}$, which may result in tissue accumulation (88).

The combination of non-pegylated IFN-α with IL-2 has been reviewed above. Studies evaluating this combination have demonstrated marginal improvements in objective tumor responses with significant toxicity limiting dose escalation. Single-agent trials of PEG IFN-α in RCC resulted in dose-limiting toxicity at a much higher-equivalent non-pegylated IFN dose without compromising efficacy. The potential of PEG IFN to be administered at higher doses when used concurrent with IL-2, or alternatively, the potential for a higher IL-2 dose to be administered, has resulted in the evaluation of the combination of PEG IFN with IL-2 in patients with metastatic RCC. In a phase I trial by Clark et al. (89), 28 patients received weekly PEG IFN-α$_{2b}$ subcutaneously concurrent with IL-2 (5.0 MIU/m² subcutaneous every 8 hours for 3 days then daily for 5 days a week for a total of 4 weeks). Overall, 7 patients responded to treatment. In another phase I trial reported by Hutson et al. (90,91), a total of 34 patients received between 1.5 and 4.5 μg/kg/wk subcutaneous PEG IFN-α$_{2b}$ concurrent with 10.0 to 20.0 MIU/m² subcutaneous IL-2 three times weekly for

6 of 8 weeks per cycle. Partial response was seen in 5 patients. Although these results are preliminary, it is possible to administer PEG IFN-α_{2b} at doses near the maximal tolerated dose as a single agent with IL-2.

Based on the clinical trials reported to date, treatment of metastatic RCC with PEG IFN is feasible. The toxicity profile and antitumor activity compare favorably to non-pegylated IFN, with the advantage of less frequent administration. Randomized trials are now required to determine the role of pegylated interferon as a therapy for patients with metastatic RCC.

Novel Interferon Combinations

A variety of novel agents are currently being evaluated as therapy for patients with metastatic RCC. These agents include small molecules, monoclonal antibodies, and new cytostatic agents that may inhibit angiogenesis or interfere with unique signaling pathways associated with the pathogenesis of RCC. Two of these, bevacizumab and thalidomide, have demonstrated single-agent antitumor activity in RCC and are currently being evaluated in combination with IFN-α_{2b} (92,93).

Bevacizumab, an antivascular endothelial growth factor antibody, has been studied as a single agent in patients with metastatic RCC. In a recently reported phase II study (92), 116 patients were randomized to placebo, low-dose antibody, or high-dose antibody. The trial was stopped after the first interim analysis demonstrated a significant prolongation in the time to progression of disease in patients receiving bevacizumab compared with those receiving placebo (high-dose antibody HR 2.55, $P < .001$; low-dose antibody HR 1.26, $P = .053$). These results have prompted interest in evaluating this agent in combination with cytokine therapy. A large phase III trial (CALGB 90206) comparing the combination of bevacizumab and IFN-α_{2b} to IFN-α_{2b} monotherapy is ongoing.

The antiangiogenic activity of thalidomide has been demonstrated in a variety of human cancers including RCC. *In vitro* studies suggest that the combination of IFN-α_{2b} and thalidomide may synergistically inhibit tumor-induced angiogenesis (94) and this combination is currently being studied as treatment of patients with metastatic RCC. In a recently reported phase II study by Hornberg et al. (95), 30 patients were treated with IFN-α_{2b} and thalidomide. The response rate in the 27 assessable patients was 22% (95% CI, 6% to 38%) with a median survival of 14.9 months. Results from a large phase III study (ECOG 2898) of IFN-α_{2b} as a single agent or in combination with thalidomide need to be analyzed before this combination can be recommended for routine use.

OTHER CYTOKINES

In addition to IFN and IL-2, several other cytokines have been investigated both as single agents and in combination with either IFN, IL-2, or, in some cases, with both IFN and IL-2, for the treatment of metastatic RCC. The most investigated cytokines include the hematopoietic growth factor, granulocyte-macrophage colony-stimulating factor (GM-CSF) and interleukin-12. However, studies of interleukin-4 (96), interleukin-6 (97) and tumor-infiltrating lymphocytes (TIL) primed *ex vivo* with various cytokines (98–100) have been reported and continue to be under investigation. Other cytokines including tumor necrosis factor and several interleukins (IL-7, -8, -9, -10, and -11) have been evaluated for antitumor activity; however, these investigations have failed to demonstrate reproducible activity against RCC (101).

Interleukin 12

Interleukin-12 (IL-12) is a pleiotropic cytokine with diverse immunomodulating activity and significant antitumor activity against RCC tumor models (102–104). Initially identified by two groups in 1986 (105) and 1989 (106), IL-12 has been evaluated in several phase I and II trials both as monotherapy (107–111) and combined with either IL-2 (112,113) or IFN-α (114). IL-12 exerts a number of regulatory effects on numerous cell types, particularly on T-lymphocytes and NK-cells, where it enhances NK/LAK cell lytic activity, facilitates specific cytolytic T-lymphocyte responses, induces IFN-γ secretion by both T cells and NK-cells, and supports cell-mediated immune responses by promoting Th$_1$-type helper T-cell development (115–117). In addition, IL-12 may have anti-angiogenic properties through induction of IFN-γ (118–120). The exact antitumor mechanism(s) remain unclear; however, preliminary studies suggest IL-12 may mediate its effect in part via induction of IFN-γ and the IFN-γ-dependent chemokines IP-10 and Mig (121,122).

Several clinical trials have been conducted to determine both the toxicity and the efficacy of subcutaneous and intravenous IL-12 in patients with RCC. In the two initial phase I trials (107,109), 118 patients with RCC were treated with various doses of either intravenous or subcutaneous IL-12. There were a total of four responses (2 PR and 2 CR) with hepatic, hematologic and pulmonary toxicity limiting dose escalation. However, an exceptionally long CR duration (>18 months) was noted resulting in further study. Motzer et al. (108) recently reported a randomized phase II trial of recombinant human IL-12 compared with IFN-α in 46 patients with advanced RCC. Patients were randomly assigned 2:1 to receive either subcutaneous IL-12 weekly or 9 MU IFN-α administered subcutaneously three times per week. Of the 30 patients treated with IL-12, only two patients achieved a partial response.

Preclinical studies suggest that IL-12 may synergize with either IFN α or IL-2 via modulation of IFN-γ-induced chemokine (IP-10 and Mig) production by T- and NK-cells (112,119). On the basis of this data, clinical trials of subcutaneous and intravenous IL-12 with either IFN-α or IL-2 have been conducted. Gollob et al. (113) recently reported the results of a phase I trial of concurrent twice weekly intravenous recombinant human IL-12 and low-dose subcutaneous IL-2 in 28 patients with either melanoma or RCC. There were no responses in the 15 RCC patients treated with this regimen. In a phase I trial by Hutson et al. (114), 26 patients with either melanoma or RCC were treated with subcutaneous recombinant human IL-12 and subcutaneous IFN-α (1 to 3 MU/m^2 three times weekly). Two of 19 patients with RCC had a partial response and the median survival was 13.3 months. Adverse events reported in these two trials were similar to other cytokine combination trials, with constitutional, hematologic, and hepatic toxicity being most common.

Despite the disappointing results from several clinical trials, correlative immunologic studies demonstrate significant activity when IL-12 is administered to patients with RCC as a single agent or in combination with other cytokines. These observations along with the results from ongoing studies will help clarify the role of IL-12 as therapy for metastatic RCC.

Granulocyte-Macrophage Colony-Stimulating Factor (GM-CSF)

GM-CSF is a multilineage hematopoietic growth factor with pleiotropic effects including stimulation of T-cell proliferation and induction of tumor necrosis factor (123). Although its specific antitumor properties remain unclear, evidence from clinical trials suggest that GM-CSF may help promote a host specific immunologic response to tumor antigens. Phase I trials of this cytokine have demonstrated profound monocytosis and enhanced activation of mononuclear phagocytes (124). In a phase II trial by Wos et al. (98), 28 patients with metastatic RCC were treated with GM-CSF. Clinical responses were seen in 2 patients with metastatic lung lesions. Toxicity to subcutaneous injections of GM-CSF is usually mild; however, a capillary leak syndrome and hypotension have been described, which may be partly explained by induction of endogenous cytokines (125, 126). Most randomized studies that used the standard dose (250 $\mu g/m^2/d$) have shown only mild adverse effects (126).

Recently, GM-CSF has been combined with IL-2 and IFN-α and administered to patients with RCC (127,128). In a phase I trial reported by de Gast et al. (127), 18 patients (11 with metastatic RCC) were treated with subcutaneous IL-2 (1, 4, or 8 MIU/m^2), a fixed dose of subcutaneous IFN-α (5 MU) and subcutaneous GM-CSF (2.5 or 5 $\mu g/kg$) for 12 days every 3 weeks. Of 8 patients with progressive metastatic RCC after nephrectomy, 3 achieved a complete remission. Side effects included fever, hypotension requiring intravenous fluid support, and fatigue. Agrawal et al. (129) recently reported the results of a phase I/II study of GM-CSF, IL-2 and IFN-α_{2b} in 61 patients with metastatic RCC. Overall, eight patients (13%) responded to treatment, and the most common side effects were nausea, vomiting, and fatigue. These reports suggest clinical responses are seen when GM-CSF is combined with other cytokines but overall resemble the trials using IL-2 and IFN-α.

BIOCHEMOTHERAPY

The therapeutic effects of cytokines administered with chemotherapy have also been investigated. In patients with RCC, the two most widely used cytotoxic agents are vinblastine and 5-fluorouracil (5-FU). Initial pilot studies of vinblastine combined with IFN-α reported response rates ranging from 0% to 30% (130–143), which were confirmed in several phase II trials in Europe (144). Subsequently, several randomized trials were conducted. Niedhart et al. (145) found no benefit with the addition of vinblastine to IFN-α, whereas Fossa et al. (146), in a series of 178 patients, noted a response rate of 24% for the combination compared with 11% for vinblastine alone. In a large phase III trial reported by Pyrhonen et al. (55), the response rate of IFN-α_{2a} and vinblastine was superior to vinblastine alone (16% vs. 2.5%). In addition, the overall median survival was nearly

doubled in the biochemotherapy arm (15.8 months vs. 8.8 months, $P < .01$). These trials suggest that IFN-α plus vinblastine are superior to chemotherapy alone (55). However, given the lack of activity of vinblastine as a single agent in metastatic RCC, these studies suggest that IFN-α may have a favorable effect on patient survival.

The fluoropyrimidine, 5-FU, has also been investigated in combination with IFN-α and IL-2 based on strong evidence of *in vitro* synergy (147–149). The combination of 5-FU and IFN-α has been reported to have minimal activity, but combination regimens using 5-FU, IFN-α, and IL-2 were reported to produce tumor regression in >30% of patients (150). A summary of larger (>50 patients) recently reported phase II trials (151–157) is provided in Table 48C.6. Significant disparity in response rate is apparent. Recently, the preliminary results of a randomized trial investigating the addition of 5-FU to subcutaneous IFN-α and IL-2 was reported (155). In this study, the response rate to IFN-α and IL-2 was 1.4% and to the biochemotherapy regimen, 8.2%. The two groups were balanced, except for a higher number of metastatic sites in the IL-2 and IFN-α-treated patients. A larger randomized trial conducted by the Medical Research Council (MRC) comparing IFN-α alone and combined with 5-FU and IL-2 is ongoing. The toxicity of biochemotherapy regimens such as these is moderate to severe, and in the absence of data confirming improvement in clinical outcomes, this form of therapy should remain investigational.

CONCLUSION

Metastatic RCC is a tumor refractory to standard cytotoxic chemotherapy regimens. The rationale for the use of cytokines in this cancer is based upon compelling evidence that RCC is sensitive to immunologic manipulation. Cytokine-based therapy with either IL-2 or IFN-α can result in objective tumor responses in up to 15% of patients, and in selected patients, these responses may be durable. Improvements in survival for patients receiving IFN-α has been demonstrated in several randomized trials. This has not been documented in patients receiving IL-2, but appropriately controlled trials have not been performed. The patients most likely to respond are those with limited pulmonary disease who are asymptomatic. Recent evidence suggests that a variety of clinical factors (serum LDH, prior nephrectomy, number and location of metastatic sites, calcium level, and hemoglobin level), as

---

TABLE 48C.6

SUMMARY OF SELECTED PHASE II/III TRIALS USING 5-FLUOROURACIL, IL-2 AND IFA-α IN METASTATIC RENAL CELL CARCINOMA

Author	n	%			m
		CR	PR	ORR	
Kirchner et al. (151)	246	10.5	22.1	32.6	21.0
Hanninen et al. (150)	120	10.8	28.2	39.1	NS
Atzpodien et al. (152)	41	17.0	22.0	39.0	>42.0
Ravaud et al. (153)	105	0.0	1.8	1.8	11.9
Ellerhost et al. (154)	55	7.2	21.8	1.0	22.9
Negrier et al. (155)	61	0.0	8.2	8.2	NS
Dutcher et al. (156)	50	4.0	12.0	16.0	16.7
Tourani et al. (157)	62	1.6	17.7	19.3	16.0

CR, complete response; PR, partial response; ORR, overall response rate; NS, not stated; m, median survival; n, number of patients.
Adapted from Bukowski RM. Cytokine therapy for metastatic renal cell carcinoma. *Semin Urol Oncol* 2001;19(2):148–154, with permission.

well as histology (clear cell, papillary, or sarcomatoid) also influence the likelihood of response to cytokine-based therapies. Attempts to identify surrogate markers that can identify responding patients have been unsuccessful.

Based on the results of two randomized trials, it is now clear that adjunctive nephrectomy is beneficial prior to commencing cytokine therapy; however, the optimal duration of therapy remains uncertain. Individuals with complete responses can be observed without maintenance treatment; in partial responders, it is uncertain whether continuation of therapy is beneficial. Encouraging results from phase I and II trials of pegylated IFN-α and IL-12 require further study to determine their role in the management of metastatic RCC. Further investigations using cytokines in combination with new targeted and cytostatic approaches, such as the antiangiogenic agents, are under way.

References

1. Yagoda A, Abi-Rached B, Petrylak D. Chemotherapy for advanced renal cell carcinoma: 1983-1993. *Semin Oncol* 1995;22:42–60.
2. Motzer RJ, Vogelzang NJ. Chemotherapy for renal cell carcinoma. In: Raghaven D, Scher HI, Leibel SA et al., eds. *Principles and practice of genitourinary oncology.* Philadelphia, PA: Lippincott–Raven, 1997: 885–896.
3. Voglezang NJ, Priest FR, Borden L. Spontaneous regression of histologically proved pulmonary metastases from renal cell carcinoma: a case with 5-year follow-up. *J Urol* 1992;148:1247–1248.
4. Finke JH, Rayman P, Hart L, et al. Characterization of TIL subsets from human renal carcinoma: specific reactivity defined by cytotoxicity, IFN γ secretion, and proliferation. *J Immunother* 1994;15:91–104.
5. Oliver RTD, Mehta A, Barnett MJ. A phase 2 study of surveillance in patients with metastatic renal cell carcinoma and assessment of response of such patients to therapy on progression. *Mol Biother* 1998;1:14–20.
6. Montie JE, Stewart BH, Straffon RA, et al. The role of adjunctive nephrectomy in patients with metastatic renal cell carcinoma. *J Urol* 1977; 117: 272–277.
7. Gleave M, Eihilali M, Prodet Y, et al. Interferon gamma-1b compared with placebo in metastatic renal cell carcinoma. *N Engl J Med* 1998;338:1265.
8. Motzer RJ, Mazumdar M, Bacik J, et al. Survival and prognostic stratification of 670 patients with advanced renal cell carcinoma. *J Clin Oncol* 1999;17:2530–2540.
9. Negrier S, Escudier B, Gomez F, et al. Prognostic factors of survival and rapid progression in 782 patients with metastatic renal carcinomas treated by cytokines: a report from the groupe Francais d'Immunotherapie. *Ann Oncol* 2002;13:1460–1468.
10. Wu J, Caliendo G, Hu XP, et al. Impact of histology on the treatment outcome of metastatic or recurrent renal cell carcinoma. *Med Oncol* 1998; 15: 44–49.
11. Sreevalsan T. Biologic therapy with interferon-alfa and beta: preclinical studies. In: DeVita VT, Hellman S, Rosenberg SA, eds. *Biologic therapy of cancer.* Philadelphia, PA: JB Lippincott Co, 1995:347–364.
12. Nagano Y, Kojima Y. Pouvoir immunisant du virus vaccinal inactive par des rayons ultraviolet. *R Soc Biol* 1954;148:1700.
13. Isaacs A, Linderman J. Virus interface. I. The interferon. *Proc R Soc Lond* 1957;147:258.
14. Motzer RJ, Berg WJ. Role of interferon in metastatic renal cell carcinoma. In: Bukowski RM, Novick AC, eds. *Current clinical oncology: renal cell carcinoma.* Totowa, NJ: Humana Press, 2001:319–329.
15. Tretter CPG, Ernstoff MS. Chemotherapy, hormonal therapy, and interferons. In: Voglezang NJ, Scardino PT, Shipley WU et al., eds. *Comprehensive textbook of genitourinary oncology,* 2nd ed. Philadelphia, PA: Lippincott Williams & Wilkins, 2000:248–259.
16. Choudhury M, Efros M, Mittelman A. Interferons and interleukins in metastatic renal cell carcinoma. *Urology* 1993;41:67–72.
17. Bukowski RM, Novick AC. Clinical practice guidelines: renal cell carcinoma. *Cleve Clin J Med* 1997;64:S1–48.
18. Kirkwood JM. Interferons. In: DeVita VT, Hellman S, Rosenberg S, eds. *Cancer: principles and practice of oncology,* 6th ed. Philadelphia, PA: Lippincott Williams & Wilkins, 2001:461–471.
19. Dorr RT. Interferon-alpha in malignant and viral diseases: a review. *Drugs* 1993;45:177–211.
20. Welsh RM, Yang H, Bukowski JF. The role of interferon in regulation of virus infections by cytotoxic lymphocytes. *Bioessays* 1998;8:10.
21. Fellous M, Nir U, Wallach D, et al. Interferon-dependent induction of mRNA for the major histocompatability antigens in human fibroblasts and lymphoblastoid cell lines. *Proc Natl Acad Sci U S A* 1982;79:3082.
22. van Schie R, Verstraten HG, Tax WJ, et al. Effect of rIFN-gamma on antibody-mediated cytotoxicity via human monocyte IgG Fc receptor II (CD32). *Scand J Immunol* 1992;36:385.
23. te Velde A, de Waal Malefijt R, Huijbens RJ, et al. IL-10 stimulates monocyte Fc gamma R surface expression and cytotoxic activity. Distinct regulation of antibody-dependent cellular cytotoxicity by IFN-gamma, IL-4 and IL-10. *J Immunol* 1992;149:4048.
24. Vuist WM, Visseren MJ, Otsen M, et al. Enhancement of the antibody-dependent cellular cytotoxicity of human peripheral blood lymphocytes with interleukin-2 and interferon alpha. *Cancer Immunol Immunother* 1993; 36:163.
25. Robertson MJ, Manley TJ, Donahue C, et al. Costimulatory signals are required for optimal proliferation of human natural killer cells. *J Immunol* 1993;150:1705.
26. Minato N, Reid L, Cantor H, et al. Mode regulation of natural killer cell activity by interferon. *J Exp Med* 1980;152:124.
27. Saksela E, Timonen T, Cantell K. Cellular interactions in the augmentation of human NK activity by interferon. *Ann N Y Acad Sci* 1980;350: 102.
28. Sato N, Nariuchi H, Tsuruoka N, et al. Actions of TNF and IFN-gamma on angiogenesis *in vitro. J Invest Dermatol* 1990;95(Suppl. 6):858.
29. White CW. Treatment of hemangiomatosis with recombinant interferon alfa. *Semin Hematol* 1990;27(Suppl. 4):15.
30. Billington DC. Angiogenesis and its inhibition: potential new therapies in oncology and non-neoplastic diseases. *Drug Des Discov* 1991;8:3.
31. Maheshwari RK, Srikantan V, Bhartiya D, et al. Differential effects of interferon gamma and alpha on *in vitro* model of angiogenesis. *J Cell Physiol* 1991;146:164.
32. Folkman J, Ingber D. Inhibition of angiogenesis. *Semin Cancer Biol* 1992; 3:89.
33. Saiki I, Sato K, Yoo YC, et al. Inhibition of tumor-induced angiogenesis by the administration of recombinant interferon-gamma followed by a synthetic lipid-A subunit analogue (GLA-60). *Int J Cancer* 1992;51:641.
34. Gruss HJ, Brach MA, Mertelsmann RH, et al. Interferon-gamma interrupts autocrine growth mediated by endogenous interleukin-6 in renal cell carcinoma. *Int J Cancer* 1991;49:770.
35. Garbe C, Krasagakis K. Effects of interferons and cytokines on melanoma cells. *J Invest Dermatol* 1993;100(Suppl. 2):2395.
36. Quesada JR, Swanson DA, Trindale A, et al. Renal cell carcinoma: antitumor effects of leukocyte interferon. *Cancer Res* 1983;43:940–947.
37. DeKernion JB, Sarna JB, Figlin R, et al. The treatment of renal cell carcinoma with human leukocyte alpha-interferon. *J Urol* 1983;130: 1063–1066.
38. Bukowski RM. Cytokine therapy for metastatic renal cell carcinoma. *Semin Urol Oncol* 2001;19(2):148–154.
39. Coppin C, Porzsolt F, Kumpf J, et al. Immunotherapy for advanced renal cell cancer. *Cochrane Database Syst Rev* 2003;3:1–46.
40. Minassian LM, Motzer RJ, Gluck L, et al. Interferon- alpha 2a in advanced renal cell carcinoma: treatment results and survival in 159 patients with long-term follow-up. *J Clin Oncol* 1993;11:1368–1375.
41. Kirkwood JM, Ernstoff MS, Davis CA, et al. Comparison of intramuscular and intravenous recombinant alpha-2 interferon in melanoma and other cancers. *Ann Intern Med* 1985;103:32.
42. Eisenhauer EA, Silver HK, Venner PM, et al. Phase II study of high dose weekly intravenous human lymphoblastoid interferon in renal cell carcinoma. *Br J Cancer* 1987;55:541.
43. Muss HB, Costanzi JJ, Leavitt R, et al. Recombinant alfa interferon in renal cell carcinoma: a randomized trial of two routes of administration. *J Clin Oncol* 1987;5:286.
44. Quesada JR, Swanson DA, Gutterman JU. Phase II study of interferon alpha in metastatic renal cell carcinoma: a progress report. *J Clin Oncol* 1985;3:1086–1092.
45. Umeda T, Niijima T. Phase II study of alpha interferon on renal cell carcinoma. Summary of three collaborative trials. *Cancer* 1986;58:1231–1235.
46. Schnall SF, Davis C, Ziyadeh T, et al. Treatment of metastatic renal cell carcinoma with intramuscular (IM) recombinant interferon alpha (IFN, Hoffman-LaRoche). *Proc Am Soc Clin Oncol* 1986;5:227.
47. Kempf RA, Grunberg SM, Daniels JR, et al. Recombinant interferon alpha-2 (Intron A) in a phase II study of renal cell carcinoma. *J Biol Resp Mod* 1999;5:27–35.
48. Fossa SD. Is interferon with or without vinblastine the "treatment of choice" in metastatic renal cell carcinoma. *Semin Surg Oncol* 1988;4: 178–183.
49. Foon JK, Doroshow J, Bonnem E, et al. A prospective randomized trial of alpha 2B-interferon/gamma-interferon or the combination in advanced metastatic renal cell carcinoma. *J Biol Resp Mod* 1988;7:540–545.
50. Steineck G, Strander H, Carbin BE, et al. Recombinant leukocyte interferon alpha-ea and medroxyprogesterone in advanced renal cell carcinoma. A randomized trial. *Acta Oncol* 1990;29:155–162.
51. Marshall ME, Simpson H, Carbin BE, et al. Treatment of renal cell carcinoma with daily low-dose alpha interferon. *J Biol Resp Mod* 1989;8: 453–461.
52. Levens W, Ruebben H, Ingenhag W. Long-term interferon treatment in metastatic renal cell carcinoma. *Eur Urol* 1989;16:378–381.
53. Bono AV, Reali L, Bevenuti C, et al. Recombinant alpha interferon in metastatic renal cell carcinoma. *Urology* 1991;38:60–63.
54. Buzaid AC, Robertone A, Kisala C, et al. Phase II study of interferon alpha-2a, recombinant (Roferon A) in metastatic renal cell carcinoma. *J Clin Oncol* 1987;5:1083–1089.
55. Pyrhonen S, Salminen E, Ruuru M, et al. Prospective randomized trial of interferon alfa-2a plus vinblastine versus vinblastine alone in patients with advanced renal cell cancer. *J Clin Oncol* 1999;17:2859–2867.

56. Medical Research Council Renal Cancer Collaborators. Interferon α and survival in metastatic renal cell carcinoma: early results of randomized trial. *Lancet* 1999;353:14–17.
57. Flannigan RC, Salmon E, Blumenstein BA, et al. Nephrectomy followed by interferon alfa-2b compared with interferon alfa-2b alone for metastatic renal-cell carcinoma. *N Engl J Med* 2001;345(23):1655–1659.
58. Mickisch GH, Garin A, van Poppel H, et al. Radical nephrectomy plus interferon-alfa-based immunotherapy compared with interferon alfa alone in metastatic renal-cell carcinoma: a randomized trial. *Lancet* 2001; 358 (9286):966–970.
59. Creagan ET, Twito DI, Johansson SL, et al. A randomized prospective assessment of recombinant leukocyte A human interferon with or without aspirin in advanced renal adenocarcinoma. *J Clin Oncol* 1991;9:2104.
60. Rinehart JJ, Young D, Laforge J, et al. Phase I/II trial of interferon-beta-serine in patients with renal cell carcinoma: immunological and biological effects. *Cancer Res* 1987;47:2481–2485.
61. Kish J, Ensley J, Al-Sarraf M, et al. Activity of serine inhibited recombinant DNA beta interferon (IFN beta) in patients with metastatic and recurrent renal cell carcinoma. *Proc Am Assoc Cancer Res* 1986;27:184.
62. Nelson KA, Wallenberg JC, Todd MB. High-dose intravenous therapy with beta-interferon in patients with renal cell cancer. *Proc Am Assoc Cancer Res* 1989;30:260.
63. Kinney P, Triozzi P, Young D, et al. Phase II trial of interferon-beta-serine in metastatic renal cell carcinoma. *J Clin Oncol* 1990;8:881–885.
64. Quesada JR, Kuzrock R, Sherwin SA, et al. Phase II studies of recombinant human interferon gamma in metastatic renal cell carcinoma. *J Biol Resp Mod* 1987;6:20–27.
65. Koiso K, Recombinant Human Interferon Gamma Research Group. Phase II study of recombinant interferon gamma on renal cell carcinoma. *Cancer* 1987;60:929–933.
66. Takaku F, Machida T, Koiso K, et al. Phase II study of recombinant human interferon gamma (S-6810) in renal cell carcinoma. *Gan to Kagaku Ryoho* 1987;14:440–445.
67. Rinehart JJ, Young D, Laforge J, et al. Phase I/II trial of recombinant gamma-interferon in patients with metastatic renal cell carcinoma: immunologic and biologic effects. *J Biol Resp Mod* 1987;6:302–312.
68. Garnick MB, Reich SD, Maxwell B, et al. Phase I/II study of recombinant interferon gamma in advanced renal cell carcinoma. *J Urol* 1988;139:251–255.
69. Kuebler J, Brown T, Goodman P, et al. Continuous infusion recombinant gamma interferon (Clr-GIFN) for metastatic renal cell carcinoma. *Proc Am Soc Clin Oncol* 1989;8:140.
70. Aulitzky W, Gastl G, Aulitzky WE, et al. Successful treatment of metastatic renal cell carcinoma with a biologically active dose of recombinant interferon-gamma. *J Clin Oncol* 1989;7:1875–1884.
71. Grups JW, Frohmuller G. Cyclin interferon gamma treatment of patients with metastatic renal cell carcinoma. *Br J Urol* 1989;64:218–220.
72. Bruntsch U, de Mulder PH, ten Bokkel Huinink WW, et al. Phase II study of recombinant human interferon-gamma in metastatic renal cell carcinoma. *J Biol Resp Mod* 1999;9:335–338.
73. Foon K, Doroshow J, Bonnem J, et al. A prospective randomized trial of alpha-2B-interferon/gamma-interferon or the combination in advanced metastatic renal cell carcinoma. *J Biol Resp Mod* 1988;7:540–545.
74. Ellerhorst JA, Kilbourn RG, Amato RJ, et al. Phase II trial of low dose gamma-interferon in metastatic renal cell carcinoma. *J Urol* 1994;152: 841–845.
75. Small EJ, Weiss GR, Malik UK, et al. The treatment of metastatic renal cell carcinoma patients with recombinant human gamma interferon. *Cancer J Sci Am* 1998;4:162–167.
76. Chikkala NF, Lewis I, Ulchaker J, et al. Interactive effects of α interferon A/D and interleukin-2 on murine lymphokine-activated killer activity: analysis at the effector and precursor level. *Cancer Res* 1990;50: 1176–1182.
77. Bukowski RM. Natural history and therapy of metastatic renal cell carcinoma: role of interleukin-2. *Cancer* 1997;80:1198–1220.
78. Bukowski RM, Dutcher JP. Low dose interleukin-2. In: Voglezang NJ, Scardino PT, Shipley WW et al., eds. *Genitourinary oncology*. Philadelphia, PA: Lippincott William & Wilkins, 2000:218–233.
79. Henriksson R, Nilsson S, Colleen S, et al. Survival in renal cell carcinoma–a randomized evaluation of tamoxifen vs interleukin-2, α interferon (leukocyte) and tamoxifen. *Br J Cancer* 1998;77:1311.
80. Negrier S, Escudier B, Lasset C, et al. Recombinant interleukin-2, recombinant interferon alfa-2a, or both in metastatic renal cell carcinoma. *N Engl J Med* 1998;338:1273–1278.
81. Voglezang NJ, Lipton A, Figlin RA. Subcutaneous interleukin-2 plus interferon alfa-2a in metastatic renal cancer: an outpatient multicenter trial. *J Clin Oncol* 1993;11:1809–1816.
82. Atkins MB, Sparano J, Fisher RI, et al. Randomized phase II trial of high-dose interleukin-2 either alone or in combination with interferon alfa-2b in advanced renal cell carcinoma. *J Clin Oncol* 1993;11:661–670.
83. Crawford J. Clinical uses of pegylated pharmaceuticals in oncology. *Cancer Treat Rev* 2002;28(Suppl.):7–11.
84. Bukowski RM, Tendler C, Cutler D, et al. Treating cancer with PEG Intron: pharmacokinetic profile and dosing guidelines for an improved interferon alpha-2b formulation. *Cancer* 2002;95:386–396.
85. Motzer RJ, Rakhit A, Ginsberg M, et al. Phase I trial of 40-kDa branched pegylated interferon alfa-2a for patients with advanced renal cell carcinoma. *J Clin Oncol* 2001;19:1312–1319.
86. Motzer RJ, Rakhit A, Thompson J, et al. Phase II trial of branched peginterferon-alpha 2a (40 kDa) for patients with advanced renal cell carcinoma. *Ann Oncol* 2002;13(11):1799–1805.
87. Bukowski R, Ernstoff MS, Gore M, et al. Pegylated interferon alfa-2b treatment for patients with solid tumors: a phase I/II study. *J Clin Oncol* 2002;20:3841–3849.
88. He XH, Shaw PC, Tam SC. Reducing the immunogenicity and improving the *in vivo* activity of trichosanthin by site-directed pegylation. *Life Sci* 1999;65:355–368.
89. Clark JI, Gollob J, Sosman J, et al. Phase I trial of polyethylene glycol (PEG) interferon alpha-2b (IFN) + interleukin-2 (IL-2) in renal cancer (RCC). *Proc Am Soc Clin Oncol* 2002:2419.
90. Hutson TE, Mekhail T, Messerli E, et al. Phase I trial of PEG-Intron and rIL-2 in patients with metastatic renal cell carcinoma. *Proc Am Soc Clin Oncol* 2002:2406.
91. Hutson TE, Leschinsky A, Moon C, et al. Toxicity and apoptotic effects of PEG-Intron and rIL-2 in patients with metastatic renal cell carcinoma. *Proc Am Assoc Cancer Res* 2003;44:2540.
92. Yang JC, Haworth BSN, Sherry RM, et al. A randomized trial of bevacizumab, an anti-vascular endothelial growth factor antibody, for metastatic renal cancer. *N Engl J Med* 2003;349(5):427–434.
93. Amato RJ. Thalidomide therapy for renal cell carcioma. *Crit Rev Oncol Hematol* 2003;46(Suppl.):59–65.
94. Bauer JA, Morrison BH, Grane RW, et al. IFN-alpha2b and thalidomide synergistically inhibit tumor-induced angiogenesis. *J Interferon Cytokine Res* 2003;23(1):3–10.
95. Hernberg M, Virkkunen P, Bono P, et al. Interferon alfa-2b three times daily and thalidomide in the treatment of metastatic renal cell carcinoma. *J Clin Oncol* 2003;21(20):3770–3776.
96. Stadler WM, Rybak ME, Voglezang NJ. A phase II study of subcutaneous recombinant human interleukin-4 in renal cell carcinoma. *Cancer* 1995; 76:1629–1633.
97. Stouthard JML, Goey H, de Vries EGE, et al. Recombinant human interleukin 6 in metastatic renal cell cancer: a phase II trial. *Br J Cancer* 1996; 73:789–793.
98. Wos E, Olencki T, Tuason L, et al. Phase II trial of subcutaneous administered granulocyte-macrophage colony-stimulating factor coadministered with interleukin 2: a phase IB study. *Cancer* 1996;77:1149–1153.
99. Schiller JH, Hank JA, Khorsand M, et al. Clinical and immunological effects of granulocyte-macrophage colony stimulating factor coadministered with interleukin-2: a phase IB study. *Clin Cancer Res* 1996;2:319–330.
100. Steger GG, Kaboo R, Figlin P, et al. The effects of granulocyte-macrophage colony-stimulating factor on tumour-infiltrating lymphocytes from renal cell carcinoma. *Br J Cancer* 1995;72:101–107.
101. Hill ADK, Redmond HP, Croke DT, et al. Cytokines in tumour therapy. *Br J Surg* 1992;79:990–997.
102. Cavallo F, Di Carlo E, Butera M, et al. Immune events associated with the cure of established tumors and spontaneous metastases by local and systemic interleukin 12. *Cancer Res* 1999;59:414–421.
103. Majewski S, Marczak M, Szmurlo A, et al. Interleukin-12 inhibits angiogenesis induced by human tumor cell lines in vivo. *J Invest Dermatol* 1996;106:114–1118.
104. Tan J, Newton CA, Djeu JY, et al. Injection of complementary DNA encoding interleukin-12 inhibits tumor establishment at a distant site in a murine renal carcinoma model. *Cancer Res* 1996;56:3399–3403.
105. Gately MK, Wilson DE, Wong HL. Synergy between recombinant interleukin 2 (rIL 2) and IL 2-depleted lymphokine-containing supernatants in faciliatating allogeneic human cytolytic T lymphocyte responses in vitro. *J Immunol* 1986;136:1274–1282.
106. Kobayashi M, Fitz L, Ryan M, et al. Identification and purification of natural killer cell stimulatory factor (NKSF), a cytokine with multiple biologic effects on human lymphocytes. *J Exp Med* 1989;170:827–845.
107. Motzer RJ, Rakhit A, Schwartz LH, et al. Phase I trial of subcutaneous recombinant human interleukin-12 in patients with advanced renal cell carcinoma. *Clin Cancer Res* 1998;4:1183–1191.
108. Motzer RJ, Rakhit A, Thompson JA, et al. Randomized multicenter phase II trial of subcutaneous recombinant human interleukin-12 versus interferon-alpha 2a for patients with advanced renal cell carcinoma. *J Interferon Cytokine Res* 2001;21(4):257–263.
109. Atkins M, Robertson M, Gordon M, et al. Phase I evaluation of intravenous recombinant human interleukin 12 in patients with advanced malignancies. *Clin Cancer Res* 1997;3:409–417.
110. Gollob JA, Mier JW, Veenstra K, et al. Phase I trial of twice weekly intravenous interleukin 12 in patients with metastatic renal cell cancer or malignant melanoma: ability to maintain IFN-gamma induction is associated with clinical response. *Clin Cancer Res* 2000;6:1678–1692.
111. Portielje JE, Kruit WH, Schuler M, et al. Phase I study of subcutaneously administered recombinant human interleukin 12 in patients with advanced renal cell cancer. *Clin Cancer Res* 1999;5(12):3983–3989.
112. Wigginton JM, Komschlies KL, Back TC, et al. Administration of interleukin 12 with pulse interleukin-2 and the rapid and complete eradication of murine renal carcinoma. *J Natl Cancer Inst* 1996;88:38–43.
113. Gollob JA, Veenstra KG, Parker RA, et al. Phase I trial of concurrent twice-weekly recombinant human interleukin-12 plus low-dose IL-2 in patients with melanoma or renal cell carcinoma. *J Clin Oncol* 2003;21(13): 2564–2573.

114. Hutson TE, Mekhail T, Molto L, et al. Phase I trial of subcutaneously administered rHuIL-12 and rHuIFN-a2b in patients with metastatic renal cell carcinoma or malignant melanoma. *Proc Am Soc Clin Oncol* 2001; 20:258a.

115. Brunda MJ. Interleukin-12. *J Leukoc Biol* 1994;55:280–288.

116. Gately MK. Interleukin-12: a recently discovered cytokine with potential for enhancing cell-mediated immune responses to tumors. *Cancer Invest* 1993;11:500–506.

117. Brunda MJ, Luistro L, Warrier RR, et al. Antitumor and antimetastatic activity of interleukin 12 against murine tumors. *J Exp Med* 1993;178: 1223–1230.

118. Hayakawa Y, Takeda K, Yagita H, et al. IFN-gamma-mediated inhibition of tumor angiogenesis by natural killer T-cell ligand, alpha-galactosylceramide. *Blood* 2002;100:1728–1733.

119. Wigginton JM, Gruys E, Geiselhart L, et al. IFN-gamma and Fas/FasL are required for the antitumor and antiangiogenic effects of IL-12/pulse IL-2 therapy. *J Clin Invest* 2001;108:51–62.

120. Voest EE, Kenyon BM, O'Reilly MS, et al. Inhibition of angiogenesis in vivo by interleukin 12. *J Natl Cancer Inst* 1995;87:581–586.

121. Tannenbaum CS, Tubbs R, Armstrong D, et al. The CXC chemokines IP-10 and Mig are necessary for IL-12-mediated regression of the mouse RENCA tumor. *J Immunol* 1998;161:927–932.

122. Bukowski RM, Rayman P, Molto L, et al. Interferon-gamma and CXC chemokine induction by interleukin 12 in renal cell carcinoma. *Clin Cancer Res* 1999;5(10):2780–2789.

123. Bagby GC, Meinrich MC. Cytokines, growth factors and hematopoiesis. In: Wingard JR, Demetri GD, eds. *Clinical applications of cytokines and growth factors.* Norwell, MA: Kluwer Academic Publishers, 1999:2–55.

124. Bukowski RM, Murthy S, Sergi J, et al. Phase I trial of recombinant granulocyte-macrophage colony stimulating factor in patients with metastatic renal cell carcinoma. *Cancer* 1996;77:639–644.

125. Lieschke GJ, Cebon J, Morstyn G. Characterization of the clinical effects after the first dose of bacterially synthesized recombinant human granulocyte-macrophage colony-stimulating factor. *Blood* 1989;74:2634–2643.

126. Petros WP. Colony-stimulating factors. In: Chabner BA, Longo DL, eds. *Cancer chemotherapy and biotherapy: principles and practice.* Philadelphia, PA: Lippincott Williams & Wilkins, 2001:829–850.

127. deGast GC, Klumpen HJ, Vyth-Dreese FA, et al. Phase I trial of combined immunotherapy with subcutaneous granulocyte macrophage colony-stimulating factor, low dose interlukin-2 and interferon α in progressive metastatic melanoma and renal cell carcinoma. *Clin Cancer Res* 2000;6: 1267–1272.

128. Schornagel JH, Kersten M, Mallo H, et al. Combined immunotherapy with subcutaneous GM-CSF, low dose IL-2, and IFN α can induce complete remissions in metastatic renal cell carcinoma. *Proc Am Soc Clin Oncol* 2000; 19:344a.

129. Agrawal NR, Olencki T, Mekhail T, et al. A phase I/II study of GM-CSF, interleukin-2 (IL-2) and interferon-alpha (INF-α) in metastatic renal carcinoma (MRCC). *Proc Am Soc Clin Oncol* 2002:1829a.

130. Schornagel JH, Verweij J, ten Bokkel Huinink WW, et al. Phase II study of recombinant interferon alpha 2a and vinblastine in advanced renal cell carcinoma. *J Urol* 1989;142(2 Pt 1):253.

131. Figlin RA, deKernion JB, Maldazys J, et al. Treatment of renal cell carcinoma with alpha (human leukocyte) interferon and vinblastine combination: a phase I-II trial. *Cancer Treat Rep* 1985;69:263.

132. Fossa SD, de Garis ST. Further experience with recombinant interferon alfa-2a with vinblastine in metastatic renal cell carcinoma: a progress report. *Int J Cancer* 1987;(Suppl. 1):36.

133. Sertoli MR, Brunetti I, Ardizzoni A, et al. Recombinant alpha-2a interferon plus vinblastine in the treatment of metastatic renal carcinoma. *Am J Clin Oncol* 1989;12:43.

134. Fossa SD, Raabe N, Moe B. Recombinant interferon-alpha with or without vinblastine in metastatic renal carcinoma. Results of a randomized phase II study. *Br J Urol* 1989;64:468.

135. Trump DL, Ravdin PM, Borden EC, et al. Interferon-alpha-n1 and continuous infusion vinblastine for treatment of advanced renal cell carcinoma. *J Biol Resp Modif* 1990;9:108.

136. Palmeri S, Gebbia V, Russo A, et al. Vinblastine and interferon-alpha-2a regimen in the treatment of metastatic renal cell carcinoma. *Tumori* 1990;76:64.

137. Kellokumpu LP, Nordman E. Recombinant interferon-alpha 2a and vinblastine in advanced renal cell cancer: a clinical phase I-II study. *J Biol Resp Modif* 1990;9:439.

138. Rizzo M, et al. Interferon alpha-2a and vinblastine in the treatment of metastatic renal carcinoma. *Eur Urol* 1989;16:271.

139. Merimsky O, Chaitchik S. Interferon plus vinblastine in renal carcinoma patients who failed on interferon alone [Letter]. *Eur J Cancer* 1990;26:921.

140. Merimsky O, Shnider BI, Chaitchik S. Does vinblastine add to the potency of alpha interferon in the treatment of renal cell carcinoma? *Mol Biother* 1991;3:34.

141. Massidda B, Migliari R, Padovani A, et al. Metastatic renal cell cancer treated with recombinant alpha 2a interferon and vinblastine. *J Chemother* 1991;3:387.

142. Ojea CA, Castro IAM, Rodriguez IB, et al. [Results of treatment with interferon and vinblastine in renal cancer]. *Actas Urol Esp* 1992;16:507.

143. Schuster D, Schneider G, Ade N, et al. [Combination of recombinant interferon alpha-2A and vinblastine in advanced renal cell cancer]. *Onkologie* 1990;13:359.

144. Bollack C, Jacqmin D, Bergerat JP, et al. Recombinant interferon alpha plus vinblastine in renal cell cancer: updated results. In: Debruyne FMJ, Bukowski RM, Pontes JE et al., eds. *Immunotherapy of renal cell carcinoma.* Berlin, Springer-Verlag New York 1991;75–81.

145. Neidhart JA, Anderson SA, Harris JE, et al. Vinblastine fails to improve response of renal cancer to interferon alfa-n1: high response rate in patients with pulmonary metastases. *J Clin Oncol* 1991;9:832.

146. Fossa SD, Martinelli G, Otto U, et al. Recombinant interferon alfa-2a with or without vinblastine in metastatic renal cell carcinoma: results of a European multi-center phase III study. *Ann Oncol* 1992;3:301.

147. Elias L, Crissman HA. Interferon effects upon the adenocarcinoma 38 and HL-60 cell lines: antiproliferative responses and synergistic interactions with halogenated pyrimidine antimetabolites. *Cancer Res* 1988;48:4868.

148. Elias L, Blumenstein BA, Kish J, et al. A phase II trial of interferon-alpha and 5-fluorouracil in patients with advanced renal cell carcinoma: a Southwest Oncology Group study. *Cancer* 1996;78:1085.

149. Reiter Z, Ozes ON, Blatt LM, et al. A dual anti-tumor effect of interferon-alpha or interleukin-2 and 5-fluorouracil on natural killer cell mediated cytotoxicity. *Clin Immunol Immunopathol* 1992;62:103.

150. Hanninen EL, Krichner H, Atzpodien J. Interleukin-2 based home therapy of metastatic renal cell carcinoma: risks and benefits in 215 consecutive single institution patients. *J Urol* 1996;155:9–25.

151. Kirchner H, Buer J, Probst-Kepper M, et al. Risk and long-term outcome in metastatic renal cell carcinoma patients receiving SC interleukin-2, SC interferon-alfa 2A, and IV 5-fluorouracil. *Proc Am Soc Clin Oncol* 1998; 17:310a.

152. Atzpodien J, Kirchner H, Franzke A, et al. Results of a randomized clinical trial comparing SC interleukin-2, SC alpha-2a-interferon, and IV bolus 5-fluorouracil against oral tamoxifen in progressive metastatic renal cell carcinoma patients. *Proc Am Soc Clin Oncol* 1997;16:32a.

153. Ravaud A, Audhuy B, Gomez F, et al. Subcutaneous interleukin-2, interferon alfa-2a, and continuous infusion of fluorouracil in metastatic renal cell carcinoma: a multicenter phase II trial. *J Clin Oncol* 1998;16:2728.

154. Ellerhost JA, Sella A, Amato RJ, et al. Phase II trial of 5-fluorouracil, interferon α and continuous infusion interleukin-2 for patients with metastatic renal cell carcinoma. *Cancer* 1997;80:2128–2132.

155. Negrier S, Escudier B, Dovillard YU, et al. Randomized study of interleukin-2 (IL-2) and interferon (IFN) with or without 5-FU (FUCY study) in metastatic renal cell carcinoma (MRCC). *Proc Am Soc Clin Oncol* 1997;16:32a.

156. Dutcher JP, Atkins M, Fisher R, et al. Interleukin-2 based therapy for metastatic renal cell cancer: the Cytokine Working Group experience, 1989–1997. *Cancer J Sci Am* 1997;3:573.

157. Tourani JM, Pfister C, Berdah JF, et al. Outpatient treatment with subcutaneous interleukin-2 and interferon alfa administration in combination with fluorouracil in patients with metastatic renal cell carcinoma: results of a sequential nonrandomized phase II study. *J Clin Oncol* 1998;16:2505.

CHAPTER 48D
Allogeneic Stem Cell Transplantation for Renal Cell Carcinoma

Andrew Artz and Richard W. Childs

INTRODUCTION

Spontaneous tumor regressions and sensitivity to various immunotherapeutic approaches have identified renal cell carcinoma (RCC) as an immune-sensitive epithelial tumor. Although some patients with metastatic disease treated with Interleukin-2 (IL-2) achieve durable remissions, the activity of conventional immune therapy remains modest at best. Allogeneic hematopoietic stem cell transplant is now recognized as a powerful form of immunotherapy that can cure some hematologic malignancies. The advent of low-intensity conditioning regimens with reduced toxicity that maintain graft-versus-malignancy effects has recently permitted investigational allogeneic transplantation to be performed in patients with treatment-refractory solid tumors.

Nonmyeloablative allogeneic transplants for cytokine-refractory advanced RCC have demonstrated feasibility and response rates in the range of 25% to 30% with occasional complete responses (CRs). Ongoing research has shed light on the potential immunologic mechanisms that account for these powerful antitumor effects. Importantly, second-generation nonmyeloablative transplant regimens that incorporate mechanisms to bolster the donor immune response against the tumor through the adoptive infusion of tumor-reactive T cell or natural killer (NK)–cell infusions or through posttransplant cancer immunization will likely be forthcoming.

IMMUNE SENSITIVITY OF RENAL CELL CARCINOMA

As early as 1928, spontaneous regression of metastatic RCC was reported, raising the intriguing possibility of immune-mediated tumor control (1). Long periods of stable disease in some patients with advanced metastasis further supported the concept that RCC might be susceptible to the host's immune system (2,3). In one randomized trial of placebo versus interferon-γ the placebo response rate was 6.6%, an observation that supported spontaneous tumor regression as occurring more commonly than previously appreciated (4). Several lines of *in vitro* data have provided additional evidence that kidney cancer cells may be killed by activated T cells and NK cells. The isolation of tumor infiltrating lymphocytes from renal cell tumors provides *in vivo* evidence supporting the concept that host immunity may have a role in the treatment of this malignancy (5,6).

IMMUNOTHERAPEUTIC APPROACHES

Cytokines are protein molecules produced and secreted by host cells that bind to cytokine receptors resulting in either the stimulation or inhibition of immune cells. The binding of a cytokine to its receptor target results in cell signaling through a variety of different intracellular pathways. Cytokines that typically up-regulate immune responses include IL-2 and interferon, whereas cytokines that may inhibit the immune response include transforming growth factor β, interleukin-6, and interleukin-10.

The activity of IL-2 or interferon-α against metastatic RCC underscores the immunoresponsive nature of this malignancy. Interferon-α has several potential modes of activity including direct tumor lysis, up-regulation of human leukocyte antigen (HLA) class-I on tumor cells and antigen presenting cells, and enhancement of NK cell function. IL-2 has multiple potential therapeutic mechanisms as well, including NK-cell and T-cell proliferation and activation. IL-2 is currently the only drug approved by the U.S. Food and Drug Administration (FDA) for the treatment of advanced RCC. Multiple trials administering IL-2 or interferon alone or in combination have demonstrated real, albeit modest, response rates in the range of 15% with about 3% to 5% of patients achieving CRs (7,8). Data exists that suggests that interferon-α may improve survival slightly in the metastatic and adjuvant setting (9–11). Combinations of IL-2 and interferon are associated with higher response rates, although toxicity is greater and there appears to be no clear beneficial impact on survival compared to either cytokine alone (7).

Over the past two decades, a variety of alternative immune-based approaches have been explored that were intended to capitalize on the immune sensitivity of RCC (12). Several groups have pursued efforts to boost host immunity against tumor cells by vaccinating patients with dendritic cells pulsed with tumor antigens. Although responses have been observed following "cancer vaccine" approaches, the vast majority of patients treated to date have failed to benefit from such therapies (13,14).

LIMITATIONS OF AUTOLOGOUS IMMUNE THERAPY

Immunotherapy approaches designed to boost the host's immune system against cancer have limitations that may preclude efficacy. First and foremost, the mere existence of metastatic disease immediately implies host immune tolerance has already developed. A number of vaccine therapies have focused on immunizing to a single peptide antigen, significantly limiting the scope of the antitumor immune response, which ultimately may promote the escape of tumor variants with selective antigen loss or "dropout" (15). Finally, exposure to systemic therapies that may be immunosuppressive (i.e., chemotherapy, radiation therapy, etc.) may engender a degree of immune dysfunction, limiting the ability to enhance an autologous immune response (16).

Unfortunately, most patients fail to respond to conventional cytokine-based immunotherapy, and the majority of patients achieving a partial response (PR) ultimately will relapse. Retreatment with cytokines after initial cytokine failure has virtually no activity (17,18). Chemotherapy has been similarly disappointing, with nondurable response occurring in the range of 10% or less (19). The recent demonstration by Yang et al. that an antibody to vascular endothelial growth factor (VEGF-bevacizumab) may prolong the time of disease progression suggests that tumor angiogenesis inhibition may hold promise in this malignancy (20). New clinical data on targeted small molecules with excellent oral bioavailability that inhibit a variety of tyrosine kinases including VEGF appear promising, with PR rates in the range of 30%. Nevertheless, the modest activity of cytokines and no reliable second-line therapy with curative potential highlights the need for alternative investigational therapeutic options.

ADVANCES IN ALLOGENEIC HEMATOPOIETIC STEM CELL TRANSPLANTATION

The last several decades have witnessed continued growth in the use of allogeneic hematopoietic stem cell transplantation (HSCT) for both malignant and nonmalignant diseases. Historically, high-dose myeloablative chemotherapy with or without total body radiotherapy, followed by infusion of major HLA-matched donor stem cells (a.k.a. the allograft), was administered for refractory hematologic malignancies in an effort to overcome chemo resistance and to rescue the patient from chemotherapy-induced aplasia. Myeloablative "conditioning therapy" also eradicates the recipient's immune system, preventing rejection of the allograft. The stem cells repopulate the recipient's lympho-hematopoietic system, providing a new immune system. Although major HLA loci are typically matched, minor HLA loci minor histocompatibility antigens (MHA) are not matched with such transplants. As a consequence, the allograft may recognize recipient tissue as being foreign, mounting a T-cell-mediated immune attack known as graft-versus-host disease (GVHD). GVHD develops in approximately 50% of patients after HSCT and contributes considerably to morbidity and mortality. GVHD is temporally classified as acute graft-versus-host disease (aGVHD) if it occurs within the first 100 days and chronic graft-versus-host disease (cGVHD) if it occurs more than 100 days after stem cell infusion. Recipient organs commonly affected by aGVHD include the skin, liver, and gut. Most transplants employ immunosuppression with agents such as cyclosporine A or tacrolimus for a period of 3 to 9 months after transplant to reduce the incidence and severity of GVHD. Recently, stem cell collections have been facilitated by using hematopoietic progenitor cells that have been mobilized peripherally into the circulation following treatment with granulocyte-colony stimulating factor (G-CSF), in contrast to bone marrow harvesting.

ALLOGENEIC HEMATOPOIETIC STEM CELL TRANSPLANT AS IMMUNOTHERAPY

The ability of HSCT to cure patients with refractory hematologic malignancies was initially attributed to the high-dose "conditioning agents" utilized before stem cell transplantation (21). Multiple observations led to the realization that the efficacy of HSCT is partly attributable to immune-mediated attack by the allograft against recipient cancer cells, a phenomenon referred to as graft-versus leukemia (GVL) or, more broadly, graft-versus-tumor (GVT). The first clinical observation that suggested a GVL effect was the association of GVHD with decreased leukemic relapse among patients with chronic myeloid leukemia (CML) following HSCT (22). Additional clinical observations that affirmed the concept of GVL included a higher risk of relapse with both syngeneic transplants (i.e., identical siblings) and transplants with T-cell depleted grafts compared to traditional allografts (23–25). Similarly, the risk of leukemia relapse is increased following autologous transplantation compared to allogeneic HSCT (26). Most compelling, donor lymphocyte infusions (DLI), without any additional chemotherapy for patients relapsing after allogeneic transplantation, are capable of inducing leukemic remission (27,28). Hematologic malignancies vary in their sensitivity to GVT effects, with CML being most sensitive, although lymphoma, myeloma, and acute leukemias all demonstrate some sensitivity to this antitumor effect.

The molecular mechanisms through which GVT effects occur are being increasingly understood. Cytotoxic T-lymphocytes of donor origin with *in vitro* antileukemic activity have been isolated from patients in remission following HSCT (29). Furthermore, such T-cell populations have been expanded *in vitro* and reinfused into relapsed patients resulting in a recurrent leukemic remission in some patients (30). Isolating T-cell populations that induce GVT without GVHD remains one of the "holy grails" of allo-transplantation as immunotherapy for malignancies.

HSCT as an investigational form of immunotherapy for RCC is appealing in several respects. HSCT avoids some of the limitations of autologous immune therapy by providing a new and competent immune system, thus circumventing tumor tolerance. Unlike autologous immunity, the donor immune system may evoke tumor responses against mHA expressed on tumor cells (31,32). Murine *in vivo* evidence exists that allogeneic immune cells can eradicate mammary adenocarcinoma cells (33). More recently, GVT effects against multiple different types of solid tumors besides RCC have been reported, including breast (34,35), pancreas (36), ovarian (37,38), and colon carcinoma (39).

REDUCED INTENSITY CONDITIONING REGIMENS

The association of "high-dose" myeloablative chemotherapy, with potentially life-threatening acute toxicities affecting the liver, gut, and lung, restricts conventional allogeneic transplantation to reasonably fit patients under 60 years of age. Over the past decade, low-dose, nonmyeloablative regimens were developed in an effort to retain the GVT effects of HSCT while reducing the acute conditioning-related toxicities; such regimens permit older and less fit patients to undergo allogeneic transplantation (40,41). Nonmyeloablative stem cell transplants (NST) using reduced intensity preparative regimens employ conditioning agents that are sufficiently immunosuppressive to enable durable engraftment of donor stem cells and immune cells. Because the recipient's marrow is not ablated, both donor and recipient lympho-hematopoietic cells initially exist together in a state referred to as mixed chimerism. Chimerism is assessed in myeloid and T-cell lineages from the peripheral blood or bone marrow using molecular techniques that distinguish the patient's cells from the donors. Because the effector cells mediating antitumor effects are donor T-lymphocytes, manipulations such as withdrawal of immunosuppression or DLI often are incorporated into NST to expedite conversion to full donor T-cell chimerism.

TRANSPLANTATION FOR RENAL CELL CARCINOMA

Allogeneic transplants for RCC were initially pioneered at the National Institutes of Health (NIH) in the late 1990s. The first patient treated with metastatic disease that was refractory to interferon-α achieved a complete response that is ongoing more than 6 years after the procedure. Subsequently, the results of the first 19 patients with cytokine-refractory disease were reported, in which 10 patients were observed to have delayed regression of tumor (three CRs) with a GVT effect (42). Over the last 3 years, several groups have confirmed that GVT effects can be induced against this malignancy using a variety of different nonmyeloablative transplant approaches (Table 48D.1).

The NIH regimen approach employed 125 mg per m^2 of fludarabine divided over 5 days and cyclophosphamide 120 mg per kg given over 2 days before transplantation (Fig. 48D.1). Antithymocyte globulin was added when HLA-mismatched donors were used in order to decrease the risk of graft rejection and GVHD. G-CSF mobilized hematopoietic progenitor cells were collected by an apheresis procedure from the donor and infused intravenously on day 0. Cyclosporine was given either alone or with mycophenolate mofetil or low-dose methotrexate to prevent GVHD.

Donor Source

As with most modern allogeneic transplant regimens, G-CSF mobilized hematopoietic progenitor cells have been used as the primary donor stem cell source. Related donors have comprised the vast majority of allografts, although two groups have recently published the results of unrelated transplants in RCC (44,45). Although transplants using unrelated donors have historically been associated with a higher incidence of GVHD and lower overall survival, better immunosuppression and improved HLA typing using molecular techniques have significantly reduced differences in outcome related to donor stem cell source (47,48). Unrelated donor transplants could theoretically offer the possibility of additional antitumor activity mediated through enhanced minor-antigen disparity. However, the lengthy process (typically 2 to 4 months) of obtaining confirmatory molecular typing and collecting stem cells from volunteer donors potentially hinders the use of unrelated donor allografts.

TABLE 48D.1

PUBLISHED SERIES OF NONMYELOABLATIVE ALLOGENEIC TRANSPLANT FOR RENAL CELL CARCINOMA

First author	N	Donor	Median age (yr)	Regimen	Immuno-suppresion	aGVHD >.1 (%)	PR/CR	OR (%)
Childs (43)	19	Rel	48	F/C +/− ATG	CsA	10 (53)	7/3	10 (53)
Bregni (34)	7	Rel	48	F/T	CsA, Mtx	6 (86)	4/0	4 (57)
Pedrazolli (44)	7	Rel	44	F/C	CsA, Mtx	0 (0)	0	0 (0)
Rini (50)	12	Rel	55	F/C	Tac, MMF	2 (17)	4/0	4 (33)
Ueno (45)	15	Rel = 13 MUD = 2	52	F/M	Tac, Mtx	7 (47)	2/2[a]	4 (27)
Hentschke (39)	10	Rel = 5 MUD = 5	59	F/TBI	CsA, MMF +/ATG	5 (50)	0	0 (0)
Blaise (46)	25	Rel	45[b]	F/Bu	ATG CsA	24 (42)[b]	2/0	2 (8)
Total	95					31 (41)	19/5	24 (25)

aGVHD, acute graft-versus-host disease; CR, complete response; PR, partial response; OR, overall response; F, Fludarabine; T, thiotepa; C, Cyclophosphamide; M, Melphalan; Bu, Busulfan; ATG, Antithymocyte globulin (usually used with HLA mismatched donors); TBI, total body irradiation; CsA, cyclosporine; Tac, tacrolimus (FK506); Mtx, mini-methotrexate; MMF, mycophenolate mofetil; Rel- HLA, matched related donor; MUD-HLA, matched unrelated donor.
[a]Metastatectomy converted one PR to CR.
[b]Mean age and acute GVHD for all 57 patients as data for the 25 RCC patients not provided.

Response

Responses following NST for RCC have typically been delayed in onset, occurring at a median 3 to 5 months following transplantation (Fig. 48D.1). Disease regression has ranged from transient and mixed to durable and complete. Furthermore, not all groups have employed standard tumor regression criteria, making an assessment of response more difficult. Moreover, mixed response and stable disease lack standardized definition, further confusing their interpretation. A summary of the published literature shows an average response rate (partial plus complete) of 25% with a range from 0% to over 50% (Table 48D.1). The initial NIH series among 19 patients demonstrated an overall response (OR) rate of 53% (7 partial, 3 complete). In a follow-up abstract, a 42% response rate among 65 patients (19 partial, 6 complete) was observed (49). Rini et al. studied a fludarabine-and-cyclophosphamide-based regimen similar to that utilized at the NIH. Four responses were observed among 12 evaluable patients (50). An updated abstract continued to show four responses (all surviving) among a total of 18 treated patients. Bregni et al. observed four responses among seven treated patients using a Thiotepa-based NST approach (35). Blaise et al. investigated a T-cell- depleted regimen with fludarabine, busulfan, and antithymocyte globulin in a cohort of 57 patients with metastatic solid tumors (46). Among the 25 RCC patients in the series, only two responded, raising the possibility that in vivo T-cell depletion with ATG may have had a deleterious effect on donor immune-mediated antitumor effects. Other than the NIH, only the M.D. Anderson Cancer Center has reported CRs (45). They studied 15 patients conditioned with fludarabine/melphalan and observed 4 responses, including 2 CRs (1 CR obtained following a metastatectomy after an initial PR).

As mentioned earlier, responses tend to be delayed in onset, occurring anywhere from 3 to 6 months after transplantation; this delay to an antitumor effect may be related to the prolonged interval required for patients to convert from mixed to predominantly donor T-cell chimerism. The vast majority of responses have occurred in the context of acute or chronic GVHD; however, the occasional observation of disease regression in the absence of GVHD (42,45,51) raises the possibility that GVT effects may be separate in some cases from nonspecific alloimmune responses that occur during GVHD. With extended follow-up, all four responders remained alive with a median response duration of 20 months (52). As with cytokine therapy, lung disease tended to be the most responsive metastatic tumor site; furthermore, mixed responses associated with regression of pulmonary lesions and progression of extra-pulmonic disease has been observed (42,43, 45). Importantly, early disease progression within the first several months after transplantation does not preclude a delayed response, further illustrating the immune-mediated nature of tumor regression.

Disease progression late after transplantation (e.g., 6 to 8 months) represents a challenging situation requiring individualized decisions. Critical factors include the timing of progressive disease (PD), chimerism, presence of GVHD, and whether or not a prior response to cytokine-based therapy has occurred. Most important, the transplant should not be abandoned solely because early disease progression has occurred, mostly in light of the fact that responses are typically delayed and may occur following immunosuppression withdrawal, DLI, or treatment with posttransplant interferon. Donor chimerism analysis is mandatory to ensure complete

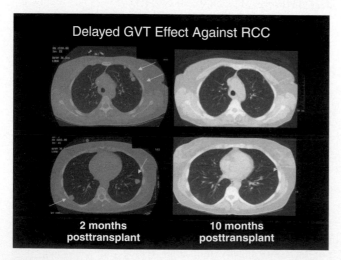

FIGURE 48D.1. Delayed graft versus tumor effect against renal cell carcinoma.

donor T-cell chimerism has been achieved. The presence and degree of GVHD may make a critical impact on posttransplant therapeutic options. For patients on immunosuppression, the withdrawal of cyclosporine or tacrolimus may achieve a response, sometimes in association with GVHD (45). For patients with mild GVHD who are off immunosuppression, both interferon-α and DLI have been reported to induce disease regression. Overall, DLI appears only modestly effective for RCC with occasional responses reported (34,42). In contrast, DLI for CML in chronic-phase relapsing after HSCT is associated with a high remission rate (27,53). DLI is frequently complicated by acute GVHD, and therefore can only be administered to patients who do not have significant GVHD. No data are currently available on second transplants, chemotherapy, or angiogenesis inhibition in patients who have a functioning allograft after NST.

Engraftment

The rate of graft failure has been less than 10% with NST in RCC. Further reductions in the intensity of immunosuppression used with the conditioning regimen may not be feasible. In the University of Chicago series, a less intensive conditioning regimen of 30 mg per m^2 of Fludarabine over 3 days (90 mg/m^2 total) with 1 day of cyclophosphamide at 2 gm per m^2 led to graft failure in 3 of the first 4 (75%) patients (50). Interestingly, the patient who engrafted had previously received temozolomide, an oral alkylating agent. Subsequent intensification of immunosuppression using fludarabine 30 mg per m^2 over 5 days (150 mg/m^2 total) and cyclophosphamide 2 gm per m^2 (4 gm/m^2 total) resulted in no engraftment failure in the subsequent 15 transplants, although a few patients died early before complete donor engraftment was achieved.

Regimens

Many groups have used a reduced-intensity conditioning regimen similar to that first described at the NIH. As shown in Table 48D.1, fludarabine-based conditioning has been the standard with the addition of one or more immunosuppressive agents including low-dose total-body irradiation. Posttransplant immunosuppression has also been fairly similar, usually consisting of cyclosporine or tacrolimus.

One of the major differences among regimens has been manipulation of immunosuppression based upon the kinetics of engrafting donor cells. Factors influencing conversion to complete donor T-cell chimerism include pretransplant chemotherapy, conditioning intensity, use of T-cell depletion, and timing of immunosuppression withdrawal. Additionally, DLI may convert mixed chimerism to complete donor chimerism. Rapid conversion to complete donor chimerism theoretically reduces tumor tolerance and increases tumor sensitivity, although higher rates of aGVHD may be observed (54–56). For example, the two series reporting the highest response rates in RCC following allogeneic transplantation (Childs et al. and Bregni et al.) also had the highest incidence of acute GVHD. The protocol utilized at the NIH (response rates >40%) emphasizes rapid complete donor T-cell chimerism by early withdrawal of immunosuppression or DLI based on chimerism analysis. The M.D. Anderson Cancer Center also incorporated methods to achieve rapid induction of full donor chimerism, but with a more modest response rate of 27% among RCC patients (45). Both NIH and M.D. Anderson Cancer Center have reported CRs. Nevertheless, the precise benefit of strategies designed to achieve rapid donor immune engraftment remain incompletely defined. It is clear that other factors such as tumor volume, metastatic sites, tumor kinetics also will impact

the ability to achieve a GVT effect. At the University of Chicago, manipulations to promote early complete donor chimerism were not incorporated into the transplant approach, yet the response rate was similar to the M.D. Anderson Cancer Center (22% vs. 27%, respectively). Interestingly, complete donor chimerism was delayed by more than 100 days in all responding patients in the Chicago series. Moreover, early conversion to complete donor chimerism must be counterbalanced by the morbidity and mortality associated with an increased risk of acute GVHD (57). In the University of Chicago series, significant aGVHD correlated with reduced survival ($P = .03$), although it is important to note that the cases of aGVHD in this series were all severe in nature (52). Therefore, rapid complete donor chimerism is not a biologic necessity for success, although data would suggest that response rates including CRs occur more often when rapid donor T-cell chimerism is achieved.

Blaise and colleagues are the only group that systematically incorporated T-cell depletion in their regimen (i.e., *in vivo* T-cell depletion using antithymocyte globulin) (46). In their series, antithymocyte globulin was incorporated with a fludarabine/busulfan conditioning followed by immunosuppression with cyclosporine in a group of 57 solid tumor patients, 25 of which were RCC. The rate of aGVHD was 24% among all patients, but only two of 25 subjects with RCC responded, raising the possibility that T-cell depletion reduced tumor responsiveness.

Histologic Subtype

As with cytokine-based therapy, preliminary data would suggest clear cell histology RCC appears more sensitive to NST. In the NIH series, responses arose only in association with pure clear cell carcinoma, whereas no responses were documented among 10 patients with other histologic subtypes. One small series indicated "transient" responses were observed among three patients with papillary histology (58). Some protocols have restricted eligibility for NST to clear cell histology, which potentially could preclude inferences about the sensitivity of less common histologic subtypes to the GVT effect.

Nephrectomy

The vast majority of RCC patients eligible for transplant have undergone prior nephrectomy, either as cytoreduction or initial treatment of apparent renal-confined disease. Cyto-reductive therapy has recently been utilized as a standard therapy for patients with RCC that have low-volume metastatic disease and a good performance status (PS) before receiving cytokine therapy (59,60). Data on the impact of cyto-reductive nephrectomy before NST is lacking. However, as cyto-reductive nephrectomy appears to be of benefit before cytokine-based immunotherapy, it is reasonable to pursue a similar strategy in patients being considered for allogeneic transplantation. Absence of a nephrectomy does not, however, preclude a durable response; the only patient at the University of Chicago with a primary renal lesion left intact obtained a durable PR, including tumor regression in the primary renal lesion.

Survival

Infections and GVHD are the primary nonrelapse causes of death among stem cell transplant recipients. Transplant-associated mortality has varied across transplant series for RCC, falling in the range of 10% to 30%. Despite concerns about the risk of transplant-related mortality (TRM) and the effects of GVHD, disease progression remains the major cause of death for RCC following NST (52), emphasizing the need for additional strategies to control the tumor following the procedure.

The early nature of NST for RCC in select patients with a lack of long-term follow precludes an accurate determination of the impact of transplantation on survival. In general, median overall survival for previously treated patients with metastatic RCC is 12.7 months, ranging from 5 months for those with several adverse risk factors to 22 months in those with no adverse risk factors (61). At the University of Chicago, the overall survival for 18 patients on an NST protocol was 14 months. The University of Chicago, M.D. Anderson, and NIH data reveal a strong positive association with response and long-term survival. However, one cannot conclude based on such evidence alone that NST prolongs survival, as responding patients could have had potentially fewer pretreatment adverse prognostic factors. Motzer et al. reviewed the Memorial Sloan-Kettering Cancer Center experience for advanced RCC after cytokines and found only 12 patients among 670 (1.7%) were disease free after 5 years (62). In this context, therefore, the observation of any durable CRs in cytokine-refractory RCC following NST is made even more provocative.

Adjuvant Transplant

No data are available applying NST in the adjuvant setting for patients at high risk of RCC relapse. As with other forms of immunotherapy, NST may be more effective with low-volume disease (63). Nevertheless, the difficulty of identifying a subset of patients at high risk of relapse, the lack of benefit from cytokine therapy in the adjuvant setting (11), the possibility of prolonged survival in a subset of patients with metastatic disease, and the risk of death associated with allogeneic transplantation taken together preclude the use of NST as adjuvant therapy for (64) for RCC.

Chronic Graft-Versus-Host Disease

Following HSCT, cGVHD develops in 30% to 70% of recipients of an HLA-matched transplant (65,66). A prior history of acute GVHD, older donor/recipient age, HLA mismatching, and prior treatment with DLI predispose to cGVHD. Limited cGVHD requires no treatment, whereas extensive cGVHD can be debilitating, mandating therapy (67,68). Standard therapy consists of prednisone, although the armamentarium of immunosuppressive therapies to treat this complication has grown recently. Balancing the need for appropriate GVHD treatment against the risks that immunosuppression may allow the tumor to escape the immune system's anticancer effects represents a challenging dilemma for transplant physicians. Frequent disease reassessment may assist the transplant team in balancing the amount of immunosuppressive therapy required to manage this complication.

Patient Selection

To date, NST for RCC has been applied to a relatively small subset of patients (Table 48D.2). Eligibility criteria have routinely included advanced RCC refractory or intolerant to cytokine therapy, age less than 65 years, adequate organ function, lack of central nervous system (CNS) disease, and good PS (i.e., PS of 0 or 1). Some, but not all protocols, have excluded nonclear cell histologic subtypes.

Adverse prognostic factors previously identified for patients with metastatic RCC include advanced PS, anemia, elevated

TABLE 48D.2

PATIENT CRITERIA PREFERRED FOR NONMYELOABLATIVE TRANSPLANTATION—GOOD

Performance status
Adequate end-organ function
Reasonable life-expectancy (e.g., >6 mo)
Clear cell histology
HLA matched sibling donor
Slow disease progression
Absence of CNS metastasis

HLA, human leukocyte antigen; CNS, central nervous system.

corrected serum calcium, tumor histology, time to the development of metastasis, elevated serum lactate dehydrogenase levels, and advanced age (61,64,67,69,70). The high degree of patient selectivity among RCC patients undergoing NST was captured by Rini et al. in their pilot NST protocol (50). Among 284 patients considered, only 15 eventually underwent allogeneic transplantation. Many series have not reported the prognostic factors that impact on survival with metastatic RCC, limiting comparisons of response and survival across studies.

Several practical issues exist in selecting patients for allogeneic transplantation. In addition to determining whether transplant is reasonable, a donor source must be procured. Because families are smaller in Western countries and because each sibling has a 25% chance of being HLA identical, only 25% to 30% of patients will have a sibling donor who could serve as a stem cell donor. Furthermore, the process of HLA typing the patient and siblings, insurance approval, and consultation with the transplant team may delay the procedure by weeks to months. Thus, early consideration and proactive planning for transplantation is paramount.

Mechanisms of Graft Versus Tumor/Future Directions

A large body of evidence exists supporting donor T cells as playing a critical role in mediating disease regression following NST (Table 48D.3). The inactivity of the chemotherapy agents used in the conditioning regimen (71–73), the observation that tumor responses are delayed or do not occur until T-cell chimerism is predominantly donor, and the correlation of GVHD response, all support donor immune-mediated GVT

TABLE 48D.3

EVIDENCE FOR ALLOGENEIC T-CELLS MEDIATING DISEASE REGRESSION IN RENAL CELL CARCINOMA

Allogeneic transplantation mediates tumor responses against a variety of hematologic malignancies
Conditioning chemotherapy inactive
Responses are delayed by months
Tumor regression occurs after full donor T-cell chimerism and immunosuppression withdrawn
Responses frequently occur in association with GVHD
T-lymphocytes cytotoxic against RCC can be isolated from responding patients

GVHD, graft-versus-host disease; RCC, renal cell carcinoma.

effects as the mechanism of tumor regression. At the NIH, cytotoxic CD8+ T cells have been isolated from patients during tumor regression that kill RCC cells *in vitro*. In some cases, these cells also kill recipient hematopoietic cells, implicating MHA as potential targets for a GVT effect in some responders. An increase in donor-derived CD8 T cells has also been associated with disease response (74). Elucidating the mechanism(s) of GVT may lead to more targeted allogeneic transplant approaches in the future. It is also reasonable to expect novel transplant strategies in the near future that incorporate the use of posttransplant tumor vaccines as well as adoptive infusions of tumor-reactive donor T cells and NK cells. Such strategies have shown promising activity *in vitro* and, if effective following transplantation, could significantly improve transplant outcome. Angiogenesis inhibition through the use of monoclonal antibodies or targeted small molecules after transplantation could potentially prevent early tumor progression, thus prolonging survival in some patients and allowing a potentially curative GVT effect to ultimately occur.

References

1. Bumpus HC. The apparent dissappearance of pulmonary metastasis in a case of hypernephoroma following nephrectomy. *J Urol* 1928;20:185.
2. Vogelzang NJ, Priest ER, Borden L. Spontaneous regression of histologically proved pulmonary metastases from renal cell carcinoma: a case with 5-year followup. *J Urol* 1992;148:1247–1248.
3. Fairlamb DJ. Spontaneous regression of metastases of renal cancer: a report of two cases including the first recorded regression following irradiation of a dominant metastasis and review of the world literature. *Cancer* 1981;47:2102–2106.
4. Gleave ME, Elhilali M, Fradet Y et al. Canadian Urologic Oncology Group. Interferon gamma-1b compared with placebo in metastatic renal-cell carcinoma. *N Engl J Med* 1998;338:1265–1271.
5. Caignard A, Guillard M, Gaudin C, et al. In situ demonstration of renal-cell-carcinoma-specific T-cell clones. *Int J Cancer* 1996;66:564–570.
6. Boon T, Coulie PG, Van den Eynde B. Tumor antigens recognized by T cells. *Immunol Today* 1997;18:267–268.
7. Negrier S, Escudier B, Lasset C, et al. Recombinant human interleukin-2, recombinant human interferon alfa-2a, or both in metastatic renal-cell carcinoma. Groupe Francais d'Immunotherapie. *N Engl J Med* 1998; 338: 1272–1278.
8. Fossa SD. Interferon in metastatic renal cell carcinoma. *Semin Oncol* 2000;27:187–193.
9. Pyrhonen S, Salminen E, Ruutu M, et al. Prospective randomized trial of interferon alfa-2a plus vinblastine versus vinblastine alone in patients with advanced renal cell cancer. *J Clin Oncol* 1999;17:2859–2867.
10. Medical Research Council Renal Cancer Collaborators. Interferon-alpha and survival in metastatic renal cell carcinoma: early results of a randomised controlled trial. *Lancet* 1999;353:14–17.
11. Messing EM, Manola J, Wilding G, et al. Phase III study of interferon alfa-NL as adjuvant treatment for resectable renal cell carcinoma: an Eastern Cooperative Oncology Group/Intergroup trial. *J Clin Oncol* 2003;21:1214–1222.
12. Graham S, Babayan RK, Lamm DL, et al. The use of ex vivo-activated memory T cells (autolymphocyte therapy) in the treatment of metastatic renal carcinoma: final results from a randomized, controlled, multisite study. *Semin Urol* 1993;11:27–34.
13. Holtl L, Zelle-Rieser C, Gander H, et al. Immunotherapy of metastatic renal cell carcinoma with tumor lysate-pulsed autologous dendritic cells. *Clin Cancer Res* 2002;8:3369–3376.
14. Kugler A, Stuhler G, Walden P, et al. Regression of human metastatic renal cell carcinoma after vaccination with tumor cell-dendritic cell hybrids. *Nat Med* 2000;6:332–336.
15. Marincola FM, Shamamian P, Alexander RB, et al. Loss of HLA haplotype and B locus down-regulation in melanoma cell lines. *J Immunol* 1994; 153:1225–1237.
16. Antonia SJ, Extermann M, Flavell RA. Immunologic nonresponsiveness to tumors. *Crit Rev Oncog* 1998;9:35–41.
17. Lee DS, White DE, Hurst R, et al. Patterns of relapse and response to retreatment in patients with metastatic melanoma or renal cell carcinoma who responded to interleukin-2-based immunotherapy. *Cancer J Sci Am* 1998;4:86–93.
18. Escudier B, Chevreau C, Lasset C, et al. Cytokines in metastatic renal cell carcinoma: is it useful to switch to interleukin-2 or interferon after failure of a first treatment? Groupe Francais d'Immunotherape. *J Clin Oncol* 1999;17:2039–2043.
19. Rini BI, Vogelzang NJ, Dumas MC, et al. Phase II trial of weekly intravenous gemcitabine with continuous infusion fluorouracil in patients with metastatic renal cell cancer. *J Clin Oncol* 2000;18:2419–2426.
20. Yang JC, Sherry RM, Steinberg SM, et al. Randomized study of high-dose and low-dose interleukin-2 in patients with metastatic renal cancer. *J Clin Oncol* 2003;21:3127–3132.
21. Thomas ED, Storb R, Clift RA, et al. Bone-marrow transplantation (second of two parts). *N Engl J Med* 1975;292:895–902.
22. Weiden PL, Flournoy N, Thomas ED, et al. Antileukemic effect of graft-versus-host disease in human recipients of allogeneic-marrow grafts. *N Engl J Med* 1979;300:1068–1073.
23. Gale RP, Horowitz MM, Ash RC, et al. Identical-twin bone marrow transplants for leukemia. *Ann Intern Med* 1994;120:646–652.
24. Apperley JF, Jones L, Hale G, et al. Bone marrow transplantation for patients with chronic myeloid leukaemia: T-cell depletion with Campath-1 reduces the incidence of graft-versus-host disease but may increase the risk of leukaemic relapse. *Bone Marrow Transplant* 1986;1:53–66.
25. Goldman JM, Gale RP, Horowitz MM, et al. Bone marrow transplantation for chronic myelogenous leukemia in chronic phase. Increased risk for relapse associated with T-cell depletion. *Ann Intern Med* 1988; 108: 806–814.
26. Zittoun RA, Mandelli F, Willemze R et al, European Organization for Research and Treatment of Cancer (EORTC) and the Gruppo Italiano Malattie Ematologiche Maligne dell'Adulto (GIMEMA) Leukemia Cooperative Groups. Autologous or allogeneic bone marrow transplantation compared with intensive chemotherapy in acute myelogenous leukemia. *N Engl J Med* 1995;332:217–223.
27. Kolb HJ, Mittermuller J, Clemm C, et al. Donor leukocyte transfusions for treatment of recurrent chronic myelogenous leukemia in marrow transplant patients. *Blood* 1990;76:2462–2465.
28. Kolb HJ, Schattenberg A, Goldman JM et al. European Group for Blood and Marrow Transplantation Working Party Chronic Leukemia. Graft-versus-leukemia effect of donor lymphocyte transfusions in marrow grafted patients. *Blood* 1995;86:2041–2050.
29. Falkenburg JH, Faber LM, van den Elshout M, et al. Generation of donor-derived antileukemic cytotoxic T-lymphocyte responses for treatment of relapsed leukemia after allogeneic HLA-identical bone marrow transplantation. *J Immunother* 1993;14:305–309.
30. Falkenburg JH, Wafelman AR, Joosten P, et al. Complete remission of accelerated phase chronic myeloid leukemia by treatment with leukemia-reactive cytotoxic T lymphocytes. *Blood* 1999;94:1201–1208.
31. Goulmy E. Human minor histocompatibility antigens: new concepts for marrow transplantation and adoptive immunotherapy. *Immunol Rev* 1997;157:125–140.
32. Warren EH, Greenberg PD, Riddell SR. Cytotoxic T-lymphocyte-defined human minor histocompatibility antigens with a restricted tissue distribution. *Blood* 1998;91:2197–2207.
33. Morecki S, Moshel Y, Gelfend Y, et al. Induction of graft vs. tumor effect in a murine model of mammary adenocarcinoma. *Int J Cancer* 1997; 71:59–63.
34. Bregni M, Dodero A, Peccatori J, et al. Nonmyeloablative conditioning followed by hematopoietic cell allografting and donor lymphocyte infusions for patients with metastatic renal and breast cancer. *Blood* 2002; 99: 4234–4236.
35. Ueno NT, Rondon G, Mirza NQ, et al. Allogeneic peripheral-blood progenitor-cell transplantation for poor-risk patients with metastatic breast cancer. *J Clin Oncol* 1998;16:986–993.
36. Omuro Y, Matsumoto G, Sasaki T, et al. Regression of an unresectable pancreatic tumor following nonmyeloablative allogeneic peripheral-blood stem-cell transplantation. *Bone Marrow Transplant* 2003;31:943–945.
37. Hanel M, Bornhauser M, Muller J, et al. Evidence for a graft-versus-tumor effect in refractory ovarian cancer. *J Cancer Res Clin Oncol* 2003; 129:12–16.
38. Bay JO, Fleury J, Choufi B, et al. Allogeneic hematopoietic stem cell transplantation in ovarian carcinoma: results of five patients. *Bone Marrow Transplant* 2002;30:95–102.
39. Hentschke P, Barkholt L, Uzunel M, et al. Low-intensity conditioning and hematopoietic stem cell transplantation in patients with renal and colon carcinoma. *Bone Marrow Transplant* 2003;31:253–261.
40. Giralt S, Estey E, Albitar M, et al. Engraftment of allogeneic hematopoietic progenitor cells with purine analog-containing chemotherapy: harnessing graft-versus-leukemia without myeloablative therapy. *Blood* 1997; 89: 4531–4536.
41. Slavin S, Nagler A, Naparstek E, et al. Nonmyeloablative stem cell transplantation and cell therapy as an alternative to conventional bone marrow transplantation with lethal cytoreduction for the treatment of malignant and nonmalignant hematologic diseases. *Blood* 1998;91:756–763.
42. Childs R, Chernoff A, Contentin N, et al. Regression of metastatic renal-cell carcinoma after nonmyeloablative allogeneic peripheral-blood stem-cell transplantation. *N Engl J Med* 2000;343:750–758.
43. Childs R, Srinivasan R. Advances in allogeneic stem cell transplantation: directing graft-versus-leukemia at solid tumors. *Cancer J* 2002;8:2–11.
44. Pedrazzoli P, Da Prada GA, Giorgiani G, et al. Allogeneic blood stem cell transplantation after a reduced-intensity, preparative regimen: a pilot study in patients with refractory malignancies. *Cancer* 2002;94: 2409–2415.
45. Ueno NT, Cheng YC, Rondon G, et al. Rapid induction of complete donor chimerism by the use of a reduced-intensity conditioning regimen composed

of fludarabine and melphalan in allogeneic stem-cell transplantation for metastatic solid tumors. *Blood* 2003;102:3829–3836.

46. Blaise D, Bay JO, Faucher C, et al. Reduced-intensity preparative regimen and allogeneic stem cell transplantation for advanced solid tumors. *Blood* 2004;103:435–441.

47. Giebel S, Giorgiani G, Martinetti M, et al. Low incidence of severe acute graft-versus-host disease in children given haematopoietic stem cell transplantation from unrelated donors prospectively matched for HLA class I and II alleles with high-resolution molecular typing. *Bone Marrow Transplant* 2003;31:987–993.

48. Zander AR, Kroger N, Schleuning M, et al. ATG as part of the conditioning regimen reduces transplant-related mortality (TRM) and improves overall survival after unrelated stem cell transplantation in patients with chronic myelogenous leukemia (CML). *Bone Marrow Transplant* 2003; 32:355–361.

49. Takahashi Y, Mena O, Srinivasan R, et al. *Minor histocompatibility antigen (mHa) specific T-cells with cytotoxicity against autologous tumor cells can be isolated from patients with renal cell carcinoma having a GVT effect after nonmyeloablative hematopoietic cell transplantation (HCT).* San Diego, CA: American Society for Hematology, 2003.

50. Rini BI, Zimmerman T, Stadler WM, et al. Allogeneic stem-cell transplantation of renal cell cancer after nonmyeloablative chemotherapy: feasibility, engraftment, and clinical results. *J Clin Oncol* 2002;20:2017–2024.

51. Appelbaum FR, Sandmaier B. Sensitivity of renal cell cancer to nonmyeloablative allogeneic hematopoietic cell transplantations: unusual or unusually important? *J Clin Oncol* 2002;20:1965–1967.

52. Artz AS, van Besien K, Zimmerman T, et al. *Long-term follow up of nonmyeloablative allogeneic stem cell transplantation for renal cell carcinoma.* The University of Chicago Experience. *Bone Marrow Transplant* 2005; 35(3):253–260.

53. Mackinnon S, Papadopoulos EB, Carabasi MH, et al. Adoptive immunotherapy evaluating escalating doses of donor leukocytes for relapse of chronic myeloid leukemia after bone marrow transplantation: separation of graft-versus-leukemia responses from graft-versus-host disease. *Blood* 1995;86:1261–1268.

54. Hill RS, Petersen FB, Storb R, et al. Mixed hematologic chimerism after allogeneic marrow transplantation for severe aplastic anemia is associated with a higher risk of graft rejection and a lessened incidence of acute graft-versus-host disease. *Blood* 1986;67:811–816.

55. Mattsson J, Uzunel M, Remberger M, et al. T cell mixed chimerism is significantly correlated to a decreased risk of acute graft-versus-host disease after allogeneic stem cell transplantation. *Transplantation* 2001;71: 433–439.

56. Childs R, Clave E, Contentin N, et al. Engraftment kinetics after nonmyeloablative allogeneic peripheral blood stem cell transplantation: full donor T-cell chimerism precedes alloimmune responses. *Blood* 1999;94: 3234–3241.

57. Gratwohl A, Brand R, Apperley J, et al. Graft-versus-host disease and outcome in HLA-identical sibling transplantations for chronic myeloid leukemia. *Blood* 2002;100:3877–3886.

58. Takaue Y. Mini-transplantation strategy for solid tumors. *Int J Hematol* 2002;76(Suppl. 2):13–14.

59. Flanigan RC, Salmon SE, Blumenstein BA, et al. Nephrectomy followed by interferon alfa-2b compared with interferon alfa-2b alone for metastatic renal-cell cancer. *N Engl J Med* 2001;345:1655–1659.

60. Flanigan RC, Mickisch G, Sylvester R, et al. Cytoreductive nephrectomy in patients with metastatic renal cancer: a combined analysis. *J Urol* 2004;171:1071–1076.

61. Motzer RJ, Bacik J, Schwartz LH, et al. Prognostic factors for survival in previously treated patients with metastatic renal cell carcinoma. *J Clin Oncol* 2004;22:454–463.

62. Motzer RJ, Mazumdar M, Bacik J, et al. Effect of cytokine therapy on survival for patients with advanced renal cell carcinoma. *J Clin Oncol* 2000; 18:1928–1935.

63. Lee CK, Badros A, Barlogie B, et al. Prognostic factors in allogeneic transplantation for patients with high-risk multiple myeloma after reduced intensity conditioning. *Exp Hematol* 2003;31:73–80.

64. Mejean A, Hopirtean V, Bazin JP, et al. Prognostic factors for the survival of patients with papillary renal cell carcinoma: meaning of histological typing and multifocality. *J Urol* 2003;170:764–767.

65. Socie G, Stone JV, Wingard JR et al, Late Effects Working Committee of the International Bone Marrow Transplant Registry. Long-term survival and late deaths after allogeneic bone marrow transplantation. *N Engl J Med* 1999;341:14–21.

66. Sullivan KM, Agura E, Anasetti C, et al. Chronic graft-versus-host disease and other late complications of bone marrow transplantation. *Semin Hematol* 1991;28:250–259.

67. Motzer RJ, Mazumdar M, Bacik J, et al. Survival and prognostic stratification of 670 patients with advanced renal cell carcinoma. *J Clin Oncol* 1999;17:2530–2540.

68. Simpson D. Drug therapy for acute graft-versus-host disease prophylaxis. *J Hematother Stem Cell Res* 2000;9:317–325.

69. Ljungberg B, Landberg G, Alamdari FI. Factors of importance for prediction of survival in patients with metastatic renal cell carcinoma, treated with or without nephrectomy. *Scand J Urol Nephrol* 2000;34: 246–251.

70. Naito S, Kimiya K, Sakamoto N, et al. Prognostic factors and value of adjunctive nephrectomy in patients with stage IV renal cell carcinoma. *Urology* 1991;37:95–99.

71. Shevrin DH, Lad TE, Kilton LJ, et al. Phase II trial of fludarabine phosphate in advanced renal cell carcinoma: an Illinois Cancer Council Study. *Invest New Drugs* 1989;7:251–253.

72. Quan WD Jr, Dean GE, Lieskovsky G, et al. Phase II study of low dose cyclophosphamide and intravenous interleukin-2 in metastatic renal cancer. *Invest New Drugs* 1994;12:35–39.

73. Lupera H, Theodore C, Ghosn M, et al. Phase II trial of combination chemotherapy with dacarbazine, cyclophosphamide, cisplatin, doxorubicin, and vindesine (DECAV) in advanced renal cell cancer. *Urology* 1989;34:281–283.

74. Harlin H, Artz AS, Mahowald M, et al. Clinical responses following nonmyeloablative allogeneic stem cell transplantation for renal cell carcinoma are associated with expansion of CD8(+) IFN-gamma-producing T cells. *Bone Marrow Transplant* 2004;33:491–497.

CHAPTER 48E
Chemotherapy and Other Approaches in the Management of Metastatic Renal Cell Carcinoma
Walter M. Stadler

INTRODUCTION

Metastatic renal cancer historically has been considered resistant to chemotherapy. This has led to a certain degree of therapeutic nihilism for these patients and a lack of enthusiasm for studying new compounds. Such pessimism may not necessarily be warranted because low-level activity has been demonstrated with certain nucleoside analogs, and because a number of vascular endothelial growth factor (VEGF)–targeted compounds and kinase inhibitors are showing promise. A major challenge with development of these new compounds is that many are expected to lead to growth inhibition and disease stabilization. The natural history of metastatic renal cell cancer (RCC) is however highly variable, and up to 10% of patients are long-term 5- and 10-year survivors, even in the absence of any systemic therapy (1,2). It is therefore difficult to predict the expected time-to-progression in a small patient cohort, and the observation of stable disease in short-term, single-arm, uncontrolled clinical trials with a new agent is probably not meaningful. Even low-level objective responses, as defined by standard tumor shrinkage criteria, may be subject to interpretation, as response rates as high as 7% have been reported in the placebo arm of randomized trials (3). Similar problems plague discussions of the value of local therapies to one or several metastatic sites. Although a discussion of clinical trial designs is beyond the scope of this chapter, clearly more emphasis must be placed on outcomes from controlled and randomized trials.

Interpretation of clinical trials of systemic agents in metastatic renal cancer also must take into account that "renal cell cancer" is not one disease but represents the most common clear cell variant, as well as other less common histologic subtypes, such as papillary and chromophobe variants (see Chapter 44). Historically, histologic distinctions for patients entered into clinical treatment trials have not been made or have been made on the basis of subtypes that are no longer recognized (e.g., granular cell). Nevertheless, 90% to 95% of patients with metastatic renal cancer have a clear cell variant (4,5), and thus, the data from trials of systemic therapy are most applicable to this subtype. This means, however, that the number of patients with non–clear cell histologies typically enrolled in these trials is too small to make any conclusions regarding activity.

This chapter will focus on the role of non–immune-based systemic therapy and localized therapy for isolated metastases in metastatic clear cell RCC. Following a discussion of resistance mechanisms, a review of cytotoxic approaches will be presented, followed by an overview of newer compounds under investigation. Finally, the role of aggressive local therapy to specified sites of metastatic disease will be discussed briefly.

MECHANISMS OF RESISTANCE

RCC resistance to classic cytotoxic drugs is due to a number of factors. The most studied and cited mechanism is overexpression of the multidrug resistance protein MDR-1 (also known as P-glycoprotein), which is the founding member of a class of membrane efflux pumps termed "adenosine triphosphate binding cassette (ABC) transporters" (6,7). The expression of MDR-1 in RCC likely reflects the normal expression of this protein in the proximal tubule from which these cancers arise (8,9). It is thus surprising that vinblastine, which is an MDR-1 substrate, was once considered a useful therapy. More modern studies have, however, demonstrated that objective responses to vinblastine are rare and likely not above those expected with placebo (10,11).

The expression of MDR-1 also has prompted a large number of studies aimed at reversing resistance through inhibition of the MDR efflux pump. To date, however, the addition of putative MDR-1 reversing agents has not altered the response rate to agents susceptible to MDR-1 mediated resistance (11–13). Most instructive is a Cancer and Leukemia Group B (CALGB) study in which patients first received vinblastine alone, followed by vinblastine plus high-dose cyclosporin or tamoxifen (11). Only 1 of 80 patients responded to vinblastine alone, and only 1 of 68 patients responded to the combination of vinblastine and the MDR modulator.

These clinical observations likely arise because a number of additional chemotherapy resistance mechanisms have been identified in RCC. For example, the MDR-1 related protein MRP2, which is also a membrane efflux pump in the ABC transporter family, has also been reported to be expressed in proximal renal tubules and renal cell carcinoma (14,15). Overexpression of glutathione may contribute to platinum resistance in this disease (16). In addition, and as in many other malignancies, RCC may have multiple mechanisms for downregulating proapoptotic pathways and activating antiapoptotic pathways. Reported examples include overexpression of BCL2 and $BCLX_L$ (17–20), overexpression of survivin (21), inefficient activation of caspase-9 (22), and activated NF-κ B pathways (23).

CLASSIC CYTOXIC THERAPY

A number of reviews of cytotoxic agent clinical trials in renal cancer have been published (24–28). The extensive list of single-agents with minimal to no activity is quite impressive (Table 48E.1). More careful perusal of these lists suggests, though, that nucleoside analogs lead to consistent, albeit low, response rates even in modern studies. Obviously, the most studied nucleoside analogs are 5-fluorouracil (5-FU) and FUDR. It is not clear that any of the classic 5-FU modulators, such as leucovorin, have an appreciable effect on overall response rate, which in the largest multi-institutional study

with 5-FU was only 5%. Although not as well studied, a low response rate has been observed as well with the nucleoside analogs gemcitabine and troxacitabine (29–31). These observations, as well as preclinical data suggesting synergistic activity (32), have led to investigations of combination gemcitabine and 5-FU (33–36). Single institution studies suggest that the overall objective response rate is 11% (4), which is the same as that observed in a multi-institutional trial of gemcitabine and the oral 5-FU analog capecitabine (37). The confidence interval on these response rates obviously overlaps those seen with 5-FU alone, and it is too low to justify the necessarily large phase III trial to test the hypothesis that the combination is more efficacious than 5-FU. A comparison of survival adjusted for risk factors to a historical control suggested a benefit of combination gemcitabine and 5-FU over classical cytotoxic therapy (4), but whether any nucleoside analog therapy in renal cancer provides a true patient benefit in terms of improvement in quality or quantity of life remains speculative.

HORMONAL THERAPIES

The use of hormonal therapies in renal cancer is based largely on observations of estrogen-mediated renal carcinogenesis in the Syrian hamster (120). This prompted a relatively large series of studies with various hormonal agents, most prominently antiestrogens and progestins (26). The objective response to the most commonly used progestin, medroxyprogesterone, in a large randomized trial versus interferon-α was only 2%, which is not significantly different from background and less than the 14% observed in the interferon arm (121). Importantly, this trial also demonstrated a statistically significant improved survival in the interferon arm. High-dose tamoxifen leads to objective responses in less than 5% of patients in well-organized modern studies with no suggestion of improvement in survival to historical or concurrent control groups (11,122–124). Similarly, reports of high-response rates to toremifine have not been replicated by other studies (125–127). Thus, at the current time, no hormonal therapy for metastatic renal cancer can be recommended for its antitumor efficacy.

RECEPTOR TYROSINE KINASE PATHWAY INHIBITORS

Laboratory studies in cancer biology have made it clear that autonomous growth is a critical cancer phenotype (128). Typically, this is the result of autocrine, paracrine, or aberrant activation of normal endogenous growth factor receptor signaling pathways. Growth factors generally bind and activate a membrane tyrosine kinase receptor, which in turn activates a series of cytoplasmic kinases that eventually activate nuclear transcription factors.

The clearest case for activation of such a pathway in kidney cancer is the activation of the MET pathway in patients with papillary renal cancer (129,130). MET is a classical receptor tyrosine kinase activated by hepatocyte growth factor (HGF) (131). Activating MET mutations were first described in patients with a familial papillary cancer, but studies suggest that MET pathway activation is important in at least some sporadic papillary cancers as well (129,132). A number of MET pathway inhibitors are in preclinical development (133–136), but to date, clinical studies with these compounds have not been reported. If further studies suggest that the MET pathway is not important in clear cell cancer, one obvious challenge for developing such compounds is that only 5% to 10% of patients with metastatic disease have a papillary

TABLE 48E.1

PHASE II TRIALS OF SELECTED CYTOTOXIC AGENTS IN RENAL CELL CARCINOMA

Agent	Year and reference	N	Response rate (%)
2-Deoxycoformycin	1991 (38)	18	0
(Pentostatin)	1992 (39)	25	0
5-Fluorouracil	1989 (40)	14	0
	1991 (41)	27	7
	1993 (42)	35	11
	1994 (43)	61	5
Altretamine	2001 (44)	30	0
Arsenic trioxide	2002 (45)	14	0
Bleomycin	1975 (46)	15	0
	1976 (47)	8	37
	1977 (48)	7	0
Bryostatin	2000 (49)	30	2
	2003 (50)	32	2
	2003 (51)	16	0
Capecitabine	2002 (52)	23	2
Carboplatin	1988 (53)	19	0
	1990 (54)	18	0
Cisplatin	1978 (55)	23	0
	1979 (56)	10	0
Cyclophosphamide	1975 (57)	10	0
	1979 (58)	44	4
	1980 (59)	12	0
Dactinomycin	1981 (60)	61	2
Docetaxel	1994 (61)	18	0
Doxorubicin	1977 (62)	38	5
Edatrexate	1997 (63)	37	2
Epirubicin	1982 (64)	20	0
	1983 (65)	19	0
Estramustine	1981 (66)	16	0
Etoposide	1979 (58)	43	2
Flavopiridol	2000 (67)	35	2
Floxuridine/FUDR	1990 (68)	68	20
	1990 (69)	42	14
	1991 (70)	14	0
	1991 (71)	40	10
	1991 (72)	15	0
	1991 (73)	29	0
	1992 (74)	26	8
	1993 (75)	28	14
Fludarabine	1987 (76)	30	0
	1989 (77)	15	0
	1992 (30)	30	10
Gemcitabine	1993 (31)	18	6
	1996 (78)	37	8
Hydroxyurea	1981 (79)	19	5
Irinotecan	2003 (80)	42	0
Ifosfamide	1980 (81)	11	9
	1981 (82)	10	20
	1987 (83)	16	0
	1988 (84)	9	0
Irofulvin	2002 (85)	20	0
	2001 (86)	12	0
KW-2189	2000 (87)	40	0
Liposomal encapsulated doxorubicin	1994 (88)	14	0
Melphalan	1993 (89)	8	0
Methotrexate	1980 (90)	8	25
Mitomycin	1987 (91)	12	25
Mitotane	1981 (92)	12	0

(Continued)

TABLE 48E.1

CONTINUED

Agent	Year and reference	N	Response rate (%)
Mitoxantrone	1984 (93)	20	0
	1984 (94)	49	0
	1984 (95)	29	0
	1986 (96)	48	0
Ranpirnase	2001 (97)	14	0
PALA	1982 (98)	15	0
Paclitaxel	1991 (99)	18	0
Pyrazoloacridine	2001 (100)	18	1
	1998 (101)	12	0
Razoxane	2000 (102)	38	0
Suramin	1991 (103)	10	0
	1992 (104)	26	4
	1999 (105)	13	0
Temozolomide	2002 (106)	12	0
Thiotepa	1977 (48)	7	14
Titanocene dichloride	1998 (107)	14	0
Topotecan	1994 (108)	14	0
Treosulfan	1999 (109)	15	0
Troxacitabine	2003 (29)	33	6
Vinblastine	1977 (48)	10	0
	1984 (110)	19	16
	1984 (111)	10	0
	1985 (112)	14	0
	1987 (113)	21	9
	1988 (114)	35	9
	1992 (115)	26	4
Vindesine	1977 (116)	17	0
	1983 (117)	24	0
Vinorelbine	1991 (118)	14	0
	1993 (119)	24	4

N = number

variant, and thus clinical trials focused only on such patients would be a challenge to complete.

To date, no growth factor pathway is known to be consistently activated in clear cell RCC. In fact, inhibitors of the most commonly activated growth factor receptor in solid tumors, the epidermal growth factor receptor (EGFR), have not had appreciable activity in RCC (137). Interestingly, however, most growth factor kinase receptor pathways activate the cellular serine/threonine kinase c-RAF. A compound developed as a c-RAF kinase inhibitor, BAY 43-9006 (sorafenib), has had impressive activity in patients with metastatic renal cancer. The drug was initially evaluated in renal cancer using a novel clinical trial design termed a randomized discontinuation phase II study. This trial suggested that sorafenib has potent disease stabilizing or growth inhibitory properties (138). Preliminary results from a more standard double-blind placebo controlled phase III trial confirmed this contention by revealing a doubling in the median time to progression from 3 to 6 months (139). Final survival data are thus eagerly awaited. Interestingly, RAF activation has been reported to be critical for tumor angiogenesis (140), and BAY 43-9006 has been reported to be a potent VEGF and a platelet-derived growth factor (PDGF) receptor inhibitor as well (141). Thus, the molecular mechanism for the clinical activity of BAY 43-9006 in RCC remains a subject of investigation. Interestingly, another VEGF and PDGF receptor tyrosine kinase inhibitor, SU11248 (sunitinib), also has impressive activity

in RCC. Two sequential single arm phase II studies reported response rates of 40% and 39% with additional patients experiencing tumor shrinkage not sufficient for classification as an "objective" response (142). Once again, more definitive phase III trials are in progress and both of these drugs are under review at the FDA for marketing approval in the United States.

Another signal transduction inhibitor that has some activity in renal cancer is CCI-779 [temsirolimus], a mammalian target of rapamycin (mTOR) inhibitor. The downstream effectors of mTOR are eukaryotic translation initiation factor 4E binding protein-1 and the 40 S ribosomal protein p70 S6 kinase, which are important for cell cycle progression (143). Activation of mTOR also enhances HIF1-α expression (144). HIF1-α, which activates the proangiogenic factors VEGF and PDGF, is already up-regulated in clear cell renal cancers due to von Hippel-Lindau (VHL) inactivation (145). Thus, mTOR inhibition could theoretically inhibit angiogenesis as well (see also "Antiangiogenic and Stromal Targeted Agents," which follows). A randomized phase II study of CCI-779 in renal cancer revealed that 6% of patients experienced an objective response with an additional 29% experiencing a minor response (146). There was no apparent dose–response effect, but there was a suggestion that survival was improved over a risk-factor–adjusted historical control, especially in patients with more aggressive disease. A phase III study is in progress, and additional mTOR inhibitors are in clinical development.

ANTIANGIOGENIC AND STROMAL TARGETED AGENTS

Given the apparent resistance of RCC to a number of agents, strategies to target the associated tumor stroma have been considered. One theoretical advantage of such a strategy is that the genetically stable stromal elements are expected to be less prone to development of resistance than the tumor cell. As noted previously, clear cell renal cancers are characterized by inactivation of the VHL pathway with associated up-regulation of HIF1-α and subsequent overexpression of various proangiogenic molecules, including VEGF and PDGF (145). This certainly explains the long clinical observation that these tumors are highly vascular and provides a rationale for testing antiangiogenic strategies.

This strategy was partially validated by a randomized phase II study with the VEGF antibody Bevacizumab in patients who had failed prior IL-2 (147). This study showed that a high dose of Bevacizumab (10 mg/kg every 2 weeks) led to a 10% objective response rate and improvement in time-to-progression in comparison to placebo. Phase III studies are in progress to assess the effects of Bevacizumab on survival in the second-line setting and to assess its effect on survival when combined with interferon. A number of small molecule PDGF and VEGF receptor inhibitors, in addition to BAY 43-9006 and SU11248 (previously noted), also have been developed, and early phase I and II trials suggest that these have activity in patients with metastatic renal cancer as well (148). It is thus likely that targeting the VEGF and PDGF pathways will become a useful strategy in this disease.

Other antiangiogenic approaches also have been investigated but not necessarily with the same success. Thalidomide has many reported mechanisms of action, but its antiangiogenic effects have garnered the most attention (149). Although some initial reports suggested high response rates in patients with metastatic RCC (150), the combined experience suggests that the objective response rate is only on the order of 5% (151). The only randomized study conducted to assess its putative disease-stabilizing effect is a study of low-dose interferon with or without thalidomide, which failed to demonstrate a survival advantage in the investigational arm (152). A randomized discontinuation study of the antiangiogenic nonvoltage dated calcium channel inhibitor carboxyamidoimadazole (CAI) also did not reveal any significant activity (153), nor did studies with the VEGFR inhibitor SU5416 (154,155). TNP-470, another antiangiogenic drug, lead to objective responses in only 1 of 33 patients, but the trial design was inadequate to assess disease stabilizing activity (156). It must be determined whether these failures are due to pharmaceutical properties of the tested drug or due to the lack of appropriate targeting. Nevertheless, these trials serve as a caution against blanket acceptance of "antiangiogenic" approaches in this disease. Individual compounds, as well as putative antiangiogenic targets, must be carefully evaluated.

LOCAL THERAPY FOR ISOLATED METASTASES

Metastatic RCC is occasionally characterized by solitary or few metastases (157). Although such patients typically should be observed for a period of time to ensure that more diffuse metastatic disease does not develop, they may experience long-term disease-free survival with aggressive local therapy (see also Chapter 48A). In addition, certain metastatic sites, such as bones or the brain can cause significant morbidity, and thus aggressive therapy to prevent local complications is also indicated. Aggressive surgical resection of lung and other soft tissue metastases has been discussed in Chapter 48A. Here, aggressive surgical and radiotherapy approaches for bone and brain metastases will be discussed.

TREATMENT OF OSSEOUS METASTASES

Radiation therapy can be used to palliate bone pain from osseous metastases, thereby improving a patient's quality of life. The few studies that have analyzed specifically the role of radiation therapy in metastatic renal cell carcinoma have done so retrospectively. In one analysis, which includes 86 bony sites, 67% of the patients receiving higher doses of radiation experienced significant relief of symptoms compared with 30% in the lower dose group (158). Similar results have been reported in other studies, but these have not necessarily noted a dose–response relationship (159,160). Notably, the duration of response is only on the order of 2 to 3 months, and benefit for patients with spinal cord compression is minimal. Other retrospective series document greater than 2-year survival in 50% or more of patients with single osseous sites and minimal visceral disease (161,162).

Therefore, for good prognosis patients with expected prolonged survival—and especially for patients with cord compression (163)—most centers recommend aggressive orthopedic resection and reconstruction, when technically feasible, followed by radiation to the surgical site. When surgical resection in such patients is not feasible, high radiation doses, with 1 cm to 2 cm field margin to doses of 60 Gy to 66 Gy at 2 Gy per fraction, should be considered. Other radiotherapeutic regimens include 50 Gy in 20 fractions and 39 Gy in 13 fractions. The choice of the fractionation schedule will be influenced by the patients, expected survival time, the site being treated, and normal tissue constraints. Similar schedules can be used in the postoperative setting, although the total radiation dose is decreased somewhat to 40 to 45 Gy in patients with no macroscopic residual disease.

Systemic agents specific for bone metastases should also be considered. Little data are available on the use of radiopharmaceuticals such as strontium-89, and the relatively low energy emissions would suggest minimal benefit in this relatively radioresistant disease. Bisphosphonates are, however, gaining a larger role. The best data are from a retrospective analysis of a randomized study of zoledronate versus placebo in patients with bony metastases from a variety of solid tumors (164). Of the 74 patients with RCC enrolled on this study, 55 were treated with 4 or 8 mg of zoledronate and 19 with placebo. The incidence of a skeletal-related event, which included fracture or the need for palliative radiotherapy or surgery, was significantly lower in the treated groups. Despite the limitations of this analysis, the low toxicity profile of zoledronate suggests that its use should be considered in patients with multiple osseous metastases.

TREATMENT OF BRAIN METASTASES

Because RCC metastases to the brain are relatively less sensitive to chemotherapy and immunotherapy, localized techniques should be emphasized. As is the case with osseous metastases, aggressive local therapy not only palliates the symptoms from brain metastases, but may also improve overall survival (165, 166). In general, and as for most solid tumors, whole brain therapy is the treatment of choice. Neurologic dysfunction is improved in 50% to 70%, and median survival is increased by 3 to 6 months. The Radiation Therapy Oncology Group

(RTOG) has conducted several investigations evaluating the efficacy of various radiation fractionation schedules. None of these innovative schedules appeared superior to the standard radiation treatment schedules used in most centers, which is to give a total dose of 30 Gy administered in 10 fractions.

However, whole brain radiotherapy has significant limitations. Median survival for patients with RCC is only on the order of 4 to 7 months but is heavily influenced by the number of metastatic lesions in the brain and the burden of systemic disease (167,168). This poor median survival is not apparently affected by whole brain radiation (168). As such, aggressive local treatment by surgical resection or by radiosurgery is now used more commonly, especially in patients with good prognostic features, who are at risk for neurocognitive toxicity of whole-brain radiotherapy. Radiosurgery is a single-day procedure that produces a focal distribution of radiation to obliterate or control relatively small tumors. Metastases are often an ideal target for radiosurgery because they are radiographically discrete and are usually noninvasive from the surrounding brain tissue. There are no clear guidelines from randomized studies comparing surgery with radiosurgery to appropriately choose one approach or the other, but the location of the tumor and the expected morbidity of a surgical resection are of paramount importance.

The success and long-term survival of patients with RCC and brain metastases treated with radiosurgery, the frequent presentation of RCC with single or few metastases, and the neurocognitive toxicity of whole brain radiotherapy has once again raised the question of whether whole brain radiotherapy is necessary in all these patients. Retrospective series suggest median survival times of greater than 1 year, and many but not all conclude that the addition of whole brain radiation therapy had no effect on overall survival or recurrence in the brain, especially in patients with only a single metastatic brain lesion (169–172). In the absence of randomized data, it is reasonable to treat single metastases with radiosurgery or surgery alone, whereas the addition of whole brain radiotherapy is reasonable in patients with multiple metastases.

CONCLUSION

Metastatic renal cancer continues to be a frustrating disease to treat. It remains refractory to the majority of agents that have been tested or are regularly available. Therapeutic nihilism that has been generated by such observations, however, is giving way to new hope. There is increasing recognition that aggressive local therapy for single metastatic sites provides significant patient benefit and may improve survival. The further development of nucleoside analogs, VEGF pathway inhibitors, and other signal transduction inhibitors suggests that systemic therapeutic approaches will be useful for patients with this disease. Nevertheless, significant basic and clinical research still must be performed. Metastatic renal cancer is clearly not one disease, and approaches for clear cell carcinoma are not necessarily going to be effective in patients with other histologic subtypes. Even within one subtype, heterogeneity in both biology and response to any agent will be seen. Clarification of these biologic issues, selection of the best candidate compounds for further study, and well-designed clinical trials do, however, hold promise for finally creating treatment approaches that will have significant clinical impact.

References

1. Guinan PD, Vogelzang NJ, Fremgen AM, et al. Renal cell carcinoma: Tumor size, stage and survival. Members of the Cancer Incidence and End Results Committee. *J Urol* 1995;153:901–903.

2. Motzer RJ, Mazumdar M, Bacik J, et al. Survival and prognostic stratification of 670 patients with advanced renal cell carcinoma. *J Clin Oncol* 1999;17:2530–2540.

3. Gleave ME, Elhilali M, Fradet Y, et al. Canadian Urologic Oncology Group. Interferon gamma-1b compared with placebo in metastatic renal-cell carcinoma. [See comments.] *N Engl J Med* 1998;338:1265–1271.

4. Stadler WM, Huo D, George C, et al. Prognostic factors for survival with gemcitabine plus 5-fluorouracil based regimens for metastatic renal cancer. *J Urol* 2003;170:1141–1145.

5. Motzer RJ, Bacik J, Mariani T, et al. Treatment outcome and survival associated with metastatic renal cell carcinoma of non-clear-cell histology. *J Clin Oncol* 2002;20:2376–2381.

6. Duensing S, Dallmann I, Grosse J, et al. Immunocytochemical detection of P-glycoprotein: initial expression correlates with survival in renal cell carcinoma patients. *Oncology* 1994;51:309–313.

7. Fojo AT, Shen DW, Mickley LA, et al. Intrinsic drug resistance in human kidney cancer is associated with expression of a human multidrug-resistance gene. *J Clin Oncol* 1987;5:1922–1927.

8. Fojo AT, Ueda K, Slamon DJ, et al. Expression of a multidrug-resistance gene in human tumors and tissues. *Proc Natl Acad Sci U S A* 1987;84: 265–269.

9. Ernest S, Rajaraman S, Megyesi J, et al. Expression of MDR1 (multidrug resistance) gene and its protein in normal human kidney. *Nephron* 1997; 77:284–289.

10. Pyrhonen S, Salminen E, Ruutu M, et al. Prospective randomized trial of interferon alfa-2a plus vinblastine versus vinblastine alone in patients with advanced renal cell cancer. *J Clin Oncol* 1999;17:2859–2867.

11. Samuels BL, Hollis DR, Rosner GL, et al. Modulation of vinblastine resistance in metastatic renal cell carcinoma with cyclosporine A or tamoxifen: a cancer and leukemia group B study. *Clin Cancer Res* 1997;3:1977–1984.

12. Warner E, Tobe SW, Andrulis IL, et al. Phase I–II study of vinblastine and oral cyclosporin A in metastatic renal cell carcinoma. *Am J Clin Oncol* 1995; 18:251–256.

13. Motzer RJ, Lyn P, Fischer P, et al. Phase I/II trial of dexverapamil plus vinblastine for patients with advanced renal cell carcinoma. *J Clin Oncol* 1995; 13:1958–1965.

14. Sandusky GE, Mintze KS, Pratt SE, et al. Expression of multidrug resistance-associated protein 2 (MRP2) in normal human tissues and carcinomas using tissue microarrays. *Histopathology* 2002;41:65–74.

15. Schaub TP, Kartenbeck J, Konig J, et al. Expression of the MRP2 gene-encoded conjugate export pump in human kidney proximal tubules and in renal cell carcinoma. *J Am Soc Nephrol* 1999;10:1159–1169.

16. Ahn H, Lee E, Kim K, et al. Effect of glutathione and its related enzymes on chemosensitivity of renal cell carcinoma and bladder carcinoma cell lines. *J Urol* 1994;151:263–267.

17. Gobe G, Rubin M, Williams G, et al. Apoptosis and expression of Bcl-2, Bcl-XL, and Bax in renal cell carcinomas. *Cancer Invest* 2002;20:324–332.

18. Huang A, Fone PD, Gandour-Edwards R, et al. Immunohistochemical analysis of BCL-2 protein expression in renal cell carcinoma. *J Urol* 1999; 162:610–613.

19. Tomita Y, Bilim V, Kawasaki T, et al. Frequent expression of Bcl-2 in renal-cell carcinomas carrying wild-type p53. *Int J Cancer* 1996;66:322–325.

20. Uchida T, Gao JP, Wang C, et al. Clinical significance of p53, mdm2, and bcl-2 proteins in renal cell carcinoma. *Urology* 2002;59:615–620.

21. Griffith TS, Fialkov JM, Scott DL, et al. Induction and regulation of tumor necrosis factor-related apoptosis-inducing ligand/Apo-2 ligand-mediated apoptosis in renal cell carcinoma. *Cancer Res* 2002;62:3093–3099.

22. Ramp U, Caliskan E, Mahotka C, et al. Apoptosis induction in renal cell carcinoma by TRAIL and gamma-radiation is impaired by deficient caspase-9 cleavage. *Br J Cancer* 2003;88:1800–1807.

23. Oya M, Ohtsubo M, Takayanagi A, et al. Constitutive activation of nuclear factor-kappaB prevents TRAIL-induced apoptosis in renal cancer cells. *Oncogene* 2001;20:3888–3896.

24. George CM, Stadler WM. The role of systemic chemotherapy in the treatment of kidney cancer. In: Figlin R, ed. *Kidney cancer.* Norwell, MA: Kluwer Academic Publishers, 2003.

25. Amato RJ. Chemotherapy for renal cell carcinoma. *Semin Oncol* 2000;27: 177–186.

26. Harris DT. Hormonal therapy and chemotherapy of renal-cell carcinoma. *Semin Oncol* 1983;10:422–430.

27. Yagoda A, Petrylak D, Thompson S. Cytotoxic chemotherapy for advanced renal cell carcinoma. *Urol Clin North Am* 1993;20:303–321.

28. Yagoda A, Abi-Rached B, Petrylak D. Chemotherapy for advanced renal-cell carcinoma: 1983–1993. *Semin Oncol* 1995;22:42–60.

29. Townsley CA, Chi K, Ernst DS, et al. Phase II study of troxacitabine (BCH-4556) in patients with advanced and/or metastatic renal cell carcinoma: a trial of the National Cancer Institute of Canada–Clinical Trials Group. *J Clin Oncol* 2003;21:1524–1529.

30. Weissbach L, de Mulder P, Osieka R, et al. Phase II study of gemcitabine in renal cancer. *Proc Am Soc Clin Oncol* 1992;11:219.

31. Mertens WC, Eisenhauer EA, Moore M, et al. Gemcitabine in advanced renal cell carcinoma: a phase II study of the National Cancer Institute of Canada–Clinical Trials Group. *Ann Oncol* 1993;4:331–332.

32. Ren Q, Kao V, Grem JL. Cytotoxicity and DNA fragmentation associated with sequential gemcitabine and 5-fluoro-2'-deoxyuridine in HT-29 colon cancer cells. *Clin Cancer Res* 1998;4:2811–2818.

33. Desai AA, Vogelzang NJ, Rini BI, et al. A high rate of venous thromboembolism in a multi-institutional phase II trial of weekly intravenous gemcitabine with continuous infusion fluorouracil and daily thalidomide in patients with metastatic renal cell carcinoma. *Cancer* 2002;95:1629–1636.

34. Ryan CW, Vogelzang NJ, Stadler WM. A phase II trial of intravenous gemcitabine and 5-fluorouracil with subcutaneous interleukin-2 and interferon-alpha in patients with metastatic renal cell carcinoma. *Cancer* 2002; 94:2602–2609.

35. George CM, Vogelzang NJ, Rini BI, et al. A phase II trial of weekly intravenous gemcitabine and cisplatin with continuous infusion fluorouracil in patients with metastatic renal cell carcinoma. *Ann Oncol* 2002;13:116–120.

36. Rini BI, Vogelzang NJ, Dumas MC, et al. Phase II trial of weekly intravenous gemcitabine with continuous infusion fluorouracil in patients with metastatic renal cell cancer. *J Clin Oncol* 2000;18:2419–2426.

37. Stadler WM, Halabi S, Ernstoff MS, et al. A phase II study of gemcitabine and capecitabine in patients with metastatic renal cell cancer: a report of Cancer and Leukemia Group B #90008. *Proc Am Soc Clin Oncol* 2004; 23:384 abst 4515.

38. Venner P, Eisenhauer EA, Wierzbicki R et al. A National Cancer Institute of Canada–Clinical Trials Group study. Phase II study of 2'-deoxycoformycin in patients with renal cell carcinoma. *Invest New Drugs* 1991;9:273–275.

39. Witte RS, Walsh C, Fisher H, et al. Evaluation of deoxycoformycin in patients with advanced renal cell carcinoma: an ECOG pilot study. *Invest New Drugs* 1992;10:49–50.

40. Zaniboni A, Simoncini E, Marpicati P, et al. Phase II trial of 5-fluorouracil and high-dose folinic acid in advanced renal cell cancer. *J Chemother* 1989;1:350–351.

41. Schulof R, Lokich J, Wampler G, et al. Phase II trial of protracted infusional 5-FU (PIF) for metastatic renal cell carcinoma. *Proc Am Soc Clin Oncol* 1991;10:170.

42. Ahlgren JD, Lokich J, Auerbach M, et al. Protracted infusional 5FU (PIF): a well tolerated regimen in metastatic renal cell carcinoma (MRC). A Mid-Atlantic Oncology Program (MOAP) study. *Proc Am Soc Clin Oncol* 1993;12:244.

43. Kish JA, Wolf M, Crawford ED, et al. A Southwest Oncology Group Study. Evaluation of low dose continuous infusion 5-fluorouracil in patients with advanced and recurrent renal cell carcinoma. *Cancer* 1994;74: 916–919.

44. Zon RT, McClean J, Helman D, et al. Altretamine for the treatment of metastatic renal cell carcinoma. A Hoosier Oncology Group trial. *Invest New Drugs* 2001;19:229–231.

45. Vuky J, Yu R, Schwartz L, et al. Phase II trial of arsenic trioxide in patients with metastatic renal cell carcinoma. *Invest New Drugs* 2002;20:327–330.

46. Johnson DE, Chalbaud RA, Holoye PY, et al. Clinical trial of bleomycin (NSC-125066) in the treatment of metastatic renal carcinoma. *Cancer Chemother Rep* 1975;59:433–435.

47. Haas CD, Coltman CA Jr, Gottlieb JA, et al. A Southwest Oncology Group study. Phase II evaluation of bleomycin. *Cancer* 1976;38:8–12.

48. Hahn DM, Schimpff SC, Ruckdeschel JC, et al. Single-agent therapy for renal cell carcinoma: CCNU, vinblastine, thioTEPA, or bleomycin. *Cancer Treat Rep* 1977;61:1585–1587.

49. Pagliaro L, Daliani D, Amato R, et al. A phase II trial of bryostatin-1 for patients with metastatic renal cell carcinoma. *Cancer* 2000;89:615–618.

50. Haas NB, Smith M, Lewis N, et al. Weekly bryostatin-1 in metastatic renal cell carcinoma: a phase II study. *Clin Cancer Res* 2003;9:109–114.

51. Madhusudan S, Protheroe A, Propper D, et al. A multicentre phase II trial of bryostatin-1 in patients with advanced renal cancer. *Br J Cancer* 2003; 89:1418–1422.

52. Wenzel C, Locker GJ, Schmidinger M, et al. Capecitabine in the treatment of metastatic renal cell carcinoma failing immunotherapy. *Am J Kidney Dis* 2002;39:48–54.

53. Tait M, Abrams J, Egorin MJ, et al. Phase II carboplatin (CBDCA) for metastatic renal cell cancer with a standard dose (SD) and a calculated dose (CD) according to renal function. *Proc Am Soc Clin Oncol* 1988;7: 125.

54. Trump DL, Elson P. Evaluation of carboplatin (NSC 241240) in patients with recurrent or metastatic renal cell cancer. *Invest New Drugs* 1990;8:201–203.

55. Rodriguez LH, Johnson DE. Clinical trial of cisplatinum (NSC 119875) in metastatic renal cell carcinoma. *Urology* 1978;11:344–346.

56. Merrin CE. Treatment of genitourinary tumours with cis- dichlorodiammineplatinum(II): experience in 250 patients. *Cancer Treat Rep* 1979; 63:1579–1584.

57. Kiruluta G, Morales A, Lott S. Response of renal adenocarcinoma to cyclophosphamide. *Urology* 1975;6:557–558.

58. Hahn RG, Bauer M, Wolter J, et al. Phase II study of single-agent therapy with megestrol acetate, VP-16-213, cyclophosphamide, and dianhydrogalactitol in advanced renal cell cancer. *Cancer Treat Rep* 1979;63:513–515.

59. Wajsman Z, Beckley S, Madajewicz S. High dose cyclophosphamide in metastatic renal cell cancer. *Proc Am Soc Clin Oncol* 1980;21:423.

60. Hahn RG, Begg CB, Davis T. Phase II study of vinblastine-CCNU, triazinate, and dactinomycin in advanced renal cell cancer. *Cancer Treat Rep* 1981;65:711–713.

61. Mertens WC, Eisenhauer EA, Jolivet J, et al. Docetaxel in advanced renal carcinoma. A phase II trial of the National Cancer Institute of Canada Clinical Trials Group. *Ann Oncol* 1994;5:185–187.

62. O'Bryan RM, Baker LH, Gottlieb JE, et al. Dose response evaluation of adriamycin in human neoplasia. *Cancer* 1977;39:1940–1948.

63. Dreicer R, Propert KJ, Kuzel T et al. An Eastern Cooperative Oncology Group study. A phase II trial of edatrexate in patients with advanced renal cell carcinoma. *Am J Clin Oncol* 1997;20:251–253.

64. Fossa SD, Wik B, Bae E, et al. Phase II study of 4'-epi-doxorubicin in metastatic renal cancer. *Cancer Treat Rep* 1982;66:1219–1221.

65. Benedetto P, Ahmed T, Needles B, et al. Phase II trial of 4'epi-adriamycin for advanced hypernephroma. *Am J Clin Oncol* 1983;6:553–554.

66. Swanson DA, Johnson DE. Estramustine phosphate (Emcyt) as treatment for metastatic renal carcinoma. *Urology* 1981;17:344–346.

67. Stadler WM, Vogelzang NJ, Amato R, et al. Flavopiridol: A novel cyclin-dependent kinase inhibitor, in metastatic renal cancer. A University of Chicago Phase II Consortium study. *J Clin Oncol* 2000;18:371–375.

68. Hrushesky WJ, von Roemeling R, Lanning RM, et al. Circadian-shaped infusions of floxuridine for progressive metastatic renal cell carcinoma. *J Clin Oncol* 1990;8:1504–1513.

69. Damascelli B, Marchiano A, Spreafico C, et al. Circadian continuous chemotherapy of renal cell carcinoma with an implantable, programmable infusion pump. *Cancer* 1990;66:237–241.

70. Merrouche Y, Negrier S, Lanier F, et al. Phase II study of continous circadian infusion FUDR in metastatic renal cell cancer (RCC). *Eur J Cancer Clin Oncol* 1991;27.

71. Dexeus FH, Logothetis CJ, Sella A, et al. Circadian infusion of floxuridine in patients with metastatic renal cell carcinoma. *J Urol* 1991;146: 709–713.

72. Dimopoulous MA, Dexeus FH, Jones E, et al. Evidence for additive antitumor activity and toxicity for the combination of FUDR and interferon alpha2B in patients (pts) with metastatic renal cell carcinoma (RCC). *Proc Am Assoc Cancer Res* 1991;32:186.

73. Richards F, Cooper MR, Jackson DV, et al. Continuous 5-day (D) intravenous (IV) FUDR infusion for renal cell cancer (RCC): a phase I–II trial of the Piedmont Oncology Association. *Proc Am Soc Clin Oncol* 1991;10:170.

74. Budd GT, Murthy S, Klein E, et al. Time-modified infusion of floxuridine in metastatic renal cell carcinoma (mRCC). *Proc Am Assoc Cancer Res* 1992;33:220.

75. Conroy T, Geoffrois L, Guillemin F, et al. Simplified chronomodulated continuous infusion of floxuridine in patients with metastatic renal cell carcinoma. *Cancer* 1993;72:2190–2197.

76. Balducci L, Blumenstein B, Von Hoff DD, et al. Evaluation of fludarabine phosphate in renal cell carcinoma. A Southwest Oncology Group Study. *Cancer Treat Rep* 1987;71:543–544.

77. Shevrin DH, Lad TE, Kilton LJ, et al. Phase II trial of fludarabine phosphate in advanced renal cell carcinoma. An Illinois Cancer Council study. *Invest New Drugs* 1989;7:251–253.

78. Rohde D, De Mulder PH, Weissbach L, et al. Experimental and clinical efficacy of 2', 2'-difluorodeoxycytidine (gemcitabine) against renal cell carcinoma. *Oncology* 1996;53:476–481.

79. Stolbach LL, Begg CB, Hall T, et al. Treatment of renal carcinoma: a phase III randomized trial of oral medroxyprogesterone (Provera), hydroxyurea, and nafoxidine. *Cancer Treat Rep* 1981;65:689–692.

80. Fizazi K, Rolland F, Chevreau C, et al. A phase II study of irinotecan in patients with advanced renal cell carcinoma. *Cancer* 2003;98:61–65.

81. Fossa SD, Talle K. Treatment of metastatic renal cancer with ifosfamide and mesnum with and without irradiation. *Cancer Treat Rep* 1980;64: 1103–1108.

82. Heim ME, Fiene R, Schick E, et al. Central nervous system side effects following ifosfamide monotherapy of advanced renal carcinoma. *J Cancer Res Clin Oncol* 1981;100:113–116.

83. De Forges A, Droz JP, Ghosn M, et al. Phase II trial of ifosfamide/mesna in metastatic adult renal carcinoma. *Cancer Treat Rep* 1987;71:1103.

84. Bodrogi I, Baki M, Sinkovics I, et al. Ifosfamide chemotherapy of metastatic renal cell cancer. *Semin Surg Oncol* 1988;4:95–96.

85. Amato RJ, Perez C, Pagliaro L. Irofulven, a novel inhibitor of DNA synthesis, in metastatic renal cell cancer. *Invest New Drugs* 2002;20:413–417.

86. Berg WJ, Schwartz L, Yu R, et al. Phase II trial of irofulven (6-hydroxymethylacylfulvene) for patients with advanced renal cell carcinoma. *Invest New Drugs* 2001;19:317–320.

87. Small EJ, Figlin R, Petrylak D, et al. A phase II pilot study of KW-2189 in patients with advanced renal cell carcinoma. *Invest New Drugs* 2000;18: 193–197.

88. Law TM, Mencel P, Motzer RJ. Phase II trial of liposomal encapsulated doxorubicin in patients with advanced renal cell carcinoma. *Invest New Drugs* 1994;12:323–325.

89. Falkson CI. New formulation intravenous melphalan in the treatment of patients with metastatic renal cancer. *Invest New Drugs* 1993;11:93.

90. Baumgartner G, Heinz R, Arbes H, et al. Methotrexate-citrovorum factor used alone and in combination chemotherapy for advanced hypernephromas. *Cancer Treat Rep* 1980;64:41–46.

91. Stewart DJ, Futter N, Irvine A, et al. Mitomycin-C and metronidazole in the treatment of advanced renal-cell carcinoma. *Am J Clin Oncol* 1987; 10:520–522.

92. Hogan TF, Citrin DL, Freeberg BL. A preliminary report of mitotane therapy of advanced renal and prostate cancer. *Cancer Treat Rep* 1981;65: 539–540.

93. De Jager R, Cappelaere P, Armand JP, et al. An EORTC phase II study of mitoxantrone in solid tumors and lymphomas. *Eur J Cancer Clin Oncol* 1984;20:1369–1375.

94. Taylor SA, Von Hoff DD, Baker LH, et al. Phase II clinical trial of mitoxantrone in patients with advanced renal cell carcinoma. A Southwest Oncology Group study. *Cancer Treat Rep* 1984;68:919–920.

95. Van Oosterom AT, Fossa SD, Pizzocaro G, et al. Mitoxantrone in advanced renal cancer: a phase II study in previously untreated patients from the EORTC Genito-Urinary Tract Cancer Cooperative Group. *Eur J Cancer Clin Oncol* 1984;20:1239–1241.

96. Gams RA, Nelson O, Birch R. Phase II evaluation of mitoxantrone in advanced renal cell carcinoma. A Southeastern Cancer Study Group trial. *Cancer Treat Rep* 1986;70:921–922.

97. Vogelzang NJ, Aklilu M, Stadler WM, et al. A phase II trial of weekly intravenous ranpirnase (Onconase), a novel ribonuclease in patients with metastatic kidney cancer. *Invest New Drugs* 2001;19:255–260.

98. Natale RB, Yagoda A, Kelsen DP, et al. Phase II trial of PALA in hypernephroma and urinary bladder cancer. *Cancer Treat Rep* 1982;66:2091–2092.

99. Einzig AI, Gorowski E, Sasloff J, et al. Phase II trial of taxol in patients with metastatic renal cell carcinoma. *Cancer Invest* 1991;9:133–136.

100. Kuebler JP, King GW, Triozzi P, et al. Phase II study of pyrazoloacridine in metastatic renal cell carcinoma. *Invest New Drugs* 2001;19:327–328.

101. Berg WJ, McCaffrey J, Schwartz LH, et al. A phase II study of pyrazoloacridine in patients with advanced renal cell carcinoma. *Invest New Drugs* 1998;16:337–340.

102. Braybrooke JP, O'Byrne KJ, Propper DJ, et al. A phase II study of razoxane, an antiangiogenic topoisomerase II inhibitor, in renal cell cancer with assessment of potential surrogate markers of angiogenesis. *Clin Cancer Res* 2000;6:4697–4704.

103. La Rocca RV, Stein CA, Danesi R, et al. A pilot study of suramin in the treatment of metastatic renal cell carcinoma. *Cancer* 1991;67:1509–1513.

104. Motzer RJ, Nanus DM, O'Moore P, et al. Phase II trial of suramin in patients with advanced renal cell carcinoma: treatment results, pharmacokinetics, and tumor growth factor expression. *Cancer Res* 1992;52:5775–5779.

105. Dreicer R, Smith DC, Williams RD, et al. Phase II trial of suramin in patients with metastatic renal cell carcinoma. *Invest New Drugs* 1999;17:183–186.

106. Park DK, Ryan CW, Dolan ME, et al. A phase II trial of oral temozolomide in patients with metastatic renal cell cancer. *Cancer Chemother Pharmacol* 2002;50:160–162.

107. Lummen G, Sperling H, Luboldt H, et al. Phase II trial of titanocene dichloride in advanced renal-cell carcinoma. *Cancer Chemother Pharmacol* 1998;42:415–417.

108. Law TM, Ilson DH, Motzer RJ. Phase II trial of topotecan in patients with advanced renal cell carcinoma. *Invest New Drugs* 1994;12:143–145.

109. Rigos D, Wechsel HW, Bichler KH. Treosulfan in the treatment of metastatic renal cell carcinoma. *Anticancer Res* 1999;19:1549–1552.

110. Kuebler JP, Hogan TF, Trump DL, et al. Phase II study of continuous 5-day vinblastine infusion in renal adenocarcinoma. *Cancer Treat Rep* 1984;68:925–926.

111. Zeffren J, Yagoda A, Kelsen D, et al. Phase I–II trial of a 5-day continuous infusion of vinblastine sulfate. *Anticancer Res* 1984;4:411–413.

112. Tannock IF, Evans WK. Failure of 5-day vinblastine infusion in the treatment of patients with renal cancer. *Cancer Treat Rep* 1985;69:227–228.

113. Crivellari D, Tumolo S, Frustaci S, et al. Phase II study of five-day continuous infusion of vinblastine in patients with metastatic renal-cell carcinoma. *Am J Clin Oncol* 1987;10:231–233.

114. Elson PJ, Kvols LK, Vogl SE, et al. Phase II trials of 5-day vinblastine infusion (NSC 49842), L-alanosine (NSC 153353), acivicin (NSC 163501), and aminothiadiazole (NSC 4728) in patients with recurrent or metastatic renal cell carcinoma. *Invest New Drugs* 1988;6:97–103.

115. Fossa SD, Droz JP, Pavone-Macaluso MM, et al. Vinblastine in metastatic renal cell carcinoma: EORTC phase II trial 30882. The EORTC Genitourinary Group. *Eur J Cancer* 1992;28A:878–880.

116. Wong PP, Yagoda A, Currie VE, et al. Phase II study of vindesine sulfate in the therapy for advanced renal carcinoma. *Cancer Treat Rep* 1977;61:1727–1729.

117. Fossa SD, Denis L, van Oosterom AT, et al. Vindesine in advanced renal cancer. A study of the EORTC Genito-Urinary Tract Cancer Cooperative Group. *Eur J Cancer Clin Oncol* 1983;19:473–475.

118. Canobbio L, Boccardo F, Guarneri D, et al. Phase II study of navelbine in advanced renal cancer. *Eur J Cancer* 1991;27:804–805.

119. Wilding G, Kirkwood J, Clamon G, et al. Phase II trial of navelbine in metastatic renal cancer. *Proc Am Soc Clin Oncol* 1993;12:253.

120. Li JJ, Li SA. Estrogen carcinogenesis in Syrian hamster tissues: role of metabolism. *Fed Proc* 1987;46:1858–1863.

121. Medical Research Council Renal Cancer Collaborators. Interferon-alpha and survival in metastatic renal carcinoma: early results of a randomised controlled trial. *Lancet* 1999;353:14–17.

122. Huland E, Heinzer H. Survival in renal cell carcinoma: a randomized evaluation of tamoxifen vs interleukin-2, alpha-interferon (leucocyte) and tamoxifen. *Br J Cancer* 2000;82:246–247.

123. Schomburg A, Kirchner H, Fenner M, et al. Lack of therapeutic efficacy of tamoxifen in advanced renal cell carcinoma. *Eur J Cancer* 1993;29A:737–740.

124. Atzpodien J, Kirchner H, Illiger HJ, et al. IL-2 in combination with IFN-alpha and 5-FU versus tamoxifen in metastatic renal cell carcinoma: long-term results of a controlled randomized clinical trial. *Br J Cancer* 2001;85:1130–1136.

125. Gershanovich MM, Moiseyenko VM, Vorobjev AV, et al. High-dose toremifene in advanced renal-cell carcinoma. *Cancer Chemother Pharmacol* 1997;39:547–551.

126. Braybrooke JP, Vallis KA, Houlbrook S, et al. Evaluation of toremifene for reversal of multidrug resistance in renal cell cancer patients treated with vinblastine. *Cancer Chemother Pharmacol* 2000;46:27–34.

127. Oh WK, Manola J, George DJ, et al. A phase II trial of interferon-alpha and toremifene in advanced renal cell cancer patients. *Cancer Invest* 2002;20:186–191.

128. Hahn WC, Weinberg RA. Rules for making human tumor cells. *N Engl J Med* 2002;347:1593–1603.

129. Sweeney P, El-Naggar AK, Lin SH, et al. Biological significance of c-met over expression in papillary renal cell carcinoma. *J Urol* 2002;168:51–55.

130. Schmidt L, Duh FM, Chen F, et al. Germline and somatic mutations in the tyrosine kinase domain of the MET proto-oncogene in papillary renal carcinomas. *Nat Genet* 1997;16:68–73.

131. Ma PC, Maulik G, Christensen J, et al. c-Met: structure, functions and potential for therapeutic inhibition. *Cancer Metastasis Rev* 2003;22:309–325.

132. Schmidt L, Junker K, Nakaigawa N, et al. Novel mutations of the MET proto-oncogene in papillary renal carcinomas. *Oncogene* 1999;18:2343–2350.

133. Christensen JG, Schreck R, Burrows J, et al. A selective small molecule inhibitor of c-Met kinase inhibits c-Met-dependent phenotypes in vitro and exhibits cytoreductive antitumor activity in vivo. *Cancer Res* 2003;63:7345–7355.

134. Sattler M, Pride YB, Ma P, et al. A novel small molecule Met inhibitor induces apoptosis in cells transformed by the oncogenic TPR-MET tyrosine kinase. *Cancer Res* 2003;63:5462–5469.

135. Wang X, Le P, Liang C, et al. Potent and selective inhibitors of the Met [hepatocyte growth factor/scatter factor (HGF/SF) receptor] tyrosine kinase block HGF/SF-induced tumor cell growth and invasion. *Mol Cancer Ther* 2003;2:1085–1092.

136. Cao B, Su Y, Oskarsson M, et al. Neutralizing monoclonal antibodies to hepatocyte growth factor/scatter factor (HGF/SF) display antitumor activity in animal models. *Proc Natl Acad Sci U S A* 2001;98:7443–7448.

137. Drucker B, Bacik J, Ginsberg M, et al. Phase II trial of ZD1839 (IRESSA) in patients with advanced renal cell carcinoma. *Invest New Drugs* 2003;21:341–345.

138. Ratain MJ, Eisen T, Stadler WM. Final findings from a Phase II, placebo-controlled, randomized discontinuation trial (RDT) of sorafenib (BAY 43-9006) in patients with advanced renal cell carcinoma (RCC). *Proc Amer Soc Clin Oncol* 2005;23:388s (Abstract 4544).

139. Escudier B, Szczylik C, Eisen T. Randomized Phase III trial of the Raf kinase and VEGFR inhibitor BAY 43-9006 (sorafenib) in patients with advanced renal cell carcinoma (RCC). *Proc Amer Soc Clin Oncol* 2005;23:380s (Abstract LBA4510).

140. Alavi A, Hood JD, Frausto R, et al. Role of Raf in vascular protection from distinct apoptotic stimuli. *Science* 2003;301:94–96.

141. Wilhelm S, Carter C, Tang L, et al. BAY 43-9006 exhibits broad spectrum anti-tumor activity and targets raf/MEK/ERK pathway and receptor tyrosine kinases involved in tumor progression and angiogenesis. *Clin Cancer Res* 2003;9:6088s (Abstract).

142. Motzer RJ, Rini BI, Michaelson MD, et al. Phase 2 trials of SU11248 show antitumor activity in second-line therapy for patients with metastatic renal cell carcinoma. *Proc Amer Soc Clin Oncol* 2005;23:380s (Abstract 4508).

143. Harris TE, Lawrence JC Jr. TOR signaling. *Sci STKE* 2003;212:re15–re15.

144. Hudson CC, Liu M, Chiang GG, et al. Regulation of hypoxia-inducible factor 1alpha expression and function by the mammalian target of rapamycin. *Mol Cell Biol* 2002;22:7004–7014.

145. Turner KJ, Moore JW, Jones A, et al. Expression of hypoxia-inducible factors in human renal cancer: relationship to angiogenesis and to the von Hippel-Lindau gene mutation. *Cancer Res* 2002;62:2957–2961.

146. Atkins M, Hidalgo M, Stadler WM, et al. Randomized phase II study of multiple dose levels of CCI-779, a novel mTOR kinase inhibitor, in patients with advanced refractory renal cell carcinoma. *J Clin Oncol* 2004;22:909–918.

147. Yang JC, Haworth L, Sherry RM, et al. A randomized trial of bevacizumab, an anti-vascular endothelial growth factor antibody, for metastatic renal cancer. *N Engl J Med* 2003;349:427–434.

148. George D, Michaelson D, Oh WK, et al. Phase I study of PTK787/ZK 222584 (PTK/ZK) in metastatic renal cell carcinoma. *Proc Am Soc Clin Oncol* 2003;22:385 (Abstract 1548).

149. D'Amato RJ, Loughnan MS, Flynn E, et al. Thalidomide is an inhibitor of angiogenesis. *Proc Natl Acad Sci U S A* 1994;91:4082–4085.

150. Eisen T. Thalidomide in solid malignancies. *J Clin Oncol* 2002;20:2607–2609.

151. Motzer RJ, Berg W, Ginsberg M, et al. Phase II trial of thalidomide for patients with advanced renal cell carcinoma. *J Clin Oncol* 2002;20:302–306.

152. Gordon MS, Manola J, Fairclough D, et al. Low dose interferon-alpha-2b + thalidomide in patients with previously untreated renal cell cancer: improvement in progression-free survival but not quality of life or overall

survival. A phase III study of the Eastern Cooperative Oncology Group (E2898). *Proc Am Soc Clin Oncol* 2004;23:384 (abstract 4516).

153. Stadler WM, Rosner G, Rini B, et al. A Cancer and Leukemia Group B (CALGB) Study. Successful implementation of the randomized discontinuation trial design (RDTD) with the putative antiangiogenic agent carboxyaminoimidazole (CAI) in renal cell carcinoma (RCC). *Proc Am Soc Clin Oncol* 2003;22:193 (abstract 773).

154. Lara PN Jr, Quinn DI, Margolin K, et al. SU5416 plus interferon alpha in advanced renal cell carcinoma: a phase II California Cancer Consortium Study with biological and imaging correlates of angiogenesis inhibition. *Clin Cancer Res* 2003;9:4772–4781.

155. Kuenen BC, Tabernero J, Baselga J, et al. Efficacy and toxicity of the angiogenesis inhibitor SU5416 as a single agent in patients with advanced renal cell carcinoma, melanoma, and soft tissue sarcoma. *Clin Cancer Res* 2003;9:1648–1655.

156. Stadler WM, Kuzel T, Shapiro C, et al. Multi-institutional study of the angiogenesis inhibitor TNP-470 in metastatic renal carcinoma. *J Clin Oncol* 1999;17:2541–2545.

157. Hellman S, Weichselbaum RR. Oligometastases. *J Clin Oncol* 1995;13:8–10.

158. Onufrey V, Mohiuddin M. Radiation therapy in the treatment of metastatic renal cell carcinoma. *Int J Radiat Oncol Biol Phys* 1985;11 2007–2009.

159. Huguenin PU, Kieser S, Glanzmann C, et al. Radiotherapy for metastatic carcinomas of the kidney or melanomas: An analysis using palliative end points. *Int J Radiat Oncol Biol Phys* 1998;41:401–405.

160. Halperin EC, Harisiadis L. The role of radiation therapy in the management of metastatic renal cell carcinoma. *Cancer* 1983;51:614–617.

161. Kollender Y, Bickels J, Price WM, et al. Metastatic renal cell carcinoma of bone: indications and technique of surgical intervention. *J Urol* 2000;164:1505–1508.

162. Durr HR, Maier M, Pfahler M, et al. Surgical treatment of osseous metastases in patients with renal cell carcinoma. *Clin Orthop* 1999;367:283–290.

163. Patchell R, Tibbs PA, Regine WF, et al. A randomized trial of direct decompressive surgical resection in the treatment of spinal cord compression caused by metastasis. *Proc Am Soc Clin Oncol* 2003;22:1 (abstract 2).

164. Lipton A, Zheng M, Seaman J. Zoledronic acid delays the onset of skeletal-related events and progression of skeletal disease in patients with advanced renal cell carcinoma. *Cancer* 2003;98:962–969.

165. Andrews DW, Scott CB, Sperduto PW, et al. Whole brain radiation therapy with or without stereotactic radiosurgery boost for patients with one to three brain metastases: phase III results of the RTOG 9508 randomised trial. *Lancet* 2004;363:1665–1672.

166. Patchell RA, Tibbs PA, Walsh JW, et al. A randomized trial of surgery in the treatment of single metastases to the brain. *N Engl J Med* 1990;322:494–500.

167. Culine S, Bekradda M, Kramar A, et al. Prognostic factors for survival in patients with brain metastases from renal cell carcinoma. *Cancer* 1998;83:2548–2553.

168. Wronski M, Maor MH, Davis BJ, et al. External radiation of brain metastases from renal carcinoma: a retrospective study of 119 patients from the M. D. Anderson Cancer Center. *Int J Radiat Oncol Biol Phys* 1997;37:753–759.

169. Hernandez L, Zamorano L, Sloan A, et al. Gamma knife radiosurgery for renal cell carcinoma brain metastases. *J Neurosurg* 2002;97:489–493.

170. Sheehan JP, Sun MH, Kondziolka D, et al. Radiosurgery in patients with renal cell carcinoma metastasis to the brain: long-term outcomes and prognostic factors influencing survival and local tumor control. *J Neurosurg* 2003;98:342–349.

171. Hoshi S, Jokura H, Nakamura H, et al. Gamma-knife radiosurgery for brain metastasis of renal cell carcinoma: results in 42 patients. *Int J Urol* 2002;9:618–625; discussion 626; author reply 627.

172. Goyal LK, Suh JH, Reddy CA, et al. The role of whole brain radiotherapy and stereotactic radiosurgery on brain metastases from renal cell carcinoma. *Int J Radiat Oncol Biol Phys* 2000;47:1007–1012.

CHAPTER 49 ■ PENILE CANCER: CLINICAL SIGNS AND SYMPTOMS

SHAHIN TABATABAEI AND W. SCOTT MCDOUGAL

PENILE CANCER: CLINICAL SIGNS AND SYMPTOMS

Carcinoma of the penis is an uncommon malignancy in the United States, comprising less than 1% of all malignancies in men. Approximately one to two cases per 100,000 population occur per annum. The peak incidence is in the sixth and seventh decades of life. In other parts of the world, particularly Asia, Africa, and South America, however, it is a more common disease. There appear to be no racial predilections.

The etiology is somewhat controversial; however, several facts are quite clear. The presence of a foreskin and exposure to human papilloma virus (HPV) appear to have the most evidence suggesting that they may play a role in the development of this disease. Indeed, it is rare to find cancer of the penis in a patient who has been circumcised at birth. One half of individuals with cancer of the penis have had a phimosis; many have had multiple sex partners, and a prior history of sexually transmitted diseases. HPV-16 and -18 have been identified in patients with squamous cell carcinoma of the penis by polymerase chain reaction (PCR) in approximately 60% to 70% of samples tested. There also is an association of penile cancer and cervical cancer in partners of patients with penile cancer, although this association has been questioned.

PREMALIGNANT LESIONS

A number of lesions of the penis are clearly premalignant, whereas others have an association with squamous cell carcinoma. Carcinoma *in situ* (CIS), balanitis xerotica obliterans (BXO), leukoplakia, and cutaneous horn all are well-established premalignant lesions. Whether condyloma acuminata and giant condyloma are premalignant is unclear.

Carcinoma *In Situ*, Bowen Disease, Erythroplasia of Queyrat

Bowen disease and erythroplasia of Queyrat are identical histologically but occur in different locations. Erythroplasia of Queyrat is CIS of the glans, whereas Bowen disease is CIS of the shaft and remainder of the genitalia and perineal area. It is a velvety red, well-circumscribed lesion that usually involves the glans. Up to one-third of patients with CIS of the penis also have invasive carcinoma of the penis (1).

Diagnosis is based on adequate biopsies of the lesion with sufficient depth to rule out invasion. These lesions respond well to limited local excision with minimal interference with penile anatomy. Circumcision is usually an adequate treatment of CIS of the prepuce. Local fulguration with electrocautery is not appropriate. Topical use of 5-fluorouracil at 5% concentration has shown good results (2). However, 5-fluorouracil is cumbersome to use and will burn scrotal tissue if it is not protected. The carbon dioxide laser and liquid nitrogen also have been used successfully (3,4). Local excision of the lesion when limited provides the best pathologic specimen and the lowest recurrence rate, provided the surgical margins are negative. Excellent cosmetic results may be obtained on both the shaft and glans when properly executed.

Bowenoid Papulosis

Bowenoid papulosis, although histologically similar to CIS, usually has a benign course (5). Lesions occur most commonly in younger men on the shaft of the penis and are usually pigmented multicentric papules. The etiology of bowenoid papulosis is unknown, although viral (particularly HPV), chemical, and immunologic causes have been suggested. The diagnosis is confirmed by excisional biopsy. Treatment includes surgical excision or elimination of the lesion by electrodesiccation, cryotherapy, laser fulguration, or topical 5-fluorouracil cream. Spontaneous regression has been reported (6).

Balanitis Xerotica Obliterans

BXO is the term applied to lichen sclerosis et atrophicus of the glans penis and prepuce. This disorder most often occurs in uncircumcised, middle-aged men and may precede, coexist with, or progress to squamous cell carcinoma.

Although initially asymptomatic, most patients complain of penile discomfort or pain, difficult urination secondary to meatal stricture, and painful erection. On examination, BXO presents as a well-defined marginated white patch on the glans penis or prepuce that may involve the urethral meatus. In chronic cases, the lesion is firm because of a thick underlying fibrosis. It is often associated with a meatal stricture. The treatment of BXO depends on the severity of the disease and consists of surgical excision, topical steroid cream, or laser therapy. Meatal stenosis requiring more than one or two dilatations is best approached by meatoplasty.

Leukoplakia

Leukoplakia is recognized by its whitish plaque-like appearance. The lesions are often multiple and usually occur about the meatal area. A history of chronic irritation is often elicited. It has been associated with CIS and verrucous carcinoma. The disease is treated by excision or by Nd-YAG laser ablation.

Cutaneous Horn

A cutaneous horn is an overgrowth and cornification of the epithelium that forms a solid protuberance. This is characterized by severe hyperkeratosis, dyskeratosis, and acanthosis. Penile horn is a rare form of cutaneous horn, with only 18 cases reported in North America (7). These lesions are considered premalignant and one-third of cases reported have been malignant at presentation (8). Surgical excision with a margin of normal tissue around the base of the lesion has been very successful in treating the disorder. Most malignant penile horns are of low grade, but metastases have been reported. Therefore, wide local excision and close follow-up to detect early metastasis is suggested for malignant forms.

Buschke-Löwenstein Tumor, Verrucous Carcinoma, Giant Condyloma Accuminatum

Whether the Buschke-Löwenstein tumor or giant condyloma and verrucous carcinoma are the same or different lesions is controversial. Their gross appearance is that of a large fungating mass. These lesions are locally invasive and may be quite aggressive. They destroy adjacent structures by local invasion. They rarely, if ever, metastasize. Treatment is directed at eradicating the local disease. This can be achieved by wide local excision of the tumor to normal penile tissue. In rare cases, total penectomy is indicated for large, infiltrative lesions.

PATHOLOGY

Ninety-five percent of cancers of the penis are squamous cell carcinoma. Histologically, the lesion contains heavy keratinization, epithelial pearl formation, increased mitotic activity and hyperchromatic, enlarged nuclei. Various histologic patterns, such as classic, basaloid, verrucous, sarcomatoid, and adenomatoid may be present. Squamous cell carcinoma may be divided histologically into well, moderately and poorly differentiated, according to the classification of Broaders (9). The distinction as to degree of differentiation is particularly important as a potential predictor for metastatic disease to the groin. It is even more powerful when combined with tumor depth of invasion (10). The remaining 5% of malignancies involving the penis include the sarcomas (angiosarcoma, fibrosarcoma, myelosarcoma, Kopasi sarcoma), melonoma, basal cell carcinoma, and lymphoma. Other tumors that have been reported on very rare occasions include rabdomyosarcoma, epithelial sarcoma, malignant schwanoma, myxosarcoma, and neurofibrosarcoma.

Approximately 50% of squamous cell carcinomas are well differentiated, approximately 30% are moderately differentiated, and 20% are poorly differentiated (10,11). Nine percent of lesions are found on the glands and prepuce, 21% on the prepuce, 48% on the glands, and 14% on the prepuce, glands, and shaft. Therefore, 92% of squamous cell carcinomas of the penis involve the glands or prepuce. Approximately, 6% involve the coronal sulcus and only 2% of squamous cell carcinomas are found on the shaft with no lesions elsewhere.

CLINICAL SYMPTOMS

The penile lesion at presentation may be quite variable, ranging from a small papule or pustule that does not heal to a large exophytic, fungating lesion. These lesions occur most commonly on the glans and prepuce and less commonly on the coronal sulcus and penile shaft. Often the foreskin, which is phimotic, results in an unrecognized lesion that becomes apparent only after it becomes quite extensive. These lesions are usually painless.

DIAGNOSIS

Unfortunately, there is usually a significant delay in diagnosis often because the patient does not wish to confront the problem. A thorough physical examination is crucial for the diagnosis and accurate staging. The penile lesion should be evaluated with regard to location, appearance, and size. Fixation of the lesion to the adjacent structures, such as corporal bodies, should be documented. The scrotum, base of the penis, and perineum should be examined for any possible tumor extension. Rectal examination complements the exam and rules out gross involvement of the perineal body or the presence of a pelvic mass. The inguinal area must be inspected and palpated thoroughly for any possible lymph node enlargement. This is a critical part of the physical examination.

Biopsy

Histologic confirmation of penile cancer should be obtained by a biopsy from the penile lesion. The biopsy is important to evaluate the depth of invasion, tumor differentiation (grade), and the presence of vascular invasion. This information is very helpful in accurately staging the tumor and allows the surgeon to discuss the therapeutic options with the patient. Although it is possible to perform the biopsy (with frozen section diagnosis) and partial or total penectomy in one session, we do not advocate this approach. Loss of a part or all of the phallus is devastating to many patients and most need some time to cope with that prospect. In order to minimize any psychological problem the patient might develop, it is important to have an interval between the biopsy and the definitive radical surgery, which will allow the patient and his physician to establish a relationship. This allows the physician time to address the psychological aspects of the treatment, thereby decreasing the tension and stress that ensues following therapy.

Imaging

Knowledge of the extent and depth of the primary tumor and the involvement of inguinal lymph nodes before any surgical intervention are important in planning the treatment. In practice, this decision usually is based on findings from a physical examination. Various imaging modalities have been used for this purpose, including ultrasonography, computed tomography (CT) scan, and magnetic resonance imaging (MRI). Because of the poor soft tissue resolution of CT scan, ultrasound and MRI are superior in the evaluation of primary tumor extension.

Ultrasound cannot precisely detect tumor extension in the glans penis area. Ultrasound, however, has shown adequate resolution to detect corpus cavernosum invasion, owing to the thick tunica albuginea that is readily visible with a 7.5 MHz linear array small parts transducer (12). In extensive infiltrating tumors, ultrasound's ability to delineate corporal invasion is compromised significantly (13).

MRI has been used in several studies, and it appears that it is the most sensitive method for determining corpus cavernosal infiltration but at the cost of lower specificity (14). In practice, none of these modalities are particularly helpful clinically.

Recently we reported the use of lymphotropic superparamagnetic nanoparticles, as an MRI contrast agent, in evaluating lymph node metastasis in patients with prostate cancer (15). Our early experience in applying this noninvasive technique in

TABLE 49.1

JACKSON STAGING SYSTEM

Stage I	Tumor confined to glans or prepuce.
Stage II	Tumor invasive into the shaft or corpora. No palpable adenopathy.
Stage III	Palpable metastases to the groin, which are resectable.
Stage IV	Inoperable groin nodes or distant metastases.

TABLE 49.2

INTERNATIONAL UNION AGAINST CANCER STAGING SYSTEM

T0	No primary tumor
Tis	CIS
Ta	Verroucus carcinoma, noninvasive
T-1	Tumor invades subepithelial connective tissue
T-2	Tumor invades corpora
T-3	Tumor invades urethra or prostate
T-4	Tumor invades other adjacent structures
N-0	No regional node metastases
N-1	Single superficial node metastasis
N-2	Multiple or bilateral superficial inguinal nodes
N-3	Deep inguinal or pelvic node metastases

CIS, carcinoma *in situ*.

several patients with penile cancer is encouraging. This modality has the potential to stage the inguinal and pelvic nodes with an accuracy that far exceeds clinical evaluation or sentinel node biopsy. More studies are required to establish the role of this technique in patients with penile cancer.

STAGING

Proper staging of carcinoma of the penis is extremely important in determining the likelihood of regional lymph node metastases. Indeed, the presence of metastasis in the ileo-inguinal or pelvic lymph nodes is the most important determinant of prognosis. Moreover, surgical excision of these nodes may be curative, and, therefore, it is extremely important to determine the likelihood of whether or not they are involved. The current method used to stage patients with penile cancer involves the pathologic stage of the primary lesion combined with a clinical assessment of the inguinal and pelvic lymph nodes. The original Jackson system (Table 49.1) is not particularly helpful clinically in selecting who is most likely to have groin disease. The tumor-node-metastasis (TNM) system is a bit better (Table 49.2), but again suffers from inability to predict the incidence of positive regional lymph nodes. Combining the TNM system with differentiation improves the predictive ability for regional nodal involvement (Table 49.3).

It has been suggested that a sentinel node biopsy would be predictive of the status of the groin so that an unnecessary groin dissection could be avoided. As originally described by Cabanas, however, it proved to be very unreliable. The positive predictive value of sentinel node biopsy may be increased by injecting the primary lesion with blue dye and technetium and then biopsy the node/nodes which scan for the technetium and take up the blue dye. In a recent report, 55 patients were scanned and biopsied (16). One-third were found not to have surgical findings that correlated with scintigraphy. Twenty percent had a positive sentinel node biopsy; 6% of patients found to have a negative sentinel node within a 3-year period were found to develop evidence of positive groin nodes.

Therefore, this methodology does eliminate a number of patients who would needlessly undergo a groin dissection at the expense of subjecting all patients to groin sentinel node biopsies. The number of false negatives is at least 6% as the follow-up in the current contemporary series is too short to determine the true false-negative rate. New modalities of lymph node imaging particularly contrast agents used with MRI are extremely exciting and in all likelihood will have a diagnostic efficacy sufficient to predict who should and who should not receive a groin dissection. Unfortunately, at this time, tumor differentiation and stage of tumor combined are more predictive than sentinel node biopsies either with or without blue dye. Therefore, poorly differentiated tumors have an 80% to 100% incidence of metastatic disease, moderately differentiated tumors a 46% incidence, and well-differentiated tumors have a 24% incidence of groin metastasis. If the corpora is not invaded, there is a 5% to 11% incidence of metastatic disease. If the corpora is invaded, there is a 61% to 75% incidence of groin metastases. Therefore, we have proposed a classification combining stage and grade (Table 49.3) to help predict the likelihood of nonpalpable metastatic groin disease. Stage I and IIA disease have an extremely low likelihood of metastatic groin disease (0% to 12%). Patients with Stage IIB disease have a 78% to 88% incidence of groin metastases. Stage III disease or those with persistently palpable groin nodes following 6 weeks of antibiotic treatment after eradication of the primary tumor and closure of the wound have a 78% to 80% likelihood of metastatic disease to the nodes. Simply put, patients with poorly differentiated tumors irrespective of T stage, those with T-2 or greater lesions, and those with persistently palpable lymph nodes require groin dissections.

TABLE 49.3

DEPTH OF INVASIVE/GRADE CLASSIFICATION SYSTEM

		T stage
Stage I	The tumor is superficial with no extension into the subcutaneous tissue	T0, Tis, Ta, N0
Stage IIA	Locally invasive tumor without involvement of the corpora, well or moderately well differentiated	T1, N0
Stage IIB	The tumor invades the corpora or it is poorly differentiated	T1, T2, N0
Stage III	Persistent palpable inguinal nodes	N-1, N-2
Stage IV	Bulky groin nodes with invasion extending outside the node, pelvic node involvement, distant metastases	N-3, N-4

References

1. Mikhail GR. Cancers, precancers, and pseudocancers on the male genitalia. A review of clinical appearances, histopathology, and management. *J Dermatol Surg Oncol* 1980;6(12):1027–1035.

2. Goette DK, Carson TE. Erythroplasia of Queyrat: treatment with topical 5-fluorouracil. *Cancer* 1976;38(4):1498–1502.

3. Rosemberg SK, Fuller TA. Carbon dioxide rapid superpulsed laser treatment of erythroplasia of Queyrat. *Urology* 1980;16(2):181–182.

4. Madej G, Meyza J. Cryosurgery of penile carcinoma. Short report on preliminary results. *Oncology* 1982;39(6):350–352.

5. Su CK, Shipley WU. Bowenoid papulosis: a benign lesion of the shaft of the penis misdiagnosed as squamous carcinoma. *J Urol* 1997;157(4):1361–1362.

6. Patterson JW, Kao GF, Graham JH, et al. Bowenoid papulosis. A clinicopathologic study with ultrastructural observations. *Cancer* 1986;57(4):823–836.

7. Lowe FC, McCullough AR. Cutaneous horns of the penis: an approach to management. Case report and review of the literature. *J Am Acad Dermatol* 1985;13(2 Pt 2):369–373.

8. Fields T, Drylie D, Wilson J. Malignant evolution of penile horn. *Urology* 1987;30(1):65–66.

9. Broders AC. Squamous cell epithelium of the skin. *Ann Surg* 1921;73:141–143.

10. McDougal WS. Carcinoma of the penis: improved survival by early regional lymphadenectomy based on the histological grade and depth of invasion of the primary lesion. *J Urol* 1995;154(4):1364–1366.

11. McDougal WS, Kirchner FK Jr, Edwards RH, et al. Treatment of carcinoma of the penis: the case for primary lymphadenectomy. *J Urol* 1986;136(1):38–41.

12. Horenblas S, Kroger R, Gallee MP, et al. Ultrasound in squamous cell carcinoma of the penis; a useful addition to clinical staging? A comparison of ultrasound with histopathology. *Urology* 1994;43(5):702–707.

13. Lont AP, Besnard AP, Gallee MP, et al. A comparison of physical examination and imaging in determining the extent of primary penile carcinoma. *BJU Int* 2003;91(6):493–495.

14. de Kerviler E, Ollier P, Desgrandchamps F, et al. Magnetic resonance imaging in patients with penile carcinoma. *Br J Radiol* 1995;68(811):704–711.

15. Harisinghani MG, Barentsz J, Hahn PF, et al. Noninvasive detection of clinically occult lymph-node metastases in prostate cancer [comment]. *N Engl J Med* 2003;348(25):2491–2499.

16. Horenblas S, Jansen L, Meinhardt W, et al. Detection of occult metastasis in squamous cell carcinoma of the penis using a dynamic sentinel node procedure. *J Urol* 2000;163(1):100–104.

CHAPTER 50 ■ SURGICAL MANAGEMENT OF PENILE CANCER

PAUL RUSSO AND SIMON HORENBLAS

INTRODUCTION

Approximately 95% of penile carcinomas are squamous cell cancers. Penile carcinomas are rare in Western countries and the overall annual experience even in tertiary referral centers is extremely limited. Despite this, there is no doubt that effective surgical intervention, fundamental throughout the natural history of this malignancy, plays an essential role in both the diagnosis and management of the primary penile cancer (1). In addition, operative intervention is essential for accurate staging and therapy for regional inguinal and pelvic lymph nodes. The main principle of surgical treatment of the primary tumor is to resect the penile cancer with adequate margins and attempt to leave as much functional penis as possible for upright voiding and sexual function (2–4). Delayed or incomplete surgical interventions can have adverse effects on patient survival, a situation made worse by the absence of effective systemic chemotherapy once metastatic disease occurs. Regional inguinal and pelvic lymph node dissection (LND) remains an integral component of the treatment of invasive penile cancer with evidence mounting that a survival advantage exists for patients undergoing early as opposed to therapeutic groin dissection. Lymphoscintigraphy to identify the sentinel lymph node, a new technique found highly effective in the management of melanoma and breast cancer, has an evolving role in patients with invasive penile cancer presenting without adenopathy. For patients with bulky metastatic groin disease, myocutaneous flap coverage increases the role of surgical intervention to provide local tumor control and effective disease palliation.

DIAGNOSIS OF THE PRIMARY PENILE LESION

When a suspicious penile tumor or ulcer is encountered, a decision concerning the extent of the biopsy procedure is made depending on the location of the lesion. Any penile lesion that is not healing after a period of 2 to 3 weeks of careful observation, meticulous hygiene, and skin care should be biopsied. For small discrete lesions, the biopsy procedure can be at the same time diagnostic and therapeutic. The biopsy specimen, regardless of location, must contain adequate underlying tissue to allow the pathologist to determine the depth of tumor invasion, an important predictor of local tumor recurrence and regional nodal metastases (5,6). Patients with noninvasive cancers [i.e., carcinoma *in situ* (CIS)] that are completely excised with negative margins must be carefully monitored with frequent physical examinations to determine any early signs of local recurrence (7).

For tumors involving only the prepuce, circumcision can be both diagnostic and therapeutic. Tumors involving the glans,

glans and prepuce, coronal sulcus, or shaft are best approached with an initial excisional biopsy that includes ample underlying soft tissue to accurately determine the depth of invasion. Tumor stage, the presence of vascular invasion, and the percentage of poorly differentiated cancer each serve as independent prognosticators for inguinal lymph node metastases in penile cancer (8). Once the diagnosis of an invasive penile cancer (T1, T2, T3) has been made, an extent of disease evaluation is ordered. Depending on stage at presentation, this evaluation includes the following if the serum calcium level is elevated: computed tomography (CT) scan of chest, abdomen, pelvis, and bone. A full discussion with the patient concerning the degree of penile resection required, the anticipated functional deficit, and the necessary reconstruction required is prudent. Occasionally, plastic surgical consultation is requested if a wide local excision with complex rotational flap coverage is contemplated. If total penectomy is planned, a psychiatric consultation is recommended to be certain the patient has the emotional capacity to tolerate such a procedure.

While adhering to basic surgical and oncological principles, a tumor free margin after resection is an essential goal. As in many other primary tumors (e.g., melanoma, prostate cancer, colon cancer, breast cancer), the extent of the negative margin required is controversial in penile cancer. If a surgeon were to adhere strictly to the generally accepted 2-cm margin, almost no penile cancers would be amenable to a penis-conserving operation. Recent studies have shown that patients treated with margins less than 2 cm also can obtain long-term recurrence-free survival. Hoffman et al. reported, after a mean follow-up of 32.4 months, no local recurrences and one inguinal metastasis in seven patients with T1 or greater tumors with microscopic margins of 10 mm or less, suggesting that a 1-cm margin is sufficient to achieve local tumor control (9). The question of what is the required surgical margin could easily be answered in a contemporary, multi-institutional, randomized trial. It is our practice to send a frozen section of the proximal margin at the time of tumor resection to assure a microscopically negative margin.

TREATMENT OF THE PRIMARY PENILE CARCINOMA

Ablative Techniques

The choice of surgical therapy is dictated by the primary tumor characteristics including size, location, and depth of invasion; and the surgeon's desire to achieve effective local tumor control while at the same time retaining maximal function of the penis. *In situ* penile lesions, such as erythroplasia of Queryat and Bowen disease, are amenable to local excision, circumcision, tissue ablative techniques such as CO_2 and Nd:

Yttrium Aluminum Garnet (YAG) lasers (10,11), and topical 5-fluorouracil cream application (12,13). Occasionally, surgeons may use surgical excision in conjunction with laser therapy to provide an additional 4-mm margin with the intent of achieving a more cosmetically appealing result. With careful case selection and close clinical follow-up, it appears that laser therapy can effectively treat some patients. The effectiveness of laser therapy for overtly invasive penile cancers is uncertain and laser treatment should not be considered an alternative to standard resection. Wound healing after the use of the laser is by secondary intention with full re-epithelialization, usually complete after 8 to 10 weeks. Wound infections are rare following laser therapy. There are also favorable reports of Mohs micrographic surgery for carefully selected *in situ* and superficially invasive lesions of the glans or shaft (14,15). A specially trained dermatologist performs serial resections until the histologic findings are tumor free. If the treating dermatologist or urologist selects an ablative technique to treat *in situ* lesions of the penis, careful physician follow-up and patient self-examinations to seek early signs of recurrence are essential.

Penile Conservation Techniques

For tumors of the prepuce, circumcision is an effective surgical treatment. Careful examination of the fully exposed glans for evidence of CIS is recommended and a low threshold for additional biopsy should exist. Local excision with adequate underlying soft tissue of invasive penile cancer without partial or total penectomy must be carefully approached. In determining which patient is a candidate for penile conservation procedures, knowledge of the true extent of the local tumor is vital. Physical examination has been shown to be quite reliable in determining the extent of disease and degree of local infiltration into the deeper structures of the penis (16). Operations must be designed to assure negative surgical margins with the goal to achieve a cosmetic result that is acceptable and not cosmetically or functionally worse than a partial penectomy. Intraoperative frozen section must assure negative margins. Local recurrence, an uncommon event following partial or total penectomy, is more common in penile-conserving operations and can be as high as 10% to 15% (17). Patients should be instructed to inspect the remaining epithelium of the glans for recurrence or a new primary, as they remain at lifelong risk (18).

Most local recurrences can be treated either with a delayed partial amputation or another attempt at penile conserving surgery. The degree to which local tumor recurrence translates into degradation in overall survival is not known. Extensive local resections by removing a part of the corona of the glans penis can improve the tumor-free margins and can aid in decreasing local recurrences. Resection of a part of the glans is also feasible. This is advised only if the lesion does not infiltrate deeply into the cavernous tissue and does not extend more than half of the glans. Otherwise, these conservative operations can lead to serious deformation and deviation of the penis during erections with the patient clearly better served with a formal partial penectomy. Larger lesions restricted to the glans penis only can be managed by resection of the glans, instead of standard partial amputation, leading to minimal loss of length of the penis. Verrucous carcinomas, which are of low to intermediate grade and have an exophytic growth pattern, are particularly amenable to local tumor excision (19). If penile conservational techniques are used, it is still necessary to frequently monitor the inguinal nodes that remain at risk for the development of metastatic disease (20).

Partial Penectomy

For invasive tumors of the distal penis, partial penectomy with at least a 1-cm margin of resection is recommended (Fig. 50.1). The operation should be designed, if possible, to allow the patient to void in the upright position and without the need to push away the scrotum; otherwise a perineal urethrostomy should be created. Partial penectomy achieves excellent tumor control with local recurrence as low as 6% reported (21). At the time of operation, a latex glove is placed over the primary tumor and distal shaft and is secured to the penis with a suture. A sterile marking pen is used to circumferentially outline the planned incision with care taken to provide at least a 1-cm margin. A medium Penrose drain is placed around the base of the penis and tightened to function as a tourniquet. The incision is circumferentially carried through the skin and Buck's fascia to the tunic of the corpora. On the dorsum of the penis, the dorsal veins and arteries are individually ligated with absorbable suture. As the resection is carried ventrally, a 1-cm stump urethra is created and spatulated to prevent stenosis of the neourethra. The tunic of corpora cavernosa is closed with 2-0 absorbable sutures that provide hemostasis. The urethra is sutured to the ventral penile skin and a sterile dressing is applied.

Total Penectomy

For bulky T3 or T4 proximal tumors involving the base of the penis, total penectomy with perineal urethrostomy is done

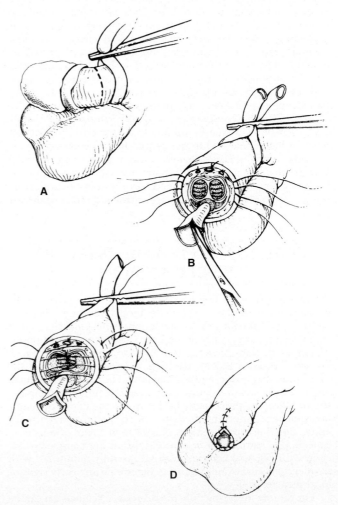

FIGURE 50.1. Technique of partial penectomy.

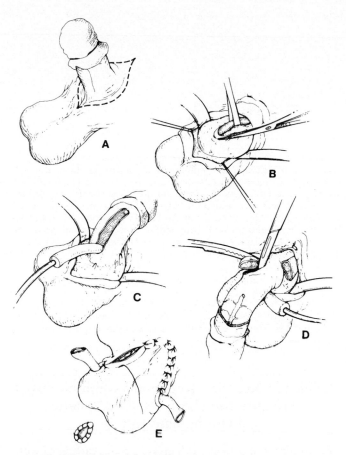

FIGURE 50.2. Technique of total penectomy.

(Fig. 50.2) Total penectomy for proximal tumors that are locally advanced and associated with painful local symptoms and bulky regional metastatic disease can provide effective palliation for these patients. Psychiatric input is recommended for patients undergoing total penectomy to be certain that the patient has the necessary emotional capacity to undergo the operation and endure its postoperative implications. During total penectomy, an incision is outlined circumferentially at the base of the penis with extension into the median raphe of the scrotum. At the base of the penis, the suspensory ligament of the penis is identified and divided. The urethra and corpora spongiosa are mobilized from the corpora between clamps and divided. A 2-cm margin of perineal urethra is preserved for construction of a perineal urethrostomy. The urethral remnant is passed through the scrotum to the midline perineum and the urethrostomy is performed. An 18-French Foley catheter is left in urethrostomy. In rare cases, the site of attachment of the corpus cavernosum to the pubic bone may need to be resected in order to achieve a clear margin.

POSTOPERATIVE MANAGEMENT AND COMPLICATIONS

Early complications after partial or total penectomy include wound infection and hematoma, and stricture of the neomeatus. Stricture of the neomeatus can be managed by simple dilatation or meatotomy. Recurrent strictures may need some form of meatoplasty to correct (i.e., Blandly inlaypasty). Needless to say, penectomy can adversely affect a patient's quality of life; however, there is little published on this subject. For previously potent men, erectile function is unaffected, however, intromission may be disturbed. A normal sense of orgasm and ejaculation can persist even after total penectomy.

MANAGEMENT OF REGIONAL LYMPH NODES

General Considerations

Like all squamous cell carcinomas, penile cancer has a propensity for locoregional dissemination, whereas hematogenous dissemination in the absence of lymphatic invasion is very uncommon. Metastases in penile carcinoma occur in a sequential manner with tumor cells embolizing through first-echelon regional inguinal nodes and then on to second-echelon deep pelvic nodes (22). Some surgeons advocate a conservative approach to the groin nodes at the time of presentation wishing not to inflict the potential morbidity of groin dissection (cellulitis, flap necrosis, lymph edema) without the certainty of a therapeutic dissection. Others advocate an immediate surgical approach toward regional node dissection at a point earlier in the course of the disease when a potential survival advantage may be realized, even at the expense of perioperative morbidity or the finding of negative nodes. Between 30% and 60% of patients presenting with squamous cell carcinoma of the penis have enlarged lymph nodes in the groin. With rare exceptions, all patients with pelvic node involvement always have inguinal node involvement first (23–34).

Nodal metastasis will develop in approximately 20% of patients presenting without any clinical sign of lymphadenopathy and unfortunately, physical examination and contemporary imaging with CT scan or magnetic resonance imaging (MRI) are not able to reliably detect minimal metastatic disease. The management of this group of patients with invasive penile cancer who are initially node negative remains difficult and controversial and may be improved by the evolving use of radio nuclide-based lymphoscintigraphy of the sentinel nodes (SNs). This evolving technique has the potential to identify early metastatic disease and at the same time spare the side effects of groin dissection in patients who are node negative. Unlike other genitourinary tumors (e.g., prostate, renal), in which nodal involvement is often synonymous with incurable disease, nodal metastases in penile cancer are highly curable and therapeutic nihilism is not justified, even in patients with locally advanced lymphatic involvement.

Anatomic Considerations

The regional lymph nodes of the penis are located in the inguinal region (Fig. 50.3) (35–37). Some urologic oncologists have divided the inguinal nodes into two groups, a superficial group and a deep group. The superficial nodes are located beneath the subcutaneous fascia and above the fascia lata covering the muscles of the upper leg. Eight to 25 nodes are found. The deep inguinal nodes are the nodes around the fossa ovalis, the opening in the fascia lata in which the saphenous vein drains into the femoral vein. Three to five nodes are usually found. These nodes intercommunicate and then drain to the pelvic nodes. From a clinical point of view, this distinction is meaningless because at the time of operation the superficial nodes cannot be distinguished from the deep nodes. This point of anatomic confusion has led some surgeons to perform operations that may be incomplete and contribute later to local recurrence. Therefore, complete groin dissection should in all cases remove both of these nodal drainage basins. The most constant and usually largest node is the node found medial to the femoral vein and just underneath the inguinal ligament, the so-called node of Cloquet or Rosenmuller. This node may be missed during either incomplete groin or pelvic dissection and can represent a common site of local recurrence following

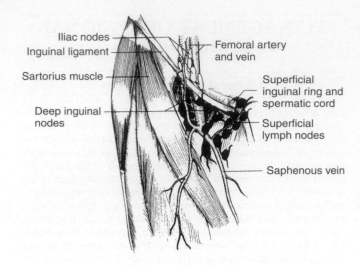

Iliac nodes
Inguinal ligament
Sartorius muscle
Deep inguinal nodes
Femoral artery and vein
Superficial inguinal ring and spermatic cord
Superficial lymph nodes
Saphenous vein

FIGURE 50.3. The pattern of lymphatic drainage of the penis involves three sequential groups of lymph nodes: the superficial inguinal lymph nodes that are superficial to the fascia lata, the deep inguinal nodes that are deep to the fascia lata and surrounded femoral vessels, and the iliac lymph nodes that surrounded the external iliac artery and vein cephalad to the inguinal ligament. (From Colberg JW, Andriole GL, Catalona WJ. Penectomy and inguinal lymphadenectomy for carcinoma of the penis. In: Marshall FF, ed. *Operative urology.* Philadelphia: WB Saunders, 1996:639, with permission.)

lymphadenectomy. It is customary to divide the inguinal region into four sections by drawing a horizontal and a vertical line through the point where the saphenous vein drains into the femoral vein. The nodes that are involved primarily in penile cancer mainly are located in the superomedial segment. However, individual variation exists, and therefore all groin nodes should be removed. The penis drains to both inguinal sides in at least 12% of the patients as evidenced by lymphographic studies and in 60% of patients as evidenced by studies utilizing lymphoscintigraphy (38,39). The pelvic nodal package consists of nodes around the iliac artery and vein as well as the obturator fossa and consists of between 12 and 20 nodes. Crossover from one pelvic nodal basin to the other has not been observed clinically or by lymphoscintigraphy.

Management of Clinically Positive Regional Nodes

Comparison of findings at physical examination and histopathology in modern series show false-positive rate for physical examination of approximately 50% (specificity 50%) (40–42). The traditional approach to patients with invasive penile cancer and enlarged lymph was to administer oral antibiotics for 4 to 6 weeks and then reevaluate the patient (40). Persistent lymph node enlargement was considered an indication for *therapeutic* groin dissection with 30% to 60% of such patients found to have regional metastatic disease. In patients with surgically resected metastatic inguinal lymph nodes, 5-year survival rates range from 57% to 66%. In the presence of unilateral inguinal lymphadenopathy, bilateral groin dissection is recommended as there is a 60% rate of bilateral disease because of the rich communications in lymphatics at the base of the penis. Recently, urologic oncologists have adopted a more invasive approach to the diagnosis of metastatic regional lymph node metastases including the use of fine-needle aspiration cytology and open lymph node biopsy. False negative rates for aspiration biopsy have been reported up to 15%. If the clinician remains suspicious and repeat needle aspiration cytology is still inconclusive, then excisional biopsy can be done. Care must be taken to position the biopsy needle or open biopsy in such a way that, if positive, the needle tract or biopsy incision will be removed with the LND. The substitution of a more aggressive biopsy approach to the suspicious inguinal node may enhance the patient's chance for survival and limit the need for protracted antibiotic administration in the absence of clinical signs of infection or cellulitis. The role of CT scan or MRI is of limited value and only serves to confirm locally advanced disease in the form of bulky groin,

pelvic nodes, or retroperitoneal nodes. Sentinel lymph node dynamic lymphoscintigraphy should not be used to determine whether persistently enlarged regional nodes require biopsy or resection.

Clinically Negative Regional Lymph Nodes at Presentation (Early vs. Therapeutic Lymphadenectomy)

The treatment of patients with invasive penile carcinoma without lymphadenopathy at the time of presentation is made difficult because of published studies subjected to selection biases, small patient numbers, and the absence of randomized trials. Despite a negative result of a physical examination, as many as 20% of such patients undergoing *early lymphadenectomy* (node dissection in the absence of clinically palpable regional lymph nodes) will be found to harbor nodal metastasis. McDougall et al. argued a shift in philosophy toward early lymphadenectomy and reported a 5-year survival rate for patients treated with early LND of 88% as opposed to 38% for those undergoing a delayed therapeutic LND (43). Comparing these results with a composite analysis from the literature, the authors found a 5-year survival rate of 83% in patients for whom inguinal lymphadenectomy had revealed metastasis in nodes that were believed to be clinically benign, compared to a 5-year survival rate of 42% for patients with invasive penile cancer who underwent delayed therapeutic groin dissection. In a subsequent report that pooled patients from four different teaching institutions, McDougall again described a survival advantage for patients undergoing early groin dissection versus therapeutic groin dissection (44). Further evidence that therapeutic groin dissection may not provide the best chance for long-term survival came from a report from Memorial Sloan-Kettering Cancer Center (MSKCC), which described the outcome of patients undergoing delayed *therapeutic groin dissections* for patients with invasive penile cancer (T1-T3). Between 1980 and 1994, 42 of 60 patients with invasive penile cancer and clinically negative groin nodes were managed with an initial surveillance-only strategy. Twenty-six of 42 (62%) patients developed inguinal recurrences after resection of the primary tumor, 50% within 1.4 years and 75% within 2.8 years. The only significant factor predictive of nodal relapse was the primary tumor grade. Despite careful follow-up, 2 patients developed inoperable inguinal recurrences and 4 patients (10%) developed metastatic disease without clinically evident groin metastasis. Somewhat surprisingly, patients with grade 1 primary tumors, traditionally felt to be at low risk for the development of systemic disease, had just a 45% long-term actuarial relapse-free survival, whereas, all other patients had a 100% relapse rate in the groin. Once there was inguinal relapse, overall long-term survival was achieved in 71% of patients undergoing therapeutic groin dissection (24). The fact that there are no curative chemotherapeutic regimens currently available for the treatment of disseminated disease enhances the appeal of a preemptive surgical approach to patients at risk for metastatic penile cancer. Although the argument for early groin dissection is based on a relatively limited number of patients from retrospective studies, it makes intuitive sense that the early intervention in the face of minimal metastatic disease would lead to an improved probability of survival, if based only on a lead-time bias.

Sentinel Lymph Node Biopsy and Lymphoscintigraphy Biopsy: Role in Patients Without Lymphadenopathy

The possibility that selective inguinal lymph node sampling of the SN could be done with sufficient precision to accurately identify patients with clinically negative lymph nodes in need of a therapeutic groin dissection was first introduced by Cabanas at MSKCC in 1977 (35,37). The SN, identified following lymphangiographic dye injections of the dorsal penile lymphatics, was located medial to the saphenous-epigastric venous junction. In his initial experience, Cabanas found 15 of 46 sentinel biopsies positive for metastatic disease leading to complete inguinal LNDs. In 12 of 15 cases, the SN was the only site of metastatic disease. Despite this initial enthusiasm, other investigators reported a disturbingly high rate of local relapse after SN biopsy, thereby making it difficult for many to fully accept the technique (45–47). Subsequent investigators argued that rather than a single, fixed anatomic SN, up to seven nodes in the area between the superficial epigastric vein and the external pudendal vein could be the SN and more closely accounted for individual variability in drainage of the penis. Yet even resecting a sentinel area or region in what amounted to a modified groin dissection did not prevent node recurrence, as was seen in 5 of 20 cases operated on at M.D. Anderson Cancer Center (48).

Despite its apparent inaccuracies, the SN biopsy concept has great appeal in principle as a method to avoid an unnecessary and potentially morbid groin dissection. The pursuit of the SN and reemergence of this strategy to spare patients nontherapeutic lymphadenectomy was lead by surgical oncologists working in melanoma and breast cancer seeking the SN first using injections of the primary tumor first with vital blue dye (49) and later using a combination of vital blue dye and technetium-99 sulfur colloid (50). This approach created a *dynamic lymphoscintigraphy*, whereby the sentinel lymph node could be directly identified both visually and by the use of a hand-held γ probe (51–53). This technique more effectively accounted for patient variability in lymphatic drainage. If a frozen section biopsy of the otherwise clinically normal-appearing SN reveals metastatic disease, then complete regional lymphadenectomy is performed. If the frozen section is negative, then the procedure is terminated. The accuracy of the lymphoscintigraphy appears greater than the blue dye alone with the best results reported in the axilla and groin, in which the anatomic lymphatic drainage is more predictable. Clinical researchers also have applied the molecular diagnostic techniques of polymerase chain reaction (PCR) and immunohistochemistry (IHC) to detect submicroscopic lymph node metastasis following sentinel lymphoscintigraphy and biopsy and incorporate this "molecular information" into algorithms using early LND (51–53). Radioactive lymphoscintigraphy with SN biopsy is now a standard surgical strategy in the treatment of breast cancer and malignant melanoma.

The application of these lymphoscintigraphy techniques in invasive penile carcinoma was first described by Horenblas et al. from the Netherlands in a report of 55 patients with T2 or greater tumors without palpable inguinal adenopathy (38). The primary tumor was injected intradermally with ^{99m}Tc colloid. The following day the SN was identified with the γ detection probe and visually by also injecting vital blue dye (Fig. 50.4). Regional LND was performed only in patients in whom the SN biopsy revealed metastatic carcinoma. A total of 125 SNs in 107 inguinal regions were identified including two patients in whom no SN was identified, one or more unilateral nodes in 10 patients, and bilateral drainage in 43 patients. In 17 of 55 patients (31%), the sentinel lymph node biopsy was deemed unsuccessful for a variety of reasons. Eleven patients (20%) had SN metastasis, 2 of which also had a contralateral sentinel lymph node metastasis, and underwent groin dissection of the involved region 1 to 2 weeks later. One patient later developed metastatic disease in a lymph node region previously declared negative using SN lymphoscintigraphy.

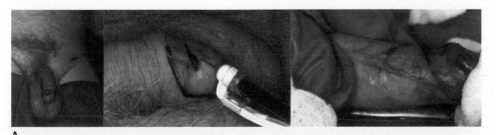

A

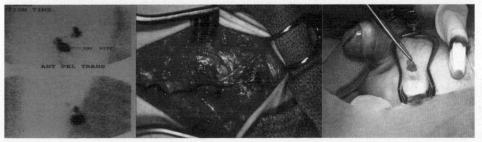

B

FIGURE 50.4. A: Technique of lymphoscintigraphy: injection of primary tumor site and absorption by local lymphatics. B: Lymphoscintigram, blue dye in lymphatics, and identification of sentinel lymph. (See color insert.)

The Dutch investigators published follow-up studies describing 80% sensitivity with dynamic SN biopsy but insisted on subsequent careful surveillance over SN-negative patients (54,55). This group recently reported a comparison of 85 patients with T2-T3 N0 M0 squamous cell carcinoma initially by managed surveillance and who then developed adenopathy and required therapeutic lymphadenectomy to 68 patients who underwent dynamic SN biopsy. In the surveillance group, 20 of 85 patients (24%) developed inguinal metastases at a median of 6 months (range 1 to 24 months). Subsequent inguinal and pelvic LNDs were performed and, despite this, 13 of 20 patients died of their disease. In the SN group, 14 of 68 patients (21%) were diagnosed with lymph node metastases and then underwent subsequent complete lymphadenectomy on the side of the positive node. Additional metastatic nodes were detected in 5 patients, including 2 with deep pelvic nodes, and 2 patients developed contra lateral lymph node metastases despite the absence of lymphoscintigraphy evidence of a SN. Four patients died of disease in the SN biopsy group. The disease-specific 3-year survival for the patients undergoing dynamic SN biopsy was significantly better (91% vs. 79%) than those undergoing initial surveillance. Although this study was not randomized and the surveillance groups were historical controls, it lends credence to the concept of a more aggressive diagnostic and therapeutic approach to the patient with invasive penile cancer and clinically negative regional nodes with the added appeal of attempting to limit the likelihood of a negative and potentially morbid lymphadenectomy (56). Despite a negative SN study, clinicians using dynamic lymphscintigraphy must continue vigilant follow-up of the inguinal nodal basins at 2-month intervals for 2 years and 3-month intervals for the third year.

Despite its promise, concerns that dynamic lymphoscintigraphy may be subject to technical problems that render it less effective have been raised. Recently, an analysis of false negative SNs was published. Modifications and suggestions for an improved methodology were given (57).

However, unanswered questions remain to be answered before dynamic lymphoscintigraphy is fully integrated into the treatment of penile cancer. Could the SN pathology be misread? Should each case have additional PCR or IHC to identify microscopic metastases? Could an inadequate dermal injection of tracer lead to a false negative identification a contralateral SN? Could inflammatory reactions or in-transit metastatic disease in the regional lymphatics obstruct the proper tracer flow and thereby render a falsely negative study? The most effective way to determine the best means of managing the inguinal nodes would be to design a national or international prospective and randomized clinical trial with three arms: a surveillance and therapeutic groin dissection group, a prophylactic groin dissection group, and a dynamic lymphoscintigraphy SN dissection group. These concerns underscore the fact that SN biopsy should not be used to determine whether node dissection is needed in patients with clinically positive nodes; it should be done only in patients without clinical signs of nodal involvement. The probability of false negative results underlines a strict follow-up scheme. During the first 2 years after a dynamic SN procedure, patients are seen every second month; in the third year, every third month. Salvage procedures can then be undertaken at the earliest possible moment. Patients who cannot comply with this follow-up should not be submitted to this procedure.

Groin Dissection: Techniques and Perioperative Care

The technique of inguinal (groin) dissection used by most uro-oncologists today was that described at MSKCC by Dr. Willet

Whitmore and is characterized by thick skin flaps that are designed to reduce the perioperative morbidity of leg lymph edema (58) and remains the operation of choice today performed by surgeons experienced in the surgical management of penile cancer (59). The patient is positioned supine on the operating table with the side to be operated on in the frog leg position. A curved transverse incision is made approximately three finger breadths below the inguinal ligament. Thick skin flaps are developed to the level of the superficial fascia with care exercised not to bruise or damage the flaps. In groin dissection for melanoma, thin skin flaps have traditionally been employed, but this is not necessary for groin dissection in carcinoma of the penis, which does not have a cutaneous or subcutaneous method of spread. The boundaries of the dissection are as follows: superiorly inguinal ligament, laterally the sartorius muscle, inferiorly to the base of the femoral triangle, and medially to the adductor longus muscle (Figs. 50.5 to 50.7).

The saphenous vein is identified at the base of the femoral triangle, ligated, and divided. Small branches of the femoral artery and vein as well as lymphatic vessels are meticulously tied and clipped as the dissection proceeds toward the sapheno-femoral junction and the fossa ovales. The undersurface of the inguinal ligament is dissected and the artery, and vein identified. There is no need to attempt to dissect beneath this neurovascular complex because all nodal tissue rests above. At the sapheno-femoral junction multiple branches of the femoral vein will be encountered (circumflex iliac, superficial epigastric, superficial external pudendal) and each need to be ligated and divided. The node package is usually delivered when the saphenous vein is ligated as it enters the femoral vein (Fig. 50.8). Following a check for hemostasis, the sartorius muscle is sharply divided from its attachment at the iliac spine, mobilized 8 to 10 cm on its fascial pedicle, rotated medially to cover the femoral vessels, and sutured to the Cooper's ligament with from two to zero nonabsorbable sutures. A closed suction drain is placed above the sartorius muscle and brought out through a separate stab wound. Prophylactic antibiotics are given shortly before the start of operation and discontinued afterward. Compression stockings and support hose are routinely used in the perioperative period. Although some surgeons have advocated strict bed rest for patients undergoing lymphadenectomy, it is not our practice. Instead, we recommend early ambulation with strict orders to avoid sitting in a chair (lying and walking, but no sitting). This approach lessens the risk of postoperative deep venous thrombosis and pulmonary embolism. Careful monitoring of the wound is done twice daily. Should signs of wound cellulitis develop, therapeutic antibiotics are begun. Any serum clots within the drain need to be carefully milked free. When drainage is down to 30 to 50 mL per shift, the drain can be discontinued. Once the drain is removed, the patient should return for a postoperative visit within 1 week, to check for signs of cellulitis or seroma. If seroma is detected, sterile needle aspiration can be done. Despite careful surgical technique in the hands of experienced surgeons, perioperative complications of cellulitis, flap necrosis, or leg edema can occur in up to 30% of patients with host factors such as nutritional status, hygiene, and the presence of diabetes strongly influencing the clinical course (60).

A modification to groin dissection has been advocated as a means to decrease postoperative complications and includes a shorter skin incision, not dissecting lateral to the femoral artery and caudad to the fossa ovalis, preservation of the saphenous vein, and not transposing the sartorius muscle (61). Long-term follow-up also has suggested that this approach is effective (62). If a frozen section biopsy reveals disease, complete inguinal lymphadenectomy should be performed. Concerns that the modified dissection may understage patients with clinically negative nodes have been reported. Lopes et al. reported recurrences within the

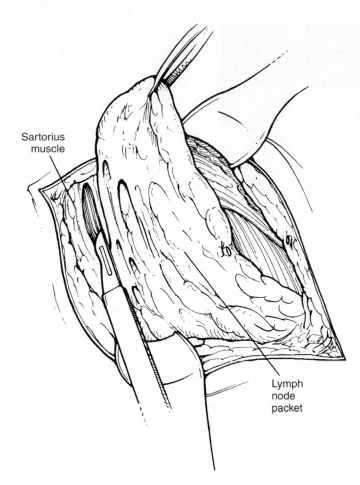

Sartorius
muscle

Lymph
node
packet

FIGURE 50.5. Standard inguinal lymphadenectomy, and showing the outer limit of dissection at the lateral margin of the femoral triangle. (From Colberg JW, Andriole GL, Catalona WJ. Penectomy and inguinal lymphadenectomy for carcinoma of the penis. In: Marshall FF, ed. Operative urology. Philadelphia: WB Saunders, 1996:643, with permission.)

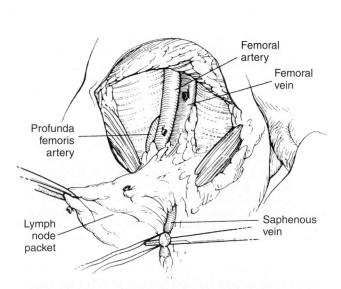

Femoral
artery

Femoral
vein

Profunda
femoris
artery

Lymph
node
packet

Saphenous
vein

FIGURE 50.6. Standard inguinal lymphadenectomy, showing the distal limit of dissection at the apex of the femoral triangle. (From Colberg JW, Andriole GL, Catalona WJ. Penectomy and inguinal lymphadenectomy for carcinoma of the penis. In: Marshall FF, ed. *Operative urology*. Philadelphia: WB Saunders, 1996:644, with permission.)

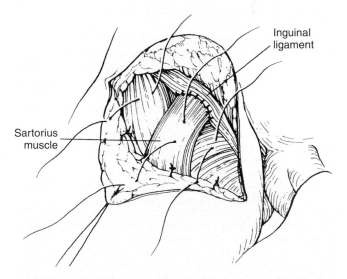

Inguinal
ligament

Sartorius
muscle

FIGURE 50.7. Standard inguinal lymphadenectomy. The sartorius muscle is divded from its origin at the anterosuperior iliac spine and rotated medially, where it is sutured to the inguinal ligament over the femoral vessels. (From Colberg JW, Andriole GL, Catalona WJ. Penectomy sund inguinal lymphadenectomy for carcinoma of the penis. In: Marshall FF, ed. *Operative urology*. Philadelphia: WB Saunders, 1996:641, with permission.)

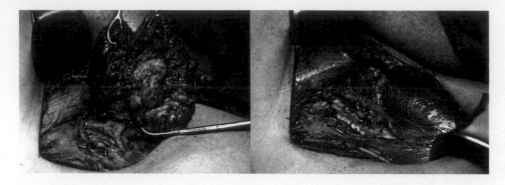

FIGURE 50.8. Groin dissection removal of nodal package and exposure of femoral vessels.

operative field in 2 of 13 patients (63). This modified operation removes the first echelon nodes in patients that are clinically free of adenopathy and is equivalent to a sentinel area biopsy, but in an era of lymphocintigraphy its future is limited. Modified node dissection should never be performed in patients with clinical adenopathy.

Complications of Lymph Node Dissection

There is a long list of potential complications after node dissection that can occur even in the most experienced of surgical hands. This explains the reluctance to propagate node dissection in every patient presenting with penile cancer. The most common complications are wound infection (10% to 20%), skin necrosis with or without wound dehiscence (14% to 65%), lymphocele/seroma (19% to 45%), and lymph edema (2% to 100%) (59,60). Choice of surgical incisions may decrease wound complications and it is important to realize the course of the vasculature of the inguinal skin in order to plan the incision as rationally as possible. In a series from Brazil, three types of incision were compared: a large bi-iliac incision, a transverse S-shaped incision, and a skin bridge technique with two separate incisions. The last showed the lowest percentage of skin necrosis and the least amount of lymph edema (32). Utmost care must be given to handling of the skin in order to preserve its viability. Antibiotic prophylaxis venodyne boots, and thrombosis prevention with low molecular heparin is strongly recommended. Individually fit stockings should be available immediate after surgery. Results with groin dissection are vastly improved when the operation is performed at tertiary centers with a significant experience. Investigators from M.D. Anderson Cancer Center described a contemporary experience with 106 lymphadenectomies in 53 patients operated on at their center between 1989 and 1998. They reported an overall rate of 68% minor and 32% major complications with incidence of major complications lower in patients undergoing prophylactic groin as opposed to therapeutic or palliative, suggesting that the extent of disease can impact on perioperative complications (64).

Pelvic Node Dissection

The role of pelvic (deep) node dissection in the surgical management of penile carcinoma is controversial. The position we generally take is as follows. If early inguinal node dissection is done and nodes are negative in the groins bilaterally, pelvic lymphadenectomy may be omitted because metastatic disease involving deep pelvic nodes and not inguinal nodes has not been reported (65). If therapeutic inguinal LND is done and metastatic disease is confirmed in one or both groins, we proceed with bilateral pelvic node dissection. Some have argued that metastatic pelvic nodes represent incurable cancer and that if such nodes are encountered in a preliminary exploration, then no further

dissection should be done (66). We proceed with pelvic dissection because of the absence of effective systemic therapy for advanced disease as well as concerns regarding local disease control. Metastatic squamous cell carcinoma can become a massive local problem creating leg edema, wound disruption, and vascular erosion that may cause significant patient morbidity or death in the absence of clinically detectable distant metastases. To that end, whenever possible, complete bilateral pelvic and bilateral inguinal LND is performed and all gross disease removed. Depending on the amount of lymph node metastases, 5-year survival can reach up to 25% (6). Anecdotally, long-term survivors with bulky pelvic nodal metastasis have been reported. Pelvic lymphadenectomy can be performed simultaneously with the inguinal dissection or as a separate procedure. In the first case, removal of the nodes through one or two incisions has been described. Most authors prefer two separate incisions. Comparison of various types of incisions showed the lowest complication rate when two incisions were used. The pelvic node dissection is either performed through a lower abdominal midline incision or a unilateral muscle- splitting incision. The boundaries of the pelvic node dissection are more extended than usual for staging prostate or bladder cancer. The rationale being that surgical removal of microscopic metastasis is of therapeutic benefit. Proximally the boundaries are the common iliac vessels, distally the passage of lymphatic vessels to the groin, laterally the ilio-inguinal nerve, medially the bladder and prostate and the bottom is the deepest part of the obturator fossa. The surgeon must dissect below the inguinal ligament to be certain that the Cloquet node is removed. Care must be given to a complete removal of the obturator fossa especially the space behind the external iliac vessels all the way to the exit place of the obturator nerve. A large node can usually be found there, and if left alone this node is prone to recurrence with intractable pain because of neural in growth. After the dissection, suction drains are left in place and removed if spontaneous drainage is less than 30 to 50 mL per shift.

Initial laparoscopic pelvic node dissection has been advocated for patients with inguinal adenopathy and if pelvic nodes are found to be metastatic, no further operative intervention is recommended. We do not agree with this approach, because achieving local tumor control, as mentioned earlier, is a worthy goal that may effectively palliate patients not yet experiencing distant metastatic disease. In addition, the absence of effective systemic chemotherapy for such patients means that their fate will be sealed without any attempt to cure (66).

Operation for Bulky Inguinal Metastasis: The Role of Myocutaneous Flaps

When a patient presents with a bulky groin metastasis with or without a draining nodal sinus, a substantial portion of overlying skin needs to be removed in order to achieve local tumor

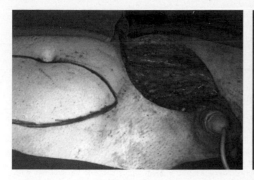
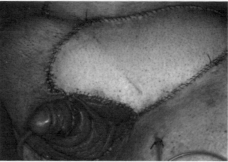

FIGURE 50.9. Use of contralateral rectus abdominus flap for myocutaneous coverage following resection of bulky groin metastasis.

control. Previously, many of these patients were considered inoperable and given palliative radiation therapy and local wound care, only to experience a miserable demise, often with local wound infections made worse by radiation or tumor erosion into vascular structures and exsanguination. The evolution of plastic surgical techniques utilizing skin stretching or myocutaneous flaps has given surgeons another option to achieve local control with minimal morbidity (67,68). Flaps that are especially effective in covering groin defects are the *tensor fascia lata* and *rectus abdmoninis flap*. The design of the overlying skin island can completely cover the wound defect without the need for a skin graft. These flaps are indicated for coverage of large wounds that cannot be closed primarily, fistulized groin wounds, and for wounds in previously irradiated fields subjected to salvage operations. Although few if any of these patients are cured, resection and myocutaneous wound coverage provides important palliation for patients with locally advanced penile cancer (Fig. 50.9).

Treatment of Inoperable Local Recurrence and Metastatic Disease

Following definitive surgical treatment of the primary and regional lymph nodes, patients with poor prognostic, high-grade, high-stage tumors are at risk for the development of regional recurrence and metastatic disease. Unfortunately, options are limited when this occurs and operative intervention usually plays no role.

CONCLUSION

In penile cancer, operative intervention is essential in the diagnosis and treatment of the primary lesion, management of the regional nodes, and effective palliation of bulky metastatic nodes. Effective local control of *in situ* or T1 tumors can be achieved by excision, laser ablation, and Mohs microsurgery. As the T stage increases, surgical resection with circumcision, partial penectomy, or total penectomy plays an increasingly important role in the management of these patients. Regional lymph nodes can be enlarged because of inflammation or early metastatic disease. A strong argument for aggressive diagnosis with aspiration cytology and biopsy or prophylactic groin dissection can be made for patients with high-grade invasive primary tumors as opposed to the traditional approach of protracted antibiotic administration and surveillance. The potential role of sentinel lymph node biopsy using lymphoscintigraphy for patients with invasive tumors and negative regional nodes is expanding as investigators gain more experience with the technique. This approach has the advantage of early detection of metastatic disease while at the same time sparing patients the unwanted morbidity of a negative groin dissection. The early data, however, indicates that if an SN biopsy is negative, careful clinical follow-up of the patient

remains necessary to detect either an ipsilateral or contralateral groin metastasis. For patients with bulky groin metastases or for patients who have recurred after groin irradiation, groin dissection with myocutaneous flaps can effectively cover large skin defects created during the resection of bulky inguinal nodes, draining sinuses, or previously irradiation groin wounds. Surgical intervention plays no role in the treatment of distant metastases from penile cancer.

References

1. Burgers JK, Badalament RA, Drago JR. Penile cancer: clinical presentation, diagnosis, and staging. *Urol Clin North Am* 1992;19:247–256.
2. Skinner DG, Leadbetter WF, Kelley SB. The surgical management of squamous cell carcinoma of the penis. *J Urol* 1972;107:273–277.
3. Gilliland FD, Key CR. Male genital cancers. *Cancer* 1995;75:295–315.
4. Lindegaard JC, Nielsen OS, Lundbeck FA, et al. A retrospective analysis of 82 cases of cancer of the penis. *Br J Urol* 1996;77:883–890.
5. Horenblas S, van Tinteren H. Squamous cell carcinoma of the penis, IV: prognostic factors of survival; analysis of tumor, nodes and metastasis classification system. *J Urol* 1994;151:1239–1243.
6. Emerson RE, Ulbright TM, Eble JN, et al. Predicting cancer progression in patients with penile squamous cell carcinoma: the importance of depth of invasion and vascular invasion. *Mod Pathol* 2001;14:963–968.
7. Horenblas S, van Tinteren H, Delemarre JF, et al. Squamous cell carcinoma of the penis, II: treatment of the primary tumor. *J Urol* 1992;147:1533–1538.
8. Slaton JW, Morgenstern N, Levy DA, et al. Tumor stage, vascular invasion and the percentage of poorly differentiated cancer: independent prognosticators for inguinal lymph node metastasis in penile squamous cancer. *J Urol* 2001;165:1138–1142.
9. Hoffman MA, Renshaw AA, Loughlin KR. Squamous cell carcinoma of the penis and microscopic pathological margins. *Cancer* 1999;85:1565–1568.
10. Bandieramonte G, Lepera P, Marchesini R, et al. Laser microsurgery of superficial lesions of the penis. *J Urol* 1987;138:315–319.
11. Windahl T, Hellsten S. Laser treatment of localized squamous cell carcinoma of the penis. *J Urol* 1995;154:1020–1023.
12. Tolia BM, Castro VL, Mouded IM, et al. Bowen's disease of the shaft of the penis: successful treatment with 5-fluorouracil. *Urology* 1976;7: 617–619.
13. van Bezooijen BP, Horenblas S, Meinhardt W, et al. Laser therapy for carcinoma in situ of the penis. *J Urol* 2001;166:1670–1671.
14. Brown MD, Zachary CB, Grekin RC, et al. Penile tumors: their management by Mohs micrographic surgery. *J Dermatol Surg Oncol* 1987;13: 1163–1167.
15. Mohs FE, Snow SN, Larson PO. Mohs micrographic surgery for penile tumors. *Urol Clin North Am* 1992;19:291–304.
16. Lont AP, Besnard AP, Gallee MP, et al. A comparison of physical examination and imaging in determining the extent of primary penile carcinoma. *BJU Int* 2003;91:493–495.
17. Horenblas S, van Tinteren H, Delemarre JFM, et al. Squamous cell carcinoma of the penis: treatment of the primary lesion. *J Urol* 1992;147: 1533–1538.
18. Horenblas S, Newling DW. Local recurrent tumour after penis-conserving therapy: a plea for long-term follow-up. *Br J Urol* 1993;72:976.
19. Seixas AL, Ornellas AA, Marota A, et al. Verrucous carcinoma of the penis: retrospective analysis of 32 cases. *J Urol* 1994;152:1476–1479.
20. Bissada NK, Yakout HH, Fahmy WE, et al. Multi-institutional long-term experience with conservative surgery for invasive penile carcinoma. *J Urol* 2003;169:500–502.
21. Horenblas S, van Tinteren H, Delemarre JFM, et al. Squamous cell carcinoma of the penis, II: treatment of the primary tumor. *J Urol* 1992;147: 1533–1538.
22. Willis RA. *The spread of tumors in the human body*, 3rd ed. London: Butterworth, 1973.

23. Demkow T. The treatment of penile carcinoma: experience in 64 cases. *Int Urol Nephrol* 1999;31:525–531.

24. Theodorescu D, Russo P, Zhang ZF, et al. Outcomes of initial surveillance of invasive squamous cell carcinoma of the penis and negative nodes. *J Urol* 1996;155:1626–1631.

25. Ayyappan K, Ananthakrishnan N, Sankaran V. Can regional lymph node involvement be predicted in patients with carcinoma of the penis? *Br J Urol* 1994;73:549–553.

26. Bouchot O, Auvigne J, Peuvrel P, et al. Management of regional lymph nodes in carcinoma of the penis. *Eur Urol* 1989;16:410–415.

27. Kamat MR, Kulkarni JN, Tongaonkar HB. Carcinoma of the penis: the Indian experience. *J Surg Oncol* 1993;52:50–55.

28. Lynch DF, Schellhammer PF. Penectomy and ilioinguinal dissection. In: Scher HI, Oesterling J, eds. *Urol Oncol*. Philadelphia, PA: WB Saunders, 1997:618–633.

29. Kulkarni JN, Kamat MR. Prophylactic bilateral groin node dissection versus prophylactic radiotherapy and surveillance in patients with N0 and N1-2A carcinoma of the penis. *Eur Urol* 1994;26:123–128.

30. Lopes A, Hidalgo GS, Kowalski LP, et al. Prognostic factors in carcinoma of the penis: multivariate analysis of 145 patients treated with amputation and lymphadenectomy. *J Urol* 1996;156:1637–1642.

31. Mukamel E, deKernion JB. Early versus delayed lymph-node dissection versus no lymph-node dissection in carcinoma of the penis. *Urol Clin North Am* 1987;14:707–711.

32. Ornellas AA, Seixas AL, Marota A, et al. Surgical treatment of invasive squamous cell carcinoma of the penis: retrospective analysis of 350 cases. *J Urol* 1994;151:1244–1249.

33. Solsona E, Iborra I, Ricos JV, et al. Corpus cavernosum invasion and tumor grade in the prediction of lymph node condition in penile carcinoma. *Eur Urol* 1992;22:115–118.

34. Catalona WJ. Role of lymphadenectomy in carcinoma of the penis. *Urol Clin North Am* 1980;7:785–792.

35. Cabanas RM. Anatomy and biopsy of sentinel lymph nodes. *Urol Clin North Am* 1992;19:267–276.

36. Colberg JW, Andriole GL, Catalona WJ. Penectomy and inguinal lymphadenectomy for carcinoma of the penis. In: Marshall FF, ed. *Operative Urology*. Philadelphia, PA: WB Saunders, 1996:634–646.

37. Cabanas RM. An approach for the treatment of penile carcinoma. *Cancer* 1977;39:456–466.

38. Horenblas S, Jansen L, Meinhardt W, et al. Detection of occult metastasis in squamous cell carcinoma of the penis using a dynamic sentinel node procedure. *J Urol* 2000;163:100–104.

39. Aboard AS, deKernion JB. Controversies in ilioinguinal lymphadenectomy for cancer of the penis. *Urol Clin North Am* 1992;19:319–324.

40. Horenblas S, van Tinteren H, Delemarre JF, et al. Squamous cell carcinoma of the penis: accuracy of tumor, nodes and metastasis classification system, and role of lymphangiography, computerized tomography scan and fine needle aspiration cytology. *J Urol* 1991;146:1279–1283.

41. Scappini P, Piscioli F, Pusiol T, et al. Penile cancer: aspiration biopsy cytology for staging. *Cancer* 1986;58:1526–1533.

42. Johnson DE, Lo RK. Management of regional lymph nodes in penile carcinoma: five-year results following therapeutic groin dissections. *Urology* 1984;24:308–311.

43. McDougall WS, Kirchner FK, Edwards RH, et al. Treatment of carcinoma of the penis. The case for primary lymphadenectomy. *J Urol* 1986;136: 38–41.

44. McDougall WS. Carcinoma of the penis: improved survival by early regional lymphadenectomy based on the histological grade and depth of invasion of the primary lesion. *J Urol* 1995;154:1364–1366.

45. Perinetti E, Crane DB, Catalona WJ. Unreliability of sentinel lymph node biopsy for staging of penile carcinoma. *J Urol* 1980;124:734–735.

46. Fowler JE. Sentinel lymph node biopsy for staging penile cancer. *Urology* 1984;23:352–354.

47. Wespes E, Simon J, Schulman CC. Cabanas approach: is sentinel node biopsy reliable for staging penile carcinoma? *Urology* 1986;28:278–279.

48. Pettaway CA, Pisters LL, Dinney CP, et al. Sentinel lymph node dissection for penile carcinoma: the MD Anderson Cancer Center experience. *J Urol* 1995;154:1999–2003.

49. Morton DL, Wen D-R, Wong JH, et al. Technical details of intraoperative lymphatic mapping for early stage melanoma. *Arch Surg* 1992;127: 392–399.

50. Alex JC, Weaver DL, Fairbank JT, et al. Gamma-probe-guided lymph node localization in malignant melanoma. *Surg Oncol* 1993;2:303–308.

51. Reintgen DS. Chaining standards of surgical care the melanoma patient. *Ann Surg Oncol* 1996;3:327–328.

52. Wang X, Heller R, VanVoorheis N, et al. Detection of submicroscopic lymph node metastasis with polymerase chain reaction in patients with malignant melanoma. *Ann Surg* 1994;220:768–774.

53. Essner R. The role of lymphoscintigraphy and sentinel node mapping in assessing patient risk in melanoma. *Sem Oncol* 1997;24S:8–10.

54. Tanis PJ, Lont AP, Meinhardt W, et al. Dynamic sentinel node biopsy for penile cancer: reliability of a staging technique. *J Urol* 2002;168: 76–80.

55. Horenblas S. Lymphadenectomy for squamous cell carcinoma of the penis, Part 1: diagnosis of lymph node metastasis. *BJU Int* 2001;88:467–472.

56. Lont AP, Horenblas S, Tanis PJ, et al. Management of clinically node negative penile carcinoma: improved survival after the introduction of dynamic sentinel node biopsy. *J Urol* 2003;170:783–786.

57. Kroon BK, Horenblas S, Estourgie SH, et al. How to avoid false negative dynamic sentinel node procedures in penile carcinoma. *J Urol* 2004;171: 2191–2194.

58. Whitmore WF, Vagaiwala MR Jr. A technique of ilioinguinal lymph node dissection for carcinoma of the penis. *Surg Gynecol Obstet* 1984;159: 573–578.

59. Horenblas S. Lymphadenectomy for squamous cell carcinoma of the penis, part 2: the role and technique of lymph node dissection. *BJU Int* 2001;88: 473–483.

60. Ravi R. Morbidity following groin dissection for penile carcinoma. *Br J Urol* 1993;72:941–945.

61. Catalona WJ. Modified inguinal lymphadenectomy for cancer of the preservation of saphenous veins: technique and preliminary results. *J Urol* 1988;140:306–310.

62. Colberg JW, Andriole GL, Catalona WJ. Long-term follow up of men undergoing modified inguinal lymphadenectomy for carcinoma of the penis. *Br J Urol* 1997;79:54–57.

63. Lopes A, Rossi BM, Fonseca FP, et al. Unreliability of modified inguinal lymphadenectomy for clinical staging of penile carcinoma. *Cancer* 1996; 77:2099–2102.

64. Bevan-Thomas R, Slaton J, Pettaway CA. Contemporary morbidity from lymphadenectomy for penile squamous cell carcinoma: the MD Anderson Cancer Center Experience. *J Urol* 2002;167:1638–1642.

65. Srinivas V, Morse MJ, Herr HW, et al. Penile cancer: relation of the extent of nodal metastasis to survival. *J Urol* 1987;137:880–882.

66. Rutstalis DB, Gerber GS, Vogelzang NJ, et al. Laparoscopic pelvic lymph node dissection: a review of 102 consecutive cases. *J Urol* 1994;151: 670–674.

67. Melis P, Bos KE, Horenblas S. Primary skin closure of a large groin defect after inguinal lymphadenectomy for penile cancer using a skin stretching device. *J Urol* 1998;159:185–187.

68. Russo P, Saldana EF, Yu S, et al. Myocutaneous flaps in genitourinary oncology. *J Urol* 1994;151:920–924.

CHAPTER 51 ■ RADIATION THERAPY FOR PENILE CANCER

JUANITA M. CROOK

INTRODUCTION

Carcinoma of the penis is rare, with an estimated incidence of approximately 1 in 100,000 men in North American and Western European countries, and accounts for a total of <1% of cancers in men. Extirpative surgery is highly effective, especially for early-stage disease, but can be associated with considerable psychosexual morbidity. Opjordsmoen reported on 30 men successfully treated for penile cancer with an average of 80 months of follow-up. A semistructured interview and self-administered questionnaire were used to evaluate the state of their sexual health. Men treated by irradiation had the fewest problems with posttreatment sexual activity, whereas those treated with partial penectomy frequently reported sexual activity that was severely reduced or completely lacking (1,2). Other series include reports of suicide or attempted suicide following partial penectomy (3–5).

Radiotherapy, either external or interstitial, is an organsparing alternative that preserves penile morphology and functions without compromising disease control or survival in select patients. Unfortunately, many urologists do not routinely offer this penis-conserving option. A recent study by Harden and Tan surveyed 289 urologists and 237 oncologists in the United Kingdom (6). Participants were presented with four case scenarios of penile cancer. Even for a small, distally situated lesion on the glans, 43% of urologists suggested amputative surgery. For a 4-cm lesion located distally on the glans, 82% preferred surgery. Quality of life and sexual health following such surgery is rarely studied or reported. Although some men might, if necessary, sacrifice sexual activity in favor of improved long-term survival, the converse may equally well apply. Posttreatment sexuality and expectations should be discussed when deciding on primary management.

Penis-conserving surgical techniques such as laser or Moh surgery may be suitable for carcinoma in situ (CIS) or very superficial tumors. These techniques are discussed in detail in the chapter on surgical management of penile cancer.

Because of the rarity of carcinoma of the penis, many series span several decades, and treatment reflects the evolution of techniques over this time span. No fewer than three different staging systems are encountered in a review of the literature of the past two decades (Table 51.1). However, despite the medley of techniques, doses, and staging systems, a common theme throughout the radiotherapy literature is the lack of accurate pathologic staging (5,7). Clinical staging of carcinoma of the penis is very subjective and, in many cases, it is impossible to distinguish T1 (invasion of subepithelial connective tissue) from T2 (invasion of corpus spongiosum or cavernosum). For this reason, techniques that treat less than the full thickness of the penis must be restricted to very carefully selected cases.

RADIOTHERAPY TECHNIQUES

External

External radiotherapy has several advantages as the radiation modality of choice for carcinoma of the penis. It is widely available, delivers a reliably homogeneous dose, and does not require the specific expertise of brachytherapy. Well-localized CIS (Tis) may be treated effectively to a depth of less than full thickness of the penile shaft using 125 to 250 kV orthovoltage beams, or 13 MeV electrons (11), using fractionation schemes commonly employed for skin cancer such as 35 Gy in 10 fractions over 2 weeks. However, most penile cancers, because of uncertainty of the depth of invasion, require irradiation to the full thickness of the penis with full dose to the skin surface. Various techniques have been devised for this purpose. Fraction sizes <2 Gy (4) may be associated with higher recurrence rates, whereas fraction sizes >2 Gy (12) may be associated with greater long-term sequelae such as urethral strictures. The most commonly prescribed dose is 60 Gy in 30 fractions over 6 weeks. Treatment interruptions because of acute reactions (edema, pain, desquamation) should be avoided (4). Circumcision should be done before definitive radiotherapy to prevent acute radiation balanitis. A setup that is easily reproducible over a 6-week period, comfortable for the patient despite increasing local reaction, and easily verified by technologists is desirable.

Wax Block

A 10 × 10 cm to 10 × 15 cm wax block is used to encompass the penis for each treatment (11,13). The block is constructed in two halves, with a central cylindrical chamber fashioned internally. The patient is positioned supine on the treatment couch, and the penis is supported in a vertical position, encased in the wax block. A tissue-equivalent "cork" must be placed in the opening. Parallel opposed beams treat the entire length of the penis. External radiation using ^{60}Co, or 4 to 6 MV photons can be used (Fig. 51.1).

The disadvantages of this technique are that it becomes increasingly uncomfortable for the patient as the treatment progresses. Penile swelling may require modification of the wax block to fit it over the penis. Furthermore, it is impossible for technicians to verify penile position within the wax. Unless the patient is catheterized throughout the 6 weeks of treatment, the penis may "slump" inside the wax, resulting in treatment of a shorter length of the shaft than planned.

TABLE 51.1

STAGING SYSTEMS FOR CARCINOMA OF THE PENIS COMMONLY SEEN IN THE LITERATURE

A. *Jackson staging system for carcinoma of the penis (8)*
1. Tumor limited to the glans or prepuce
2. Tumor extending into the shaft or corpora, without node involvement
3. Tumor confined to the shaft, with malignant but operable lymph nodes
4. Invasion beyond the shaft, with inoperable lymph nodes or distant metastases

B. *TNM staging UICC 1978 (9)*
Tis: CIS
T1: ≤2 cm
T2: >2 cm and ≤5 cm
T3: >5 cm or deep invasion including urethra
T4: tumor invades adjacent structures
N1: metastases in unilateral inguinal lymph nodes
N2: metastases in bilateral inguinal lymph nodes
N3: fixed inguinal lymph nodes

C. *TNM staging UICC 1987–2002 (10)*
T1: subepithelial connective tissue
T2: corpus spongiosum/cavernosum
T3: urethra/prostate
T4: other adjacent structures
N1: one superficial inguinal lymph node
N2: multiple/bilateral superficial inguinal lymph nodes
N3: deep inguinal or pelvic lymph nodes

UICC, union internationale contre le cancer; CIS, carcinoma *in situ*; TNM, tumor, nodes, metastases.

Perspex Block

The use of a Perspex block (4) follows the same principles as the wax block technique, providing full buildup to the skin surface and allowing treatment by parallel opposed beams. Blocks can

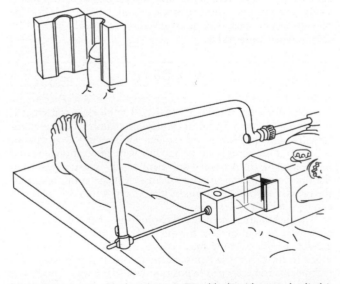

FIGURE 51.1. Wax block technique. Wax block with central cylindrical chamber for penis provides full buildup of dose to skin surface for parallel opposed mega voltage beams. (From McLean M, Akl AM, Warde P, et al. The results of primary radiation therapy in the management of squamous cell carcinoma of the penis. *Int J Radiat Oncol Biol Phys* 1993;25:623–628, with permission.)

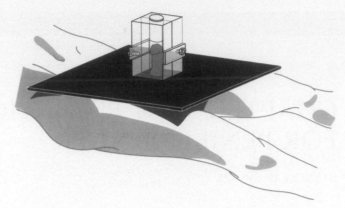

FIGURE 51.2. Perspex block technique. Blocks provide full buildup as in the wax block technique but are transparent for verification of penile position. The blocks are bivalved and can be made in a range of sizes to accommodate penile swelling as treatment progresses.

be preconstructed with a range of sizes of the central cylindrical chamber and be sterilized for reuse. They have several advantages over wax blocks. Penile swelling can be accommodated easily by choosing the next larger size, and penile position within the transparent block can be easily verified visually before each treatment (Fig. 51.2).

Water Bath

Sagerman et al. (14) and Vujovic and Stewart (15) have reported a technique for external beam irradiation of the penis using a water bath in place of wax or Perspex to provide full dosage to the penile surface. A watertight rectangular box (9 × 9 15.5 cm) can be constructed out of 4 mm thick acrylic sheet and bonded with solvent cement to a square base with sides to catch the water overflow. The patient is positioned prone on the treatment couch, the upper and lower portions of his body supported on Styrofoam slabs, with the water bath positioned to contain the suspended penis (Fig. 51.3). This technique has the advantages of easy visual inspection of correct positioning and does not require daily manipulation of the penis by technologists. It results in the least discomfort for the patient during a protracted course of radiotherapy as the acute reaction intensifies. Beam arrangement and fractionation are the same as for wax or Perspex blocks.

Brachytherapy

The penis is well suited to brachytherapy. For centers with appropriate expertise, either surface molds or interstitial techniques can be used with good effect. Circumcision should be performed before brachytherapy to ensure complete exposure of the tumor and prevent subsequent phimosis or annular fibrosis of the foreskin.

Molds

Neave et al. (12) has reported experience with iridium molds for Jackson stage 1 or 2 (8) (Table 51.1) penile carcinoma. A hollow cylindrical Perspex tube is fitted over the penis along its long axis and is held in place by a girdle fitting around the patient's groin and upper thighs. Iridium 192 wire is arranged circumferentially in concentric rings in a second outer source-carrying tube, which is positioned daily by the patient and is worn for approximately 12 hours each day until the prescribed dosage is reached. Hospitalization for the duration of

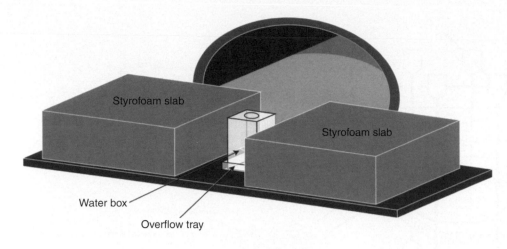

FIGURE 51.3. Water bath technique. The patient lies prone on the Styrofoam slabs such that the penis will be suspended in the water bath. The overflow tray catches the runoff. Transparent sides on the water bath permit visual check of penile position.

treatment is required, and the patient must be cooperative, with good eyesight and coordination. One advantage of the mold technique over external beam radiation therapy (EBRT) is that the acute reaction develops after the treatment is finished. Unlike interstitial brachytherapy, a mold is not invasive and dosage does not require anesthesia. A surface dose of 55 to 60 Gy (16) is prescribed, with a central axis dose of 46 to 50 Gy. Although the authors did not describe the dosage rate, the total treatment duration is approximately 1 week.

Akamoto et al. (17) has reported a custom mold technique using silicon monomer. The penis is suspended using traction on a catheter to hold it centrally in a plastic cylinder. Silicon monomer mixed with a catalyst is poured into the cylinder, around the penis, and hardens into a spongelike material within 10 minutes. The material can be removed easily after it has set, and hollow catheters are inserted longitudinally for after-loading sources. The authors describe using a variety of sources over the duration covered by their report, including ^{226}Ra, ^{137}Cs, and ^{192}Ir. Patients were treated with one to three fractions. Fraction size ranged from 10.7 to 40 Gy (median 20 Gy), with total dosages ranging from 32 to 74 Gy.

Interstitial Brachytherapy

There is a wide experience with interstitial brachytherapy for T1 and T2 penile carcinoma, with reports from many European countries, from Canada, and from India. Implants are generally performed under general anesthesia but also are possible under local or spinal anesthesia. The Paris system of dosimetry (18) is most commonly employed and is applicable to both manually after-loaded implants and remote after-loading pulse dose rate (PDR), although for the latter, some optimization can be introduced.

Penile brachytherapy is generally performed as a volume implant delivering treatment to the full thickness of the glans, although well-selected, very superficial tumors, or T1s disease, may be treated with a single-plane implant. For volume implants, two or three parallel planes of sources are inserted, with intersource and interplane spacing being equal and ranging from 12 to 18 mm.

The distribution, spacing, and total number of needles depend on tumor size. Four (2 × 2), six (2 × 3) or nine (3 × 3) needles may be required. Planes are usually oriented with the needles passing from the dorsal to the ventral surface of the glans, but a left–right orientation may be acceptable depending on tumor location. Needle placement requires 30 to 45 minutes in the operating room. Catheterization of the patient during the procedure aids in identification of the urethra so as

to avoid transfixing it with implant needles. The 19.5-gauge needles are used in association with manually after-loaded ^{192}Ir wire, and 17.5-gauge needles are compatible with a PDR remote after-loader. The needles are held in place through the duration of the implant with predrilled plexiglass templates. The prescribed dose is generally 60 Gy at a classic low dose rate (LDR) of 50 to 60 cGy/hr (<1 Gy/hr). No dosage rate correction is required for PDR as compared with continuous LDR. The total duration is 100 to 120 hours (4 to 5 days). A Styrofoam collar is positioned around the base of the penis proximal to the needles to support the penis and to thereby minimize unnecessary irradiation of the adjacent abdominal wall, thigh, or scrotal skin. If preservation of fertility is a concern, a thin sheet of lead can be inserted into the Styrofoam collar to minimize transmitted dosage to the testicles.

The brachytherapy needles are remarkably well tolerated. The patient remains catheterized and in bed for the duration of the implant, although with PDR the source cables can be disconnected from the needles to allow the patient to mobilize for a brief period between fractions if desired. Sufficient analgesia is usually provided by acetaminophen, with or without codeine. Leg exercises and subcutaneous heparin (5,000 U q12h) are recommended as prophylaxis against deep vein thrombosis. Removal of the needles occurs at the bedside following premedication with a narcotic analgesic.

Interstitial brachytherapy has the advantage of being completed within 4 to 5 days, and, like mold therapy, the acute reaction peaks after the treatment is finished. Interstitial brachytherapy treats the least amount of the penile shaft, and because the lesion is clearly visible as the needles are being placed, visual verification of coverage can be readily accomplished. Care must be taken to adhere to the rules of the Paris system (18) and to be aware of the relation of the treated volume to the needles such that all needles are placed to contain the entire tumor and desired margin within the high-dose volume (Fig. 51.4).

RESULTS OF TREATMENT

Results for several recent series in the literature are summarized in Table 51.2. Except for the collaborative report of Rozan et al. from several centers in France (7), the number of patients in each series is relatively small. Often series span several decades, during which treatment techniques evolve and dose prescription changes. Staging systems also undergo major modifications. The three most commonly seen in the select literature [Jackson (8), TNM 1978 (9) and TNM 1992 (10)] are shown in Table 51.1.

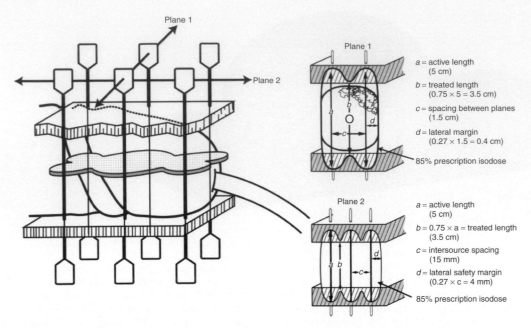

FIGURE 51.4. Interstitial brachytherapy according to Paris system of dosimetry. A two-plane, six-needle implant is shown.

TABLE 51.2

COMPARATIVE RESULTS FROM RADIOTHERAPY SERIES

Author (ref.) yr	n	Type RT	Dose, Gy	F/up, mo	LC by RT 5 yr	CSS[a] 5 yr	Complications	Penile preservation
Chaudhary et al. (19) 1999	23	BT	50	21 (4–117)	70% (8 yr)		No necrosis 2/23 stenosis	70% (8 yr)
Crook et al. (20) 2002	30	BT	60	34 (6–103)	76%	85.4%	1/30 necrosis 3/30 stenosis	83% Crude
Delannes et al. (21) 1992	51	BT	50–65	65 (12–144)	86% crude	85%	23% necrosis 45% stenosis	75%
Kiltie et al. (22) 2000	31	BT	63.5	61.5	81%	85.4%	8% necrosis 44% stenosis	75%
Mazeron et al. (23) 1984	50	BT	60–70	36–96	78% crude		6% necroses 19% stenoses	74%
Rozan et al. (7) 1995	184	BT	63	139	86%	88%	21% necrosis 45% stenosis	78%
Soria et al. (5) 1997	102	BT	61–70	111	77%	72%	Not stated	72% (6 %)
Gotsadze et al. (24) 2000	155	Ext	40–60	4 decades experience	65%	86%	Necrosis: 1 Stenosis: 5	65%
McLean et al. (11) 1993	26	Ext	35/10–60/25	116 (84–168) —	61.5%	69% CSS	7/26 unspec.	66% Crude
Neave et al. (12) 1993	24 20	Mold Ext Ext	55.6 50–55 /20–22	36 min 36 min	69.7%	67% 58%	13% stenosis 10% stenosis	55% 60%
Sarin et al. (4) 1997	59	Ext	60/30	62 (2–264)	55%	66%	3% necrosis 9/59 stenosis	50% crude
Zouhair et al. (13) 2001	23	Ext	45–74 @1.8–2 Gy/ fraction	12 (5–139)	41%		2/23 stenosis	36%

RT, radiotherapy; F/up, follow-up; LC, local control; BT, brachytherapy; Ext, external radiotherapy.
[a]Corrected for intercurrent deaths.

TABLE 51.3

TYPE OF SALVAGE SURGERY FOR LOCAL RECURRENCE AFTER RADIOTHERAPY

Study	Local excision	Partial penectomy	Total penectomy
Chaudhary et al. (19)		4	every case
Crook et al. (20)		3	2
Delannes et al. (21)		4	3
Kiltie et al. (22)		2	3
Rozan et al. (7)	3	16	12
Zouhair et al. (13)	1	6	7

From Table 51.2 it can readily be appreciated that radical radiotherapy, as either brachytherapy or EBRT, is effective in achieving local control in a high percentage of patients. Surgery for salvage is highly effective with success rates in excess of 80% (7,13). As in primary management, local excision is rarely appropriate as surgical salvage. Salvage operations are equally divided between total and partial penectomy (7,13,21,22,25) (Table 51.3. The type of salvage procedure depends on penile length and the proportion of the shaft irradiated by the primary treatment. Brachytherapy, because of the more localized treatment volume, should lend itself to a less radical salvage operation, but this is not reflected in the literature.

Interstitial brachytherapy results in 5-year local tumor–control rates of 70% to 86% and results in penile preservation rates at 5 years that range from 72% to 83%. External radiotherapy does not appear to be quite as effective in local control of the primary tumor (41% to 70% at 5 years), but local failures are readily salvaged by surgery. Penile preservation rates reflect the more frequent need for second line surgery after external radiation as compared with brachytherapy and range from 36% to 66%. Careful extended follow-up is recommended, as local failures can occur several years after treatment. Mazeron et al. reported that of the 11 local failures in his series of 50 patients treated by interstitial brachytherapy, only 36% were in the first 2 years, whereas 45% occurred between years 2 and 5, and 18% between years 5 and 8 (23).

PATIENT SELECTION

Several factors have been identified to predict for successful penile preservation. For external radiotherapy, failures are dose-related. Sarin et al. identified that a total dose <60 Gy, a protracted treatment time of >45 days or a daily fraction size of <2 Gy were all associated with an increased risk of local failure (4). The report of Zouhair et al. included a range of doses from 45 Gy to 74 Gy and fraction sizes of 1.8 Gy to 2 Gy. The authors explain their inferior local control rate (41%) as likely dose related. Only 5 of the 14 patients with local failures in this series received a dose ≥64 Gy (13).

For patients treated with brachytherapy, the size or volume of the tumor, and the depth of invasion (5,7,22,23) are predictive of local control. The ideal tumor for brachytherapy should be <4 cm in maximum diameter (5,20,22,23), with <1 cm of invasion (5,23) Kiltie et al. reported a local failure rate of 60% for tumors ≥4 cm and 14% for those <4 cm. Those that required more than six brachytherapy needles to encompass their volume were associated with a 75% failure rate (22). Rozan et al. found that tumor volumes >8 mL were associated with an increased risk of failure (7). Mazeron et al. reported 11% local failure for T1 (<2 cm), 22% for T2 (2 to 5 cm), and 29% for T3 (TNM 1979) (23). Soria et al. found that invasion of the corpora was an independent predictor of both overall and disease-free survival in multivariate analysis (5).

Histopathology does not appear to be a factor in local control. Most penile cancers are well-differentiated squamous cell carcinomas. Soria reported a more favorable outcome for the 9% verrucous cancers in his experience, but most series do not report on this pathology subtype. Although moderate to poor differentiation influences overall survival and the risk of nodal involvement (20), it does not preclude a penile conserving approach to treatment.

TOXICITY: ACUTE REACTION

The acute reaction (moist desquamation) after brachytherapy peaks in 2 to 3 weeks, but it may take 2 to 3 months to heal completely. Local hygiene is important, including frequent soaks in baking soda and water. An open-ended telfa tube over the penis and glans is helpful until re-epithelialization is complete. Sterile distal urethritis is common. Adhesions, causing a divided or deviated urinary stream, should be separated by passing an 18-French Foley catheter partway into the penis. Intercourse can be resumed as soon as the patient is comfortable, but as the healing epithelium is fragile, additional water based lubricant is recommended.

The acute reaction to EBRT peaks during treatment and may involve edema of the penile shaft and more extensive desquamation, but otherwise management is similar to that for patients undergoing brachytherapy.

LATE REACTIONS

The two most common late complications of radiotherapy for penile cancer are soft tissue necrosis and urethral stenosis. Both can occur with either EBRT or brachytherapy (Table 51.2).

Soft Tissue Necrosis

Soft tissue necrosis is reported in 0% to 23% of patients and is related to dose and type of treatment. It is reported with greater frequency after brachytherapy than after external radiation. Necrosis is the most common reason for failure of penile conservation in a tumor-free penis. Rozan reported that 11 of 34 total or partial amputations were performed because of posttreatment soft tissue necrosis and found that the risk of necrosis/fibrosis increased with increasing dosages of more than 60 Gy (7). No cases were seen in the series by Chaudhary et al. where the brachytherapy dose was limited to 50 Gy (19). Mazeron has reported an increased risk of necrosis with T3 tumors (TNM 1979) (23). Rozan et al. reported that both implant volume (>30 mL, $P = .01$) and number of needle planes (no. of planes >2, $P = .001$) were predictive of subsequent necrosis (7).

Prevention and Management

The peak time for soft tissue ulceration is 7 to 18 months after brachytherapy (21), but it can occur much later. Causative factors include trauma and cold exposure. Patients should be counseled to use additional water-based lubricant for intercourse and to dress appropriately in cold winter climates. The poorly vascularized tissue of the irradiated glans is more prone to frostbite. Areas of ulceration should be treated conservatively with attention to good hygiene, antibiotic, and steroid creams. Biopsy should be avoided unless there is a strong suspicion of concomitant tumor. A deeper or painful area of necrosis may respond well to hyperbaric oxygen treatment (26). If such treatment is available, it should be tried before resorting to amputation.

Urethral Stenosis

Urethral stenosis is reported in 10% to 45% of patients and tends to occur later in the follow-up period but usually before 3 years. It appears to be dose-related for external beam radiation, seen in 30% of the series studied by Duncan and Jackson (27) where a hypofractionated treatment regimen was used (50 to 57.5 Gy in 16 fractions). Rozan et al. reported that, for brachytherapy, the only factor predictive of urethral stenosis was the number of needle planes used in the implant ($P = .001$ for >2 planes) (7).

Prevention and Management

When a three-plane implant is indicated because of tumor size or morphology, needle positions are, of necessity, much closer to the urethra. When using PDR remote after-loading rather than manually loaded iridium wires, optimization of dwell times can limit the urethral dose under these circumstances.

Urethral adhesions in the acute reaction phase should be separated and the distal urethra dilated with an 18- to 20-Fr Foley catheter. With proper management, these will not become a chronic problem. Many late urethral stenoses are low grade and can be managed with repeat dilatations, often at infrequent intervals. In more troublesome cases, patients also can be taught to perform this themselves at regular intervals. Severe cases may require reconstructive surgery, such as urethroplasty or meatoplasty (21–23).

SEXUAL FUNCTION

There is no systematic study available in the literature dealing with sexual function and satisfaction following radiotherapy for penile cancer. The impact on sexual function is often not routinely documented in these retrospective reports (4,5,22). Crook et al. reported that "sexually active men resumed intercourse in a few weeks. Two men reported a loss of potency after implantation" (20). Delannes et al. noted that apart from a patient who developed painful erections due to sclerosis, "sexual function did not appear to be altered by the implant" (21). Sarin et al. provided details for only 14 of the 59 patients, noting that 12 were normal and 2 had minor impairment (4). Mazeron et al. stated that for noninfiltrating or moderately infiltrating tumors <4 cm, "sexual function remained the same as before treatment" (23).

Thermoluminescent dosimeters (TLD) measurements for PDR penile brachytherapy after incorporation of a layer of 2 mm of lead into the Styrofoam collar around the penis indicate a total dose of 53 to 58 cGy to the anterior testicle and of 26 cGy to the posterior testicle (Crook, personal experience). No data is available on postbrachytherapy sperm counts.

OTHER SEQUELAE

Other commonly observed sequelae are not usually of consequence. Mottled hypo- or hyperpigmentation can occur in the treated area, as can telangiectasia and mild to moderate focal fibrosis. Some atrophy of the glans may occur, especially in areas of deep tumor infiltration. Sandeman reported disappointing cosmetic results for 26 patients with T1-T2 tumors treated with EBRT using a wax block technique, but no details were provided as to the total dosage or fractionation scheme employed (28).

LYMPH NODE MANAGEMENT: THE N0 PATIENT

Treatment of the patients with clinically negative groins remains controversial. Most radiotherapy series report, and continue to recommend, a "wait and see" policy with no systematic staging investigations such as computed tomography (CT) scans or final needle aspiration (5,7,21–23). Overall, only approximately 20% of clinically negative nodes will harbor micrometastases (5,29), a figure that does not warrant the morbidity of staging lymph node dissection for all patients.

Furthermore, only 50% of clinically palpable suspicious nodes actually will be histologically positive (30). Inguinal node dissection may be complicated in one-third of cases by infection, skin flap necrosis requiring a secondary skin graft, deep vein thrombosis (31–33), or severe leg edema that interferes with ambulation.

However, nodal status is known to be the strongest predictive factor for overall survival (5,34,35). Lymph node dissection may be a curative procedure for men with microscopic regional spread. Several surgical series have identified that therapeutic node dissection is associated with an inferior survival rate than prophylactic node dissection. McDougal found a 5-year survival following inguinal node dissection in Jackson stage 2 patients who were clinically N0 of 92%, whereas for those with clinically involved nodes, 5-year survival was only 33% (36). Parra has reported reduced morbidity for a technique of modified inguinal lymphadenectomy that spares the saphenous vein and limits the dissection laterally, distally, and proximally. In 12 cases, there was no incidence of flap necrosis or leg edema (33).

The surgical literature has established histopathologic factors that allow prophylactic inguinal node dissection to be offered to select patients at high risk for microscopic regional spread. Theodorescu reported on a series of 42 patients who were initially clinically node negative, 62% of whom became node positive, 50% within 1.4 years and 75% within 2.8 years. Grade was the strongest predictive factor for regional failure, which occurred in only 30% of well differentiated tumors but in 81% of moderately to poorly differentiated primary tumors (32). Slaton et al. reported on 48 patients, 18 of whom demonstrated regional failure. He found that T stage, vascular invasion and the presence of >50% poorly differentiated cancer in the primary tumor predicted for nodal relapse. None of the pathologic T1 cancers had vascular invasion or subsequent nodal failure (35). McDougal also found that tumor grade and the presence of corporeal invasion (T stage) were the strongest predictors of nodal relapse. Patients initially presenting with clinically negative nodes, but who had either poorly differentiated cancers or invasion of the corpora, had a 78% rate of node positivity. On the contrary, patients with well or moderately differentiated tumors and no invasion of the corpora had only a 4% rate of regional spread (36).

The difficulty with applying this information to decision making in radiotherapy is that the primary tumor is not available for complete histopathologic examination. The all-important presence of invasion of the corpora may be under-appreciated clinically. Lopez et al. reported on 145 patients and found that the presence of tumor emboli in venous or lymphatic channels was the strongest predictor for regional spread (37). This factor, and tumor differentiation, can be assessed on biopsy material. Even for a clinical T1 primary tumor, if tumor emboli are present in lymphovascular spaces, or the tumor is less than well differentiated, more careful assessment of regional lymph nodes is warranted. It is our practice to recommend a bilateral modified inguinal node dissection for staging for these cases, and for all clinical T2 tumors that are either moderately or poorly differentiated. The specificity and sensitivity of CT scans are not sufficiently reliable (38), and fine needle aspiration is only applicable to nodes that are already under suspicion of harboring micrometastases.

Dynamic sentinel node mapping using a γ probe after intradermal injection of technetium 99m around the primary tumor is a promising staging technique to detect early lymph node involvement (38). Recent reports indicate a false-negative rate of 11% to 22% (38–40). This procedure is not yet an accepted alternative to modified inguinal node dissection.

NODE-POSITIVE DISEASE AND THE ROLE OF RADIOTHERAPY

Involved nodes should be resected wherever possible. If one is guided by the experience with squamous cell cancers of other sites that drain to the inguinal regions (41), then patients with pathologic findings of multiple positive nodes or extracapsular spread should be offered postoperative radiotherapy. If dissection was extended to the deep pelvic nodes and these are known to be negative, treatment can be limited to the involved groin. A direct anterior electron field of suitable energy to deliver a dose of 45 to 50 Gy to the depth of the nodes over 5 weeks is appropriate. If the status of the pelvic nodes is unknown, then these should be included in the treatment volume.

Unresectable nodes will rarely be controlled by radiotherapy but can be treated palliatively. A combined approach with systemic chemotherapy may be warranted if the patient's general condition permits an aggressive approach. Reports using combination chemotherapy, either 5-fluorouracil and mitomycin C (42) or various cisplatin-based regimens (43) indicate limited success. Intra-arterial chemotherapy for locally advanced or recurrent penile cancer using cisplatin, methotrexate, and bleomycin (CMB) (25) or CMB plus 5-fluorouracil and mitomycin C (44) has shown promise. The Southwest Oncology Group (45) has reported a trial using CMB in locally advanced or metastatic penile cancer in 40 men with a response rate of 32.5%. Surgery or radiotherapy can be used following a response to chemotherapy.

CONCLUSION

Penile cancer is a rare but psychologically devastating disease. The functional and sexual implications of treatment should be discussed with patients. For T1 and T2 tumors <4 cm in diameter, a penile-conserving approach as primary management is warranted. Interstitial brachytherapy is the treatment of choice and results in penile preservation in 70% to 80% of cases. If brachytherapy expertise is not available, external radiotherapy can prevent amputation in 50% to 60% of patients. With either modality, close and extended follow-up is necessary as surgical salvage of local failures can be curative.

Observation of regional nodes is acceptable for low-risk T1 and T2 tumors that are well differentiated with no evidence of lymphovascular space invasion. Moderately or poorly differentiated tumors and all T3 tumors should have regional lymph node staging.

References

1. Opjordsmoen S, Fossa SD. Quality of life in patients treated for penile cancer. A follow-up study. *Br J Urol* 1994;74:652–657.
2. Opjordsmoen S, Waehre H, Aass N, et al. Sexuality in patients treated for penile cancer: patients' experience and doctors' judgement. *Br J Urol* 1994;73:554–560.
3. Hanash KA, Furlow WL, Utz DC, et al. Carcinoma of the penis: a clinico-pathologic study. *J Urol* 1970;104:291–297.
4. Sarin R, Norman AR, Steel GG, et al. Treatment results and prognostic factors in 101 men treated for squamous carcinoma of the penis. *Int J Radiat Oncol Biol Phys* 1997;38:713–722.
5. Soria JC, Fizazi K, Piron D, et al. Squamous cell carcinoma of the penis: multivariate analysis of prognostic factors and natural history in monocentric study with a conservative policy. *Ann Oncol* 1997;8:1089–1098.
6. Harden SV, Tan LT. Treatment of localized carcinoma of the penis: a survey of current practice in the UK. *Clin Oncol (R Coll Radiol)* 2001;13:284–287, quiz 288.
7. Rozan R, Albuisson E, Giraud B, et al. Interstitial brachytherapy for penile carcinoma: a multicentric survey (259 patients). *Radiother Oncol* 1995;36:83–93.
8. Jackson S. The treatment of carcinoma of the penis. *Br J Surg* 1966;53:33–35.
9. Harmer M. Penis (ICD-0187), *TNM classification of malignant tumours*, 3rd ed. Geneva, 1978:126–128.
10. Hermanek PS. Penis (ICD-0 187). In: *TNM classification of malignant tumours*, 4th ed. Berlin, Heidelberg: Springer-Velag, 1987.
11. McLean M, Akl AM, Warde P, et al. The results of primary radiation therapy in the management of squamous cell carcinoma of the penis. *Int J Radiat Oncol Biol Phys* 1993;25:623–628.
12. Neave F, Neal AJ, Hoskin PJ, et al. Carcinoma of the penis: a retrospective review of treatment with iridium mould and external beam irradiation. *Clin Oncol (R Coll Radiol)* 1993;5:207–210.
13. Zouhair A, Coucke PA, Jeanneret W, et al. Radiation therapy alone or combined surgery and radiation therapy in squamous-cell carcinoma of the penis? *Eur J Cancer* 2001;37:198–203.
14. Sagerman RH, Yu WS, Chung CT, et al. External-beam irradiation of carcinoma of the penis. The treatment of early cancer of the penis with megavoltage x rays. *Radiology* 1984;152:183–185.
15. Vujovic OGJB, Stewart D. Carcinoma of the penis: a treatment technique with external beam radiation. *Ann R Coll Physicians Surg Can* 2001;34:495–497.
16. el-Demiry MI, Oliver RT, Hope-Stone HF, et al. Reappraisal of the role of radiotherapy and surgery in the management of carcinoma of the penis. Carcinoma of the penis: a clinicopathologic study. Is conservative organ-sparing treatment of penile carcinoma justified? *Br J Urol* 1984;56:724–728.
17. Akimoto T, Mitsuhashi N, Takahashi I, et al. Brachytherapy for penile cancer using silicon mold. *Oncology* 1997;54:23–27.
18. Pierquin B, Chassagne D, Wilson F. *Modern brachytherapy*. New York: Masoom Pub, 1987.
19. Chaudhary AJ, Ghosh S, Bhalavat RL, et al. Interstitial brachytherapy in carcinoma of the penis. *Strahlenther Onkol* 1999;175:17–20.
20. Crook J, Grimard L, Tsihlias J, et al. Interstitial brachytherapy for penile cancer: an alternative to amputation. *J Urol* 2002;167:506–511.
21. Delannes M, Malavaud B, Douchez J, et al. Iridium-192 interstitial therapy for squamous cell carcinoma of the penis. *Int J Radiat Oncol Biol Phys* 1992;24:479–483.
22. Kiltie AE, Elwell C, Close HJ, et al. Iridium-192 implantation for node-negative carcinoma of the penis: the Cookridge Hospital experience. *Clin Oncol (R Coll Radiol)* 2000;12:25–31.
23. Mazeron JJ, Langlois D, Lobo PA, et al. Interstitial radiation therapy for carcinoma of the penis using iridium 192 wires: the Henri Mondor experience (1970–1979). *Int J Radiat Oncol Biol Phys* 1984;10:1891–1895.
24. Gotsadze D, Matveev B, Zak B, et al. Is conservative organ-sparing treatment of penile carcinoma justified? *Eur Urol* 2000;38:306–312.
25. Huang XY, Kubota Y, Nakada T, et al. Intra-arterial infusion chemotherapy for penile carcinoma with deep inguinal lymph node metastasis. *Urol Int* 1999;62:245–248.
26. Evans AW, Levin W, Crook J. Brachy therapy induced penile necrosis treated with hyperboric oxygen. Presented at the undersea & Medical Hyperboric Society, Sydney, Australia, 2004. Abst. available on-line http://www.uhmsassociates.org.
27. Duncan W, Jackson SM. The treatment of early cancer of the penis with megavoltage x-rays. *Clin Radiol* 1972;23:246–248.
28. Sandeman TF. Carcinoma penis. *Australas Radiol* 1990;34:12–16.

29. Lindegaard JC, Nielsen OS, Lundbeck FA, et al. A retrospective analysis of 82 cases of cancer of the penis. *Br J Urol* 1996;77:883–890.
30. Narayana AS, Olney LE, Loening SA, et al. Carcinoma of the penis: analysis of 219 cases. *Cancer* 1982;49:2185–2191.
31. Bevan-Thomas R, Slaton JW, Pettaway CA. Contemporary morbidity from lymphadenectomy for penile squamous cell carcinoma: the M.D. Anderson Cancer Center Experience. *J Urol* 2002;167:1638–1642.
32. Theodorescu D, Russo P, Zhang ZF, et al. Outcomes of initial surveillance of invasive squamous cell carcinoma of the penis and negative nodes. *J Urol* 1996;155:1626–1631.
33. Parra RO. Accurate staging of carcinoma of the penis in men with nonpalpable inguinal lymph nodes by modified inguinal lymphadenectomy. *J Urol* 1996;155:560–563.
34. Horenblas S, van Tinteren H. Squamous cell carcinoma of the penis. IV. Prognostic factors of survival: analysis of tumor, nodes and metastasis classification system. *J Urol* 1994;151:1239–1243.
35. Slaton JW, Morgenstern N, Levy DA, et al. Tumor stage, vascular invasion and the percentage of poorly differentiated cancer: independent prognosticators for inguinal lymph node metastasis in penile squamous cancer. *J Urol* 2001;165:1138–1142.
36. McDougal WS. Carcinoma of the penis: improved survival by early regional lymphadenectomy based on the histological grade and depth of invasion of the primary lesion. *J Urol* 1995;154:1364–1366.
37. Lopes A, Hidalgo GS, Kowalski LP, et al. Prognostic factors in carcinoma of the penis: multivariate analysis of 145 patients treated with amputation and lymphadenectomy. *J Urol* 1996;156:1637–1642.
38. Horenblas S, van Tinteren H, Delemarre JF, et al. Squamous cell carcinoma of the penis. II. Treatment of the primary tumor. *J Urol* 1992;147:1533–1538.
39. Tanis PJ, Lont AP, Meinhardt W, et al. Dynamic sentinel node biopsy for penile cancer: reliability of a staging technique. *J Urol* 2002;168:76–80.
40. Valdes Olmos RA, Tanis PJ, Hoefnagel CA, et al. Penile lymphoscintigraphy for sentinel node identification. *Eur J Nucl Med* 2001;28:581–585.
41. Katz A, Eifel PJ, Jhingran A, et al. The role of radiation therapy in preventing regional recurrences of invasive squamous cell carcinoma of the vulva. *Int J Radiat Oncol Biol Phys* 2003;57:409–418.
42. Pedrick TJ, Wheeler W, Riemenschneider H. Combined modality therapy for locally advanced penile squamous cell carcinoma. *Am J Clin Oncol* 1993;16:501–505.
43. Kattan J, Culine S, Droz JP, et al. Penile cancer chemotherapy: twelve years' experience at Institut Gustave-Roussy. *Urology* 1993;42:559–562.
44. Roth AD, Berney CR, Rohner S, et al. Intra-arterial chemotherapy in locally advanced or recurrent carcinomas of the penis and anal canal: an active treatment modality with curative potential. *Br J Cancer* 2000;83:1637–1642.
45. Haas GP, Blumenstein BA, Gagliano RG, et al. Cisplatin, methotrexate and bleomycin for the treatment of carcinoma of the penis: a Southwest Oncology Group study. *J Urol* 1999;161:1823–1825.

CHAPTER 52 ■ CHEMOTHERAPY FOR PENILE CANCER

GIORGIO PIZZOCARO, WINSTON W. TAN, AND ROBERT DREICER

Penile cancer is a rare cancer in the United States, accounting for 500 to 1,000 cases each year (1). Although subsets of men with localized or local-regional disease may be cured with surgery or radiotherapy, metastatic penile carcinoma presents a major therapeutic dilemma. With the limitations of our current armamentarium, the goals of managing the patient with advanced penile cancer are primarily palliative.

Given the clinical significance of nodal disease in the management of penile cancer, patients with nodal disease appreciated either on physical examination or on radiographic assessment preoperatively, and those at high risk postoperatively are at times referred to medical oncology for consideration of neoadjuvant or adjuvant therapy. In some series, up to 50% of palpable lymph nodes are secondary to an inflammatory process (2), emphasizing the need for a thorough evaluation including histologic/cytologic confirmation of the presence of nodal metastases before committing the patient to chemotherapy.

In the patient deemed appropriate to undergo curative intent resection, various pathologic features have been identified as having prognostic value in predicting risk of occult nodal disease. These features include local tumor size and grade and have been prospectively validated in one small study (3). Patients at highest risk for nodal recurrence are those with poorly differentiated or locally advanced primary lesions. It is widely recognized that 10% to 20% of patients with clinically negative groins have microscopic lymph-node metastasis (4–6). Five-year survival in patients with regional lymph-node involvement is in the 10% to 30% range (7,8). The inordinate risk of systemic failure and poor long-term outcome for high-risk patients, irrespective of curative-intent local therapy, has provided some investigators a rationale for an evaluation of the role of adjuvant chemotherapy.

Penile cancer is a moderately chemotherapy-sensitive neoplasm. Some drugs demonstrated to be effective 20 to 30 years ago—mainly bleomycin, methotrexate, and cisplatin—have been clinically tested as single agents or in multidrug schedules. Other combination chemotherapy regimens evaluated to date include cisplatin/5-fluorouracil (PF) and vincristine/bleomycin/methotrexate (VBM). Newer agents have been studied only rarely in penile cancer. As is common with rare cancers, the literature is filled with case series and the occasional phase II trial. Our goal is to provide the reader with a focused review of the current database and to place into clinical context the role of chemotherapy in advanced penile cancer.

SINGLE AGENTS

Bleomycin as a single agent has a response rate of approximately 21% apparently irrespective of schedule (daily or weekly). Dosages and schedules that have been evaluated include those in the 3 to 20 mg/m² range administered as a continuous infusion or 10 to 30 mg/m² daily or weekly as intravenous push (IVP). Objective and partial responses with bleomycin alone were observed in nearly one-third of cases, as summarized by Eisenberger (9). Bleomycin was employed at a level very close to the maximum tolerated dosage, and side effects such as skin rashes, fever, chills, and pulmonary interstitial fibrosis were reported. In the series of 14 patients treated by Ahmed et al. three objective responses were recorded, all belonging to the group of 8 patients with inguinal metastases only. Responses were independent of previous chemotherapy. The authors also reported two cases of severe pulmonary toxicity, with one death (10).

Methotrexate has been reported as the most effective single agent for squamous cell carcinoma of the penis. Administered at dosages of 30 to 40 mg/m² per week, overall responses in the 38% to 62% range were reported in two series (11,12). Ahmed et al. treated 13 patients with methotrexate at the dosage of either 250 mg/m² every 2 to 4 weeks or 30 to 40 mg/m² weekly, producing 1 complete and 7 partial responders. Responses did not depend on metastatic sites and, although responses were typically brief, 2 patients had durable responses over 1 year (10). Severe granulocytopenia was seen in 2 of 13 patients, one of whom died of sepsis. Hepatic and renal toxicities were less common.

Cisplatin in doses ranging from 50 to 120 mg/m² has produced objective responses in the 15% to 27% range. Ahmed et al. administered cisplatin at either 70 or 120 mg/m² every 21 days to 14 patients heavily pretreated with other drugs. Three of 12 evaluable patients (25%) achieved an objective response, including 1 complete responder. All of the responses were in patients previously treated with bleomycin (n = 1) or methotrexate (n = 2) (10). The Southwest Oncology Group (SWOG) conducted a multicenter phase II trial in 26 patients with advanced disease who were chemotherapy naïve. Cisplatin was administered at 50 mg/m² on days 1 and 8 every 28 days. Eleven (42%) of the patients had received prior radiotherapy. As would be anticipated from single-agent cisplatin, toxicity was primarily nausea and vomiting (preserotonin antagonist) and renal insufficiency. There were 4 partial responders (15%). Unfortunately, the median duration of response was less than 3 months with a very poor median survival of 4.7 months (13).

COMBINATION CHEMOTHERAPY

Among the most widely used combination regimens in advanced penile cancer is cisplatin and 5-fluorouracil. Several investigators, extrapolating from the experience with this combination in squamous cell carcinoma of the head and neck, have reported their institutional experiences with this doublet. Hussein et al. treated six patients with advanced disease with cisplatin 100 mg/m² followed by a 120-hour infusion of 5-fluorouracil at 960 mg/m². Five (83%) objective responses were achieved, four of which were partial and one complete.

Two patients were able to undergo radical resection, with histologic evidence of residual disease in both cases. One of these patients relapsed and was treated with further PF chemotherapy in combination with radiotherapy: He was alive at 32 months and rendered disease-free. The other patient operated upon received adjuvant radiotherapy and survived for 26 months (14). Shammas et al. treated eight patients with cisplatin 100 mg/m² on day 1 and 5-fluorouracil 1,000 mg/m² administered as a 24-hour infusion days 1 to 5. Two of eight patients were responders, and these two patients were reported to be disease-free at 32 and 57 months, respectively (15). Fisher et al. reported four responses [two pathologic complete responses (CRs) and two partial responses (PRs)] in five previously untreated patients for locally advanced penile cancer prior to lymph-node dissection (16).

Cisplatin/Bleomycin/Methotrexate

Using standard combination chemotherapy principles, Dexeus et al. combined the three most widely investigated agents into a three-drug combination and treated 14 patients with locally advanced or metastatic penile cancer with cisplatin 20 mg/m² on days 2 to 5; methotrextate 200 mg/m² on days 1, 8, and 15 with leucovorin rescue; and bleomycin 10 mg/m² on days 2 to 5. Three patients received cisplatin and bleomycin intra-arterially. Although the toxicity was considerable (myelosuppression, neurotoxicity, nephrotoxicity, and pulmonary fibrosis), they reported a 72% response rate including two CRs and eight PRs. Only three of the eight PRs could undergo surgery. The median duration of response was 6 months (17).

A confirmatory trial, which was the largest multi-institutional prospective clinical trial ever performed in penile cancer, was reported by SWOG (18). The regimen was modified to contain 75 mg/m² cisplatin on day 1, 25 mg/m² methotrexate on days 1 and 8, and 10 U/m² bleomycin on days 1 and 8. Therapy was repeated every 21 days. Forty-five patients from 31 institutions were enrolled over an 8-year period, emphasizing both the difficulty and the need for the cooperative group structure to conduct trials in this disease. Five patients were deemed ineligible, having received prior chemotherapy. Of 40 evaluable patients, only 6 completed all planned courses of therapy. This study showed a response rate of 32.5% (5 CRs and 8 PRs among 40 evaluable patients), but toxicity was formidable, with 11% treatment-related mortality and 17% of the remaining patients experiencing life-threatening toxicity. Of the 5 treatment-related deaths, 1 was due to infection and 4 were due to pulmonary complications. Severe myelosuppression was common, as were gastrointestinal toxicity and mucositis. The level of toxicity observed overshadowed the promising activity, and the regimen was neither adopted as standard care nor moved forward in clinical trials.

Vincristine/Bleomycin/Methotrexate

The intriguing activity achieved with a combination of low-dose vincristine, bleomycin, and methotrexate (VBM) in advanced squamous cell carcinoma of the head and neck (19) encouraged Pizzocaro and Piva (20) to use this easily administered combination chemotherapy in patients with squamous cell carcinoma of the penis in the following schedule:

— vincristine, 1 mg intravenously on day 1
— bleomycin, 15 mg intramuscularly 6 and 12 hours after vincristine
— methotrexate, 30 mg orally on day 3

This regimen was repeated weekly for 12 weeks. In elderly patients and in patients with chronic bronchitis, only the first dose of bleomycin was administered, and methotrexate was given on day 1. The first series of 5 patients with fixed inguinal nodes and 12 patients with radically resected inguinal metastases were submitted to either primary or adjuvant VBM chemotherapy. Three of the five patients with unresectable inguinal metastases achieved partial remission and could undergo surgery; only 1 of the 12 patients who received adjuvant VBM relapsed after a median follow-up of 42 months (20). Updated results showed only 4 relapses among 25 patients treated with adjuvant VBM for radically resected nodal metastases. Treatment was generally well tolerated, although fever, lung fibrosis, and skin hyperpigmentation were seen.

Intra-arterial Chemotherapy

Roth et al. reported 16 patients (8 with penile carcinomas and 8 with anal cancer) treated with intra-arterial chemotherapy (21). Fifteen of them were treated for locally advanced or recurrent disease, and the chemotherapy was administered via a femoral intra-arterial catheter with its tip located above the aortic bifurcation and under the inferior mesenteric artery. It consisted of eight push injections, given over a 48-hour period, of the following drug combination: cisplatin 8.5 mg/mq, 5-fluorouracil 275 mg/mq, methotrexate 27.5 mg/mq, mitomycin C 1.2 mg/mq, and bleomycin 4 mg/mq. Leucovorin was given p.o., 4×15 mg/day/mq during the chemotherapy and for three days thereafter. A total of 52 cycles of treatment were administered. Of the 15 patients evaluated for response, 6 obtained a CR (three penile, three anal cancer) and 8 a PR. Among the complete responders, 4 are alive and disease-free 15 years after treatment. The other patients enjoyed an objective response lasting 3 to 25 months (median 7 months). Four patients developed grade III hematological toxicity with three episodes of febrile neutropenia, one of them with a fatal outcome, one a grade III mucositis of the glands, and four a grade III/IV cutaneous toxicity, the latter caused by the intra-arterial administration of bleomycin.

BIOLOGICAL RESPONSE MODIFIERS

Based on both preclinical activity in human squamous cell carcinoma cell lines and in phase II trials of patients with squamous cell carcinoma of the skin and cervix, the Eastern Cooperative Oncology Group (ECOG) performed a phase II trial of 13-cis Retinoic acid (13-cRA) plus interferon α-2a. Eighteen patients with advanced disease were treated with 3 MU/day of interferon α-2a and 1 mg/kg 13-cRA. Although therapy was relatively well tolerated (only grade 3 hypertriglyceridemia was common), only 1 of 16 evaluable patients demonstrated an objective response. The investigators concluded that this combination did not warrant further evaluation in penile cancer (22).

COMBINED MODALITY THERAPY

Chemotherapy became part of the combined treatment modalities for squamous cell carcinoma of the penis in an attempt to improve the results of surgery or radiotherapy, and some successful results allowed oncologists to design new therapeutic strategies. These new strategies focused on organ-sparing treatments in selected patients with organ-confined disease and on the improvement of cure rates in patients with metastatic disease.

CHEMOTHERAPY IN CONSERVATIVE TREATMENT OF PRIMARY TUMOR FOR ORGAN-CONFINED DISEASE

Contact Chemotherapy

Very superficial carcinoma of the penis, such as penile intraepithelial neoplasia or Queyrat eritroplasia, can be successfully treated with 5-fluorouracil cream, and a case of squamous cell carcinoma successfully treated with imiquimod 5% cream has been recently reported (23).

Chemotherapy with Radiotherapy

Some reports explored the combination of chemotherapy and radiotherapy, mainly relying on the synergism between bleomycin and irradiation. Edsmyr et al. submitted 42 patients with T1–T2 squamous cell carcinoma of the penis to radiotherapy (4,500 to 5,800 rads to the whole penis by opposed fields with a conventional x-ray device over 5 to 6 weeks) combined with bleomycin 15 mg intramuscularly on days 3 to 5 of weeks 1, 3, and 5. Complete remission was achieved in 39 (93%) patients, and 4 patients required a salvage amputation. The overall 5-year survival was 77%, and conservatively treated patients maintained both normal micturition and sexual function if they were normal before therapy. No major side effects were recorded, and in particular no pulmonary fibrosis occurred (24). Perez-Tamayo et al. were not able to repeat such excellent results with the same combination therapy in 10 patients (25). Modig et al. reported a series of 25 patients with T1N0 squamous cell carcinoma of the penis who were treated with a combination of irradiation and bleomycin. Radiotherapy to the whole penis was given from two opposed portals with a daily dose of 1.8 Gy up to a total dosage of 56 Gy to 58 Gy over a period of 6 weeks. The patients received 2.5 mg (13 cases) or 5 mg (12 cases) of bleomycin intramuscularly 1 hour before each treatment. The total dose of bleomycin was of 70 to 140 mg. Five (20%) patients had a local recurrence and underwent partial amputation. After a minimum follow-up of 8 years, no patient had died of the disease. The combination of irradiation and bleomycin was well tolerated, and patients who entered treatment with sexual activity retained this ability. Minor reversible local reactions occurred, and only 1 patient had a late stricture of urethral meatus that required repeated meatotomy operations (26).

Chemotherapy and Laser CO_2 Surgery

At the National Cancer Institute in Milan between 1981 and 1990, 27 patients with strictly exophytic T1N0 squamous cell carcinoma of the penis were selected to enter a program of primary (neoadjuvant) VBM chemotherapy followed by CO_2 laser excision of the glans penis surface and circumcision. The CO_2 laser excision was carried out to a depth of 2.5 mm, and a histologic evaluation of the resected specimen was performed in all cases. Patients were seen every 4 weeks in the outpatient department during chemotherapy, which was administered at home with the cooperation of the family doctor. Twelve weekly courses were to be administered, but some complete responders were operated on after 8 weeks. Twelve (44%) patients achieved a pathologic complete remission and 9 had an incomplete response, for an overall response rate of 78%. Seventeen of the 21 responsive patients remained disease-free following CO_2 laser and excisional surgery, whereas 4 had

a recurrence. Recurrences were cured conservatively in three cases, and only 1 patient needed a partial amputation. Of the 6 poorly responsive patients, 2 were cured conservatively and 4 required penile amputation. Overall, 23 (85%) of the 27 selected patients could avoid penile amputation. After a minimum follow-up of 4 years, no patient had progression and 2 patients died disease-free from unrelated causes. Skin rashes occurred in 5 (19%) patients, and only 1 patient had to withdraw from bleomycin therapy because of early lung fibrosis. Cosmetic results of laser CO_2 surgery were excellent. Normal micturition and sexual function were preserved in all patients undergoing the conservative approach (27).

Chemotherapy for Nodal Metastases

Radical surgical excision represents the therapeutic milestone for nodal metastases from squamous cell carcinoma of the penis. Chemotherapy is used in the adjuvant setting to improve the disease-free survival after radical dissection, or in the neoadjuvant setting to induce resectability of fixed inguinal nodes (28,29).

Adjuvant Chemotherapy after Radical Resection of Nodal Metastases

Adjuvant chemotherapy after resection of nodal metastases has been reported in a few heterogeneous series in which concomitant groin irradiation has been used. Between 1979 and 1990, 25 consecutive patients with radically resected inguinal metastases from squamous cell carcinoma of the penis were to receive 12 weekly courses of adjuvant VBM at our institution. All patients underwent radical inguinopelvic lymph-node dissection, and pelvic nodes were involved in 7 cases. Only 4 (16%) patients showed relapse, with a 5-year disease-free actuarial survival of 82%. These findings compare favorably with a previous series of 31 patients submitted to radical inguinopelvic lymph-node dissection alone, whose 5-year disease-free survival was only 37%. A more accurate analysis of these two series allowed the identification of some risk factors in patients with metastatic nodes. In the series of 31 patients who did not receive adjuvant chemotherapy, only the involvement of a single node was associated with good prognosis, whereas in the series of 25 patients treated with adjuvant VBM, only bilaterality of metastases and pelvic nodes involvement remained significantly associated with poor prognosis ($P = .006$). None of the patients who had a single intranodal metastasis suffered any relapse, regardless of postoperative treatment (category N1 patients). This small subset of patients seems to have no need for adjuvant chemotherapy, whereas patients with pelvic or bilateral nodal involvement are now treated with three courses of adjuvant PF chemotherapy (30).

Neoadjuvant Chemotherapy for Fixed Inguinal Nodes

Historically, primary chemotherapy often meant palliation for unresectable metastases from squamous cell carcinoma of the penis, and it has been associated with radiotherapy. Nonetheless, important results have been obtained with neoadjuvant chemotherapy in the early 1990s. By combining the experiences of Hussein et al. Shammas et al. Dexeus et al. and Kattan et al. it is possible to consider a population of 29 patients who have been treated with various cisplatin-based combination chemotherapies for primary or recurrent fixed inguinal metastases from squamous cell carcinoma of the penis (14,15,17,31). Objective responses were achieved in 19 (66%) cases, of which 11 (38%) could be radically resected: 5 patients (17%) were reported to be alive and disease-free at 12, 24, 32, and 57 months.

The potential advantage of neoadjuvant chemotherapy in patients with resectable inguinal metastases was evaluated by Fisher et al. in five patients with Jackson's stage 3 squamous cell carcinoma of the penis (16). Two courses of PF combination chemotherapy were administered before inguinopelvic dissection. One patient who was unresponsive to the first cycle refused any further treatment and died of progressive disease. Four patients achieved an objective remission and underwent surgery: Two had no viable tumor in the specimen, and two had residual disease. No relapses were recorded after a follow-up of 6 to 40 months.

Since 1979, 16 consecutive patients with fixed nodal metastases from squamous cell carcinoma of the penis were treated with neoadjuvant chemotherapy at the National Cancer Institute in Milan. The first 13 patients received 12 weekly courses of VBM combination chemotherapy. Seven of the first 13 cases achieved a partial remission and underwent surgery, but only 5 could be radically resected. Two of the 5 radically resected patients are alive and disease-free after 5 and 13 years, respectively (30). Of the 6 patients treated with PF—3 previously treated with VBM and 3 chemotherapy naïve—5 achieved a partial remission and underwent surgery, which was radical in 4 patients. Three (50%) of the 4 radically resected patients were alive and disease-free after 3, 8, and 10 years. PF has since become the standard neoadjuvant chemotherapy at Milan for patients with fixed nodal metastasis.

CHEMOTHERAPY AND SURGERY

Neoadjuvant Chemotherapy

Culkin and Beer recently reviewed the management of penile cancer identified responses in 24 of 35 patients with fixed inguinal nodes treated with neoadjuvant cisplatin-based combinations. Of these responding patients, 15 underwent complete resection of disease, with 8 being alive and disease-free for intervals ranging from 1 to 10 years (32). As noted earlier, Pizzocaro et al. demonstrated activity in the neoadjuvant setting with the vincristine, bleomycin, and methotrextate regimen (33).

Bermejo et al. treated 11 patients with large pelvic and inguinal metastases (defined as >4 cm) over a 7-year period with several different drug combinations, including ifosfamide, paclitaxel, and cisplatin; carboplatin and paclitaxel; and bleomycin, methotrextate, and cisplatin. Three patients achieved a CR, with 8 others a PR. Of 8 patients with no evidence of disease 1 month after therapy, 6 remain alive and disease-free with a median follow-up of 19 months (2 to 72 months) (34).

Adjuvant Chemotherapy

The systematic evaluation of newer cytotoxics (i.e., gemcitabine, pemetrexed, and docetaxel) or any of the emerging small molecules in penile cancer presents a daunting challenge to the international urologic oncology community. In the United States, phase II clinical trials conducted by cooperative groups sponsored by the National Cancer Institute represent the only viable mechanism to perform meaningful evaluations of new therapies in uncommon cancers (Table 52.1). Both SWOG and ECOG have performed multicenter phase II trials, which represent the most important contributions to the literature. The SWOG is currently conducting a phase II trial evaluating the activity of docetaxel in patients with locally advanced or metastatic penile cancer.

TABLE 52.1

MULTICENTER PHASE II TRIALS IN PENILE CANCER

Group	Agents studied	Number of pts	Overall response rate
SWOG (13)	Cisplatin	26	15%
SWOG (18)	CMB	40	33%
ECOG (22)	13-cRA + interferon α-2a	18	6%

13-cRA, 13-cis retinoic acid; CMB, cisplatin, methotrexate, bleomycin; ECOG, eastern cooperative Oncology Group; pts, patients; SWOG, southwest oncology group

CONCLUSION

Sufficient data are available to conclude that penile cancer is moderately sensitive to cisplatin, bleomycin, and methotrexate. Several small reports suggest that the combination of cisplatin with 5-fluorouracil, a workhorse of head and neck cancer chemotherapy, is also active in penile cancer. The combination of cisplatin, bleomycin, and methotrexate is active, but it is associated with prohibitive toxicity. The single-agent activity of many important classes of new agents has not yet been evaluated.

In selected cases with organ-confined disease, the combination of chemotherapy with radiotherapy or minimally invasive surgery can avoid the heavy psychosocial consequences of amputation of the penis in approximately 80% of patients. The relatively poor prognosis of patients with radically resected nodal metastases has been transformed into a 5-year expected disease-free survival of approximately 80% with adjuvant chemotherapy (30).

Unresectable nodal metastases from squamous cell carcinoma of the penis are a challenging issue. Nonetheless, combination chemotherapy seems able to produce major responses in approximately 60% of patients, resulting in resectability in about 50% of cases and durable disease-free survival in 15% to 30% of cases. Of the three reported regimens, VBM is the easiest to administer but is probably also the least active. The two cisplatin-containing regimens seem to be more effective, but the methotrexate-bleomycin-cisplatin combination seems excessively toxic. The PF regimen is probably advisable as first-line therapy in patients with fixed inguinal nodes, whereas intra-arterial therapy deserves further investigation.

Occasionally, patients treated in the neoadjuvant setting for "resectable" nodal metastases progressed to unresectability during the therapy, and no patient with metastatic disease was cured by chemotherapy alone. Radical surgery remains the milestone to achieve cure in patients with nodal metastases from squamous cell carcinoma of the penis, whereas combination chemotherapy may improve the cure rate.

Advanced disease may occasionally benefit from palliative-intent chemotherapy; however, the management of the majority of such patients involves aggressive symptomatic supportive care.

References

1. Jemal A, Murray T, Ward E, et al. Cancer statistics, 2005. CA Cancer J Clin 2005;55:10–30.
2. Slaton J, Morgenstern N, Levy D, et al. Tumor stage, vascular invasion and the percentage of poorly differentiated cancer: Independent prognosticators for inguinal lymph node metastasis in penile squamous cancer. J Urol 2001;165:1138–1142.
3. Solsona E, Iborra I, Rubi J, et al. Prospective validation of the association of local tumor stage and grade as a predictive factor for occult lymph node

micrometastasis in patients with penile carcinoma and clinically negative inguinal lymph nodes. *J Urol* 2001;165:1506–1509.

4. Horenblas S, VanTinteren H, Delemarre J, et al. Squamous cell carcinoma of the penis: III. Treatment of regional nodes. *J Urol* 1993;149:492–497.

5. Fraley E, Zhang G, Manivel C, et al. The role of ileoinguinal lymphadenectomy and significance of histological differentiation in treatment of carcinoma of the penis. *J Urol* 1989;142:1478–1482.

6. McLean M, Akl A, Warde P, et al. The results of primary radiation therapy in the management of squamous cell carcinoma of the penis. *Int J Radiat Oncol Biol Phys* 1993;25:623–628.

7. Kulkarni J, Kamat M. Prophylactic bilateral groin node dissection versus prophylactic radiotherapy and surveillance in patients with N0 and N1-2A carcinoma of the penis. *Eur Urol* 1994;26:123–128.

8. Ornellas A, Seixas A, Marota A, et al. Surgical treatment of invasive squamous cell carcinoma of the penis: Retrospective analysis of 350 cases. *J Urol* 1994;151:1244–1249.

9. Eisenberger MA. Chemotherapy for carcinomas of the penis and urethra. *Urol Clin North Am* 1992;19:333–338.

10. Ahmed T, Sklaroff R, Yagoda A. Sequential trials of methotrexate, cisplatin and bleomycin for penile cancer. *J Urol* 1984;132:465–468.

11. Sklaroff R, Yagoda A. Methotrexate in the treatment of penile cancer. *Cancer* 1980;45:214–216.

12. Garnick M, Skarin A, Steele G. Metastatic carcinoma of the penis: Complete remission after high dose methotrexate chemotherapy. *J Urol* 1979;122:265–266.

13. Gagliano R, Blumenstein B, Crawford E, et al. Cis-diamminedichloroplatinum in the treatment of advanced carcinoma of the penis: A Southwest Oncology Group study. *J Urol* 1989;141:66–67.

14. Hussein AM, Benedetto P, Sridar KS. Chemotherapy with cisplatin and 5-fluorouracil for penile and urethral squamous cell carcinomas. *Cancer* 1990;65:433–438.

15. Shammas F, Ous S, Fossa S. Cisplatin and 5-fluorouracil in advanced cancer of the penis. *J Urol* 1992;147:630–632.

16. Fisher HA, Barada JH, Horton H, et al. Neoadjuvant therapy with cisplatin and 5-fluorouracil for stage III squamous cell carcinoma of the penis (Abstract 653). *J Urol* 1990;143(Suppl. 4):352A.

17. Dexeus F, Logothetis C, Sella A, et al. Combination chemotherapy with methotrexate, bleomycin and cisplatin for advanced squamous cell carcinoma of the male genital tract. *J Urol* 1991;146:1284–1287.

18. Haas G, Blumenstein B, Gagliano R, et al. Cisplatin, methotrexate and bleomycin for the treatment of carcinoma of the penis: A Southwest Oncology Group study. *J Urol* 1999;161:1823–1825.

19. Molinari R, Mattavelli F, Cantu G, et al. Results of a low-dose combination with vincristine, bleomycin and methotrexate in the palliative treatment of head and neck squamous cell carcinoma. *Eur J Cancer* 1980;16:469–472.

20. Pizzocaro G, Piva L. Adjuvant and neoadjuvant vincristine, bleomycin and methotrexate for inguinal metastases from squamous cell carcinoma of the penis. *Acta Oncol* 1988;27:823–824.

21. Roth AD, Berney CR, Rohner S, et al. Intra-arterial chemotherapy in locally advanced or recurrent carcinomas of the penis and anal canal: An active treatment modality with curative potential. *Br J Cancer* 2000;83:1637–1642.

22. Skeel R, Huang J, Manola J, et al. A phase II study of 13-cis Retinoic acid plus interferon alpha-2a in advanced stage penile carcinoma: An Eastern Cooperative Oncology Group study (E3893). *Cancer Invest* 2003;21:41–46.

23. Schroeder TL, Sengelmann RD. Squamous cell carcinoma in situ of the penis successfully treated with imiquimod 5% cream. *J Am Acad Dermatol* 2002;46:545–548.

24. Edsmyr F, Anderson L, Espositi PL. Combined bleomycin and radiotherapy in carcinoma of the penis. *Cancer* 1985;56:1257–1263.

25. Perez-Tamayo C, Wijnmaalen A, Pomp J, et al. Combined approach to squamous cell carcinoma of the penis (SCP). (Abstract 428). *Pro Am Soc Clin Onc* 1987;6:109.

26. Modig H, Duchek M, Sjodin AG. Carcinoma of the penis: Treatment by surgery or combined bleomycin and radiation therapy. *Acta Urol Ital* 1993;32:653–655.

27. Bandieramonte G, Lepera P, Marchesini R, et al. Laser microsurgery for superficial lesions of the penis. *J Urol* 1987;138:315–319.

28. Maiche AG. Adjuvant treatment using bleomycin in squamous cell carcinoma of the penis: Study of 19 cases. *Br J Urol* 1983;55:542–544.

29. Fossa SD, Hall KS, Johannesses NB, et al. Cancer of the penis. *Eur Urol* 1987;13:372–377.

30. Pizzocaro G, Piva L, Nicolai N. Treatment of lymphatic metastases of squamous cell carcinoma of the penis: Experience at the National Cancer Institute in Milan. *Arch Ital Urol Androl* 1996;68:169–172.

31. Kattan J, Culine S, Droz JP, et al. Penile cancer chemotherapy: Twelve years' experience at Institut Gustave-Roussy. *Urology* 1993;42:559–562.

32. Culkin D, Beer T. Advanced penile carcinoma. *J Urol* 2003;170:359–365.

33. Pizzocaro G, Piva L, Bandieramonte G, et al. Up-to-date management of carcinoma of the penis. *Eur Urol* 1997;32:5–15.

34. Bermejo C, Sanchez-Ortiz R, Kamat A, et al. Neoadjuvant chemotherapy followed by aggressive surgical consolidation for metastatic penile cancer (Abstract 683). *J Urol* 2003;169:177.

CHAPTER 53 ■ ADRENAL NEOPLASMS

SAREENA MALHI, ALIREZA MOINZADEH, INDERBIR S. GILL, AND RONALD M. BUKOWSKI

HISTORICAL PERSPECTIVE

The adrenal glands play a prominent role in maintaining normal homeostasis. Bartholomeo Eustachi first recognized them as organs that are distinct from the kidneys in 1563 (1). Knowledge of structure and function of the adrenal glands originated in 1805 when Currier recognized the presence of a cortex and medulla within the gland. In 1855, almost 300 years after the original description of these glands, Thomas Addison described the clinical effects of adrenal insufficiency (2). The demonstration by Brown-Sequard that death occurred following adrenalectomy firmly established the importance of the adrenal gland (3).

Sir William Osler reported the beneficial effects of adrenal extracts for the treatment of Addison disease and thus began attempts at studying and using crude adrenal extracts. Isolation of cortisol from the adrenal cortex and adrenaline from the medulla was accomplished in the first half of the 20th century, and the modern era of adrenal physiology can be dated from the time of these significant research efforts. In view of the central and complex role of this gland in normal homeostasis, a discussion of adrenal neoplasms, their diagnosis, and treatment requires an introduction to normal as well as pathologic adrenal physiology.

ADRENAL PHYSIOLOGY

Adrenal Cortex

The adrenal cortex comprises the bulk of the adrenal gland and is the site of synthesis of many types of steroid hormones. The steroid synthesis pathway is a complex sequence of enzymatically mediated biochemical steps by which adrenal steroids are derived from cholesterol. Clinical manifestations of steroid excess result from autonomous production of various steroid compounds and precursors. The terms *functional* and *nonfunctional* have been applied to cortical neoplasms based on their clinical manifestations and/or excess hormone production. This may be misleading as adrenocortical tumor steroidogenesis differs from normal steroidogenesis in several aspects. Adrenal tumors often synthesize steroids that are not normally major adrenal products; instead these steroids may be early precursors such as Δ5-pregnenolone, dehydroepiandrosterone (DHEA), or similar compounds (4–6). These steroids may not have glucocorticoid/androgenic activity or may have only weak activity and, therefore, clinical syndromes of excess may not be seen. Many tumors and probably most malignant tumors do not respond to adrenocorticotropin (ACTH), another cardinal characteristic of constitutive steroidogenesis in adrenal neoplasms (5).

Adrenal Medulla

The adrenal medulla consists of chromaffin tissue originating from neuroectoderm. This portion of the adrenal gland is the major source of catecholamines, including epinephrine. Synthesis of these compounds proceeds through a series of enzymatic reactions involving tyrosine to epinephrine. Catecholamine synthesis occurs predominantly in chromaffin cells but also occurs in parts of the central nervous system (CNS) and postganglionic nerves (7).

The major portion of plasma catecholamine is composed of norepinephrine, with dopamine and epinephrine accounting for less than 30% (8). The metabolic products of these catecholamines include homovanillic acid (dopamine), metanephrines, and vanillylmandelic acid (epinephrine, norepinephrine). Only small amounts of epinephrine, norepinephrine, and dopamine are excreted unchanged in the urine.

The metabolic and physiologic effects of catecholamines include promotion of hepatic glycogenolysis and inhibition of hepatic glyconeogenesis plus insulin release (9). Cardiovascular effects include positive inotropy of the heart and a mixture of vasoconstriction and vasodilation. The overproduction of various catecholamines by tumors of chromaffin tissue (e.g., pheochromocytoma) is responsible for syndromes typically associated with these neoplasms.

ADRENOCORTICAL TUMORS—PATHOLOGY

In autopsy series, the prevalence of clinically inapparent adrenal masses is about 2.1%, which increases to about 7% in patients older than 70 years (10,11). In contrast, the prevalence of adrenocortical carcinoma (ACC) is rare. The National Cancer Institute's Surveillance, Epidemiology, and End Results database suggests an incidence of 0.5 to 2.0 per million populations per year (12). A review of the same database from 1973 to 1987 reported 552 cases of adrenocortical tumors forming 3.6% of all endocrine malignancies. The age-adjusted incidence rates were reported to be 0.1 to 0.2 per 100,000 over this period (13).

The relation between adrenal adenoma and carcinoma is unclear. Progression from a benign adenoma to carcinoma was felt to be unlikely in view of the wide disparity in incidence. On the basis of clonal analysis and many studies with comparative genomic hybridization, data have been emerging that suggest adrenal tumorigenesis is a multistep process, and that sequential progression from normal to adenomatous cells and then to malignant cells occurs in some tumors (14,15).

The Association of Directors of Anatomic and Surgical Pathology recommended guidelines for the histologic classification of neoplasms or tumorlike lesions of the adrenal cortex and medulla (16). These guidelines are illustrated in Table 53.1.

TABLE 53.1

HISTOLOGIC CLASSIFICATIONS OF NEOPLASMS OR TUMORLIKE LESIONS OF ADRENAL CORTEX AND MEDULLA

Adrenal cortical tumors
Adenoma
Carcinoma
Myelolipoma
Tumorlike adrenocortical nodules
Other

Adrenal medullary tumors
Pheochromocytoma
Neuroblastoma, ganglioneuroblastoma
Other

Miscellaneous neoplasms and tumorlike lesions
Adrenal cyst
Primary mesenchymal or neural tumors
Metastatic tumors
Other

Recommendations for reporting of tumors of the adrenal cortex and medulla. Association of Directors of Anatomic and Surgical Pathology. *Am J of Clin Pathol* 1999;112 (4):451;1991 American Society of Clinical pathologists. Reprinted with permission.

Adrenocortical Adenoma Pathology

Adrenocortical adenomas are benign tumors of the adrenal cortex, and on cross-section are often well defined with apparent encapsulation. Occasionally on cut section, there may be areas of hemorrhage, but confluent tumor necrosis is unusual (17). Microscopically, adenomas typically contain nests and cords of cohesive vacuolated cells with abundant cytoplasm (Fig. 53.1A). They are composed of lipid-rich spongiocytes or of compact cells that are devoid of lipid. Generally, mitoses are lacking, but focal nuclear atypism and hyperchromasia may be seen (18). Vascular and capsular invasion are also absent. The histologic and anatomic differences distinguishing benign and malignant adrenal tumors are still controversial (19,20).

Adrenocortical Carcinoma Pathology

ACCs are usually large tumors as compared with adenomas, but very small adrenocortical tumors (i.e. <40 g) can metastasize and some very large tumors (1,400 g) fail to behave in a malignant fashion (21). Grossly, ACC has a coarse nodular structure with areas of necrosis, hemorrhage, and, occasionally, cystic degeneration. Microscopically (Fig. 53.1B), the architecture can be trabecular, alveolar (nested), diffuse (solid), or a combination of these patterns (17,21).

Reliable differentiation of ACC from adenoma or benign lesions may be difficult. To address this problem, large series of patients diagnosed in the 1980s with long-term clinical follow-up have been assessed. Three sets of criteria have been proposed by Hough et al. (22), Weiss et al. (19), and Van Slooten et al. (23). Hough et al. (22) evaluated 41 patients with ACC for the presence of 15 histologic and 5 nonhistologic features that had been associated with malignant behavior. Twelve criteria were statistically significant in predicting subsequent metastasis. The most significant among those were evidence of weight loss, broad fibrous bands, diffuse pattern, vascular invasion, necrosis, and tumor mass. Van Slooten et al. (23) assessed the discriminatory value of seven histologic parameters: regressive changes likes necrosis and hemorrhage, preservation of architecture, nuclear atypia, nuclear hyperchromasia, nuclear structure, mitotic activity, and invasion into blood vessels or capsule. In their series of 45 patients with more than 10 years of follow-up, tumor weight and mitotic activity as single parameters had the highest discriminating value. The calculated histologic index (based on the sum of the numeric value of each parameter) had a critical value of 8, such that tumors with a histologic index less than 8 were smaller and less likely to be malignant. However, absolute differentiation between adenoma and carcinoma was not possible.

A third set of criteria proposed by Weiss et al. (19) on evaluation of 43 adrenocortical tumors is listed in Table 53.2. In a review by Medeiros and Weiss (20), it is noted that the following characteristics are seen only in malignant adrenocortical tumors: mitotic rate of 5 or more per 50 high-power field, atypical mitotic figures, and venous invasion. It appears that all three sets of criteria are useful in predicting the behavior of adrenocortical neoplasms. Each system has some unique features, and a study comparing all three has been recommended to develop a common set of criteria.

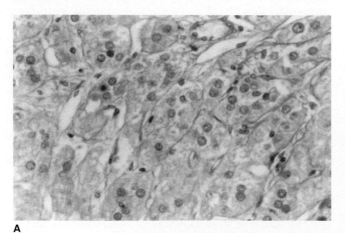

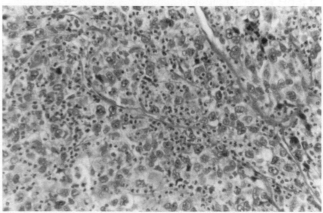

A   B

FIGURE 53.1. Histologic comparison of a benign adrenocortical adenoma and a carcinoma. **A:** *Benign adenoma.* Adenomas are characterized by nests and cords of clear cells with abundant cytoplasm separated by fibrovascular trabeculae. Mitoses are absent or rare, and cells have an orderly, monotonous appearance. **B:** *Adrenocortical carcinoma (ACC).* This cancer retains the fibrovascular trabeculae, but the cells demonstrate marked pleomorphism, enlarged and hyperchromatic nuclei, and obvious nucleoli.

TABLE 53.2

HISTOLOGIC CRITERIA OF MALIGNANCY IN ADRENOCORTICAL CARCINOMA

1. High nuclear grade
2. Mitotic rate of 5 or more per 50 high-power field
3. Atypical mitoses
4. Eosinophilic tumor cell cytoplasm (≥75% cells)
5. Diffuse pattern/architecture
6. Presence of necrosis
7. Vascular invasion
8. Sinusoidal invasion
9. Invasion of capsule

Adapted from Medeiros LJ, Weiss LM. New developments in the pathologic diagnosis of adrenal cortical neoplasms: A review. *Am J Clin Pathol* 1992;97:73.

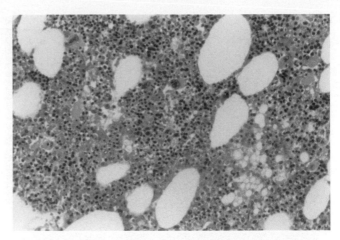

FIGURE 53.2. Histologic appearance of a myelolipoma showing fat (white areas) intermixed with myeloid tissue.

There does not appear to be a diagnostic immunoprofile for ACC, but immunohistochemistry still plays some role in its evaluation (18,24,25). Keratin and vimentin expression have been studied; keratin positivity, however, varies with the methods of tissue fixation and preparation. Vimentin expression appears to have an inverse relation with cytokeratin. Most carcinomas express this protein intensely: Normal cortical cells are negative and adenomas demonstrate intermediate expression. Another study has reported positive staining for neuron-specific enolase, synaptophysin, and neurofilament protein (26). The oncogene p53 and MIB-1 (a marker of cell proliferation) may be overexpressed in carcinomas compared to normal adrenal tissue, and benign adenomas (27). Immunostaining for chromogranin is positive in pheochromocytomas and negative in ACC. Similarly, the monoclonal antibody D11 has utility in distinguishing adrenocortical tumors from other tumors, but not benign from malignant. It therefore appears that immunohistochemical studies are useful in distinguishing adrenal neoplasms from other tumors but are of limited value in differentiating benign and malignant adrenal tumors.

Early studies suggested that carcinomas are aneuploid (28); in one series, however, 6 of 30 (20%) adenomas also contained aneuploid cell lines (29). Similarly, studies of telomerase, which is an enzyme that adds repeated telomere sequences to the ends of chromosomes arms maintaining cell proliferation, have shown conflicting results (30,31).

Myelolipoma

Myelolipomas are benign endocrine-inactive tumors (Fig. 53.2) composed of mature adipose tissue and fatty elements (32). The hematopoietic cells include granulocytic, erythroid, and, rarely, megakaryocytic precursors. Sparse adrenocortical tissue may also be found. These tumors are thought to arise from metaplasia of undifferentiated stromal tissue (33). Myelolipomas are usually small, nonfunctional, and discovered incidentally (33). They may occasionally reach an extremely large size and cause symptoms. The recommended treatment is conservative in asymptomatic patients. Such individuals can be clinically monitored, with periodic radiographic assessment every few years.

Adrenal Cysts

Adrenal cysts are rare, usually asymptomatic lesions occurring more frequently in women. Endothelial-lined cysts of lymphatic origin account for almost one-half of all adrenal cysts. The next most common cysts are pseudocysts, which result from old adrenal hemorrhages. These are usually thick walled and unilocular and contain red–brown fluid. Least common are epithelial cysts derived from cystic cortical adenomas (Fig. 53.3). Adrenal cysts are benign and generally treated by simple excision. Because adrenal cancers and pheochromocytomas may bleed and give rise to pseudocysts, frozen section examination of the cyst wall should be obtained at the time of excision.

Evaluation of the Incidental Adrenal Mass

Given the increased use of radiologic imaging, incidental adrenal masses are detected in 0.6% to 1.3% of abdominal computed tomography (CT) scans and in 2% to 9% of autopsy series (34,35). Histologically, most of these tumors are benign and nonfunctional adenomas. The masses are typically serendipitously discovered on an abdominal ultrasound or CT scan performed for an unrelated cause. The clinical challenge is to differentiate between clinically important entities that require therapy versus the nonfunctioning adenomas that can be safely observed. Table 53.3 outlines the differential diagnosis of an adrenal mass lesion. Figure 53.4 illustrates a useful algorithm in the workup and treatment of incidentally discovered adrenal masses. The history and physical examination should include a careful survey for subtle manifestations of hyperfunctioning tumors. The syndromes associated with functional adrenal masses include hypercortisolism or Cushing syndrome (Tables 53.3, 53.4, Fig. 53.5), hyperaldosteronism or Conn syndrome, pheochromocytomas (see subsequent text and Fig. 53.6), and feminization or virilization syndromes. A careful search for occult primary tumors of other sites should be made, with special attention to the lung and breast cancers as the most common source of adrenal metastases. Hypertension is nonspecific and may be associated with Cushing syndrome, aldosterone-secreting tumors, and pheochromocytoma. A history of upper abdominal or flank trauma may suggest adrenal hemorrhage.

Biochemical Assessment of the Incidental Adrenal Mass

The initial biochemical assessment of an incidental adrenal mass is straightforward, with more detailed confirmatory tests reserved for equivocal cases or those in which the initial functional evaluation is normal but the clinical suspicion of a

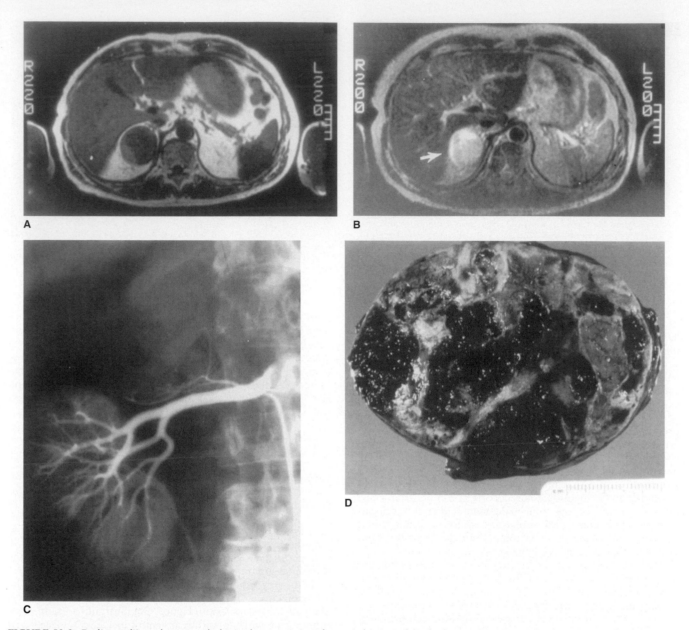

FIGURE 53.3. Radiographic and gross pathologic characteristics of a cystic benign adrenal adenoma. **A:** T1-weighted magnetic resonance image in a 57-year-old woman performed after incidental binding of an adrenal mass on computed tomographic (CT) scan obtained because of vague abdominal discomfort. A 5-cm homogeneous mass isodense with the liver replaces the right adrenal gland. **B:** T2-weighted magnetic resonance image (MRI) in the same patient. The tumor (*arrow*) appears hyperintense compared with the liver, a finding suggestive of malignancy. **C:** Selective right renal angiogram in the same patient. The tumor is hypovascular and displaces branches of the right adrenal artery. The upper pole of the right kidney is displaced interiorly and laterally. **D:** Gross specimen revealing multiple hemorrhagic pseudocysts arising from a benign cortical adenoma.

functional tumor is high. An initial biochemical screen should include measurement of serum levels of electrolytes and of 24-hour urine metanephrines, catecholamines, and free cortisol. A positive result from any screening test or high clinical suspicion based on a patient's history/physical examination should prompt a full functional screening. This tailored style of screening helps lessen costs without negatively affecting accuracy (36). In settings where initial tests are normal, the tumor is less than 3 cm, the patient is asymptomatic, no evidence of occult primary tumor exists, and the radiographic appearance is compatible with a benign nonfunctioning adrenocortical adenoma, the patient may be safely followed radiographically with serial CT scanning.

An elevated urinary cortisol level suggests the presence of Cushing syndrome. The rationale for recommending the

dexamethasone suppression test is the detection of subclinical glucocorticoid excess (Table 53.5). This subclinical syndrome is not well characterized and its impact on long-term morbidity of patients with benign adrenal masses is unclear. The reader is referred to an article by Boscaro et al. (37) for a detailed review of the diagnosis and management of Cushing syndrome. A finding of hypokalemia suggests an aldosterone-secreting tumor. This suspicion should be confirmed by a plasma aldosterone concentration to plasma renin activity (PAC:PRA) ratio. A ratio greater than 30 and a PAC of greater than 0.5 nmol/L are highly suggestive of autonomous aldosterone production. For a detailed review of the diagnosis and management of adrenal aldosterone-secreting tumors, the reader is referred to an outstanding review (38). Elevated 24-hour urinary catecholamines are

TABLE 53.3

DIFFERENTIAL DIAGNOSIS OF AN ADRENAL MASS

Benign masses	Malignant masses
Adenoma	ACC
Amyloidosis	Angiosarcoma
Adrenal cyst	Leiomyosarcoma
Congenital hyperplasia	Malignant scwannoma
Ganglioneuroma	Malignant melanoma (primary)
Granuloma	Metastatic carcinoma
Hamartoma	Malignant pheochromo cytoma
Hemorrhage	Neuroblastoma
Hemangioma	
Infection	
Leiomyoma	
Lipoma	
Myelolipoma	
Neurofibroma	
Nodular hyperplasia	
Pheochromocytoma	

ACC, adrenocortical carcinoma.

indicative of pheochromocytoma. For diagnosis of pheochromocytoma, plasma-free metanephrines (normetanephrine and metanephrine) should be measured. These combined tests have a sensitivity of 99% and specificity of 89%.

Radiologic Assessment of Incidental Adrenal Masses

Ultrasound

The diagnosis of adrenal tumors using ultrasonography is nonspecific because both benign and malignant tumors can be solid or contain cystic areas due to hemorrhage or necrosis. Ultrasound has a low sensitivity for detection of small adrenal lesions and has poor characterization of extension to adjacent structures for larger lesions.

Computed Tomography Scan

CT imaging of adrenal incidentalomas has been used to assess the risk of malignancy. Adrenal cysts, myelolipomas, and adrenal hemorrhage have CT features that are diagnostic and seldom require further evaluation. Myelolipomas have large amounts of fat, which produces low-signal-intensity on CT scans (Fig. 53.7). CT scans also define adrenal cysts better than ultrasound studies, especially with contrast enhancement. In a review of 37 benign cysts, 19 had mural and 7 had central calcifications, 28 were unilocular and 7 had high attenuation values (39). The wall thickness was less than 3 mm in 31 lesions. The authors concluded that the finding of a nonenhancing mass with or without calcifications could distinguish a cyst from an adenoma (Fig. 53.8). The high attenuation value of a hemorrhage is also readily apparent on a nonenhanced CT scan. Benign adenomas are usually homogeneous lesions with smooth, regular, encapsulated margins that do not increase in size over time.

Using data from multiple published studies, the optimal sensitivity (71%) and specificity (98%) for the diagnosis of adenoma results from choosing a threshold attenuation of less than 10 Hounsfield units (HU) on a nonenhanced CT scan (40). Several studies have also reported high sensitivity and specificity of density readings on a delayed post–contrast CT scan. In a study

of 166 adrenal masses on nonenhanced CT scans, those with attenuation values greater than 10 HU were prospectively evaluated with contrast-enhanced CT scans and contrast-enhanced CT scans with 15-minute delays (41). The sensitivity and specificity of diagnosing an adrenal adenoma versus metastasis were 98% (124/127) and 97% (33/34), respectively. Primary ACCs usually have a more aggressive appearance on CT scan, characterized by irregular contour, large size, invasion of surrounding structures, and heterogeneous internal architecture (Fig. 53.9). Central necrosis is common, and calcification is seen in 20% to 30% of cases (42).

Magnetic Resonance Imaging

Magnetic resonance imaging (MRI) has the advantage of avoiding ionizing radiation and has been used in several studies in an attempt to differentiate benign from malignant adrenal masses (43). Adenomas typically show low signal intensity on T2-image sequence, whereas both pheochromocytomas and adrenal metastases have a bright signal intensity on T2-weighted images (Figs. 53.8, 53.9, 53.10). Carcinomas are typically heterogeneously hyperintense on both T1- and T2-weighted images, reflecting frequent internal hemorrhage and necrosis. Intravenous extension is very well depicted on MRIs, and they can be helpful in defining the cephalad extension of the tumor (44). Chemical-shift MRI imaging results in a decrease in signal intensity of tissue containing both lipid and water as compared to lipid alone. Benign adenoma exhibits a signal drop on T2-weighted images and can be distinguished from metastases. There is no conclusive data using this technique with ACC and, therefore, its use cannot be justified in the differentiation of adenoma from ACC (44).

Adrenocortical Scintigraphy

Adrenocortical scintigraphy with ^{131}I-labeled 6β-iodomethyl-norcholesterol (NP59) and adrenal medullary imaging with ^{131}I-labeled or ^{123}I labeled metaiodobenzylguanidine (MIBG) provide functional metabolic information for characterization of adrenal lesions (45,46). NP59 is a cholesterol analogue and as a radiotracer is taken up by functional adrenocortical cells. If the uptake corresponds to a lesion on a CT or MRI, the diagnosis of adenoma is specific (44). Nonfunctioning malignancies or other lesions demonstrate decreased or absent (discordant) uptake. MIBG has high specificity for pheochromocytomas. These techniques, however, are expensive, time consuming, and not readily available. Therefore, data on their clinical usefulness are insufficient.

Positron Emission Tomography Scan

Data are emerging on the use of [18]FDG positron emission tomography (PET) in characterization of adrenal lesions. In one reported series of 50 adrenal lesions in 41 patients, PET identified 18/18 malignant lesions with 100% sensitivity and 94% specificity (46). However, as more data mature, it is becoming evident that adenomas can also have increased FDG uptake and give false-positive results (47). The value of PET scans for differentiating various adrenal lesions remains uncertain.

Treatment of the Incidental Adrenal Mass

The major treatment issue is whether an incidentally discovered adrenal lesion is functional or nonfunctional and whether it is benign or malignant. If the history, physical examination, and radiologic and biologic assessment confirm the presence of a unilateral functioning lesion, the treatment of choice even for smaller lesions is surgical excision. The long-term effects of mild biochemical derangement in the absence of clinical symptoms are unknown; therefore, adrenalectomy or careful

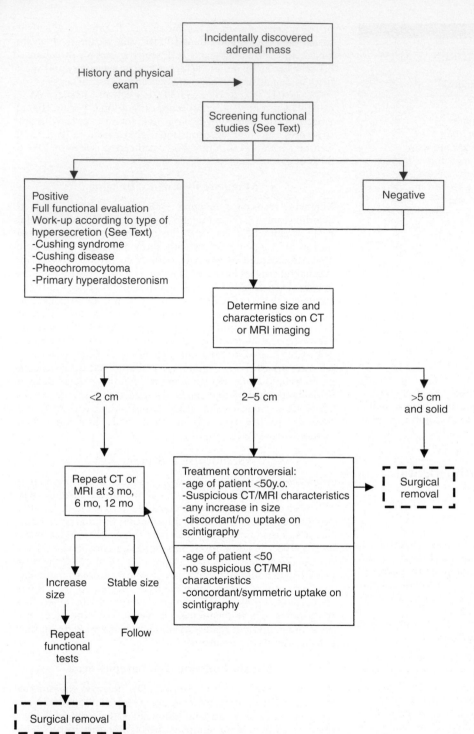

FIGURE 53.4. Algorithm illustrating the stepwise clinical evaluation and treatment of a patient with an incidentally discovered adrenal mass. (Modified from Moinzadeh A, Libertino JA. Asymptomatic adrenal mass. In: Resnick MI, Elder JS, Spirnak JP, eds. *Critical decisions in urology*, 3rd ed. Hamilton, Ontario: BC Decker Inc, 2004: 381, with permission.)

observation remain options for such patients. In patients with nonfunctioning tumors, consideration should be given to size, imaging characteristics, and growth rate to help in distinguishing benign from malignant tumors. Tumors larger than 6 cm have a high likelihood of malignancy. These large tumors should therefore be removed surgically. The incidence of ACC in adrenal masses less than 6 cm in diameter has varied from 35% to 98% in the literature (43). In a review of 630 cases of incidentalomas, 26 ACCs were found, and 85% of these were larger than 6 cm (48). In another retrospective review of 210 patients with adrenal masses, 15 adrenocortical cancers were discovered that formed 13% of their adrenal masses in patients who were operated upon. Using a cutoff of 5.0 cm yielded

a specificity of 93% and sensitivity of 64% for the diagnosis of malignant lesion (49).

The treatment of nonfunctioning tumors of 3 cm to 6 cm in diameter remains controversial because of insufficient data on their natural history in untreated patients. Management options include surgical removal, percutaneous biopsy, and observation with serial radiographs. Surgical excision offers the certainty of histologic diagnosis and the potential for cure of the occasional small primary tumor. Since the first description of laparoscopic adrenalectomy by Gagner in 1992 (50), numerous series have been reported supporting the advantages of the laparoscopic approach for the excision of the adrenal gland (51,52). Studies have documented that laparoscopy is safe, feasible, and capable

TABLE 53.4

CLINICAL FEATURES OF HYPERCORTISOLISM

General	Neuropsychiatric
Weight gain[a]	Emotional liability[a]
Hypertension[a]	Psychosis
General skin disorders	Metabolic changes
Plethora[a]	Glucose intolerance[a]
Hirsutism[a]	Hyperlipidemia[a]
Striae	Polyuria
Acne	Hypokalemia
Bruising	Kidney stones
Musculoskeletal	Gonadal dysfunction
Osteopenia[a]	Menstrual disorders[a]
Weakness/fatigue[a]	Impotence/decreased libido

[a]Noted in more than 50% of patients.

of removing large tumors (53). Established advantages of this approach over the conventional "open" approach include less postoperative pain, shorter hospital stay, better cosmesis, and earlier postoperative convalescence (53,54). Laparoscopy has been applied to functional and nonfunctional adenomas, ACCs, adrenal metastases, and pheochromocytomas with acceptable morbidity (50,54). At this writing, laparoscopic adrenalectomy may be considered the standard approach for benign surgical tumors of the adrenal gland. As with any surgical procedure, proper patient selection and laparoscopic expertise are necessary for successful surgical outcomes. The laparoscopic approach may be contraindicated in patients with large tumors (>10 cm), malignant pheochromocytoma with adenopathy, and suspected ACCs with invasion of surrounding structures.

Percutaneous needle biopsy is limited by difficulties in distinguishing benign from malignant adrenocortical tumors, but it has a role in confirming the presence of metastatic tumors. In one series of 28 patients with metastatic tumors to the adrenal gland, 26 (94%) were accurately diagnosed by percutaneous biopsy (55). However, biopsy of an incidental adrenal mass without suspicion of metastatic disease is not indicated. In summary, decisions for management should be individualized

Clinical suspicion of hypercortisolism
1. Overnight dexamethasone suppression test
2. 24 hr urinary free cortisol, 17 hydroxy steroids
3. Plasma AM/PM cortisol
Elevated Values
Nature of excessive cortisol production
Pituitary-Independent versus Dependent
1. High dose dexamethasone suppression test (2 to 8 mg/d)
2. Plasma ACTH levels
3. Corticotropin–releasing hormone stimulation test
Adrenal Source Indicated
Localization studies
1. Imaging studies: CT, MRI, U/S
2. Adrenal vein sampling

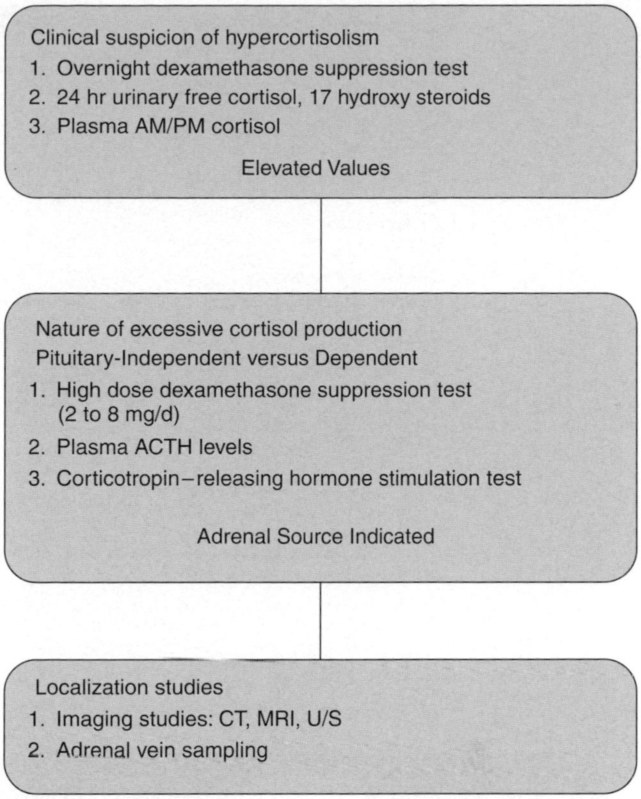

FIGURE 53.5. Nomogram illustrating the stepwise clinical evaluation of patients with suspected hypercortisolism.

Pheochromocytoma suspected
Biochemical diagnosis
Result: Normal
Result: Equivocal biochemical studies
Result: Elevated biochemical studies
Provocative test:
-Glucogon stimulation
-Clonodine suppression
Localization:
-CT
-MRI
-MIBG
Result: Normal
Seek other causes
Surgical removal of tumor

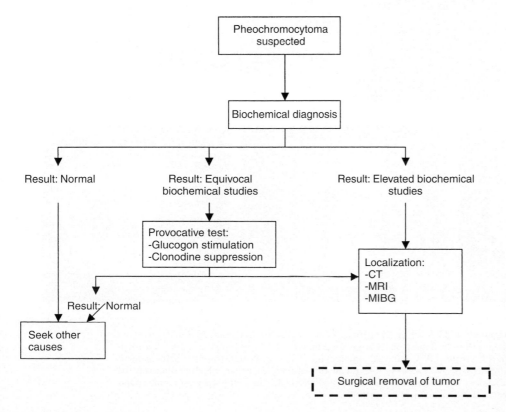

FIGURE 53.6. Algorithm illustrating the stepwise clinical evaluation and treatment of a patient with pheochromocytoma. (Modified from Moinzadeh A, Libertino JA. Pheochromocytoma. In: Resnick MI, Elder JS, Spirnak JP, eds. *Critical decisions in urology,* 3rd ed. Hamilton, Ontario: BC Decker Inc, 2004:381, with permission.)

TABLE 53.5

DEXAMETHASONE SUPPRESSION TESTS: INTERPRETATION OF RESULTS

	Diagnosis	Additional studies
Low-dose suppression test		
Serum cortisol level decreases	Normal pituitary-adrenal axis	Recheck serum cortisol level; obtain 24-hour urine sample for free cortisol level
No change in serum cortisol level	—	Perform high-dose dexamethasone suppression
High-dose suppression test		
Serum cortisol decreases	Cushing disease (pituitary adenoma)	Surgical/medical management
No change in serum cortisol	—	Check ACTH level; if low, consider functional adenoma or carcinoma; if high, consider ectopic sources of production

ACTH, adrenocorticotropic hormone.

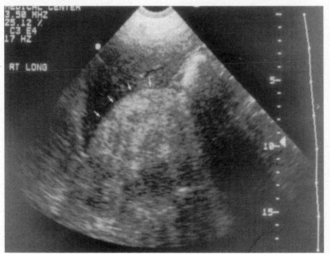

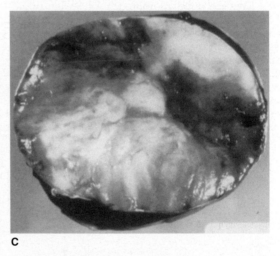

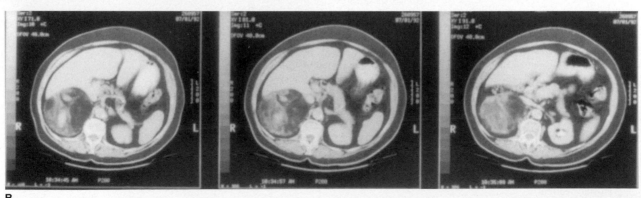

FIGURE 53.7. Radiographic and pathologic appearance of an adrenal myelolipoma. **A:** Renal ultrasound in a 47-year-old woman with right flank pain. A large, solid tumor with the hyperechoic appearance typical of fat is demonstrated (*arrows*). **B:** Computed tomographic (CT) scan demonstrating a heterogeneous tumor in the right adrenal gland with areas of low attenuation also typical of fat. Myelolipoma was suspected based on these studies. The tumor measured 10 cm in diameter. **C:** Gross appearance of a myelolipoma after removal, demonstrating heterogeneous nature.

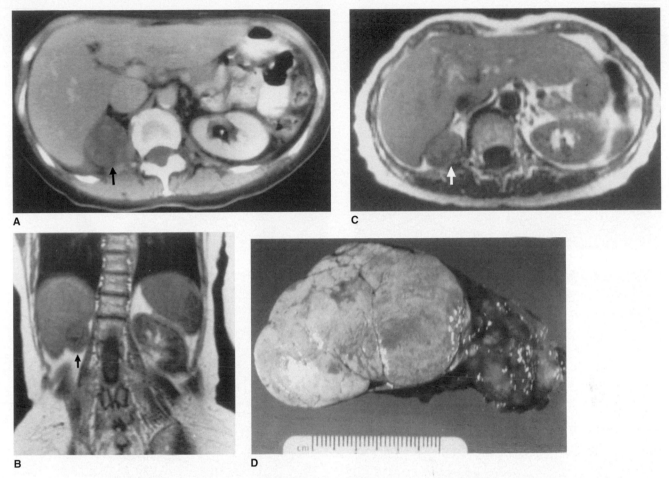

FIGURE 53.8. Radiographic and gross pathologic appearance of a benign functioning adrenocortical adenoma. A: Computed tomographic (CT) scan in a 64-year-old woman with hypercortisolism. A 4.5-cm mass replaces the right adrenal gland (*arrow*). B: T1-weighted magnetic resonance image in the same patient in the coronal plane. The right upper quadrant mass (*arrow*) appears isodense with liver. C: T2-weighted magnetic resonance image (MRI) in the same patient in a transverse plane. The tumor appears homogeneous and remains isodense with liver (*arrow*). D: Gross specimen after surgical removal, with the typical smooth, lobulated, and homogeneous appearance of a benign cortical adenoma.

based on the patient's age, medical status, and willingness to undergo surgery versus tolerating uncertainty of diagnosis, as well as the size and functional status of the adrenal mass.

Prognosis

Most adrenal incidentalomas are nonfunctional adenomas that do not require surgery. In a series of 27 patients with 30 incidentalomas followed up for 7 years, none of the nine deaths were attributed to the incidentaloma (56). Five of the 21 adrenal masses had increased in size and none had developed hormonal production on evaluation. Young (57) reported on four studies that included a total of 238 patients with adrenal incidentalomas followed for an average of 4.2 years. The adrenal masses enlarged in 8% and decreased in size in 1.3%, and none of the lesions proved to be malignant.

ADRENOCORTICAL CARCINOMAS

Carcinoma of the adrenal cortex is a rare neoplasm that may present with symptoms of endocrine hyperfunction or symptoms suggestive of advanced malignancy. Evaluation and therapy for these tumors involve endocrinologic evaluation, as well as radiologic and nuclear medicine studies. Therapeutic approaches may involve surgical removal of the primary and/or metastatic tumors and administration of various systemic agents to palliate symptoms.

Epidemiology

The incidence of adrenocortical carcinomas in the United States is approximately 0.5 to 2.0 cases per million population yearly (12). It has been estimated that 75 to 115 new cases are seen each year, and that 0.05% or less of all malignant tumors are of adrenal origin (58).

Occurrence is bimodal, with an initial peak in children younger than 5 years and the second peak in adults in the fourth and fifth decades of life (59). In a review of 1,891 cases reported in literature in the English language, Wooten and King (60) noted a similar distribution, with more than 855 tumors in children being functional. This neoplasm is more common in women (4:3) and appears to be functional more frequently in women (7:3) than in men (3:2). Several studies have shown a left-sided prevalence, while a few have shown right-sided preponderance. Approximately 2% to 10% of patients with adrenal cancer have bilateral disease (61).

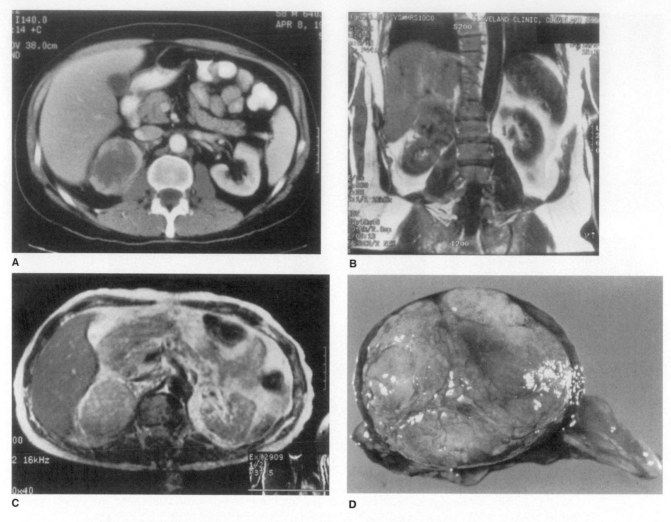

FIGURE 53.9. Radiographic and pathologic characteristics of an adrenocortical carcinoma (ACC). **A:** Computed tomographic (CT) scan in a 46-year-old man performed because of malaise and fever. A 7 cm × 5 cm heterogeneous mass with an irregular border replaces the right adrenal gland. **B:** T1-weighted magnetic resonance image (MRI) in the same patient in a coronal plane. The tumor is isodense with liver and displaces right kidney. **C:** Transverse T2-weighted MRI in the same patient demonstrating a slight increase in the tumor image intensity compared with the liver. **D:** Adrenal tumor after excision, demonstrating an irregular lobulated surface and areas of hemorrhage suggestive of ACC.

Although the incidence of adrenal incidentalomas seems to be higher in some familial neoplasia syndromes—such as multiple endocrine neoplasia, type I (MEN-I) , familial adenomatous polyposis (FAP), Li-Fraumeni syndrome—it is not entirely clear whether this is accompanied by a higher predisposition to adrenal cancer (62). In some areas of the world, like southern Brazil, the incidence of adrenal cancer is high, especially in children. The role of environmental mutagens is postulated in these geographic areas (63).

Molecular Pathogenesis

Genetic Tumor Syndromes

Several hereditary tumor syndromes are associated with the formation of benign or malignant adrenocortical tumors. The discovery of genetic events involved in these syndromes, and further characterization of these candidate genes in sporadic carcinomas, has increased the understanding of adrenal tumorigenesis. Sandrini et al. (63) investigated malividuals with childhood adrenal cancers from several cancer-prone families. Novel p53 mutations in exon 8 were detected. Germline mutations in

p53 are responsible for autosomal dominant Li-Fraumeni syndrome, and 5% of such patients develop ACCs (63). Germline mutations of p53 have been found in children with ACCs without classic family history of Li-Fraumeni syndrome, as well (63). The complete loss of one insulinlike growth factor type II (IGF-II) allele, which maps to 11p15.5 locus, and a duplication of the remaining allele in association with IGF-II overexpression has been demonstrated in tumors with Beckwith-Wiedemann syndrome and in sporadic adrenocortical tumors (63,64). In a report by Gicquel et al. (65), IGF-II was overexpressed in 27 of the 29 malignant adrenocortical tumors compared to 3 of 35 benign adenomas. Carney complex is another hereditary syndrome that is associated with primary pigmented nodular adrenocortical disease in 20% to 30% of patients (66). Two chromosomal loci have been identified (2p16 and 17q22–17q24); however, no deletions at these loci have been identified, implying that the responsible gene may be an oncogene rather than a tumor- suppressor gene (66,67). Approximately 35% of patients with MEN I have adrenal nodules, and the syndrome is related to germline mutations in the tumor-suppressor menin gene (11q13). In a series of 33 patients with MEN I, 12/33 had adrenocortical tumors, with loss of constitutional heterozygosity reported in 1 patient with ACC and not in

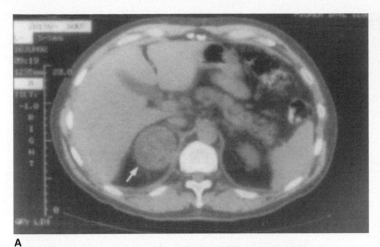

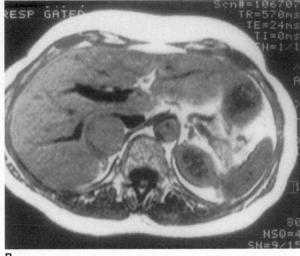

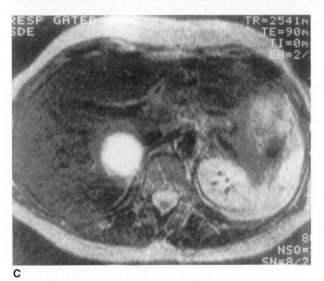

FIGURE 53.10. Computed tomographic (CT) and magnetic resonance imaging (MRI) of a pheochromocytoma. **A:** An abdominal CT in a 45-year-old patient with hypertension and elevated serum catecholamine level demonstrates a rounded homogeneous tumor replacing the right adrenal gland (*arrow*). **B:** T1-weighted MRI of the 45-year-old patient illustrated in (A). The tumor is isodense with the liver. **C:** T2-weighted MRI in the same patient. The tumor has a very high signal intensity and appears bright white, which is pathognomonic of a pheochromocytoma.

11 patients with benign adenomas (68). The genes involved in familial adenomatous polyposis coli (APC)gene and McCune Albright syndrome (activating mutations in the GNAS1 gene) have also been investigated as possible candidates in view of the presence of adrenal lesions in patients with these genetic syndromes.

Sporadic Adrenocortical Tumors

The genetic abnormalities in nonfamilial adrenal cancers are complex. Several studies have investigated the clonal composition of adrenocortical tumors using X chromosome inactivation. Gicquel et al. (69) found a monoclonal pattern in four carcinomas. Most data thus suggest that ACCs are monoclonal as a result of oncogenic mutations in single cells. Yano et al. (70) studied loss of heterozygosity (LOH) in one primary and eight recurrent ACCs and in eight sporadic benign lesions. The carcinomas showed LOH on 17p, 11p, and 13q with no changes in benign lesions. Using comparative genomic hybridization (CGH), a high frequency of genetic aberrations, involving losses on chromosome 2, 11q, and 17p and gains on chromosome 4 and 5 have been reported (14). Subsequent studies using CGH have shown equal distributions of chromosomal gains and losses in benign and malignant adrenocortical

tumors, although the specific genetic events have been different (15). In a recent case, Bernard et al. (71) suggested multi-step tumorigenesis. They studied a patient with malignant and benign sections in a tumor. This was confirmed by molecular analysis (expressions of IGF II and allelic status of 11p15 and 17p13 loci) and CGH. Using the "candidate gene approach," several studies have looked at putative oncogenes and tumor-suppressor genes such as p53, IGF II, APC, MEN I, and Ras; however, a low prevalence of mutations were found (72). Mutations of ACTH receptors and constitutive activations of regulatory proteins of cAMP such as G-protein coupled receptors have also been implicated in adrenal tumorigenesis. Mutational analysis of the coding region of the receptor in 41 adrenocortical tumors, however, did not demonstrate presence of any mutation (73).

Staging

The staging commonly used for adrenal cancer is outlined in Table 53.6 (74). Stages I and II include tumors confined to the adrenal gland; stages III and IV represent tumors with local and distant metastases, respectively. In different series, 40% to 50% of patients have advanced disease when the diagnosis is

TABLE 53.6

TABLE 53.6

STAGING SYSTEM FOR ADRENOCORTICAL CARCINOMA

Tumor characteristics, disease extent	
T1	Tumor ≤5cm no capsule invasion
T2	Tumor >5cm, no capsule invasion
T3	Tumor with invasion into periadrenal fat
T4	Tumor invading adjacent organs
N0	Negative lymph nodes
N1	Positive regional lymph nodes
M0	No metastases
M1	Distant metastases
Staging categories	
I	T1, N0, M0
II	T2, N0, M0
III	T1–T2, N1, M0; T3, N0, M0
IV	Any T, any N, M1; T3–T4, N1, M0

Adapted from Norton JA. Cancer of the endocrine system: Adrenal tumors. In: DeVita VT, Hellman S, Rosenberg SA, eds. *Cancer principles and practices of oncology.* Philadelphia: Lippincott–Raven Publishers, 1997:1,659.

made, and the median survival of these individuals is less than 1 year. In an analysis of 602 patients with adrenal carcinoma treated between 1936 and 1999 at seven institutions, Ng and Libertino (75) found the 5-year survival by stage was as follows: stage I, 30% to 45%; stage II, 12.5% to 57%; stage III, 5% to 18%; and stage IV 0%. Median survival in unresectable tumors was 3 to 9 months, whereas after complete surgical resection it ranged from 13 to 28 months.

Clinical Presentation

The biochemical basis and the various syndromes resulting from the excessive production of corticosteroids, androgens, estrogens, or mineralocorticoids have been described. In patients with adrenal cancers, the most common syndrome is Cushing syndrome. This syndrome has been reported in 30% to 40% of patients with cancer (76). Virilization alone or in combination with excess cortisol has been found in 20% to 25% of patients. Feminization or aldosterone excess is rarely reported (76,77). Both functional and nonfunctional adrenal cancers have been described. Reviews of various case series in patients with adrenal carcinoma demonstrate that clinical presentation varies based on whether the report comes from an oncologic or endocrine clinic. Functional carcinomas are more frequent in the endocrinologic literature. In a review of 1,480 patients in which functional status was mentioned, Wooten and King (60) noted that 60% of the cases were associated with evidence of function. In large retrospective series of patients with adrenal cancers, functional tumors have been reported in 34% to 72% (78). Some authors (10) have speculated that cancers are less efficient in steroidogenesis and are therefore less likely to be associated with clinical syndromes of steroid excess. Methods of screening for steroid precursors are not standard, and the excessive production of early precursors such as Δ5-pregnenolone or DHEA may not be detected. The method of study or screening patients who lack clear clinical syndromes may vary, and studies indicating a functional tumor will vary with the vigor with which such studies are pursued.

In patients with nonfunctioning tumors, the diagnosis is generally made when a neoplasm produces symptoms by virtue of its size or disease spread. Nonfunctional ACCs can be more difficult to diagnose because they remain clinically silent. These tumors typically present late in their natural history and are more often of advanced stage than are functional tumors. Typical symptoms of nonfunctional tumors include abdominal mass, pain on the affected side, and constitutional symptoms of weight loss, fever, anorexia, nausea, and myalgia, owing to advanced malignancy (79). Some patients will have symptoms of metastatic disease before a primary diagnosis, whereas others present with incidental findings on abdominal CT scans performed for unrelated reasons.

Diagnostic Evaluation of Adrenal Cancer

The diagnostic evaluation of ACC is a two-step process and includes (a) biochemical assessment and (b) radiographic localization and staging.

Biochemical Assessment

Studies in patients with adrenal cancers have demonstrated the following well-documented biochemical abnormalities: elevated levels of urinary free cortisol; loss of circadian rhythm of cortisol secretion; loss of suppressibility of pituitary–adrenal axis; elevated urinary levels of steroid precursors; and low levels of ACTH in the serum due to high levels of circulating cortisol. Decisions on specific components of biochemical parameters depend to some degree on the clinical presentation of the patient.

In patients who present with Cushing syndrome, a 24-hour urinary free cortisol level determination is the most sensitive measure of excess cortisol production. Levels of cortisol metabolites in the urine, including 17-hydroxycorticosteroids and 17-ketosteroids, may also be elevated. Serum studies in a patient with suspected Cushing syndrome should include cortisol levels measured early in the morning and in the late afternoon or early evening. The normal adrenal cortex exhibits a circadian rhythm such that the morning cortisol levels are approximately two to three times higher than late afternoon/evening levels; hypersecreting adrenal tumors lose this diurnal variation and produce high levels at all times.

In patients with virilization, serum measurements of levels of androstenedione, testosterone, and DHEA and its sulfate, are appropriate. In men with feminization, estradiol levels are often elevated. In patients with hypertension and hypokalemia, the PAC:PRA ratio should be measured. Finally, in patients with an uncertain etiology, a dexamethasone suppression test should be considered, as previously outlined in the section "Evaluation of the Incidental Adrenal Mass."

Radiographic Localization and Staging

In addition to the biochemical studies, radiographic evaluation of the adrenal glands and possible metastatic sites should be performed for the purpose of clinical staging and operative planning. The radiographic evaluation should include a chest x-ray as a screen for pulmonary metastases. CT of the abdomen and pelvis will define the location and local extent of the tumor, as well as associated nodal and visceral metastases. CT will allow an evaluation of local invasion into the ipsilateral kidney and an assessment of the function of the contralateral kidney. This is important because it is often necessary to remove large adrenal tumors *en bloc* with the ipsilateral kidney.

MRI is also useful in defining the extent of ACCs. Typically, these tumors appear isodense to liver on T1-weighted images and hyperintense with a bright white appearance on T2-weighted images. Coronal MRI cuts may be useful for establishing the presence or absence of liver invasion in right-sided tumors and for defining the presence, absence, or extent of tumor thrombi extending into the inferior vena cava (Fig. 53.9).

Prognostic Factors

Multiple authors have investigated the relation between various pathologic and clinical characteristics and survival in patients with adrenal cancer. Stage appears to be one of the most important factors, with stages I and II (localized disease) having the best chance of cure with surgical removal (79,80). Patients with metastatic disease have median survivals of less than 1 year (81). The relation between prognosis and various characteristics of primary tumor has been investigated, including mitotic activity, grade, vascular invasion, various architectural features, and tumor size (20). In most studies, none of these factors was independently associated with disease-free survival. Deoxyribonucleic acid (DNA) content has been examined, but in individual cases, it is not a reliable indicator of prognosis (82).

Clinical features have also been studied, and it has been suggested that functional status is associated with enhanced survival. In most studies (80,81,83), however, this has not been confirmed. The Southwest Oncology Group (81) investigated the clinical features of 37 patients with metastatic adrenal cancer using a Cox model and found that prior adrenal surgery and performance status were associated with improved survival.

Therapy of Adrenocortical Carcinoma

The primary treatment of ACC is complete surgical removal of tumor when feasible. *En bloc* resection of the tumor and, in selected instances, removal of isolated metastatic disease are indicated. On occasion, this may include resection of adjacent organs or great vessels, including ipsilateral kidney, a portion of the pancreas, and sections of the liver. When indicated, renal vein or inferior vena cava (IVC) tumor thrombus may be removed at the time of surgical resection with cardiopulmonary bypass (84). In general, lower-stage tumors are managed by surgical excision, while more advanced tumors may require a debulking procedure. The incision used to perform the surgery is dependent on a number of factors, including size and location of tumor, appearance on radiographic imaging, and the experience level of the surgeon. In most instances, a thoracoabdominal or Chevron incision is utilized. This incision allows access to the more cephalad location of the gland within the abdomen and the vessels supplying it. An attempt is always made to excise the tumor in its entirety. However, even with complete excision, a 35% to 85% recurrence rate has been reported (75).

Although the safety and efficacy of laparoscopy have been documented for benign tumors, uncertainty still exists about the role of laparoscopy in the treatment of primary or metastatic malignant tumors of the adrenal gland. A number of reports have suggested caution in the use of the laparoscopic approach for malignant adrenal tumors. These case reports totaling seven patients describe recurrent malignancy shortly after laparoscopic adrenalectomy (85–91). Except for two cases of metastatic lung cancer to the adrenal gland, all other cases were initially thought to be benign and were only later diagnosed as ACC. This underscores the difficulty of diagnosing ACC even with the entire pathologic specimen. Although laparoscopy is hypothesized potentially to have played a role in the dissemination of tumor in each case, no clear evidence as such is provided. Other important factors, such as the innate aggressive nature of the tumor and the potential techniques used in resection, should be considered.

On the other hand, there have been nine published reports totaling 74 patients with short to intermediate follow-up that lend credence to the use of laparoscopic adrenalectomy for selected patients having adrenal malignancy (92–99). A recent review of the Cleveland Clinic experience with laparoscopic adrenalectomy for malignancy was conducted. Of 250 total cases, 31 patients were identified with pathologically confirmed adrenal malignancy. The cohort included patients with preoperative suspicion of solitary metastasis to the adrenal gland and those found incidentally to have primary adrenal malignancy. A total of 33 procedures were performed in these 31 patients. There were 19 men and 12 women, mean age 60.7 years (range, 38 to 79). Mean adrenal tumor size on preoperative CT scan was 5 cm (range, 1.8–10 cm). Mean operative time was 181 minutes, estimated blood loss was 258 mL, and hospital stay was 2.1 days. There was no operative mortality. The cohort consisted primarily of patients with metastatic cancer to the adrenal gland ($n = 25$) and primary adrenocrotical carcinoma ($n = 6$). Follow-up data were available for 30 (97%) patients with a median follow-up of 28 months (range 1 to 65). Thirteen (42%) of these patients were alive with no evidence of disease at a median follow-up of 42 months. Fourteen patients (45%) died of recurrent disease, and 1 patient died of other causes. Local recurrence was noted in 7 (22%) patients. Three of these patients are currently alive with disease. We believe contemporary series, including ours, demonstrate that laparoscopy in carefully selected patients is suitable for the treatment of a small, organ-confined, primary adrenal malignancy or metastasis to the adrenal gland.

Surgical Therapy for Recurrent Disease

Given the relative poor results of systemic chemotherapy for ACC, aggressive resection remains a valid option. This surgical philosophy has been used for other malignancies (100). In addition, at least theoretically, removal of the recurrent adrenal cancer may decrease hormonal symptoms (101). This aggressive approach has been used in select patients, some with surprisingly long-term survival (102,103). Bellantone et al. (103) retrospectively reviewed 179 cases of ACC from a national registry. Fifty-two cases (37%) were found to have local recurrence. Of those patients, 20 underwent a second resection while the remaining 32 received chemotherapy. Mean survival in the operative patients was 15.8 months relative to 3.2 months in the nonoperative group. On the basis of these results, the authors recommend an aggressive surgical strategy for recurrent ACC. The best candidates remain those without distant metastasis (the exception being lung metastasis). The role of debulking surgery remains unclear.

Chemotherapy

Chemotherapeutic agents have been used in patients with functional syndromes to control excess steroid production or, alternatively, for their cytotoxic activity to selectively destroy residual and/or metastatic tumor cells. In patients presenting with florid Cushing syndrome, preoperative suppression of tumor-hormone production may decrease associated operative risks. Improvements in tissue fragility and wound healing may occur. Agents used in the past include metyrapone, aminoglutethimide, ketoconazole, and mitotane [o,p'-DDD (1,1-dichloro-2,2-bis(p-chlorophenyl)ethane)]. This latter agent has a slow onset of action and is, therefore, of limited use preoperatively.

Metyrapone. Metyrapone inhibits 11-β-hydroxylation in adrenocortical cells and blocks the conversions of substance S to cortisol and 11-desoxycorticosterone to corticosterone (4). It is used to control symptoms in patients with all types of Cushing syndrome (104). In patients with cancer and excessive cortisol production, metyrapone also has been used to control clinical symptoms. When used for extended periods, however, this agent causes hypokalemic alkalosis and hypertension (2), which are secondary to increased production of desoxycorticosterone by tumor cells, which then has potent mineralocorticoid effects. It can also enhance androgen synthesis and produce hirsutism and virilism.

Prolonged use of metyrapone has had limited success (4). Doses of 1.0 g to 3.0 g daily can be used. When administered in combination with other drugs that inhibit mineralocorticoid production such as aminoglutethimide, lower doses of each agent may be used. In patients with bulky tumors, metyrapone is of limited value in controlling the manifestations of hypercortisolism (4).

Aminoglutethimide. Aminoglutethimide inhibits cholesterol side chain cleavage (105) and blocks steroid aromatization by its actions on cytochrome p-450 reduction and other steps involved in steroidogenesis (106). This agent has, therefore, been used to inhibit estrogen production in patients with estrogen-responsive metastatic breast cancer and to inhibit steroid production in patients with Cushing syndrome. It has been reported to decrease the plasma cortisol levels by 50% in patients with adrenal cancer (107) and may be more effective than o,p'-DDD in producing adrenal insufficiency (106). Aminoglutethimide also alters extraadrenal metabolism of cortisol (107,108) and, therefore, disproportionately decreases urinary 17-hydroxycorticosteroid excretion. In view of this, plasma cortisol levels are best used to gauge therapy and assess patient status.

The dose of aminoglutethimide utilized in this setting is 250 mg to 500 mg four times daily. It is effective in decreasing cortisol secretion in patients with adrenal cancer after 10 to 14 days of administration; however, it has no effects on tumor progression (109). Schmoll (110) also reported use of aminoglutethimide in a patient with an estrogen-producing adrenal cancer in whom hormone levels normalized and tumor size stabilized. Because adrenal insufficiency may develop with its use, prophylactic administration of cortisone preparations is advisable. Additionally, aldosterone secretion may be inhibited, and addition of mineralocorticoid preparations may be required. At doses of 2.0 g daily, aminoglutethimide has variable toxicity, including anorexia, vomiting, fever, somnolence, skin rash, and ataxia (4).

Mitotane. Development of o,p'-DDD evolved from observations that the insecticide DDD, if administered chronically to dogs, produced atrophy and necrosis of the adrenal glands (111). DDD was then fractionated into two isomers, and the o,p'-DDD compound contained all the adrenolytic activity. Administration of o,p'-DDD to dogs for 4 days blocked the response to ACTH (111). This combination of steroid inhibition and adrenolytic activity suggested the possibility that o,p'-DDD could be useful in patients with adrenal cancers. In 1960, Bergenstal et al. (112) reported the initial clinical experience with o,p'-DDD and demonstrated regression of metastatic lesions and decreases of urinary steroid excretion in patients with adrenocortical cancers. After this report, the agent became standard therapy for both functional and nonfunctional metastatic adrenocortical tumors.

The mechanisms of o,p'-DDD action on the adrenal cortex is not clear, but it appears to involve inhibition of several enzyme systems, including Δ5-pregnenolone,11-β-hydroxylation, and 18-hydroxylation (113). Inhibition of the 11-β-hydroxylase reaction may lead to increase in plasma 11-deoxycortisol and sub-

sequent reduction in urinary free cortisol (114). Additionally, glucocorticoids are excreted as 6-β-hydroxysteroids, a category of compounds not detected in the 17-hydroxycorticoid fraction. These changes can occur in the absence of objective tumor regression.

Oral administration is standard for o,p'-DDD, and bioavailability studies indicate that approximately 40% is absorbed (115). Between 20% and 30% of an oral dose is stored in body fat; concentrates in liver, brain, and adrenal tissue; and may be released over a period of months after it is discontinued. The maximal plasma concentration is reached in 3 to 5 hours, and the serum half-life is 2 to 3 hours (116). After prolonged o,p'-DDD therapy, serum half-life after discontinuation has varied from 18 to 159 days (117).

In the intial report by Bergenstal et al. (112), objective remissions were noted in 7 of 18 (39%) patients with metastatic adrenal cancer, and 7 additional patients had significant suppression of steroid excretion. The average doses used in this trial were 8 to 10 g/d for 6 to 8 weeks. The National Cancer Institute then sponsored the production and distribution of o,p'-DDD for therapy for patients with histologically proven ACC. This experience was summarized by Hutter and Kayhoe (118). Table 53.7 summarizes clinical results with mitotane. Control of steroid production was noted in 70% to 90% of patients; tumor regression was noted in 34% to 61%. These studies were uncontrolled and represent retrospective analyses of data from multiple investigators. Criteria for objective tumor regression were variable, doses used inconsistent, and duration of therapy not standardized. No randomized trials comparing o,p'-DDD to another agent or regimen have been performed.

In a 1990 report, Luton et al. (80) summarized the findings in 59 patients receiving o,p'-DDD, and the responses in 37 individuals with objectively measurable disease. Endocrine hypersecretion was controlled in 75% of patients. Objective tumor regressions were noted in 8 of 37 patients, and 5 instances (13%), were characterized as 50% or more. The site of response in these latter patients was the lung, with a median response duration of 12 months (range 5 to 25 months). In this study, the relationship of o,p'-DDD therapy to overall survival also was examined, and no relation was noted. The only factors that independently influenced cumulative survival were age and presence of metastases.

Van Slooten et al. (120) investigated the relationship of serum levels of o,p'-DDD to response. Among patients with measurable disease, 34 were treated and objective responses were seen in 8 (29%). In 7 of the 8 responding patients, serum levels of o,p'-DDD were 14 μg/mL or more for more than 6 months. In 19 of 20 nonresponders in whom serum levels were determined, values of less than 10 μg/mL were present. Serum o,p'-DDD levels and 50% survival times were also compared, and levels of 14 μg/mL or more were associated with significant increases in survival rates ($P < .01$). The authors concluded that no therapeutic effects can be expected at serum levels of less than 10 μg/mL, and levels should be maintained as high as tolerated, with a minimum of 14 μg/mL. The dose levels, dose modification scheme, and schedule for o,p'-DDD in this report are, however, unclear. In another prospective study where mitotane (6 to 12 g) was used in 13 patients with metastatic ACC and 11 patients as adjuvant therapy, serum levels were monitored to achieve levels of o,p'-DDD between 14 mg/L and 20 mg/L (121). Of the 6 patients with metastatic disease who achieved these levels, 4 had objective tumor responses. Of the 11 patients who received mitotane as adjuvant therapy, 8 had disease recurrence, although plasma levels were greater than 14 mg/L in 6. Grade 3/4 neurologic toxicity was observed in 3 patients, all with an o,p'-DDD level greater than 20 mg/L. Use of low-dose mitotane (2 to 3 g/d) to achieve the same therapeutic range has also been reported by Terzolo et al. though efficacy data are not available (122).

TABLE 53.7

RESULTS OF MITOTANE THERAPY IN PATIENTS WITH ADVANCED ADRENOCORTICAL CARCINOMA

Author	yr	Number of patients in report	Mitotane therapy Adjuvant	Measurable disease	Response (%) objective (CR + PR)
Hutter and Kayhoe (118)	1996	138	—	59	34
Lubitz et al. (119)	1973	115	—	75	61
Schteingart et al. (123)	1982	23	4	9	33
Venkatesh et al. (124)	1989	110	7	72	29
Luton et al. (80)	1990	105	45	37	21
Decker et al. (133)	1991	52	—	36	22
Icard et al. (77)	1992	156	—	15	20
Pommier and Brennan (214)	1992	73	7	29	24
Vassieopoulou et al. (125)	1993	19	13	—	—
Haak et al. (126)	1994	96	11	52	29
Kasperlik-Zaluska et al. (215)	1995	50	36	2	NR
Barzon et al. (216)	1997	45	27	23	17

CR, complete response; NR, not reported; PR, partial response.

Wooten and King (60) in 1993 reviewed 64 reports of o,p'-DDD use in patients with adrenal cancer and noted that partial or complete responses were reported in 194 of 551 patients (35%). The variability of response criteria was discussed and included tumor measurements, biochemical findings, and various clinical findings.

In view of its apparent activity in advanced disease, o,p'-DDD also has been used as an adjuvant after surgical resection of stages I, II, and III (localized and regional disease) adrenal carcinoma. Schteingart et al. (123) studied patients after resection or/and radiation, where mitotane was given to 17 patients and 6 received no treatment. Survival appeared longer in the treated group. Venkatesh et al. (124) reported that 6 of 7 patients on adjuvant mitotane were alive 1 to 4 years after surgery. Retrospective reviews (80,83,125,126) did not demonstrate differences in survival rates for patients receiving o,p'-DDD after surgery. In a more recent series reported by Barzon et al. (127) 26 patients were divided into two comparable groups given mitotane or not given mitotane after tumor resection. Cumulative disease-free interval and survival were not different in the two groups. Evidence for positive effects of o,p'-DDD in the adjuvant setting is lacking. In summary, use of mitotane in nonresectable cases and long-term therapy in the presence of a clinical response is reasonable.

The toxicity of o,p'-DDD is substantial and often requires dose reduction or discontinuation. Doses of 6.0 to 12.0 g daily are recommended, but most patients do not tolerate more than 6.0 g/d for more than 2 months (128). Usually o,p'-DDD is begun at a dose of 500 mg three to four times daily, with gradual increases until patient intolerance occurs. The most common side effects are gastrointestinal, with nausea, vomiting, anorexia, and diarrhea occurring in more than 50% of individuals. Moolenarr et al. (129) suggested that administration of o,p'-DDD and powdered milk, mixed in water, may enhance absorption and diminish the gastrointestinal toxicity. Neurologic toxicity is also frequent and is seen in more than 40% of patients (119). Lethargy, dizziness, confusion, myalgia, and headache are common. Serum levels of 20 μg/mL or more increase the neuromuscular toxicity, and at levels of 30 μg/mL or more, the symptoms become intolerable (120). Other reported indications of CNS toxicity include psychiatric abnormalities, such as depression, and nonspecific electroencephalogram (EEG) abnormalities. Skin rashes, hematuria, hemorrhagic

cystitis, and proteinuria have been reported. In addition, o,p'-DDD can decrease total serum thyroxine concentrations (130) and prolong bleeding times by production of an aspirin-like defect of platelet function (131). Adrenal and extra-adrenal metabolism of steroids are affected by o,p'-DDD, and concomitant therapy with hydrocortisone is generally suggested. Addition of mineralocorticoids should be considered, especially if prolonged treatment is planned.

Cytotoxic Chemotherapy. Table 53.8 presents a summary of the chemotherapeutic agents and regimens that have been used in patients with metastatic adrenal carcinoma. Most reported series are small, include fewer than 20 patients, and present anecdotal results. The most commonly used agent has been cisplatin, either alone (132) or in combination with other agents. The majority of patients who respond have partial regressions; however, occasionally prolonged responses (more than 24 months) are seen. Two of the largest series (81,133) used o,p'-DDD with cisplatin or doxorubicin (DOX) as single agents and reported response rates of 30% and 19%, respectively. Cisplatin in combination with etoposide and/or DOX (135–141) also has been used.

The Southwest Oncology Group (81) investigated the factors associated with enhanced survival in patients receiving o,p'-DDD and cisplatin. Previous surgery for removal of the primary adrenal tumor ($P = .0005$) and performance status ($P = .04$) were predictive of survival, with the former also associated with performance levels. Interestingly, functional status of the tumor was not significant. The Eastern Cooperative Oncology Group (133) treated 16 patients with DOX and noted this agent was ineffective in patients with well-differentiated tumors.

A 170- to 180-kDa membrane-associated protein, p-Glycoprotein (PGP) appears to mediate multidrug resistance by enhancing the efflux of natural chemotherapeutic agents (142). The normal adrenal cortex expresses mRNA for mdr-1/PGP, the multidrug resistance gene (143). High levels persist in adrenocortical tumors (141,143,144). No correlations with clinical stage, survival, functional status, or histologic index were found (141). Additionally, no relation of PGP expression and responses to o,p'-DDD was noted (144). *In vitro*, o,p'-DDD can reverse the multidrug resistance of cultured adrenal cancer cell lines and provides a basis for investigating o,p'-DDD with agents such as etoposide or DOX.

TABLE 53.8

RESULTS REPORTED WITH CYTOTOXIC CHEMOTHERAPY IN PATIENTS WITH ADRENOCORTICAL CARCINOMA

Regimen	Number of patients	Response data			
		CR	PR	Percent PR + CR	Response duration (mo)
CDDP (132)	14	—	5	36	4.0–9.0
CDDP + o,p′-DDD (81)	37	1	10	30	7.9
CDDP + VP-16 (155) (135)	15	0	8	53	NR
CDDP + VP-16 + bleomycin (136)	4	1	1	50	3.5–12.0
CDDP + VP-16 + DOX (137)	2	0	2	100	7.0,21+
CDDP + DOX + 5-FU (138)	6	1	1	33	6+ to 38.0
CDDP + DOX + CTX (139)	11	0	2	18	NR
Carboplatin + VP-16 (140)	1	1	—	100	10+
DOX (134) (217)	35	1	3	11	3.5–78.0
Suramin (146) (147)	16	0	2	13	2.0–6.8
CDDP + VP-16 + DOX + o,p′-DDD (218)	28	2	13	53.5	NR
Dox + VP-16 + Vinc + mitotane (145)	36	1	7	22	12.4
Streptozocin + o,p′-DDD (219)	22	NR	NR	36.4	NR
CDDP + VP-16 + o,p′-DDD (220)	18	3	3	33	NR
Total	245	11	57	28%	—

5-FU, fluorouracil; CDDP, cisplatin; CR, complete response; CTX, cyclophosphamide; DOX, doxorubicin; NR, not reported; o,p′-DDD, mitotane; PR, partial response; VP-16, etoposide; Vinc, Vincristine.

Berruti et al. (137) reported a phase II trial of o,p′-DDD (up to 4 g/d) in combination with etoposide (100 mg/m^2 on days 5 and 7), DOX (20 mg/m^2 on days 1 and 8), and cisplatin (40 mg/m^2 on days 1 and 9). Of 28 patients, 15 responded (2 CRs). The median time to progression was 24.4 months. In 16 patients with functioning tumors, a complete hormonal response was noted. Toxicity with this regimen was reported as moderate; however, only 9 patients took 4.0 g of o,p′-DDD daily. In a phase II trial, Abraham et al. (145) gave daily oral mitotane (4 to 6 g/d), 96 hours infusional DOX (10 mg/m^2/d), vincristine(0.4 mg/m^2/d) and etoposide (75 mg/m^2/d) to 36 patients. Responses were observed in 8 (22%) patients. The median survival of patients who did not respond to chemotherapy was 11.6 months, whereas it was 34.3 months in patients who responded to chemotherapy (from a point 4 months after initiation of chemotherapy). Neutropenia was observed in 66% of cycles, but febrile neutropenia was present in only 3% of 190 cycles administered. Grade 1 to grade 2 toxicity secondary to mitotane, including nausea, diarrhea, fatigue, and neuropsychiatric changes, was observed in 31 of 36 patients and made administration of therapy difficult.

Miscellaneous Agents. Other agents investigated include suramin (146,147). This agent appears to have multiple effects, including displacement of growth factors (146) and inhibition of various cellular enzyme systems (146). Trials in 16 patients with adrenal cancer demonstrated 2 partial responders (146,147).

Gossypol, derived from crude cottonseed oil, has been reported to inhibit growth of adrenal cancer in nude mice (148). Oral gossypol (30 to 70 mg) was used to treat 21 patients with metastatic adrenal cancer, and responses similar to those observed with o,p′-DDD were noted (149). The toxicity of this agent was substantially less than o,p′-DDD.

The antifungal agent ketoconazole is a potent inhibitor of the p-450 cytochrome enzyme system, participating in gonadal and adrenal steroid synthesis (150), which has led to its use in patients with excess cortisol secretion and Cushing syndrome (151). It also has been used in patients with virilizing adrenal cancers (152), with tumor regression noted in one instance.

Doses of 600 to 1,200 mg daily have been administered, and this agent appears to represent another method for controlling the excessive steroid production associated with functional adrenal cancers. The overall efficacy associated with its use is unclear, and the reported experience is anecdotal.

Radiation Therapy

The role of radiation therapy in patients with adrenal cancer has received minimal attention. Percarpio and Knowlton (153) reviewed 11 patients receiving 15 to 51 Gy of radiation for palliation of symptoms. In all instances, symptom relief was reported. The experience with radiation preoperatively or as a postoperative adjuvant is quite limited (153, 154); however, the possibility that postoperative radiotherapy administered to the tumor bed and nodal areas in stage III disease may improve local control has been suggested (154). Data to support this are lacking, however. The use of radiation in doses of approximately 30 to 40 Gy delivered over 2 to 3 weeks for palliation of symptoms is reasonable (155).

Embolization and Radiofrequency Ablation

Use of transarterial embolization has been reported in patients with only partially resectable or unresectable hepatic metastases (156). Use of hepatic artery occlusion or embolization may be of value for control of symptoms in carefully selected patients. Wood et al. (157) report on image-guided percutaneous radiofrequency ablation (RFA) of 15 primary and metastatic neoplasms in eight patients. All patients had unresectable tumors or were poor candidates for surgery. Eight of the 15 lesions showed evidence of stable disease at median follow-up of 10 months. Three lesions were reported to have nearly disappeared. There was no significant short-term morbidity from the procedure; however, its long-term efficacy and impact on survival, if any, are unknown.

PHEOCHROMOCYTOMAS

Tumors of the adrenal medulla are uncommon and may be either benign or malignant. Neuroblastomas arise from sympathetic neuroblasts and occur almost exclusively in infancy or childhood. Approximately one third of these tumors arise in the adrenal gland (158). Ganglioneuromas are rare tumors of sympathetic nerve fibers that may occur in the adrenal or in extra-adrenal locations (128). These tumors are generally benign and inactive, but reports have noted the presence of Leydig cells with production of testosterone and subsequent virilization (159). Preganglionic fibers of the autonomic nervous system synapse on chromaffin cells of the adrenal medulla. These cells secrete catecholamines (epinephrine 80% and norepinephrine 20%) into the circulation. Pheochromocytomas are tumors that arise from these chromaffin cells within the adrenal gland 90% of the time. If the tumor is derived from chromaffin cells outside of the adrenal gland (10%), the term "paragangliomas" is applied. These tumors may arise anywhere from the neck down to the pelvis. Most pheochromocytomas are benign; however, approximately 10% are reported as malignant (159). The malignant tumors are also functional and represent the counterpart of ACCs in the medullary portion of the gland. Sporadic and familial forms occur; however, the latter are uncommon, accounting for 10% or fewer of these tumors (160). Finally, a rare variety of adrenal medullary tumor is the compound tumor characterized by a mixture of pheochromocytoma and ganglioneuroma (155). These neoplasms are benign, and approximately 75% are functional.

Epidemiology and Genetics

The frequency of pheochromocytomas has been estimated to be approximately 0.1% in patients with hypertension whose urinary catecholamines are measured (161). In autopsy series, this tumor is found in 0.005% to 0.100% of individuals (162).

Approximately 10% of pheochromocytomas are familial, and these tumors are usually benign (163). Several distinct syndromes have been described in which the incidence of this neoplasm is increased and include (a) neurofibromatosis, (b) von Hippel-Lindau (VHL) disease, (c) MEN, and (d) familial pheochromocytoma. In patients with von Recklinghausen disease (neurofibromatosis), the frequency of this neoplasm has been reported as less than 1%, whereas in patients with VHL disease it has been estimated as 25% (164). The multiple endocrine neoplasia syndromes (MEN-2a and MEN-2b) may include bilateral adrenal medullary pheochromocytomas (165). Table 53.9 compares the characteristics of patients with hereditary or sporadic tumors.

Cytogenetic and molecular genetic studies of sporadic and hereditary pheochromocytomas have demonstrated various abnormalities. LOH for loci on chromosome arms 1p, 3p, 3q, 11p, 13q, 17p, and 22q were reported by Mulligan et al. (166) in tumors from patients with MEN-2 syndromes (medullary thyroid carcinoma, pheochromocytomas). Other studies of pheochromocytomas have demonstrated LOH on chromosome arms 1p and/or 22q in both sporadic and familial variants (167). In patients with neurofibromatosis, loss of NF1 alleles in pheochromocytomas has been noted (168).

MEN-2 is a dominantly inherited syndrome resulting from mutations in the RET proto-oncogene (chromosome 10q 11.2). The RET protein is a receptor tyrosine kinase related to platelet-derived growth factor. The function of this protein is unclear. The germline mutations associated with MEN-2 are found in one of the eight codons distributed among the five exons in this gene (169). Nineteen different mutations in families with pheochromocytomas have been described, and in one family, a codon 634 mutation has been associated with the development of this tumor (170).

TABLE 53.9

CHARACTERISTICS OF PATIENTS WITH PHEOCHROMOCYTOMA-ASSOCIATED SYNDROMES

Type	Associated lesions	Mean age at diagnosis (yr)	Inheritance	Frequency Multiple pheochromocytoma	Frequency Extra-adrenal pheochromocytoma
Sporadic	None	46	Autosomal dominant	8%	16%
Multiple endocrine neoplasia					
Type 2A	CCH, MTC, HPT	37	Autosomal dominant	75%	13%
Type 2B	CCH, MTC, developmental abnormalities				
VHL	Retinal angiomatosis, CNS hemangioblastomas, RCC (uncommon), pancreatic cysts	27	Autosomal dominant	44%	30%
NF-1	Cutaneous neurofibroma	Unknown	Autosomal dominant	Possible	Unknown

CCH, c-cell hyperplasia; CNS, central nervous system; HPT, hyperparathyroidism; MTC, medullary thyroid cancer; NF, neurofibromatosis; RCC, renal cell carcinoma; VHL, von Hippel-Lindau syndrome.
Adapted from Neumann HPH, Berger DP, Sigmund G, et al. Pheochromocytomas, multiple endocrine neoplasia type 2, and von Hippel-Lindau disease. *N Engl J Med* 1993; 329: 1531; Neumann HPH, Bender BU, Januszewicz A, et al. Inherited pheochromocytoma. *Adv Nephrol* 1998;27:361.

In VHL disease, mutations in the VHL gene (chromosome 3 p25 to p26) have been detected (171). The reader is referred to the renal cell carcinoma (RCC) chapter of this book for an excellent review of this topic.

Patients with pheochromocytomas should be considered initially to have an inherited type of this tumor. Patients with multiple tumors are more likely candidates, and those with malignant pheochromocytomas are less likely to be carriers of a genetic disorder. Current molecular genetic techniques can clarify the status of these individuals. Formerly, clinical screening was used in at-risk individuals; however, current genetic testing is noninvasive and less expensive. Van der Horst et al. (172) retrospectively screened a group of 68 patients presenting with pheochromocytomas, and VHL gene mutations were found in 8.8%. These studies indicate inherited forms of pheochromocytoma are common in patients presenting with sporadic tumors and also that families of identified individuals should be considered at risk and screened. Positive genetic studies occur in 70% of VHL and in 95% of MEN-2 families (165).

Pathology

The average size of pheochromocytoma is 5.0 cm, and weight is approximately 75 to 150 g (173). Pathologically, it is almost impossible to differentiate between benign and malignant pheochromocytomas. Instead, the clinician must rely on the presence or absence of metastasis. Malignant pheochromocytomas originate more frequently in extra-adrenal sites (174) and may be larger in size (173). Microscopically, these tumors are composed of chromaffin-like cells arranged in cords or alveolar patterns (Fig. 53.11). Capsular invasion, vascular invasion, or both have been noted in benign tumors (173). Cellular atypia and pleomorphism likewise do not predict malignant behavior of these tumors (173).

The correlation of clinical behavior with nuclear DNA content has also been examined (174). Diploid DNA content generally is associated with a benign course (175). Abnormal DNA ploidy is more frequently associated with malignancy (174), but aneuploid or tetraploid patterns can occur in benign tumors. Hosaka et al. (176) proposed using a proliferation index derived from DNA histograms as another alternative for classifying these tumors as potentially malignant. However, at this time, no definitive predictions can be made on the sole basis of DNA ploidy.

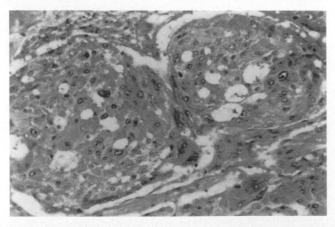

FIGURE 53.11. Histologic appearance of a pheochromocytoma. This tumor is characterized by pleomorphic pink-staining polyhedral cells separated by abundant vascular channels and sinusoidal spaces.

Clinical Syndromes

Due to secretion of catecholamines by pheochromocytomas, hypertension is the hallmark clinical finding. Other signs and symptoms may include frontal headache, diaphoresis, palpitation, facial pallor, and apprehension. If ongoing severe hypertension is not diagnosed, disastrous results may ensue, including myocardial infarction and stroke (177). Approximately 50% of patients will have sustained hypertension (178). Headache, sweating, and palpitation have been noted in 75% of patients in one large series (159). If all three symptoms are present, a patient may be diagnosed with pheochromocytoma with a specificity and sensitivity approaching 90%.

Clinical Evaluation

Biochemical Studies

An algorithm for the diagnosis and treatment of pheochromocytomas is presented in Figure 53.6. The biochemical work-up for pheochromocytomas is straightforward. The clinical diagnosis of pheochromocytoma is based on the demonstration of increased levels of catecholamines in the urine or blood. Measurement of serum epinephrine, norepinephrine (179), urinary free catecholamine, or urinary metanephrine levels (180) may serve as screening tests. In patients suspected of having pheochromocytomas, 24-hour urinary determinations of levels of catecholamines and their metabolites are the tests of choice for screening (181).

In patients with paroxysmal hypertension or borderline elevated values of plasma or urinary catecholamines, provocative tests may be required. The Glucogon Stimulation Test (0.5 to 1.0 mg intravenously) causes a pressor response, which may be hazardous in patients with a high basal blood pressure. In general, a 3-fold increase in plasma catecholamine is diagnostic of pheochromocytoma (160). The clonidine suppression test may also be used in patients with borderline levels of plasma or urinary catecholamines (182). Baseline levels of plasma epinephrine and norepinephrine are obtained, followed by administration of 0.3 mg of clonidine orally. The plasma samples are repeated in 3 hours. In patients with pheochromocytomas (clonidine being a centrally acting α-agonist), administration does not suppress catecholamine levels, whereas in patients with idiopathic hypertension, these levels will decrease 50% or more.

Imaging Studies

Given the bilateral or extraadrenal nature of pheochromocytomas, radiologic localization is necessary. Both CT scan and MRI are useful in the localization of clinically suspected pheochromocytomas. The appearance on a CT scan is typically that of a nonspecific homogeneous adrenal mass (Fig. 53.10) that cannot be reliably differentiated from other benign or malignant tumors. CT scanning has a sensitivity of approximately 95% and specificity over 70% (183). Occasionally, pheochromocytomas may be quite large, with areas of cystic necrosis. On MRI, pheochromocytomas have a characteristically high signal intensity on T2-weighted images (Fig. 53.10), which is pathognomonic and only rarely seen in other situations such as adrenal hemorrhage. Because of this characteristic appearance, MRI scan is more specific than CT scan and more sensitive for demonstrating extra-adrenal lesions.

Extra-adrenal pheochromocytomas or paragangliomas arising from the sympathetic chain appear as retroperitoneal masses and, if large, may displace adjacent organs (Fig. 53.12). CT scan, MRI, and angiography are useful in planning the operative approach.

In clinical use for more than 20 years, ^{131}I-MIBG is a catecholamine precursor that localizes with high specificity to tissue actively synthesizing catecholamines, including primary adrenal pheochromocytomas, extra-adrenal lesions, and metastases (Fig. 53.13). It localizes approximately 85% of primary adrenal pheochromocytomas and is especially useful in identifying small tumors at extra-adrenal sites (184). It has been shown to have high sensitivity (more than 85%) and specificity (more than 95%) for all types and locations of pheochromocytomas (185). In one study, ^{131}I-MIBG disclosed unsuspected lesions in the lung, bone, and abdominal nodes not apparent on CT scan in 40% of patients with known metastatic tumors (186).

PET is being investigated as an alternate to ^{131}I-MIBG scanning, specifically for those tumors that are not imaged by ^{131}I-MIBG scans. Early results with this technology demonstrate high sensitivity and specificity (187).

Surgical Therapy

Preoperative Preparation

Optimal preoperative management is critical for successful outcome of surgery. The close integration of surgical, anesthetic, and medical specialties is required for optimal preoperative management. The main aims of preoperative management include normalization of blood pressure and expanding the volume contracted state in order to ensure a smooth intraoperative course with minimal postoperative complications. Chronic catecholamine excess leads to hypertension and plasma volume contraction. Cardiomyopathy that is reversible may occur. Therefore, a preoperative cardiology consultation is useful. Although various pharmacologic agents have been used, α-blockers play a major role. Phenoxybenzamine, a nonselective α-blocker, was classically utilized. Other agents include selective α_1-blockers (prazosin), calcium-channel blockers (verapamil-SR and nifedipine-XL), β-blockers (propanolol), and α-methylparatyrosine. The reversible blockade created by prazosin can be overcome by intraoperative catecholamine surges. Therefore, the use of prazosin as monotherapy is inadequate. Calcium-channel blockers normalize blood pressure without any of the side effects of chronic α blockade. They may also prevent catecholamine-induced vasospasm and myocarditis. Preoperative β-blockade (such as with propranolol, 20 to 120 mg/d) is indicated only in the presence of significant supraventricular tachyarrhythmias or angina. β-blockers should not be used without prior α-blockade because they

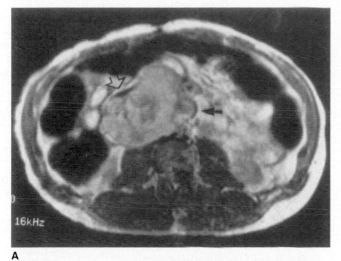

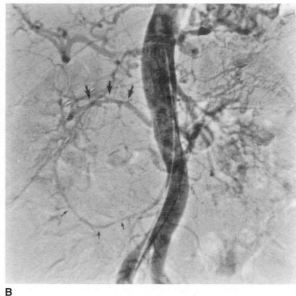

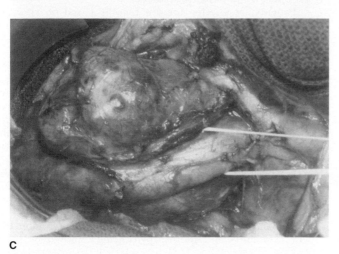

FIGURE 53.12. Paraganglioma in a 45-year-old hypertensive man. **A:** T2-weighted magnetic resonance image of the retroperitoneum demonstrating a moderately bright tumor arising in the right retroperitoneal space. The tumor is adjacent to the aorta (*solid arrow*) and displaces the inferior vena cava (IVC) anteriorly (*open arrow*). **B:** Angiogram shows a hypovascular tumor with lateral displacement of the aorta, superior displacement of the right renal artery (*large arrows*), and inferior displacement of a lumbar artery (*small arrows*). **C:** Operative photograph demonstrating a 15-cm tumor in the interaortocaval region. Vessel loop surrounds the aorta. The patient became normotensive when the blood supply to the tumor was ligated.

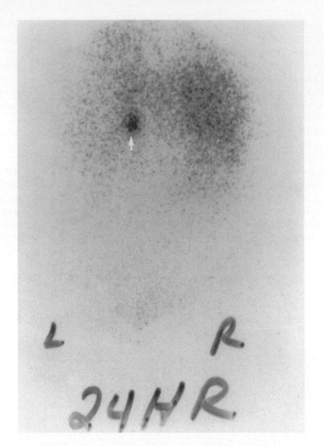

FIGURE 53.13. A ^{131}I-MIBG scan in a hypertensive patient, demonstrating increased uptake in the area of the left adrenal gland (*arrow*). At surgery, this finding proved to be a pheochromocytoma.

block the vasodilatory effect of epinephrine and can result in severe hypertension (160). β-blockers are only required in the presence of tachyarrhythmias.

Operative Considerations

AnestheticManagement. Given the potential wide rage of intraoperative blood pressures, routine invasive monitoring including intraarterial line, central venous pressure monitoring, and occasionally Swan-Ganz monitoring is employed. Induction may be performed with intravenous thiopental, followed by isoflurane as the agent of choice for maintenance. This agent decreases myocardial irritability. Episodic hypertension is controlled by intravenous drips of phentolamine or nitroprusside. Bolus infusion of esmolol, a β-blocker, is helpful if nitroprusside provides insufficient blood pressure control (188).

Operative Technique

Surgical extirpation remains the main treatment of identified pheochromocytomas. As with other benign tumors of the adrenal gland, pheochromocytomas can be efficaciously removed laparoscopically (189–193). Initially, concern existed over the hemodynamic stability of patients undergoing removal of pheochromocytomas laparoscopically. We retrospectively compared 14 laparoscopic and 20 open adrenalectomies done for pheochromocytoma (188). Laparoscopy was superior in terms of blood loss (100 vs. 400 cc, $P <.05$), hospital stay (3 vs. 7.5 days, $P <.05$), and surgical time (177 vs. 196 mins). Patients in the laparoscopic group had fewer hypotensive episodes (0 vs. 2, $P = .05$). Thus, the feasibility and safety of laparoscopy

appears to be comparable if not superior to open surgery. Laparoscopic adrenalectomy for pheochromocytomas has usually been performed via the transperitoneal approach. The same goals/dicta of open surgery are stressed with laparoscopic pheochromocytoma surgery, namely, "Dissect the patient away from the tumor" and early ligation of the main adrenal vein to minimize dangerous catecholamines surges. As stated in the section "Adrenocortical Cancer," malignant-appearing pheochromocytomas, which are usually adherent to surrounding structures, are resected *en bloc*. One of the basic principles in the treatment of malignant pheochromocytomas is the surgical resection of metastases whenever possible (194). Surgical excision of metastatic pheochromocytoma may be indicated in select cases in which isolated metastases exist or in which symptoms cannot be effectively palliated medically. Sites amenable to surgical excision include liver, bone, lung, and retroperitoneal lymph nodes. Although long-term cures are rare, normalization or reduction in the levels of circulating catecholamines have been reported for up to 18 months, with improved symptom control (186). The preoperative and intraoperative management of these lesions is similar to that described for removal of primary pheochromocytomas.

Radiopharmaceuticals

The development of ^{131}I-MIBG not only improved diagnostic techniques but also was used as therapy for patients with metastatic pheochromocytomas. This agent accumulates in catecholamine storage granules and can produce antitumor effects in this fashion (195). Malignant pheochromocytomas generally show uptake of ^{131}I-MIBG in more than 90% of cases (196). Most patients receive several courses of therapy, and dosimetric studies indicate delivered doses range from 12.5 to 80.0 Gy. Therapeutic responses in published series have been reviewed (196,197). Responses were reported in approximately 30% of patients, with complete tumor eradication uncommon (complete responses 2% to 4%). The frequency of hormonal improvement is more common. Loh et al. (197) estimated 13% of patients will demonstrate complete normalization, and 32% will demonstrate partial improvement in catecholamine levels. Symptomatic improvement such as relief of catecholamine-related symptoms or pain occur in more than 75% of treated patients.

Patients are selected for this therapy based on visualized uptake of ^{131}I-MIBG on scans. They receive thyroid blockage with an iodine preparation during therapy, as well as hydration to decrease bladder toxicity. In the series reviewed by Loh et al. (197), patients received from 1 to 11 doses (mean 3.3) of ^{131}I-MIBG, and the cumulative dose delivered was from 96 to 2,322 mCi (mean of 490 ± 350 mCi). The radiation doses delivered ranged from 1 to 198 Gy (mean of 59 ± 51 Gy).

The toxicity of this treatment includes nausea and vomiting (23%) and exacerbation of pheochromocytoma-related symptoms (19%) (83). Myelosuppression is also noted, and variable degrees are seen in 40% of treated patients.

Symptomatic and radiologic tumor response appears to be more common in soft tissue metastases than in osseous metastases. The duration of response is variable and ranges from 4 to more than 100 months (197). Use of this modality after surgery, in patients receiving chemotherapy, and in combination with external-beam radiotherapy is being explored.

Chemotherapy

Use of chemotherapy in patients with metastatic pheochromocytoma has received little attention, and most reports are anecdotal experiences in single patients using either single agents or

TABLE 53.10

COMBINATION CHEMOTHERAPY REGIMENS USED IN PATIENTS WITH METASTATIC PHEOCHROMOCYTOMA

Author(s)	Regimen	Number of patients	Biochemical	Responses Objective (CR + PR)/Total	Response duration[a] (mo)
Scott et al. (209)	CTX/VCR	3	NS	1/2	NS/6.0
Phillips et al. (206)	CTX/VCR	1	NS	0/1	—
Schlumberger et al. (186)	VP–16/CDDP	4	0/4	0/4	—
	5–FU/STZ	1	1/1	0/1	—
	VCR/DOX/CTX	1	0/1	0/1	—
Bukowski and Vidt (205)	5–FU/CTX/STZ	2	1/2	0/2	4.0/NS
Averbuch et al. (208)	CTX/VCR/DTIC	14	11/14	8/14	>22.0/21.0
Senan et al. (207)	CTX/VCR/DTIC	2	2/2	NS	—
Total		28 (62%)	15/24 (37%)	9/24	

5-FU, fluorouracil; CDDP, cisplatin; CR, complete response; CTX, cyclophosphamide; DTIC, dacarbazine; DOX, doxorubicin; NR, no response; NS, not stated; PR, partial response; STZ, streptozotocin; VCR, vincristine; VP-16, etoposide.
[a]Biochemical/objective response duration.

various drug combinations (198). Agents that have been used in this neoplasm include thiotepa (199), cyclophosphamide (179,200), DOX (201,202), streptozotocin (203,204), and dacarbazine (205). Combination regimens that have been used in two or more patients are outlined in Table 53.10 (186, 205–209). In view of the similarities between pheochromocytomas and neuroblastoma, Averbuch et al. (208) used a regimen that has an 80% response rate in the latter neoplasm (198). This three-drug regimen consisted of cyclophosphamide (750 mg/m^2 intravenously on day 1), vincristine (1.4 mg/m^2 intravenously on day 1), and dacarbazine (600 mg/m^2 on days 1 and 2). Cycles were repeated every 3 to 4 weeks. The reported response rates were a 57% objective regression (one complete) and 79% biochemical response rate. These results have not been confirmed by other investigators, but appear superior to those reported with other regimens. Another report by Rao et al. (210), using a similar regimen of chemotherapy, showed a clinical response in five out of nine patients. In the five responders to chemotherapy, there were statistically significant declines in chromogranin A and norepinephrine when compared to nonresponders.

Reports (205) of hypertensive crises or exacerbation of existing hypertension during chemotherapy administration exist. In the series reported by Averbuch et al. (208), adequate administration of α-adrenergic blockers prevented this problem. The role of chemotherapy in this tumor is not clear. The results and response durations reported with the cyclophosphamide, vincristine, and dacarbazine combination regimen are promising but require confirmation.

Radiation Therapy and Miscellaneous Approaches

A frequent metastatic site in patients with adrenal cancer is bone and, therefore, palliation with external-beam radiation therapy has been used. It is reported to be as effective for palliation of bone lesions (211), with doses of 2,500 to 3,060 cGy used. Yu et al. (212) suggested that this dose may be inadequate and indicated that doses of 40 to 50 Gy delivered over 4 to 5 weeks may be preferable. The use of higher initial doses may result in longer disease control. Another approach has involved transarterial embolization (213) of accessible lesions with alcoholic emulsion. Although this was successful in a small group of patients, long-term follow-up is required as concern exists over malignant lesions with local or distant metastasis.

References

1. Eustatchi B, Fallopio G. Opuscula anatomica. Venice, 1563.
2. Addison T. On the constitutional and local effects of disease of suprarenal capsules. London. Samual Highly, 1855.
3. Brown-Sequard C. Recherches experimentales sur la physiologie et la pathologie des capsules surrenalse. C R Acad Sci IIb Mec 1856; 43:422–425.
4. Plager JE. Carcinoma of the adrenal cortex: Clinical description, diagnosis, and treatment. Int Adv Surg Oncol 1984;7:329–353.
5. Freeman D. The biochemistry of adrenal cortical tumors. Comprehensive Endocrinology: The Adrenal Gland. 1992: 451–463.
6. Dluhy RG, Barlow JJ, Mahoney EM, et al. Profile and possible origin of an adrenocortical carcinoma. J Clin Endocrinol Metab 1971;33(2):312–317.
7. Daly PA, Landsberg L. Phaeochromocytoma: diagnosis and management. Baillieres Clin Endocrinol Metab 1992;6(1):143–166.
8. Manger W. In: Rankel R, ed. Pheochormocytoma: Conn's current therapy. Philadelphia, PA: WB Saunders, 1991:612.
9. Lefor AT. The role of laparoscopy in the treatment of intra-abdominal malignancies. Cancer J 2000;6(Suppl. 2):S159–S168.
10. Brennan MF. Adrenocortical carcinoma. CA Cancer J Clin 1987;37(6): 348–365.
11. Grumbach MM, Biller BM, Braunstein GD, et al. Management of the clinically inapparent adrenal mass ("incidentaloma"). Ann Intern Med 2003; 138(5):424–429.
12. Third National Cancer Survey. National Cancer Institute Monogram 1975;41:1.
13. Correa P, Chen VW. Endocrine gland cancer. Cancer 1995;75(Suppl. 1): 338–352.
14. Dohna M, Reincke M, Mincheva A, et al. Adrenocortical carcinoma is characterized by a high frequency of chromosomal gains and high-level amplifications. Genes Chromosomes Cancer 2000;28(2):145–152.
15. Sidhu S, Marsh DJ, Theodosopoulos G, et al. Comparative genomic hybridization analysis of adrenocortical tumors. J Clin Endocrinol Metab 2002;87(7):3,467–3,474.
16. Association of Directors of Anatomic and Surgical Pathology. Recommendations for reporting of tumors of the adrenal cortex and medulla. Am J Clin Pathol 1999;112(4):451–455.
17. Lack E. Tumors of the adrenal gland. In: Fletcher CDM, ed. Diagnostic histopathology of tumors. London: Churchill Livingstone, 2000:1,058.
18. Wick MR, Cherwitz DL, McGlennen RC, et al. Adrenocortical carcinoma: An immunohistochemical comparison with renal cell carcinoma. Am J Pathol 1986;122(2):343–352.
19. Weiss LM, Medeiros LJ, Vickery AL Jr. Pathologic features of prognostic significance in adrenocortical carcinoma. Am J Surg Pathol 1989; 13(3): 202–206.

20. Medeiros LJ, Weiss LM. New developments in the pathologic diagnosis of adrenal cortical neoplasms: A review. *Am J Clin Pathol* 1992;97(1):73–83.
21. Lack E, Travis W, Oertel J. Adrenal cortical neoplasms. In: *Pathology of the adrenal glands*. New York: Churchill Livingstone, 1990:115–171.
22. Hough AJ, Hollifield JW, Page DL, et al. Prognostic factors in adrenal cortical tumors: A mathematical analysis of clinical and morphologic data. *Am J Clin Pathol* 1979;72(3):390–399.
23. Van Slooten H, Schaberg A, Smeenk D, et al. Morphologic characteristics of benign and malignant adrenocortical tumors. *Cancer* 1985;55(4):766–773.
24. Miettinen M, Lehto VP, Virtanen I. Immunofluorescence microscopic evaluation of the intermediate filament expression of the adrenal cortex and medulla and their tumors. *Am J Pathol* 1985;118(3):360–366.
25. Gaffey MJ, Traweek ST, Mills SE, et al. Cytokeratin expression in adrenocortical neoplasia: An immunohistochemical and biochemical study with implications for the differential diagnosis of adrenocortical, hepatocellular, and renal cell carcinoma. *Hum Pathol* 1992;23(2):144–153.
26. Miettinen M. Neuroendocrine differentiation in adrenocortical carcinoma. New immunohistochemical findings supported by electron microscopy. *Lab Invest* 1992;66(2):169–174.
27. Bernini GP, Moretti A, Viacava P, et al. Apoptosis control and proliferation marker in human normal and neoplastic adrenocortical tissues. *Br J Cancer* 2002;86(10):1,561–1,565.
28. Camuto P, Schinella R, Gilchrist K, et al. Adrenal cortical carcinoma: Flow cytometric study of 22 cases, an ECOG study. *Urology* 1991;37(4):380–384.
29. Cibas ES, Medeiros LJ, Weinberg DS, et al. Cellular DNA profiles of benign and malignant adrenocortical tumors. *Am J Surg Pathol* 1990; 14 (10):948–955.
30. Hirano Y, Fujita K, Suzuki K, et al. Telomerase activity as an indicator of potentially malignant adrenal tumors. *Cancer* 1998;83(4):772–776.
31. Bamberger CM, Else T, Bamberger AM, et al. Telomerase activity in benign and malignant adrenal tumors. *Exp Clin Endocrinol Diabetes* 1999; 107(4):272–275.
32. Lam KY, Lo CY. Adrenal lipomatous tumours: A 30 year clinicopathological experience at a single institution. *J Clin Pathol* 2001;54(9):707–712.
33. Sanders R, Bissada N, Curry N, et al. Clinical spectrum of adrenal myelolipoma: Analysis of 8 tumors in 7 patients. *J Urol* 1995;153(6):1,791–1,793.
34. Glazer HS, Weyman PJ, Sagel SS, et al. Nonfunctioning adrenal masses: Incidental discovery on computed tomography. *AJR Am J Roentgenol* 1982;139(1):81–85.
35. Kloos RT, Gross MD, Francis IR, et al. Incidentally discovered adrenal masses. *Endocr Rev* 1995;16(4):460–484.
36. Ross NS, Aron DC. Hormonal evaluation of the patient with an incidentally discovered adrenal mass. *N Engl J Med* 1990;323(20):1,401–1,405.
37. Boscaro M, Barzon L, Fallo F, et al. Cushing's Cushing'syndrome. *Lancet* 2001;357(9258):783–791.
38. Ganguly A. Primary aldosteronism. *N Engl J Med* 1998;339(25):1,828–1,834.
39. Rozenblit A, Morehouse HT, Amis ES Jr. Cystic adrenal lesions: CT features. *Radiology* 1996;201(2):541–548.
40. Boland GW, Lee MJ, Gazelle GS, et al. Characterization of adrenal masses using unenhanced CT: An analysis of the CT literature. *AJR Am J Roentgenol* 1998;171(1):201–204.
41. Caoili EM, Korobkin M, Francis IR, et al. Adrenal masses: Characterization with combined unenhanced and delayed enhanced CT. *Radiology* 2002;222(3):629–633.
42. Fishman EK, Deutch BM, Hartman DS, et al. Primary adrenocortical carcinoma: CT evaluation with clinical correlation. *AJR Am J Roentgenol* 1987;148(3):531–535.
43. Brunt LM, Moley JF. Adrenal incidentaloma. *World J Surg* 2001; 25(7):905–913.
44. Lockhart ME, Smith JK, Kenney PJ. Imaging of adrenal masses. *Eur J Radiol* 2002;41(2):95–112.
45. Kurtaran A, Traub T, Shapiro B. Scintigraphic imaging of the adrenal glands. *Eur J Radiol* 2002;41(2):123–130.
46. Yun M, Kim W, Alnafisi N, et al. 18F-FDG PET in characterizing adrenal lesions detected on CT or MRI. *J Nucl Med* 2001;42(12):1,795–1,799.
47. Erasmus JJ, Patz EF Jr, McAdams HP, et al. Evaluation of adrenal masses in patients with bronchogenic carcinoma using 18F-fluorodeoxyglucose positron emission tomography. *AJR Am J Roentgenol* 1997;168(5):1,357–1,360.
48. Siren JE, Haapiainen RK, Huikuri KT, et al. Incidentalomas of the adrenal gland: 36 operated patients and review of literature. *World J Surg* 1993; 17(5):634–639.
49. Terzolo M, Ali A, Osella G, et al. Prevalence of adrenal carcinoma among incidentally discovered adrenal masses. A retrospective study from 1989 to 1994. Gruppo Piemontese Incidentalomi Surrenalici. *Arch Surg* 1997; 132(8):914–919.
50. Gagner M, Lacroix A, Bolte E. Laparoscopic adrenalectomy in Cushing's syndrome and pheochromocytoma. *N Engl J Med* 1992;327(14):1,033.
51. Sung GT, Gill IS. Laparoscopic adrenalectomy. *Semin Laparosc Surg* 2000;7(3):211–222.
52. Thompson GB, Grant CS, van Heerden JA, et al. Laparoscopic versus open posterior adrenalectomy: A case-control study of 100 patients. *Surgery* 1997;122(6):1,132–1,136.
53. Porpiglia F, Destefanis P, Fiori C, et al. Does adrenal mass size really affect safety and effectiveness of laparoscopic adrenalectomy? *Urology* 2002; 60(5):801–805.
54. Vargas HI, Kavoussi LR, Bartlett DL, et al. Laparoscopic adrenalectomy: A new standard of care. *Urology* 1997;49(5):673–678.
55. Karstrup S, Torp-Pedersen S, Nolsoe C, et al. Ultrasonically guided fine-needle biopsies from adrenal tumors. *Scand J Urol Nephrol Suppl* 1991; 137:31–34.
56. Siren J, Tervahartiala P, Sivula A, et al. Natural course of adrenal incidentalomas: Seven-year follow-up study. *World J Surg* 2000;24(5):579–582.
57. Young WF Jr. Management approaches to adrenal incidentalomas: A view from Rochester, Minnesota. *Endocrinol Metab Clin North Am* 2000; 29(1):159–185.
58. Greenberg PH, Marks C. Adrenal cortical carcinoma: A presentation of 22 cases and a review of the literature. *Am Surg* 1978;44(2):81–85.
59. Cagle PT, Hough AJ, Pysher TJ, et al. Comparison of adrenal cortical tumors in children and adults. *Cancer* 1986;57(11):2,235–2,237.
60. Wooten MD, King DK. Adrenal cortical carcinoma. Epidemiology and treatment with mitotane and a review of the literature. *Cancer* 1993; 72(11):3,145–3,155.
61. Latronico AC, Chrousos GP. Extensive personal experience: Adrenocortical tumors. *J Clin Endocrinol Metab* 1997;82(5):1,317–1,324.
62. Li FP, Fraumeni JF Jr, Mulvihill JJ, et al. A cancer family syndrome in twenty-four kindreds. *Cancer Res* 1988;48(18):5,358–5,362.
63. Sandrini R, Ribeiro RC, DeLacerda L. Childhood adrenocortical tumors. *J Clin Endocrinol Metab* 1997;82(7):2,027–2,031.
64. Henry I, Jeanpierre M, Couillin P, et al. Molecular definition of the 11p15.5 region involved in Beckwith-Wiedemann syndrome and probably in predisposition to adrenocortical carcinoma. *Hum Genet* 1989;81(3):273–277.
65. Gicquel C, Raffin-Sanson ML, Gaston V, et al. Structural and functional abnormalities at 11p15 are associated with the malignant phenotype in sporadic adrenocortical tumors: Study on a series of 82 tumors. *J Clin Endocrinol Metab* 1997;82(8):2,559–2,565.
66. Koch CA, Pacak K, Chrousos GP. The molecular pathogenesis of hereditary and sporadic adrenocortical and adrenomedullary tumors. *J Clin Endocrinol Metab* 2002;87(12):5,367–5,384.
67. Casey M, Vaughan CJ, He J, et al. Mutations in the protein kinase A R1alpha regulatory subunit cause familial cardiac myxomas and Carney complex. *J Clin Invest* 2000;106(5):R31–R38.
68. Skogseid B, Larsson C, Lindgren PG, et al. Clinical and genetic features of adrenocortical lesions in multiple endocrine neoplasia type 1. *J Clin Endocrinol Metab* 1992;75(1):76–81.
69. Gicquel C, Leblond-Francillard M, Bertagna X, et al. Clonal analysis of human adrenocortical carcinomas and secreting adenomas. *Clin Endocrinol (Oxf)* 1994;40(4):465–477.
70. Yano T, Linehan M, Anglard P, et al. Genetic changes in human adrenocortical carcinomas. *J Natl Cancer Inst* 1989;81(7):518–523.
71. Bernard MH, Sidhu S, Berger N, et al. A case report in favor of a multistep adrenocortical tumorigenesis. *J Clin Endocrinol Metab* 2003; 88(3):988–1,001.
72. Reincke M, Beuschlein F, Slawik M, et al. Molecular adrenocortical tumourigenesis. *Eur J Clin Invest* 2000;30(Suppl. 3):63–68.
73. Latronico AC, Reincke M, Mendonca BB, et al. No evidence for oncogenic mutations in the adrenocorticotropin receptor gene in human adrenocortical neoplasms. *J Clin Endocrinol Metab* 1995;80(3):875–877.
74. Norton J. In: Rosenberg R, ed. *Cancer principles and practice of oncology.* Philadelphia : Lippincott–Raven Publishers, 1997:1,659.
75. Ng L, Libertino JA. Adrenocortical carcinoma: Diagnosis, evaluation and treatment. *J Urol* 2003;169(1):5–11.
76. Dackiw AP, Lee JE, Gagel RF, et al. Adrenal cortical carcinoma. *World J Surg* 2001;25(7):914–926.
77. Icard P, Chapuis Y, Andreassian B, et al. Adrenocortical carcinoma in surgically treated patients: A retrospective study on 156 cases by the French Association of Endocrine Surgery. *Surgery* 1992;112(6):972–979; discussion 979–980.
78. Xiao XR, Ye LY, Shi LX, et al. Diagnosis and treatment of adrenal tumours: A review of 35 years' experience. [see comment]. *Br J Urology* 1998;82(2):199–205.
79. Wajchenberg BL, Albergaria Pereira MA, Medonca BB, et al. Adrenocortical carcinoma: Clinical and laboratory observations. *Cancer* 2000; 88(4):711–736.
80. Luton JP, Cerdas S, Billaud L, et al. Clinical features of adrenocortical carcinoma, prognostic factors, and the effect of mitotane therapy. *N Engl J Med* 1990;322(17):1,195–1,201.
81. Bukowski RM, Wolfe M, Levine HS, et al. Phase II trial of mitotane and cisplatin in patients with adrenal carcinoma: A Southwest Oncology Group study. *J Clin Oncol* 1993;11(1):161–165.
82. Moore L, Bramwell NH, Byard RW. DNA analysis and clinical outcome in pediatric adrenal cortical tumors. *Pathology* 1993;25(2):144–147.
83. Bodie B, Novick AC, Pontes JE, et al. The Cleveland Clinic experience with adrenal cortical carcinoma. *J Urol* 1989;141(2):257–260.
84. Hedican SP, Marshall FF. Adrenocortical carcinoma with intracaval extension. *J Urol* 1997;158(6):2,056–2,061.
85. Ushiyama T, Suzuki K, Kageyama S, et al. A case of Cushing's syndrome due to adrenocortical carcinoma with recurrence 19 months after laparoscopic adrenalectomy. *J Urol* 1997;157(6):2,239.

86. Suzuki K, Ushiyama T, Mugiya S, et al. Hazards of laparoscopic adrenalectomy in patients with adrenal malignancy. *J Urol* 1997;158(6):2227.

87. Hofle G, Gasser RW, Lhotta K, et al. Adrenocortical carcinoma evolving after diagnosis of preclinical Cushing's syndrome in an adrenal incidentaloma: A case report. *Horm Res* 1998;50(4):237–242.

88. Hamoir E, Meurisse M, Defechereux T. Is laparoscopic resection of a malignant corticoadrenaloma feasible? Case report of early, diffuse and massive peritoneal recurrence after attempted laparoscopic resection. *Ann Chir* 1998;52(4):364–368.

89. Deckers S, Derdelinckx L, Col V, et al. Peritoneal carcinomatosis following laparoscopic resection of an adrenocortical tumor causing primary hyperaldosteronism. *Horm Res* 1999;52(2):97–100.

90. Foxius A, Ramboux A, Lefebvre Y, et al. Hazards of laparoscopic adrenalectomy for Conn's adenoma: When enthusiasm turns to tragedy. [comment]. *Surg Endosc* 1999;13(7):715–717.

91. Chen B, Zhou M, Cappelli MC, et al. Port site, retroperitoneal and intra-abdominal recurrence after laparoscopic adrenalectomy for apparently isolated metastasis. *J Urol* 2002;168(6):2,528–2,529.

92. Feliciotti F, Paganini AM, Guerrieri M, et al. Laparoscopic anterior adrenalectomy for the treatment of adrenal metastases. *Surg Laparosc Endosc Percutan Tech* 2003;13(5):328–333.

93. Lombardi CP, Raffaelli M, Boscherini M, et al. [Laparoscopic adrenalectomy in the treatment of malignant adrenal lesions]. *Tumori* 2003;89 (Suppl. 4): 255–256.

94. Sarela AI, Murphy I, Coit DG, et al. Metastasis to the adrenal gland: The emerging role of laparoscopic surgery. *Ann Surg Oncol* 2003;10(10): 1,191–1,196.

95. Rassweiler J, Tsivian A, Kumar AV, et al. Oncological safety of laparoscopic surgery for urological malignancy: Experience with more than 1,000 operations. *J Urol* 2003;169(6):2,072–2,075.

96. Valeri A, Borrelli A, Presenti L, et al. Adrenal masses in neoplastic patients: The role of laparoscopic procedure. *Surg Endosc* 2001;15(1):90–93.

97. Heniford BT, Arca MJ, Walsh RM, et al. Laparoscopic adrenalectomy for cancer. *Semin Surg Oncol* 1999;16(4):293–306.

98. Henry JF, Sebag F, Iacobone M, et al. Results of laparoscopic adrenalectomy for large and potentially malignant tumors. *World J Surg* 2002;26(8): 1,043–1,047.

99. Kebebew E, Siperstein AE, Clark OH, et al. Results of laparoscopic adrenalectomy for suspected and unsuspected malignant adrenal neoplasms. *Arch Surg* 2002;137(8):948–951; discussion 952–953.

100. Creagan ET, Fleming TR, Edmonson JH, et al. Pulmonary resection for metastatic nonosteogenic sarcoma. *Cancer* 1979;44(5):1,908–1,912.

101. Norton JA, Sugarbaker PH, Doppman JL, et al. Aggressive resection of metastatic disease in selected patients with malignant gastrinoma. *Ann Surg* 1986;203(1):352–359.

102. Fujii Y, Kageyama Y, Kawakami S, et al. Successful long-term disease-free survival following multimodal treatments in a patient with a repeatedly recurrent refractory adrenal cortical carcinoma. *Int J Urol* 2003; 10(8): 445–448.

103. Bellantone R, Ferrante A, Boscherini M, et al. Role of reoperation in recurrence of adrenal cortical carcinoma: Results from 188 cases collected in the Italian National Registry for Adrenal Cortical Carcinoma. *Surgery* 1997;122(6):1,212–1,218.

104. Verhelst JA, Trainer PJ, Howlett TA, et al. Short- and long-term responses to metyrapone in the medical management of 91 patients with Cushing's syndrome. *Clin Endocrinol (Oxf)* 1991;35(2):169–178.

105. Salhanick HA. Basic studies on aminoglutethimide. *Cancer Res* 1982; 42 (Suppl. 8):3,315s–3,321s.

106. Schteingart DE, Cash R, Conn JW. Amino-glutethimide and metastatic adrenal cancer: Maintained reversal (six months) of Cushing's syndrome. *JAMA* 1966;198(9):1,007–1,010.

107. Bledsoe T, Island DP, Ney RL, et al. An effect of O,P'-DDD on the extra-adrenal metabolism of cortisol in man. *J Clin Endocrinol Metab* 1964;24: 1,303–1,311.

108. Fishman LM, Liddle GW, Island DP, et al. Effects of amino-glutethimide on adrenal function in man. *J Clin Endocrinol Metab* 1967;27(4): 481–490.

109. Bochner F, Lloyd HM, Roeser HP, et al. Effects of o,p'DDD and aminoglutethimide on metastatic adrenocortical carcinoma. *Med J Aust* 1969; 1(16):809–812.

110. Schmoll H. Treatment of estrogen producing adrenal carcinoma with aminoglutethimide. 2004.

111. Vilar O, Tullner WW. Effects of o,p' DDD on histology and 17-hydroxy-corticosteroid output of the dog adrenal cortex. *Endocrinology* 1959; 65 (1):80–86.

112. Bergenstal D, Hertz R, Lipsett M, et al. Chemotherapy of adrenocortical cancer with o,p'-DDD. *Ann Intern Med* 1960;53:672.

113. Hoffman DL, Mattox VR. Treatment of adrenocortical carcinoma with o,p'-DDD. *Med Clin North Am* 1972;56(4):999–1,012.

114. Freeman DA. Adrenal carcinoma. *Curr Ther Endocrinol Metab* 1997; 6: 173–175.

115. Moy RH. Studies of the pharmacology of o,p'DDD in man. *J Lab Clin Med* 1961;58:296–304.

116. Moolenaar A, Setters Av. o,p'-DDD values in plasma and tissue during and after chemotherapy of adrenocortical carcinoma. *Acta Endocrinol Suppl* 1975;199:226.

117. May CA, Garnett WR. Treatment of adrenocortical carcinoma: A case report and review of the literature. *Drug Intell Clin Pharm* 1986;20(1): 24–32.

118. Hutter AM Jr, Kayhoe DE. Adrenal cortical carcinoma: Results of treatment with o,p'DDD in 138 patients. *Am J Med* 1966;41(4):581–592.

119. Lubitz JA, Freeman L, Okun R. Mitotane use in inoperable adrenal cortical carcinoma. *JAMA* 1973;223(10):1,109–1,112.

120. Van Slooten H, Moolenaar AJ, van Seters AP, et al. The treatment of adrenocortical carcinoma with o,p'-DDD: Prognostic implications of serum level monitoring. *Eur J Cancer Clin Oncol* 1984;20(1):47–53.

121. Baudin E, Pellegriti G, Bonnay M, et al. Impact of monitoring plasma 1,1-dichlorodiphenildichloroethane (o,p'DDD) levels on the treatment of patients with adrenocortical carcinoma. *Cancer* 2001;92(6):1,385–1,392.

122. Terzolo M, Pia A, Berruti A, et al. Low-dose monitored mitotane treatment achieves the therapeutic range with manageable side effects in patients with adrenocortical cancer. *J Clin Endocrinol Metab* 2000;85(6): 2,234–2,238.

123. Schteingart DE, Motazedi A, Noonan RA, et al. Treatment of adrenal carcinomas. *Arch Surg* 1982;117(9):1,142–1,146.

124. Venkatesh S, Hickey RC, Sellin RV, et al. Adrenal cortical carcinoma. *Cancer* 1989;64(3):765–769.

125. Vassilopoulou-Sellin R, Guinee VF, Klein MJ, et al. Impact of adjuvant mitotane on the clinical course of patients with adrenocortical cancer. *Cancer* 1993;71(10):3,119–3,123.

126. Haak HR, Hermans J, van de Velde CJ, et al. Optimal treatment of adrenocortical carcinoma with mitotane: Results in a consecutive series of 96 patients. *Br J Cancer* 1994;69(5):947–951.

127. Barzon L, Fallo F, Sonino N, et al. Comment: Is there a role for low doses of mitotane (o,p'-DDD) as adjuvant therapy in adrenocortical carcinoma? *J Clin Endocrinol Metab* 1999;84(4):1,488–1,489.

128. Bulger AR, Correa RJ. Experience with adrenal cortical carcinoma. *Urology* 1977;10(1):12–18.

129. Moolenaar AJ, van Slooten H, van Seters AP, et al. Blood levels of o,p'-DDD following administration in various vehicles after a single dose and during long-term treatment. *Cancer Chemother Pharmacol* 1981; 7(1):51–54.

130. Gutierrez ML, Crooke ST. Mitotane (o,p'-DDD). *Cancer Treat Rev* 1980; 7(1):49–55.

131. Haak HR, Caekebeke-Peerlinck KM, van Seters AP, et al. Prolonged bleeding time due to mitotane therapy. *Eur J Cancer* 1991;27(5):638–641.

132. Chun HG, Yagoda A, Kemeny N, et al. Cisplatin for adrenal cortical carcinoma. *Cancer Treat Rep* 1983;67(5):513–514.

133. Decker RA, Elson P, Hogan TF, et al. Eastern Cooperative Oncology Group study 1879: Mitotane and adriamycin in patients with advanced adrenocortical carcinoma. *Surgery* 1991;110(6):1,006–1,013.

134. Johnson DH, Greco FA. Treatment of metastatic adrenal cortical carcinoma with cisplatin and etoposide (VP-16). *Cancer* 1986;58(10):2,198–2,202.

135. Burgess M, Legha S, Sellin R. Chemotherapy with cis-platinum and etoposide (VP-16) for patients with advanced adrenal cortical-carcinoma. *Proc Am Soc Clin Oncol* 1993;12:188.

136. Hesketh PJ, McCaffrey RP, Finkel HE, et al. Cisplatin-based treatment of adrenocortical carcinoma. *Cancer Treat Rep* 1987;71(2):222–224.

137. Berruti A, Terzolo M, Paccotti P, et al. Favorable response of metastatic adrenocortical carcinoma to etoposide, adriamycin and cisplatin (EAP) chemotherapy: Report of two cases. *Tumori* 1992;78(5):345–348.

138. Schlumberger M, Ostronoff M, Bellaiche M, et al. 5-Fluorouracil, doxorubicin, and cisplatin regimen in adrenal cortical carcinoma. *Cancer* 1988; 61(8):1,492–1,494.

139. Van Slooten H, van Oosterom AT. CAP (cyclophosphamide, doxorubicin, and cisplatin) regimen in adrenal cortical carcinoma. *Cancer Treat Rep* 1983;67(4):377–379.

140. Ayass M, Gross S, Harper J. High-dose carboplatinum and VP-16 in treatment of metastatic adrenal carcinoma. *Am J Pediatr Hematol Oncol* 1991; 13(4):470–472.

141. Haak HR, van Seters AP, Moolenaar AJ, et al. Expression of P-glycoprotein in relation to clinical manifestation, treatment and prognosis of adrenocortical cancer. *Eur J Cancer* 1993;29A(7):1,036–1,038.

142. Bradley G, Juranka PF, Ling V. Mechanism of multidrug resistance. *Biochim Biophys Acta* 1988;948(1):87–128.

143. Bates SE, Shieh CY, Mickley LA, et al. Mitotane enhances cytotoxicity of chemotherapy in cell lines expressing a multidrug resistance gene (mdr-1/P-glycoprotein) which is also expressed by adrenocortical carcinomas. *J Clin Endocrinol Metab* 1991;73(1):18–29.

144. Flynn SD, Murren JR, Kirby WM, et al. P-glycoprotein expression and multidrug resistance in adrenocortical carcinoma. *Surgery* 1992;112(6): 981–986.

145. Abraham J, Bakke S, Rutt A, et al. A phase II trial of combination chemotherapy and surgical resection for the treatment of metastatic adrenocortical carcinoma: Continuous infusion doxorubicin, vincristine, and etoposide with daily mitotane as a P-glycoprotein antagonist. *Cancer* 2002;94(9):2,333–2,343.

146. Stein CA, LaRocca RV, Thomas R, et al. Suramin: An anticancer drug with a unique mechanism of action. *J Clin Oncol* 1989;7(4):499–508.

147. La Rocca RV, Stein CA, Danesi R, et al. Suramin in adrenal cancer: Modulation of steroid hormone production, cytotoxicity in vitro, and clinical antitumor effect. *J Clin Endocrinol Metab* 1990;71(2):497–504.

148. Wu YW, Chik CL, Knazek RA. An in vitro and in vivo study of antitumor effects of gossypol on human SW-13 adrenocortical carcinoma. *Cancer Res* 1989;49(14):3,754–3,758.

149. Flack MR, Pyle RG, Mullen NM, et al. Oral gossypol in the treatment of metastatic adrenal cancer. *J Clin Endocrinol Metab* 1993;76(4): 1,019–1,024.

150. Nagai K, Miyamori I, Ikeda M, et al. Effect of ketoconazole (an imidazole antimycotic agent) and other inhibitors of steroidogenesis on cytochrome P450-catalyzed reactions. *J Steroid Biochem* 1986;24(1):321–323.

151. Loli P, Berselli ME, Tagliaferri M. Use of ketoconazole in the treatment of Cushing's syndrome. *J Clin Endocrinol Metab* 1986;63(6):1,365–1,371.

152. Contreras P, Rojas A, Biagini L, et al. Regression of metastatic adrenal carcinoma during palliative ketoconazole treatment. *Lancet* 1985;2(8447): 151–152.

153. Percarpio B, Knowlton AH. Radiation therapy of adrenal cortical carcinoma. *Acta Radiol Ther Phys Biol* 1976;15(4):288–292.

154. Markoe AM, Serber W, Micaily B, et al. Radiation therapy for adjunctive treatment of adrenal cortical carcinoma. *Am J Clin Oncol* 1991;14(2): 170–174.

155. Moore PJ, Biggs PJ. Compound adrenal medullary tumor. *South Med J* 1995;88(4):475–478.

156. Koh M, Lee M, Hong S, et al. Partial remission with transarterial embolization in a case of metastatic adrenal cortical carcinoma. *J Korean Med Sci* 1991;6:173.

157. Wood BJ, Abraham J, Hvizda JL, et al. Radiofrequency ablation of adrenal tumors and adrenocortical carcinoma metastases. *Cancer* 2003;97(3): 554–560.

158. Green D, Tarbell N, Shamberger R. In: DeVita V, Hellman S, Rosenberg S, eds. *Solid tumors of childhood neuroblastoma*. Philadelphia: Lippincott–Raven Publishers, 1997:2,099.

159. Keiser H. Pheochromocytoma and other diseases of the sympathetic nervous system. In: Becker K, ed. *Principles and practice of endocrinology and metabolism,* 2nd ed. Philadelphia, PA: JB Lippincott Co, 1995: 763–770.

160. Manger WM, Gifford RW Jr. Pheochromocytoma: Current diagnosis and management. *Cleve Clin J Med* 1993;60(5):365–378.

161. Beard CM, Sheps SG, Kurland LT, et al. Occurrence of pheochromocytoma in Rochester, Minnesota, 1950 through 1979. *Mayo Clin Proc* 1983; 58(12):802–804.

162. Sutton MG, Sheps SG, Lie JT. Prevalence of clinically unsuspected pheochromocytoma: Review of a 50-year autopsy series. *Mayo Clin Proc* 1981;56(6):354–360.

163. Green D, Tarbell N, Shamberger R. Solid tumors of childhood neuroblastoma. *Cancer principles and practices of oncology.* Philadelphia: Lippincott–Raven Publishers, 1997:2,099.

164. Maher ER, Kaelin WG Jr. Von Hippel-Landau disease. *Medicine*. Baltimore. 1997;76(6):381–391.

165. Neumann HP, Bender BU, Januszewicz A, et al. Inherited pheochromocytoma. *Adv Nephrol Necker Hosp* 1997;27:361–376.

166. Mulligan LM, Gardner E, Smith BA, et al. Genetic events in tumour initiation and progression in multiple endocrine neoplasia type 2. *Genes Chromosomes Cancer* 1993;6(3):166–177.

167. Tanaka N, Nishisho I, Yamamoto M, et al. Loss of heterozygosity on the long arm of chromosome 22 in pheochromocytoma. *Genes Chromosomes Cancer* 1992;5(4):399–403.

168. Xu W, Mulligan LM, Ponder MA, et al. Loss of NF1 alleles in phaeochromocytomas from patients with type I neurofibromatosis. *Genes Chromosomes Cancer* 1992;4(4):337–342.

169. Ponder BA. Mutations of the RET proto-oncogene in multiple endocrine neoplasia type 2. *Cancer Surv* 1995;25:195–205.

170. Frank-Raue K, Hoppner W, Frilling A, et al. Mutations of the RET protooncogene in German multiple endocrine neoplasia families: Relation between genotype and phenotype. German Medullary Thyroid Carcinoma Study group. *J Clin Endocrinol Metab* 1996;81(5):1,780–1,783.

171. Linehan WM, Walther MM, Zbar B. The genetic basis of cancer of the kidney. *J Urol* 2003;170(6 Pt 1):2,163–2,172.

172. Van der Horst E, de Krijger RR, Dinjens WN, et al. Germline mutations in the VHL gene in patients presenting with phaeochromocytomas. *Int J Cancer* 1998;77(3):337–340.

173. Page D, DeLellis D, Hough A. Tumors of the adrenal. *Atlas of tumor pathology.* Washington, DC: Armed Forces Institute of Pathology, 1986.

174. Nativ O, Grant CS, Sheps SG, et al. The clinical significance of nuclear DNA ploidy pattern in 184 patients with pheochromocytoma. *Cancer* 1992;69(11):2,683–2,687.

175. Pang LC, Tsao KC. Flow cytometric DNA analysis for the determination of malignant potential in adrenal and extra-adrenal pheochromocytomas or paragangliomas. *Arch Pathol Lab Med* 1993;117(11):1,142–1,147.

176. Hosaka Y, Aso Y, Rainwater LM, et al. Flow cytometric DNA histograms of paraffin-embedded pheochromocytomas. *Urol Int* 1991;47(Suppl. 1): 100–103.

177. Manger WM, Gifford RW. Pheochromocytoma. *J Clin Hypertens (Greenwich)* 2002;4(1):62–72.

178. Gifford RW Jr, Manger WM, Bravo EL. Pheochromocytoma. *Endocrinol Metab Clin North Am* 1994;23(2):387–404.

179. Hengstmann JH. Evaluation of screening tests for pheochromocytoma. *Cardiology* 1985;72(Suppl. 1):153–156.

180. Kremer R, Crawhall JC, Kolanitch R. Rapid and reliable estimation of urinary free catecholamines in patients with pheochromocytoma: Comparison with plasma catecholamines and vanillylmandelic acid excretion. *J Chromatogr* 1985;344:313–318.

181. Young WF Jr. Phaeochromocytoma: how to catch a moonbeam in your hand. *Eur J Endocrinol* 1997;136(1):28–29.

182. Karlberg BE, Hedman L. Value of the clonidine suppression test in the diagnosis of pheochromocytoma. *Acta Med Scand Suppl* 1986;714:15–21.

183. Shimazui T, Kikuchi K, Sato K, et al. Detectability and characteristics of the primary adrenal tumor by ultrasonography: Comparison with CAT scan and adrenal scintigraphy. *Nippon Hinyokika Gakkai Zasshi* 1989; 80(7):1,031–1,036.

184. Sisson JC, Frager MS, Valk TW, et al. Scintigraphic localization of pheochromocytoma. *N Engl J Med* 1981;305(1):12–17.

185. Shapiro B, Sisson JC, Shulkin BL, et al. The current status of metaiodobenzylguanidine and related agents for the diagnosis of neuro-endocrine tumors. *Q J Nucl Med* 1995;39(4 Suppl. 1):3–8.

186. Schlumberger M, Gicquel C, Lumbroso J, et al. Malignant pheochromocytoma: Clinical, biological, histologic and therapeutic data in a series of 20 patients with distant metastases. *J Endocrinol Invest* 1992;15(9):631–642.

187. Hoegerle S, Nitzsche E, Altehoefer C, et al. Pheochromocytomas: Detection with 18F DOPA whole body PET: Initial results. *Radiology* 2002; 222(2):507–512.

188. Sprung J, O'Hara JF Jr, Gill IS, et al. Anesthetic aspects of laparoscopic and open adrenalectomy for pheochromocytoma. *Urology* 2000;55(3): 339–343.

189. Fernandez-Cruz L, Taura P, Saenz A, et al. Laparoscopic approach to pheochromocytoma: Hemodynamic changes and catecholamine secretion. *World J Surg* 1996;20(7):762–768; discussion 768.

190. Janetschek G, Finkenstedt G, Gasser R, et al. Laparoscopic surgery for pheochromocytoma: Adrenalectomy, partial resection, excision of paragangliomas. *J Urol* 1998;160(2):330–334.

191. Gagner M, Breton G, Pharand D, et al. Is laparoscopic adrenalectomy indicated for pheochromocytomas? *Surgery* 1996;120(6):1,076–1,079; discussion 1,079–1,080.

192. Mobius E, Nies C, Rothmund M. Surgical treatment of pheochromocytomas: Laparoscopic or conventional? *Surg Endosc* 1999;13(1):35–39.

193. Col V, de Canniere L, Collard E, et al. Laparoscopic adrenalectomy for phaeochromocytoma: Endocrinological and surgical aspects of a new therapeutic approach. *Clin Endocrinol (Oxf)* 1999;50(1):121–125.

194. Lewi HJ, Reid R, Mucci B, et al. Malignant phaeochromocytoma. *Br J Urol* 1985;57(4):394–398.

195. Shapiro B, Sisson JC, Eyre P, et al. 131I-MIBG: A new agent in diagnosis and treatment of pheochromocytoma. *Cardiology* 1985;72(Suppl. 1): 137–142.

196. Troncone L, Rufini V. 131I-MIBG therapy of neural crest tumours (review). *Anticancer Res* 1997;17(3B):1,823–1,831.

197. Loh KC, Fitzgerald PA, Matthay KK, et al. The treatment of malignant pheochromocytoma with iodine-131 metaiodobenzylguanidine (131I-MIBG): A comprehensive review of 116 reported patients. *J Endocrinol Invest* 1997;20(11):648–658.

198. Keiser HR, Goldstein DS, Wade JL, et al. Treatment of malignant pheochromocytoma with combination chemotherapy. *Hypertension* 1985; 7(3 Pt 2):I18–I24.

199. Moloney GE, Cowdell RH, Lewis CL. Malignant phaeochromocytoma of the bladder. *Br J Urol* 1966;38(4):461–470.

200. Scharf Y, Nahir AM, Better OS, et al. Prolonged survival in malignant pheochromocytoma of the organ of Zuckerkandl with pharmacological treatment. *Cancer* 1973;31(3):746–750.

201. Drasin H. Treatment of malignant pheochromocytoma. *West J Med* 1978; 128(2):106–111.

202. DeAsis DN Jr, Ali MK, Soto A, et al. Acute cardiac toxicity of antineoplastic agents as the first manifestation of pheochromocytoma. *Cancer* 1978;42(4):2,005–2,008.

203. Feldman JM. Treatment of metastatic pheochromocytoma with streptozocin. *Arch Intern Med* 1983;143(9):1,799–1,800.

204. Gross DJ, Schlank E, Ipp E. Streptozotocin therapy for malignant pheochromocytoma. *Arch Intern Med* 1985;145(2):367–368.

205. Bukowski RM, Vidt DG. Chemotherapy trials in malignant pheochromocytoma: Report of two patients and review of the literature. *J Surg Oncol* 1984;27(2):89–92.

206. Philipps AF, McMurtry RJ, Taubman J. Malignant pheochromocytoma in childhood. *Am J Dis Child* 1976;130(11):1,252–1,255.

207. Senan S, Reed N, Connell J. Palliation of malignant phaeochromocytoma with combination chemotherapy. *Eur J Cancer* 1992;28A(4-5): 1,006–1,007.

208. Averbuch SD, Steakley CS, Young RC, et al. Malignant pheochromocytoma: Effective treatment with a combination of cyclophosphamide, vincristine, and dacarbazine. *Ann Intern Med* 1988;109(4):267–273.

209. Scott HW Jr, Reynolds V, Green N, et al. Clinical experience with malignant pheochromocytomas. *Surg Gynecol Obstet* 1982;154(6):801–818.

210. Rao F, Keiser HR, O'Connor DT. Malignant pheochromocytoma: Chromaffin granule transmitters and response to treatment. *Hypertension* 2000; 36(6):1,045–1,052.

211. Olson JJ, Loftus CM, Hitchon PW. Metastatic pheochromocytoma of the cervical spine. *Spine* 1989;14(3):349–351.

212. Yu L, Fleckman AM, Chadha M, et al. Radiation therapy of metastatic pheochromocytoma: Case report and review of the literature. *Am J Clin Oncol* 1996;19(4):389–393.

213. Wang P, Zuo C, Qian Z, et al. Computed tomography guided percutaneous ethanol injection for the treatment of hyperfunctioning pheochromocytoma. *J Urol* 2003;170(4 Pt 1):1,132–1,134.

214. Pommier RF, Brennan MF. An eleven-year experience with adrenocortical carcinoma. *Surgery* 1992;112(6):963–970; discussion 970–971.

215. Kasperlik-Zaluska AA, Migdalska BM, Zgliczynski S, et al. Adrenocortical carcinoma: A clinical study and treatment results of 52 patients. *Cancer* 1995;75(10):2,587–2,591.

216. Barzon L, Fallo F, Sonino N, et al. Adrenocortical carcinoma: Experience in 45 patients. *Oncology* 1997;54(6):490–496.

217. Haq MM, Legha SS, Samaan NA, et al. Cytotoxic chemotherapy in adrenal cortical carcinoma. *Cancer Treat Rep* 1980;64(8-9):909–913.

218. Berruti A, Terzolo M, Pia A, et al. Mitotane associated with etoposide, doxorubicin, and cisplatin in the treatment of advanced adrenocortical carcinoma. Italian Group for the Study of Adrenal Cancer. *Cancer* 1998;83(10):2,194–2,200.

219. Khan TS, Imam H, Juhlin C, et al. Streptozocin and o,p′DDD in the treatment of adrenocortical cancer patients: Long-term survival in its adjuvant use. *Ann Oncol* 2000;11(10):1,281–1,287.

220. Bonacci R, Gigliotti A, Baudin E, et al. Cytotoxic therapy with etoposide and cisplatin in advanced adrenocortical carcinoma. Reseau Comete IN-SERM. *Br J Cancer* 1998;78(4):546–549.

CHAPTER 54 ■ GENITOURINARY SARCOMAS AND CARCINOSARCOMAS IN ADULTS

TOHRU NAKAGAWA, IGOR FRANK, SATORU TAKAHASHI, TAIJI TSUKAMOTO, AND MICHAEL M. LIEBER

Extraskeletal soft tissue sarcomas are malignant neoplasms that arise in the mesenchymal connective tissues. The genitourinary system is an uncommon origin for soft tissue sarcomas (1,2). In the last century, approximately 1,000 cases have been reported in the English-language medical literature, which account for no more than 1% to 2% of all malignant tumors of the genitourinary system (Table 54.1). Because of the rarity of these neoplasms, their exact characteristics, including pathologic features and natural history, remain uncertain. Although combined treatment with surgery plus adjuvant chemotherapy and radiation therapy has been more widespread and has contributed to improved disease-free survival from rhabdomyosarcomas in children, the prognosis for adult patients with genitourinary sarcomas is still poor, and optimum treatment guidelines have not been established (3).

In this chapter, sarcomas of the kidney, urinary bladder, prostate, spermatic cord, testis, and paratestis are reviewed first. The extremely rare carcinosarcomas of the adult genitourinary system are discussed separately at the end of the chapter.

The most common genitourinary sarcomas in adults are those of the spermatic cord, testis, and paratestis, with 393 cases reported in the English-language medical literature until 1998. Sarcomas of the kidney are the second most common (259 cases), followed by those of the urinary bladder and prostate gland (Table 54.1).

SARCOMA OF THE KIDNEY

Sarcomas of the kidney are uncommon, with just 259 cases being reported in the English-language medical literature from 1950 through 1998 (1,3–42). This accounting excludes retroperitoneal sarcomas arising from an uncertain anatomic origin and sarcomatoid renal cell carcinoma (3). Approximately 1% of primary renal cell tumors are true sarcomas. A greater variety of histologic types of sarcomas arise in the kidney than in other genitourinary organs (Table 54.2). The most common renal sarcoma in adults is leiomyosarcoma, which accounts for 38.2% of reported cases. The second most common type is liposarcoma (8.5%), which is very rare in the bladder and the prostate gland. Most other histologic types of sarcomas, including hemangiopericytoma, osteosarcoma, and malignant fibrous histiocytoma, also have been reported in the kidney but in smaller percentages. In addition, recently several cases of synovial sarcoma of the kidney (43–49) and Ewing sarcoma/primitive neuroectodermal tumor of the kidney (50–53) have been reported. The establishment of these new entities among the renal neoplasms is mainly based on the molecular detection of the fusion gene transcript identical with their counterparts in the other soft tissues by reverse-transcription PCR (RT-PCR), namely SYT/SSX fusion gene in synovial sarcoma (43–47,49) and EWS/FLI-1 in Ewing sarcoma/primitive neuroectodermal tumor (50–52).

Age and sex distribution of 126 cases of renal sarcoma is presented in Figure 54.1. The ratio of men to women is 1:1.2. The age distribution for all renal sarcomas is slightly younger than that seen with renal cell carcinoma, with a peak incidence in the fifth decade (mean age 49 years). For 125 cases, the common symptoms and signs of renal sarcoma were pain (65%), a palpable renal mass (55%), hematuria (35%), and weight loss (28%) (Table 54.3). Hematuria, the most common symptom of renal cell carcinoma, is relatively less common for renal sarcoma. The high prevalence of a palpable renal mass, flank pain, and weight loss is attributed to the advanced stage at diagnosis. Some cases with

TABLE 54.1

UROGENITAL SARCOMAS IN ADULTS (1,027 CASES)

Sarcoma type	Kidney (1950–1998)	Bladder (1954–1998)	Prostate (1938–1998)	Spermatic cord, testis, paratestis (1950–1998)
Sarcoma of fibrous tissue	28 (11%)	9 (5%)	6 (3%)	55 (14%)
Sarcoma of adipose tissue	22 (8%)	7 (4%)	1 (0.5%)	139 (35%)
Sarcoma of muscle	111 (43%)	132 (69%)	143 (78%)	183 (47%)
Sarcoma of vessels	41 (16%)	7 (4%)	2 (1%)	0 (0%)
Sarcoma of peripheral nerve	1 (0.4%)	1 (0.5%)	0 (0%)	0 (0%)
Extraskeletal bone sarcoma	19 (7%)	30 (16%)	1 (0.5%)	2 (0.5%)
Miscellaneous	37 (14%)	6 (3%)	30 (16%)	14 (4%)
Total	259	192	183	393

TABLE 54.2

SARCOMA OF THE KIDNEY IN ADULTS

Sarcoma type	Total number	Number by subtype (%)
Sarcoma of fibrous tissue	28	
Fibrosarcoma		12 (4.6)
Malignant fibrous histiocytoma		16 (6.2)
Sarcoma of adipose tissue	22	
Liposarcoma		22 (8.5)
Sarcoma of muscle	111	
Leiomyosarcoma		99 (38.2)
Rhabdomyosarcoma		12 (4.6)
Sarcoma of vessels	41	
Hemangiopericytoma		14 (5.4)
Angiosarcoma		19 (7.3)
Angiomyoliposarcoma		1 (0.4)
Kaposi sarcoma		7 (2.7)
Sarcoma of peripheral nerves	1	
Malignant schwannoma		1 (0.4)
Extraskeletal bone sarcoma	19	
Osteogenic sarcoma		17 (6.6)
Chondrosarcoma		2 (0.8)
Miscellaneous	37	
Malignant mesenchymoma		2 (0.8)
Mixed sarcoma		6 (2.3)
Round cell sarcoma		1 (0.4)
Spindle cell sarcoma		5 (1.9)
Clear cell sarcoma		14 (5.4)
Undifferentiated sarcoma		9 (3.5)
Total	259	

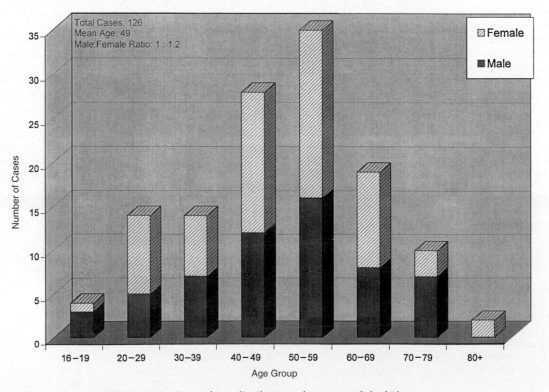

FIGURE 54.1. Age and sex distribution of sarcoma of the kidney.

TABLE 54.3

MAJOR SYMPTOMS AND SIGNS IN SARCOMA OF THE KIDNEY (125 CASES)

Symptom/Sign	Number of occurrences (%)
Pain	81 (65)
Mass	69 (55)
Hematuria	44 (35)
Gastrointestinal symptoms	
Vomiting	8 (6)
Nausea	6 (5)
Diarrhea	2 (2)
General nonspecific symptoms	
Weight loss	35 (28)
Fever	14 (11)
Anorexia	13 (10)
No symptoms	5 (4)

incidental tumor rupture also have been reported (54–56). However, an increasing number of asymptomatic cases have been diagnosed incidentally (5–7,9); one such case was a patient whose sarcoma was detected by computed tomographic (CT) scan study for liver dysfunction (6).

Sarcomas can arise from both the renal parenchyma and the renal capsule. Three cases of a leiomyosarcoma of the renal capsule have been reported (27). CT scan is usually accurate in suggesting the site of origin. Smooth muscle fibers of renal pelvis (24,57), artery (58), and vein (4,8,59) also can serve as the origins of leiomyosarcoma.

The etiology of soft tissue sarcomas of the kidney is not known. Sarcomas at other sites occur with increased incidence in fields of previous irradiation or after the use of alkylating agents (60). No such cause has been identified for renal sarcomas. One paper has argued the possible role of Epstein-Barr virus infection in the pathogenesis of leiomyosarcoma arising in the organ transplant patients (61).

Although the development of renal sarcomas does not seem to have a clear hereditary component, renal angiosarcoma has been reported to occur in a familial distribution. One case report described two brothers, 3 years apart in age, who developed angiosarcoma of the left kidney at the ages of 52 and 69 years. Both rapidly developed metastatic disease and died 6 weeks and 3 months, respectively, after nephrectomy. No common carcinogen or hereditary or other causal factor was identified (40).

Kaposi sarcoma of the kidney is a relatively new entity that is becoming progressively more prevalent in the era of human immunodeficiency virus. Human herpes virus 8 (HHV8) is known to be the pathogen of Kaposi sarcoma in immunosuppressed patients, such as patients with acquired immunodeficiency syndrome (AIDS) or those who have had organ transplants (62). Seven cases of Kaposi sarcoma of the kidney have been reported (one symptomatic and six asymptomatic) (33). All cases of renal involvement documented in the English-language medical literature occurred in homosexual men with AIDS and documented cutaneous disease. The presence of cutaneous disease in all reported cases makes the origin of Kaposi sarcoma in the kidney controversial. Some argue that it arises from the arcuate vessels; however, others maintain that hematogenous spread from other sites and subsequent trapping in the renal vascular bed may be occurring (34).

Diagnosis

Renal sarcoma typically presents as a large solid-mass lesion of the kidney indistinguishable by standard radiologic techniques from the much more common renal cell carcinomas. No particular findings by ultrasonography or CT scan distinguish renal sarcomas, and virtually all renal sarcomas have been diagnosed postoperatively. Inferior vena caval (IVC) and right atrial thrombus, often seen in renal cell carcinomas, cannot exclude the possibility of clear cell sarcoma (54,63–65), synovial sarcoma (47), or Ewing sarcoma/primitive neuroectodermal tumor (49). Renal leiomyosarcoma also may mimic transitional cell carcinoma because of its hypovascularity, and appear on CT scan, intravenous urography, or retrograde pyelography as a filling defect consistent with transitional cell carcinoma (24,57).

The presence on magnetic resonance imaging (MRI) of multiple regions of low-signal-intensity in renal leiomyosarcomas, representing areas of predominantly fibrous tissue, has been reported (20) and may be helpful in the differential diagnosis. The hypervascularity seen on angiography for the majority of renal cell carcinomas is usually not seen with renal sarcomas. Angiographic findings in 32 patients have been reported. Of these, 12 showed hypervascularity or neovascularity or both, and 20 (63%) showed hypovascularity. Six of 12 patients with hypervascular tumors had leiomyosarcoma. All fibrous sarcomas and liposarcomas were hypovascular. Although preoperative diagnosis of renal sarcomas by radiologic imaging techniques is not usually possible, identification of a large hypovascular tumor infiltrating adjacent organs, but without distant metastasis, may raise the suspicion of a renal sarcoma. Hypercalcemia and the hepatic dysfunction syndrome seen with renal cell carcinoma have not been reported with renal sarcomas. Although rare, hemangiopericytomas are sometimes associated with hypoglycemia; nine such cases have been reported, three of which were renal (3).

Additional diagnostic clues may be present in osteogenic sarcoma of the kidney. Radiographic examination of the abdomen may reveal a sunburstlike pattern along with some distortion of the calyceal system on excretory urography. This pattern may be present in up to 82% of patients with osteogenic sarcoma of the kidney (39). Diagnosis of primary renal osteogenic sarcoma also may be suggested preoperatively by marked elevation of serum alkaline phosphatase level in the absence of bone disease (36), although many patients with the disease do not exhibit this elevation.

Although routine biopsy of solid renal lesions is not recommended, sarcoma of the kidney can be diagnosed with fine-needle aspiration cytology and electron microscopy. Five cases of clear cell sarcoma (41,42), two cases of leiomyosarcoma (25,26), and one case each of fibromyxoid sarcoma (66), angiosarcoma (67), and synovial sarcoma (68) diagnosed by fine-needle aspiration biopsy have been reported. This technique may be useful in the diagnosis of select cases of unresectable sarcomas and may help guide nonsurgical therapy.

Treatment

The treatment selected for a renal sarcoma in general is that which is indicated for a similar stage of renal cell carcinoma, because preoperative tissue diagnosis is unlikely. In the absence of evidence of metastatic disease by preoperative evaluation, radical nephrectomy is the treatment of choice. On rare occasions, nephron-sparing surgery could be considered (69). At present, no reason exists to recommend a formal retroperitoneal lymph node dissection for renal sarcoma (3). Nephrectomy also should be offered to patients experiencing severe unrelenting symptoms, such as flank pain, fever, or hematuria.

For patients who have obvious metastatic disease, usually in the chest, but with a renal primary tumor visualized radiologically, a tissue diagnosis must be made at some site. This is particularly important because renal sarcoma is more likely to be responsive to radiotherapy or cytotoxic chemotherapy than is renal cell carcinoma.

Multimodality therapy consisting of surgery, chemotherapy, and radiotherapy should be considered for the treatment of locally advanced and metastatic or recurrent renal sarcoma. In sarcoma of the other soft tissues, doxorubicin hydrochloride and ifosfamide are the key drugs, and dacarbazine (DTIC), gemcitabine, and taxane seem to have activity in at least a subset of sarcomas (70,71). However, in renal sarcomas, the efficacy of adjuvant and therapeutic chemotherapies and/or radiotherapy for salvage treatment of patients with recurrent disease has not been established.

Prognosis

Death for most patients with sarcoma of the kidney is caused by the tumor. Survival curves for renal sarcomas in adults are shown in Figure 54.2. Liposarcoma and hemangiopericytoma have a more favorable prognosis, and the 5-year survival rate for both groups is approximately 90%. One patient with renal liposarcoma, however, was reported to have recurrent disease 14 years after nephrectomy (11). The 5-year survival rate for the fibrosarcoma group (e.g., fibrosarcoma and malignant fibrous histiocytoma) is <50%. Leiomyosarcoma, the most common renal sarcoma, has a much poorer prognosis, with 5-year and 10-year survival rates of 32% and 8%, respectively. Nuclear grade has been reported to be correlated with prognosis of leiomyosarcoma (72). Osteosarcoma has an even poorer prognosis, with 75% of patients having died from metastatic disease within 2 years. Rhabdomyosarcoma is the most unfavorable, with all patients dying of the disease within 2 years. Overall, the prognosis for 115

renal sarcomas was worse than that for renal cell carcinoma (73). The average 5-year survival rate is approximately 32%. No obvious improvement in survival was seen in the last decade when compared with the previous three decades, despite the increasing popularity of aggressive multimodal therapy.

In an attempt to identify a prognostic marker for sarcoma of the kidney, flow cytometric studies have been reported for 17 renal sarcoma cases. No correlation with clinical outcome has been found (10).

SARCOMA OF THE URINARY BLADDER

Whereas sarcoma of the bladder is a common pediatric malignancy, sarcomas of the bladder in adults are quite rare, with only 192 such cases being reported in the English-language medical literature since 1954 until 1998 (1,3,16,74–94) (Tables 54.1 and 54.4). Because carcinomas of the bladder are among the most common urinary tract tumors in adults, with approximately 60,240 new cases being reported annually in the United States alone (73), the relative scarcity of sarcomas of the bladder is readily apparent. The incidence of bladder sarcoma is often estimated to be 0.2% to 0.3% of all primary bladder tumors (3) but is probably even lower. Rhabdomyosarcoma is the most common histologic type of bladder neoplasm in children. In contrast, almost half of sarcomas of the bladder in adults are leiomyosarcomas and one-fifth are rhabdomyosarcomas (Table 54.4). The remaining histologic types make up just a small fraction of tumor types observed. Carcinosarcoma is also relatively common in this organ and is discussed at the end of the chapter. Age and sex distribution of patients with bladder sarcomas are shown in Figure 54.3. Bladder sarcomas are most common in the sixth decade (mean age 54 years) and occur predominantly in men (the ratio of men to women is 1:0.7). A review of 91 cases revealed that

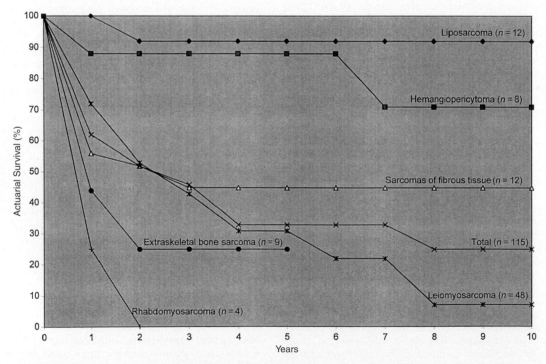

FIGURE 54.2. Actuarial survival curves for 115 patients with sarcoma of the kidney according to histologic type. The total number includes patients with miscellaneous sarcomas whose survival curve is not shown separately (From Herr HW. Sarcoma of the urinary tract. In: deKernion JB, Paulson DF, eds. *Genitourinary cancer management*, Philadelphia, PA: Lea & Febiger, 1987:259–270).

TABLE 54.4

SARCOMA OF THE BLADDER IN ADULTS

Sarcoma type	Total number	Number by subtype (%)
Sarcoma of fibrous tissue	9	
Fibrosarcoma		5 (2.6)[a]
Malignant fibrous histiocytoma		4 (2.1)
Sarcoma of adipose tissue	7	
Myxoid liposarcoma		7 (3.6)
Sarcoma of muscle	132	
Leiomyosarcoma		89 (46.3)[b]
Rhabdomyosarcoma		40 (20.8)[c]
Myosarcoma		1 (0.5)
Leiomyosarcoma plus rhabdomyosarcoma		2 (1.0)
Extraskeletal bone sarcoma	30	
Osteogenic sarcoma		28 (14.6)[d]
Osteochondrosarcoma		1 (0.5)
Chondrosarcoma		1 (0.5)
Sarcoma of peripheral nerves	1	
Plexosarcoma		1 (0.5)
Sarcoma of blood vessels	7	
Angiosarcoma		7 (3.6)[e]
Miscellaneous	6	
Mixed sarcoma		2 (1.0)
Spindle-cell sarcoma		1 (0.5)
Undifferentiated sarcoma		3 (1.6)
Total	192	

[a]Including two cyclophosphamide-induced sarcomas.
[b]Including seven cyclophosphamide-induced sarcomas.
[c]Including one radiation-induced sarcoma.
[d]Including one patient with radiation-induced tumor and three. patients with previous history of schistosomiasis.
[e]Including two radiation-induced tumors.

hematuria and irritative voiding symptoms are the most common symptoms of this malignancy (Table 54.5).

Other rare bladder sarcomas include osteosarcoma (95,96), plexosarcoma (93), angiosarcoma (94,97,98), osteochondrosarcoma (91), pleomorphic sarcoma (99), and granulocytic sarcoma (100,101). Among them, plexosarcoma, osteochondrosarcoma, and pleomorphic sarcoma are even rarer, with only one case of each sarcoma having been reported to date. Plexosarcoma is a tumor that arises from the autonomic nerve plexus of the bladder. Plexosarcomas have previously been reported in association with gastrointestinal autonomic nerve plexus (93).

TABLE 54.5

MAJOR SYMPTOMS AND SIGNS IN SARCOMA OF THE BLADDER (91 CASES)

Symptom/Sign	Number of occurrences (%)
Gross hematuria	72 (79)
Painless	40 (44)
Urinary frequency	24 (26)
Dysuria	23 (25)
Urinary urgency	6 (7)
Urinary retention	2 (2)
Pain	9 (10)

Granulocytic sarcoma is also rare. It is composed of myeloid precursor cells presenting as a extramedullary mass lesion, and usually occur in clinical settings of acute or chronic myeloid leukemia. However, two cases of primary granulocytic sarcoma of the bladder without hematologic disorder have been reported (100,101).

Several causative agents have been implicated in the pathogenesis of some cases of bladder sarcoma. Several well-documented cases have been reported of cyclophosphamide-induced leiomyosarcoma of the bladder occurring 7 to 14 years after therapy for an unrelated neoplasm (74,79,82,84,102–105). These cases of secondary leiomyosarcoma, combined with two cases of cyclophosphamide-induced fibrosarcoma as well as 54 transitional cell carcinomas, 12 squamous cell carcinomas, and one adenocarcinoma that developed after cyclophosphamide therapy, indicate a specific association between therapy with cyclophosphamide and subsequent development of the mesodermal-derived malignancies (84). Urinary formation and excretion of acrolein, a metabolite of cyclophosphamide, is thought to be the direct causative factor (84). In addition, radiation and schistosomiasis have been implicated in the pathogenesis of this malignancy, with at least six reported cases of radiation-induced bladder sarcoma (75,76,78,94–107) and three cases occurring in patients with a previous history of schistosomiasis (108). In addition, two cases of leiomyosarcoma of the bladder have been reported recently among survivors of hereditary retinoblastoma with no history of radiation or chemotherapy (109,110). These cases raise the possibility of genetic predisposition of the germline mutation of Rb gene toward the bladder leiomyosarcoma.

Diagnosis

The presence of gross hematuria usually prompts urologic referral and then cystoscopy. Diagnosis of bladder sarcoma is therefore commonly made by cystoscopic biopsy. Bladder sarcomas usually have a different cystoscopic appearance than the typical low-grade papillary transitional cell carcinomas. These tumors, however, often are indistinguishable from sessile invasive transitional cell carcinomas or squamous cell carcinomas. Bladder sarcoma usually occurs as sessile mass with or without ulceration involving the bladder wall. No location within the bladder for sarcomas is predominant. In men, differentiation between a sarcoma of the prostate and a sarcoma of the bladder sometimes can be difficult, because sarcomas in these organs usually have locally extensive disease (3). In women, localization of the exact origin to the bladder, urethra, or urethrovaginal septum may be difficult.

Endoscopic biopsy of the tumor mass generally yields a valid tissue diagnosis. Standard radiologic imaging techniques for staging sarcomas of the bladder are similar to those used to stage invasive transitional cell carcinoma of the bladder. CT or MRI scan is most useful for evaluating the local extent and potential resectability of the tumor. Excretory urography to show the upper urinary tract anatomy is also important, because many sarcoma cases demonstrate evidence of upper tract obstruction at the time of initial diagnosis. Osteosarcoma of the bladder may exhibit marked calcifications on CT scan (88).

Treatment

For patients with no evidence of metastatic disease, wide local surgical excision is indicated. Sarcomas of the bladder normally arise in the muscular layer and cannot be treated successfully by endoscopic resection. Therefore, open surgery is indicated as initial surgical resection. Because bladder sarcoma

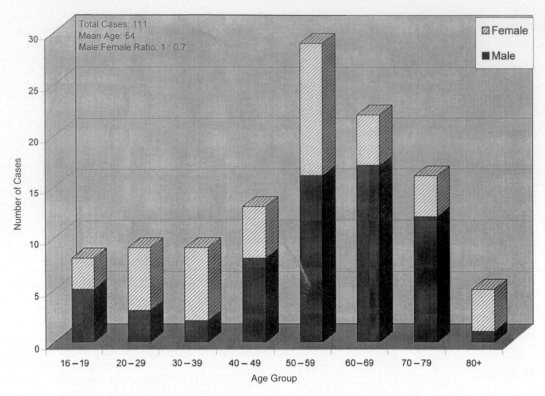

FIGURE 54.3. Age and sex distribution of sarcoma of the bladder.

is not a field-change disease, like transitional cell carcinoma, every attempt should be made, depending on the histologic type, size, and location of the tumor, to perform a partial cystectomy to save a functional bladder (3). The operation of choice is a wide local excision, in which the overlying perivesical fat is taken and the ureter is reimplanted if necessary. If the tumor involves the bladder neck or trigone or both, formal radical cystectomy should be performed. The only exception to this general rule is angiosarcoma. It has a particularly high rate of local recurrence (greater than 30%), frequently extends beyond the lesion grossly apparent at surgery, and is not responsive to radiation therapy (107). Therefore, radical cystectomy appears to be the treatment of choice for local bladder angiosarcoma (94). Regardless of treatment, however, mean survival rate for these patients is less than 12 months (94).

A formal pelvic lymph node dissection is also recommended in this setting because pelvic nodes are often involved, and nodal metastases, if present, would indicate the need for systemic adjuvant chemotherapy.

Multimodality therapy should be considered, especially in locally advanced or metastatic cases, as well as in high-grade or positive surgical-margin cases. Neoadjuvant chemotherapy with doxorubicin and ifosfamide may allow the curative resection even in the locally advanced or metastatic cases (111). Postoperative radiotherapy in the tumor bed is recommended for patients with relatively low-grade leiomyosarcomas in which local recurrence is apt to be the most common problem. For patients with high-grade leiomyosarcomas, rhabdomyosarcomas, and other more anaplastic tumors, aggressive combined treatment is recommended, including adjuvant radiotherapy and doxorubicin hydrochloride–based chemotherapy (16,70,71,77,111). Bone marrow transplant may have a role (16,112), but rarity of the disease precludes definitive statements.

Interestingly, one 25-year-old man underwent debulking surgery for an unresectable leiomyosarcoma of the bladder and had no response to salvage chemotherapy. He had a spontaneous regression of the tumor 5 months after cessation

of therapy and is still alive without evidence of disease 51 months after the diagnosis (85).

Prognosis

Survival curves for 112 patients with sarcoma of the bladder are presented in Figure 54.4. Overall, the prognosis is not as poor as that of renal sarcoma. The 5-year survival rate for all patients with bladder sarcomas is 58%. Rhabdomyosarcomas of the bladder have a much poorer prognosis than leiomyosarcomas. The 5-year survival rate for patients with rhabdomyosarcomas is 28% and for those with leiomyosarcomas is 67%. Patients with angiosarcoma or osteosarcoma of the bladder do particularly poorly, with a mean survival of less than 12 months; 6 out of 7 patients with angiosarcoma and 19 out of 24 patients with osteosarcoma died within 6 months irrespective of treatment modality. Patients with low-grade bladder sarcoma seem to have favorable long-term outcome (113). A series of 36 patients with bladder leiomyosarcoma represents the largest single-instituion experiences, which has reported tumor stage as the only significant predictor of survival with multivariate analysis (111).

SARCOMA OF THE PROSTATE

Prostate sarcoma is rare, with only 183 cases reported in the English-language medical literature from 1938 to 1998 (1,3,16, 114–133). By contrast, adenocarcinoma of the prostate is now the most common malignancy for men in the United States, with an estimated 230,110 new cases diagnosed in 2004 (73). Although the incidence of sarcoma of the prostate has been estimated to be 0.1% to 0.3% of malignant prostate tumors (3), this must be a significant overestimation. The histologic types of sarcoma seen in the adult prostate are presented in Table 54.6. The distribution of tumor types reported is quite similar to that seen for sarcoma of the bladder. Leiomyosarcoma is the most

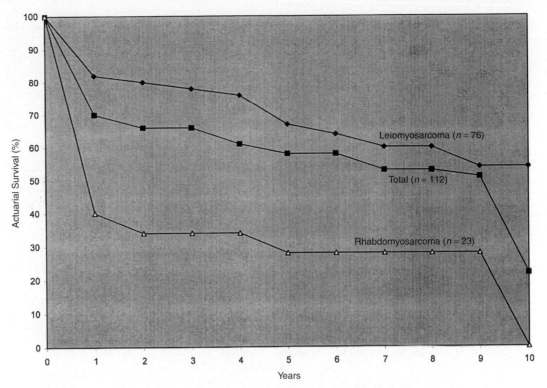

FIGURE 54.4. Actuarial survival curves for 112 patients with sarcoma of the bladder according to histologic type (From Herr HW. Sarcoma of the urinary tract. In: deKernion JB, Paulson DF, eds. *Genitourinary cancer management*, Philadelphia, PA: Lea & Febiger, 1987:259–270).

TABLE 54.6

SARCOMA OF THE PROSTATE IN ADULTS

Sarcoma type	Total number	Number by subtype (%)
Sarcoma of fibrous tissue	6	
Fibrosarcoma		5 (2.7)
Myxofibrosarcoma		1 (0.5)
Sarcoma of adipose tissue	1	
Myxoid liposarcoma		1 (0.5)
Sarcoma of muscle	143	
Leiomyosarcoma		88 (48.1)
Rhabdomyosarcoma		49 (26.8)
Myosarcoma		6 (3.3)
Sarcoma of vessels	2	
Angiosarcoma		2 (1.1)
Extraskeletal bone sarcoma	1	
Osteogenic sarcoma		1 (0.5)
Miscellaneous	30	
Spindle-cell sarcoma		10 (5.5)[a]
Undifferentiated sarcoma		2 (1.1)
Sarcoma (unknown origin)		4 (2.2)[b]
Cystosarcoma phyllodes		14 (7.6)
Total	**183**	

[a]Including one case of radiation-induced sarcoma.
[b]Including one case of radiation-induced sarcoma.

common tumor type, accounting for approximately 50% of cases. The next most common type is rhabdomyosarcoma, occurring in 27% of patients. The other types of sarcoma are rare. The age distribution of 109 patients with sarcoma of the prostate is shown in Figure 54.5. Mean age was 48 years, roughly 15 years younger than that of patients with adenocarcinoma of the prostate. Leiomyosarcoma, the most common tumor, is seen more frequently in older patients, with the majority being older than 50 years (mean age, 54 years). Rhabdomyosarcoma is much more common in younger patients and shows a peak of incidence in the second decade (only four patients with rhabdomyosarcoma of the prostate were older than 60 years). In addition to the other prostate sarcomas with rare histopathology described in Table 54.6, one case of chondrosarcoma and two cases of synovial sarcoma of the prostate have been reported recently (134–136).

Radiation to the prostate may confer significantly increased risk for the development of subsequent sarcoma. In fact, several cases of radiation-induced sarcoma of the prostate have been reported, although most of them were after definitive radiation therapy against adenocarcinoma of the prostate (110,137–139). To date, only one case of postradiation sarcoma without previous history of adenocarcinoma of the prostate has been reported (137).

Cystosarcoma phyllodes of the prostate is a special case that deserves a brief discussion (131–133,140–144). First described by Cox in 1960 (132), it is an extremely rare neoplasm that is characterized by hyperplastic and neoplastic glandulostromal proliferation that mimics cystosarcoma phyllodes of the breast. Although it is considered benign, the tumor occasionally recurs after resection. Surgical resection is curative in 75% of cases, with the remainder experiencing local recurrences (140,141). Metastatic diseases also have been reported (142–144).

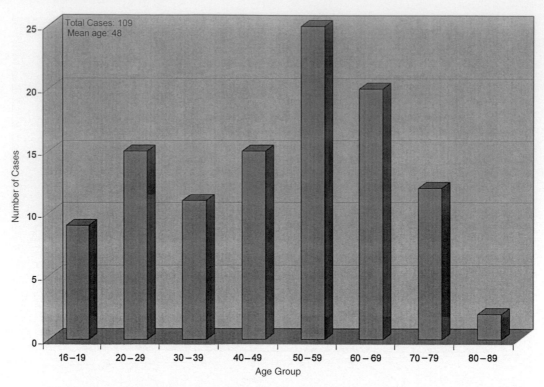

FIGURE 54.5. Age distribution of sarcoma of the prostate.

Diagnosis

Most patients with sarcoma of the prostate have symptoms related to bladder outlet obstruction (Table 54.7). In 103 informative cases, 89% of patients reported symptoms of urinary obstruction. In 18% of cases, symptoms related to rectal obstruction were observed. On digital rectal prostate examination, sarcomas are often found to be smooth and globular or soft and elastic, in contrast to the usual findings with adenocarcinoma of the prostate (Table 54.7).

TABLE 54.7

MAJOR SYMPTOMS AND CHARACTERISTICS OF THE PROSTATE ON PALPATION IN SARCOMA OF THE PROSTATE

Symptoms/Characteristics	Number of occurrences (%)
Symptoms	103
Related to bladder outlet	
obstruction	91 (89)
Related to rectal obstruction	19 (18)
Others	
Pain	6 (6)
Hematuria	4 (4)
Weight loss	1 (1)
Characteristics on palpation	
Surface	33
Smooth	21 (65)
Globular	2 (6)
Irregular	10 (29)
Consistency	40
Soft or boggy	8 (21)
Elastic or tense	6 (16)
Firm or hard	26 (63)

Diagnosis is usually made by needle biopsy. Prostatic sarcoma may show an irregular hypoechoic prostatic mass with an anechoic area by ultrasonography (137). Evaluation for local extension of a prostate sarcoma would normally include a careful bimanual examination under anesthesia, cystoscopy to check for involvement of the bladder base, and CT or MRI scan. In skillful hands, transrectal ultrasonography may be useful not only in guiding transrectal biopsies but also in delineating local extent of the disease. A study involving three patients with rhabdomyosarcoma revealed that local extent of the disease could be delineated at the time of transrectal needle biopsy (145).

Generally, most prostate sarcomas are locally extensive but not metastatic at the time of diagnosis. Among 20 patients, 4 (20%) showed metastatic disease at the time of diagnosis. The organ sites of metastases were lung [2 cases (115,118)], bone [2 cases (118,119)], and liver [1 case (114)].

Treatment

In the absence of evidence of metastatic disease, aggressive local surgical excision should be performed. Occasionally, a small, low-grade leiomyosarcoma may be confined within the prostate capsule and can be treated with radical prostatectomy. Most prostate sarcomas are usually quite large at the time of diagnosis, however, and radical cystoprostatectomy is the local extirpative option. For locally extensive sarcomas involving the rectum, a total pelvic exenteration is indicated. The authors usually perform bilateral pelvic lymphadenectomy combined with radical prostatectomy (cystoprostatectomy) for the staging information it yields. Patients with low-grade leiomyosarcomas with positive resection margins should receive postoperative radiotherapy to lower the risk of local recurrence. Patients with high-grade leiomyosarcomas or rhabdomyosarcomas and those with nodal metastases should generally receive adjuvant chemotherapy. Once again, a combination chemotherapy regimen that includes doxorubicin hydrochloride seems most advisable, despite no clear evidence of benefit (3). In the report of one of the largest single-institution experiences, among six cases treated with neoadjuvant chemotherapy or chemoradiotherapy, three achieved size reduction of the primary tumor (146). One case of unresectable high-grade prostate leiomyosarcoma has been reported to demonstrate a more than 60% tumor reduction after combination doxorubicin hydrochloride–based chemotherapy followed by radiotherapy (120). Such chemotherapy, however, did not achieve durable remission in any patients with metastatic disease. Although many initial treatment regimens have been reported, no strong support for any one treatment can be gleaned from the literature at this time.

Prognosis

Patients with prostate sarcomas do less well than those with sarcomas of the urinary bladder, with a 5-year survival rate of 28% for 97 patients overall (Fig. 54.6). This is most likely secondary to the fact that prostate sarcomas reach a much larger size before causing symptoms, whereas sarcomas of the bladder cause symptoms at a smaller size and earlier stage. Leiomyosarcomas of the prostate have a better prognosis than rhabdomyosarcomas, with a 5-year survival rate of 42% for 53 cases of leiomyosarcoma in contrast to a 13% 5-year survival rate for 21 cases of rhabdomyosarcoma (Fig. 54.6). No obvious improvement in survival rates for patients with prostate sarcoma was identified through this review of the reports covering more than 50 years. Two reports of the largest single-instituion experience have revealed the existence of occasional long term survivors (122,146). Negative surgical margin and absence of metastatic disease at presentation have been reported as predictive of long-term survival (146).

SARCOMAS OF THE SPERMATIC CORD, TESTIS, AND PARATESTIS

Sarcomas of the spermatic cord, testis, and paratestis are the most common genitourinary tract sarcomas in adults, with 393

TABLE 54.8

SARCOMA OF SPERMATIC CORD, TESTIS, AND PARATESTIS IN ADULTS

Sarcoma type	Total number	Number by subtype (%)
Sarcoma of fibrous tissue	55	
Fibrosarcoma		27 (6.9)
Myxofibrosarcoma		2 (0.5)
Malignant fibrous histiocytoma		26 (6.6)
Sarcoma of adipose tissue	139	
Liposarcoma		119 (30.3)
Myxoliposarcoma		16 (4.1)
Fibroplastic liposarcoma		2 (0.5)
Lipoblastic liposarcoma		1 (0.2)
Lipofibromyosarcoma		1 (0.2)
Sarcoma of muscle	183	
Leiomyosarcoma		89 (22.6)
Rhabdomyosarcoma		89 (22.6)
Myosarcoma		5 (1.3)
Extraskeletal bone sarcoma	2	
Osteogenic sarcoma		2 (0.5)
Miscellaneous	14	
Mixed sarcoma		4 (1.0)
Spindle-cell sarcoma		4 (1.0)
Undifferentiated sarcoma		5 (1.3)
Mesothelioma		1 (0.2)
Total	393	

cases reported in adults from 1950 through 1998 (1,3,16, 147–178) (Table 54.8). As a group, sarcomas of muscle origin make up slightly less than 50% of these tumors. Liposarcoma is the most common single histologic type of sarcoma of the

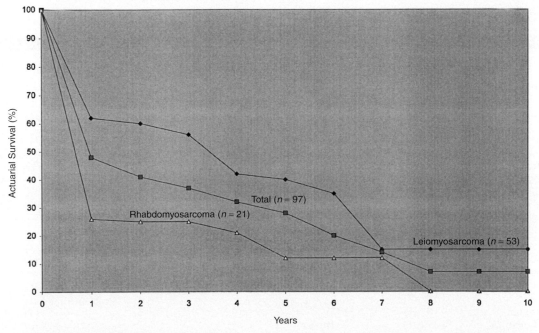

FIGURE 54.6. Actuarial survival curves for 97 patients with sarcoma of the prostate according to histologic type (From Herr HW. Sarcoma of the urinary tract. In: deKernion JB, Paulson DF, eds. *Genitourinary cancer management*, Philadelphia, PA: Lea & Febiger, 1987:259–270).

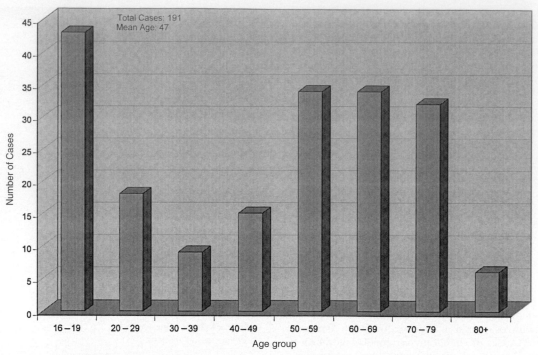

FIGURE 54.7. Age distribution of sarcoma of the spermatic cord, testis, and paratestis.

spermatic cord, testis, and paratestis, however, accounting for 30.3% of cases. Leiomyosarcoma and rhabdomyosarcoma follow, with 22.6% of cases each. Fibrosarcomas and malignant fibrous histiocytomas make up 6.9% and 6.6% of cases, respectively. The age distribution is shown in Figure 54.7. Two obvious peaks of incidence are observed at age 16 years through 19 years and at older than 50 years. Almost all of the large number of patients younger than 30 years had rhabdomyosarcomas. Leiomyosarcomas, liposarcomas, and fibrosarcomas were most common in the fifth, sixth, and seventh decades. Rhabdomyosarcomas occurred only rarely after 40 years of age. Table 54.9 presents the spectrum of anatomic locations of these

tumors. Rhabdomyosarcoma, leiomyosarcoma, and liposarcoma were most common on the right side of the scrotum. Fibrosarcomas generally occurred in the spermatic cord, with an equal number in the intrascrotal region and inguinal canal. Most liposarcomas also involved the spermatic cord or paratestis in the intrascrotal region, with one-third being found in the inguinal canal. The majority of leiomyosarcomas involved the spermatic cord in the intrascrotal or inguinal region, but a substantial number of cases arose in the epididymis (20%). Almost all rhabdomyosarcomas were found in the intrascrotal region and occurred in the spermatic cord, testis, epididymis, tunica vaginalis, or paratestis area. Recently, synovial sarcoma (179) and

TABLE 54.9

LOCATION OF SPERMATIC CORD, TESTIS, AND PARATESTIS SARCOMAS

Sarcoma type	Sides			Inguinal region spermatic cord (%)
	Right (%)	Left (%)	Unknown (%)	
Fibrosarcoma	18 (51)	16 (46)	1 (3)	14 (40)
Liposarcoma	20 (53)	16 (42)	2 (5)	12 (32)
Leiomyosarcoma	25 (56)	13 (30)	6 (14)	9 (20)
Rhabdomyosarcoma	32 (47)	24 (35)	12 (18)	4 (6)
Miscellaneous	2 (33)	1 (17)	3 (50)	—
Total	97 (51)	70 (37)	24 (12)	39 (20)

Sarcoma type	Intrascrotal region					
	Spermatic cord (%)	Testis (%)	Epididymis (%)	Tunica vaginalis (%)	Paratestis (%)	Total cases
Fibrosarcoma	14 (40)	1 (3)	5 (14)	—	1 (3)	35
Liposarcoma	18 (47)	—	—	—	8 (21)	8
Leiomyosarcoma	18 (42)	1 (2)	9 (20)	2 (5)	5 (11)	44
Rhabdomyosarcoma	21 (31)	7 (10)	7 (10)	5 (7)	24 (36)	68
Miscellaneous	2 (33)	2 (33)	—	—	2 (33)	6
Total	73 (38)	11 (6)	21 (11)	7 (4)	40 (21)	191

granulocytic sarcoma (180,181) have been added to the wide spectrum of histopathology of sarcoma of this region.

Sarcomas may occur either alone or in combination with a testicular germ cell tumor. Forty-one cases of rhabdomyosarcoma combined with a testicular germ cell tumor have been reported (182,183). Although other histologic patterns occur, sarcoma is the most common type of non–germ cell tumor associated with teratoma. In a study of 46 patients with testicular teratoma, 26 (63%) had an associated sarcoma (182). Accurate histologic diagnosis in such cases is important and can be complicated in some instances because the features of sarcoma may resemble those of undifferentiated teratoma. In doubtful cases, definitive diagnosis can be made with immunohistochemical studies, which are positive for myoglobin in the presence of rhabdomyosarcoma (184). The origin of non–germ cell malignancies within germ cell tumors is uncertain, but these may occur by malignant transformation of preexisting teratomatous elements or through differentiation of totipotential germ cells (183).

Diagnosis

Sarcomas of the spermatic cord, testis, and paratestis normally occur as a firm, painless, palpable mass. Therefore, if a hard mass is palpated in the paratestis area or in the spermatic cord, either within the scrotum or in the inguinal canal, sarcoma should be suspected. Germ cell tumors of the testis usually form a hard mass in the substance of the testis (within the tunica albuginea), whereas a sarcoma is normally felt as a hard mass outside the tunica albuginea. Nevertheless, primary intratesticular sarcomas, which are extremely rare, should be diagnosed only after surgical exploration (147,185). Sarcomas (especially liposarcomas) of the inguinal canal are sometimes mistaken for inguinal hernias or hydrocele. Liposarcomas occasionally transmit light, which adds to diagnostic confusion. Because most lesions in the scrotum are benign and include such common findings as spermatoceles and cysts of various kinds, the use of high-resolution scrotal ultrasonography for delineating the solid or cystic character of intrascrotal pathology is particularly important.

Although ultrasonography is reliable in distinguishing between solid and cystic lesions as well as in identifying the extratesticular location of a mass, it cannot definitively distinguish benign from malignant solid lesions (186,187). Frates et al. (186) correlated the sonographic findings for 17 extratesticular masses with surgical pathologic findings. The authors found that size, distinctness of borders, relation to the epididymis, and echotexture were not useful criteria for distinguishing benign from malignant lesions. Eighteen percent of the lesions in the study were malignant. Therefore, any noncystic abnormal lesion in the scrotum, external to the tunica albuginea, should be surgically explored and a biopsy performed. Although adenomatoid tumors of the epididymis and paratestis are the most common solid lesions in an extratesticular scrotal location (188), their diagnosis cannot be made with confidence preoperatively and requires surgical exploration.

CT scan and MRI also may be useful in evaluation of patients with a scrotal mass. Preoperatively, these imaging modalities can be used to evaluate tumors that extend to the internal inguinal ring. Postoperatively, they can be used for staging.

Treatment and Prognosis

As with most other urologic sarcomas, many modalities have been used to treat patients with sarcomas of the spermatic cord, testis, and paratestis. No definitive conclusion about treatment can be made from this varied experience. Nevertheless, the recommendation is that patients with a suspicious lesion of the

spermatic cord, testis, or paratestis be formally explored through an inguinal incision for an operative biopsy. Transscrotal biopsy and excision of tumor are not recommended (189). If a sarcoma is diagnosed at the time of inguinal exploration, radical orchiectomy with high ligation of the cord should be performed. One study has shown that microscopic residual disease was identified after wide repeat excision in 3 of 11 macroscopically completely excised cases (190), which may highlight the importance of local therapy with adequate resection with or without radiotherapy when the most predominant form of recurrence is local (191).

Additional therapy would depend on the histologic type of tumor. Liposarcomas are an especially favorable group in that they rarely metastasize or cause death (Fig. 54.8). The 5-year survival rate of 31 patients with liposarcoma was greater than 90%, and only a few cases of death caused by this disease have been reported in the last 10 years (192). Thus, liposarcoma of the spermatic cord may be treated only with aggressive local excision. In the patients with leiomyosarcoma, nuclear grade has reported to be predictive of prognosis (193). In patients with rhabdomyosarcomas, leiomyosarcomas, or the fibrosarcoma group, the retroperitoneal lymph nodes must be staged by CT scan. In the presence of obvious metastatically involved retroperitoneal lymph nodes, aggressive cytotoxic chemotherapy is recommended. Patients with rhabdomyosarcoma of these areas have the poorest prognosis, with a 5-year survival rate of approximately 40% (Fig. 54.8).

If the lymph nodes appear normal on CT scan, a formal retroperitoneal lymph node dissection is recommended. In this review, reports were found of 19 patients with rhabdomyosarcoma in whom retroperitoneal lymph node dissection had been performed. Of these, 11 patients (61%) had metastatic disease of the lymph nodes. Another review of 101 patients revealed 29 cases (29%) of lymph node involvement discovered after a retroperitoneal lymph node dissection, of which 17 had isolated lymphatic dissemination (194). Patients with positive lymph nodes (even microscopically) should receive aggressive doxorubicin hydrochloride–based combination chemotherapy. Because most patients with rhabdomyosarcoma of these regions are men who are under age 30, an aggressive surgical approach and adjuvant chemotherapy seem indicated, much as in the treatment of patients with germ cell testis tumors (3). One patient with paratesticular rhabdomyosarcoma received multimodal treatment on the T6 protocol (195) for metastatic retroperitoneal nodes after resection of the primary tumor and then underwent retroperitoneal lymph node dissection. He was alive at 70 months (16).

A small study has suggested that radiation therapy combined with wide surgical resection may offer longer survival than local resection alone. In this study, all recurrences occurred in the group that was treated with local resection alone (five of nine vs. zero of nine in the radiation-treated group) (156). The other study representing the largest single-instituion experience, however, has failed to demonstrate the therapeutic effect of adjuvant radiation or chemotherapy (196). Further research in this area is needed to make any definitive conclusions.

GENITOURINARY CARCINOSARCOMAS

Carcinosarcoma is a mixed malignant tumor that contains carcinomatous and sarcomatous components. It is not to be confused with sarcomatoid carcinoma, which is a tumor that consists of a carcinoma and a carcinomatous spindle cell component. Many different sarcomatous and carcinomatous components have been described (Table 54.10). The most common epithelial component in carcinosarcoma of the bladder is transitional cell carcinoma, whereas the most common epithelial component in

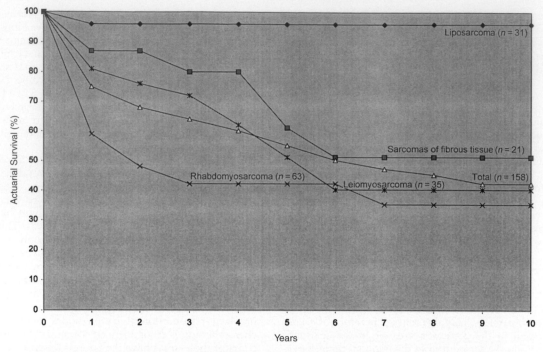

FIGURE 54.8. Actuarial survival curves for 158 patients with sarcoma of the spermatic cord, testis, and paratestis according to histologic type. The total number includes patients with miscellaneous sarcomas, whose survival curve is not shown separately (From Herr HW. Sarcoma of the urinary tract. In: deKernion JB, Paulson DF, eds. *Genitourinary cancer management*, Philadelphia, PA: Lea & Febiger, 1987: 259–270).

the prostate is adenocarcinoma. The origin of carcinosarcoma is unknown, and various interpretations have been proposed (3). Three papers have suggested that both the carcinomatous and sarcomatous elements have a common monoclonal origin by examining the alellic status of the genome (197–199).

One hundred twenty-seven cases of carcinosarcoma of the kidney, bladder, prostate, ureter, and penis have been reported in the English-language medical literature through 1998 (1,3,4,200–225) (Table 54.11). The most common site of these tumors was the urinary bladder (65.4%), followed by

TABLE 54.10

SARCOMATOUS AND EPITHELIAL COMPONENTS IN CARCINOSARCOMA OF KIDNEY, BLADDER, AND PROSTATE (70 CASES)

	Location			
Component	Kidney (11 cases)[a]	Bladder (41 cases)	Prostate (18 cases)	Total (70 cases)
Sarcomatous				
Fibrosarcoma	3 (27%)	6 (15%)	1 (6%)	10 (14%)
Malignant fibrous histiocytoma	—	1 (2%)	1 (6%)	2 (3%)
Liposarcoma	—	1 (2%)		1 (1%)
Leiomyosarcoma	—	5 (12%)	4 (22%)	9 (13%)
Rhabdomyosarcoma	3 (27%)	4 (10%)	2 (11%)	9 (13%)
Angiosarcoma	—	—	1 (6%)	1 (1%)
Osteosarcoma	5 (45%)	10 (24%)	8 (44%)	23 (33%)
Chondrosarcoma	2 (18%)	14 (34%)	12 (67%)	28 (40%)
Spindle cell sarcoma	1 (9%)	6 (15%)	—	7 (10%)
Undifferentiated sarcoma	—	4 (10%)	1 (6%)	5 (7%)
Epithelial				
Adenocarcinoma	8	7	13	—
Transitional cell carcinoma	4	23	—	—
Squamous cell carcinoma	—	9	1	—
Undifferentiated carcinoma	—	4	4	—

[a]Including four patients with carcinosarcoma of the renal pelvis.

TABLE 54.11

UROGENITAL CARCINOSARCOMA IN ADULTS

Type	Number of cases (%)
Kidney (1950–1998)	12 (9.4)
Bladder (1954–1998)	83 (65.4)
Prostate (1938–1998)	20 (15.7)
Ureter (1966–1998)	10 (7.9)
Penis (1966–1998)	2 (1.6)
Total	127

the prostate (15.7%), kidney (9.4%), ureter (7.9%), and penis (1.6%). No obvious gender predominance was observed in carcinosarcomas of the kidney, whereas carcinosarcoma of the bladder is much more common in men (occurring in 30 men vs. 12 women in one review). The age distribution for a group of 72 well-described cases of carcinosarcoma of the kidney, bladder, and prostate is shown in Figures 54.9 and 54.10. Carcinosarcomas of the kidney, bladder, and prostate were seen more commonly in elderly patients; mean age was 67 years in this review. Many patients were in the eighth decade of life.

Radiation exposure (216,218,219) and long-standing chemotherapy with cyclophosphamide (199,219,226) for the treatment of unrelated diseases have been suggested as predisposing factors for the development of carcinosarcoma of the urinary bladder. Many patients with carcinosarcoma of the prostate have a preceeding treatment history with radiation (207,227) or hormonal therapy (207,225–228) for the known diagnosis of adenocarcinoma of the prostate. A case with carcinosarcoma of the renal pelvis was associated with nephrolithiasis (229).

The diagnosis of carcinosarcoma in the anatomic sites mentioned in the preceding text is unusual, unsuspected, and normally determined by the diagnostic methods described

previously. MRI may be helpful in differential diagnosis of carcinosarcoma of the bladder from transitional cell carcinoma: carcinosarcoma shows heterogenous signal intensity on T2-weighted and contrast-enhanced MR imaging (230). In prostate carcinosarcomas, in general, the serum prostatic acid phosphatase (PAP) and prostate-specific antigen (PSA) levels are normal or slightly elevated. Of 11 cases with a mention of serum levels of PAP or PSA or both, 10 cases (91%) showed normal levels.

Many different initial treatment regimens have been used, but so few cases have been seen that no definite recommendations can be drawn. Because the prognosis for patients with carcinosarcoma of the kidney, bladder, and prostate is so poor (Fig. 54.11), an aggressive treatment regimen, modified in keeping with the chronologic and physiologic age of the patient, is recommended.

Patients with renal carcinosarcoma should be treated with radical nephrectomy and adjuvant chemotherapy. Patients with carcinosarcoma of the bladder and prostate without evidence of metastatic disease should be treated with radical cystoprostatectomy and bilateral pelvic lymphadenectomy. In general, endocrine therapy for prostate carcinosarcoma is not effective. The exact role of preoperative radiotherapy for patients with carcinosarcoma has yet to be defined. One patient was reported to have been treated with 50-Gy external-beam radiotherapy for a local recurrence of bladder carcinosarcoma after partial cystectomy and to be free of disease 8 years after initial surgical treatment (60). Patients with positive lymph nodes should receive adjuvant chemotherapy, which should be chosen according to the histologic findings of the metastatic lesion (i.e., either carcinoma or sarcoma or both).

The study by Lopez-Beltran et al. represents the largest single-institution experience with carcinosarcoma of the bladder (219): all the 15 cases were at T2b disease or more, and among 14 cases whose follow-up data were available, 11 died of carcinosarcoma at a mean of 17.2 months (219). Only a few patients with tumor showing limited invasion into the bladder wall (pT1) may survive long (218,231). Pathologic

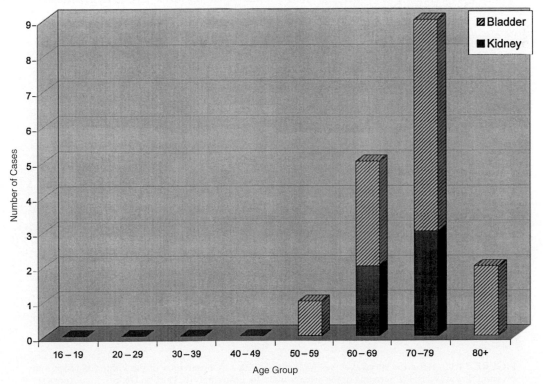

FIGURE 54.9. Age distribution of female patients with carcinosarcoma of the kidney and bladder.

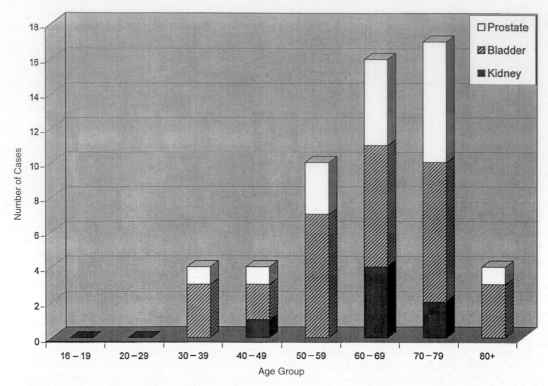

FIGURE 54.10. Age distribution of male patients with carcinosarcoma of the kidney, bladder, and prostate.

stage has been reported to be the only predictor of patient survival (218,219).

The prognosis of the prostate carcinosarcoma is also poor. In a report of the largest single-instituion experience by Dundore et al. 18 out of 21 patients died of carcinosarcoma from 2 to 107 months (mean 34 months, median 9.5 months) after diagnosis (227). According to an extensive literature review of 42 cases (232), common metastastatic sites were the lung

(43%), bone (26%), lymph nodes (19%), liver (17%), and brain (10%).

CONCLUSION

Genitourinary sarcomas in adults are so uncommon that no individual institution has much experience with these tumors.

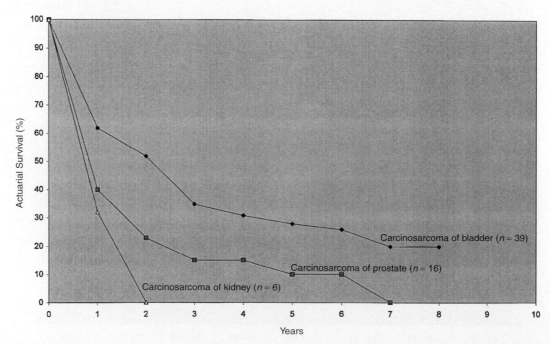

FIGURE 54.11. Actuarial survival curves for patients with carcinosarcoma of the kidney, bladder, and prostate (From Herr HW. Sarcoma of the urinary tract. In: deKernion JB, Paulson DF, eds. *Genitourinary cancer management*, Philadelphia, PA: Lea & Febiger, 1987:259–270).

Nevertheless, gathering the reported experience with these tumors in the literature allows for the formulation of some general guidelines about their natural history and treatment. Clearly, each histologic type of sarcoma in these anatomic sites has a different natural history, so the treatment of sarcoma in these organs should be modified accordingly. Without question, some histologic types are more favorable, and thus carry a better prognosis than others. Although most patients with unfavorable tumors do poorly despite aggressive therapy, in the last decade, several patients have been reported to obtain long-term survival without evidence of disease with multimodal treatment. This raises much hope and calls for more research in the area of multimodal therapy in general and chemotherapy in particular. Patients with intermediate types of tumors, such as low-grade and intermediate-grade leiomyosarcomas, deserve the best individualized approach to obtain a good chance of cure while avoiding radical exenterative surgery if anatomically feasible. Because some histologic types of sarcoma are sensitive to chemotherapeutic agents, the hope is that new active compounds will be identified and a curative chemotherapy regimen will be established.

References

1. Frank I, Takahashi S, Tsukamoto T. Genitourinary sarcomas and carcinosarcomas in adults. In: Vogelzang NJ, Scardino PT, Shipley WU et al., eds. *Comprehensive textbook of genitourinary oncology.* 2nd ed. Baltimore, MD: Williams & Wilkins, 2000:1102–1119.
2. Herr HW. Sarcoma of the urinary tract. In: deKernion JB, Paulson DF, eds. *Genitourinary cancer management,* Philadelphia, PA: Lea & Febiger, 1987: 259–270.
3. Tsukamoto T, Lieber MM. Sarcomas of the kidney, urinary bladder, prostate, spermatic cord, paratestis, and testis in adults. In: Raaf JH. ed. *Soft tissue sarcomas. Diagnosis and treatment.* St. Louis, MO: Mosby, 1993;201–226.
4. Herman C, Morales P. Leiomyosarcoma of renal vein. *Urology* 1981;18: 395–398.
5. Srinivas V, Sogani PC, Hajdu SI, et al. Sarcoma of the kidney. *J Urol* 1984;132:13–16.
6. Takashi M, Murase T, Kato K, et al. Malignant fibrous histiocytoma arising from the renal capsule: report of a case. *Urol Int* 1987;42: 227–230.
7. Krech RH, Loy V, Dieckmann KP, et al. Leiomyosarcoma of the kidney. Immunohistological and ultrastructural findings with special emphasis on the growth fraction. *Br J Urol* 1989;63:132–134.
8. Martin J, Garcia M, Duran A, et al. Renal vein leiomyosarcoma: a case report and literature review. *Urol Radiol* 1989;11:25–29.
9. Geng P, Liu T, Ye Q. Adult clear cell sarcoma of the kidney: case report and review of literature. *Chin Med J* 1989;102:457–460.
10. Grignon DJ, Ayala AG, Ro JY, et al. Primary sarcoma of the kidney. A clinicopathologic and DNA flow cytometric study of 17 cases. *Cancer* 1990;65:1611–1618.
11. Mayes DC, Fechner RE, Gillenwater JY. Renal liposarcoma. *Am J Surg Pathol* 1990;14:268–273.
12. Thirumavalavan VS, Kennedy CL, Alrufaie HK. Leiomyosarcoma of kidney. *Br J Urol* 1991;68:659–660.
13. O'Malley FP, Grignon DJ, Shepherd RR, et al. Primary osteosarcoma of the kidney. *Arch Pathol Lab Med* 1991;115:1262–1265.
14. Yokose T, Fukuda H, Ogiwara A, et al. Myxoid leiomyosarcoma of the kidney accompanying ipsilateral ureteral transitional cell carcinoma. A case report with cytological, immunohistochemical and ultrastructural study. *Acta Pathol Jpn* 1991;41:694–700.
15. Taccagni G, Terreni MR, Caputo V, et al. Nondifferentiated-type small cell sarcoma of kidney in a young woman. *Ultrastruct Pathol* 1991;15:291–299.
16. Russo P, Brady MS, Conlon K, et al. Adult urological sarcoma. *J Urol* 1992;147:1032–1037.
17. Ah-chong AH, Yip AWC. Primary osteogenic sarcoma of the kidney presenting as staghorn calculus. *Br J Urol* 1993;71:223–224.
18. Oda H, Shiga J, Machinami R. Clear cell sarcoma of kidney. Two cases in adults. *Cancer* 1993;71:2286–2291.
19. Sugimura Y, Yamamoto I, Tochigi H, et al. Multimodality therapy for advanced clear cell sarcoma of the kidney in young adults. *Urol Int* 1993;51: 39–42.
20. Ochiai K, Onitsuka H, Honda H, et al. Leiomyosarcoma of the kidney: CT and MR appearance. *J Comput Assist Tomogr* 1993;17:656–658.
21. Berkmen F, Celebioglu AS. Adult genitourinary sarcomas: a report of seventeen cases and review of the literature. *J Exp Clin Cancer Res* 1997;16: 45–48.
22. Fernandez Acenero MJ, Hernandez Gomez MJ, Blanco Gonzalez J, et al. Sarcomas of the kidney. *Minerva Urol Nefrol* 1997;49:145–149.
23. Lewis DJ, Moul JW, Williams SC, et al. Perirenal liposarcoma containing extramedullary hematopoiesis associated with renal cell carcinoma. *Urology* 1994;43:106–109.
24. Chen JH, Lee SK. Renal leiomyosarcoma mimicking transitional cell carcinoma [Letter]. *AJR Am J Roentgenol* 1997;169:312–313.
25. Chow LT, Chan SK, Chow WH. Fine needle aspiration cytodiagnosis of leiomyosarcoma of the renal pelvis. A case report with immunohistochemical study. *Acta Cytol* 1994;38:759–763.
26. Villanueva RR, Nguyen-Ho P, Nguyen GK. Leiomyosarcoma of the kidney. Report of a case diagnosed by fine needle aspiration cytology and electron microscopy. *Acta Cytol* 1994;38:568–572.
27. Roy C, Pfleger D, Tuchmann C, et al. Small leiomyosarcoma of the renal capsule: CT findings. *Eur Radiol* 1998;8:224–227.
28. Buchman AL, Truong LD. Colonic metastasis from a primary renal leiomyosarcoma: an unusual cause of gastrointestinal hemorrhage. *South Med J* 1997;90:1238–1240.
29. Mordkin RM, Dahut WL, Lynch JH. Renal angiosarcoma: a rare primary genitourinary malignancy. *South Med J* 1997;90:1159–1160.
30. Hiratsuka Y, Nishimura H, Kajiwara I, et al. Renal angiosarcoma: a case report. *Int J Urol* 1997;4:90–93.
31. Tsuda N, Chowdhury PR, Hayashi T, et al. Primary renal angiosarcoma: a case report and review of the literature. *Pathol Int* 1997;47:778–783.
32. Martinez-Pineiro L, Lopez-Ferrer P, Picazo ML, et al. Primary renal angiosarcoma. Case report and review of the literature. *Scand J Urol Nephrol* 1995;29:103–108.
33. Pollok RC, Francis N, Cliff S, et al. Kaposi's sarcoma in the kidney. *Int J STD AIDS* 1995;6:289–290.
34. Mazbar SA, Schoenfeld PY, Humphryes M. Renal involvement in patient infected with HIV: experience at San Francisco General Hospital. *Kidney Int* 1990;37:1325–1332.
35. Vogelzang NJ, Fremgen AM, Guinan PD, et al. Primary renal sarcoma in adults: a natural history and management study by the American Cancer Society, Illinois Division. *Cancer* 1993;71:804–810.
36. Watson R, Kanowski P, Ades C. Primary osteogenic sarcoma of the kidney. *Aust N Z J Surg* 1995;65:622–623.
37. Leventis AK, Stathopoulos GP, Boussiotou AC, et al. Primary osteogenic sarcoma of the kidney—a case report and review of the literature. *Acta Oncol* 1997;36:775–777.
38. Weingartner K, Gerharz EW, Neumann K, et al. Primary osteosarcoma of the kidney. Case report and review of literature. *Eur Urol* 1995;28:81–84.
39. Messen S, Bonkhoff H, Bruch M, et al. Primary renal osteosarcoma. Case report and review of the literature. *Urol Int* 1995;55:158–161.
40. Kern SB, Gott L, Faulkner J II. Occurrence of primary renal angiosarcoma in brothers. *Arch Pathol Lab Med* 1995;119:75–78.
41. Srinivasan R, Nijhawan R, Dey P, et al. Fine needle aspiration cytology of clear cell sarcoma of the kidney and its distinction from Wilms' tumor [Letter]. *Acta Cytol* 1997;41:950–951.
42. Drut R, Pomar M. Cytologic characteristics of clear cell sarcoma of the kidney (CCSK) in fine needle aspiration biopsy (FNAB): a report of 4 cases. *Diagn Cytopathol* 1991;7:611–614.
43. Argani P, Faria PA, Epstein JI, et al. Primary renal synovial sarcoma: molecular and morphologic delineation of an entity previously included among embryonal sarcomas of the kidney. *Am J Surg Pathol* 2000;24:1087–1096.
44. Kim DH, Sohn JH, Lee MC, et al. Primary synovial sarcoma of the kidney. *Am J Surg Pathol* 2000;24:1097–1104.
45. Koyama S, Morimitsu Y, Morokuma F, et al. Primary synovial sarcoma of the kidney: report of a case confirmed by molecular detection of the SYT-SSX2 fusion transcripts. *Pathol Int* 2001;51:385–391.
46. Bella AJ, Winquist EW, Perlman EJ. Primary synovial sarcoma of the kidney diagnosed by molecular detection of SYT-SSX fusion transcripts. *J Urol* 2002;168:1092–1093.
47. Chen PC, Chang YH, Yen CC, et al. Primary renal synovial sarcoma with inferior vena cava and right atrium invasion. *Int J Urol* 2003;10: 657–660.
48. Park SJ, Kim HK, Kim CK, et al. A case of renal synovial sarcoma: complete remission was induced by chemotherapy with doxorubicin and ifosfamide. *Korean J Intern Med* 2004;19:62–65.
49. Jun SY, Choi J, Kang GH, et al. Synovial sarcoma of the kidney with rhabdoid features: report of three cases. *Am J Surg Pathol* 2004;28:634–637.
50. Karnes RJ, Gettman MT, Anderson PM, et al. Primitive neuroectodermal tumor (extraskeletal Ewing's sarcoma) of the kidney with vena caval tumor thrombus. *J Urol* 2000;164:772.
51. Kuroda M, Urano M, Abe M, et al. Primary primitive neuroectodermal tumor of the kidney. *Pathol Int* 2000;50:967–972.
52. Jimenez RE, Folpe AL, Lapham RL, et al. Primary Ewing's sarcoma/primitive neuroectodermal tumor of the kidney: a clinicopathologic and immunohistochemical analysis of 11 cases. *Am J Surg Pathol* 2002;26:320–327.
53. Dogra PN, Goel A, Kumar R, et al. Extraosseous Ewing's sarcoma of the kidney. *Urol Int* 2002;69:150–152.
54. Chen HT, Chen JT, Hung SW, et al. Primary renal sarcoma with inferior vena cava thrombus presenting with tumor rupture. *Zhonghua Yi Xue Za Zhi (Taipei)* 2001;64:183–186.
55. Moazzam M, Ather MH, Hussainy AS. Leiomyosarcoma presenting as a spontaneously ruptured renal tumor-case report. *BMC Urol* 2002;2:13.

56. Aksoy Y, Gursan N, Ozbey I, et al. Spontaneous rupture of a renal angiosarcoma. *Urol Int* 2002;68:60–62.
57. Moudouni SM, En-Nia I, Rioux-Leclerq N, et al. Leiomyosarcoma of the renal pelvis. *Scand J Urol Nephrol* 2001;35:425–427.
58. Gill IS, Hobart MG, Kaouk JH, et al. Leiomyosarcoma of the main renal artery treated by laparoscopic radical nephrectomy. *Urology* 2000;56:669.
59. Kaushik S, Neifeld JP. Leiomyosarcoma of the renal vein: imaging and surgical reconstruction. *AJR Am J Roentgenol* 2002;179:276–277.
60. Vogelzang NJ, Yang X, Goldman S, et al. Radiation-induced renal cell cancer: a report of four cases and review of the literature. *J Urol* 1998;160:1987–1990.
61. Ashfaq A, Haller JE, Mossey R, et al. Recurrent membranous nephropathy and leiomyosarcoma in the renal allograft of a lupus patient. *J Nephrol* 2004;17:134–138.
62. Antman K, Chang Y. Kaposi's sarcoma. *N Engl J Med* 2000;342:1027–1038.
63. Toyoda Y, Yamashita C, Sugimoto T, et al. Clear cell sarcoma of kidney with tumor extension into the right atrium. *J Cardiovasc Surg (Torino)* 1998;39:489–491.
64. Bhayani SB, Liapis H, Kibel AS. Adult clear cell sarcoma of the kidney with atrial tumor thrombus. *J Urol* 2001;165:896–897.
65. Rosso D, Ghignone GP, Bernardi D, et al. Clear cell sarcoma of the kidney with invasion of the inferior vena cava. *Urol Int* 2003;70:251–252.
66. Silverman JF, Nathan G, Olson PR, et al. Fine-needle aspiration cytology of low-grade fibromyxoid sarcoma of the renal capsule (capsuloma). *Diagn Cytopathol* 2000;23:279–283.
67. Johnson VV, Gaertner EM, Crothers BA. Fine-needle aspiration of renal angiosarcoma. *Arch Pathol Lab Med* 2002;126:478–480.
68. Vesoulis Z, Rahmeh T, Nelson R, et al. Fine needle aspiration biopsy of primary renal synovial sarcoma. A case report. *Acta Cytol* 2003;47:668–672.
69. Lacquaniti S, Destito A, Candidi MO, et al. Two atypical cases of renal leiomyosarcoma: clinical picture, diagnosis and therapy. *Arch Ital Urol Androl* 1998;70:199–201.
70. Maki RG. Role of chemotherapy in patients with soft tissue sarcomas. *Expert Rev Anticancer Ther* 2004;4:229–236.
71. Fanucchi M. Update on the management of connective tissue malignancies. *Semin Oncol* 2004;31:16–19.
72. Deyrup AT, Montgomery E, Fisher C. Leiomyosarcoma of the kidney: a clinicopathologic study. *Am J Surg Pathol* 2004;28:178–182.
73. Jemal A, Tiwari RC, Murray T, et al. Cancer Statistics, 2004. *CA Cancer J Clin* 2004;54:8–29.
74. Seo IS, Clark SA, McGovern FD, et al. Leiomyosarcoma of the urinary bladder, 13 years after cyclophosphamide therapy for Hodgkin's disease. *Cancer* 1985;55:1597–1603.
75. Kanno J, Sakamoto A, Washizuka M, et al. Malignant mixed mesodermal tumor of bladder occurring after radiotherapy for cervical cancer: report of a case. *J Urol* 1985;133:854–856.
76. Berenson RJ, Flynn S, Freiha FS, et al. Primary osteogenic sarcoma of the bladder. *Cancer* 1986;57:350–355.
77. Taylor RE, Busuttil A. Case report: adult rhabdomyosarcoma of bladder, complete response to radiation therapy. *J Urol* 1989;142:1321–1322.
78. Kerr KM, Grigor KM, Tolley DA. Rhabdomyosarcoma of the adult urinary bladder after radiotherapy for carcinoma. *Clin Oncol* 1989;1:115–116.
79. Thrasher JB, Miller GJ, Wettlaufer JN. Bladder leiomyosarcoma following cyclophosphamide therapy for lupus nephritis. *J Urol* 1990;143:119–121.
80. Oesterling JE, Epstein JI, Brendler CB. Malignant fibrous histiocytoma of the bladder. *Cancer* 1990;66:1836–1842.
81. Özteke O, Demirel A, Aydin NE, et al. Bladder leiomyosarcoma: report of three cases. *Int Urol Nephrol* 1992;24:393–396.
82. Kawamura J, Sakurai M, Tsukamoto K, et al. Leiomyosarcoma of the bladder eighteen years after cyclophosphamide therapy for retinoblastoma. *Urol Int* 1993;51:49–53.
83. Aydoganli L, Tarhan F, Atan A, et al. Rhabdomyosarcoma of the urinary bladder in an adult. *Int Urol Nephrol* 1993;25:159–161.
84. Pedersen-Bjergaard J, Jonsson V, Pedersen M, et al. Leiomyosarcoma of the urinary bladder after cyclophosphamide [Letter]. *J Clin Oncol* 1995;13:532–533.
85. Lei KI, Gwi E, Ma L, et al. "Spontaneous" regression of advanced leiomyosarcoma of the urinary bladder. *Oncology* 1997;54:19–22.
86. De Berardinis E, Giulianelli R, Zarrelli G, et al. Leiomyosarcoma of urinary bladder: personal experience in 3 cases over a 10-year period. *Arch Ital Urol Androl* 1997;69(Suppl. 1):73–80.
87. Lauro S, Lalle M, Scucchi L, et al. Rhabdomyosarcoma of the urinary bladder in an elderly patient. *Anticancer Res* 1995;15:627–629.
88. Abbas AM, Katz DS, Sommer FG. CT findings of primary osteosarcoma of the bladder [Letter]. *AJR Am J Roentgenol* 1996;167:535–536.
89. Okada E, Hasegawa Y, Takahashi K, et al. Primary osteosarcoma of the urinary bladder. *Int Urol Nephrol* 1997;29:437–440.
90. Phan CN, Wilkinson M, Cohen MB, et al. Primary osteogenic sarcoma of the urinary bladder successfully treated with combination therapy. *Urology* 1994;44:771–774.
91. Tzakas E, Ioannidis S, Dimitriadis G, et al. Primary osteochondrosarcoma of the urinary bladder. *Br J Urol* 1994;73:320–321.
92. Kingsley KL, Peier AM, Meloni-Ehrig AM, et al. Cytogenetic findings in a bladder chondrosarcoma. *Cancer Genet Cytogenet* 1997;96:183–184.
93. Reid I, Suvarna SK, Wagner BE, et al. Plexosarcoma of the bladder. *Eur J Surg Oncol* 1997;23:463–465.
94. Navon JD, Rahimzadeh M, Wong AK, et al. Angiosarcoma of the bladder after therapeutic irradiation for prostate cancer. *J Urol* 1997;157:1359–1360.
95. Kato T, Kubota Y, Saitou M, et al. Osteosarcoma of the bladder successfully treated with partial cystectomy. *J Urol* 2000;163:548–549.
96. Ghalayini IF, Bani-Hani IH, Almasri NM. Osteosarcoma of the urinary bladder occurring simultaneously with prostate and bowel carcinomas: report of a case and review of the literature. *Arch Pathol Lab Med* 2001;125:793–795.
97. Engel JD, Kuzel TM, Moceanu MC, et al. Angiosarcoma of the bladder: a review. *Urology* 1998;52:778–784.
98. Schindler S, De Frias DV, Yu GH. Primary angiosarcoma of the bladder: cytomorphology and differential diagnosis. *Cytopathology* 1999;10:137–143.
99. Hama Y, Okizuka H, Kusano S. Pleomorphic sarcoma of the adult urinary bladder: sonographic findings. *J Clin Ultrasound* 2004;32:215–217.
100. Aki H, Baslar Z, Uygun N, et al. Primary granulocytic sarcoma of the urinary bladder: case report and review of the literature. *Urology* 2002;60:345.
101. Hasegeli Uner A, Altundag K, Saglam A, et al. Granulocytic sarcoma of the urinary bladder. *Am J Hematol* 2004;75:262–263.
102. Rowland RG, Eble JN. Bladder leiomyosarcoma and pelvic fibroblastic tumor following cyclophosphamide therapy. *J Urol* 1983;130:344–346.
103. Motta L, Porcaro AB, Ficarra V, et al. Leiomyosarcoma of the bladder fourteen years after cyclophosphamide therapy for retinoblastoma. *Scand J Urol Nephrol* 2001;35:248–249.
104. Parekh DJ, Jung C, O'Conner J, et al. Leiomyosarcoma in urinary bladder after cyclophosphamide therapy for retinoblastoma and review of bladder sarcomas. *Urology* 2002;60:164.
105. Tanguay C, Harvey I, Houde M, et al. Leiomyosarcoma of urinary bladder following cyclophosphamide therapy: report of two cases. *Mod Pathol* 2003;16:512–514.
106. Ferrie BG, Imrie JEA, Peterson PJ. Osteosarcoma of bladder 27 years after local radiotherapy. *J R Soc Med* 1984;77:962–963.
107. Morgan MA, Moutos DM, Pippitt CH, et al. Vaginal and bladder angiosarcoma after therapeutic irradiation. *South Med J* 1989;82:1434.
108. El Boulkainy MN, Ghoneim MA, Mansour MA. Carcinoma of the bilharzial bladder in Egypt. *Br J Urol* 1972;44:561–570.
109. Liang SX, Lakshmanan Y, Woda BA, et al. A high-grade primary leiomyosarcoma of the bladder in a survivor of retinoblastoma. *Arch Pathol Lab Med* 2001;125:1231–1234.
110. Venkatraman L, Goepel JR, Steele K, et al. Soft tissue, pelvic, and urinary bladder leiomyosarcoma as second neoplasm following hereditary retinoblastoma. *J Clin Pathol* 2003;56:233–236.
111. Rosser CJ, Slaton JW, Izawa JI, et al. Clinical presentation and outcome of high-grade urinary bladder leiomyosarcoma in adults. *Urology* 2003;61:1151–1155.
112. Dallorso S, Manzitti C, Morreale G, et al. High dose therapy and autologous hematopoietic stem cell transplantation in poor risk solid tumors of childhood. *Haematologica* 2000;85:66–70.
113. Froehner M, Lossnitzer A, Manseck A, et al. Favorable long-term outcome in adult genitourinary low-grade sarcoma. *Urology* 2000;56:373–377.
114. Baker ME, Silverman PM, Korobkin M. Computed tomography of prostatic and bladder rhabdomyosarcomas. *J Comput Assist Tomogr* 1985;9:780–783.
115. Yao JC, Wang WCC, Tseng HH, et al. Primary rhabdomyosarcoma of the prostate: diagnosis by needle biopsy and immunocytochemistry. *Acta Cytol* 1988;32:509–512.
116. Scully JM, Uno JM, McIntyre M, et al. Radiation-induced prostatic sarcoma: a case report. *J Urol* 1990;144:746–748.
117. Yum M, Miller JC, Agarwal BL. Leiomyosarcoma arising in atypical fibromuscular hyperplasia (phyllodes tumor) of the prostate with distant metastasis. *Cancer* 1991;68:910–915.
118. Bos SD, Slaa ET. An adult man with a rhabdomyosarcoma of the prostate: a case report. *Scand J Urol Nephrol* 1991;25:329–330.
119. Waring PM, Newland RC. Prostatic embryonal rhabdomyosarcoma in adults. *Cancer* 1992;69:755–762.
120. Russo P, Demas B, Reuter V. Adult prostatic sarcoma. *Abdom Imaging* 1993;18:399–401.
121. Palmer MA, Viswanath S, Desmond D. Adult prostatic rhabdomyosarcoma. *Br J Urol* 1993;71:489–490.
122. Cheville JC, Dundore PA, Nascimento AG, et al. Leiomyosarcoma of the prostate. Report of 23 cases. *Cancer* 1995;76:1422–1427.
123. Germiyanoglu C, Ozkardes H, Kurt U, et al. Leiomyosarcoma of the prostate. A case report. *Int Urol Nephrol* 1994;26:189–191.
124. Terris MK, Eigner EB, Briggs EM, et al. Transrectal ultrasound in the evaluation of rhabdomyosarcoma involving the prostate. *Br J Urol* 1994;74:341–344.
125. Lazar EB, Whitman GJ, Chew FS. Embryonal rhabdomyosarcoma of the prostate. *AJR Am J Roentgenol* 1996;166:72.
126. Moroz K, Crespo P, de las Morenas A. Fine needle aspiration of prostatic rhabdomyosarcoma. A case report demonstrating the value of DNA ploidy. *Acta Cytol* 1995;39:785–790.
127. Beyzadeoglu M, Balkan M, Ozgok Y, et al. Prostate rhabdomyosarcoma in a young adult: a case study. *Radiat Med* 1997;15:199–201.
128. Berkmen F, Celebioglu AS. Adult genitourinary sarcomas: a report of seventeen cases and review of the literature. *J Exp Clin Cancer Res* 1997;16:45–48.

129. Atherton PJ, Stockdale AD, Rennie CD. Sarcoma of the prostate treated with radiotherapy. *Clin Oncol (R Coll Radiol)* 1994;6:269–270.

130. Nghiem HV, Sommer FG, Moretto JC. MRI of radiation-induced prostate sarcoma. *Clin Imaging* 1995;19:54–56.

131. Cacic M, Petrovic D, Tentor D, et al. Cystosarcoma phyllodes of the prostate. *Scand J Urol Nephrol* 1996;30:501–502.

132. Cox R, Dawson IMP. A curious prostatic tumor: probably a true mixed tumor (cystadeno-leiomyofibroma). *Br J Urol* 1960;32:306.

133. Reese JH, Lombard CM, Krone K, et al. Phyllodes type of atypical prostatic hyperplasia: a report of 3 new cases. *J Urol* 1987;138:623–626.

134. Dogra PN, Aron M, Rajeev TP, et al. Primary chondrosarcoma of the prostate. *BJU Int* 1999;83:150–151.

135. Iwasaki H, Ishiguro M, Ohjimi Y, et al. Synovial sarcoma of the prostate with t(X;18)(p11.2;q11.2). *Am J Surg Pathol* 1999;23:220–226.

136. Williams DH, Hua VN, Chowdhry AA, et al. Synovial sarcoma of the prostate. *J Urol* 2004;171:2376.

137. Terris MK. Transrectal ultrasound appearance of radiation-induced prostatic sarcoma. *Prostate* 1998;37:182–186.

138. Nishiyama T, Ikarashi T, Terunuma M, et al. Osteogenic sarcoma of the prostate. *Int J Urol* 2001;8:199–201.

139. Chandan VS, Wolsh L. Postirradiation angiosarcoma of the prostate. *Arch Pathol Lab Med* 2003;127:876–878.

140. Olson EM, Trambert MA, Mattrey RF. Cystosarcoma phyllodes of the prostate: MRI findings. *Abdom Imaging* 1994;19:180–181.

141. Kim HS, Lee JH, Nam JH, et al. Malignant phyllodes tumor of the prostate. *Pathol Int* 1999;49:1105–1108.

142. Yamamoto S, Ito T, Miki M, et al. Malignant phyllodes tumor of the prostate. *Int J Urol* 2000;7:378–381.

143. Lam KC, Yeo W. Chemotherapy induced complete remission in malignant phyllodes tumor of the prostate metastasizing to the lung. *J Urol* 2002;168:1104–1105.

144. Agrawal V, Sharma D, Wadhwa N. Malignant phyllodes tumor of prostate. *Int Urol Nephrol* 2003;35:37–39.

145. Terris MK, Eigner EB, Briggs EM, et al. Transrectal ultrasound in the evaluation of rhabdomyosarcoma involving the prostate. *Br J Urol* 1994;74:341–344.

146. Sexton WJ, Lance RE, Reyes AO, et al. Adult prostate sarcoma: the M. D. Anderson Cancer Center Experience. *J Urol* 2001;166:521–525.

147. Zukerberg LR, Young RH. Primary testicular sarcoma: a report of two cases. *Hum Pathol* 1990;21:932–935.

148. Palma PD, Barbazza R. Well-differentiated liposarcoma of the paratesticular area: report of a case with fine-needle aspiration preoperative diagnosis and review of the literature. *Diagn Cytopathol* 1990;6:421–426.

149. Sønksen J, Hansen EF, Colstrup H. Liposarcoma of the spermatic cord. *Scand J Urol Nephrol* 1991;25:239–240.

150. Hellstöm PA, Mäkäräinen H, Tammela TLJ, et al. Spermatic cord liposarcoma: ultrasound for diagnosis and follow-up. *Scand J Urol Nephrol* 1991;25:321–324.

151. Maguire BM, Lewis SB, Cooke SL. Malignant fibrous histiocytoma: review and case report. *Aust N Z J Surg* 1991;61:636–639.

152. Heyn BR, Raney RB, Hays DM, et al. Late effects of therapy in patients with paratesticular rhabdomyosarcoma. *J Clin Oncol* 1992;10:614–623.

153. Ciancio G, Civantos F, Block NL. Malignant fibrous histiocytoma of spermatic cord. *Urology* 1993;41:55–58.

154. Gore RL, Auber AE. Ultrasonographic appearance of malignant fibrous histiocytoma of the spermatic cord: a case report. *Mil Med* 1993;158:631–633.

155. Soosay GN, Parkinson MC, Paradinas J, et al. Paratesticular sarcomas revisited: a review of cases in the British Testicular Tumour Panel and Registry. *Br J Urol* 1996;77:143–146.

156. Fagundes MA, Zietman AL, Althausen AF, et al. The management of spermatic cord sarcoma. *Cancer* 1996;77:1873–1876.

157. Bulbul MA, Saker G, Salem-Shabb N, et al. Liposarcoma of the spermatic cord. *Scand J Urol Nephrol* 1996;30:333–335.

158. Rao CR, Srinivasulu M, Naresh KN, et al. Adult paratesticular sarcomas: a report of eight cases. *J Surg Oncol* 1994;56:89–93.

159. Anjum MI, Eccersley J, Bhat A, et al. Liposarcoma of the spermatic cord: a report of two cases. *Int Urol Nephrol* 1997;29:227–232.

160. Bauer JJ, Sesterhenn IA, Costabile RA. Myxoid liposarcoma of the scrotal wall. *J Urol* 1995;153:1938–1939.

161. Schwartz SL, Swierzewski SJ III, Sondak VK, et al. Liposarcoma of the spermatic cord: report of 6 cases and review of the literature. *J Urol* 1995;153:154–157.

162. Soosay GN, Parkinson MC, Paradinas J, et al. Paratesticular sarcomas revisited: a review of cases in the British Testicular Tumour Panel and Registry. *Br J Urol* 1996;77:143–146.

163. Berkmen F, Celebioglu AS. Adult genitourinary sarcomas: a report of seventeen cases and review of the literature. *J Exp Clin Cancer Res* 1997;16:45–48.

164. Kitamura K, Kiyomatsu K, Nonaka M, et al. Liposarcoma developing in the paratesticular region: report of a case. *Surg Today* 1996;26:842–845.

165. Katsuno S, Hibi H, Takashi M, et al. Two cases of intrascrotal liposarcoma. *Hinyokika Kiyo* 1996;42:751–754.

166. Yol S, Tavli S, Tavli L, et al. Retroperitoneal and scrotal giant liposarcoma: report of a case. *Surg Today* 1998;28:339–342.

167. Ikinger U, Westrich M, Pietz B, et al. Combined myxoid liposarcoma and angiolipoma of the spermatic cord. *Urology* 1997;49:635–637.

168. Dalla Palma P, Barbazza R. Well-differentiated liposarcoma of the paratesticular area: report of a case with fine needle aspiration preoperative diagnosis and review of the literature. *Diagn Cytopathol* 1990;6:421.

169. Lehmann K, Stock U, Musy JP, et al. Primary paratesticular liposarcoma. *Urol Int* 1993;51:54.

170. Lipset RE, Kirpekar M, Cooke KS, et al. US case of the day. Myxoid liposarcoma of the spermatic cord. *Radiographics* 1997;17:1316–1318.

171. Washecka RM, Mariani AJ, Zuna RE, et al. Primary intratesticular sarcoma. Immunohistochemical ultrastructural and DNA flow cytometric study of three cases with a review of the literature. *Cancer* 1996;77:1524–1528.

172. Koh KB, Joyce A, Boon AP. Leiomyosarcoma of the scrotum. *Br J Urol* 1994;73:717–718.

173. Konety BR, Singh J, Lyne JC, et al. Leiomyosarcoma with osteoclast-like giant cells of the spermatic cord. A case report and review of the literature. *Urol Int* 1996;56:259–262.

174. Jeddy TA, Vowles RH, Southam JA. Leiomyosarcoma of the dartos muscle. *Br J Urol* 1994;74:129–130.

175. Bhushan B, Mohan V, Salker DM. Ultrasound diagnosis of para-testicular neoplasm. *J Clin Ultrasound* 1996;24:375–377.

176. Ofiaeli RO, Mbonu OO. Recurrent paratesticular rhabdomyosarcoma reported from Nigeria. *Trop Doct* 1997;27:171–172.

177. Banfield GK, Brookstein R. Rhabdomyosarcoma arising in teratoma of the testis. *J R Army Med Corps* 1995;141:167–168.

178. Beiswanger JC, Woodruff RD, Savage PD, et al. Primary osteosarcoma of the spermatic cord with synchronous bilateral renal cell carcinoma. *Urology* 1997;49:957–959.

179. Chan JA, McMenamin ME, Fletcher CD. Synovial sarcoma in older patients: clinicopathological analysis of 32 cases with emphasis on unusual histological features. *Histopathology* 2003;43:72–83.

180. Miyoshi I, Saito T, Taguchi H, et al. Granulocytic sarcoma of the testis. *Br J Haematol* 2004;124:695.

181. Eggener SE, Abrahams A, Keeler TC. Granulocytic sarcoma of the testis. *Urology* 2004;63:584–585.

182. Motzer RJ, Amsterdam A, Prieto V, et al. Teratoma with malignant transformation: diverse malignant histologies arising in men with germ cell tumors. *J Urol* 1998;159:133–138.

183. Ulbright TM, Loehrer PJ, Roth LM, et al. The development of non-germ malignancies within germ cell tumors. *Cancer* 1984;54:1824–1833.

184. Banfield GK, Brookstein R. Rhabdomyosarcoma arising in teratoma of the testis. *J R Army Med Corps* 1995;141:167–168.

185. Yachia D, Auslander L. Primary leiomyosarcoma of the testis. *J Urol* 1989;141:955–956.

186. Frates MC, Benson CB, Disalvo DN, et al. Sonographically solid extratesticular masses: not necessarily benign. *J Ultrasound Med* 1997;16(Suppl.):S19 abst.

187. Akbar SA, Sayyed TA, Jafri SZ, et al. Multimodality imaging of paratesticular neoplasms and their rare mimics. *Radiographics* 2003;23:1461–1476.

188. Mostofi FK, Price EB. *Campbell's urology*, 5th ed. Philadelphia, PA: WB Saunders, 1986:1609.

189. Dall'Igna P, Bisogno G, Ferrari A, et al. Primary transcrotal excision for paratesticular rhabdomyosarcoma: is hemiscrotectomy really mandatory? *Cancer* 2003;97:1981–1984.

190. Catton C, Jewett M, O'Sullivan B, et al. Paratesticular sarcoma: failure patterns after definitive local therapy. *J Urol* 1999;161:1844–1847.

191. Ballo MT, Zagars GK, Pisters PW, et al. Spermatic cord sarcoma: outcome, patterns of failure and management. *J Urol* 2001;166:1306–1310.

192. Montgomery E, Fisher C. Paratesticular liposarcoma: a clinicopathologic study. *Am J Surg Pathol* 2003;27:40–47.

193. Fisher C, Goldblum JR, Epstein JI, et al. Leiomyosarcoma of the paratesticular region: a clinicopathologic study. *Am J Surg Pathol* 2001;25:1143–1149.

194. Banowsky LH, Schultz GN. Sarcoma of the spermatic cord and tunics: review of literature, case report and discussion of the role of retroperitoneal lymph node dissection. *J Urol* 1970;103:628.

195. Ghavimi F, Exelby PR, Jereb B, et al. Multidisciplinary treatment of advanced stages of embryonal rhabdomyosarcoma in children. *Natl Cancer Inst Monogr* 1981;56:103–109.

196. Coleman J, Brennan MF, Alektiar K, et al. Adult spermatic cord sarcomas: management and results. *Ann Surg Oncol* 2003;10:669–675.

197. Halachmi S, Farhat W, Metcalfe P, et al. Efficacy of polydimethylsiloxane injection to the bladder neck and leaking diverting stoma for urinary continence. *J Urol* 2004;171:1287–1290.

198. Gronau S, Menz CK, Melzner I, et al. Immunohistomorphologic and molecular cytogenetic analysis of a carcinosarcoma of the urinary bladder. *Virchows Arch* 2002;440:436–440.

199. Mukhopadhyay S, Shrimpton AE, Jones LA, et al. Carcinosarcoma of the urinary bladder following cyclophosphamide therapy: evidence for monoclonal origin and chromosome 9p allelic loss. *Arch Pathol Lab Med* 2004;128:e8–11.

200. Zenklusen HR, Weymuth G, Rist M, et al. Carcinosarcoma of the prostate in combination with adenocarcinoma of the prostate and adenocarcinoma of the seminal vesicles. *Cancer* 1990;66:998–1001.

201. Bloxham CA, Bennett MK, Robinson MC. Bladder carcinomas: three cases with diverse histogenesis. *Histopathology* 1990;16:63–67.

202. Nazeer T, Barada JH, Fisher HA, et al. Prostatic carcinosarcoma: case report and review of literature. *J Urol* 1991;146:1370–1373.
203. Kaneko Y, Yoshiki T, Fukumoto M, et al. Carcinosarcoma of the prostate. *Urol Int* 1992;48:105–107.
204. Lindboe CF, Mjønes J. Carcinosarcoma of prostate: immunohistochemical and ultrastructural observations. *Urology* 1992;40:376–380.
205. Mazzucchelli L, Kraft R, Gerber H, et al. Carcinosarcoma of the urinary bladder: a distinct variant characterized by small cell undifferentiated carcinoma with neuroendocrine features. *Virchows Arch A Pathol Anat Histopathol* 1992;421:477–483.
206. Orsatti G, Corgan FJ, Goldberg SA. Carcinosarcoma of urothelial organs: bladder, ureter, and renal pelvis. *Urology* 1993;41:289–291.
207. Lauwer GY, Schevchuk M, Armenakas N, et al. Carcinosarcoma of the prostate. *Am J Surg Pathol* 1993;17:342–349.
208. Kubosawa H, Matsuzaki O, Kondo Y, et al. Carcinosarcoma of the prostate. *Acta Pathol Jpn* 1993;43:209–214.
209. Nagayoshi J, Kawakami T, Maruyama Y. Sarcomatoid carcinoma of the ureter: a case report. *Int J Urol* 1997;4:618–620.
210. Burt JD, Murphy D, Heffernan EB. Carcinoma of the ureter presenting as biliary colic. *Aust N Z J Surg* 1995;65:63–64.
211. Ishikura H, Kumagai F, Yoshiki T. Carcinosarcoma of the ureter with unusual histologic features. *Jpn J Clin Oncol* 1994;24:175–180.
212. Tsutsumi M, Kamiya M, Skamoto M, et al. A ureteral small cell carcinoma mixed with malignant mesodermal and ectodermal elements: a clinopathological, morphological, and immunohistochemical study. *Jpn J Clin Oncol* 1993;23:325–329.
213. Orsatti G, Corgan FJ, Goldberg SA. Carcinosarcoma of urothelial organ: sequential involvement of urinary bladder, ureter, and renal pelvis. *Urology* 1993;41:289–291.
214. Xu YM, Cai RX, Wu P, et al. Urethral carcinosarcoma following total cystectomy for bladder carcinoma. *Urol Int* 1993;50:104–107.
215. Nuwahid F, German K, Campbell F, et al. Carcinosarcoma in a bladder diverticulum. *Urology* 1994;44:775–778.
216. Lahoti C, Schinella R, Rangwala AF, et al. Carcinosarcoma of urinary bladder: report of 5 cases with immunohistologic study. *Urology* 1994;43:389–393.
217. Crisan D, Olinici CD, Coman I. Carcinosarcoma (malignant mesodermal mixed tumor) of urinary bladder. *Rom J Morphol Embryol* 1997;43(1–2):69–73.
218. Perret L, Chaubert P, Hessler D, et al. Primary heterologous carcinosarcoma (metaplastic carcinoma) of the urinary bladder: a clinicopathlogic, immunohistochemical, and ultrastructural analysis of eight cases and a review of the literature. *Cancer* 1998;82:1535–1549.
219. Lopez-Beltran A, Pacelli A, Rothenberg HJ, et al. Carcinosarcoma and sarcomatoid carcinoma of the bladder: clinicopathological study of 41 cases. *J Urol* 1998;159:1497–1503.
220. Kamishima T, Fukuda T, Usuda H, et al. Carcinosarcoma of the urinary bladder: expression of epithelial markers and different expression on heat shock proteins between epithelial and sarcomatous elements. *Pathol Int* 1997;47(2–3):166–173.
221. Gedikoglu G, Sokmensuer C, Soylemezoglu F, et al. Carcinosarcoma of the urinary bladder. *Int Urol Nephrol* 1996;28:333–336.
222. Swaminathan I, Yang TL, Ong BH. Carcinosarcoma of the urinary bladder—case report and literature review. *Ann Acad Med Singapore* 1995;24:640–643.
223. Sakkas G, Kastriotis I, Karagiannis A, et al. Carcinosarcoma of the bladder. *Int Urol Nephrol* 1995;27:57–60.
224. Carter C, Lesna M, Rundle J. Carcinosarcoma of the penis. *J Pathol* 1995;175(Suppl.):132A; (meeting abst).
225. Sak SD, Orhan D, Yaman O, et al. Carcinosarcoma of the prostate. A case report and a possible evidence on the role of hormonal therapy. *Urol Int* 1997;59:50–52.
226. Sigal SH, Tomaszewski JE, Brooks JJ, et al. Carcinosarcoma of bladder following long-term cyclophosphamide therapy. *Arch Pathol Lab Med* 1991;115:1049–1051.
227. Dundore PA, Cheville JC, Nascimento AG, et al. Carcinosarcoma of the prostate. Report of 21 cases. *Cancer* 1995;76:1035–1042.
228. Poblet E, Gomez-Tierno A, Alfaro L. Prostatic carcinosarcoma: a case originating in a previous ductal adenocarcinoma of the prostate. *Pathol Res Pract* 2000;196:569–572.
229. Kayaselcuk F, Bal N, Guvel S, et al. Carcinosarcoma and squamous cell carcinoma of the renal pelvis associated with nephrolithiasis: a case report of each tumor type. *Pathol Res Pract* 2003;199:489–492.
230. Tekes A, Kamel IR, Szarf G, et al. Carcinosarcoma of the urinary bladder: dynamic contrast-enhanced MR imaging with clinical and pathologic correlation. *AJR Am J Roentgenol* 2003;181:139–142.
231. Baschinsky DY, Chen JH, Vadmal MS, et al. Carcinosarcoma of the urinary bladder—an aggressive tumor with diverse histogenesis. A clinicopathologic study of 4 cases and review of the literature. *Arch Pathol Lab Med* 2000;124:1172–1178.
232. Fukawa T, Numata K, Yamanaka M, et al. Prostatic carcinosarcoma: a case report and review of literature. *Int J Urol* 2003;10:108–113.

CHAPTER 55 ■ MALIGNANT LYMPHOMA OF THE GENITOURINARY TRACT

ANN S. LACASCE, M. DROR MICHAELSON, AND GEORGE P. CANELLOS

INTRODUCTION

Non-Hodgkin lymphoma (NHL) comprises 5% of all malignancies and represents the fifth most common cancer in the United States. The annual incidence rate is approximately 56,200 cases per year. NHL may involve any extranodal organ. Although it may disseminate to the genitourinary tract from other systemic sites, NHL usually involves primarily the testicle. In 1877, the first case of lymphoma involving the testes was described by Malassez. Autopsy series have demonstrated a higher rate of secondary involvement of the urogenital tract ranging from approximately 20% to 30%, particularly in high-grade lymphomas, such as Burkitt lymphoma (1–3).

TESTICULAR NON-HODGKIN LYMPHOMA

Epidemiology

Primary testicular lymphoma is a rare entity, representing 1% to 2% of all cases of lymphoma and 1% to 7% of all testicular neoplasms. The overall rate of testicular neoplasms is estimated at 3.7 per 100,000 (4), whereas testicular lymphoma is estimated at 0.0015 per 100,000 men (5). It is a disease of older men, with 85% of cases presenting in men older than 60 years (4,6–8). In men older than 50 years, it represents the most common testicular neoplasm (4,6–8). Predisposing factors including undescended testicles, trauma, or infection, are unclear (5), but a higher incidence has been noted in men who are HIV-positive (9–12).

Pathology

Nearly all cases of lymphoma involving the testis are NHL, although rare cases of Hodgkin lymphoma have been reported in the literature (4). More than 80% of all cases of lymphoma of the testis are classified as diffuse large B-cell lymphoma (DLBCL) (6,7,13,14). Burkitt and Burkitt-like lymphoma rarely have been reported to present with testicular involvement (2,3). Low-grade histologies, including follicular and follicular mixed lymphoma, are very infrequent (14). Several cases of Epstein-Barr virus (EBV) positive CD56+ natural killer (NK) cell lymphoma, which histologically resembles the nasal/nasal-type disease, have been reported to involve the testis in Asian men (15).

Molecular studies on a series of 20 primary testicular lymphoma specimens failed to demonstrate either EBV or human herpes virus 8 (16). Translocations typical for follicular lymphoma t (14,17) and mantle cell lymphoma t (11,14) were not identified in any specimens. Rearrangement of V-D-J heavy chain compared with germline suggested extensive somatic hypermutation in tumor samples, raising the possibility of antigenic stimulation in the pathogenesis of the disease. Another study in nine specimens confirmed the absence of t (14,17) translocation despite the presence of bcl-2 protein in all of the samples (18).

Presentation

Lymphoma of the testis commonly presents as a painless, unilateral testicular mass. Bilateral involvement has been reported in up to 35% of cases (6,7). Pain is unusual and more suggestive of infection. Approximately 25% of patients present with systemic symptoms, such as weight loss, fevers, and night sweats, which correlate with disease that is more extensive. Central nervous system (CNS) involvement at presentation occurs in approximately 10% of patients. Other rare sites of involvement at presentation include Waldeyer ring, skin, and pulmonary disease (7).

The diagnostic procedure of choice is radical inguinal orchiectomy. Trans scrotal needle aspirates may obtain insufficient tissue for diagnosis. The concern for tumor seeding is also a consideration, especially when the differential can include germ cell tumors (17).

Staging

Staging work-up is similar to NHL involving other nodal or other extranodal groups. Physical examination should include careful examination of Waldeyer ring, skin, and the CNS (5). Routine staging for NHL should include computed tomography (CT) scans of the chest, abdomen, and pelvis and a bone marrow biopsy, and possibly an ultrasound of the contralateral testis. Gallium 67-citrate or 2-[^{18}F]-fluoro-2-deoxy-D-glucose/positron emission tomography (FDG-PET) scanning may provide useful prognostic information both with early restaging and following the completion of therapy (19). Laboratory studies should include complete blood count, chemistries, and a serum lactate dehydrogenase (LDH) level.

Most men present with "early stage" disease as defined by the Ann Arbor staging classification, with 80% having stage IE or IIE disease; the remaining 20% present in stages III and IV. Patients with stage IV disease typically have bone, skin, or CNS involvement at presentation (8).

Treatment

Although patients with primary testicular lymphoma present in an apparently localized, extranodal stage, the median survival is significantly worse than predicted by the International Prognostic Index (IPI) (20). Early series of patients treated with orchiectomy, even those patients with stage IE disease, showed disappointing results, with the disease relapsing in most patients (up to 90%) within 2 years of orchiectomy. Major sites of relapse included the contralateral testicle, the regional lymph nodes, and the CNS (4,7).

The addition of radiotherapy to retroperitoneal lymph nodes after orchiectomy has also yielded disappointing results, with approximately 70% of patients relapsing, typically outside the radiation field, although some patients who received less than 35 Gy did experience local relapse (7,21–23).

Most retrospective studies of combination chemotherapy in testicular lymphoma have also yielded disappointing results (24). In the M.D. Anderson series of 22 patients with large-cell testicular lymphoma, all received doxorubicin-based therapy, and 5 also received radiotherapy. Complete remission was attained in 73% of patients. At 153 months, failure-free survival was only 16% for all patients. The IPI score was not predictive of outcome, with only 32% of patients who were alive presented with IPI scores of less than or equal to one. No patients with an IPI score of greater than 1 survived. All patients who failed to respond to primary therapy, and 50% of patients who relapsed from complete remission, had CNS and/or contralateral testicular involvement.

The Mayo Clinic experience entailed a retrospective review of 62 patients whose median age was 68 (25). Following orchiectomy, 37% received combination chemotherapy, and 16% received combined modality therapy plus radiotherapy. At 2.7 years of follow-up, 80% of patients had relapsed, with 60% of patients dead from disease. Contrary to a number of previous reports, in which nearly all relapses occurred within 2 years, late recurrences were common in this series, with no plateau of the relapse-free survival curve. Thirteen patients relapsed in the CNS, and, in 8 patients, it was the sole site of relapse. Eleven of 13 patients had parenchymal disease without meningeal involvement.

In another large series, Lagrange described 84 cases with a median age of 67, 75% of whom were categorized as DLBCL (26). Following surgery, 40% of patients received chemotherapy and 33% received combined modality therapy. Complete response was attained in 73% of patients who were stratified according to stage as follows: 100% stage I, 68% stage II, and 33% stages III–IV disease. Relapse occurred in 38%, 9 of whom had CNS disease. The median overall survival was 32 months for the entire group, with 52 months for stage I disease; 32 months for stage II; and 12 months for stages III–IV. As in all the previously described studies, CNS prophylaxis was not used.

A small series from the British Columbia group, however, reported more encouraging results (23). Fourteen historical controls who underwent surgery (and 11 of these 14 also received radiotherapy) were compared to 15 patients treated with brief chemotherapy and involved field radiotherapy. The chemotherapy consisted of either three cycles of cyclophosphamide, adriamycin, hydrochloride, oncovin, prednisone (CHOP) or 6 weeks of ACOB—Adriamycin, cyclophosphamide, oncovin (vincristine), and bleomycin. The overall survival at 4 years in the chemotherapy group was 93% compared to 50% for the historical controls. Despite the lack of prophylaxis, no CNS relapses occurred in the chemotherapy group, and only two occurred in the historical controls.

The largest series to date is a retrospective analysis of 373 cases of primary diffuse large B-cell lymphoma of the testis from 23 tertiary cancer centers by the International Extranodal Lymphoma Study Group (IELSG) (8). The median age at diagnosis was 66, ranging from 19 to 91 years. Approximately 80% of patients had stage I or II disease, which correlated with low and low-to-intermediate IPI scores. Ninety percent of patients had no B symptoms. Ninety-five percent of patients underwent orchiectomy. In 75% of patients, surgery was followed by intensive doxorubicin-containing chemotherapy. CNS prophylaxis with intrathecal chemotherapy was administered to 68 of 73 patients. Eight percent received high-dose systemic methotrexate,

and only 39% had radiation therapy to the contralateral testis. Nine percent of patients were treated with anthracycline-based chemotherapy combined with CNS prophylaxis and scrotal irradiation, which is the current recommended approach.

At a median follow-up of 7.6 years, 52% of patients had relapsed, with a short median survival of 4.5 months after relapse. As predicted, survival was significantly worse than that predicted by the IPI, with most patients having low or low-to-intermediate stage disease. Extranodal relapse occurred in most patients (72%), with CNS relapse occurring in 15% of patients, primarily as parenchymal involvement. The likelihood of CNS relapse continued up to 10 years following presentation. Of those with CNS relapse, 20% had received prior intrathecal prophylaxis, which correlated with delayed relapse but did not impact survival. Too few patients received intravenous methotrexate to determine its effect on subsequent CNS relapse. However, of the 34 patients who were treated with intensive, systemic chemotherapy and CNS prophylaxis with contralateral scrotal irradiation, 88% were alive at 3 years. Multivariate analysis identified IPI score, absence of B symptoms, anthracycline-based chemotherapy, and prophylactic scrotal irradiation as associated with improved outcomes.

The only report of a prospectively treated group of patients was published by the French Goelams group in 2002 (27). In a prospective trial of 494 patients with stage I–II aggressive NHL, 16 patients with primary testicular lymphoma were evaluated separately. The median age was 62, and all cases were classified as DLBCL. They were treated with three cycles of anthracycline-based chemotherapy; radiotherapy to the inguinal, iliac, para-aortic nodes (40 Gy); CNS prophylaxis with intrathecal chemotherapy; and whole brain radiotherapy (24 Gy). All 16 patients achieved a complete response. At a median follow-up of 73.5 months, disease-free survival was 70%, and overall survival was 65%. For patients younger than 60 years, disease-free and overall survival were 66% and 84%, respectively, and 74% and 56% for those patients older than 60. Four patients relapsed in extranodal sites. Prognosis was not affected by extent of testicular involvement, stage, IPI score, or serum LDH. Among the many unknowns in lymphoma biology, the propensity for CNS relapse in testicular lymphoma.

Because 10% to 25% of patients relapse in the CNS, the optimal management of patients with primary testicular lymphoma must include CNS prophylaxis. Most patients relapse with parenchymal brain disease, and it is uncertain whether intrathecal prophylaxis is adequate. Systemic high-dose methotrexate has been used in only a few patients. The use of whole brain radiotherapy is an issue, particularly with the risk of cognitive dysfunction in this typically older group of patients. The value of prophylactic radiotherapy to the contralateral testis is, however, better documented. In the absence of radiotherapy, 5% to 35% of patients will relapse in this site. Radiotherapy to the contralateral testis is now recommended and can greatly reduce the risk of subsequent relapse (8,24,28).

PRIMARY RENAL NON-HODGKIN LYMPHOMA

Primary renal lymphoma is an extremely rare entity, accounting for 0.7% of all extranodal lymphomas in North America (29). Renal involvement by systemic disease is significantly more common and has been reported in up to 50% of cases at autopsy (30,31). Approximately 65 cases have been reported in the literature (31), but given that lymphoma may originate in the kidney and disseminate systemically or originate elsewhere and involve the kidneys secondarily, it is difficult to determine whether these cases truly represent primary renal lymphoma. Some investigators dispute the existence of primary renal lymphoma because the kidney does not contain lymphatic tissue (30,32). Given the infrequency of primary renal lymphoma, specific criteria have been suggested to establish the diagnosis. They include renal failure as the initial presentation, enlarged kidney without obstruction or involvement of other lymph nodes or organs, no other identifiable cause of renal failure, biopsy-proven involvement of the kidney by lymphoma, and rapid improvement of renal function following the administration of therapy (31).

DLBCL is the predominant subtype. Ferry et al. reported a series of 11 patients from a single institution in which 7 were classified as DLBCL, 1 follicular mixed, 2 small lymphocytic plasmacytoid, and 1 small noncleaved non-Burkitt lymphoma (33). A Japanese series of 8 patients demonstrated that 6 cases were DLBCL, with mixed cell type in 1 and small lymphocytic lymphoma in the other. Five cases reported from the Mayo Clinic showed 4 were DLBCL and 1 was Burkitt lymphoma (34). In Stallone's review of single case reports, however, most cases were high-grade lymphomas, Burkitt lymphoma, and lymphoblastic lymphoma (35).

Primary renal NHL typically presents with flank pain or hematuria. Systemic symptoms such as fever, night sweats, and weight loss, are common. Renal insufficiency is often present, although the mechanism is not clear. Other possible etiologies include secondary lymphomatous infiltration of the kidney parenchyma with subsequent loss of tubules and alteration in renal vasculature. The interstitium is primarily involved, which is consistent with the lack of proteinuria and the often-rapid normalization of renal function following the initiation of therapy (36–38).

Prognosis is generally poor in published case reports. In the Japanese series, no patient survived past 2 years. Although the therapy was not well described, only three patients were confirmed to have received intensive combination chemotherapy (38). Five patients treated at the Mayo Clinic all received combination chemotherapy (34). The overall median survival was only 8 months, but two patients, who underwent surgical removal of gross disease before chemotherapy, were in remission at 80 months. In the Ferry series, four patients died of disease between 1 and 23 months and five patients were alive with short follow-up (median 15 months) (33). Of the two remaining patients, one had not completed therapy and one had not been treated for an asymptomatic indolent lesion.

LYMPHOMA OF OTHER GENITOURINARY SITES

In addition to testis and kidney lymphoma, every other structure of the genitourinary system can also be involved with lymphoma. The bladder is the next most commonly described site of primary genitourinary (GU) lymphoma (39–42), but prostate, adrenal, ureteral, urethral, seminal vesicular, and renal allograft involvement have also been described (13,43–49).

B-cell mucosa-associated lymphoid tissue (MALT) lymphoma is the most common primary bladder lymphoma (39). Of 36 cases in the Mayo Clinic Tissue Registry with lymphomas involving the bladder, 6 were thought to be primary bladder lymphomas, and all were of the MALT type. None of these patients died from lymphoma. In a recent review from Princess Margaret Hospital, four cases were identified from a 30-year period, adding to a total of 84 prior cases covered in the English-language literature (50). In another series of 6 primary bladder lymphomas, half were MALT and half were DLBCL, with evidence in 1 case of transformation from low-grade MALT to aggressive large cell lymphoma (40). Most patients are women, generally older than 60 years, and many, but not all, have a history of recurrent infectious cystitis (50,51). The most common presenting symptom is hematuria, occasionally accompanied by dysuria, urinary frequency, or suprapubic discomfort. Diagnosis

is made with cystoscopy and biopsy (52). MALT lymphomas, often stage IE at presentation, may appear only as focal thickening of the bladder wall. DLBCL of the bladder is characterized as bulky, polypoid tumors that are associated with areas of focal hemorrhage that extend into muscularis propria. Because these lesions are submucosal, urine cytology is rarely helpful.

There are at least two reports of long-term remission of bladder MALT lymphoma following antibiotic therapy for *Helicobacter pylori*, suggesting that this is an appropriate initial treatment (53,54). Others have successfully treated such patients with standard chemotherapy (55). In older series, treatment has included radical surgery or radiation, with uniformly good outcome in terms of lymphoma treatment (51,56); however, less radical treatment is likely to be sufficient for MALT lymphomas of the bladder. DLBCL and other aggressive lymphomas of the bladder should be treated the same as malignancies arising at other sites.

More common than primary bladder lymphoma is secondary involvement of the bladder from systemic lymphoma. In one large postmortem analysis, 13% of patients with lymphoma were found to have bladder involvement (57). Clinical symptoms from bladder involvement are unusual, and these patients will also often have involvement of the kidney or ureter. Because primary bladder lymphoma is uncommon, any finding of lymphoma in the bladder should prompt a thorough search for other sources of systemic disease.

A series of 62 prostate lymphomas found that 22 of these were primary prostate lymphomas, including a wide variety of histologic subtypes (48). Of the remaining cases, 30 were patients with systemic lymphoma and secondary involvement of the prostate, and the remainder could not be classified. Symptoms were similar to those of benign prostatic hyperplasia, including urinary urgency and frequency. Cystoscopic examination often showed changes consistent with partial outflow obstruction, including extraluminal narrowing and bladder trabeculation, with no characteristic features. Hodgkin lymphoma of the prostate was extremely rare, with only 2 cases described. There was no major difference in histologic subtype or in clinical outcome between patients with primary or secondary lymphoma. A report from Stanford analyzing 1,092 specimens from radical prostatectomies performed between 1988 and 1995 revealed that 13 of these (1.2%) were incidentally noted lymphoma in the prostate or pelvic lymph nodes (58). Of these, 9 were indolent lymphomas thought not to require specific therapy.

In the series from the Mayo Clinic, disease-specific survival was 64% at 1 year, 50% at 2 years, and 33% at 5 and 10 years (48). Aggressive lymphomas require standard systemic chemotherapy. Individual cases of MALT lymphoma of the prostate have been successfully treated with relatively low doses of external beam radiation therapy (4,400 cGy) or with standard CHOP chemotherapy (59–61).

Lymphomatous involvement of all other genitourinary sites has been reported, but no important distinguishing features have been noted. External ureteral compression is more common than lymphomatous infiltration of the ureter and may require mechanical relief of obstruction to preserve renal function. In an autopsy series, 16% of cases had ureteral involvement, and most of these had ureteral obstruction (43). Primary adrenal lymphomas are rare, most often are DLBCL, and are commonly accompanied by adrenal insufficiency suggestive of bilateral involvement (49).

Patients who have undergone renal allograft transplantation are at increased risk of lymphoma, estimated at 30- to 40-fold greater than that of the general population (62). The risk of lymphoma is greatly influenced by the use of immunosuppressive agents, with the highest risk in patients receiving anti-CD3 monoclonal antibodies (63). Extranodal involvement, including allograft involvement, is common, although primary lymphoma of the allograft is rare. While occasional remissions are observed with removal of immunosuppression, most of these patients require systemic combination chemotherapy.

CONCLUSION

Among primary extranodal sites of lymphoma, clinical involvement of the GU system is very rare. Most cases are large cell B-cell lymphoma and generally have a poor prognosis. The clinical biology of testicular large cell lymphoma differs from the other extranodal presentations with its high propensity for CNS relapse despite the absence of bone marrow involvement at diagnosis. The therapeutic challenge for testicular lymphoma resides in CNS prophylaxis. The case studies enumerated in this chapter have too few patients to draw conclusions, except that a comprehensive plan for the challenge of CNS prophylaxis is needed. The biologic issues explaining high predilection of testicular lymphoma for parenchymal CNS involvement remain an enigma because this is in contradistinction to the situation in nodal presentations of large cell lymphoma. Primary presentations of renal, adrenal, and bladder large cell lymphoma require both optimal local therapy where possible and systemic combination chemotherapy. In these presentations, CNS relapse is less of an issue, but relapse in other systemic sites remains a challenge for systemic chemotherapy.

References

1. Givler RL. Testicular involvement in leukemia and lymphoma. *Cancer* 1,969;23:1290–1295.
2. Banks PM, Arseneau JC, Gralnick HR, et al. American Burkitt's lymphoma: a clinicopathologic study of 30 cases. II. Pathologic correlations. *Am J Med* 1975;58:322–329.
3. Root M, Wang TY, Hescock H, et al. Burkitt's lymphoma of the testicle: report of 2 cases occurring in elderly patients. *J Urol* 1990;144:1239–1241.
4. Doll DC, Weiss RB. Malignant lymphoma of the testis. *Am J Med* 1986; 81:515–524.
5. Baldetorp LA, Brunkvall J, Cavallin-Stahl E, et al. Malignant lymphoma of the testis. *Br J Urol* 1984;56:525–530.
6. Moller MB, d'Amore F, Christensen BE, The Danish Lymphoma Study Group, LYFO. Testicular lymphoma: a population-based study of incidence, clinicopathological correlations and prognosis. *Eur J Cancer* 1994; 30A:1760–1764.
7. Shahab N, Doll DC. Testicular lymphoma. *Semin Oncol* 1999;26:259–269.
8. Zucca E, Conconi A, Mughal TI, et al. Patterns of outcome and prognostic factors in primary large-cell lymphoma of the testis in a survey by the International Extranodal Lymphoma Study Group. *J Clin Oncol* 2003; 21:20–27.
9. Leibovitch I, Goldwasser B. The spectrum of acquired immune deficiency syndrome-associated testicular disorders. *Urology* 1994;44:818–824.
10. Buzelin F, Karam G, Moreau A, et al. Testicular tumor and the acquired immunodeficiency syndrome. *Eur Urol* 1994;26:71–76.
11. Armenakas NA, Schevchuk MM, Brodherson M, et al. AIDS presenting as primary testicular lymphoma. *Urology* 1992;40:162–164.
12. Kaplan LD, Abrams DI, Feigal E, et al. AIDS-associated non-Hodgkin's lymphoma in San Francisco. *Jama* 1989;261:719–724.
13. Salem YH, Miller HC. Lymphoma of genitourinary tract. *J Urol* 1994;151: 1,162–1,170.
14. Ferry JA, Harris NL, Young RH, et al. Malignant lymphoma of the testis, epididymis, and spermatic cord: a clinicopathologic study of 69 cases with immunophenotypic analysis. *Am J Surg Pathol* 1994;18:376–390.
15. Chan JK, Tsang WY, Lau WH, et al. Aggressive T/natural killer cell lymphoma presenting as testicular tumor. *Cancer* 1996;77:1198–1205.
16. Hyland J, Lasota J, Jasinski M, et al. Molecular pathological analysis of testicular diffuse large cell lymphomas. *Hum Pathol* 1998;29:1231–1239.
17. Donahue JP. Surgical management of testicular cancer. In: Einhorn L, ed. *Testicular tumors, management and treatment.* New York: Masson, 1980: 29–46.
18. Lambrechts AC, Looijenga LH, van't Veer MB, et al. Lymphomas with testicular localisation show a consistent BCL-2 expression without a translocation (14;18): a molecular and immunohistochemical study. *Br J Cancer* 1995;71:73–77.
19. Kida T, Andoh M. Testicular involvement of malignant lymphoma diagnosed by Ga-67 scintigraphy. *Clin Nucl Med* 1994;19:238–239.
20. The International Non-Hodgkin's Lymphoma Prognostic Factors Project. A predictive model for aggressive non-Hodgkin's lymphoma. *N Engl J Med* 1993;329:987–994.
21. Tondini C, Ferreri AJ, Siracusano L, et al. Diffuse large-cell lymphoma of the testis. *J Clin Oncol* 1999;17:2854–2858.
22. Ostronoff M, Soussain C, Zambon E, et al. Localized stage non-Hodgkin's lymphoma of the testis: a retrospective study of 16 cases. *Nouv Rev Fr Hematol* 1995;37:267–272.
23. Connors JM, Klimo P, Voss N, et al. Testicular lymphoma: improved outcome with early brief chemotherapy. *J Clin Oncol* 1988;6:776–781.
24. Touroutoglou N, Dimopoulos MA, Younes A, et al. Testicular lymphoma: late relapses and poor outcome despite doxorubicin-based therapy. *J Clin Oncol* 1995;13:1361–1367.
25. Fonseca R, Habermann TM, Colgan JP, et al. Testicular lymphoma is associated with a high incidence of extranodal recurrence. *Cancer* 2000;88: 154–161.
26. Lagrange JL, Ramaioli A, Theodore CH, et al. Non-Hodgkin's lymphoma of the testis: a retrospective study of 84 patients treated in the French anticancer centres. *Ann Oncol* 2001;12:1313–1319.
27. Linassier C, Desablens B, Lefrancq T, et al. Stage I–IIE primary non-Hodgkin's lymphoma of the testis: results of a prospective trial by the GOELAMS Study Group. *Clin Lymphoma* 2002;3:167–172.
28. Read G. Lymphomas of the testis: results of treatment 1960–77. *Clin Radiol* 1981;32:687–692.
29. Freeman C, Berg JW, Cutler SJ. Occurrence and prognosis of extranodal lymphomas. *Cancer* 1972;29:252–260.
30. Kandel LB, McCullough DL, Harrison LH, et al. Primary renal lymphoma. Does it exist? *Cancer* 1987;60:386–391.
31. Da'as N, Polliack A, Cohen Y, et al. Kidney involvement and renal manifestations in non-Hodgkin's lymphoma and lymphocytic leukemia: a retrospective study in 700 patients. *Eur J Haematol* 2001;67:158–164.
32. Paganelli E, Arisi L, Ferrari ME, et al. Primary non-Hodgkin's lymphoma of the kidney. *Haematologica* 1989;74:301–304.
33. Ferry JA, Harris NL, Papanicolaou N, et al. Lymphoma of the kidney: a report of 11 cases. *Am J Surg Pathol* 1995;19:134–144.
34. Okuno SH, Hoyer JD, Ristow K, et al. Primary renal non-Hodgkin's lymphoma: an unusual extranodal site. *Cancer* 1995;75:2258–2261.
35. Stallone G, Infante B, Manno C, et al. Primary renal lymphoma does exist: case report and review of the literature. *J Nephrol* 2000;13:367–372.
36. Arranz Arija JA, Carrion JR, Garcia FR, et al. Primary renal lymphoma: report of 3 cases and review of the literature. *Am J Nephrol* 1994;14:148–153.
37. Truong LD, Soroka S, Sheth AV, et al. Primary renal lymphoma presenting as acute renal failure. *Am J Kidney Dis* 1987;9:502–506.
38. Yasunaga Y, Hoshida Y, Hashimoto M, et al. Malignant lymphoma of the kidney. *J Surg Oncol* 1997;64:207–211.
39. Kempton CL, Kurtin PJ, Inwards DJ, et al. Malignant lymphoma of the bladder: evidence from 36 cases that low-grade lymphoma of the MALT-type is the most common primary bladder lymphoma. *Am J Surg Pathol* 1997;21:1324–1333.
40. Bates AW, Norton AJ, Baithun SI. Malignant lymphoma of the urinary bladder: a clinicopathological study of 11 cases. *J Clin Pathol* 2000;53: 458–461.
41. Maghfoor I, Koontz P, Weaver-Osterholtz D, et al. Primary extra-nodal lymphoma of the urinary bladder. *South Med J* 2000;93:317–318.
42. Cohen DD, Lamarre C, Lamarre L, et al. Primary low-grade B-cell lymphoma of the urinary bladder: case report and literature review. *Can J Urol* 2002;9:1694–1697.
43. Scharifker D, Chalasani A. Ureteral involvement by malignant lymphoma: ten years' experience. *Arch Pathol Lab Med* 1978;102:541–543.
44. Bostwick DG, Mann RB. Malignant lymphomas involving the prostate: a study of 13 cases. *Cancer* 1985;56:2932–2938.
45. Shea TC, Spark R, Kane B, et al. Non-Hodgkin's lymphoma limited to the adrenal gland with adrenal insufficiency. *Am J Med* 1985;78:711–714.
46. Carey RW, Harris N, Kliman B. Addison's disease secondary to lymphomatous infiltration of the adrenal glands: recovery of adrenocortical function after chemotherapy. *Cancer* 1987;59:1087–1090.
47. Olcott EW, Gozldstein RB, Salvatierra O. Lymphoma presenting as allograft hematoma in a renal transplant recipient. *J Ultrasound Med* 1990;9: 239–241.
48. Bostwick DG, Iczkowski KA, Amin MB, et al. Malignant lymphoma involving the prostate: report of 62 cases. *Cancer* 1998;83:732–738.
49. Wang J, Sun NC, Renslo R, et al. Clinically silent primary adrenal lymphoma: a case report and review of the literature. *Am J Hematol* 1998;58: 130–136.
50. Al-Maghrabi J, Kamel-Reid S, Jewett M, et al. Primary low-grade B-cell lymphoma of mucosa-associated lymphoid tissue type arising in the urinary bladder: report of 4 cases with molecular genetic analysis. *Arch Pathol Lab Med* 2001;125:332–336.
51. Ohsawa M, Aozasa K, Horiuchi K, et al. Malignant lymphoma of bladder: report of three cases and review of the literature. *Cancer* 1993;72: 1969–1974.
52. Downs TM, Kibel AS, DeWolf WC. Primary lymphoma of the bladder: a unique cystoscopic appearance. *Urology* 1997;49:276–278.
53. Van den Bosch J, Kropman RF, Blok P, et al. Disappearance of a mucosa-associated lymphoid tissue (MALT) lymphoma of the urinary bladder after treatment for Helicobacter pylori. *Eur J Haematol* 2002;68: 187–188.
54. Oscier D, Bramble J, Hodges E, et al. Regression of mucosa-associated lymphoid tissue lymphoma of the bladder after antibiotic therapy. *J Clin Oncol* 2002;20:882.

55. Wazait HD, Chahal R, Sundurum SK, et al. MALT-type primary lymphoma of the urinary bladder: clinicopathological study of 2 cases and review of the literature. *Urol Int* 2001;66:220–224.

56. Bhansali S, Cameron K. Primary malignant lymphoma of the bladder. *Br J Urol* 1960;32:440–454.

57. Sufrin G, Keogh B, Moore RH, et al. Secondary involvement of the bladder in malignant lymphoma. *J Urol* 1977;118:251–253.

58. Terris MK, Hausdorff J, Freiha FS. Hematolymphoid malignancies diagnosed at the time of radical prostatectomy. *J Urol* 1997;158:1457–1459.

59. Tomikawa S, Okumura H, Yoshida T, et al. Primary prostatic lymphoma of mucosa-associated lymphoid tissue. *Intern Med* 1998;37:628–630.

60. Tomaru U, Ishikura H, Kon S, et al. Primary lymphoma of the prostate with features of low grade B-cell lymphoma of mucosa associated lymphoid tissue: a rare cause of urinary obstruction. *J Urol* 1999;162:496–497.

61. Mermershtain W, Benharroch D, Lavrenkov K, et al. Primary malignant lymphoma of the prostate: a report of three cases. *Leuk Lymphoma* 2001;42:809–811.

62. Hoover R, Fraumeni JF Jr. Risk of cancer in renal-transplant recipients. *Lancet* 1973;2:55–57.

63. Swinnen LJ, Costanzo-Nordin MR, Fisher SG, et al. Increased incidence of lymphoproliferative disorder after immunosuppression with the monoclonal antibody OKT3 in cardiac-transplant recipients. *N Engl J Med* 1990;323:1723–1728.

CHAPTER 56 ■ CANCER OF THE URETHRA

ANTHONY H. RUSSELL AND GUIDO DALBAGNI

INTRODUCTION

Primary malignancies of the urethra are infrequent, constituting a fraction of 1% of genitourinary malignancies in both men and women. This rarity is the major factor contributing to the lack of standardized assessment and treatment algorithms. Tertiary cancer referral institutions in North America may treat two or three patients annually, and most centers will see fewer. Clinical reports retrospectively detail limited numbers of patients spanning multiple decades during which diagnostic techniques and management philosophies have evolved rather than remained static.

As a consequence of the diversity of histologic types, the spectrum of clinical stage at presentation, and the heterogeneity of the patient population afflicted with these rare neoplasms, it is clearly imprudent to advocate rigid treatment algorithms and nearly impossible to compare survival outcomes from different therapeutic modalities or combinations of modalities.

In the absence of compelling prospective data, treatment inevitably represents some measure of extrapolation from general principles of oncologic management tailored on the basis of histology, tumor location and extent, and the constraining comorbidities of an individual patient.

Despite the considerably shorter length of the female urethra, female urethral cancer is approximately threefold more prevalent than male urethral cancer. Median age for both men and women is approximately 60 years, with reported cases including teenagers and nonagenarians.

ETIOLOGY

No definitive etiologic factors have been identified in the pathogenesis of epithelial tumors of the female urethra. Etiologic factors in the development of transitional and squamous malignancies of the bladder urothelium are believed to be common to the development of these cell types in the posterior (proximal) urethra. Urothelial neoplasms of the bladder may precede, follow, or, rarely, be detected synchronously with urethral tumors suggesting "field cancerization" in some patients. Chronic inflammation and infection have been associated with urethral cancer, but no clear linkage has been established. Presence of oncogenic genotypes of human papillomavirus (HPV) (types 16 and 18) have been documented in 59% of cases in one series with HPV limited to squamous and transitional cancers and not found in adenocarcinomas (1). Malignancies in women may arise in urethral diverticula, particularly clear cell carcinomas, prompting the speculation that focal urinary stasis may contribute to the initiation of malignancy in some patients.

In men, no definitive etiologic factors have been identified; however, chronic inflammation seems to play a significant role in the development of carcinoma of the urethra. Urethral strictures have been reported in 25% to 70% of patients, sexually transmitted diseases in 24% to 37% of patients, and trauma in 7% to 10% of patients (2–5). Herpes simplex virus has been associated with carcinoma of the urethra (6), and human papillomavirus type 16 may play a role in the development of carcinoma of the pendulous urethra (7,8).

ANATOMY

The female urethra (Fig. 56.1) is variable in length (2 to 6 cm), but 3 to 4 cm is the average. Transitional epithelium lines the proximal third of the urethra, with the distal two thirds lined by squamous epithelium. Surrounding the urethra are the para-urethral glands and ducts (Skene glands) that are the female homolog of the prostate gland. The muscular wall of the urethra has an inner longitudinal layer and outer circular layers continuous with the bladder detrusor. Except during micturition, the lumen is a virtual space. Arterial supply is from the branches of the pudendal artery.

Lymphatic drainage of the distal third or anterior urethra, distal vagina, and anterior vulva, is to the medial, superficial inguinal nodes. Subsequent lymphatic flow is to nodes deep in the cribriform fascia, then under the inguinal ligaments to the caudal external iliac nodes. From the proximal two thirds of the urethra and the proximal vagina, lymphatic flow is to the obturator, hypogastric, and external iliac nodes. However, there are no discrete boundaries between these lymphatic drainage basins, and the lymphatic net is rich with interconnections. Additionally, normal lymphatic drainage patterns may be distorted or blocked by the presence of disease. When planning a treatment strategy for an individual patient, it is prudent to assess both the inguinofemoral and pelvic nodal chains, particularly in patients with locally extensive disease, and to consider therapy which will address both potential avenues of lymphatic dissemination.

The urethra in men can be divided anatomically into three parts: prostatic, membranous, and penile (spongiose) (Fig. 56.2). The prostatic urethra is approximately 3 to 4 cm long. It begins at the internal urethral orifice located in the bladder neck and extends the entire length of the prostate to the prostatic apex. Within the prostatic urethra is the urethral crest, an elevation of the mucous membrane. The ejaculatory ducts open on each side of the prostatic utricle, a slitlike opening located on an elevation called the *colliculus seminalis* (verumontanum) in the middle of the urethral crest (10). The urethral crest is flanked on both sides by a depression called the *prostatic sinus*, the floor of which is perforated by the prostatic ducts. The membranous urethra is the shortest portion, measuring only 1 cm in length. It goes from the apex of the prostate to the bulb of the penis, traversing through the musculature of the urethral sphincter and inferior fascia of the urogenital diaphragm. One small bulbourethral gland (Cowper gland) is located on either side of this portion of the urethra (10). The penile (spongiose) urethra is the longest segment, measuring approximately 15 cm and extending from the distal surface of the urogenital diaphragm to urethral orifice in the glans penis.

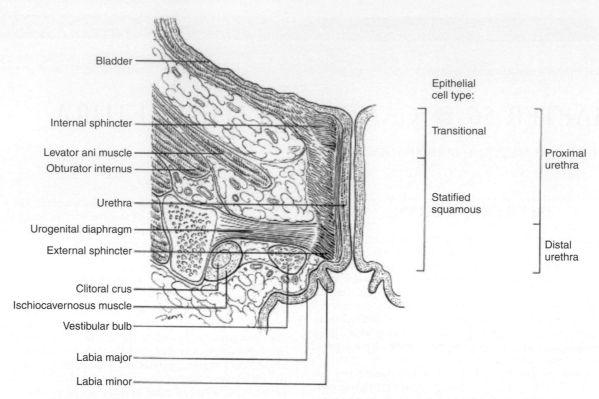

FIGURE 56.1. Anatomy of the female urethra. (From Carroll PR: Surgical management of urethral carcinoma. In: Crawford ED, Das S, eds. *Current Genitourinary Cancer Surgery*. Philadelphia: Lea & Febiger, 1990, with permission.)

The penile urethra can be further subdivided into the bulbous and pendulous urethra. The bulbourethral glands open on the lateral surfaces of the bulbous portion of the penile urethra. The penile urethra is surrounded by the corpus spongiosum along its entire length.

The membranous and prostatic urethra make up the posterior urethra, and the bulbous and pendulous portion of the penile urethra make up the anterior urethra. However, clinically and pathologically, the bulbous segment of the penile urethra is included in the posterior urethra as a result of a similar prognosis for carcinoma in the bulbous and membranous urethra, whereas only the pendulous segment of the penile urethra is referred to as the anterior urethra.

The lining epithelium is derived from endoderm of the urogenital sinus except distally in the area of the fossa navicularis, the epithelial lining of which is formed by canalization of ectodermal cells extending into the glans from its tip. The type of epithelium lining the prostatic urethra is of the transitional cell type as far as the ejaculatory ducts, then of the pseudostratified columnar epithelium along the membranous and most of the penile urethra, and nonkeratinized stratified squamous epithelium near the external urethral orifice (9,10). This epithelial lining corresponds to a healthy urethra, whereas in the diseased state, or after instrumentation, metaplastic changes can be noted.

The lymphatic drainages of the urethra and of the penis are closely interconnected. One or more major collecting trunks that receive the lymphatic drainage from the glans and the pendulous urethra run with the deep dorsal vein and drain into a presymphyseal plexus. Two or more trunks drain from this plexus into the inguinal nodes and occasionally into the external iliac nodes (11). The bulbous segment of the penile urethra and the membranous urethra drain into the external iliac nodes. The lymphatic drainage of the prostatic urethra follows one of the three routes. The first is along the prostatic artery to the obturator and internal iliac nodes, the second is with lymphatics over the seminal vesicle to the external iliac nodes, and the third is from the posterior part of the prostate to the sacral nodes (11).

SYMPTOMS

In women, urinary frequency and dysuria are common. Erratic bleeding will occur in most patients. Obstructive symptoms may progress to urinary retention in some patients. Extension to the vulva may result in pain, pruritus, and inflammation. Erosion into the vagina with ulceration may result in foul-smelling vaginal discharge. Proximal lesions extending to the bladder neck and upper vagina can result in formation of a vesico-vaginal fistula with incontinence. Only rarely are urethral cancers diagnosed by surveillance physical examination in asymptomatic patients. Ninety-eight percent of patients are symptomatic at the time of diagnosis, with a median interval of 4.5 months between onset of symptoms and diagnosis (12).

The diagnosis of carcinoma of the male urethra is often delayed, as a result of the nonspecific nature of the symptoms. The median interval from the onset of symptoms to diagnosis has been reported to be 7.5 months (3). The most common mode of presentation is obstructive urinary symptoms, followed by a perineal mass (2,3,13,14). Patients may also present with an abscess, a fistula, hematuria, spotting, irritative symptoms, urethral discharge, or pain. New onset of a urethral stricture in a middle-aged man who has not undergone prior urethral instrumentation should arouse a suspicion of malignancy and should be thoroughly investigated. Rare cases of carcinoma of the male urethra with hypercalcemia have been reported (15,16).

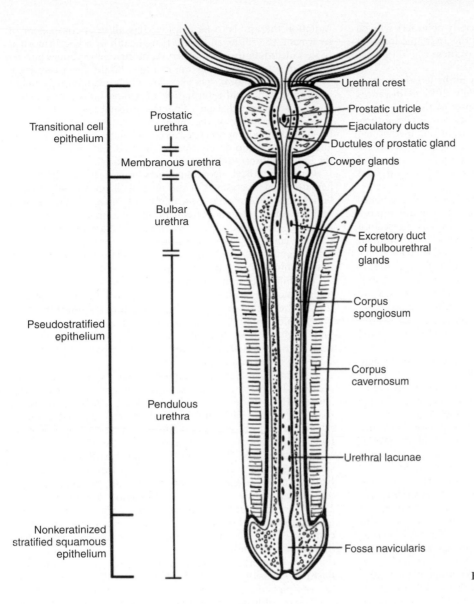

Transitional cell epithelium

Prostatic urethra

Membranous urethra

Bulbar urethra

Pseudostratified epithelium

Pendulous urethra

Nonkeratinized stratified squamous epithelium

Urethral crest

Prostatic utricle

Ejaculatory ducts

Ductules of prostatic gland

Cowper glands

Excretory duct of bulbourethral glands

Corpus spongiosum

Corpus cavernosum

Urethral lacunae

Fossa navicularis

FIGURE 56.2. Anatomy of the male urethra.

PATHOLOGY

Urethral neoplasms in women and men are both histopathologically different as well as somewhat different in clinical behavior, phenomena attributed to differences between the sexes in normal anatomy and the histology of the urethra (17).

In women, transitional epithelium lines the proximal third of the urethra, and squamous epithelium the distal two thirds. These areas give rise to carcinomas morphologically derivative from those epithelial cell lines, which, in aggregate, account for approximately 80% of primary urethral tumors in women. Squamous carcinomas constitute most primary urethral tumors in women, comprising from 50% to 65% of cases in clinical series (18–20). Transitional cell cancers comprise approximately 15% of cases (12,19).

Adenocarcinomas account for 10% to 12% of primary female urethral neoplasms (17,19) but may account for 35% to 57% of cases in referral institutions (12,21). The submucosa of the urethra contains periurethral glands (Skene glands) that are the female homolog to prostatic ductal and glandular tissue in the male. The ducts are lined by pseudostratified and stratified columnar epithelium in which may be found intraepithelial mucous-secreting glands. Skene glands give rise to adenocarcinomas morphologically similar to prostate cancer that may stain immunohistochemically for prostate-specific antigen (PSA) and prostate-specific acid phosphatase (PSAP), and occasionally may produce serologically detectable levels of PSA (22).

Clear cell adenocarcinomas of the urethra characteristically originate in urethral diverticula and are morphologically similar to clear cell adenocarcinomas arising from Mullerian tissues elsewhere in the female genitourinary tract including the ovaries, fallopian tubes, endometrium, and foci of malignant degeneration in endometriosis. Clear cell cancers comprise approximately 40% of adenocarcinomas of the urethra (23). These generally do not stain for PSA or PSAP (24), although a rare instance has been reported of such staining properties. Immunoreactivity for cancer-associated antigen 125 (CA-125) has been reported for this cell type (25).

Other primary urethral adenocarcinomas include mucinous/columnar or colloid cancers that resemble primary colorectal or endometrial cancers and that may stain positively for carcinoembryonic antigen (CEA) (26) and signet ring cell adenocarcinomas.

Cancers with neuroendocrine features including carcinoid and small cell cancers are anecdotally seen. Carcinosarcoma, plasmacytoma, and Hodgkin and non-Hodgkin lymphoma have been reported as primary within the urethra. In general, management of rare histologic types of urethral neoplasia more commonly associated with other anatomic structures (neuroendocrine tumors, plasmacytoma, lymphoma) will be predicated on the histology rather than the anatomic location of origin and will parallel management of these cell lines diagnosed at other primary sites.

Malignant melanoma can be primary in the female urethra, and may be amelanotic in approximately 20% of instances (27). Therapy is generally surgical because of the relative insensitivity of melanoma to radiation and cytotoxic chemotherapy. Often more deeply invasive than cutaneous melanoma, possibly as a result of delayed diagnosis, prognosis for these lesions is grim, with a propensity to fail rapidly after surgical therapy with local recurrence, regional nodal spread, and hematogenous dissemination (28).

In men, squamous cell carcinoma is the predominant histologic type, representing 50% to 90% of all urethral tumors (2,3,13,14,29–31). Transitional cell carcinoma is the second most common histologic type, followed by adenocarcinoma. The histology of tumors originating in the urethra tends to coincide with the morphology of the urothelial lining: tumors originating in the prostatic urethra are transitional cell carcinomas, whereas tumors originating in the penile urethra are squamous in origin. However, there have been numerous reports of transitional cell carcinoma originating in the pendulous urethra (32–37) which could be explained by urothelial metaplasia.

Adenocarcinoma may arise from the surface mucosa through a process of metaplasia or from periurethral glands. The possibility of direct extension from rectal adenocarcinoma should be entertained. Stage for stage, adenocarcinomas in men have the same prognosis as primary tumors of other histologies.

Sixty percent of tumors originate in the membranous urethra and bulbous portion of the penile urethra (bulbomembranous urethra), 30% in the pendulous segment of the penile urethra, and 10% in the prostatic urethra (3–5,14,38).

Cowper glands are small mucous tubuloalveolar bulbourethral glands located on either side of the membranous urethra (10) (Fig. 56.2). They drain through separate excretory ducts in the bulbous urethra after traversing the corpus spongiosum. Cowper glands are the homolog of Bartholin glands in women. However, pathologic conditions such as infections or carcinoma associated with Cowper glands are much less common than those associated with Bartholin glands (39). This might reflect the difficulty in making an early diagnosis because of the inaccessible location and lack of early clinical symptoms.

Documented cases of adenocarcinoma of Cowper glands are extremely rare. The patients' ages have ranged from 19 to 70 years. Patients present with perineal pain, lower urinary tract symptoms, and a mass in the perineum (39–43). The tumors have a tendency for local invasion and less propensity for metastasis (41,43,44). Microscopically, these neoplasms share many of the same features with adenocarcinomas arising from the urethral surface mucosa. The patients have been managed either by local resection (39) or by radical excision (42) with and without radiation. Local control has been achieved in a few patients, with most progressing locally with or without metastatic sites within a short period of time. The prognosis is poor with no documented survivors beyond 5 years.

Adenoid cystic carcinoma, morphologically similar to similar tumors arising in major and minor salivary glands and Bartholin glands, has been reported arising in Cowper glands with anecdotal long-term survival after combined modality therapy (45).

EVALUATION AND STAGING

In women, as a consequence to the accessibility to examination, there can be no substitute for the information gleaned by obtaining a history and performing a careful physical examination. If radiation therapy is to be employed as all or a component of treatment, the status and underlying health of adjacent normal tissues including the vagina, cervix, uterus, pelvic bones and femurs, major vessels, and anorectum should be ascertained. Physical examination, possibly including examination under anesthesia, will yield information regarding both tumor extent and the status of adjacent vulnerable normal tissues that is beyond the capability of the most sensitive imaging techniques. Imaging should be appreciated as complementary to physical examination and should be used to assess disease extent beyond the limits of direct visualization and palpation.

Female urethral neoplasms very rarely have identifiable hematogenous metastasis at the time of diagnosis (46). Lungs, bones, and liver are the most commonly affected distant sites, with the lungs being most frequent. In the absence of bone pain, a chest x-ray constitutes an adequate assessment for patients with the common epithelial histologies. A more thorough search for disseminated disease may be appropriate for patients with unusual histology (lymphoma, melanoma, sarcoma).

Techniques that may be helpful to define the extent of local disease include urethroscopy, cystoscopy, and direct visualization of the vagina and cervix by speculum examination possibly supplemented by colposcopy. With extensive lesions, it may be difficult to determine the precise location of the primary site that will necessarily be somewhat arbitrarily assigned to the apparent tumor epicenter.

Diagnostic imaging techniques include vaginal ultrasound, computed tomography (CT) scan, and magnetic resonance imaging (MRI). Gadolinium-enhanced MRI will be more useful than CT scan in discriminating tumor from normal tissue in the assessment of local extent but may overestimate tumor extent in the context of inflammatory changes (47).

Approximately 10% to 30% of women will have clinically suspicious groin nodes at the time of diagnosis (12,20,48–51). Evaluation of regional lymph nodes can be accomplished using several different imaging modalities. Lymphaniograms are notoriously difficult to interpret in the inguinofemoral nodes, and lymphography has largely been supplanted by contrast-enhanced CT scan and gadolinium-enhanced MRI that can additionally assess lymph nodes not routinely visualized by lymphangiograms (internal iliacs, presacral nodes). Positron emission tomography (PET) and PET/CT scan have been employed to assess both nodal and hematogenous spread of disease, although their use remains anecdotal. Given the rarity of urethral neoplasms, it is unlikely that routine deployment of such expensive new imaging modalities will be approved by regulatory agencies and insurance entities based on prospective data.

Lymph node enlargement is nonspecific and may represent an inflammatory response to infection within necrotic tumor rather than metastasis. It is usually feasible to confirm regional node metastasis by imaging-guided needle biopsy for pelvic nodes or deep inguinal nodes, direct needle biopsy of palpable inguinal nodes, or local excision of a clinically suspicious node. Presence or absence of proven regional node metastasis may impact the selection, sequencing, scope, and intensity of treatment modalities. The extent and intent of surgery (radical monotherapy or component of multimodality therapy) will be influenced by this information. Potential radiation target volumes, total dose, and fractionation will also be impacted by this knowledge. Therefore, histologic confirmation of lymph node status should be attempted whenever clinically or radiographically suspicious nodes are encountered.

In men, the diagnosis of urethral cancer is generally made by transurethral biopsy. Needle biopsy is occasionally helpful in determining the local extent of neoplasm. A voided urine cytology has been suggested as a diagnostic tool (29). The sensitivity of a voided urine cytology was 55% in a cohort of 29 patients (52). It is important to palpate for the presence of

TABLE 56.1

TNM STAGING AMERICAN JOINT COMMITTEE ON CANCER 2002

Stage	Symtptom
Primary Tumor	
TX	Primary tumor cannot be assessed
T0	No evidence of primary tumor
Ta	Noninvasive papillary, polypoid, or verrucous carcinoma
Tis	CIS
T1	Tumor invades subepithelial connective tissue
T2	Tumor invades any of the following: corpus spongiosum, prostate, periurethral muscle
T3	Tumor invades any of the following: corpus cavernosum, beyond prostatic capsule, anterior vagina, bladder neck
T4	Tumor invades other adjacent organs
Regional Lymph Nodes (N)	
NX	Regional lymph nodes cannot be assessed
N0	No regional lymph node metastasis
N1	Metastasis in a single lymph node, 2 cm or less in greatest dimension
N2	Metastasis in a single node more than 2 cm in greatest dimension, or in multiple nodes
Distant Metastasis (M)	
MX	Distant metastasis cannot be assessed
M0	No distant metastasis
M1	Distant metastasis

CIS, carcinoma *in situ.*
From AJCC Cancer Staging Manual. In: Green FL, Page DL, Fleming ID et al., eds. *American Joint Committee On Cancer. American Cancer Society,* 6th ed. New York: Springer-Verlag, 2002.

positive lymph nodes in the inguinal area, particularly with tumors of the pendulous urethra. As in women, CT scan or MRI may help to evaluate the pelvic and para-aortic nodes. Most tumors in men are at high stage at presentation. A series of pathologically staged patients from Memorial Sloan-Kettering Cancer Center (MSKCC) in New York reported 30% pT2, 37% pT3, and 11% pT4, with positive lymph nodes in 22% of patients overall and 40% of patients who underwent a lymph node dissection (3).

Urethral cancer is assigned a stage according to the 2002 American Joint Committee on Cancer (AJCC) Tumor-Node-Metastasis (TNM) formalism (53) based on the depth of invasion, presence or absence of regional node metastases, and the presence or absence of remote nodal or hematogenous metastases (Table 56.1).

TREATMENT

The dual but competitive objectives of cancer therapy are to maximize the probability of tumor control while minimizing chronic functional and cosmetic loss to the afflicted patient. Because of proximity to functionally important structures (bladder, vagina, anterior vulva and clitoris, femoral necks, and anterior pubic rami) treatment of female urethral neoplasms is frequently multimodality in an effort to spare patients the late morbidities associated with radical monotherapy. Selection and sequencing of treatment modalities will depend on assessment of initial disease extent and the presence or absence of limiting patient comorbidities.

Surgical excision is the primary therapy for carcinoma of the male urethra, although alternative, penile-preserving treatment strategies based on chemoradiation alone or coordinated with conservative surgery may be appropriate in select patients with squamous or epidermoid carcinomas.

Surgery in Women

Removal of the distal third of the female urethra can be accomplished surgically with conservation of urinary continence. Distal urethrectomy is appropriate monotherapy for carefully selected patients with small volume distal tumors with minimal, if any, extension to adjacent structures (Tis, T1, T2, and minimal T3 with clinically negative groin nodes). Electrofulguration or laser vaporization have been utilized to treat small, superficial cancers, particularly those involving the meatus; however, these techniques compromise the ability to assess histopathologic margins and thereby the adequacy of local therapy.

Surgery for invasive lesions should generally encompass bilateral groin nodes as these will be a frequent site of subsequent failure if not addressed with initial therapy. Techniques for identification of sentinel lymph nodes (blue dye injection, radio-colloid injection) that have been employed with clinical utility in the treatment of breast, vulvar, and other neoplasms might theoretically be useful in tailoring the level and extent of groin dissection in patients with distal urethral cancer. Application of these techniques has not been studied prospectively in this rare group of malignancies, and their clinical use can only be justified by extrapolation.

When clinically apparent groin node metastases are present, radical surgery as monotherapy will no longer be sensible. Conservative surgery for resection limited to grossly enlarged groin nodes or gross primary disease may be helpful in coordination with a course of preoperative or postoperative radiation. Complete superficial and deep inguinofemoral node dissection in the setting of known groin node metastases will substantially escalate the risk of debilitating leg lymphedema if combined with radiation therapy, and should be avoided.

Surgery (generally anterior exenteration or total urethrectomy with continent conduit connected to the bladder) is rarely appropriate as initial therapy when cancer involves the proximal two thirds of the female urethra and should usually be reserved for salvage of local radiation failure. Exceptions include cases in which a patient has free-flowing incontinence based on fistula formation or other nonremedial cause. Under such circumstances, selection of conservative treatment to preserve urinary continence becomes moot.

When cancer of the distal urethra extends to involve the vulva in limited fashion, conservative local surgical therapy may still be possible. In a sexually active woman, or a patient who may become sexually active, this should not be undertaken if tumor extends grossly to within 1 cm of the clitoris or if surgery would imply extensive loss of the venereal fat pad. Under such circumstances, carefully planned radiation or chemoradiation, possibly supplemented by limited surgery, affords a better opportunity for a patient to remain sexually active and orgasmic without dyspareunia.

Results of surgery as monotherapy are good when limited to carefully selected patients of low stage, and may approach 80% survival at 5 years (54). Survival with surgery alone in patients with locally advanced disease is reported to be less than 20% at 5 years (54). Surgical failures almost invariably involve at least a component of local or regional (nodal) disease, frequently in the absence of distant dissemination. This observation sensibly leads to rational combinations of surgical therapy for variable extent coupled with adjuvant radiation in modest dose.

Surgery in Men

Early series supported the use of radical surgery for tumors of the posterior urethra, with a 30% 5-year disease-free survival for patients undergoing surgery versus 3% for those who did not undergo radical surgery (4).

Carcinoma of the anterior (pendulous) urethra has a better prognosis than posterior urethral carcinoma due to a lower stage at presentation (55) and better local control (56).

A noninvasive superficial papillary tumor is best managed by transurethral resection and fulguration. Invasive carcinoma of the pendulous urethra is best managed by a partial or total penectomy, which results in excellent local control (2,5,14, 38,56–58). In the presence of inguinal metastasis, a bilateral inguinal lymphadenectomy may be therapeutic (5). However, the role of prophylactic lymphadenectomy is controversial (14). Because of the high incidence of undetected microscopic positive lymph nodes (56), a bilateral inguinal lymphadenectomy with pelvic lymph node dissection is appropriate surgical therapy for all patients with invasive carcinoma of the pendulous urethra.

Transurethral or segmental resection may be adequate for treatment of early superficial tumors involving the bulbomembranous urethra, but such cases are rare. Most patients present at an advanced stage, and radical excision has been the treatment of choice (2,3,38). In a compilation of several major series, 5-year disease-free survival was 30% (4). The primary cause of failure is lack of local disease control. Experience suggests that when local control of the tumor can be achieved, overall long-term results are favorable. Such tumors tend to be locally extensive and are apt to recur locally with inadequate local treatment. Metastasis appears to be a late event. This has led to aggressive combined therapy approaches in patients with bulky posterior urethral carcinoma. In Gheiler's series from Wayne State University in Detroit, four patients with high-stage tumors were treated with neoadjuvant chemotherapy and radiation before surgery, and two of them were rendered disease-free (55). Klein et al. from MSKCC reported a 58% disease-free survival when total penectomy and cystectomy were combined with preoperative radiation and excision of the inferior or pubic rami (59). However, the number of patients is limited and paucity of data precludes any strong recommendation.

Primary carcinoma arising from the prostatic urethra is rare; it accounts for 9% of carcinomas of the urethra (2). Superficial lesions of the prostatic urethra carry a good prognosis and are treated endoscopically by transurethral resection. It is extremely important to make a distinction between primary carcinoma of the prostatic urethra and primary transitional cell carcinoma of the prostate, which carries a poor prognosis. The patients with primary carcinoma of the prostatic urethra usually present with gross hematuria or irritative lower tract symptoms (14). In most instances, the tumor involves the bulk of the prostate with variable extension to the bulbomembranous urethra or to the bladder neck and trigone. In this situation, cystoprostatectomy and urethrectomy are the treatments of choice.

Radiation Therapy in Women

Radiation has been employed preoperatively and postoperatively in coordination with conservative surgery in an effort to control microscopic, clinically occult disease extension at the periphery of a surgical margin or within regional nodes. Sensible combinations of surgery and modest-dose adjuvant radiation (4500 cGy to 5400 cGy) may permit conservative surgical therapy with narrower margin (5 to 10 mm) than traditional (1 to 2 cm) surgical margins of functionally important normal tissue. Whether radiation should be administered preoperatively or postoperatively will depend on whether or not all gross tumor can be excised by initial conservative excision, as well as on the

basis of patient age, comorbidities, and anticipated difficulties with wound healing. There exists no randomized data demonstrating the superiority of one approach over another, although outcome analysis from MSKCC suggested substantial improvement in local control when radiation was administered prior to surgery (12). A combined surgical-radiotherapeutic approach has been reported to show better efficacy in patients with more locally advanced disease when compared to patients selected for surgery as monotherapy based on limited disease extent (49).

The volume chosen for radiation should include elective or "prophylactic" treatment of inguinal or pelvic lymph nodes in analogy to the successful use of radiation to control clinically occult regional micrometastases in lymph nodes of patients with cancers of the anus, vulva, vagina, and other sites (20,48). With such treatment, the incidence of subsequent groin failure is reduced by approximately 80% from 52% to 10% (49).

When radiation therapy is used alone, or combined with synchronous, radiopotentiating chemotherapy, available techniques include brachytherapy (intersitial or intracavitary placement of radioisotopes) alone or in combination with teletherapy (external radiation).

Brachytherapy can be accomplished with either low-dose-rate (LDR; 50 to 80 cGy/hr) or high-dose-rate (HDR; 50 to 150 cGy/min) inpatient or outpatient techniques. Brachytherapy has been accomplished using intraurethral sources in combination with intravaginal sources employing high dose-rate technique (60). More commonly, brachytherapy will be done with temporary interstitial needle insertions usually inserted using a guide template for optimal spatial placement of needles to avoid excessive "hot" spots or "cold" areas of underdosage (61–63).

Teletherapy will generally include treatment of an initial large area addressing the primary, local extensions of the primary, and potential sites of occult micrometastases in regional nodes. This volume will be conventionally treated to 4,500 cGy to 5,040 cGy in 25 to 28 treatment fractions, five treatment fractions weekly. This will be followed by focused "boost" radiation to reduced volumes comprising the primary tumor with a narrow margin of clinically normal tissue and gross lymph node metastases. These reduced volumes will be treated to a cumulative dose between 6,500 cGy and 7,500 cGy. Treatment of a boost volume encompassing the primary disease may be treated using a variety of techniques, including interstitial brachytherapy (Fig. 56.3) or reduced-volume teletherapy which possibly employs an en-face perineal port using low-energy photons or high-energy electrons. The potential advantage of brachytherapy techniques include an overall shorter treatment time (which may be biologically more effective) as well as tighter confinement of high radiation dose to tissues directly infiltrated by cancer with a steeper gradient or "fall-off" in radiation dose within surrounding normal tissues. This allows, in theory, prescription of a higher total radiation dose. In contrast, teletherapy is generally less operator-dependent and will give greater radiation dose homogeneity within the treatment volume, avoiding the potential "hot" and "cold" areas associated with brachytherapy that can be the cause of inadvertent radiation complications or local tumor persistence. Generally, boost therapy to inguinal node metastases will be accomplished with teletherapy using electron beam.

Clinical series reporting outcomes of these variable approaches in patients allocated to different treatment techniques by unspecified selection criteria simply do not justify endorsement of one radiation technique over another. In general, smaller and better-defined tumors in the distal urethra have been selected for treatment, thereby emphasizing brachytherapy. More extensive tumors, particularly those extending proximally to the bladder outlet, will be treated with radiation techniques emphasizing teletherapy. Prognosis under such circumstances is probably better defined by tumor location and

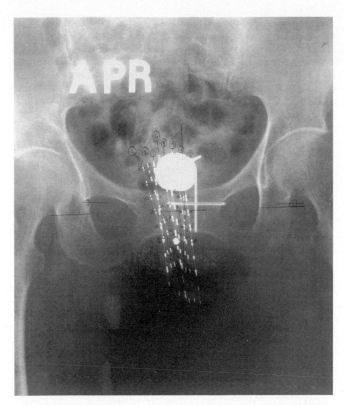

FIGURE 56.3. Interstitial radioactive implant covering the primary tumor in the distal urethra.

extent (stage) than by radiation treatment technique. However, retrospective outcomes analysis in several series of patients treated with radiation suggests that patients treated with a combination of teletherapy and brachytherapy appear to have significantly improved local control and survival compared to patients treated with teletherapy alone (49,64), although this observation is not uniform (51).

Complications of primary radiation include urethral stenosis and stricture, necrosis with possible fistula formation, and radiation cystitis. Radiation complications have been correlated with radiation dose. Escalating cumulative radiation dose (the sum of teletherapy dose and LDR brachytherapy dose) beyond approximately 7,500 cGy appears to increase the incidence of severe late complications without improving local control (51).

When radiation is administered with synchronous, radiopotentiating cytotoxic chemotherapy, the total dose of radiation has been reduced by 10% to 25% by extrapolation from the chemoradiation data generated from treating squamous cancers of the esophagus, anus, and vulva. In general, dose reduction has been undertaken by reducing the total number of treatments rather than by reducing the daily treatment dose, which is conventionally 180 cGy or 200 cGy per treatment fraction. For chemoradiation treatment of primary squamous or transitional cell tumors of the female urethra, a cumulative radiation dose of 5,400 to 6,300 cGy may suffice in contrast to 6,500 to 7,500 cGy that would generally be recommended with radiation as monotherapy. In theory, this reduced radiation dose will result in diminished late radiation sequelae (complications) in normal tissues. However, use of chemoradiation in this clinical context has been very limited, consisting of favorable case reports and small series, sometimes treating patients with advanced local-regional disease (55,65–69). No prospective comparison of radiation alone versus chemoradiation has been done (or would seem logistically feasible) such as have been accomplished for more

common cancers of the anus, esophagus, cervix, and squamous cancers of the upper aero-digestive tracts. Therefore, for the foreseeable future, the question of whether chemoradiation is superior to radiation alone as definitive or surgical adjuvant therapy will remain a judgment based on clinical impression rather than clinical science.

Radiation Therapy in Men

Radiation therapy in men has the advantage of preserving the penis. It is not, however, very effective as the sole modality (5,14), and may result in urethral stricture and chronic edema. The most common approach has been external-beam radiation therapy (EBRT), using a variety of techniques to deliver 5,000 to 6,000 cGy in 5 to 9 weeks. The integration of chemotherapy and radiation therapy has yielded excellent results in squamous cell carcinoma of the anal canal with the rate of complete response approaching 90% (70). This led to the exploration of concurrent chemotherapy and radiation, followed in some cases by limited surgery, as a penile-preserving treatment of urethral carcinoma. Baskin, from the University of California, San Francisco, reported the first case of penile-preserving surgery for squamous cell carcinoma of the pendulous urethra (71). Combined 5-fluorouracil (5-FU) plus mitomycin C and 4,000 cGy to downstage the tumor was followed by distal urethrectomy with *en bloc* resection of the adjacent corpora cavernosa and a perineal urethrostomy. Lutz et al. (69) from the Medical College of Virginia, Richmond, reported the first case of squamous cell carcinoma of the bulbous urethra to be treated with the Nigro (70) regimen (72). Licht et al. (69) from the Cleveland Clinic Foundation in Ohio reported complete response in a patient with a squamous cell carcinoma of the bulbous urethra. The patient received 5-FU and mitomycin C concurrent with 4,320 cGy, followed by chemotherapy alone. Licht et al. also reported partial response in a patient given a similar treatment of squamous cell carcinoma of the anterior urethra (69). Oberfield et al. from the Lahey Hitchcock Medical Center in Burlington, Massachusetts, confirmed the efficacy of the Nigro (70) regimen in the treatment of squamous cell carcinoma of the male urethra (73). Although promising, those results are based on a very small number of patients. Furthermore, this approach was used in patients with squamous cell carcinoma, which is the major histologic type, but it has not been investigated in patients with transitional cell carcinoma or adenocarcinoma.

Chemotherapy

Cytotoxic chemotherapy for the common forms of disseminated epithelial malignancy of the urethra (squamous and transitional cell cancers) has paralleled the use of chemotherapy for primary urothelial cancers originating in the bladder. As a single agent, cisplatin is probably the most active drug. The MVAC regimen (methotrexate, vinblastine, doxirubicin, and cisplatin) has been the most commonly employed multiagent combination (74). The combination of cisplatin and gemcitabine is active in metastatic urothelial (transitional cell) cancers and is being compared with cisplatin/gemcitabine/paclitaxel in a phase III, intergroup cooperative trial (European Organization for Research and Treatment of Cancer EORTC 30987, Southwest Oncology Group SWOG 30987, National Cancer Institute of Canada NCIC-BL7).

There is no standard approach to the treatment of metastatic adenocarcinoma of the female urethra, although extrapolation from the treatment of adenocarcinomas arising elsewhere in the upper female reproductive tract would suggest that the combination of a platinum compound with a taxane would be a reasonable choice. Carboplatin and paclitaxel as used in the treatment of ovarian, fallopian tube, and, increasingly, endometrial cancer would be a logical extrapolation. Doxirubicin and liposomal doxirubicin might also be expected to be active agents in adenocarcinoma.

Data on chemotherapy response is anecdotal, and must be interpreted with the understanding that most treatment failures in patients with urethral cancer involve a component of local or regional disease, often lying within irradiated tissues. Distant failure alone is uncommon, and distant disease may be present in 30% or less of patients at death (21). Therefore, both response rates to chemotherapy and tolerance for chemotherapy might be expected to be reduced compared to results observed while treating previously unirradiated patients with metastatic bladder cancers or Mullerian derived adenocarcinomas of the upper female reproductive tract.

Chemotherapy used to potentiate local radiation effect should be given synchronously with radiation. Concurrent radiation and chemotherapy has been reported using regimens commonly employed in the treatment of anal canal, vulvar, and cervical cancer. Prolonged venous infusion 5-FU at 1,000 to 1250 mg/m^2/24 hr for 96 to 120 hours in combination with mitomycin C or cisplatin has been the most frequently reported approach. At this time, limited numbers of case reports suggest that results from this approach will parallel the accomplishments of chemoradiation at other primary sites. The number of treated patients and the duration of surveillance follow-up are too limited to permit more than the speculative conclusion that this approach appears promising but unproven (55,65–69,71,72).

Weekly cisplatin at 40 mg/m^2 concurrently with radiation for treatment of primary squamous cancers by extrapolation from the treatment of cervical cancer might be an alternative chemoradiation strategy. Results from such an approach have not been reported.

Although the concept of using neoadjuvant chemotherapy before local therapy is theoretically appealing and has been advocated as a mechanism to reduce the rate of eventual distant failure (12) there are no published data currently that support the routine use of neoadjuvant cytotoxic drugs in the treatment of urethral cancer. Neoadjuvant carboplatin, paclitaxel, and gemcitabine followed by concurrent cisplatin and radiotherapy is presently under phase II cooperative group investigation for treatment of patients with locally advanced or locally recurrent urothelial cancers (Southwest Oncology Group SWOG SO121).

Results

Therapeutic outcomes as reported in the literature are challenging to interpret. Series spanning patients collected over multiple decades report diverse treatment techniques often without detailing selection criteria. Patients with *in-situ* disease are included with patients treated for invasive disease, and clinical series report group outcomes for patients with histologically diverse tumors. Given these limitations, it is impossible to dogmatically endorse one treatment algorithm as superior to another.

There is no uniformity of opinion regarding whether histology of the primary tumor is prognostically important. In a series of 44 patients reported from Washington University in St. Louis, substantially less favorable outcomes were observed in 13 patients with adenocarcinoma than in patients with squamous carcinoma or transitional cell cancer (20). Others have not observed a significant difference in outcome based on adenocarcinoma histology (12,49,64). There is general consensus regarding the poor prognosis of patients with melanoma (28,46).

The majority opinion is that cancers confined to the distal (anterior) urethra are prognostically more favorable than cancers arising in the proximal (posterior) urethra or those involving the full length of the urethra (12,20,50,51). Primary tumor size (≤2 cm, 2 to 4 cm, or >4 cm) can be correlated with prognosis, and most authors agree that increasing primary size correlates with progressive decrements in cancer-free survival (20). Length of urethral involvement, which may be a surrogate for tumor volume and T category, is predictive of increased risk of local failure in patients managed with radiation therapy (51).

There is also consensus that the presence of lymph node metastases adversely affects prognosis (12), although this is not uniformly reported to be the case.

In multivariate analysis of a series of 72 patients spanning 36 years reported from MSKCC, primary (T) stage, nodal status, and site of disease (anterior vs. proximal) were independent predictors of survival (12).

Inability to identify consistent prognostic factors from reports in the literature likely represents the small number of heterogenous patients reported over multiple decades from single institutions with variable referral intake patterns, evolving diagnostic assessments over time, and different management philosophies.

Overall survival at 5 to 10 years is in the range of 30% to 40% in larger series, with cause-specific survival in the 40% to 50% range. Regardless of treatment modalities employed, most patients who fail therapy will manifest local or regional recurrence as at least a component of the pattern of initial failure. Use of combined modality therapy (preoperative radiation coordinated with surgery) appears to improve local control (12), but this has not translated clearly into improved overall or cause-specific survival.

Trimodality therapy (preoperative chemoradiation followed by conservative surgery) would appear to offer several theoretic advantages: simultaneous treatment directed at local, regional, and distant disease from the time of initiation of therapy, diminished late radiation complications from reduction in total radiation dose made feasible by the radiosensitization of synchronous chemotherapy, and a decrease in surgical sequelae by enabling less extensive margins than would be desirable when surgery is employed as monotherapy. Although this is an attractive concept, the efficacy of such an approach remains unproven.

The prognosis of carcinoma of the male urethra depends on the location of the tumor and the stage at presentation. Dalbagni et al. from MSKCC reported an overall survival rate of 83% for superficial disease (Ta, Tis, T1) versus 36% for invasive tumors (T3, T4), and 26% for tumors of the bulbomembranous urethra versus 69% for tumors of the anterior urethra (3).

SUMMARY

Urethral cancers are rare and heterogeneous. Clinical series span across multiple decades during which diagnostic assessments, staging, and treatment methods have evolved. Therapy is necessarily individualized based on location, extent, histology, patient comorbidities, and patient preferences. Historically, radiation therapy has been the mainstay of treatment of all but the earliest female urethral cancers, whereas surgery has been the basis of treatment of most male urethral cancer. Current trends seem to favor multimodality therapy designed to address all components of historical patterns of failure (local, regional, and distant). Chemoradiation, alone or coordinated with conservative surgery, is a treatment approach that may offer select patients their best opportunity for local-regional control with preservation of function and cosmesis.

References

1. Wiener JS, Walther PJ. A high association of oncogenic human papillomaviruses with carcinomas of the female urethra: polymerase chain reaction-based analysis of multiple histological types. *J Urol* 1994;151:49–53.
2. Kaplan GW, Bulkey GJ, Grayhack JT. Carcinoma of the male urethra. *J Urol* 1967;98:365–371.
3. Dalbagni G, Zhang ZF, Lacombe L, et al. Male urethral carcinoma: analysis of treatment outcome. *Urology* 1999;53:1126–1132.
4. Farrer JH, Lupu AN. Carcinoma of deep male urethra. *Urology* 1984;24:527–531.
5. Bracken RB, Henry R, Ordonez N. Primary carcinoma of the male urethra. *South Med J* 1980;73:1003–1005.
6. Grussendorf-Conen EI, Deutz FJ, de Villiers EM. Detection of human papillomavirus-6 in primary carcinoma of the urethra in men. *Cancer* 1987;60:1832–1835.
7. Wiener JS, Liu ET, Walther PJ. Oncogenic human papillomavirus type 16 is associated with squamous cell cancer of the male urethra. *Cancer Res* 1992;52:5018–5023.
8. Cupp MR, Malek RS, Goellner JR, et al. Detection of human papillomavirus DNA in primary squamous cell carcinoma of the male urethra. *Urology* 1996;48:551–555.
9. Carroll PR. Surgical management of urethral carcinoma. In: Crawford ED, Das S, eds. *Current genitourinary cancer surgery*. Malvern, PA: Lea & Febiger, 1990:380–400.
10. Warwick R, Williams PL. *Gray's anatomy*, 35th ed. Edinburgh: Longman, 1973.
11. Hinman FJ. Structure and function of the penis and male urethra. *Atlas of urosurgical anatomy*. Philadelphia, PA: WB Saunders, 1993:430–447.
12. Dalbagni G, Zhang ZF, Lacombe L, et al. Female urethral carcinoma: an analysis of treatment outcome and a plea for a standardized management strategy. *Br J Urol* 1998;82:835–841.
13. Mullin EM, Anderson EE, Paulson DF. Carcinoma of the male urethra. *J Urol* 1974;112:610–613.
14. Mandler JI, Pool TL. Primary carcinoma of the male urethra. *J Urol* 1966;96:67–72.
15. Saito R. An adenosquamous carcinoma of the male urethra with hypercalcemia. *Hum Pathol* 1981;12:383–385.
16. Mittal VK, Ghosh P, Mohindra R. Carcinoma of male urethra with pseudohyperparathyroidism. *Br J Urol* 1983;55:127–128.
17. Amin MB, Young RH. Primary carcinomas of the urethra. *Semin Diagn Pathol* 1997;14:147–160.
18. Narayan P, Konety B. Surgical treatment of female urethral carcinoma. *Urol Clin North Am* 1992;19:373–382.
19. Sailer SL, Shipley WU, Wang CC. Carcinoma of the female urethra: a review of results with radiation therapy. *J Urol* 1988;140:1–5.
20. Grigsby PW. Carcinoma of the urethra in women. *Int J Radiat Oncol Biol Phys* 1998;41:535–541.
21. Mayer R, Fowler JE, Clayton M Jr. Localized urethral cancer in women. *Cancer* 1987;60:1548–1551.
22. Dodson MK, Cliby WF, Keeney GL, et al. Skene's gland adenocarcinoma with increased serum level of prostate-specific antigen. *Gynecol Oncol* 1994;5:304–307.
23. Meis JM, Ayala AG, Johnson DE. Adenocarcinoma of the urethra in women. A clinicopathologic study. [erratum appears in *Cancer* 1987;60:2900]. *Cancer* 1987;60:1038–1052.
24. Oliva E, Young RH. Clear cell adenocarcinoma of the urethra: a clinicopathologic analysis of 19 cases. *Mod Pathol* 1996;9:513–520.
25. Drew PA, Murphy WM, Civantos F, et al. The histogenesis of clear cell adenocarcinoma of the lower urinary tract. Case series and review of the literature. *Hum Pathol* 1996;27:248–252.
26. Kato H, Ogihara S, Kobayashi Y, et al. Carcinoembryonic antigen positive adenocarcinoma of a female urethral diverticulum: case report and review of the literature. *Int J Urol* 1998;5:291–293.
27. Oliva E, Quinn TR, Amin MB, et al. Primary malignant melanoma of the urethra: a clinicopathologic analysis of 15 cases. *Am J Surg Pathol* 2000;24:785–796.
28. DiMarco DS, DiMarco CS, Zincke H, et al. Outcome of surgical treatment for primary malignant melanoma of the female urethra. *J Urol* 2004;171:765–767.
29. King LR. Carcinoma of the urethra in male patients. *J Urol* 1964;91:555–559.
30. Grabstald H. Proceedings: tumors of the urethra in men and women. *Cancer* 1973;32:1236–1255.
31. Hopkins SC, Nag SK, Soloway MS. Primary carcinoma of male urethra. *Urology* 1984;23:128–133.
32. Shivde AV, Kher AV, Hardas UD, et al. Transitional cell carcinoma of male urethra (a case report). *J Postgrad Med* 1973;19:48–50.
33. Robles JE, Luzuriaga J, Ponz M, et al. Transitional cell carcinoma of the anterior urethra. *Eur Urol* 1985;11:139–140.
34. Ono Y, Matsumoto K, Kosaku N, et al. Transitional cell carcinoma in the fossa navicularis of the male urethra: a case report. *Int J Urol* 1998;5:294–295.
35. Bans LL, Eble JN, Lingeman JE, et al. Transitional cell carcinoma of the fossa navicularis of the male urethra. *J Urol* 1983;129:1055–1056.
36. Harty JI, Mojsejenko IK. Transitional cell carcinoma of the anterior urethra. *J Surg Oncol* 1982;21:121–124.
37. Genta RM, Rosen MA. Transitional cell carcinoma of fossa navicularis in a man with three other synchronous malignancies. *Urology* 1994;43:251–254.
38. Ray B, Canto AR, Whitmore WF Jr. Experience with primary carcinoma of the male urethra. *J Urol* 1977;117:591–594.
39. Guttierrez R. Primary carcinoma of Cowper's gland. *Surg Gynecol Obstet* 1937;65:238–248.
40. Bourque JL, Charghi A, Gauthier GE, et al. Primary carcinoma of Cowper's gland. *J Urol* 1969;103:758–761.
41. Griesau WA, Lipphard D. Carcinoma of Cowper's gland. *J Urol* 1951;65:460–466.
42. Arduino LJ, Nuesse WE. Carcinoma of Cowper's gland: case report. *J Urol* 1969;102:224–229.
43. LeDuc E. Carcinoma of Cowper's gland: report of the eleventh case. *Calif Med* 1962;96:44–47.
44. Bourque JL, Charghi A, Gauthier GE, et al. Primary carcinoma of Cowper's gland. *J Urol* 1970;103:758–761.
45. Small JD, Albertsen PC, Graydon RJ, et al. Adenoid cystic carcinoma of Cowper's gland. *J Urol* 1992;147:699–701.
46. Turner AG, Hendry WF. Primary carcinoma of the female urethra. *Br J Urol* 1980;52:549–554.
47. Hricak H, Secaf E, Buckley DW, et al. Female urethra: MR imaging. *Radiology* 1991;178:527–535.
48. Hahn P, Krepart G, Malaker K. Carcinoma of female urethra. Manitoba experience: 1958-1987. *Urology* 1991;37:106–109.
49. Foens CS, Hussey DH, Staples JJ, et al. A comparison of the roles of surgery and radiation therapy in the management of carcinoma of the female urethra. *Int J Radiat Oncol Biol Phys* 1991;21:961–968.
50. Weghaupt K, Gerstner GJ, Kucera H. Radiation therapy for primary carcinoma of the female urethra: a survey over 25 years. *Gynecol Oncol* 1984;17:58–63.
51. Garden AS, Zagars GK, Delclos L. Primary carcinoma of the female urethra. Results of radiation therapy. *Cancer* 1993;71:3102–3108.
52. Touijer AK, Dalbagni G. Role of voided urine cytology in diagnosing primary urethral carcinoma. *Urology* 2004;63:33–35.
53. AJCC Cancer Staging Manual. In: Green FL, Page DL, Fleming ID et al., eds. *American Joint Committee On Cancer. American Cancer Society*, 6th ed. New York: Springer-Verlag, 2002.
54. Grabstald H, Hilaris B, Henschke U, et al. Cancer of the female urethra. *JAMA* 1966;197:835–842.
55. Gheiler E, Tefilli M, Tiguert R, et al. Management of primary urethral cancer. *Urology* 1998;52:487–493.
56. Dinney CP, Johnson DE, Swanson DA, et al. Therapy and prognosis for male anterior urethral carcinoma: an update. *Urology* 1994;43:506–514.
57. Anderson KA, McAninch JW. Primary squamous cell carcinoma of anterior male urethra. *Urology* 1984;23:134–140.
58. Thompson IM, Bivings FG. Aspects of urethral carcinoma. *J Urol* 1962;87:891–895.
59. Klein FA, Whitmore WF, Herr HW, et al. Inferior pubic rami resection with en bloc radical excision for invasive proximal urethral carcinoma. *Cancer* 1983;51:1238–1242.
60. Kuettel MR, Parda DS, Harter KW, et al. Treatment of female urethral carcinoma in medically inoperable patients using external beam irradiation and high dose rate intracavitary brachytherapy. *J Urol* 1997;157:1669–1671.
61. Martinez A, Edmundson GK, Cox RS, et al. Combination of external beam irradiation and multiple-site perineal applicator (MUPIT) for treatment of locally advanced or recurrent prostatic, anorectal, and gynecologic malignancies. *Int J Radiat Oncol Biol Phys* 1985;11:391–398.
62. Micaily B, Dzeda MF, Miyamoto CT, et al. Brachytherapy for cancer of the female urethra. *Semin Surg Oncol* 1997;13:208–214.
63. Gupta AK, Vicini FA, Frazier AJ, et al. Iridium-192 transperineal interstitial brachytherapy for locally advanced or recurrent gynecological malignancies. *Int J Radiat Oncol Biol Phys* 1999;43:1055–1060.
64. Milosevic MF, Warde PR, Banerjee D, et al. Urethral carcinoma in women: results of treatment with primary radiotherapy. *Radiother Oncol* 2000;56:29–35.
65. Shah AB, Kalra JK, Silber L, et al. Squamous cell cancer of female urethra. Successful treatment with chemoradiotherapy. *Urology* 1985;25:284–286.
66. Tran LN, Krieg RM, Szabo RJ. Combination chemotherapy and radiotherapy for a locally advanced squamous cell carcinoma of the urethra: a case report. *J Urol* 1995;153:422–423.
67. Johnson DW, Kessler JF, Ferrigni RG, et al. Low-dose combined chemotherapy/radiotherapy in the management of locally advanced urethral squamous cell carcinoma. *J Urol* 1989;141:615–616.
68. Eng TY, Naguib M, Galang T, et al. Retrospective study of the treatment of urethral cancer. *Am J Clin Oncol* 2003;26:558–562.
69. Licht MR, Klein EA, Bukowski R, et al. Combination radiation and chemotherapy for the treatment of squamous cell carcinoma of the male and female urethra. *J Urol* 1995;153:1918–1920.
70. Nigro ND, Vaitkevicius VK, Considine B Jr. Combined therapy for cancer of the anal canal: a preliminary report. *Dis Colon Rectum* 1974;17:354–356.
71. Baskin LS, Turzan C. Carcinoma of male urethra: management of locally advanced disease with combined chemotherapy, radiotherapy, and penile-preserving surgery. *Urology* 1992;39:21–25.

72. Lutz ST, Huang DT. Combined chemoradiotherapy for locally advanced squamous cell carcinoma of the bulbomembranous urethra: a case report. *J Urol* 1995;153:1616–1618.

73. Oberfield RA, Zinman LN, Leibenhaut M, et al. Management of invasive squamous cell carcinoma of the bulbomembranous male urethra with co-ordinated chemo-radiotherapy and genital preservation. *Br J Urol* 1996;78:573–578.

74. Scher HI, Yagoda A, Herr HW, et al. Neoadjuvant M-VAC (methotrexate, vinblastine, doxorubicin and cisplatin) for extravesical urinary tract tumors. *J Urol* 1988;139:475–477.

CHAPTER 57 ■ URACHAL TUMORS

S. MACHELE DONAT AND HARRY W. HERR

Urachal tumors are rare, accounting for less than 1% of bladder neoplasms. Fewer than 300 cases are documented in the literature, and most are individual case reports or small case series. Most urachal tumors are adenocarcinomas arising from the urachal ligament at the dome of the bladder. Urachal cancers are associated with a poor prognosis because of their obscure anatomic location, advanced local stage at presentation, propensity for extravesical growth, and high risk of distant metastases. The biologic behavior of urachal cancers favors a long silent course before detection that belies its aggressive nature. This chapter discusses the anatomic considerations, clinical features, current treatment, and outcome of urachal tumors.

THE URACHUS

The urachus is a thick tubelike structure formed in the embryo as the allantois involutes (1). It extends from the bladder dome to the umbilicus. After birth, it becomes a fibrous cord called the *median umbilical ligament*. A patent urachus is rare; however, persistence of urachal remnants is common. Such remnants are found in one third of bladders, usually in the dome, but also along the anterior and rarely along the posterior bladder wall. They may persist as simple tubules with focal cystic dilatation or complex tubules with multiloculated cysts.

Urachal remnants may develop into cysts and epithelial neoplasms. The epithelium lining the urachus is usually transitional, but one third of cases harbor glandular epithelium. Glandular epithelium originates either from embryologic enteric rests or from metaplasia. Divergent differentiation (metaplasia) of transitional cells lining the urachal ligament most likely explains the development of adenocarcinoma and other diverse types of malignant urachal neoplasms. The urachus has intramucosal, intramuscular, and supravesical segments. Urachal tumors may arise from any of these segments (2).

OCCURRENCE

The estimated annual incidence of urachal cancer in the general population is 1 in 5 million, or 0.01% of all cancers in adults. There is approximately 1 case of urachal carcinoma per 600 treated bladder tumors. Urachal carcinoma is estimated to account for 0.17% to 0.34% of all bladder tumors and 34% of adenocarcinomas of the bladder (3). Urachal cancer presents generally in younger individuals (median age, 46 years) than do primary bladder tumors, but it may appear at any age (range, 16 to 88 years). Two thirds of patients are between 38 and 70 years at the time of diagnosis. Urachal tumors affect men and women with equal frequency (4).

PATHOLOGY

Urachal neoplasms may be benign or malignant (5). Benign neoplasms are extremely rare and include simple or multilocular cysts, adenomas, fibromas, and leiomyomas. Urachal cysts are lined with benign epithelium or varying degrees of dysplasia. Adenocarcinoma or papillary transitional cell carcinoma may be found in urachal cysts (6,7). Rare cases of villous or tubulovillous adenoma of the urachus have been reported, and they may give rise to mucin-producing invasive adenocarcinoma (8).

Malignant urachal neoplasms are usually (84%) adenocarcinomas (2,9). Most have enteric features and are mucinous. Mucin-positive adenocarcinomas (69%) may be colonic (the most common), colloid, or signet ring cell type (7%). Mucin-negative adenocarcinomas (15%) include small cell carcinomas (3%) and undifferentiated carcinomas (2%) that are not of urothelial origin. Less common malignant urachal neoplasms include sarcoma (8%), squamous cell cancer (3%), transitional cell carcinoma (3%), and anaplastic tumors (2%). Mixed-cell types may occur in as many as 17% of cases. Clear cell carcinoma (Mullerian derivation) does not arise from the urachus (10).

Urachal tumors may be classified as either low grade or high grade. Prognosis of urachal cancer is not dependent on tumor grade or histologic cell type (9), although signet ring cell adenocarcinomas and small cell carcinomas tend to display insidious local invasion and dissemination even when they appear to be clinically localized (11).

A clinical and pathologic diagnosis of urachal carcinoma is based upon the following criteria: (a) location in the dome of the bladder, (b) absence of cystitis cystica or cystitis glandularis, (c) predominant involvement of the muscularis rather than submucosa, (d) a urachal remnant connected with the neoplasm, (e) presence of a suprapubic mass, (f) sharp demarcation between tumor and surface epithelium, and (g) tumor growth in the bladder wall branching into the space of Retzius (12,13).

These criteria are arguably too restrictive because not all urachal cancers are associated with urachal remnants and some occur in the presence of cystitis cystica or glandularis. In practice, among the criteria listed in the preceding text, only (a) and (f) are clinically relevant, and indeed they may be the only indications of urachal cancer. If a tumor is located within the bladder wall beneath a layer of normal urothelium, it is clearly urachal carcinoma. Often this layer has been destroyed, making it difficult to distinguish urachal carcinoma from bladder dome adenocarcinoma. Urachal carcinoma has a predilection for local invasion, most often to the bladder wall, space of Retzius, anterior abdominal wall, peritoneum, or umbilicus. Any solitary tumor, particularly adenocarcinoma, located in the dome of the bladder, and without evidence of urothelial carcinoma *in situ*, should be treated as urachal cancer.

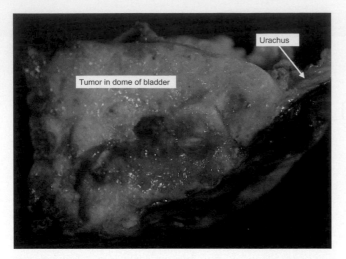

FIGURE 57.1. Gross specimen of a typical mucinous (colloid) urachal carcinoma.

Figures 57.1 and 57.2 show typical gross appearance and microscopic histology of a mucin-producing adenocarcinoma of the urachus.

CLINICAL FEATURES

Urachal tumors tend to produce few symptoms until advanced in stage. Hematuria is the presenting symptom in 80% of cases. Dysuria (40% to 60%) and suprapubic pain (21% to 42%) are common. Mucosuria is found in 25% of cases. A palpable suprapubic mass is present in only 3% of patients (3). Rarely, patients have presented with pseudomyxoma peritonei (14). Although these tumors arise in the urachus, more than 90% involve the bladder.

The most common radiologic finding is a mass or filling defect in the region of the bladder dome on computed tomography (CT) scan or magnetic resonance imaging (MRI) scan. Stippled calcification within a mass is a characteristic radiologic finding of urachal cancer. CT scanning is useful in differentiating urachal cancer from bladder dome tumors. CT scan evidence of extravesical growth along the course of the urachus is found exclusively in urachal cancers, whereas bladder

tumors exhibit intravesical growth. Some authors feel that MRI is better than CT scanning in defining tissue planes and local invasion of adjacent organs. In our experience, both CT scan and MRI are useful in detecting and staging urachal cancer.

DIAGNOSIS

The diagnosis is established by cystoscopy and biopsy of a tumor in the dome or anterior wall of the bladder. Although these tumors arise in the urachus, 90% have a visible lesion at cystoscopy. For practical purposes, any solitary tumor, especially adenocarcinoma confined to the dome of the bladder, should be suspected as urachal tumor. Percutaneous needle biopsy should be avoided because of a risk of tumor seeding. If a histologic diagnosis cannot be obtained preoperatively, a mass detected in the urachus or dome of the bladder should be surgically excised (*en bloc* removal of the mass, urachus, and a cuff of bladder) because of a high likelihood of urachal cancer (15).

Other sites of adenocarcinoma secondarily involving the bladder should be excluded. However, "drop" metastases from upper gastrointestinal primaries or ovarian cancers are more likely in the *cul-de-sac* rather than the dome and are exceedingly rare. Colon cancers may erode into the bladder, but that is usually obvious from CT scan, colonoscopy, and clinical symptomatology (i.e., pneumaturia). More commonly, large urachal carcinomas invade into the colon or adjacent small bowel. Therefore, it is not necessary to search for occult primary adenocarcinoma as part of the clinical evaluation of suspected urachal cancers.

There is no universally accepted staging system for urachal cancer that is validated by survival data. Table 57.1 shows the staging system proposed by Sheldon et al. (3) Although the Sheldon staging system is the most commonly used, other than the rare *in situ* urachal tumor, most urachal carcinomas are locally invasive (stages III–IV). Because of the silent nature of early lesions and their propensity for local growth, 83% of patients present with stage III disease. All suspected urachal tumors should be considered locally invasive and treated surgically with wide local excision.

NATURAL HISTORY

The clinical behavior and prognosis of urachal tumors are directly related to pathologic stage and aggressive natural history.

TABLE 57.1

SHELDON STAGING SYSTEM OF URACHAL CARCINOMA

Stage	Description
I	No invasion beyond urachal mucosa
II	Invasion confined to urachus
III	Local extension
A	Into bladder
B	Into abdominal wall
C	Into peritoneum
D	Into viscera other than bladder
IV	Metastatic
A	To regional lymph nodes
B	To distant sites

From Sheldon CA, Clayman RV, Gonzalez R, et al. Malignant urachal lesions. *J Urol* 1984;131:1–7.

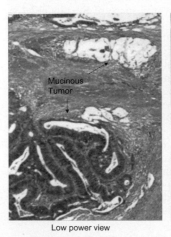 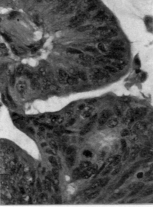

FIGURE 57.2. Histology of a mucin-positive adenocarcinoma of the urachus.

Extravesical, abdominal, and intravesical growth is characteristic of urachal cancers, favoring local recurrence. The frequency of local relapse is important in the natural history of urachal cancer. Urachal cancers recur in 20% to 38% of patients (16). The most common sites of recurrence are the pelvis (21%), bladder (16%), and the surgical incision or abdominal wall (6%). Local recurrence is noted most often (80%) within 2 years and is rare after more than 4 years following excision of the primary tumor. Only a few patients have distant metastases without local recurrence after surgical excision of clinically localized disease. Local recurrences are rarely salvaged by additional surgery, chemotherapy, or radiation.

Distant metastases from urachal carcinoma are usually a late event (17). The most common sites are bone (50%), particularly the spine; lung (46%); liver (27%); peritoneum (carcinomatosis) (23%); lymph nodes (20%); brain (19%); and various other sites (27%).

The fact that urachal cancers typically show an enteric-type pattern and share antigens with colon cancer suggests that carcinoembryogenic antigen (CEA) or carbohydrate antigen (CA 125) levels may play a clinical role. Neither has proved useful in the diagnosis, follow-up, or determination of response to therapy for urachal cancer. Immunohistochemistry of tumor tissue aids in understanding the pathogenesis of urachal carcinoma, but it is not useful for determining prognosis or for direct treatment (17,18).

TREATMENT

Surgery

As the natural history of urachal cancer indicates, complete surgical excision and local control of the primary tumor are crucial to success. *En bloc* excision with contiguous removal of the involved bladder segment offers the best prospects for survival, and most treatment failures occur because the tumor is not controlled locally by the initial operation. Microscopic soft tissue extension beyond a palpable tumor is common, and lymph node metastases may be present in up to 20% of cases. Prognosis is largely determined by tumor stage, and currently only 50% to 60% of patients are cured by surgery alone.

Any mass in the region of the urachus or dome of the bladder, either benign or malignant, should undergo complete surgical excision. Benign urachal cysts and adenomas are resected because they may contain foci of adenocarcinoma or transform into invasive cancers if left alone. Resection of benign cysts or *in situ* (stage 0) urachal tumors is curative.

Although the literature supports surgery as the best initial treatment for urachal cancer, controversy continues about what surgery is best: radical or partial cystectomy. What is not debated is that, in every surgery, a total urachectomy is required. This entails removal of the umbilicus, which is involved in 7% of cases, and the urachus together with the posterior rectus fascia and a generous portion of peritoneum overlying the bladder, extending lateral to the median umbilical ligaments down to their origin at the internal iliac artery. A bilateral pelvic lymphadenectomy is performed to include the tissue around the bifurcation of the common iliac artery where the median umbilical ligament inserts. The superior vesical arteries are sacrificed and, in cases of partial cystectomy, the entire upper half of the bladder above this level is removed. A wide margin of the bladder is incorporated in the specimen not only to ensure removal of tumor in the bladder wall but also to excise microscopic tumor involving perivesical fat. This operation is properly regarded as an extended partial

cystectomy to emphasize that removal of a portion of the bladder entails substantially more than segmental resection of only the bladder dome (19).

An extended partial cystectomy is the bladder surgery of choice for most patients with limited disease. A partial cystectomy provides excellent control of most urachal cancers because of their supravesical location and limited bladder involvement. The rationale for an extended partial cystectomy is that urachal tumors arise from embryonic rests outside the bladder and are prone to extravesical, rather than multifocal intravesical growth. The entire length of the median umbilical ligament may harbor urachal remnants that may develop carcinoma synchronously or metachronously. Urachal tumors often push into the bladder lumen without invading the bladder wall and demonstrate a sharp demarcation between the tumor and adjacent bladder epithelium. Both features of urachal carcinoma suggest that the entire tumor with a wide soft tissue margin is feasible without sacrificing the entire bladder. We submit three or four specimens of the full thickness of the bladder wall for frozen section to ensure at least a 2- or 3-cm negative surgical margin has been obtained.

Figure 57.3 shows a gross surgical specimen of an extended partial cystectomy.

Radical cystectomy is indicated for urachal carcinoma when a partial cystectomy is considered unlikely to provide complete anatomic resection of the tumor. The goal is to achieve a negative soft-tissue surgical margin using whatever extent of surgery is appropriate for individual cases. Radical cystectomy is advised for most signet cell carcinomas because

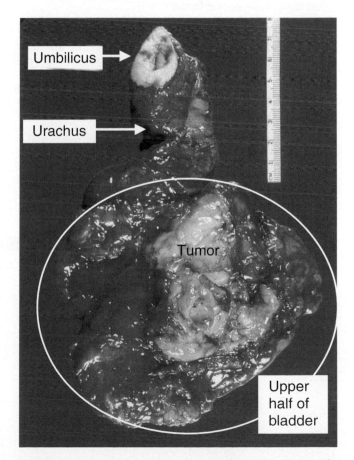

FIGURE 57.3. Surgical specimen of extended partial cystectomy for urachal cancer (urachus, umbilicus, upper half of bladder). Entire specimen measured 17 × 9 cm, and contained a 6 × 3.7 × 2.5 cm urachal carcinoma.

of their propensity for lateral involvement of the bladder wall and extensive pelvic soft-tissue invasion (20). Some adenocarcinomas extending along the posterior wall of the bladder or anteriorly toward the bladder neck are also better treated by radical cystectomy. Resection of involved adjacent organs, such as the large or small bowel, uterus and ovaries, or abdominal wall may be necessary (21). A bilateral pelvic lymph node dissection is recommended with either radical or partial cystectomy because 10% to 20% of cases may have regional nodal metastases. A few patients may be surgically cured with limited nodal metastases. Effective adjuvant chemotherapy is currently unavailable, although chemotherapy similar to that used adjuvantly for colon cancer is used in anecdotal cases.

Radical cystectomy does not offer a survival advantage over an extended partial cystectomy if all disease is resected with negative surgical margins. Survival free of disease is enhanced when *en bloc* excision of the urachus, posterior rectus fascia, and peritoneum is performed, coupled with either an extended partial or total cystectomy.

Bladder augmentation may be employed to restore functional bladder capacity in cases requiring extensive resection of the bladder. Orthotopic neobladder construction may be used in both men and women after radical cystectomy (22) or in rare cases after prostate-sparing total cystectomy.

Because of the rarity of urachal cancers, few surgeons and institutions concentrate on enough cases to provide meaningful treatment recommendations and outcome data for all patients, and those who have assembled more than a handful of cases span decades of experience. Table 57.2 shows current outcomes after initial surgical treatment of urachal cancer collected from the larger, more recent series.

Of a total of 210 patients, 121 (58%) survived for 5 years or more, but survival rates varied between 33% and 86% among different series. Most patients had locally advanced disease (stage III or IV) that directly invaded the bladder, peritoneum, abdominal wall, or local viscera. Survival rates vary little from the earliest to the most recent series, suggesting that patient selection and stage of disease most likely account for differences in outcome.

Most patients underwent partial cystectomy (170 cases), and 40 patients (20%) underwent radical cystectomy. Survival was associated with negative surgical margins and absence of nodal involvement ($P = .01$). Survival was not associated with age, gender, race, histologic grade, tumor type, or extent of bladder surgery. The 5-year survival rate was 55% after radical cystectomy compared to 62% after partial cystectomy.

The M.D. Anderson Cancer Center (MDACC) reported 42 patients with urachal carcinoma (35 localized and 7 metastatic) who were treated from 1985 to 2001. Overall survival from diagnosis for all 42 patients was 46 months, with 40% surviving 5 years. Of the 35 with resectable disease that was managed initially with surgery, 16 (46%) survived. This surgical outcome is deceptively low, however, because 19 patients did not have a total urachectomy. All but several of these patients died, including 7 of 8 with positive surgical margins. Of the 16 who had complete resection of the urachal ligament and umbilicus, 13 (81%) were long-term survivors. These data emphasize that wide resection of the tumor above the bladder, inclusive of the urachus and umbilicus, attempting to achieve negative surgical margins is critical to a successful outcome.

In our recent Memorial Sloan-Kettering Cancer Center (MSKCC) series, all patients were treated by extended partial cystectomy with *en bloc* resection of the urachus and umbilicus. Of the 21 patients, 18 (86%) survived for a median of 11 years (range, 1 to 24 years), including 12 patients alive beyond 8 years. Recurrent disease occurred in the bladder in 4 (19%) patients (3 patients were salvaged with additional surgery and 1 eventually died), and 2 patients had extravesical relapse. Recurrence occurred within a median of 1 year following partial cystectomy (range, 0.5 to 2 years). Two patients with abdominal wall or adjacent colon involvement (Sheldon IIIB, IIIC) survived after complete resection without adjuvant treatment for 11 and 13 years.

Chemotherapy

Patients who present with or develop metastatic disease have a uniformly poor prognosis. Currently, there is no established chemotherapeutic regimen for metastatic urachal carcinoma. A review of the meager literature detailing only a handful of cases reveals a few major responses to 5-fluorouracil and ifosfamide-based regimens (17). There are no reported responses or survival with methotrexate, vinblastine, doxorubicin, cisplastin (M-VAC) chemotherapy used effectively against transitional cell carcinoma of the bladder.

Chemotherapy appropriate for enteric-type adenocarcinoma can induce objective responses, but meaningful improvement in survival is not yet achieved. When 5-fluorouracil was combined with doxorubicin and mitomycin C, tumor remissions were produced lasting up to 19 months in 2 of 8 patients with unresectable urachal adenocarcinoma (30). The MDACC recently reported that chemotherapy produced only 4 (15%) significant

TABLE 57.2

SURGICAL OUTCOME OF URACHAL CARCINOMA

Series	Year	Number of patients	Number alive (%)	Follow-up (yr)
Sheldon et al. (3)	1984	5	3 (60%)	5
Johnson et al. (23)	1985	14	7 (50%)	6
Grignon et al. (9)	1991	24	15 (61%)	5
Herr et al. (19)	1993	12	10 (83%)	1–13
Zincke et al. (24)	1993	34	15 (43%)	5
Asano et al. (25)	1994	15	9 (60%)	7
Santucci et al. (26)	1997	17	15 (88%)	1–10
Dandekar et al. (27)	1997	21	9 (46%)	5
Shou et al. (28)	1999	12	4 (33%)	5
MDACC (17)	2001	35	16 (46%)	.2–13
MSKCC (29)	2003	21	18 (86%)	1–24
Totals		210	121 (58%)	

MDACC, M.D. Anderson Cancer Center; MSKCC, Memorial Sloan-Kettering Cancer Center; N, number.

responses among 26 patients with metastatic urachal cancer, including 3 of 9 patients (33%) treated with 5-fluorouracil and cisplatin regimens. Median survival from recognition of metastatic disease was 20 months. Although there were no long-term survivors, 1 patient remained alive and free of disease 29 months after chemotherapy. Survival was not dependent on the site of metastases. Seven patients who received adjuvant chemotherapy for positive surgical margins or node-positive urachal cancer and 2 patients receiving neoadjuvant chemotherapy for extensive local urachal cancers also eventually relapsed and died of disease.

The current regimen at MSKCC for nontransitional cell carcinomas of the bladder is a combination of ifosfamide, paclitaxel, and cisplatin (ITP) chemotherapy (31). The ITP regimen achieved a 22% objective (partial and complete) response rate among nine patients with metastatic urachal adenocarcinoma, with durations of response lasting up to 36 months, but there are no known cures. Lack of effective chemotherapy does not justify its routine use as neoadjuvant chemotherapy for urachal tumors.

Multimodality treatment has not been systematically investigated against advanced urachal cancer. A few patients have been treated successfully with combinations of chemotherapy (5-fluorouracil + cisplatin or (cisplatin + doxorubicin + mitomycin C), radiation, and postchemotherapy surgical resection of residual disease (32). This suggests that combined treatment strategies may improve survival of patients with locally advanced, node-positive, and even some metastatic, tumors.

Radiation

Most urachal cancers are resistant to radiation therapy (3,17). Other than anecdotal reports of occasional long-term survival, most patients who receive radiation as the principal method of treatment succumb to disease. Radiation therapy has not been investigated systematically in combination with surgery or chemotherapy to treat urachal carcinoma. Radiation may be used to palliate symptomatic local recurrence or bone metastases.

CONCLUSION

Urachal carcinomas are rare neoplasms that are usually locally advanced when diagnosed and have a relatively poor prognosis. Any tumor confined to the dome of the bladder should be approached initially as if it were urachal carcinoma and surgically removed. More than half the patients can be cured with early diagnosis and an attempt at margin-negative *en bloc* resection of the entire urachus and involved bladder segment, if possible. A pelvic node dissection is also advised because nodal involvement is frequent. There is no currently accepted or effective chemotherapy. Incompletely resected, locally recurrent or metastatic urachal tumors may respond to chemotherapy, but long-term survival is rare. Prospective studies, preferably within the context of a national registry or cooperative groups, may help develop and refine successful multimodality therapy for urachal tumors.

References

1. Begg RC. The urachus: its anatomy, histology and development. *J Anat* 1930;64:170–183.
2. Eble JN. Abnormalities of the urachus. In: Young RB, ed. *Pathology of the urinary bladder.* New York: Churchill Livingstone, 1989:213–243.
3. Sheldon CA, Clayman RV, Gonzalez R, et al. Malignant urachal lesions. *J Urol* 1984;131:1–7.
4. Santucci RA, Lange PH. Urachal carcinoma. In: Raghavan D, Scher HI, Leibel SA et al., eds. *Principles and practice of genitourinary oncology.* Philadelphia : Lippincott–Raven Publishers, 1997:331–334.
5. Bourne CW, May JE. Urachal remnants: benign or malignant? *J Urol* 1977;118:743–747.
6. Paul AB, Hunt CR, Harney JM, et al. Stage 0 mucinous adenocarcinoma in situ of the urachus. *J Clin Pathol* 1998;51:483–484.
7. Rudin JP, Kasznica JM, Davis CA, et al. Transitional cell carcinoma in a urachal cyst. *J Urol* 1999;162:1,687–1,699.
8. Ng KJ, Newman P, Price-Thomas JM. Carcinoma of the urachus associated with urachal adenoma. *Br J Urol* 1991;67:215–216.
9. Grignon RJ, Ro JY, Ayala AG, et al. Primary adenocarcinoma of the urinary bladder: aclinicopathologic analysis of 72 cases. *Cancer* 1991;67:2,165–2,172.
10. Oliva E, Amin MB, Young RH. Clear cell carcinoma of the urinary bladder. *Am J Surg Pathol* 2002;26:190–197.
11. Loggie BW, Fleming RA, Hosseinian AA. Peritoneal carcinomatosis with urachal signet-cell adenocarcinoma. *Urology* 1997;50:446–448.
12. Wheeler JD, Hill WT. Adenocarcinoma involving the urinary bladder. *Cancer* 1954;7:119–124.
13. Mostofi FK, Thomson RV, Dean AL. Mucinous adenocarcinoma of the urinary bladder. *Cancer* 1955;8:741–749.
14. Stenhouse G, McRae D, Pollock AM. Urachal adenocarcinoma in situ with pseudomyxoma peritonei. *J Clin Pathol* 2003;56:152–153.
15. McMahon R, Hunt RC. In situ adenocarcinoma of the bladder: the role of the urachus. *Am J Surg Pathol* 2002;26:271–272.
16. Besarani D, Purdie CA, Townell NH. Recurrent urachal adenocarcinoma. *J Clin Pathol* 2003;56:882–883.
17. Siefker-Radtke AO, Gee J, Shen Y, et al. Multimodality management of urachal carcinoma: the M. D. Anderson Cancer Center experience. *J Urol* 2003;169:1,295–1,298.
18. Pantuck AJ, Bancila E, Das KM, et al. Adenocarcinoma of the urachus and bladder expresses a unique colonic epithelial epitope: an immunohistochemical study. *J Urol* 1997;158:1,722–1,727.
19. Herr HW. Urachal carcinoma: the case for extended partial cystectomy. *J Urol* 1994;151:365–366.
20. Jakse G, Schneider HM, Jacobi GH. Urachal signet-ring cell carcinoma, a rare variant of vesical adenocarcinoma: incidence and pathological criteria. *J Urol* 1978;120:764–767.
21. Tamita K, Tobisu K, Kume H, et al. Long survival with extended surgery for urachal carcinoma involving adjacent organs. *J Urol* 1998;159:1,298–1,299.
22. Stein JP, Grossfeld GD, Freeman JA, et al. Orthotopic lower urinary tract reconstruction in women. *J Urol* 1997;158:400–405.
23. Johnson DE, Hodge GB, Abdul-Karim FW, et al. Urachal carcinoma. *Urology* 1985;26:218–221.
24. Henly DR, Farrow GM, Zincke H. Urachal cancer: role of conservative surgery. *Urology* 1993;42:635–639.
25. Asano K, Miki J, Yamada H, et al. Carcinoma of the urachus. *Nippon Hinyokika Gakkai Zasshi* 2003;94(4):487–494.
26. Santucci RA, True LD, Lange PH. Is partial cystectomy the treatment of choice for mucinous adenocarcinoma of the urachus? *Urology* 1997;49:536–540.
27. Dandekar NP, Dalal AV, Kamat MR. Adenocarcinoma of bladder. *Eur J Surg Oncol* 1997;23:157–160.
28. Shou J, Ma J, Xu B. Adenocarcinoma of the urinary bladder: a report of 27 cases. *Zhonghua Zhong Liu Za Zhi* 1999;21:461–463.
29. Cohen M, Bochner B, Herr HW. Urachal carcinoma: The MSKCC experience (submitted).
30. Logothetis CJ, Samuels ML, Ogden S. Chemotherapy for adenocarcinomas of bladder and urachal origin. *Urology* 1985;26:252–255.
31. Bajorin DF, McCaffrey JA, Dodd PM, et al. Ifosphamide, paclitacel, and cisplatin for patients with advanced transitional cell carcinoma of the urothelial tract. *Cancer* 2000;88:1,671–1,678.
32. Kawakami S, Kageyama Y, Yonese J, et al. Successful treatment of metastatic adenocarcinoma of the urachus: report of 2 cases with more than 10-year survival. *Urology* 2001;58:462–464.

Page numbers followed by *f* indicate figures; page numbers followed by *t* indicate tables.